Textbook of
Rheumatology

Textbook of Rheumatology

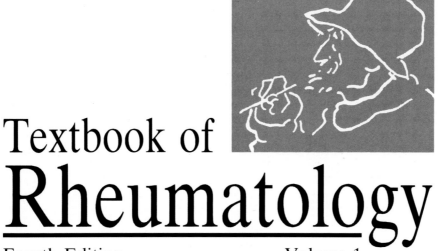

Fourth Edition   Volume 1

WILLIAM N. KELLEY, M.D.

Chief Executive Officer
University of Pennsylvania Medical Center
Executive Vice President and Robert G. Dunlop
    Professor of Medicine and Biochemistry and Biophysics
University of Pennsylvania
Dean, University of Pennsylvania School of Medicine
Philadelphia, Pennsylvania

EDWARD D. HARRIS, Jr., M.D.

Arthur L. Bloomfield Professor and Chairman
Department of Medicine
Stanford University School of Medicine
Stanford, California

SHAUN RUDDY, M.D.

Elam Toone Professor of Internal Medicine,
    Immunology, and Microbiology
Chairman
Division of Rheumatology, Allergy, and Immunology
Department of Internal Medicine
Medical College of Virginia
Virginia Commonwealth University
Richmond, Virginia

CLEMENT B. SLEDGE, M.D.

John B. and Buckminster Brown Professor of Orthopedic Surgery
Harvard Medical School
Chairman
Department of Orthopedic Surgery
Brigham and Women's Hospital
Boston, Massachusetts

W.B. SAUNDERS COMPANY
Harcourt Brace Jovanovich, Inc.
Philadelphia   London   Toronto   Montreal   Sydney   Tokyo

W.B. SAUNDERS COMPANY
Harcourt Brace Jovanovich, Inc.

The Curtis Center
Independence Square West
Philadelphia, Pennsylvania 19106

Library of Congress Cataloging-in-Publication Data

Textbook of rheumatology / William N. Kelley . . . [et al.].—
4th ed.

    p.   cm.

Includes bibliographical references and indexes.

ISBN 0–7216–3157–6 (set)

1. Rheumatology.   I. Kelley, William N., 1939–
    [DNLM: 1. Arthritis.   2. Rheumatic Diseases.
    WE 544 T355 1993]

RC927.T49 1993   616.7′23—dc20

DNLM/DLC
for Library of Congress   92–48331
                                   CIP

TEXTBOOK OF RHEUMATOLOGY, Fourth Edition   ISBN

                                  Volume I   0–7216–3155–X
                                  Volume II   0–7216–3156–8
                                  Two Volume Set 0–7216–3157–6

Printed in the United States of America.

Last digit is the print number: 9   8   7   6   5   4   3   2   1

We wish to dedicate this edition of the
Textbook of Rheumatology to our families.

Lois Kelley and children:
Paige Kelley Nath, Ginger Kelley Yost, Lori Kelley, and Mark Kelley.

Ned Harris, Tom Harris, and Chandler Harris.

Millicent Ruddy and children:
Christi Ruddy and Candace Ruddy Lau-Hansen.

Georgia Sledge and children:
Margaret Sledge Tracy, John Sledge, Matthew Sledge, and Claire Sledge.

Contributors

CAROLINE M. ALEXANDER, Ph.D.
Postdoctoral Fellow, University of California, San Francisco, School of Medicine, San Francisco, California
Proteinases and Matrix Degradation

ROY D. ALTMAN, M.D.
Professor of Medicine, Arthritis Division, University of Miami School of Medicine; Chief, Arthritis Section, Department of Veterans Affairs Medical Center; Staff Physician, University of Miami Hospital and Clinics; Staff Physician, Jackson Memorial Hospital, Miami, Florida
Hypertrophic Osteoarthropathy

WILLIAM P. AREND, M.D.
Professor of Medicine and Head, Division of Rheumatology, University of Colorado Health Sciences Center; Attending Physician, University Hospital, Denver, Colorado
Cytokines and Growth Factors

M. AMIN A. ARNAOUT, M.D.
Associate Professor of Medicine, Harvard Medical School, and Department of Medicine, Massachusetts General Hospital; Director, Leukocyte Biology and Inflammation Program, Associate Physician, Department of Medicine, Massachusetts General Hospital, Boston, Massachusetts
Cell Adhesion Molecules

WILLIAM J. ARNOLD, M.D.
Clinical Professor of Medicine, University of Chicago Pritzker School of Medicine, Chicago; Chairman, Department of Medicine, Lutheran General Hospital, Park Ridge, Illinois
Sarcoidosis

LLOYD AXELROD, M.D.
Associate Professor of Medicine, Harvard Medical School; Physician and Chief of the James Howard Means Firm, Massachusetts General Hospital, Boston, Massachusetts
Glucocorticoids

STANLEY P. BALLOU, M.D.
Associate Professor of Medicine, Case Western Reserve University; Director of Arthritis Clinic, MetroHealth Medical Center, Cleveland, Ohio
Laboratory Evaluation of Inflammation

ROBERT M. BENNETT, M.D., F.R.C.P.
Professor of Medicine and Chairman, Division of Arthritis and Rheumatic Diseases, The Oregon Health Sciences University, Portland, Oregon
The Fibromyalgia Syndrome: Myofascial Pain and the Chronic Fatigue Syndrome; Mixed Connective Tissue Disease and Other Overlap Syndromes

HÅKAN BERGSTRAND, Ph.D.
Professor, University of Lund; Assistant Director, Scientific Advisor, Pharmacology I, Astra Draco, Lund, Sweden
Neutrophils and Eosinophils

MARIE-JOSEÉ BERTHIAUME, M.D., F.R.C.P.S.
Musculoskeletal Radiologist and Associate Professor, Royal Victoria Hospital, McGill University Faculty of Medicine, Montreal, Quebec, Canada
Imaging

ALAN L. BISNO, M.D.
Professor, Department of Medicine, University of Miami School of Medicine; Chief, Medical Service, Miami Veterans Affairs Medical Center; Attending Physician, Veterans Affairs Medical Center and Jackson Memorial Hospital, Miami, Florida
Rheumatic Fever

ARTHUR L. BOLAND, M.D.
Assistant Clinical Professor of Orthopedic Surgery, Harvard Medical School; Visiting Orthopedic Surgeon, Massachusetts General Hospital, Brigham and Women's Hospital, New England Baptist Hospital, Boston, Massachusetts
Sports Medicine

KENNETH D. BRANDT, M.D.
Professor of Medicine and Head, Rheumatology Division, Indiana University School of Medicine; Attending Physician, Indiana University Hospital, Indianapolis, Indiana
Pathogenesis of Osteoarthritis; Management of Osteoarthritis

DOREEN B. BRETTLER, M.D.
Associate Professor, University of Massachusetts Medical School, Director, New England Hemophilia Center, Worcester, Massachusetts
Hemophilic Arthropathy

GREGORY W. BRICK, M.D.
Clinical Instructor in Orthopedic Surgery, Harvard Medical School; Orthopedic Surgeon at Brigham and Women's Hospital and West Roxbury Veterans Administration Hospital, Boston, Massachusetts
The Hip

REBECCA H. BUCKLEY, M.D.
J. Buren Sidbury Professor of Pediatrics, Professor of Immunology, Duke University School of Medicine; Chief, Division of Allergy and Immunology, Department of Pediatrics, Duke University Medical Center, Durham, North Carolina
Specific Immunodeficiency Diseases, Excluding AIDS

DAVID S. CALDWELL, M.D.
Associate Professor of Medicine, Division of
Rheumatology and Immunology, Department of
Medicine, Duke University; Attending Physician, Duke
University Hospital, Durham, North Carolina
Musculoskeletal Syndromes Associated with Malignancy

DENNIS A. CARSON, M.D.
Professor of Medicine, University of California, San
Diego; Director, The Sam and Rose Stein Institute for
Research on Aging, University of California, San Diego,
San Diego, California
Rheumatoid Factor

JAMES T. CASSIDY, M.D.
Professor, Division of Pediatric Rheumatology, University
of Missouri–Columbia School of Medicine; Professor of
Child Health, University of Missouri–Columbia School of
Medicine, Columbia, Missouri
*Juvenile Rheumatoid Arthritis; Systemic Lupus Erythematosus,
Juvenile Dermatomyositis, Scleroderma, and Vasculitis*

EDGAR S. CATHCART, M.D., D.Sc.
Professor of Medicine, Boston University School of
Medicine, Boston; Chief of Staff, Edith Nourse Rogers
Memorial Department of Veterans Affairs Medical Center,
Bedford, Massachusetts
Amyloidosis

PHILIP J. CLEMENTS, M.D.
Professor of Medicine, University of California, Los
Angeles, School of Medicine; Physician, Center for
Health Sciences, University of California, Los Angeles,
Los Angeles, California
Nonsteroidal Anti-inflammatory Drugs (NSAIDs)

DOYT L. CONN, M.D.
John F. Finn, Minnesota Arthritis Foundation Professor of
Medicine, Mayo Medical School; Consultant in
Rheumatology and Internal Medicine, Mayo Clinic,
Rochester, Minnesota
Vasculitis and Related Disorders

RAMZI S. COTRAN, M.D.
F. B. Mallory Professor of Pathology, Harvard Medical
School; Chairman, Department of Pathology, Brigham
and Women's Hospital, Boston, Massachusetts
Endothelial Cells

JOE CRAFT, M.D.
Associate Professor of Medicine and Chief, Section of
Rheumatology, Department of Medicine, Yale University
School of Medicine; Attending, Yale–New Haven
Hospital, New Haven, Connecticut
Antinuclear Antibodies

JODY A. DANTZIG
Department of Physiology, University of Pennsylvania
School of Medicine; Research Specialist, Pennsylvania
Muscle Institute, Philadelphia, Pennsylvania
Muscle

LAURIE S. DAVIS, Ph.D.
Assistant Professor, Department of Internal Medicine/
Division of Rheumatology, University of Texas
Southwestern Medical Center, Dallas, Texas
T Cells and B Cells

RICHARD O. DAY, M.B., M.D., F.R.A.C.P.
Professor of Clinical Pharmacology, University of New
South Wales; Director of Clinical Pharmacology, St.
Vincent's Hospital, Darlinghurst, Sydney, Australia
Aspirin and Salicylates; Sulfasalazine

JEAN-MICHEL DAYER, M.D.
Associate Professor of Medicine, Division of Immunology
and Allergy, University of Geneva; Attending Physician,
University Hospital, Geneva, Switzerland
Cytokines and Growth Factors

JONATHAN T. DELAND, M.D.
Assistant Professor of Orthopedic Surgery, Cornell
University Medical College; Orthopedic Surgeon,
Hospital for Special Surgery, New York, New York
Foot Pain; Sports Medicine

PENG THIM FAN, M.D.
Clinical Professor of Medicine, University of California,
Los Angeles; Attending Physician, V. A. Wadsworth
Medical Center, Los Angeles, California
Reiter's Syndrome

ANTHONY S. FAUCI, M.D.
Chief, Laboratory of Immunoregulation, and Director,
National Institute of Allergy and Infectious Diseases,
National Institutes of Health, Bethesda, Maryland
Immunoregulatory Agents

ANDREW P. FERRY, M.D.
Professor and Chairman, Department of Ophthalmology,
and Professor of Pathology, Medical College of Virginia,
Virginia Commonwealth University, Richmond, Virginia
The Eye and Rheumatic Diseases

IRVING H. FOX, M.D., C.M.
Vice-President, Medical Affairs, Biogen; Clinical Professor
of Medicine, Harvard Medical School; Clinical Associate,
Massachusetts General Hospital, Boston, Massachusetts
Antihyperuricemic Drugs

ROBERT I. FOX, M.D., Ph.D.
Associate Member, Department of Immunology, The
Scripps Research Institute, Department of Rheumatology,
Scripps Clinic and Research Foundation, La Jolla,
California
Sjögren's Syndrome

ANDREW G. FRANKS, Jr., M.D.
Clinical Associate Professor of Dermatology, New York
University School of Medicine; Attending Physician,
Tisch Hospital, The University Hospital of NYU;
Associate Rheumatologist, Hospital for Joint Diseases,
New York University Medical Center, New York, New
York
The Skin and Rheumatic Diseases

BRUCE FREUNDLICH, M.D.
Associate Professor of Medicine, University of
Pennsylvania School of Medicine; Chief, Clinical
Rheumatology Service, Hospital of the University of
Pennsylvania, Philadelphia, Pennsylvania
Eosinophilia-Myalgia Syndrome

WILLIAM W. GINSBURG, M.D.
Associate Professor, Mayo Medical School, Rochester, Minnesota; Consultant, St. Luke's Hospital, Jacksonville, Florida
Multicentric Reticulohistiocytosis

DON L. GOLDENBERG, M.D.
Professor of Medicine, Tufts University School of Medicine, Boston; Chief of Rheumatology, Director, Arthritis-Fibromyalgia Center, Newton-Wellesley Hospital, Newton, Massachusetts
Bacterial Arthritis

YALE E. GOLDMAN, M.D., Ph.D.
Professor, Department of Physiology, University of Pennsylvania School of Medicine; Director, Pennsylvania Muscle Institute, Philadelphia, Pennsylvania
Muscle

DUNCAN A. GORDON, M.D., F.P.C.P.C., F.A.C.P.
Professor of Medicine, University of Toronto Faculty of Medicine; Senior Rheumatologist, The Toronto Hospital Arthritis Centre, Toronto, Ontario, Canada
Gold Compounds in Rheumatic Diseases

BEVRA H. HAHN, M.D.
Professor of Medicine and Chief of Rheumatology, University of California, Los Angeles; Physician, Center for the Health Sciences, University of California, Los Angeles, Los Angeles, California
Management of Systemic Lupus Erythematosus

THEODORE J. HAHN, M.D.
Professor of Medicine, University of California, Los Angeles, School of Medicine; Chief, Geriatric Medicine, and Director, Geriatric Research, Education and Clinical Center, Veterans Administration Medical Center, West Los Angeles; Director, Osteoporosis and Metabolic Bone Disorders Center, UCLA Medical Center; Attending Physician, UCLA Medical Center, UCLA School of Medicine, Los Angeles, California
Metabolic Bone Disease

LENA HÅKANSSON, Ph.D.
Associate Professor, University of Uppsala; Research Engineer, Department of Clinical Chemistry, University Hospital, Uppsala, Sweden
Neutrophils and Eosinophils

JOHN A. HARDIN, M.D.
Professor and Chairman, Department of Medicine, School of Medicine, Medical College of Georgia, Augusta, Georgia
Antinuclear Antibodies

EDWARD D. HARRIS, Jr., M.D.
Arthur L. Bloomfield Professor and Chairman, Department of Medicine, Stanford University School of Medicine; Chief of Medical Services, Stanford University Hospital, Stanford, California
Etiology and Pathogenesis of Rheumatoid Arthritis; Clinical Features of Rheumatoid Arthritis; Treatment of Rheumatoid Arthritis

JEROME H. HERMAN, M.D.
Professor of Medicine, University of Cincinnati College of Medicine; Attending Physician, University Hospital and Holmes Division of the University of Cincinnati Medical Sciences Center; Consultant (Immunology/Rheumatology), Veterans Administration Hospital, Cincinnati, Ohio
Polychondritis

GARY S. HOFFMAN, M.S., M.D.
Head, Vasculitis and Related Diseases, National Institutes of Health, National Institute of Allergy and Infectious Diseases, Laboratory of Immunoregulation, Bethesda, Maryland
Mycobacterial and Fungal Infections

GENE G. HUNDER, M.D.
Professor of Medicine, Mayo Medical School; Chairman, Division of Rheumatology, Mayo Clinic, Rochester, Minnesota
Examination of the Joints; Vasculitis and Related Disorders; Giant Cell Arteritis and Polymyalgia Rheumatica

JOHN N. INSALL, M.D.
Clinical Professor of Orthopaedic Surgery, Mt. Sinai School of Medicine; Attending Orthopaedic Surgeon and Director of Insall Scott Kelly Institute for Orthopaedic and Sports Medicine, Beth Israel Medical Center–North Division, New York, New York
The Knee

SILVIU ITESCU, M.D., F.R.A.C.P.
Assistant Professor, Division of Autoimmune and Molecular Diseases, Columbia University College of Physicians and Surgeons; Attending Physician, Presbyterian Hospital, New York, New York
Rheumatologic Manifestations of HIV Infection

ISRAELI A. JAFFE, M.D.
Professor of Clinical Medicine, College of Physicians and Surgeons, Columbia University; Attending Physician, Presbyterian Hospital, New York, New York
Penicillamine

KENNETH A. JOHNSON, M.D.
Professor, Mayo Medical School; Consultant, Mayo Clinic Scottsdale, Scottsdale, Arizona
The Ankle and Foot

HO-IL KANG, M.D, Ph.D.
Postdoctoral Fellow, Department of Immunology, The Scripps Research Institute, La Jolla, California
Sjögren's Syndrome

WILLIAM N. KELLEY, M.D., M.A.C.P.
Chief Executive Officer, University of Pennsylvania Medical Center; Executive Vice President and Robert G. Dunlop Professor of Medicine and Biochemistry and Biophysics, University of Pennsylvania; Dean, University of Pennsylvania School of Medicine, Philadelphia, Pennsylvania
Hyperuricemia; Gout

PAUL D. KEMP, Ph.D.
Winchester, Massachusetts
Matrix Glycoproteins and Proteoglycans

JOEL M. KREMER, M.D.
Professor of Medicine, Albany Medical College;
Attending Physician, Albany Medical Center Hospital,
Albany, New York
Nutrition and Rheumatic Diseases

IRVING KUSHNER, M.D.
Professor of Medicine and Pathology, Case Western
Reserve University; Rheumatologist, MetroHealth Medical
Center, Cleveland, Ohio
Laboratory Evaluation of Inflammation

R. ELAINE LAMBERT, M.D.
Assistant Professor of Medicine, Division of Immunology
and Rheumatology, Stanford University School of
Medicine; Medical Staff, Stanford University Medical
Center, Stanford, California
*Iron Storage Disease; Arthropathies Associated with Endocrine
Disorders*

MATTHEW H. LIANG, M.D., M.P.H.
Associate Professor of Medicine, Harvard Medical School;
Lecturer in Health Policy and Management, Harvard
School of Public Health; Attending, Brigham and
Women's Hospital, Boston, Massachusetts
Psychosocial Management of Rheumatic Diseases

PETER E. LIPSKY, M.D.
Professor of Internal Medicine, University of Texas
Southwestern Medical Center of Dallas; Attending,
Parkland Memorial Hospital, Zale-Lipshy University
Hospital, Dallas, Texas
T Cells and B Cells; Monocytes and Macrophages

STEPHEN J. LIPSON, M.D.
Associate Professor of Orthopedic Surgery, Harvard
Medical School; Orthopedic Surgeon-in-Chief, Beth Israel
Hospital; Orthopedic Surgeon, Brigham and Women's
Hospital, Boston, Massachusetts
Low Back Pain; The Cervical Spine

CARLO L. MAINARDI, M.D.
Professor and Vice Chairman, Department of Medicine,
University of Tennessee; Chief, Medical Service, Veterans
Administration Medical Center, Memphis, Tennessee
Fibroblast Function and Fibrosis; Localized Fibrotic Disorders

HENRY J. MANKIN, M.D.
Edith M. Ashley Professor of Orthopedic Surgery,
Harvard Medical School; Chief of the Orthopedic Service,
Massachusetts General Hospital, Boston, Massachusetts
*Pathogenesis of Osteoarthritis; Clinical Features of
Osteoarthritis*

W. JOSEPH McCUNE, M.D.
Associate Professor, Department of Internal Medicine,
and Associate Chief for Clinical Activities, Division of
Rheumatology, University of Michigan Medical Center,
Ann Arbor, Michigan
Monarticular Arthritis

JAMES L. McGUIRE, M.D.
Associate Professor of Medicine, Associate Dean for
Clinical Affairs and Graduate Medical Education,

Stanford University School of Medicine; Chief of Staff,
Stanford University Hospital, Stanford, California
*Iron Storage Disease; Arthropathies Associated with Endocrine
Disorders*

KATHERYN MEEK, D.V.M.
Assistant Professor, Internal Medicine, University of
Texas Southwestern Medical Center, Dallas, Texas
T Cells and B Cells

JEFFERY L. MEIER, M.D.
Clinical Associate, Laboratory of Clinical Investigation,
National Institute of Allergy and Infectious Diseases; The
Warren G. Magnuson Clinical Center, National Institutes
of Health, Bethesda, Maryland
Mycobacterial and Fungal Infections

ROBERT W. METCALF, M.D.
Late Professor of Orthopedic Surgery, University of Utah
School of Medicine, Salt Lake City, Utah
Arthroscopy

CLEMENT J. MICHET, M.D., M.P.H.
Associate Professor of Medicine, Mayo Medical School;
Consultant in Rheumatology, Mayo Clinic Scottsdale,
Scottsdale, Arizona
Examination of the Joints; Psoriatic Arthritis

LEWIS H. MILLENDER, M.D.
Clinical Professor of Orthopedic Surgery, Tufts University
School of Medicine; Assistant Chief, Hand Surgery
Section, New England Baptist Hospital, Boston,
Massachusetts
The Hand

MARC L. MILLER, M.D.
Assistant Clinical Professor of Medicine, University of
Vermont College of Medicine, Burlington; Attending
Physician, Maine Medical Center, Portland, Maine
Weakness

B. F. MORREY, M.D.
Professor, Mayo Medical School; Chairman, Department
of Orthopedic Surgery, Mayo Clinic, Mayo Foundation,
Rochester, Minnesota
Reconstruction and Rehabilitation of the Elbow Joint

ROLAND W. MOSKOWITZ, M.D.
Professor of Medicine, Case Western Reserve University;
Director, Division of Rheumatic Diseases, University
Hospitals of Cleveland; Director, Northeast Ohio
Multipurpose Arthritis Center, Cleveland, Ohio
*Diseases Associated with the Deposition of Calcium
Pyrophosphate or Hydroxyapatite*

GEORGE MOXLEY, M.D.
Assistant Professor, Internal Medicine, Medical College of
Virginia, Virginia Commonwealth University, Richmond,
Virginia
Immune Complexes and Complement

KENNETH K. NAKANO, M.D., M.P.H., S.M.,
F.R.C.P.(C)
Medical Director, Straub Foundation, Honolulu, Hawaii
Neck Pain; Entrapment Neuropathies and Related Disorders

EDWARD A. NALEBUFF, M.D.

Clinical Professor of Orthopedic Surgery, Tufts University School of Medicine; Chief of Hand Surgery Section, New England Baptist Hospital, Boston, Massachusetts
The Hand

CHARLES S. NEER II, M.D.

Professor of Clinical Orthopaedic Surgery, Emeritus, and Special Lecturer in Orthopaedic Surgery, Columbia University College of Physicians and Surgeons; Consultant Orthopaedic Surgeon, Emeritus, New York Orthopaedic–Columbia–Presbyterian Medical Center, New York, New York
The Shoulder

BARBARA S. NEPOM, M.D.

Research Assistant Member, Virginia Mason Research Center, and Affiliate Assistant Professor, Division of Immunology/Rheumatology, Department of Pediatrics, University of Washington School of Medicine, Seattle, Washington
Immunogenetics and the Rheumatic Diseases

GERALD T. NEPOM, M.D., Ph.D.

Member and Director, Immunology Program, Virginia Mason Research Center, and Associate Professor (Affiliate), Department of Immunology, University of Washington School of Medicine, Seattle, Washington
Immunogenetics and the Rheumatic Diseases

ALAN P. NEWMAN, M.D.

Associate Professor of Orthopedic Surgery, University of Utah School of Medicine; Staff Orthopedic Surgeon, University Hospital, Salt Lake City, Utah
Synovectomy

JOHN J. NICHOLAS, M.D.

Professor and Chairman, Department of Physical Medicine and Rehabilitation, Rush Medical College; Senior Attending Physician, Rush–Presbyterian–St. Luke's Medical Center; Consulting Staff, Marianjoy Rehabilitation Center and Clinics, Chicago, Illinois
Rehabilitation of Patients with Rheumatic Diseases

J. DESMOND O'DUFFY, M.D.

Professor of Medicine, Mayo Medical School; Staff, Methodist Hospital, St. Mary's Hospital, Rochester, Minnesota
Vasculitis and Related Disorders; Multicentric Reticulohistiocytosis

DUNCAN S. OWEN, Jr., M.D.

Taliaferro/Scott Professor of Internal Medicine, Medical College of Virginia, Virginia Commonwealth University; Attending Physician, Medical College of Virginia Hospitals; Consultant, Hunter Holmes McGuire Department of Veterans Affairs Medical Center, Richmond, Virginia
Aspiration and Injection of Joints and Soft Tissues

HAROLD E. PAULUS, M.D.

Professor of Medicine, University of California, Los Angeles, School of Medicine; Attending Physician, Center for Health Sciences, University of California, Los Angeles, Los Angeles, California
Nonsteroidal Anti-inflammatory Drugs (NSAIDs)

ROBERT S. PINALS, M.D.

Professor of Medicine, University of Medicine and Dentistry of New Jersey–Robert Wood Johnson Medical School, New Brunswick; Chairman, Department of Medicine, The Medical Center at Princeton, Princeton, New Jersey
Felty's Syndrome

ROBERT POSS, M.D.

Professor of Orthopedic Surgery, Harvard Medical School; Vice Chairman, Department of Orthopedic Surgery, Brigham and Women's Hospital, Boston, Massachusetts
The Hip

DARWIN J. PROCKOP, M.D., Ph.D.

Chairman and Professor, Department of Biochemistry and Molecular Biology, Jefferson Medical College, Philadelphia, Pennsylvania
Collagen and Elastin

ERIC L. RADIN, M.D.

Clinical Professor of Orthopedic Surgery, University of Michigan, Ann Arbor; Director, Henry Ford Hospital Bone and Joint Center; Chairman of Orthopedic Surgery, Henry Ford Hospital, Detroit, Michigan
Biomechanics of Joints

DONALD RESNICK, M.D.

Professor of Radiology, University of California, San Diego, School of Medicine; Staff, University Hospital, Veterans Affairs Medical Center, San Diego, California
Imaging

ANDREW E. ROSENBERG, M.D.

Assistant Professor, Harvard Medical School; Assistant Pathologist, Massachusetts General Hospital, Boston, Massachusetts
Tumors and Tumor-Like Lesions of Joints and Related Structures

DAVID W. ROWE, M.D.

Professor of Pediatrics, Division of Endocrinology/Diabetes, University of Connecticut Health Center School of Medicine, Farmington, Connecticut
Heritable Disorders of Structural Proteins

CLINTON T. RUBIN, Ph.D.

Director, Musculo-Skeletal Research Laboratory; Associate Professor, Department of Orthopaedics, School of Medicine, State University of New York at Stony Brook, Stony Brook, New York
Biology, Physiology, and Morphology of Bone

SHAUN RUDDY, M.D.

Elam Toone Professor of Internal Medicine; Chairman, Division of Rheumatology, Allergy, and Immunology, Department of Internal Medicine, Medical College of Virginia, Virginia Commonwealth University, Richmond, Virginia
Immune Complexes and Complement; Complement Deficiencies and Rheumatic Diseases

RICHARD I. RYNES, M.D.
Professor of Medicine and Head, Division of Rheumatology, Albany Medical College; Attending Physician, Albany Medical Center Hospital, Albany, New York
Antimalarial Drugs

CHARLES L. SALTZMAN, M.D.
Assistant Professor, Department of Orthopaedic Surgery, University of Iowa, Iowa City, Iowa
The Ankle and Foot

DAVID J. SARTORIS, M.D.
Associate Professor of Radiology, University of California, San Diego, School of Medicine; Chief, Quantitative Bone Densitometry, University of California, San Diego, Medical Center, San Diego; Staff, Veterans Administration Medical Center, San Diego; Scripps Clinic and Research Foundation, La Jolla, California
Imaging

ALAN L. SCHILLER, M.D.
Irene Heinz Given and John LaPorte Given Professor of Pathology, Mt. Sinai School of Medicine; Professor and Chairman, Department of Pathology, Mt. Sinai Medical Center, New York, New York
Tumors and Tumor-Like Lesions of Joints and Related Structures

THOMAS J. SCHNITZER, M.D., PH.D.
Professor of Internal Medicine and Director, Sections of Rheumatology and Geriatric Medicine, Rush Medical College; Senior Attending, Rush–Presbyterian–St. Luke's Medical Center; Medical Director, Johnston R. Bowman Health Center for the Elderly, Chicago, Illinois
Viral Arthritis

H. RALPH SCHUMACHER, JR., M.D.
Professor of Medicine, University of Pennsylvania School of Medicine; Director, Arthritis-Immunology Center, Veterans Affairs Medical Center; Acting Chief, Division of Rheumatology, University of Pennsylvania School of Medicine and Hospital of the University of Pennsylvania, Philadelphia, Pennsylvania
Synovial Fluid Analysis and Synovial Biopsy; Gout; Hemoglobinopathies and Arthritis

PETER H. SCHUR, M.D.
Professor of Medicine, Harvard Medical School; Senior Physician, Brigham and Women's Hospital, Boston, Massachusetts
Clinical Features of SLE

LAWRENCE B. SCHWARTZ, M.D., PH.D.
Charles and Evelyn Thomas Professor of Medicine, Medical College of Virginia, Virginia Commonwealth University, Richmond, Virginia
The Mast Cell

RICHARD D. SCOTT, M.D.
Associate Clinical Professor of Orthopaedic Surgery, Harvard Medical School; Surgeon, Brigham and Women's Hospital, New England Baptist Hospital, Boston, Massachusetts
Surgical Management of Juvenile Rheumatoid Arthritis

JAMES R. SEIBOLD, M.D.
Director, Clinical Research Center, and Director, Program in Clinical Pharmacology, University of Medicine and Dentistry of New Jersey–Robert Wood Johnson Medical School; Chief, Clinical Pharmacology, Attending in Medicine/Rheumatology, Robert Wood Johnson University Hospital, New Brunswick, New Jersey
Scleroderma

JOHN S. SERGENT, M.D.
Professor of Medicine, Vanderbilt University School of Medicine; Chief of Medicine, St. Thomas Hospital, Nashville, Tennessee
Polyarticular Arthritis

JAY R. SHAPIRO, M.D.
Associate Professor and Program Director for the General Clinical Research Center, The Johns Hopkins University School of Medicine, Baltimore, Maryland
Heritable Disorders of Structural Proteins

BARRY P. SIMMONS, M.D.
Associate Professor of Orthopedic Surgery, Harvard Medical School; Chief, Orthopedic Hand Surgery Service, Brigham and Women's Hospital; Associate in Orthopedic Surgery, Brigham and Women's Hospital; Associate in Orthopedic Surgery, Children's Hospital Medical Center, Boston, Massachusetts
The Hand

SHELDON R. SIMON, M.D.
Professor and Chief, Division of Orthopaedics, Ohio State University; Attending Staff, Ohio State University Hospital, and Children's Hospital, Columbus, Ohio
Biomechanics of Joints

CLEMENT B. SLEDGE, M.D.
John B. and Buckminster Brown Professor of Orthopedic Surgery, Harvard Medical School; Chairman, Department of Orthopedic Surgery, Brigham and Women's Hospital, Boston, Massachusetts
Biology of the Joint; Biology, Physiology, and Morphology of Bone; Introduction to Surgical Management; Surgical Management of Juvenile Rheumatoid Arthritis

NICHOLAS A. SOTER, M.D.
Professor of Dermatology, New York University School of Medicine; Medical Director, Charles C. Harris Skin and Cancer Pavilion; Attending Physician, Tisch Hospital, The University Hospital of NYU, New York, New York
The Skin and Rheumatic Diseases

ALLEN C. STEERE, M.D.
Professor of Medicine, Tufts University School of Medicine; Chief, Rheumatology/Immunology, New England Medical Center, Boston, Massachusetts
Lyme Disease

DAVID R. STEINBERG, M.D.
Assistant Professor, Department of Orthopaedics, University of California, Davis, School of Medicine; Attending Surgeon, Department of Orthopaedics, University of California, Davis, Medical Center, Sacramento, California
Osteonecrosis

MARVIN E. STEINBERG, M.D.
Professor and Vice Chairman, Department of
Orthopaedic Surgery, University of Pennsylvania School
of Medicine; Director, Hip Clinic and Joint Reconstruction
Center, Hospital of the University of Pennsylvania,
Philadelphia, Pennsylvania
Osteonecrosis

JERRY TENENBAUM, M.D., F.R.C.P.(C), F.A.C.P.
Associate Dean of Continuing Medical Education and
Associate Professor of Medicine, University of Toronto;
Staff Physician, Mt. Sinai Hospital; Staff Consultant
(Rheumatology), Baycrest Geriatric Center, and Toronto
Hospital, Toronto, Ontario, Canada
Hypertrophic Osteoarthropathy

RANJENY THOMAS, M.B.B.S., F.R.A.C.P.
Fellow in Rheumatology, University of Texas,
Southwestern Medical Center at Dallas; Fellow, Parkland
Memorial Hospital, Dallas, Texas
Monocytes and Macrophages

THOMAS S. THORNHILL, M.D.
Associate Clinical Professor of Orthopedics, Harvard
Medical School; Staff, Brigham and Women's Hospital,
New England Baptist Hospital, Boston, Massachusetts
Shoulder Pain

ROBERT L. TRELSTAD, M.D.
Professor and Chairman, Department of Pathology,
University of Medicine and Dentistry of New Jersey–
Robert Wood Johnson Medical School; Staff, Robert
Wood Johnson University Hospital, New Brunswick,
New Jersey
Matrix Glycoproteins and Proteoglycans

PAUL J. TSAHAKIS, M.D.
Director of Arthritis Research, Carolinas Medical Center;
Orthopedic Surgeon, Miller Orthopedic Clinic, Charlotte,
North Carolina
The Hip

KATHERINE S. UPCHURCH, M.D.
Associate Professor of Medicine, University of
Massachusetts Medical School; Chief, Division of
Rheumatology, Medical Center of Central Massachusetts,
Worcester, Massachusetts
Hemophilic Arthropathy

FRANK H. VALONE, M.D.
Associate Professor of Medicine, Dartmouth Medical
School, Hanover; Attending Physician, Dartmouth-
Hitchcock Medical Center, Lebanon, New Hampshire
Platelets

PHILIPP VANDENBERG, M.D.
Research Associate, Thomas Jefferson University,
Department of Biochemistry, Philadelphia, Pennsylvania
Collagen and Elastin

PER VENGE, M.D.
Professor, University of Uppsala; Head, Department of
Clinical Chemistry, University Hospital, Uppsala, Sweden
Neutrophils and Eosinophils

MARY C. WACHOLTZ, M.D., Ph.D.
Assistant Professor in Internal Medicine (Rheumatology),
University of Texas Southwestern Medical Center at

Dallas; Medical Staff, Parkland Memorial Hospital and
Zale-Lipshy University Hospital in Dallas, Dallas, Texas
T Cells and B Cells

MICHAEL E. WEINBLATT, M.D.
Associate Professor of Medicine, Harvard Medical School;
Vice Chairman of Clinical Affairs, Department of
Rheumatology, Brigham and Women's Hospital, Boston,
Massachusetts
Methotrexate

BARBARA N. WEISSMAN, M.D.
Associate Professor of Radiology, Harvard Medical
School; Chief, Musculoskeletal Radiology Section, and
Assistant Chairman of Radiology for Ambulatory
Services, Brigham and Women's Hospital, Boston,
Massachusetts
Radiographic Evaluation of Total Joint Replacement

ZENA WERB, Ph.D.
Professor of Anatomy, Radiology, and Radiobiology,
University of California, San Francisco, School of
Medicine, San Francisco, California
Proteinases and Matrix Degradation

CHARLENE J. WILLIAMS, Ph.D.
Research Assistant Professor, Thomas Jefferson
University, Department of Biochemistry and Molecular
Biology, Philadelphia, Pennsylvania
Collagen and Elastin

ROBERT J. WINCHESTER, M.D.
Professor of Pediatrics and Head, Division of
Autoimmune and Molecular Diseases, Department of
Pediatrics, Columbia University College of Physicians and
Surgeons; Attending Physician, Presbyterian Hospital,
New York, New York
Rheumatologic Manifestations of HIV Infection

RUSSELL E. WINDSOR, M.D.
Associate Professor of Surgery (Orthopaedics), Cornell
University Medical College; Associate Chief, The Knee
Service, Hospital for Special Surgery; Associate Attending
Orthopaedic Surgeon, Hospital for Special Surgery, New
York, New York
The Knee

FRANK A. WOLLHEIM, M.D., Ph.D.
Professor of Rheumatology, University of Lund Medical
School; Professor and Chairman, Department of
Rheumatology, Lund University Hospital, Lund, Sweden
Ankylosing Spondylitis; Enteropathic Arthritis

BRUCE T. WOOD, D.P.M.
Associate in Orthopedics-Podiatry, Harvard Medical
School, and Brigham and Women's Hospital; Staff
Podiatrist, Massachusetts Institute of Technology,
Cambridge, Massachusetts
Foot Pain

VIRGIL L. WOODS, Jr., M.D.
Associate Professor of Medicine, University of California,
San Diego; Attending Physician, University of California,
San Diego, Medical Center, San Diego, California
Pathogenesis of Systemic Lupus Erythematosus

ROBERT L. WORTMANN, M.D.
Professor and Chairman, Department of Medicine, East
Carolina University School of Medicine; Chief of
Medicine, Pitt County Memorial Hospital, Greenville,
North Carolina
Inflammatory Diseases of Muscle

K. RANDALL YOUNG, JR., M.D.
Director, Division of Pulmonary and Critical Care
Medicine, Department of Medicine, University of
Alabama at Birmingham; Staff Physician, University of
Alabama Hospital, Birmingham, Alabama
Immunoregulatory Agents

DAVID TAK YAN YU, M.D.
Professor of Medicine, University of California, Los
Angeles, School of Medicine; Staff, University of
California, Los Angeles, Medical Center, Los Angeles,
California
Reiter's Syndrome

ROBERT B. ZURIER, M.D.
Professor of Medicine and Director, Division of
Rheumatology, University of Massachusetts Medical
School; Attending Physician, University of Massachusetts
Medical Center Hospital, Worcester, Massachusetts
Prostaglandins, Leukotrienes, and Related Compounds

Preface

The field of rheumatology continues to show remarkable progress. An impressive transition has occurred from the empirical approach of the nineteenth-century spas to today's multidisciplinary specialty ranging from the monumental advances in molecular biology, immunogenetics, and immunoregulation to the modern miracles of total joint replacement and the promise of gene therapy. There have been many critical contributions to this evolution. Pathologists and orthopedic surgeons such as Goldthwait, Smith-Peterson, and Wilson began important work early in the century. In the 1930s, internists such as Bauer, Cecil, Hench, Holbrooke, and Pemberton added their creative, scientific, and organizational skills to the embryonic discipline. Societies were created to stimulate the exchange of ideas, and an explosion of federal funding for research fostered expansion of essential scientific information.

Over the past three decades, consolidation of efforts in diverse disciplines has provided a truly scientific basis for rheumatology. The basic structure and function of immunoglobulins are now clarified at both the gene and the protein levels. Highly sophisticated techniques have allowed the careful study of specific lymphocyte subpopulations and their roles in controlling the immune response. Investigation of the inflammatory process has defined a multitude of effectors and their target cells. The details of how proteolytic enzymes destroy tissues in joints in inflammatory arthritis have been deciphered. The genes coding for these effectors are being cloned, as are the genes for the receptors themselves. These studies will allow not only improved understanding of their specific structure and function but also, eventually, the production of effectors, receptors, and their analogues in pharmacologic quantities or as substrates for gene therapy. The identification within the major histocompatibility complex of specific genetic polymorphisms associated with unusual predisposition to rheumatic disease represents a major breakthrough. Transgenic animals now provide critical animal models of disease. Advances in bioengineering, matched with sophisticated surgical approaches, have established metal and polymer prostheses as major components of therapy. Considering all these frontiers along which we are advancing, the outlook for a better understanding of and new effective treatments for rheumatic diseases has never been brighter.

In the First Edition, the principal goal was to include a complete spectrum of the information necessary for the understanding, differential diagnosis, and management of the patient with a rheumatic complaint. This led to the inclusion of chapters addressing areas not covered by existing reference books in rheumatology, such as the scientific basis of rheumatology, a large section on the general approach to the patient, a full evaluation of the diagnostic tests utilized in the evaluation of patients with rheumatic diseases, and extensive coverage of rehabilitation and reconstructive surgery as they relate to rheumatology. The Second and Third Editions were reorganized and revised extensively.

The Fourth Edition has been comprehensively revised beyond the improvements of the first three editions. There are new chapters in areas such as immunogenetics and the rheumatic diseases, cell adhesion molecules, fibroblast function in fibrosis, laboratory evaluation of inflammation, sulfasalazine, the eosinophilia-myalgia syndrome, rheumatologic manifestations of human immunodeficiency virus infection, and specific immunodeficiency diseases excluding acquired immunodeficiency syndrome. We have combined and consolidated a number of other chapters in order to enhance the flow of information. All of these chapters include not only the many major advances in basic science occurring during the past several years but also the discussion of their possible clinical implications.

The editors continue to believe that the quality of this textbook depends on the quality of its contributors. We also recognize the importance of regular replacement of contributors to ensure that even the best chapters will be extensively updated over a period of several editions. In the Fourth Edition, we have continued to follow this policy, with the inclusion of 53 new authors. This has allowed us to approach certain areas differently and to consolidate several areas to improve the flow of text. Even those chapters that do not have new authors were substantially updated and, when possible, improved in quality. The editors are highly pleased with the final product.

We wish to express our thanks to our teachers and to our students, from whom we have learned much, as well as to our colleagues for their patience and understanding of the time and energy the development of this textbook has required of us. Throughout the preparation of this edition, the expertise of the professionals at W.B. Saunders has continued to impress us. We benefited from the assistance of Mr. Richard Zorab, Senior Acquisitions Editor; Mr. Lawrence McGrew, Senior Developmental Editor; Mr. Peter Faber, Production Manager; Ms. Gina Scala, Senior Copy Editor; Ms. Maureen Sweeney, Designer, and Mr. Walt Verbitski, Illustrations Coordinator. Their help has been essential and is deeply appreciated. Finally, we wish to thank our editorial assistants and secretaries, including Rebecca Trumbull, Jodi Sarkisian, Mary Wisch, Carole Wonsiewicz, Jean Doran, Gloria Smith, Michelle Young, and Phyllis White. They have been of immeasurable assistance.

WILLIAM N. KELLEY, M.D.
EDWARD D. HARRIS, JR., M.D.
SHAUN RUDDY, M.D.
CLEMENT B. SLEDGE, M.D.

Contents

COLOR PLATES

PLATE I

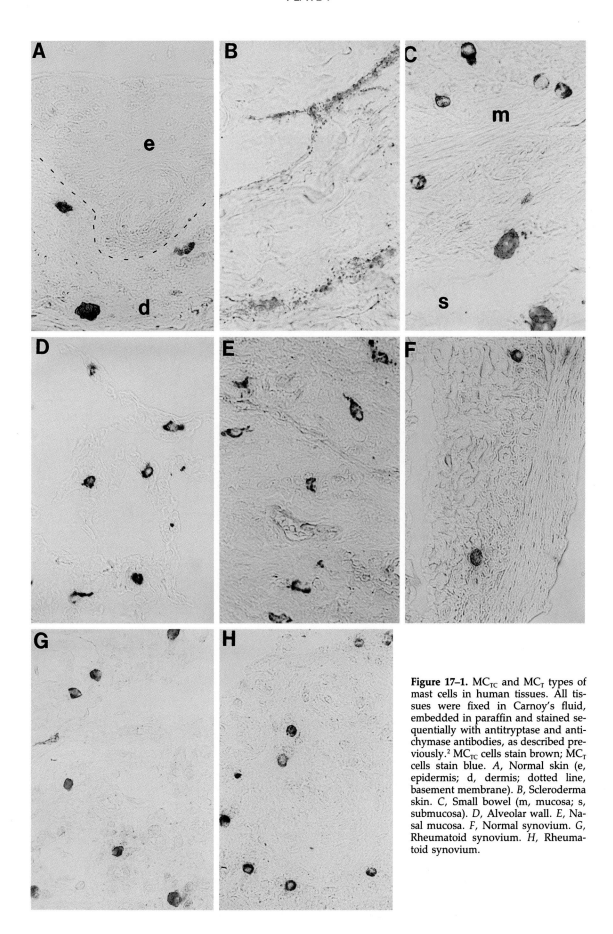

Figure 17–1. MC_{TC} and MC_T types of mast cells in human tissues. All tissues were fixed in Carnoy's fluid, embedded in paraffin and stained sequentially with antitryptase and antichymase antibodies, as described previously.[2] MC_{TC} cells stain brown; MC_T cells stain blue. *A*, Normal skin (e, epidermis; d, dermis; dotted line, basement membrane). *B*, Scleroderma skin. *C*, Small bowel (m, mucosa; s, submucosa). *D*, Alveolar wall. *E*, Nasal mucosa. *F*, Normal synovium. *G*, Rheumatoid synovium. *H*, Rheumatoid synovium.

PLATE II

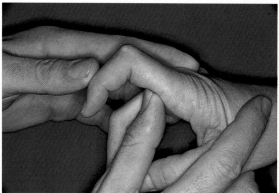

Figure 23–1A

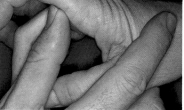

Figure 23–1B

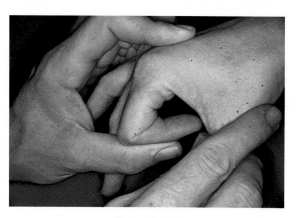

Figure 23–1C

Figure 23–1. Bunnell's sign. This sign is used to distinguish synovitis of the proximal interphalangeal joint from spasm of the intrinsic muscles due to metacarpophalangeal synovitis as the cause of decreased motion of the proximal interphalangeal joint. *A,* With the metacarpophalangeal joint extended, decreased flexion of the proximal interphalangeal joint is noted. If normal flexion is noted (i.e., the tip of the finger can touch the volar pad), then involvement of all three joints (metacarpophalangeal, proximal interphalangeal, and distal intraphalangeal) is excluded. *B,* With the metacarpophalangeal joint flexed, the contracted intrinsic muscles are relaxed. Restricted motion with the metacarpophalangeals flexed therefore is indicative of proximal interphalangeal involvement. *C,* Normal proximal interphalangeal motion when the metacarpophalangeal joints are flexed indicates that the prior proximal interphalangeal restriction was due to intrinsic muscle contracture, presumably caused by metacarpophalangeal synovitis.

PLATE III

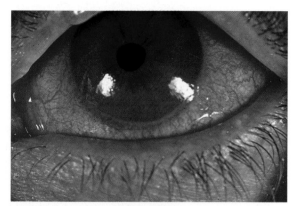

Figure 32–1

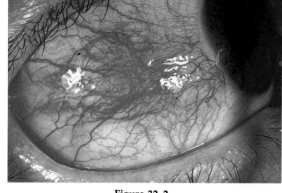

Figure 32–2

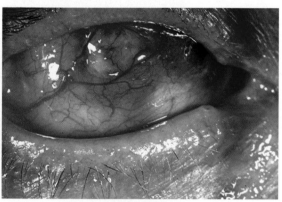

Figure 32–3

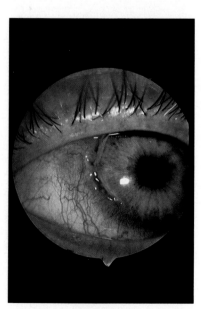

Figure 32–8

Figure 32–1. Keratoconjunctivitis sicca. Intense hyperemia of the conjunctival vessels accounts for the prominent redness. Dryness of the corneal epithelium causes the reflection from the photographic flash to be dull and irregular rather than normally sharp and highly polished.

Figure 32–2. Severe episcleritis involving the temporal aspect of the right eye in the region of the interpalpebral fissure. Congestion of the episcleral vessels accounts for the bright red appearance.

Figure 32–3. Necrotizing scleritis. The eye is adducted and slightly elevated. Destruction of sclera has rendered visible the underlying ciliary body, which has a bluish gray color.

Figure 32–8. Wegener's granulomatosis. Deep ring ulcer in corneal periphery superotemporally in patient with previously undiagnosed Wegener's granulomatosis. Note also the episcleritis adjacent to the corneal lesion. Necrotizing scleritis developed in this area within several weeks after the photograph was made.

PLATE IV

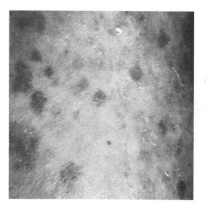

Figure 33–10B

Figure 33–11

Figure 33–10. Necrotizing venulitis. *B,* Close-up view of the lesions.

Figure 33–11. Necrotizing venulitis. Circumscribed area of edema (urticaria).

PLATE V

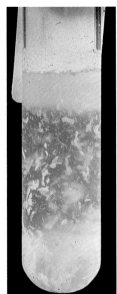

Figure 36–2

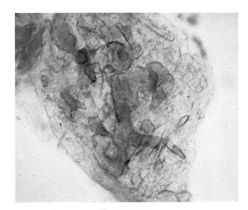

Figure 36–4

Figure 36–2. Synovial fluid rice bodies containing fibrin and debris from degenerated villi are especially common in rheumatoid arthritis but can also be seen in other conditions such as tuberculous arthritis.

Figure 36–4. Shards of golden or ochre cartilage fragments embedded in detached synovium found floating in synovial fluid in a patient with ochronotic arthropathy.

Figure 36–5. Monosodium urate crystals from a gouty synovial fluid as viewed with compensated polarized light. The crystals are yellow parallel to the axis of slow vibration marked on the compensator (negative birefringence).

Figure 36–6. CPPD crystals can be needle, rod, or rhomboid shaped but usually have blunt ends (*A*). They often have fainter birefringence than is seen with urates (*B*). CPPD are blue when aligned longitudinally with the axis of slow vibration of the compensator (positive birefringence).

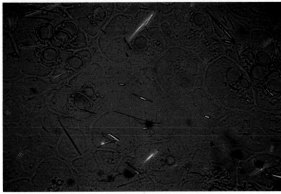

Figure 36–5

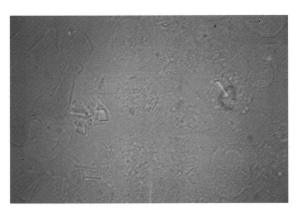

Figure 36–6A

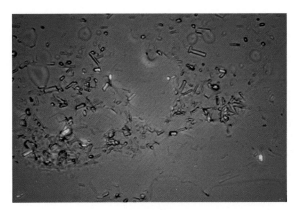

Figure 36–6B

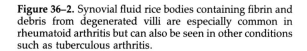

PLATE VI

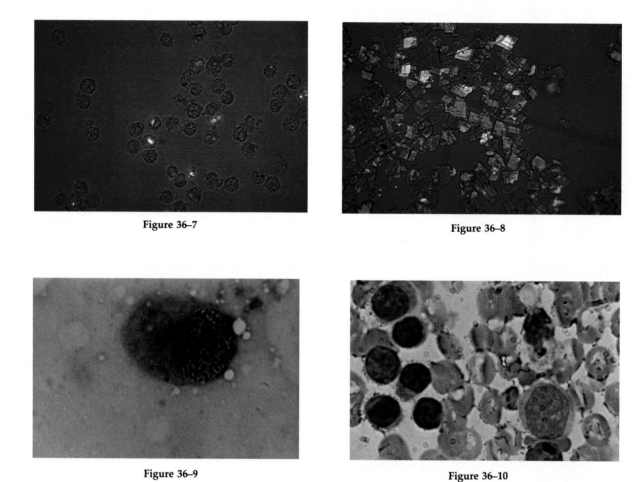

Figure 36–7

Figure 36–8

Figure 36–9

Figure 36–10

Figure 36–7. Triamcinolone acetonide (Aristospan) crystals phagocytized by synovial fluid cells after intra-articular injection.

Figure 36–8. Cholesterol crystals from a chronic rheumatoid olecranon bursal effusion. These are most often flat plates with notched corners.

Figure 36–9. Synovial lining cell. The prominent homogeneous blue cytoplasm is typical of type B or synthetic cells. Other large cells with a nucleus:cytoplasm ratio of less than 50 percent have vacuolated cytoplasm and are either phagocytic lining cells or large monocytes (macrophages).

Figure 36–10. Synovial fluid small lymphocytes with one activated lymphocyte, the larger cell with nucleus filling most of the cytoplasm.

PLATE VII

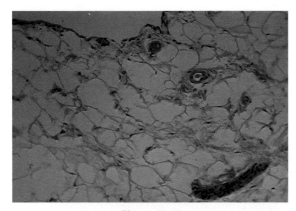

Figure 36–15

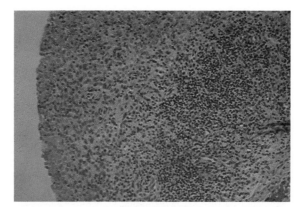

Figure 36–16

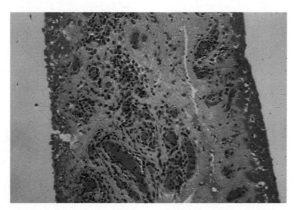

Figure 36–17

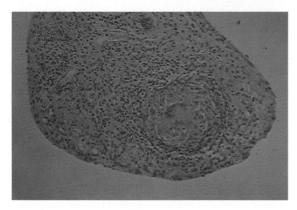

Figure 36–19

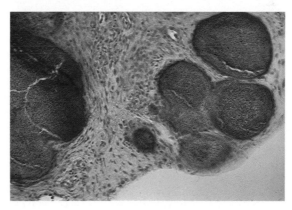

Figure 36–20

Figure 36–15. Normal synovial membrane of the knee. There is a single layer of flattened synovial cells overlying areolar connective tissue. Note the small synovial vessels immediately under the lining layer and the larger vessel in the lower right corner. × 100. Hematoxylin and eosin stain.

Figure 36–16. Rheumatoid arthritis synovium showing many layers of synovial lining cells on the left and infiltration of lymphocytes and plasma cells on the right. × 100. Hematoxylin and eosin stain.

Figure 36–17. Synovial membrane in early scleroderma shows massive superficial fibrin, loss of lining cells, and infiltration with lymphocytes and plasma cells. × 100. Hematoxylin and eosin stain.

Figure 36–19. Granuloma in superficial synovium in tuberculous arthritis. Some superficial granulomas such as this one do not show caseation. There is also scattered chronic inflammatory cell infiltration. × 100. Hematoxylin and eosin stain.

Figure 36–20. Tophus-like deposits in synovium containing positively birefringent crystals in pseudogout. × 100. Hematoxylin and eosin stain.

PLATE VIII

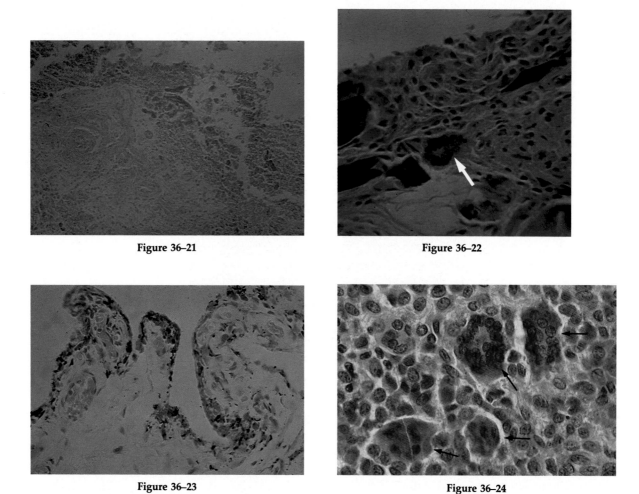

Figure 36–21

Figure 36–22

Figure 36–23

Figure 36–24

Figure 36–21. Amyloid arthritis as seen here in a patient with multiple myeloma is characterized by Congo red staining on the surface and sparing of the synovial vessels (V). × 100. Congo red stain.

Figure 36–22. Dark, angular cartilage shards pigmented brown with homogentisic acid polymer are embedded in ochronotic synovium. Note also a giant cell *(arrow)* and mild proliferation of synovial lining cells. × 400. Hematoxylin and eosin stain.

Figure 36–23. Iron stain of synovial membrane in idiopathic hemochromatosis shows blue (dark) staining predominantly in the lining cells. × 100. Prussian blue stain.

Figure 36–24. Pigmented villonodular synovitis is characterized by golden brown hemosiderin in deep macrophages, giant cells *(arrows)*, monotonous proliferation of deep cells with pale nuclei, and, not illustrated here, foam cells, lining cell hyperplasia (dark), and villous proliferation. × 400. Hematoxylin and eosin stain. (Courtesy of Schumacher, H. R.: Semin. Arthritis Rheum. 12:32, 1982.)

PLATE IX

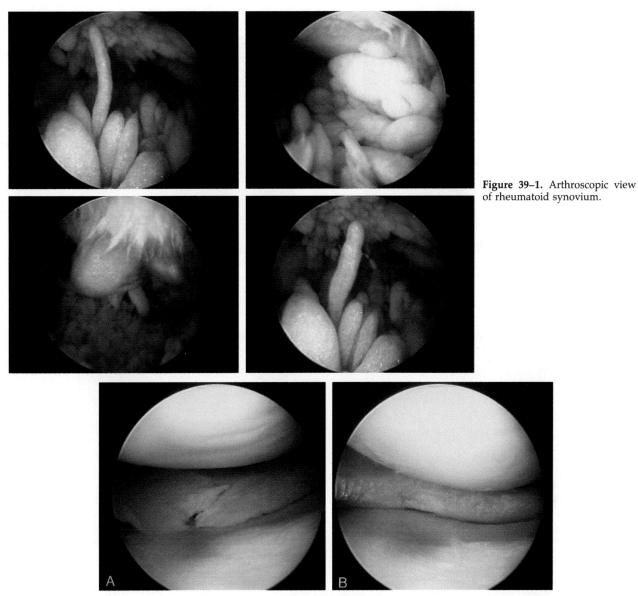

Figure 39–1. Arthroscopic view of rheumatoid synovium.

Figure 39–2. Débridement of meniscal flap tear. *A*, Flap tear of posterior aspect of medial meniscus. *B*, Arthroscopic view after resection of the tear, removing all unstable tissue and leaving behind as much normal meniscus as possible, in order to preserve the mechanical function of the joint.

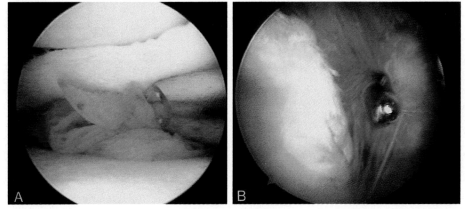

Figure 39–3. *A*, Arthroscopic view of motorized synovial resector tip approaching the perimeniscal synovium beneath the lateral meniscus (in a case of PVNS). *B*, Visualization of the posteromedial compartment of a knee with hemophilic arthropathy, with the synovial resector inserted through a separate posteromedial portal.

PLATE X

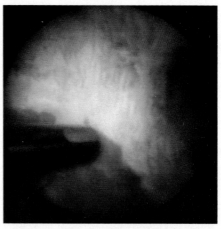

Figure 39–4. Arthroscopic view of synovial membrane in hemophilia. Note the orange pigmentation and the marked synovial hypertrophy.

Figure 39–8. Synovial resector working on the anteromedial synovial membrane. Note the boundary between the remaining abnormal synovium and the exposed subsynovial layer. It is important to make every effort to keep working at this boundary in one location rather than skipping around to different areas.

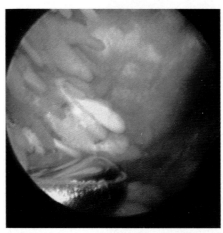

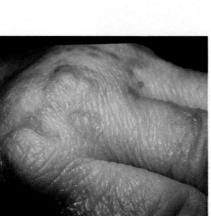

Figure 46–3. This photograph shows bullous lesions in the skin of a DP-treated patient with RA. The clinical and histologic findings are those of pemphigus. The DP was stopped, and glucocorticoids were required; the lesions gradually resolved.

Figure 57–2. Asymmetric polyarthritis of the feet. Note the sausage toes with severe redness and swelling of the phalangeal shafts and the swelling of the tarsus.

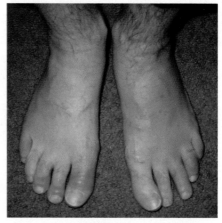

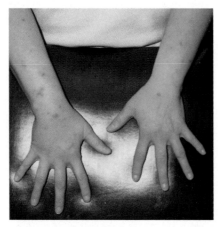

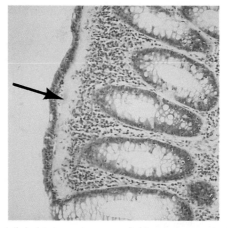

Figure 59–4. Recurrent pustular rash in a case of bypass arthritis-dermatitis.

Figure 59–5. Biopsy specimen of colon in a case of collagen colitis. Arrow indicates layer of collagen deposition. Hematoxylin-eosin stain. (Courtesy Dr. C. Lindström.)

Section I

Structure and Function of Joints, Connective Tissue, and Muscle

---

Chapter 1   Clement B. Sledge

Biology of the Joint

INTRODUCTION

The structure of each joint is closely linked to its function. Some joints have a wide range of motion but little intrinsic stability (e.g., the knee, shoulder). Others have minimal movement and need little, if any, stabilization from overlying muscle groups (e.g., the hips). It is useful to recognize two basic types of articulations: (1) *synovial* or *diarthrodial* joints (Fig. 1–1), which are articulations with free movement that have a synovial membrane lining the joint cavity; and (2) *synarthrodial* joints, which have very little movement. There are four subclassifications of synarthroses: (a) *symphyses,* in which a fibrocartilaginous disc separates bone ends that are joined by firm ligaments (e.g., symphysis pubis and intervertebral joints); (b) *synchondroses,* in which bone ends are covered with articular cartilage, but there is no synovium or significant joint cavity (e.g., sternomanubrial joint); (c) *syndesmoses,* in which bones are joined directly by fibrous ligaments without a cartilaginous interface (the distal tibiofibular articulation is the only joint of this type outside the cranial vault); and (d) *synostoses,* in which bone bridges between bones, producing ankylosis.

Among synovial joints there are great differences in function and, therefore, structure. For instance, the humeroulnar joint is a true hinge joint limited to motion in one plane, whereas the spherical hip joint, a ball (the femoral head) and socket (the acetabulum) joint, has motion in all directions and rotations. Accompanying the relative restrictions on planes of motion of the elbow is an intrinsic stability; the hinge construction needs little surrounding muscle to stabilize it. Conversely, the freedom of motion inherent in the structure of a ball-and-socket joint, such as the hip or shoulder, demands that a powerful musculature be developed to provide stability and to prevent frequent subluxation.

The appendicular skeleton of the upper extremity must be articulated to allow the prehensile hand to function in the midline of the body, from mouth to perineum. The lower extremity is articulated to allow locomotion over a variety of terrains with minimal expenditure of energy. Although many homologies exist between the upper and the lower extremities, their different functions have resulted in different adaptations of joint shape and motion.

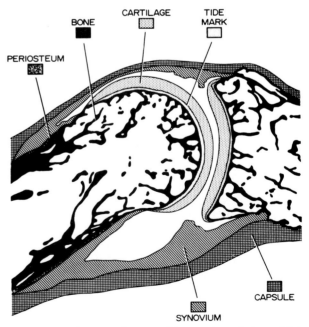

Figure 1–1. A diagram of a normal human interphalangeal joint in sagittal section, as an example of a synovial or diarthrodial joint. The "tidemark" represents the calcified cartilage that bonds articular cartilage to the subchondral bony plate. (With permission from Sokoloff, L., and Bland, J. H.: The Musculoskeletal System. Baltimore, Williams & Wilkins, 1975. © 1975, the Williams & Wilkins Co., Baltimore.)

1

(Details of structure and range of motion of individual joints are discussed in detail in Chapter 21.)

Most joints have the muscle insertion close to the fulcrum (articular surface) so that small muscle contractions produce an extensive arc of motion of the terminal member (hand or foot). Although this arrangement facilitates function, a mechanical price is paid. The muscle is at a mechanical disadvantage; for example, a small weight in the hand, given the force of the muscle contraction necessary to move it, results in a magnification in amplitude of the applied force of three to five times. To dissipate these significant forces over the largest available area, the ends of the bones are flared to increase surface area and thereby reduce the load per unit area to which the cartilage cells are exposed.

The basic structural features of the skeleton, including the articulations, are self-differentiating; the developing limb carries the genetic information to complete its differentiation from primitive mesenchyme to a normally formed structure composed of bone, cartilage, synovium, and so forth. As will be seen, it is the primary form of the cartilaginous model that is entirely self-differentiating; the bony replacement of this model is highly responsive to physical forces.

DEVELOPMENTAL BIOLOGY OF DIARTHRODIAL JOINTS

In the discussion of the events of limb development, two terms that are widely employed by embryologists but that have only loose definitions will be used. A *blastema* is a growing mass of embryonic mesenchymal tissue before definitive tissues or organs can be distinguished. The term is usually used in conjunction with a condensation of cells destined to give rise to a particular structure, for example, the blastemal condensation of the femur. An *anlage* is the first visible and identifiable precursor of a specific organ; for example, the cartilaginous anlage of the humerus refers to the cartilaginous model from the time it first becomes identifiable until it reaches the conclusion of the embryonic period.[1]

Two time gradients exist in the development of the appendicular skeleton. The first gradient is proximodistal, which implies that proximal structures develop in advance of more distal structures. Thus, the glenohumeral articulation develops before the wrist and hand. The second gradient is from craniad to caudad: this refers to the fact that the upper extremity develops approximately 24 hours earlier than homologous portions of the lower limb. The importance of this lies in understanding the influence of environmental factors on congenital anomalies; insults to embryonic development during the period of limb formation will affect a more distal portion of the upper extremity than of the lower extremity.

Early in limb development, "limb mesoderm, like the somite, contains a heterogeneous distribution of chondrogenic and myogenic cells. . . .[The] common precursor 'mesenchyme' cell ancestral to myoblasts and chondroblasts must have divided into cells in the myogenic and chondrogenic lineages at least two generations prior to the appearance of terminally differentiated muscle and cartilage cells."[2] What then determines that cartilage will form centrally and muscle peripherally? Many hypotheses have been advanced under two major categories: (1) cytodifferentiation induced by information transmitted over relatively long distances, usually by gradients of diffusible "morphogens"; and (2) the morphology results from relatively short-distance communication between cells that perhaps already are committed to their functional destinies. With either type of hypothesis, positional information is generated, and it does seem that developing limb cells recognize and respond to their position within the limb.[3]

The Saunders-Zwilling hypothesis is the prime example of the gradient theory; it postulates the elaboration of diffusible agents at the tip of the limb bud that promote the condensation of anlagen along the proximodistal axis.[4] The posterior margin of the limb bud seems to be capable of establishing a second gradient for the anteroposterior axis.

Mathematic models of the gradient theory are particularly exciting for further elucidating how diffusible agents might specify pattern within the developing limb.[5, 6] Newman and Frisch[6] proposed a theory to explain the pattern of limb elements. They address the problem of "how a field of cells that are competent to diversify along more than one pathway do so in a patterned fashion such that appropriate structures appear in the correct positions."[6] The model they propose assumes that two distinct cell populations are found in the blastema—myogenic and chondrogenic—and that these cell types, although indistinguishable microscopically, are geographically separate. The more central cells are chondrogenic and are surrounded by myogenic cells. This arrangement can be predicted on thermodynamic grounds by differences in cell-to-cell adhesion. The chondrogenic cells have three options: cartilage formation, differentiation into fibroblasts, or cell death.

Newman and Frisch also propose that a molecule that promotes cell-to-cell contact produces chondrification in competent cells.[6] They further postulate that there must also be an inhibitor of chondrification. On the basis of analysis of the size of various compartments in the developing chick embryo and the diffusion rates of various-sized molecules through the dilute hyaluronate gel of the developing limb, they have proposed that the chondrogenic molecule is fibronectin and the inhibitor is hyaluronate. These molecules meet the size requirements dictated by the mathematic model. Furthermore, both can be demonstrated in precartilage mesenchyme at the tip of the developing limb bud[5, 7]; hyaluronate has been shown to inhibit chondrogenesis,[8] and the presence of hyaluronidase in the base of the limb bud provides a mechanism to remove

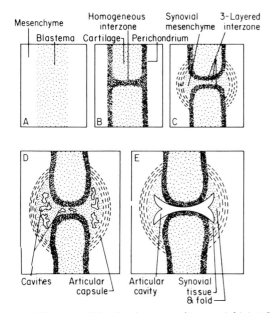

Mesenchyme   Homogeneous   Synovial   3-Layered
              interzone   mesenchyme interzone
  Blastema   Cartilage   Perichondrium

Cavites   Articular   Articular   Synovial
          capsule   cavity   tissue
                                  & fold

Figure 1–2. Diagram of the development of a synovial joint. Joints develop from the blastema, not the surrounding mesenchyme. Chondrification has occurred in *B*. The *interzone* remains avascular and highly cellular. The *synovial mesenchyme* develops from the periphery of the interzone *(C)* and becomes vascularized. Following shortly after differentiation of synovial membrane is *cavitation,* which may begin centrally in the interzone or peripherally *(D)* and merge to form the joint cavity *(E).* (From O'Rahilly, R., and Gardner, E.: The embryology of movable joints. *In* Sokoloff, L. [ed.]: The Joints and Synovial Fluid. Vol. 1. New York, Academic Press, 1978. Used by permission.)

the inhibitory hyaluronate and allow chondrogenesis to proceed from the proximal to the distal end of the limb.[9] Further physicochemical considerations allow the model to predict the arithmetic progression in the number of skeletal elements found from the proximal to the distal sites: one humerus, one radius plus one ulna, three to four carpal bones, and five digits. Furthermore, subtle changes in concentration of any of the three critical molecules or changes in the size of compartments can produce congenital anomalies such as polydactyly or intercalary defects.

Although this model answers some questions, it is neither perfect nor confirmed. Yet, it is interesting that the temporal and spatial distribution of fibronectin predicted by this model has been demonstrated by immunofluorescence.[10] Fibronectin persists in the cartilage core but is diminished in the muscle primordia. The migration of myogenic cells may be oriented by the fibronectin boundary.[11] Migration and adhesion are fundamental processes in this model as well as several others. Edelman[12] and Thiery[13] have demonstrated the existence of cell adhesion molecules that are important in the development of the nervous system. By extension, fibronectin seems to be functioning in a similar role in limb development.[14, 15]

The normal sequences of limb bud formation are well described by O'Rahilly and Gardner.[16] A summary of the stages in order of occurrence follows (Fig. 1–2).

Condensation. Condensation of mesenchyme by cellular aggregation forms a blastema. This occurs shortly after limb buds appear and before a cartilaginous matrix is formed.[17]

Chondrification. Chondrification (Fig. 1–3) begins in the regions of future bones and effectively divides the blastema into cartilaginous precursors of individual limb bones. Intercellular sulfated material accumulates and can be demonstrated by autoradiography.[18] In humans, chondrification can be detected when the embryo is as small as 11.7 mm (stage 17 of embryonic development).[19]

Interzones, the Future Joints. The spaces between segments undergoing chondrification are called *interzones* (Fig. 1–4) and remain as avascular, homogeneous, densely cellular areas where material staining intensely for polysaccharides (probably chondroitin sulfate) is secreted.[20] This extracellular material appears to force the interzone cells apart, resulting in a loose cellular area that becomes the joint cavity.

Formation of Synovial Mesenchyme. The joint capsule evolves as a dense layer of collagen deposited by fibroblasts in the mesoderm surrounding the interzone. The capsule forms at a distance from the interzone, enclosing some of the vascularized mesoderm into the future joint. It is this richly vascularized tissue that gives rise to the vascularized intra-articular structures: synovium, intracapsular ligaments and tendons, and the periphery of the menisci in joints such as the knee. The synovium differentiates at the periphery of the interzone. It probably originates from the surrounding general mesenchyme.[20, 21] In addition to the synovial lining, the joint capsule, intracapsular ligaments, menisci, and tendons all develop from the synovial mesenchyme. Unlike the central interzone or its chondrogenous borders, the synovial mesenchyme becomes vascularized. A dense capillary network develops in the subsynovial tissue with numerous capillary loops into the true synovial lining layer.

As soon as the multiple cavities within the interzone begin to coalesce, the first synovial lining cells can be distinguished. At this stage, only one type of synovial cell can be recognized. Somewhat later, there is an invasion of synovial mesenchyme by blood vessels, with macrophages and other cell types accompanying this vascular invasion. After the primitive joint cavity is formed, expansion takes place rapidly. In all large joints in humans, complete joint cavities are seen at the beginning of the fetal period. The synovial lining cells form a smooth surface, one or two cells thick, overlying a richly vascularized subjacent mesenchyme. The synovial lining cells demonstrate acid phosphatase, beta (β)-glucuronidase, and ATPase activity at this stage. As the joint cavity increases in size, significant proliferation of synovial lining cells must occur to maintain a continuous lining. With continued enlargement of the joint, the synovial cavity develops its characteristic recesses and bursae and acquires its lining of several layers

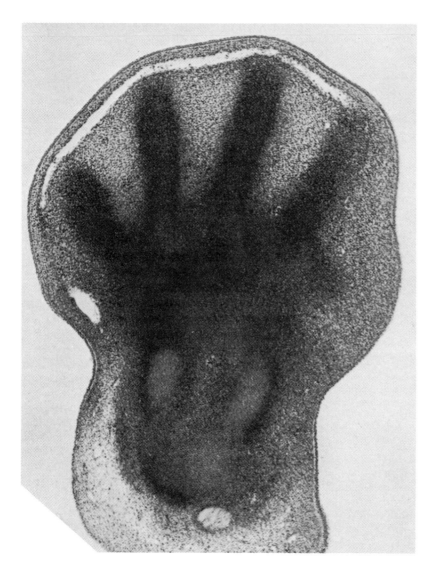

Figure 1–3. Coronal section of the hand at 11.7 mm (stage 17). The blastema with its increased cellularity serves to outline the form of the hand. Faint lightening in the region of the third and fourth metacarpals indicates very early chondrification. The radius and ulna are further along in chondrification. (From O'Rahilly, R.: The development of joints. Ir. J. Med. Sci. 6:456, 1957. Used by permission)

of rounded synovial cells interspersed with the lymphocytes, plasma cells, mast cells, and macrophages that accompanied vascular invasion. The individual synovial lining cells are not connected by means of desmosomes or tight junctions but lie loosely in a bed of hyaluronate interspersed with collagen fibrils. This meshwork of synovial cells, hyaluronate, and collagen overlies a vascular stroma surrounded by the joint capsule. In common usage, the term *synovium* refers both to the true synovial lining and to the subjacent vascular and areolar tissue, up to but excluding the capsule. As tight junctions are not found in normal human synovium, the use of the term *synovial membrane* is not entirely correct. The semipermeable nature of the synovium is imparted not by cell-to-cell junctions but by the macromolecular sieve effect of the hyaluronate surrounding the synovial lining cells.

Synovial villi do not appear until the end of the second month, early in the fetal period. They greatly increase the surface area available for exchange between the joint cavity and the vascular space.

Formation of the Joint Cavity. Cavitation occurs at about the time the synovial mesenchyme differentiates into a pseudomembrane (Figs. 1–5 and 1–6). The precise mechanisms causing cavitation have not been completely defined, but extracellular matrix destruction by enzymes is the final pathway. The interzone cells are probably programmed to release the enzymes that degrade the extracellular material. In chick embryos, it has been shown that movement of the limb is essential for normal cavitation,[22, 23] but similar experiments in developing human embryonic joints have yielded conflicting views.[24]

The cavity begins in the central interzone, the periphery of which is absorbed into each adjacent chondrogenous zone, evolving into the articular surface. Thus, when the cavity has formed, the joint is lined on all surfaces either by hyaline cartilage or by synovial membrane. These two very different tissues merge at the periphery of the joint, where the cartilage melds into bone. A potential space in the body has developed without any basement membrane below the lining cell surface. This absence of any true epithelial tissue is a major determinant of joint physiology.

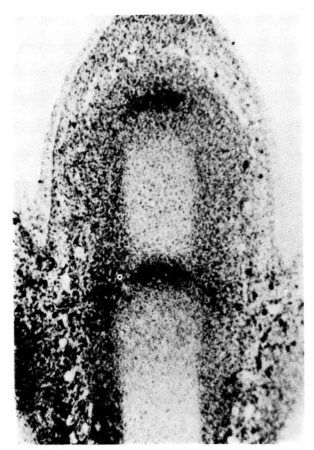

Figure 1–4. Histochemical preparation demonstrating intense localization of acid phosphatase (representing lysosomal activity) in the zone of presumptive joint formation in a mouse embryo. This enzymatic removal of matrix allows cavitation to occur, separating the limb elements. (From Milaire, J.: *In* Frantz C. H. [ed.]: Normal and Abnormal Embryological Development. Washington, DC, National Research Council, 1947, p. 61.)

rump length of 57 to 75 mm (i.e., well into the fetal stage).[25, 26] This retardation may be related to the fact that this joint develops in the absence of a continuous blastema and that its completion is related to insertion of a fibrocartilaginous disc between bone ends[25] derived from muscular and mesenchymal derivatives of the first pharyngeal arch.[26]

Synostoses (cartilaginous and fibrous joints) are presumed to evolve similarly, with the important exceptions that cavitation does not occur and synovial mesenchyme is not formed. Indeed, the "fused" peripheral joints induced in chicken embryos by paralyzing their limbs resemble symphyses, with fibrocartilaginous plates developing between hyaline cartilage at the ends of bones.[27] It may be that symphyses develop as they do because there is relatively little motion during their development.

Human vertebrae and intervertebral discs develop as units from material arising from somites that form a homogeneous blastema.[28] The embryonic intervertebral discs serve as chondrogenous zones (both rostral and caudal) for the evolving vertebral bodies. The periphery of the embryonic "disc" is replaced, after it ceases chondrifying, by the annulus fibrosus.[29] The intervertebral disc bears many similarities to the joint; the annulus is the joint capsule, the nucleus pulposus is the joint cavity, and the vertebral end-plates are the cartilage-covered bone ends comprising the articulation. As the nucleus pulposus contains proteoglycans as well as type II (cartilaginous) collagen,[30–32] it is thought to represent segmented inclusions of the original embryonic disc still active in chondrification.

Direct experimental evidence is lacking as to when hyaluronate (characteristic of joint fluid) first appears in the newly formed cavity. Synovial fibroblasts synthesize and release hyaluronate, which is admixed with a protein-rich filtrate of blood to form synovial fluid. Thus, true synovial fluid cannot form until the synovial mesenchyme has vascularized and cellular differentiation in lining cells has progressed sufficiently to result in hyaluronate synthesis.

The entire development from a cellular but undifferentiated blastema to structures resembling an adult joint occurs in humans from about 4 1/2 to 7 weeks after fertilization.[1] By this time, all large synovial joints have recognizable cavities and are, functionally, true joints. Formation of joints occurs prior to many other crucial phases of musculoskeletal development, including vascularization of epiphyseal cartilage (8 to 12 weeks), appearance of villous folds in synovium (10 to 12 weeks), evolution of bursae (3 to 4 months), and appearance of fat pads (4 to 5 months).

In contrast to other joints, the temporomandibular joint develops slowly, with cavitation at a crown-

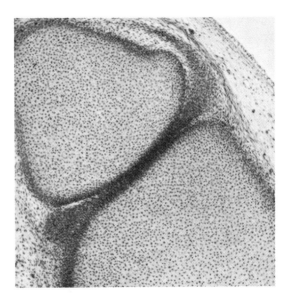

Figure 1–5. The embryonic joint developing between the femur and tibia at 31 mm (stage 23). The lateral meniscus is outlined by cavitation on the femoral side. Cavitation will subsequently spread in a medial direction as well as developing spontaneously at other foci. (From Gardner, E., and O'Rahilly, R.: The early development of the knee joint in staged human embryos. J Anat. 102:289, 1968. Used by permission of Cambridge University Press.)

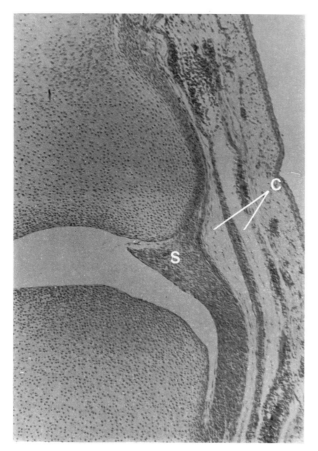

Figure 1–6. Adjacent phalanges in a human embryo hand are separated by a clearly demarcated joint space containing early synovial tissue. The densely collagenous joint capsule lying exterior to the synovium is clearly demonstrated. *S*, Synovium; *C*, capsule. (From Sledge, C. B.: *In* Resnick, D., and Niwayana, G. [eds.]: Diagnosis of Bone and Joint Disorders. 2nd ed. Philadelphia, W. B. Saunders Company, 1988, p. 618. Used by permission.)

ORGANIZATION OF THE MATURE JOINT

The mature diarthrodial joint is a complex structure. Understanding it demands consideration of biomechanics (see Chapter 99) and analysis of the different function of each joint, which is determined in turn by the anatomy peculiar to each joint. In the following section, components of the "typical" synovial joint will be described.

Muscles, Tendons, and Ligaments. The physiology of muscle is described in detail in Chapter 5. It is sufficient here to mention only the direct correlation between muscle *mass* around a joint and the normal *motion* of the joint in different planes. The shoulder, for example, is surrounded by bulky musculature with multiple components. This is essential to allow control of its many extensive arcs of motion: forward flexion, 160 degrees; backward extension, 50 degrees; abduction, 170 degrees; adduction, 50 degrees; and rotation (internal, 70 degrees; external, 70 to 90 degrees). In contrast, more peripheral joints are not stabilized by muscle mass but rather by their conforming anatomy and by dense ligaments that are structurally part of the joint capsule; this arrangement results in a restricted range of motion. The ankle, for example, moves in one plane through limited arcs: flexion, 50 degrees; and extension, 20 degrees.

Individual variability in passive joint motion has a broad range, from the muscled athlete often at risk for muscle "pulls and strains" to the "loose-jointed" asthenic person who suffers frequent joint sprains and who may have a predisposition to developing osteoarthritis[33] and to resembling patients with Ehlers-Danlos type III syndrome (see Chapter 95).

Joint effusions produce reflex inhibition of muscle contraction,[34] and muscle atrophy around a painful (and therefore hypomobile) joint occurs within days; this is especially evident around the knee.

Tendons. Tendons[35] act as functional and anatomic bridges between muscle and bone. As described by Canoso, in addition to focusing the force of a large mass of muscle into a localized area on bone, tendons can, by splitting to form numerous insertions on different bones, transmit the force of a single muscle to different bones (e.g., the multiple insertions of the tibialis posterior).[36] In development, muscle is not necessary for early differentiation of tendons, but without muscle (and possibly muscle contraction), sustained development of tendons fails.[37] Tendons are formed of longitudinally arranged type I collagen bundles interlaced by a delicate reticular network of type III collagen, blood vessels, lymphatics, and possibly thin cellular processes of fibroblasts, which can provide cell-to-cell contact.[38] The principal cell product for export from tendon fibroblasts is type I collagen, although they also synthesize proteoglycans (always a part of the connective tissue matrix) and other proteins (e.g., metalloproteinases and collagenase inhibitors that have implications in the breakdown and repair of tendon components).

Most tendon attachments to bone are a highly specialized complex of transitions through which collagen fibers blend into fibrocartilage, mineralize, then merge into bone.[37] Sharpey's perforating fibers, the tendon fibrils that run through the periosteum and become continuous with outer bone lamellae, may be important at tendon insertions where there are no intervening tiers of fibrocartilage. An example of this is the insertion of the pectoralis major tendon into the humerus.[39] It is unusual for the muscle-tendon apparatus to fail, but when it does, it is secondary to enormous, quickly generated forces across a joint. The site of failure is usually near the tendon insertion into bone.

Many tendons, particularly those with a large range of motion, run through vascularized, discontinuous sheaths of collagen lined with mesenchymal cells resembling synovium. Tendon sheaths provide gliding function, which probably is enhanced by hyaluronic acid produced by the lining cells.[40] Loss of gliding function by formation of fibrous adhesions between tendons and their sheaths occurs when inflammation or surgical incision is followed by long periods of immobilization.

Tendon calcification and tendon rupture are complex pathophysiologic processes that have not been thoroughly evaluated. Factors involved at different times to a greater or lesser degree are (1) aging processes, including loss of extracellular water and an increase in intermolecular cross-links of collagen; (2) traumatically induced ischemic areas in tendon; (3) iatrogenic factors, including intratendon injection of glucocorticoids; and (4) deposition of calcium hydroxyapatite crystals—perhaps enhanced by presence of the calcium-binding amino acid gamma (γ)-carboxyglutamic acid.[41]

There are few anatomic and structural differences between ligaments and tendons. The obvious difference is that one end of tendon collagen fibrils is intertwined and braided among the fibrillar endomysium that surrounds each individual muscle fiber, whereas both ends of ligaments insert into bone on either side of a joint. Ligaments often are recognized only as hypertrophied components of the fibrous joint capsule. Some ligaments have a much higher ratio of elastin to collagen (1:4) than do tendons (1:50).[36] The ligamentum flavum, which holds adjacent vertebral laminae in place and stretches with spine flexion, is an example of a ligament with a high concentration of elastin. Ligaments and tendons synthesize substances that regulate connective tissue metabolism locally. For example, in addition to collagen, tendon cells produce collagenase in latent form as well as inhibitors of collagenolytic enzymes.

Ligaments. Ligaments[42] play a major role in the passive stabilization of joints, aided by the capsule and, when present, menisci. In the knee (the most studied of all joints), the collateral and cruciate ligaments provide stability when there is little or no load on the joint. During load-bearing conditions, there is an increasing contribution to stability from the joint surfaces themselves as compressive load increases. The components that provide surface stability are friction (minimal) between the joint surfaces, deformation of the cartilage, and geometric conformity of the condyles.

Bursae. The many bursae in the human body serve to facilitate gliding function much as a tendon sheath facilitates movement of the tendon within, enabling low-friction motion of one tissue over another. Bursae are closed sacs, lined sparsely with mesenchymal cells similar to synovial cells. Although most bursae differentiate concurrently with synovial joints during embryogenesis, during life new bursae may develop in response to stress and previously existing ones may become hypertrophied.[43] During life, again in response to stress (i.e., inflammation or trauma), deep bursae often develop communications with joints.[36] Examples of this include (1) iliopsoas bursa–hip joint; (2) subacromial bursae–glenohumeral joint; and (3) gastrocnemius or semimembra-nous bursae–knee joint. It is unusual for subcutaneous bursae (e.g., the prepatellar bursa or olecranon bursa) to develop communication with the underlying joint. Bursal fluid, even when the bursa is infected or host to an attack of gout, rarely generates an inflammatory response (measured by number of polymorphonuclear leukocytes) that a similar process does within a joint.[44] This may be related to a lesser degree of vascularization of bursae.

Menisci. Menisci[45] are fibrocartilaginous, wedge-shaped structures that are best developed in the knee but are also found in the acromioclavicular and sternoclavicular joints, the ulnocarpal joint, and the temporomandibular joint. Until recently, these structures were believed to have little function and an indolent metabolism with no capability of repair. Removal of menisci from the knee was found to lead to premature arthritic changes in the joint,[46] and, thus, there has been increased attention directed toward preserving the meniscus by repair of tears. To understand why some tears heal and others do not, investigators have examined the blood supply of the meniscus and found the outer one third to have a good enough perfusion to mount a repair response.[47] The microanatomy of the meniscus is complex and age dependent. The characteristic shape of both the lateral and medial menisci is obtained early in prenatal development. At that time, they are very cellular and highly vascularized throughout their substance. Vascularity then decreases, progressing from central to the peripheral margin with alterations in the collagen fiber arrangement. After skeletal maturity, the peripheral portion constitutes from 10 to 30 percent of the total structure. It is highly vascularized, dense connective tissue that contains type I and type II nerve endings. Blood vessels arborize and form a capillary plexus that is mainly circumferential with radial branches directed centrally. The remaining portion of the meniscus is made up of an avascular, aneural, and alymphatic fibrocartilage consisting of cells surrounded by an abundant extracellular matrix. The matrix is comprised of 60 percent chondroitin-6 sulfate, 25 percent chondroitin-4 sulfate, 10 percent nonsulfated chondroitin, and 5 percent dermatan sulfate. Hyaluronic acid comprises 6 percent of the total uronate of the tissues. Collagen, mostly type I, constitutes 60 to 70 percent of the dry weight of the meniscus. There are trace quantities of type III and type V collagen and a small but significant quantity of type II in the inner avascular portion of the meniscus. There is also some type VI collagen found, presumably in pericellular lacunar capsules where it anchors the larger fibrils together. Collagen fibers in the periphery are mostly circumferentially oriented, with radial fibers extending toward the central portion.[48] The cells of the meniscus are able to repair wounds and remodel the matrix after injury when such injury occurs in the vascularized peripheral zone.

Articular Cartilage

The following discussion is a brief synthesis of the structure and function of articular cartilage. Details of its structural components can be found in Chapter 2 (collagen) and Chapter 3 (glycoproteins).

Organization of Articular Cartilage. Articular cartilage is the unique structure of joints; it is highly differentiated and has physical properties that no other tissue or synthetic product of bioengineering laboratories can equal. Articular cartilage must provide a smooth, resilient surface for joint motion under conditions of intense pressure or high velocity, or both. At the same time, the cartilage must retain capacity for maintenance without morphologic change and, in the absence of any blood vessels, for transport of nutrients and removal of products of chondrocyte metabolism and matrix turnover. Even though endowed with a capacity for maintenance, articular cartilage cannot effectively regenerate itself, and this imposes a limitation on the organism—a need to protect articular cartilage from destruction.

Figure 1–7 is a diagrammatic representation of the various zones and regions of cartilage.

The *superficial zone* (5 to 10 percent of total thickness) has a reduced metachromatic staining for glycosaminoglycans and a rich content of immunoreactive proteoglycan core protein and link protein. Called the *lamina splendens,* this is probably composed of hyaluronic acid or absorbed glycoproteins, or both.[49] The superficial zone is covered at the cartilage surface by a layer of thin fibrils (4 to 10 mm in diameter), which are arranged in a random fashion up to several microns in depth. Early studies using scanning electron microscopy showed ridges and undulations in the cartilage surface.[50, 51] Other investigators believe that these undulations are artifacts of cutting and fixation.[52, 53] However, there is evidence that there are shallow pits or round undulations in the surface contour (10 to 40 nm in diameter and 1 to 6 nm deep), which may represent underlying lacunae of chondrocytes[54, 55] (Fig. 1–8). It is not known whether these depressions exist in vivo, although researchers who study joint lubrication have often used the existence of undulations as evidence of crucial "trapped" reservoirs for squeeze-film lubrication.

Collagen. The collagen fibrils within articular cartilage are arranged with some degree of order: on the surface, the fibrils are parallel to the surface and have a preferential orientation at an angle to the usual direction of motion of the joint, much like the reinforcing fibers in a radial tire. In the deeper portion of the cartilage, fibrils originate in the calcified layer and form plates that sweep vertically through the middle or "radial" zone, then curve to blend into the surface fibrils. Pericellular collagen capsules, probably type V collagen, interdigitate with the vertical fibers, tying the whole structure, with its contained chondrocytes, into a coherent structure capable of resisting shear forces.[56–58] Type II collagen comprises 90 percent of this fibrillar network. There are also minor collagens such as types III, VI, IX, and XI.[59] In pericellular areas, collagen fibril diameters are much less than in territorial and interterritorial areas. Type V collagen is found primarily in a pericellular location near chondrocytes.[60]

Proteoglycans. Proteoglycans are organized in territorial and pericellular regions of the deep zone in a manner similar to that of comparable regions in the superficial and middle zones.[60] Immunoelectron microscopic studies have revealed that the interterritorial regions of the deep zone differ markedly in organization from the territorial regions of the deep zone.[61] The territorial regions revealed minimal evidence for link protein, whereas only the interterritorial regions of the deep zone revealed staining patterns consistent with structural organization of hyaluronate, link protein, proteoglycan core protein, and glycosaminoglycans as large aggregates.

These large aggregates and the large amount of water bound to them form a massive polyanionic complex that has a large domain and the capacity to resist compressive force; compression shrinks the domain of each aggregate, increasing the electronegative repellent force. In addition, the charge effects cause a resistance to bound water flow. The effect, in biomechanical terms, is to make the cartilage elastic, so that after compression is released, the aggregated proteoglycans return to their fully extended state from forces generated by mutual repulsion of negatively charged groups.[62]

It has been suggested that because the interterritorial regions have widely spaced, thick collagen fibrils and large amounts of link-stabilized proteoglycans, it is this area of cartilage that has the greatest compressibility.[61] The nature of the association of proteoglycans and hyaluronic acid with collagen is complex.[63] Certain fractions of proteoglycans may affect the formation of fibrils,[64] whereas others may inhibit calcification in articular cartilage.[65] Significantly, fractions of proteoglycans capable of inhibiting mineral crystal formation are absent from calcifying cartilage.[66]

Glycoproteins. Glycoproteins are present in cartilage in a concentration inverse to that of collagen.[67] Lysozyme and other cationic glycoproteins of low molecular weight are present in cartilage, probably synthesized by chondrocytes. Some of these cationic proteins have the capacity to inhibit proteolytic enzymes[68–70] and tumor neovascularization[71] and retard the development of osteoclasts.[72] These factors are of particular interest because avascular cartilage is generally resistant to invasion by tumors. The proteinase (trypsin) inhibitors in cartilage appear to be identical to the well-known bovine pancreatic trypsin inhibitor.[70] The collagenase inhibitor found in cartilage is a molecular species separate from the serine or thiol proteinase inhibitors.[73] (See Chapter 14 for discussion of the enzymes and enzyme inhibitors of cartilage.)

Water. Amid collagen fibers is a heterogeneous

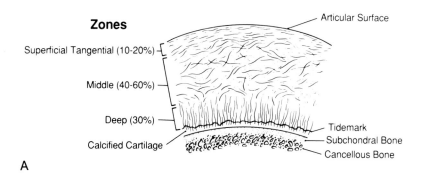

Zones

Superficial Tangential (10-20%)

Middle (40-60%)

Deep (30%)

Calcified Cartilage

Articular Surface

Tidemark

Subchondral Bone

Cancellous Bone

A

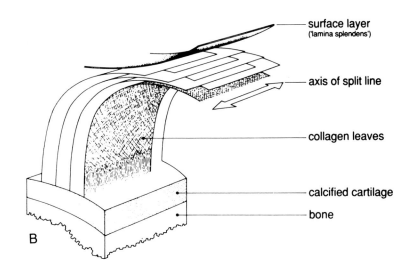

surface layer
('lamina splendens')

axis of split line

collagen leaves

calcified cartilage

bone

B

Figure 1–7. *A,* Zones of articular cartilage showing apparent random organization of collagen fibrils. *B,* Three-dimensional view of collagen plates in articular cartilage illustrating how the appearance of the collagen changes from ''arcades'' to random to plates, depending upon the orientation of the section. *C,* Diagrammatic representation of the zones and regions of bovine articular cartilage. (Part A reprinted with permission from Mow, V. C., et al. *In* Nordin, M., and Frankel, V. H. [eds.]: Basic Biomechanics of the Musculoskeletal System. 2nd ed. Philadelphia, Lea & Febiger, 1989. Part B from Jeffery, A. K., et al.: Three-dimensional collagen architecture in bovine articular cartilage. J. Bone Joint Surg. [Br.] 73-B:795, 1991. Part C reproduced from Poole, A. R., et al.: An immuno–electron microscope study of the organization of proteoglycan monomer, link protein, and collagen in the matrix of articular cartilage. *Journal of Cell Biology* 93:921, 1982. By copyright permission of the Rockefeller University Press.)

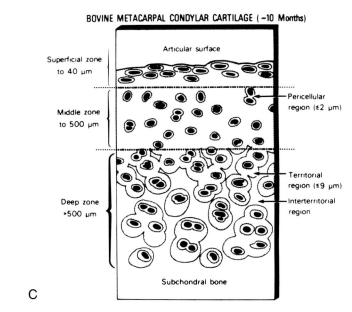

BOVINE METACARPAL CONDYLAR CARTILAGE (~10 Months)

Articular surface

Superficial zone
to 40 μm

Middle zone
to 500 μm

Deep zone
>500 μm

Pericellular
region (≤2 μm)

Territorial
region (≤9 μm)

Interterritorial
region

Subchondral bone

C

collection of water and ground substance. Water content is about 70 to 75 percent of the wet weight, and, in many instances, this rises to over 80 percent near the surface.[74]

Micropuncture studies of articular cartilage have revealed an electrolyte concentration in this extracel-lular fluid similar to that in plasma except for a pH of 7.1 to 7.2.[75] Interestingly, at the growth area of articular cartilage around hypertrophic cells, the pH is higher, a factor that may facilitate calcification near the tidemark.

As reviewed by Mankin,[76] most of the water of

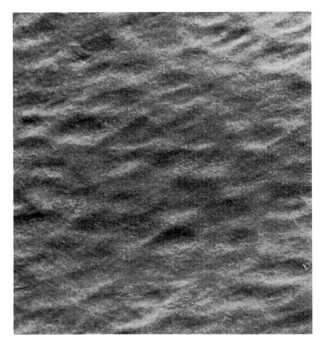

Figure 1–8. Scanning electron microscopic view of the "pits" found on the surface of articular cartilage. This view of adult rabbit cartilage at ~500 magnification. It is not known whether the depressions are present in vivo or whether they represent artifacts produced by desiccation and shrinkage during preparation for microscopy. Prominent ridgings of the surface of articular cartilage reported by earlier investigators are probably true cutting artifacts. Surface irregularity of some magnitude is essential for the full development of the hypothesis of squeeze-film lubrication in which, during weight bearing, interstitial fluid from cartilage matrix would be trapped in surface depressions (or between ridges) and prevent direct cartilage-cartilage contact. (From Ghadially, F. N., et al.: Experimental production of ridges on rabbit articular cartilage: A scanning electron microscopic study. J. Anat. 121:119, 1976. Used by permission of Cambridge University Press.)

articular cartilage is bound loosely within the matrix and exchanges readily with water in synovial fluid. The cartilage glycosaminoglycans do not appear to be essential for water binding; in osteoarthritis, when proteoglycan content is decreased, water content in cartilage can be increased by as much as 8 percent, owing to loss of restraint of glycosaminoglycans and to collagen network defects.[77]

It is of interest that movement of uncharged small solutes, such as glucose, is not impaired by diffusion through matrices containing large amounts of glycosaminoglycans, and Hadler has reviewed studies indicating that diffusivity of small molecules through hyaluronate is actually enhanced.[78] If applicable to articular cartilage in vivo, this phenomenon would facilitate nutrient exchange during compressive force on cartilage.

Chondrocytes. Chondrocytes exist in relative isolation, living singly or in pairs or with a few other cells in clusters. They are highly specialized and express the capacity to synthesize matrix components (e.g., collagen, proteoglycans, noncollagenous acidic glycoproteins, chondronectin, small cationic polypeptides, and other glycoproteins) as well as en-

zymes (e.g., collagenase, neutral proteinases, and cathepsins) capable of breaking down matrix components. Chondrocytes lie in a zone of finely textured matrix containing abundant ground substance but only a few collagen fibers.[79] Taking into consideration mean cell size and density, Stockwell and Meachim have estimated that the volume of cartilage occupied by cells is between 0.4 and 2 percent of total cartilage volume.[3] The "lacunae" seen around chondrocytes prepared for light microscopy are shrinkage artifacts.[80]

Preparations of articular cartilage made for transmission electron microscopy show cells with rounded or oval nuclei that sometimes contain fibrous laminae (up to 95 nm thick, particularly in chondrocytes involved, apparently, in repair of tissue defects).[81] Rough endoplasmic reticulum and the Golgi complex are most developed in chondrocytes of zones II and III. Short cell processes are seen on all chondrocytes but are better developed in cells of deeper zones and may play a role in transport of cellular enzymes to the extracellular space or in pinocytotic function, or both.[82] Chondrocytes certainly have a phagocytic function and can be shown to take up red blood cell products in chronic hemarthrosis[83] (see Chapter 90). Cartilage cells die in situ from time to time. Necrotic remnants of cells are found adjacent to healthy cells. As data by Stockwell have shown that the cell density of the full thickness of human adult femoral condylar cartilage is $(14.5 + 3.0) \times 10^3$ cells per mm^3 from age 20 through 80 years, it follows that new chondrocytes arise by mitosis to replace dead ones.[84] Despite this logical extrapolation of data, mitoses are not observed in normal adult articular cartilage.[3]

Nutrition. Since William Hunter's observations in 1743 that adult articular cartilage contains no blood vessels,[85] there has been debate about how chondrocytes receive nutrients, although numerous studies have confirmed an early study by Bywaters[86] that articular cartilage principally utilizes anaerobic glycolysis for energy production.

In the growing child, active enchondral ossification occurs at the base of articular cartilage just as it does at the growth plate (primary epiphysis). Here, in the hypertrophic zone of cartilage, blood vessels penetrate between columns of chondrocytes. The cartilage is calcified and, subsequently, is replaced by true bone. It is likely that diffusion from these tiny end capillaries through matrix to chondrocytes occurs. This mechanism is unlikely in the adult, because the tidemark (the dense, calcified lower layer of articular cartilage) is not bridged by capillaries, although some studies have described partial defects in the osteocartilaginous barrier.[87, 88] Collins has suggested that the existence of this calcified barrier is characteristic of a "stable" joint, and, whether in a diarthrodial joint, rib, or intervertebral disc, it prevents passage of material across the barrier.[89]

In contrast, morphologic, physiologic, and pathologic studies have confirmed that solutes pass easily from the synovial fluid into cartilage and that cartilage does not survive without contact with synovial fluid in vivo. Strangeways provided early support for the concept of nutrition by diffusion by noting that loose bodies of cartilage in joints actually grow in size.[90] In experimental systems it has been shown that sufficient agitation of synovial fluid results in nourishment of even the deepest layers of articular cartilage.[91]

There are three potential mechanisms for nutrient transfer within cartilage matrix: diffusion, active transport by chondrocytes, and pumping by intermittent compression of cartilage matrix. Maroudas and associates have demonstrated that molecules the size of hemoglobin (M_r 65,000) are the largest that can diffuse through normal articular cartilage.[91] Fortunately, the molecular weight of solutes needed for cellular metabolism is small enough to permit adequate diffusion within the cartilage of mobilized, healthy joints.

Intermittent compression serving as a pump mechanism for solute exchange in cartilage is a concept that has arisen from observations that joint immobilization[92] or dislocation[93] or other events that interfere with normal movement of one articular surface on its counterpart lead to degenerative changes in cartilage. Exercise, in contrast, increases solute penetration into cartilage in experimental systems.[91] Pressing filter paper against cartilage squeezes out liquid that has the ionic composition of extracellular fluid.[94] McCutchen suggested that during weight bearing, fluid escapes from the load-bearing region by flow to other cartilage sites and into grooves in the slightly irregular cartilage surface.[95] When the load was removed, cartilage would re-expand and draw back fluid. Nutrients could be exchanged with waste materials during such a process. Whether diffusion, even boosted by pressure, could occur fast enough for this weeping lubrication to facilitate solute exchange and penetration is hotly debated but is supported by studies showing free exchange of water between cartilage and synovial fluid and the enhanced diffusivity of solutes in a matrix of hyaluronate.

Mechanical Properties of Cartilage. Articular cartilage, which has little capability of repair, functions for the lifetime of the organism only if the physical demands placed on it are kept within a narrow range, around 25 kg per cm². The most important physical parameter is unit load—the force applied divided by the area over which the load is spread. There are four mechanisms available to protect joints, one active (muscle contraction) and three passive: (1) transfer of forces into surrounding soft tissue, ligaments, and muscles; (2) joint incongruency, which allows increasing contact area with increasing load; and (3) compliance of the cartilage–cancellous bone unit. The articular ends of the bones are flared to provide the largest articular surface for joint contact, thereby minimizing the unit load on articular cartilage. The flared end is composed of trabecular bone aligned along stress lines, minimiz-

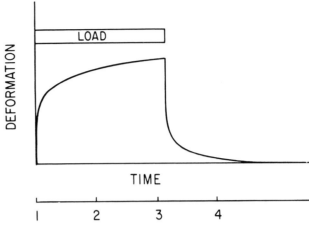

Figure 1–9. A typical curve of deformation of articular cartilage by a load as a function of time. The four phases expressed as a function of time are as follows: 1 = instantaneous deformation coincident with application of the load; 2 = slow deformation that gradually slows in rate of deformation; 3 = instantaneous recovery; 4 = time-dependent recovery to normal cartilage thickness. (After Bär, E.: Elasticitätsprufungen der Gelenkkorpel. Arch. J. Entwicklungsmech. Organ. 108:739, 1926; and Kempson, G. E.: Mechanical properties of articular cartilage. *In* Freeman, M. A. R. [ed.]: Adult Articular Cartilage. New York, Grune & Stratton, 1974, p. 196. Used by permission.)

ing weight while providing optimal strength and resilience to absorb joint impact forces.

The demands placed on each joint dictate the precise relationships among the three mechanisms of force dissipation. The shoulder, having an enormous range of motion, must have a small area of contact and minimal constraint. Stress overload is prevented by two mechanisms: (1) dissipation of forces into the soft tissues supporting the mechanically unstable articulation, and (2) high compliance conferred by virtue of having one side of the articulation (the scapula) "floating" in a highly compliant mass of muscle. The ankle, which provides limited and essentially uniaxial motion, experiences enormous forces but must remain small, with limited contact areas, because of its distance from the fulcrum (the hip) and the inertia that would prevent the acceleration of a large, heavy body segment through a distance. Here the solution is by significant dissipation of forces to the fibula and, to a lesser extent, by incongruency and expansion of the articulation with increasing force.

The most important function of cartilage—its ability to be compressed by a load and recover from this deformity—has been an object of research since Bar's studies in 1926[96] (Fig. 1–9). When a load is applied to cartilage, there is a rapid ("instantaneous") indentation that is followed by a time-dependent compression (called *creep*) phase, during which indentation increases while load remains constant. On removal of the load, there is an initial immediate recovery, followed by a long, sustained recovery to normal volume. The initial rapid deformation results from a bulk movement of water and compression of collagen fibers. In the second, time-dependent compression, water flows through the matrix.

From studies of the bone-bone contact in the absence of cartilage, it has become apparent that a function of cartilage, in addition to providing low-friction movement at high speeds, may be to absorb some of the energy of impact loading by deforming and effectively spreading a load over a broad area. Freeman and Kempson have put forth the argument that in normal cartilage both collagen and proteoglycans contribute to load carriage.[97] Tensile strength of the collagen resists deformation and maintains the basic structural framework to allow proteoglycans to remain in place. The proteoglycans, through strong charge interactions with water, control solute flow and, therefore, the absolute and time-dependent deformation by weight bearing.

Studies of matrix-depleted cartilage have helped clarify the relative roles of collagen and proteoglycans in the function of cartilage. With the use of canine articular cartilage slices, it was demonstrated that cartilage incubated with collagenase became filmy, flimsy, and transparent; it was devoid of tensile strength.[98] Similar slices incubated with trypsin sufficient to deplete matrix proteoglycans did not change in gross appearance; however, the physical qualities changed. Control slices were relatively rigid, whereas trypsin-treated slices were easily bent in half. More detailed studies to measure deformation revealed that proteoglycan-depleted cartilage had lost its ability to rebound from a deforming load; it had lost compressive stiffness.[99, 100] In similar experiments, using cathepsin D, British investigators freed 50 percent of tissue uronic acid without releasing any hydroxyproline (a collagen marker).[101] This produced a 50 percent reduction in compressive stiffness.

Repair of Articular Cartilage.[102] Healing of cartilage defects that do not penetrate the subchondral bone plate is dependent entirely on surviving chondrocytes near the margins of injury. In humans, essentially no repair is generated by these cells.[103] Occasionally, the chondrocytes proliferate to form clones or "brood capsules," but the clefts in cartilage do not heal. Defects will remain without progression so long as the subchondral bone plate remains intact.

In deeper injury through the subchondral plate, there is extensive fibroblastic proliferation into the defect, but seldom is true hyaline cartilage produced. More often, a fibrocartilaginous scar results from this extrinsic repair effort.[103, 104] Thus, repair of articular cartilage is not programmed well in human biologic systems; the emphasis is on protection from damage. In the early stages of osteoarthritis, however, there is considerable increase in new matrix synthesis, which may retard progression of destructive disease (see Chapter 78).

Aging of Articular Cartilage. The thickness of articular cartilage in mammalian limbs has been found to be related to body weight, hip-to-shoulder length, and the area of the tibial plateau.[105] Cartilage thickness is asymmetric over the surface of weight-bearing joints.[106] On the surface of the human femoral head, cartilage is thickest on the anterosuperior surface of the femoral head and increases with age. The increased thickness has not been related to fibrillation of the cartilage and cannot be interpreted as a change associated with early osteoarthrosis.[107]

The overall cellularity of cartilage does not change with age, nor does the fluid content or total amount of collagen and glycosaminoglycan.[97] Changes in color appear; adult cartilage develops a yellow tinge, but there is no evidence that this pigment has any functional significance. As mentioned earlier, cartilage collagen fibers in aged articular cartilage are thicker than those in cartilage of younger people.

In areas of articular cartilage that are not in habitual contact with an opposing cartilage surface, fibrillation develops with age.[108] This type of fibrillation cannot be considered as necessarily leading to osteoarthritis and may best be considered a "regressive change." It often occurs first at the periphery of joint surfaces.[104, 107] Fibrillation is initially confined to the superficial layers of cartilage. Here the cartilage shows foci of mild splitting and fraying. Surface "pits" develop, and grossly the surface develops a matte instead of a gloss appearance.

Chemical analysis of fibrillated areas of cartilage has shown a depletion of glycosaminoglycans with normal collagen concentration.[77, 109] Comparative stiffness of the cartilage is decreased. If fibrillation progresses into deeper layers of cartilage, an abnormal multicellular cluster of chondrocytes that stain intensely for glycosaminoglycans is found at the base of clefts.[108] The fibrillated areas by this time are noticeably softer or malacic. Freeman and Kempson[97] have presented a reasonable argument for the hypothesis that fibrillation begins with fatigue fracture of superficial collagen bundles. This results in superficial clefts, which deepen if the process continues. (See Chapter 78 for a detailed discussion of the changes in osteoarthritis.)

Subchondral Bone. The microstructure of bone in the plate beneath the calcified base of articular cartilage may have many effects on the cartilage above it. The subchondral bone of the knee is formed from a meshwork of fine trabeculae of less than 0.2-mm diameter and in a density of fewer than two trabeculae per millimeter of bone. The stiffness of subchondral bone, and thus the impact transmitted to cartilage during weight bearing or effort, may be a factor in the health of normal articular cartilage.[110, 111]

VASCULAR AND NERVE SUPPLY

Arterial and venous networks of the joint are complex and are characterized by arteriovenous anastomoses that communicate freely with the vascular supply to periosteum and to periarticular bone.[112] As large synovial arteries enter the deep layers of the

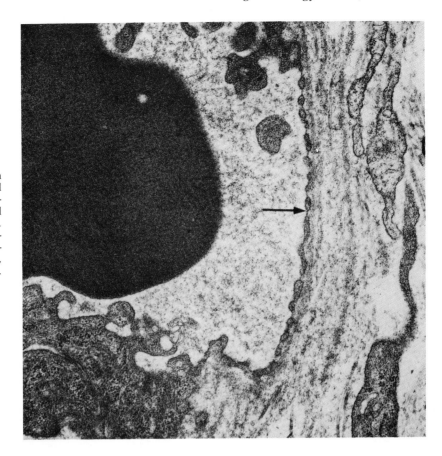

Figure 1–10. Fenestrated blood capillary in human synovium. This capillary is situated just beneath the lining layer. Pores in endothelium are indicated by the arrow. A red blood cell lies in the lumen of the capillary. × 11,000. (From Bassleer, R., et al.: *In* Franchimont, P. [ed.]: Articular Synovium: Anatomy, Physiology, Pathology, Pharmacology, and Therapy. Basel, Karger, 1982, pp. 1–26. Used by permission.)

synovium near the capsule, they give off branches, which branch again to form microvascular units in the subsynovial layers. As in other tissues, precapillary arterioles probably play a major role in controlling circulation to the lining layer. The surface area of the synovial capillary bed is very large and, as it runs only a few cell layers deep to the surface, it has a role in trans-synovial exchange of molecules, which may explain the propensity of diarthrodial joints to develop effusions and hemarthroses.

Heat (up to an intra-articular temperature of 40°C) increases blood flow through synovial capillaries.[113] Exercise, although resulting in an increase in periarticular muscle blood flow, may actually result in a decrease in the clearance rate of small molecules.[114] Immobilization, in experimental animals, actually decreases the number of capillary plexi as well as blood flow in joints.[113] Pressure also has an effect on blood flow. Effusions can act to tamponade blood supply, and it is possible that large effusions could virtually shut off blood flow to superficial lining layers.[115]

Synovial capillaries are fenestrated; they contain small pores covered by a thin membrane[114, 116] (Fig. 1–10). These fenestrations may facilitate rapid exchange of small molecules (e.g., glucose, lactate, and so on) with the synovial fluid.

Dissection studies have shown that each joint has a dual nerve supply: (1) specific articular nerves that penetrate the capsule as independent branches of adjacent peripheral nerves; and (2) articular branches that arise from related muscle nerves.[116] The definition of joint position and the detection of joint motion are monitored separately and by a combination of multiple inputs from different receptors in varied systems. Dee has summarized data indicating that nerve endings in muscle as well as in the joint capsule are involved in articular kinesthetic sensation.[117] Patients who have had capsulectomy along with total hip replacement[118] or surgical removal of proximal interphalangeal or metacarpophalangeal joints of the hand[119] still retain good awareness of joint position.

SYNOVIUM

The synovial "membrane" covers all intra-articular structures except for articular cartilage and the central portions of fibrocartilaginous menisci, and localized "bare areas" where bone is exposed.[89] Although it lines a closed space in the body, there is no epithelial tissue in the synovium and, therefore, no basement membrane or structural barrier between synovial fluid and synovial blood vessels (Fig. 1–11).

Organization of the Synovium. The absence of a basement membrane assures a continuation of morphology as well as of function. Although the outer layers of the joint capsule are relatively acellular and formed of thick, intertwining bands of collagen

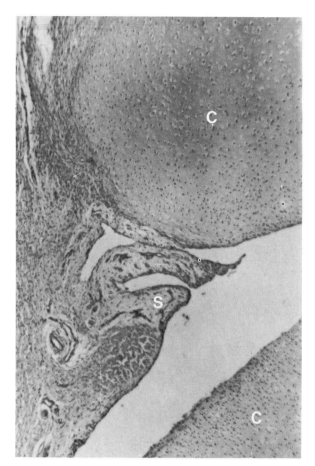

Figure 1–11. With further development of the synovial lining, the surface is thrown up into multiple folds or villi, which greatly increase the surface area available for diffusion from the subsynovial vessels into the joint space and vice versa. *S*, Synovium; *C*, cartilage. (From Sledge, C. B.: *In* Resnick, D., and Niwayana, G. [eds.]: Diagnosis of Bone and Joint Disorders. 2nd ed. Philadelphia, W. B. Saunders Company, 1988, p. 619. Used by permission.)

fibers that do not resemble the highly cellular synovial lining, the change from one to the other is not abrupt. The cells below the lining layers resemble lining cells, but there is more connective tissue. Continuing centrifugally, the cells appear more as fibroblasts. Fat cells increase in number, larger blood vessels are seen, and dense bands of collagen appear. The ligaments that span joints and confer stability on them are continuous with the outer layers of capsule in many joints. With this concept of a structural continuum established, however, it is convenient to divide the lining into (1) the intima or synovial lining, (2) subsynovial tissue, and (3) the joint capsule.

The synovial lining layer may be discontinuous in some locations. In areas where the synovium is subjected to pressure and over ligaments and tendons, the cells are widely separated; at these loci, the extracellular connective tissue, not synovial cells, constitutes the lining layer.[120] Intra-articular fat pads are usually covered by a single layer of synovial cells.

In other areas not subject to trauma, the synovial cells often accumulate in layers three to four cells deep. Viewed under a tangential light source, a faint pebbling that represents microvilli can be seen.

Synovial Lining Cells. Barland and colleagues[119a] defined two principal types of synovial lining cells, (Fig. 1–12), and the cells' existence has been confirmed by others.[120, 121] *Type A cells* (macrophage-like) contain a prominent Golgi complex and many microvesicles, various and heterogeneous inclusions (residual bodies), and lysosomes. The nucleus contains dense chromatin. Microfilaments are abundant, lying in the long axis of the cell. Frequent, thin cell processes stretching into the adjacent matrix are seen. *Type B cells* (fibroblast-like) have a prominent, rough endoplasmic reticulum with few cell processes and vacuoles. Nuclear chromatin is less dense, and nu-

A

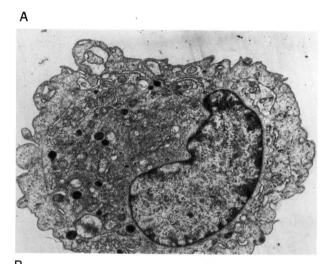

B

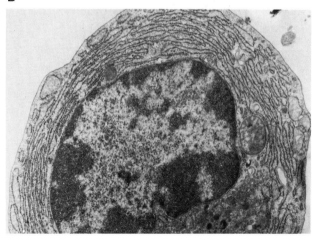

Figure 1–12. *A*, Type A human synovial cell with many undulations in the cell membrane, vacuoles, and inclusions. This cell presumably has phagocytic capabilities and is thought of as a macrophage. × 11,200. (Courtesy of Donald Gates.) *B*, Type B human synovial cell with a very well-developed endoplasmic reticulum. This cell presumably has capabilities for synthesis of protein. × 17,500. (Courtesy of Donald Gates.) It must be emphasized that there are many synovial cells with organelles developed for both synthetic and phagocytic function. In addition, it is possible that individual cells may be modulated from cells with synthetic to ones with phagocytic function.

cleoli are more developed. Cytoplasmic vacuoles and vesicles are rare.

It has been natural to ascribe phagocytic and, therefore, macrophage-like function to type A cells and synthetic or fibroblast-like function to type B cells.[122, 123] This, however, may be a naive assumption. It ignores the facts that one cell may have more than one function and that in response to different stimuli, cells can modulate their internal structure as their function changes. A number of observations support these principles. First, type C cells or intermediate synovial cells have been described that have endoplasmic reticulum and Golgi complexes and vacuoles.[123] Second, using stains for RNA on ribosomes (an acceptable index of synthetic function in cells), only a few cells stain positively in normal synovium. Staining increases in intensity and appears in increased numbers of cells if a joint has been traumatized; in severe inflammatory states, no cells without a developed endoplasmic reticulum are observed.[124] Synovial cells that appear morphologically to be fibroblasts nevertheless demonstrate macrophage-like function in response to certain stimuli. Rabbit synovial "fibroblasts," for example, actively phagocytose latex particles.[125] Gold salts injected into the synovial cavity are rapidly taken up in pinocytotic vesicles,[126] and iron pigment is readily engulfed after intra-articular hemorrhage in hemophilia.[127] Evidence is mounting that type A cells may synthesize and secrete hyaluronic acid. The firmest data are the demonstrations by ultrastructural studies that hyaluronic acid is found both in the Golgi complex and in the large secretory vacuoles of these phagocytic cells.[128]

It may be reasonable to consider the synovial lining cell as one with multiple phenotypic possibilities and to resist categorizing it by its morphologic resemblance at certain stages to other, better characterized cells. As noted by Ghadially, "Type A and B may be cells whose difference in morphology reflects the function they are performing at a given moment."[79] In the normal human knee, there is a vascular, wedge-shaped tongue of tissue covering the articular surface at the margin. This is in continuity with and immunohistochemically similar to the adjacent synovial tissue and contains cells possessing both class II HLA antigens and antigens present on macrophages and type B synoviocytes.[129]

Fibronectin[130] and probably laminin[131] are secreted by synovial cells. These glycoproteins may aid in attachment of cells to underlying matrix.[132–135]

Type VI collagen is found in the extracellar matrix of the lining cell layer of normal synovium, and there is type III collagen in the lining and sublining cell layers. It has been suggested that type VI collagen, with the ability to bind cells to interstitial collagen, plays an important role in binding the synovial lining cells together in the absence of tight junctions or desmosomes.[136] In cell culture, synovial cells synthesize collagen (types I and III), latent collagenase, latent proteinases, an activator of colla-

genase, inhibitors of neutral metalloproteinases, hyaluronic acid, proteoglycans, and many other minor and unidentified matrix constituents.

Normal synovium in culture can be induced to produce interleukin-1 (IL-1), which stimulates chondrocytes to release enzymes that degrade the cartilage matrix.[137–139] This cytokine also stimulates the production of prostaglandin E_2 as well as fibronectin and types I and III collagen.[140] Synovial fibroblasts respond to stimulation by IL-1β, tumor necrosis factor-α (TNF-α), and interferon-γ (IFN-γ) by increasing the expression of intercellular adhesion molecule-1 and also by increased expression of HLA class II antigen.[141]

Synovial Fluid. Fluid in normal joints is present in small quantities sufficient to coat multiple folds of synovial membrane. Small pools collect in recesses in the joint, but in the normal state there is never sufficient volume to distend the joint or to separate redundant surfaces of synovium one from the other.

As in other systems, more is known about abnormal synovial fluid than about normal because there is an excess of the former. Truly normal synovial fluid is rarely analyzed. The largest accumulation of data was by Ropes and Bauer,[142] and their treatise is still a valuable reference. Synovial fluid is a filtrate of plasma that passes through the fenestrations of subsynovial capillary endothelium into the extracellular space, where it joins with hyaluronic acid that is secreted by synovial cells and achieves an equilibrium with free fluid in the joint space. Rates of transfer from capillaries to the interstitial fluid and of diffusion through this tissue are affected by many factors. Each component of synovial fluid must be considered separately.

Components of Synovial Fluid Originating in Plasma

Small Molecules. As has been pointed out, synovial cells lack tight junctions and have no underlying basement membrane. As a result, synovial fluid is continuous with, and in most respects an extension of, the interstitial fluid in synovial tissue; the interstitial forces may be considered to be those measurable in synovial fluid. The oncotic pressure of synovial fluid is thus related to plasma proteins and, to a lesser extent, hyaluronic acid.[115]

The regulation of intra-articular pressure is also influenced by the rate of egress of fluid from the joint. There are valves in synovial veins and lymphatics; with motion and muscle contraction, there can be a gradient from one end of the capillary to the other as in most tissues. It is proposed that slight decompression effectively pumps venous return and sustains an arterial-venous pressure lower than that in the adjacent collecting system. This decompression, plus a similar mechanism in the lymphatics, would clear extravascular plasma proteins from the synovium, lowering the oncotic pressure and promoting fluid passage.[115] Most small molecules pass through synovial interstitium by a process of free

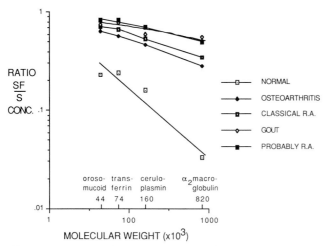

Figure 1–13. Ratio of the concentration of proteins in synovial fluid to that found in serum, plotted as a function of molecular weight. (From Kushner, I., and Somerville, J.A.: Permeability of human synovial membrane to plasma proteins. Arthritis Rheum. 14:560, 1971. Used by permission.)

diffusion.[143] The concentration of electrolytes is the same as in plasma. Cations that bind significantly to protein are present in concentrations consistent with the lower concentrations of serum proteins present in synovial fluid (see following). The concentration of glucose in synovial fluid is close to that in plasma.[144] However, in the nonsteady state, glucose enters the joint space at a rate faster than expected from its molecular size, indicating facilitated diffusion or active transport of this molecule into (but not out of) joints.[143] It seems likely, therefore, that to explain low levels of glucose in sepsis or severe inflammation, one must invoke both impaired delivery and increased utilization by synovial components.

Large Molecules. Proteins are present in synovial fluid in concentrations inversely proportional to molecular size.[145] This selective retardation of large molecule influx into synovial fluid is due in part to regulation by the extracellular matrix of synovium; when plasma is filtered through hyaluronic acid, an ultrafiltrate is produced with a composition similar to that found in normal synovial fluid.[146] Hyaluronic acid in interstitial tissues acts as a molecular filter; by its large domain, it excludes large solute molecules from passing through into synovial fluid. Because of their large size, molecules such as α_2-macroglobulin (the principal proteinase inhibitor of plasma), fibrinogen, and IgM are present in only small quantities in noninflammatory synovial fluid. In inflammatory synovial fluids, this selective exclusion is altered, perhaps because of increased size of endothelial cell fenestrations or because interstitial hyaluronate-protein complexes are fragmented by enzymes associated with the inflammatory process.[145] Thus, larger proteins enter synovial fluid, enabling it to form fibrin clots and to have higher concentrations of proteinase inhibitors (Fig. 1–13).

Removal of Material from Synovial Fluid. The

synovial lining cells phagocytize debris presented at the fluid-cell interface. In addition, the lymphatic system can enhance removal of synovial fluid macromolecules.[147] All large molecules appear to leave the joint at equivalent rates, unlike the rate (inversely proportional to molecular weight) at which they enter the joint space.[15] There is indirect evidence to suggest that this clearing mechanism is inadequate to the task presented in severe inflammation of joints. For instance, the synovial fluid appears to act as a "sink" for complement components in rheumatoid arthritis.[148] In severe inflammation, proteinases released by leukocytes drawn by chemotactic factors accumulate within the joint fluid and soon saturate the inhibitors present there.[149, 150]

LUBRICATION

Lubrication is a complicated subject that has been reviewed by Wright and Dowson[151] and in more detail by McCutchen,[152] Swanson,[153] and, most recently, by Mow and Rosenwasser.[62]

Although there have been at least 12 distinct mechanisms put forth to explain part or all of joint lubrication, most fall into two basic categories: (1) *fluid-film lubrication,* in which cartilage surfaces are separated by a fluid film; and (2) *boundary lubrication,* in which surface-to-surface contact exists, with protection and a decreased coefficient of friction offered by special molecules attached to cartilage surfaces. Variants of these may evolve as follows: (1) *squeeze-film lubrication,* in which, as discussed earlier, a film of fluid is trapped between opposing cartilage surfaces and, because the fluid film is noncompressible, prevents the surfaces from touching[154]—this is similar, of course, to weeping lubrication[155]; (2) *boosted lubrication,* in which pools of synovial fluid are compressed, as in weeping lubrication, but at high load the low-molecular-weight solute is driven back into cartilage or to non–weight-bearing fluid, leaving hyaluronate ("mucin") concentrates to bear weight[156, 157]; and (3) *elastohydrodynamic lubrication,* in which the viscosity and shear rate (hence, the coefficient of friction) are reduced because cartilage surfaces are deformable by a combination of tangential stretching and compression of the opposing surfaces.[158]

In all likelihood, several of these mechanisms and mixtures of them are involved in lubrication at both high and low loads and velocity imposed by daily activities. In walking, the load on weight-bearing joints (hip and knee) rises to three or four times body weight yet is reduced to a fraction of body weight moments later. Thus, during the walking cycle, three distinct modes may lubricate the knee: (1) as the heel hits the walking surface, impact is high and load maximal; squeeze-film lubrication could protect the surfaces from direct contact and attenuate the force of impact[151] (Fig. 1–14); (2) as the point of contact shifts from heel to toe, a combination

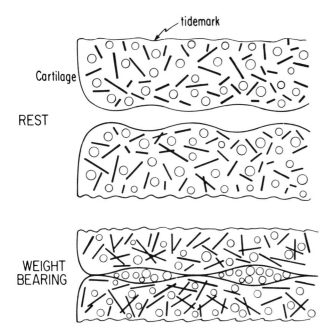

Figure 1–14. A scheme of a possible mechanism for both cartilage lubrication and provision of nutrition to chondrocytes. Two opposing articular surfaces are shown at rest and during weight bearing. The lines indicate collagen fibrils within cartilage. The circles represent solute, the interstitial fluid. Proteoglycans are not included for the sake of clarity. During weight bearing the cartilage is compressed. Fluid is driven out of the cartilage into the intercondylar space. When weight bearing is released, solute (presumably having exchanged cellular metabolites for nutrients) is resorbed as cartilage re-expands.[118]

of many mechanisms may apply; cartilage may be deformed by shear forces that minimize surface-to-surface motion (elastohydrodynamic lubrication); and (3) boundary lubrication is always available if cartilage surfaces approximate each other sufficiently, although the evidence suggests that boundary lubrication mechanisms fail during high load.

Hyaluronate, the extremely large and viscous molecule found in abundance in synovial fluid, is probably not involved in cartilage-cartilage lubrication. Hyaluronidase treatment did not inhibit the lubrication capability of synovial fluid at low load, whereas trypsin (with the capability of digesting glycoproteins) in synovial fluid did eliminate lubricating ability.[159] The compound responsible for cartilage-cartilage lubrication has been purified. It is a glycoprotein of molecular weight of 225,000 d and has been named *lubricin*.[40] This molecule, synthesized by synovial cells, is 200 nm in length and 1 to 2 nm in diameter.[160] The exact structure-function relationships of this molecule remain unknown, but it appears to be the primary boundary lubricant in mammalian joints.[161] Another boundary lubricant may be fat. Lipid is reported to compose 1 to 2 percent of dry weight of cartilage,[162] and experimental treatment of cartilage surfaces with fat solvents impairs lubrication qualities.[163]

It is also important to realize that articular surfaces are protected by other mechanisms not involv-

ing lubrication. During impact loading, muscles and bone absorb the great majority of force and energy, leaving only a small amount to be absorbed by cartilage itself.[164] Finely tuned neuromuscular reflexes are essential for this system to work effectively.[165] It is possible that small failures in these reflex arcs may lead to insufficient attenuation of impact loading, resulting in degenerative changes in joints and subchondral bone (i.e., Charcot's arthropathy).

Other Aspects of Synovial Physiology

Intra-articular Temperature. The vascular system of the extremities acts as a countercurrent distribution system for temperature of tissues. Although core body temperature in most humans varies little from the mean of 37°C, it is likely that temperatures within joints reflect more the temperature of overlying soft tissues. For example, the metacarpophalangeal joint, one with very little overlying insulation of fat or muscle, has intra-articular temperatures that parallel those of skin closely between the resting temperatures and 39° to 40°C created by insertion of the hand into an electric mitten.[166] The knee joint temperature is not so simple a function. Although intra-articular temperatures are always below 36°C (at ambient temperatures of around 20°C), there are wide variations noted between joint and skin temperature.[167] In addition, cold or hot packs reflexly change knee joint temperatures in the opposite direction.[168] Similarly, painful stimuli (e.g., apprehension or alarm) and smoking lower the skin temperature and elevate the joint temperature. Non–weight-bearing active movements increase intra-articular temperature as much as 1°C, a phenomenon probably best explained by an increased subsynovial tissue blood flow. The reason for interest in these data is that rates of enzyme action are a direct function of temperature. Connective tissue metabolism is generally studied in vitro at 37°C, yet tissues in joints do not reach this temperature except during inflamed states. Biochemical reactions that proceed vigorously at 37°C may at 32°C be altered sufficiently so that the net effect would be movement of a metabolic pathway in the opposite direction, or retardation of rates of reaction. For instance, the rate of destruction of articular cartilage collagen fibers by synovial collagenase is significant at 37°C; at 32°C it is imperceptible.[169] In addition, large increases in the rate of hyaluronic acid synthesis occur over an 8°C temperature change (30° to 38°C) in both normal and rheumatoid cell lines in culture, whereas glucose utilization and lactate production increase only slightly.[170]

Intra-articular Pressure. The joint cavity is a *potential* space. The small amount of synovial fluid present lines synovial surfaces but does not separate them. Indeed, the pressure within normal joints is negative (-5.7 cm H_2O) compared with ambient atmospheric pressure.[171] During the procedure of pulling rapidly on a relaxed phalanx ("knuckle cracking"), a gas bubble is created within the joint, which cavitates with a cracking sound, liberating energy in the form of heat and sound.[172] This cavitation is the same process that destroys propellers of steamships; presumably, if repeated frequently enough, it could destroy a joint. The normal negative pressure in the joint plays a role in stabilizing articular surfaces against one another. The presence of a synovial effusion changes all this. Intra-articular pressure becomes positive, and roentgenograms may show a widening of the apparent joint space as the articulating surfaces are forced apart. Pressure within a joint is perceived by humans as an uncomfortable sensation; a patient with a knee effusion rests it in a position of slight flexion, the position at which pressure is minimal.[173] Full flexion or extension increases pressures within joints containing effusions and may be sufficient to rupture a joint capsule.[174] High intra-articular pressure may compromise synovial blood flow. Inflamed, chronic proliferative synovitis generates a thickened joint capsule, which gradually, perhaps secondary to increased joint pressure, becomes redundant and stretched and demonstrates decreased compliance.[175] Pressure in these joints may be minimal until a critical volume at which the noncompliant capsule stretches no more, and intra-articular pressure soars to produce rupture or even penetration through weakened bone to form subchondral cysts.[173, 176]

The ease with which fluid passes across the synovial lining is enhanced when the intra-articular fluid pressure is raised acutely to pathologic levels. This is related to a reduction of synovial thickness as the synovium is "stretched," with increased proximity of the synovial capillaries to the joint lumen and therefore the distance for perfusion. Capillary depth is proposed as the major factor governing fluid exchange in joints.[177]

It is likely that increased intra-articular pressure in the presence of effusions affects synovial blood flow.[175] One study reports that synovial blood flow is compromised by modest elevations in intra-articular pressure in the range of those encountered in daily activities in patients with knee effusions. Intra-articular pressures exceeded 45 mm Hg during standing and the stance phase of walking, and this was shown to diminish the blood flow and aggravate the tendency to hypoxia and lactic acidosis.[178]

Neuropeptides. Neuropeptides, including substance P, are found in normal and inflamed synovium, as well as in synovial fluid of patients following trauma and in patients with rheumatoid arthritis.[179] It has been suggested that neuropeptides may potentiate inflammatory synovitis and account for the symmetry of rheumatoid arthritis involvement.[180]

References

1. Sledge, C. B., and Zaleske, D. J.: Developmental anatomy of joints. *In* Resnick, D., and Niwayama, G. (eds.): Diagnosis of Bone and Joint Disorders. Philadelphia, W. B. Saunders Company, 1988, pp. 604–624.
2. Dienstman, S. R., Biehl, J., Holtzer, S., et al: Myogenic and chondrogenic lineages in developing limb buds grown in vitro. Dev. Biol. 39:83, 1974.
3. Stockwell, R. A., and Meachim, G.: The chondrocytes. *In* Freeman, M. A. R. (ed.): Adult Articular Cartilage. London, Pitman Medical, 1979, pp. 69–145.
4. Zwilling, E., Saunders, J. W., Jr., and Gasseling, J. T.: Involvement of the apical ectodermal ridge in chick limb development. Anat. Rec. 136:307, 1960.
5. Vaheri, A., Ruoslahti, E., and Mosher, D. (eds.): Fibroblast Surface Protein. Vol. 312. New York, New York Academy of Sciences, 1978.
6. Newman, S. A., and Frisch, H. L.: Dynamics of skeletal pattern formation in developing chick limb. Science 205:662, 1979.
7. Felts, W. J.: In vivo implantation as a technique in skeletal biology. Int. Rev. Cytol. 12:243, 1961.
8. Toole, B. P., Jackson, G., and Gross, J.: Hyaluronate in morphogenesis: Inhibition of chondrogenesis in vitro. Proc. Natl. Acad. Sci U.S.A. 69:1384, 1972.
9. Toole, B. P.: Hyaluronate turnover during chondrogenesis in the developing chick limb and axial skeleton. Dev. Biol. 29:321, 1972.
10. Kosher, R. A., Walker, K. H., and Ledger, P. W.: Temporal and spatial distribution of fibronectin during development of the embryonic chick limb bud. Cell Differ. 11:217, 1982.
11. Turner, D. C., Lawton, J., Dollenmeier, P., et al: Guidance of myogenic cell migration by oriented deposits of fibronectin. Dev. Biol. 95:497, 1983.
12. Edelman, G. M.: Cell-adhesion molecules: A molecular basis for animal form. Sci. Am. 250:118, 1984.
13. Thiery, J. P.: Mechanisms of cell migration in the vertebrate embryo. Cell Differ. 15:1, 1984.
14. Newman, S. A., Frenz, D. A., Tomasek, J. J., et al: Matrix-driven translocation of cells and non-living particles. Science 228:885, 1985.
15. Brown, P. J., and Juliano, R. L.: Selective inhibition of fibronectin-mediated cell adhesion by monoclonal antibodies to a cell-surface glycoprotein. Science 228:1448, 1985.
16. O'Rahilly, R., and Gardner, E.: The embryology of movable joints. *In* Sokoloff, L. (ed.): The Joints and Synovial Fluid. Vol. 1. New York, Academic Press, 1978.
17. O'Rahilly, R.: The development of joints. Ir. J. Med. Sci. 6:456, 1957.
18. Thorogood, P. V., and Hinchcliffe, J. R.: An analysis of the condensation process during chondrogenesis in the embryonic chick hind limb. J. Embryol. Exp. Morphol. 33:581, 1975.
19. Friberg, V., and Ringertz, N. R.: An autoradiographic study on the uptake of radiosulfate in the rat embryo. J. Embryol. Exp. Morphol. 4:313, 1956.
20. Anderson, H., and Bro-Rasmussen, F.: Histochemical studies on the histogenesis of the joints in human fetuses with special reference to the development of the joint cavities in the hand and foot. Am. J. Anat. 108:111, 1961.
21. Warsilev, W.: Elektronenmikroskopische und histochemische Untersuchungen zur Entwicklung des Kniegelenkes der Ratte. Z. Anat. Entwicklungsgest 137:221, 1972.
22. Drachman, D. B., and Sokoloff, L.: The role of movement in embryonic joint development. Dev. Biol. 14:401, 1966.
23. Murray, P. D. F., and Drachman, D. B.: The role of movement in the development of joints and related structures: The head and neck in the chick embryo. J. Embryol. Exp. Morphol. 22:349, 1969.
24. Yasuda, Y.: Differentiation of human limb buds in vitro. Anat. Rec. 175:561, 1973.
25. Symons, N. B. B.: The development of the human mandibular joint. J. Anat. 86:326, 1952.
26. Moffett, B. C.: The prenatal development of the human temporomandibular joint. Contrib. Embryol. Carnegie Inst. 36:19, 1957.
27. Bradley, S. J.: An analysis of self-differentiation of chick limb buds in chorio-allantoic grafts. J. Anat. 107:479, 1970.
28. Bauer, R.: Zur Problem der Neugliederung der Wurbelsaule. Acta Anat. (Basel) 72:321, 1969.
29. Walmsley, R.: The development and growth of the intervertebral disc. Edinburgh Med. J. 60:341, 1983.
30. Linsenmeyer, T. F., Trelstad, R. L., and Gross, J.: The collagen of chick embryonic notochord. Biochem. Biophys. Res. Commun. 3:39, 1973.
31. Eyre, D. R., and Muir, H.: Collagen polymorphism: Two molecular species in pig intervertebral discs. FEBS Lett. 42:192, 1974.
32. Herbert, C. M., Lindberg, K. A., Jayson, M. I. V., et al: Changes in the collagen of human intervertebral discs during aging and degenerative joint disease. J. Mol. Med. 1:79, 1975.
33. Bird, H. A., Tribe, D. R., and Bacon, P. A.: Joint hypermobility leading to osteoarthritis and chondrocalcinosis. Ann. Rheum. Dis. 37:203, 1978.
34. Jayson, M. I. V.: Intra-articular pressure. Clin. Rheum. Dis. 7:149, 1981.
35. Gelberman, R., Goldberg, V., An, K.-N., et al: Tendon. *In* Woo, S. L.-Y., and Buckwalter, J. A. (eds.): Injury and Repair of the Muscu-

loskeletal Soft Tissues. Park Ridge, IL, American Academy of Orthopaedic Surgeons, 1988, p. 5.

36. Canoso, J. J.: Bursae, tendons and ligaments. Clin. Rheum. Dis. 7:189, 1981.

37. Kieny, M., and Chevallier, A.: Autonomy of tendon development in the embrvonic duck wing. J. Embryol. Exp. Morphol. 49:153, 1979.

38. Gay, S., and Miller, E. J.: Collagen in the Physiology and Pathology of Connective Tissue. Stuttgart, Gustav Fisher, 1978, pp. 51–54.

39. Cooper, R. R., and Misol, S.: Tendon and ligament insertion: A light and electron microscopic study. J. Bone Joint Surg. 82A:1, 1970.

40. Swann, D. A.: Macromolecules of synovial fluid. In Sokoloff, L. (ed.): The Joints and Synovial Fluid. New York, Academic Press, 1978, pp. 407–435.

41. Glimcher, M. J., Brickley-Parsons, D., and Kossiva, D.: Phosphopeptides and γ-carboxyglutamic acid–containing peptides in calcified turkey tendon: Their absence in uncalcified tendon. Calcif. Tissue Int. 27:281, 1979.

42. Frank, C., Woo, S., Andriacchi, T., et al: Normal ligament: Structure, function, and composition. In Woo, S. L.-Y. and Buckwalter, J. A. (eds.): Injury and Repair of the Musculoskeletal Soft Tissues. Park Ridge, IL, American Academy of Orthopaedic Surgeons, 1988, p. 45.

43. Kuhns, J. G.: Adventitious bursa. Arch. Surg. 46:687, 1943.

44. Canoso, J. J., and Yood, R. A.: Reaction of superficial bursae to specific disease stimuli. Arthritis Rheum. 22:1361, 1979.

45. Arnoczky, S., Adams, M., DeHaven, K., et al: Meniscus. In Woo, S. L.-Y., and Buckwalter, J. A. (eds.): Injury and Repair of the Musculoskeletal Soft Tissues. Park Ridge, IL, American Academy of Orthopaedic Surgeons, 1988, p. 487.

46. Fairbank, T. J.: Knee joint changes after meniscectomy. J. Bone Joint Surg. 30B:664, 1948.

47. Arnoczky, S. P., and Warren, R. F.: The microvasculature of the meniscus and its response to injury: An experimental study in the dog. Am. J. Sports Med. 11:131, 1983.

48. McDevitt, C. A., and Webber, R. J.: The ultrastructure and biochemistry of meniscal cartilage. Clin. Orthop. Rel. Res. 252:8, 1990.

49. Balacz, E. A., Bloom, G. D., and Swann, D. A.: Fine structure and glycosaminoglycan content of the surface layer of articular cartilage. Fed. Proc. 28:1813, 1966.

50. Redler, I., and Zimmy, M. L.: Scanning electron microscopy and abnormal articular cartilage and synovium. J. Bone Joint Surg. 52A:139, 1970.

51. Gardner, D. L.: The influence of microscopic technology on knowledge of cartilage surface structure. Ann. Rheum. Dis. 31:235, 1972.

52. Clarke, I. C.: Human articular surface contours and related surface depression frequency studies. Ann. Rheum. Dis. 30:15, 1971.

53. Clarke, I. C.: Surface characteristics of human articular cartilage: A scanning electron microscope study. J. Anat. 108:23, 1971.

54. Gardner, D. L., and McGilliwray, D. C.: Living articular cartilage is not smooth. Ann. Rheum. Dis. 30:3, 1971.

55. Ghadially, F. N., Ghadially, J. A., Oryschak, A. F., et al: Experimental production of ridges on rabbit articular cartilage: A scanning electron microscopic study. J. Anat. 121:119, 1976.

56. Clark, J. M.: The organization of collagen in cryofractured rabbit articular cartilage. J. Orthop. Rel. Res. 3:17, 1985.

57. Clark, J. M.: The organization of collagen fibrils in the superficial zones of articular cartilage. J. Anat. 171:117, 1990.

58. Clark, J. M.: Variation of collagen fiber alignment in a joint surface: A scanning electron microscope study of the tibial plateau in dog, rabbit, and man. J. Orthop. Rel. Res. 9:246, 1991.

59. Bossier, M.-C., Chiocchia, G., Ronziere, M.-C., et al: Arthrigenicity of minor cartilage collagens (types IX and XI) in mice. Arthritis Rheum. 33:1, 1990.

60. Poole, A. R., Pidoux, I., Reiner, A., et al: Localization of proteoglycan monomer and link protein in the matrix of bovine articular cartilage: An immunohistochemical study. J. Histochem. Cytochem. 28:621, 1980.

61. Poole, A.R., Pidoux, I., Reiner, A., et al: An immunoelectron microscope study of the organization of proteoglycan monomer, link protein, and collagen in the matrix of articular cartilage. J Cell. Biol. 93:921, 1982.

62. Mow, V., and Rosenwasser, M.: Articular cartilage: Biomechanics. In Woo, S. L.-Y., and Buckwalter, J. A. (eds.): Injury and Repair of the Musculoskeletal Soft Tissues. Park Ridge, IL, American Academy of Orthopaedic Surgeons, 1988, p. 427.

63. Hardingham, T. E., and Muir, H.: The specific interaction of hyaluronic acid with cartilage proteoglycans. Biochim. Biophys. Acta 279:401, 1972.

64. Poole, B. P., and Lowther, D. A.: The effect of chondroitin sulfate protein on the formation of collagen fibrils in vitro. Biochem. J. 109:857, 1968.

65. DiSalvo, J., and Schubert, M.: Specific interaction of some cartilage protein polysaccharides with freshly precipitating calcium phosphate. J. Biol. Chem. 242:705, 1967.

66. Howell, D. S., Pita, J. C., Marquez, J. F., et al: Demonstration of macromolecular inhibitors of calcification and nucleation factor(s) in fluid from calcifying sites in cartilage. J. Clin. Invest. 48:630, 1969.

67. Muir, H., Bullough, P., and Maroudas, A.: The distribution of collagen in human articular cartilage with some of its physiological implications. J. Bone Joint Surg. 52B:554, 1970.

68. Kuettner, K. E., Hiti, J., Eisenstein, R., et al: Collagenase inhibition by cationic proteins derived from cartilage and aorta. Biochem. Biophys. Res. Commun. 72:40, 1976.

69. Kuettner, K. E., Soble, L., Croxen, R. L., et al: Tumor cell collagenase and its inhibition by a cartilage-derived protease inhibitor. Science 196:653, 1977.

70. Rifkin, D. B., and Crowe, R. M.: Isolation of a protease inhibitor from tissues resistant to tumor invasion. Hoppe Seyler Z. Physiol. Chem. 358:152, 1977.

71. Langer, R., Brem, H., Flaterman, K., et al: Isolation of a cartilage factor that inhibits tumor neovascularization. Science 193:70, 1976.

72. Horton, J. E., Wezeman, F. H., and Kuettner, K. E.: Inhibition of bone resorption in vitro by a cartilage-derived anticollagenase factor. Science 199:1342, 1978.

73. Roughley, P. J., Murphy, G., and Barrett, A. J.: Proteinase inhibitors of bovine nasal cartilage. Biochem. J. 169:721, 1978.

74. Linn, F. C., and Sokoloff, L.: Movement and composition of interstitial fluid of cartilage. Arthritis Rheum. 8:481, 1965.

75. Pita, J. C., and Howell, D. S.: Micro-biochemical studies of cartilage. In Sokoloff, L. (ed.): The Joints and Synovial Fluid. Vol. 1. New York, Academic Press, 1978, pp. 273–330.

76. Mankin, H.J.: The water of articular cartilage. In Simon, W. H. (ed.): The Human Joint in Health and Disease. Philadelphia, University of Pennsylvania Press, 1978, pp. 37–42.

77. Bollet, A. J., and Nance, J. L.: Biochemical findings in normal and osteoarthritic articular cartilage: II. Chondroitin sulfate concentration and chain length, water and ash content. J. Clin. Invest. 4:1170, 1966.

78. Hadler, N. M.: The biology of the extracellular space. Clin. Rheum. Dis. 7:71, 1981.

79. Ghadially, F. N.: Fine structure of joints. In Sokoloff, L. (ed.): The Joints and Synovial Fluid. New York, Academic Press, 1978, p. 140.

80. Davies, D. V., Barnett, C. H., Cochrane, W., et al: Electron microscopy of articular cartilage in the young adult rabbit. Ann. Rheum. Dis. 21:11, 1962.

81. Ghadially, F. N.: Waxing and waning of nuclear fibrous lamina. Arch. Pathol. 94:303, 1972.

82. Ghadially, F. N., Meachim, G., and Collins, D. H.: Extracellular lipid in the matrix of human articular cartilage. Ann. Rheum. Dis. 24:196, 1965.

83. Ghadially, F. N., Orvyshak, A. F., Ailsby, R. L., et al: Electronprobe x-ray analysis of siderosomes in haemarthrotic articular cartilage. Virchows Arch. [B] 16:43, 1974.

84. Stockwell, R. A.: The cell density of human articular and costal cartilage. J. Anat. 10:753, 1967.

85. Hunter, W.: On the structure and diseases of articulating cartilage. Philos. Trans. R. Soc. Lond. [Biol.] 42:514, 1743.

86. Bywaters, E. G. L.: The metabolism of joint tissues. J. Pathol. Bacteriol. 44:247, 1937.

87. Woods, G. C., Greenwald, A. J., and Haynes, D. W.: Subchondral vascularity in the human femoral head. Ann. Rheum. Dis. 29:138, 1970.

88. Mitul, M. A., and Millington, P. F.: Osseous pathway of nutrition to articular cartilage of the human femoral head. Lancet 1:842, 1970.

89. Collins, D. H.: The Pathology of Articular and Spinal Disease. London, Arnold, 1949.

90. Strangeways, T. S. P.: The nutrition of articular cartilage. Br. Med. J. 1:661, 1920.

91. Maroudas, A., Bullough, P., Swanson, S. A. V., et al: The permeability of articular cartilage. J. Bone Joint Surg. 50B:166, 1968.

92. Sood, S. C.: A study of the effects of experimental immobilization on rabbit articular cartilage. J. Anat. 108:497, 1971.

93. Bennett, G., and Bauer, W.: Joint changes resulting from patellar displacement and their relation to degenerative hip disease. J. Bone Joint Surg. 19A:667, 1937.

94. Lewis, P. R., and McCutchen, C. W.: Experimental evidence for weeping lubrication in mammalian joints. Nature 184:1285, 1959.

95. McCutchen, C. W.: An approximate equation for weeping lubrication, solved with an electrical analogue. Ann. Rheum. Dis. 34:85, 1975.

96. Bar, E.: Elasticitätsprufungen der Gelenkkorpel. Arch. J. Entwicklungsmech. Organ. 108:739, 1926.

97. Freeman, M. A. R., and Kempson, G. E.: Load carriage. In Freeman, M. A. R. (ed.): Adult Cartilage. New York, Grune & Stratton, 1974, pp. 228–246.

98. Harris, E. D., DiBona, D. R., and Krane, S. M.: A mechanism for cartilage destruction in rheumatoid arthritis. Trans. Assoc. Am. Phys. 83:267, 1970.

99. Harris, E. D., Jr., Parker, H. G., Radin, E. L., et al: Effects of proteolytic enzymes on structural and mechanical properties of cartilage. Arthritis Rheum. 15:497, 1972.

100. Kempson, G. E., Muir, H., Swanson, S. A. V., et al: Correlations between stiffness and the chemical constituents of cartilage on the human femoral head. Biochim. Biophys. Acta 215:70, 1970.

101. Kempson, G. E.: Mechanical properties of articular cartilage. In Freeman, M. A. R. (ed.): Adult Articular Cartilage. New York, Grune & Stratton, 1974, p. 196.

102. Buckwalter, J., Rosenberg, L., Coutts, R., et al: Articular cartilage: Injury and repair. In Woo, S. L.-Y, and Buckwalter, J. A. (eds.): Injury and Repair of the Musculoskeletal Soft Tissues. Park Ridge, IL, American Academy of Orthopaedic Surgeons, 1988, p. 465.

103. Landells, J. W.: The reactions of injured human articular cartilage. J. Bone Joint Surg. 39B:548, 1957.

104. Meachim, G., and Osborne, G. V.: Repair at the femoral articular cartilage surface in osteoarthritis of the hip. J. Pathol. 102:1, 1970.

105. Simon, W. H.: Scale effects in animal joints: I. Articular cartilage thickness and compressive stress. Arthritis Rheum. 13:244, 1970.

106. Armstrong, C. G., and Gardner, D. L.: Thickness and distribution of human femoral head articular cartilage: Changes with age. Ann. Rheum. Dis. 36:407, 1977.

107. Byers, P. D., Contepomi, C. A., and Farker, T. A.: A postmortem study of the hip joint. Ann. Rheum. Dis. 29:15, 1970.

108. Collins, D. H., and Meachim, G.: Sulphate ($^{35}SO_4$) fixation by human articular cartilage compared in the knee and shoulder joints. Ann. Rheum. Dis. 20:117, 1961.

109. Mankin, H. J., and Lippiello, L.: Biochemical and metabolic abnormalities in articular cartilage from osteoarthritic human hips. J. Bone Joint Surg. 52A:424, 1970.

110. Burr, D. B., and Radin, E. L.: Trauma as a factor in the initiation of osteoarthritis. In Brandt, K. D. (ed.): Cartilage Changes in Osteoarthritis. Indianapolis, Indiana University School of Medicine, 1990, p. 73.

111. Oegema, T. R., and Thompson, R. C. J.: Cartilage-bone interface (tidemark). In Brandt, K. D. (ed.): Cartilage Changes in Osteoarthritis. Indianapolis, Indiana University School of Medicine, 1990, p. 43.

112. Liew, M., and Dick, C.: The anatomy and physiology of blood flow in a diarthrodial joint. Clin. Rheum. Dis. 7:131, 1981.

113. Lindstrom, J.: Microvascular anatomy of synovial tissue. Acta Rheum. Scand. 7:1, 1963.

114. Suter, J., and Majno, G.: Ultrastructure of the joint capsule in the rat: Presence of two kinds of capillaries. Nature 202:920, 1964.

115. Simkin, P., and Benedict, R. S.: Hydrostatic and oncotic determinants of microvascular fluid balance in normal canine joints. Arthritis Rheum. 33:80, 1990.

116. Schumacher, H. R.: The microvasculature of the synovial membrane of the monkey: Ultrastructural studies. Arthritis Rheum 112:387, 1969.

117. Dee, R.: Structure and function of hip joint innervation. Ann. R. Coll. Surg. Engl. 45:357, 1969.

118. Griff, P., Finerman, G. A., and Riley, L. H. R.: Joint position sense after total hip replacement. J. Bone Joint Surg. 55:1016, 1973.

119. Cross, M. J., and McCloskey, D.: Position sense following surgical removal of joints in man. Brain Res. 55:443, 1973.

119a. Barland, P., Novikoff, A. B., and Hamerman, D.: Electron microscopy of the human synovial membrane. J. Cell Biol. 14:207, 1962.

120. Bassleer, R., Lhoest-Ganthier, M.-P., Renard, A.-M., et al: Histological structure and functions of synovium. In Franchimont, P. (ed.): Articular Synovium. Basel, Karger, 1982, pp. 1–26.

121. Ghadially, F. N., and Roy, S.: Ultrastructure of Synovial Joints in Health and Disease. London, Butterworth, 1969.

122. Hirohata, K., and Kobayashi, I.: Fine structure of the synovial tissue in rheumatoid arthritis. Kobe J. Med. Sci. 10:195, 1964.

123. Krey, P. R., Cohen, A. S., Smith, C. B., et al: The human fetal synovium: Histology, fine structure and changes in organ culture. Arthritis Rheum. 14:319, 1971.

124. Roy, S., Ghadially, F. N., and Crane, W. A. J.: Synovial membrane in traumatic effusion: Ultrastructure and autoradiography with tritiated leucine. Ann. Rheum. Dis. 25:259, 1966.

125. Werb, Z., and Reynolds, J. J.: Stimulation by endocytosis of the secretion of collagenase and neutral proteinases from rabbit synovial fibroblasts. J. Exp. Med. 140:1482, 1976.

126. Norton, W. L., Lewis, D. C., and Ziff, M.: Electron-dense deposits following injection of gold sodium thiomalate and thiomalic acid. Arthritis Rheum. 11:436, 1968.

127. Ghadially, F. N., Ailsby, R. L., and Yong, N. K.: Ultrastructure of the hemophilic synovial membrane and electron-probe x-ray analysis of haemosiderin. J. Pathol. 120:201, 1976.

128. Roy, S., and Ghadially, F. N.: Synthesis of hyaluronic acid by synovial cells. J. Pathol. Bacteriol. 93:555, 1967.

129. Allard, S. A., Bayliss, M. T., and Maini, R. N.: The synovium-cartilage junction of the normal human knee. Arthritis Rheum. 33:1170, 1990.

130. Hynes, R. O.: Cell surface proteins and malignant transformation. Biochim. Biophys. Acta 458:73, 1976.

131. Clemmensen, I., Holund, B., and Andersen, R. B.: Fibrin and fibronectin in rheumatoid synovial membrane and rheumatoid synovial fluid. Arthritis Rheum. 26:497, 1983.

132. Hynes, R. O.: Alteration of cell-surface proteins by viral transformation and proteolysis. Proc. Natl. Acad. Sci. U. S. A. 70:3170, 1973.

133. Yamada, K. M., and Weston, J. A.: Isolation of a major cell surface glycoprotein from fibroblasts. Proc. Natl. Acad. Sci. U. S. A. 71:3492, 1974.

134. Ali, I. V., Mautner, V., Lanza, R., et al: Restoration of normal morphology, adhesion and cytoskeleton sensitive surface protein. Cell 11:115, 1977.

135. Scott, D. L., Wainwright, A. C., Walton, K. W., et al: Significance of fibronectin in rheumatoid arthritis and osteoarthritis. Ann. Rheum. Dis. 40:142, 1981.

136. Okada, Y., Naka, K., Minamoto, T., et al: Localization of type VI collagen in the lining cell layer of normal and rheumatoid synovium. Lab. Invest. 63:647, 1990.

137. Fell, H. B., and Jubb, R. W.: The effect of synovial tissue on the breakdown of articular cartilage in organ culture. Arthritis Rheum. 20:1359, 1977.

138. Dingle, J. T., Saklatvata, J., Hembry, R., et al: A cartilage catabolic factor from synovium. Biochem. J. 184:177, 1979.

139. Steinberg, J., Sledge, C. B., Noble, J., et al: A tissue-culture model of cartilage breakdown in rheumatoid arthritis. Biochem. J. 180:403, 1979.

140. Krane, S. M., Dayer, J. M., Simon, L. S., et al: Mononuclear cell-conditioned medium containing mononuclear cell factor (MCF), homologous with interleukin 1, stimulates collagen and fibronectin synthesis by adherent rheumatoid synovial cells: Effects of protaglandin E_2 and indomethacin. Coll. Rel. Res. 5:99, 1985.

141. Chin, J. E., Winterrowd, G. E., Krzesicki, R. F., et al: Role of cytokines in inflammatory synovitis. Arthritis Rheum. 33:1776, 1990.

142. Ropes, M. W., and Bauer, W.: Synovial Fluid Changes in Joint Diseases. Cambridge, Harvard University Press, 1953.

143. Simkin, P. A., and Pizzoro, J. E.: Transsynovial exchange of small molecules in normal human subjects. J. Appl. Physiol. 36:581, 1974.

144. Ropes, M. W., Muller, A. F., and Bauer, W.: The entrance of glucose and other sugars into joints. Arthritis Rheum. 3:496, 1960.

145. Kushner, I., and Somerville, J. A.: Permeability of human synovial membrane to plasma proteins. Arthritis Rheum. 14:560, 1971.

146. Nettelbladt, E., Sundblad, L., and Jonsson, B.: Permeability of the synovial membrane to proteins. Acta Rheum. Scand. 9:28, 1963.

147. Noble, J., Jones, A. G., Davies, M. A., et al: Leakage of radioactive particle systems from a synovial joint studied with a gamma camera: Its application to radiation synovectomy. J. Bone Joint Surg. 65A:381, 1983.

148. Ruddy, S.: Synovial fluid: Mirror of the inflammatory lesion in rheumatoid arthritis. In Harris, E. D., Jr. (ed.): Rheumatoid Arthritis. New York, Medcom Press, 1974, pp. 58–71.

149. Abe, S., and Nagai, Y.: Evidence for the presence of a complex of collagenase with α_2-macroglobulin in human rheumatoid synovial fluid: A possible regulatory mechanism of collagenase activity in vivo. J. Biochem. 73:897, 1973.

150. Harris, E. D., Jr., Faulkner, C. S., II, and Brown, F. E.: Collagenolytic systems in rheumatoid arthritis. Clin. Orthop. Rel. Res. 110:303, 1975.

151. Wright, V., and Dowson, D.: Lubrication and cartilage. J. Anat. 121:107, 1976.

152. McCutchen, C. W.: Lubrication of joints. In Sokoloff, L. (ed.): The Joints and Synovial Fluid. Vol. I. New York, Academic Press, 1978, pp. 437–477.

153. Swanson, S. A. V.: Lubrication. In Freeman, M. A. R. (ed.): Adult Articular Cartilage. New York, Grune & Stratton, 1977, pp. 247–277.

154. Fein, R. S.: Are synovial joints squeeze-film lubricated? Proc. Inst. Mech. Eng. 181:125, 1967.

155. Skantze, K. A., Brinckerhoff, C. E., Cololier, J. P., et al: Modulation of chrondrocyte function in agar culture (Abstract). Arthritis Rheum. 26:41, 1983.

156. Walker, P. S., Dowson, D., Longfield, M. D., et al: "Boosted lubrication" in synovial joints by fluid entrapment and enrichment. Ann. Rheum. Dis. 27:512, 1968.

157. Dowson, D., Unsworth, A., and Wright, V.: Analysis of boosted lubrication in human joints. J. Mech. Eng. Sci. 12:364, 1970.

158. Dintenfass, L.: Lubrication in synovial joints. Nature 197:496, 1963.

159. Radin, E. L., Swann, D. A., and Weisser, P. A.: Separation of hyaluronate-free lubricating fraction from synovial fluid. Nature 288:377, 1970.

160. Swann, D. A.: Structure and function of lubricin, the glycoprotein responsible for the boundary lubrication of articular cartilage. In Franchimont, P. (ed.): Articular Synovium. Basel, Karger, 1982, pp. 45–58.

161. Swann, D. A., Silver, F. H., Slayter, H. S., et al: The molecular structure and lubricating activity of lubricin isolated from bovine and human synovial fluids. Biochem. J. 225:195, 1985.

162. Stockwell, R. A.: Lipid content of human costal and articular cartilage. Ann. Rheum. Dis. 26:481, 1967.

163. Little, T., Freeman, M. A. R., and Swanson, S. A. V.: Experiments on friction in the human hip joint. In Wright, V. (ed.): Lubrication and Wear in Joints. London, Sector, 1969, p. 110.

164. Radin, E. L., and Paul, I. L.: A consolidated concept of joint lubrication. J. Bone Joint Surg. 54A:607, 1972.
165. Ito, H., Nagasaki, H., Hashizume, K., et al: Time-course of force production by fast isometric contraction of the knee extensor in young and elderly subjects. J. Hum. Ergol. 19:23, 1990.
166. Mainardi, C. L., Walter, J. M., Spiegel, P. K., et al: The lack of effect of daily heat therapy on the progression of rheumatoid arthritis. Arch. Phys. Med. Rehabil. 60:390, 1979.
167. Horvath, S. M., and Hollander, J. L.: Intra-articular temperature as a measure of joint reaction. J. Clin. Invest. 28:469, 1949.
168. Hollander, J. L., and Horvath, S. M.: The influence of physical therapy procedures on the intra-articular temperature of normal and arthritic subjects. Am. J. Med. Sci. 218:543, 1949.
169. Harris, E. D., Jr., and McCroskery, P. A.: The influence of temperature and fibril stability on degradation of cartilage collagen by rheumatoid synovial collagenase. N. Engl. J. Med. 290:1, 1974.
170. Castor, C. W., and Yaron, M.: Connective tissue activation: VIII. The effects of temperature studied in vitro. Arch. Phys. Med. Rehabil. 57:5, 1976.
171. Mueller, W.: Uber den negativen Lufdruck im Gelenkram. Dtsch. Z. Chir. 218:395, 1929.
172. Unsworth, A., Dowson, D., and Wright, V.: "Cracking joints": A bioengineering study of cavitation in the metacarpophalangeal joint. Ann. Rheum. Dis. 30:348, 1971.
173. Jayson, M. I. V., Rubenstein, D., and Dixon, A. S. J.: Intra-articular pressure and rheumatoid geodes (bone "cysts"). Ann. Rheum. Dis. 29:496, 1970.
174. Jayson, M. I. V., and Dixon, A. S. J.: Valvular mechanisms in juxta-articular cysts. Ann. Rheum. Dis. 29:415, 1970.
175. Myers, D. B., and Palmer, D. G.: Capsular compliance and pressure-volume relationships in normal and arthritic knees. J. Bone Joint Surg. 54B:710, 1972.
176. Magyer, E., Talerman, A., Feher, M., et al: The pathogenesis of the subchondral pseudocysts in rheumatoid arthritis. Clin. Orthop. Rel. Res. 100:341, 1974.
177. McDonald, J. N., and Levick, J. R.: Pressure induced deformation of the interstitial route across synovium and its relation to hydraulic conductance. J. Rheum. 17:341, 1990.
178. James, M. J., Cleland, L. G., Rolfe, A. M., et al: Intraarticular pressure and the relationship between synovial perfusion and metabolic demand. J. Rheum. 17:521, 1990.
179. Marshall, K. W., Chiu, B., and Inman, R. D.: Substance P and arthritis: Analysis of plasma and synovial fluid levels. Arthritis Rheum. 33:87, 1990.
180. Kidd, B. L., Gibson, S. J., O'Higgens, F., et al: A neurogenic mechanism for symmetrical arthritis. Lancet 2:1128, 1989.

Chapter 2
Collagen and Elastin

Charlene J. Williams
Philipp Vandenberg
Darwin J. Prockop

INTRODUCTION

Connective tissue and extracellular matrix are loosely defined as the compartments and components that provide the structural support of the body and bind together its cells, organs, and tissues. The major connective tissues are bone, skin, tendons, ligaments, and cartilage. The term connective tissue is also applied to blood vessels and to synovial spaces and fluids. In effect, however, all organs and tissues contain connective tissue in the form of membranes and septa.

All connective tissues contain large amounts of water, salt, albumin, and other components of plasma. The characteristic feature of connective tissues, however, is that they contain a series of specific macromolecules that are assembled into large and complex structures that define the size and shape of most organs. Two of the most characteristic macromolecules of connective tissue are the fibrous proteins collagen and elastin. Connective tissues also contain a series of proteoglycans and related molecules.

The differences among connective tissues such as bone, skin, and cartilage are in part attributable to differences in their contents of specific macromolecules (Table 2–1). Tendons and ligaments, for example, consist primarily of fibrils of type I collagen bound together into large fibers. They also contain small amounts of other types of collagen that bind to and probably help organize the fibrils of type I collagen. Cartilage contains large amounts of type II collagen, a protein very similar to type I collagen. The fibrils of type II collagen in cartilage form an arcade-like network that is distended by the presence of highly charged proteoglycans that trap large amounts of water and salts. Blood vessels such as the aorta contain large amounts of another fibrillar collagen known as type III and large amounts of elastin. The differences among connective tissues also depend on variations in the size, orientation, and packing of collagen fibrils. Fibrils and fibers of type I collagen in tendon are in a parallel orientation. Whereas the type I collagen fibrils of skin are randomly oriented in the plane of the skin, the type I collagen fibrils in cortical bone are deposited in complex helical rays around haversian canals. Accordingly, the differences in the morphology and function of connective tissues are based in part on their content of specific macromolecules and in part

on the organization of the macromolecules in the extracellular spaces.

Collagen and elastin, the subjects of this chapter, are similar in that they are tough fibrous proteins. At the same time, they are dramatically different in that the monomers of most collagens spontaneously self-assemble into highly ordered structures, whereas elastin forms amorphous fibrils in which it is difficult to find any evidence of an ordered structure.

COLLAGENS

More than 15 different kinds of collagens have now been identified in different tissues of vertebrates (for reviews, see references 1 to 3). This family of collagens can be divided into four subclasses: fibrillar collagens, basement membrane–associated collagens, fibril-associated collagens, and short-chain collagens (Table 2–2).

All the fibrillar collagens form fibrils that appear similar by electron microscopy. They vary in diameter and probably length but have a characteristic cross-striated pattern that reflects the gaps between the ends of the molecules found on the surface of the fibrils (Fig. 2–1, *Panel A*). The major fibrillar proteins (types I, II, and III) are among the most abundant proteins in the body. Fibrils and fibril bundles or fibers of type I collagen account for 60 to 90 percent of the dry weight of skin, ligaments, and bone (demineralized). Type I collagen is also found in many thin tissues, including the lungs and dentin and the sclerae of the eyes. In addition, it is the major constituent of mature scars. Type II collagen accounts for over half the dry weight of cartilage, and it is found in the vitreous gel of the eye. Type II collagen is also transiently present in many tissues during embryonic development. Type III collagen is abundant in large blood vessels and is found in small amounts in most tissues that contain type I collagen, but it is not present in bone. Of special interest is that a large fraction of the type III collagen found in some tissues, particularly skin, is found as a partially processed precursor form that retains the N-propeptides (see later). The partially processed form defined as type III pNcollagen binds to the surface of type I collagen fibrils and thereby limits their lateral growth.[5] The less abundant fibrillar collagen known as type V collagen is found as thin fibrils in synovial membranes, lung, skin, and a few other tissues.

22

Table 2–1. CONSTITUENTS OF CONNECTIVE TISSUE IN VARIOUS TISSUES

Connective Tissue	Known Constituents	Approximate Amounts (% dry weight)	Characteristics
Skin (dermis), ligaments, tendons	Type I collagen	80	Bundles of fibers of high tensile strength
	Type III collagen	5 to 15	Thin fibrils
	Type IV collagen, laminin, nidogen	<5	In basal laminae under epithelium and in blood
	Types V to VII	<5	Distributions and functions unclear
	Fibronectin	<5	Associated with collagen fibers and cell surfaces
	Proteoglycans*	0.5	Provides resiliency
	Hyaluronate	0.5	Provides resiliency
Bones (demineralized)	Type I collagen	90	Complex organization of fibrils
	Type V collagen	1 to 2	Function unclear
	Proteoglycans	1	Function unclear
	Sialoproteins	1	Function unclear
	Osteonectin	2 to 3	Role in ossification
	Osteocalcin	1	Probable role in ossification
	α_2-Glycoprotein	1	Possible role in ossification
Aorta	Type I collagen	20 to 40	
	Type III collagen	20 to 40	Thin fibrils
	Elastin, microfibrillar protein	20 to 40	Amorphous, elastic fibrils
	Type IV collagen, laminin, nidogen	<5	In basal lamina
	Types V and VI collagens	<2	Functions unclear
	Proteoglycans	<3	Mucopolysaccharides, mainly chondroitin sulfate and dermatan sulfate; heparan sulfate in basal lamina
Cartilage	Type II collagen	40 to 50	Thin fibrils
	Types IX and XI collagen	5 to 25	Possible flexible spacers
	Type X collagen	5	Undefined role in hypertrophic region
	Proteoglycans	15 to 50	Provides resiliency
	Hyaluronate	0.5 to 2	Provides resiliency

*Proteoglycan structures are incompletely defined. About five different protein cores have been identified, and each has one or more kinds of mucopolysaccharides attached. Major mucopolysaccharides of skin and tendon are dermatan sulfate and chondroitin-4-sulfate; of aorta, chondroitin-4-sulfate and dermatan sulfate; of cartilage, chondroitin-4-sulfate, chondroitin-6-sulfate, and keratan sulfate. Basal lamina contains a heparan sulfate.

Type XI collagen is uniformly distributed in articular cartilage, where it can account for 5 to 20 percent of the total collagen. The fibrils formed by type V and type XI collagens appear to be similar to those of the major fibrillar collagens, but they have not been studied as extensively.[3]

Type IV collagen is a major constituent of all basement membranes. Monomers of the protein bind to one another through globular extensions found at both ends of the molecules to form large structures resembling a wire network (Fig. 2–2). The network-like structures serve as filtration barriers and as a scaffolding for the binding of other basement membrane constituents such as laminin, nidogen, and a large heparan sulfate proteoglycan. The decorated scaffold then serves as an important barrier for fluids and solutes and as an important surface for the attachment and movement of cells. Type VII collagen is found in the upper layers of the dermis, where it forms thin and short structures that serve as "anchoring fibrils" between the basement membrane of the skin, and the dermis.

The fiber-associated collagens (types VIII, IX, and XIV) are found on the surface of fibrils of type I and type II collagens, where they probably serve as flexible spacers among the fibrils. The structures assembled from the short-chain collagens (types VIII and X) and a number of other recently identified collagens are poorly defined, but they may form specialized networks among specific cell types.[3]

Structure of Collagen Fibrils

The fibrils formed by the fibrillar collagens consist almost entirely of monomers of the protein tightly packed in a quarter-stagger array (see Fig. 2–1). The molecular structure of type I collagen is composed of two identical polypeptide chains called α1(I) and one slightly different polypeptide chain called α2(I) (see Table 2–2). Type II collagen is a homotrimer made up of three identical α1(II)-chains, and type III collagen is a homotrimer composed of three α1(III)-chains. The structure of all the α-chains of the fibrillar collagens is highly repetitive. Glycine is every third amino acid, and each α-chain has about 1000 amino

Table 2–2. MAJOR TYPES OF COLLAGEN AND THEIR α-CHAIN COMPOSITIONS*

Classes	α-Chain Composition
Fibrillar	
Type I	Two α1(I) and one α2(I)
Type II	Three α1(II)
Type III	Three α1(III)
Type V	α1(V), α2(V), and α3(V)
Type XI	α1(XI), α2(XI), and α3(XI)
Basement Membrane–Associated	
Type IV	α1(IV), α2(IV), ± α3(IV), ± α4(IV), and ± α5(IV)
Type VII	α1(VII)
Fiber-Associated†	
Type IX	α1(IX), α2(IX), and α3(IX)
Type XII	α1(XII)
Short-Chain	
Type VIII	α1(VIII)
Type X	α1(X)

*For more complete descriptions, see references 2 to 4.
†Chain composition apparently varies in different tissues, with α3(IV), α4(IV), and α5(IV) prominent in kidney.

acids. Therefore the sequence of each α-chain can be defined as $(Gly-X-Y)_{333}$. The X-position in the sequence is frequently occupied by proline, and the Y-position is frequently occupied by hydroxyproline, an unusual amino acid that is abundant in collagen but rare in any other protein. An important feature of the triple helix of collagen is that the glycine residues are packed into a restricted space near the center of the triple helix that can accommodate only glycine, the smallest amino acid residue.[2] Because proline and hydroxyproline are saturated ring amino acids, they keep the α-chains in an extended configuration that stabilizes the structure of the triple helix. Some of the X- and Y-positions in each α-chain contain hydrophobic or charged amino acids that appear in clusters. The clusters of hydrophobic and charged amino acids on the surface of the triple helix direct binding of one molecule to another so that each is quarter-staggered relative to a nearest neighbor in a fibril (see Fig. 2–1). Each of the α-chains of a fibrillar collagen also contains short sequences of about 25 amino acids at each end (telopeptides) that do not have a triple-helical structure and that play an important but incompletely defined role in assembly of the proteins into fibrils.

All collagens have at least one triple-helical domain similar to the large triple-helical domain that accounts for most of the structure of a fibrillar collagen. In the nonfibrillar collagens, however, the repetitive Gly-X-Y sequences are frequently interrupted by short regions of other amino acid sequences that introduce more flexible hinge regions into the proteins.[13] Type IV collagen, for example, has numerous short interruptions of its large triple-helical domain that are probably important for its assembly into network-like structures (see Fig. 2–2) or binding of other basement membrane constituents. One of the hinge regions of type IX collagen is an attachment site for a mucopolysaccharide chain (chondroitin sulfate).

Structure of Collagen Genes

The genes for collagens have several unusual features. Each of the genes for the major fibrillar collagens (types I, II, and III) has 52 to 54 exons that code for the large triple-helical domain of the protein.[1, 3, 6] The most common exon size is 54 base pairs (bp); some exons are 108 bp (twice 54), and one is 162 (three times 54). Still other exons are variations on the 54-bp theme in that they are 99 bp (54 plus 45). With one exception, the sizes of specific exons are identical in the two genes for type I procollagen (*COL1A1* and *COL1A2*), the gene for type II procollagen (*COL2A1*), and the gene for type III procollagen (*COL3A1*). In addition, the same exons have the same sizes in the genes from humans, rodents, and chickens. The unusual 54-bp motif of the genes for fibrillar collagens has been interpreted as suggesting either that the genes arose by duplication of a 54-bp exon

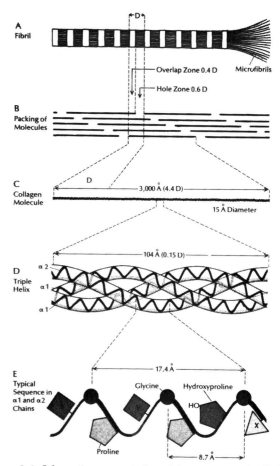

Figure 2–1. Schematic representation of the structure of a fibril of type I collagen. (From Prockop, D. J., and Guzman, N. A.: Collagen diseases and the biosynthesis of collagen. Hosp. Pract. 12[12]:61–68, 1977. Reproduced by permission from the Hospital Practice.)

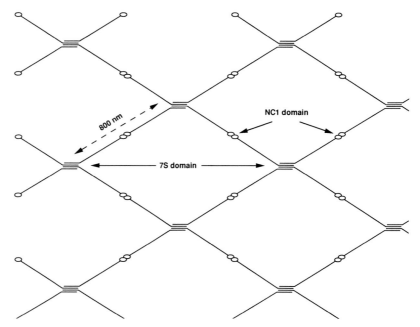

Figure 2–2. Schematic representation of the network-like structures formed by the assembly of type IV collagen in basement membranes. The NC1 domains are the globular extensions at the C terminal of the molecule. The 7S domains are noncollagenous domains at the N terminal of the protein.

or that the molecular mechanisms for replication of the genes specifically perpetuate a 54-bp motif.

The same 54-bp motif is seen in parts of the structures for nonfibrillar collagens. However, some of the exons of the genes for these other collagens have varying structures, and many of the exons begin with the second base for a glycine codon, rather than a complete codon for glycine as seen in the exons for fibrillar collagens.

BIOSYNTHESIS

The biosynthesis of collagen involves a large number of post-translational processing steps (for review, see reference 1).

The major fibrillar collagens (types I, II, and III) are first assembled as large precursor procollagens that have additional N-terminal and C-terminal propeptides not found in the nonfibrillar collagens (Fig. 2–3). The three proα-chains of a procollagen are initially synthesized with N-terminal signal sequences that direct their binding to the ribosomes of the cisternae of the rough endoplasmic reticulum. As the proα-chains pass into the cisternae, the signal peptides are cleaved and the proα-chains undergo a series of hydroxylations and glycosylations. About 100 prolyl residues in the Y-positions are hydroxylated to hydroxy-4-proline, and about 10 lysyl residues in the Y-positions are hydroxylated to hydroxylysine. Some of the hydroxylysyl residues are subsequently modified by the addition of galactose or both galactose and glucose to the epsilon-hydroxyl (ε-hydroxyl) group. Both the hydroxylation of proline and that of lysine require ascorbic acid. Of the two hydroxylations, the hydroxylation of proline to hydroxyproline is more critical, since a stable collagen triple helix cannot be formed at body temperature unless each α-chain contains about 100 hydroxyprolyl residues. The requirement for ascorbic acid in the enzymatic hydroxylation of proline probably explains the failure of wounds to heal in scurvy. In addition to the modifications of the prolyl and lysyl residues, a mannose-rich carbohydrate is added to the C-terminal propeptide of each proα-chain. As these modifications of the proα-chains are occurring, the three chains come together through their globular C-propeptides and become disulfide linked. After the three chains associate and acquire the necessary content of hydroxyproline, a nucleus of triple helix forms near the C terminal of the α-chain domains. The triple-helical conformation is then propagated from the C to the N terminals of the molecule.

An unusual relationship is found between the folding of procollagen into a triple-helical conformation and the post-translational modifications that introduce hydroxyproline, hydroxylysine, and glycosylated hydroxylysine.[1] The two hydroxylases and the two glycosyl transferases involved in the reactions can modify only proα-chains or α-chains that are in a random coil conformation. As soon as the protein folds into a triple helix, the enzymes no longer interact with the proα-chains. Since the protein cannot fold into a triple helix until most of the Y-position prolyl residues are hydroxylated to hydroxyproline, the content of hydroxyproline in most fibrillar collagens is essentially the same. The contents of hydroxylysine and glycosylated hydroxylysine, however, vary and depend on several poorly controlled factors, such as the relative concentrations of the proα-chain substrates, the enzymes, and the cofactors for the enzymes in the cisternae of the rough endoplasmic reticulum. The lack of precise control of these factors probably explains why the contents of hydroxylysine and glycosylated hydroxy-

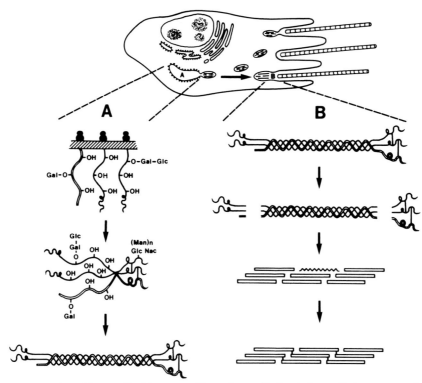

Figure 2–3. Schematic representation of how a fibroblast assembles collagen fibrils. *A*, Intracellular post-translational modifications of proα-chains, association of C-propeptide domains, and folding into the triple-helical conformation. *B*, Enzymatic cleavage of procollagen to collagen, self-assembly of collagen monomers into fibrils, and cross-linking of fibrils into fibers. (From Prockop, D. J., and Kivirikko, K. I.: Heritable diseases of collagen. N. Engl. J. Med. 311:376–386, 1984. Reprinted with permission from the New England Journal of Medicine.)

lysine are higher in embryonic tissues than in adult tissues. The content of glycosylated hydroxylysine in collagen affects its biologic function, since the glycosylated hydroxylysyl residues project from the surface of the triple helix and interfere with lateral packing of the molecule into fibrils. Therefore, an increase in glycosylated hydroxylysine decreases the diameter of the fibrils formed. Any condition that delays folding of the proα-chains into a triple helix increases the contents of hydroxylysine and glycosylated hydroxylysine. As a result, most mutations that change the amino acid sequences of proα-chains increase the content of hydroxylysine and glycosylated hydroxylysine in procollagen and collagen (see later).

The folding of procollagen into a triple-helical conformation is also intimately related to its secretion from cells. Under normal conditions, secretion begins only after the protein is correctly folded. In a condition such as ascorbate deficiency, the rate of hydroxylation of prolyl residues, and hence the rate of protein folding, is decreased. Consequently, there is an accumulation of nonhelical proα-chains in the rough endoplasmic reticulum and an overall decrease in the secretion of helical procollagen molecules from the cell. Accumulation of nonhelical proα-chains is also seen with agents that inhibit prolyl hydroxylase and with mutations in the structure of the proα-chains that delay folding (see later).

As soon as the protein folds into a triple-helical conformation, it is transported from the rough endoplasmic reticulum to Golgi vesicles, from which it is secreted. The protein is then further processed extracellularly by a specific procollagen N-proteinase that cleaves the N-propeptides and a separate procollagen C-proteinase that cleaves the C-propeptides. After the propeptides are cleaved, the solubility of the protein decreases over 1000-fold to less than 1 μg per ml at 37°C, and it spontaneously self-assembles into fibrils.[1, 7, 8] The fibers initially assembled have the same morphology as mature fibers of collagen, but they do not achieve their optimal tensile strength until some of the lysyl and glycosylated hydroxylysyl residues are enzymatically deaminated by the enzyme lysyl oxidase to generate aldehydes that project from the surfaces of the molecules. The aldehydes then spontaneously form covalent cross-links among adjacent molecules in the fibril. The formation of the cross-links stabilizes the fibril structure so that it acquires a tensile strength that approximates that of a steel wire.

The biosynthetic pathways for nonfibrillar collagens are similar to those for the fibrillar collagens, but they have not been as extensively studied. Most of the nonfibrillar collagens have globular extensions at both ends, but there is no evidence that the globular ends of the proteins are cleaved in a manner comparable to that of the globular ends of fibrillar procollagens. Instead, the globular ends persist in tissues and appear to be involved in the assembly of matrix structures (see Fig. 2–2).

Metabolic Turnover

The collagens in adult tissues are highly stable structures. However, there is dramatic degradation and resynthesis of collagen fibrils during embryonic development as tissues change their shape and increase in size.[1] Considerable metabolic turnover of collagens continues throughout the growth of the organism. After maturity of the skeleton, the collagen fibrils and fibers in most tissues become stable metabolically so that they have half-lives of many weeks or months. In bone, however, collagen continues to be degraded and resynthesized as remodeling continues throughout life. In addition, large amounts of collagen can be lost from the skin and other connective tissues during periods of malnutrition or starvation. The collagen in many tissues, therefore, is a replenishable source of amino acids for gluconeogenesis. Also, diseases of connective tissue produce marked increases in collagen turnover. For example, there are marked increases in the metabolic turnover of collagen in bone in Paget's disease, hyperparathyroidism, and metastatic diseases. There are large increases in the turnover of collagen as well as most other proteins in hyperthyroidism. Increases in collagen turnover are accompanied by increases in the excretion in urine of peptide-bound hydroxyproline and hydroxylysine that arise from incomplete degradation of collagen polypeptides. Assays of the urinary excretion of hydroxyproline and glycosylated hydroxylysine have therefore been used clinically to measure turnover of collagen. Also, immunoassays of serum levels of procollagen propeptides have been used to follow changes in rates of collagen biosynthesis. The most widely used have been assays of the serum levels of the N-propeptide of type III procollagen and the 7S fragment of type IV, and they have been particularly useful in following liver fibrosis.[9, 10]

The degradation of the collagen in tissues is initiated by cleavage of the molecule by one of several specific collagenases. The collagenases cleave the molecule at a site that is about three quarters of the distance from the N to the C terminal. The resulting three-quarter and one-quarter fragments then partially unfold so that they are further degraded by nonspecific proteases such as gelatinases and stromelysin. In addition to the extracellular degradation of collagen fibrils, part of the newly synthesized proα-chains in cells appears to be degraded before they are incorporated into functional procollagen or collagen molecules. The intracellular degradation of the newly synthesized chains may represent a mechanism for correcting errors in biosynthesis.

Principle of Nucleated Growth in Collagen Biosynthesis

One of the unusual features of collagen biosynthesis is that it extensively employs a principle of nucleated growth whereby a few molecules first assemble into a structure defined as a nucleus, and the structure of the nucleus is then propagated by the orderly and rapid addition of thousands of the same molecules.[7, 8] The principle of nucleated growth is used extensively in nature in the formation of crystals by many inorganic materials, including the formation of snowflakes by water. In collagen biosynthesis, the principle of nucleated growth is used in folding of the protein in that a nucleus of triple helix is formed near the C terminal of the procollagen molecule and is then rapidly propagated to the N terminal (see Fig. 2–3). In addition, the principle of nucleated growth is employed in the assembly of fibrils in that a few molecules of the protein first form a nucleus of a fibril, and then the nucleus grows by the orderly and rapid addition of many collagen molecules.

Nucleated growth is a highly efficient mechanism for assembly of large structures with a precisely defined architecture. Nucleated growth, however, requires that all the molecules or subunits in the system have the same structure. As illustrated by the growth of inorganic crystals, a few molecules with a defective structure prevent propagation of the nucleus and "poison" the system. Because it extensively employs the principle of nucleated growth, collagen biosynthesis is markedly disturbed by mutations that change the amino acid sequence of the protein. In particular, single-base mutations that convert a glycine codon to a codon for an amino acid with a bulkier side residue can prevent propagation of the triple helix so that the molecule cannot form a functional protein. The presence of one proα-chain with a single glycine substitution can prevent folding and cause degradation of both the abnormal proα-chain and two normal proα-chains in a process referred to as "procollagen suicide" (Fig. 2–4). Surprisingly, however, some mutations substituting bulkier amino acids for glycine residues have little effect on the folding of the protein but produce subtle changes in conformation such as a flexible "kink" in the triple helix that is visible by electron microscopy (Fig. 2–5). The presence of conformational kinks in the molecule can poison fibril assembly so as to generate fibrils with highly distorted morphology (Fig. 2–6) or markedly decrease the amount of collagen incorporated in the fibrils.

Mutations in Collagen Genes That Produce Human Diseases

Mutations in collagen genes were first encountered in studies on osteogenesis imperfecta (OI), a heritable disorder characterized by brittleness of

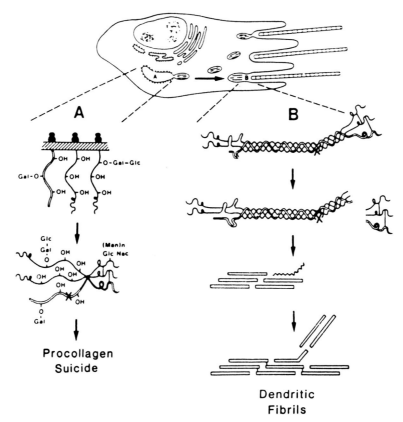

Figure 2–4. Schematic representation of how mutations that change the structure of type I collagen can interfere with either the intracellular assembly of the protein or the subsequent assembly of collagen fibrils. As discussed in the text, a mutation that converts a codon for a glycine residue to a codon for a bulkier amino acid can prevent the folding of the protein into a triple-helical conformation. If folding is prevented, both the normal proα-chains and the mutated proα-chains are degraded through a process referred to as "procollagen suicide." Alternatively, a glycine substitution or other mutation can allow folding into a triple-helical conformation but introduces a subtle change in conformation of the protein such as a "kink." Monomers with an altered conformation can interfere with fibril assembly so that highly abnormal fibrils are generated. (From Prockop, D. J., and Kivirikko, K. I.: Heritable diseases of collagen. N. Engl. J. Med. 311:376–386, 1984. Reprinted with permission from the New England Journal of Medicine.)

bones that is frequently associated with changes in other tissues rich in collagen. More than 90 percent of patients with OI have a mutation in the gene for the proα1(I)-chain (*COL1A1*) or the gene for the proα2(I)-chain (COL1A2) of type I procollagen (for recent reviews, see references 13 and 14). As yet, no patient with OI has been shown to have a mutation in any other gene-protein system. Mild forms of OI are caused primarily by mutations that decrease the synthesis of proα1(I)-chains. More severe variants of OI, however, are caused by mutations that produce synthesis of abnormal but partially functional proα1(I)- or proα2(I)-chains of type I procollagen. Unrelated patients and families rarely have the same mutation, and more than 70 different mutations have now been defined.

The devastating effects of mutations that change the structure of a proα1(I)- or proα2(I)-chain are explained by the extensive use of nucleated growth in collagen biosynthesis.[7, 8] Of special interest has been a large number of single-base mutations that convert a codon for glycine to a codon for a bulkier amino acid. The glycine substitutions are highly position-specific in that a substitution of one glycine

position can produce procollagen suicide, whereas a substitution of the same or a similar amino acid for a nearby glycine position has essentially no effect on the folding of the triple helix but can markedly alter fibril assembly (Fig. 2–7 and Table 2–3). Also, the glycine substitutions are position-specific in the sense that substitutions for some glycine residues produce severe OI that is lethal in utero or shortly after birth, whereas others cause only mild forms of the disease. The results suggest that some regions of the α-chains are more critical to the stability of triple helix than are others. They also suggest that some regions of the molecule may be important for its normal function in tissues such as bone, whereas other regions are more important for its function elsewhere. Such generalizations probably explain why some patients with moderately severe OI have fragile bones, together with evidence of decreased collagen in other tissues such as blue sclerae, severe dentinogenesis imperfecta, and strikingly thin skin, whereas other patients with equally fragile bones have apparently normal sclerae, teeth, and skin.

The large number of mutations in the type I procollagen genes causing OI prompted a search for

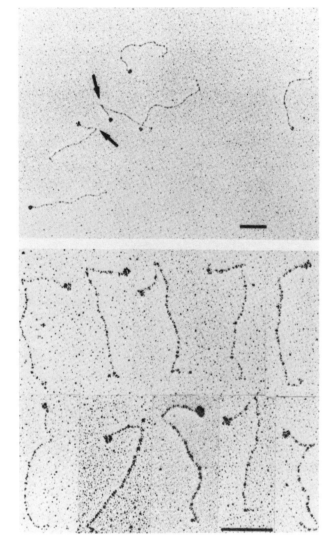

Figure 2–5. Rotary shadowing electron microscopy of mutated type I procollagen molecules. A panel of individual molecules is presented. The C terminal of the protein can be identified because the globular C-propeptide is larger than the globular N-propeptide. The molecules demonstrate the presence of a flexible kink at the site of a mutation that has converted the codon for glycine at position α1-748 to a codon for cysteine. (From Vogel, B. E., et al.: A substitution of cysteine for glycine 748 of the α1 chain produces a kink at this site in the procollagen I molecule and an altered N-proteinase cleavage site over 225 nm away. J. Biol. Chem. 263:19249–19255, 1988.)

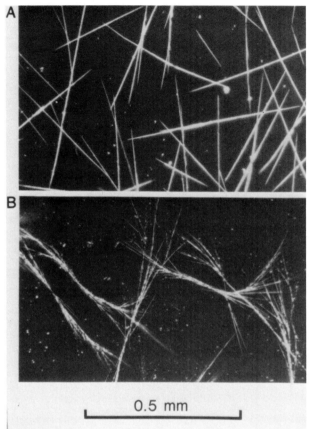

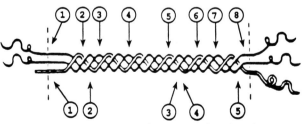

Figure 2–6. Collagen fibrils assembled from normal human type I collagen *(A)* and collagen from a proband with a heterozygous mutation that converted the codon for glycine at position α1-748 to a codon for cysteine *(B)*. About 10 percent of the protein in the fibrils is the mutated type I collagen, and 90 percent is normal type I collagen. As indicated, the presence of the mutated protein generates fibrils that are abnormally branched. (From Kadler, K. E., Torre-Blanco, A., et al.: A type I collagen with substitution of a cysteine for glycine-748 in the α1(I) chain copolymerizes with normal type I collagen and can generate fractal-like structures. Biochemistry 30:5081–5088, 1991. Reproduced by permission from Biochemistry. Copyright 1991, American Chemical Society.)

reditary disorder characterized by hematuria and nephritis frequently associated with deafness. Linkage studies[16] suggest that a mutation in the gene for type VII collagen may cause the dystrophic form of epidermolysis bullosa, in which blistering occurs

mutations in other procollagen genes that might cause other heritable disorders of connective tissue. A series of mutations in the gene for type II procollagen have been found to cause severe chondrodysplasias.[13, 14] Similarly, mutations in the gene for type III procollagen have been shown to cause the potentially lethal form of Ehlers-Danlos syndrome known as type IV, a disease that produces marked changes in tissues rich in type III collagen, such as thinness and scarring of skin and rupture of large arteries and other whole organs. Mutations in the gene for the α5(IV)-chain of type IV collagen have been shown to cause X-linked forms of Alport's syndrome,[15] a he-

Figure 2–7. Approximate sites of mutations that alter the primary structure of type I procollagen. *Numbers Above the Molecule,* Approximate sites of mutations in the proα1(I)-chain. *Numbers Below the Molecule,* Approximate sites of mutations in the proα2(I)-chain. Effects of the mutations are summarized in Table 2–3.

Table 2–3. MUTATIONS IN TYPE I PROCOLLAGENS, THEIR EFFECTS ON THE PROTEIN, AND THE PHENOTYPES THEY PRODUCE (SEE FIG. 2–6)*

Mutation	Molecular Mechanism		Disease Phenotype
	Procollagen Suicide	Abnormal Fibrils	
Proα1-Chain			
(1) Splicing of exon 6		+	Loose joints (EDS VIIA)†
(2) Gly^{175}→Cys	±	+	Moderate OI
(3) Gly^{244}→Cys	0	(+)	Lethal OI
(4) Gly^{391}→Arg	±	(+)	Lethal OI
(5) Gly^{598}→Ser	+		Lethal OI
(6) Gly^{748}→Cys	+	+	Lethal OI
(7) Gly^{832}→Ser	±	(+)	Moderate OI
(8) Gly^{988}→Cys	+	+	Lethal OI
Proα2-Chain			
(1) Splicing of exon 6		+	Loose joints (EDS VIIA)†
(2) Partial deletion of IVS10/exon 11	+	+	Loose joints or fragile bones
(3) Gly^{646}→Cys	±	(+)	Mild OI
(4) Gly^{661}→Ser	0	(+)	Osteoporosis
(5) Gly^{907}→Asp	+	(?)	Lethal OI

*For recent summaries of mutations and their effects, see Kuivaniemi et al.[13] and Byers.[14]
†Mutations that prevent cleavage of the N-propeptide.
Symbols: +, proven mechanism; ±, secondary mechanism; (+), probable mechanism; EDS, Ehlers-Danlos syndrome; OI, osteogenesis imperfecta. Superscript numbers indicate amino acid position in the α1(I)- or α2(I)-chains.

below the basement membrane of the skin associated with a decrease in the anchoring fibrils[17] formed by type VII collagen.

In addition, recent data suggest that mutations in collagen genes may be a cause of more common diseases of connective tissues. A glycine substitution in type III procollagen was shown to cause aortic aneurysms in a family without any of the characteristic features of Ehlers-Danlos syndrome type IV or Marfan's syndrome.[18] Linkage studies suggested that a mutation in the gene for type II procollagen was the cause of osteoarthritis in two large Finnish families.[19] In addition, a mutation that converted an arginine codon to a codon for cysteine[20] was shown to cause osteoarthritis associated with a mild chondrodysplasia in one family (Figs. 2–8, 2–9, and 2–10). Similarly, several reports indicate that mutations in the genes for type I procollagen may be the cause

of some forms of postmenopausal osteoporosis.[21–23] The results demonstrate that mutations in genes for fibrillar collagens are the cause of at least subsets of these common diseases (Table 2–4). The data are still too preliminary, however, to establish whether such mutations account for a large fraction of the common forms of postmenopausal osteoporosis, aortic aneurysms, or primary generalized osteoarthritis.

ELASTIN

The elastic properties of tissues such as skin, large blood vessels, lung, and large ligaments depend largely on the presence of rubber-like elastic fibers.[24–27] In contrast with collagen fibrils and fibers, elastic fibers are amorphous structures in the sense that their molecular components are not assembled

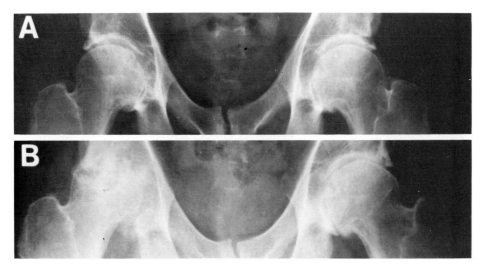

Figure 2–8. Radiographs from an affected member of the family with primary generalized osteoarthritis associated with mild chondrodysplasia. *A,* Radiograph showing osteoarthritis in both hips, but no apparent dysplasia. *B,* Radiograph of same patient 3 years later. There is a progressive increase in osteoarthritis-induced changes that are more pronounced on the right. (From Knowlton, R. G., et al.: Genetic linkage of a polymorphism in the type II procollagen gene (COL2A1) to primary osteoarthritis associated with mild chondrodysplasia. N. Engl. J. Med. 322:526, 1990. Reprinted with permission from the New England Journal of Medicine.)

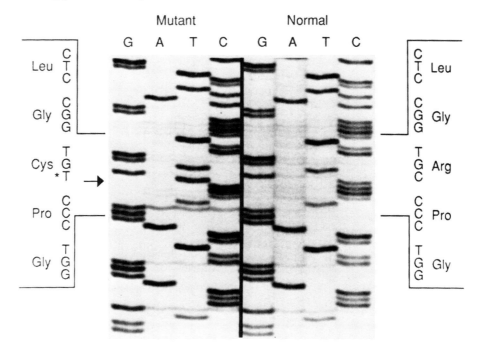

Figure 2–9. DNA sequencing film of an appropriate region of the cosmid clone containing the mutation from an affected member of the family with osteoarthritis and mild chondrodysplasia. An asterisk marks the single-base change that converts the codon CGT for arginine at position 519 of the α1(II)-chain to TGT, a codon for cysteine. The sequences are from the appropriate allele of the patient shown in Figure 2–8. (From Ala-Kokko, L., et al.: Single base mutation in the type II procollagen gene (COL2A1) as a cause of primary osteoarthritis associated with a mild chondrodysplasia. Proc. Natl. Acad. Sci. U.S.A. 87:6565–6568, 1990.)

in a regular pattern that can be detected by electron microscopy or x-ray diffraction. The major constituent of elastic fibers is elastin, an unusual protein composed of a single polypeptide chain of 72,000 daltons. The protein has large domains of hydrophobic amino acids joined by shorter sequences that are rich in alanine and lysine. The amino acid sequences of the hydrophobic domains are similar to the α-chains of collagen in that they frequently have sequences of Gly-X-Y. A few of the prolines in the Y-position of the sequences are hydroxylated to hydroxyproline, but the presence of hydroxyproline in elastin appears to have no functional significance. The regions rich in alanine and lysine are sites for covalent cross-links among different regions of the same chain and among different chains of the protein. The elastic properties of the protein derive from the marked tendency of the hydrophobic domains to fold in on themselves and from coil-like compartments within the fibers.[24] Stretching the fibers unfolds the hydrophobic domains and extends the polypeptide chains so that they are held together primarily by the cross-links. As soon as the stretching force is released, the hydrophobic domains spontaneously refold. Detailed studies on elastin, however, are hampered by the fact that the protein is among the most insoluble proteins in nature and cannot be extracted from tissues with solvents as harsh as 8 M urea or hot alkali.

In addition to elastin, the elastic fibers in tissues contain poorly defined microfibrillar structures. The microfibrillar structures are seen early in embryonic development as elastic fibers are first formed. They are also seen at the edges of elastic fibrils in mature tissues. The composition of the microfibrillar structures has not been fully defined, but a major component has recently been shown to be fibrillin, a large glycoprotein of about 300,000 daltons that appears to be associated with most elastin fibrils.[28]

The Gene for Elastin and Fibrillin

The human gene for elastin contains 34 exons that range in size from 27 to 186 bp and code for a polypeptide chain of 786 amino acids.[29] The hydrophobic and the cross-linking domains of the protein are coded by separate exons. The introns of the gene are relatively large compared with genes for collagens and other proteins, and they contain a large number of Alu repetitive sequences, particularly at the 3' end of the gene.

One of the most interesting features of the elastin gene is that RNA transcripts are spliced by a large

Table 2–4. TYPES OF COLLAGENS AND DISEASES CAUSED BY MUTATIONS IN COLLAGEN GENES

	Human Disorder	
Collagen	*Most severe*	*Mildest*
Fibrillar		
Type I	Lethal OI	A subset of osteoporosis
Type II	Lethal chondrodysplasias	A subset of osteoarthritis
Type III	Ehlers-Danlos syndrome IV (lethal)	A subset of aortic aneurysms
Basement-Membrane Associated		
Type IV	Alport's syndrome	
Type VII	Epidermolysis bullosa (dystrophic form)	

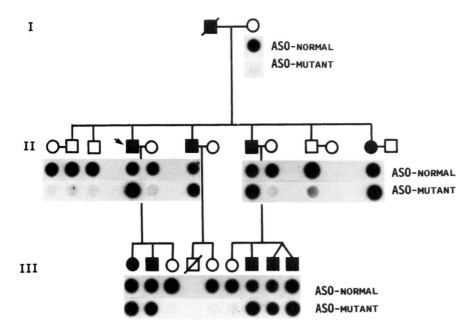

Figure 2–10. Hybridization assays for the presence of the normal allele for type II collagen and the mutated allele for type II collagen containing cysteine at position 519 of the α1(II)-chain. Genomic DNA from members of the family was amplified with a polymerase chain reaction. Products of the polymerase chain reaction were blotted on nitrocellulose filters and hybridized with ^{32}P-labeled DNA probes specific for either the normal base sequence (ASO-normal) or the mutated sequence (ASO-mutant). Black squares and circles in the pedigree indicate affected members of the family. (From Ala-Kokko, L., et al.: Single base mutation in the type II procollagen gene (COL2A1) as a cause of primary osteoarthritis associated with a mild chondrodysplasia. Proc. Natl. Acad. Sci. 87:6565–6568, 1990.)

number of alternative pathways to generate a large series of mRNAs that differ because they lack the codons from one or more exons of the gene.[29, 30] As a result, cells synthesizing elastin produce a variety of polypeptide chains of different sizes and amino acid composition. The reasons for these variations are not known.

Genes for fibrillin have only recently been isolated, and they have not been fully characterized.[31, 32] The first gene isolated was located on the long arm of chromosome 15 (see later). In the course of screening libraries of genomic DNA, two other similar genes were isolated. The two additional genes have chromosomal locations different from those of the first gene, and the relationships among the three genes have not yet been defined.

Biosynthesis and Metabolic Turnover

Elastin is synthesized by smooth muscle cells and, to a lesser extent, by fibroblasts. Initial studies suggested that the protein was first synthesized as a larger and more soluble precursor protein, but this possibility was subsequently excluded by more detailed biosynthetic studies.[33] Therefore, it is not apparent how this highly insoluble protein is synthesized without premature aggregation in cells. Also, little information is available about the biosynthesis of fibrillin.

After elastin is secreted, it undergoes extensive cross-linking reactions.[27] The cross-linking reactions (Fig. 2–11) begin with removal of the ε-amino group of lysine by lysyl oxidase, the same enzyme involved in collagen cross-linking. About 40 lysine residues in elastin are deaminated to generate aldehydes that undergo a series of apparently spontaneous interactions to form complex aromatic structures. The parent

compound is desmosine, but a number of variations on the structure are also found, including reduced aldehyde condensation products.

Elastases that degrade elastin are present in polymorphonuclear leukocytes and in the pancreas.[34, 35] Since desmosine is metabolized poorly, if at all, the urinary excretion of desmosine has been used to assay metabolic turnover of elastin. The results suggest that only about 1 percent of total body elastin is degraded per year in a normal adult.[36]

Diseases Related to Elastin and Fibrillin

Genetic defects in elastin that cause human disease have long been suspected, but none have been definitively identified.

The extreme looseness of skin seen in cutis laxa is probably caused by a genetic defect in elastin.[37] Decreased levels of mRNA for elastin were found in fibroblasts from a few patients with the disease. However, no gene defect has yet been defined, and some forms of the disease may be explained by an increase in elastase activity. Similarly, defects in elastin may well be the cause of pseudoxanthoma elasticum, which is characterized by abnormal accumulations of calcified elastic fibers in the mid-dermis.[37] Also, defects in the elastin gene may explain the skin tumors rich in elastic fibers and the osteopoikilotic bone lesions of Buschke-Ollendorff syndrome.[37] Studies with cultured fibroblasts from patients with the syndrome suggest that there is an unexplained increase in elastin biosynthesis.

Deficiencies in serum α₁-antitrypsin cause a heritable form of emphysema that is sometimes associated with hepatitis and cirrhosis.[38] Serum α₁-antitrypsin is the major inhibitor of neutrophil elastase in the lower respiratory tract, and deficiencies of the inhib-

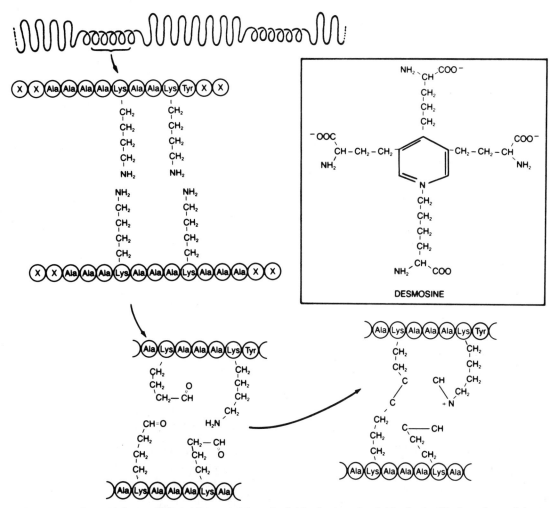

Figure 2–11. Formation of peptidyl cross-links in the conversion of soluble elastin to insoluble elastin. The large loop of the tropoelastin structure represents hydrophilic stretchable areas composed primarily of the amino acids, glycine, proline, valine, phenylalanine, isoleucine, and leucine. The small coiled areas represent the alanine-rich areas that surround the lysine residues involved in cross-link formation. This is an α-helical region containing two lysine residues separated by two and three alanine residues. Two peptide chains are parallel such that the side chains of lysine or allysine after oxidative deamidation can spontaneously condense to form the stable peritoneum ring structure with three double bonds (as depicted). The desmosine molecule, therefore, is composed of three allysine residues and one lysine residue in a peritoneum ring structure to form the tetrafunctional amino acid that participates in both inter- and intrachain cross-linking.

itor apparently cause destruction of lung tissue because of increased elastase activity. The causal relationship between deficiency of the inhibitor and the disease is strongly supported by the observation that similar emphysematous changes are seen in experimental animals in which elastase is introduced into the lungs. The hepatic injury seen in some forms of the disease is related to mutations that change the structure of α_1-antitrypsin so that it is not secreted by hepatocytes, in which it is normally synthesized. Several different defects in the gene for α_1-antitrypsin have now been identified.[39]

Recently, linkage studies demonstrated that Marfan's syndrome was linked to the long arm of chromosome 15.[40, 41] Also, a gene for fibrillin was cloned and also located to the long arm of chromosome 15.[31] In addition, two unrelated patients with spontaneous Marfan's syndrome were shown to have the same sporadic mutation that changed an arginine codon to a codon for proline.[32] The results suggest that most forms of the disease are caused by mutations in the fibrillin gene(s). The importance of two similar genes for fibrillin located on two different chromosomes is still not apparent.

References

1. Prockop, D. J., and Kivirikko, K. I.: Heritable diseases of collagen. N. Engl. J. Med. 311:376, 1984.
2. Piez, K.: Molecular and aggregate structures of the collagens. *In* Piez, K. A., and Reddi, A. H. (eds.): Extracellular Matrix Biochemistry. New York, Elsevier, 1984, pp. 1–40.
3. Van der Rest, M., and Garrone, R.: Collagen family of proteins. FASEB J. 5:2814, 1991.
4. Prockop, D. J., and Guzman, N. A.: Collagen diseases and the biosynthesis of collagen. Hosp. Pract. 12(12):61, 1977.
5. Romanic, A. M., Adachi, E., Kadler, K. E., Hojima, Y., and Prockop, D. J.: Copolymerization of pNcollagen III and collagen I. pNcollagen

III decreases the rate of incorporation of collagen I into fibrils, the amount of collagen incorporated, and the diameter of fibrils formed. J. Biol. Chem. 266:12703, 1991.

6. Chu, M.-L., and Prockop, D. J.: Collagen: Gene structures. In Royce, P. M., and Steinmann, B. (eds.): Extracellular Matrix and Inheritable Disorders of Connective Tissue. New York, Alan R. Liss, Inc. (in press).

7. Prockop, D. J.: Mutations that alter the primary structure of type I collagen. The perils of a system for generating large structures by the principle of nucleated growth. J. Biol. Chem. 265:15349, 1990.

8. Engel, J., and Prockop, D. J.: The zipper-like folding of collagen triple helices and the effects of mutations that disrupt the zipper. Annu. Rev. Biophys. Biophys. Chem. 20:137, 1991.

9. Rohde, H., Vargas, L., Hahn, E., Kalbfleisch, H., Bruguera, M., and Timpl, R.: Radioimmunoassay for type III procollagen peptide and its application to human liver disease. Eur. J. Clin. Invest. 9:451, 1979.

10. Ala-Kokko, L., Günzler, V., Hoek, J. B., Rubin, E., and Prockop, D. J.: Hepatic fibrosis in rats produced by carbon tetrachloride and dimethylnitrosamine. Observations suggesting immunoassays of serum for the 7S fragment of type IV collagen are a more sensitive index of liver damage than immunoassays for the NH$_2$-terminal propeptide of type III procollagen. Hepatology (in press).

11. Vogel, B. E., Doelz, R., Kadler, K. E., Hojima, Y., Engel, J., and Prockop, D. J.: A substitution of cysteine for glycine-748 of the α1 chain produces a kink at this site in the procollagen I molecule and an altered N-proteinase cleavage site over 225 nm away. J. Biol. Chem. 263:19249, 1988.

12. Kadler, K. E., Torre-Blanco, A., Adachi, E., Vogel, B. E., Hojima, Y., and Prockop, D. J.: A type I collagen with substitution of a cysteine for glycine-748 in the α1(I) chain copolymerizes with normal type I collagen and can generate fractal-like structures. Biochemistry 30:5081, 1991.

13. Kuivaniemi, H., Tromp, G., and Prockop, D. J.: Mutations in collagen genes: causes of rare and some common diseases in humans. FASEB J. 5:2052, 1991.

14. Byers, P. H.: Brittle bones–fragile molecules: Disorders of collagen gene structure and expression. Trends Genet. 6:293, 1990.

15. Barker, D. F., Hostikka, S. L., Zhou, J., Chow, L. T., Oliphant, A. R., Gerken, S. C., Gregory, M. C., Skolnick, M. H., Atkin, C. L., and Tryggvason, K.: Identification of mutations in the COL4A5 collagen gene in Alport syndrome. Science 248:1224, 1990.

16. Ryynänen, N., Knowlton, R. G., Parente, M. G., Chung, L. C., Chu, M.-L., and Uitto, J.: Human type VII collagen. Genetic linkage of the gene (COL7A1) on chromosome 3 to dominant dystrophic epidermolysis bullosa. Am J. Hum. Genet. 49:797, 1991.

17. Bachinger, H. P., Morris, N. P., Lunstrum, G. P., Keene, D. R., Rosenbaum, L. M., Compton, L. A., and Burgeson, R. E.: The relationship of the biophysical and biochemical characteristics of type VII collagen to the function of anchoring fibrils. J. Biol. Chem. 265:10095, 1990.

18. Kontusaari, S., Tromp, G., Kuivaniemi, H., Romanic, A., and Prockop, D. J.: A mutation in the gene for type III procollagen (COL3A1) in a family with aortic aneurysms. J. Clin. Invest. 86:1465, 1990.

19. Palotie, A., Vaisanen, P., Ott, J., Ryhanen, L., Ilma, K., Vikkula, M., Cheah, K., Vuorio, E., and Peltonen, L.: Predisposition to familial osteoarthrosis linked to type II collagen gene. Lancet 1:924, 1989.

20. Ala-Kokko, L., Baldwin, C. T., Moskowitz, R. W., and Prockop, D. J.: Single base mutation in the type II procollagen gene (COL2A1) as a cause of primary osteoarthritis associated with a mild chondrodysplasia. Proc. Natl. Acad. Sci. U.S.A. 87:6565, 1990.

21. Spotila, L. D., Constantinou, C. D., Sereda, L., Ganguly, A., Riggs, B. L., and Prockop, D. J.: Mutation in a gene for type I procollagen (COL1A2) in a woman with post-menopausal osteoporosis. Evidence for phenotypic and genotypic overlap with mild OI. Proc. Natl. Acad. Sci. U.S.A. 88:6624, 1991.

22. Constantinou, C. D., Pack, M., and Prockop, D. J.: A mutation in the type I procollagen gene on chromosome 17q21.31-q22.05 or 7q21.3-q22.1 that decreases the thermal stability of the protein in a woman with ankylosing spondylitis and osteopenia. Cytogenet. Cell Genet. 51:979, 1990.

23. Shapiro, J. R., Burn, V. E., Chipman, S. D., Velis, K. P., and Bansal, M.: Osteoporosis and familial idiopathic scoliosis: Association with an abnormal α2(I) collagen. Connect. Tissue Res. 21:117, 1989.

24. Urry, D. W.: Molecular prospectives of vascular wall structure and disease—elastin component. Perspect. Biol. Med. 21:265, 1978.

25. Sandberg, L. B., Soskel, N. J., and Solt, M. S.: Structure of the elastin fiber: An overview. J. Invest. Dermatol. 79:128, 1982.

26. Rucker, R. B., and Dubick, M. A.: Elastin metabolism and chemistry: Potential roles in lung development and structure. Environ. Health Perspect. 55:179, 1984.

27. Siegel, R. C.: Lysyl oxidase. Int. Rev. Connect. Tissue Res. 8:73, 1979.

28. Sakai, L. Y., Keene, D. R., Glanville, R. W., and Bachinger, H. P.: Purification and partial characterization of fibrillin, a cysteine-rich structural component of connective tissue microfibrils. J. Biol. Chem. 266:14763, 1991.

29. Rosenbloom, J., Bashir, M., Yeh, H., Rosenbloom, J., Ornstein-Goldstein, N., Fazio, M., Kahari, F.-M., and Uitto, J.: Regulation of elastin gene expression. Ann. N.Y. Acad. Sci. 624:116, 1991.

30. Indik, Z., Yeh, H., Ornstein-Goldstein, N., Sheppard, P., Anderson, N., Rosenbloom, J. C., Peltinen, L., and Rosenbloom, J.: Alternate splicing of human elastin mRNA indicated by sequence analysis of cloned genomic and complementary DNA. Proc. Natl. Acad. Sci. U.S.A. 84:5680, 1987.

31. Maslen, C. L., Corson, G. M., Maddox, B. K., Glanville, R. W., and Sakai, L. Y.: Partial sequence of a candidate gene for the Marfan syndrome. Nature 353:334, 1991.

32. Dietz, H. C., Cutting, G. R., Pyeritz, R. E., Maslen, C. L., Sakai, L. Y., Corson, G. M., Puffenberger, E. G., Hamosh, A., Nanthakumar, E. J., Curristin, S. M., Stetten, G., Meyers, D. A., and Francomano, C. A.: Marfan syndrome caused by a recurrent de novo missense mutation in the fibrillin gene. Nature 353:337, 1991.

33. Bressan, G. M., and Prockop, D. J.: Synthesis of elastic in aortas from chick embryos. Conversion of newly secreted elastin to cross-linked elastin without apparent proteolysis of the molecule. Biochemistry 16:1406, 1977.

34. Shapiro, S. D., Campbell, E. J., Welgus, H. G., and Senior, R. M.: Elastin degradation by mononuclear phagocytes. Ann. N. Y. Acad. Sci. 624:69, 1991.

35. Snider, G. L., Ciccolella, D. E., Morris, S. M., Stone, P. J., and Lucey, E. C.: Putative role of neutrophil elastase in the pathogenesis of emphysema. Ann. N.Y. Acad. Sci. 624:45, 1991.

36. Partridge, S. M., Elsden, D. F., and Thomas, J.: Biosynthesis of the desmosine and isodesmosine cross-bridges in elastin. Biochem. J. 93:30, 1964.

37. Uitto, J., Christiano, A. M., Veli-Matti, K., Bashir, M. M., and Rosenbloom, J.: Molecular biology and pathology of human elastin. Biochem. Soc. Trans. 19:824, 1991.

38. Cox, D. W.: α1-Antitrypsin deficiency. In Scriber, C. R., Beaudet, A. L., Sly, W., and Valle, D. (eds.): The Metabolic Basis of Inherited Disease. 6th ed. New York, McGraw-Hill, 1989, pp. 2409–2437.

39. Okayama, H., Brantly, M., Holmes, M., and Crystal, R. G.: Characterization of the molecular basis of the α1-antitrypsin F allele. Am. J. Hum. Genet. 48:1154, 1991.

40. Kainulainen, K., Pulkkinen, L., Savolainen, A., Kaitila, I., and Peltonen, L.: Location on chromosome 15 of the gene defect causing Marfan syndrome. N. Engl. J. Med. 323:935, 1990.

41. Lee, B., Godfrey, M., Vitale, E., Hori, H., Mattel, M.-G., Sarfarazi, M., Tsipouras, P., Ramirez, F., and Hollister, D. W.: Linkage of Marfan syndrome and a phenotypically related disorder to two different fibrillin genes. Nature 352:330, 1991.

42. Knowlton, R. G., Katzenstein, P. L., Moskowitz, R. W., Weaver, E. J., Malemud, C. J., Pathria, M. N., Jimenez, S. A., and Prockop, D. J.: Genetic linkage of a polymorphism in the type II procollagen gene (COL2A1) to primary osteoarthritis associated with mild chondrodysplasia. N. Engl. J. Med. 322:526, 1990.

Chapter 3

Robert L. Trelstad
Paul D. Kemp

Matrix Glycoproteins and Proteoglycans

INTRODUCTION

The proteins in the extracellular matrix with covalently bound carbohydrates have classically been categorized as structural components composed of glycoproteins, proteoglycans, and collagens. Integral membrane proteins with extracellular domains have not traditionally been included with matrix glycoproteins, nor have proteins that are present in the circulation. However, cell surface macromolecules, with functions as receptors, adhesion molecules, and regulators, are similar chemically to the classic matrix macromolecules such that the logical and functional boundaries between the matrix and the cell surface have blurred. Glycoproteins, proteoglycans, and glycosaminoglycans are also present inside the cell in secretory granules or as free molecules.

This presentation of matrix glycoproteins and proteoglycans considers three matrix phases: (1) a solid phase, as exemplified by tissues such as tendon, bone, cartilage, and ligament; (2) a fluid phase, exemplified by macromolecules that circulate in blood, lymph, and tissue fluids as well as inside the cell; and (3) a cell surface phase, exemplified by molecules on the cell surface that are both integral membrane components and noncovalently associated as a basement membrane or cell lamina. Readers wishing more details about these matrix constituents may consult a number of reviews.[1–14, 24, 72, 134, 136, 157, 168]

SOLID PHASE MATRIX

The solid phase connective tissue matrix is well known. It is the stuff of which the animal kingdom is constructed, and it is often the subject of clinical disorders. The components of the solid phase matrix include collagens, proteoglycans, structural glycoproteins, and elastins. The space-filling character of these materials is a major feature of their functions at a macroscopic level as a biomaterial, and at a cellular level, as an adhesive, biomaterial, filter, receptor, signal, and a message recording device, or text.

FLUID PHASE MATRIX

Many of the components of the solid phase matrix are also present in soluble forms, either within the blood or in tissue fluids. Hyaluronan, fibronectin, vitronectin, thrombospondin, cartilage matrix protein, and laminin are found intact or as fragments, in blood, lymph, synovial fluid, and bronchoalveolar lavage fluid. There is reason to believe that all matrix components, as fragments, can enter the circulation, where they serve new functions.[15–19, 21, 22, 78, 79, 197]

CELL SURFACE MATRIX

The location of matrix components at the cell's surface is effected, in part, by specific receptors in the cell membrane.[7] Once bound, these polyvalent matrix molecules can then bind other ligands and thereby extend the linkage between the surface of the cell and the pericellular space (Fig. 3–1). Typical examples of this are the integrins, which bind a number of matrix components at the cell surface. The intracellular portions of these receptors interact with cytoplasmic structures via a variety of cytoskeletal elements providing a direct linkage, physically and functionally, with the interior of the cell.[7, 168] A new finding is that matrix macromolecules are present at the cell surface as integral membrane components and can serve as receptors. Some of these molecules, such as syndecan, betaglycan, and glypican, contain glycosaminoglycan chains that are capable of interactions with other ligands, including growth factors, other matrix components, and other cell surface materials.[4, 5] Matrix macromolecules are thus primary and secondary receptors on the cell surface with linkages to intracellular structures.

CELL LAMINA (BASEMENT MEMBRANE)

At the surface of most animal cells there is a matrix that is noncovalently linked to the plasma membrane and is called the basement membrane (Figs. 3–1 and 3–2). The term *basement membrane* (BM) is well engrained, but the term *cell lamina* may be more inclusive. The BM covers nearly the entire surface of smooth, cardiac, and skeletal muscle cells, fat cells, Schwann's cells, and the basal surface of most epithelia.[11, 12, 23, 24] It is a coat or lamina on a majority of cells, filtering and protecting the surface

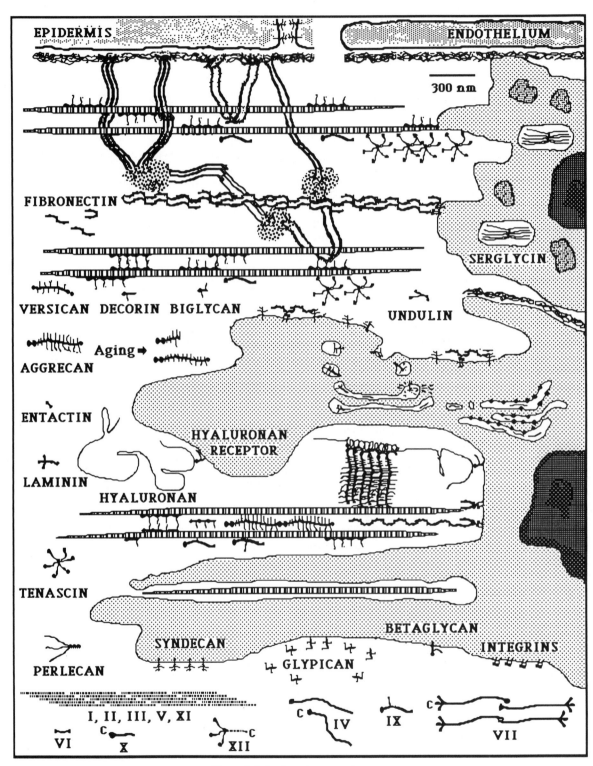

Figure 3–1 *See legend on opposite page*

Figure 3–2. The components of the cell lamina/basement membrane include type IV collagen, laminin, perlecan, sparc, entactin, and calcium ions. The capacities of various components to engage in homotypic interactions are indicated. The network formed from type IV interactions involves both lateral and end-to-end associations that are more complex than is illustrated because the individual molecules and pairs of molecules twist on each other.[11, 24] Laminin can form a gel through purely homotypic interactions,[29] and perlecan interacts by its core protein and through the three extended GAG chains to form various multimers. These three components along with entactin and sparc interact in the presence of charged species, including calcium, to form a network, illustrated at the lower left, that begins to approximate the pore and charge selective filter that covers the surface of many cells.

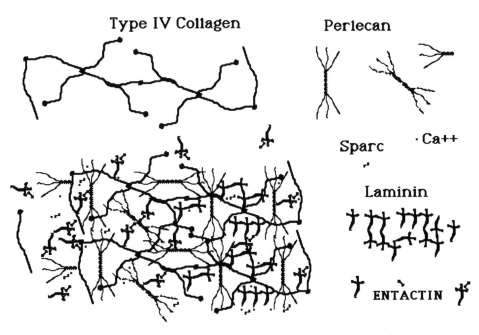

CELL LAMINA/BASEMENT MEMBRANE

of the cell, binding temporarily a variety of regulators and factors, and all the while being involved in the active exchange that represents daily nutrition, respiration, and waste disposal. The cell lamina is a heteropolymeric mixture of molecules including type IV collagen, laminin, perlecan, entactin, and sparc (see Fig. 3–2).[11, 12, 23] These relatively constant molecular constituents undergo a variety of self-assembly reactions of both a homopolymeric and a heteropolymeric nature to produce a felt-like coat. This ranges from 50 to 200 nm in thickness with linkages to the cell surface that are noncovalent and calcium dependent and are probably mediated via its constituents acting individually and/or together.[6, 7, 11, 12, 24–29] While the filtration functions of the cell lamina are well known, particularly in the glomerulus, it plays additional important binding and storage roles for materials such as osteogenin,[30] lipoprotein lipase (LPL),[31, 32] and numerous growth factors.[33, 34]

The progress in the molecular dissection of these cell coats has led to more explicit identification of potentially causal reactants. For example, a monoclonal IgM kappa (κ) from a patient with Waldenström's macroglobulinemia (IgM-Rod) has been identified that is directed against heparan sulfate and that also cross-reacts with the mitotic spindle.[35] Recently a number of patients with various types of glomerulonephritis have been shown to have antibodies to bovine entactin, suggesting this component as a non-Goodpasture glomerular BM antigen involved in the pathogenesis of certain forms of autoimmune glomerulonephritis.[36] Matzner and colleagues[37] have shown that when unstimulated neutrophils contact the BM and/or subendothelial extracellular matrix,

Figure 3–1. The extracellular matrix in a two-dimensional projection drawn to scale for both the cells and the macromolecular components in the extracellular space. At the top of the diagram is the basal portion of an epithelial *(left)* or endothelial *(right)* cell, covered along its basal surface by the basement membrane (BM). In situ these cells are not contiguous. The dense structures linked to the basal surface of the BM are aggregates of type VII collagen, the major component of anchoring fibrils. Type VII collagen forms a long (nearly 1 µm) dimer *(bottom corner right)* in which the COOH-terminals have a trident structure composed of globular domains with affinities for type IV collagen. The anchoring fibrils form "loops" attached noncovalently to the basal surface of the epithelium and entrap collagen and other fibronectin fibrils. This "velcro-like" architecture is important in the anchorage of some epithelia to the matrix. Assorted other macromolecules are shown decorating the surfaces of the collagen fibrils. The cell beneath the endothelium at the upper right is a generic white blood cell showing secretory vacuoles, including one that contains serglycin. Were this a mast cell, the granules might also include laminin and type IV collagen. The fibroblast shows a convoluted topography with a number of cell surface receptors and matrix components. Note that hyaluronan, either bound to the cell surface by a receptor or penetrating the cell during biosynthesis, could form a large pericellular coat if present at high density. A cell lamina is shown on a portion of the upper surface of the fibroblast at the right, as would be expected were this a smooth muscle cell. In the lower portion of the fibroblast, a forming collagen fibril is present in an extracellular compartment. Portions of the extracellular space are under direct control by the cell through formation of compartments surrounded by cellular processes. Matrix components are illustrated both in the extracellular matrix and bound to the cell surface. At the cell surface, matrix components are either bound by receptors or present as integral membrane components. The extended configurations of the matrix components indicate that a wide variety of interactions are geometrically possible. Most of the interactions indicated have been demonstrated.

Cell-Lamina/Basement Membrane	Linked Oligosaccharides	Linked Glycosaminoglycans	Receptor	Solid Phase Matrix	Fluid Phase Matrix	Cell Surface Matrix		GAG Chain Type	Sequence Homology Group	Core Protein Size (kD)	Size (nM) 300 nM
	■	■		■	■	■	Aggrecan	CS/KS	LP, LB, CC	320	
	■		■			■	Betaglycan				
	■	■		■			Biglycan	CS/DS	LR	40	
		■	■			■	CD44	CS*	LP	85	
	■			■	■		Cartilage Matrix Pr.		EG,IN	150	
■	■			■		■	Collagen Type IV			525	
	■			■			Collagen Type VI		IN	500	
	■	■		■			Collagen Type IX	CS		270	
	■	■	■	■	■	■	Decorin	CS/DS	LR	40	
	■		■			■	EGF Receptor		EG		
■	■			■			Entactin/Nidogen		LN,EG	120	
	■			■			Fibrillin			350	
	■	■		■			Fibromodulin	CS/DS	LR	60	
	■			■	■	■	Fibronectin		F1, F2,F3	500	
	■	■	■		■	■	Glypican	HS		65	
				■	■	■	Hyaluronan				
	■		■			■	IgG Superfamily		IG		
	■		■			■	Integrins		IN	220	
		■				■	Invariant Chain	CS*			
■	■			■	■	■	Laminins		LN, EG	840	
	■			■	■		Link		IG, LP	40	
	■			■			Osteocalcin		GC	6	
	■			■		■	Osteopontin			35	
■	■	■		■	■		Perlecan	HS	LN,EG	600	
		■			■		Serglycin	CS/DS			
■	■			■			Sparc/Osteonectin		EF	40	
	■	■	■	■	■	■	Syndecan	HS/CS		35	
				■	■		tPA/uPA		F1 EG CC		
	■			■	■		Tenascin		EG	320	
		■				■	Thrombomodulin	CS*			
	■	■			■		Thrombospondin	HS*	TS, EF,EG	450	
	■			■			Undulin			640	
	■	■		■			Versican	CS/DS	EG, LP	250	
	■				■		Vitronectin		SB	50	

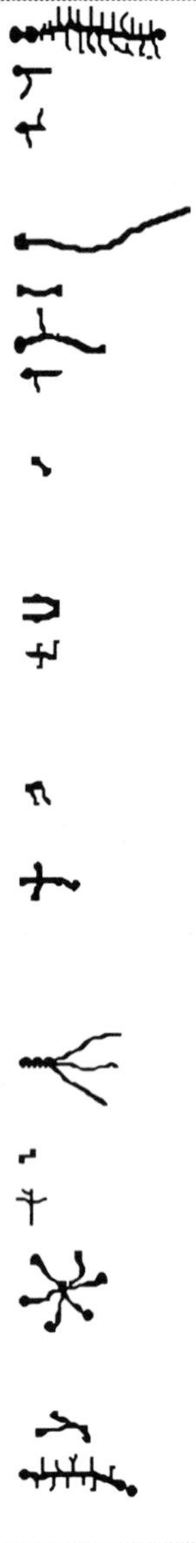

Figure 3–3 *See legend on opposite page*

they release endoglycosidases or heparanases that may play a role in the diapedesis of cells through vessels as well as in the release of bound growth factors. An interesting correlation between BMs and amyloid deposits in Alzheimer's disease has been suggested, particularly with respect to perlecan.[38, 39]

NOMENCLATURE

There is no historical consensus definition of matrix glycoproteins, and in this chapter they are proteins to which may be attached one or more of three classes of carbohydrate polymers: simple hexoses, branched oligosaccharides, and unbranched glycosaminoglycans. The hexose chains on collagen are simple monosaccharides and disaccharides linked to hydroxylysine. The oligosaccharides are branched structures, often rich in mannose and sialic acid, that undergo extensive alterations during synthesis and postsynthetic modifications. The glycosaminoglycans are unbranched, long chains that are highly sulfated and have a motif of a disaccharide repeat.[1, 2, 4, 5]

This broad definition of glycoproteins thus includes the proteoglycans, proteins in which the major carbohydrate is a glycosaminoglycan (GAG). The logic of this taxonomy, however, will not eliminate the term *proteoglycan* from common usage, and, in fact, it seems likely that as more proteins containing occasional GAG chains are discovered (e.g., type IX collagen, CD44, betaglycan),[5] the term will continue to be used. The names of the matrix glycoproteins have changed significantly during the past several years. The large aggregating proteoglycan of cartilage has become aggrecan; the small proteoglycans of the tendon, PG(I) and PG(II), have become biglycan and decorin, respectively; the low-density, high molecular weight heparan sulfate proteoglycan of BM has become perlecan. A group of cell surface proteins to which glycosaminoglycan chains are intermittently linked have been termed *part-time* proteoglycans.[5] These include the invariant chain, the transferrin receptor, thrombomodulin, and the CD44/hyaluronan receptor/lymphocyte homing receptor.

Understanding cellular, cell surface, circulating, and matrix glycoproteins and their multimolecular aggregates in current terms thus acknowledges structural and functional redundancies. The structural redundancies at the carbohydrate level are based on the presence of similar types of carbohydrate chains on different core proteins and the presence within these carbohydrate chains of disaccharide motifs.[1, 2] Redundancies at the protein level are based on sequence similarities or homologies and structural repeats in primary structure both within the same protein and between "different" proteins.[40–42] These structural redundancies in both protein and carbohydrate structure are reflected in functional redundancies such that the biologic effects of one particular glycoprotein may be mimicked, modified, or blocked by a similar sequence in another (Fig. 3–3).

CHEMICAL STRUCTURE

The chemical structures of the glycoproteins and proteoglycans are deceptively simple while yielding a multiplicity of final products. To a protein core of variable size and character, carbohydrate polymers are covalently linked at one of four amino acids: asparagine, threonine, serine, and hydroxylysine. The linkage at the asparagine residues occurs through a nitrogen atom and is termed N-linked; those linkages through threonine, serine, and hydroxylysine are through an oxygen atom and termed O-linked (Fig. 3–4).[2] The size of the protein cores of the glycoproteins and proteoglycans varies from approximately 40 kilodaltons (kD) to 600 kD and from less than 30 nM to greater than 300 nM in greatest dimension (see Fig. 3–3). The core protein of perlecan, for example, is 50 percent greater than type IV collagen in mass (600 kD vs. 400 kD) but is about one-quarter its size (100 nM vs. 400 nM) in linear dimension. Such size/mass considerations are partic-

---

Figure 3–3. This chart presents the major matrix components discussed in this chapter along with a number of other relevant extracellular and cell surface molecules to which they are related structurally and/or functionally. Each of the components is identified in respect to parameters listed in the heading on the figure. The scaled size of a number of molecules is illustrated at the right, along with the approximate mass of the core protein in kilodaltons (kD). The sequence homologies of these various components (see text) indicate considerable interrelationships. GAG Chain Types: CS, chondroitin sulfate; KS, keratan sulfate; DS, dermatan sulfate; HS, heparan sulfate. The * indicates a "part time" proteoglycan.[5] CC, Complement control protein (Clr, Cls, C2, ELAM-1, factor H, human beta-2 glycoprotein 1, human complement receptor); CN, collagen non–triple helix (cartilage matrix protein, type VI collagen, von Willebrand factor); EF, EF-hand/calcium-binding (sparc, thrombospondin); EG, epidermal growth factor (Clr, Cls, cartilage matrix protein, ELAM-1, epidermal growth factor, factor VII, factor IX, factor X, factor XII, LDL-receptor, LDL-receptors, laminin, Mel-14/ LHR, protein C, protein S, TGF alpha, tenascin, thrombospondin, tPA); F1, first found in fibronectin (factor XII, fibronectin, tPA); F2, first found in fibronectin (factor XII, fibronectin); F3, first found in fibronectin (fibronectin, N-CAM, twitchin); GC, gamma-carboxyglutamic acid (factor VII, factor IX, factor X, protein C, protein S, sparc); IG, immunoglobulin superfamily (contactin, faciclin II, immunoglobulins, L-1, link, N-CAM, PDGF receptor, twitchin); IN, integrin (alpha 1 type VI collagen, alpha 2 type VI collagen, cartilage matrix protein, complement factor B, integrins, von Willebrand factor); LB, lectin binding (ELAM-1, hepatic lectin, mannose-binding protein, Mel-14/LHR, surfactant apoprotein, tetranectin); LN, laminin (epithelial glycoprotein [HEA 125], placental protein 12, entactin, laminin, thyroglobulin precursor); LP, link protein (CD/44, gp 90 Hermes, hyaluronan receptor); LR, leucine-rich glycoprotein (biglycan, chaoptin, decorin, fibromodulin); LR, LDL-receptor and complement (LDL-receptor); PA, plasminogen activator (factor XII, tPA); SB, somatomedin B (vitronectin); TS, first found in thrombospondin (properdin, thrombospondin). (Modified from Goetinck, P., and Winterbottom, N.: Proteoglycans: Modular macromolecules of the extracellular matrix. *In* Goldsmith, L. [ed.]: Biochemistry and Physiology of the Skin. 2nd ed. New York, Oxford University Press, 1991; and Baron, M., Norman, D. G., and Campbell, I. D.: Protein modules. Trends Biochem. Sci. 16:13, 1991. Used by permission.)

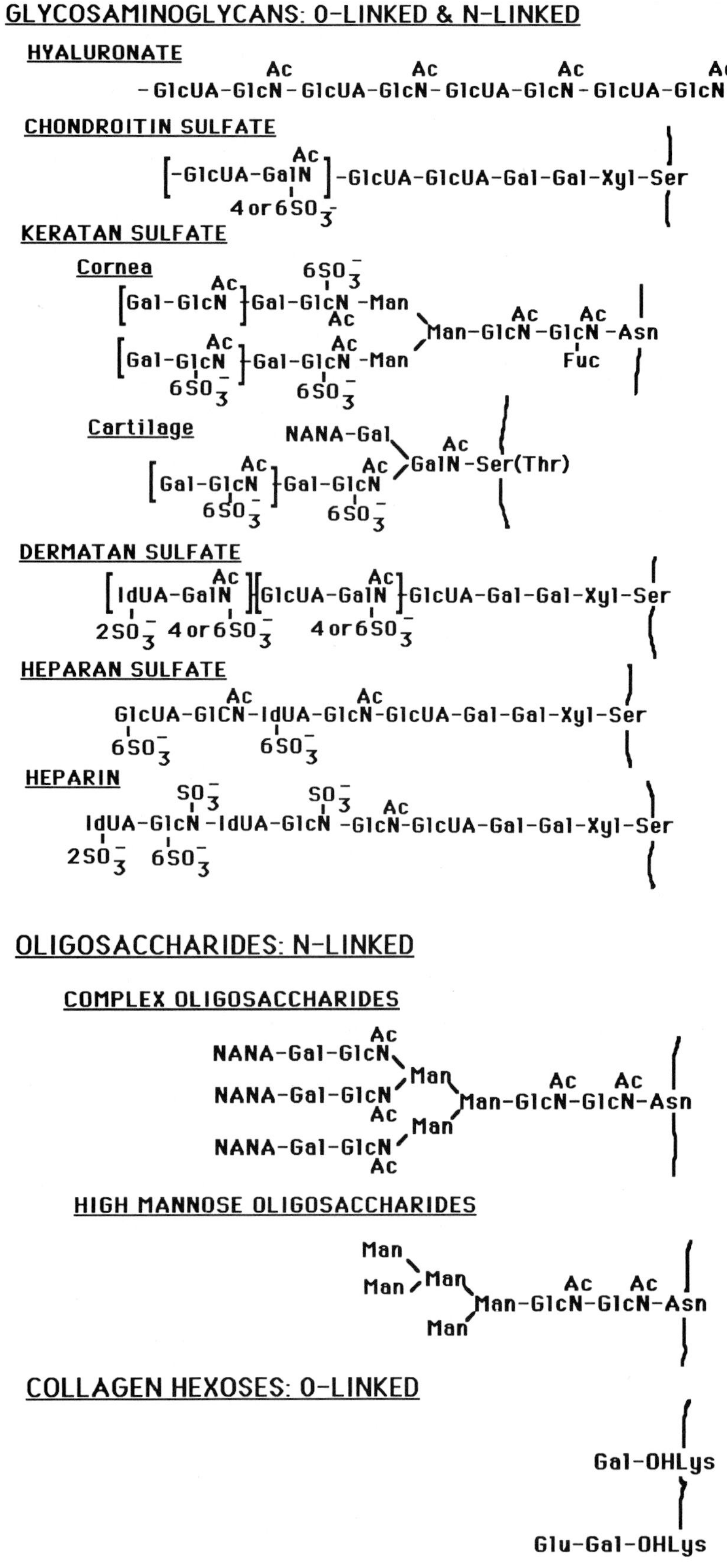

GLYCOSAMINOGLYCANS: O-LINKED & N-LINKED

HYALURONATE

$$-GlcUA\overset{Ac}{-}GlcN-GlcUA\overset{Ac}{-}GlcN-GlcUA\overset{Ac}{-}GlcN-GlcUA\overset{Ac}{-}GlcN-$$

CHONDROITIN SULFATE

$$\left[-GlcUA\overset{Ac}{\underset{4\,or\,6SO_3^-}{-GalN}}\right]-GlcUA-GlcUA-Gal-Gal-Xyl-Ser$$

KERATAN SULFATE

Cornea

$$\left[Gal\overset{Ac}{-}GlcN\right]Gal\overset{Ac}{-}GlcN\overset{6SO_3^-}{-}Man$$
$$Man\overset{Ac}{-}GlcN\overset{Ac}{-}GlcN-Asn$$
$$\left[Gal\overset{Ac}{\underset{6SO_3^-}{-}}GlcN\right]Gal\overset{Ac}{\underset{6SO_3^-}{-}}GlcN-Man$$
$$Fuc$$

Cartilage

$$NANA-Gal$$
$$\overset{Ac}{GalN}-Ser(Thr)$$
$$\left[Gal\overset{Ac}{\underset{6SO_3^-}{-}}GlcN\right]Gal\overset{Ac}{\underset{6SO_3^-}{-}}GlcN$$

DERMATAN SULFATE

$$\left[IdUA\overset{Ac}{\underset{2SO_3^-\;4\,or\,6SO_3^-}{-}}GalN\right]\left[GlcUA\overset{Ac}{\underset{4\,or\,6SO_3^-}{-}}GalN\right]GlcUA-Gal-Gal-Xyl-Ser$$

HEPARAN SULFATE

$$GlcUA\overset{Ac}{\underset{6SO_3^-}{-}}GlcN-IdUA\overset{Ac}{\underset{6SO_3^-}{-}}GlcN-GlcUA-Gal-Gal-Xyl-Ser$$

HEPARIN

$$IdUA\overset{SO_3^-}{\underset{2SO_3^-}{-}}GlcN-IdUA\overset{SO_3^-}{\underset{6SO_3^-}{-}}GlcN\overset{Ac}{-}GlcN-GlcUA-Gal-Gal-Xyl-Ser$$

Figure 3–4. Diagram indicating linkage patterns in N-linked and O-linked oligosaccharides; in O-linked hexoses in the collagens; and the O-linked and N-linked (keratan sulfate) patterns in the glycosaminoglycans. The vertical lines attached to the amino acids indicate the protein chain. IdUA, iduronic acid; GlcUA, glucuronic acid; GlcN, glucosamine; GalN, galactosamine; Gal, galactose; Glu, glucose; Man, mannose; Fuc, fucose; Xyl, xylose; Ser, serine; Thr, threonine; Asn, asparagine; OHLys, hydroxylysine; 2-SO3, O-sulfation at position 2; 6-SO3, O-sulfation at position 6; SO3, N-sulfation; Ac, N-acetylation.

OLIGOSACCHARIDES: N-LINKED

COMPLEX OLIGOSACCHARIDES

$$NANA-Gal\overset{Ac}{-}GlcN$$
$$Man$$
$$NANA-Gal\overset{Ac}{-}GlcN$$
$$Man\overset{Ac}{-}GlcN\overset{Ac}{-}GlcN-Asn$$
$$Man$$
$$NANA-Gal\overset{Ac}{-}GlcN$$

HIGH MANNOSE OLIGOSACCHARIDES

$$Man$$
$$Man\,Man$$
$$Man\overset{Ac}{-}GlcN\overset{Ac}{-}GlcN-Asn$$
$$Man$$

COLLAGEN HEXOSES: O-LINKED

$$Gal-OHLys$$

$$Glu-Gal-OHLys$$

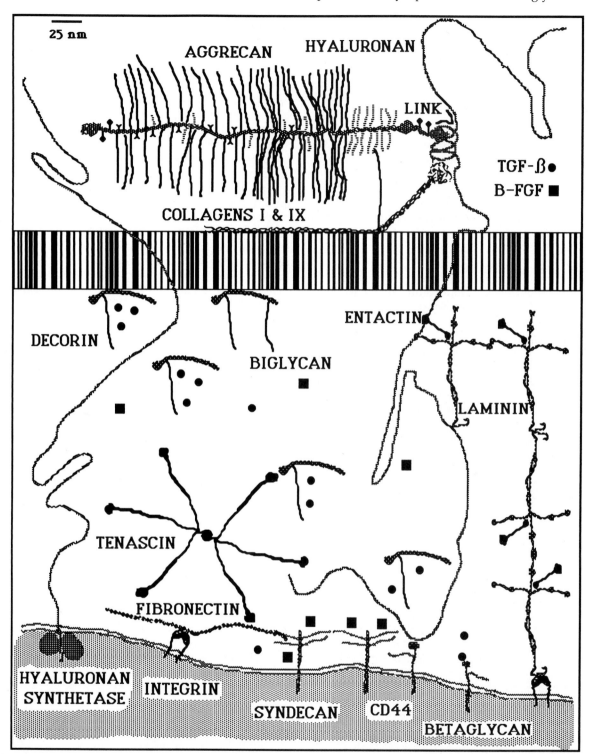

Figure 3–5. A detailed view of the cell surface and the pericellular matrix drawn to scale. The type I collagen fibril is presented in a typical view as a 67-nm striated structure. The fibril-associated components, such as decorin, biglycan, and a type IX molecule, while seemingly "plastered" onto the fibril surface are likely to be more integrated with the type I molecules at the surface than is indicated. It is known that chains from the type IX molecule covalently cross-link with those of type I.[95] Decorin and biglycan both interact with the fibril, and conceivably the bound GAG chains of these and type IX might intercalate into the type I fibril structure. Decorin and biglycan can influence fibril formation and probably postdepositional fusion.[96, 97] The immediately external surface of the cell shows a single fibronectin molecule bound to an integrin receptor; syndecan interacting with the end of the same fibronectin molecule as well as with some bFGF; hyaluronan bound to the cell via CD44 as well as anchored through the membrane during synthesis; and laminin forming an extended coat, anchored by an integrin. The large size of tenascin, possibly interacting in and with a variety of components, indicates that this large molecule might interfere in relatively nonspecific manners with this pericellular "calyx." The binding of TGF-β to both decorin and betaglycan is indicated. Given the complex relationships of TGF-β to these elements (see text), it is likely that the regulation of the matrix by agents that also bind to it and may be dependent on that binding for transport, storage, and entrance into the cell will be a multifactorial, iterative process with unexpected regulatory features.

ularly relevant when attempting to understand and present the real size and shape of multimolecular aggregates, and the reader can inspect Figures 3–1, 3–2, and 3–5 to appreciate a number of examples.

Carbohydrate Structures

The character of the carbohydrate chain is dictated by the intrinsic properties of the individual sugars, the specific sites and stereochemistry of the linkages between adjacent sugars, the order in which they are added and/or removed during biosynthesis, and postsynthetic modifications that include epimerization and sulfation.

Epimerization and Sulfation

The structures of chondroitin sulfate (CS) and dermatan sulfate (DS) glycosaminoglycan chains are similar because of the *epimerization* of glucuronic acid in CS to iduronic acid in DS, a conversion that occurs after the oligosaccharide is synthesized and that is dependent, in part, on the degree of sulfation of the substrate. The biologic and possible pharmacologic importance of the epimerizations that occur in the iduronic acid–to–glucuronic acid shift should not be underestimated. A variety of "nutritional deficiencies" from sulfate to vitamin A and agents such as chlorate, an inhibitor of sulfate adenylyltransferase, cause a decreased epimerization of D-glucuronic to L-iduronic acid.[43-45] This decreased epimerization leads to an increase in the CS character of the GAG with a concomitant decrease in its DS character; in patients with aspartylglycosaminuria, this phenotype of "epimerization block" is associated with abnormal skin collagen fibril formation,[46] and in human colonic tumors the increase of chondroitin sulfate chains relative to dermatan sulfate occurs through an effect of the malignant epithelial cells on the biosynthetic activities of the underlying smooth muscle.[47, 48]

Sulfation, in general, appears to provide a form of stored energy for enthalpic interactions with other macromolecules, with the potential for leading to what are known as dissipative structures.[49] Dissipative structures are structures that require energy for their nonequilibrium state and that usually have unique morphologies.[50] Of interest in this regard is that the synergistic effects of heparin on acidic fibroblast growth factor are dependent on both the size and the degree of sulfation of the heparin,[51] and the modulation of laminin polymerization is significantly influenced by heparin in a sulfation-dependent manner.[29]

Protein Structures

Post-translation modification of matrix proteins includes glycosylation to form the various N- or O-linked oligosaccharides or glycosaminoglycans, acy-lation by the long-chained fatty acids myristate and palmitate,[52] and tyrosine-O-sulfation.[53]

The primary structures of many of the structural glycoproteins and core proteins of the proteoglycans have been elucidated in the past several years, primarily by gene sequencing. Structural themes of protein structure include the presence of *consensus sequences* (short stretches of amino acids that have specific functions) and *modules* or *domains* or *sequence homologies,* in which relatively long stretches (40 to 100 amino acids) have a common domain structure.

Consensus sequences are usually less than 20 amino acids and are sites of interactions with other macromolecules. One of the best examples is that originally described in fibronectin, the RGD (Arg-Gly-Asp) sequence, which is one of the binding sequences for the integrin receptors.[54] A large number of matrix-related and non–matrix-related proteins contain this sequence. Another matrix consensus sequence is the XBBSBX or XBBBXXBX, in which B is a basic amino acid and X is any other. This sequence has a relatively high affinity for GAG chains and has been found in fibronectin, vitronectin, thrombospondin, LPL, basic fibroblast growth factor (bFGF), and acidic FGF (aFGF).[55] A third example of a consensus sequence is the linkage sites of glycosaminoglycan chains, which are usually either Ser-Gly-X-Gly (SGXG) or (Glu/Asp)-Gly-Ser-Gly-(Glu/Asp) (E/DGSGE/D)[2, 5]; and a fourth consensus sequence is the linkage sites for N-linked oligosaccharides of Asn-X-Ser/Thr (DXS/T), where X cannot be Asp or Pro.[2, 5]

Modular Protein Substructure

The sequencing of a large number of proteins has revealed that they are composed, in part, of modular units. The modular unit is based on sequence similarities or homologies among polypeptide stretches of 45 to 90 amino acids, and the modules frequently contain intramodule disulfide cross-links. Modules presumably arise within one protein by exon duplication and among unrelated proteins by exons that have shuffled from one gene to another.[41, 42] Matrix proteins have an extensive modular character. Through these modules, the structure and possible function of one macromolecule may be duplicated by another region of the same molecule or by an apparently unrelated macromolecule, as, for example, the epidermal growth factor (EGF) domains in laminin that can stimulate cells with EGF receptors.[59] The examples of shared modules are now extensive, and the examples diagrammed in Figure 3–3 emphasize the involvement and extent of such "cross-modularity" in matrix proteins. The purpose in presenting such a list in this context is to suggest that new kinds of cross-reactivities are to be expected among heretofore seemingly unrelated macromolecules, and their understanding will possibly address puzzling biologic and clinical phenomena such as cross-reactivity of immune reactions.

MATRIX FUNCTIONS

The matrix fills a variety of functions covered under the general categories of adhesives, biomaterials, filters, receptors, signals, and texts. The matrix acts as an adhesive, binding cells to cells and cells to the matrix; as a biomaterial, providing the major structural determinants of human form from the cellular to organ levels; as a filter, both in the glomerulus and at the cell level as a cell lamina or cell surface coat; as a receptor for small ligands with signaling potential, such as growth factors, and large ligands, such as other matrix components; as a signal itself, both in macromolecular form and as small molecular weight derivatives; and as a text, a substratum on which is recorded a history of prior activities, a history written by oxidations, reductions, glycosylations, epimerizations, sulfations, phosphorylations, other adductions and cross-linkages.

Adhesives

In and of themselves, matrix components are adhesives that bind to each other in both native and denatured forms, in homotypic and heterotypic combinations. It is the receptor-matrix functions that are new to the adhesive considerations of the matrix. The major groups of adhesive molecules identified during the past ten years include the calcium-independent cell adhesion molecules, or CAMs; calcium-dependent cadherins; selectins; desmosomes; and a variety of receptors on lymphocytes, some belonging to the immunoglobulin superfamily, others not.[3, 7, 134] Many are reviewed in Chapter 12. A major class of cell-matrix receptors is the integrins.[7, 168] The overlaps among these various sets of receptors at both structural and functional levels exist, and it is now apparent that matrix-matrix and cell-matrix adhesive interactions are not part of separate classes but, through the integrins, possibly one of the primary mechanisms of biologic adhesion.

Biomaterials

The biomechanical aspects of the matrix are well understood at macroscopic levels of bones, joints, tendons, skin, and other organs and at cellular levels, where the matrix serves similar functions as well as being a substrate for cell attachment and locomotion. The matrix components can be reassembled in a theoretically limitless number of combinations, in differing sizes and shapes, to form implantable devices or substrates for cells at sites of injury. It is reasonable to predict that biomaterials, composed of the components described in this and other chapters, will be available for clinical use in a significant manner before the turn of the century.

Filters

All nutrients, gases, regulators, hormones, factors, and cell processes must penetrate or pass through the extracellular matrix in moving from one tissue or compartment to another. Matrix components bind, select, inhibit, facilitate, release, and probably irreversibly remove components with which they come in contact. Accordingly, when attention is directed to intercellular exchanges of information, from neural transmission to secreted factors, the role of the matrix must be considered. Moreover, it should be expected that the matrix at one site in one tissue is not the same as the matrix in a seemingly comparable tissue elsewhere.[5]

Receptors

The usual connotation of a receptor is that of a nondiffusible substance that engages in specific binding with either a diffusible or nondiffusible ligand and transduces a signal to the intracellular environment. Solid phase matrix glycoproteins and proteoglycans are not receptors of this type, but they have a binding, storage, and protective function for growth factors and other regulatory factors. The release of such ligands bound to the matrix may occur through matrix degradation (e.g., a heparanase rendering the ligand free), through competitive interactions with other ligands, or through some change in the ligand itself.[202] This storage-receptor activity in the matrix shows considerable specificity and is likely to be a major matrix role. At the same time that the solid phase matrix is a storage-receptor, matrix elements in the cell surface phase are typical signal-transducing receptors. There are now a number of full-time or part-time proteoglycans that are integral membrane elements, such as syndecan, betaglycan, transferrin receptor, and invariant chain; or lipid-anchored proteoglycans, such as glypican; or intercalated glycosaminoglycans, such as hyaluronan. Each acts as a receptor using transduction mechanisms that must be clarified.

Signals

The roles of the matrix in signaling and mediating cell-cell interactions were apparent in early studies of developing embryos and in cell culture studies in which collagen was shown to support and promote differentiation in vitro. Later studies on hyaluronic acid and fibronectin opened a new view of the broad biologic effects of matrix components as signals.[9, 57] The signaling functions of matrix macromolecules are dependent on information encoded within the linear sequences of their amino acids or carbohydrates. Such information may be detected by cells when the molecules are in a complex macroaggregate, and as small polypeptides or oligosaccharides released from the parent molecule by hydrolysis. Examples of the phenomena include the solid phase signals operative during cell migration during development[66] and the oxygen-mediated bactericidal efforts of neutrophils when adherent to the matrix.[63] Laminin, for example, either intact or in fragments containing the inner segments of the short arms, segments with EGF-like modules, can stimulate cells bearing EGF receptors to proliferate.[59] The RGDS (Arg-Gly-Asp-Ser) peptide in solid phase in intact fibronectin or released from fibronectin can effectively inhibit cell binding to a number of serum and matrix components.[54] Short sequences of carbohydrates or oligosaccharides have similar regulatory effects. The replication of smooth muscle cells is significantly inhibited by oligosaccharides derived from heparin, and this effect is dependent on both the size and the charge of the oligosaccharide.[60] The mechanism of the heparin inhibition of smooth muscle cell proliferation is effected by inhibition of a protein kinase C–dependent pathway.[61, 204] The matrix also has "positional information" sufficient to influence the homing and orientation of cells, as shown by the effects of matrix on neural crest cell migration[66] or the polarizing influence of the COOH-terminal of the A chain of laminin on nephrogenic mesenchyme.[67]

Texts

Finally, the matrix is a text, a record of events that transpire around a cell and within a tissue. It is a repository of information and a historical document, recording local events from the time of synthesis inside the cell to events much later in the extracellular spaces in which other events such as cell migrations, homing, inflammation, and cross-linking are occurring. These postdepositional events involve deliberate and/or accidental glycosylation,[64] cross-linking,[122] oxidation,[65] phosphorylation,[159] and epimerization,[47] to name but a few.

BIOSYNTHESIS AND CELLULAR PROCESSING

Solid Phase Matrix

The biosynthesis of the glycoproteins and proteoglycans that predominantly remain as solid phase matrix elements involves a stepwise progression through a series of intracellular and extracellular compartments. The intracellular sequence begins in the cisterns of the endoplasmic reticulum, where the protein is synthesized, following which oligosaccharides are covalently N-linked via a dolichol intermediate. The dolichol serves as the site of synthesis of the oligosaccharides and then transfers the oligosaccharides to asparagine residues. The formation of O-linked oligosaccharides to threonine, serine, and hydroxylysine residues occurs by the sequential addition of individual uridine nucleotide sugar precursors and the actions of glycosyltransferases at a consensus site.[68, 69]

Both the termination and the processing of the carbohydrate polymers are continued in the Golgi apparatus, where a series of deletions and additions are made to both the oligosaccharides and the glycosaminoglycans. These modifications include the removal of glucose by glucosidases; the addition of sialic acid; the epimerization of glucuronic acid to iduronic acid; and the sulfation of certain sugars.[1, 2]

The biosynthesis of hyaluronan is unique in that it does not follow the pathways previously described but rather is synthesized by an enzyme complex that is in the cytoplasm and that links the disaccharides together into an extended polymer that penetrates the plasma membrane and directly enters the extracellular space. In this configuration, the hyaluronan is anchored into the membrane, and its mass and length of extension into the pericellular space are determined by the rate and extent of activity of the hyaluronan synthetase complex.[9]

Fluid Phase Matrix

The biosynthesis of matrix elements destined to become part of the fluid phase matrix follows much the same pattern as that previously described for solid phase matrix elements. There are differences, however, that render one product relatively insoluble or destined for polymerization and others more soluble and less polymerized. One mechanism by which this is effected is to produce isoforms of the molecule with unique attributes through alternative RNA splicing during the production of mRNA from the primary gene transcript.[70, 71] In the production of plasma fibronectin mRNA, the exon encoding for one type III repeat is spliced out, producing a smaller mRNA from that used for cell-associated fibronectin. There are three exons encoding for fibronectin that are candidates for alternative splicing, making it possible to construct more than 20 different proteins from one gene.[71] The fluid phase matrix elements that are produced by circulating cells are probably stored in intracellular compartments for a significantly longer period of time than are those destined to become solid phase components, as for example, the laminin B1 and B2 chains and type IV collagen that are produced by mast cells.[19]

Cell Surface Phase Matrix

The synthesis of the cell-associated matrix elements follows the general theme for solid phase matrix previously outlined, with several exceptions. The intracellular processing of those components that will become integral membrane components is different from that of excreted products in that membrane intercalation is a major step in the process.[135] Accordingly, the intracellular processing of syndecan and perlecan, for example, will follow different pathways, the former becoming membrane intercalated, the latter not.[77] Glypican is one of the new matrix receptors that are anchored to the membrane by a phospholipid linkage, a process that involves unique biosynthetic steps and another biosynthetic pathway relevant to matrix proteins.[72, 73] Receptors for the matrix can also be stored in secretory vacuoles for various periods of time before exposure on the surface. Singer and colleagues[74] have recently shown that a number of matrix receptors are present in the specific granules of human leukocytes, including receptors for laminin, fibronectin, vitronectin, fibrinogen, and endotoxin.

MATRIX RELATED REGULATORS

The regulatory factors that impact on matrix synthesis, degradation, and function are many and include growth factors, cytokines, hormones, vitamins, and autocrine and paracrine factors.[199, 200] The logic of matrix regulation may be somewhat different from that for other proteins in that the matrix is more distant from the genetic and biosynthetic machinery inside the cell. Nonetheless, the matrix is directly and indirectly involved in feedback on its production, polymerization, and/or degradation. Matrix binding of growth factors and the integration of that binding into local and distant cellular physiology promise to provide a new area of biologic regulation. At present, the best examples of this phenomenon are the interplay between growth factors and proteoglycans, as exemplified by transforming growth factor-β (TGF-β) binding to decorin,[4, 99] or bFGF and syndecan,[76, 177] or aFGF and the subendothelial matrix.[203]

Generically, the binding of regulatory factors to the matrix has a number of consequences: (1) the agonist/inhibitor is restricted by such binding and is unable to interact with its specific receptor[4, 99]; (2) the agonist/inhibitor is protected by binding from degradation[201]; and (3) the diffusion of the agonist/inhibitor through the matrix is altered by the binding.[80] These and other possible relationships are illustrated in Figure 3–5, which shows the surface of the cell and the pericellular environment.

MATRIX COMPONENTS

The following are the various macromolecules related to the multiple phases of the matrix about which there is now extensive structural and emerging functional information. The macromolecules are presented in alphabetical order. To have done otherwise would have been to impose old, less useful, or new less understood, organizational schemes. Following the name of the proteoglycans, the chemical classes of the GAG chains are listed as CS, chondroitin sulfate; DS, dermatan sulfate; HS, heparan sulfate; and KS, keratan sulfate.

Aggrecan CS/KS

The major proteoglycan from a variety of cartilages was one of the first to be studied in detail and was most recently known as the "large aggregating cartilage proteoglycan." The molecular structure of aggrecan consists of a long core protein (350 nm) with three distinct globular domains: two near the NH$_2$ terminal and one at the COOH terminal (see Fig. 3–1). The amino terminal globular domain shows sequence similarity to link, and the carboxy terminal globule to lectin binding proteins. The amino terminal globule binds to hyaluronan and forms a macroaggregate that contributes to the three-dimensional organization of most cartilages. The GAG chains as well as the core protein undergo shortening in the tissues long after synthesis and deposition, possibly accounting for some of the changes that occur in cartilages with age (see Fig. 3–1).[1, 2]

Betaglycan

Betaglycan is an integral membrane protein as well as soluble matrix element that is in its membrane phase the type III receptor for TGF-β. Betaglycan is one of the part-time proteoglycans in that it does not always contain a GAG chain.[75]

Biglycan CS/DS

Biglycan, decorin, and fibromodulin are members of a proteoglycan family from cartilage, tendon, skin, cornea, and sclera as well as from organs such as the kidney and several tumors. Biglycan was previously known as PG(I), decorin as PG(II). The GAG chains are of the chondroitin-dermatan sulfate class. Sequence studies show significant homologies among the core proteins of these three molecules, and it is probable that other molecules of this group will be identified.[81–84] These relatively small proteoglycans are involved in widely different kinds of regulatory phenomena and exemplify the dynamic role that matrix components play in the regulation of cellular physiology and tissue architecture, presumably simultaneously.[85, 86]

CD44 CS

CD44 is a lymphocyte-homing receptor that has been shown to interact with hyaluronan and to be the hyaluronan receptor. The interactions of the CD44-hyaluronan receptor with hyaluronan are inhibited by low concentrations of hyaluronan and high concentrations of chondroitin sulfate, suggesting that the receptor ligand interaction may mimic the interactions of aggrecan, link, and hyaluronan in the matrix.[87] This suggestion is supported by the identification of sequence homologies among the hyaluronan-binding domains in aggrecan and versican with the protein core of the hyaluronan receptor. The hyaluronan receptor on lymphocytes is responsible for their homing to high-endothelium during the process of physiologic and pathologic extravasation (see Chapter 51). Miyake and colleagues[58] have recently shown that hyaluronan recognition accounts for the adhesion between B lineage hybridoma cells and stromal cells in long-term marrow cultures in a calcium-independent manner.

Cartilage Matrix Protein

Cartilage matrix protein is a 148-kD protein that is present in nonarticular cartilages. The functions of this protein are not well understood, but it is released into the serum in some, but not all rheumatoid conditions.[88] The gene for the protein contains eight exons and seven introns, is located on chromosome 1p35, and codes for a protein of approximately 50 kD with potential N-glycosylation sites.[89] The protein has a modular organization with one epidermal growth factor–like domain and two domains that have homologies with the type A repeats of von Willebrand factor, complement factors B and C2, alpha-chains (α-chains) of the integrins Mac-1, p150,95, and LFA-1,[89, 90, 94] and a globular domain on type VI collagen.[91] In the chick limb during development, the expressions of the genes for cartilage matrix protein, type II collagen, link protein, and aggrecan all are independent.[92]

Collagens CS

The collagens are discussed in Chapter 2, but the chemical overlaps of some of the collagens with the structural glycoproteins and proteoglycans deserve mention here. As noted earlier, the collagens, structural glycoproteins, and proteoglycans all may contain any of the three major classes of carbohydrate additions, hydroxylysine-linked neutral hexoses, N-linked high mannose or branched oligosaccharides, and O-linked glycosaminoglycans; the $\alpha 3$ type IX chain contains all three.[93]

Type IX collagen is the only collagen known at present that contains a GAG chain, but many of the others contain various N-linked carbohydrates. The non–triple helical domains of several of the collagens contain modules found in other noncollagenous matrix proteins, as for example, an EGF-like module in type VI collagen, cartilage matrix protein, and a leukocyte integrin α-subunit[94], and a module in a propeptide of type II collagen with one in thrombospondin and von Willebrand factor.[91]

Decorin CS/DS

Decorin has a 45-kD protein core to which is attached a single CS/DS GAG chain.[81–83] Significant sequence similarities occur with the core proteins of biglycan and fibromodulin. Decorin binds to type I collagen fibrils with relatively high affinity via the core protein, not the GAG chain,[95, 96] and affects the assembly process and mechanical properties of collagen fibrils.[85] When decorin is present during collagen fibril assembly, fibrils of smaller diameter are formed; such fibrils will have less biomechanical strength, since tensile properties of woven polymers such as collagen are dependent, in part, on the fibril diameter.[96–98] While the solid-phase functions of decorin as a structural element are important, its newly described binding of TGF-β in a regulatory manner is likely to be of equal or greater importance.[4, 13, 99] The TGF-β binding by decorin presumably involves decorin in both its solid phase and its fluid phase. This effect is coupled with the binding of decorin to TGF-β and to the stimulatory effects of TGF-β on decorin synthesis by the cells, in an autoregulatory process[4, 13, 99] (see Fig. 3–5).

The recent descriptions of decorin gene deficiencies in humans[100] with a Marfan syndrome–like phenotype suggest that further explorations of the roles of decorin will provide new avenues for clinical studies and therapies. The gene for decorin has been cloned, and it is probable that studies by site-directed mutagenesis and homologous recombination will lead to a rapid increase in our understanding of its various structures and physiologies.[101] Decorin is located on human chromosome 12 (12q).[84]

Entactin

Entactin, also known as nidogen, is a major constituent of the cell lamina and is a dumbbell-shaped molecule with three domains, a NH$_2$-terminal globular domain linked by a relatively rigid rod to a COOH-terminal globular domain. The rod-like domain consists of EGF modules and a thyroglobulin module and has an overall size of about 150 kD.[6, 102] Entactin also shows homologies with a newly described intestinal epithelial glycoprotein.[103] Entactin is a structural element binding laminin to type IV collagen. The COOH-terminal domain of entactin has a high affinity for laminin near the intersection of the laminin arms, and the NH$_2$-terminal domain a high affinity for calcium. Of potential clinical interest is that the human entactin gene is a single copy with multiple restriction fragment length polymorphisms (RFLPs) that may be of use in evaluating various clinical phenotypes.[104] Recently Saxena and colleagues[36] have proposed that entactin is a BM antigen potentially involved in the pathogenesis of autoimmune glomerulonephritis (non-Goodpasture anti-GBM glomerulonephritis) and that the immunoglobulin deposition in these circumstances is granular, rather than linear, despite the likelihood that the immunogen is a structural component of the BM.

Fibrillin

Fibrillin is a structural glycoprotein of about 350 kD, initially identified in association with the amorphous core of elastin, but found also as isolated bundles of microfibrils 10 nm in diameter in skin, bronchioles, glomeruli, blood vessels, cartilage, tendon, corneal stroma, Descemet's membrane, muscle perimysium, muscle endomysium, suspensory ligament of the lens, bone, placenta, heart, and aorta.[105, 106] In the heart, fibrillin is distributed at the interface of the cardiac muscle cell surface and matrix, transferring tension from the contracting myocardial cells to the cardiac matrix.[107] At the dermal-epidermal junction, fibrillin penetrates into the lamina densa of the BM. In bone, fibrillin is found in conjunction with type III collagen, and at the bone-periosteum interface it is associated with linking the mineralized bone cortex to ligaments and tendons.[108] In a recent study of patients with Marfan's syndrome, 24 of 27 were shown to have a decreased content of fibrillin in skin fibroblast cultures and/or in their skin directly.[109] In an unusual case of a patient with phenotypic manifestations of Marfan's syndrome unilaterally, the affected side showed alterations of fibrillin, but not type III collagen, whereas the normal side did not.[110]

Fibromodulin CS/DS

Fibromodulin is a 59-kD protein isolated from a number of connective tissues that has homologous structures to those found in decorin and biglycan. Fibromodulin is functionally similar to decorin in that it binds to collagen types I and II during fibrillogenesis. The fibromodulin isolated from cartilage contains at least one keratan sulfate chain, suggesting that this group of molecules might show structural heterogeneities from tissue to tissue based on their GAG adducts.[111]

Fibronectin

Fibronectin is an adhesive, a solid phase element, a cell surface matrix protein, and a fluid phase element in the blood serving as an opsonin and chemoattractant. It is a polyvalent molecule with affinities for fibrin, collagen, heparin, the cell surface, components in bacterial cell coats, and itself. The forms of fibronectin include one in serum, synthesized by the liver, and a cell-associated form that aggregates near the cell surface and in the extracellular matrix. Fibronectin is produced early in embryogenesis and plays an important role in guiding migratory cells during early morphogenesis.[66] In wound healing, fibronectin, as an intact molecule and as peptide fragments, is chemotactic.[17] It also forms a substrate to which the cells involved in the repair reaction can adhere. Elevated levels of fibro-

nectin in the joint fluid of patients with arthritis have been reported, although a good correlation between these levels and indices of inflammatory activity has not been found.[112]

The polyfunctional binding of fibronectin is accomplished by the presence of unique domains along the axis of the two approximately 200-kD polypeptide chains. There are three types of such repeating sequences in fibronectin, types I, II, and III (listed as F1, F2, and F3 in Figure 3–3), and more than 30 of these three repeats are arranged along one fibronectin chain. The absence of a single type III repeat near the carboxy terminal determines the differences between the serum- and cell-associated forms of fibronectin. The repeating domains are grouped into larger functional domains that have binding affinities for heparin, fibrin, collagen, and cell surfaces. The binding of fibronectin to the cell is mediated by the sequence Arg-Gly-Asp (RGD). This sequence was first discovered in fibronectin and has now been found in a relatively large number of proteins (see Fig. 3–3).[7]

The production of the plasma form of fibronectin, with the missing type III repeat, involves alternative RNA splicing during the production of mRNA from the primary gene transcript. In the production of plasma fibronectin mRNA, the exon encoding for one type III repeat is spliced out, producing a mRNA smaller than that used for cell-associated fibronectin. Indeed, there are three exons in fibronectin that are candidates for alternative splicing, making it possible to construct more than 20 different proteins from one gene.[40, 70, 71] The stimulation of collagen synthesis by TGF-β can be abrogated by simultaneous treatment with gamma-interferon (γ-IFN).[114] Interestingly, this combined treatment does not similarly reduce fibronectin production, but rather increases it. Accordingly, cells exposed to both agents are stimulated to make fibronectin, but not type I collagen, whereas those exposed only to TGF-β make both.

The multiplicities of interactions possible because of the domain structure of monomers and/or multimers of the matrix components are well illustrated with the apparently contradictory effects fibronectin and its proteolytic fragments have on cell migration and anchorage. For example, fibroblasts interact with the integrin-binding domain and both heparin-binding domains of plasma fibronectin, and this combination of interactions determines whether a cell adheres to the matrix or migrates upon it.[113] Perris and coworkers[66] have demonstrated a clear relationship between the migration of neural crest cells and the underlying matrix and have shown that both fibronectin and laminin have complex influences on this process. The multiplicities of effects obtained with heparin-fibronectin combinations is likely to reflect not only the surface characteristics of such multimers but also their capacities to engage in complex matrix reactions such as "matrix-driven translocations."[115]

Marks and colleagues[116] have recently demonstrated that the attachment and migration of human neutrophils is quite sensitive to the presence of vitronectin or fibronectin as both a solid phase substrate and a soluble phase component and that there is a complex interaction of these two phases of the matrix with the surrounding calcium concentration to influence the behavior of the PMN in either a stimulatory or inhibitory manner. The autoregulatory role of the matrix is also likely to operate in this situation, since it has been shown by Kreis and coworkers[117] that both fibronectin and thrombospondin are synthesized by PMNs in inflamed human joints. It seems likely that most circulating cells will synthesize matrix components either for export or for storage-related functions (see serglycin), and also for interactions with the matrix in chemotactic and stimulatory manners.[118]

In a study of the fluid and solid phase fibronectins in human fibroblast cultures, Peters and colleagues[119] have shown that both components can be co-localized at the cell surface, but not in an entirely random manner. Assembly reactions at the cell surface are essential to linking the matrix with the contractile machinery of the cell, and their importance is readily seen in experimental wound healing studies in which contraction of the wound is dependent on fibronectin–receptor-actin linkages.[97, 120, 121] The macromolecular aggregates that constitute fibronectin fibrils are heteropolymeric with respect to the type of fibronectin and also with respect to the presence of other secondarily covalently linked components, including proteoglycans.[122]

In the fluid phase, fibronectin has long been known to act as an opsonin, binding to various surface components of microorganisms and also to collagen and other protein-derived polypeptides.[123] Cederholm and associates[124] have demonstrated that patients with primary IgA nephropathy have circulating complexes of fibronectin and IgA that bind to tissues, mediated with respect to collagen binding through the fibronectin component. Measurements of fluid phase fibronectin and other matrix components are now regularly reported in bronchoalveolar lavage,[79] joint fluids,[78] and wound fluids.[112]

Werb and colleagues[125] have shown that the fibronectin receptor not only is responsible for binding solid and fluid phase fibronectin but also by that process is a signal to the cell to induce collagenase and stromelysin gene expression. This transduction does not involve changes in the cell shape as occurs with other inducers of these matrix degrading enzymes, inducers such as phorbol esters and growth factors.[126] Other examples of the role of integrins in the transduction of signals, involving fibronectin and/or its derivatives, as ligands include the activation of human CD4 T lymphocytes.[127]

Free GAG

The idea of "free GAG," that is, glycosaminoglycan chains not attached to a protein core, has only recently been given attention. Studies from several laboratories have shown that free sulfated GAG can be found in tissues, on the cell surface, and inside the cell.[129–131] In some circumstances it would appear that the synthesis of free GAGs does not involve degradation of proteoglycans, as in the case of human keratinocytes,[130] whereas in other circumstances such as those found with human T lymphocytes, it may.[132] In keratinocytes the majority of the cell-associated GAG synthesis is in a free form, whereas that in the matrix is linked to protein. That portion associated with the cell is not accessible to degradative enzymes, indicating a protected environment on the cell surface, in vacuoles, or in the cytoplasm.[130] In fibroblast cultures, in contrast, the cell surface–associated free chains are susceptible to enzymatic attack.[129] In hepatocytes, the free heparan sulfate chains found in the cell nucleus or associated with the nuclear membrane are 10 percent of the total GAG produced by the cells, and their chemistry is distinctly different from that of the GAG chains associated with a protein core.[128]

Glypican HS

Glypican is a new cell surface heparan sulfate proteoglycan, with a core protein of approximately 64 kD, linked to the cell surface by a glycosyl-phosphatidylinositol linkage. The core protein has both N-linked carbohydrate and four potential sites for O-linked heparan sulfate. The anchorage of the core protein to the cell surface via a phosphoinositol linkage renders it susceptible to cleavage by phospholipases, and glypican is readily shed from the cell surface.[73, 133] In adult rat sciatic nerve, glypican may play a role in binding the Schwann's cell plasma membrane to the adjacent BM.[73]

Hyaluronan

Hyaluronan was the first glycosaminoglycan recognized that is not covalently bound to protein and is the only GAG that is not sulfated. It consists of a repeating disaccharide of glucuronic acid and N-acetylglucosamine.[1, 2] It is involved in biologic situations as varied as embryonic development, wound healing, and tumor invasion, and it is an important constituent of many tissues ranging from the eye to the joint space. Because of its extended conformation, it is highly hydrated and is usually associated with edematous, loosely organized matrices.[57]

Hyaluronan is simultaneously a solid phase matrix element in association with aggrecan and link proteins forming the compressible structure of cartilage; a fluid phase matrix element, circulating in the plasma and flowing in the synovial space under normal and abnormal conditions; and one of the most important of the interface matrix elements,

Figure 3–6. The integrins are dimeric cell surface receptors composed of two noncovalently linked subunits. The alpha (α) and beta (β) classes of subunits and their various names are listed. The abbreviations used by some of the subunits include LFA (leukocyte function antigen), VLA (very late activation antigen), CD (cluster designation), and GP (platelet glycoprotein). The binding ligands for each of the α-β combinations are indicated using the following abbreviations: FN (fibronectin, solid phase), LN (laminin), FN (alt) (fibronectin, fluid phase), VN (vitronectin), VW (von Willebrand factor), TS (thrombospondin), CN (collagen), and FB (fibrinogen). The dependence of the interactions on the RGD sequence is indicated.

β Subunits	α Subunits	Ligands	RGD
β1 Chicken integrin band 3	α1 = VLA-1 (CD49a)	LN (CN)	−
Fibronectin receptor β	α2 = VLA-2 (CD49b)	CN (LN)	−
VLA – β	α3 = VLA-3 (CD49c)	FN LN CN	−
CD29	α4 = VLA-4 (CD49d)	FN (alt)	−
Platelet GP IIa			−
	α5 = VLA-5 (CD49e)	FN	+
	α6 = VLA-6 (CD49f)	LN	−
	αv = CD51	FN	+
β2	αL = LFA-1 (CD11a)	I-CAM	−
LFA-1	αM = MAC-1 (CD11b)	C3bi FB	+
Mac-1/p150.95			
β3 CD18	αIIb = GP IIb (CD41)	FN FB VN VW	+
	αv = CD51	VN FB VW TS	
Platelet GP IIIA			
Vitronectin receptor β			
β4 CD61	α6 = CD49f	?LN	?
β5	αv = CD51	VN FN	+

present on the cell surface both in a receptor form and as an integral membrane component.[9, 58, 87]

Hyaluronan was the first matrix component for which a receptor was identified.[87] This receptor has recently been detected on a broad spectrum of cells from fibroblasts to lymphocytes,[58, 87, 134] where hyaluronan is the ligand for the CD44 homing receptor on lymphocytes.[137] Hyaluronan is present in the serum of humans and is cleared by the liver. The serum levels are elevated in a variety of clinical disorders, including liver disease and arthritis. Patients with rheumatoid arthritis show elevations in plasma levels, particularly early in the day in association with morning stiffness.[9]

Hyaluronan Receptor (See CD44)

Integrins

The integrins are a class of cell surface receptors that consist of heterodimers of noncovalently associated α- and β-subunits. The integrins are involved in both cell-cell and cell-matrix interactions. There are nearly a dozen α-subunits and half as many β that can associate in a variety of combinations leading to various binding affinities. A full review of the integrins is beyond the scope of this chapter, but understanding of their structures and functions is essential to comprehending the new physiologies of the matrix. The integrins and their various families and ligands are shown in Figure 3–6, which follows the organization proposed by Hynes[168] and was adopted from the review by Albelda and Buck.[7] A series of selected references pertaining to the interactions of matrix with the integrins is provided.[25–27, 67, 127, 134–139]

Invariant Chain CS

The invariant chain is a part-time proteoglycan that is a component of the class II histocompatibility antigens.[140] The role(s) of the GAG chain on the invariant chain in intracellular interactions, after presentation on the cell surface or possibly after release from the cell, is unknown.

Laminins

The laminins are a class of polyvalent structural glycoproteins first isolated from the EHS sarcoma and shown to be a promient component of most BMs. The monomer is composed of three separate polypeptide chains, A, B1, and B2, each representing unique gene products and each likely to have multiple isoforms. The three chains are entwined to form a cross-shaped structure made up of both globular and nonglobular regions (Figs. 3–1 to 3–3 and 3–5). Receptor-mediated cell attachment promotion of neurite outgrowth and heparin binding reside in the terminal region of the long arm, while in the short arm are a separate cell attachment site, a solid phase signaling site with mitogenic capacity, binding sites for entactin, and the calcium-dependent sites involved in aggregation. These various sites are composed principally of cysteine-rich regions with EGF and perlecan homologies.[10, 23, 29, 59, 64, 66, 67, 141–148]

Recently a number of different laminin variants have been described in which distinct A or B chains are present within the molecule or in which a chain may be missing. Merosin is one such isoform of laminin found in placenta, striated muscle, and peripheral nerves in which the A chain is a different gene product from that originally described.[144]

S-laminin isoform has a unique B1 chain and has been identified in relatively high levels in synaptic neuromuscular junctions.[56]

Laminin interacts strongly with other matrix components, including heparan sulfate proteoglycan, type IV collagen, and itself. The self-assembly of laminin into higher-ordered structures involves the globular ends of both the short and the long arms and is a calcium- and heparin-dependent process.[11, 29] Laminin also interacts with perlecan via the carboxy terminal globular end of the A chain, the same site at which the major binding of neurites occurs.[142]

Interactions of cells with laminin occur at two sites: the carboxy terminal of the long arm or A chain and an internal portion of the B1 chain.[141] Laminin-cell interactions are important in a spectrum of events from normal development[66, 145] to tumor invasion.[146] The binding of cells to laminin and to fragments containing the sites of interaction are mediated by Arg-Gly-Asp (RGD)–independent interactions with integrin class receptors.[143]

The list of functions of the laminins grows rapidly and ranges from the structural to the regulatory. As a structural element, it is a major constituent of the cell-lamina or BM; it is a major constituent of the neuromuscular junction, where its structural functions are matched by its solid phase signaling; and it is a major constituent of the glomerulus, where its structural functions are closely related to its being a filter. As a regulatory element, laminin is a major promoter of neurite outgrowth; it is significantly increased on the surfaces of transformed cells[149] and is a stimulant of metastasis.[146] The metastasis-promoting activity also stimulates the production of collagenase IV activity, and both of these effects reside in a 19-residue polypeptide. The loss or gain of binding to laminin during transformation can also be influenced by TGF-β, which switches the integrins in osteosarcoma cells to selectively lose binding to laminin.[25] Other proteolytic fragments of the laminin A chain are strongly chemotactic for mast cells[18] that, having been attracted to a site of A chain degradation, are able to produce B chains, type IV collagen, and a heparan sulfate proteoglycan, presumably perlecan.[19]

Neurite outgrowth on laminin is a complex process that likely involves several different cellular receptors on the neurite; different biosynthetic products of the neurite, including laminin-binding proteoglycans[150]; and a variety of intracellular mechanisms from physical to chemical transductions of external signals with consequent influence on intracellular protein kinase C activity.[62] Begovac and Shur[64] have demonstrated an interaction via a cell surface galactosyltransferase, and their data could be interpreted to indicate that as cells move and attach to laminin they glycosylate the substrate, thereby leaving a trail, or text, behind. This "text writing" receptor on neurites is clearly different from the major RGD-independent cell binding site, also at the

end of the long arm.[142] While neurite outgrowth has received considerable attention, it should be noted that laminin also promotes the polarization of nephrogenic mesenchyme[67]; the formation of cell cords in cultures of Sertoli's cells[145]; the formation of capillary-like structures[141]; and the formation of canalicular structures in bone cell cultures.[148]

Link

Link, a protein isolated from cartilage, is involved in the interactions of the NH$_2$-terminal of aggrecan with hyaluronan. This interaction, which stabilizes the extracellular macromolecules, might begin within the compartments of the cell during biosynthesis and packaging.[69] The structure of link shows similarities to the receptor for hyaluronan and is similar to the lymphocyte-homing receptor, CD44.[151] Link is not restricted to cartilaginous structures but has also been found in the embryonic chick mesonephros.[152]

Merosin (See Laminin)

Nidogen (See Entactin)

Osteocalcin

The proteins in the organic matrix of bone are many, including those made by bone such as type I collagen, alkaline phosphatase, sparc, biglycan, decorin, osteocalin, osteopontin, and others such as α$_2$-HS-glycoprotein, TGF-β, platelet-derived growth factor (PDGF), insulin-like growth factor-1 (IGF-1), aFGF, bFGF, and interleukin-1 (IL-1), which are synthesized elsewhere and which bind secondarily to the bone matrix.[1, 30, 82, 108, 153, 157] Osteocalcin is seemingly a specific bone cell product and is one of the few matrix proteins that contain a high content of γ-carboxyglutamic acid (GLA).

Osteocalcin and alkaline phosphatase in bone are expressed only by nonproliferating osteoblasts, whereas type I collagen is expressed in proliferating cells. The regulation of the genes for osteocalcin, alkaline phosphatase, and type I collagen is related to two proto-oncogenes, fos and jun, and to their interactions with the vitamin D–responsive element (VDRE)[154] in a manner suggesting that vitamin D influences collagen, but not osteocalcin and alkaline phosphatase expression in proliferating osteoblasts. TGF-β inhibits osteocalcin production by rat osteoblasts while at the same time stimulating the synthesis of type I collagen, sparc, and osteopontin.[153, 155]

Interestingly, while osteocalcin is relatively restricted to bone, its release by bone fragments does not stimulate mononuclear cells to release IL-1 and is likely not to play a role in the increased IL-1 secretion by circulating monocytes in patients with high-turnover osteoporosis. Rather it appears that the collagen fragments, detected by integrin receptors on the monocytes, are responsible for IL-1 release.[156]

Osteonectin (See Sparc)

Osteopontin

Osteopontin, originally called bone sialoprotein, is an acidic glycoprotein that is prominent in bone and teeth but is also found in hypertrophic chondrocytes, brain, kidney, deciduum, and placenta. The protein is about 42 kD and contains the RGD sequence. It binds to both an integrin receptor, shared with vitronectin, and the inorganic hydroxyapatite in the mineral phase of bone. Its synthesis is increased by both TGF-β and 1,25-dihydroxyvitamin D$_3$.[158] In cell cultures from normal and transformed osteocytes, various forms of osteopontin are produced, the transformed cell product being highly phosphorylated.[159, 162] Reinholt and colleagues[160, 161] have shown that osteopontin is a possible adhesion protein for osteoclasts in that it is highly enriched at sites of bone resorption; at such sites there is colocalization with the vitronectin receptor.

Osteopontin is selectively bound by staphylococci isolated from patients with osteomyelitis. The binding of the organisms is to the protein core and not to the carbohydrate side chains and cannot be inhibited by fibronectin, type I collagen, staphylococcal protein A, IgG, or fibrinogen.[163]

Perlecan HS

Perlecan is a high molecular weight, low-density proteoglycan, best characterized from the EHS sarcoma. The protein core consists of five to six globular domains, to the last of which are linked one to three GAG chains of the heparan sulfate type.[24, 164] Perlecan plays an integral role in the structure of cell laminae or BMs.[24] As a structural element, it plays a major charge-dependent sieving function in the BM. It interacts with itself, through both protein core and GAG chain interactions, and also interacts with type IV collagen, laminin, basic fibroblast growth factor,[76] and extracellular superoxide dismutase C.[165] The linkage of perlecan to the cell surface is not well understood, but a possible receptor for the core protein has been described.[28]

The glycosaminoglycan chains of heparin and heparan sulfate can serve as potent signals if released by endoglycosidases. In addition to known effects on hemostasis, the fragments of these glycosaminoglycan chains can dampen the stimulus to replication of smooth muscle cells that have been subjected to stimulation by PDGF.[15, 16, 60, 61]

Recently some unexpected relationships between perlecan and amyloidosis have developed. Schubert and colleagues have suggested that the amyloid β protein precursor is similar to the heparan sulfate proteoglycan core protein secreted by PC12, a nerve cell line,[160, 167] and Snow and colleagues[38] have presented immunocytochemical evidence linking the amyloid in a variety of neurodegenerative conditions, including Gerstmann-Straussler syndrome, Creutzfeldt-Jakob disease, and scrapie, to the presence of heparan sulfate proteoglycan.

Serglycin CS/DS

All types of hematopoietic cells produce a secretory form of proteoglycan, the best known of which is serglycin, named because of the frequent sequences Ser-Gly, the consensus sequences for O-linkage of GAG chains.[4, 5, 21] Serglycin is produced by all types of hematopoietic cells in both a regulated and a constitutive fashion, including mast cells, basophils, T lymphocytes, and natural killer (NK) cells.[21, 132] Serglycin is a proteinase-resistant proteoglycan whose function is to store and protect a variety of agonists with which it is copackaged. The serglycin protein core is highly glycosylated by a variety of GAG chains, and this secretory, fluid phase matrix component has been implicated in the regulation of inflammation, immune responses, and coagulation of blood. In circulating cells such as mast cells, platelets, and NK cells, there is evidence that serglycin is complexed with cationic proteins and pharmacologic amines such as histamine. Presumably, the interactions of serglycin with these agonists, both within the cell and after discharge into the matrix, represent a means for regulating the release and rates of degradation of bioactive reagents.

Solid Phase Derivatives

All the matrix components discussed in this chapter are likely to be found as breakdown products in and around the cells, in lymphatic fluids, in the serum, in the joint space—virtually in all spaces open to diffusion. Many of these fragments will be rapidly cleared by fixed and mobile macrophages. Others are likely to exert significant biologic effects prior to their final removal. As further exploration of matrix molecules progresses, it is apparent that breakdown products have significant effects and that this fluid phase matrix set will require more attention in the future.[75, 146, 156]

Sparc

Sparc, also called osteonectin and BM-40, is a solid, fluid, and cell-surface phase matrix glycoprotein, found in solid phase in abundance in bone; in fluid phase in the serum; and in the cell-surface phase as part of the cell lamina or BM. The protein was originally described in bone as osteonectin, where it is the most abundant noncollagenous protein.[169] However, it is widely distributed outside bone, and the acronym SPARC, for *secreted protein acidic rich in cysteine*, was coined. The name sparc is less restrictive than osteonectin. The protein is produced by a variety of cells, including parietal endoderm cells, osteoblasts, odontoblasts, Schwann's cells, decidual cells, endothelial cells, Leydig's cells, Sertoli's cells, and cells of the corpus luteum and adrenal cortex.[171–174] It is present in platelets and is released by collagen or thrombin from platelets in a dose-dependent manner; it is also present on the platelet cell surface. The platelet form of sparc appears to be larger than that found in bone.[175]

In vitro, sparc induces cell rounding, as does thrombospondin and tenascin, and all three thus can act to inhibit cell spreading. Sparc interacts with collagen types III and V and with thrombospondin.[173] The affinities of sparc for the matrix are calcium dependent and act in concert with other regions of the molecule to inhibit cellular spreading.[175] Endothelial cells, for example, fail to adhere to type III collagen gels that contain sparc.[173] It has been suggested that cell shape influences might also operate in cells such as Leydig's and Sertoli's cells in the testis.[172] Sparc is released from endothelial cells when they are injured, and Sage and colleagues[174] view sparc as modulating extracellular calcium-dependent processes, including proteinases involved in injury reactions as well as cell-matrix adhesive relationships. When sparc is added to cells in culture, the effects on cell anchorage and migration are not inhibited by the RGD peptide.[173] The biologic effects of sparc are dependent on calcium binding at both NH_2- and COOH-terminal "E-F" hand modules.[169, 171, 175, 176] The 90-kD protein contains a high percentage of cysteine, and there is high homology among sparc proteins obtained from various species.[169, 170]

Syndecan HS/CS

Syndecan is a cell surface proteoglycan that is found primarily on epithelial cells but is also transiently present on mesenchyme at sites of epithelial-mesenchymal interactions.[177, 178] It is probably a family of integral membrane proteoglycans that share cytoplasmic domains but have unique extracellular domains containing linked chondroitin sulfate and heparan sulfate glycosaminoglycan chains.[177, 179] The cytoplasmic domain interacts with the actin cytoskeleton, and the extracellular domain binds to a variety of other macromolecules including matrix components such as fibronectin, collagen types I, III, and V, and thrombospondin, but not to laminin or vitronectin. Syndecan binds regulatory macromolecules, including basic fibroblast growth factor (bFGF).

In embryonic tissues, under circumstances of epithelial-mesenchymal interactions as in the tooth and limb, syndecan is transiently expressed on mesenchyme.[178, 179] Syndecan is expressed on the surface of plasma cells,[180] initially when present as pre-B cells in the marrow, but not when circulating in the blood, and then again when present in tissues such as the lymph nodes and spleen.[182]

The syndecan on mouse mammary epithelial cells shows preferential increase in chondroitin sulfate when treated with TGF-β,[179] and that on the vaginal epithelium of the mouse is significantly modulated by either endogenous or exogenous estrogens and progesterones.[183]

Tenascin

Tenascin is a large matrix glycoprotein prominent in states of high tissue remodeling and morphogenesis.[14] It was originally described at the myotendinous junction, at which site it presumably plays an important biomechanical function.[184] The binding of tenascin to fibronectin has been questioned, but recent studies indicate a weak affinity that nonetheless is sufficient to block cell binding and migration on fibronectin.[185] This effect of tenascin is probably based on its capacity to block or mask the fibronectin and/or its receptors. Review of Figure 3–5 demonstrates that the large extended configuration of tenascin could have significant, nonspecific effects on not only fibronectin-cell surface interactions but also other ligand-receptor interactions. In the developing chick limb, a tenascin-rich sheet has been identified that extends from the ectodermal BM to the proximally located muscle anlage. This sheet lies in the position in which the tendons form, and Hurle and colleagues[186] have suggested that it represents a template that influences the spatial organization of the tendons in the limb.

Thrombomodulin

Thrombomodulin is an endothelial cell surface part-time proteoglycan that, in rabbits, influences coagulation by (1) acting as a cofactor for thrombin-induced protein C activation, (2) altering the procoagulant activity of thrombin, and (3) accelerating antithrombin III inhibition of thrombin.[187, 188] The second and third of these activities are dependent on a solitary chondroitin sulfate chain; the first is not. The GAG-dependent actions are inhibited by the GAG binding region of a vitronectin-derived peptide. Human thrombomodulin from placenta has only a slight influence on the second and third activities previously described. Whether this species difference is due to masking, absence, or chemically different GAG chains is not known.

Thrombospondin

Thrombospondin is a large, 450-kD homotrimeric glycoprotein formed from three subunits of approximately equal size, each terminating in a globular domain.[189] It is produced by monocytes, and endothelial cells and is released by activated platelets.[117] It interacts with the cell surface through an integrin and syndecan; and it interacts with matrix macromolecules, including fibronectin and fibrinogen. It influences platelet aggregation, fibrin formation and lysis, cell adhesion and migration, and cell proliferation. A module in thrombospondin is homologous with a cysteine-rich region of the globular domain of the NH_2-terminal of type II collagen and with von Willebrand factor.[190]

Undulin

Undulin is a matrix glycoprotein of relatively large size composed of three polypeptides, called A, B1, and B2. The protein shows sequence homologies with fibronectin and tenascin and is distributed in tissues at sites at which tenascin is absent. It binds to collagen fibrils, particularly those of a diameter greater than 60 nM in areas where fibril packing is dense. It has been described in skin, uterus, liver, large intestine, blood vessels, and placenta. It is not found in bone or in significant amounts in scar tissue.[191]

Versican CS/DS

Versican is a large proteoglycan found in fibrous tissues with a structure and a probable function similar to those of aggrecan.[5, 192]

Vitronectin

Vitronectin (VN), also known as serum spreading factor, complement S protein, or epibolin, is an adhesive glycoprotein that interacts with complement, coagulation, and fibrinolytic and immunologic components as well as cells and platelets.[193–197] It is present in plasma as a single chain 75-kD polypeptide or as two chains of 65 and 10 kD linked by a disulfide bond. Many of the interactions of VN with complement derivatives C7, C8, and C9 occur via a heparin-binding domain near the COOH-terminal that binds to glycosaminoglycan chains. Vitronectin also binds to collagens and elastins, but it does not bind to laminin and fibronectin. Vitronectin interacts with the integrin class receptors through an RGD consensus sequence, and vitronectin receptor also has specificity for osteopontin.[160] The cross-linked forms of VN retain binding affinities to heparin, platelets, and plasminogen activator inhibitor type-1 (PAI-1).[20]

CONCLUSIONS

In 1985 it was apparent that matrix physiology was much broader than traditionally presented in standard texts and in traditional graduate and medical education.[208] An integrated view of the injury, inflammatory, immune, regeneration, and repair reactions is emerging as we recognize that prior boundaries of these disciplines were drawn by narrow perspectives and insufficient information.

References

1. Heinegard, D., and Oldberg, A.: Structure and biology of cartilage and bone matrix noncollagenous macromolecules. FASEB J. 3:2042, 1989.
2. Gallagher, J. T.: The extended family of proteoglycans: social residents of the pericellular zone. Curr. Opin. Cell Biol. 1:1201, 1989.
3. Buck, C. A., and Horwitz, A. F.: Cell surface receptors for extracellular matrix molecules. Annu. Rev. Cell Biol. 3:179, 1987.
4. Ruoslahti, E., and Yamaguchi, Y.: Proteoglycans as modulators of growth factor activities. Cell 64:867, 1991.
5. Ruoslahti, E.: Proteoglycans in cell regulation. J. Biol. Chem. 264:13369, 1989.
6. Chung, A. E., and Durkin, M. E.: Entactin: structure and function. Am. J. Respir. Cell Mol. Biol. 3:275, 1990.
7. Albelda, S. M., and Buck, C. A.: Integrins and other cell adhesion molecules. FASEB J. 4:2868, 1990.
8. Goetinck, P., and Winterbottom, N.: Proteoglycans: Modular macromolecules of the extracellular matrix. In Goldsmith, L. (ed.): Biochemistry and Physiology of the Skin. 2nd ed. New York, Oxford University Press, 1991.
9. Laurent, T. C., and Fraser, J. R.: The properties and turnover of hyaluronan. Ciba Found. Symp. 124:9, 1986.
10. Beck, K., Hunter, I., and Engel, J.: Structure and function of laminin: anatomy of a multidomain glycoprotein. FASEB J. 4:148, 1990.
11. Schittny, J. C., and Yurchenco, P. D.: Basement membranes: molecular organization and function in development and disease. Curr. Opin. Cell Biol. 1:983, 1989.
12. Timpl, R.: Structure and biological activity of basement membrane proteins. Eur. J. Biochem. 180:487, 1989.
13. Massague, J.: The transforming growth factor-β family. Annu. Rev. Cell Biol. 6:597, 1990.
14. Erickson, H. P., and Bourdon, M. A.: Tenascin: An extracellular matrix protein prominent in specialized embryonic tissues and tumors. Annu. Rev. Cell Biol. 5:71, 1989.
15. Castellot, J. J., Jr., Choay, J., Lormeau, J. C., Petitou, M., Sache, E., and Karnovsky, M. J.: Structural determinants of the capacity of heparin to inhibit the proliferation of vascular smooth muscle cells. II. Evidence for a pentasaccharide sequence that contains a 3-0 sulfate group. J. Cell Biol. 102:1979, 1986.
16. Castellot, J. J., Jr., Hoover, R. L., and Karnovsky, M. J.: Glomerular endothelial cells secrete a heparinlike inhibitor and a peptide stimulator of mesangial cell proliferation. Am. J. Pathol. 125:493, 1986.
17. Clark, R. A. F.: Wound repair. Curr. Opin. Cell Biol. 1:1000, 1989.
18. Thompson, H. L., Burbelo, P. D., Yamada, Y., Kleinman, H. K., and Metcalfe, D. D.: Mast cells chemotax to laminin with enhancement after IgE-mediated activation. J. Immunol. 143:4188, 1989.
19. Thompson, H. L., Burbelo, P. D., Gabriel, G., Yamada, Y., and Metcalfe, D. D.: Murine mast cells synthesize basement membrane components. A potential role in early fibrosis. J. Clin. Invest. 87:619, 1991.
20. Sane, D. C., Moser, T. L., Parker, C. J., Seiffert, D., Loskutoff, D. J., and Greenberg, C. S.: Highly sulfated glycosaminoglycans augment the cross-linking of vitronectin by guinea pig liver transglutaminase. Functional studies of the cross-linked vitronectin multimers. J. Biol. Chem. 265:3543, 1990.
21. Kolset, S. O., and Gallagher, J. T.: Proteoglycans in haemopoietic cells. Biochim. Biophys. Acta 1032:191, 1990.
22. Kaufman, O. D., Seidman, R. J., Phillips, M. E., and Gruber, B. L.: Cutaneous manifestations of the L-tryptophan–associated eosinophilia-myalgia syndrome: a spectrum of sclerodermatous skin disease. J. Am. Acad. Dermatol. 23:1063, 1990.
23. Desjardins, M., and Bendayan, M.: Heterogenous distribution of type IV collagen, entactin, heparan sulfate proteoglycan, and laminin among renal basement membranes as demonstrated by quantitative immunocytochemistry. J. Histochem. Cytochem. 37:885, 1989.
24. Yurchenco, P. D., and Schittny, J. C.: Molecular architecture of basement membranes. FASEB J. 4:1577, 1990.
25. Heino, J., and Massague, J.: Transforming growth factor-beta switches the pattern of integrins expressed in MG-63 human osteosarcoma cells and causes a selective loss of cell adhesion to laminin. J. Biol. Chem. 264:21806, 1989.

26. Larson, R. S., Corbi, A. L., Berman, L., and Springer, T.: Primary structure of the leukocyte function-associated molecule-1 alpha sub-unit: an integrin with an embedded domain defining a protein super-family. J. Cell Biol. 108:703, 1989.

27. Sonnenberg, A., Linders, C. J., Modderman, P. W., Damsky, C. H., Aumailley, M., and Timpl, R.: Integrin recognition of different cell-binding fragments of laminin (P1, E3, E8) and evidence that alpha 6 beta 1 but not alpha 6 beta 4 functions as a major receptor for fragment E8. J. Cell Biol. 110:2145, 1990.

28. Clement, B., Segui Real, B., Hassell, J. R., Martin, G. R., and Yamada, Y.: Identification of a cell surface-binding protein for the core protein of the basement membrane proteoglycan. J. Biol. Chem. 264:12467, 1989.

29. Yurchenco, P. D., Cheng, Y. S., and Schittny, J. C.: Heparin modulation of laminin polymerization. J. Biol. Chem. 265:3981, 1990.

30. Paralkar, V. M., Nandedkar, A. K., Pointer, R. H., Kleinman, H. K., and Reddi, A. H.: Interaction of osteogenin, a heparin-binding bone morphogenetic protein, with type IV collagen. J. Biol. Chem. 265:17281, 1990.

31. Chajek Shaul, T., Friedman, G., Bengtsson Olivecrona, G., Vlodavsky, I., and Bar Shavit, R.: Interaction of lipoprotein lipase with subendo-thelial extracellular matrix. Biochim. Biophys. Acta 1042:168, 1990.

32. Cisar, L. A., Hoogewerf, A. J., Cupp, M., Rapport, C. A., and Bensadoun, A.: Secretion and degradation of lipoprotein lipase in cultured adipocytes. Binding of lipoprotein lipase to membrane hepa-ran sulfate proteoglycans is necessary for degradation. J. Biol. Chem. 264:1767, 1989.

33. Morton, K., Hutchinson, C., Jeanny, J. C., Karpouzas, I., Pouliquen, Y., and Courtois, Y.: Colocalization of fibroblast growth factor binding sites with extracellular matrix components in normal and keratoconus corneas. Curr. Eye Res. 8:975, 1989.

34. Rogelj, S., Klagsbrun, M., Atzmon, R., Kurokawa, M., Haimovitz, A., Fuks, Z., and Vlodavsky, I.: Basic fibroblast growth factor is an extracellular matrix component required for supporting the prolifera-tion of vascular endothelial cells and the differentiation of PC12 cells. J. Cell Biol. 109:823, 1989.

35. Roussel, B., Arvieux, J., Jacob, M. C., Lorimier, P., and Cavigioli, E.: A human monoclonal IgM with autoantibody activities against heparan sulphate and the mitotic spindle. Clin. Exp. Immunol. 82:294, 1990.

36. Saxena, R., Bygren, P., Butkowski, R., and Wieslander, J.: Entactin: a possible auto-antigen in the pathogenesis of non-Goodpasture anti-GBM nephritis. Kidney Int. 38:263, 1990.

37. Matzner, Y., Vlodavsky, I., Michaeli, R. I., and Eldor, A.: Selective inhibition of neutrophil activation by the subendothelial extracellular matrix: possible role in protection of the vessel wall during diapedesis. Exp. Cell Res. 189:233, 1990.

38. Snow, A. D., Wight, T. N., Nochlin, D., Koike, Y., Kimata, K., DeArmond, S. J., Prusiner, S. B.: Immunolocalization of heparan sulfate proteoglycans to the prion protein amyloid plaques of Gerstmann-Straussler syndrome, Creutzfeldt-Jakob disease, and scra-pie. Lab. Invest. 63:601, 1990.

39. Perlmutter, L. S., and Chui, H. C.: Microangiopathy, the vascular basement membrane and Alzheimer's disease: a review. Brain Res. Bull. 24:677, 1990.

40. Hynes, R.: Molecular biology of fibronectin. Annu. Rev. Cell Biol. 1:67, 1985.

41. Doolittle, R. F., Feng, D. F., Johnson, M. S., and McClure, M. A.: Relationships of human protein sequences to those of other organisms. Cold Spring Harb. Symp. Quant. Biol. 51:447, 1986.

42. Baron, M., Norman, D. G., and Campbell, I. D.: Protein modules. Trends Biochem. Sci. 16:13, 1991.

43. Greve, H., Cully, Z., Blumberg, P., and Kresse, H.: Influence of chlorate on proteoglycan biosynthesis by cultured human fibroblasts. J. Biol. Chem. 263:12886, 1988.

44. Twining, S. S.: Wilson, P. M., and Hatchell, D. L.: Characterization of corneal proteoglycans under vitamin A deficiency. Biochim. Bio-phys. Acta. 992:181, 1989.

45. Silbert, C. K., Humphries, D. E., Palmer, M. E., and Silbert, J. E.: Effects of sulfate deprivation on the production of chondroitin/der-matan sulfate by cultures of skin fibroblasts from normal and diabetic individuals. Arch. Biochem. Biophys. 285:137, 1991.

46. Nanto Salonen, K., Larjava, H., Saamanen, A. M., Heino, J., Pentti-nen, R., Pelliniemi, L. J., and Tammi, M.: Abnormal dermal proteo-glycan in aspartylglycosaminuria: a possible mechanism for ultrastruc-tural changes of collagen fibrils in a glycoprotein storage disorder. Connect. Tissue Res. 16:367, 1987.

47. Iozzo, R. V.: Neoplastic modulation of extracellular matrix: Colon carcinoma cells release polypeptides that alter proteoglycan metabo-lism in colon fibroblasts. J. Biol. Chem. 260:7464, 1985.

48. Iozzo, R. V.: Presence of unsulfated heparan chains on the heparan sulfate proteoglycan of human colon carcinoma cells. Implications for heparan sulfate proteoglycan biosynthesis. J. Biol. Chem. 264:2690, 1989.

49. Comper, W. D. Extracellular matrix interactions: sulfation of connective

50. Prigogine, I.: From Being to Becoming. San Francisco, Freeman, C., 1980.

51. Sudhalter, J., Folkman, J., Svahn, C. M., Bergendal, K., and D'Amore, P.A.: Importance of size, sulfation, and anticoagulant activity in the potentiation of acidic fibroblast growth factor by heparin. J. Biol. Chem. 264:6892, 1989.

52. Iozzo, R. V., Kovalszky, I., Hacobian, N., Schick, P. K., Ellingson, J. S., and Dodge, G. R.: Fatty acylation of heparan sulfate proteoglycan from human colon carcinoma cells. J. Biol. Chem. 265:19980, 1990.

53. Rauch, U., Hollmann, J., Schmidt, A., Buddecke, E., and Kresse, H.: Tyrosine O-sulfate ester in proteoglycans. Biol. Chem. Hoppe-Seyler 369:595, 1988.

54. Dedhar, S., and Ruoslahti, E., and Pierschbacher, M. D.: A cell surface receptor complex for collagen type I recognizes the Arg Gly Asp sequence. J. Cell Biol. 104:585, 1987.

55. Cardin, A. D., and Weintraub, H. J.: Molecular modeling of protein-glycosaminoglycan interactions. Arteriosclerosis 9:21, 1989.

56. Sanes, J. R., Engvall, E., Butkowski, R., and Hunter, D. D.: Molecular heterogeneity of basal laminae: isoforms of laminin and collagen IV at the neuromuscular junction and elsewhere. J. Cell Biol. 111:1685, 1990.

57. Toole, B. P., Goldberg, R. L., Chi-Rosso, G., Underhill, C. B., and Orkin, R. W.: Hyaluronate-cell interactions. In Trelstad, R. L. (ed.): The Role of Extracellular Matrix in Development. New York, Alan R. Liss, 1984, pp. 43–66.

58. Miyake, K., Underhill, C. B., Lesley, J., and Kincade, P. W.: Hyalu-ronate can function as a cell adhesion molecule, and CD44 participates in hyaluronate recognition. J. Exp. Med. 172:69, 1990.

59. Panayotou, G., End, P., Aumailley, M., Timpl, R., and Engel, J.: Domains of laminin with growth-factor activity. Cell 56:93, 1989.

60. Wright, T. C., Jr., Castellot, J. J., Jr., Petitou, M., Lormeau, J. C., Choay, J., and Karnovsky, M. J.: Structural determinants of heparin's growth inhibitory activity. Interdependence of oligosaccharide size and charge. J. Biol. Chem. 264:1534, 1989.

61. Castellot, J. J., Jr., Pukac, L. A., Caleb, B. L., Wright, T. C., Jr., and Karnovsky, M. J.: Heparin selectively inhibits a protein kinase C–dependent mechanism of cell cycle progression in calf aortic smooth muscle cells. J. Cell. Biol. 109:3147, 1989.

62. Bixby, J. L., and Jhabvala, P.: Extracellular matrix molecules and cell adhesion molecules induce neurites through different mechanisms. J. Cell Biol. 111:2725, 1990.

63. Hermann, M. Jaconi, M. E., Dahlgren, C., Waldvogel, F. A., Stendahl, O., and Lew, D. P.: Neutrophil bactericidal activity against Staphylo-coccus aureus adherent on biological surfaces. Surface-bound extracel-lular matrix proteins activate intracellular killing by oxygen-dependent and -independent mechanisms. J. Clin. Invest. 86:942, 1990.

64. Begovac, P. C., and Shur, B. D.: Cell surface galactosyltransferase mediates the initiation of neurite outgrowth from PC12 cells on laminin. J. Cell. Biol. 110:461, 1990.

65. Bernstein, R. E.: Nonenzymatically glycosylated proteins. Adv. Clin. Chem. 26:1, 1987.

66. Perris, R., Paulsson, M., Bronner-Fraser, M.: Molecular mechanisms of avian neural crest cell migration on fibronectin and laminin. Dev. Biol. 136:222, 1989.

67. Sorokin, L., Sonnenberg, A., Aumailley, M., Timpl, R., and Ekblom, P.: Recognition of the laminin E8 cell-binding site by an integrin possessing the alpha 6 subunit is essential for epithelial polarization in developing kidney tubules. J. Cell Biol. 111:1265, 1990.

68. Farquhar, M. G.: Progress in unraveling pathways of Golgi traffic. Annu. Rev. Cell Biol. 1:447, 1985.

69. Vertel, B. M., Velasco, A., LaFrance, S., Walters, L., Kaczman-Daniel, K.: Precursors of chondroitin sulfate proteoglycan are segregated within a subcompartment of the chondrocyte endoplasmic reticulum. J. Cell Biol. 109:1827, 1989.

70. Andreadis, A., Gallego, M. E., and Nadal-Ginard, B.: Generation of protein isoform diversity by alternative splicing: Mechanistic and biological implication. Annu. Rev. Cell Biol. 3:207, 1987.

71. Hynes, R. O., Schwarzbauer, J. E., and Tamkun, J. W.: Isolation and analysis of cDNA and genomic clones of fibronectin and its receptor. Methods Enzymol. 144:447, 1987.

72. Cross, G. A. M.: Glycolipid anchoring of plasma membrane proteins. Annu. Rev. Cell Biol. 6:1, 1990.

73. Carey, D. J., and Stahl, R. C.: Identification of a lipid-anchored heparan sulfate proteoglycan in Schwann cells. J. Cell Biol. 111:2053, 1990.

74. Singer, I. I., Scott, S., Kawka, D. W., and Kazazis, D. M.: Adhesomes: specific granules containing receptors for laminin, C3bi/fibrinogen, fibronectin, and vitronectin in human polymorphonuclear leukocytes and monocytes. J. Cell Biol. 109:3169, 1989.

75. Andres, J. L., Stanley, K., Cheifetz, S., and Massague, J.: Membrane-anchored and soluble forms of betaglycan, a polymorphic proteoglycan that binds transforming growth factor-beta. J. Cell Biol. 109:3137, 1989.

76. Vigny, M., Ollier Hartmann, M. P., Lavigne, M., Fayein, N., Jeanny, J. C., Laurent, M., and Courtois, Y.: Specific binding of basic fibroblast

tissue polysaccharides creates macroion binding templates and condi-tions for dissipative structure formation. J. Theor. Biol. 145:497, 1990.

growth factor to basement membrane–like structures and to purified heparan sulfate proteoglycan of the EHS tumor. J. Cell. Physiol. 137:321, 1988.

77. Mooradian, D. L., Lucan, R. C., Weatherbee, J. A., and Furcht, L. T.: Transforming growth factor-beta 1 binds to immobilized fibronectin. J. Cell. Biochem. 41:189, 1989.

78. Walle, T. K., Vartio, T., Helve, T., Virtanen, I., and Kurki, P.: Cellular fibronectin in rheumatoid synovium and synovial fluid: a possible factor contributing to lymphocytic infiltration. Scand. J. Immunol. 31:535, 1990.

79. Blaschke, E., Eklund, A., and Hernbrand, R.: Extracellular matrix components in bronchoalveolar lavage fluid in sarcoidosis and their relationship to signs of alveolitis. Am. Rev. Respir. Dis. 141:1020, 1990.

80. Flaumenhaft, R., Moscatelli, D., and Rifkin, D. B.: Heparin and heparan sulfate increase the radius of diffusion and action of basic fibroblast growth factor. J. Cell Biol. 111:1651, 1990.

81. Neame, P. J., Choi, H. U., and Rosenberg, L. C.: The primary structure of the core protein of the small, leucine-rich proteoglycan (PG I) from bovine articular cartilage. J. Biol. Chem. 264:8653, 1989.

82. Fedarko, N. S., Termine, J. D., Young, M. F., and Robey, P. G.: Temporal regulation of hyaluronan and proteoglycan metabolism by human bone cells in vitro. J. Biol. Chem. 265:12200, 1990.

83. Schwarz, K., Breuer, B., and Kresse, H.: Biosynthesis and properties of a further member of the small chondroitin/dermatan sulfate proteoglycan family. J. Biol.Chem. 265:22023, 1990.

84. McBride, O. W., Fisher, L. W., and Young, M. F.: Localization of PGI (biglycan, BGN) and PGII (decorin, DCN, PG-40) genes on human chromosomes Xq13-qter and 12q, respectively. Genomics 6:219, 1990.

85. Vogel, K. G., and Koob, T. J.: Structural specialization in tendons under compression. Int. Rev. Cytol. 115:267, 1989.

86. Border, W. A., Okuda, S., Languino, L. R., and Ruoslahti, E.: Transforming growth factor-beta regulates production of proteoglycans by mesangial cells. Kidney Int. 37:689, 1990.

87. Aruffo, A., Stamenkovic, I., Melnick, M., Underhill, C. B., Seed, B.: CD44 is the principal cell surface receptor for hyaluronate. Cell 61:1303, 1990.

88. Saxne, T., and Heinegard, D.: Involvement of nonarticular cartilage, as demonstrated by release of a cartilage-specific protein, in rheumatoid arthritis. Arthritis Rheum. 32:1080, 1989.

89. Kiss, I., Deak, F., Holloway, R. G., Jr., Delius, H., Mebust, K. A., Frimberger, E., Argraves, W. S., Tsonis, P. A., Winterbottom, N., and Goetinck, P. F.: Structure of the gene for cartilage matrix protein, a modular protein of the extracellular matrix. Exon/intron organization, unusual splice sites, and relation to alpha chains of beta 2 integrins, von Willebrand factor, complement factors B and C2, and epidermal growth factor. J. Biol. Chem. 264:8126, 1989.

90. Jenkins, R. N., Osborne-Lawrence, S. L., Sinclair, A. K., Eddy, R. L., Jr., Byers, M. G., Shows, T. B., and Duby, A. D: Structure and chromosomal location of the human gene encoding cartilage matrix protein. J. Biol. Chem. 265:19624, 1990.

91. Koller, E., Winterhalter, K. H., and Trueb, B.: The globular domains of type VI collagen are related to the collagen-binding domains of cartilage matrix protein and von Willebrand factor. EMBO J. 8:1073, 1989.

92. Stirpe, N. S., and Goetinck, P. F.: Gene regulation during cartilage differentiation: temporal and spatial expression of link protein and cartilage matrix protein in the developing limb. Development 107:23, 1989.

93. Muller-Glauser, W., Humbel, B., Glatt, M., Strauli, P., Winterhalter, K. H., and Bruckner, P.: On the role of type IX collagen in the extracellular matrix of cartilage: type IX collagen is localized to intersections of collagen fibrils. J. Cell Biol. 102:1931, 1986.

94. Corbi, A. L., Garcia Aguilar, J., and Springer, T. A.: Genomic structure of an integrin alpha subunit, the leukocyte p150,95 molecule. J. Biol. Chem. 265:2782, 1990.

95. Brown, D. C., and Vogel, K. G.: Characteristics of the in vitro interaction of a small proteoglycan (PG II) of bovine tendon with type I collagen. Matrix 9:468, 1990.

96. Scott, J. E.: Proteoglycan: collagen interactions and subfibrillar structure in collagen fibrils. Implications in the development and ageing of connective tissues. J. Anat. 169:23, 1990.

97. Birk, D. E., Silver, F. H., and Trelstad, R. L.: Matrix assembly. In Hay, E. D. (ed.): Biology of the Extracellular Matrix. New York, Plenum Press, 1991, pp. 221–254.

98. Silver, F. H.: Biological Materials: Structure, Mechanical Properties, and Modeling of Soft Tissues. New York, New York University Press, 1987.

99. Yamaguchi, Y., Mann, D. M., and Ruoslahti, E.: Negative regulation of transforming growth factor-beta by the proteoglycan decorin. Nature 346:281, 1990.

100. Pulkkinen, L., Kainulainen, K., Krusius, T., Makinen, P., Schollin, J., Gustavsson, K. H., and Peltonen, L.: Deficient expression of the gene coding for decorin in a lethal form of Marfan syndrome. J. Biol. Chem. 265:17780, 1990.

101. Mann, D. M., Yamaguchi, Y., Bourdon, M. A., and Ruoslahti, E.: Analysis of glycosaminoglycan substitution in decorin by site-directed mutagenesis. J. Biol. Chem. 265:5317, 1990.

102. Chakravarti, S., Tam, M. F., and Chung, A. E.: The basement membrane glycoprotein entactin promotes cell attachment and binds calcium ions. J. Biol. Chem. 265:10597, 1990.

103. Simon, B., Podolsky, D. K., Moldenhauer, G., Isselbacher, K. J., Gattoni Celli, S., and Brand, S. J.: Epithelial glycoprotein is a member of a family of epithelial cell surface antigens homologous to nidogen, a matrix adhesion protein. Proc. Natl. Acad. Sci. U.S.A. 87:2755, 1990.

104. Nagayoshi, T., Sanborn, D., Hickok, N. J., Olsen, D. R., Fazio, M. J., Chu, M. L., Knowlton, R., Mann, K., Deutzmann, R., Timpl, R., et al.: Human nidogen: complete amino acid sequence and structural domains deduced from cDNAs, and evidence for polymorphism of the gene. DNA 8:581, 1989.

105. Sakai, L. Y., Keene, D. R., and Engvall, E.: Fibrillin, a new 350-kD glycoprotein, is a component of extracellular microfibrils. J. Cell Biol. 103:2499, 1986.

106. Maddox, B. K., Sakai, L. Y., Keene, D. R., and Glanville, R. W.: Connective tissue microfibrils. Isolation and characterization of three large pepsin-resistant domains of fibrillin. J. Biol. Chem. 264:21381, 1989.

107. Vracko, R., Thorning, D., and Frederickson, R. G.: Spatial arrangements of microfibrils in myocardial scars: application of antibody to fibrillin. J. Mol. Cell. Cardiol. 22:749, 1990.

108. Keene, D. R., Sakai, L. Y., and Burgeson, R. E.: Human bone contains type III collagen, type VI collagen, and fibrillin: type III collagen is present on specific fibers that may mediate attachment of tendons, ligaments, and periosteum to calcified bone cortex. J. Histochem. Cytochem. 39:59, 1990.

109. Hollister, D. W., Godfrey, M., Sakai, L. Y., and Pyeritz, R. E.: Immunohistologic abnormalities of the microfibrillar-fiber system in the Marfan syndrome. N. Engl. J. Med. 323:152, 1990.

110. Godfrey, M., Olson, S., Burgio, R. G., Martini, A., Valli, M., Cetta, G., Hori, H., and Hollister, D. W.: Unilateral microfibrillar abnormalities in a case of asymmetric Marfan syndrome. Am. J. Hum. Genet. 46:661, 1990.

111. Oldberg, A., Antonsson, P., Lindblom, K., and Heinegard, D.: A collagen-binding 59-kd protein (fibromodulin) is structurally related to the small interstitial proteoglycans PG-S1 and PG-S2 (decorin). EMBO J. 8:2601, 1989.

112. Wysocki, A. B., and Grinnell, F.: Fibronectin profiles in normal and chronic wound fluid. Lab. Invest. 63:825, 1990.

113. Couchman, J. R., Austria, M. R., and Woods, A.: Fibronectin-cell interactions. J. Invest. Dermatol. 94:7S, 1990.

114. Varga, J., Olsen, A., Herhal, J., Constantine, G., Rosenbloom, J., and Jimenez, S. A.: Interferon-gamma reverses the stimulation of collagen but not fibronectin gene expression by transforming growth factor-beta in normal human fibroblasts. Eur. J. Clin. Invest. 20:487, 1990.

115. Jaikaria, N. S., Rosenfeld, L., Khan, M. Y., Danishefsky, I., and Newman, S. A.: Interaction of fibronectin with heparin in model extracellular matrices: role of arginine residues and sulfate groups. Biochemistry 30:1538, 1991.

116. Marks, P. W., Hendey, B., and Maxfield, F. R.: Attachment to fibronectin or vitronectin makes human neutrophil migration sensitive to alterations in cytosolic free calcium concentration. J. Cell Biol. 112:149, 1991.

117. Kreis, C., La Fleur, M., Menard, C., Paquin, R., and Beaulieu, A. D.: Thrombospondin and fibronectin are synthesized by neutrophils in human inflammatory joint disease and in a rabbit model of in vivo neutrophil activation. J. Immunol. 143:1961, 1989.

118. Somersalo, K., and Saksela, E.: Fibronectin facilitates the migration of human natural killer cells. Eur. J. Immunol. 21:35, 1991.

119. Peters, D. M., Portz, L. M., Fullenwider, J., and Mosher, D. F.: Co-assembly of plasma and cellular fibronectins into fibrils in human fibroblast cultures. J. Cell Biol. 111:249, 1990.

120. Birk, D. E., Zycband, E. I., Winkelmann, D. A., and Trelstad, R. L.: Collagen fibrillogenesis in situ: Fibril segments are intermediates in matrix assembly. Proc. Natl. Acad. Sci. U.S.A. 86:4549, 1989.

121. Welch, M. P., Odland, G. F., and Clark, R. A.: Temporal relationships of F-actin bundle formation, collagen and fibronectin matrix assembly, and fibronectin receptor expression to wound contraction. J. Cell Biol. 110:133, 1990.

122. Kinsella, M. G., and Wight, T. N.: Formation of high molecular weight dermatan sulfate proteoglycan in bovine aortic endothelial cell cultures. Evidence for transglutaminase-catalyzed cross-linking to fibronectin. J. Biol. Chem. 265:17891, 1990.

123. Raja, R. H., Raucci, G., and Hook, M.: Peptide analogs to a fibronectin receptor inhibit attachment of Staphylococcus aureus to fibronectin-containing substrates. Infect. Immun. 58:2593, 1990.

124. Cederholm, B., Wieslander, J., Bygren, P., and Heinegard, D.: Circulating complexes containing IgA and fibronectin in patients with primary IgA nephropathy. Proc. Natl. Acad. Sci. U.S.A. 85:4865, 1988.

125. Werb, Z., Tremble, P. M., Behrendtsen, O., Crowley, E., and Damsky,

C. H.: Signal transduction through the fibronectin receptor induces collagenase and stromelysin gene expression. J. Cell Biol. 109:877, 1989.

126. Alexander, C. M., and Werb, Z.: Proteinases and extracellular matrix remodeling. Curr. Opin. Cell Biol. 1:974, 1989.

127. Yamada, A., Nikaido, T., Nojima, Y., Schlossman, S. F., and Morimoto, C.: Activation of human CD4 T lymphocytes. Interaction of fibronectin with VLA-5 receptor on CD4 cells induces the AP-1 transcription factor. J. Immunol. 146:53, 1991.

128. Fedarko, N. S., and Conrad, H. E.: A unique heparan sulfate in the nuclei of hepatocytes: structural changes with the growth state of the cells. J. Cell Biol. 102:587, 1986.

129. Piepkorn, M., Hovingh, P., and Linker, A.: Glycosaminoglycan free chains. External plasma membrane components distinct from the membrane proteoglycans. J. Biol. Chem. 264:8662, 1989.

130. Piepkorn, M., Fleckman, P., Carney, H., Hovingh, P., and Linker, A.: The distinctive pattern of proteoglycan and glycosaminoglycan free chain synthesis by cultured human epidermal keratinocytes. J. Invest. Dermatol. 94:107, 1990.

131. Platt, J. L., Trescony, P., Lindman, B., and Oegema, T. R.: Heparin and heparan sulfate delimit nephron formation in fetal metanephric kidneys. Dev. Biol. 139:338, 1990.

132. Steward, W. P., Christmas, S. E., Lyon, M., and Gallagher, J. T.: The synthesis of proteoglycans by human T lymphocytes. Biochim. Biophys. Acta 1052:416, 1990.

133. David, G., Lories, V., Decock, B., Marynen, P., Cassiman, J. J., and Van den Berghe, H.: Molecular cloning of a phosphatidylinositol-anchored membrane heparan sulfate proteoglycan from human lung fibroblasts. J. Cell Biol. 111:3165, 1990.

134. Springer, T. A.: The sensation and regulation of interactions with the extracellular environment: The cell biology of lymphocyte adhesion receptors. Annu. Rev. Cell Biol. 6:359, 1990.

135. Singer, S. J.: The structure and insertion of integral proteins in membranes. Annu. Rev. Cell Biol. 6:247, 1990.

136. Shimizu, Y., van Seventer, G. A., Horgan, K. J., and Shaw, S.: Roles of adhesion molecules in T-cell recognition: fundamental similarities between four integrins on resting human T cells (LFA-1, VLA-4, VLA-5, VLA-6) in expression, binding, and costimulation. Immunol. Rev. 114:109, 1990.

137. Holzmann, B., and Weissman, I. L.: Integrin molecules involved in lymphocyte homing to Peyer's patches. Immunol. Rev. 108:45, 1989.

138. Altruda, F., Cervella, P., Tarone, G., Botta, C., Balzac, F., Stefanuto, G., and Silengo, L.: A human integrin beta 1 subunit with a unique cytoplasmic domain generated by alternative mRNA processing. Gene 95:261, 1990.

139. Carter, W. G., Kaur, P., Gil, S. G., Gahr, P. J., and Wayner, E. A.: Distinct functions for integrins alpha 3 beta 1 in focal adhesions and alpha 6 beta 4/bullous pemphigoid antigen in a new stable anchoring contact (SAC) of keratinocytes: relation to hemidesmosomes. J. Cell Biol. 111:3141, 1990.

140. Simonis, S., Miller, J., and Cullen, S. E.: Biosynthesis and intracellular transport of MHC class II molecules associated with a mutated, glycosaminoglycan-negative invariant chain. Mol. Immunol. 27:413, 1990.

141. Kleinman, H. K., and Weeks, B. S.: Laminin: structure, functions and receptors. Curr. Opin. Cell Biol. 1:964, 1989.

142. Deutzmann, R., Aumailley, M., Wiedemann, H., Pysny, W., Timpl, R., and Edgar, D.: Cell adhesion, spreading and neurite stimulation by laminin fragment E8 depends on maintenance of secondary and tertiary structure in its rod and globular domain. Eur. J. Biochem. 191:513, 1990.

143. Forsberg, E., Paulsson, M., Timpl, R., and Johansson, S.: Characterization of a laminin receptor on rat hepatocytes. J. Biol. Chem. 265:6376, 1990.

144. Ehrig, K., Leivo, I., Argraves, W. S., Ruoslahti, E., and Engvall, E.: Merosin, a tissue-specific basement membrane protein, is a laminin-like protein. Proc. Natl. Acad. Sci. U.S.A. 87:3264, 1990.

145. Hadley, M. A., Weeks, B. S., Kleinman, H. K., and Dym, M.: Laminin promotes formation of cord-like structures by Sertoli cells in vitro. Dev. Biol. 140:318, 1990.

146. Kanemoto, T., Reich, R., Royce, L., Greatorex, D., Adler, S. H., Shiraishi, N., Martin, G. R., Yamada, Y., and Kleinman, H. K.: Identification of an amino acid sequence from the laminin A chain that stimulates metastasis and collagenase IV production. Proc. Natl. Acad. Sci. U.S.A. 87:2279, 1990.

147. Mohan, P. S., Chou, D. K., and Jungalwala, F. B.: Sulfoglucuronyl glycolipids bind laminin. J. Neurochem. 54:2024, 1990.

148. Vukicevic, S., Luyten, F. P., Kleinman, H. K., and Reddi, A. H.: Differentiation of canalicular cell processes in bone cells by basement membrane matrix components: regulation by discrete domains of laminin. Cell 63:437, 1990.

149. Bober, F. J., Birk, D. E., Shenk, T., and Raska, K.: Tumorigenicity of adenovirus-transformed cells: Collagen interaction and cell surface laminin are controlled by the serotype origin of the E1A and E1B genes. J. Virol. 62:580, 1988.

150. Dow, K. E., and Riopelle, R. J.: Specific effects of ethanol on neurite-promoting proteoglycans of neuronal origin. Brain Res. 508:40, 1990.

151. Stamenkovic, I., Amiot, M., Pesando, J. M., and Seed, B.: A lymphocyte molecule implicated in lymph node homing is a member of the cartilage link protein family. Cell 56:1057, 1989.

152. Stirpe, N. S., Dickerson, K. T., and Goetinck, P. F.: The chicken embryonic mesonephros synthesizes link protein, an extracellular matrix molecule usually found in cartilage. Dev. Biol. 137:419, 1990.

153. Noda, M., and Rodan, G. A.: Type beta transforming growth factor regulates expression of genes encoding bone matrix proteins. Connect. Tissue Res. 21:71, 1989.

154. Owen, T. A., Bortell, R., Yocum, S. A., Smock, S. L., Zhang, M., Abate, C., Shalhoub, V., Aronin, N., Wright, K. L., van Wijnen, A. J., et al.: Coordinate occupancy of AP-1 sites in the vitamin D–responsive and CCAAT box elements by Fos-Jun in the osteocalcin gene: model for phenotype suppression of transcription. Proc. Natl. Acad. Sci. U.S.A. 87:9990, 1990.

155. Stein, G. S., Lian, J. B., and Owen, T. A.: Relationship of cell growth to the regulation of tissue-specific gene expression during osteoblast differentiation. FASEB J. 4:3111, 1990.

156. Pacifici, R., Carano, A., Santoro, S. A., Rifas, L., Jeffrey, J. J., Malone, J. D., McCracken, R., and Avioli, L. V.: Bone matrix constituents stimulate interleukin-1 release from human blood mononuclear cells. J. Clin. Invest. 87:221, 1991.

157. Termine, J. D.: Non-collagen proteins in bone. Ciba Found. Symp. 136:178, 1988.

158. Butler, W. T.: The nature and significance of osteopontin. Connect. Tissue Res. 23:123, 1989.

159. Wrana, J. L., Kubota, T., Zhang, Q., Overall, C. M., Aubin, J. E., Butler, W. T., Sodek, J.: Regulation of transformation-sensitive secreted phosphoprotein (SPPI/osteopontin) expression by transforming growth factor-beta. Comparisons with expression of SPARC (secreted acidic cysteine-rich protein). Biochem. J. 273:523, 1991.

160. Reinholt, F. P., Hultenby, K., Oldberg, A., and Heinegard, D.: Osteopontin—a possible anchor of osteoclasts to bone. Proc. Natl. Acad. Sci. U.S.A. 87:4473, 1990.

161. Swanson, G. J., Nomura, S., and Hogan, B. L.: Distribution of expression of 2AR (osteopontin) in the embryonic mouse inner ear revealed by in situ hybridisation. Hear. Res. 41:169, 1989.

162. Fet, V., Dickinson, M. E., and Hogan, B. L.: Localization of the mouse gene for secreted phosphoprotein 1 (Spp-1) (2ar, osteopontin, bone sialoprotein 1, 44-kDa bone phosphoprotein, tumor-secreted phosphoprotein) to chromosome 5, closely linked to Ric (Rickettsia resistance). Genomics 5:375, 1989.

163. Ryden, C., Yacoub, A. I., Maxe, I., Heinegard, D., Oldberg, A., Franzen, A., Ljungh, A., and Rubin, K.: Specific binding of bone sialoprotein to Staphylococcus aureus isolated from patients with osteomyelitis. Eur. J. Biochem. 184:331, 1989.

164. Noonan, D. M., Horigan, E. A., Ledbetter, S. R., Vogeli, G., Sasaki, M., Yamada, Y., and Hassell, J. R.: Identification of cDNA clones encoding different domains of the basement membrane heparan sulfate proteoglycan. J. Biol. Chem. 263:16379, 1988.

165. Karlsson, K., and Marklund, S. L.: Binding of human extracellular-superoxide dismutase C to cultured cell lines and to blood cells. Lab. Invest. 60:659, 1989.

166. Schubert, D., LaCorbiere, M., Saitoh, T., and Cole, G.: Characterization of an amyloid beta precursor protein that binds heparin and contains tyrosine sulfate. Proc. Natl. Acad. Sci. U.S.A. 86:2066, 1989.

167. Klier, F. G., Cole, G., Stallcup, W., and Schubert, D.: Amyloid beta-protein precursor is associated with extracellular matrix. Brain Res. 515:336, 1990.

168. Hynes, R. O.: Integrins, a family of cell surface receptors. Cell 48:549, 1987.

169. Bolander, M. E., Young, M. F., Fisher, L. W., Yamada, Y., and Termine, J. D.: Osteonectin cDNA sequence reveals potential binding regions for calcium and hydroxyapatite and shows homologies with both a basement membrane protein (SPARC) and a serine proteinase inhibitor (ovomucoid). Proc. Natl. Acad. Sci. U.S.A. 85:2919, 1988.

170. Kluge, M., Mann, K., Dziadek, M., and Timpl, R.: Characterization of a novel calcium-binding 90-kDa glycoprotein (BM-90) shared by basement membranes and serum. Eur. J. Biochem. 193:651, 1990.

171. McVey, J. H., Nomura, S., Kelly, P., Mason, I. J., and Hogan, B. L.: Characterization of the mouse SPARC/osteonectin gene. Intron/exon organization and an unusual promoter region. J. Biol. Chem. 263:11111, 1988.

172. Vernon, R. B., and Sage, H.: The calcium-binding protein SPARC is secreted by Leydig and Sertoli cells of the adult mouse testis. Biol. Reprod. 40:1329, 1989.

173. Sage, H., Vernon, R. B., Funk, S. E., Everitt, E. A., and Angello, J.: SPARC, a secreted protein associated with cellular proliferation, inhibits cell spreading in vitro and exhibits Ca^{+2}-dependent binding to the extracellular matrix. J. Cell Biol. 109:341, 1989.

174. Sage, H., Decker, J., Funk, S., and Chow, M.: SPARC: a Ca^{2+}-binding extracellular protein associated with endothelial cell injury and proliferation. J. Mol. Cell. Cardiol. 21(Suppl. 1):13, 1989.

175. Kelm, R. J., Jr., and Mann, K. G.: Human platelet osteonectin: release, surface expression, and partial characterization. Blood 75:1105, 1990.

176. Lane, T. F., and Sage, E. H.: Functional mapping of SPARC: peptides from two distinct Ca+(+)-binding sites modulate cell shape. J. Cell Biol. 111:3065, 1990.

177. Bernfield, M., and Sanderson, R. D.: Syndecan, a developmentally regulated cell surface proteoglycan that binds extracellular matrix and growth factors. Philos. Trans. R. Soc. Lond. [Biol.] 327:171, 1990.

178. Solursh, M., Reiter, R. S., Jensen, K. L., Kato, M., and Bernfield, M.: Transient expression of a cell surface heparan sulfate proteoglycan (syndecan) during limb development. Dev. Biol. 140:83, 1990.

179. Rapraeger, A.: Transforming growth factor (type beta) promotes the addition of chondroitin sulfate chains to the cell surface proteoglycan (syndecan) of mouse mammary epithelia. J. Cell Biol. 109:2509, 1989.

180. Hayashi, K., Hayashi, M., Jalkanen, M., Firestone, J. H., Trelstad, R. L., and Bernfield, M.: Immunocytochemistry of cell surface heparan sulfate proteoglycan in mouse tissues. A light and electron microscopic study. J. Histochem. Cytochem. 35:1079, 1987.

181. Vainio, S., Jalkanen, M., and Thesleff, I.: Syndecan and tenascin expression is induced by epithelial-mesenchymal interactions in embryonic tooth mesenchyme. J. Cell Biol. 108:1945, 1989.

182. Sanderson, R. D., Lalor, P., and Bernfield, M.: B lymphocytes express and lose syndecan at specific states of differentiation. Cell Regulation 1:27, 1989.

183. Hayashi, K., Hayashi, M., Boutin, E., Cunha, G. R., Bernfield, M., and Trelstad, R. L.: Hormonal modification of epithelial differentiation and expression of cell surface heparan sulfate proteoglycan in the mouse vaginal epithelium. An immunohistochemical and electron microscopic study. Lab. Invest. 58:68, 1988.

184. Chiquet, M., and Fambrough, D. M.: Chick myotendinous antigen II. A novel extracellular glycoprotein complex consisting of large disulfide-linked subunits. J. Cell Biol. 98:1937, 1984.

185. Lightner, V. A., and Erickson, H. P.: Binding of hexabrachion (tenascin) to the extracellular matrix and substratum and its effect on cell adhesion. J. Cell Sci. 95:263, 1990.

186. Hurle, J. M., Ros, M. A., Ganan, Y., Macias, D., Critchlow, M., and Hinchliffe, J. R.: Experimental analysis of the role of ECM in the patterning of the distal tendons of the developing limb bud. Cell Differ. Dev. 30:97, 1990.

187. Preissner, K. T., Koyama, T., Muller, D., Tschopp, J., and Muller Berghaus, G.: Domain structure of the endothelial cell receptor thrombomodulin as deduced from modulation of its anticoagulant functions. Evidence for a glycosaminoglycan-dependent secondary binding site for thrombin. J. Biol. Chem. 265:4915, 1990.

188. Bourin, M. C., Lundgren Akerlund, E., and Lindahl, U.: Isolation and characterization of the glycosaminoglycan component of rabbit thrombomodulin proteoglycan. J. Biol. Chem. 265:15424, 1990.

189. Mosher, D. F.: Physiology of thrombospondin. Annu. Rev. Med. 41:85, 1990.

190. Ryan, M. C., and Sandell, L. J.: Differential expression of a cysteine-rich domain in the amino-terminal propeptide of type II (cartilage) procollagen by alternative splicing of mRNA. J. Biol. Chem. 265:10334, 1990.

191. Schuppan, D., Cantaluppi, M. C., Becker, J., Veit, A., Bunte, T., Troyer, D., Schuppan, F., Schmid, M., Ackermann, R., and Hahn, E. G.: Undulin, an extracellular matrix glycoprotein associated with collagen fibrils. J. Biol. Chem. 265:8823, 1990.

192. Zimmermann, D. R., and Ruoslahti, E.: Multiple domains of the large fibroblast proteoglycan, versican. EMBO J. 8:2975, 1989.

193. Biesecker, G.: The complement SC5b-9 complex mediates cell adhesion through a vitronectin receptor. J. Immunol. 145:209, 1990.

194. Ciambrone, G. J., and McKeown Longo, P. J.: Plasminogen activator inhibitor type I stabilizes vitronectin-dependent adhesions in HT-1080 cells. J. Cell Biol. 111:2183, 1990.

195. Seiffert, D., Wagner, N. N., and Loskutoff, D. J.: Serum-derived vitronectin influences the pericellular distribution of type 1 plasminogen activator inhibitor. J. Cell Biol. 111:1283, 1990.

196. Ehrlich, H. J., Gebbink, R. K., Keijer, J., Linders, M., Preissner, K. T., and Pannekoek, H.: Alteration of serpin specificity by a protein cofactor. Vitronectin endows plasminogen activator inhibitor 1 with thrombin inhibitory properties. J. Biol. Chem. 265:13029, 1990.

197. Bhakdi, S., Hugo, F., and Tranum Jensen, J.: Functions and relevance of the terminal complement sequence. Blut. 60:309, 1990.

198. Weiner, H. L., and Swain, J. L.: Acidic fibroblast growth factor mRNA is expressed by cardiac myocytes in culture and the protein is localized to the extracellular matrix. Proc. Natl. Acad. Sci. U.S.A. 86:2683, 1989.

199. Sporn, M. B., and Roberts, A. B.: TGB-β: problems and prospects. Cell Regulation 1:875, 1990.

200. Habenicht, A. (ed.): Growth Factors, Differentiation Factors, and Cytokines. Berlin, Heidelberg, Springer-Verlag, 1990, pp. 3–476.

201. Saksela, O., Moscatelli, D., Sommer, A., and Rifkin, D. B.: Endothelial cell–derived heparan sulfate binds basic fibroblast growth factor and protects it from proteolytic degradation. J. Cell Biol. 107:743, 1988.

202. Burgess, W. H., Bizik, J., Mehlman, T., Quarto, N., and Rifkin, D. B.: Direct evidence for methylation of arginine residues in high molecular weight forms of basic fibroblast growth factor. Cell Regulation. 2:87, 1991.

203. Ishai-Michaeli, R., Eldor, A., and Vlodavsky, I.: Heparanase activity expressed by platelets, neutrophils, and lymphoma cells releases active fibroblast growth factor from extracellular matrix. Cell Regulation 1:833, 1990.

204. Feige, J. J., Bradley, J. D., Fryburg, K., Farris, J., Cousens, L. C., Barr, P. J., and Baird, A.: Differential effects of heparin, fibronectin, and laminin on the phosphorylation of basic fibroblast growth factor by protein kinase C and the catalytic subunit of protein kinase. A. J. Cell. Biol. 109:3105, 1989.

205. Kiss, I., Bosze, Z., Szabo, P., Altanchimeg, R., Barta, E., and Deak, F.: Identification of positive and negative regulatory regions controlling expression of the cartilage matrix protein gene. Mol. Cell. Biol. 10:2432, 1990.

206. Valles, A. M., Tucker, G. C., Thiery, J. P., and Boyer, B.: Alternative patterns of mitogenesis and cell scattering induced by acidic FGF as a function of cell density in a rat bladder carcinoma cell line. Cell Regulation 1:975, 1990.

207. Morgelin, M., Paulsson, M., Malmstrom, A., and Heinegard, D.: Shared and distinct structural features of interstitial proteoglycans from different bovine tissues revealed by electron microscopy. J. Biol. Chem. 264:12080, 1989.

208. Trelstad, R. L.: Glycosaminoglycans: mortar, matrix, mentor. Lab. Invest. 53:1, 1985.

Chapter 4

Biology, Physiology, and Morphology of Bone

Clinton T. Rubin
Clement B. Sledge

Bone is an extremely complex tissue that regulates its mass and architecture to meet two critical and competing responsibilities: one structural and the other metabolic. In the first case, the skeleton provides a sophisticated framework for the body; it protects vital organs and facilitates locomotion. Second, it serves as a mineral reservoir containing 99 percent of the body's total calcium, 85 percent of its phosphorus, and 66 percent of its magnesium. It is this dual responsibility that creates conflicting goals and competing stimuli in the regulation of skeletal tissues. Metabolic aberrations such as hypocalcemia, hyperparathyroidism, endocrinopathy, and aging will put the skeleton's structural integrity at risk to ensure calcium homeostasis. On the other hand, altered functional responsibilities, such as exercise or bed rest, will stimulate the skeleton to adapt (i.e., to add or remove tissue) to these new mechanical demands. This adaptation occurs to retain a structurally optimized skeleton yet ignores the potential consequences of rapid fluctuations in serum calcium (e.g., renal lithiasis) or the metabolic burden of producing and transporting all the mineralized tissue. While metabolic processes may occur independently of the skeleton's structural functions, and vice versa, the viability of an organism is critically dependent on an intricate balance between these responsibilities. This balance is achieved via the complex and tightly regulated process of the formation and resorption of bone tissue. Beginning at the level of the cell, this chapter will cover local and systemic factors that influence bone turnover, the composition and mineralization of the matrix, the architecture and material properties of the tissue, and finally, the adaptive capacity of the skeleton. This multilevel, multidisciplinary overview is intended to provide the reader with an appreciation of both the complexity of bone and its success in serving both structural and mineral responsibilities. Ultimately, as more is known of the normal biology, physiology, and morphology of bone, an understanding of the pathogenesis and etiology of metabolic bone disease will follow.

CELLULAR BASIS OF BONE REMODELING

Bone tissue is a highly specialized, mineralized connective tissue, metabolically active and intrinsi-

cally capable of adapting to subtle changes in its physical (i.e., mechanical or electrical) environment. While the bone's toughness, hardness, and resilience to fatigue belies an inert material, the constant modeling and remodeling that occurs at the tissue level allows the obliteration of the scars left by fracture and infection, the rapid mobilization of mineral for metabolic homeostasis, and the fine adjustment of skeletal mass and morphology toward an optimal supporting structure.

The skeleton's capacity to adapt to changes in both its mechanical and its metabolic milieus is achieved through its sophisticated and integrated network of osteoregulatory cells. These cells, the osteoblasts, osteoclasts, and osteocytes, are found on all bone surfaces except those of the sinuses of the adult skull, a structure perhaps too specialized to accommodate metabolic or physical fluctuation. This cell network, or syncytium, mediates the remodeling balance of the skeleton.

It was once believed that a common stem cell ancestry existed for osteoblasts and osteoclasts. How-

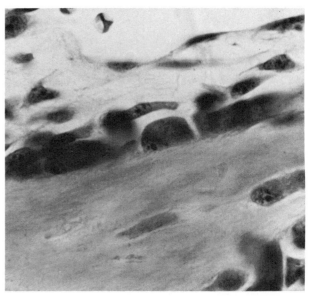

Figure 4–1. Polyhedral osteoblasts lying on the surface of newly formed bone matrix. (Courtesy of Dr. B. Boothroyd.)

ever, rather than the generic mesenchymal stem cell requiring only one level of differentiation, distinct precursors have now been identified for the differentiated cells of bone. In essence, the biphyletic origin of osteoregulatory cells ascribes a mesenchymal cell origin for the osteoblast,[1] whereas the multinucleated osteoclast arises from the fusion of mononuclear precursors of hematopoietic tissue.[2] Interestingly, it appears that the osteoclast precursor is limited to a specific hematopoietic subpopulation that markers suggest are marrow-derived cells, and is blood monocytes and tissue macrophages cannot give rise to either osteoclasts or osteoblasts.[3]

Osteoblast

These plump, cuboidal cells are connected to one another via extended cell processes connected by gap junctions[4] and morphologically exist as a single continuous cell layer on bone surfaces (Fig. 4–1). These features help distinguish osteoblasts from the mesenchymal osteoprogenitor cells (preosteoblasts), which are flat, not polygonal, but are also found on bone surfaces. Together, these two cell types are known as "bone-lining" cells. Morphologically, the tight canopy of the lining cells enables the selective isolation of the mineralized surface from the extracellular milieu, which is critical for the site-specific initiation of mineralization or resorption.[5] The cytoplastic elements of the osteoblast include abundant endoplasmic reticulum with cisternae, a well-developed Golgi body, and numerous free ribosomes; the latter are responsible for the basophilia seen in hematoxylin and eosin–stained sections. The preosteoblast lining cells contain fewer organelles and are considered inactive osteoblasts with the *potential* to modulate to the active cell type.[6]

The major function of the osteoblast is to synthesize osteoid, which is composed primarily of type I collagen and proteoglycans. The fundamental "protocollagen" is synthesized within the osteoblast on the rough endoplasmic reticulum, followed by the hydroxylation and glycosylation of lysine and proline residues to facilitate cross-linking and the formation of procollagen trimers.[7] As this step requires both vitamin C and alpha(α)-ketoglutarate,[8] a Krebs cycle by-product, collagen synthesis is directly affected by changes in the cell's level of metabolic activity. The procollagen trimers are then transported to Golgi vesicles and secreted from the dilated cisternae onto the "bone" side of the osteoblast canopy.[9] Outside the cell, the N and C terminal regions of the procallagen are cleaved, and tropocollagen is formed, organized in sheets of parallel fibers.[10] Within each sheet, or lamella, these fibers will lie predominantly parallel to each other,[11] whereas the fibril orientations on adjacent lamellae run in directions distinct from this axis (Fig. 4–2).

The functional life of the osteoblast varies, depending on the vertebrate species, ranging from 3 days in young rabbits[12] to reports of the human osteoblast surviving up to 8 weeks.[13] In humans, the typical active osteoblast will produce a seam of osteoid about 15 μm thick, at a rate of 0.5 to 1.5 μm per day,[14] suggesting the average osteoblast life in humans to be 15 days. While seams have been reported to exceed 70 μm, suggesting that the osteoblast can actively secrete osteoid throughout its life span,[15] such a seam width can also indicate a disruption or flaw in the mineralization process (e.g., rickets, osteomalacia).

As mineralization proceeds, the osteoblast may not remain an osteoblast. The osteoblast may itself become engulfed in its own osteoid matrix and, with time, will become further and further removed from the active site of secretion separated by newly recruited osteoblasts moving en masse along the mineralization front.[16] These osteoblasts that remain behind diminish their secretions of collagen and alkaline phosphatase and become osteocytes.[17]

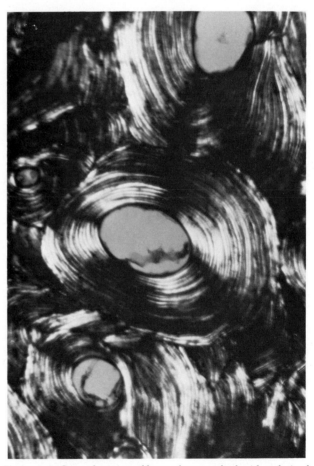

Figure 4–2. Ground section of bone photographed with polarized light showing the concentric lamellar structure of the basic unit of mature bone, the osteon. The central vascular canal (empty in this preparation) is surrounded by multiple lamellae of bone. The adjacent lamellae are composed of collagen bundles with differing orientations, giving rise to alternating light and dark bands in polarized light.

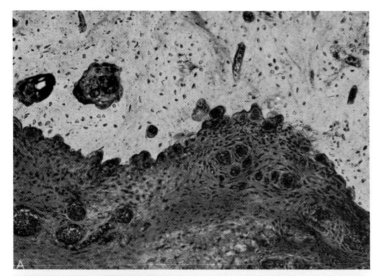

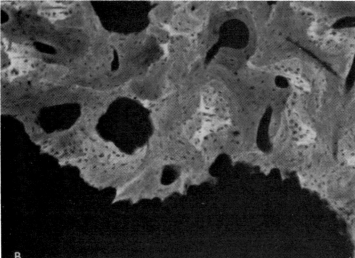

Figure 4–3. *A,* Paragon-stained mineralized section with large multinucleate osteoclasts lying along the pale-staining bone surface. *B,* Microradiograph of the same area showing Howship's lacunae in the areas of osteoclastic resorption. (From Jowsey, J., and Gordan, G.: *In* Bourne, G. H. [ed.]: The Biochemistry and Physiology of Bone. Vol. III. 2nd ed. New York, Academic Press, 1972, pp. 201–238. Used by permission.)

Osteocyte

Once presumed to be effete, aged, impotent osteoblasts entombed in their own osteoid, osteocytes are now recognized as essential to the metabolic regulation of bone tissue. Although the sequestered osteoblast entrenched in its lacuna will lose cell organelles and actually shrink as it modulates to an osteocyte, it retains a sophisticated communication network with other osteocytes and bone lining cells through an extensive system of cytoplasmic extensions that pass through a network of catacombs radiating outward from the central vascular canal (see Fig. 4–4). These interconnecting canaliculi are ideal pathways for chemical, electrical, and stress-generated fluid communication through the dense bone matrix.[18] The volume of bone occupied by this syncytium is approximately 5 percent by the canaliculi network and 2 percent for the lacunar spaces.[19] The surface area of the lacunar and canalicular system has been estimated to be at least 250 meters^2 (m^2) per liter of calcified bone matrix and communicates with a submicroscopic, interfibrillar space representing 35,000 mm^2 per mm^3. Thus, exchange of minerals, nutrients, and chemical and physical stimuli through this enormous network could be both rapid and substantial and is certainly essential to the homeostatic control of the skeleton. With such critical regulatory responsibility, and boasting such an extensive communication network, the osteocyte's reputation as irrelevant and "dilettantish" is clearly inappropriate.

Osteoclast

Where existing bone tissue is being removed, these large, motile, multinucleate cells are found proliferating in irregular scalloped cavities known as Howship's lacunae or cutting cones (Fig. 4–3). Although derived from hematopoietic mononuclear cells, by the time these cells have differentiated to the ravenous bone consumer, they can be as large as 200,000 μm^2 and contain as many as 100 nuclei, many derived from pre-existing cells in the area.[20] An osteoclast's speed is matched only by its appetite.

These giant multinucleated cells can travel up to 100 μm per day and can resorb a cavity 300 μm in diameter, containing 200,000 $μm^3$ of bone. Within this volume of bone, three to six osteocytes will vanish and require seven to ten generations of osteoblasts to follow and fill the resorption space.[21]

Clinical[22] and laboratory[23] observations have confirmed a two-stage link between marrow progenitor cells and osteoclasts. Some believe that the circulating monocyte, which can be the precursor of the tissue macrophage, may subsequently become an osteoclast.[24] As they are formed from mononuclear cells and require a steady supply of new nuclei, the life span and ultimate fate of the osteoclast are uncertain. While tissue culture experiments suggest a life span of approximately 2 or 3 days,[25] experiments in the rat[26] and dog[27] suggest that the mean life span of the osteoclast nuclei can be as long as 12 days. Interestingly, these studies suggest that the constant supply of new precursor cells is derived locally, perhaps from osteocytes, rather than from circulating cells, the original source of the giant cell precursor.[28] Whatever their origin, they certainly must be readily accessible. Increased numbers of osteoclasts can be seen within 17 to 24 hours after injection of parathyroid hormone into experimental animals.[29] In less volatile skeletal alterations such as disuse, it may take as long as 7 days to recruit these cells.[30]

The portion of this polarized giant cell that is actively consuming the bone matrix is called the subosteoclastic space and is characterized by a ruffled border comprising many cytoplasmic folds. This active site of bone resorption is encompassed by a clear zone, where it is believed that the osteoclast uses integrins[31] to anchor to matrix-bound proteins, such as osteopontin,[32] to encase and seal the zone of bone destruction. It appears that osteoclasts are unable to bind to either the unmineralized osteoid surfaces or the bone tissue still enveloped by the osteoblast canopy.[33] This suggests that for resorption to progress the bone mineral itself must be exposed and therefore vulnerable to the giant cell. Considering the damage that a population of unregulated osteoclasts could induce on a bone surface, it is fortunate that such site-specific control of resorption is possible.

The cytoplasm of an active osteoclast is often foamy, owing to the large number of digestive vacuoles and vesicles and the numerous lysosomal bodies that contain histochemically demonstrable acid hydrolases.[34] When these acids contact the bone matrix, they leach out the mineral scaffold via a complex chemical dissolution process.[35] Briefly, intracellular carbonic anhydrase degrades carbonic acid to produce hydrogen ions. These protons are actively removed from the cell via a proton pumping ATPase. The protons accumulate within the confined subosteoclastic space, lowering the pH of this micromilieu to a level sufficient to dissolve the mineral phase of the matrix (pH of 2 to 4) and activate osteoclastic hydrolytic enzymes. The organic matrix that remains is subsequently dissolved by lysosomal enzymes (e.g., cathepsin B) released across the ruffled border, leaving only the osteoclast's signature scalloped resorption cavities.[36] As the excavation proceeds, the ionized calcium levels just beyond the clear zone will elevate from a basal level of 1 to 2 mM to as high as 20 mM.[37] This increase in extracellular calcium stimulates mobilization of osteoclast intracellular calcium,[38] decreasing the cell's motility and facilitating its detachment. Thus, not only is the site of osteoclastic resorption carefully controlled by osteoblasts, but also the extent of their resorption is autoregulated by factors such as the level of calcium adjacent to the periphery of the subosteoclastic space.

SYSTEMIC REGULATION OF BONE CELL METABOLISM

Bone formation and resorption not only is regulated at the local level but also is controlled by systemic factors. For example, as already discussed, osteoclasts are incapable of independently resorbing bone unless the osteoid lining is first removed. This denuding is typically accomplished via proteases such as collagenase, an enzyme that osteoclasts do not produce. However, in the presence of the systemic parathyroid hormone (PTH), osteoblasts will produce collagenase and may actually secrete it complexed with a peptide inhibitor of collagenase,[39] further facilitating the *resorptive* process.

PTH

Many systemic factors play a critical role in the regulation of bone metabolism, even though it could easily be argued that the principal responsibility of these peptide or steroid hormones is to regulate mineral homeostasis rather than to focally control skeletal morphology. For example, a primary function of PTH is to maintain serum ionized calcium levels within a narrow physiologic range. Serum calcium levels below 6 mg/dl elevate PTH stimulation, whereas levels above 10 mg/dl suppress secretion and indicate primary hyperparathyroidism.[40] Considering that the major reservoir of the body's calcium is the skeleton, the most expedient avenue for PTH to regulate calcium levels is to directly target bone tissue. By stimulating osteoclast activity and, in turn, bone resorption, PTH will ultimately release calcium and phosphate into the metabolic milieu. Ironically, attempts to stimulate osteoclast activity solely with PTH and independent of osteoblasts have not been successful.[41] However, PTH receptors do exist on the the membrane of *osteoblasts*, and their exposure to this hormone will stimulate substantial morphologic and metabolic changes in both osteoblasts and osteoclasts.[42] PTH elevates osteoblast activity by stimulating accumulation of cAMP and by mobilization of cytosolic calcium ion, both of which serve as second messengers.[43] Although PTH receptors do not exist on osteoclasts,[44] these cells are activated within minutes of osteoblast exposure to PTH. Elevated PTH will also convert vitamin D into 1,25-dihydroxyvitamin D, its physiologically relevant metabolite, which in turn stimulates intestinal calcium absorption. Thereby, PTH contributes to maintaining serum calcium level via both direct and indirect interactions with the skeleton.

Vitamin D

Vitamin D is another systemic factor that plays a critical role in both bone remodeling and calcium homeostasis. Brief exposure of the skin (10 to 20 minutes) to ultraviolet light (sun) will endogenously produce sufficient quantities of vitamin D_3 from 7-dehydrocholesterol. Diet is the principal source of its isomer, vitamin D_2. In a series of steps, these fat-soluble vitamins are first hydroxylated to 25-hydroxyvitamin D, biologically inactive but the most abundant of the vitamin D metabolites. In the kidney, 25-hydroxyvitamin D is further hydroxlyated to 1,25-dihydroxyvitamin D. Often referred to as calcitriol, 1,25-dihydroxyvitamin D stimulates intestinal absorption of calcium, thereby elevating serum calcium concentrations and establishing a positive milieu for the mineralization of new bone. It is important to emphasize that the principal role of vitamin D is to regulate calcium levels in the serum—its concern with the maintenance of bone mass appears secondary. Even though the presence of vitamin D may promote bone formation via elevated serum calcium, it also facilitates bone *resorption* by stimulating differentiation of osteoclast precursors to the mature osteoclast.[45] Clearly, by influencing both the calcium levels and the resident bone cell population, vitamin D has a complex but important role in both the formation and the resorption of bone.[46]

Estrogen

The rapid decline of skeletal mass following the menopause underscores the critical regulatory role of estrogens in bone cell metabolism. Indeed, recent identification of estrogen receptors within osteoblasts[47, 48] demonstrates these bone cells to be a direct target of this steroid. Elevated estrogen levels will both increase osteoblast proliferation[49] and attenuate the osteoblast response to PTH.[50] In addition, estrogens will increase both osteoblastic collagen gene expression[49] and insulin growth factor$_2$ (IGF$_2$) production.[51] Although estrogen interactions are not so relevant to the skeletons of males, androgen receptors have been identified within the osteoblast of males,[52] and androgens will affect these cells in a manner similar to that of estrogens.[53] Considering the ever-escalating percentage of our population that is elderly, and the severe social, clinical, and eco-

nomic burden caused by type I and II osteopenia,[54] it is clear that an improved understanding of the effects of estrogen-androgen interactions on the formation and resorption of bone will benefit the treatment of these skeletal disorders.

Prostaglandins

In response to hormonal stimuli, osteoblasts also secrete prostaglandin E_2 (PGE$_2$), a stimulator of both bone formation and resorption, as well as serving as an osteoclast-tactic factor.[55] Although PGE$_2$ and PTH stimulate the same second messengers in osteoblasts, PGE$_2$ can also influence osteoclasts directly. PGE$_2$ stimulates several second messenger responses in bone cells, including an increase in cytosolic calcium, elevated cAMP production, and activation of the phosphatidylinositol pathway.[56] Therefore, variable levels of PGE$_2$ directly modulate the response of both forming and resorbing cells both locally and systemically.

Calcitonin

Calcitonin is a calcium regulatory hormone that works independently of either PTH or vitamin D levels and possesses a potent capacity to modulate serum calcium and phosphate levels.[57] Similar to the regulation of PTH secretion from parathyroid cells, serum calcium levels regulate the secretion of calcitonin from parafollicular, or "C," cells of the thyroid. In contrast with PTH secretion, which is inversely proportional to serum calcium levels, calcitonin secretion is directly related to serum calcium; as serum Ca goes up, calcitonin secretion follows.[58] Unlike the case with PTH or 1,25-dihydroxyvitamin D, receptors for calcitonin do exist on osteoclasts.[59] A marked decrease in osteoclast metabolic activity will result following exposure to calcitonin,[60] an effect potentiated by phosphodiesterase inhibitors such as theophylline, which inhibit the degradation of cAMP.[61] Calcitonin also increases cytosolic calcium in osteoclasts, which contributes to considerable contraction of these cells following exposure.[62] Therefore, calcitonin effects are mediated by two second messengers, cAMP and cytosolic calcium, are specific for osteoclasts, are mediated by serum calcium levels, and work essentially by defusing the cell. The efficacy of calcitonin in inhibiting osteoclast activity in vitro has been used as a basis to consider this peptide as a prophylaxis for osteopenia. While the potential use of calcitonin as treatment for metabolic bone disease is high, its efficacy in vivo remains controversial.[63]

Growth Factors

Osteoblasts also produce a number of growth factors that are critical to the process of bone formation, remodeling, and repair. For example, insulin-like growth factor I (somatomedin C) directly stimulates osteoblast replication and function.[64] Another osteoblast stimulator, transforming growth factor-beta (TGF-β), is released by the matrix during the process of bone resorption,[65] establishing a protective feedback loop, or coupled response, for osteoblast and osteoclast activity. Not only does this growth factor increase levels of osteoblast activity,[66] but also it appears to inhibit differentiation and maturation of osteoclast precursors.[67] Although our understanding of growth factors is only embryonic, considering their potency in the remodeling process and the possibility of using recombinant techniques to produce them, these peptides are certain to make a major contribution to the treatment of skeletal disorders.

T Lymphocytes

While the actual signals responsible for the control of stem cell modulation and progenitor differentiation have not been identified, there is clear evidence that both physical and chemical cues can influence these processes. Vitamin D not only affects the differentiation of pleuripotential stem cells along osteoblast or osteoclast lines but also influences the production of T lymphocytes in the immune system.[68] This suggests normal T cell function to be necessary for the regulation of calcium. In support of this postulation, many congenital osseous abnormalities have been shown to be associated with disorders of the immune system.[69] Thus, vitamin D seems to "coax" marrow cells along a specific monocyte line that also expresses receptors for the vitamin. At some point, these receptors disappear and the monocytes coalesce into osteoclasts.[70] Concurrent with this modulation, the presence of vitamin D on T lymphocytes also stimulates the production of kinins, PGE$_2$, and osteoclast activating factors,[71] which catalyze osteoblast shrinkage via microtubule disaggregation, which, in turn, exposes the underlying matrix. The resorptive process is accelerated by the osteoblastic production of plasminogen activator, which initiates a cascade via plasminogen, plasmin, and precollagenase to produce collagenase.[72]

Biophysical Stimuli

Vitamin D, PGE$_2$, steroids and other systemic "chemical" factors play vital roles in the determination of the modulation of cell types and skeletal modeling and remodeling. However, one of the most potent influences in the development and maintenance of the skeleton is physical (mechanical-electrical) factors. To put the role of these chemical mediators in perspective, it is appropriate to acknowledge physical factors as a critical control mechanism in the regulation of tissue differentiation and in tissue growth, repair, and remodeling.[73] Physical stimuli as potent determinants of skeletal morphology have even been postulated as a primary regulator of chondro-osseous morphogenesis.[74] The influence of physical stimuli on the formation and resorption of bone is discussed in detail later in this chapter.

In summary, while seemingly contradictory, *osteoblasts* are required for the site-specific regulation of bone *resorption*, while *deposition* of bone is often preceded by a period of *osteoclast* recruitment and activity. Thus, a cellular symbiosis exists in which an integrated "activation, resorption, reversal, and formation," or ARRF, occurs that reflects intricate control of both cell lines,[75] coupling the turnover of bone (Fig. 4–4). To initiate this sequence, monocyte "preosteoclasts" are chemotactically attracted to remodeling areas via specific receptors for chemical factors.[76] Remodeling of bone begins by mononuclear preosteoclasts activating an otherwise quiescent site populated by inactive lining cells that have exposed some portion of the matrix.[77] The multinucleated osteoclasts begin the resorption cycle, creating Howship's lacunae. When resorption is completed, new bone formation begins, leaving a boundary that is visible in histologic sections as a "reversal line." When the resorbed bone is replaced by new bone, the reversal line clearly demarcates this junction.[78] This "pocket" of new bone is known as a bone modeling unit (BMU).[79] A similar line, called a "cement line," is seen between the adjacent lamellae of bone (Fig. 4–5).

COMPOSITION OF THE BONE MATRIX

Bone is composed of inorganic mineral (70 percent of weight), organic matrix and cells (25 percent), and water (5 percent). Before its calcification, newly synthesized bone matrix is essentially completely organic and is called osteoid. Collagen is the predominant organic component in bone, accounting for approximately 94 percent of the unmineralized matrix. Other noncollagenous proteins unique to bone are found in osteoid, accounting for approximately 4 percent of its weight. These include glycoproteins and phosphoproteins such as osteonectin,[80] sialoproteins, which are predominantly osteopontin,[81] bone Gla protein, also called BGP or osteocalcin,[82] and bone morphogenetic protein.[83] Extracts of bone also include enzymes, hormones, growth factors, and other metabolites essential for bone metabolism.[84] Bone cells, for all their responsibility to mineral and structural homeostasis, constitute only 2 percent of the organic tissue's constituents. While beyond the scope of this chapter, an extensive review by Robey[85] on the biochemistry of bone provides a detailed discussion of the function and inter-relatedness of these matrix components.

Collagen

Bone collagen (see Chapter 2) is essentially all type I and resembles other type I collagens found in

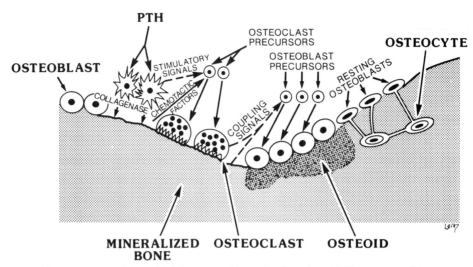

Figure 4–4. Sequence of bone turnover (*left to right*): Bone-resorbing stimuli such as PTH cause osteoblasts to retract from the bone surface and secrete collagenase, thereby initiating bone breakdown. Mononuclear osteoclast precursors are activated by chemotactic factors and by stimulatory signals from the osteoblasts. Multinucleated osteoclasts then form and begin to resorb bone. Coupling signals from the osteoclasts and bone matrix stimulate the formation of new osteoblasts from precursors. These new osteoblasts deposit bone protein matrix (osteoid) oriented along lines of physical stress. The osteoid is then mineralized to form mature bone. "Retired" osteoblasts remain either as resting osteoblasts (lining cells) on the bone surface or as osteocytes embedded within lacunae. The osteocytes and osteoblasts are interconnected by an extensive network of cytoplasmic extensions.

skin and tendon. The basic unit of bone collagen, the tropocollagen molecule, is a triple helix of three polypeptide (α) chains, each of approximately 1000 amino acids.[86] By stabilizing these soluble molecules with cross-links of hydroxylysine and lysine, the bone collagen fibrils become essentially insoluble.[87] Type I collagen differs from the type II collagen of cartilage in several salient aspects. All of the three α-chains of type II collagen are identical to each other, yet their amino acid composition is different from that of any of the three (one pair, one unique) α-chains of the type I tropocollagen of bone.[88] As

compared with type I, the chains of type II contain much more glycosylated hydroxylysine, making cartilage all the more resistant to degradation by collagenase.

The triple helix of type I collagen forms a linear molecule approximately 300 nm long.[89] Each molecule is aligned parallel to the next, producing a collagen fibril. Within the collagen fibril, gaps called "hole zones" exist between the end of one molecule and the beginning of the next. It is thought that noncollagenous proteins reside in these spaces, which chemotactically attract and initiate the miner-

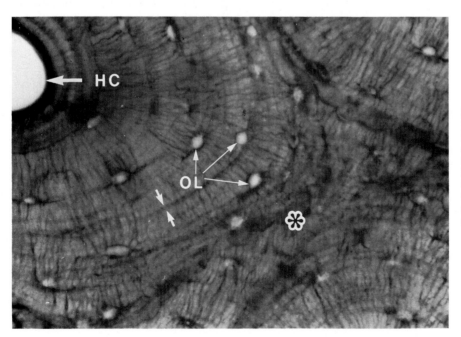

Figure 4–5. Ground section of bone photographed in normal light showing empty osteocyte lacunae (OL) connected by fine darkly stained canaliculi. The central haversian canal (HC) is seen in the upper left hand corner; the reversal line (*) marking the junction between two adjacent osteons and the cement line ($\rightarrow \leftarrow$) separating adjacent lamellae are seen.

alization process.[90] The fibrils are further grouped in bundles to form the collagen fiber.

Proteoglycans

Proteoglycans are the principal noncollagenous protein in the mineralized matrix (see Chapter 3). They are the major macromolecule of the ground substance, consisting of approximately 95 percent polysaccharide (glycosaminoglycans) and 5 percent protein. This molecule, similar in structure to the cartilage proteoglycan, consists of a thin protein core with multiple covalently bound glycosaminoglycan chains[91] composed of repeating disaccharide units of the amino sugars chondroitin sulfate, keratan sulfate, and hyaluronate.[92] While the role of these proteins in bone has not been determined, it has been proposed that they may actually store load information following functional activity, serving as a form of strain memory.[93] Proteoglycans protrude into canalicular spaces and even touch osteocyte membranes. These molecules deform rapidly in response to load, yet re-establish their original orientation relatively slowly. Although somewhat speculative, this matrix-cell interaction may well serve as a signal transduction mechanism to transfer mechanical information from the matrix to the adjacent osteocytes.

Osteonectin

Glycoprotein matrix molecules such as osteonectin serve as binding catalysts between the extracellular matrix and cell processes.[94] The acidic PO_4 complexes on these glycoproteins bind to collagen and have a high affinity for calcium and hydroxyapatite,[95] suggesting their direct role in mineral formation. It is thought that the acidic phospholipids of osteonectin first form on matrix vesicles to facilitate collagen-mediated nucleation and perhaps serve as seeding sites for mineralization at the collagen fibril "hole zones."[96]

Osteocalcin

Also present in the matrix are substantial quantities of osteocalcin, constituting 1 to 2 percent of the total bone protein. Osteocalcin synthesis takes place in the osteoblasts during the carboxylation of glutamate, a vitamin K–dependent reaction.[97] 1,25-Dihydroxyvitamin D will enhance the synthesis of this noncollagenous protein, further evidence that vitamin D has a direct stimulatory effect on osteoblasts.[98] The function of this protein remains unclear, but it has been postulated to play a role in both osteoclast recruitment and bone formation.[99] As osteocalcin is the only protein known to be made exclusively by osteoblasts, serum osteocalcin levels are considered an accurate reflection of bone formation activity.[100]

Hydroxyapatite

Bone mineral is generically referred to as hydroxyapatite $[Ca_{10}(PO_4)_6(OH)_2]$, a plate-like crystal 20 to 80 nm long and 2 to 5 nm thick. Bone hydroxyapatite is quite different from naturally occurring apatite, containing a number of impurities, including sodium, fluorine, strontium, lead, and radium. It is smaller than natural apatites (100 vs. 400 angstroms [Å]) and more reactive and soluble because of its less perfect atomic arrangement. The nucleation sites of bone mineral may not be the plates of hydroxyapatite but more energetically favorable crystal spicules such as amorphous calcium phosphate (ACP) or octacalcium phosphate (OCP).[101] It is believed that these unstable precursors are formed first and are gradually transformed to the more crystalline hydroxyapatite. The enormous surface area of ACP, with its hydration shell, provides an immense face for mineral exchange. This is reflected in the greater avidity of new bone for "bone-seeking" isotopes (technetium, fluorine, strontium) and perhaps explains the greater rate of calcium exchange in young as opposed to old subjects. It has also been demonstrated that bone mineral continues to mature through an individual's lifetime,[102] becoming more and more "perfect" and thus exposing less surface area for a given volume of mineral. The process of crystal maturity has been suggested as contributing to the etiology of osteopenia[103]; not only will greater levels of systemic factors be needed to liberate calcium from the more stable crystal, but stress-generated zeta potentials will attenuate as a function of the diminished surface area of the mineral constituents. The magnitude of these potentials, generated by the ionic constituents of the fluid flowing by the charged phase of the mineral, will proportionally drop as less mineral is exposed at the micro-boundary layer.

MINERALIZATION OF BONE TISSUE

The mineralization of bone normally begins only after the organic osteoid matrix has been laid down for a period of 10 to 15 days. At this point, mineral increases almost immediately to 70 percent of the ultimate content, whereas deposition of the final 30 percent takes several months.[104] The process of mineralization is an extremely complex, temporally dynamic process, and is a subject of intense study.[105] There is emerging evidence that hydroxyapatite deposition and seeding of mineralization is strongly dependent on both cartilage- and bone-derived macromolecules such as osteonectin, phosphoproteins, and proteolipids. Surprisingly, the initial sites of calcium-phosphate nucleation in growing bone fracture callus, and calcifying cartilage appear not to be at the bone surface but on the processes of matrix vesicles.[106] Matrix vesicles are small, round, extracellular lipid-bilaminar bound organelles that bud from hypertrophic chondrocytes or osteoblasts undergoing the process of apoptosis[107] as well as from cell processes originating from the plasma membrane.[108] There is a definite polarity to the vesicles, with mineralization occurring in a predictable and organized way adjacent to the requisite phosphatases on the inner leaflet of the membrane.[109] The matrix vesicles contain alkaline phosphatase, ATPase, inorganic pyrophosphatase, 5'-nucleotidase, and ATP-pyrophosphohydrolase[110] in addition to phospholipids (especially phosphatidylserine), which have a strong affinity for calcium ions.[111] It is believed that these ions accumulate in the matrix vesicle because of their affinity for the phospholipids and a membrane-bound calcium pump. At a point of supersaturation, nucleation of the mineral begins.[112]

Nucleation

Alkaline phosphatase, a biosynthetic product of osteoblasts, is present in very high concentrations during development and osteoid production.[113] While the regulatory role of this disulfide-linked dimer is not known, it has been postulated that its presence may increase local concentrations of P and thereby facilitate hydroxyapatite deposition.[114] Increasing the concentration of P in the micromilieu will exceed the local solubility product and catalyze deposition along the inner leaflet of the vesicle. Following this accretion, the destruction of the membrane has been attributed to an increasing concentration of lysophospholipids within the matrix vesicles, suggesting that they are programmed to self-destruct.[115] Following dissolution of the matrix vesicle membrane, the hydroxyapatite crystals are exposed to the extravesicular environment, where additional mineral accretes to the newly formed crystal.[116] The crystal is then believed to chemotactically move toward and preferentially bind at the hole zones between collagen fibrils, precipitated by the nesting osteonectin[117] and fibronectin.[118] Mineralization proceeds and extends over the collagen matrix, with the long axis of the hydroxyapatite crystal parallel to the collagen fiber. The arrangement of the collagen matrix that is synthesized during osteoblast activity ultimately determines the orientation of the bone mineral crystals.[88]

In the extravesicular milieu, glycosaminoglycans *inhibit* the calcification process by modulating the advancing mineral front.[119] Indeed, it may be just these proteoglycan macromolecules, found in high concentrations in noncalcifying collagenous structures such as ligament, tendon, and skin, that may prevent mineral deposition.[120] Other theories for the noncalcification of dense connective tissues include the tighter packing of their collagen fibrils, impeding the access of phosphate ions to the interfibrillar nucleation sites, and the existence of crystallization inhibitors such as pyrophosphate, present in synovial fluid, plasma, and urine at concentrations sufficient to prevent deposition of calcium carbonates.[121] Once

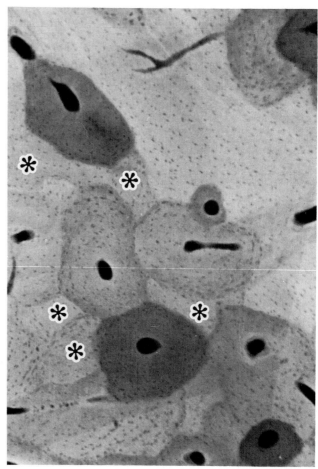

Figure 4–6. Microradiograph of cortical bone showing osteons in varying degrees of mineralization with numerous interstitial fragments (*).

the concentration of these inhibitors reaches a threshold, mineralization is halted, leaving a thin layer of osteoid between the lining cells and the mineralization front. This establishes the syncytium, or cellular canopy, that must be retracted to reinitiate ARRF.

Turnover

In undecalcified ground sections, microradiography demonstrates subtle differences in the calcium content of the bone tissue, thus allowing separation into "old" or "new" bone based on contrast intensity (Fig. 4–6). For example, young osteons, in the process of formation, have large central vascular canals that narrow with infilling, showing progressively less mineralization toward the center. This contrasts sharply with the active tunneling process of resorption, in which case the inside rim of the osteon appears as equally mineralized as the outer rings. Static remodeling parameters such as osteoid seam width, number of resorptive events, and number of formative events can thus be inferred from these morphologic characteristics. By using double fluorescent labels (e.g., tetracyclines), administered at spe-

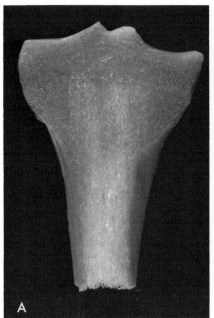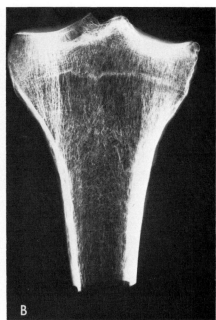

Figure 4–7. *A*, Macerated preparation of the human knee showing the trabecular structure that supports the flared articular surface. *B*, Radiograph of the specimen shown in *A*.

cific intervals, dynamic parameters of bone remodeling can be determined (i.e., rates of turnover, infilling, and formation). Static and dynamic histomorphometry, quantified via biopsy specimens harvested from areas such as the iliac crest, are extremely powerful means of evaluating the systemic state of the skeleton.[122]

The complex composite nature of bone achieved through the secretion of the collagen matrix and its subsequent mineralization is a product of the synergistic inter-relationships of the cell types, the systemic regulators of calcium metabolism, and the matrix-bound proteins that locally control bone remodeling. The product of this sophisticated and interdependent process is an extremely successful tissue that serves as both a structural organ and a mineral reservoir.

ARCHITECTURE OF BONE

Bones are remarkably well suited for their structural role. At the gross level, as hollow tubes they derive maximal strength from minimal weight.[123] Descending to the next structural level, cortical and cancellous morphology is strategically arranged to evenly distribute functional stresses.[124] Lower still, the arrangement of the collagen within the cancellous or cortical bone, combined with the two-phase composite matrix of the collagen and mineral, provides both tensile and compressive strength.[125] The ultimate tensile strength of bone approaches that of cast iron, its capacity to absorb and release energy is twice that of oak, yet the weight of bone is only one third that of steel. And while proving a resilient and resistant material, this tissue's capacity to remodel, adapt, and repair itself is what identifies bone as the ultimate biomaterial. The structural success of skeletal morphology can be examined at a series of levels:

1. its gross anatomy and functional responsibility,
2. its ultrastructural morphology (cortical or cancellous),
3. its microscopic organization (lamellar or woven), and
4. its mineralization process (enchondral or intramembranous).

Macroscopic Organization

At the gross, structural level, each bone has a diverse and distinct morphology. Regardless of function, each bone is composed of dense cortical bone (e.g., diaphyseal shaft), and cancellous bone such as the trabecular cascades found in the neck of the femur or the metaphysis of the proximal tibia (Fig. 4–7). At the microscopic level, two types of bone are identified: the disorganized, hypercellular woven bone and the highly organized, relatively hypocellular lamellar bone. Essentially all bone tissue can be described by either of these two morphologies, whether mature, growing, pathologic, or healing.

Woven bone is a product of rapid bone formation and architecturally has an irregular, disorganized pattern of collagen orientation and osteocyte distribution (Fig. 4–8). While woven bone is characteristic of embryonic and fetal development, it is also found in the healthy adult skeleton at ligament and tendon insertions as well as in specific disease states such as Paget's disease, osteogenic sarcoma, and metastases. Under less severe pathologic conditions (fracture callus, inflammatory responses, stress fractures),

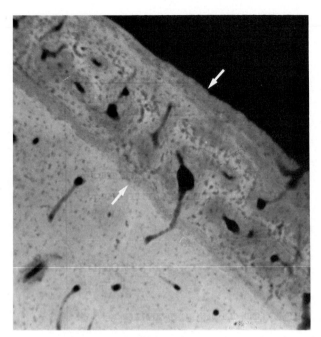

Figure 4–8. Outer cortex of bone showing the results of rapid periosteal bone formation producing woven bone, followed by the slower formation of primary osteons surrounding blood vessels.

woven bone will usually be reabsorbed and replaced by lamellar bone within a few weeks of its deposition.[126]

Microscopic Organization

Lamellar, or mature, bone may be packed tightly to form the dense cortex of a bone or may be organized as the trabecular struts in cancellous bone (Fig. 4–9). In contrast with the random and disorganized structure of woven bone, the lamellar appearance of this mature bone is the product of highly organized mineralized plates. In trabecular bone, the lamellae run parallel to the trabeculae. In cortical bone, several patterns occur. The predominant one is that found in osteons, which are made up of small concentric lamellar cylinders surrounding a central vascular channel, not unlike the rings in a tree trunk. Osteons are typically 200 to 300 μm in diameter, consisting of as many as six or seven concentric osteocyte rings composed of up to 20 lamellar plates.[127] Canaliculi in lamellar bone are consistent in diameter and orientation and in toto contain fewer osteocytes per unit volume than does woven bone (20,000 cells per μm^3 vs. 80,000 cells per μm^3).

During growth in diameter, new bone must be added appositionally. Following formation of the periosteal cuff about the primary center of ossification, bone increases its diameter by one of two methods. During rapid growth, spicules of new woven bone are formed perpendicular to the surface, allowing maximal radial expansion with minimal material. The gaps between the spicules are subsequently filled in and consolidated by the formation of lamellar bone.[128] In this process, individual periosteal blood vessels that lay in the valley of the spicules are surrounded by the encroaching new lamellar formation, creating primary osteons parallel to the long axis of the bone. An osteon that has formed de novo, as in the woven bone consolidation process just referred to, is known as a primary osteon. If this occurs intracortically via a resorptive

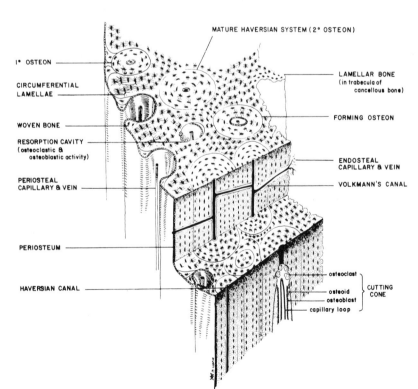

Figure 4–9. Diagrammatic representation of the structure of human cortical bone.

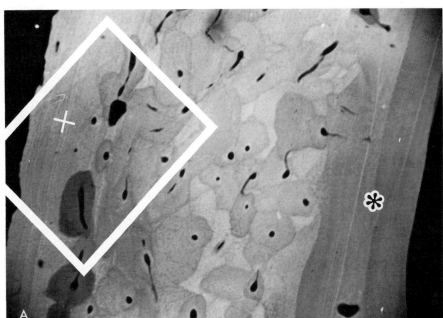

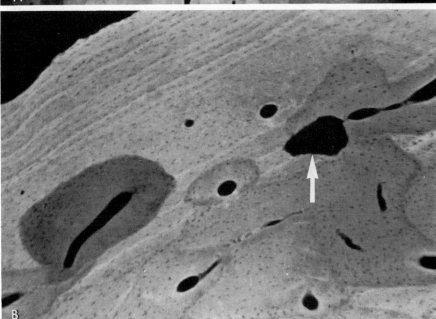

Figure 4–10. *A*, Microradiograph of the full thickness of cortical bone showing outer (+) and inner (*) circumferential lamellae with concentric (osteonal) bone in the center. *B*, Enlarged section of a portion of *A* showing resorption cavity (→) with irregular margins "burrowing" into the older circumferential lamellar bone.

process to *replace* pre-existing bone tissue, it is referred to as a secondary osteon, or haversian system, and constitutes the bulk of adult human bone[129] (Fig. 40–10*A*).

When slow diametric growth occurs, seams of new bone are laid appositionally on the existing surface (Fig. 4–10*B*). As discussed previously, the birefringent pattern of both circumferential lamellae and single osteons is believed to be produced by the altering of collagen bundle direction from one layer to the next, therefore maximizing strength in a number of different planes. Although the collagen bundles within each of these lamellar plates are highly oriented, individual fibers will often traverse inter-

lamellar spaces. Such a composite integration will increase both the individual osteon's resistance to external loads and the effective strength of the bone structure.[130] An alternative theory for the polarized light birefringence of an osteon is based on fiber-rich, fiber-poor lamellar rings, in which the thinner (1 to 2 μm) plates contain a greater degree of glycosaminoglycans (ground substance) than the adjacent 5- to 7-μm collagen-rich layers.[131] These glycosaminoglycans are thought to be continuous from the "thin" lamellar plate, through the cement line, to interdigitate with the ground substance of the "thick" plate. This architecture, with a true continuity between plates, would produce an increase in the stiffness of each osteon or each circumferential plate. Perhaps the morphology of lamellar bone will prove to be some combination of these two postulations, thus maximizing both the stiffness of the material (continuity of ground substance) and its toughness (integration of collagen layers).

Cortical Drifts

If periosteal surface modeling were to occur in the absence of endosteal resorption, the overall thickness of the cortex would increase with increasing age, leaving too much bone and too little marrow space. Fortunately, the increasing periosteal diameter is directly coordinated with a concomitant increase in the diameter of the endosteal envelope, achieved through resorption at this inner surface.[132] Although these rapid surface drifts diminish in the mature skeleton, they rise again in the elderly population. In the aged skeleton, the rate of surface erosion of the endosteal surface exceeds the formation rate of the periosteum, resulting in a net decrease in total bone mass. However, this age-related expansion of the cortex establishes a biomechanical compensatory mechanism via the concurrent increase in the cross-sectional moments of inertia, resulting in an increased capacity of the bone to resist bending loads.[133]

Metaphyseal Reshaping

During growth in length, the inverse to the above can occur. As the metaphysis and diaphysis elongate, resorption at the *periosteal* surface must be closely coordinated with deposition at the endosteum, a process known as metaphyseal reshaping.[134] Under these circumstances, some of the cortical bone within the epiphyseal shell is spared and subsequently becomes a component of the cancellous structure within the metaphysis (Fig. 4–11). Where fragments of osteons as well as new lamellae and abundant cement lines are seen, the ultrastructural organization of trabeculae reflects their cortical origin (Fig. 4–12).

Haversian Remodeling

Bone remodeling is a process of "real time" tissue replacements. In places, trabeculae are covered with osteoblasts making new bone, while in others osteoclasts are eroding the surface. By this process of resorption and formation, orientation of the trabeculae can be rapidly altered to accommodate changes in manner of loading or shifts in alignment secondary to disease or fracture.[135] To remodel cortical bone such that intracortical damage or dead tissue can be replaced, the cortex must first be

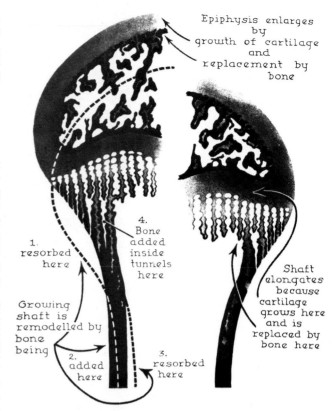

Figure 4–11. Diagram of the articular end of the bone showing the process of addition of new bone and removal of old bone that allows the articular end to increase in size while maintaining its shape during longitudinal growth. (From Ham, A. W.: Some histophysiological problems peculiar to calcified tissues. J. Bone Joint Surg. 34A:701, 1952. Used by permission.)

resorbed from within, thus creating a surface for apposition. Haversian systems' replacement or remodeling of existing bone is not necessarily achieved through the identical pathway of the original osteon. Indeed, these secondary osteons can persist directly through an existing arrangement of osteons and circumferential lamellae, leaving only remnants of these pre-existing structures. These fragments of lamellar or woven bone are called interstitial lamellae (see Fig. 4–6). As the structural integrity of the bone must be preserved during this remodeling, this replacement process must be undertaken with close integration between resorption and formation. For the strength of each skeletal element to be retained, the cutting cone of the osteoclast must be followed rapidly by a capillary and the simultaneous intrusion of a population of osteoblasts infilling the lamellar rings of the secondary osteon (see Fig. 4–10B). As discussed previously, matrix bound proteins such as TGF-β that are released via the resorption process are critical to the close integration of this coupling process.

Although levels of intracortical remodeling may be elevated by changes in the organism's nutritional status (calcium deficiency),[136] endocrine balance (hy-

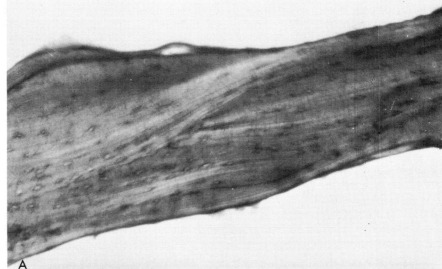

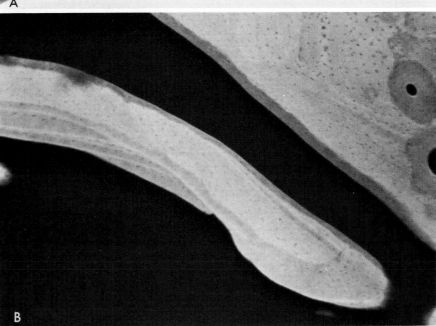

Figure 4–12. *A,* Ground section of cancellous bone showing a single trabecula composed of multiple lamellae of bone and numerous osteocytes. *B,* Microradiograph of a trabecula adjacent to the inner cortex of bone. Growth of the trabecula by the addition of new seams of lamellar bone is clearly seen.

perparathyroidism),[137] or even aging (type II osteopenia),[103] one of the most potent stimuli for remodeling is alterations in the organism's level of physical activity.[138] If physical demands are altered (e.g., increase or decrease in level of activity), or the manner in which the bone is loaded is changed (e.g., distribution of strain or loading rate), the bone remodels internally to adapt to the new demands.[139] Experimental evidence of this osteonal turnover has been presented by Radin and coworkers,[140] who demonstrated in rabbits a 150 percent increase in the number of labeled secondary osteons in the subchondral plate of the proximal tibia subjected to repetitive impulsive loads as compared with their contralateral quiescent knee. In addition, O'Connor and coworkers[141] demonstrated that one of the strongest correlates to elevated intracortical turnover was increased strain rate.

MECHANICAL PROPERTIES OF BONE

The mechanical strength of fully mature osteonal bone is greater than that of immature bone composed of circumferential lamellae and a few osteons that may be only partially mineralized.[142] Values for the mechanical properties of individual osteons range from tensile elastic modulus of 120,000 kg per μm^2 and almost 12 kg per μm^2 per meter (m) ultimate tensile strength for a fully mature, mineralized osteon to less than half that modulus and only 75 percent the ultimate tensile strength for a younger, less mineralized osteon. For normal tensile or compressive loading, the stiffness of the material, or elastic modulus, shows human haversian bone to be about 17.0 GPa (Gigapascals) in the longitudinal direction, 11.5 GPa in the transverse direction, and 3.3 GPa in shear.[143] The degree of mineralization (young bone) or porosity (old bone) will compromise the stiffness of the bone and thereby lower the elastic modulus.

Strength

The true strength of bone, however, is derived from its composite structure of haversian, circumferential, and interstitial lamellae, which works synergistically to avoid yield or ultimate strain. Strain, a dimensionless unit of change in length divided by original length, is used in bone physiology as 10^{-6} strain, or microstrain. The yield strain of bone, or that degree of deformation reached where the bone will not elastically recover, is approximately 7000 microstrain; i.e., a 0.7 percent change in length will cause irreversible damage to the tissue. Ultimate strain in bone, or that degree of deformation where the material actually fractures, is 15,000 microstrain.[144] An analogy of a bundle of straws versus a solid stick illustrates how a composite structure such as bone can prove more successful in resisting loads by avoiding yield and ultimate strain of the material. The solid stick breaks with relatively little bending, because relatively high strains are generated within the material. However, the bundle of straws composed of the same mass and subjected to the same bending conditions will continue to deform (strain) rather than break, as each independent element slips relative to adjacent bundles. By dissipating the strains generated by identical forces, the chance of exceeding yield strains, or ultimate failure, is greatly diminished. This analogy is often put into practice with the use of multistranded wire chosen over the use of single strand wire. During flexion, each individual strand will slip relative to its neighbor rather than strain, thus minimizing the generation of potentially damaging levels of strain. In the same manner, individual lamellae will "slip" relative to adjacent lamellae, dissipating energy and minimizing strain levels within the material, thus allowing the entire system to react in a more elastic manner rather than sustain brittle failure or ultimate fracture.

Toughness

Bone, as an organ, has a requirement to be both stiff (to resist deformation) and tough (to prevent crack propagation). However, there is a compromise between these two objectives, as they are attained through a balance of the composite between collagen and mineral. Comparatively small changes in the mineral content of bone tissue can have substantial effects on its properties as a material, as demonstrated by Curry[145] in his determination of the mechanical properties of diverse types of bone. By comparing the bovine femur, the deer antler, and the whale tympanic bulla, he illustrated that as the morphologic responsibility of the skeletal element changed, so did its mineral content. In the extreme, the mineral content ranged from 86 percent in the bulla, which requires a high acoustic impedance, to 59 percent in the antler, which must be resilient to high impact loads. The consequence of this high mineral content is revealed by comparing the relative work to fracture of these bones: the bulla is only 3 percent that of the antler.

The material properties of the appendicular skeleton, however, remain remarkably consistent through a wide range of animals (see reference 146 for a review). Over an animal mass range of 0.09 to 700.0 kg, the bending strength of those bones relegated to traditional load-bearing responsibilities remains approximately 200 to 250 MPa, with an elastic modulus consistently approaching 20 GPa. To adapt to changes in the physical demands placed upon it, the appendicular skeleton appears to respond not by changing its material properties but by altering its shape and morphology.[147]

STRUCTURAL ADAPTATION IN BONE

Bone tissue has the capacity to adapt to its functional environment such that its morphology is "optimized" for its mechanical demand. Indeed, the concept proposed in 1892 that the course and balance of bone remodeling can be affected by mechanical function is one of the oldest in modern medicine and is widely referred to as Wolff's law.[148] But what component of the functional environment is osteoregulating, and what is the structural objective of bone morphology? Strains measured during functional activity should indicate what the architecture of the skeleton is trying to amplify or suppress. Loads can be sustained with the smallest strains if they are applied axially. However, the axial component of functional activity is responsible for only a small percentage of the total strain measured at the bone surface; the femur, humerus, radius, ulna, and tibia all show that well over 80 percent of the measured strain is caused by bending moments.[149] As the neutral axis of strain typically passes across the marrow cavity, a significant portion of the tissue is in fact subjected to tension.[150] Although bending moments cannot be extinguished, their effect would be minimized if the bone's longitudinal curvature were oriented such that they counteracted those externally imposed by activity. Surprisingly, long bone curvature does not appear directed toward the neutralization of bending, and in some cases this curvature is oriented such that bending is increased.[151] Perhaps bone curvature, a morphologic modification attributable to functional loading,[152] actually acts to accentuate bone strain rather than cancel it.

Dynamic Strain Similarity

Contrary to our normal interpretation of Wolff's law, it appears that minimizing strain is not the ultimate goal of adaptation, but instead skeletal morphology strives to generate a certain *type* of strain. What kind of strain is morphology trying to achieve? Although vertebrate design and function is diverse, at the level of small volumes of tissue all loads and bending moments resolve into strain. Peak strain magnitudes measured in adult species, including horses, humans, lizards, sheep, goat, geese, pigs, macaques, turkeys, sunfish, and dogs, are remarkably similar, ranging from 2000 to 3500 microstrain. This relationship has been called "dynamic strain similarity" and suggests that skeletal morphology and locomotion character combine to elicit a very specific and perhaps beneficial level of strain.[153]

This limited range of strain has implications beyond the maintenance of a two-times safety factor within the bone material. While the structural benefit of a safety factor cannot be denied, it is difficult to imagine a cellular process that could monitor how close to deleterious strain levels the skeleton came during activity and then adjust the tissue's mass simply to avoid them. It seems reasonable that the cell population responsible for adjusting skeletal mass can respond only to the strains to which it is subjected, not the potential strain it might see should an aberrant loading incident occur. Instead, perhaps the safety factors within bone are simply a valuable by-product of a tissue that strives for some cytologic benefit generated by this common strain milieu. The interspecies similarities in strain magnitudes are strong evidence for the existence of a common strain-sensitive cellular population within the skeletal tissues of each of these animals. Further, it suggests that a generic cellular mechanism exists that strives toward a common, strain-determined structural goal that is beneficial to the bone cell population.

Strain Regulated Adaptation

While the nature of this structure-function relationship is only poorly understood, it has been proposed that bone remodeling is continually influenced by the level and distribution of the functional strains within the bone.[154] One striking example of the skeleton's capacity to adapt to its functional environment was demonstrated in professional tennis players.[155] By comparing the humeral mass of the racquet arm with that of the arm that simply throws the ball into the air, they observed a 35 percent increase in men and a 28 percent increase in women in the cortical thickness of the more active humerus.

The converse can also be demonstrated, as immobilization and bed rest can cause negatively balanced bone remodeling either locally or within the entire skeleton. Healthy adult males restricted to complete bed rest for up to 36 weeks showed a total body calcium loss during that period averaging 4.2 percent. However, bone mineral content measurements of the calcaneus showed a mean decrease of 34 percent, and in one case 45 percent of bone

mineral was lost,[156] demonstrating that at specific weight-bearing sites the negatively balanced bone remodeling stimulated by diminished demand can be quite severe.

Optimal Strain Stimulus

Attempts to identify those aspects of the skeleton's functional milieu that are responsible for generating and controlling this adaptive response have demonstrated that alterations in bone mass, turnover, and internal replacement are sensitive to changes in the magnitude,[157] distribution,[158] and rate of strain[141] generated within the bone tissue. A loading regimen must be dynamic in nature; static loads do not influence bone morphology.[159] However, full osteogenic potential is achieved following only an extremely short exposure to this stimulus.[160] The potency of the stimulus is proportional to the magnitude of the strain.[157] The fact that strain levels that are acceptable in one location induce adaptive remodeling in others would suggest that each region of each bone is genetically programmed to accept a particular amount and pattern of intermittent strain as normal. Deviation from this optimal strain environment will stimulate changes in the bone's remodeling balance, resulting in adaptive increases or decreases in its mass. It is not yet clear whether this strain discrepancy is picked up at the level of each individual osteocyte and the cell has the ability to manipulate the structural milieu of its adjacent space, or whether the osteocyte network somehow spatially integrates the load information across the cortex. But it does demonstrate that bone mass is substantially influenced by strain situations engendered by short periods of particularly osteogenic activity, for example, vigorous and diverse exercise, rather than by the strain situation experienced during a predominant activity, for example, walking, or by the fatigue damage that this might produce.

Isolating specific components of the physical milieu that actually regulate skeletal morphology has been difficult; no single parameter of the mechanical environment has been shown to reliably predict bone remodeling in all naturally observed or experimentally created conditions.[161] Perhaps our limited success in identifying these elusive stimuli has been due in part to our presumption that structural efficiency, that is, minimal strain with minimal mass, is an essential goal of skeletal morphology. That the skeleton has "optimized" its structure is supported by the similarity in peak strains generated in the cortex regardless of animal or activity (2000 to 3000 microstrain), indicating a common peak-strain–determined goal. Contrasting with this perspective, however, is the nonuniform but consistent distribution of normal and shear strains that exist throughout the stance phase, leaving large areas of the diaphyseal shaft subjected only to extremely low levels of strain energy density.[150] Further, rather than a signal to repair accumulated damage, a new strain milieu need be applied only for a very short time to maximize the tissue response.[160] Perhaps the engineering perspective that strain is harmful to bone and that remodeling is a repair drive process needs to be reconsidered. Instead, there may be some by-product of strain, such as stress-generated potentials, piezoelectric currents, or increased perifusion, that enhances the cell population's vitality.

Perhaps a principal objective of tissue adaptation is to promote and regulate some specific aspect of the functional milieu such that the matrix or cells within the tissue enjoy some direct or indirect benefit of strain.[162] Indeed, it may not even be the predominant components of the physical milieu that regulate these processes. We have found that extremely low-intensity electric fields (<1 mV per cm)[163] as well as low-magnitude strains (<500 microstrain)[164] when induced within a specific hyperphysiologic (10 to 50 Hz) frequency band influence bone mass as effectively as stimuli of greater intensity induced at more "physiologic" frequencies. Perhaps we should be more hesitant to presume skeletal morphology to be a product of dominant strain parameters with the structural goal of minimizing strain and instead consider the matrix and cellular advantages of a tissue exposed to a dynamic functional milieu.

Bioelectric Stimuli

While these data demonstrate some relationship of function to form, they do not suggest the means by which the physical signal is transduced by the cell and extracellular matrix into the adaptive process. A potential mechanism for the coupling of mechanical deformation and control of cellular metabolic activity may be the stress-generated electric potential (SGP). A change in the bone's level or type of activity will, in turn, alter the magnitude of this potential charge at the bone-fluid interface. Vascular channels within haversian systems, combined with the lacunae and canaliculi occupied by cells and the microporosity of the matrix, may consume as much as 10 percent of the bone tissue's volume and are filled with fluids and/or cellular components. The deformation, or straining, of the skeleton caused by functional activity will initiate this fluid to flow, similar to water flowing through a sponge that is stretched or compressed. While at one level this fluid behavior may contribute to increased perifusion and nutrient delivery, the ionic constituents of the fluid will interact with the charged nature of the mineral to generate electrokinetic potentials.[165] In 1962, Bassett and Becker[166] proposed that a primary step in translating functional load-bearing to an adaptive cellular response was linked to the electric potential generated by the mechanical deformation of the bone tissue. This postulation has been fully supported by many subsequent investigators showing the relationship between electric potential and regulation of bone cell

activity, with a number of excellent reviews available to the interested reader.[167, 168] As fluid pressure gradients and the resultant streaming potentials would affect primarily those cells confined within the cortices of the extracellular matrix (osteocytes), and changes in the "normal" electrokinetic signal would be generated by alterations in the type and/or amplitude of function, this intracortical syncytium could be a key regulator of osteoblast or osteoclast activity. This potential, in turn, may act to effect proliferation of osteoprogenitor cells[169] or to catalyze the production[170] or mineralization[171] of the extracellular matrix.

A final example of the transduction of mechanical loading to a cellular response is an accelerated prostaglandin synthesis and release following mechanical deformation of osteoblast cultures grown on collagen ribbons.[172] Whatever the signal transduction pathway of transforming physical information to something the cell population can perceive and respond to, it is clear that the capacity of bone tissue to adapt to its functional demands is critical to the skeleton's structural success. Indeed, as we attempt to evaluate the cellular mechanisms responsible for the positive control of bone mass, the osteogenic potential of physical stimuli cannot be ignored.

DEVELOPMENT OF THE SKELETON

Most of the bones of the skeleton are first formed in the embryo as cartilaginous models, which are later resorbed and replaced by bone tissue. This cartilage template, or anlage, is formed by the condensation of mesenchymal cells in the developing limb bud. While the shape of the anlage resembles that of the adult bone and appears to be genetically determined, the bone that replaces the cartilage template is greatly influenced by physical factors (e.g., weight bearing, muscle pull) and is constantly modeled and remodeled as these forces change according to the dictums of Wolff's law.[148]

The cartilage anlage expands and elongates by interstitial growth in which chondrocytes divide, enlarge, and surround themselves with the new matrix.[173] At about the same time, cells in the connective tissues surrounding the anlage (perichondrium) begin to lay down bone tissue and form a collar of bone around the center of the cartilage model. At the time it is formed, the anlage is pierced by a capillary that invades the calcified cartilage matrix and begins to hollow out its center, replacing the excavated cartilage with bone and creating the primitive marrow space. This process of vascular invasion of the cartilage model, followed by bone deposition, is referred to as enchondral ossification. The process continues until the entire shaft of the anlage is replaced by marrow and bone, confining the growth process of chondrocyte multiplication to the epiphyseal ends of the bone, away from the primary center of ossification. As the epiphysis

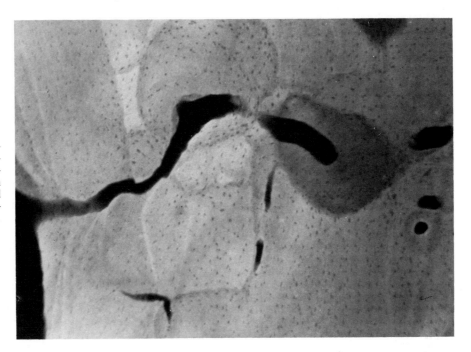

Figure 4–13. Endosteal capillary penetrating the inner cortex to communicate with two haversian canals, providing an anastomotic communication between the nutrient artery, periosteal arteries, and capillaries traveling longitudinally within the haversian canal.

swells, the central chondrocytes find themselves too remote from the blood supply to survive solely by means of diffusion. Cartilage canals facilitate diffusion of nutrients[174] and provide conduits for subsequent capillary ingrowth. The hypertrophic chondrocytes survive[175] and elaborate angiotrophic substances.[176]

Rosenberg and coworkers[177] have characterized the changes that occur in the lower hypertrophic bone, demonstrating the deposition of a 35,000 dalton protein (probably osteocalcin) and the modification of existing proteoglycans. Mineral deposition begins in the matrix vesicles located in the columns between the last hypertrophic chondrocytes on the extreme metaphyseal end of the physis.[178] Invasion by osteoblasts and osteoclasts results in the resorption of this woven bone and its replacement by mature lamellar bone.[179] The hydroxyapatite formed during primary ossification is a rather rough crystal whose imperfections may render it more vulnerable to attack and resorption,[180] suggesting the facility with which woven bone is removed.

The controlling mechanism for the mineralization and morphogenesis of the cartilage anlage is unknown, but this process is typically considered templated by genetic determinants. Alternative regulatory machanisms include that first proposed by Roux[181] in 1895, in which he hypothesized that the differentiation of connective tissues was controlled by mechanical stresses. More recently, this general "stress" postulation has been refined by Carter and coworkers,[182] proposing that intermittently applied shear stresses will promote enchondral ossification and that intermittent hydrostatic compression inhibits cartilage degeneration and ossification. Therefore, the mechanical stress environment to which the

anlage is exposed would contribute heavily to the bone's ultimate shape.

While growth in length occurs at the growth plate, growth in diameter occurs by the centrifugal proliferation of cartilage cells along the groove of Ranvier,[183] an anatomic structure bordered outwardly by a continuation of the fibrous periosteum and inwardly by the physeal cartilage. When swelling of the cartilaginous anlage first begins, a condensed layer of mesenchyme develops around it as a membrane of cells and collagen, called perichondrium. As the cartilage is replaced by bone, this membrane is renamed periosteum. In the growing skeleton, this periosteum is clearly divided into an inner cellular layer and an outer fibrous layer that merges gradually into the surrounding muscle. Muscles take origin from the periosteum, while collagen bundles can be traced from tendon and ligament, through the periosteum, to anchor directly into the bone via Sharpey's fibers.[184]

BLOOD SUPPLY OF BONE

Bone is extremely vascular and requires approximately 10 percent of the cardiac output.[185] Blood supply to the cortical diaphysis is derived from the nutrient artery and the periosteal vessels. The nutrient artery (or arteries) represents the original capillary that pierced the cartilaginous anlage to form the primitive marrow cavity. With continued longitudinal and circumferential growth, this vessel enlarges and arborizes to supply the marrow and inner two thirds of the cortex.[186] These periosteal capillaries are especially abundant at sites of tendon and ligament insertion and muscle origin (Fig. 4–13). In the

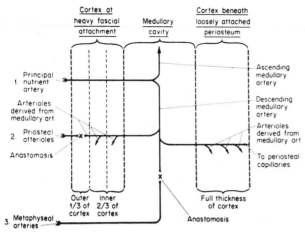

Figure 4–14. Diagrammatic representation of the circulation of bone emphasizing the multiple communications seen at the site of heavy fascial attachment contrasted with the sparse communication in other areas. (From Rhinelander, F. W.: *In* Bourne, G. H. [ed.]: The Biochemistry and Physiology of Bone. Vol. II. 2nd ed. New York, Academic Press, 1972. Used by permission.)

metaphyseal ends of the bone, where metabolism is most active, the periosteal vessels are large and abundant, and they are also referred to as metaphyseal arteries, although they are entirely analogous to the periosteal capillaries. The third set of vessels, the epiphyseal arteries, supply the subarticular ends of the bones and assume special importance because of the growth process in this area and the vulnerability of these vessels to injury (Fig. 4–14).

During infancy and adolescence, the epiphyseal plate serves as a barrier separating the epiphysis from the metaphysis. Although a few vessels crossing the plate have been described, it is widely accepted that there is no effective circulation across the plate. Essentially, therefore, the epiphyses have an isolated blood supply via the epiphyseal arteries, but those few vessels do present a potential route for spread of infection or tumor from metaphysis into the epiphysis. In most joints, there are abundant soft tissue attachments to the epiphyses (muscles, ligaments, capsule), so that numerous vessels supply the bone through these attachments (Fig. 4–15A). In a few locations, such as the proximal femur, the entire epiphysis may be intra-articular and therefore covered by articular cartilage. Since neither the articular nor the growth cartilage is penetrated by vessels, the few epiphyseal arteries must pass alongside the growth plate, covered by a thin layer of periosteum, to perforate the epiphysis[187] (see Fig. 4–15B). This route of blood supply is extremely vulnerable to trauma (fractures through the growth plate), increased intra-articular pressure (joint infections or bleeding into the joint), or idiopathic interruption (Legg-Perthes disease in children, avascular necrosis in adults (see Chapter 97).

Epiphyseal vessels arborize within the bony nucleus to supply the marrow, cancellous bone, and the crucial dividing chondrocytes in the microepiphyseal plates in the depths of the articular cartilage

and the growth plate itself (see Fig. 4–15C). Because of this, interruption of the vessels leads to cessation of longitudinal growth and loss of further diametric growth of the epiphysis and joint surface.

In contrast with the critical role of epiphyseal vessels during growth, the metaphyseal vessels are responsible only for resorption of the growth plate prior to its replacement by bone. Interruption of these vessels therefore will lead only to temporary loss of this function with increased thickness of the growth plate owing to accumulation of chondrocytes and matrix. Upon re-establishment of the metaphyseal blood supply, the thickened plate is resorbed to its normal thickness, and growth is not affected.[188]

Even in growing bones there is an abundant system of anastomoses between metaphyseal, periosteal, and nutrient arteries. Interruption of a single system results in limited changes in bone. With termination of longitudinal growth and obliteration of the growth plate, anastomoses are also established between the metaphyseal system and the epiphyseal system, thereby interconnecting the entire blood sup-

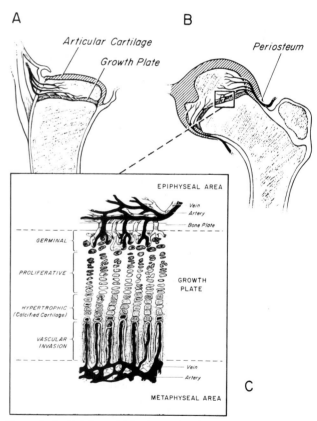

Figure 4–15. Epiphyseal blood supply of growing bone. *A,* The blood supply of most secondary centers of ossification is abundant by virtue of the numerous soft tissue attachments. *B,* Certain secondary centers, such as the proximal femur, are devoid of soft tissue attachments, and the blood supply therefore follows a tenuous route through the joint where it is liable to injury. *C,* Diagrammatic representation of the blood supply to the growth plate showing the contribution of the epiphyseal artery to the germinal portion of the growth plate. (From Sledge, C. B.: *In* Cave, E. F. [ed.]: Trauma Management. Chicago, Mosby-Year Book Medical Publishers, 1974. Used by permission.)

ply of the bone. For this reason, elevation of the periosteum (dissecting infection or surgical approaches) or obliteration of the nutrient artery (intraarticular fixation devices or infection) has only limited effects on the blood supply to the entire bone.[186]

Within the cortex of bone, capillaries travel primarily in the longitudinal direction within haversian canals. Occasional branching is seen, and lateral communications with the periosteal vessels through Volkmann's canals provide collateral circulation. The usual haversian system is 100 μm or less in diameter; thus, individual osteocytes are not more than 50 μm from their blood supply. The rich system of canaliculi radiating out from the central canal enhances microcirculation to the most distant osteocytes.

Although the periosteum and marrow have long been shown to be innervated with sensory and autonomic fibers, there is only limited information regarding the existence of nerves within the haversian canals.[189] Neural, hormonal, and metabolic factors affecting the blood supply to bone have been discussed by Shim[185] and the effects of loss of blood to cortical and cancellous bone are discussed in Chapter 97.

SUMMARY

This chapter has provided a brief overview of the cellular mechanisms and systemic and physical factors that contribute to the skeleton's capacity to serve as both mineral reservoir and structural entity. The processes of cell differentiation and modulation, matrix synthesis and mineralization, growth and adaptation have been discussed. If anything, perhaps this chapter has managed to diminish the skeleton's reputation as a static entity and has demonstrated its critical responsibility in the very dynamic process of mineral homeostasis, and its unmatched capacity to facilitate locomotion. It is not solely a reservoir of mineral or uniquely a mechanical structure. The skeleton represents an extremely complex and successful combination of these responsibilities.

References

1. Marks, S. C., and Popoff, S. N.: Bone cell biology: The regulation of development, structure, and function in the skeleton. Am. J. Anat. 183:1, 1988.
2. Roodman, G. D., Ibbotson, K. J., MacDonald, B. R., Kuehl, T. J., and Mundy G. R.: 1,25(OH)2 vitamin D3 causes formation of multinucleated cells with osteoclast characteristics in cultures of primate marrow. Proc. Natl. Acad. Sci. U.S.A. 82:8213, 1985.
3. Van Furth, R., Dresselhoff dan Durk, M., Suiter, W., and van Dissell, J. T.: New perspectives on the kinetics of mononuclear phagocytes. In van Furth, R. (ed.): Mononuclear Phagocytes: Characteristics, Physiology and Function. The Hague, Nijhoff, 1985, pp. 201–208.
4. Doty, S. B.: Morphological evidence of gap junctions between bone cells. Calcif. Tissue Int. 33:509, 1981.
5. Rodan, G. A., and Martin, T. J.: Role of osteoblasts in hormonal control of bone resorption—a hypothesis. Calcif. Tissue Int. 33:349, 1981.
6. Raisz, L. G., and Kream, B. E.: Regulation of bone formation—part I. N. Engl. J. Med. 309(1):29, 1983.
7. Rosenbloom, J., and Prockop, D. J.: Biochemical aspects of collagen biosynthesis. Repair and regeneration. In Dunphy, J. S., and Van Winkle, W. (eds.): Scientific Basis of Surgical Practice. New York, McGraw-Hill, 1969, pp. 117–135.
8. Rhoades, R. E., and Udenfriend, S.: Decarboxylation of alpha-ketoglutarate coupled to collagen proline hydroxylase. Proc. Natl. Acad. Sci. U.S.A. 60:1473, 1968.
9. Prockop, D. J., Kivirikko, K. I., Tuderman, L., and Guzman, N. A.: The biosynthesis of collagen and its disorders. N. Engl. J. Med. 301:13, 77, 1979.
10. Pritchard, J. J.: General histology of bone. In Bourne, G. H. (ed.): The Biochemistry and Physiology of Bone. Vol. I. 2nd ed. New York, Academic Press, 1972, p. 15.
11. Ascenzi, A., and Bonucci, E.: Relationship between ultrastructure and "pin test" in osteons. Clin. Orthop. 121:275, 1976.
12. Owen, M.: Cellular dynamics of bone. In Bourne, G. H. (ed.): The Biochemistry and Physiology of Bone, Vol. III. 2nd ed. New York, Academic Press, 1972, p. 271.
13. Jaworski, Z. F. G.: Lamellar bone turnover system and its effector organ. Calcif. Tissue Int. 36S:46, 1984.
14. Jowsey, J.: Metabolic Diseases of Bone. Philadelphia, W. B. Saunders Company, 1977, p. 61.
15. Parfitt, A. M.: Osteomalacia and related disorders. In Avioli, L. V., and Krane, S. M. (eds.): Metabolic Bone Disease and Clinically Related Disorders. Philadelphia, W. B. Saunders Company, 1990, p. 329.
16. Menton, D. N., Simmons, D. J., Chang, S. L., and Orr, B. Y.: From bone lining cell to osteocyte—an SEM study. Anat. Rec. 209:29, 1984.
17. Rodan, G. A., and Rodan, S. B.: Expression of the osteoblastic phenotype. In Peck, W. A. (ed.): Bone and Mineral Research Annual II. Amsterdam, Excerpta Medica, 1984, pp. 244–285.
18. Curtis, T. A., Ashrafi, S. H., and Weber, D. F.: Canalicular communication in the cortices of human long bones. Anat. Rec. 212:336, 1985.
19. Robinson, R. A.: Observations regarding compartments for tracer calcium in the body. In Frost, H. M. (ed.): Bone Biodynamics. Boston, Little, Brown & Company, 1964.
20. Parfitt, A. M.: The cellular basis of bone remodeling: The quantum concept re-examined in light of recent advances in cell biology of the bone. Calcif. Tissue Int. 36S:537, 1984.
21. Albright, J. A., and Skinner, C.: Bone: Structural organization and remodeling dynamics. In Albright, J. A., and Brand, R. A. (eds.): The Scientific Basis of Orthopaedics. 2nd ed. East Norwalk, CT, Appleton & Lange, 1987, pp. 161–198.
22. Vaughan, J.: Osteogenesis and haematopoiesis. Lancet 2:133, 1981.
23. Chambers, T. J.: The cellular basis of bone resorption. Clin. Orthop. 151:283, 1980.
24. Bonucci, E.: New knowledge on the origin, function and fate of osteoclasts. Clin. Orthop. 158:252, 1981.
25. Hancox, N. M.: The osteoclast. In Willmer, E. N. (ed.): Cells and Tissues in Culture. Vol. 2 New York, Academic Press, 1965, p. 261.
26. Owen, M.: The origin of bone cells in the postnatal organism. Arthritis Rheum. 23:1073, 1980.
27. Jaworski, Z. F. G., Duck, B., and Sekaly, G.: Kinetics of osteoclasts and their nuclei in evolving secondary haversian systems. J. Anat. 133:397, 1981.
28. Baron, R., Vignery, A., and Horowitz, M.: Lymphocytes, macrophages and the regulation of bone remodeling. In Peck, W. A. (ed.): Bone and Mineral Research: Annual. Vol. 2. New York Elsevier, 1983, pp. 175–243.
29. Bingham, P. J., Brazell, I. A., and Owen, M.: The effect of parathyroid extract on cellular activity and plasma calcium levels in vivo. J. Endocrinol. 45:387, 1969.
30. Bain, S., and Rubin, C.: Temporal nature of osteoclast resorption in response to disuse. J. Bone Miner. Res. 5(1):573, 1990.
31. Reinholt, F. P., Hultenby, K., Oldberg, A., and Heinegard, D.: Osteopontin—a possible anchor of osteoclasts to bone. Proc. Natl. Acad. Sci. U.S.A. 87:4473, 1990.
32. Horton, M. A., and Davies, J.: Perspectives: Adhesion receptors in bone. J. Bone Miner. Res. 4(6):803, 1989.
33. VanderWiel, C. J., Grubb, S. A., and Talmage, R. V.: The presence of lining cells on surfaces of human trabecular bone. Clin. Orthop. 134:350, 1978.
34. Walker, D. G.: Enzymatic and electron microscopic analysis of isolated osteoclasts. Calcif. Tissue Res. 9:296, 1972.
35. Blair, H. C., Teitelbaum, S. L., Ghiselli, R., and Gluck, S.: Osteoclastic bone resorption by a polarized vacuolar proton pump. Science 245:855, 1989.
36. Jones, S. J., Boyde, A., Ali, N. N., and Maconnachie, E.: A review of bone cell substratum interactions. Scanning 7:5, 1985.
37. Silver, A., Murrills, R. J., and Etherington, D. J.: Microelectrode studies on the acid microenvironment beneath adherent macrophages and osteoclasts. Exp. Cell Res. 175:266, 1988.
38. Malgaroli, A., Meldolesi, J., Zallone, A. Z., and Teti, A.: Control of cytosolic free calcium in rat and chicken osteoclasts. J. Biol. Chem. 264(24):14342, 1989.
39. Partridge, N. C., Jeffrey, J. J., Ehlich, L. S., Teitelbaum, S. L., Fliszar,

C., Welgus, H. G., and Kahn, A. J.: Hormonal regulation of the production of collagenase and a collagenase inhibitor activity by rat osteogenic sarcoma cells. Endocrinology 120(5):1956, 1987.

40. Diagnosis and Management of Asymptomatic Primary Hyperparathyroidism: Consensus Development Conference Statement. Ann. Intern. Med. 114:593, 1991.

41. McSheehy, P. M. J., and Chambers, T. J.: Osteoblastic cells mediate osteoclastic responsiveness to parathyroid hormone. Endocrinology 118:824, 1986.

42. McSheehy, P. M. J., and Chambers, T. J.: Osteoblast-like cells in the presence of parathyroid hormone release soluble factor that stimulates osteoclastic bone resorption. Endocrinology 119:1654, 1986.

43. Donahue, H. J., Fryer, M. J., Eriksen, E. F., and Heath, H., III: Differential effects of parathyroid hormone and its analogues on cytosolic calcium ion and cAMP levels in cultured rat osteoblast-like cells. J. Biol. Chem. 263(27):13522, 1988.

44. Rouleau, M. F., Warshawsky, H., and Goltzman, D.: Parathyroid hormone binding in vivo to renal, hepatic, and skeletal tissues of the rat using a radioautographic approach. Endocrinology 118:919, 1986.

45. Pharoah, M. J., and Heersche, J. N. M.: 1,25-dihydroxyvitamin D_3 causes an increase in the number of osteoclastlike cells in cat bone marrow cultures. Calcif. Tissue Int. 37:276, 1985.

46. Stern, P. H.: Vitamin D and bone. Kidney Int. 38(29):S17, 1990.

47. Eriksen, E. F., Colvard, D. S., Berg, N. J., Graham, M. L., Mann, K. G., Spelsberg, T. C., and Riggs, L.: Evidence of estrogen receptors in normal human osteoblast-like cells. Science 241:84, 1988.

48. Komm, B. S., Terpening, C. M., Benz, D. J., Graeme, K. A., Gallegos, A., Korc, M., Greene, G. L., O'Malley, B. W., and Haussler, M. R.: Estrogen binding, receptor mRNA, and biologic response in osteoblast-like osteosarcoma cells. Science 241:81, 1988.

49. Ernst, M., Schmid, Ch., and Froesch, E. R.: Enhanced osteoblast proliferation and collagen gene expression by estradiol. Proc. Natl. Acad. Sci. U.S.A. 85:2307, 1988.

50. Fukayama, S., and Tashjian, A. H.: Direct modulation by estradiol of the response of human bone cells (SaOS-2) to human parathyroid hormone (PTH) and PTH-related protein. Endocrinology 124(1):397, 1989.

51. Gray, T. K., Mohan, S., Linkhart, T. A., and Baylink, D. J.: Estradiol stimulates in vitro the secretion of insulin-like growth factors by the clonal osteoblastic cell line, UMR106. Biochem. Biophys. Res. Comm. 158(2):407, 1989.

52. Colvard, D. S., Eriksen, E. F., Keeting, P. E., Wilson, E. M., Lubahn, D. B., French, F. S., Riggs, B. L., and Spelsberg, T. C.: Identification of androgen receptors in normal human osteoblast-like cells. Proc. Natl. Acad. Sci. U.S.A. 86:854, 1989.

53. Fukayama, S., and Tashjian, A. H.: Direct modulation by androgens of the response of human bone cells (SaOS-2) to human parathyroid hormone (PTH) and PTH-related protein. Endocrinology 125(4):1789, 1989.

54. NIH Consensus Development Conference on Osteoporosis. J.A.M.A. 252(6):799, 1984.

55. Raisz, L. G., and Niemann, I.: Effect of phosphate, calcium and magnesium on bone resorption and hormonal responses in tissue culture. Endocrinology 85:446, 1969.

56. Yamaguchi, D. T., Hahn, T. J., Beeker, T. G., Kleeman, C. R., and Muallem, S.: Relationship of cAMP and calcium messenger systems in prostaglandin-stimulated UMR-106 cells. J. Biol. Chem. 263(22):10745, 1988.

57. Austin, L. A., and Heath, H., III: Calcitonin: physiology and pathophysiology. N. Engl. J. Med. 304:269, 1981.

58. Arnaud, C. D., and Kolb, F. O.: The calciotropic hormones and metabolic bone disease. In Greenspan, F. S., and Forsham, P. H. (eds.): Basic and Clinical Endocrinology. Los Altos, CA, Lange Medical Publications, 1983, pp. 187–250.

59. Nicholson, G. C., Moseley, J. M., Sexton, P. M., Mendelsohn, F. A. O., and Martin, T. J.: Abundant calcitonin receptors in isolated rat osteoclasts—biochemical and autoradiographic characterization. J. Clin. Invest. 78:355, 1986.

60. Chambers, T. J., Athanasou, N. A., and Fuller, K.: Effect of parathyroid hormone and calcitonin on the cytoplasmic spreading of isolated osteoclasts. J. Endocrinol. 102:281, 1984.

61. Murrills, R. J., and Dempster, D. W.: The effects of stimulators of intracellular cyclic AMP on rat and chick osteoclasts in vitro: Validation of a simplified light microscope assay of bone resorption. Bone 11:333, 1990.

62. Deftos, L. J., and Roos, B.: Medullary thyroid carcinoma and calcitonin gene expression. In Peck, W. A. (ed.): Bone and Mineral Research. Amsterdam, Excerpta Medica, 1989, pp. 267–316.

63. Raisz, L. G.: Local and systemic factors in the pathogenesis of osteoporosis. N. Engl. J. Med. 318(13):818, 1988.

64. Canalis, E., McCarthy, T., and Centrella, M.: Growth factors and the regulation of bone remodeling. J. Clin. Invest. 81:277, 1988.

65. Pfeilschifter, J. P., Seyedin, S., and Mundy, G. R.: Transformed growth factor B inhibits bone resorption in fetal rat long bone cultures. J. Clin. Invest. 82:680, 1988.

66. Noda, M., and Camilliere, J. J.: In vivo stimulation of bone formation by transforming growth factor-beta. Endocrinology 124:2991, 1989.

67. Chenu, C., Pfeilschifter, J., Mundy, G. R., and Roodman, G. D.: Transforming growth factor B inhibits formation of osteoclast-like cells in long-term human marrow cultures. Proc. Natl. Acad. Sci. U.S.A. 85:5683, 1988.

68. Mundy, G. R., Varani, J., Orr, W., Gondek, M. D., and Ward, P. A.: Resorbing bone is chemotactic for monocytes. Nature 275:132, 1978.

69. Labat, M. L., and Milhaud, G.: Osteoporosis and the immune deficiency syndrome. In Peck, W. A. (ed.): Bone and Mineral Research. New York, Elsevier, 1986, pp. 131–212.

70. Baron, R., Vignery, A., and Tran Van, P.: The significance of lacunar erosion without osteoclasts: Studies on the reversal phase of the remodelling sequence. Metab. Bone Dis. Rel. Res. 2S:35, 1980.

71. Manolugas, S. C., Povvedini, D. M., and Tsoukas, C.: Interactions of 1,25-dehydroxyvitamin D_3 and the immune system. Mol. Cell. Endocrinol. 43:113, 1985.

72. Rodan, G. A., and Martin, T. J.: Role of osteoblasts in hormonal control of bone resorption—a hypothesis. Calcif. Tissue Int. 33:349, 1981.

73. Rubin, C. T., and Hausman, M. R.: The cellular basis of Wolff's law—transduction of physical stimuli to skeletal adaptation. Rheum. Dis. Clin. North Am. 14(3):503, 1988.

74. Carter, D., and Wong, A.: Mechanical stresses and endochondral ossification in chondroepiphysis. J. Orthop. Res. 6:148, 1988.

75. Parafitt, A. M.: The coupling of bone resorption to bone formation: A critical analysis of the concept and of its relevance to the pathogenesis of osteoporosis. Metab. Bone Dis. Rel. Res. 4:1, 1982.

76. Bingham, P. J., Brazell, I. A., and Owen, M.: The effect of parathyroid extract on cellular activity and plasma calcium levels in vivo. Endocrinology 45:387, 1969.

77. Baron, R., Vignery, A., and Horowitz, M.: Lymphocytes, macrophages and the regulation of bone remodeling. In Peck, W. (ed.): Bone and Mineral Research 2. Amsterdam, Elsevier, 1984.

78. Bain, S. D., Impeduglia, T. M., and Rubin, C. T.: Cement line staining in undecalcified thin sections of cortical bone. Stain Technol. 65(4):159, 1990.

79. Parfitt, A. M.: The cellular basis of bone remodeling. The quantum concept re-examined in light of recent advances in cell biology of bone. Calcif. Tissue Int. 36:S37, 1984.

80. Fisher, L. W., Robey, P. G., Tuross, N., Otsuka, A. S., Tepen, D. A., Esch, F. S., Shimasaki, S., and Termine, J. D.: The M_r 24,000 phosphoprotein from developing bone is the NH_2-terminal propeptide of the α1 chain of type I collagen. J. Biol. Chem. 262:13457, 1987.

81. Noda, M., Yoon, K., Prince, C. W., Butler, W. T., and Rodan, G. A.: Transcriptional regulation of osteopontin production in rat osteosarcoma cells by type B transforming growth factor. J. Biol. Chem. 263:13916, 1988.

82. Price, P. A., Wetekam, W., Poser, J. W., et al.: Characterization of gamma-carboxyglutamic acid–containing protein from bone. Proc. Natl. Acad. Sci. U.S.A. 73:1447, 1976.

83. Urist, M. R., Huo, Y. K., Brownell, A. G., Hohl, W. M., Buyske, J., Lietze, A., Tempst, P., et al.: Purification of bovine bone morphogenetic protein by hydroxyapatite chromatography. Proc. Natl. Acad. Sci. U.S.A. 81:371, 1984.

84. Termine, J. D., Belcourt, A. B., Conn, K. M., and Kleinman, H. K.: Mineral and collagen-binding proteins of fetal calf bone. J. Biol. Chem. 256:10403, 1981.

85. Robey, P. G.: The biochemistry of bone. Endocrinol. Metab. Clin. North Am. 18(4):859, 1989.

86. Eyre, D. R.: Collagen: Molecular diversity in the body's protein scaffold. Science 207:1315, 1980.

87. Boskey, A. L., and Posner, A. S.: Bone structure, composition and mineralization. Orthop. Clin. North Am. 15:597, 1984.

88. Veis, A., Sharkey, M., and Dickson, I.: Non-collagenous proteins of bone and dentin extracellular matrix and their role in organized mineral deposition. In Wasserman, R. H. (ed.): Calcium Binding Proteins and Calcium Function. New York, Elsevier, 1977, pp. 409–418.

89. Glimcher, M. J.: Studies of the structure, organization and reactivity of bone collagen. In Gibson, T. (ed.): Proceedings of the International Symposium on Wound Healing. New York, Montreaux Found. Intern. Coop. Med. Sci., 1975, p. 253.

90. Termine, J. D., Belcourt, A. B., Conn, K. M., and Kleinman, H. K.: Mineral and collagen-binding proteins of fetal calf bone. J. Biol. Chem. 256:10403, 1981.

91. Herring, G. M.: The chemical structure of tendon cartilage, dentin and bone matrix. Clin. Orthop. 60:261, 1968.

92. Herring, G. M.: The organic matrix of bone. In Bourne, G. H. (ed.): The Biochemistry and Physiology of Bone. Vol. I. 2nd ed., New York, Academic Press, 1972, p. 127.

93. Skerry, T. M., Suswillo, R., El Haj, A. J., Ali, N. N., Dodds, R. A., and Lanyon, L. E.: Load-induced proteoglycan orientation in bone tissue in vivo and in vitro. Calcif. Tissue Int. 46:318, 1990.

94. Termine, J. D., Kleinman, H. K., Whitson, S. W., Conn, K. M.,

McGarvey, M. L., and Martin, G. R.: Osteonectin, a bone-specific protein linking mineral to collagen. Cell 26:99, 1981.

95. Romberg, R. W., Werness, P. G., Lollar, P. , Riggs, B. L., and Mann, K. G.: Isolation and characterization of native adult osteonectin. J. Biol. Chem. 260:2728, 1985.

96. Termine, J. D., Eanes, E. D., and Conn, K. M.: Phosphoprotein modulation of apatite crystallization. Calcif. Tissue Int. 31:247, 1980.

97. Hauschka, P. V., Lian, J. B., Cole, D. E. C., and Gundberg, C. M.: Osteocalcin and matrix Gla protein: vitamin K–dependent protein in bone. Phys. Rev. 69:990, 1988.

98. Lian, J. B., Coutts, M., and Canalis, E.: Studies of hormonal regulation of osteocalcin synthesis in cultured fetal rat calvariae. J. Biol. Chem. 260:8706, 1985.

99. Canalis, E., McCarthy, T., and Centrella, M.: Growth factors and the regulation of bone remodeling. J. Clin. Invest. 81:277, 1988.

100. Lian, J. B., and Gundberg, C. M.: Osteocalcin: biochemical considerations and clinical applications. Clin. Orthop. 262:267, 1988.

101. Posner, A. S.: Crystal chemistry of bone mineral. Physiol. Rev. 49:760, 1969.

102. Bonar, L. C., Roufosse, A. H., Sabine, W. K., Grynpas, M. D., and Glimcher, M. J.: X-ray diffraction studies of the crystallinity of bone mineral in newly synthesized and density fractionated bone. Calcif. Tissue Int. 35:202, 1983.

103. Rubin, C. T., Bain, S., and McLeod, K. J.: Suppression of the osteogenic response in the aging skeleton. Calcif. Tissue Int. 50:306, 1992.

104. Jowsey, J.: Microradiography: A morphologic approach to quantitating bone turnover. In Excerpta Medica International Congress Series No. 270. Amsterdam, Excerpta Medica Foundation, 1972, p. 114.

105. Glimcher, M. J., and Lian, J. B.: The Chemistry and Biology of Mineralized Tissues. Proceedings of the Third International Conference on the Chemistry and Biology of Mineralized Tissues. New York, Gordon & Breach Science Publishers, 1988.

106. Wuthier, R. E., Jajeska, R. J., and Collins, G. M.: Biosynthesis of matrix vesicles in epiphyseal cartilage. 1. In vivo incorporation of 32P-orthophosphate into phospholipid of chondrocyte, membrane and matrix vesicle fractions. Calcif. Tissue Res. 23:135, 1977.

107. Kerr, J. F. R., Wyllie, A. H., and Currie, A. R.: Apoptosis: a basic biological phenomenon with wide-ranging implications in tissue kinetics. Br. J. Cancer 26:239, 1972.

108. Russell, R. G. G., Caswell, A. M., Hearn, P. R., and Sharrard, R. M.: Calcium in mineralized tissues and pathological cacification. Br. Med. Bull. 42(4):435, 1986.

109. Anderson, H. C.: Electron microscopic studies of induced cartilage development and calcification. J. Cell Biol. 35:81, 1967.

110. Anderson, H. C.: Matrix vesicle calcification: Review and update. In Peck, W. A. (ed.): Bone and Mineral Research/3. New York, Elsevier, 1985.

111. Wuthier, R. E.: Lipid composition of isolated cartilage cells, membranes and matrix vesicles. Biochim. Biophys. Acta 409:128, 1975.

112. Endo, A., and Glimcher, M. J.: The potential role of phosphoproteins in the in vitro calcification of bone collagen. Trans. Orthop. Res. Soc. 11:221, 1986.

113. Puzas, J. E.: Phosphotyrosine phosphatase activity in bone cells: an old enzyme with a new function. Adv. Prot. Phosphatases 3:237, 1986.

114. Anderson, H. C.: Biology of disease: Mechanism of mineral formation in bone. Lab. Invest. 60:320, 1989.

115. Wuthier, R. E.: The role of phospholipids in biological calcification: distribution of phospholipase activity in calcifying epiphyseal cartilage. Clin. Orthop. 90:191, 1973.

116. Peress, N. S., Anderson, H. C., and Sajdera, S. W.: The lipids of matrix vesicles from bovine fetal epiphyseal cartilage. Calcif. Tissue Res. 14:275, 1974.

117. Termine, J. D., Belcourt, A. B., Conn, K. M., and Kleinman, H. K.: Mineral and collagen-binding proteins of fetal calf bone. J. Biol. Chem. 256:10403, 1981.

118. Hynes, R. O.: The molecular biology of fibronectin. Annu. Rev. Cell Biol. 1:67, 1985.

119. Glimcher, M. J., and Krane, S. M.: The organization and structure of bone and the mechanism of calcification. In Ramachandran, G. N., and Gould, B. S. (eds.): Treatise on Collagen. Vol. 11B, Biology of Collagen. New York, Academic Press, 1968, p. 68.

120. Baylin, D., Wengedal, J., and Thompson, E.: Loss of protein polysaccharides at sites where bone mineralization is initiated. J. Histochem. Cytochem. 20:279, 1972.

121. Glimcher, M. J.: Composition, structure and organization of bone and other mineralized tissues and the mechanism of calcification. In Greep, R. O., and Astwood, E. B. (eds.): Handbook of Physiology: Endocrinology, VII. Baltimore, Williams & Wilkins Company, 1976, p. 25.

122. Parfitt, A. L.: Bone histomorphometry: Proposed system for standardization of nomenclature, symbols and units. Calcif. Tissue Int. 42:284, 1988.

123. Hayes, W. C., and Gerhart, T. N.: Biomechanics of bone: applications for assessment of bone strength. In Peck, W. A. (ed.): Bone and Mineral Research/3. 1985, p. 259.

124. Lanyon, L. E.: Analysis of surface bone strain in the calcaneus of sheep during normal locomotion. Strain analysis of the calcaneus. J. Biomech. 6:41, 1973.

125. Ascenzi, A.: The micromechanics versus the macromechanics of cortical bone—a comprehensive presentation. J. Biomech. Eng. 110:357, 1988.

126. Jones, B. H., Harris, J. McA., Vinh, T. N., and Rubin, C. T.: Exercise-induced stress fractures and stress reactions of bone: Epidemiology, etiology, and classification. Exerc. Sport Sci. Rev. 17:379, 1989.

127. Albright, J. A., and Skinner, H. C. W.: Bone: structural organization and remodeling dynamics. In Albright, J. A., and Brand, R. A. (eds.): The Scientific Basis of Orthopaedics. 2nd ed. East Norwalk, CT, Appleton & Lange, 1987, pp. 161–198.

128. Rubin, C. T., Bain, S. D.: Long-term remodeling bone response to potent osteogenic stimuli: Stages in the achievement of lamellar bone. Trans. Orthop. Res. Soc. 16:419, 1991.

129. Frost, H. M.: Secondary osteon population densities. An algorithm for estimating the missing osteons. In Yearbook of Physical Anthropology. Vol. 30. Washington, D.C., American Anthropological Assn., 1987, pp. 221–238.

130. Ascenzi, A., and Benvenuti, A.: Orientation of collagen fibers at the boundary between two successive osteonic lamellae and its mechanical interpretation. J. Biomech. 19:455, 1986.

131. Schaffler, M. B., Burr, D. B., and Fredrickson, R. G.: Morphology of the osteonal cement line in human bone. Anat. Rec. 217:223, 1987.

132. Garn, S. M.: The course of bone gain and the phases of bone loss. Orthop. Clin. North Am. 3:503, 1972.

133. Ruff, C. V., and Hays, W. C.: Subperiosteal expansion and cortical remodeling of the human femur and tibia with aging. Science 217:945, 1982.

134. Enlow, D. H.: Principles of Bone Remodeling. Springfield, IL, Charles C Thomas, 1963.

135. Koch, J. C.: The laws of bone architecture. Am. J. Anat. 21:177, 1917.

136. Lanyon, L. E., Rubin, C. T., and Baust, G.: Modulation of bone loss during calcium insufficiency by controlled dynamic loading. Calcif. Tissue Int. 38:209, 1986.

137. Bain, S. D., and Rubin, C. T.: Metabolic modulation of disuse osteopenia: Endocrine-dependent site specificity of bone remodeling. J Bone Miner. Res. 5(10):1069, 1990.

138. Rubin, C. T.: The benefits and consequences of structural adaptation in bone. In Fitzgerald, R. (ed.): Non-Cemented Total Hip Arthroplasty. 1988, pp. 41–48.

139. Brown, T. D., Pedersen, D. R., Gray, M. L., Brand, R. A., and Rubin, C. T.: Toward an identification of mechanical parameters initiating periosteal remodeling: A combined experimental and analytic approach. J. Biomech. 23(9):893, 1990.

140. Radin, E. L., Martin, R. B., Burr, D. B., Caterson, B., Boyd, R. D., and Goodwin, C.: Effects of mechanical loading on the tissues of the rabbit knee. J. Orthop. Res. 2:221, 1984.

141. O'Connor, J. A., Lanyon, L. E., and MacFie, H.: The influence of strain rate on adaptive bone remodeling. J. Biomech. 15:767, 1982.

142. Ascenzi, A., and Bell, G. H.: Bone as a mechanical engineering problem. In Bourne, G. H. (ed.): The Biochemistry and Physiology of Bone. Vol. 1. Structure. New York, Academic Press, 1972, p. 311.

143. Reilly, D. T., and Burstein, A. H.: The elastic and ultimate properties of compact bone tissue. J. Biomech. 8:393, 1975.

144. Carter, D. R., Harris, W. H., and Caler, W. E.: The mechanical and biological response of cortical bone to in vivo strain histories. In Cowin, S. C. (ed.): Mechanical Properties of Bone. Vol. 45. New York, The American Society of Mechanical Engineers, 1981, pp. 81–92.

145. Curry, J. D.: Mechanical properties of bone with greatly differing functions. J. Biomech. 12:313, 1979.

146. Lanyon, L. E., and Rubin, C. T.: Functional adaptation in skeletal structures. In Hildebrand, M., Bramble, D. M., Leim, K. F., and Wake, D. B. (eds.): Functional Vertebrate Morphology. Cambridge, Harvard University Press, 1985, pp. 1–25.

147. Woo, S. L. Y.: The relationships of changes in stress levels on long bone remodeling. In Cowen, S. (ed.): Mechanical Properties of Bone. Vol. 45. New York, The American Society of Mechanical Engineers, 1981, p. 107.

148. Wolff, J.: The Law of Bone Remodeling. Translated by Maquet, P., and Furlong, R., Berlin, Springer-Verlag, 1986 (original manuscript 1892).

149. Rubin, C. T., and Lanyon, L. E.: Limb mechanics as a function of speed and gait: A study of functional strains in the radius and tibia of horse and dog. J. Exp. Biol. 101:187, 1982.

150. Gross, T. S., McLeod, K. J., and Rubin, C. T.: Normal and shear strain distributions of the equine third metacarpal during locomotion: A characterization of bone's functional milieu. J. Biomech. 1992 (in press).

151. Rubin, C. T.: Skeletal strain and the functional strain significance of bone architecture. Calcif. Tissue Int. 36:S11, 1984.

152. Lanyon, L. E.: The influence of function on the development of bone curvature. An experimental study on the rat tibia. J. Zool. (Lond.) 192:457, 1980.

153. Rubin, C. T., and Lanyon, L. E.: Dynamic strain similarity in vertebrates; an alternative to allometric limb bone scaling. J. Theor. Biol. 107:321, 1984.
154. Rubin, C. T., and Lanyon, L. E.: Osteoregulatory nature of mechanical stimuli: Function as a determinant for adaptive remodeling in bone. J. Orthop. Res. 5:300, 1987.
155. Jones, H. H., Priest, J. D., Hayes, W. C., Tichenor, C. C., and Nagel, D. A.: Humeral hypertrophy in response to exercise. J. Bone Joint Surg. 59A:204, 1977.
156. Donaldson, C. L., Hulley, S. B., Vogel, J. M., Hattner, R. S., Bayers, J. H., and McMillan, D. E.: Effect of prolonged bed rest on bone mineral. Metabolism 19:1071, 1970.
157. Rubin, C. T., and Lanyon, L. E.: Regulation of bone mass by mechanical loading: The effect of peak strain magnitude. Calcif. Tissue Int. 37:411, 1985.
158. Lanyon, L. E., Goodship, A. E., Pye, C., and MacFie, H.: Mechanically adaptive bone remodeling: A quantitative study on function adaptation in the radius following ulna osteotomy in sheep. J. Biomech. 15:141, 1982.
159. Lanyon, L. E., and Rubin, C. T.: Static versus dynamic loads as an influence on bone remodeling. J. Biomech. 17:897, 1984.
160. Rubin, C. T., and Lanyon, L. E.: Regulation of bone formation by applied dynamic loads. J. Bone Joint Surg. 66A:397, 1984.
161. Brown, T. D., Pedersen, D. R., Gray, M. L., Brand, R. A., and Rubin, C. T.: Toward identification of mechanical parameters initiating periosteal remodeling: A combined experimental and analytic approach. J. Biomech. 23(9):893, 1990.
162. Rubin, C. T., and McLeod, K. J.: Biologic modulation of mechanical influences in bone remodeling. In Mow, V. C., Ratcliffe, A., and Woo, S. L. Y. (eds.): Biomechanics of Diarthrodial Joints. Vol. II. 1990, pp. 97–118.
163. McLeod, K. J., and Rubin, C. T.: Stimulation of new bone formation by low-frequency sinusoidal electric fields. Trans. 34th Orthop. Res. Soc. 13:123, 1988.
164. McLeod, K. J., and Rubin, C. T.: Predictions of osteogenic mechanical loading paradigms from electrical response data. Trans. Bio. Growth Rep. Soc. 9:20, 1989.
165. Pollack, S. R., Korostoff, E., Fineberg, M., Steinberg, D., and Brighton, C.: Stress-generated potentials in bone: Effects of collagen modification. Biomed. Mater. Res. 11:677, 1962.
166. Bassett, C., and Becker, R.: Generation of electric potentials by bone in response to mechanical stress. Science 137:1063, 1962.
167. Brighton, C. T., and McCluskey, W. P.: Cellular response and mechanisms of action of electrically induced osteogenesis. In Peck, W. A. (ed.): Bone and Mineral Research/4. New York, Elsevier Science Publishers, 1986.
168. Bassett, C. A.: Fundamental and practical aspects of therapeutic uses of pulsed electromagnetic fields (PEMFs). Crit. Rev. Biomed. Eng. 17(5):451, 1989.
169. Ashihara, T., Kagawa, K., Kamich, M., et al.: 3H-Thymidine autoradiographic studies of the cell proliferation and differentiation in electrically stimulated osteogenesis. In Brighton, C. T., Black, J., and Pollack, S. R. (eds.): Electrical Properties of Bone and Cartilage. New York, Grune & Stratton, 1979.
170. McLeod, K. J., Lee, R. D., and Ehrlich, H. P.: Frequency dependence of electric field modulation of fibroblast protein synthesis. Science 236:1465, 1987.
171. Bassett, C. A. L., Chokshi, H. R., Hernandez, E., et al.: The effect of pulsing electromagnetic fields on cellular calcium and calcification of nonunions. In Bright, C. T., Black, J., and Pollack, S. R. (eds.): Electrical Properties of Bone and Cartilage. New York, Grune & Stratton, 1979.
172. Yeh, C. K., and Rodan, G. A.: Tensile forces enhance prostaglandin E synthesis in osteoblastic cells grown on collagen ribbons. Calcif. Tissue Int. 36:S67, 1984.
173. Gardner, E.: Osteogenesis in the human embryo and fetus. In Bourne, G. H. (ed.): The Biochemistry and Physiology of Bone. Vol. III. 2nd ed. New York, Academic Press, 1972.
174. Brookes, M.: The Blood Supply of Bone. An Approach to Bone Biology. London, Butterworths, 1971, pp. 123–132.
175. Hunziker, E. B., Schenk, R. K., and Cruz-Orive, L. M.: Quantitation of chondrocyte performance in growth-plate cartilage during longitudinal bone growth. J. Bone Joint Surg. 69A(2):162, 1987.
176. Hurrell, D. J.: The vascularisation of cartilage. J. Anat. 69:47, 1934.
177. Rosenberg, L. C., Choi, H. U., and Poole, A. R.: Biological processes involved in endochondral ossification. In Rubin, R. T., Weiss, G. B., and Putney, J. B. (eds.): Calcium in Biological Systems. New York, Plenum Publishing Corp., 1985, pp. 617–624.
178. Eggli, P. S., Herrmann, W., Hunziker, E. B., and Schenk, R. K.: Matrix compartments in the growth plate of the proximal tibia of rats. Anat. Rec. 211:246, 1985.
179. Floyd, W. E., Zaleske, D. J., Schiller, A. L., Trahan, C., and Mankin, H. J.: Vascular events associated with the appearance of the secondary center of ossification in the murine distal femoral epiphysis. J. Bone Joint Surg. 69A:185, 1987.
180. Trelstad, R. L., and Silver, F. H.: Matrix assembly. In Hay, E. D. (ed.): Cell Biology of Extracellular Matrix. New York, Plenum Publishing Corp., 1981, pp. 179–215.
181. Roux, W.: Gesammelte Abhandlungen uber Entwicklungsmechanik der Organismen, Vols. I and II. Leipzig, Wilhelm Engelmann, 1895. Terminologie der Entwicklungsmechanik der Tiere und Pflanzen. Leipzig, Wilhelm Engelmann, 1912. Anpassungslehre, Histomechanik und Histochemie. Berichtigungen zu R. Thomas gleichnamigem Aufsatz. Mit Bemerkungen uber die Entwicklung und Formestaltung der satz. Mit Bemerkungen uber die Entwicklung und Formgestaltung der Gelenke. Virchows Arch. (A) 209:168, 1912.
182. Carter, D. R., Orr, T. E., Fyhrie, D. P., and Schurman, D. J.: Influences of mechanical stress on prenatal and postnatal skeletal development. Clin. Orthop. 219:237, 1987.
183. Shapiro, F., Holtrop, M. E., and Glimcher, M. J.: Organization and cellular biology of the perichondrial ossification groove of Ranvier. J. Bone Joint Surg. 59A:703, 1977.
184. Cooper, R. R., and Misol, S.: Tendon and ligament insertion: A light and electron microscopic study. J. Bone Joint Surg. 52A:1, 1970.
185. Shim, S. S.: Physiology of blood circulation of bone. J. Bone Joint Surg. 50A:812, 1968.
186. Rhinelander, F. W.: Circulation of bone. In Bourne, G. H. (ed.): The Biochemistry and Physiology of Bone. Vol. II. 2nd ed. New York, Academic Press, 1972.
187. Sledge, C. B.: Epiphyseal injuries. In Cave, E. F., Burke, J. F., and Boyd, R. J. (eds.): Trauma Management. Chicago, Year Book Medical Publishers, 1974.
188. Trueta, J.: Studies of the Development and Decay of the Human Frame. Philadelphia, W. B. Saunders Company, 1968.
189. Cooper, R. R., James, M. D., Milgram, J. W., and Robinson, R. A.: Morphology of the osteon. J. Bone Joint Surg. 48A:1239, 1966.

Jody A. Dantzig
Yale E. Goldman

Chapter 5
Muscle

INTRODUCTION

Approximately 640 muscles constituting up to 40 percent of the adult body mass make up the skeletal muscle system that supports and moves the body under control of the central nervous system (CNS). The specialization of muscle cells for this task is evident in the complex structure and biochemistry of the contractile apparatus and internal membrane systems. Muscle cells are normally subjected to wide variations in their levels of activity and are able to adapt in size, isoenzyme composition, and membrane organization. This "plasticity" can be surprisingly swift and extensive. This chapter outlines the development, structure, and function of muscle and introduces the basis for its highly adaptive response to altered demands.

MUSCLE DEVELOPMENT

Connective tissue, bone, and muscle are all derived from mesodermal mesenchyme cells. The complex program that controls the differentiation of mesenchymal cells into these tissues is beginning to yield to genetic investigation. In the case of presumptive muscle cells, several transcriptional regulatory factors have been identified that control expression of muscle-type specific genes.[1] These myogenic regulatory factors have a basic helix-loop-helix (HLH) tertiary structural motif homologous to a variety of regulatory gene products.[1a] Homodimers or heterodimers of HLH proteins bind to a consensus DNA sequence (CANNTG, "E-box") present in many gene enhancers, such as those of the immunoglobulin gene and many muscle-specific genes. An example of a myogenic regulatory factor is MyoD,[2] which can initiate muscle differentiation when transfected *in vitro* into several nonmuscle cell types.[1] Members of the MyoD family are expressed only in muscle cells, appear at specific stages in development, and tend to promote expression of each other. The interrelationship of these regulatory factors, the potential for differential control by heterodimerization with more promiscuously expressed HLH proteins, and the "master switch" in this genetic program all remain to be elucidated.

Presumptive myoblasts derived from mesenchymal cells proliferate and migrate throughout the embryo into regions that will give rise to muscle.

They withdraw from the cell cycle and differentiate into spindle-shaped myoblasts. The myoblasts align and fuse to produce multinucleated myotubes (Fig. 5–1), which synthesize embryonic muscle-specific proteins. Myofibrils are assembled near the periphery of these myotubes, and continued synthesis fills the cytoplasm, at which point the nuclei migrate to the periphery. Secondary generations of myoblasts elongate, fuse, and differentiate into secondary myotubes within the basal lamina of the primary myotube.[3] The secondary myotubes separate and form independent fibers. Myotubes mature into phenotypically distinct types of muscle fibers by sequentially expressing a series of discrete embryonic, neonatal, and mature type-specific isoforms of the contractile proteins. Axons of α-motor neurons grow out from the ventral horn of the spinal column and branch near the muscle to innervate several fibers simultaneously.

A pool of myogenic stem cells remains in mature muscles, forming a cellular reservoir for muscle repair and growth. These *satellite cells* are situated between the muscle cell membrane (sarcolemma) and basal lamina of the muscle fibers. The number of muscle fibers remains roughly constant throughout life, but when a cell is structurally damaged or necrotic, satellite cells migrate into the affected area and fuse to form a new myotube. This process is under control of mitogenic factors and peptide regulators released from the damaged cells.[4]

STRUCTURE

Approximately 85 percent of the mass of a muscle corresponds to the muscle fibers, the remainder being innervation, blood supply, and connective tissue structures providing support, elasticity, and force transmission to the skeleton. Variation of mechanical properties arises from several geometric arrangements of fibers in the muscle: parallel, fan shaped, fusiform (spindle-like), or pennate (feather-like). As an example, for a given size of the muscle and consequent metabolic load, the tilt of the fibers in pennate muscles increases force generation, at the expense of speed and range of movement, compared with a muscle having fibers arranged parallel to the force axis.[5]

Human skeletal muscle fibers are cylindrical cells 10 to 150 μm in diameter, ranging in length from a

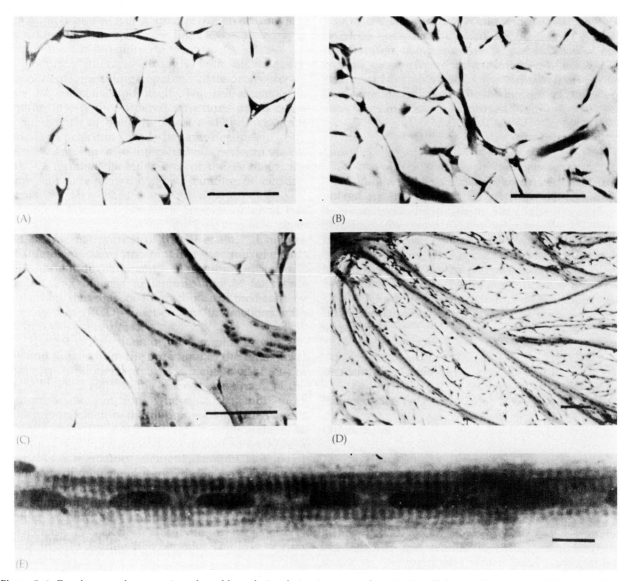

Figure 5–1. Developmental progression of myoblasts during fusion into myotubes. *A,* Unicellular myoblasts, bar = 0.1 mm. *B,* Initial fusion of myoblasts. *C,* Multinucleated myotubes. *D,* Lower magnification micrograph of multinucleated myotubes showing extent of cell fusion. *E,* Multinucleated myotube with cross-striations; bar = 0.01 mm. (From Buckley, P. A., and Konigsberg, I. R.: Myogenic fusion and the duration of the post-mitotic gap (G1). Dev. Biol. 37:198, 1974. Used by permission.)

few to more than 300 mm. The muscle cell membrane invaginates at regular intervals to form the transverse tubule (*T tubule*) network, which consists of connected longitudinal and lateral components that pervade the fiber. The lumen of the T tubule network is contiguous with the extracellular space and contains the high Na^+ and low K^+ concentrations of the interstitial fluid.[6] A high K^+ and low Na^+ intracellular compartment, the sarcoplasmic reticulum (SR), contains the Ca^{2+}-binding protein calsequestrin in its terminal cisternae and serves as a reservoir for Ca^{2+} ions. The dihydropyridine receptor of the T tubules[7] (homologous to plasma membrane Ca^{2+} channels in other cells) is juxtaposed to the cytoplasmic domain of the SR Ca^{2+} release channel[8] (foot protein) in the SR terminal cisternae membrane, thus linking the two membrane systems. Figure 5–2 shows the rela-

tionship of the intracellular membrane systems to the contractile apparatus.

The organelles responsible for production of force or shortening are *myofibrils* (Fig. 5–3), cylindrical protein arrays approximately 1 μm in diameter that usually extend the entire length of the fiber. The basic contractile unit, the *sarcomere*, periodically repeats approximately every 2.5 μm along the length of the myofibril and is delineated by densely packed Z-lines at each end containing α-actinin. The contractile and structural proteins are arranged within the myofibril in a highly ordered, nearly crystalline lattice of interdigitating filaments[9] (Fig. 5–3). The locations and putative functions of these proteins are listed in Table 5–1.

Thick myosin-containing filaments, 1.6 μm long, are located in the center of the sarcomere, in the

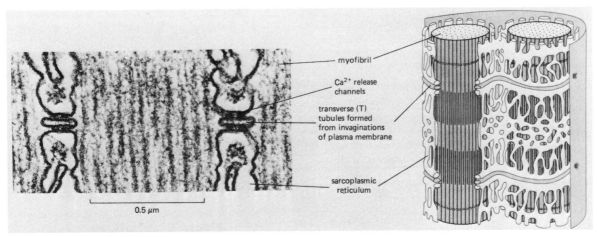

Figure 5–2. Membrane systems that relay the excitation signal from the sarcolemma to the cell interior. In the electron micrograph, two T tubules are cut in cross-section. The electron densities spanning the gap between the T tubules and sarcoplasmic reticulum are channels that release calcium into the myoplasm. (From Alberts, B., et al.: Molecular Biology of the Cell. 2nd ed. New York, Garland Publishers, 1989, p. 622. Micrograph courtesy of Dr. Clara Franzini-Armstrong.)

optically anisotropic A-band. Myosin is an asymmetric molecule with an α-helical coiled-coil portion (rod) at one end and a globular portion (cross-bridge) at the other end. Each myosin molecule contains two 220-kD heavy chains and four light chain subunits of approximately 20 kD each. The rod portions of approximately 300 myosin molecules polymerize in a three-stranded helix with a 14.3 nm subunit spacing and a 42.9 nm axial repeat to form the backbone of a thick filament. The cross-bridges protrude from the filament backbone (Fig. 5–3, diagram 12) and contain adenosine triphosphatase (ATPase) activity as well as an actin-binding region. Thick filaments are positioned laterally in a hexagonal lattice and are stabilized by M-filaments[10] and muscle-specific creatine phosphokinase[11] (MM CPK) in the centrally located M-line.

Thin filaments extend 1.1 μm from each side of the Z-line forming the more isotropic I-band and are positioned within the hexagonal lattice of the A-band equidistant from three thick filaments. Thin filaments are double-stranded helical polymers of actin with 5.1, 5.9, and 72 nm helical pitches. A regulatory complex of three troponin subunits (C, T, and I) and

Table 5–1. SIGNALING AND CONTRACTILE PROTEINS OF SKELETAL MUSCLE

Protein	Molecular Weight (kD)	Subunits (kD)	Location	Function
Acetylcholine receptor	~250	5 × ~50	Postsynaptic membrane of neuromuscular junction	Neuromuscular signal transmission
Dihydropyridine receptor	~380	1 × ~160 1 × ~130 1 × ~60 1 × ~30	T tubule membrane	Voltage sensor
SR calcium-release channel foot protein	1800	4 × 450	Terminal cisternae of SR	SR Ca^{2+} release
Troponin	78	1 × 18 1 × 30 1 × 30	Thin filament	Regulation of contraction
Tropomyosin	64	2 × 32	Thin filament	Regulation of contraction
Myosin	500	2 × 220 4 × 20	Thick filament	Chemomechanical energy transduction
Actin	42	—	Thin filament	Chemomechanical energy transduction
MM CPK	40	—	M-line	ATP buffer Structural protein
α-Actinin	190	2 × 95	Z-line	Structural protein
Titin	3000	—	Entire sarcomere	Structural protein
Nebulin	600	—	I-band	Structural protein
Dystrophin	400	—	Subsarcolemma	Maintenance of membrane Structural integrity

SR, sarcoplasmic reticulum; CPK, creatine phosphokinase.

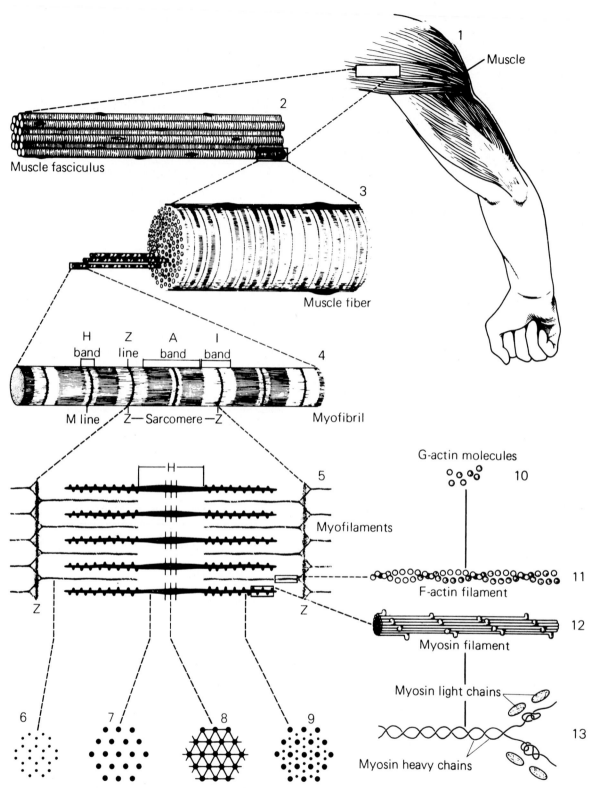

Figure 5–3. Diagram of the components of the contractile apparatus in successively magnified views from the tissue to the molecular levels. The myofibril (4) shows the band pattern and extent of the sarcomere between two Z-lines. Diagrams 6 to 9 show cross-sections of the hexagonal filament lattice at various points within the sarcomere. (From Junqueira, L. C., et al.: Basic Histology. 5th ed. Norwalk, CT, Appleton-Lange Publishers, 1986. Modified from Bloom, W., and Fawcett, D. W.: A Textbook of Histology. 10th ed. Philadelphia, W. B. Saunders, 1975.)

a tropomyosin molecule is associated with each group of seven successive actin monomers along the thin filament.[9]

The sarcomeric filaments are remarkably uniform in length and lateral registration even during activation. This highly regular organization has facilitated biophysical studies of muscle by sophisticated structural[9] and spectroscopic techniques.[13] The lateral alignment of the filaments within each sarcomere and the alignment between sarcomeres of adjacent myofibrils leads to the cross-striated histologic appearance of both skeletal and cardiac muscle.

Two recently identified sets of sarcomeric filaments consist of the giant proteins titin and nebulin. Individual titin molecules extend from the M-line to the Z-line and associate with the thick filaments in the A-band. Nebulin is restricted to the I-band and associates with thin filaments.[12] In addition to the proteins arrayed in the myofibrils, the cytoskeleton of muscle fibers is composed of cytoplasmic actin, microtubules, intermediate filaments,[14] and membrane-associated proteins such as *dystrophin*. Duchenne's muscular dystrophy results from mutations in the dystrophin gene,[15, 15a] emphasizing the importance of cytoskeletal elements for the structural integrity of the cell.

EVENTS DURING CONTRACTIONS

A skeletal muscle fiber is normally activated briefly, after which it relaxes. This brief contraction, called a *twitch*, is initiated by propagation of an action potential along a myelinated α-motor neuron from the CNS to the motor end-plate at the neuromuscular junction. An individual α-motor neuron can establish synapses with 5 to 1600 muscle fibers to form a *motor unit*. The level of activity in a muscle is controlled by varying the rate of the twitches and the number of active motor units. As the level of activity increases, more and larger motor units are recruited. Afferent feedback pathways from Golgi tendon organs and spindle receptors modulate activity to produce the desired movement. The same feedback system generates the stretch reflex.

When the nerve action potential reaches the presynaptic terminal of the neuromuscular junction, the membrane depolarization switches local calcium channels open. Extracellular Ca^{2+} enters through these channels, triggering fusion of acetylcholine (ACh) loaded membrane vesicles with the presynaptic junctional membrane, releasing the transmitter into the junctional cleft. Synapsin I, a phosphoprotein associated with these vesicles, synaptophysin, an integral vesicular membrane protein, and other recently identified proteins participate with cytoplasmic actin in the transport of the vesicles to the terminal membrane and subsequent exocytosis of the neurotransmitter.[16] ACh rapidly diffuses across the cleft to the postsynaptic region of the sarcolemma, where it binds to nicotinic ACh receptors that function as ACh-gated ion channels. Cloning and sequencing of the ACh receptor[17] and description of the molecular structure in two-dimensional crystals[18] have launched a productive era in structure-function studies of membrane proteins.

When ACh binds to the sarcolemmal receptors, increased permeability to cations depolarizes the postsynaptic membrane, initiating a regenerative action potential that propagates via voltage-gated Na^+ and K^+ channels over the entire sarcolemma and T tubule network. The dihydropyridine receptor in the T tubule membrane serves as a voltage sensor to transmit the activation signal directly to the foot protein of the SR membrane, which then releases Ca^{2+} into the myoplasm, activating the contractile machinery. The twitch is ended when Ca^{2+} is transported back into the SR by an adenosine triphosphate (ATP) driven Ca^{2+} pump located in the longitudinal regions of the SR membranes. In cultured cells from a dysgenic strain of mice with phenotypically absent coupling between excitation and Ca^{2+} release, coupling of excitation and contraction is rescued by transfection with complementary DNA encoding for the major subunit of the dihydropyridine receptor.[19] Expression of chimeras of the skeletal and cardiac dihydropyridine receptors in this system demonstrated that a cytoplasmic domain determines the tissue-specific phenotype.[20] Mutations in the SR Ca^{2+} release channel probably result in malignant hyperthermia.[21]

A cyclic interaction between actin in the thin filaments and myosin in the thick filaments leads to a relative sliding force between the two filaments, with energy derived from hydrolysis of ATP to adenosine diphosphate (ADP) and orthophosphate (P_i). The regulatory proteins troponin and tropomyosin in the thin filaments inhibit the actomyosin ATPase, but when the Ca^{2+} released from the SR binds to troponin, this inhibition is relieved. The molecular events in the actomyosin interaction (cross-bridge cycle) are shown in more detail in Fig. 5–4. As long as Ca^{2+} is present, a complex of myosin, ADP, and P_i can attach to the thin filament (step a), and a structural change associated with P_i release generates the sliding force.[22, 22a] After ADP is released, ATP binds to the myosin and dissociates it from actin (step d). The ATP is then hydrolyzed to form the myosin-ADP-P_i complex, completing the cycle (step e). The structural change in actomyosin that leads to force generation is often depicted as a tilting motion (Fig. 5–4), but this point has not been firmly established.[23, 23a, 23b]

If the mechanical load on the activated muscle fiber is high, the cross-bridge cycle produces force to support the load (isometric contraction), but if the load is moderate, the thin filaments slide toward the center of the sarcomere, resulting in work production and shortening of the muscle. An elevation in the energy requirement for the work performed during shortening is reflected by an increase of the ATPase rate. The ATP concentration in skeletal muscle is

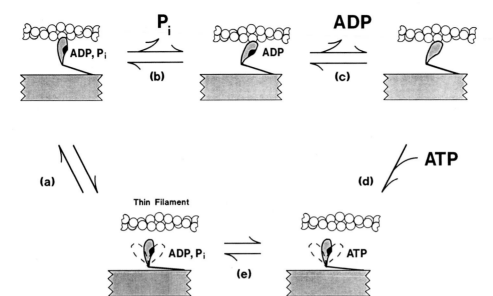

Figure 5–4. The actomyosin cross-bridge cycle. Myosin molecules have two globular head regions (cross-bridges), but for clarity only one head is shown. The sequence of reactions is attachment (a), P_i release and the force generating transition (b), ADP release (c), ATP binding and detachment (d), and ATP hydrolysis (e). The state of bound nucleotide is shown next to each head. The dashed lines near the myosins on the bottom row indicate that the detached cross-bridges are highly mobile.

buffered effectively by MM CPK, which catalyzes the transfer of phosphate from creatine phosphate to ADP, forming ATP in the myofibrils and bulk cytoplasm. Glycolysis and mitochondrial oxidative phosphorylation re-establish metabolic conditions on a slower time scale.

During intense or prolonged activity, muscle fatigue is caused by alterations of metabolite levels that suppress the contractile apparatus or excitation-contraction coupling, or both. Marked increases in myoplasmic P_i and H^+ concentrations can be detected by magnetic resonance spectroscopy.[24] The chemomechanical linkage between P_i release and force generation shown in Figure 5–4 implies that the increased myoplasmic P_i concentration in fatigue will reduce the force of contraction.[22]

PLASTICITY

Muscle fibers are classified according to their size, speed of contraction, balance between aerobic and glycolytic metabolism, and fatigue resistance, as shown in Table 5–2. Isoenzymes of the contractile and regulatory proteins and the surface area of the SR membranes are key features that distinguish functional properties. For instance, the duration of the twitch is established by the SR Ca^{2+} release and reuptake mechanisms, and the velocity of shortening is determined by the different myosin isoenzymes. Each motor unit is composed of a homogeneous population of fibers and, thus, they can be classified according to the same criteria. However, classification schemes are not absolute because some motor units can be found that have composite functional, ultrastructural, and histochemical characteristics.

Classic cross-innervation experiments demonstrated that the innervation can specify and modify muscle fiber type.[25] All of the functional and histologic properties listed in Table 5–2 shift toward the target muscle type over several weeks following cross-innervation, clearly indicating that muscles are in a dynamic state of adaptation and remodeling due to the demands placed on their activity. Control of this plasticity is not fully understood, but the rate and pattern of neuronal firing are influential, and trophic substances from the neuron may also be involved. There is evidence that during development, fiber type specificity is partly determined prior to innervation.[26]

Plasticity of muscle is expressed in many physiologic and clinical situations. The adaptations to exercise include alterations in specific contractile, regulatory, structural, and metabolic proteins. The frequency, intensity, and duration of a training stimulus mediate the adaptive response,[27] but the roles of neural trophic and growth factors have not been fully characterized. Strength training leads to hypertrophy of fast, type IIB muscle fibers, whereas endurance training enhances metabolism in type I and IIA fibers. Long-term hyperplasia does not usually occur following training. There is also little evidence that voluntary training regimens can switch fibers between the major categories. Reduction of physical activity, for instance in limb immobilization, results in a decreased cross-section of muscle fibers and a reduction in endurance due to a decreased metabolic reserve. Exercise hypertrophy and disuse atrophy are both reversible, but after extensive alterations the reversion may be incomplete.[28]

The endocrine system also participates in plasticity. For instance, normal levels of circulating thyroid hormones are required during muscle development and differentiation.[29] Experimental alterations of thyroid hormone promote changes in the levels of myosin and regulatory protein isoforms within the

Table 5–2. CLASSIFICATION OF MUSCLE FIBER TYPES

Characteristic	Fiber Type			
	I	IIA	IIB	IIC
Size	Moderate	Small	Large	Small
Color	Red	White	White	White
Mitochondria	Many	Intermediate	Few	Intermediate
Capillary blood supply	Extensive	Sparse	Sparse	Sparse
SR membrane	Sparse	Extensive	Extensive	Extensive
Z-line	Wide	Wide	Narrow	Narrow
Protein isoforms				
MHC	MHCI	MHCIIA	MHCIIB	MHCI and MHCIIA
MLC	MLC1s	MLC1f	MLC1f	MLC1f and MLC1s
MPLC	MPLC2s	MPLC2f	MPLC2f	MPLC2f and MPLC2s
Regulatory proteins	Slow	Fast	Fast	Fast
Mechanical properties				
Contraction time	Slow and sustained	Fast twitch	Fast twitch	Moderate twitch
SR calcium ATPase rate	Low	High	High	High
Shortening velocity	Slow	Fast	Fast	Moderate
Actomyosin ATPase rate	Low	High	High	Moderate
Resistance to fatigue	High	Moderate	Low	Moderate
Metabolic profile				
Oxidative capacity	High	Intermediate	Low	High
Glycolytic capacity	Moderate	High	High	High
NADH-TR/SDH/MDH	High	Moderate	Low	Moderate
LDH and phosphorylase	Low	Medium	High	NA
Glycogen	Low	High	High	Variable
Myoglobin	High	Medium	Low	NA

MHC, myosin heavy chain; MLC, myosin alkali light chain; MPLC, myosin phosphorylatable light chain (regulatory); NADH-TR, nicotinamide adenine dinucleotide tetrazolium reductase; SDH, succinate dehydrogenase; MDH, malate dehydrogenase; LDH, lactate dehydrogenase; NA, not available from the literature.

myofibrils as well as in the activity of some metabolic enzymes.[30] An intact nerve supply is required for these effects, but mediation through growth factors, such as somatomedins and fibroblast growth factor, has not been excluded.

SUMMARY

The complex functional capacity of muscle to produce finely tuned and coordinated movements is ultimately expressed as transduction of chemical to mechanical energy by actomyosin. A twitch is initiated via an action potential propagated from the CNS along an α-motor neuron, neuromuscular chemical transmission, direct protein-protein communication at the T tubule–SR junction, Ca^{2+} ion diffusion in the myoplasm, and Ca^{2+} binding to thin-filament regulatory proteins. Because the CNS controls activity only through recruitment of motor units, gradation and coordination of movement depend critically on the pattern of connections between the α-motor neurons and the muscle fibers and the variation of properties among motor units. Development and maintenance of the muscular system involve a complex series of genetic programs and cellular interactions just beginning to be understood at the molecular level. Plasticity of motor unit properties is evident not only in training regimens but also in reduced activity due to pain or joint immobilization and in compromised metabolic, hormonal, or nutri-

tional conditions. Hence, plasticity impacts on the clinical course of many diseases. In addition to its importance in pathophysiology, muscle serves as an excellent substrate for understanding the molecular basis of development, protein structure-function, cell signaling, and energy transduction processes.

References

1. Weintraub, H., Davis, R., Tapscott, S., Thayer, M., Krause, M., Benezra, R., Blackwell, T. K., Turner, D., Rupp, R., Hollenberg, S., Zhuang, Y., and Lassar, A.: The *myoD* gene family: Nodal point during specification of the muscle cell lineage. Science 251:761, 1991.
1a. Schwarz, J. J., Chakraborty, T., Martin, J., Zhou, J., and Olson, E. N.: The basic region of myogenin cooperates with the two transcription activation domains to induce muscle-specific transcription. Mol. Cell. Biol. 12:266, 1992.
2. Tapscott, S. J., Davis, R. L., Thayer, M. J., Cheng, P.-F., Weintraub, H., and Lassar, A. B.: MyoD1: A nuclear phosphoprotein requiring a *Myc* homology region to convert fibroblasts to myoblasts. Science 242:405, 1988.
3. Kelly, A. M., and Rubenstein, N. A.: Development of neuromuscular specialization. Med. Sci. Sports Exerc. 18:292, 1986.
4. Florini, J. R.: Hormonal control of muscle growth. Muscle and Nerve 10:577, 1987.
5. Gowitzke, B. A., and Milner, M.: Scientific Bases of Human Movement, 3rd ed. Baltimore, Williams and Wilkins, 1988, pp. 144–145.
6. Somlyo, A. V., Gonzalez-Serratos, H., Shuman, H., McClellan, G., and Somlyo, A. P.: Calcium release and ionic changes in the sarcoplasmic reticulum of tetanized muscle: An electron-probe study. J. Cell Biol. 90:577, 1981.
7. Schwartz, L. M., McCleskey, E. W., and Almers, W.: Dihydropyridine receptors in muscle are voltage-dependent but most are not functional calcium channels. Nature 314:747, 1985.
8. Block, B. A., Imagawa, T., Campbell, K. P., and Franzini-Armstrong, C.: Structural evidence for direct interaction between the molecular components of the transverse tubule/sarcoplasmic reticulum junction in skeletal muscle. J. Cell Biol. 107:2587, 1988.

9. Squire, J.: The Structural Basis of Muscular Contraction. New York, Plenum Press, 1981.
10. Chowrashi, P. K., and Pepe, F. A.: M-band proteins: Evidence for more than one component. *In* Pepe, F. A., Sanger, J. W., and Nachmias, V. T. (eds.): Motility in Cell Function. New York, Academic Press, 1979, pp. 419–422.
11. Wallimann, T., Pelloni, G., Turner, D. C., and Eppenberger, H. M.: Removal of the M-line by treatment with Fab' fragments of antibodies against MM-creatine kinase. *In* Pepe, F. A., Sanger, J. W., and Nachmias, V. T. (eds.): Motility in Cell Function. New York, Academic Press, 1979, pp. 415–418.
12. Wang, K.: Sarcomere-associated cytoskeletal lattices in striated muscle. *In* Shay, J. W. (ed.): Cell and Muscle Motility, vol. 6. New York, Plenum Press, 1985, pp. 315–369.
13. Thomas, D. D.: Spectroscopic probes of muscle cross-bridge rotation. Annu. Rev. Physiol. 49:691, 1987.
14. Toyama, Y., Forry-Schaudies, S., Hoffman, B., and Holtzer, H.: Effects of taxol and colcemid on myofibrillogenesis. Proc. Natl. Acad. Sci. U.S.A. 79:6556, 1982.
15. Hoffman, E. P., Brown, R. H., Jr., and Kunkel, L. M.: Dystrophin: The protein product of the Duchenne muscular dystrophy locus. Cell 51:919, 1987.
15a. Ibraghimov-Beskrovnaya, O., Eruasti, J. M., Leveille, C. J., Slaughter, C. A., Sernett, S. W., and Campbell, K. P.: Primary structure of dystrophin-associated glycoproteins linking dystrophin to the extracellular matrix. Nature 355:696, 1992.
16. Torri-Tarelli, F., Villa, A., Valtorta, F., De Camilli, P., Greengard, P., and Ceccarelli, B.: Redistribution of synaptophysin and synapsin I during α-latrotoxin–induced release of neurotransmitter at the neuromuscular junction. J. Cell Biol. 110:449, 1990.
17. Mishina, M., Takai, T., Imoto, K., Noda, M., Takahashi, T., Numa, S., Methfessel, C., and Sakmann, B.: Molecular distinction between fetal and adult forms of muscle acetylcholine receptor. Nature 321:406, 1986.
18. Brisson, A., and Unwin, P. N. T.: Quaternary structure of the acetylcholine receptor. Nature 315:474, 1985.
19. Tanabe, T., Beam, K. G., Powell, J. A., and Numa, S.: Restoration of excitation-contraction coupling and slow calcium current in dysgenic muscle by dihydropyridine receptor complementary DNA. Nature 336:134, 1988.
20. Tanabe, T., Beam, K. G., Adams, B. A., Niidome, T., and Numa, S.: Regions of the skeletal muscle dihydropyridine receptor critical for excitation-contraction coupling. Nature 346:567, 1990.
21. Gillard E. F., Otsu, K., Fujii, J., Khanna, V. K., De Leon, S., Derdemezi, J., Britt, B. A., Duff, C. L., Worton, R. G., and MacLennan, D. H.: A substitution of cysteine for arginine 614 in the ryanodine receptor is potentially causative of human malignant hyperthermia. Genomics 11:751, 1991.
22. Goldman, Y. E.: Kinetics of the actomyosin ATPase in muscle fibers. Annu. Rev. Physiol. 49:637, 1987.
22a. Dantzig, J. A., Goldman, Y. E., Millar, N. C., Lacktis, J., and Hornsher, E.: Reversal of the cross-bridge force-generating transition by photogeneration of phosphate in rabbit psoas muscle fibres. J. Physiol. 1992 (in press).
23. Cooke, R., Crowder, M. S., Wendt, C. H., Barnett, V. A., and Thomas, D. D.: Muscle cross-bridges: Do they rotate? *In* Pollack, G. H., and Sugi, H. (eds.): Contractile Mechanisms in Muscle. Advances in Experimental Medicine and Biology. vol. 170. New York, Plenum Press, 1984, p. 413.
23a. Tanner, J. W., Thomas, D. D., and Goldman, Y. E.: Transients in orientation of a fluorescent cross-bridge probe following photolysis of caged nucleotides in skeletal muscle fibres. J. Mol. Biol. 223:185, 1992.
23b. Irving, M., Lombardi, V., Piazzesi, G., and Ferenczi, M.: Myosin head movements are synchronous with the elementary force-generating process in muscle. Nature, 1992 (in press).
24. Meyer, R. A., Brown, T. R., and Kushmerick, M. J.: Phosphorus nuclear magnetic resonance of fast- and slow-twitch muscle. Am. J. Physiol. 248:C279, 1985.
25. Buller, A. J., Eccles, J. C., and Eccles, R. M.: Differentiation of fast and slow muscles in the cat hind limb. J. Physiol. 150:399, 1960.
26. Miller, J. B., and Stockdale, F. E.: What muscle cells know that nerves don't tell them. Trends Neurosci. 10:325, 1987.
27. Faulkner, J. A., and White, T. P.: Adaptations of skeletal muscle to physical activity. *In* Bouchard, C., Shephard, R. J., Stephens, T., Sutton, J. R., and McPherson, B. D. (eds.): Exercise, Fitness, and Health, Champaign, IL, Human Kinetics Publishers, 1990, pp. 265–279.
28. Appell, H.-J.: Muscular atrophy following immobilisation: A review. Sports Med. 10:42, 1990.
29. Rubenstein, N. A., Lyons, G. E., and Kelly, A. M.: Hormonal control of myosin heavy chain genes during development of skeletal muscles. Ciba Found. Symp. 138:35, 1989.
30. Nwoye, L., and Mommaerts, W. F. H. M.: The effects of thyroid status on some properties of rat fast-twitch muscle. J. Muscle Res. Cell Motil. 2:307, 1981.

Section II

Immune and Inflammatory Responses

Chapter 6

Barbara S. Nepom
Gerald T. Nepom

Immunogenetics and the Rheumatic Diseases

INTRODUCTION

Genetic control of the immune response is governed by a limited set of genes, which are variable among different individuals. This variation, or genetic polymorphism, is a key element used by the immune system to discriminate self from non-self; in other words, to regulate the recognition of foreign antigens. In the autoimmune disorders, including the rheumatic diseases, the variation among these genes is also a primary genetic determinant of disease susceptibility. Particular genetic variants are responsible for an individual's predisposition to a particular disease. The genetic and structural basis for these predisposing genes, and the insight into the mechanisms of pathogenesis gained from the study of these genes, are discussed in this chapter.

Genetic Susceptibility

For many of the rheumatic diseases, genetic susceptibility is an important member of a triad of triggering factors implicated in pathogenesis. As schematically illustrated in Figure 6–1, this genetic contribution is an important determinant of disease susceptibility but does not act alone. Environmental contributions—unknown for most of the rheumatic diseases—and developmental factors, possibly including additional genetic elements, act in concert with the immunogenetic contribution to trigger disease. Thus, disease susceptibility genes are best viewed as "permissive" for disease, interacting with other etiologic factors in pathogenesis.

Because of this requirement for other interactions, most individuals who carry disease susceptibility genes do not get clinical disease. In other words, many individuals are genetically "at risk" but fall outside the intersecting triad of triggering factors. In this sense, disease susceptibility genes can be regarded as naturally occurring genetic variations that, by themselves, are not sufficient for clinical disease.

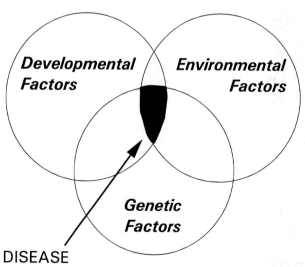

Figure 6–1. Schematic illustration of the role of genetic factors in susceptibility to autoimmune disease, and interactions with other triggering factors. The genetic susceptibility factors are "permissive" for disease and identify at-risk individuals, although in most people who carry such genes disease does not occur.

The degree of penetrance of such disease susceptibility genes is hard to generalize, as the contributions of environmental and developmental factors vary for different diseases. However, a rough estimate of the genetic contribution within the framework of this susceptibility triad can be estimated from studies of monozygotic twin pairs in which one of the twins carries a rheumatic disease. In rheumatoid arthritis (RA), for example, several such studies have been performed and suggest that the concordance rate for RA among monozygotic twins is approximately one in six.[1, 2] Thus, while the appropriate susceptibility genes are permissive for disease, the other interacting elements are major determinants of pathogenesis.

Two other related issues are frequently considered in discussions of disease susceptibility: Is susceptibility dominant or recessive? Does the presence of such genes confer susceptibility, or does their absence confer protection? These issues will be considered in more detail in some of the examples discussed later. In general, however, the notion of a permissive susceptibility gene, whose penetrance is dependent on environmental and developmental interactions, lends itself best to a model of incomplete, but dominant, susceptibility. With a few exceptions, most immunogenetic models in the rheumatic diseases can be satisfactorily explained by considering one or more susceptibility genes, inherited as a single copy in an individual, as providing the essential susceptibility trait within the framework of a triad of interacting triggering factors.

Genetic Polymorphism

As previously indicated, disease susceptibility genes are examples of variations within important genetic elements that regulate the immune response. They represent individual branches on a complex evolutionary tree that has a large number of other genetic members. This genetic variation within a family of closely related genes, which occur at the same locus in the genome, is referred to as *polymorphism*. When multiple polymorphic variants of a single gene occur in the population, each variant is referred to as an allele, and thus individual disease susceptibility genes are allelic with respect to other closely related genes that themselves are not disease susceptibility genes. An understanding of this simple genetic relationship forms the basis for much of the immunogenetic analysis of disease susceptibility.

Two basic insights into pathogenesis derive from studies of polymorphism. First, simple genetic detection of a disease susceptibility allele provides a way of determining an individual's disease predisposition, and, second, comparisons of the disease susceptibility allele with closely related alleles not involved with disease provide important clues as to the primary genetic basis for mechanisms of disease. These concepts are best understood for several of the rheumatic diseases in which the primary disease susceptibility genes lie within a region of chromosome 6 known as the HLA complex. The next section will briefly outline the structure and organization of the human leukocyte antigen (HLA) gene complex and then will discuss the immunogenetics of this complex in relationship to specific rheumatic diseases.

THE HLA COMPLEX

The HLA genes, which encompass approximately 4000 kilobases of DNA on chromosome 6, compose the major histocompatibility complex (MHC) in humans. These genes encode the HLA molecules, which are the essential and central molecular contributors to the specificity of immune recognition; in other words, the primary determinants of what is self and what is non-self in terms of immune activation. The function of these molecules is intimately tied to their structure, and in this section we will first consider the gene organization and structure as a means of introducing the molecular basis for their association with disease.

Gene Organization

The HLA complex is located on the short arm of chromosome 6, approximately 15 centimorgans (recombination map distance) from the centromere (Fig. 6–2). The HLA class I genes lie at the telomeric end of this complex and include at least six known HLA class I loci, three of which encode highly polymorphic HLA class I proteins, known as the class I histocompatibility antigens. A number of other possibly significant genes lie in this region as well, including a collagen type 4 gene and genes for the cytokines tumor necrosis factor-alpha (TNF-α) and lymphotoxin (also called TNF-β) near the HLA-B locus, as well as a number of other as yet unidentified genes.[3-8]

Centromeric of the class I region of the HLA complex lies a cluster of genes encoding complement components C2, C4, and Bf, as well as the structural gene for 21-hydroxylase.[9 &10] This region, sometimes referred to as the HLA class III region, separates the class I region from the HLA class II genes, which cluster at the centromeric end of the HLA region.

The number of HLA class II genes is variable among different haplotypes but averages approximately 14 loci, of which many are pseudogenes (see Fig. 6–2). On most haplotypes, seven of these loci encode functionally important class II polypeptides, as discussed later. As with the class I genes, other non-HLA genes are interspersed among the class II loci and are of possible importance in disease susceptibility, including genes that play a role in antigen processing.

Class I Genes. The gene organization of the

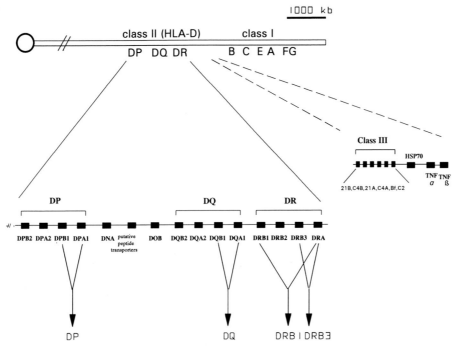

Figure 6–2. Gene organization of the MHC located on chromosome 6. HLA genes segregate into the class I and class II clusters, separated by the non-HLA class III cluster. Several additional non-HLA genes that map into the MHC are also shown; disease susceptibility associated with particular HLA genes may be due to an HLA structural gene or to a non-HLA gene linked to other genes within the complex. Vertical arrows denote HLA class II *expressed* genes that encode the major DR, DQ, and DP molecules; other class II genes are pseudogenes or have unknown function. Genes are illustrated with the centromere on the left; 21A and 21B: 21-hydroxylase genes; C4B, C4A, C2: complement component genes; Bf: properdin factor B; TNF: tumor necrosis factor; HSP70: heat shock protein 70.

HLA class I complex is illustrated in Figure 6–2. Three loci, termed *HLA-A, B,* and *C,* encode the principal HLA class I molecules, which are expressed on all nucleated cells. Each of these three loci is highly polymorphic, with more than 80 alleles so far described for *HLA-A* and *B,* and additional alleles undoubtedly yet to be described (Table 6–1). These loci are often called the "classic" transplantation antigens, since they form the major histocompatibility barrier to allogeneic transplantation. Even minor allelic variation can be functionally important; for example, a single amino acid difference has been implicated in the allorecognition seen in a case of bone marrow graft rejection.[11]

Early definition of class I alleles depended on serologic recognition by serum from multiparous women or monoclonal antibodies. Many of the original specificities defined, such as *HLA-B27,* have since been shown by biochemical and DNA sequence studies to be families of several related alleles. Six alleles carrying the B27 specificity have been defined to date.[12, 13]

The *HLA-E, F,* and *G* genes, as well as additional class I–like loci of unknown function, are often referred to as the "non-classic" class I genes. Like the *HLA-A, B,* and *C* genes, which are expressed in most nucleated cells, transcription of the *HLA-E* and *F* genes has been seen in most cells where it has been investigated.[14] Expression of the *HLA-G* gene, on the other hand, appears restricted to placental tropho-

blasts, an intriguing observation implying potentially interesting functional consequences.[15] Heavy chains of all three genes, *HLA-E, F,* and *G,* are somewhat truncated relative to other class I genes, owing to shortened cytoplasmic tails.[16]

Class II Genes. Genes of the HLA class II complex are of two types, those that encode α-polypeptides and those that encode β-polypeptides, which together, as an α-β heterodimer, constitute the mature class II molecule. Although there are multiple class II genes, the gene organization reflects an evolutionary history in which certain clusters of genes correspond to discrete patterns of α- and β-polypeptide pairs. Thus, three major subregions of the class II complex are described, known as HLA-DR, DQ, and DP. This nomenclature replaces the previous description of this complex as the HLA-D region. In the HLA-DR region, a single α gene, *HLA-DRA,* is linked to one or more β genes, known as *HLA-DRB1, DRB3, DRB4,* or *DRB5.* On most haplotypes, some of these *HLA-DRB* genes are nonfunctional, or pseudogenes, so that in most cases only two of these genes are expressed. The resulting HLA-DR molecule encoded by the *HLA-DR* gene complex is a heterodimeric product of two such genes (e.g., *HLA-DRA/DRB1,* or *HLA-DRA/DRB3*). The *DRB1* locus encodes the β-chains comprising the alleles DR1 (currently *DRB1*0101*), DR2, DR3, etc., while the second expressed gene varies on different haplotypes, such that most *DR3* haplotypes, for example,

Table 6–1. CURRENT NOMENCLATURE OF HLA-A, B, AND C ALLELES RECOGNIZED BY THE WHO COMMITTEE FOR FACTORS OF THE HLA SYSTEM, AS OF 1990[49]

"Classic" HLA Class I Alleles					
HLA-A Alleles		HLA-B Alleles		HLA-C Alleles	
1990 NOMENCLATURE	PREVIOUS DESIGNATIONS	1990 NOMENCLATURE	PREVIOUS DESIGNATIONS	1990 NOMENCLATURE	PREVIOUS DESIGNATIONS
A*0101	A1	B*0701	B7, B7.1	Cw*0101	Cw1
A*0201	A2, A2.1	B*0702	B7, B7.2	Cw*0201	Cw2, Cw2.1
A*0202	A2, A2.2F	B*0801	B8	Cw*02021	Cw2, Cw2.2
A*0203	A2, A2.3	B*1301	B13, B13.1	Cw*02022	Cw2, Cw2.2
A*0204	A2	B*1302	B13, B13.2	Cw*0301	Cw3
A*0205	A2, A2.2Y	B*1401	B14	Cw*0501	Cw5
A*0206	A2, A2.4a	B*1402	Bw65 (14)	Cw*0601	Cw6
A*0207	A2, A2.4b	B*1501	Bw62 (15)	Cw*0701	Cw7
A*0208	A2, A2.4c	B*1801	B18	Cw*0702	Cw7, JY328
A*0209	A2, A2-0ZB	B*2701	B27,27f	Cw*1101	Cw11
A*0210	A2, A2-LEE	B*2702	B27, 27e, 27K, B27.2	Cw*1201	C×52
A*0301	A3, A3.1	B*2703	B27, 27d, 27J	Cw*1202	Cb-2
A*0302	A3, A3.2	B*2704	B27, 27b,27C,B27.3	Cw*1301	CwBL18
A*1101	A11, A11E	B*2705	B27, 27a, 27W, B27.1	Cw*1401	Cb-1
A*1102	A11, A11K	B*2706	B27, 27D, B27.4		
A*2401	A24 (9)	B*3501	B35		
A*2501	A25 (10)	B*3502	B35		
A*2601	A26 (10)	B*3701	B37		
A*2901	A29 (w19)	B*3801	B38 (16), B16.1		
A*3001	A30 (w19), A30.3	B*3901	B39 (16), B16.2		
A*3101	A31 (w19)	B*4001	Bw60 (40)		
A*3201	A32 (w19)	B*4002	B40, B40*		
A*3301	Aw333 (w19), Aw33.1	B*4101	Bw41		
A*6801	Aw68 (28), Aw68.1	B*4201	Bw42		
A*6802	Aw68 (28), Aw68.2	B*4401	B44 (12), B44.1		
A*6901	Aw69 (28)	B*4402	B44 (12), B44.2		
		B*4601	Bw46		
		B*4701	Bw47		
		B*4901	B49 (21)		
		B*5101	B51 (5)		
		B*5201	Bw52 (5)		
		B*5301	Bw53		
		B*5701	Bw57 (17)		
		B*5801	Bw58 (17)		
		B*7801	B'SNA'		

also express DRw52 (currently *DRB3*0101*) (Table 6–2).

The HLA-DQ complex consists of two pairs of linked α and β genes: the genes, *DQA2* and *DQB2*, encode an as yet unidentified and uncharacterized "DX" product.

The HLA-DP region is the most centromeric of the class II regions in the HLA complex. There is one set of functional α and β genes in this region, known as *HLA-DPA1* and *DPB1*, which encode the functional DP molecule. The *HLA-DPA2* and *DPB2* genes are pseudogenes, apparently evolutionary remnants from some ancient gene duplication event.

Additional class II genes that lie between the DQ and DP regions encode an α gene known as *HLA-DNA* and a β gene known as *HLA-DOB*, as well as an interesting vestigial α-β pair known as HLA-DMA and DMB.[16a] Transcripts for each have been identified, but the function of molecules encoded by these loci, if any, is yet unknown.

The different HLA class II loci differ in terms of sites of expression, which may indicate functional differences among the products. *HLA-DR* and *DP*

genes are constitutively expressed on many lymphoid cells, particularly B lymphocytes, monocytes, and other antigen-presenting cells. They are inducible in many somatic tissue types, including activated T lymphocytes and vascular endothelium at sites of cytokine-mediated inflammation. The HLA-DQ molecules have a more restricted distribution of constitutive expression but are similarly inducible on multiple lymphoid and nonlymphoid tissue types.[17]

As with the HLA class I molecules, allelic polymorphism is the predominant structural feature of the class II genes. With the exception of the *HLA-DRA* and *DPA* loci, each of the other expressed class II genes is highly polymorphic, with from 10 to 30 alleles or more so far identified (see Table 6–2).

Identification of Class II Alleles. Like class I molecules, many class II alleles were originally identified as serologically recognized specificities (Fig. 6–3). Mixed lymphocyte cultures (MLC) allowed finer discrimination of allelic differences, by cellular recognition by cultured T lymphocytes of foreign MHC antigens. In this way, for example, MLC could identify Dw4, Dw10, Dw13, Dw14, and Dw15 "subtypes"

Table 6–2. CURRENT NOMENCLATURE OF HLA-DR, DQ, AND DP ALLELES RECOGNIZED BY THE WHO COMMITTEE FOR FACTORS OF THE HLA SYSTEM AS OF 1990[49]

HLA Class II Alleles			
1990 NOMENCLATURE	PREVIOUS DESIGNATIONS	1990 NOMENCLATURE	PREVIOUS DESIGNATIONS
DRB1 Alleles		*DQA1 Alleles*	
DRB1*0101	DR1,Dw1	DQA1*0101	DQA 1.1, 1.9
DRB1*0102	DR1, Dw20	DQA1*0102	DQA 1.2, 1.19, 1.AZH
DRB1*0103	DR' BR', Dw' BON'	DQA1*0103	DOA 1.3, 1.18, DRw8–Dqw1
DRB1*1501	DRw15 (2), Dw2	DQA1*0201	DQA 2, 3.7
DRB1*1502	DRw15 (2), Dw12	DQA1*03011	DOA 3, 3.1, 3.2
DRB1*1601	DRw16 (2), Dw21	DQA1*03012	DQA 3, 3.1, 3.2, DR9–DQw3
DRB1*1602	DRw16, (2), Dw22	DQA1*0302	DQA 3, 3.1, 3.2, DR9–DQw3
DRB1*0301	DRw17 (3), Dw3	DQA1*0401	DQA 4.2, 3.8
DRB1*0302	DRw18 (3), Dw' RSH'	DQA1*0501	DQA 4.1, 2
DRB1*0401	DR4, Dw4	DQA1*05011	DQA 4.1, 2
DRB1*0402	DR4, Dw10	DQA1*05012	DQA 4.1, 2
DRB1*0403	DR4, Dw13, 13.1	DQA1*05013	DQA 4.1, 2
DRB1*0404	DR4, Dw14, 14.1	DQA1*0601	DQA 4.3
DRB1*0405	DR4, Dw15		
DRB1*0406	DR4, Dw' KT2'	*DQB1 Alleles*	
DRB1*0407	DR4, Dw13, 13.2	DQB1*0501	DQw5 (w1), DQB 1.1, DRw10–DQw1.1
DRB1*0408	DR4, Dw14, Dw14.2	DQB1*0502	DQw5 (w1), DQB 1.2, 1.21
DRB1*0409	DR4	DQB1*05031	DQw5 (w1), DQB 1.3, 1.9, 13.1
DRB1*0410	DR4	DQB1*05032	DQw5 (w1), DQB 1.3, 1.9, 13.2
DRB1*0411	DR4	DQB1*0504	DQB 1.9
DRB1*1101	DRw11 (5), Dw5, DRw11.1	DQB1*0601	DQw6 (w1), DQB 1.4, 1.12
DRB1*1102	DRw11 (5), Dw' JVM', DRw11.2	DQB1*0602	DQw6 (w1), DQB 1.5, 1.2
DRB1*1103	DRw11 (5), DRw11.3	DQB1*0603	DQw6 (w1), DQB 1.6, 1.18
DRB1*1104	DRw11 (5), Dw' FS'	DQB1*0604	DQw6 (w1), DQB 1.7, 1.19
DRB1*1201	DRw12 (5), Dw 'DB6'	DQB1*0605	DQw6 (w1), DQB 1.8, 1.19b
DRB1*1202	DRw12 (5), DRw12b	DQB1*0201	DQw2, DQB 2
DRB1*1301	DRw13 (w6), Dw18 DRw6a	DQB1*0301	DQw7 (w3), DQB 3.1
DRB1*1302	DRw13 (w6), Dw19, DRw6c	DQB1*0302	DQw8 (w3), DQB 3.2
DRB1*1303	DRw13 (w6), Dw 'HAG'	DQB1*03031	DQw9 (w3), DQB 3.3
DRB1*1304	DRw13 (w6)	DQB1*03032	DQw9 (w3), DQB 3.3
DRB1*1305	DRw13 (w6)	DQB1*1401	DQw4, DQB 4.1, Wa
DRB1*1401	DRw14 (w6), Dw9, DRw6b	DQB1*0402	DQw4, DQB 4.2, Wa
DRB1*1402	DRw14 (w6), Dw16		
DRB1*1403	DRw14 (w6)	*DPA1 Alleles*	
DRB1*1404	DRw6b.2	DPA1*0101	LB14/LB24, DPA1
DRB1*1405	DRw14 (w6)	DPA1*0102	pSBα-318
DRB1*0701	DR7, Dw17	DPA1*0103	DPw4α1
DRB1*0702	DR7, Dw' DB1'	DPA1*0201	DPA2, pDAα13B
DRB1*0801	DRw8, Dw8.1		
DRB1*08021	DRw8, Dw8.2	*DPB1 Alleles*	
DRB1*08022	DRw8, Dw8.2	DPB1*0101	DPw1, DPB1, DPw1a
DRB1*08031	DRw8, Dw8.3	DPB1*0201	DPw2, DPB2.1
DRB1*08032	DRw8, Dw8.3	DPB1*02011	DPw2, DPB2.1
DRB1*0804	DRw8	DPB1*02012	DPw2, DPB2.1
DRB1*09011	DR9, Dw23	DPB1*0202	DPw2, DPB2.2
DRB1*09012	DR9, Dw23	DPB1*0301	DPw3, DPB3
DRB1*1001	DRw10	DPB1*0401	DPw4, DPB4.1, DPw4a
		DPB1*0402	DPw4, DPB4.2, DPw4b
Other DRB Alleles		DPB1*0501	DPw5, DPB5
DRB3*0101	DRw52a, DW24	DPB1*0601	DPw6, DPB6
DRB3*0201	DRw52b, Dw25	DPB1*0801	DPB8
DRB3*0202	DRw52b, Dw25	DPB1*0901	DPB9
DRB3*0301	DRw52c, Dw26	DPB1*1001	DPB10
DRB4*0101	DRw53	DPB1*1101	DPB11
DRB5*0101	DRw15 (2), Dw2	DPB1*1301	DPB13
DRB5*0102	DRw15 (2), Dw12	DPB1*1401	DPB14
DRB5*0201	DRw16 (2), Dw21	DPB1*1501	DPB15
DRB5*0202	DRw16 (2), Dw22	DPB1*1601	DPB16
		DPB1*1701	DPB17
		DPB1*1801	DPB18
		DPB1*1901	DPB19

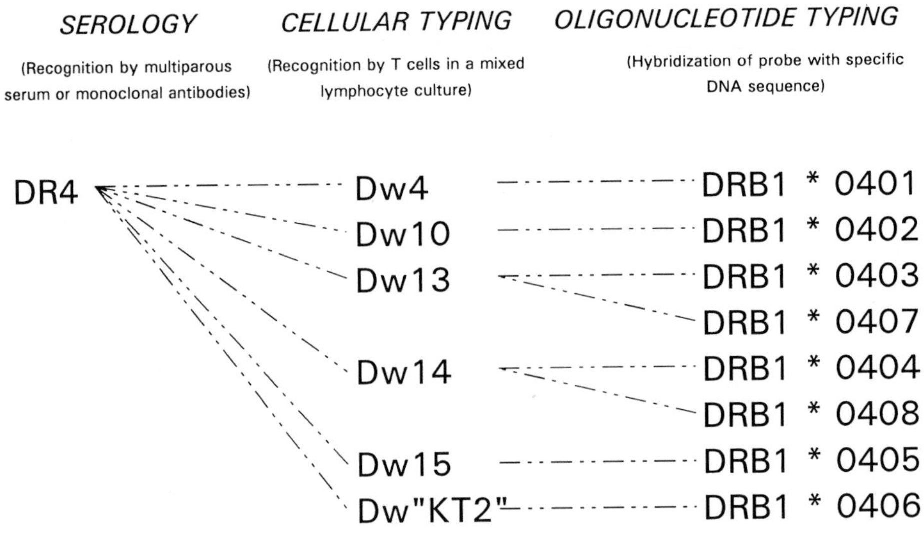

Figure 6–3. The spectrum of HLA class II typing. Serologic reactivity patterns identify traditional antibody-defined HLA "types," which represent public specificities present on the HLA class II molecule. The major allogeneic determinants on HLA molecules are defined by mixed lymphocyte culture, or HLA-D "typing," and represent an additional set of cellularly defined specificities on the same molecules. The relationship between such serologically and cellularly defined determinants, and specific genes within the HLA complex, can be quite complicated. This is illustrated for members of the *HLA-DR4* family of alleles: *HLA-DR4* is defined by antibody reactivity; this type can be "split" into six identifiable specificities by T cell recognition in mixed lymphocyte cultures. Synthetic oligonucleotide typing takes advantage of individual nucleotide differences to identify each gene on the basis of its DNA sequence, distinguishing further alleles, some of which are listed here.

SEROLOGY	CELLULAR TYPING	OLIGONUCLEOTIDE TYPING
(Recognition by multiparous serum or monoclonal antibodies)	(Recognition by T cells in a mixed lymphocyte culture)	(Hybridization of probe with specific DNA sequence)

of the serologically defined DR4 specificity common to all the subtypes. Nucleotide sequencing has detailed the fine differences among these alleles,[18] now permitting exquisitely sensitive oligonucleotide typing to identify alleles.[19, 19a] Amino acid sequences of a number of recognized class II *DRB1* alleles are shown in Figure 6–4.

Haplotype Organization. The high degree of polymorphism, or allelic variability, at different class I and class II loci creates the potential for an astounding degree of HLA gene diversification within a single individual. However, the relationship between different alleles at the *HLA-DP, DQ, DR, HLA-B, HLA-C,* and *HLA-A* loci is not actually random, and the lack of randomness, or "linkage disequilibrium" between these loci, results in a large but finite number of distinct haplotypes. For example, one of the alleles at the *HLA-B* locus, known as *HLA-B8*, is most often found on haplotypes that also carry a particular allele, *DR3*, at the *HLA-DRB1* locus, as well as an allele called *DQ2* at the *DQB1* locus and the allele *DP1* at the *DPB1* locus. Another example is seen in the linkage between *HLA-B44, DR4,* and *DQ7*, so that an individual with *B44* is very likely also to have *DR4*, while an individual with *B8* is very likely to have *DR3*.[20] These haplotypic relationships indicate that recombination between the HLA loci is not random and becomes an important consideration in the interpretation of HLA genetic contributions to diseases in two respects: first, the assignment of genetic susceptibility to a particular HLA gene must be done cautiously in cases in which there is linkage

Figure 6–4. Amino acid sequences, using the single letter amino acid code, encoded by several of the most common alleles within the *HLA-DRB1* locus. The sequence shown spans the first domain of the β chain of the HLA-DR class II molecule, demonstrating regions of "hypervariability" interspersed among conserved regions. The variable sequences are responsible for functional differences among different alleles, primarily by restricting the binding of antigenic peptides and the T cell receptor.

on the same haplotype to other HLA alleles. Thus, for example, the association of rheumatoid arthritis with the *HLA-B44* allele is now known to be secondary to a primary linkage with *DR4*-positive alleles at the *HLA-DRB1* locus, as discussed more fully later. A second issue raised by the presence of linkage disequilibrium within HLA genes is that polymorphic genes that lie between HLA loci (i.e., some of the non-HLA "peptide transporter" genes or the TNF genes [see later]) may themselves be implicated in disease susceptibility on haplotypes in which the polymorphic HLA gene acts as a marker gene, rather than as a primary disease susceptibility determinant.

Regulation of HLA Genes. Transcription of the HLA genes is tightly regulated. An ordered set of promoter and enhancer elements controls basal levels of transcription as well as inducible expression.[21]

The class I *HLA-A, B,* and *C* genes appear to be coordinately regulated, although this has not yet been exhaustively studied. Their expression is constitutive on all nucleated cells. The class II genes, on the other hand, have multiple levels of regulatory control. On the one hand, there is some coordinate regulation among all class II genes, as best illustrated by examples of immunodeficiency associated with the "bare lymphocyte syndrome." In this rare disorder, class I genes are expressed, but all class II genes are transcriptionally silent, apparently as a result of a rare autosomal defect.[22–24] Class II expression in cells from these patients can be "rescued" by fusion with normal lymphocytes, implying the deficiency of a key coordinated transcription factor.[25]

In addition to this coordinate regulation, however, class II genes are differentially regulated. There are interlocus differences among the *DR, DQ,* and *DP* loci in terms of constitutive and inducible expression, tissue specificity, and the specificity of nuclear proteins that bind to promoter elements associated with each of these genes.[26, 27] Another level of complexity is seen among different alleles of class II genes. In studies of the DQB promoter elements, DNA sequence allelic polymorphism has been observed, with resulting differences in both nuclear protein binding to different alleles at the same *DQB1* locus and concurrent effects on transcriptional activity of the promoter.[28] The interplay between these regulatory factors in relation to the effect of the HLA genes in autoimmunity is not yet known.

HLA Molecules

The genetic organization and polymorphism of the HLA genes have direct structural repercussions that are critical for function. The HLA class II molecules and the classic class I molecules are expressed as membrane-bound surface proteins in which their polymorphic features are oriented toward the outside of the cell.

Class I Molecules. The HLA class I molecule is a dimeric protein composed of a 44,000-dalton heavy

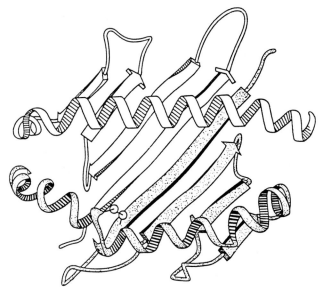

Figure 6–5. Three-dimensional view of the antigen-recognition domains of an HLA molecule, looking down into the antigen-binding groove, with α-helices forming the walls and β-pleated sheets forming the floor of the groove. The antigen-recognition domains are adjacent to additional membrane-proximal domains in both class I and class II molecules, which provide for signal transduction and co-recognition properties of the molecule. HLA polymorphisms—the amino acids that uniquely identify each allele—consist of structural variation focused primarily along the inner faces of the antigen-binding groove in positions suitable for direct contact with antigenic peptides. (Adapted from Bjorkman, P. J., Saper, M. A., Samraoui, B., et al.: Structure of the human class I histocompatibility antigen, HLA-A2. Nature 329:506, 1987. Reprinted by permission from Nature, vol. 329, p. 506. Copyright © 1987 Macmillan Magazines, Ltd.).

chain glycoprotein encoded by the class I gene, complexed with a 12,000-dalton subunit, β₂-microglobulin, encoded outside the MHC. The structure of a class I molecule is illustrated in Figure 6–5, derived from an x-ray crystallographic analysis of the HLA-A2 molecule,[29] in good agreement with a subsequent structural determination for the Aw68 allele.[30] There are several characteristic features of the class I molecule that relate directly to function. The class I heavy chain is folded into three distinct structural domains, referred to as α1, α2, and α3. The primary known function of class I gene products is to present peptide antigens to T cells of the immune system, which is directly accomplished by the α1 and α2 domains, which form a peptide-binding groove. External loops of the α1 and α2 domains, as well as the peptides bound in the groove, form the recognition surface for specific T cell receptors.

The polymorphism that is so characteristic of the HLA complex at the genetic level is reflected in the protein structure by a number of amino acid substitutions, predominantly in the regions of the α1 and α2 domain that border the peptide-binding groove.[31] As a consequence, the polymorphism is responsible for differences in peptide binding among different class I molecules. Such amino acid variations deter-

Peptide binding groove

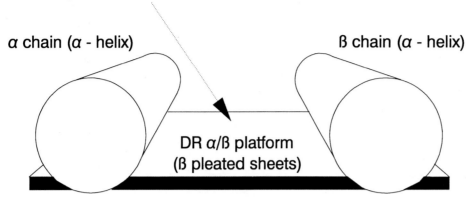

α chain (α - helix)

ß chain (α - helix)

DR α/ß platform
(ß pleated sheets)

Figure 6–6. Schematic representation of the peptide binding groove of an HLA-DR molecule, modeled by analogy with conserved elements of the HLA class I structure. The α- and the β-chains of the DR molecule each contribute an α-helical wall of the groove, and each chain also forms part of the β-pleated sheets on the floor of the groove. The HLA-DRα molecule is nonpolymorphic, so that variation among HLA-DR molecules is predominantly contributed by DRβ-chain polymorphisms, both along the α-helical loop and the β-pleated sheet platform of the antigen-recognition domain.

mine whether or not a certain peptide will bind to a particular class I molecule and also dictate the conformation that the peptide assumes when it does bind. These points are emphasized by the recent description of the structure of the HLA-B27 molecule derived by x-ray crystallography.[31a] Two deep "pockets" within the peptide binding groove appear to dictate the specific residues of an antigen that are necessary for binding[31a, 31b]; indeed, peptides directly purified from the HLA-B27 binding groove were of uniform length and all shared the same arginine amino acid residue at the second position of the peptide, in a position to fit inside one of the "pockets."[31c] Since peptide binding by the HLA molecule is a requirement for T cell recognition, T cells are said to be "restricted" by the nature of the polymorphic variation of the HLA molecule (i.e., the allele).

In addition to all the polymorphic residues on class I molecules, there are many conserved sites. While most of these conserved regions probably serve to maintain the overall architecture of the molecule, one site in the α3 domain has an additional functional role. When a T cell comes in contact with a target cell containing a class I molecule, the affinity of the interaction between T cell receptor and its target is dramatically enhanced by a second intercellular interaction, between the CD8 co-receptor molecule on the T cell, and the α3 domain of the HLA class I molecule.[32] Thus, the class I molecule actually binds to two T cell surface molecules, the antigen-specific T cell receptor and the CD8 molecule. It is this intermolecular interaction that is responsible for the functional dichotomy of T cell subsets (discussed more thoroughly in Chapter 2); namely, that CD8-positive T cells are usually restricted by HLA class I molecules, while CD4-positive T cells are restricted by HLA class II–positive molecules (see later).

Class II Molecules. HLA class II molecules are glycoprotein dimers with an α-chain and a β-chain. The 31,000-dalton α-chain and the 27,000-dalton β-chain assemble as an intracellular dimer in association with a third polypeptide called the invariant chain, which is encoded outside the MHC.[33] The

invariant chain apparently helps in the assembly and stability of the class II complex, as well as being responsible for chaperoning the class II complex through various intracellular compartments on its way to the cell surface.[34, 35] The invariant chain does not bind HLA class I molecules, and this difference may be responsible for some of the key functional differences that distinguish class I– and class II–mediated immune recognition, as discussed in the next section.

The precise structure of a class II molecule is not yet known; however, a high degree of overall homology with the class I structure is likely, based on similarities in a number of conserved amino acids important for the tertiary structure of the protein.[36] However, whereas the peptide-binding cleft of a class I molecule was formed by the class I α1 and α2 domains, the comparable peptide-binding cleft in an HLA class II molecule is formed by distinct domains contributed by both the α- and the β-polypeptides. The amino terminal domains of the class II molecules, the α1 domain of the class II α-chain, together with the β1 domain of the class II β-chain, form the critical peptide-recognition and binding compartment.

A large number of structural studies involving site-directed mutagenesis have been performed on HLA class II molecules, all of which are consistent with the notion that the class II structure is very similar to that of the class I molecule, with parallel peptide-binding functions.[37–40] Also similar are the location and role of polymorphic residues in the class II structure: Sites of allelic variation among class II genes occur at positions that are predicted to interact with peptides bound in the class II binding pocket and at sites on the external surface of the α1 and β1 domains that apparently contact the T cell receptor.[36, 39] As shown in Figure 6–6, the peptide-binding pocket is envisaged as a deep cleft, whose walls are formed by the α-helices contributed by portions of the α1 and β1 domains, and whose floor is formed by β-pleated sheets contributed by different portions of the α1 and β1 domains. Thus, the recognition of a class II molecule along with a bound

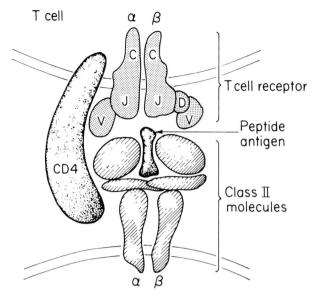

Antigen presenting cell

Figure 6–7. Molecular interactions in the triggering of antigen-specific immune responses. Illustrated are the components of the tri-molecular complex essential for T cell activation—the HLA class II molecule, a peptide antigen, and the T cell antigen-specific receptor—as well as the CD4 co-receptor molecule. The HLA molecule is anchored in the membrane of an antigen-presenting cell, with the antigen-recognition domain and its bound peptide accessible to the T cell receptor. The T cell receptor recognizes the processed peptide antigen in the context of its HLA class II molecule, while a CD4 molecule enhances the binding interaction and assists with signal transduction into the T cell compartment. The orientation of the variable segments of the T cell receptor, V, D, and J, and the structural interactions of the CD4 molecule are modeled after indirect experimental evidence and are not yet precisely known.

peptide is accomplished by direct contact and interactions with a T cell antigen receptor to residues of the α1 domain, the β1 domain, and the bound peptide (Fig. 6–7).

As with HLA class I molecules and the CD8 molecule in the T cell, there is also an important co-receptor relationship for the HLA class II molecules. Some T cell subsets carry a CD4 molecule (more thoroughly discussed in Chapter 2). The CD4 molecule directly binds to HLA class II molecules on antigen-presenting cells, increasing the affinity of the T cell receptor–class II interaction and assisting in intercellular communication of activation signals.[41] This special affinity of the class II molecule for the CD4 molecule is responsible for the preference of CD4-positive T cells to recognize HLA class II–positive cells.

Intercellular Interactions

The structural features previously outlined have important functional correlates. As the primary function of HLA molecules is to bind and present peptides to the T cell receptor, the nature of this class II–peptide interaction must be tightly regulated; in-

deed, failure of the peptide presentation pathways to distinguish self from non-self recognition accurately is a central feature in concepts of triggering events in autoimmunity.

Peptides that are potentially immunogenic challenge the immune system from several sources. External antigens, such as circulating toxins or phagocytosed remnants of foreign cells or tissue, often make their entry into the immune system via endocytic compartments in B cells, monocytes, and macrophages. On the other hand, other potential antigens, such as viral proteins, may be synthesized de novo in the cytoplasm of an infected cell and thus bypass the endosomal pathways. Finally, of course, a whole host of self-proteins continuously arrive in the internal and external environments of the cell. It now appears that class I and class II HLA molecules display preferential patterns of activity to monitor these different types of potential antigens (reviewed in reference 42). This is schematically illustrated in Figure 6–8.

When class II molecules are first synthesized, structural constraints introduced by polymorphic amino acid residues on both the α- and the β-chains establish a hierarchy of relative affinities determining which α-chains pair with which β-chains.[43] The α-β dimer is stabilized by the association of the invariant chain polypeptide, which carries important subcellular localization signals and is responsible for transporting the class II molecule into endosomal compartments.[35] It is also probable that the invariant chain bound to the class II molecule actually occupies or blocks the peptide-binding pocket during this transport step, thus preventing self-peptides from the cytoplasm from binding the class II molecule at this time.[44] Endosomes containing class II molecules participate in additional trafficking pathways, apparently intersecting pathways of endosomes that have carried external antigens into the intracellular compartment.[45] Thus, it appears that class II molecules first contact external antigens within the milieu of endosomal compartments (see Fig. 6–8). Acidification of the endosome and proteolytic cleavage of the invariant chain combine to provide access to the class II binding pocket for such foreign peptides.[46] By the time the endosomal trafficking cycle deposits the class II molecule on the cell surface, then, the binding pocket of most class II molecules is presumably occupied by potentially immunogenic peptides.

The experimental description of antigen-presenting cells that are defective in this class II processing pathway raises the possibility that important control mechanisms may be found that influence the nature or efficiency of class II antigen presentation. Indeed, one intriguing element of these studies is the suggestion that genes for such regulatory elements may themselves lie within the same region of chromosome 6 as the HLA complex itself.[8, 46a]

The interaction of HLA class I molecules and antigenic peptides is similarly compartmentalized. Cytoplasmic peptides apparently contact class I pep-

Figure 6–8. Pathways of HLA class I and class II molecule assembly and antigen processing. HLA molecules are preferentially compartmentalized during their synthesis and transport within the cell, resulting in selective pathways for contact with antigens. In the class I pathway, putative peptide transporter molecules may carry processed peptide antigens to the endoplasmic reticulum (ER), where they are thought to interact with and bind the class I molecule, formed from the polymorphic class I α or heavy chain and the conserved, non–MHC-encoded β₂-microglobulin. This compartment presumably facilitates the presentation of endogenously synthesized antigens, such as viral polypeptides, by the class I pathway. The peptide–class I complex moves to the cell surface after trafficking through the Golgi and post-Golgi compartments.

In the class II pathway, invariant chain complexes with both the HLA α- and β-chains in

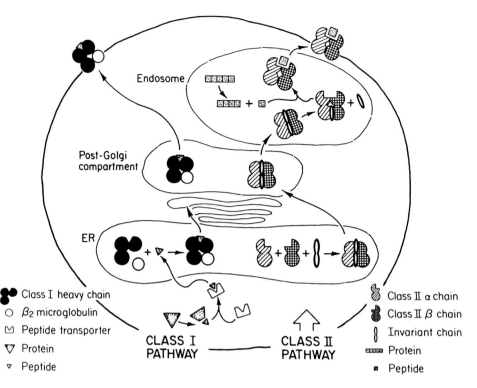

the ER and may play a role in stabilizing the class II dimer. This class II–invariant chain complex then trafficks through the Golgi and post-Golgi compartments; binding of the invariant chain to the class II molecule is thought to interfere with peptide binding, thus discouraging binding to self-peptides in these compartments. Invariant chain does not bind to class I molecules. The class II–invariant chain complex is then transported to an acidic endosomal compartment, where "foreign" proteins, transported from phagolysosomes or recycling endosomes, are digested to peptides. In this same compartment, the invariant chain is cleaved and released from the class II dimer, now allowing peptide to bind to the antigen-binding groove. The peptide–class II complex then moves to the cell surface, where it is available for T cell recognition.

tide-binding molecules in the endoplasmic reticulum or Golgi compartment, soon after synthesis of the class I heavy chain.[47] Indeed, a "peptide transporter" protein may be essential for translocation of appropriate peptides across the membrane of the endoplasmic reticulum to facilitate this interaction. Studies of cell lines defective in the class I pathway of antigen presentation indicate that such a peptide transporter is encoded by genes that lie near the class II *HLA-DO* gene within the HLA complex.[7, 8, 47a] Subsequent to peptide–class I interaction, movement of the complex to the cell membrane in association with β₂-microglobulin occurs; as with the class II molecules, it is likely that under normal circumstances most of the class I molecules already on the cell surface have their peptide-binding pockets occupied.

Regulation of the Immune Response

The role of HLA molecules in regulating the immune response is determined by the structural and genetic features previously described. The main determinant of immunologic specificity lies in the nature of the specific amino acid polymorphisms within the peptide-binding groove and T cell receptor contact sites on the HLA molecule. These are the residues that directly determine whether a particular

peptide will be bound and presented to antigen-specific T cells. When this occurs, the immune system interprets the recognition as either a self or a non-self signal, leading to immune activation or tolerance, respectively. Such events are the culmination of a large number of highly variable biologic events, beginning with transcription of the HLA gene and progressing through various intracellular stages involving transport, proteolysis, peptide binding, and intermolecular signaling.

Viewed in this way, the antigen-presenting role of HLA molecules helps clarify the concept of HLA as a "permissive" genetic element in autoimmune disease. The presence of a particular disease susceptibility gene within the HLA complex is a key part (but certainly not all) of the molecular ensemble needed for autoimmune activation. The HLA gene is permissive in the sense that it plays the key genetically variable role in the intermolecular interactions leading to immune activation, but the other events relating to peptide presentation and T cell recognition must also occur.

HLA AND DISEASE ASSOCIATIONS

Numerous population and family studies have documented the association of certain HLA compo-

TAble 6–3. ASSOCIATIONS BETWEEN HLA ALLELES AND SUSCEPTIBILITY TO SOME RHEUMATIC DISEASES

Disease	HLA Marker	Frequency (%) in Patients (Whites)	Frequency (%) in Controls (Whites)	Relative Risk
Ankylosing spondylitis	B27	90	9	87
Reiter's syndrome	B27	79	9	37
Psoriatic arthritis	B27	48	9	10
Inflammatory bowel disease with spondylitis	B27	52	9	10
Adult rheumatoid arthritis	DR4	70	30	6
Polyarticular juvenile rheumatoid arthritis	DR4	75	30	7
Pauciarticular juvenile rheumatoid arthritis	DR8	30	5	5
	DR5	50	20	4.5
	DP2.1	55	20	4
Systemic lupus erythematosus	DR2	46	22	3.5
	DR3	50	25	3
Sjögren's syndrome	DR3	70	25	6

nents with specific rheumatic disorders. Up to the last decade, these studies relied on the association between serologically and cellularly defined markers that were present on some HLA molecules in patients with disease. More recently, through the use of molecular genetic techniques, it has become standard practice to identify individual haplotypes or individual HLA genes that are more prevalent in patients than in unaffected control individuals. In this section, we will present an overview of the HLA markers, both serologically defined and gene-specific markers, that are known to be associated with rheumatic disorders. In a few examples, it has recently been possible to develop more detailed genetic models for the contribution of specific HLA genes to a disease, and we will briefly discuss these examples as illustrations of the insight into pathogenesis offered by detailed immunogenetic analysis.

Table 6–3 lists some of the most significant associations between HLA markers and specific rheumatic diseases. The associations are indicated as "relative risk," which is an odds ratio reflecting the relative frequency of each disease in individuals with a particular HLA marker compared with the frequency of the disease in individuals not carrying that marker.[48]

Class I–Associated Diseases

The prototypic example of an HLA class I disease association is the B27 specificity, which has a striking association with a number of spondyloarthropathies (see Table 6–3). The B27 specificity is a serologically defined marker present on at least six different alleles of the class I HLA-B locus.[12, 13] Historically, these alleles have been referred to as B27a, B27b, B27c, etc., or B27.1, B27.2, B27.3, etc., and have been recently renamed by the World Health Organization (WHO) as HLA-B*2701, B*2702, B*2703, etc.[49] All members of this family of class I molecules react with antisera defining the HLA-B27 specificity and so are often considered together in population studies. In a limited number of detailed genetic analyses, it appears that each of the B27 "subtypes" is found in patients with ankylosing spondylitis (AS), suggesting that a feature of the B27 family common to all the different alleles is critical for disease (reviewed in reference 50).

The different B27 alleles differ from each other by one to six amino acids scattered throughout the peptide-binding groove of the class I molecule.[12] These members of the B27 family share a sequence motif that includes a combination of cystine at residue 67, lysine at residue 70, and asparagine at residue 97.[51] This combination of residues is not found in any other HLA-A, B, or C class I molecule and may be responsible for the high correlation with susceptibility to B27-associated diseases. For the same reason, these residues are also likely to contribute to the serologically recognized site that defines the B27 family of alleles. As seen in Table 6–3, the frequency of HLA-B27 in patients with AS is 90 percent, compared with less than 10 percent in control subjects. In all populations and racial groups studied, B27 is associated with AS, as well as with Reiter's disease, psoriatic arthritis, and acute anterior uveitis.[48]

While this association between the spondyloarthropathies and HLA-B27 has been recognized for many years, it has been difficult to test directly whether the B27 molecule itself is responsible for disease or whether the B27 genes involved are markers for a linked gene, as yet unidentified, which itself is the primary pathogenic determinant of disease. This uncertainty seems likely to be resolved in favor of the former concept, that the B27 molecule itself is directly involved in disease, for several reasons. As previously mentioned, different racial groups, with diverse HLA "background genes," all are associated with the spondyloarthropathies if they carry an HLA-B27 gene; this argues indirectly for a contribution of HLA-B27 itself. When molecular genetic studies identified multiple B27-positive alleles, it was initially anticipated that only some of these alleles would be associated with disease. However, since numerous B27 alleles are found in patients with AS,[52] it now

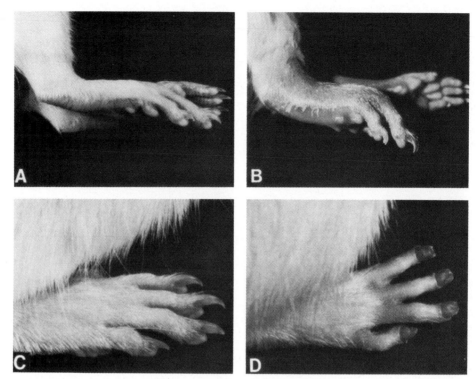

Figure 6–9. Peripheral joint and nail pathology seen in *HLA-B27* transgenic rats. Genes for both the heavy chain *HLA-B27* gene and the human β_2-microglobulin were inserted into Lewis rats to create transgenic animals expressing the human HLA-B27 molecule. In some rats with high copy numbers inserted, a spontaneous inflammatory condition developed, with features similar to those of human spondyloarthropathies. *A*, Normal distal hindlimb from control Lewis rat. *B*, Distal hindlimb of a 6-month-old *B27* transgenic rat showing swelling and erythema. *C*, Normal hindlimb digits and nails from control rat. *D*, hindlimb digits and nails of a 3.5-month-old *B27* transgenic rat, showing hyperkeratosis and dystrophy of the nails and alopecia over the digits. (From Hammer, R. E., Maika, S. D., Richardson, J. A., et al.: Spontaneous inflammatory disease in transgenic mice expressing HLA-B27 and human β2m: an animal model of HLA-B27–associated human disorders. Cell 63:1099, 1990. Copyright © 1990 Cell Press. Used by permission.)

seems likely that it is a feature of the B27 molecule itself, possibly an epitope dependent on the three amino acids at positions 63, 70, and 92, which provides a peptide-binding or immune-activation property directly contributing to disease.

Finally, a recent demonstration of the generation of spondyloarthritis in an animal model may be the most direct test to date of the hypothesis that the B27 molecule itself is pathogenic. In these studies, a human *HLA-B27* gene, and the gene for human β_2-microglobulin, were introduced as transgenes into rat oocytes, which, following in vitro fertilization, were grown into adult rats carrying multiple copies of the introduced human genes. These rats not only expressed the B27 molecule but also displayed marked clinical signs and symptoms characteristic of human B27-associated spondyloarthropathies[53] (Fig. 6–9).

Class II–Associated Disease

Detailed genetic studies have implicated specific class II alleles, and residues within those alleles, as directly contributing to disease pathogenesis in a number of rheumatic diseases. Rheumatoid arthritis is one of the most thoroughly studied and well-documented examples of genetic susceptibility to an autoimmune disease. The most striking feature of this association is the high prevalence (from 65 to 80 percent in different population studies) of HLA-DR4 in patients with RA.[54–61] As with the other HLA serotypes, HLA-DR4 is a serologically defined specificity present on multiple different class II molecules[18, 62 &63] (see Fig. 6–3). There are at least 11 different alleles at the *HLA-DRB1* locus that encode DR4-positive polypeptides. The different *DRB1* alleles that serologically type as HLA-DR4 are often, for historical reasons, referred to by nomenclature based on allogeneic recognition of alleles by T cells in an MLC and are known as Dw4, Dw10, Dw13, Dw14, Dw15, etc. Recent revisions by the WHO Nomenclature Committee have renamed this set of alleles *DRB1*0401, *0402, *0403*, etc. (see Table 6–2).

In contrast with the situation with HLA-B27, not all the DR4 subtypes are responsible for the association with RA. As shown in Figure 6–10, only those haplotypes that carry a *DRB1*0401* (Dw4) or *DRB1*0404* (Dw14) allele are increased in white patients with RA. Dw4 is found in approximately 50 percent of patients with RA, and Dw14 is found in as many as 35 percent.[60, 61, 64]

The same *HLA-DRB1* alleles, Dw4 and Dw14, identified as probable susceptibility genes in adult

Rheumatoid Arthritis:

HLA-DRB1 genes containing the "shared epitope" confer susceptibility in different populations

DRB1 Susceptibility Gene	Prevalence in RA	Relative Risk
Caucasians:		
DR4, Dw4 (*0401)	50%	6
DR4, Dw14 (*0404)	35%	5
DR1, Dw1 (*0101)	24%	1
Japanese:		
DR4, Dw15 (*0405)	71%	3.5
Yakima Indians:		
DR6, Dw16 (*1402)	83%	3.3
Israeli Jews:		
DR1, Dw1 (*0101)	28%	6

Figure 6–10. Summary of *HLA-DR* susceptibility genes for rheumatoid arthritis in different ethnic populations. While the HLA serotype differs in different populations, each allele listed contains the "shared epitope" formed by identical amino acids in a portion of the *DRB1*-encoded polypeptide, as described in the text. The relative risk represents an odds ratio reflecting the risk of disease in an individual carrying the susceptibility gene compared with an individual from the same ethnic group not carrying the susceptibility gene.

RA are also found in children with one form of juvenile rheumatoid arthritis (JRA), rheumatoid factor–positive disease. This seropositive JRA is clinically very similar to classic adult RA, with polyarticular, erosive, symmetrical arthritis. Not only do most of these patients carry the Dw4 and Dw14 genes, but also the majority are heterozygous for one of each allele; in other words, they are DR4 homozygous, but heterozygous for one Dw4 and one Dw14 gene.[65, 66] This raises the intriguing speculation that a "double-dose" of these two susceptibility genes may predispose to earlier expression of this form of JRA, which is probably an early-onset form of the classic RA common in older individuals.

Evidence that these two *DRB1* genes, Dw4 and Dw14, are themselves implicated in disease pathogenesis comes from two lines of investigation, comparison among different DR4-positive alleles and comparison of DR4 with non-DR4 genes associated with RA. The nucleotide and amino acid sequences of the Dw4 and Dw14 genes are very similar, with only two amino acid differences, at codons 71 and 86. However, some of the *DRB1* alleles that are not associated with RA are also remarkably similar in sequence but have a limited set of important differences. For example, the Dw10 allele, also encoding a DR4-positive molecule, differs from the Dw4 and Dw14 genes in just three codons, at residues 67, 70, and 71. Similarly, the Dw13 allele, also a DR4 subtype, differs from Dw4 and Dw14 at residue 74. These comparisons suggest that a discrete region of the DRβ polypeptide, between residues 67 and 74, might be particularly relevant in distinguishing alleles associated with RA from alleles that are not (Fig. 6–11). This prediction is verified in two key populations: patients with RA who do not have HLA-DR4, and patients with RA who, because of different ethnic backgrounds, come from populations with a low prevalence of the Dw4 and Dw14 genes.

In white patients who do not have HLA-DR4 (approximately 15 percent of all patients with RA), the majority are found to be positive for HLA-DR1.[58, 61, 67] They carry a *DRB1*0101* allele, which is markedly different in primary sequence from Dw4 and Dw14, except for a portion of the β1 domain extending from residues 50 to 80.[68] This region of identity encompasses the sequence from codons 67 to 74 thought to be important for RA and suggests that a primary sequence in this region of the DRβ molecule is present in most white patients with RA, both DR4-positive and DR4-negative patients.

In other populations, some ethnic groups have very low frequencies of the Dw4 and Dw14 genes. Remarkably, patients with RA from these populations also share the same sequence within their DRβ molecules. In studies of Ashkenazi Jews in Israel, *DR1* was again the most prevalent HLA-associated gene.[69] In Japan, the HLA-Dw15 gene is the most highly associated HLA allele,[70] and, in a recent study of Native American Indians, an HLA-DR6–related allele known as Dw16 was found in more than 80 percent of patients with RA[71] (see Fig. 6–10). All these alleles, Dw1, Dw15, and Dw16, are genes at the *DRB1* locus that encode the same amino acid residues from codons 67 to 74 as those found in the HLA-Dw14 gene[18, 68, 71] (see Fig. 6–11). Since these disparate *DRB1* genes are otherwise quite different, this suggests that the amino acid sequence within this portion of the DRβ molecule itself is implicated in pathogenesis.[72, 73]

A model for the role of this shared DRβ sequence, or "shared epitope," derives from experiments using site-directed mutagenesis to change the amino acids within this key set of residues.[38] Amino acid residues at 67, 70, and 71 were found to play key roles in peptide and T cell interactions critical for immune activation.[38, 40, 74, 75] This is consistent with the predicted three-dimensional model for class II

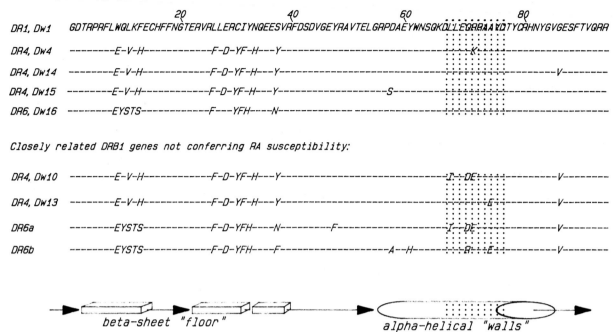

Figure 6–11. Comparison of amino acid sequences, using the single letter amino acid code, for *HLA-DRB1* genes conferring susceptibility to RA in different populations. The shaded area indicates the ''shared epitope'' region, which is conserved among all the susceptibility alleles. In contrast, sequences of selected nonsusceptibility alleles are also shown, illustrating that although their sequences may be nearly identical to a susceptibility allele, they differ in the critical epitope region. A linear representation of the antigen-binding domain of the HLA-DR molecule is shown under the sequence alignments, illustrating the position of the shared epitope within a very specific region of the HLA molecule in the α-helical loop that forms one wall of the antigen-binding groove. In this location, amino acid residues within the shared epitope associated with RA are situated in a position suitable for direct interaction with the T cell receptor as well as with bound peptide.

molecules in which these residues lie on one of the boundaries of the peptide-binding groove in positions likely to have direct intermolecular contact both with bound peptide and with the T cell receptor[76] (see Fig. 6–11).

These two examples, *B27* (for the spondyloarthropathies) and *DR4* (for RA) are the best studied and most thoroughly documented examples of specific candidate genes likely to be directly involved in the pathogenesis of HLA-associated rheumatic disease. Other examples listed in Table 6–3 are not currently as thoroughly understood but may yet provide some insights into the mechanisms of pathogenesis. Two that will be briefly considered here are the association of *DR3* with systemic lupus erythematosus (SLE) and Sjögren's syndrome and the association of multiple HLA genes with pauciarticular-onset JRA.

HLA-DR3 is found with increased frequency in patients with SLE and with Sjögren's syndrome.[77–86] However, detailed studies of HLA associations in the context of clinical subsets of each of these diseases have suggested an interesting correlation: When patients are subdivided based on the spectrum of autoantibody specificities associated with the disease, the HLA associations are much more striking. Thus, when anti-Ro (SS-A) antibodies are accompanied by anti-La (SS-B) antibodies, a strong correlation with the *DR3* haplotype is found, compared with patients

without this combination of autoantibodies.[87] Patients heterozygous for *DR2* and *DR3* haplotypes show higher relative risks (7 to 15) for the presence of anti-Ro (SS-A) than nonheterozygotes. This latter finding is also seen in Sjögren's syndrome, where *DR2/DR3* heterozygotes produce the highest levels of anti-Ro (SS-A).[87] Thus, the production of certain autoantibodies characteristic of each of these syndromes appears to be more closely associated with specific HLA class II alleles than the disease itself. This illustrates one of the confounding issues likely to be of importance in many clinically heterogeneous syndromes.

Pauciarticular-onset juvenile rheumatoid arthritis, a form of inflammatory arthritis marked by involvement of a small number of usually large joints primarily in pre-school-aged females and frequently associated with chronic anterior uveitis and circulating antinuclear antibodies, is another interesting example of genetic heterogeneity. Associations with at least three *HLA-DRB1* markers, *DR5*, *DR6*, *DR8*, have been reproducibly reported in pauciarticular-onset JRA patients (reviewed in references 88 and 89). Recent molecular genetic studies have shown that a set of *HLA-DQA1* alleles closely linked to the *DR* locus on *DR5-* and *DR8-*positive haplotypes is also prevalent.[90] Thus, it is difficult to distinguish between the contributions of different *DRB1* alleles versus different *DQA1* alleles in these patients. In addition, there have been several reports of *HLA-DP* associations with pauciarticular JRA.[91-94] An allele of the *DPB1* locus known as *DP2.1* appears to be an independent HLA marker associated with pauciarticular-onset JRA, often appearing either in *cis* or *trans* in the same patients who also carry a *DR5-*, *DR6-*, or *DR8-*positive *DRB1* allele. Whether this indicates genetic synergy between multiple class II genes in a single disease, or whether it merely reflects the contribution of as yet unknown genes on these haplotypes remains to be seen.

T CELL RECEPTOR GENES

Structure and Function

The human antigen-specific T cell receptor (TcR) is expressed on mature T cells, in combination with other T cell membrane-bound polypeptides such as CD3 and CD4 or CD8.[95, 96] The TcR is a disulfide-linked heterodimer made up of two chains, each of approximately 45,000 daltons. These are called TcRα and TcRβ and are encoded separately: The TcRα genes are encoded in a complex on chromosome 14, and the TcRβ genes are encoded in a complex on chromosome 7.

The TcR molecules within a single individual display an extremely high degree of structural diversity. This diversity is responsible for the fact that mature T cells are capable of responding to a wide universe of potential antigens. Recent understanding of the gene organization for the TcRα and β gene complexes has clarified the structural basis for this diversity and, at the same time, has made it possible to evaluate the contributions of these diverse genes in autoimmune diseases.

Both the TcRα and β genes are arranged as discontinuous gene segments in germline DNA. Functional genes are constructed during T cell maturation by the juxtaposition of different sets of these discontinuous gene segments through a process of specific chromosomal rearrangement. A functional TcRα gene is assembled from three of the discontinuous gene segments, called variable (Vα), joining (Jα), and constant (Cα). There are somewhere between 50 and 100 Vα gene segments to choose from, and approximately 50 Jα segments. Thus, through combinatorial rearrangements, a large number of different functional TcRα genes may be assembled, each in a different mature T cell.

In similar fashion, a functional TcRβ gene is assembled from discontinuous gene segments, with one additional diversity segment (Dβ) inserted between Vβ and Jβ. There are approximately 70 Vβ segments to choose from, as well as two Dβ segments, 13 Jβ segments, and two Cβ segments. Thus, as with TcRα, a high degree of diversification is generated through combinatorial reassembly. Even greater variation is achieved by some junctional diversification between V, D, and J, known as N-region

diversity, in which additional nucleotides are inserted during rearrangement.

Because of this genomic rearrangement mechanism to generate a functional receptor, there are two quite distinct genetic mechanisms by which TcR genes may be associated with rheumatic disorders. On the one hand, naturally occurring polymorphic variation in the germline gene segments exists in the population. Although not as marked as the high degree of allelic polymorphism for HLA genes, there is variation within the TcRα and β complexes, both in terms of gene number and in terms of allelic polymorphism. Thus, the inherited repertoire of potential TcR gene segments differs in different individuals and may be an important disease predisposition factor.

On the other hand, because of the genomic rearrangement events leading to a functional receptor, the specific usage of a particular V, D, or J segment or the combination of VDJ rearrangement is a potential significant determinant of genetic susceptibility. In other words, the usage of a particular rearranged T cell receptor, which can differ between different individuals with the same germline TcR gene segments (even among identical twins), may be the critical mechanism whereby TcR genes contribute to pathogenesis.

In addition to the receptors encoded on T cells by these TcR α and β genes, there is a class of receptors on a distinct subset of T cells known as γδ receptors, encoded by different gene segments. Whether these receptors contribute to pathogenesis is not yet known.

Consideration of the TcR genetic contribution to rheumatic diseases, then, is addressed in two distinct experimental approaches. One issue is the nature of inherited gene segments that may predispose to disease, and a second issue is the nature of the actual rearranged VDJ segments that are utilized in patients compared with unaffected individuals who may or may not have the identical germline gene segments. We will briefly review recent studies in these two areas.

TcR-Disease Association. Studies of T cell receptor genes in population and disease studies are usually performed by following genetic markers known as restriction fragment length polymorphisms (RFLPs). RFLPs are a useful technical tool for characterizing specific haplotypes and linkage patterns. In a complex set of genes such as TcRα or TcRβ, RFLPs provide the best currently available technology to apply to large groups of patients.

RFLPs identify variation that is within or linked to the gene complex of interest, such as the Vβ complex, or the Cα complex. There are two major limitations to this type of RFLP study. First is the fact that the genetic source of an RFLP (e.g., of genomic variation) may or may not lie within an actual segment of DNA that encodes part of the T cell receptor. Frequently, the RFLP arises in a piece of flanking DNA that does not directly encode the molecule. Therefore, the RFLP serves, at best, as a marker for the presence of a set of unknown linked genes. The second problem with RFLP analysis of a multigene complex such as Vβ or Vα is that different members of these gene families are separated by large genetic distances. In addition, there are frequent recombination events that occur between members of the same family (i.e., within the Vβ complex). Thus, an RFLP present at one end of the gene complex may not provide a marker for genes near the other end of the complex.

As might be expected, given these difficulties, RFLP analyses of TcR associations with rheumatic disorders are, to date, inconclusive. Rheumatoid arthritis[97] and SLE[98, 99] have been studied, and some investigators, though not all, suggest the possibility that preferential associations of particular TcR haplotypes could be contributing to disease predisposition. Further studies in this area await more detailed and specific genetic probes for different portions of the TcR gene complex to resolve this issue.

TcR Usage in RA. An alternative approach to the analysis of TcR contributions in rheumatic disorders is to attempt to identify the VDJ gene segments that are utilized by T cells in patients and, preferably, by T cells involved in the pathogenesis of the disease. Most such studies have focused on RA, anticipating that some of the T cells in or near inflamed synovium might carry rearranged receptors with specific VDJ usage.

These studies have, to date, been hindered by both clinical and technical variables. Probably the most daunting concern is the question of sampling of the T cell population in patients with RA under conditions where it is likely that these T cells are contributing to disease. Thus, while large numbers of investigators have recovered for analysis T lymphocytes from synovial fluid in acute and chronically inflamed joints, it is not clear whether this is the key population of cells to investigate. Some of these studies report an oligoclonal distribution of TcR. In other words, populations of T cells are recovered that look to be clonally expanded from a limited number of precursors, displaying characteristic VDJ rearrangements.[100, 101] However, several difficulties pertain: different individuals display evidence of different rearrangements, most of the samples obtained were from late-stage disease and may not be reflective of causally relevant T cells, and very few of the studies simultaneously sample synovial tissue for comparison. Thus, while it appears that there is some T cell amplification in synovial fluid in these patients, it is not yet known whether the TcR usage patterns relate specifically to pathogenesis or are secondary to other inflammatory stimuli.

Recent improvements in molecular technology using gene amplification now make it possible to analyze much smaller amounts of cells and tissue and provide an opportunity to identify directly, and with more precision, the TcR usage pattern in small numbers of T cells, potentially early in disease.

Indeed, in the first such study to be reported, there is a small but significant alteration in preferential Vβ gene segment utilization in synovial T cells compared with peripheral T cells in the same patient.[102]

MECHANISMS TO ACCOUNT FOR THE GENETIC ASSOCIATION WITH RHEUMATIC DISEASES

As previously outlined, recent advances have greatly clarified the basic immunogenetic basis for two of the major gene complexes critically involved in the activation of the immune response. Particularly in the case of the HLA complex, with the longstanding and well-characterized evidence for genetic association with several rheumatic diseases, this molecular and genetic information is leading directly to molecular models of immune activation events relevant to the pathogenesis of disease. Current mechanistic models to account for the genetic associations fall into three broad categories: *tolerance models*, in which physiologic mechanisms to prevent autoreactivity are defective in disease; *antigen presentation models*, in which exogenous antigen triggers disease in an MHC-restricted fashion; and *molecular mimicry models*, in which an exogenous event such as a viral infection activates certain lymphocytes whose receptors cross-react on self-antigens. The general aspects of each of these three models will be briefly discussed here, although it is not yet known for any of the rheumatic diseases which model, if any, adequately explains pathogenesis.

MHC–T Cell Interactions in Tolerance Induction. During the development of the immune system in an individual, a bias is introduced into the T cell repertoire in favor of T cells expressing receptors capable of recognizing a molecular complex of self-HLA molecule and antigen. Two types of selection events are thought to occur as T cells develop. In an event known as "negative selection," T cells that undergo VDJ rearrangement and express autoreactive T cell receptors are apparently triggered to "self-destruct" before they mature. This programmed cell death is triggered by contact between such an autoreactive T cell receptor and the host MHC molecules.[103, 104] Therefore, this negative selection plays a critical role in establishing self-tolerance; that is, the concept that mature T cells should preferentially not react with self-tissue.

During T cell development, T cells that are not negatively selected, but whose receptors still maintain the ability to interact with a complex of self-MHC molecules and antigen, are assisted by specialized antigen-presenting cells, usually in the thymus, to undergo a final maturation step known as "positive selection."[105, 106] It is these cells that establish the peripheral T cell repertoire.

As is apparent from this brief synopsis of T cell development, the nature of the MHC polymorphism that influences both negative and positive selection in an individual is of critical importance for establishing and maintaining tolerance. One of the models to account for HLA associations with autoimmunity postulates that, in individuals with a particular polymorphic susceptibility allele, the nature of those polymorphisms on the HLA molecule are defective in efficient negative selection and permit the escape of potentially autoreactive T cells.

MHC–T Cell Interactions in Antigen Presentation. The direct contact between TcR and HLA molecules during antigen-specific T cell activation provides an obvious setting in which polymorphisms associated with HLA susceptibility alleles might be a crucial triggering factor in autoimmunity. As described earlier in this chapter, the specific amino acid polymorphisms on class II molecules determine whether or not particular antigenic peptides will be bound and subsequently presented for T cell recognition. Preferential binding of a pathogenic peptide or, indeed, a "self" peptide by a particular susceptibility gene product could directly account for the HLA contribution to disease. Such an event likely occurs in the peripheral immune system—perhaps in the target organ, such as the synovium—itself and may be the primary inciting event leading directly to localized disease. Pathogenic models based on the notion that this trimolecular complex—between TcR, peptide, and MHC molecule—is the critical induction event that precedes disease also lead to potential novel therapeutic approaches, although these have not yet been applied to rheumatic disorders. In other autoimmune disease models it has been possible to attempt specific immunosuppression by interrupting the MHC-peptide interaction or the TcR-MHC interaction with specific synthetic peptide drugs.[107]

Mimicry. In proposed mimicry mechanisms, an exogenous event such as a viral infection may activate clones of T and B lymphocytes whose receptors cross-react on self-antigens. Evidence to indicate the plausibility of this model in rheumatic disorders comes from multiple examples of primary sequence homology between different infectious agents and some putative target antigens or, indeed, some HLA molecules themselves. For example, the target antigen of some anti-SMP antibodies apparently shares cross-reactive epitopes with capsid proteins of several herpesviruses.[108] In RA, there is some sequence homology between an EBV coding region sequence and the Dw14 epitope on the DRB1 molecule described earlier, although there is as yet no direct evidence for immunologic cross-reactivity in patients.[109] Perhaps the best known example of a candidate rheumatic disease in which molecular mimicry might be a possible mechanism relates to the B27-associated spondyloarthropathies. Amino acid sequences characteristic of the HLA-B27 molecule are found with great frequency in the prokaryotic world. Different proteins from *Klebsiella*, *Shigella*, and a number of other organisms show similarity with the B27 sequence and, in experimental models, are able to elicit antibodies that will cross-react against peptides de-

rived from the B27 sequence, although, again, a direct cross-reactivity in patients has not been demonstrated.[110, 111]

Each of these three models would appear to be a satisfactory mechanistic explanation to account for the known immunogenetic contributions to disease susceptibility. Indeed, it is likely that different rheumatic disorders with genetic associations in the MHC may actually be mediated through different mechanisms. As stressed earlier in this chapter, however, each of these mechanistic models shares a central focus: that is, that the nature of the specific structural polymorphisms on the MHC molecules implicated in disease, and to a lesser extent on TcR molecules as well, accounts for the known immunogenetic contributions. Polymorphism in the MHC, the hallmark of specific immune recognition, is the primary structural determinant of the disease predisposition and susceptibility.

References

1. Lawrence, J. S.: Genetics of rheumatoid factor and rheumatoid arthritis. Clin. Exp. Immunol. S2:769, 1967.
2. Myerowitz, S., Jacox, R. F., and Hers, D. W.: Monozygotic twins discordant for rheumatoid arthritis. Arthritis Rheum. 11:1, 1968.
3. Carroll, M. C., Katzman, P., Alicot, E. M., et al.: Linkage map of the human major histocompatibility complex including the tumor necrosis factor genes. Proc. Nat. Acad. Sci. U.S.A. 84:8535, 1987.
4. Sargent, C. A., Dunham, I., Trowsdale, J., et al.: Human major histocompatibility complex contains genes for the major heat shock protein HSP70. Proc. Natl. Acad. Sci. U.S.A. 86:1968, 1989.
5. Spies, T., Blanck, G., Bresnahan, M., et al.: A new cluster of genes within the human major histocompatibility complex. Science 243:214, 1989.
6. Deverson, E. V., Gow, I. R., Coadwell, W. J., et al.: MHC class II region encoding proteins related to multidrug resistance family of transmembrane transporters. Nature 348:738, 1990.
7. Trowsdale, J., Hanson, I., Mockridge, I., et al.: Sequences encoded in the class II region of the MHC related to the "ABC" superfamily of transporters. Nature 348:741, 1990.
8. Spies, T., Bresnahan, M., Bahram, S., et al.: A gene in the human major histocompatibility complex class II region controlling the class I antigen presentation pathway. Nature 348:744, 1990.
9. Carroll, M. C., Campbell, R. D., Bentley, D. R., et al.: A molecular map of the human major histocompatibility complex class III region linking complement genes C4, C2, and factor B. Nature 307:237, 1984.
10. White, P. C.: Molecular genetics of the class III region of the HLA complex. In Dupont, B. (ed.): Immunobiology of HLA. Immunogenetics and Histocompatibility. New York, Springer-Verlag, 1989, pp. 62–69.
11. Fleischhauer, K., Kernan, N. A., O'Reily, R. J., et al.: Bone marrow–allograft rejection by T lymphocytes recognizing a single amino acid different in HLA-B44. N. Engl. J. Med. 323:1818, 1990.
12. Rojo, S., and Lopez de Castro, J. A.: Structure of HLA-B27 subtypes: evolutionary implications. In Dupont, B. (ed.): Immunobiology of HLA. Immunogenetics and Histocompatibility. New York, Springer-Verlag, 1989, pp. 111–112.
13. Choo, S. Y., Antonelli, P., Nisperos, B., et al.: Six variants of HLA-B27 identified by isoelectric focusing. Immunogenetics 23:23, 1986.
14. Wei, X., and Orr, H. T.: Differential expression of HLA-E, HLA-F, and HLA-G transcripts in human tissue. Hum. Immunol. 29:131, 1990.
15. Kovats, S., Main, E. K., Librach, C., et al.: A class I antigen, HLA-G, expressed in human trophoblasts. Science 248:220, 1990.
16. Geraghty, D. E., Koller, B. H., and Orr, H. T.: A human major histocompatibility complex class I gene that encodes a protein with a shortened cytoplasmic segment. Proc. Natl. Acad. Sci. U.S.A. 84:9145, 1987.
16a. Trowsdale, J., Ragoussis, J., and Campbell, R.: Map of the human MHC. Immunology Today 12:443, 1991.
17. Lee, J. S.: Regulation of HLA Class II gene expression. In Dupont, B. (ed.): Immunobiology of HLA. New York, Springer-Verlag, 1989, pp. 49–62.

18. Gregersen, P. K., Shen, M., Song, Q. L., et al.: Molecular diversity of HLA-DR4 haplotypes. Proc. Natl. Acad. Sci. U.S.A. 83:2642, 1986.

19. Scharf, S. J., Griffith, R. L., and Erlich, H. A. : Rapid typing of DNA sequence polymorphism at the HLA-DRB1 locus using polymerase chain reaction and nonradioactive oligonucleotide probes. Hum. Immunol. 30:190, 1991.

19a. Petersdorf, E., Smith, A., Mickelson, E., et al.: Tel HLA-DR4 alleles defined by sequence polymorphisms within the DRB1 first domain. Immunogenetics 33:267, 1991.

20. Egea, G. E., Yunis, I., Spies, T., et al.: Association of polymorphisms in the HLA-B region with extended haplotypes. Immunogenetics 33:4, 1991.

21. Sullivan, K. E., Calman, A. F., Nakanishi, M., et al.: A model for the transcriptional regulation of MHC class II genes. Immunol. Today 8:289, 1987.

22. Lisowska-Grospierre, B., Charron, D. J., dePreval, C., et al.: Defect of expression of MHC genes responsible for an abnormal HLA class I phenotype and the class II negative phenotype of lymphocytes from patients with combined immunodeficiency. In Albert, E. D., et al. (eds.): Histocompatibility Testing 1984. Berlin, Springer-Verlag, 1984, pp. 650–655.

23. Touraine, J. L., Marseglia, G. L., and Betuel, H.: Thirty international cases of bare lymphocyte syndrome: biological significance of HLA antigens. Exp. Hematol. 13:86, 1985.

24. Hume, C. R., Shookster, L. A., Collins, N., et al.: Bare lymphocyte syndrome: Altered HLA class II expression in B cell lines derived from two patients. Hum. Immunol. 25:1, 1989.

25. Yang, Z., Accolla, R. S., Pious, D., et al.: Two distinct loci regulating class II gene expression are defective in human mutant and patient cell lines. EMBO J. 7:1965, 1988.

26. Boothby, M., Liou, H. C., and Glimcher, L. H.: Differences in DNA sequence specificity among MHC class II X box binding proteins. J. Immunol. 142:1005, 1989.

27. Benoist, C., and Mathis, D.: Regulation of major histocompatibility complex class-II genes: X, Y, and other letters of the alphabet. Annu. Rev. Immunol. 8:681, 1990.

28. Andersen, L. C., Beaty, J. S., Nettles, J. W., et al.: Allelic polymorphism in transcriptional regulatory regions of HLA-DQβ genes. J. Exp. Med. 173: 181, 1991.

29. Bjorkman, P. J., Saper, M. A., Samraoui, B., et al.: Structure of the human class I histocompatibility antigen, HLA-A2. Nature 329:506, 1987.

30. Garrett, T. P., Saper, M. A., Bjorkman, P. J., et al.: Specificity pockets for the side chains of peptide antigens in HLA-Aw68. Nature 342:692, 1989.

31. Bjorkman, P. J., Saper, M. A., Samraoui, B., et al.: The foreign antigen binding site and T cell recognition regions of class I histocompatibility antigens. Nature 329:512, 1987.

31a. Madden, D., Gorga, J., Strominger, J., et al.: The structure of HLA-B27 reveals nonamer self-peptides bound in an extended conformation. Nature 353:321, 1991.

31b. Buxton, S., Benjamin, R., Clayberger, C., et al.: Anchoring pockets in HLA class I molecules: analysis of the conserved B "45" pocket of HLA-B27. J. Exp. Med. 175:809, 1992.

31c. Jardetzky, T., Lane, W., Robinson, R., et al.: Identification of self-peptides bound to purified HLA-B27. Nature 353:326, 1991.

32. Rosenstein, Y., Ratnofsky, S., Burakoff, S. J., et al.: Direct evidence for binding of CD8 to HLA class I antigens. J. Exp. Med. 169:149, 1989.

33. Claesson-Welsh, L., Barker, P. E., Larhammar, D., et al.: The gene encoding the human class II antigen–associated τ chain is located on chromosome 5. Immunogenetics 20:89, 1984.

34. Cresswell, P., Blum, J., Kelner, D. N., et al.: Biosynthesis and processing of class II histocompatibility antigens. CRC Crit. Rev. Immunol. 7:31, 1987.

35. Lotteau, V., Teyton, L., Peleraux, A., et al.: Intracellular transport of class II MHC molecules directed by invariant chain. Nature 348:600, 1990.

36. Brown, J. H., Jardetzky, T., Saper, M. A., et al.: A hypothetical model of the foreign antigen binding site of class II histocompatibility molecules. Nature 332:845, 1988.

37. Kwok, W. W., Lotshaw, C., Milner, E. C., et al.: Mutational analysis of the HLA-DQ3.2 IDDM susceptibility gene. Proc. Natl. Acad. Sci. U.S.A. 86:1027, 1989.

38. Hiraiwa, A., Yamanaka, K., Kwok, W. W., et al.: Structural requirements for recognition of the HLA-Dw14 class II epitope—a key HLA determinant associated with rheumatoid arthritis. Proc. Natl. Acad. Sci. U.S.A. 87:8051, 1990.

39. Peccoud, J., Dellabona, P., Allen, P., et al.: Delineation of antigen contact residues on an MHC class II molecule. EMBO J. 9:4215, 1990.

40. Krieger, J. I., Karr, R. W., Grey, H. M., et al.: Single amino acid changes in DR and antigen define residues critical for peptide-MHC binding and T cell recognition. J. Immunol. 146:2331, 1991.

41. Mittler, R. S., Goldman, S. J., Spitalny, G. L., et al.: T-cell receptor-CD4 physical association in a murine T-cell hybridoma: induction by antigen receptor ligation. Proc. Natl. Acad. Sci. U.S.A. 86:8531, 1989.

42. Brachiale, T. J., and Brachiale, V. L.: Antigen presentation: structural themes and functional variations. Immunol. Today 12:124, 1991.

43. Kwok, W. W., Schwarz, D., Nepom, B., et al.: HLA-DQ molecules form α-β heterodimers of mixed allotype. J. Immunol. 141:3123, 1988.

44. Roche, P. A., and Cresswell, P.: Invariant chain association with HLA-DR molecules inhibits immunogenic peptide binding. Nature 345:615, 1990.

45. Cresswell, P.: Intracellular class II HLA antigens are accessible to transferrin-neuraminidase conjugates internalized by receptor-mediated endocytosis. Proc. Natl. Acad. Sci. U.S.A. 82:8188, 1985.

46. Blum, J. S., and Cresswell, P.: Role for intracellular proteases in the processing and transport of class II HLA antigens. Proc. Natl. Acad. Sci. U.S.A. 85:3975, 1988.

46a. Mellins, E., Kempin, S., and Smith, L.: A gene required for class II–restricted antigen presentation maps to the major histocompatibility complex. J. Exp. Med. 174:1707, 1991.

47. Carbone, F. R., and Bevan, M. J.: Class I–restricted processing and presentation of exogenous cell–associated antigen in vivo. J. Exp. Med. 171:377, 1990.

47a. Spies, T., and DeMars, R.: Restored expression of major histocompatibility class I molecules by gene transfer of a putative peptide transporter. Nature 351:323, 1991.

48. Tiwari, J., and Terasaki, P.: HLA and Disease Associations. New York, Springer-Verlag, 1985, p. 375.

49. Bodmer, J. G., Marsh, S. G. E., Albert, E. D., et al.: Nomenclature for factors of the HLA system, 1990. Tissue Antigens 37:97, 1991.

50. Khan, M. A.: Ankylosing spondylitis and heterogeneity of HLA-B27. Semin. Arthritis Rheum. 18:134, 1988.

51. Parham, P., Lawlor, D. A., Salter, R. D., et al.: HLA-A, B, C: Patterns of polymorphism in peptide-binding proteins. In Dupont, B. (ed.): Immunobiology of HLA. New York, Springer-Verlag, 1989, pp. 10–32.

52. Breur-Vriesendorp, B. S., Dekker-Saeys, A. J., and Ivany, P.: Distribution of HLA-B27 subtypes in patients with ankylosing spondylitis: the disease is associated with a common determinant of the various B27 molecules. Ann. Rheum. Dis. 46:353, 1987.

53. Hammer, R. E., Maika, S. D., Richardson, J. A., et al.: Spontaneous inflammatory disease in transgenic rats expressing HLA-B27 and human β2m: an animal model of HLA-B27–associated human disorders. Cell 63:1099, 1990.

54. McMichael, S. J., Sasazuki, T., McDevitt, H. O., et al.: Increased frequency of HLA-Cw3 and HLA-Dw4 in rheumatoid arthritis. Arthritis Rheum. 20:1037, 1977.

55. Stastny, P.: Association of the B-cell alloantigen DRw4 with rheumatoid arthritis. N. Engl. J. Med. 298:869, 1978.

56. Thomsen, M., Morling, N., Snorrason, E., et al.: HLA-Dw4 and rheumatoid arthritis. Tissue Antigens 13:56, 1979.

57. Young, A., Jaraquemada, D., Awad, J., et al.: Association of HLA-DR4/Dw4 and DR2/Dw2 with radiologic changes in a prospective study of patients with rheumatoid arthritis. Arthritis Rheum. 27:20, 1984.

58. Duquesnoy, R. J., Marrari, M., Hackbarth, S., et al.: Serological and cellular definition of a new HLA-DR–associated determinant, MC1, and its association with rheumatoid arthritis. Hum. Immunol. 10:165, 1984.

59. Nepom, G. T., Seyfried, C. E., Holbeck, S. L., et al.: Identification of HLA-Dw14 genes in DR4+ rheumatoid arthritis. Lancet 2:1002, 1986.

60. Zoschke, D., and Segall, M.: Dw subtypes of DR4 in rheumatoid arthritis: evidence for a preferential association with Dw4. Hum. Immunol. 15:118, 1986.

61. Nepom, G. T., Byers, P., Seyfried, C., et al.: HLA genes associated with rheumatoid arthritis. Arthritis Rheum. 32:15, 1989.

62. Reinsmoenn, N., and Bach, F.: Five HLA-D clusters associated with HLA-DR4. Hum. Immunol. 4:249, 1982.

63. Nepom, B. S., Nepom, G. T., Michelson, E., et al.: Electrophoretic analysis of human HLA-DR antigens from HLA-DR4 homozygous cell lines: Correlation between beta-chain diversity and HLA-D. Proc. Natl. Acad. Sci. U.S.A. 80:6962, 1983.

64. Wordsworth, B., Lanchbury, J. S. S., Sakkas, L. I., et al.: HLA-DR4 subtype frequencies in rheumatoid arthritis indicate that DRB1 is the major susceptibility locus within the HLA class II region. Proc. Natl. Acad. Sci. U.S.A. 86:10049, 1989.

65. Nepom, B., Nepom, G. T., Schaller, J., et al.: Characterization of specific HLA-DR4–associated histocompatibility molecules in patients with juvenile rheumatoid arthritis. J. Clin. Invest. 74:287, 1984.

66. Vehe, R. K., Begovich, A. B., and Nepom, B. S.: HLA susceptibility genes in rheumatoid factor–positive juvenile rheumatoid arthritis. J. Rheumatol. 17 (Suppl. 26):11, 1990.

67. Legrand, L., Lathrop, G. M., Marcelli-Barge, A., et al.: HLA-DR genotype risks in seropositive rheumatoid arthritis. Am. J. Hum. Genet. 36:690, 1984.

68. Bell, J. I., Estess, P., St. John, T., et al.: DNA sequence and characterization of human class II major histocompatibility complex β chains from the DR1 haplotype. Proc. Natl. Acad. Sci. U.S.A. 82:3405, 1985.

69. Schiff, B., Mizrachi, Y., Orgad, S., et al.: Association of HLA-Aw31 and HLA-DR1 with adult rheumatoid arthritis. Ann. Rheum. Dis. 41:403, 1982.

70. Ohta, N., Nishimura, Y. K., Tanimoto, K., et al.: Association between HLA and Japanese patients with rheumatoid arthritis. Hum. Immunol. 5:123, 1982.

71. Willkens, R. F., Nepom, G. T., Marks, C. R., et al.: The association of HLA-Dw16 with rheumatoid arthritis in Yakima Indians: Further evidence for the "shared epitope" hypothesis. Arthritis Rheum. 34: 43, 1991.

72. Gregersen, P. K., Silver, J., and Winchester, R. J.: The shared epitope hypothesis: An approach to understanding the molecular genetics of susceptibility to rheumatoid arthritis. Arthritis Rheum. 30:1205, 1987.

73. Seyfried, C. E., Mickelson, E., Hansen, J. A., et al.: A specific nucleotide sequence defines a functional T cell recognition epitope shared by diverse HLA-DR specificities. Hum. Immunol. 21:289, 1988.

74. Weyand, C. M., and Goronzy, J. J.: Disease-associated human histocompatibility leukocyte antigen determinants in patients with seropositive rheumatoid arthritis. J. Clin. Invest. 85:1051, 1990.

75. Lombardi, G., Sidhu, S., Batchelor, J. R., et al.: Allorecognition of DR1 by T cells from a DR4/DRw13 responder mimics self-restricted recognition of endogenous peptides. Proc. Natl. Acad. Sci. U.S.A. 86:4190, 1989.

76. Nepom, G. T.: Reverse immunogenetics: Investigations of HLA-associated disease based on the structural and genetic identification of candidate susceptibility genes. In Melchers, F. (ed.): Progress in Immunology, Vol. VII. New York, Springer-Verlag, 1989, pp. 805–812.

77. Reinertsen, J. L., Klippel, J. H., Johnson, A. H., et al.: B lymphocyte alloantigens associated with systemic lupus erythematosus. N. Engl. J. Med. 299:515, 1978.

78. Ahearn, J. M., Provost, T. T., Dorsch, C. A., et al.: Interrelationships of HLA-DR, MB, and MT phenotypes, autoantibody expression, and clinical features in systemic lupus erythematosus. Arthritis Rheum. 25:1031, 1982.

79. Hochberg, M. C., Boyd, R. E., Ahearn, J. M., et al.: Systemic lupus erythematosus: a review of clinico-laboratory features and immunogenetic markers in 150 patients with emphasis on demographic subsets. Medicine 64:285, 1985.

80. Arnett, F. C., Reveille, J. D., Wilson, R. W., et al.: Systemic lupus erythematosus. Semin. Arthritis Rheum. 14:24, 1984.

81. Fronek, Z., Timmerman, L. A., Alper, C. A., et al.: Major histocompatibility complex genes and susceptibility to systemic lupus erythematosus. Arthritis Rheum. 33:1542, 1990.

82. Chused, T. M., Kassan, S. S., Opelz, G., et al.: Sjögren's syndrome associated with HLA-Dw3. N. Engl. J. Med. 296:895, 1977.

83. Hinzova, E., Ivanyi, D., Sula, K., et al.: HLA-Dw3 in Sjögren's syndrome. Tissue Antigens 9:8, 1977.

84. Fye, K. H., Terasaki, P. I., Michalski, J. P., et al.: Relationship of HLA-Dw3 and HLA-B8 to Sjögren's syndrome. Arthritis Rheum. 21:337, 1978.

85. Mann, D. L., and Moutsopoulos, H. M.: HLA DR alloantigens in different subsets of patients with Sjögren's syndrome and in family members. Ann. Rheum. Dis. 42:533, 1983.

86. Wilson, R. W., Provost, T. T., Bias, W. B., et al.: Sjögren's syndrome. Influence of multiple HLA-D region alloantigens on clinical and serologic expression. Arthritis Rheum. 27:1245, 1984.

87. Arnett, F. C., Bias, W. B., and Reveille, J. D.: Genetic studies in Sjögren's syndrome and systemic lupus erythematosus. J. Autoimmun. 2:403, 1989.

88. Maksymowych, W. P., and Glass, D. N.: Population genetics and molecular biology of the childhood chronic arthropathies. Bailliere's Clin. Rheumatol. 2:649, 1988.

89. Nepom, B. S.: The immunogenetics of juvenile rheumatoid arthritis. Rheum. Dis. Clin. North Am. 17:825, 1991.

90. Nepom, B. S., Malhotra, U., Schwarz, D. A., et al.: HLA and T cell receptor polymorphisms in pauciarticular juvenile rheumatoid arthritis. Arthritis Rheum. 34:1260, 1991.

91. Hoffman, R. W., Shaw, S., Francis, L. C., et al.: HLA-DP antigens in patients with pauciarticular juvenile rheumatoid arthritis. Arthritis Rheum. 29:1057, 1986.

92. Odum, N., Morling, N., Friis, J., et al.: Increased frequency of HLA-DPw2 in pauciarticular onset juvenile chronic arthritis. Tissue Antigens 28:245, 1986.

93. Begovich, A. B., Bugawan, T. L., Nepom, B. S., et al.: A specific HLA-DPβ allele is associated with pauciarticular juvenile rheumatoid arthritis but not adult rheumatoid arthritis. Proc. Natl. Acad. Sci. U.S.A. 86:9489, 1989.

94. Fernandez-Vina, M. A., Fink, C. W., and Stastny, P.: HLA antigens in juvenile arthritis: pauciarticular and polyarticular juvenile arthritis are immunogenetically distinct. Arthritis Rheum. 33:1787, 1990.

95. Allison, J. P., and Lanier, L. L.: Structure, function, and serology of the T-cell antigen receptor complex. Annu. Rev. Immunol. 5:503, 1987.

96. Clevers, H., Alarcon, B., Wileman, T., et al.: The T cell receptor/CD3 complex: a dynamic protein ensemble. Annu. Rev. Immunol. 6:629, 1988.

97. Gao, X., Ball, E. J., Dombrausky, L., et al.: Class II human leukocyte antigen genes and T cell receptor polymorphisms in patients with rheumatoid arthritis. Am. J. Med. 85:14, 1988.

98. Fronek, Z., Lents, D., Berliner, N., et al.: Systemic lupus erythematosus is not genetically linked to the beta chain of the T cell receptor. Arthritis Rheum. 29:1023, 1986.

99. Perl, A., Divincenzo, J. P., Gergely, P., et al.: Detection and mapping of polymorphic KpnI alleles in the human T-cell receptor constant beta-2 locus. Immunology 67:135, 1989.

100. Stamenkovic, I., Stegagno, M., Wright, K. A., et al.: Clonal dominance among T-lymphocyte infiltrates in arthritis. Proc. Natl Acad. Sci. U.S.A. 85:1179, 1988.

101. Savill, C. M., Delves, P. J., Kioussis, D., et al.: A minority of patients with rheumatoid arthritis show a dominant rearrangement of T cell receptor β chain genes in synovial lymphocytes. Scand. J. Immunol. 25:629, 1987.

102. Paliard, X., West, S. G., Lafferty, J. A., et al.: Evidence for the effects of a superantigen in rheumatoid arthritis. Science 253:325, 1991.

103. Kappler, J. W., Wade, T., White, J., et al.: A T cell receptor Vβ segment that imparts reactivity to a Class II major histocompatibility complex product. Cell 49:263, 1987.

104. Marrack, P., Lo, D., Brinster, R., et al.: The effect of thymus environment on T cell development and tolerance. Cell 53:627, 1988.

105. Kisielow, P., Teh, H. S., Blüthmann, H., et al.: Positive selection of antigen-specific T cells in thymus by restricting MHC molecules. Nature 335:730, 1988.

106. Teh, H. S., Kisielow, P., Scott, B., et al.: Thymic major histocompatibility complex antigens and the αβ T-cell receptor determine the CD4/CD8 phenotype of T cells. Nature 335:229, 1988.

107. Wraith, D. C., McDevitt, H. O., Steinman, L., et al.: T cell recognition as the target for immune intervention in autoimmune disease. Cell 57:709, 1989.

108. Oldstone, M. B. A.: Molecular mimicry as a mechanism for the cause and as a probe uncovering etiologic agent(s) of autoimmune disease. In Melchers, F. (ed.): Current Topics in Microbiology and Immunology. Vol. 145. Berlin-Heidelberg, Springer-Verlag, 1989, pp. 127–135.

109. Roudier, J., Rhodes, G., Petersen, J., et al.: Hypothesis: The Epstein-Barr virus glycoprotein gp110, a molecular link between HLA DR4, HLA DR1, and rheumatoid arthritis. Scand. J. Immunol. 27:367, 1988.

110. Edwing, C., Ebringer, R., Tribbick, G., et al.: Antibody activity in ankylosing spondylitis sera to two sites on HLA B27.1 at the MHC groove region (within sequence 65-85), and to a Klebsiella pneumoniae nitrogenase reductase peptide (within sequence 181-199). J. Exp. Med. 171:1635, 1990.

111. Keat, A.: Is spondylitis caused by Klebsiella? Immunol. Today 70:144, 1986.

Chapter 7
T Cells and B Cells

Peter E. Lipsky
Laurie S. Davis
Katheryn Meek
Mary C. Wacholtz

INTRODUCTION

The salient features of the immune system are (1) the capacity to respond specifically to the universe of foreign antigens, (2) the capacity to develop enhanced responsiveness to encountered antigens during the first exposure (priming), (3) the capacity to retain specific memory of an encountered antigen and respond more vigorously and quickly to a second exposure, and (4) the capacity to discern self from nonself. All these characteristic features can be accounted for by the activities of thymus-derived lymphocytes (T cells) and bone marrow–derived lymphocytes (B cells), the antigen-specific cellular elements of the immune system.

Both T cells and B cells express clonally distributed antigen receptors that endow these cells with the ability to respond to all the antigens that an organism will encounter during its lifetime. T cells differ from B cells in the nature of their antigen receptors, the nature of the antigens they recognize, the mechanisms by which they recognize antigens, and their responses to such antigens.

B cells utilize a membrane form of immunoglobulin (Ig) as their receptors to recognize soluble antigens. After stimulation, they respond by clonal expansion and differentiation into Ig-secreting cells. In contrast, T cells express one of two types of antigen receptors that recognize cell-associated antigenic peptides bound to polymorphic determinants of the products of either class I or class II major histocompatibility complex (MHC) molecules. After stimulation, T cells acquire a number of effector functions, such as the capacity to kill specific target cells, as well as regulatory activities, many of which are accomplished by a variety of secreted, antigen-nonspecific molecules, or cytokines. In concert, the actions of antigen-specific T and B cells and their various secreted effector molecules account for the exquisite specificity, acquired reactivity, memory, and self-nonself discrimination that are hallmarks of the immune system.

CELLS OF THE IMMUNE SYSTEM

B Lymphocytes

B lymphocytes are the cells in the body that are specialized to produce Ig. Their name denotes their origin in the bone marrow in mammals and the bursa of Fabricius in birds.[1] The most characteristic feature of B lymphocytes is the capacity to synthesize Ig and both to express it as an integral membrane protein and to secrete it. Developmentally, B lymphocytes constitute a distinct lineage of cells, whose various members differ in degree of maturation and activation and extent of differentiation.[2, 3] Distinct stages of B cell maturation and development can be recognized, including early B lineage precursors (pro-B cells, pre-pre-B cells), pre-B cells, immature and mature B cells, and plasma cells (Fig. 7–1). In general, these can be distinguished by the status of Ig gene rearrangements and the production of Ig gene products, as well as the expression of other B lineage markers.[4, 5]

Most mature peripheral B lymphocytes express two Igs on their surface, IgM and IgD, each with identical light chains and antigen-binding capabilities.[6] More immature B cells only express surface membrane IgM, whereas pre-B cells express cytoplasmic mu (μ) heavy chains but neither kappa (κ) nor lambda (λ) light chains and no surface Ig. After activation, B cells rapidly lose surface IgD expression and, if they undergo switch recombination, IgM expression as well. Postswitch memory B cells can therefore be identified by the expression of membrane-associated IgG, IgA, or IgE. When B lineage cells undergo terminal differentiation to high-rate Ig-secreting plasma cells, they cease to express all surface membrane–associated Ig.

B Cell Surface Markers. Besides Ig, B cells express a number of non-Ig surface proteins, some of which appear to be B lineage specific or uniquely expressed by B cell subpopulations. Many of these markers are expressed in a developmentally regulated way or are altered as a result of activation stimuli (Table 7–1).

CD19 is the first of the B cell–specific differentiation markers to be expressed. It is found on pro-B cells, the earliest committed precursors of the B cell lineage.[7, 8] Its expression is up-regulated after activation and is lost only at the terminal stages of B cell maturation. CD19 is a 90-kD, heavily glycosylated transmembrane glycoprotein that is a member of the Ig supergene family. Although the physiologic function of CD19 is unknown, cross-linking with monoclonal antibodies dramatically inhibits B cell proliferation whereas coligation of surface IgM and CD19 markedly enhances B cell proliferation.[9, 9a]

108

HUMAN B LYMPHOCYTE DIFFERENTIATION

Stage of B Cell Maturation

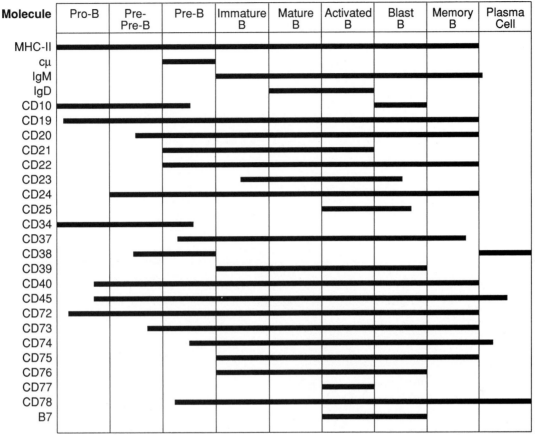

Figure 7–1. Sequential expression of B lineage–specific or –associated molecules during B cell maturation and differentiation. The stages of B cell ontogeny are defined by the rearrangement patterns and expression of immunoglobulin genes. Immunoglobulin genes are in germline configuration in pro-B cells but are rearranged in pre-pre-B, pre-B, and B cells. Pre-pre-B cells do not express cytoplasmic μ (cμ) heavy chains or surface IgM. Pre-B cells express cytoplasmic μ heavy chains but do not express surface IgM. Immature B cells and memory B cells express surface IgM but not surface IgD. Mature and activated B cells may coexpress surface IgM and surface IgD. (Modified from Uckun, F. M.: Regulation of human B-cell ontogeny. Blood 76:1908, 1990. Used by permission.)

CD20 is a 33-kD transmembrane glycoprotein that has several transmembrane-spanning regions.[10–12] CD20 is expressed exclusively on B cells. It is expressed by pre-pre-B cells, after CD19 can first be detected but before the appearance of cytoplasmic μ-chains. CD20 expression is lost after B cells differentiate into Ig-secreting cells. Engaging CD20 on B cells induces cell cycle entry, suggesting that this molecule may also play a role in the functional activation of B cells.[13]

CD21 is a 140-kD B cell–specific glycoprotein molecule. It is the receptor for the C3d subunit of complement as well as a receptor for Epstein-Barr virus.[14–16] The expression of CD21 can first be noted on pre-B cells, after CD19 and CD20. Cross-linking CD21 with its natural ligand or with monoclonal antibodies can enhance T cell–supported proliferation and differentiation of B cells,[17] suggesting that this receptor can also play a role in signal transduction.

CD22 is a B cell–specific 135-kD member of the Ig supergene family,[18, 19] whose expression parallels that of CD21. Initially after activation, the expression of CD22 increases and then is lost. Engagement of CD22 can also deliver a costimulatory signal to B cells.[20]

CD72 is a 43-kD transmembrane protein that is expressed at all stages of B cell maturation, except by plasma cells when it is lost.[21, 22] It belongs to a gene family that contains a lectin-homology domain in its external C-terminal domain.[23] CD72 is the human equivalent of the murine Lyb-2 molecule. Engagement of this molecule on either human or murine B cells generates an activation signal.[24] Recent evidence indicates that CD72 is a receptor for CD5 expressed by all T cells and a subset of B cells.[25]

B cells express a number of other molecules that are not B lineage specific but can be useful in identifying the stage of B cell differentiation and may play a role in regulating B cell activation. Among

Table 7–1. HUMAN B CELL DIFFERENTIATION MOLECULES

Molecule	Other Designation	Molecular Weight (kD)	Function	Distribution	Comments
CD5	T1, Leu-1, Ly-1	67	Signaling molecule	B cell subset, T cells	? Identifies autoantibody-producing cells
CD9	—	24	Unknown	Pre-B cells, monocytes, platelets	Induction of homotypic adhesion
CD19	B4	90	Signaling molecule	B cells	Modulation of B cell proliferation
CD20	B1	35–37	Signaling molecule	B cells	Activation or inhibition of B cell function
CD21	B2	140	C3d receptor (CR2) EBV receptor	B cell subset	Stimulation of B cell proliferation
CD22	—	135	Signaling molecule	B cells	Augmentation of B cell activation
CD23	Blast-2	45–50	Low-affinity IgE receptor	B cell subset, activated monocytes, eosinophils	Induced by IL-4, shed as 33 kD B cell growth factor
CD24	—	38–41	Signaling molecule	B cells, granulocytes	Costimulates B cell proliferation, inhibits differentiation
CD40	—	45–50	Receptor for ligand on activated T cells	B cells, some carcinomas	Facilitates B cell growth and IgE production with IL-4
CD72	Lyb-2	45	Signaling molecule	B cells	Receptor for CD5
B7	BB-1	46	Facilitate T-B collaboration	Activated B cells	Receptor for CD28

EBV, Epstein-Barr virus.

these is CD23, the low-affinity receptor for IgE on human B cells, which is distinct from the high-affinity IgE receptor on mast cells and basophils.[26, 27] CD23 is also expressed by platelets, eosinophils, macrophages, natural killer (NK) cells, dendritic cells, and possibly T cells. Expression of CD23 on B cells is limited to IgM-IgD–bearing B cells and is increased by activation and regulated by the action of cytokines.[28, 29] CD23 is not a member of the Ig supergene family but belongs to the same primitive supergene family of lectin-containing molecules as CD72.[23, 27] A feature of this molecule is that proteolysis cleaves it, generating a fragment that may have B cell growth factor activity.[30] Moreover, monoclonal antibodies to CD23, but not IgE itself, costimulate B cell proliferation, suggesting that this molecule may be able to deliver stimulatory signals to B cells.

CD40 is a 45- to 50-kD integral membrane protein whose expression is largely, but not completely, limited to B lineage cells.[31, 32] CD40 is a member of a family of cell-surface receptors, including the tumor necrosis factor (TNF) receptors and the receptor for nerve growth factor.[33, 34] Engagement of CD40 on B cells costimulates growth with interleukin-4 (IL-4) as well as the production of IgE.[35–38]

B Cell Subsets. A subpopulation of B cells expresses the pan-T cell marker, CD5.[39] These cells constitute 10 to 20 percent of the total circulating B cells in healthy adults. Larger numbers of CD5+ B cells are present in fetal spleen, neonatal blood, and the blood of patients following bone marrow trans-

plantation. The CD5 marker is also expressed on most chronic lymphocytic leukemia B cells. In the mouse, CD5+ B cells and their progenitors constitute a major fraction of peritoneal B cells.[40] That CD5+ B cells represent a distinct population is suggested by the findings that levels of CD5+ B cells are genetically regulated in the mouse and human. It has been suggested that the CD5+ B cell subpopulation is a distinct B cell lineage, because adult bone marrow precursors do not give rise to CD5+ B cells. A role for these cells in the pathogenesis of autoimmune disease has been suggested because elevated levels of CD5+ B cells are found in autoimmune mice, where they produce IgM autoantibodies constitutively.[41] Studies in humans indicate that CD5+ B cell levels are elevated in patients with rheumatoid arthritis and Sjögren's syndrome and that these cells produce autoantibodies.[42] However, in humans, CD5+ B cells do not preferentially produce autoantibodies.[43] Moreover, CD5 may not identify a unique lineage of B cells in humans, as this marker is induced by activation of CD5– B cells.[44] Therefore, the role of CD5+ B cells in the pathogenesis of autoimmunity in humans is unclear.

T Lymphocytes

T Cell Surface Markers. A number of cell surface molecules are uniquely expressed by T lineage cells (Table 7–2). The earliest of these is CD7, a 40-kD

Table 7–2. HUMAN T CELL DIFFERENTIATION MOLECULES

Molecule	Other Designation	Molecular Weight (kD)	Function	Distribution	Comments
CD1a,b,c	T6	43–46	Unknown	Thymocytes, dendritic cells, some B cells	Associated with β_2 microglobulin
CD2	T11	50	Receptor for LFA-3	T cells, some NK cells	Triggers alternative activation pathway
CD3	T3	5 chains of 16–25	Components of T cell antigen receptor	Thymocytes, T cells	Generates activation signals from TCR
TCR	Ti	Heterodimer of 42 and 45	Antigen recognition	Thymocytes, T cells	Polymorphic receptor for antigen-MHC complex
CD4	T4	59	Binds MHC class II	Thymocytes, helper-inducer T cells, monocytes	Receptor for HIV, associated with p56[lck]
CD5	T1, Leu-1, Ly-1	67	Signaling molecule	Thymocytes, T cells, B cell subset	Receptor for CD72
CD7	—	40	Unknown	Prethymocytes, thymocytes, T cells	Earliest T cell marker
CD8	T8	Heterodimer of 32	Binds MHC class I	Thymocytes, suppressor/cytotoxic T cells, some NK cells	Associated with p56[lck]

HIV, human immunodeficiency virus.

transmembrane glycoprotein with an extracellular portion composed of a single Ig variable region–like domain.[45–47] CD7 is expressed by all T cells, including prethymic precursor T cells in the bone marrow, although it may be transiently modulated after stimulation, engaging its ligand, or entry into tissues.[48] It is also expressed at diminished density on memory T cells.[49] CD2[50, 51] and CD5[52] are also expressed on all peripheral blood T cells, although neither is specific because CD2 is expressed on NK cells[53] and CD5 on a subset of B cells.[39]

From a functional point of view, the most characteristic T cell surface molecule is the T cell receptor (TCR) heterodimer.[54–60] The TCR is an 80- to 90-kD disulfide-linked heterodimer that is noncovalently associated with as many as five invariant chains of the CD3 complex (Fig. 7–2).[61] The TCR is composed of a 48- to 54-kD acidic alpha (α)-chain and a 37- to 42-kD more basic beta (β)-chain. Each chain is an integral membrane protein with both constant and variable domains. Both chains are members of the Ig supergene family. A small subpopulation of T cells expresses a similar, but distinct TCR composed of gamma (γ)- and delta (δ)-chains, also associated with the CD3 molecular complex. The γ-chains range in size from 35 to 55 kD and are disulfide bonded to the 45- to 52-kD δ-chain. T cells expressing the $\gamma\delta$ TCR usually fail to express either CD4 or CD8, whereas the vast majority of the $\alpha\beta$ TCR expressing T cells are either CD4+ or CD8+.[62] The structural variability and antigenic specificity of the TCR are explained by the organization, recombination, and expression of the genes encoding these chains.

In contrast to Ig molecules, TCRs occur only as membrane-bound molecules. Each T cell expresses only a single TCR consisting of either an $\alpha\beta$ or $\gamma\delta$ heterodimer. All four TCR polypeptides consist of two Ig domains, one variable, and one constant. The one exception is the Cγ2 molecule, which has undergone duplication.[63] Each polypeptide has transmembrane and cytoplasmic domains encoded by separate exons. The $\alpha\beta$ and $\gamma\delta$ heterodimers are covalently bound via disulfide bonds C-terminal to the constant region domains. As in the case of Ig, TCRs are glycosylated proteins.

The function of the TCR is to recognize antigenic peptides. However, the TCR does not recognize free antigen but rather cell-associated antigenic fragments bound to molecules of the MHC on the surface of specialized antigen-presenting cells. Although three-dimensional structures of TCRs are not yet available, there has been considerable speculation concerning the means by which the TCR recognizes antigen and the structure of the TCR-MHC–antigenic peptide complex.[64] Similar to Ig molecules, sequence analysis of TCR has revealed regions of hypervariability between different TCR molecules that, by analogy to Ig, have been termed *hypervariable regions* or *complementarity-determining regions* (CDRs). As is the case with Ig, there are three CDRs in each polypeptide chain. Molecular modeling analysis of the TCR based on the three-dimensional structure of Ig molecules predicts that CDR1 and CDR2, which are encoded in the variable portion of the TCR polypeptides, contact the polymorphic residues of the α-helices of MHC molecules, whereas the CDR3s of both polypeptides, which are derived during V(D)J recombination, interact with the antigenic peptide found in the antigen-binding cleft of the MHC molecule. This model predicts that T cell recognition of the antigenic uni-

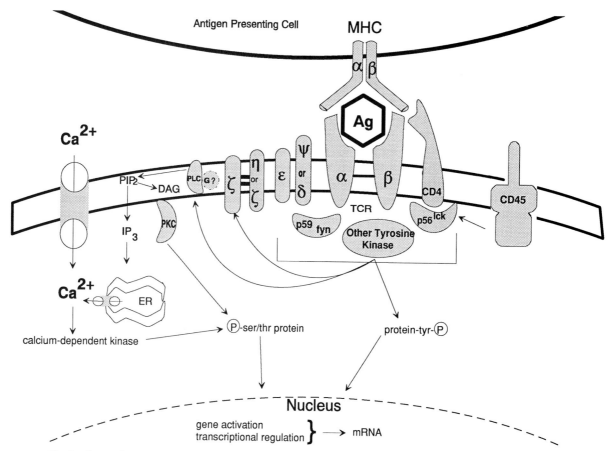

Figure 7–2. The biochemical events stimulated by T cell receptor (TCR) occupancy. The TCR recognizes antigen (Ag) complexed with an MHC molecule, here class II, on the surface of an antigen-presenting cell. The TCR is associated with the CD3 complex ($\gamma,\delta,\epsilon,\zeta,\eta$). PLC, phospholipase C; G, G protein; PIP_2, phosphatidylinositol-4,5-bisphosphate; IP_3, inositol trisphosphate; DAG, diacylglycerol; PKC, protein kinase C; ER, endoplasmic reticulum (intracellular Ca^{2+} store).

verse would be very great because it is governed by the most diverse portion of the TCR molecule, the CDR3. It should be pointed out, however, that the model of the interaction of these three molecules, the TCR, MHC molecule, and antigenic peptide, remains hypothetical.

Both $\alpha\beta$ and $\gamma\delta$ TCRs are expressed on the cell surface in association with the CD3 complex. CD3 is not a single protein but rather a multichain complex of 16- to 28-kD subunits, consisting of γ, δ, epsilon (ϵ), zeta (ζ), and eta (η)-chains.[65–68] Each chain is the product of an individual gene,[69–72] except for ζ and η, which are alternatively spliced forms of the same gene.[73] γ, δ, and ϵ are present as single chains, whereas ζ and η form dimers. ζ is found primarily as a disulfide-linked homodimer but may also form a heterodimer with the η-chain. Recently, functional η-η homodimers have also been identified.[74] The exact organization of the CD3 complex has not been determined, although it appears that separate complexes may contain γ or δ associated with one or more ϵ-chains.[75]

CD3 and the TCR appear to be physically associated on the surface of T cells.[76–78] Moreover, both the TCR and the components of the CD3 complex are necessary for surface expression of both

structures.[79, 80] Association of the TCR with the CD3 complex appears to relate to the presence of charged amino acids in the transmembrane domains of the molecules.[81] CD3 is thought to play a central role in T cell activation after engagement of the TCR. Because CD3 components are not polymorphic, the role of CD3 does not involve antigen recognition. Rather, CD3 appears to function by transmitting signals from the TCR to the interior of the cell (Fig. 7–2). Of the components of the CD3 molecular complex, the cytoplasmic domain of the ζ-chain appears to play a particularly critical role.[82]

CD2 is another transmembrane protein that identifies T cells and may play a role in signal transduction. Originally recognized as a receptor for sheep erythrocytes, CD2 is a 50-kD glycoprotein that binds to leukocyte function–associated molecule-3 (LFA-3, CD58) expressed by a variety of cell types.[50, 51, 83] CD2 is expressed by the vast majority of thymocytes and all peripheral T cells, as well as by some NK cells.[52] The possibility that CD2 provides an alternative activation pathway, which could be important during ontogeny before the TCR-CD3 complex is expressed, has been suggested by the finding that monoclonal antibodies to this molecule induce T cell activation.[84] Alternatively, interactions between

CD2 and LFA-3, expressed by a variety of accessory cells, may serve to costimulate T cell activation after antigen recognition.[85]

CD4 is a 59-kD member of the Ig supergene family[86, 87] expressed by specific subsets of thymocytes, one of the two major subsets of αβ expressing peripheral T cells, and some monocyte-macrophages, especially those capable of serving as antigen-presenting cells.[88] CD4 was originally thought to denote T cells with the capacity to function as helper cells for B cell responses or as inducer cells for the maturation of other T cell subsets, but more recent information indicates that CD4 is expressed by T cells whose capacity to recognize antigen is restricted by class II molecules of the MHC.[89–91] CD4 plays at least two roles in this process. First, CD4 directly binds to nonpolymorphic determinants on class II MHC molecules, increasing the avidity of the interaction between the TCR and the antigenic peptide bound to the antigen-binding groove of class II MHC molecules displayed on the surface of an antigen-presenting cell.[92] Second, engagement of CD4 provides a co-stimulatory signal that amplifies T cell activation induced by recognition of antigen.[93–95] For many T cells, the binding and costimulatory roles of CD4 are critical to allow antigen recognition to result in T cell activation. With some T cells, apparently with very high avidity TCRs, interactions with CD4 do not appear to play a necessary role in T cell activation. In some circumstances, engaging CD4 may deliver a negative signal that inhibits T cell activation.[85] This may be important in the immunosuppression that follows infection with the human immunodeficiency virus, which utilizes its envelope glycoprotein gp120 to bind to the CD4 molecule.[96, 97] The signaling capacity of the CD4 molecule relates to the fact that the cytoplasmic domain of this molecule associates with a lymphocyte-specific tyrosine kinase, p56[lck].[98–101] Association of CD4 with the TCR-CD3 molecular complex apparently brings this kinase into association with new substrates whose phosphorylation appears to be important in the cascade of biochemical events involved in T cell activation.

CD8 is expressed by specific subsets of thymocytes, a subpopulation of peripheral T cells that generally does not express CD4, and also by many NK cells.[86, 102] Whereas the human CD4 molecule is present on the cell surface as a monomer, the CD8 molecule is expressed on the T cell surface as a dimer consisting of 32- to 34-kD monomers. There are two forms of CD8 expressed on T cells, either CD8α/α homodimers or CD8α/β heterodimers.[103] Both the α- and β-chains are similar in size and are members of the Ig supergene family. They are encoded by two closely linked genes. T cells expressing αβ TCRs may express both CD8α/α and CD8α/β on the same cell, although coexpression of the two forms varies between individuals. CD8+ T cells expressing the γδ TCR and CD8+ NK cells express only the CD8α/α homodimer.[104] Although the expression of CD8 was originally thought to denote T cells with suppressor or cytotoxic activity, more recent information indicates that CD8 is expressed by T cells whose capacity to recognize antigen is restricted by class I MHC molecules.[91, 105, 106] CD8 binds to nonpolymorphic amino acids of the α3 domain of class I MHC molecules.[107] Such binding not only increases the avidity of interactions between CD8+ T cells and antigen-presenting cells expressing antigenic peptides bound into the antigen-binding cleft of class I MHC molecules but also delivers a costimulatory signal to the T cell.[95] Associations between the cytoplasmic domain of CD8 and p56[lck] appear to play an important role in the capacity of CD8 to costimulate T cell activation.[98–100, 108]

There are many other molecules expressed by T cells, some of which play a role in modulating the function of these cells (Table 7–3). One of these is CD28, a homodimeric transmembrane glycoprotein consisting of two 44-kD polypeptide chains.[109, 110] This member of the Ig supergene family is expressed on nearly all CD4+ and about 50 percent of CD8+ T cells. One of the natural ligands of CD28 is the B7/BB1 molecule, another member of the Ig supergene family expressed by activated B cells.[110] Engagement of CD28 provides an activation signal to T cells that is unique in that it is not dependent on the expression of the TCR-CD3 complex.[111]

T Cell Subsets. A wide variety of activities have been attributed to T cells. Early studies suggested that CD4+ cells represented helper-inducer cells and that CD8+ cells represented cytolytic-suppressor cells. Subsequent studies documented that these activities were not strictly related to the expression of CD4 and CD8. Rather, the CD4+ or CD8+ phenotype of the T cell related more closely to its capacity to recognize antigen in the context of either class II or class I MHC molecules, respectively.[89–91, 105, 106] It is clear that recognition of antigen by T cells is fundamentally distinct from antigen recognition by B cells. Cell-bound antigen, rather than soluble antigen, is the form recognized by T cells. Cell-bound antigenic peptides are recognized by T cells after association with molecules of the MHC. A direct physical interaction between antigenic peptides and class I and class II MHC molecules has been demonstrated.[112–116] Class I MHC molecules play the major role as restricting elements for peptides derived endogenously within antigen-presenting cells, whereas class II MHC molecules restrict T cell responses to exogenous proteins that are taken up and degraded in the lysosomes of antigen-presenting cells to reveal antigenic peptides.[117] The strong association between class I and class II MHC restriction and the CD8+ and CD4+ subsets of T cells, respectively, is likely to reflect a fundamental role of the CD4 and CD8 molecules during T cell activation and also during the selection of the T cell repertoire in the thymus.

CD4+ T cells comprise approximately 60 percent of the circulating T cell population. These cells seem to be the most effective but not the only cells

Table 7–3. T CELL SURFACE MOLECULES THAT PLAY A ROLE IN SIGNAL TRANSDUCTION

Surface Antigens	Early Activation Events	Comments
CD1	$[Ca^{2+}]_i$	Costimulates with PMA; CD3 independent
CD2	$[Ca^{2+}]_i$, PI, Tyr P	APC ligand-LFA-3 (CD58); surface CD3 required
CD3-TCR	$[Ca^{2}]_i$, PI, Tyr P, PKC	APC ligand–polymorphic MHC
CD4/CD8	$[Ca^{2+}]_i$, Tyr P via p56^{lck}	APC ligand–class II/I MHC; costimulates with CD3
CD5	$[Ca^{2+}]_i$, PI	B cell ligand–CD72; surface CD3 required; costimulates with CD3
CD6	Modest $[Ca^{2+}]_i$	Costimulates with CD3
CD7	Modest $[Ca^{2+}]_i$	Absence is associated with immunodeficiency
CD11a/CD18 (LFA-1)	Augment $[Ca^{2+}]_i$	APC ligand–ICAM-1(CD54), ICAM-2; costimulates with CD3
CD26	Unknown	Costimulates with CD2, CD3
CD28	Tyr P	Ligand on B cells–B7/BB1; costimulates with PMA, CD3; CD3 independent
VLA-4 (CD49d/CD29)	Unknown	Ligand-fibronectin, VCAM-1; costimulates with CD3
CD43 (sialophorin)	$[Ca^{2+}]_i$, PI, PKC	Costimulates with CD3, PMA; absence is associated with immunodeficiency; ligand–ICAM-1
CD44	Unknown	Ligand-addressins; costimulates with CD2 or CD3
CD45	Tyrosine phosphatase	Various isoforms expressed by cells at different maturation states
CD55 (DAF)	Augment $[Ca^{2+}]_i$	Ligand–complement components; costimulates with CD3, AC + PMA
CDw60	Unknown	Costimulates with AC or PMA
CD69	$[Ca^{2+}]_i$	Costimulates with PMA
CD73	Unknown	Costimulates with PMA
MHC class I	$[Ca^{2+}]_i$	Ligand-CD8; requires cross-linking and CD3 expression

PI, phosphatidylinositol; PKC, protein kinase C; PMA, phorbol myristate acetate; APC, antigen-presenting cell; AC, accessory cell; Tyr P, tyrosine kinase activity.

that can provide help for B cell differentiation and that mediate delayed-type hypersensitivity reactions.[118, 119] In addition, these cells appear to play a major role in mediating graft-versus-host disease and allograft rejection when class II MHC molecules are the major alloantigenic stimulus.[120] Of importance, these cells appear to play a major immunopathogenic role in a number of autoimmune diseases in experimental animals, including experimental allergic encephalomyelitis, insulin-dependent diabetes mellitus, murine lupus, collagen-induced arthritis, and autoimmune thyroiditis, as evidenced by the finding that these experimental diseases can be successfully treated with monoclonal antibodies to CD4.[121–125] Much of the functional activity of these cells appears to relate to their capacity to produce a variety of cytokines that affect the function of a myriad of other cell types. In addition, CD4+ T cells can exert a variety of effector functions, including the capacity to kill targets expressing appropriate class II MHC molecules and the ability to down-modulate the function of B lymphocytes.

Recent studies in the mouse have suggested that CD4+ T cell clones can be generated that express specific functional activities (Table 7–4), although differences in the expression of differentiation markers have not been appreciated.[126, 127] T helper-1 (TH-1) cells are effective mediators of delayed-type hypersensitivity reactions and are the primary producers of IL-2 and interferon-γ (IFN-γ), whereas TH-2 cells produce IL-4, IL-5, and IL-6 and are effective helper cells for B cell differentiation and especially the secretion of IgE. Of note, TH-1 cells appear to regulate the activities of TH-2 cells by producing IFN-γ, whereas TH-2 cells interfere with the function of TH-1 cells by secreting IL-10, which limits the capacity of antigen-presenting cells to activate TH-1 cells.

The unique actions of TH-1 and TH-2 cells may bias the immune response toward delayed-type hypersensitivity or humoral immunity and especially IgE production, respectively. It has been difficult to identify TH-1 and TH-2 type clones in humans[128] and, therefore, the possibility that human CD4+ T cells differentiate into such functionally defined subsets remains to be determined.

In both the human and the mouse, as well as other species, CD4+ T cells have been separated into "memory" and "naive" subsets based on the expression of a variety of markers (Table 7–5).[129–131] Although these subsets differ in the expression of a number of markers, the most useful ones to separate them have proven to be the isoforms of CD45, with the higher-molecular-weight form, CD45RA, expressed by naive T cells and the lower-molecular-weight CD45RO by memory T cells. These isoforms differ only in the extracellular portion of the molecule and are generated by alternative splicing. In general,

Table 7–4. FUNCTIONAL PROPERTIES OF MURINE CD4 SUBSETS

Function	TH1	TH2
Lymphokine secretion		
IL-2	+	−
IFN-γ	+	−
IL-3	+	+
GM-CSF	+	+
IL-4	−	+
IL-5	−	+
IL-6	−	+
IL-10	−	+
Help for B cells		
IgM, IgG	+	+
IgE	−	+
Delayed type hypersensitivity	+	−

Table 7–5. SURFACE MARKERS ON NAIVE AND MEMORY T CELLS

Molecule	Other Designation	Molecular Weight (kD)	Characteristic	Expression	
				Memory	*Naive*
CD58	LFA-3	45–66	Ligand for CD2	+ +	+
CD2	T11	50	Alternative activation pathway	+ + +	+ +
CD11a/CD18	LFA-1	180–195	Receptor for ICAM1/2	+ + +	+ +
CD29	—	130	β-chain of $β_1$(VLA) integrins	+ + + +	+
CD45RO	—	180	Isoform of CD45	+ + + +	—
CD45RA	—	220	Isoform of CD45	—	+ + + +
CD44	Pgp-1	80–95	HCAM	+ + +	+ +
CD54	ICAM-1	90	Counter-receptor for LFA-1	+	—
CD26	—	120	Dipeptidyl peptidase IV	+	—
CD7	—	40	T cell lineage marker	+ / −	+ +
CD3	—	Multichain complex	Part of TCR complex	+	+

VLA, very late antigen; HCAM, homing cell adhesion molecule.

monoclonal antibodies against CD45RA or CD45RO recognize reciprocal populations of resting T cells. After activation, there is a predominantly unidirectional transition from expression of CD45RA to CD45RO, which is thought to parallel the differentiation from naive to memory T cells. A number of other observations support the conclusion that CD45RA and CD45RO are expressed on naive and memory T cells, respectively. First, neonatal T cells are largely CD45RA+, with the percentage of CD45RO+ cells progressively increasing with age. Moreover, responses to recall antigens are largely exhibited by CD45RO+ cells, whereas both populations can respond to mitogenic stimulation and allogeneic stimulator cells. The capacity of CD45RO+ memory cells to produce certain cytokines is also enhanced compared with that of CD45RA+ naive cells. Thus, memory cells produce IL-4, IFN-γ, and IL-6, whereas both populations can secrete IL-2 after appropriate stimulation. There is evidence that the activation requirements of naive T cells are more stringent than for memory T cells. Previously reported discrepancies in the functional activities of these two subsets are likely to result from these differences in activation requirements and cytokine production.

The CD8-expressing subset comprises approximately 35 percent of peripheral T cells. These cells recognize antigenic peptides that are bound to class I MHC molecules.[105, 106] Because this pathway of peptide presentation is most important in the recognition of endogenously synthesized proteins, CD8+ T cells are particularly involved in host defense to intracellular pathogens, such as viruses and other intracellular microorganisms.[117, 132] In some situations, the response of CD8+ T cells to microbial peptides may be sufficiently vigorous not only to eradicate the organism but also to cause tissue pathology.[133]

Prominent among the activities of CD8+ T cells is the capacity to differentiate into cytolytic effector cells.[134] This activity is not unique to CD8+ T cells in that CD4+ T cells can also differentiate into killer cells.[128] However, the specificity of CD4+ cytolytic

cells is different, with the activity directed toward class II MHC molecules or peptides presented by class II MHC molecules. Moreover, CD8+ T cells are not limited in their effector functions and are also able to produce a variety of cytokines, including IL-2, TNF-α, and IFN-γ and, under certain circumstances, can also support B cell differentiation.[119] Although it was previously believed that the differentiation of cytolytic effector cells from CD8+ T cell precursors required an interaction with CD4+ T cells, more recent evidence indicates that in many circumstances this is not necessary.[135]

The mechanism by which cytolytic effector cells kill their targets involves a complex series of steps. Initially, there is TCR-mediated recognition of the target, which is facilitated by adhesion molecules on the killer cell, such as LFA-1 (CD11a/CD18) and CD2, which recognize intercellular adhesion molecule-1 (ICAM-1, CD54) and LFA-3 (CD58), respectively, on the target cell.[83] Subsequently, the lytic mechanism is activated.[136–142] This involves the action of a number of preformed granule-associated proteins, including several serine esterases (granzymes) and a membrane pore-forming protein, perforin. The action of these various secreted granule components leads to direct lysis of non-nucleated targets and a more complex form of death of nucleated targets that involves DNA fragmentation similar to that noted with apoptosis, or programmed cell death. In certain circumstances, secreted cytokines such as TNF-α or lymphotoxin may contribute to target cell death.

T cells expressing the γδ TCR represent a distinct set of peripheral T cells.[143, 144] Most of these cells express neither CD4 nor CD8. They represent a minor percentage of T cells in the peripheral blood (2 to 5 percent), but appear to be enriched at epithelial surfaces, including the skin, reproductive tract, respiratory system, and gastrointestinal tract.[145] In general, their capacity to recognize antigens appears to be more limited than that of αβ T cells, recognizing bacterial antigens, heat shock proteins, and MHC or MHC-related proteins.[146–148] As opposed to αβ T cells, recognition of some antigens by γδ T cells does not appear to be restricted by class I or class II MHC molecules. Functionally, γδ cells can act as cytolytic effector cells and also secrete a variety of cytokines.[149] Some γδ cells appear to mature in extrathymic sites as opposed to αβ cells that exclusively develop in the thymus.[150–152]

The function of γδ cells is not yet completely delineated. However, their capacity to respond to specific bacterial antigens as well as their tissue distribution at epithelial surfaces and their cytolytic potential have suggested that they may play a unique role as the first line of defense against invasion by certain bacterial pathogens. A potential role of γδ cells in perpetuating certain autoimmune diseases has also been suggested.[153] Thus, there are increased numbers of γδ T cells in the synovial fluid of patients with rheumatoid arthritis and other inflammatory arthritides.[154] Similarly, increased numbers of γδ T cells have been noted in the mucosal lesions of patients with Behçet's syndrome[155] and in the inflamed muscle of a patient with polymyositis.[156] Finally, a role for γδ T cells in lupus nephritis has been suggested.[157] The nature of the involvement of γδ cells in the pathogenesis of these diseases is unknown, but the presence of increased numbers of these cells at the site of inflammation suggests that they might play an important part in the autoimmune process.

EFFECTOR MOLECULES OF THE IMMUNE SYSTEM

Cytokines

Cytokines are soluble protein or glycoprotein molecules secreted by a variety of cells in response to a challenge by a foreign antigen or other stimulus. Cytokines regulate the growth, differentiation, and function of cells in an autocrine, paracrine, and endocrine manner and are primarily involved in regulating immune and inflammatory responses. Although cytokines are primarily involved in immune surveillance, they can also be responsible for tissue injury and even death that occur in response to some infections and autoimmune diseases.

Initial characterizations of cytokines were carried out using crude supernatants from stimulated peripheral blood cells, spleen cells, or cell lines. Several of the cytokines were first produced by murine cells and, subsequently, human cells were tested for similar activities. The genes for these various molecules have been cloned from the human and the mouse, and many human recombinant cytokines are now available for study or therapeutic applications. By comparing recombinant products with purified natural products, it was learned that most of the cytokines exhibited activities in more than one bioassay. Moreover, a number of the functional activities ascribed to various natural products were found to result from the action of a single recombinant cytokine (Table 7–6). Because the cytokines were thought to be primarily the products of leukocytes and to function to communicate regulatory signals to other leukocytes, the name *interleukin* was coined to simplify the categorization of these molecules.[158] Other cytokines continue to be grouped into functional families such as the interferons, growth factors, and colony-stimulating factors (CSFs).[159] Despite their original designations, many of the cytokines exhibit a number of additional activities, including the ability to regulate the growth and differentiation of lymphocytes, to regulate hematopoiesis, or to participate in promoting inflammation and destruction of infected cells or tissue. The cytokines that regulate the growth and differentiation of mature leukocytes include IL-1, IL-2, IL-4, IL-5, TNF-α, lymphotoxin, and transforming growth factor-β (TGF-β). Cytokines that promote hematopoiesis include IL-3, IL-7, granulocyte-macrophage colony-stimulating factor (GM-CSF), monocyte CSF, and granulocyte CSF. Some cytokines affect many different cell types and participate in regulating inflammatory responses. These include IL-1, IL-5, IL-6, IL-8, IFN-γ, TNF-α, and lymphotoxin. Other cytokines function to down-regulate immune responses, such as TGF-β, and IL-10. In addition, a number of other nonimmune mediators such as hormones and prostaglandins can up-regulate or dampen systemic or local development of an immune response, primarily by altering or disrupting cytokine production. T cells produce some cytokines exclusively and, along with other cells, may produce several other cytokines.

Interleukin-1. Two forms of IL-1 (IL-1α and IL-1β) have been cloned and sequenced, and their functional activities have been reassessed using recombinant products.[160–163] IL-1 is produced by a variety of cell types, including keratinocytes, Langerhans' cells, smooth muscle cells, endothelial cells, and T cells.[164, 165] However, monocytes are responsible for producing most of both the secreted and membrane-bound forms of IL-1.[159, 165–168] Although T cells recently have been reported to produce IL-1α, the mRNA for this cytokine is not detected until the fourth day after activation, indicating that IL-1α produced by T cells does not participate in the initial response but rather may promote ongoing responses.[168] By contrast, monocyte-derived IL-1α and IL-1β are more important for early augmentation of T cell activation and amplification of T cell proliferative responses.[165, 169] Both IL-1α and IL-1β bind the same receptors and have similar activities.[170, 171] IL-1 receptors are found on most cells of the body.[170–175] IL-1 receptors have been cloned from a T cell line and belong to the Ig supergene family.[176] The T cell IL-1 receptor has a higher affinity for IL-1β than IL-1α, whereas B cells express an IL-1 receptor that has the reciprocal affinities.[177] IL-1 also enhances the growth and differentiation of B cells and enhances the cytotoxic activity of NK cells and monocytes.[178–180] IL-1 facilitates the growth or protein synthesis, or both, of many other cell types, including hematopoietic cells, smooth muscle cells, endothelial cells, fibroblasts, hepatocytes, osteoblasts, and chondrocytes.[159, 164, 165, 175] IL-1 and TNF-α cause fever and induce the synthesis of acute-phase plasma proteins by the liver and also cachexia.[159, 175, 181]

Several inhibitors of IL-1 have been described. Most of the inhibitors function by competing with IL-1 for binding to the IL-1 receptor.[159, 182] IL-1 inhibitors are produced by monocytes, macrophages, neutrophils, keratinocytes, and B lymphoblastoid cell lines.[159, 182, 183] IL-1 receptor antagonist protein (IRAP) has been sequenced, cloned, and a recombinant product expressed.[182] The IRAP has about 70 percent amino acid sequence homology with both forms of IL-1 and appears to belong to the same gene family as IL-1. However, the mRNA lacks the motifs found in IL-1 and many other cytokine mRNAs that render them susceptible to rapid enzymatic degradation. IRAP binds to the IL-1 receptor but has no agonist activity; therefore, it functions as a competitive inhibitor with IL-1. It is produced by monocytes and other cell types, and its production is enhanced by GM-CSF. IRAP can inhibit the action of IL-1 in vivo as indicated by its capacity to prevent IL-1–induced hypotension and production of acute-phase proteins. The inhibitor is specific and cannot compete with other cytokines such as TNF-α. Thus, the natural IRAP may act as a negative feedback regulator of IL-1 responses. The possibility that recombinant IRAP may be useful in controlling inflammatory responses is currently being tested.

Interleukin-2. IL-2 was first named *T cell growth factor* and is produced exclusively by activated T cells.[184] IL-2 has been cloned and sequenced.[185–188] In the mouse, only some CD4+ T cell clones produce IL-2 (TH-1 cells), whereas other clones produce IL-4, IL-5, and IL-6 (TH-2 cells).[127] In the human, many freshly isolated peripheral blood T cells have the capacity to produce IL-2.[128] IL-2 appears to be the most important growth factor for human T and B cells.[184, 189, 190] Recent studies have suggested that a lack of sufficient IL-2 to drive a proliferative response may cause activated T cells to enter an anergic state and, therefore, be unable to respond to subsequent antigenic challenge (anergy).[191] Both CD4+ and CD8+ T cells can produce IL-2.[128] However, only a small subset of cells in a T cell population may produce IL-2 in response to a given stimulus, whereas many nearby cells may become activated to express high-avidity IL-2 receptors and respond to IL-2.

IL-2 receptor expression is limited to a few types of cells of hematopoietic origin as compared with receptors for many other cytokines.[192] IL-2 receptors are expressed by activated T cells, activated B cells, activated monocytes, and NK cells.[189] As is shown in Table 7–6, the receptor for IL-2 is composed of two chains, which together comprise the high-affinity receptor for IL-2.[189] The p55 chain, originally named *Tac* and now designated CD25, binds IL-2 with low avidity but does not transmit an activation signal, whereas p70 binds IL-2 with higher avidity and conveys an activation signal after being engaged. Together, the molecules form the high-avidity IL-2 receptor, with the capacity to transmit growth signals to the cells. T and B cells express both the p70 and the p55 chains of the IL-2 receptor in response to activation. NK cells express the intermediate-avidity p70 chain but do not express the low-avidity p55 chain.[193] Therefore, NK cells always require higher levels of IL-2 to proliferate than do activated T and B cells. Engagement of the IL-2 receptor on monocytes, which is up-regulated by stimulation with IFN-γ, leads to enhanced functional activation.[159, 194] Although the IL-2 receptor has been shown to be associated with several other cell surface molecules, its role in transducing the growth signal and the biochemical events initiated by receptor occupancy remains unknown. It has been suggested that signals transmitted through the IL-2 receptor may be mediated by a protein kinase activity. Recent studies indicate that the IL-2 receptor is associated with a lymphocyte tyrosine kinase (p56[lck]) that also may play an important role in T cell antigen receptor–mediated signaling.[195]

A soluble form of the p55 chain of the IL-2 receptor, probably produced by proteolytic cleavage of the membrane-bound form, is found in the serum and synovial fluid of patients with rheumatoid arthritis and other inflammatory diseases.[159, 196] Recent attempts have been made to associate the amount of circulating IL-2 receptor with disease activity.[159] Although inhibitors for IL-2 have been reported, it is doubtful that the soluble p55 form of the IL-2 receptor has the ability to compete with cell-bound high- and intermediate-avidity IL-2 receptors. It has also been suggested that antibodies to IL-2 might act as IL-2 inhibitors.

Interleukin-3. IL-3 is produced exclusively by activated T cells and is a member of the family of cytokines that stimulate the growth and differentiation of bone marrow progenitor cells called the *colony-stimulating factors*.[197–200] IL-3 promotes the growth and differentiation of almost all murine immature hematopoietic precursors.[197–200] In humans, the effects of IL-3 may be more limited, and other CSFs produced by T cells, such as GM-CSF, may be more important for maturation of bone marrow progenitor cells.[200]

Interleukin-4. IL-4 is a 14-kD growth factor that is produced by activated T cells and mast cells.[201–204] As mentioned earlier, in the mouse, IL-4 is produced by a distinct subset of CD4+ cells that also produce IL-5 and IL-6 in response to antigen stimulation.[127] In the human, IL-4 production appears to be restricted to the subpopulation of CD4+ memory T cells.[205] A wide variety of cells bear receptors for IL-4, including cells in brain and muscle.[159, 206–208] However, most of the work with IL-4 has focused on the effects of IL-4 on bone marrow–derived cells. IL-4 was first described as a growth factor for B cells and is the only factor known to date that can induce murine B cells to switch to IgE production.[208] IL-4 can also increase production of IgE from human B

Table 7–6. T CELL–DERIVED CYTOKINES

Cytokine	Other Names*	M$_r$ of Natural Protein	Amino Acids of Mature Protein	Chromosome	Receptor	Activities
IL-1α	Lymphocyte activating factor (LAF) B cell activating factor (BAF) Leukocyte endogenous mediator (LEM) Endogenous pyrogen (EP) Hemopoietin I Catabolin Mononuclear cell factor (MCF) Osteoclast activating factor (OAF) Epidermal cell derived thymocyte Activating factor (ETAF)	17,500	159	2	80 kD; single chain; type 1 receptor	Costimulates T and B cell activation and the secretion of cytokines (IL-2, IFN-γ) and antibody; increases killing by NK cells; myriad of effects on nonlymphoid cells
IL-2	T cell growth factor (TCGF)	15,000–17,000	133	4	Low affinity, CD25, IL-2Rα, p55; intermediate affinity, IL-2Rβ, p75; high affinity, p55 + p75; other associated chains: CD54; p95–105; tyrosine kinase; p35 homodimer; p22; MHC Class I; non-IL-2 binding p75	Promotes growth and differentiation of activated T and B cells; activates killer cells, macrophages
IL-3	Multipotential colony stimulating factor (Multi-CSF) Hematopoietic cell growth factor (HCGF) P-cell growth factor (PSP) Mast cell growth factor (MCGF) Erythroid colony stimulating factor (ECSF) Megakaryocyte colony stimulating factor (Meg-CSF) Eosinophil colony stimulating factor (Eo-CSF)	20,000–26,000	133	5	135 kD; single chain	Stimulates proliferation and differentiation of precursors of all hemopoietic cell lineages
IL-4	Burst-promoting activity (BPA) B cell-stimulatory factor I (BSF-1) B cell differentiation factor-γ (BCDF-γ) T cell growth factor-2 (TCGF-2) Mast cell growth factor-2 (MCGF-2)	14,000	120	5	138–145 kD; single chain	Promotes growth and differentiation of T cells, B cells; enhances tumoricidal activity of macrophages, but inhibits IL-1 and TNF-α production

Abbreviation	Synonyms	Molecular weight	No. amino acids	Receptor	Function
IL-5	B cell growth factor II (BCGF-II) T cell replacing factor (TRF) Killer helper factor (KHF) Eosinophil differentiation factor (EDF) Eosinophil-colony stimulating factor (Eo-CSF)	45,000–50,000	123	Low affinity, 60 kD; no information on high affinity form (two chains?)	Promotes growth of cytotoxic cells and differentiation of B cells
IL-6	IgA-enhancing factor (IgA-EF) Interferon-β_2 (IFN-β_2) B cell stimulatory factor-2 (BSF-2) Hepatocyte stimulatory factor II (HSF-II) Hybridoma plasmacytoma growth factor (HPGF, IL-HP1) Myeloma cell growth factor (MCGF) 26-kD protein	26,000	7	80 kD; single chain (associated gp130 possibly signal transducing chain)	Enhances IL-2 production from T cells and Ig production by B cells; myriad of effects on nonlymphoid cells
IL-10	Cytokine synthesis inhibition factor (CSIF) B cell derived T cell growth factor (B-TCGF)	18,700	1	No information	Stimulates T cell and thymocyte growth; inhibits IL-2 and IFN-γ production; inhibits macrophage cytokine production
GM-CSF	Colony stimulating factor-α Pluripoietin Colony stimulating factor 2 Neutrophil migration inhibitory factor from T cells (NIF-Δ)	22,000	5	Low affinity, 80 kD; Intermediate affinity, 120 kD; high affinity, 80 kD + 120 kD	Activates macrophages
IFN-γ	Macrophage-activating factor (MAF)	20,000	12	70–80 kD; single chain	Enhances differentiation of T and B cells; counteracts effects of IL-4; enhances killing by NK cells; activates macrophages; induces class II MHC molecules on many nonimmune cells
LT	Tumor necrosis factor-β (TNF-β)	25,000	6	60 kD homodimer; 60 kD + 80 kD	LT and TNF-α have the same activities; enhance T and B cell
TNF-α	Cachectin	17,000	6	60 kD monomers and homodimers; 60 kD + 80 kD (same as for LT)	proliferation; enhance B cell differentiation; increase killing by NK cells
TGF-β		25,000	2×112	565 kD; two chains	Inhibits T cell growth and cytokine secretion; inhibits B cell growth and differentiation; counteracts effects of IFN-γ on nonimmune cells.

*Abbreviations in parentheses.

119

cells but does not appear to be unique in this capacity.[190] IL-4 stimulates a subset of T cells to grow and promotes the generation of cytotoxic T cells.[159, 208] IL-4 up-regulates some macrophage functions while down-regulating others, and is a growth factor for murine mast cells.[159, 208]

Interleukin-5. IL-5 is a 45- to 50-kD molecule produced by a subset of T cells and mast cells.[208–210] IL-5 was originally described as a B cell growth factor and appears to facilitate B cell growth and differentiation in combination with other cytokines.[208, 211] IL-5 enhances Ig production by murine B cells and especially appears to induce enhanced production of IgA by facilitating the growth of postswitch IgA-expressing B cells.[208, 210] IL-5 promotes the generation of murine cytotoxic T cells and also the growth, differentiation, and activation of eosinophils.[210–214] Thus, in murine models, IL-5 has been shown to play an important role in limiting parasitic infection.[208] The role of IL-5 in human immune responses is much less well delineated.

Interleukin-6. IL-6 has many biologic activities and is produced by activated T cells, monocyte-macrophages, and TNF-α or IL-1–stimulated fibroblasts and endothelial cells.[159, 215–221] It is produced constitutively by monocytes, Epstein-Barr virus–transformed B cells, and some tumor cells.[159, 215–222] Receptors for IL-6 have been found on T cells, activated B cells, hematopoietic stem cells, astrocytes, hepatocytes, and fibroblasts.[222, 223] Two of the most important roles of IL-6 appear to be the ability to effect B cell differentiation and myeloma cell growth and the ability to induce acute-phase proteins. IL-6 stimulates the terminal maturation of activated B cells and induces Epstein-Barr virus–transformed B cells to produce antibody.[222] One of its earliest recognized properties was as a myeloma or hybridoma growth factor.[221] IL-6 potentiates the growth and differentiation of murine T cells and stimulates hematopoietic progenitors.[159, 215, 222] Fibroblast growth is inhibited by IL-6; however, expression of class I MHC molecules is enhanced. Importantly, IL-6 induces hepatocytes to produce some of the acute-phase plasma proteins, including haptoglobin, fibrinogen, and α_1-antitrypsin.[159, 215]

Interleukin-10. IL-10, or cytokine synthesis inhibitory factor, is a recently discovered cytokine produced by both murine and human T cells.[224–226] It is produced by a subset of murine T cells (TH-2 cells) and promotes growth of these cells.[226] IL-10 inhibits IL-2 and IFN-γ production by a distinct subset of murine T cells (TH-1), resulting in inhibition of the growth of these cells. Inhibition of TH-1 cell responses is indirect, resulting from a direct action on antigen-presenting cells that are rendered incompetent to activate TH-1, but not TH-2, cell growth. IL-10 also inhibits the production of cytokines by macrophages.

Granulocyte-Macrophage Colony-Stimulating Factor. GM-CSF is produced by activated T cells, IL-1– or TNF-α–stimulated monocytes, endothelial cells, and fibroblasts.[227] The gene for GM-CSF has been cloned and recombinant material produced.[228] It is also produced by some virally transformed cell lines. Human GM-CSF promotes the growth and differentiation of noncommitted and committed bone marrow progenitor cells.[229] For example, human GM-CSF can act on red blood cell as well as leukocyte progenitors. Thus, in the human, GM-CSF may replace the activity of IL-3, whereas in the mouse, GM-CSF has restricted activity to only the committed progenitor cells. GM-CSF also activates human and murine macrophages and increases their expression of class II MHC molecules. GM-CSF inhibits migration and enhances the activity of neutrophils as well as eosinophil-mediated leukotriene production and cytotoxicity.

Interferon-γ. The structure and sequence of the IFN-γ gene have been determined, and studies have been carried out with the recombinant protein.[230–232] IFN-γ is produced by both CD4+ and CD8+ subsets of T cells and, to a lesser extent, by NK cells.[233, 234] After stimulation of T cells, IFN-γ is produced largely by memory and not naive cells.[235] Like other IFNs, IFN-γ has antiviral and antiproliferative activities.[234] However, IFN-γ has several other important functions in an inflammatory response. IFN-γ is the most potent macrophage-activating cytokine produced by T cells.[236, 237] It enhances macrophage MHC class I and class II expression and production of reactive oxygen molecules, thereby increasing tumoricidal activity.[233, 234] IFN-γ also increases macrophage production of IL-1 and TNF-α. T cells and NK cells exposed to IFN-γ are enhanced in their capacity to differentiate into cytotoxic cells.[233, 234] IFN-γ also enhances the production of all isotypes of Ig from stimulated human B cells.[190] IFN-γ modulates the activity of many different cell types, suppressing T cell–induced up-regulation of hematopoiesis, up-regulating MHC class I expression, and inducing MHC class II expression on many of these cells.[233, 234, 238]

Tumor Necrosis Factor-α. TNF-α has been cloned and sequenced and is linked to the MHC on chromosome 6.[239–241] TNF-α has both a secreted and a membrane-bound form.[183] TNF-α is produced by activated T cells, mast cells, and macrophages[242–244]; however, monocyte-macrophages produce the majority of TNF-α. TNF-α was first described as a factor that caused hemorrhagic necrosis of solid tumors in vivo.[245] TNF-α, like IL-1, can induce a number of effects in vivo, including shock, fever, cachexia, and production of some of the acute phase–response plasma proteins.[246] TNF-α has two receptors, both with similar abilities to bind to the TNF-α molecule.[247, 248] TNF-α receptors have been found on many cell types, including activated T and B cells, macrophages, neutrophils, fibroblasts, endothelial cells, NK cells, and many other cells.[242, 245, 246] TNF-α receptor expression can be up-regulated by IFN-γ. TNF-α enhances IL-2 receptor expression but not IL-2 secretion by activated T cells and augments proliferative responses of T cells.[169, 249] TNF-α also augments proliferation and differentiation of B cells and the cytotoxic activity of NK cells. Macrophages produce IL-1 and prostaglandins in response to TNF-α. TNF-α is chemotactic for neutrophils and is a more potent activator of neutrophils than IFN-γ. Endothelial cell MHC class I molecules, cytokines, and adhesion molecules that are important for cell trafficking into tissues are also up-regulated by TNF-α, as well as by IL-1.

The TNF-α receptor is cleaved from activated cells and may act as an important inhibitor of TNF-α activity in vivo.[183, 250] In contrast to the IL-2 receptor, the TNF-α receptor can compete with the cell-bound TNF-α receptor and thus acts as an inhibitor of TNF-α activity. Although TNF-α shares many activities with IL-1, the soluble TNF-α receptor does not compete with IL-1 receptors and therefore does not alter the action of IL-1.[183]

Lymphotoxin. Lymphotoxin is a 25-kD molecule whose gene is found next to TNF-α on chromosome 6. Because of its structural similarity to TNF-α, it has been designated *TNF-β*.[159, 251] Lymphotoxin is produced by activated T cells and B lymphoblastoid cell lines.[252, 253] Lymphotoxin has about 30 percent homology with TNF-α but binds to the same receptors and therefore shares many of the same activities.[251, 254] Lymphotoxin is produced in soluble form, and the amounts produced by activated T cells are much less than the amounts of TNF-α produced by activated monocytes. Many of the effects of lymphotoxin and TNF-α can be further enhanced by IFN-γ.

Transforming Growth Factor-β. TGF-β is a potentially important negative regulator of immune and inflammatory responses.[255, 256] TGF-β is produced by activated T cells and macrophages, platelets, osteocytes, synovial fibroblasts, and almost all cultured cell lines.[159, 183] Although T cells and macrophages produce an active form of TGF-β, most cells produce an inactive form that must be activated by proteases. TGF-β was first described as a growth factor that induced anchorage-independent growth typical of malignant cells. Although TGF-β indirectly promotes the growth of fibroblasts, it inhibits the growth of many other cells, including B cells, T cells, and endothelial cells. TGF-β also inhibits the differentiation of T cells and B cells.[190] However, in the mouse, TGF-β has been shown to induce B cells to produce IgA.[190] TGF-β is chemotactic for macrophages and may induce IL-1 production in some circumstances, but it inhibits macrophage activation and neutrophil function under other conditions. TGF-β antagonizes IFN-γ–induced class II MHC molecule expression and inhibits the production of a variety of cytokines, including IL-2.[183]

Cytokine Regulation. Most T cell–derived cytokines are secreted only after T cells have been stimulated via a TCR-specific mechanism. Monocytes and other cells will secrete cytokines in response to microbial products or other cytokines. There are several features of cytokines that contribute to the complexity of an immune response. For example, the same stimulus may induce different cytokines from T cells, depending on the state of differentiation of the T cells. Thus, when T cells are activated with monoclonal antibodies to the TCR-CD3 complex or potent mitogens, human memory T cells produce more IFN-γ and IL-4 than naive T cells, and murine TH-1 cells secrete IL-2, lymphotoxin, and IFN-γ, whereas TH-2 cells secrete IL-4, IL-5, IL-6, and IL-10.[127, 235] Moreover, the presence of additional cytokines or other immunomodulatory molecules also influence cytokine production. For example, monocyte-derived IL-1 augments T cell IL-2 production.[179] However, IL-1 can also induce monocytes to produce prostaglandins that have been shown to inhibit both IL-1 and IL-2 production.[159, 179] By contrast, prostaglandins have no effect on IL-4 production and have been reported to enhance IL-5 and GM-CSF production.[257, 258]

Several other general principles appear to apply to understanding most cytokines. Cytokine production is highly regulated and self-limited. The production of each cytokine is under the control of several regulatory elements in the 5′ promoter region of the gene. These elements bind specific proteins that either up- or down-regulate transcription of the gene. For example, glucocorticoid response elements have been identified in the 5′ promoter region of several cytokine genes.[222] The immunosuppressive agents cyclosporin A and FK-506 prevent IL-2, IL-3, IL-4, and GM-CSF production by interacting with distinct cytosolic proteins (cyclophilin and FK-binding protein, respectively, each of which is a *cis-trans* prolyl isomerase) and subsequently regulating gene transcription.[259] Even after stimulation, cytokine gene transcription is tightly regulated and is usually limited to a brief period. Moreover, the mRNA produced is usually very unstable. For example, the half-life of IL-2 mRNA is approximately 30 minutes.[260] Once the cytokines are secreted, they usually have a short half-life in vivo. The activity of each cytokine is determined by the presence of specific receptors on the responding cells. There is little or no cross-reactivity of cytokines such that each cytokine is recognized by its specific receptor. For example, although IL-1 and TNF-α have many similar activities, the receptors for each cytokine are specific and cells bearing only IL-1 receptors will not respond to TNF-α and vice versa. In general, activated cells bear increased numbers of cytokine receptors and different cytokines may up- or down-regulate their own or each other's receptors.[159, 175, 177, 190] In addition, different cytokines may affect the same cell in similar ways. For example, several cytokines, such as IL-4, IL-6, and IFN-γ, can all promote B cell growth.[190] Alternatively, the same cytokine may affect different cells in different ways, although the intracellular signaling is induced through the same receptor. Thus, IL-1 promotes the growth of many cells, including lymphocytes and fibroblasts, but is cytotoxic for other cells such as β cells of the human pancreatic islets and thyrocytes.[165] Finally, there are probably other T cell cytokines that have yet to be identified, cloned, and tested for function.

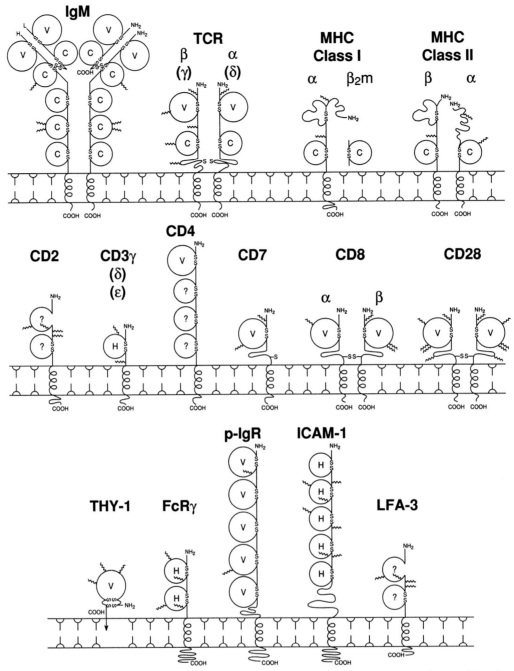

Figure 7–3. Cell membrane members of the immunoglobulin supergene family involved in the regulation of lymphocyte function. (Modified from Hunkapillar, T., and Hood, L.: Diversity of the immunoglobulin gene superfamily. Adv. Immunol. 44:1, 1989. Used by permission.)

Immunoglobulin

Antibody molecules were the first members of the Ig supergene family described[261] and now often serve as prototypes in discussing molecules of this multigene family (Fig. 7–3). The Ig supergene family includes not only many different molecules of immunologic importance but also many other molecules, especially of the nervous system. Characteristically, these proteins share amino acid sequence

homology encompassing a fundamental structure, the Ig "domain," which is duplicated in various forms that provide the basic subunits to generate a variety of large macromolecules. The Ig domain is a compact, globular structure made up of seven antiparallel β-pleated sheets ("immunoglobulin fold" or "β-barrel").[262] In most members of the Ig supergene family, each domain is encoded by a separate exon. In general, there is a single intrachain disulfide bond per domain.

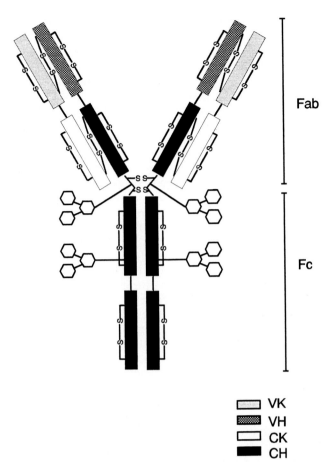

Figure 7–4. Schematic representation of a prototypic immunoglobin monomer. Individual Ig domains (intrachain disulfide bonded) are represented by rectangles. Interchain disulfide bonds (between heavy and light and between the two heavy chains) have also been demonstrated. Carbohydrate moieties are depicted attached in C_H2 and C_H3, although carbohydrate can be found attached at other locations.

Figure 7–4 depicts a prototypic Ig molecule.[263] Ig molecules consist of two identical heavy chains disulfide bonded to two identical light chains. In general, heavy chains contain four domains—a variable domain, encoded by the variable region exon that is derived by bringing together three separate genetic elements during ontogeny, the V_H or variable segment, the D_H or diversity segment, and the J_H or joining region; and three constant region domains C_H1, C_H2, and C_H3. Light chains (either κ or λ) have two domains, variable (V_κ or V_λ) and constant (C_κ or C_λ). Each domain is approximately 110 amino acids.[264]

In the complete antibody molecule, the two light chains pair with the variable and C_H1 domains of the two heavy chains, whereas the C_H2 and C_H3 domains pair with each other. Early studies using various proteolytic enzymes demonstrated that Ig monomers could be cleaved into two functional units, termed *Fab* and *Fc*, for fraction antigen binding and fraction crystallizable, respectively.[265] It is now known that the Fab consists of V_L and C_L paired with V_H and C_H1, whereas the Fc is comprised of dimers of C_H2

and C_H3. There is an interchain disulfide bond between each C_L and C_H1 domain. The Fc portion of the molecule is the site of all known effector functions, whereas the Fab gives an antibody molecule its capacity to recognize a specific antigen. Because Igs have two Fab fragments per Fc, each antibody molecule can bind two identical antigenic moieties simultaneously and, thus, are bivalent.

Crystal structures of antigen-specific antibody molecules demonstrate that the portions of the molecule that are involved in antigen recognition are the loops between the β-pleated sheets.[266] By analyzing sequence data from a large number of expressed and germline V regions, it is clear that these portions of the molecule are more variable than the parts that encode the β-pleated sheets.[267] There are three of these regions in both Ig heavy and light chains, and they have been termed the *hypervariable regions* or *complementarity-determining regions* (CDR1 to 3). The third hypervariable region of both heavy and light chains is encoded by the portion of the variable region exon that is generated by V(D)J joining. Generally, the most variable portion of any of the immune receptor molecules is the CDR3, and variations in this region often engender different antigenic specificities.

In the heavy chain, there is an additional exon between the exons encoding C_H1 and C_H2, which encodes the hinge region. This relatively short protein sequence connects the two Fab fragments to the Fc portion of the molecule and allows for considerable flexibility between the antigen-binding part of the molecule and the effector region.[264] The IgM and IgE constant regions do not have hinge regions but, instead, have four constant domains (C_H1 to 4). The IgG3 hinge region is much longer than the hinge regions of the other isotypes, giving the IgG3 molecule added flexibility. Interchain disulfide bonds between the two heavy chains are located in the hinge region. Both N-linked and O-linked carbohydrate groups are found in antibody molecules, primarily modifying the heavy chain, although the position and type are variable among different Ig heavy chain isotypes.

Certain constant region isotypes allow for the formation of Ig multimers. Specifically, secreted IgM generally occurs as a pentamer, whereas secreted IgA is usually a dimer. In both instances, an accessory molecule, the J (for joining) chain, is involved in multimer formation.[268] The J chain, which is synthesized by IgM- and IgA-secreting B cells, is not a member of the Ig supergene family. Obviously, multimeric Ig molecules have higher valences than their monomeric counterparts. Another accessory molecule that is secreted by epithelial cells, secretory component, now known as the *poly-Ig receptor* and also a member of the Ig supergene family, associates with IgA and facilitates transport of IgA across epithelial cells.[269]

Ig molecules all have numerous effector functions, and the capacity of each heavy chain isotype

Legend (from figure):
- □ VK
- ▨ VH
- □ CK
- ■ CH

for each effector function is quite different.[264] IgM is the isotype produced in primary immune responses. As a surface receptor, monomeric IgM is an important signaling molecule. Even though IgM antibodies have often not proceeded through affinity maturation via the process of antigen selection, because of the pentameric nature of the molecule, antigen-antibody complexes can be formed with high avidity. Furthermore, IgM is a potent activator of complement. IgG antibodies are the predominant antibodies formed in secondary immune responses and are important in a multiplicity of different functions, including phagocytosis and antibody-dependent cellular cytotoxicity. These functions are mediated in an antigen-specific manner by a variety of different cells such as macrophages, mast cells, or polymorphonuclear leukocytes, which specifically bind secreted IgG via a series of Fc receptors. IgA is found predominantly in mucosal secretions, including tears, saliva, nasal mucus, or milk. Finally, IgE is the primary defense against parasitic infections. Dysregulation of IgE synthesis results in allergic disease. Table 7–7 summarizes the characteristics of the different heavy chain isotypes.

ANTIGEN-SPECIFIC RECOGNITION: THE ORIGIN OF DIVERSITY

The efficiency with which higher organisms can defend themselves from pathogens is, in large part, a consequence of the ability to generate an enormous variety of antigen receptor molecules.

B Lymphocytes

It has been estimated that the number of different antibody molecules in an individual at any given time is approximately 10^7. The origin of such enormous antibody diversity was not understood for decades because it was thought that each protein was encoded by a separate gene. Because it was known that the approximate total number of genes in the human genome is only about 10^6, this represented a puzzle. The mechanism by which this enormous diversity is generated from a limited number of genes has now been delineated. The genes of the immune receptor molecules are not encoded within the germline as functional genes but rather as gene segments that have to be juxtaposed by a somatic recombination event to create a functional gene. Thus, different combinations of germline gene segments can generate many different antigen receptors from a limited amount of germline information.[270, 271] Furthermore, because imprecisions exist in the recombination process, significant additional differences can be generated at the sites at which the genetic elements are rejoined. This results in the generation of antigen receptor molecules that can differ in their antigen specificity even though they derive from the same germline information. Whereas recombination generates antigen receptor diversity in both TCRs and Ig, B cells also generate their effector function diversity via an additional somatic recombination event called *switch recombination*, in which the same set of genes encoding antigen binding is used to encode antibody molecules of different heavy chain classes and, therefore, different functional activities.[272]

There are seven immune receptor loci: TCR-α, -β, -γ, and -δ, and Ig heavy chain, κ, and λ. T cells express TCRs for antigen composed of either αβ heterodimers or γδ heterodimers in conjunction with the CD3 complex.[273, 274] B cells express Ig heterodimers consisting of a heavy chain and a light chain. These molecules are expressed in association with a complex of nonpolymorphic proteins that appear to play analogous roles to CD3 in T cells.[275] Ig not only serves as the B cell antigen receptor (membrane-bound Ig) but also is itself an immune mediator as a

Table 7–7. PROPERTIES OF HUMAN IG CLASSES

Property	IgG	IgA	IgM	IgD	IgE
Molecular form (usual)	Monomer	Monomer, dimer	Pentamer	Monomer	Monomer
Subclasses	IgG1, IgG2, IgG3, IgG4	IgA1, IgA2	–	–	–
Molecular weight	150,000	160,000	950,000	175,000	190,000
Serum level, approximate (mg/ 100 ml, adult)	1250	210	125	4	0.03
Half-life (days)	23	5.8	5.1	2.8	2.5
Valence	2	2	5 or 10	?	?
Complement fixation classic	+ (IgG1/IgG2/ IgG3)	–	+	—	—
Alternative	+ (IgG4)	+ (IgA1/IgA2)	—	+	—
Binding to cells	Macrophages; neutrophils	—	—	—	Mast cells
Biologic properties	Secondary response; placental transfer	Secretions	Primary response	Surface molecule	Anaphylaxis; allergy

secreted form. There are nine Ig heavy chain isotypes (IgM, IgD, IgG1 to 4, IgA1 and 2, and IgE), all encoded at the IgH locus on chromosome 14, and two light chain isotypes (κ and λ) encoded at distinct loci on chromosome 2 and 22, respectively. The TCRs are encoded by separate genes on chromosome 14 (α, δ), and 7 (β, γ), with the δ locus residing within the α-chain locus.

In general, the organization of the immune receptor loci is analogous. At the IgH, TCR-β, and TCR-δ, the general order of the gene segments is V (for variable), D (for diversity), and J (for joining), although there are exceptions. The Igκ, Igλ, TCR-α, and TCR-γ are similar, except there are no D segments. In B and T cells, somatic recombination events juxtapose two or three gene segments (V, + or − D, and J) to create a functional gene that generates a single exon encoding the "variable" region of the mature immune receptor molecule. This rearrangement is illustrated in Figure 7–5. The functional variable region exon is expressed in conjunction with downstream exons that encode the nonvariable or "constant" region of the immune receptor molecule. A schematic representation of the gene organization at each locus is depicted in Figure 7–6. For the purpose of describing V(D)J recombination, the IgH locus will be used as an example. Analogous events occur during recombination of the light chain and TCR loci.

There are about 150 different V_H gene segments, 30 different D_H gene segments, and 6 different J_H gene segments. Because any J_H gene segment can recombine with any of the D_H gene segments, which in turn can rearrange with any of the V_H gene segments, the number of possible VDJ combinations to generate a heavy chain variable region exon is about 200 × 30 × 6, or 36,000. In addition, it is thought that any heavy chain can pair with any light chain (κ or λ), which are also derived by somatic recombination of distinct gene segments. Even though random combination of gene segments has an enormous capacity for the derivation of a very large number of unique receptor molecules, in some situations, utilization of different gene segments is not completely random. For example, certain V_H, D_H, and J_H gene segments are overexpressed in fetal B cells.[276] The reason for this bias is not currently understood. Although there is clearly some bias of gene segment use in certain situations, the potential for generating adequate diversity is probably not compromised.

Additional diversity is generated during DNA rearrangement because the recombination event is not precise in that there is deletion or addition of non–germline-encoded nucleotides at the joining sites of recombination. The portion of the antibody molecule that is encoded by the nucleotides in the region where the gene segments (V_H-D_H-J_H) are joined is often crucial for binding antigen. Thus, variations in the recombination joints can produce antibodies that recognize different antigens. There-

fore, antibodies that are reactive to different antigens can be derived from identical genetic information, a result of the addition or deletion of non–germline-encoded nucleotides that occurs during recombination. This explains how the immune system can generate antibodies to virtually any antigen using only a limited amount of genetic information.

The DNA elements involved in the rearrangement process have been well characterized.[277] Immune receptor genes have palindromic heptamer and A/C or T/G rich nonamer sequences immediately adjacent to their coding sequences (Fig. 7–7). The heptamer is separated from the nonamer by a non-conserved spacer of either 12 (±1) or 23 (±1) base pairs, approximately one or two turns of the DNA helix. This highly conserved sequence motif is found flanking the rearranging elements in the immune receptor genes of all species that have been studied. These sequences are evidently the binding or recognition sites, or both, of the enzyme or enzymes involved in the rearrangement process.

At each receptor locus, the organization of the genes is such that a recombination signal sequence with a 12–base-pair spacer rearranges to a recombination signal sequence with a 23–base-pair spacer (Fig. 7–7). At the Ig heavy chain locus, variable region gene segments (the most 5' gene segments) have signal sequences with 23–base-pair spacers immediately 3' of their coding sequences. D_H segments are flanked by signal sequences with 12–base-pair spacers, and J_H segments have signal sequences with 23–base-pair spacers 5' of their coding sequences. Thus, V_H-D_H (23-12) and D_H-J_H (12-23) recombinations are allowed, whereas V_H-J_H (23-23) and D_H-D_H (12-12) are precluded. This 12/23 base-pair recombination rule has been maintained at all seven of the immune receptor loci (IgH, Igκ, Igλ, TCR-α, TCR-β, TCR-γ, TCR-δ), although less common rearrangements (for example, D_H-D_H rearrangements) that violate the 12/23 rule do occur, but at a lower frequency.[278] Even these less common rearrangements can contribute to the generation of additional diversity. Considerable experimental data have demonstrated that the heptamer element is the most important of the two sequence motifs in that much more sequence variability is tolerated in the nonamer than in the heptamer motif.[279] In fact, authentic V-D-J recombination events can be mediated by the heptamer motif alone, although recombination is much more efficient if both the heptamer and nonamer are present.

The recombination reaction involves two double-stranded DNA cuts and subsequent religations (Fig. 7–7). This results in the formation of two new DNA joints: coding joints, which contain the coding information, and reciprocal joints, which contain the two recombination signal sequences. The DNA between the two rearranging gene segments can be either deleted from the chromosome or inverted, and thus maintained on the chromosome but in opposite orientation (see Fig. 7–5).[280] In vivo, the relative transcriptional orientation of the two rearranging genes

1. Germline Configuration

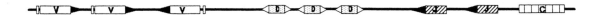

2. D-J Rearrangement (Deletion)

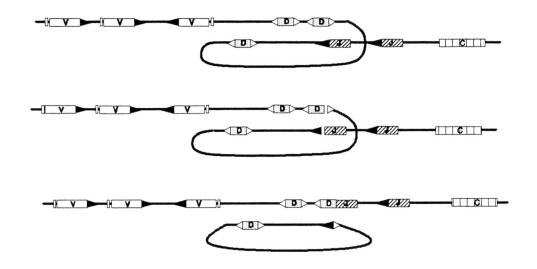

3. V-DJ Rearrangement (Inversion)

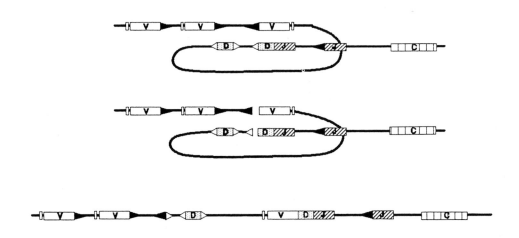

4. Transcription and processing

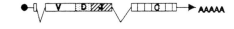

Figure 7–5. Schematic representation of V-D-J rearrangement. In this example, so that both direct and inverted rearrangements could be demonstrated, D-J rearrangement is demonstrated as deletional rearrangement, whereas V-DJ rearrangement is via inversion. Whether or not rearrangement occurs by either of these mechanisms is entirely dependent on the relative transcriptional orientation of the two rearranging gene segments. The constant region in this example is depicted as a single exon, although in most situations the constant regions of the immune receptor molecules are encoded by multiple exons.

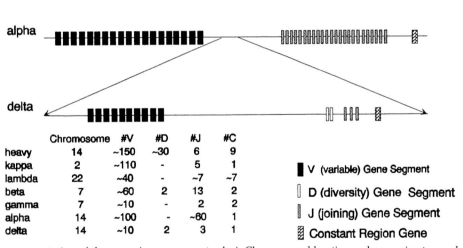

Figure 7–6. Schematic representation of the seven immune receptor loci. Chromosomal location and approximate number of each type of gene segment are listed below.

dictates whether rearrangement is by deletion or inversion. If the two rearranging gene segments are in the same transcriptional orientation, rearrangement is via deletion; if the two gene segments involved are in opposite transcriptional orientation, the intervening DNA is inverted on the chromosome. If rearrangement is by deletion, the reciprocal joint is deleted from the chromosome on a closed circular DNA by-product. If rearrangement is via inversion, the reciprocal joint remains on the chromosome. The relative efficiencies of direct and inverted rearrangement are essentially equivalent.

Reciprocal joints are generally precise in that the heptamer sequences from each gene segment are joined exactly, head to head, without addition or deletion of any nucleotides, although additional nucleotides are occasionally observed. Deletion of nucleotides from reciprocal joints is extremely rare. In contrast, joining of the coding sequences is remarkably variable.[281] Significant deletions (up to 12 nucleotides or more) of the coding region sequences can occur before coding sequence ligation. This results in a shortened third hypervariable region. The presumed mechanism, which allows for "nibbling"

VDJ Recombination Reaction

CLEAVAGE

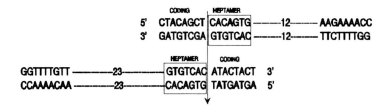

SIGNAL JOINT LIGATION

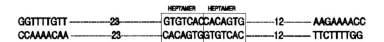

CODING JOINT MODIFICATION AND LIGATION

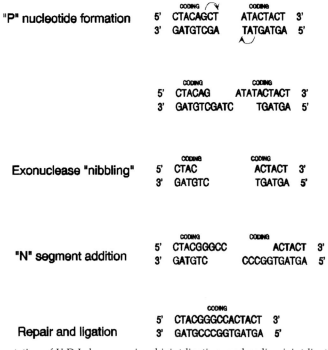

Figure 7–7. Schematic representation of V-D-J cleavage, signal joint ligation, and coding joint ligation reactions.

of coding sequences, is illustrated in Figure 7–7. First, a double-stranded cleavage occurs exactly at the coding sequence–heptamer juncture. The two heptamer sequences are ligated without modification. Subsequently, the last two nucleotides of the 5' end of each DNA strand in the coding segments are cleaved and then ligated to the opposite DNA strand, generating a short overhang that is palindromic to the last two nucleotides (termed P for palindrome nucleotides).[282] This provides a suitable template for exonuclease activity. Usually, nucleotides are cleaved from one or both coding strand ends. Occasionally, no nibbling occurs and the overhang is converted to double-stranded DNA, presumably by a DNA polymerase, and the two coding strands ligated, thus maintaining the P nucleotides in the variable region exon.

An additional coding joint modification process that significantly contributes to junctional diversity is mediated by the enzyme terminal deoxynucleotidyltransferase (TdT).[281] This enzyme is expressed in both T and B cells at the time immune receptor rearrangement is occurring. In many rearrangements, apparently random nucleotides are added at the site of V-D, D-J, and V-J joining. These have been termed N segments and are often GC rich, a reflection of the preference of TdT for certain nucleotides as substrate.

Expression of TdT is not uniform in all lymphocytes undergoing immune receptor rearrangements. Because expression of TdT in developing B cells diminishes drastically from the time of heavy chain rearrangement to the time of light chain rearrangement (see later), κ- and λ-chains, unlike the other immune receptor molecules, generally lack N segments.[267] Recent data demonstrate that TdT is also differentially regulated during development. This results in a relative lack of N segment additions in fetal Ig molecules and TCRs, limiting to some extent the early fetal repertoire.[283]

The rearrangement process itself is an ordered one, in which different receptor genes are rearranged in a defined sequence during lymphocyte development.[274] In B cells, first D_H to J_H rearrangements occur, usually on both alleles, followed by V_H to D_H-J_H rearrangements. V_H to D_H-J_H rearrangements continue until a functional product is generated on one allele. If nonfunctional V_H-D_H-J_H rearrangements are generated on both alleles, either the B cell dies, or, in some situations, a less common rearrangement (V_H region replacement) occurs.[284] V_H region replacement can occur even when there have been two aberrant V_H-D_H-J_H rearrangements, and there are no D_H segment recombination-signal sequences retained. This is because there is a heptamer sequence at the 3' end of the coding sequence in virtually all Ig V_H gene segments. Thus, upstream V_H regions can rearrange into the aberrant rearrangement at the V_H-D_H junction. Because a nonamer sequence is lacking, this type of rearrangement is less efficient than typical joining that follows the 12/23 rule.

Once a functional variable region exon is generated, μ-chain is expressed. Experimental evidence indicates that the presence of μ-chain signals both termination of rearrangement at the heavy chain locus and initiation of κ rearrangement. Recently, proteins that resemble Ig light chains (V pre-B, $\lambda 5$), but that do not undergo somatic recombination, have been discovered. These "surrogate" light chains pair with the membrane but not the secreted form of μ-chain and are expressed on the surface of pre-B cells before κ and λ rearrangement.[285]

If initial κ rearrangement on both alleles fails to result in a functional light chain exon, rearrangment can continue at both κ alleles by V_κ genes rearranging to other more downstream J_κ gene segments. Alternatively, much of the κ locus can be deleted by rearrangement to a heptamer sequence, termed the κ-deleting element, found 24 kilobases (kb) downstream of the C_κ gene.[286] In most, but not all situations, rearrangement at the λ locus begins only after C_κ is deleted. As is the case with μ-chain, expression of a functional light chain signals termination of light chain rearrangement. This provides the mechanism of allelic exclusion that dictates expression of only a single Ig molecule from any one B cell. Little is known about the precise molecular mechanism that allows for the ordered rearrangement process of D_H to J_H, followed by V_H to D_H-J_H, and finally, light chain rearrangement.

In recent years, an accessibility model for rearrangement has been proposed.[287] This model is largely based on the observation that transcription of unrearranged genes (germline transcription) often precedes rearrangement. In this model, B cell–specific factors are proposed to act on the promoters of specific variable regions, resulting in transcription of these unrearranged genes. Chromatin is in an "open" configuration during transcription. The "openness" of the chromatin may also allow the recombinase enzymes access to their substrates and, therefore, explain the correlation between transcription and recombination. Alternatively, the actual transcription process, or even the germline transcripts themselves, may have some role in recombination. The factors that initiate germline-variable region transcription by either T cells or B cells are only beginning to be understood.

B cells, but not T cells, have an additional mechanism to generate diversity. Somatic mutation allows for the generation of very high affinity antigen recognition. There is a large body of experimental evidence demonstrating hypermutation of expressed Ig genes during the maturation of an antibody response.[288] Although mutations appear to occur randomly, B cells expressing mutated antibodies, which have a higher antigen-binding avidity, are selectively expanded by a process that appears to be mediated by T cells or T cell factors (antigen selection). B cells expressing higher-avidity surface Ig antigen receptors may capture antigen more efficiently and thereby serve as more effective antigen-presenting cells to helper T cells, thus focusing the immune response and resulting in the preferential expansion of B cells with higher-avidity receptors. In secondary and tertiary responses, antigen-specific antibodies will have a high incidence of somatic mutations, with a higher than random rate of changes in coding, rather than silent nucleotides. Moreover, these mutations will be most apparent in the portion of the molecule that is directly involved in antigen binding, the CDRs. The estimated rate of somatic hypermutation in B cells is approximately 10^{-3} per base pair per cell division.

The molecular mechanism of hypermutation is still obscure.

Although the process of rearrangement has been intensely studied for the last decade, relatively little is known about the enzymes or recombinases that mediate V-D-J rearrangement. Recently, two highly conserved genes were isolated, recombinase activating genes-1 and -2 (RAG-1 and -2), which are encoded within the same genetic locus.[289] When these genes are transfected into fibroblasts, recombination of extrachromosomal recombination substrates occurs. Expression of these genes is, in general, coincident with expression of V-D-J recombinase activity. There is currently no biochemical information about the nature of the proteins encoded by these two genes or their potential enzymatic activity. However, deletion of RAG-1 or RAG-2 prevents the development of B cells and T cells.[289a, 289b] The possibility that other factors, ubiquitously expressed or activated by these genes, are necessary for recombination has not been ruled out.

In summary, unique T and B cell antigen receptors are generated by several mechanisms: (1) selection of particular V, D, and J segments to form a complete antigen combining site; (2) junctional diversity generated at the joints of V-D-J or V-J rearrangement; (3) the addition of nucleotides at the junctions of rearranged gene segments (N segments); (4) pairing of heavy, β-, or δ-chains with κ or λ-, α-, or γ-chains to form heterodimeric molecules; and (5) somatic hypermutation of rearranged gene segments in B cells. These various processes generate an enormous number of immune receptors that give the organism the potential to respond to an almost limitless number of encountered antigens. It is important to note that, except for somatic hypermutation, each of these events is intrinsically controlled and regulated and occurs in the absence of antigenic exposure.

Expression of the immune receptor genes is regulated at two levels. First, because productive rearrangement of these genes is limited to the appropriate cell lineage, this represents a major mechanism for regulation of gene expression. In addition, numerous cis and trans acting elements exist that regulate the tissue-specific expression of the immune receptor genes. In the last decade, numerous laboratories have focused extensively on the regulation of Ig gene expression. As a result, the regulation of B cell antigen receptors is much better understood than is that of the T cell antigen receptor and will be presented as an example here.[290–292]

After gene rearrangement, regulation of expression could occur at multiple different steps, including mRNA stability and translational effects, but the rate-limiting step in Ig production is at the level of transcription. There are two major DNA regulatory sequence elements that are responsible: the promoter elements found 5' of all Ig V regions, and the enhancer elements found between the J and the constant region genes. V-D-J rearrangement brings these two sequence elements into proximity with each other, which appears to facilitate Ig expression. Because the promoter elements of unrearranged V elements are not in close proximity to the enhancer elements, unrearranged V regions are generally not transcribed, although just before rearrangement, unrearranged V regions are sometimes transcribed.

The two most well-characterized sequence motifs of the Ig promoters are the TATA box and the octamer motif. TATA boxes are found in most eukaryotic promoters, whereas the octamer motif is more specific, although not completely unique, to Ig promoters. The octamer motifs of V_H and V_κ promoters are in opposite orientations. It has been demonstrated that the octamer motif is essential for B cell–specific expression of Ig as well as for optimal levels of Ig gene transcription.[293]

Ig enhancer regions are DNA sequences composed of numerous different sequence motifs that affect transcription of the Ig genes. These regions are very complex and are only now beginning to be understood. Both the IgH and κ enhancers have relatively well-characterized sequence motifs termed *E boxes*. In addition, the IgH enhancer includes an octamer motif, whereas the κ enhancer has a binding site termed *NFκB* (for nuclear factor, κ binding). Gene transcription is regulated by two *trans*-acting factors that bind to the octamer site, octamer transcription factors-1 and -2, as well as the *trans*-acting element, NFκB.[294–296] Regulation of Ig gene transcription is extremely complex, involving not only these elements but also numerous other DNA binding sites in both the promoters and enhancers of the Ig genes and *trans*-acting factors that interact with these sequences.

Transcription of fully rearranged Ig genes initiates upstream of the promoter regions, proceeds through the leader exon, the VDJ exon, through the downstream unrearranged J regions and enhancer element, and finally through the constant region exons. Generation of a mature transcript is accomplished via mRNA splicing (shown schematically in Fig. 7–5). In the case of Ig molecules, either secreted or membrane-bound forms of the mRNA can be generated by differential use of polyadenylation signals and splicing, as discussed later.

Ig switch recombination is the molecular mechanism by which functional diversity is generated. Class switching provides a mode for a variety of different biologic functions to be associated with any particular set of rearranged Ig variable regions ($V_\lambda J_\lambda$ or $V_\kappa J_\kappa$ and $V_H D_H J_H$). It is now known that the class switch involves the molecular association of a $V_H D_H J_H$ rearrangement with one of the different Ig constant region genes.

The human Ig constant region locus is composed of nine functional and two nonfunctional constant region genes. The μ and δ genes are the most J_H proximal constant regions, whereas the remaining genes are located on two duplication units (Cγ-Cγ-Cϵ-Cα) centromeric of Cμ. The ϵ gene in the more Cμ proximal unit is a pseudogene, and the two units are separated by an additional γ pseudogene. Thus, the organization of the locus is as follows: Cμ-Cδ-Cγ3-Cγ1-ψCε-Cα1-ψCγ-Cγ2-Cγ4-Cε-Cα2.

The ability of a single $V_H D_H J_H$ to be expressed with different C regions is accomplished predominantly via a DNA recombination between tandemly repeated sequences (termed *switch regions*) located 5′ of each C_H gene (except Cδ). The result of this somatic recombination event is that downstream constant regions are juxtaposed in the same relative position that the μ constant region occupies in germline configuration. This recombination is illustrated in Figure 7–8. For example, when a B cell switches from IgM to IgG production, the following events transpire: (1) a double-stranded DNA break occurs in the Cμ switch region; (2) a second break occurs in the Cγ switch region; and (3) the J_H proximal portion of Sμ and the J_H distal portion of Sγ are ligated. Thus, the original $V_H D_H J_H$ is juxtaposed to the Cγ1 gene. Recently, it has been demonstrated that the intervening DNA is also ligated as a closed circular DNA byproduct and presumably is not replicated in future cell generations.[297]

The genomic structures of the nine human Ig constant region genes are analogous. The IgG, IgD, and IgA constant regions have three constant region exons (C_H1 to 3) that encode Ig domains and a hinge exon, whereas IgE and IgM have four constant region exons that encode Ig domains (C_H1 to 4). Each isotype can be expressed as either a membrane or secreted form.[298] There are generally two additional exons downstream of C_H3 (or C_H4 for μ and ε) that encode a short transmembrane segment (usually 26 amino acids) and a cytoplasmic tail that is variable in length, depending on the isotype. The secreted or membrane form of each mRNA can be differentially expressed by utilizing one of two cleavage-polyadenylation sites, one before the transmembrane exon, or one after the cytoplasmic exon. Resting B cells express more of the membrane form of the mRNA, whereas activation and differentiation generally result in expression of more of the secreted form of the mRNA.

Unlike the other constant region genes, the δ constant region lacks a switch region. IgD and IgM are coexpressed in developing B cells via cotranscription of a single long transcript beginning 5′ of the variable exon and continuing through the δ membrane exon.[299] There is some suggestion that long transcripts may mediate expression of other downstream isotypes, but this is probably a minor mechanism.

Whereas VDJ recombination is directed by recombination signal sequences (heptamer-nonamer) that are rigidly conserved, the specific DNA sequences that direct switch recombination are very large (up to 10 kb) and are characterized by short tandem repeats that are not strictly conserved.[300] Although the human switch regions have not been completely characterized, from the data available it is clear that they are composed of pentameric sequences similar to those found in murine switch regions.

These pentameric sequence motifs have some homology to CHI sequences in prokaryotes.[300] CHI sequences are short-sequence motifs that stimulate genetic recombination in bacteria in vivo but are not essential for recombination. The name CHI derives from the fact that the DNA structure generated during recombination resembles the Greek letter chi (X). Unlike VDJ recombination, it is clear that during switch recombination, the double-stranded breaks are not always within or adjacent to a particular sequence motif.[301] The breakpoints in switch recombination seem more akin to what is observed in homologous recombination in prokaryotes. For these reasons, it was proposed that Ig switch recombination might be an accelerated example of genetic recombination, that is, homologous recombination events might occur between switch sequences. In this model, the B cells that express downstream isotypes because of these fortuitous recombinations would be selected because of an advantage conveyed by expression of the downstream isotype. Experimental results, however, have suggested an alternative explanation.

It has been demonstrated that antibody responses to various antigens are tailored in response to the eliciting antigen.[302] For example, the responses to polysaccharide antigens are generally IgG2 in humans and IgG3 in mice, whereas the response to parasitic antigens are generally IgE antibodies. Furthermore, this bias during immune responses to particular types of antigens for particular constant region utilization appears to be independent of the particular $V_H D_H J_H$ rearrangement employed. These and analogous observations suggest that isotype expression is precisely regulated and not random during immune responses. More recent experimental evidence demonstrates that switch recombination is in fact a directed and regulated process and not a stochastic or random one.

It has been proposed that switch specificity is accomplished by controlling the ability of the recombinase to interact with specific switch regions. The "accessibility" of the gene segments may be regulated by transcription factors. Thus, as with VDJ rearrangement, switch recombination is preceded by germline transcription of the gene segments involved.[303]

In recent years, the validity of the accessibility model has been supported by a large body of data, primarily, but not entirely, from murine systems, demonstrating germline transcription of unrearranged constant region genes in response to various stimuli. For example, in murine B lymphocytes, IL-4 induces germline transcription of both Cγ1 and Cε, whereas treatment with lipopolysaccharide (LPS) induces transcription of Cγ2b and Cγ3. These germline transcripts initiate 5′ of the various switch regions, continue through the constant region exons, and are spliced to generate both membrane and secreted

1. Configuration prior to class switching.

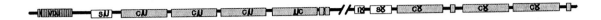

2. Transcription of downstream constant region prior to switch recombination.

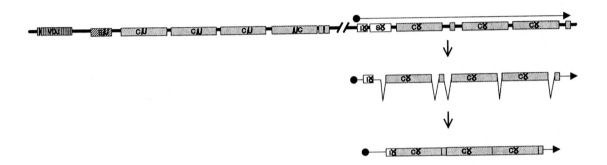

3. Switch Recombination.

Cleavage within switch regions.

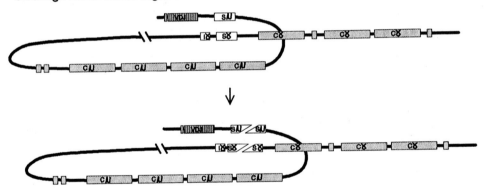

Ligation, creating hybrid switch regions, and deletion of intervening DNA.

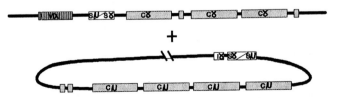

Figure 7–8. Schematic representation of switch recombination. Initially, rearranged VDJ exons are expressed in conjunction with the IgM constant region. Expression of downstream constant regions is achieved via a site-specific recombination between two switch regions. This site-specific recombination event is usually preceded by transcription of the unrearranged downstream constant region, as illustrated.

forms of the particular mRNA. Evidently, no protein product is generated. It has been clearly demonstrated that germline constant region genes are routinely transcribed before switch recombination. Thus, it is likely that T cell factors, either by inducing transcription through the constant region switch sequences or by increasing the accessibility of those regions to both transcription factors and recombination factors, direct switching to specific constant region genes.

T Lymphocytes

The genes of the TCR undergo a similar rearrangement process to generate functional genes.[304] The TCR α-chain consists of a single C_α region gene, approximately 60 J_α region genes, and approximately 100 V_α genes.[305] For α-chains, the mechanism of recombination appears to be deletion of the DNA between V_α and J_α. Allelic exclusion of α-chain genes is not as precise as for β-chain genes or Ig genes, but the mechanism has not been delineated.

There are two tandemly arranged β-chain constant region genes. There are no known functional differences between the two, and they are used interchangeably by T cells. Upstream of each C_β region are seven J_β regions and one D_β segment. The order of rearrangement of the β-chain locus is analogous to that of the Ig heavy chain locus.[306]

The γ-chain locus consists of at least 14 V_γ region genes, of which six are pseudogenes, each of which is capable of rearranging to any of five J_γ region genes.[63] There are two C_γ region genes in humans that are significantly different in that Cγ2 contains reduplicated second exons that lack the cysteine residues involved in the interchain disulfide bond, thereby giving rise to larger γ-chains that are not disulfide bonded to δ-chains. Assembly of the γ-chain gene is analogous to the TCR α-chain and λ and κ, resulting from a single V_γ to J_γ rearrangement. The δ-chain genes are located within the α-chain gene between V_α and J_α.[60] There is a single C_δ region gene and at least two J_δ and two D_δ regions. Rearrangement is comparable to that of TCR-β and V_H.

Expression of TCRs during ontogeny also occurs in a very ordered fashion with respect to the use of αβ versus γδ type receptors, and with respect to the use of specific V region gene segments.[307–312] Transcription of rearranged γδ genes begins first, increasing through days 15 to 17 of fetal life in the mouse and then decreasing so as to be barely detectable in adult thymocytes. TCR-β transcription can be detected on day 14 of fetal life in the mouse, but mRNA is truncated and incomplete (D-J only). Complete V-D-J rearrangements are first seen on day 16 and correspond to the appearance of full-length mRNA. TCR-α gene transcription is the last to begin, with full-length mRNA first detectable on day 17 of fetal life in the mouse. The level of α and β gene transcription increases from this time through birth.

Consistent with the pattern of TCR gene transcription, cell surface expression of γδ receptors occurs before that of αβ receptors. TCR-γδ + cells are detectable on day 14 of fetal life in the mouse and increase in number through day 17. The absolute number of γδ cells remains at a plateau from day 17 until birth. After day 17, γδ cells rapidly decrease as a percentage of total TCR + thymocytes. This results from a sudden expansion of αβ cells. TCR-αβ + thymocytes are occasionally detectable on day 16, rapidly expand in number on day 17 to 18 and outnumber γδ cells after day 18. In the murine adult thymus, δγ cells account for only 0.3 to 0.5 percent of all TCR + cells.[313]

In addition to the order of appearance of γδ TCRs before αβ TCRs, there is also ordered expression of V_γ and V_δ region genes. Thus, during ontogeny, particular V_γ and V_δ genes are preferentially rearranged and expressed at certain times during thymic ontogeny.[314] The physiologic explanation for this phenomenon remains to be delineated.

Based on the order of appearance of γδ TCRs before αβ TCRs in ontogeny and on the observation that many αβ T cells also have γ gene rearrangements, it was suggested that γδ and αβ cells belonged to the same lineage. According to this model, precursor cells attempt to rearrange γ and δ genes, and if successful, become γδ T cells. If unsuccessful, these same cells would go on to rearrange their α and β genes. Because the δ genes are found within the α locus, rearrangements of V_α to J_α would result in deletion of δ. If the above model is correct, the DNA deleted during V_α-J_α rearrangement would be expected to contain rearranged δ genes. However, in most instances the δ gene of αβ cells genes remain in a germline configuration,[315, 316] making this an unlikely alternative. More recently, information obtained through the use of γδ transgenic mice has led to the conclusion that γδ and αβ T cells develop along independent lines.[317, 318] In γδ transgenic mice, the extent to which αβ T cells develop was found to depend on the presence or absence of a cis-acting DNA element, called a silencer, in the flanking regions of γ.[318] If the γ transgene included the silencer, αβ T cells developed normally. If the silencer was eliminated from the γ transgene, αβ T cell development was blocked. It appears that activation of the γ silencer occurs in a portion of T cell precursors and the αβ lineage develops from these cells. In contrast, multiple cis-acting elements that silence the TCR α enhancer are active in γδ cells and a variety of non–T cell lines, but not in αβ cells.[319] Entry into the αβ T cell lineage may involve inhibition of these elements.

ONTOGENY AND SELF-NONSELF DISCRIMINATION

T Lymphocytes

Immunocompetent T cells develop in the thymus from bone marrow–derived or fetal liver–derived precursors.[320, 321] During this complex maturational process, deletion of autoreactive T cells (negative selection) and expansion of T cells whose antigen reactivity is restricted by self-MHC antigens (positive selection) occur. During the development of T cells in the thymus, more than 90 percent of immature thymocytes are eliminated, with the remainder exiting the thymus to constitute the T cell arm of the immune system. Distinct stages of thymic ontogeny have been identified by surface phenotype, rearrangement and expression of T cell receptors, and functional capability.

The ultimate thymocyte precursors are derived from multipotent precursors in the fetal liver and later in life in the bone marrow.[320, 321] The CD7 molecule is the earliest T cell–specific cell surface molecule and can be identified in human fetal liver, yolk sac, and upper thorax as early as weeks 7 to 8½ of human embryonic development.[46, 47, 322] CD7 is expressed by prethymocytes, as well as by all thymocytes and most peripheral T cells. These cells may contain cytoplasmic CD3 but have not rearranged their TCR genes and, hence, do not express the TCR-CD3 complex on their surface. In addition, they do not express either CD4 or CD8. CD7+ precursors of T cells colonize the thymus very early in fetal life (day 11 in the mouse, week 7 to 8 in the human) and continue to migrate into the thymus from the bone marrow during postnatal and adult life. Under the influence of thymic epithelium–derived chemotactic factors, thymocyte precursors localize initially to the subcapsular portion of the thymic cortex.[323]

During the process of thymic maturation, thymocytes migrate from the cortex to the medulla as they mature (Fig. 7–9). After entry of cells into the thymus and the initiation of maturation, they begin to express a variety of differentiation markers, such as CD2 and CD1.[320, 322] Although mature T cells continue to express CD2, CD1 expression is lost as T cells mature in the thymus. By contrast, mature, functionally differentiated thymocytes acquire expression of CD5.[324]

A host of other changes in the phenotype of T cells occurs in a programmed manner as they mature in the thymus (Fig. 7–9). The most characteristic changes involve expression of the TCR-CD3 complex and CD4 and CD8.[321] The induction of TCR gene rearrangement and expression occurs in the subcapsule of the thymus under the influence of the thymic epithelium. For αβ T cells, this is the exclusive site of TCR rearrangements, whereas γδ T cells may also mature in extrathymic sites.[151, 152] In the subcapsule of the thymus, TCR gene rearrangement begins as a result of direct interactions with thymic epithelium and perhaps macrophages.[325, 326] This process appears to be mediated by a number of adhesive interactions, including those involving CD2 and leukocyte function–associated antigen-1 (LFA-1) on the thymocytes and their counter-receptors on thymic stromal cells, LFA-3 (CD58), and intercellular adhesion molecule-1 (ICAM-1), respectively. These cells remain CD4−,

CD8−, and CD3− and are the likely precursors of the next stage of thymic maturation.

In the thymic cortex, the CD4−CD8− thymocytes begin to express both CD4 and CD8, as well as CD3 and the TCR. Among the CD4+CD8+CD3+TCR+ thymocytes, there is positive selection of those recognizing self-MHC molecules expressed primarily on cortical epithelium.[327] The exact nature of the thymic epithelial cells involved in positive selection remains to be completely delineated, but thymic nurse cells are likely to play a role. In the absence of positive selection, there is an accumulation of CD4+CD8+ cells followed by their elimination by means of programmed cell death, or apoptosis.[328] CD4+CD8+ cells that have undergone positive selection up-regulate expression of CD3. Negative selection of autoreactive T cells with high-avidity receptors for self-peptides follows.[327] The populations inducing negative selection include bone marrow–derived macrophages, dendritic cells, and B cells and lead to apoptosis of self-reactive T cells. Thymocytes that progress beyond negative selection continue to up-regulate CD3 and lose either CD4 or CD8, becoming mature single positive thymocytes in the medulla. Afterward, these cells exit the thymic medulla and populate peripheral lymphoid organs. As a result of positive and negative selection in the thymus, mature CD4+ and CD8+ T cells are generated, which are restricted in their capacity to recognize antigenic peptides bound to class II and class I MHC molecules, respectively, and which have been purged of cells expressing TCRs for self-antigens.

Some autoreactive T cells escape deletion in the thymus. These T cells are maintained in a state of nonresponsiveness by a process known as *peripheral anergy*.[329] In this process, potentially autoreactive T cells are rendered nonresponsive by encountering antigen displayed on the surface of inappropriate antigen-presenting cells. These cells differ from classic or "professional" antigen-presenting cells, such as macrophages, dendritic cells, or B cells, in that they lack the capacity to provide costimulatory signals necessary for antigen recognition to lead to T cell activation.[111] The exact nature of these costimulatory signals and the surface receptors involved have not been completely delineated, although interactions involving CD28 on the T cell and B7/BB1 on the antigen-presenting cell appear to play an important role.[329a] It is clear, however, that when potentially autoreactive T cells encounter antigen displayed by an antigen-presenting cell that is unable to deliver these signals, anergy and not activation results. Such induced nonresponsiveness appears to be a major mechanism in preventing autoreactive T cells that escape the thymus from causing autoimmune disease.

B Lymphocytes

B cells develop from precursors initially found in the placenta and fetal liver and subsequently in

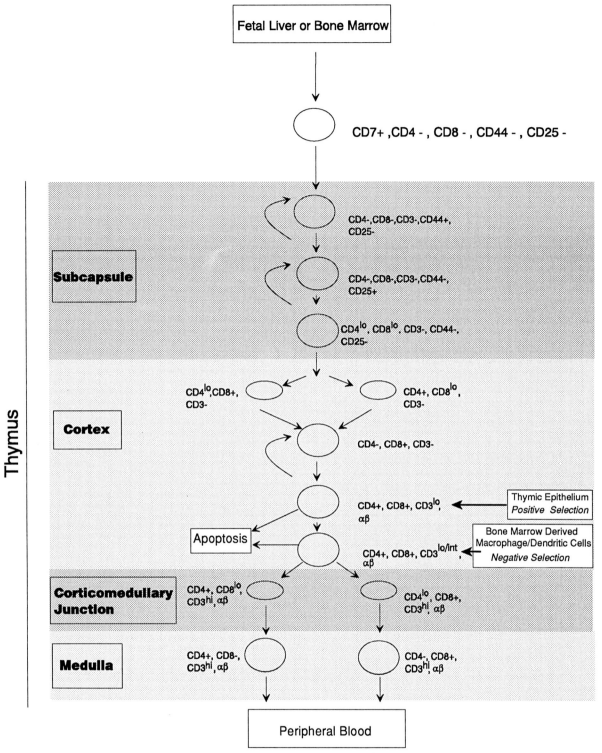

Figure 7–9. Schematic representation of the maturation of αβ T cells in the thymus.

the bone marrow.[2, 3, 330, 331] During adult life, B cell precursors reside in the bone marrow. The development of B cells involves the commitment of hematopoietic stem cells to the B cell lineage, with subsequent rearrangement of Ig genes and expression of membrane-associated Ig and other specific B cell lineage markers (see Fig. 7–1).

In prenatal and adult life, the decision to enter the B cell lineage occurs in the fetal liver and bone marrow, respectively. Adherent bone marrow stromal cells play a critical role in the commitment of precursors to the B cell lineage.[331] Stromal cells secrete growth factors for pre-B cells that appear to play a critical role in this process. Bone marrow macrophages and other stromal cells also contribute to the induction of stem cell commitment to the B cell lineage.

The maturation of stem cell precursors into functional human B lymphocytes represents a multistep process of programmed development that involves both Ig gene rearrangements and the induction of expression of a number of B lineage differentiation molecules. CD19 appears to be the earlier B lineage differentiation molecule expressed by developing B cells.[2, 3] These pro-B cells also express HLA-DR, CD10 (enkephalinase), CD34, and TdT. These early B cell precursors evolve through a complex series of maturational changes into pre-pre-B cells and then pre-B cells and immature B cells, as outlined in Figure 7–1, eventually giving rise to mature B cells that exit the bone marrow. Ig rearrangement begins in CD19+ pre-pre-B cells, before they have begun to express CD20 or CD21.[3, 4] Pre-B cells first express cytoplasmic μ-chains but do not express membrane IgM, whereas immature B cells express surface IgM but not IgD. Mature B cells express both IgD and IgM.

During the maturation of B cells, specific cytokines appear to facilitate the growth or differentiation, or both, of precursors at different stages. Thus, for example, low-molecular-weight B cell growth factor and IL-3, but not IL-1, IL-4, IL-5, or IL-6, induce proliferation of pro-B cells.[3, 331] Similarly, a subpopulation of fetal liver pro-B cells proliferate in response to IL-7, a 15-kD stromal cell–derived cytokine.[332, 333] As B cell precursors mature, the expression of cytokine receptors changes in a programmed manner. IL-7 receptors are lost during the pre-B cell stage, whereas IL-3 receptors are lost as cells become immature B cells.[3] Immature membrane IgM+ IgD− B cells first express receptors for IL-4, whereas receptors for IL-1, IL-2, IL-5, and IL-6 are first expressed by mature IgM+ IgD+ B cells.

Peripheral B cells can be classified as either naive or memory cells based on their antigenic experience. Naive B cells that have not yet encountered antigen account for the majority of mature, peripheral B cells. These cells express both membrane IgM and IgD and are continuously replenished from the maturational process in the bone marrow. Memory B cells, selected for expansion in T cell–dependent immune responses because of high-avidity binding of their target antigen, frequently express somatically mutated Ig VDJ region genes, and persist in the immune system for a long period.[334] They usually do not express IgD and may express IgM, but they usually express IgG, IgA, or IgE on their surface membranes.

The repertoire of Ig receptors expressed by peripheral B lymphocytes is influenced by positive and negative selection in a manner that is analogous to the shaping of the T cell repertoire during ontogeny. Thus, newly generated B cells appear to undergo a process of positive selection as they differentiate from pre-B cells into the mature peripheral B cell pool.[335] The nature of the cells and molecules responsible for this positive selection process is unknown. B cells expressing membrane Ig receptors that recognize autoantigens are deleted during B cell ontogeny.[336–338] This is particularly effective for B cells that recognize cell-bound antigens. Autoreactive B cells that escape into the periphery become unresponsive to the autoantigen by a process that involves down-regulation of their surface Ig receptors as well as functional anergy, which is similar to that observed with autoreactive T cells that escape the thymus.

LYMPHOCYTE ACTIVATION

T Lymphocytes

Activation is the series of steps that begins with antigen recognition and includes the biochemical events that will initiate cell cycle entry and sustain cell cycle progression to mitosis and the production of daughter cells. An important result of T cell activation is the production of a number of cytokines as activation results in up-regulation of cytokine gene transcription. Cytokines not only are required for T cell cycle progression but also have important regulatory effects on B cells, monocytes, and other cells of the immune system. T cell activation can be conveniently separated into three series of events: (1) the required cellular interactions, (2) the generation of the initial transmembrane signals, and (3) the subsequent gene activation events that occur in orderly progression to induce the production of cytokines and other proteins or cell products needed to sustain cell cycle progression and to stimulate cellular division and growth.

Cellular Interactions. Under normal circumstances, T cells recognize antigen bound to MHC molecules on the surface of specialized antigen-presenting cells. Cell surface molecules have evolved on both the T cell and the antigen-presenting cells to mediate antigen presentation and recognition. The T cell expresses the clonally distributed TCR, which recognizes antigen complexed with an MHC molecule that is present on the surface of the antigen-presenting cell (see Fig. 7–2). The TCR is a heterodimer whose ligand-binding domain is unique to each clone of T cells. Both of these chains belong to the Ig superfamily, have a single membrane-spanning region and short cytoplasmic tails (4 to 12 amino acids), and are linked by a single disulfide bond.[61] The TCR is always noncovalently associated on the cell surface with additional proteins, the CD3 complex. The CD3 complex is composed of up to five different polypeptide chains that are invariant in structure in all T cells. The association of CD3 with the TCR appears to involve interactions between charged amino acids of their transmembrane domains. The TCR structure determines the specificity of antigen recognition, and the CD3 complex mediates transduction of signals to the T cell.

Three of the proteins found in the CD3 complex, γ, δ, and ε, are coded for on human chromosome

11, are highly homologous in structure, and probably arose by gene duplication. Only γ (28 kD) and δ (20 kD) are glycosylated.[61] The CD3 complex always includes ε but may contain either γ or δ.[75] Two additional proteins, ζ (16 kD) and η, that have no structural homology to γ, δ, or ε, are independently associated with the TCR. CD3-ζ is not glycosylated, maps to human chromosome 1, and has a short extracellular domain but a cytoplasmic domain of 113 amino acids. Approximately 90 percent of ζ is found as a homodimer. This homodimer, unlike CD3-γ, δ, ε, is not unique to T cells but is also found associated with CD16, the receptor for IgG Fc, on NK cells.[339, 340] The γ-chain found in the high-affinity IgE receptor of mast cells and basophils is homologous to the ζ-chain and may have arisen by gene duplication.[341] Thus, T cell ζ,η and IgE-γ form a family of proteins. The other 10 percent of ζ exists as a heterodimer with η. CD3-η is derived by alternative splicing from the same gene locus on chromosome 1 as CD3-ζ, also has a long cytoplasmic tail, and can exist as homodimers as well as ζ-η heterodimers.[342, 343] The cytoplasmic domain of CD3-ζ appears to be the major component of the CD3 complex required for signaling T cell activation,[82] although recent evidence suggests that signaling through γ, δ, ε also occurs.[343a] Whereas CD3-ζ$_2$, CD3-ζ-η, and CD3-η$_2$ isoforms are able to transduce signals,[343] the presence of the ζ-η heterodimer seems important for efficient coupling to phosphoinositol hydrolysis.[61]

T cell–antigen-presenting cell recognition requires not only that an appropriate antigen is presented to be recognized by a unique TCR but also that the antigen is bound to the correct class I or class II MHC molecule on the antigen-presenting cell. This further restriction occurs because CD4+ T cells recognize antigen bound to class II MHC molecules on the antigen-presenting cell, whereas CD8+ T cells recognize antigen when it is presented on antigen-presenting cell class I MHC molecules.[62] CD4 can directly bind nonpolymorphic regions of class II MHC molecules, whereas CD8 can bind the nonpolymorphic regions of the α3 domain of class I MHC proteins. The restriction of the T cell–antigen-presenting cell interaction on the basis of CD4 or CD8 phenotype has been known for some time. However, it is now clear that ligation of CD4 or CD8 performs a specific signaling function for the T cell. CD4 and CD8 physically associate with the TCR when antigen is recognized, thus forming a complex in which antigen recognition and CD4 or CD8 association occurs on the same MHC molecule (see Fig. 7–2).[344] As CD4 and CD8 are associated with the lymphocyte-specific intracellular protein kinase, p56^{lck}, one result of formation of this complex is to bring p56^{lck} into proximity with one of its substrates, CD3-ζ.[345] It is clear, however, that signaling through the CD4 or CD8 molecule can also occur without complexing with CD3.[111]

An important advance in the understanding of the role of the MHC-encoded molecules has occurred

as a result of determination of the three-dimensional structure of the heterodimeric class I MHC.[346] The larger α-chain (44 kD), coded for by the MHC, is organized into three extracellular domains, an α$_1$ and α$_2$ domain that form the antigen-binding region and an α$_3$ Ig-like domain. In addition, the polypeptide has a transmembrane sequence and a cytoplasmic tail. There is one peptide-binding site per molecule, and the cleft that is formed to bind antigen is large enough to bind a peptide fragment of nine amino acids. Most of the polymorphic amino acid residues of the heavy chain are found in the α-helical sides or the β-pleated sheet floor of the peptide-binding cleft. These allelic differences in the peptide-binding cleft contribute to the ability of the molecule to bind different peptides.[347] The heavy chain is noncovalently associated with a smaller peptide (12 kD), β$_2$-microglobulin, which is not MHC encoded and is entirely extracellular. β$_2$-microglobulin is folded in an Ig-like conformation and is associated with the α$_3$ domain of the heavy chain. This association seems to be critical in maintaining the tertiary structure of the complex and in stabilizing peptide binding and expression on the cell surface.

The primary amino acid sequences of many class II MHC molecules are known, although the crystallographic structure has not been determined. The molecule is unlike the class I MHC molecule in that it is composed of two noncovalently associated chains, an α-chain and a β-chain, which are similar in structure. Although the three-dimensional structure of the class II MHC molecule has not yet been completed, the tertiary structure can be modelled in analogy to the class I MHC molecule. This hypothesized three-dimensional structure has an antigen binding cleft with α-helical sides and a β-pleated sheet forming the floor. The polymorphic amino acid residues point toward the groove where the antigenic peptide is proposed to reside. Unlike the class I MHC molecule, however, the antigen-binding site is formed by both chains.[348]

Certain bacterial enterotoxin "superantigens," including the staphylococcal enterotoxins and toxic shock syndrome–associated toxin, also bind to class II MHC molecules.[349] These bacterial enterotoxins, produced by certain staphylococci, streptococci, or mycoplasma, can stimulate a high percentage (10 to 40 percent) of T cells to divide and produce lymphokines. The presence of accessory cells that express class II MHC molecules is absolutely required for this effect. The enterotoxins recognize amino acid sequences on the antigen-presenting cell class II MHC molecules, which are distinct from the polymorphic regions that define the peptide-binding site. The superantigens also specifically recognize regions of the TCR distinct from the antigen-binding site. Most seem to bind to variable regions of the TCR β-chain, thus accounting for the ability to activate only the T cells that carry the particular V$_β$ region recognized by the individual enterotoxin. A role for superantigens in the development of the T cell repertoire and, potentially, in initiating autoimmune diseases has been suggested.[349]

Although the interactions of TCR-MHC are critical for stimulation of specific T cells, these ligand receptor interactions may not be sufficient to activate the T cell and, in isolation, can lead to subsequent T cell unresponsiveness, a form of anergy.[111, 329] A number of additional interactions with other molecules expressed on the T cell surface are important in providing a sufficient stimulus to activate the resting T cell (see Table 7–3). Antigen-presenting cells are known to express ligands for some of these T cell antigens, including CD2, CD4, CD8, and LFA-1. Many of these molecules function to increase adhesive interactions between T cells and antigen-presenting cells and also have the capacity to generate activation signals. Whether antigen-presenting cells have ligands for all of these molecules and whether they affect signal transduction during the physiologic T cell–antigen-presenting cell interaction are unknown. However, it is likely that T cells receive multiple signals from engagement of these various receptors during interactions with antigen-presenting cells that can summate and thus facilitate T cell activation.[111]

Transmembrane Signaling. Once an appropriate T cell–antigen-presenting cell couple has been formed, information must be transmitted to the T cell to initiate the cascade of biochemical events that will eventually result in cytokine receptor expression, cytokine gene expression, cell cycle progression, and clonal expansion. Phosphorylation or dephosphorylation of proteins is one of the central biochemical mechanisms used to regulate intracellular events in response to extracellular signals. In fact, the earliest detectable event that occurs after TCR-CD3 ligation is phosphorylation of a variety of polypeptides on their tyrosine residues.[350, 351] The critical role of tyrosine kinase phosphorylation is indicated by the observation that inhibition of tyrosine kinase–mediated phosphorylation prevents T cell activation and IL-2 production.[351–353] Tyrosine phosphorylation of some proteins has been detected as early as 5 seconds after ligation of the TCR-CD3 complex, and tyrosine phosphorylation of the ζ-chain of the TCR occurs within minutes. Such tyrosine phosphorylation occurs before detectable phospholipase C activation.[350]

Although tyrosine phosphorylation is initiated by ligation of the TCR-CD3 complex, the TCR is not itself a tyrosine kinase. However, CD4 and CD8 associate with a tyrosine kinase found in T cells called p56[lck], which is a member of the *src* family of protein tyrosine kinases.[345] p56[lck] binds the cytoplasmic tails of either CD4 or CD8 through a specific binding site on the N terminus of p56[lck]. Thus, engagement of the TCR, which results in physical association of CD4 or CD8 with the TCR-CD3 complex, brings p56[lck] into proximity of the CD3 proteins, including ζ, which is a substrate for p56[lck].[345] p56[lck] is itself regulated by phosphorylation. p56[lck] can autophosphorylate at Tyr394, which increases activity.

Another site of tyrosine phosphorylation, Tyr505, is constitutively phosphorylated in T cells, and this is inhibitory. Dephosphorylation at this site is an important mechanism of activation of p56[lck]. Mutants expressing constitutively dephosphorylated and therefore activated p56[lck] exhibit augmented responses to antigen activation.[354] p56[lck] is only one of several tyrosine kinases that are found in T cells. A more widely expressed tyrosine kinase, p59[fyn], is directly associated with the TCR.[355]

An important mediator of dephosphorylation is the CD45 molecule, which is expressed as different isoforms on T cell subsets, B cells, and other bone marrow–derived cells. The cytoplasmic domain of CD45 has tyrosine phosphatase activity,[130, 356, 357] and cells that fail to express CD45 cannot be activated appropriately.[358] p56[lck] is a substrate for CD45 that can dephosphorylate Tyr505, thus activating the kinase.[359, 360] CD45 can physically associate with CD3 and with CD2.[361, 362] Thus, one result of ligation of the TCR-CD3 is to bring CD4 or CD8, both of which are associated with p56[lck] tyrosine kinase, into physical association with CD45, which results in activation of p56[lck].

Physiologically, other pathways appear to be linked to surface receptors by the action of the tyrosine kinases described earlier. Tyrosine phosphorylation is required for activation of phospholipase C (PLC), with CD3 ligation resulting in tyrosine phosphorylation of the PLC-γ1 isoform.[353, 363] Inhibition of tyrosine phosphorylation prevents the activation of PLC and generation of the increase in intracellular calcium ($[Ca^{2+}]_i$) observed in response to ligation of the TCR-CD3 complex.[352, 364] Membrane-bound PLC hydrolyzes phosphatidylinositol-4,5-bisphosphate, a minor membrane lipid, to produce intracellular inositol trisphosphate (IP_3) and diacylglycerol (DAG) in response to engagement of TCR-CD3.[365] IP_3 mobilizes an intracellular store of calcium, which when released contributes to the initial increase in $[Ca^{2+}]_i$ that is observed after mitogen activation of T cells. DAG is believed to be the physiologic activator of protein kinase C, a serine-threonine kinase. Regulation of PLC activity may also involve G proteins, which are membrane-limited mediators of transmembrane signaling present in a variety of cells, including T cells.[366] Unlike other cell types, use of a G protein does not seem to be the mechanism for coupling ligation of the TCR-CD3 complex to PLC activation, however.[367]

The increase in $[Ca^{2+}]_i$ observed after mitogen stimulation is not entirely caused by mobilization of intracellular stores by IP_3, as movement of calcium from the extracellular medium into the cell is necessary both for T cell activation and for the maintenance of the sustained increase in $[Ca^{2+}]_i$ associated with T cell activation.[368, 369] How calcium moves across the T cell membrane is not yet clear, although a cation movement that is stimulated by mitogens has been detected.[370] This cation entry is not voltage gated and, thus, is unlike the classical voltage-gated calcium channels found in most other cells. Activation of T cells requires concomitant increases in $[Ca^{2+}]_i$ and activation of protein kinase C. Moreover, several hours of a sustained increase in $[Ca^{2+}]_i$ and protein kinase C activation is required to maximize the T cell proliferative response. The importance of this pathway is underscored by the observation that it can be mimicked pharmacologically by the addition of a calcium ionophore to raise $[Ca^{2+}]_i$ and a phorbol ester to activate protein kinase C, a combination that activates the vast majority of T cells. This is the minimal stimulus required to activate T cells to produce cytokines and to proliferate.[371, 372]

In addition to the tyrosine kinase phosphorylation discussed previously, many proteins have potential serine or threonine phosphorylation sites. Addition of phorbol ester, which activates protein kinase C, results in phosphorylation of a number of proteins, including the CD3-γ chain, CD4, CD8, and CD18.[373, 374] Cyclic adenosine monophosphate (AMP)-dependent protein kinase A also phosphorylates serine-threonine residues, but the pattern of phosphorylation is different. Moreover, elevation of cyclic AMP in lymphocytes is typically inhibitory.[375] The role of other serine-threonine kinases, such as calmodulin kinase or casein kinase, is poorly understood in T cell activation.

In the physiologic T cell–antigen-presenting cell interaction, multiple different surface molecules are engaged in addition to the TCR-CD3. Ligation of these additional T cell surface molecules is required for T cell activation, cytokine gene expression, and progression to mitosis after T cell recognition of antigen (see Table 7–3). Such binding of multiple surface molecules may increase the avidity of the cellular interaction. However, it is probably more important that ligation of different surface molecules stimulates transmembrane signaling events required to move the G_0 resting T cell into the cell cycle. The importance of these interactions has been inferred in several ways. First, monoclonal antibodies that recognize the specific surface antigen can either stimulate or inhibit the T cell response, usually when another surface molecule such as CD3 or CD2 is simultaneously engaged. In some instances, monoclonal antibodies to a specific determinant can partially block the accessory cell–dependent stimulation, demonstrating the importance of that interaction in T cell activation. More importantly, there are known ligands for many of these receptors on T cells. Finally, ligation of certain surface antigens can be directly shown to provide signaling information to the T cell, such as inducing an increase in $[Ca^{2+}]_i$ (see Table 7–3).

The CD2 surface antigen was the first antigen-independent activation pathway to be described.[83] The ligand for CD2 is LFA-3 (CD58), which is expressed on a variety of cell types. Ligation of CD2 can stimulate a rise in $[Ca^{2+}]_i$ and phosphatidylinositol turnover and can costimulate phosphorylation of CD3-γ or tyrosine phosphorylation of CD3-ζ.[111, 376]

Although CD2-stimulated T cell activation does not require additional signals delivered via CD3, surface CD3 expression does seem to be required for this pathway to be active, suggesting cross-talk between CD3 and CD2.[111]

The CD28 molecule mediates a distinct signaling pathway. CD28 is a 90-kD glycoprotein homodimer expressed on 80 percent of human T cells. Ligation of CD28 costimulates T cell activation, but, unlike many other T cell surface molecules that transduce signals, CD3 surface expression is not required and the resultant induction of IL-2 secretion is resistant to cyclosporine.[377] The second messengers that mediate the effects of CD28 are not completely understood, although ligation of CD28 induces phosphorylation of tyrosine residues on specific protein substrates.[377a] CD28 stimulation results in stabilization of several lymphokine mRNAs, including IL-2 mRNA,[378] and can augment IL-2 gene transcription.[379] One ligand for CD28 is the B7/BB1 molecule expressed on activated B cells.[110]

Not all of the ligands for these T cell surface antigens (see Table 7–2) are yet known, and it is not yet clear which of these interactions are critical to T cell activation. It is interesting that the absence of expression of certain of these T cell molecules is associated with immunodeficiency states. Absence of surface expression of sialophorin (CD43) or expression of defective molecules occurs in Wiskott-Aldrich syndrome.[380] Bone marrow transplantation corrects the immunologic defects in this disease. T cell activation occurs if CD43 is ligated in the presence of accessory cells, suggesting that this molecule has an important role in T cell activation. Recent evidence suggests that intercellular adhesion molecule-1 (ICAM-1) is a ligand for CD43.[380a] Absence of surface expression of CD7 has been observed in a patient with severe combined immunodeficiency.[381] The patient's T cell and B cell defects were corrected after successful bone marrow transplantation resulted in repopulation with donor T lymphocytes that expressed CD7. Although the B cells were of host origin, after transplantation, normal B cell responses were observed, including Ig and specific antibody synthesis, indicating that CD7, a T cell–specific marker, may be important in T cell–B cell collaboration.

Gene Activation and DNA Synthesis. Although the subsequent sequence of events after generation of second messengers that lead to gene activation are largely unknown, a large number of genes that are activated in an orderly sequence have been identified (Fig. 7–10). Immediate genes are expressed within minutes and do not require protein synthesis, whereas early and late genes require protein synthesis.[382] Immediate and early genes are expressed before cell division; late genes are expressed after mitosis.

The location of the IL-2 gene transcriptional enhancer has been determined and contains four regions critical to regulation by the TCR.[382] The most

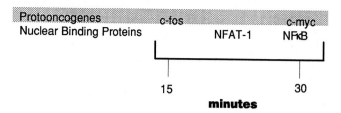

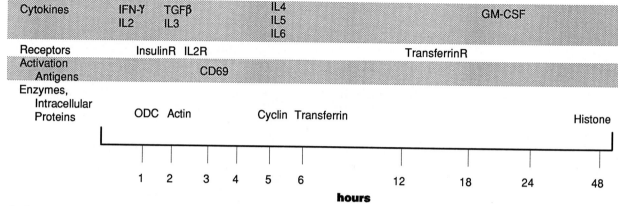

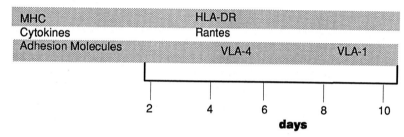

Figure 7–10. Programmed activation of genes after TCR occupancy and effective signal generation. These data are modified from Crabtree.[382]

proximal region is designated *antigen receptor response element* (ARRE-1) and binds the nuclear factor of IL-2A (NFIL-2A). A second antigen receptor response element (ARRE-2) binds the nuclear factor of activated T cells (NFAT-1). NFAT-1 is synthesized approximately 20 minutes after T cell activation and precedes appearance of IL-2 mRNA. Although IL-2 mRNA expression is dependent on NFAT-1 and NFIL-2A, binding of those proteins does not explain the striking increase in IL-2 gene transcription in response to phorbol ester. Phorbol ester sensitivity is conferred by the AP-1 binding site. AP-1 is the product of the c-*jun* proto-oncogene, and its binding affinity to DNA is enhanced when it forms a complex with protein products of the c-*fos* proto-oncogene, resulting in a "leucine zipper" structure.[383] Another factor that is inducible by phorbol ester, NFκB, also has a binding site in the IL-2 enhancer.[384] Finally, activation of T cells via CD28 in the presence of phorbol ester induces a protein complex that has a separate binding site in the IL-2 enhancer. Such

binding increases IL-2 enhancer activity and IL-2 gene transcription.[379]

IL-2 is produced specifically by T cells and is critical in maintaining the progression of events that leads to mitosis.[385] The receptor for IL-2, IL-2R, is not detected on resting T cells but is rapidly expressed after stimulation by mitogen or antigen.[192] The IL-2R is composed of at least two polypeptide chains, a low-affinity 55-kD protein (α), and an intermediate-affinity 70-kD peptide (β). Both peptides bind IL-2, but physical interaction of the p70 and p55 peptide forms the tertiary structure that binds IL-2 with high affinity. IL-2R can be detected on T cells as early as 12 hours after stimulation. IL-2 mRNA and IL-2 secretion are detected much sooner than IL-2R, and IL-2 itself stimulates an up-regulation of p55 IL-2R mRNA transcription and cell surface expression. A binding site for the phorbol ester–sensitive NFκB has been defined in the IL-2R gene transcription initiation region.[382]

Investigation of second messenger signals that

result from IL-2 binding to the IL-2R has shown that binding of IL-2 to its receptor does not increase $[Ca^{2+}]_i$ or phosphatidylinositol turnover.[386, 387] Although translocation of protein kinase C has been reported, it is not necessary for the effects of IL-2.[388] Activation of the Na^+/H^+ antiporter also occurs, but inhibition of Na^+/H^+ antiport activity does not inhibit T cell activation.[389] IL-2 binding to IL-2R does result in tyrosine phosphorylation of several proteins. The p70 (β) subunit is sufficient to transmit the signal that results in tyrosine phosphorylation, and the p70 subunit is itself a substrate for tyrosine phosphorylation.[390-392] Neither the p70 nor the p55 subunits or the complete IL-2R complex has intrinsic tyrosine kinase activity, but the IL-2R complex is associated with a tyrosine kinase activity that may be the same p56^{lck} that is associated with CD4 and CD8.[195]

B Lymphocytes

Many of the initial signaling events that have been defined in B cells are triggered in response to ligation of surface Ig. Mature B cells express surface IgM or IgD. Membrane Ig has a very short three amino acid cytoplasmic tail and no known enzymatic activity or binding domains for kinases or G proteins. Therefore, the Ig heavy chain is unlikely to mediate signal transduction directly, although the cytoplasmic tail is important in some functions because deletion eliminates calcium signaling and antigen presentation in response to ligation of surface Ig.[393] Surface IgM and IgD, however, are associated with additional transmembrane proteins.[275] IgM is associated with a heterodimer composed of IgM-α (43 kD) coded for by the mb-1 gene and Ig-β (39 kD) coded for by the B29 gene. IgM-α is required for transport of IgM to the B cell surface. Membrane IgD is associated with Ig-β, a closely related protein Ig-γ (34 kD), and an additional subunit of 33 kD, which is similar to IgM-α, called IgD-α. The heterodimer associated with IgM (IgM-α/Ig-β) is disulfide linked and has N-glycosylated Ig-like surface domains. The transmembrane sequences seem to be important for interaction with the transmembrane portion of the IgM heavy chain.

The cytoplasmic tails of both Ig-β and IgM-α contain tyrosine kinase phosphorylation sites and can be isolated as the phosphoproteins.[275] A 220-kD isoform of the tyrosine phosphatase CD45 is expressed in B cells, and CD45 can dephosphorylate both IgM- and IgD-associated heterodimers. Although the heterodimers associate with surface Ig and can themselves undergo tyrosine phosphorylation, the IgM-associated heterodimers do not seem to be responsible for transducing the calcium signal directly.

As in T cells, tyrosine phosphorylation may be critical to integrating different pathways of signal transduction. The IgM complex is associated with a tyrosine kinase, possibly the *src* family member *lyn*.[394]

Other tyrosine kinases that are proto-oncogene products are found in B cells including *blk*, which is B cell specific, and *hck*.[394-396] Stimulation of B cells with *Staphylococcus aureus*, a polyclonal B cell activator, or by cross-linking surface Ig results in tyrosine phosphorylation of a number of B cell proteins.[397-399] One of the proteins that is tyrosine phosphorylated is the γ1 form of B cell PLC. Moreover, inhibition of tyrosine phosphorylation prevents both IP_3 production and the increase in $[Ca^{2+}]_i$.[400-402] As in T cells, activation of PLC results in the production of IP_3 and DAG, with the resultant increase in $[Ca^{2+}]_i$ and the translocation of protein kinase.[403] Consistent with the importance of this pathway in B cell activation, treatment of B cells with phorbol ester and a calcium ionophore will trigger B cell proliferation.

Signal transduction in physiologic B cell activation stimulated by interaction with T cells may involve many B cell surface molecules other than surface Ig. B cells express a number of surface molecules that have signaling capacity (see Table 7–1).[5, 190, 401] Of the B cell–specific molecules, CD19, CD20, CD21, and CD23 either increase $[Ca^{2+}]_i$ when cross-linked or augment anti-IgM calcium signaling. Other molecules, including CD40 and CD72, may also play a role in signaling B cell activation. The role of the class II MHC molecules on B cells may be particularly important because they can interact with CD4 on the T cell helper population. Ligation of class II MHC molecules on B cells leads to an increase in B cell $[Ca^{2+}]_i$, phosphatidylinositol turnover, protein phosphorylation, and B cell proliferation.[404-406] Other B cell ligands are known to bind T cell surface molecules, including B7/BB1, which binds CD28,[110] CD72, which is the ligand for CD5,[25] and LFA-1 on B cells, which interacts with ICAM-1 (CD54) on CD4+ T cells.[407] It is likely that these B cell surface molecules transduce intracellular signals to B cells because anti-CD72 monoclonal antibodies induce proliferation in B cells,[24, 408] and ligating LFA-1 can increase $[Ca^{2+}]_i$ in T cells.[409] Thus, the T cell–B cell cognate interaction may result in summation of multiple signals generated by mutual interaction of cell surface ligands to lead to the initial activation of the resting B cell (Fig. 7–11).

CELL-CELL INTERACTIONS

Lymphocyte Trafficking

Newly generated lymphocytes leave their site of production, which, under usual circumstances, is the bone marrow or thymus, and subsequently migrate via the blood stream through essentially all tissues and organs. The continuous recirculation through tissues in relation to blood flow provides a constant surveillance function.[410] The resultant distribution of lymphocytes is not random, however, because lymphocytes migrate into tissues via specific homing pathways through endothelial cells. The existence of

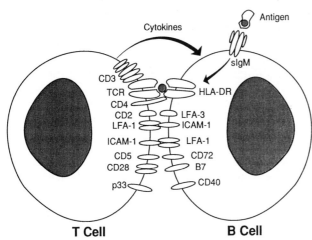

Figure 7–11. Schematic representation of T cell–B cell collaboration.

preferential pathways is suggested by the unique distribution of lymphocytes in certain tissues. For example, B cells are the predominant population in the spleen and in Peyer's patches, whereas T cells are the major population of lymphocytes in peripheral lymph node.[410, 411] Lymphocytes recirculate through tissues by two main mechanisms: (1) by entry via a specialized pathway in which lymphocytes recognize specific cell surface molecules on high endothelial venule (HEV) cells, which line postcapillary venules of lymphoid tissue; or (2) by crossing endothelium-lined blood vessels that lack specialized HEV.[412] Entry via HEV is important for the high-volume movement of lymphocytes through lymphoid tissue. Less frequent movement into other tissues such as gut or skin occurs by lymphocyte recognition of counter-receptors on flat endothelium.

Endothelium with morphology very similar to that of HEV is observed in inflamed synovium and other inflammatory sites.[413–415] These morphologic changes in endothelium can be induced in skin in response to the cytokines TNF-α and IFN-γ.[416] The HEV-like morphology may occur in response to increased lymphocyte traffic or, after induction, may augment the movement of lymphocytes into areas of inflammation. Table 7–8 lists the known lymphocyte receptors and tissue ligands (counter-receptors) that determine the specific interactions that allow lymphocytes to discriminate between HEV of different tissue sites. Lymphocytes also can home to organs such as spleen, bone marrow, lung, and liver in which HEVs are not prominent, but little is known about specific receptor-ligand interactions in these tissues.[417]

T lymphocytes have different migration patterns, depending on whether they have encountered antigen. "Naive" (CD45RA+) T cells, which originate in the thymus, express the surface receptor L-selectin, which is important for binding to lymph node HEV. Thus, naive T cells, which are the predominant population in peripheral lymph nodes, enter lymph nodes from blood by crossing HEV and leave via the efferent lymph.[412] Memory T cells (CD45RO+), which are believed to have previously encountered antigen, leave the peripheral vascular bed across flat endothelium to localize preferentially in nonlymphoid tissue and are the primary population in inflammatory sites. Thus, memory cells leave the circulation by crossing endothelium in tissue, then migrate to lymph nodes via afferent lymph, and leave peripheral lymphoid tissue via the efferent lymphatic circulation.

Migration of T cells into sites of inflammation is also directed by specific T cell–counter-receptor interactions (Table 7–9). Lymphocytes removed from sites of inflammation will migrate back to tissue-specific sites of inflammation, suggesting a specific homing receptor interaction.[417] Endothelium in inflamed synovium also can develop HEV-like postcapillary venules but bind lymphocytes by a receptor mechanism distinct from that used by lymph node or mucosa.[413, 414] The expression of the endothelial cell counter-receptors used to bind lymphocytes is induced by the cytokines IL-1 and TNF-α. These are up-regulated at sites of inflammation, such as the rheumatoid synovium.[410, 418]

ICAM-1 expression on endothelium is increased when endothelial cells are activated in culture and when endothelium is examined in inflammatory sites.[419, 420] The T cell ligand for ICAM-1, LFA-1, is important in initial binding of T cells,[421, 422] and, after initial binding, T cells migrate through the intercellular junctions of endothelial cells by a process that appears to involve progressive interactions of LFA-1 with ICAM-1 expressed by the endothelial cell.[418] ICAM-1 is also the counter-receptor for CD11b-CD18 (Mac-1, CR3) but this appears to play a more important role in the migration of neutrophils rather than lymphocytes. Expression of vascular cell adhesion molecule-1 (VCAM-1) and E-selectin (formerly known as endothelial leukocyte adhesion molecule-1, ELAM-1), both members of the Ig supergene family, is increased on endothelium activated by cytokines such as IL-1 and TNF-α.[423, 424] Both ICAM-1 and VCAM-1 expression may be important for directed migration of memory cells to inflamed sites as their respective T cell ligands, LFA-1 and very late antigen-4 (VLA-4, CD49-α/CD29) are up-regulated on memory T cells.[412] E-selectin binding may be most specific for memory T cells.[425, 426] In addition, a subset of memory T cells that carries the cutaneous lymphocyte–associated antigen (CLA) constitutes 80 to 90 percent of T cells in chronic skin lesions and is one cell population that binds E-selectin, whose expression is increased in chronically inflamed skin.[426] Finally, additional as yet unknown receptor–counter-receptor interactions are likely to contribute to the homing and migration of lymphocytes into inflamed tissues.

Endothelial cells also participate in lymphocyte migration into tissue by producing a variety of polypeptide mediators that affect this process. Endothe-

Table 7–8. ADHESION RECEPTORS MEDIATING B AND T CELL HOMING

Lymphoid Cells	Lymphocyte Receptors	Family	Counter-receptor	Tissue Expressing Counter-receptor
T cells	L-selectin (LECAM-1, Leu-8, LAM-1)	Selectin	Vascular addressin-1 (charged oligosaccharides)	Lymphoid (peripheral, mesenteric)
B cells	CD44	HCAM	Vascular addressin-2	Lymphoid (Peyer's patch, mesenteric)
T and B cells	CD11a/CD18 (LFA-1)	Integrin	ICAM-1 (CD54), ICAM-2	Many cell types (increased by cytokines and endotoxin)

LECAM, leukocyte–endothelial cell adhesion molecule; LAM, leukocyte adhesion molecule; ICAM, intercellular adhesion molecule; LFA, leukocyte function–associated antigen; HCAM, homing cell adhesion molecule.

lial cells can produce the cytokine IL-8, which is a chemotactic factor for T lymphocytes and neutrophils.[427–429] On the other hand, T cells also affect this process by producing cytokines such as TNF-α and IFN-γ that induce the expression of the counter-receptors used for transendothelial cell migration. In addition, T cells can produce chemotactic factors, such as the cytokine RANTES, which is a chemoattractant for CD4+ memory T cells[430] and may contribute to the preferential movement of memory T cells into tissues. Thus, a complicated interplay of regulatory factors governs the entry of lymphocytes into tissue.

T Cell–B Cell Collaboration

For many antigens, the induction of antibody production requires collaboration between antigen-specific T cells and B cells. Recent experimental results have provided an explanation for the observation that this interaction is restricted by class II molecules of the MHC, although the T cell and B cell respond to different aspects of the stimulating antigen.[431, 432] A variety of cells that express class II MHC molecules can function as antigen-presenting cells, but during T cell–B cell collaboration, it appears to be the B cell that acts as the antigen-presenting

Table 7–9. ADHESION RECEPTORS KNOWN TO MEDIATE ENTRY OF T CELLS INTO INFLAMMATORY SITES

Lymphocyte Receptor	Endothelial Cell Counter-receptor	Regulation of Endothelial Cell Counter-receptor
LFA-1 (CD11a/CD18)	ICAM-1 (CD54); ICAM-2	ICAM-1 (constitutive, increased with cytokine, endotoxin); ICAM-2 (constitutive)
VLA-4 (CD49d/CD29)	VCAM-1	Induced by cytokine
CLA	E-selectin	Induced by cytokine
Unknown ligands	?	?

CLA, cutaneous lymphocyte antigen; VCAM, vascular cell adhesion molecule.

cell (Fig. 7–11). Expression of membrane Ig allows B cells to recognize specific antigen effectively. In this regard, it is important that B cell Ig receptors recognize native antigen without the need for initial enzymatic degradation and, therefore, B cells can directly bind intact antigen molecules. After binding antigen by virtue of surface Ig, antigen is internalized and degraded within the lysosomal compartment. Particular antigenic peptides bind to class II MHC molecules within the lysosome, and the complexes are subsequently expressed on the surface of the B cell, where they can be recognized by CD4+ helper T cells. By virtue of the expression of surface membrane Ig, B cells are 1000 times more effective presenters of their specific antigen than they are for irrelevant antigens.[433] Moreover, engaging surface Ig with antigen may activate the B cell to become a more effective antigen-presenting cell.

After the antigen bound into the peptide-binding cleft of the class II MHC molecules is displayed on the surface of the B cell, it can be recognized by helper T cells. The requirement for helper T cells to recognize peptides bound to self–class II MHC molecules accounts for the genetic restriction of T cell–B cell collaboration. A number of receptors of B cells and counter-receptors on T cells appear to be capable of facilitating the activation of T cells during this interaction. These include LFA-1, ICAM-1, LFA-3, class II MHC, B7/BB1, CD72, and CD40 on the B cell interacting with ICAM-1, LFA-1, CD2, CD4, CD28, CD5, and a newly described 33-kD molecule on the T cell.[25, 110, 407] As a result of these various costimulatory interactions, antigen-specific T cells are activated in an antigen-specific manner restricted by class II MHC molecules.

The activated T cell develops the capacity to stimulate the antigen-presenting B cell.[119] This involves both a contact-dependent event and the action of a variety of cytokines. A similar set of receptor–counter-receptor interactions involved in initial T cell stimulation is likely to play a role in B cell activation as a result of T cell–B cell collaboration. Of note, however, once the T cells have been stimulated, their capacity to activate the antigen-presenting B cells is not restricted by class II MHC molecules but rather by the various receptor–counter-receptor interactions described earlier. Thus, B cell stimulation during T

Table 7–10. CYTOKINES INVOLVED IN HUMAN B
CELL RESPONSIVENESS

ACTIVATION	PROLIFERATION	DIFFERENTIATION
IL-2	IL-2	IL-2
L-BCGF	L-BCGF	IFN-α
IFN-γ	H-BCGF	IFN-γ
IFN-α	TNF-α/LT	IL-1
TNF-α	IL-1	IL-4
IL-1	IFN α	TNF-α/LT
	IFN γ	IL-6
		IL-3

SUPPRESSION OF CYTOKINE SUPPORT OF ACTIVATION
IL-4
TGF-β

L-BCGF, low molecular weight B cell growth factor; H-BCGF, high
molecular weight B cell growth factor; LT, lymphotoxin.

cell–B cell collaboration appears to be antigen nonspecific, influenced and focused by the proximity of
the B cell to the antigen-activated T cell and perhaps
the signals initially provided by the binding of antigen by means of surface Ig.

Stimulation of B cells is a complex process in
which resting B cells are activated to enter the cell
cycle, undergo several rounds of proliferation, and
finally undergo differentiation into high-rate Ig-secreting cells.[190] This sequence of events is tightly
modulated by activating signals provided by the
interaction with stimulated T cells and a series of
cytokines (Table 7–10).

The cytokines regulating B cell responsiveness
originate from a variety of cell types, including cells
that are not members of the immune system such as
fibroblasts and endothelial cells. However, T cells or
their products are necessary for the production of
antibody to many antigens and polyclonal B cell
activators, emphasizing the central role for T cell–
derived cytokines in regulating B cell responses. A
number of these cytokines play distinct roles in the
regulation of B cell responses.

Resting B cells express few receptors for cytokines. Therefore, activation signals that promote the
expression of cytokine receptors are necessary for
the development of B cell cytokine responsiveness.
Features of B cell biology other than receptor display
must also play an important role in governing B cell
cytokine responsiveness, however, because the same
cytokine may exert different effects at various phases
of B cell activation, proliferation, and differentiation.
The nature of these aspects of B cell physiology is
largely unknown.

Clonal expansion of the responding B lymphocyte is an integral component of the immune response. Beyond this, it has been demonstrated that
proliferation is an essential event in the subsequent
differentiation of Ig-secreting cells. After activated B
cells undergo at least one round of cell division,
some differentiate into Ig-secreting cells. It is difficult
to separate proliferation from differentiation of human B cells, because the two processes initially occur
simultaneously in the same cell. Thus, the initial Ig-

secreting cells that appear after the first few rounds
of cell division are themselves rapidly dividing cells.
Continued proliferation of these Ig-secreting cells is
necessary for ongoing Ig production.[434] Only after
many rounds of cell division by the Ig-secreting cells
do nondividing high-rate Ig-producing cells emerge
in cultures stimulated by either pokeweed mitogen
and T cells or *S. aureus* and T cell factors. Therefore,
proliferation and Ig secretion are not two discrete
events but rather processes that occur simultaneously, eventually resulting in the terminal differentiation of high-rate Ig-secreting plasma cells.

After initial activation, proliferation, and differentiation, individual B cells may cease secreting Ig of
one antibody isotype and commence producing antibody encoded for by the same VDJ gene segments
but a different, usually more 3′, heavy chain constant
region gene segment. The usual mechanism for this
isotype switch appears to be deletional recombination
induced or selected for by T cell–derived cytokines.[435]
The isotype of antibody produced may have significant effects on complement activation, microorganism opsonization, transplacental transport, and mucosal surface protection.

A number of cytokines influence human B cell
responses, of which IL-2 appears to play a central
role. After resting B cells are activated, they express
high-avidity receptors for IL-2. As a result, IL-2 can
sustain ongoing proliferation of activated human B
cells.[436–438] In humans, IL-2 also appears to play a
central role in stimulating proliferating B cells to
secrete Ig. Although cytokines such as low-molecular-weight B cell growth factor and TNF-α can support the proliferation of activated B cells in the
absence of IL-2, IL-2 appears to be necessary to
promote differentiation of activated human B cells.
The effect of IL-2 on human B cell differentiation is
not isotype specific. IL-2 can support the secretion
of IgM, IgG, IgA, and IgE by activated B cells.[439]
Several cytokines that cannot induce differentiation
of Ig-secreting cells alone can augment the Ig production induced by IL-2. These include the IFNs, IL-
1, IL-6, TNF-α, and TNF-β. Thus, IL-2 plays an
essential role in the induction of Ig secretion by
human B cells, but the effect of IL-2 can be modified
by the actions of a number of cytokines produced by
a variety of cell types.

IL-4 plays a central role in regulating murine B
cell function, with effects on activation, proliferation,
and differentiation.[440] IL-4 alone stimulates small resting murine B cells to increase their volume and
expression of class II MHC molecules and CD23. In
addition, IL-4 cofacilitates entry into the S phase by
activated B cells. Finally, IL-4 exerts a major influence
on murine B cell differentiation, promoting the production of IgG1 and IgE by appropriately costimu-
lated B cells.[441]

The effect of IL-4 on human B cell responsiveness
is somewhat different. IL-4 does not enhance the
capacity of resting human B cells to respond to
activation stimuli and does not induce cell cycle entry

by human G_0 B cells.[35] IL-4 has only a modest effect on the expression of class II MHC molecules by human B cells but does increase the expression of CD23 and CD40.[29] Expression of IgD, which is decreased on activated B cells, is not affected by IL-4. IL-4, however, can enhance proliferation of human B cells to some but not all stimuli.[442, 443] Thus, the role of IL-4 on human B cell activation or subsequent proliferation is less apparent than that observed with murine B cells. Moreover, most of the effects of IL-4 on these aspects of human B cell responsiveness are not unique and can also be accomplished by other cytokines, especially by IL-2. Finally, in the mouse, most of the effects of IL-4 are antagonized by IFN-γ.[444] However, a more varied effect of IFN-γ on IL-4–promoted responses of human B cells has been noted. Thus, IFN-γ suppresses IL-4–mediated induction of CD23 expression but enhances IL-2–supported proliferation and Ig secretion of anti-IgM–stimulated B cells.[29, 439, 443]

The effects of IL-4 on the differentiation of human B cells are quite complex. Thus, IL-4 can either inhibit or enhance Ig secretion, depending on the mode of B cell stimulation or the time during the activation cascade that it is present.[443] When present during initial activation, IL-4 can inhibit subsequent Ig production by human B cells, whereas it modestly enhances Ig secretion by previously activated B cells. These effects can modulate the production of all Ig isotypes.[439]

In the mouse, IL-4 exerts an isotype-specific effect on the differentiation of activated murine B cells, selectively inducing the secretion of IgG1 and IgE and decreasing the production of IgM, IgG3, and IgG2a.[441] The effect on IgG1 and IgE secretion is mediated by promoting Ig heavy chain switching.[445, 446]

In some situations, IL-4 may enhance human IgE and IgG4 production.[446–449] Recent data suggest that the capacity of IL-4 to promote IgE production may be most noteworthy when the cells are simultaneously stimulated with a monoclonal antibody to CD40.[36, 38]

The major role of IL-6 appears to be on the promotion of B cell differentiation.[450] IL-6 cannot stimulate resting B cells that do not express IL-6 receptors.[451] However, IL-6 is most active on terminal stages of B cell differentiation.[452] Activated B cells secrete IL-6 and may therefore amplify their ability to produce Ig.[453] The effect of IL-6 is not isotype specific.

IL-5 is produced by activated T cells and by murine mast cells.[208–210] It was first described as a murine B cell differentiation factor and was found to induce the CD25 component of the IL-2 receptor on murine B cells.[215] IL-5, like IL-4, is produced by the TH-2 subset of murine helper T cells.[208] In addition to its effects on murine B cells, IL-5 also promotes eosinophil growth and differentiation and may modulate T cell responses. High- and low-avidity receptors for IL-5 have been identified on murine cells of

the B cell lineage.[454] In humans, IL-5 is known to enhance the growth and differentiation of eosinophils.[209] However, the same recombinant IL-5 had no effect on the proliferation of human B cells.[455] IL-5 has been reported to enhance the production of IgA by LPS-stimulated murine B cells.[456] The action of IL-5 on murine IgA secretion appears not to relate to the induction of an isotype switch but rather to expansion and enhanced secretion of B cells already expressing surface IgA.[457, 458] This effect appears to be analogous to the effect of IL-5 on the secretion of other Ig isotypes and therefore is not specific for IgA.[459] It remains unclear whether IL-5 enhances the secretion of IgA by human B cells.[210]

A number of other cytokines can amplify the proliferation of human B cells, including IL-1, TNF-α, lymphotoxin, IFN-γ, and IFN-α.[190] Low-molecular-weight B cell growth factor is a 12-kD product of activated T cells that can sustain the proliferation of activated T cells and enhance Ig production by activated B cells stimulated by IL-2.[460] TGF-β inhibits the growth and differentiation of human B cells.[461, 462] TGF-β has been reported to promote the secretion of IgA by activated murine B cells[463] by promoting Ig isotype switch to IgA. A similar effect of TGF-β on production of IgA by human B cells has recently been reported.[464]

In summary, the regulation of antibody responses is dependent on the delivery of both contact-dependent and cytokine-mediated signals. The complex nature of these regulatory events is only beginning to be appreciated.

References

1. Roitt, I. M., Torrigiani, G., Greaves, M. F., Brostoff, J., and Playfair, J. H.: The cellular basis of immunological responses. Lancet 2:367, 1969.
2. Loken, M., Shah, V., Dattilio, K., and Civin, C.: Flow cytometric analysis of human bone marrow: II. Normal B cell development. Blood 70:1316, 1987.
3. Uckun, F. M.: Regulation of human B-cell ontogeny. Blood 76:1908, 1990.
4. Korsmeyer, S. J., Hieter, P. A., Ravetch, J. V., Poplack, D. G., Waldmann, T. A., and Leder, P.: Developmental hierarchy of immunoglobulin gene rearrangements in human leukemic pre B cells. Proc. Natl. Acad. Sci. U.S.A. 78:7096, 1981.
5. Clark, E. A., and Ledbetter, J. A.: Structure, function and genetics of human B cell associated surface molecules. Adv. Cancer Res. 52:81, 1989.
6. Abney, E. R., Cooper, M. D., Kearney, J. F., Lawton, A. R., and Parkhouse, R. M. E.: Sequential expression of immunoglobulin on developing B lymphocytes: A systematic survey that suggests a model for the generation of immunoglobulin isotype diversity. J. Immunol. 120:2041, 1978.
7. Nadler, L., Anderson, K., Marti, G., Bates, M., Park, E., Daley, J., and Schlossman, S.: B4, a human B lymphocyte-associated antigen expressed on normal, mitogen-activated, and malignant B lymphocytes. J. Immunol. 131:244, 1983.
8. Stamenkovic, I., and Seed, B.: CD19, the earliest differentiation antigen of the B cell lineage, bears three extracellular immunoglobulin-like domains and an Epstein-Barr virus–related cytoplasmic tail. J. Exp. Med. 168:1205, 1988.
9. Pezzutto, A., Dorken, B., Rabinovitch, P., Ledbetter, J., Moldenhauer, G., and Clark, E.: CD19 monoclonal antibody, HD37 inhibits anti-immunoglobulin–induced B cell activation and proliferation. J. Immunol. 138:2793, 1987.
9a. Carter, R. H., and Feuron, D. T.: CD19: Lowering the threshold for antigen receptor stimulation of B lymphocytes. Science 256:105, 1992.

10. Stashenko, P., Nadler, L. M., Hardy, R., and Schlossman, S. F.: Characterization of a human B lymphocyte specific antigen. J. Immunol. 125:1678, 1980.

11. Rosenthal, P., Rimm, I. J., Umiel, T., Griffin, J. D., Osathanondh, R., Schlossman, S. F., and Nadler, L. M.: Ontogeny of human hematopoietic cells: Analysis utilizing monoclonal antibodies. J. Immunol. 131:232, 1983.

12. Einfield, D. A., Brown, J. P., Valentine, M. A., Clark, E. A., and Ledbetter, J. A.: Molecular cloning of the human CD20 receptor predicts a hydrophobic protein with multiple transmembrane domains. EMBO J. 7:711, 1988.

13. Clark, E., Shu, G., and Ledbetter, J.: Role of the Bp35 cell surface polypeptide in human B cell activation. Proc. Natl. Acad. Sci. U.S.A. 82:1766, 1985.

14. Nadler, L. M., Stashhenko, P., Hardy, R., Van Agthoven, A., Terhorst, C., and Schlossman, S. F.: Characterization of a human B cell specific antigen (B2) distinct from B1. J. Immunol. 126:1941, 1981.

15. Fingeroth, J. D., Weis, J. J., Tedder, T. F., Strominger, J. L., Biro, P. A., and Fearon, D. T.: Epstein-Barr virus receptor of human B lymphocytes is the C3d receptor CR2. Proc. Natl. Acad. Sci. U.S.A. 81:4510, 1984.

16. Moore, M. D., Cooper, N. R., Tack, B. F., and Nemerow, G. R.: Molecular cloning of the cDNA encoding the Epstein-Barr virus/C3d receptor (complement receptor type 2) of human B lymphocytes. Proc. Natl. Acad. Sci. U.S.A. 84:9194, 1987.

17. Nemerow, G. R., McNaughton, M. E., and Cooper, N. R.: Binding of monoclonal antibody to the Epstein Barr Virus (EBV) CR2 receptor induces activation and differentiation of human B lymphocytes. J. Immunol. 135:3068, 1985.

18. Boue, D., and Lebien, T.: Structural characterization of the human B lymphocyte–restricted differentiation antigen CD22: Comparison with CD21 (Complement receptor type 2/Epstein-Barr Virus receptor). J. Immunol. 140:192, 1988.

19. Stamenkovic, I., and Seed, B.: The B cell antigen CD22 mediates monocyte and erythrocyte adhesion. Nature 345:74, 1990.

20. Pezzutto, D., Modenhauer, G., and Clark, E.: Amplification of human B cell activation by a monoclonal antibody to the B cell–specific antigen CD22, Bp130/140. J. Immunol. 138:98, 1987.

21. Von Hoegen, I., Nakayama, E., and Parnes, J. R.: Identification of a human protein homologous to the mouse Lyb-2 B cell differentiation antigen and sequence of the corresponding cDNA. J. Immunol. 144:4870, 1990.

22. Dorkin, B., Moller, P., Pezzutto, A., Schwartz-Albiez, R., and Moldenhauer, G.: B cells: CD72. In Knapp, W., Dorken, B., Gilks, W. R., Rieber, E. P., Schmidt, R. E., Stein, H., and von dem Borne, A. E. G. Kr. (eds.): Leukocyte Typing IV. Oxford, Oxford Press, 1989, p. 99.

23. Nakayama, E., Von Hoegen, I., and Parnes, J. R.: Sequence of the Lyb-2 B cell differentiation antigen defines a gene superfamily of receptors with inverted membrane orientation. Proc. Natl. Acad. Sci. U.S.A. 86:1352, 1989.

24. Kamal, M., Katira, A., and Gordon, J.: Stimulation of B lymphocytes via CD72 (human Lyb-2). Eur. J. Immunol. 21:1419, 1991.

25. Van de Velde, H., Von Hoegen, I., Luo, W., Parnes, J. R., and Thielemans, K.: The B cell surface protein CD72/Lyb-2 is the ligand for CD5. Nature 351:662, 1991.

26. Yukawa, K., Kikutani, H., Owaki, H., Yamasaki, K., Yokota, A., Nakamura, H., Barsumian, E. L., Hardy, R. R., Suemura, M., and Kishimoto, T.: A B cell-specific differentiation antigen, CD23, is a receptor for IgE (FcεR) on lymphocytes. J. Immunol. 138:2576, 1987.

27. Kikutani, H., Inui, S., Sato, R., Barsumain, E. L., Owaki, H., Yamasaki, K., Kaisho, T., Uchibayashi, N., Hardy, R. R., Hirano, T., Tsunasawa, S., Sakiyama, F., Suemura, M., and Kishimoto, T.: Molecular structure of human lymphocyte receptor for immunoglobulin E. Cell 47:657, 1986.

28. Thorley-Lawson, D. A., Nadler, L. M., Bhan, A. K., and Schooley, R. T.: Blast-2 [EBVCS], an early cell surface marker of human B cell activation, is superinduced by Epstein Barr virus. J. Immunol. 134:3007, 1985.

29. Defrance, T., Aubry, J., Rousset, F., Vanbervliet, B., Bonnefoy, J., Arai, N., Takebe, Y., Yokota, T., Lee, F., and Arai, K.: Human recombinant interleukin 4 induces Fc epsilon receptors (CD23) on normal human B lymphocytes. J. Exp. Med. 165:1459, 1987.

30. Gordon, J., Webb, A., Walker, L., Guy, G., and Rowe, M.: Evidence for an association between CD23 and the receptor for a low molecular weight B cell growth factor. Eur. J. Immunol. 16:1627, 1986.

31. Paulie, S., Rosen, A., Ehlin-Henriksson, B., Braesch-Andersen, S., Jakobson, E., Koho, H., and Perlmann, P.: The human B lymphocyte and carcinoma antigen, CDw40, is a phosphoprotein involved in growth signal transduction. J. Immunol. 142:590, 1989.

32. Stamenkovic, I., Clark, E. A., and Seed, B.: A B lymphocyte molecule related to the nerve growth factor receptor and induced by cytokines in carcinomas. EMBO J. 8:1403, 1989.

33. Braesch-Andersen, S., Paulie, S., Koho, H., Nika, H., Aspenstrom, P., and Perlmann, P.: Biochemical characteristics and partial amino acid sequence of the receptor-like human B cell and carcinoma antigen CDw40. J. Immunol. 142:562, 1989.

34. Smith, C. A., Davis, T., Anderson, D., Solam, L., Beckmann, M. P., Jerzey, R., Dower, S. K., Cosman, D., and Goodwin, R. G.: A receptor for tumor necrosis factor defines an unusual family of cellular and viral proteins. Science 248:1019, 1990.

35. Gordon, J., Millsum, M., Guy, G., and Ledbetter, J.: Resting B lymphocytes can be triggered directly through the CDw40 (Bp50) antigen: A comparison with IL-4–mediated signaling. J. Immunol. 140:1125, 1988.

36. Jabara, H. H., Fu, S. M., Geha, R., and Vercelli, D.: CD40 and IgE: Synergism between anti-CD40 monoclonal antibody and interleukin 4 in the induction of IgE synthesis by highly purified human B cells. J. Exp. Med. 172:1861, 1990.

37. Bancherau, J., de Paoli, P., Valle, A., Garcia, E., and Rousset, F.: Long-term human B cell lines dependent on IL-4 and anti-CD40. Science 251:70, 1991.

38. Zhang, K., Clark, E. A., and Saxon, A.: CD40 stimulation provides an IFN-γ–independent and IL-4–dependent differentiation signal directly to human B cells for IgE production. J. Immunol. 146:1836, 1991.

39. Kipps, T. J.: The CD5 B cell. Adv. Immunol. 47:117, 1989.

40. Hardy, R. R., and Hayakawa, K.: Development and physiology of Ly-1B and its human homologue, LEU-1B. Immunol. Rev. 93:54, 1986.

41. Hayakawa, K., Hardy, R. R., Honda, M., Herzenberg, L. A., Steinberg, A. D., and Herzenberg, L. A.: Ly-1 B cells: Functionally distinct lymphocytes that secrete IgM autoantibodies. Proc. Natl. Acad. Sci. U.S.A. 81:2494, 1984.

42. Hardy, R. R., Hayakawa, K., Shimizu, M., Yamasaki, K., and Kishimoto, T.: Rheumatoid factor secretion from human Leu-1+ B cells. Science 236:81, 1987.

43. Suzuki, N., Sakane, T., and Engelman, E. G.: Anti-DNA antibody production by CD5+ and CD5− B cells of patients with systemic lupus erythematosus. J. Clin. Invest. 85:238, 1990.

44. Vernino, L. A., Pisetsky, D. S., and Lipsky, P. E.: Analysis of the expression of CD5 by human B cells and correlation with functional activity. Cell. Immunol. 139:185, 1992.

45. Aruffo, A., and Seed, B.: Molecular cloning of two CD7 (T cell leukemia antigen) cDNAs by a COS cell expression system. EMBO J. 6:3313, 1987.

46. Haynes, B., Kurtzberg, J., Lobach, D., Denning, S., and Singer, K.: Phenotypic characterization of T cell precursors during human development. Fed. Proc. 46:768, 1987.

47. Haynes, B. F., Einenbarth, G. S., and Fauci, A. S.: Human lymphocyte antigens: Production of a monoclonal antibody that defines functional thymus-derived lymphocyte subsets. Proc. Natl. Acad. Sci. U.S.A. 76:5829, 1979.

48. Lazarovits, A. I., and Karsh, J.: Decreased expression of CD7 occurs in rheumatoid arthritis. Clin. Exp. Immunol. 72:470, 1988.

49. Heinrich, G., Gram, H., Kocher, H. P., Schreier, M. H., Ryffel, B., Akbar, A., Amlot, P. L., and Junossy, G.: Characterization of a human T cell–specific chimeric antibody (CD7) with human constant and mouse variable regions. J. Immunol. 143:3589, 1989.

50. Howard, F. D., Ledbetter, J. A., Wong, J., Bieber, C. P., Stinson, E. B., and Herzenberg, L. A.: A human T lymphocyte differentiation marker defined by monoclonal antibodies that block E rosette formation. J. Immunol. 126:2117, 1981.

51. Sewell, W. A., Brown, M. H., Dunne, J., Owen, M. J., and Crumpton, M. J.: Molecular cloning of the human T-lymphocyte surface CD2 (T11) antigen. Proc. Natl. Acad. Sci. U.S.A. 83:8718, 1986.

52. Jones, N. H., Clabby, M. L., Dialynas, D. P., Huang, H. -J., Herzenberg, L. A., and Strominger, J. L.: Isolation of complementary DNA clones encoding the human lymphocyte glycoprotein T1/Leu 1. Nature 323:346, 1986.

53. Siliciano, R. F., Pratt, J. C., Schmidt, R. E., Ritz, J., and Reinherz, E. L.: Activation of cytolytic T lymphocyte and natural killer cell function through the T11 sheep erythrocyte binding protein. Nature 317:428, 1985.

54. Allison, J. P., and Lanier, L. L.: Structure, function and serology of the T-cell antigen receptor complex. Annu. Rev. Immunol. 5:503, 1987.

55. Yanagi, Y., Yoshikai, Y., Leggett, K., Clark, S., Aleksander, I., and Mak, T.: A human T cell–specific cDNA clone encodes a protein having extensive homology to immunoglobulin chains. Nature 308:145, 1984.

56. Hedrik, S., Cohen, D., Nielsen, E., and Davis, M.: Isolation of cDNA clones encoding T-cell–specific membrane-associated proteins. Nature 308:149, 1984.

57. Hedrik, S., Nielsen, E., Kavaler, J., Cohen, D., and Davis, M.: Sequence relationships between putative T-cell receptor polypeptides and immunoglobulins. Nature 308:153, 1984.

58. Chien, Y., Becker, D., Lindstein, T., Okamura, M., Cohen, D., and Davis, M.: A third type of murine T-cell receptor gene. Nature 312:31, 1984.

59. Saito, H., Kranz, D., Takagaki, Y., Hayday, A., Eisen, H., and Tonegawa, S.: A third rearranged and expressed gene in a clone of cytotoxic T lymphocytes. Nature 312:36, 1984.

60. Chien, Y. H., Isashima, M., Kaplan, K. B., Elliot, J. F., and Davis, M. M.: A new T cell receptor gene located within the alpha locus and expressed early in T cell differentiation. Nature 327:677, 1987.
61. Ashwell, J. D., and Klausner, R. D.: Genetic and mutational analysis of the T-cell antigen receptor. Annu. Rev. Immunol. 8:139, 1990.
62. Parnes, J. R.: Molecular analysis and function of CD4 and CD8. Adv. Immunol. 44:265, 1989.
63. LeFranc, M. P., Forster, A., and Rabbitts, T. H.: Genetic polymorphism and exon changes of the constant regions of the human T-cell rearranging gene gamma. Proc. Natl. Acad. Sci. U.S.A. 83:9596, 1986.
64. Davis, M. M., and Bjorkman, P. J.: T-cell antigen receptor genes and T-cell recognition. Nature 334:395, 1988.
65. Borst, J., Alexander, S., Elder, J., and Terhorst, C.: The T3 complex on human T lymphocytes involves four structurally distinct glycoproteins. J. Biol. Chem. 258:5135, 1983.
66. Kanellopoulos, J. M., Wigglesworth, N. M., Owen, M. J., and Crumpton, M. J.: Biosynthesis and molecular nature of the T3 antigen of human T lymphocytes. EMBO J. 2:1807, 1983.
67. Samelson, L. E., Harford, J. B., and Klausner, R. D.: Identification of the components of the murine T cell antigen receptor complex. Cell 43:223, 1985.
68. Baniyash, M., Garcia-Morales, P., Bonifacino, J. S., Samelson, L. E., and Klausner, R. D.: Disulfide linkage of the ζ and η chains of the T cell receptor: Possible identification of two structural classes of receptors. J. Biol. Chem. 263:9874, 1988.
69. Van den Elsen, P., Shepley, B., Borst, J., Coligan, J. E., Markham, A. F., Orkin, S., and Terhorst, C.: Isolation of cDNA clones encoding the 20K T3 glycoprotein of human T cell receptor complex. Nature 312:413, 1984.
70. Gold, D. P., Puck, J. M., Petty, C. L., Cho, M., Coligan, J., Woody, J., and Terhorst, C.: Isolation of cDNA clones encoding the 20K nonglycosylated polypeptide chain of the human T cell receptor/T3 complex. Nature 321:431, 1986.
71. Krissansen, G. W., Owen, M. J., Verbi, W., and Crumpton, M. J.: Primary structure of the T3γ subunit of the T3/T cell antigen receptor complex deduced from cDNA sequences: Evolution of the T3 γ and δ subunits. EMBO J. 5:1799, 1986.
72. Weissman, A. M., Hou, D., Orloff, D. G., Modi, W. S., Seuanez, H., O'Brien, S. J., and Klausner, R. D.: Molecular cloning and chromosomal localization of the human T cell receptor zeta chain: Distinction from the molecular CD3 complex. Proc. Natl. Acad. Sci. U.S.A. 85:9709, 1988.
73. Clayton, L. K., D'Adamio, L. D., Howard, F. D., Sieh, M., Hussey, R. E., Koyasu, S., and Reinherz, E. L.: CD3η and CD3ζ are alternatively spliced products of a common genetic locus and are transcriptionally and/or post transcriptionally regulated during T cell development. Proc. Natl. Acad. Sci. U.S.A. 88:5202, 1991.
74. Clayton, L. K., Bauer, A., Jin, Y. -J., D'Adamio, L., Koyasu, S., and Reinherz, E. L.: Characterization of thymus-derived lymphocytes expressing Tiα-β CD3γδεζ-ζ, Tiα-β CD3γδεη-η or Tiα-β CD3γδεζ-ζ/ζ-η antigen receptor isoforms: Analysis by gene transfection. J. Exp. Med. 172:1243, 1990.
75. Alarcon, B., Ley, S. C., Sanchez-Madrid, F., Blumberg, R. S., Lee, S. T., Fresno, M., and Terhorst, C.: The CD3-γ and CD3-δ subunit of the T cell antigen receptor can be expressed within distinct functional TCR/CD3 complexes. EMBO J. 10:903, 1991.
76. Meuer, S. C., Fitzgerald, K. A., Hussey, R. E., Hodgdon, J. C., Schlossman, S. F., and Reinherz, E.: Clonotypic structures involved in antigen-specific human T cell function: relationship to the T3 molecular complex. J. Exp. Med. 157:705, 1983.
77. Oettgen, H. C., Kappler, J., Tax, W. J. M., and Terhorst, C.: Characterization of the two heavy chains of the T3 complex on the surface of human T lymphocytes. J. Biol. Chem. 259:12039, 1984.
78. Brenner, M. B., Trowbridge, I. S., and Strominger, J. L.: Cross-linking of human T cell receptor proteins: association between the T cell idiotype β subunit and the T3 glycoprotein heavy subunit. Cell 40:183, 1985.
79. Weiss, A., and Stobo, J. D.: Requirement for the coexpression of T3 and the T cell antigen receptor on a malignant human T cell line. J. Exp. Med. 160:1284, 1984.
80. Ohashi, P. S., Mak, T. W., Van den Elsen, P., Yanagi, Y., Yoshikai, Y., Calman, A. F., Terhorst, C., Stobo, J. D., and Weiss, A.: Reconstitution of an active surface T3/T-cell antigen receptor by DNA transfer. Nature 316:606, 1985.
81. Manolios, N., Bonifacino, J. S., and Klausner, R. D.: Transmembrane helical interactions and the assembly of the T cell antigen receptor complex. Science 249:274, 1990.
82. Irving, B. A., and Weiss, A.: The cytoplasmic domain of the T cell receptor ζ chain is sufficient to couple to receptor associated signal transduction pathways. Cell 64:891, 1991.
83. Springer, T. A., Dustin, M. L., Kishimoto, T. K., and Marlin, S. D.: The lymphocyte function-associated LFA-1, CD2, and LFA-3 molecules: Cell adhesion receptors of the immune system. Annu. Rev. Immunol. 5:223, 1987.
84. Meuer, S. C., Hussey, R. E., Fabbi, M., Fox, D., Acuto, O., Fitzgerald, K. A., Hodgdon, J. C., Protentis, J. P., Schlossman, S. F., and Reinherz, E.: An alternative pathway of T-cell activation: A functional role for the 50 kd T11 sheep erythrocyte receptor protein. Cell 36:897, 1984.
85. Geppert, T. D., and Lipsky, P. E.: Activation of T lymphocytes by immobilized monoclonal antibodies to CD3: Regulatory influences of monoclonal antibodies to additional T cell surface determinants. J. Clin. Invest. 81:1497, 1988.
86. Littman, D. R.: The structure of the CD4 and CD8 genes. Annu. Rev. Immunol. 5:561, 1987.
87. Maddon, P. J., Littman, D. R., Godfrey, M., Maddon, D. E., Chess, L., and Axel, R.: The isolation of nucleotide sequence of a cDNA encoding the T cell surface protein T4: A new member of the immunoglobulin gene family. Cell 42:93, 1985.
88. Szabo, G., Miller, C. L., and Kodys, K.: Antigen presentation by the CD4 positive monocyte subset. J. Leukoc. Biol. 47:111, 1990.
89. Biddison, W. E., Rao, P. E., Talle, M. A., Goldstein, G., and Shaw, S.: Possible involvement of the OKT4 molecule in T cell recognition of class II HLA antigens. J. Exp. Med. 156:1065, 1982.
90. Engelman, E. G., Benike, C. J., Grumet, C., and Evans, R. L.: Activation of human T lymphocyte subsets: Helper and suppressor/cytotoxic T cells recognize and respond to distinct histocompatibility antigens. J. Immunol. 127:2124, 1981.
91. Swain, S. L.: T cell subsets and the recognition of MHC class. Immunol. Rev. 74:129, 1983.
92. Doyle, C., and Strominger, J. L.: Interaction between CD4 and class II MHC molecules mediates cell adhesion. Nature 330:256, 1987.
93. Marrack, P., Endres, R., Schimonkevitz, R., Zlotnick, A., Dialynas, D., Fitch, F., and Kappler, J.: The major histocompatibility complex–restricted antigen receptor on T cells: II. Role of the L3T4 product. J. Exp. Med. 158:1077, 1983.
94. Wassmer, P., Chan, C., Lozdberg, L., and Shevach, E. M.: Role of the L3T4-antigen in T cell activation: II. Inhibition of T cell activation by monoclonal anti-L3T4 antibodies in the absence of accessory cells. J. Immunol. 135:2237, 1985.
95. Wacholtz, M. C., Patel, S. S., and Lipsky, P. E.: Patterns of costimulation of T cell clones by cross-linking CD3, CD4/CD8 and class I MHC molecules. J. Immunol 142:4201, 1989.
96. Dalgleish, A. G., Beverly, P. C. L., Clapham, P. R., Crawford, D. H., Greaves, M. F., and Weiss, R. A.: The CD4 (T4) antigen is an essential component of the receptor for the AIDS retrovirus. Nature 312:763, 1984.
97. Maddon, P. J., Dalgeish, A. G., McDougal, J. S., Clapham, P. R., Weiss, R. A., and Axel, R.: The T4 gene encodes the AIDS virus receptor and is expressed in the immune system and the brain. Cell 47:333, 1986.
98. Veillette, A., Bookman, M. A., Horak, E. M., and Bolen, J. B.: The CD4 and the CD8 T cell surface antigens are associated with the internal membrane tyrosine protein-kinase p56lck. Cell 55:301, 1988.
99. Barber, E. K., Dasgupta, J. D., Schlossman, S. F., Trevillyan, J. M., and Rudd, C. D.: The CD4 and CD8 antigens are coupled to a protein-tyrosine kinase (p56lck) that phosphorylates the CD3 complex. Proc. Natl. Acad. Sci. U.S.A. 86:3277, 1989.
100. Turner, J. M., Brodsky, M. H., Irving, B. A., Levin, S. D., Perlmutter, R. M., and Littman, D. R.: Interaction of the unique N-terminal region of tyrosine kinase p56lck with cytoplasmic domains of CD4 and CD8 is mediated by cysteine motifs. Cell 60:755, 1990.
101. Glaichenhaus, N., Shastri, N., Littman, D. R., and Turner, J. M.: Requirement for association of p56lck with CD4 in antigen specific signal transduction in T cells. Cell 64:511, 1991.
102. Littman, D. R., Thomas, Y., Maddon, P. J., Chess, L., and Axel, R.: The isolation and sequence of the gene encoding T8: A molecule defining functional classes of T lymphocytes. Cell 40:237, 1985.
103. Gorman, S. D., Sun, Y. H., Zamoyska, R., and Parnes, J. R.: Molecular linkage of the Ly-3 and Ly-2 genes: Requirement for Ly-2 and Ly-3 surface expression. J. Immunol. 140:3646, 1988.
104. Baume, D. M., Caligiuni, M. A., Manley, T. J., Daley, J. F., and Ritz, J.: Differential expression of CD8 alpha and CD8 beta associated with MHC-restricted and non–MHC-restricted cytolytic effector cells. Cell Immunol. 131:352, 1990.
105. Engleman, E. G., Benike, C. J., Grumet, C., and Evans, R. L.: Activation of human T lymphocyte subsets: Helper and suppressor/cytotoxic T cells recognize and respond to distinct histocompatibility antigens. J. Immunol. 127:2124, 1981.
106. Meuer, S. C., Schlossman, S. F., and Reinherz, E.: Clonal analysis of human cytotoxic T lymphocytes T4+ and T8+ effector T cells recognize products of different major histocompatibility complex regions. Proc. Natl. Acad. Sci. U.S.A. 79:4395, 1982.
107. Norment, A. M., Salter, R. D., Parham, P., Engelhard, V. H., and Littman, D. R.: Cell-cell adhesion mediated by CD8 and MHC class I molecules. Nature 336:79, 1988.
108. Chalupny, N. J., Ledbetter, J. A., and Kavathas, P.: Association of CD8 with p56lck is required for early T cell signalling events. EMBO J. 10:1201, 1991.

109. Aruffo, A., and Seed, B.: Molecular cloning of a CD28 cDNA by a high efficiency COS cell expression system. Proc. Natl. Acad. Sci. U.S.A. 84:8573, 1987.
110. Linsley, P. S., Clark, E. A., and Ledbetter, J. A.: T-cell antigen CD28 mediates adhesion with B cells by interacting with activation antigen B7/BB1. Proc. Natl. Acad. Sci. U.S.A. 87:5031, 1990.
111. Geppert, T. D., Davis, L. S., Gur, H., Wacholtz, M. C., and Lipsky, P. E.: Accessory cell signals involved in T cell activation. Immunol. Rev. 117:5, 1990.
112. Babbitt, B. P., Allen, P. M., Matsueda, G., Haber, E., and Unanue, E. R.: Binding of immunogenic peptides to Ia histocompatibility molecules. Natures 317:359, 1985.
113. Buus, S., Colon, S., Smith, C., Freed, J. H., Miles, C., and Grey, H. M.: Interaction between a "processed" ovalbumin peptide and Ia molecules. Proc. Natl. Acad. Sci. U.S.A. 83:3968, 1986.
114. Guillet, J. -G., Lai, M. -Z., Briner, T. J., Smith, J. A., and Gefter, M. L.: Interaction of peptide antigens and class II major histocompatibility complex antigens. Nature 324:260, 1986.
115. Townsend, A. R. M., Rothbard, J., Gotch, F. M., Bahadur, G., Wraith, D., and McMichael, A. J.: The epitopes of influenza nucleoprotein recognized by cytotoxic T lymphocytes can be defined with short synthetic peptides. Cell 44:959, 1986.
116. Benjamin, R., and Parham, P.: Guilt by association: HLA-B27 and ankylosing spondylitis. Immunol. Today 11:137, 1990.
117. Morrison, L. A., Lukacher, A. E., Braciale, V. L., Fan, D. P., and Braciale, T. J.: Differences in antigen presentation to MHC class I and class II restricted influenza virus–specific cytolytic T lymphocyte clones. J. Exp. Med. 163:903, 1986.
118. Reinherz, E. L., Kung, P. C., Goldstein, G., and Schlossman, S. F.: Separation of functional subsets of human T cells by a monoclonal antibody. Proc. Natl. Acad. Sci. U.S.A. 76:4061, 1979.
119. Hirohata, S., Jelinek, D. F., and Lipsky, P. E.: T cell–dependent activation of B cell proliferation and differentiation by immobilized monoclonal antibodies to CD3. J. Immunol. 140:3726, 1988.
120. Woodcock, J., Wofsy, D., Eriksson, E., Scott, J. H., and Seaman, W. E.: Rejection of skin grafts and generation of cytotoxic T cells by mice depleted of L3T4+ cells. Transplantation 42:636, 1986.
121. Waldor, M. K., Sriram, S., Hardy, R., Herzenberg, L. A., Herzenberg, L. A., Lanier, L., Lim, M., and Steinman, L.: Reversal of experimental allergic encephalomyelitis with monoclonal antibody to a T-cell subset marker. Science 227:415, 1985.
122. Shizuru, J. A., Taylor-Edwards, C., Banks, B. A., Gregory, A. K., and Fathman, G.: Immunotherapy of the nonobese diabetic mouse: Treatment with an antibody to T-helper lymphocytes. Science 240:659, 1988.
123. Wofsy, D., and Seaman, W. E.: Successful treatment of autoimmunity in NZB/NZW F₁ mice with monoclonal antibody to L3T4. J. Exp. Med. 161:378, 1985.
124. Ranges, G. E., Sriram, S., and Cooper, S. M.: Prevention of type II collagen-induced arthritis by in vivo treatment with anti-L3T4. J. Exp. Med. 162:1105, 1985.
125. Kong, Y. M., Waldmann, H., Cobbold, S. P., Giraldo, A. A., and Fuller, B. E.: Altered pathogenic mechanisms in murine autoimmune thyroiditis after depletion in vivo of L3T4+ and Lyt2+ cells. Immunobiology (Suppl.) 3:30, 1987.
126. Mosman, T. R., Cherwinski, H., Bond, M. W., Giedlin, M. A., and Coffman, R. L.: Two types of murine helper T cell clone: I. Definition according to profiles of lymphokine activities and secreted proteins. J. Immunol. 136:2348, 1986.
127. Street, N. E., and Mosmann, T. R.: Functional diversity of T lymphocytes due to secretion of different cytokine patterns. FASEB J. 5:171, 1991.
128. Patel, S. S., Duby, A. D., Thiele, D. L., and Lipsky, P. E.: Phenotypic and functional characterization of human T cell clones. J. Immunol. 141:3726, 1988.
129. Akbar, A. N., Salmon, M., and Janossy, G.: The synergy between naive and memory T cells during activation. Immunol. Today 12:184, 1991.
130. Sanders, M. E., Makgoba, M. W., and Shaw, S.: Human naive and memory T cells: Reinterpretation of helper-inducer and suppressor-inducer subsets. Immunol. Today 9:195, 1988.
131. Cerotini, J. C., and MacDonald, H. R.: The cellular basis of T-cell memory. Annu. Rev. Immunol. 7:77, 1989.
132. Zinkernagel, R. M., and Rosenthal, K. L.: Experiments and speculation on antiviral specificity of T and B cells. Immunol. Rev. 58:132, 1981.
133. Oldstone, M. B. A., Nerenberg, M., Southern, P., Price, J., and Lewicki, H.: Virus infection triggers insulin-dependent diabetes mellitus in a transgenic model: Role of anti-self (virus) immune response. Cell 65:319, 1991.
134. Nabholz, M., and MacDonald, H. R.: Cytolytic T lymphocytes. Annu. Rev. Immunol. 1:273, 1983.
135. Mizuochi, T., Hugin, A. W., Morse, H. C., III, Singer, A., and Buller, R. M.: Role of lymphokine-secreting CD8+ T cells in cytotoxic T lymphocyte responses against vaccinia virus. J. Immunol. 142:270, 1989.
136. Podack, E. R., and Konigsberg, P. J.: Cytolytic T cell granules: isolation, structural, biochemical, and functional characterization. J. Exp. Med. 160:695, 1984.
137. Podack, E. R., Young, J. D. -E., and Cohn, Z. A.: Isolation and biochemical and functional characterization of perforin 1 from cytolytic T-cell granules. Proc. Natl. Acad. Sci. U.S.A. 82:8629, 1985.
138. Gershenfeld, H. K., and Weissman, I. L.: Cloning of a cDNA for a T cell–specific serine protease from a cytotoxic T lymphocyte. Science 232:854, 1986.
139. Lobe, C. G., Finlay, B. B., Paranchych, W., Paetkau, V. H., and Bleackley, R. C.: Novel serine proteases encoded by two cytotoxic T lymphocyte–specific genes. Science 232:858, 1986.
140. Masson, D., and Tschopp, J.: A family of serine esterases in lytic granules of cytolytic T lymphocytes. Cell 49:679, 1987.
141. Young, J. D. -E., and Cohn, Z. A.: Cell-mediated killing: A common mechanism? Cell 46:641, 1986.
142. Tschopp, J., and Nabholz, M.: Perforin-mediated target cell lysis by cytolytic T lymphocytes. Annu. Rev. Immunol. 8:279, 1990.
143. Lanier, L. L., and Weiss, A.: Presence of Ti(WT31)-negative T lymphocytes in normal blood and thymus. Nature 324:268, 1986.
144. Lanier, L. L., Federspiel, N. A., Ruitenberg, J. J., Phillips, J. H., Allison, J. P., Littman, D., and Weiss, A.: The T cell antigen receptor complex expression on normal peripheral blood CD4−, CD8− T lymphocytes. J. Exp. Med. 165:1076, 1987.
145. Janeway, C. A., Jones, B., and Hayday, A.: Specificity and function of T cells bearing γδ receptors. Immunol. Today 9:73, 1988.
146. Bluestone, J. A., Cron, R. Q., Cotterman, M., Houlden, B. A., and Matis, L. A.: Structure and specificity of T cell receptor gamma/delta on major histocompatibility complex antigen–specific CD3+, CD4−, CD8− T lymphocytes. J. Exp. Med. 168:1899, 1988.
147. Kabelitz, D., Bender, A., Schondelmaier, S., Schoel, B., and Kaufmann, S. H.: A large fraction of human peripheral blood gamma/delta+ T cells is activated by Mycobacterium tuberculosis but not by its 65-kD heat shock protein. J. Exp. Med. 171:667, 1990.
148. Born, W., Hall, L., Dallas, A., Boymel, J., Shinnick, T., Young, D., Brennan, P., and O'Brien, R.: Recognition of a peptide antigen by heat shock-reactive gamma-delta T lymphocytes. Science 249:67, 1991.
149. Patel, S. S., Wacholtz, M. C., Duby, A. D., Thiele, D. L., and Lipsky, P. E.: Analysis of the functional capabilities of CD3+CD4−CD8− and CD3+CD4+CD8+ human T cell clones. J. Immunol. 143:1108, 1989.
150. Guy-Grand, D., Cerf-Bensussan, N., Malissen, B., Malassis-Seris, M., Briottet, C., and Vassalli, P.: Two gut intraepithelial CD8+ lymphocyte populations with different T cell receptors: A role for the gut epithelium in T cell differentiation. J. Exp. Med. 173:471.
151. Bandeira, A., Itohara, S., Bonneville, M., Burlen-DeFranoux, O., Mota-Santos, T., Coutinho, A., and Tonegawa, S.: Extrathymic origin of intestinal intraepithelial lymphocytes bearing T-cell antigen receptor gamma delta. Proc. Natl. Acad. Sci. U.S.A. 88:43, 1991.
152. Lefrancois, L., LeCorre, R., Mayo, J., Bluestone, J. A., and Goodman, T.: Extrathymic selection of TCR gamma delta T cells by class II major histocompatibility complex molecules. Cell 63:333, 1990.
153. Haregewoin, A., Singh, B., Gupta, R. S., and Finberg, R. W.: A mycobacterial heat-shock protein–responsive gamma delta T cell clone also responds to the homologous human heat-shock protein: A possible link between infection and autoimmunity. J. Infect. Dis. 163:156, 1991.
154. Soderstrom, K., Halapi, E., Nilsson, E., Gronberg, A., van Emdben, J., Klareskog, L., and Kiessling, R.: Synovial cells responding to a 65-kDa mycobacterial heat shock protein have a high proportion of a TcR gamma delta subtype uncommon in peripheral blood. Scand. J. Immunol. 32:503, 1990.
155. Fortune, F., Walker, J., and Lehner, T.: The expression of gamma delta T cell receptor and the prevalence of primed, activated and IgA-bound T cells in Behçet's syndrome. Clin. Exp. Immunol. 82:326, 1990.
156. Hohlfeld, R., Engel, A. G., Ii, K., and Harper, M. C.: Polymyositis mediated by T lymphocytes that express the gamma/delta receptor. N. Engl. J. Med. 324:877, 1991.
157. Rajagopalan, S., Zordan, T., Tsokos, G. C., and Datta, S. K.: Pathogenic anti-DNA autoantibody-inducing T helper cell lines from patients with active lupus nephritis: Isolation of CD4−8− T helper cell lines that express the gamma delta T-cell antigen receptor. Proc. Natl. Acad. Sci. U.S.A. 87:7020, 1990.
158. Aarden, L. A., Brunner, T. K., Cerottini, J. C., Dayer, J. M., deWeck, A. L., Dinarello, C. A., Disabato, G., Farrar, J. J., Gery, I., Gillis, S., Handschumacher, R. E., Henney, C. S., Hoffman, M. K., Koopman, W. J., Krane, S. M., Lachman, L. B., Lefkowitz, I., Mishell, R. I., Mizel, S. B., Oppenheim, J. J., Paetkau, V., Plate, J., Rollinghoff, M., Rosenstreich, D., Rosenthal, A. S., Rosenwasser, L. J., Schimpl, A., Shin, H. S., Simon, P. L., Smith, K. A., Wagner, H., Watson, J. D., Wecker, E., and Wood, D. D.: Revised nomenclature for antigen-nonspecific T cell proliferation and helper factors. J. Immunol. 123:2928, 1979.
159. Lipsky, P. E., Davis, L. S., Cush, J. J., and Oppenheimer-Marks, N.:

The role of cytokines in the pathogenesis of rheumatoid arthritis. Springer Semin. Immunopathol. 11:123, 1989.

160. Lomedico, P. T., Gubler, U., Hellmann, C. P., Dukovich, M., Giri, J. G., Pan, Y. -C. E., Collier, K., Semionow, R., Chua, A. O., and Mizel, S. B.: Cloning and expression of murine interleukin-1 cDNA in *Escherichia coli*. Nature 312:458, 1984.

161. Auron, P. E., Webb, A. C., Rosenwasser, L. J., Mucci, S. F., Rich, A., Wolff, S. M., and Dinarello, C. A.: Nucleotide sequence of human monocyte interleukin 1 precursor cDNA. Proc. Natl. Acad. Sci. U.S.A. 81:7907, 1984.

162. March, C. J., Mosley, B., Larsen, A., Cerretti, D. P., Braedt, G., Price, V., Gillis, S., Henney, C. S., Kronheim, S. R., Grabstein, K., Conlon, P. J., Hopp, T. P., and Cosman, D.: Cloning, sequence and expression of two distinct human interleukin-1 complementary DNAs. Nature 315:641, 1985.

163. Gubler, U., Chua, A. O., Stern, A. S., Hellmann, C. P., Vitek, M. P., Dechiara, T. M., Benjamin, W. R., Collier, K. J., Dukovich, M., Familletti, P. C., Fiedler-Nagy, C, Jenson, J., Kaffka, K., Kilian, P. L., Stremlo, D., Wittreich, B. H., Woehle, D., Mizel, S. B., and Lomedico, P. T.: Recombinant human interleukin 1α: Purification and biological characterization. J. Immunol. 136:492, 1986.

164. Oppenheim, J. J., and Gery, I.: Interleukin 1 is more than an interleukin. Immunol. Today 3:113, 1982.

165. Dinarello, C. A.: Interleukin-1 and its biologically related cytokines. Adv. Immunol. 44:153, 1989.

166. Tartakovsky, B., Kovacs, E. J., Takacs, L., and Durham, S. K.: T cell clone producing an IL-1–like activity after stimulation with antigen-presenting B cells. J. Immunol. 137:160, 1986.

167. Acres, R. B., Larsen, A., and Conlon, P. J.: IL 1 expression in a clone of human T cells. J. Immunol. 138:2132, 1987.

168. Cerdan, C., Martin, Y., Brailly, H., Courcoul, M., Flavetta, S., Costello, R., Mawas, C., Birg, F., and Olive, D.: IL-1α is produced by T lymphocytes activated via the CD2 plus CD28 pathway. J. Immunol. 146:560, 1991.

169. Hackett, R. J., Davis, L. S., and Lipsky, P. E.: Comparative effects of tumor necrosis factor-α and IL-1β on mitogen-induced T cell activation. J. Immunol. 140:2639, 1988.

170. Dower, S. K., Kronheim, S. R., Hopp, T. P., Cantrell, M., Deeley, M., Gillis, S., Henney, C. S., and Urdal, D. L.: The cell surface receptors for interleukin-1α and interleukin-1β are identical. Nature 324:266, 1986.

171. Matsushima, K., Akahoshi, T., Yamada, M., Furutani, Y., and Oppenheim, J. J.: Properties of a specific interleukin 1 (IL 1) receptor on human Epstein-Barr Virus–transformed B lymphocytes: Identity of the receptor for IL 1-α and IL 1-β. J. Immunol. 136:4496, 1986.

172. Lowental, J. W., and MacDonald, H. R.: Binding and internalization of interleukin-1 by T cells: Direct evidence for high- and low-affinity classes of interleukin-1 receptor. J. Exp. Med. 164:1060, 1986.

173. Chin, J., Cameron, P. M., Rupp, E., and Schmidt, J. A.: Identification of a high-affinity receptor for native human interleukin 1β and interleukin 1α on normal human lung fibroblasts. J. Exp. Med. 165:70, 1987.

174. Farrar, W. L., Killian, P. L., Ruff, M. R., Hill, J. M., and Pert, C. B.: Visualization and characterization of interleukin 1 receptors in brain. J. Immunol. 139:459, 1987.

175. Dinarello, C. A.: Biology of interleukin 1. FASEB J. 2:108, 1988.

176. Sims, J. E., March, C. T., Cosman, D. J., Widmer, M. B., MacDonald, H. R., MacMahan, C. J., Gruben, C. E., Wignall, J. M., Jackson, J. L., Call, S. M., Friend, D., Albert, A. A., Gillis, S., Urdal, D. L., and Dower, S. K.: cDNA expression cloning of the IL-1 receptor, a member of the immunoglobulin superfamily. Science 241:585, 1988.

177. Horuk, R., Huang, J. J., Covington, M., and Newton, R. C.: A biochemical and kinetic analysis of the interleukin-1 receptor: Evidence for differences in molecular properties of IL-1 receptors. J. Biol. Chem. 262:162, 1987.

178. Hoffman, M. K., Koenig, S., Mittler, R. S., Oettgen, H. F., Ralph, P., Galanos, C., and Hammerling, U.: Macrophage factor controlling differentiation of B cells. J. Immunol. 122:497, 1979.

179. Lipsky, P. E.: The role of interleukin 1 in human B cell activation. Contemp. Top. Mol. Immunol. 10:195, 1985.

180. Lovett, D., Kozan, B., Hadam, M., Resch, K., and Gemsa, D.: Macrophage cytotoxicity: Interleukin 1 as a mediator of tumor cytostasis. J. Immunol. 136:340, 1986.

181. Perlmutter, D. H., Dinarello, C. A., Punsal, P. I., and Colten, H. R.: Cachectin/tumor necrosis factor regulates hepatic acute-phase gene expression. J. Clin. Invest. 78:1349, 1986.

182. Carter, D. B., Deibel, M. R., Jr., Dunn, C. J., Tomich, C. -S., Laborde, A. L., Slightom, J. L., Berger, A. E., Bienkowski, M. J., Sun, F. F., McEwan, R. N., Harris, P. K. W., Yem, A. W., Waszak, G. A., Chosay, J. G., Sieu, L. C., Hardee, M. M., Zurcher-Neely, H. A., Reardon, I. M., Heinrikson, R. L., Truesdell, S. E., Shelly, J. A., Eessalu, T. E., Taylor, B. M., and Tracey, D. E.: Purification, cloning, expression, and biological characterization of an interleukin-1 receptor antagonist protein. Nature 344:633, 1990.

183. Arend, W. P., and Dayer, J. -M.: Cytokines and cytokine inhibitors or antagonists in rheumatoid arthritis. Arthritis Rheum. 33:305, 1990.

184. Smith, K. A.: T cell growth factor. Immunol. Rev. 51:337, 1980.

185. Devos, R., Plaetinck, G., Cheroutre, H., Simons, G., Degrave, W., Tavernier, J., Remaut, E., and Fiero, W.: Molecular cloning of human interleukin 2 cDNA and its expression in *E. Coli*. Nucleic Acids Res. 11:4307, 1983.

186. Taniguchi, T., Matsui, H., Fujita, T., Takaoka, C., Kashiman, N., Yoshimoto, R., and Hamuro, J.: Structure and expression of a cloned cDNA for human interleukin-2. Nature 302:305, 1983.

187. Fujita, T., Takaoka, C., Matsui, H., and Taniguchi, T.: Structure of the human interleukin 2 gene. Proc. Natl. Acad. Sci. U.S.A. 80:7437, 1983.

188. Holbrook, N. J., Smith, K. A., Fornace, A. J., Jr., Comeau, C. H., Wiskocil, R. L., and Crabtree, G. R.: T-cell growth factor: Complete nucleotide sequence and organization of the gene in normal and malignant cells. Proc. Natl. Acad. Sci. U.S.A. 81:1634, 1984.

189. Robb, R. J.: Interleukin 2: The molecule and its function. Immunol. Today 5:203, 1984.

190. Splawski, J. B., and Lipsky, P. E.: Human B-cell regulation by growth and differentiation factors. In Cambier, J. C. (ed.): Ligands, receptors, and signal transduction in regulation of lymphocyte function. Washington, D.C., American Society for Microbiology, 1990, p. 149.

191. Norton, S. D., Havinen, D. E., and Jenkins, M. K.: IL2 secretion and T cell clonal anergy are induced by distinct biochemical pathways. J. Immunol. 146:1125, 1991.

192. Waldmann, T. A.: The Interleukin-2 receptor. J. Biol. Chem. 266:2681, 1991.

193. Siegel, J. P., Sharon, M., Smith, P. L., and Leonard, W. J.: The IL2 receptor β chain (p70): Role in mediating signals for LAK, MK, and proliferative activities. Science 238:75, 1987.

194. Malkovsky, M., Loveland, B., North, M., Asherson, G. L., Gao, L., Ward, O., and Fiers, W.: Recombinant interleukin-2 directly augments the cytotoxicity of human monocytes. Nature 325:262, 1987.

195. Hatakeyama, M., Kono, T., Kobayashi, N., Kawahara, A., Levin, S. D., Perlmutter, R. M., and Taniguchi, T.: Interaction of the IL-2 receptor with the src-family kinase p56ᶦᶜᵏ. Identification of novel intermediate association. Science 252:1523, 1991.

196. Symons, J. A., Wood, N. C., DiGiovine, F. S., and Duff, G. W.: Soluble IL-2 receptor in rheumatoid arthritis: Correlation with disease activity, IL-1 and IL-2 inhibition. J. Immunol. 141:2612, 1988.

197. Yang, Y. -C., Ciarletta, A. B., Temple, P. A., Chung, M. P., Kovacic, S., Witek-Giannotti, J. S., Leary, A. C., Kriz, R., Donahue, R. E., Wong, G. G., and Clark, S. C.: Human IL-3 (multi-CSF): Identification by expression cloning of a novel hematopoietic growth factor related to murine IL-3. Cell 47:3, 1986.

198. Sieff, C. A.: Hematopoietic growth factors. J. Clin. Invest. 79:1549, 1987.

199. Clark, S. C., and Kamen, R.: The human hematopoietic colony-stimulating factors. Science 236:1229, 1987.

200. Nicola, N. A.: Hematopoietic cell growth factors and their receptors. Annu. Rev. Biochem. 58:45, 1989.

201. Arai, N., Nomura, D., Villaret, D., Malefijt, R. D., Yoshida, M., Minoshima, S., Fukuyama, R., Maekawa, M., Kudoh, J., Shimizu, N., Yokota, K., Abe, E., Yokota, T., Takeabe, Y., and Arai, K.: Complete nucleotide sequence of the chromosomal gene for human IL-4 and its expression. J. Immunol. 142:274, 1989.

202. Kishimoto, T.: B-cell stimulatory factors (BSFs): Molecular structure, biological function, and regulation of expression. J. Clin. Immunol. 7:343, 1987.

203. Paul, W. E.: Interleukin 4/B cell stimulatory factor 1: One lymphokine, many functions. FASEB J. 1:456, 1987.

204. Yokota, T., Otsuka, T., Mosmann, T., Banchereau, J., DeFrance, T., Blanchard, D., DeVries, J. E., Lee, F., and Arai, K. -I.: Isolation and characterization of a human interleukin cDNA clone, homologous to mouse B-cell stimulatory factor 1, that expresses B-cell– and T-cell–stimulating activities. Proc. Natl. Acad. Sci. U.S.A. 83:5894, 1986.

205. Bettens, F., Walker, C., Gauchat, J. F., Gauchar, D., Wyss, T., and Pichler, W. J.: Lymphokine gene expression related to CD4 T cell subset (CD45R/CDw29) phenotype conversion. Eur. J. Immunol. 19:1569, 1989.

206. Lowenthal, J. W., Castle, B. E., Christiansen, J., Schreurs, J., Rennick, D., Arai, N., Hoy, P., Takebe, Y., and Howard, M.: Expression of the high affinity receptors for murine interleukin 4 (BSF-1) on hemopoietic and nonhemopoietic cells. J. Immunol. 140:456, 1988.

207. Mosley, B., Beckmann, M. P., March, C. J., Idzerda, R. L., Gimpel, S. D., VandenBos, T., Friend, D., Alpert, A., Anderson, D., Jackson, J., Wignall, J. M., Smith, C., Gallis, B., Sims, J. E., Urdal, D., Widmer, M. B., Cosman, D., and Park, L. S.: The murine interleukin-4 receptor: Molecular cloning and characterization of secreted and membrane bound forms. Cell 59:335, 1989.

208. Street, N. E., and Mosmann, T. R.: IL4 and IL5: The role of two multifunctional cytokines and their place in the network of cytokine interactions. Biotherapy 2:347, 1990.

209. Campbell, H. D., Tucker, W. Q. J., Hort, Y., Martinson, M. E., Mayo, G., Clutterbuck, E. J., Sanderson, C. J., and Young, I. G.: Molecular cloning, nucleotide sequence, and expression of the gene encoding human eosinophil differentiation factor (interleukin 5). Proc. Natl. Acad. Sci. U.S.A. 84:6629, 1987.

210. Yokota, T., Coffman, R. L., Hagiward, H., Rennick, D. M., Takebe, Y., Yokota, K., Gemmell, L., Shrader, B., Yang, G., Meyerson, P., Luh, J., Hoy, P., Pene, J., Briere, F., Spits, H., Banchereau, J., deVries, J., Lee, F. D., Arai, N., and Arai, K. -I.: Isolation and characterization of lymphokine cDNA clones encoding mouse and human IgA-enhancing factor and eosinophil colony-stimulating factor activities: Relationship to interleukin 5. Proc. Natl. Acad. Sci. U.S.A. 84:7388, 1987.

211. Rasmussen, R., Takatsu, K., Harada, N., Takahashi, T., and Bottomly, K.: T cell-dependent hapten-specific and polyclonal B cell responses require release of interleukin 5. J. Immunol. 140:705, 1988.

212. Takatsu, K., Kikuchi, Y., Takahashi, T., Honjo, T., Matsumoto, M., Harada, N., Yamaguchi, N., and Tominaga, A.: Interleukin 5, a T-cell-derived B-cell differentiation factor also induces cytotoxic T lymphocytes. Proc. Natl. Acad. Sci. U.S.A. 84:4234, 1987.

213. Waren, D. J., and Moore, M. A. S.: Synergism among interleukin 1, interleukin 3, and interleukin 5 in the production of eosinophils from primitive hemopoietic stem cells. J. Immunol. 140:94, 1988.

214. Loughnan, M. S., Takatsu, K., Harada, N., and Nossal, G. J. V.: T-cell-replacing factor (interleukin 5) induces expression of interleukin 2 receptors on murine splenic B cells. Proc. Natl. Acad. Sci. U.S.A. 84:5399, 1987.

215. Kishimoto, T.: B-cell stimulatory factors (BSFs): Molecular structure, biological function, and regulation of expression. J. Clin. Immunol. 7:343, 1987.

216. Sehgal, P. B., May, L. T., Tamm, I., and Vilcek, J.: Human β2 interferon and B-cell differentiation factor BSF-2 are identical. Science 235:731, 1987.

217. Zilberstein, A., Ruggieri, R., Korn, J. H., and Revel, M.: Structure and expression of cDNA and genes for human interferon-beta-2, a distinct species inducible by growth-stimulatory cytokines. EMBO J. 5:2529, 1986.

218. Sehgal, P. B., Zilberstein, A., Ruggieri, R. -M., May, L. T., Ferguson-Smith, A., Slate, D. L., Revel, M., and Ruddle, F. H.: Human chromosome 7 carries the B² interferon gene. Proc. Natl. Acad. Sci. U.S.A. 83:5219, 1986.

219. Hirano, T., Yasukawa, K., Harada, H., Taga, T., Watanabe, Y., Matsuda, T., Kashiwamura, S. -I., Nakajima, K., Koyama, K., Iwamatsu, A., Tsunasawa, S., Sakiyama, F., Matsui, H., Takahara, Y., Taniguchi, T., and Kishimoto, T.: Complementary DNA for a novel human interleukin (BSF-2) that induces B lymphocytes to produce immunoglobulin. Nature 324:73, 1986.

220. Gauldie, J., Richards, C., Harnish, D., Lansdorp, P., and Baumann, H.: Interferon β²/B-cell stimulatory factor type 2 shares identity with monocyte-derived hepatocyte-stimulating factor and regulates the major acute phase protein response in liver cells. Proc. Natl. Acad. Sci. U.S.A. 84:7251, 1987.

221. Brakenhoff, J. P. J., deGroot, E. R., Evers, R. F., Pannekoek, H., and Aarden, L. A.: Molecular cloning and expression of hybridoma growth factor in Escherichia coli. J. Immunol. 139:4116, 1987.

222. Hirano, T., Akira, S., Taga, T., and Kishimoto, T.: Biological and clinical aspects of interleukin 6. Immunol. Today 11:443, 1990.

223. Taga, T., Kawanishi, Y., Hardy, R. R., Hirano, T., and Kishimoto, T.: Receptors for B cell stimulatory factor 2: Quantitation, specificity, distribution, and regulation of their expression J. Exp. Med. 166:967, 1987.

224. Fiorentino, D. F., Bond, M. W., and Mosmann, T. R.: Two types of mouse T helper cell: IV. TH2 clones secrete a factor that inhibits cytokine production by TH1 clones. J. Exp. Med. 170:2081, 1989.

225. Moore, K. W., Vieira, P., Fiorentino, D. F., Trounstine, M. L., Khan, T. A., and Mosmann, T. R.: Homology of cytokine synthesis inhibitory factor (IL-10) to the Epstein-Barr virus gene BCRFI. Science 248:1230, 1990.

226. MacNeil, I. A., Suda, T., Moore, K. W., Mosmann, T. R., and Zlotnik, A.: IL-10, a novel growth cofactor for mature and immature T cells. J. Immunol. 145:4167, 1990.

227. Metcalf, D.: The granulocyte-macrophage colony-stimulating factors. Science 229:16, 1985.

228. Wong, G. G., Witek, J. S., Temple, P. A., Wilkens, K. M., Leary, A. C., Luxenberg, D. P., Jones, S. S., Brown, E. L., Kay, R. M., Orr, E. C., Shoemaker, C., Golde, D. W., Kaufman, R. J., Hewick, R. M., Wamg, E. A., and Clark, S. C.: Human GM-CSF: Molecular cloning of the complementary DNA and purification of the natural and recombinant proteins. Science 228:810, 1985.

229. Walker, F., Nicola, N. A., Metcalf, D., and Burgess, A. W.: Hierarchical down-modulation of hemopoietic growth factor receptors. Cell 43:269, 1985.

230. Gray, P. W., and Goeddel, D. V.: Structure of the human immune interferon gene. Nature 198:859, 1982.

231. Friedman, R. L., Manly, S. P., McMahon, M., Kerr, I. M., and Stark, G. R.: Transcriptional and posttranscriptional regulation of interferon-induced gene expression in human cells. Cell 38:745, 1984.

232. Bonnem, E. M., and Oldham, R. K.: Gamma-interferon: Physiology and speculation on its role in medicine. J. Biol. Response Modifiers 6:275, 1986.

233. Paliard, X., Malefijt, R. D. W., Yssel, H., Blanchard, D., Chretien, I., Abrams, J., DeVries, J., and Spits, H.: Simultaneous production of IL-2, IL-4, and IFN-γ by activated CD4+ and CD8+ clones. J. Immunol. 141:849, 1988.

234. Pestka, S., Langer, J. A., and Zoon, K. C.: Interferons and their actions. Annu. Rev. Biochem. 56:727, 1987.

235. Andersson, U., Andersson, J., Lindfors, A., Wagner, K., Moller, G., and Heusser, C. H.: Simultaneous production of interleukin 2, interleukin 4 and interferon-γ by activated human blood lymphocytes. Eur. J. Immunol. 20:1591, 1990.

236. Nathan, C. F., Murray, H. W., Wiebe, M. E., and Rubin, B. Y.: Identification of interferon-γ as the lymphokine that activates human macrophage oxidative metabolism and antimicrobial activity. J. Exp. Med. 158:670, 1983.

237. Nathan, C. F., Prendergast, T. J., Wiebe, M. E., Stanley, E. R., Platzer, E., Remold, H. G., Welte, K., Rubin, B. Y., and Murray, H. W.: Activation of human macrophages: Comparison of other cytokines with interferon-γ. J. Exp. Med. 160:600, 1984.

238. Zoumbos, N. C., Djeu, J. Y., and Young, N. S.: Interferon is the suppressor of hematopoiesis generated by stimulated lymphocytes in vitro. J. Immunol. 133:769, 1984.

239. Shirai, T., Yamaguchi, H., Ito, H., Todd, C. W., and Wallace, R. B.: Cloning and expression in Escherichia coli of the gene for human tumour necrosis factor. Nature 313:803, 1985.

240. Pennica, D., Nedwin, G. E., Hayflick, J. S., Seeburg, P. H., Derynck, R., Palladino, M. A., Kohr, W. J., Aggarwal, B. B., and Goeddel, D. V.: Human tumour necrosis factor: Precursor structure, expression, and homology to lymphotoxin. Nature 312:724, 1984.

241. Spies, T., Morton, C. C., Nedospasov, S. A., Fiers, W., Pious, D., and Strominger, J. L.: Genes for the tumor necrosis factors α and β are linked to the human major histocompatibility complex. Proc. Natl. Acad. Sci. U.S.A. 83:8699, 1986.

242. Le, J., and Vilcek, J.: Tumor necrosis factor and interleukin 1: Cytokines with multiple overlapping biological activities. Lab. Invest. 56:234, 1987.

243. Aggarwal, B. B., Kohr, W. J., Hass, P. E., Moffat, B., Spencer, S. A., Henzel, W. J., Bringman, T. S., Nedwin, G. E., Goeddel, D. V., and Harkins, R. N.: Human tumor necrosis factor: Production, purification, and characterization. J. Biol. Chem. 260:2345, 1985.

244. Beutler, B. A., Milsark, I. W., and Cerami, A.: Cachectin/tumor necrosis factor: Production, distribution, and metabolic fate in vivo. J. Immunol. 135:3972, 1985.

245. Beutler, B., and Cerami, A.: Cachectin: More than a tumor necrosis factor. N. Engl. J. Med. 316:379, 1987.

246. Cerami, A., and Beutler, B.: The role of cachectin/TNF in endotoxic shock and cachexia. Immunol. Today 8:28, 1988.

247. Dembic, Z., Loetscher, H., Gubler, U., Pan, Y. -C. E., Lahm, H. -W., Gentz, R., Brockhaus, M., and Lesslauer, W.: Two human TNF receptors have similar extracellular, but distinct intracellular domain sequences. Cytokine 2:231, 1990.

248. Naume, B., Shalaby, R., Lesslauer, W., and Espevik, T.: Involvement of the 55- and 75-kDa tumor necrosis factor receptors in the generation of lymphokine-activated killer cell activity and proliferation of natural killer cells. J. Immunol. 146:345, 1991.

249. Scheurich, P., Thoma, B., Ucer, U., Pfizenmaier, K.: Immunoregulatory activity of recombinant human tumor necrosis factor (TNF)-alpha: Induction of TNF receptors on human T cells and TNF-alpha mediated enhancement of T cell responses. J. Immunol 138:1786, 1987.

250. Novick, D., Engelmann, H., Wallach, D., and Rubenstein, M.: Soluble cytokine receptors are present in normal urine. J. Exp. Med. 170:1409, 1989.

251. Spies, T., Morton, C. C., Nedospasov, S. A., Fiers, W., Pious, D., and Strominger, J. L.: Genes for the tumor necrosis factors α and β are linked to the human major histocompatibility complex. Proc. Natl. Acad. Sci. U.S.A. 83:8699, 1986.

252. Aggarwal, B. B., Henzel, W. J., Moffat, B., Kohr, W. J., and Harkins, R. N.: Primary structure of human lymphotoxin derived from 1788 lymphoblastoid cell line. J. Biol. Chem. 260:2334, 1985.

253. Kehrl, J. H., Alvarez-Mon, M., Delsing, G. A., and Fauci, A. S.: Lymphotoxin is an important T cell-derived growth factor for human B cells. Science 238:1144, 1987.

254. Aggarwal, B. B., Eessalu, T. E., and Hass, P. E.: Characterization of receptors for human tumour necrosis factor and their regulation by γ-interferon. Nature 318:665, 1985.

255. Sporn, M. B., Roberts, A. B., Wakefield, L. M., and Assoian, R. K.: Transforming growth factor-β: Biological function and chemical structure. Science 233:532, 1986.

256. Derynck, R., Jarrett, J. A., Chen, E. Y., Eaton, D. H., Bell, J. R., Assoian, R. K., Roberts, A. B., Sporn, M. B., and Goeddel, D. V.:

Human transforming growth factor-β complementary DNA sequence and expression in normal and transformed cells. Nature 316:701, 1985.

257. Betz, M., and Fox, B. S.: Prostaglandin E₂ inhibits production of TH1 lymphokines but not of TH2 lymphokines. J. Immunol. 146:18, 1991.

258. Quill, H., Gaur, A., and Phipps, R. P.: Prostaglandin E₂–dependent induction of granulocyte-macrophage colony-stimulating factor secretion by cloned murine helper T cells. J. Immunol. 142:813, 1989.

259. Siekierka, J. J., Hung, S. H. Y., Poe, M., Lin, C., and Sigal, N. H.: A cytosolic binding protein for the immunosuppressant FK506 has peptidyl-prolyl isomerase activity but is distinct from cyclophilin. Nature 341:755, 1989.

260. Shaw, J. P., Meerovitch, J. K., Cleackley, R. C., and Paetkau, V.: Mechanisms regulating the level of IL-2 mRNA in T lymphocytes. J. Immunol. 140:2243, 1988.

261. Hunkapillar, T., and Hood, L.: Diversity of the immunoglobulin gene superfamily. Adv. Immunol. 44:1, 1989.

262. Edmundson, A. B., Ely, K. R., Abola, E. E., Schiffer, M., and Panagiotopoulos, N.: Rotational allomerism and divergent evolution of domains in immunoglobulin light chains. Biochemistry 14:3953, 1975.

263. Saul, F. A., Amzel, L. M., and Poljak, R. J.: Preliminary refinement and structural analysis of the Fab fragment of human immunoglobulin New at 2.09 A resolution. J. Biol. Chem. 253:585, 1977.

264. Hasemann, C. A., and Capra, J. D.: Immunoglobulins: Structure and function. In Paul, W. E. (ed.): Fundamental Immunology, 2nd ed. New York, Raven Press, 1989, p. 209.

265. Fleischman, J. B., Pain, R. H., and Porter, R. R.: Reduction of gammaglobulins. Arch. Biochem. Biophys. Suppl. 1:174, 1962.

266. Amit, A. G., Mariuzza, R. A., Phillips, S. E. V., and Poljak, R. J.: Three-dimensional structure of an antigen antibody complex at 2.8 A resolution. Science 233:747, 1986.

267. Kabat, E. A., Wu, T. T., Reid-Miller, M., Perry, H. M., and Gottesman, K. S.: Sequences of Proteins of Immunologic Interest, 4th ed. Bethesda, MD, U.S. Department of Health and Human Services, 1987.

268. Mole, J. E., Bhown, A. S., and Bennett, J.: Primary structure of human J chain: Alignment of peptides from chemical and enzymatic hydrolyses. Biochemistry 16:3507, 1977.

269. Mostov, K. E., Friedlander, M., and Blobel, G.: The receptor for transepithelial transport of IgA and IgM contains multiple immunoglobulin-like domains. Nature 308:37, 1984.

270. Honjo, T.: Immunoglobulin genes. Annu. Rev. Immunol. 1:499, 1983.

271. Tonegawa, S.: Somatic generation of antibody diversity. Nature 302:575, 1983.

272. Lutzker, S., and Alt, F. W.: Immunoglobulin heavy-chain class switching. In Berg, D. E., and Howe, M. M. (eds.): Mobile DNA. Washington, DC, American Society for Microbiology, 1989, p. 691.

273. Hedrick, S. M.: T lymphocyte receptors. In Paul, W. E. (ed.): Fundamental Immunology, 2nd ed. New York, Raven Press, 1989.

274. Max, E.: Immunoglobulins: Molecular genetics. In Paul, W. E. (ed.): Fundamental Immunology, 2nd ed. New York, Raven Press, 1989, p. 235.

275. Reth, M., Hombach, J., Wienards, J., Campbell, K. S., Chien, N., Justement, L. B., and Cambier, K. S.: The B-cell antigen receptor complex. Immunol. Today 12:196, 1991.

276. Yancopoulos, G. D., Desiderio, S. V., Paskind, M., Kearney, J. F., Baltimore, D., and Alt, F.: Preferential utilization of the most J$_H$-proximal V$_H$ gene segments in pre-B cell lines. Nature 311:727, 1984.

277. Rathbun, G. A., and Tucker, P. W.: Conservation of sequences necessary for V gene recombination. In Kelsoe, G., and Shultz, D. (eds.): Evolution of the Immune Response. San Francisco, Academic Press, 1986, p. 75.

278. Meek, K. D., Hasemann, C. A., and Capra, J. D.: Novel rearrangements at the immunoglobulin D locus: Inversions and fusions add to somatic diversity. J. Exp. Med. 170:39, 1989.

279. Hesse, J. E., Lieber, M. R., Mizuchi, K., and Gellert, M.: V(D)J recombination: A functional definition of the joining signals. Genes Dev. 3:1053, 1989.

280. Lewis, S., Gifford, A., and Baltimore, D.: DNA elements are asymmetrically joined during the site specific recombination of kappa immunoglobulin genes. Science 228:677, 1985.

281. Alt, F. W., and Baltimore, D.: Joining of immunoglobulin heavy chain gene segments: Implications from a chromosome with evidence of three D-JH fusions. Proc. Natl. Acad. Sci. U.S.A. 79:4118, 1982.

282. Lafaille, J. J., DeCloux, A., Bonneville, M., Takagake, Y., and Tonegawa, S.: Junctional sequences of T cell receptor γδ genes: Implications for γδ T cell lineages and for a novel intermediate of V-(D)-J joining. Cell 59:859, 1989.

283. Meek, K.: Analysis of junctional diversity during B lymphocyte development. Science 250:820, 1990.

284. Reth, M., Gehrmann, P., Petrac, E., and Wiese, P.: A novel VH to VHDJH joining mechanism in heavy-chain–negative (null) pre-B cells results in heavy-chain production. Nature 322:840, 1986.

285. Kudo, A., and Melchers, F.: A second gene, V preB in the lambda 5 locus of the mouse, which appears to be selectively expressed in pre-B lymphocytes. EMBO J. 6:103, 1987.

286. Siminovitch, K. A., Bakhshi, A., Goldman, P., and Korsmeyer, S. J.: A uniform deleting element mediates the loss of K genes in human B cells. Nature 316:260, 1985.

287. Blackwell, T. K., Moore, M. W., Yancopoulos, G. D., Suh, H., Lutzker, S., Selsing, E., and Alt, F. W.: Recombination between immunoglobulin variable region gene segments is enhanced by transcription. Nature 324:585, 1986.

288. Clarke, S. H., Huppi, K., Ruezinsky, D., Staudt, L., Gerhard, W., and Weigert, M.: Inter- and intraclonal diversity in the antibody response to influenza hemagglutinin. J. Exp. Med. 161:687, 1985.

289. Schatz, D. G., Oettinger, M. A., and Baltimore, D.: The V(D)J recombination activating gene, RAG-1. Cell 59:1035, 1989.

289a. Shinkai, Y., Rathbun, G., Lam, K.-P., Oltz, E. M., Stewart, V., Mendelsohn, M., Charron, J., Datta, M., Young, F., Stall, A. M., and Alt, F. W.: RAG-2 deficient mice lack mature lymphocytes owing to inability to initiate V(D)J rearrangement. Cell 68:855, 1992.

289b. Mombaerts, P., Iacomini, J., Johnson, R. S., Herrup, K., Tonegawa, S., and Papaioannou, V. E.: RAG-1–deficient mice have no mature B and T lymphocytes. Cell 68:869, 1992.

290. Bergman, Y., Rice, D., Grosschedl, R., and Baltimore, D.: Two regulatory elements for immunoglobulin kappa light chain gene expression. Proc. Natl. Acad. Sci. U.S.A. 81:7041, 1984.

291. Ballard, D. W., and Bothwell, A.: Mutational analysis of the immunoglobulin heavy chain promoter region. Proc. Natl. Acad. Sci. U.S.A. 83:9626, 1986.

292. Mizushima-Sugano, J., and Roeder, R. G.: Cell-type specific transcription of an immunoglobulin kappa light chain gene in vitro. Proc. Natl. Acad. Sci. U.S.A. 83:8511.

293. Wirth, T., Staudt, L., and Baltimore, D.: An octamer oligonucleotide upstream of a TATA motif is sufficient for lymphoid-specific promoter activity. Nature 329:174, 1987.

294. Scheidereit, C., Heguy, A., and Roeder, R. G.: Purification and characterization of a human lymphoid-specific octamer-binding protein (OTF-2) that activates transcription of an immunoglobulin promoter in vitro. Cell 51:783, 1987.

295. Fletcher, C., Heintz, N., and Roeder, R. G.: Purification and characterization of OTF-1, a transcription factor regulating cell cycle expression of a human histone H2b gene. Cell 51:773, 1987.

296. Sen, R., and Baltimore, D.: Inducibility of kappa immunoglobulin enhancer-binding protein NF-kappa B by a post-translational mechanism. Cell 47:921, 1986.

297. Von Schwedler, U., Jack, H. -M., and Wable, M.: Circular DNA is a product of the immunoglobulin class switch rearrangement. Nature 345:452, 1990.

298. Early, P., Rogers, J., Davis, M., Calame, K., Bond, M., Wall, R., and Hood, L.: Two mRNAs can be produced from a single immunoglobulin mu gene by alternative RNA processing pathways. Cell 20:313, 1980.

299. Knapp, M. R., Liu, C. P., Newell, N., Ward, R. B., Tucker, P. W., Strober, S., and Blattner, F.: Simultaneous expression of immunoglobulin μ and δ heavy chains by a clones B-cell lymphoma: A single copy of the VH gene is shared by two adjacent CH genes. Proc. Natl. Acad. Sci. U.S.A. 79:2996, 1982.

300. Kenter, A., and Birshtein, B.: Chi, a promoter of generalized recombination of λ phage, is present in immunoglobulin genes. Nature 293:402, 1983.

301. Ott, D., Alt, F., and Marcu, K.: Immunoglobulin heavy chain switch recombination within a retroviral vector in murine pre-B cells. EMBO J. 6:577, 1987.

302. Perlmutter, R., Hansburg, D., Briles, D., Nicolotti, R., and Davie, J.: Subclass restriction of murine anticarbohydrate antibodies. J. Immunol. 121:566, 1978.

303. Lutzker, S., Rothman, P., Pollock, R., Coffman, R., and Alt, F. W.: Mitogen- and IL4-regulated expression of germline Ig g2b transcripts: Evidence for directed heavy chain class switching. Cell 53:177, 1988.

304. Kronenberg, M., Siu, G., Hood, L. E., and Shastri, N.: The molecular genetics of the T cell receptor and T cell antigen recognition. Annu. Rev. Immunol. 4:529, 1986.

305. Yoshikai, Y., Clark, S. P., Taylor, S., Sohn, U., Wilson, B. I., Mindon, M. D., and Mak, T. W.: Organization and sequences of the variable, joining and constant region genes of the human T cell receptor alpha chain. Nature 316:837, 1985.

306. Lai, E., Concannon, P., and Hood, L.: Conserved organization of the human and murine T cell receptor beta gene families. Nature 331:5436, 1985.

307. Raulet, D. H., Garman, R. D., Saito, H., and Tonegawa, S.: Developmental regulation of T-cell receptor gene expression. Nature 314:103, 1985.

308. Snodgrass, H. R., Dembic, Z., Steinmetz, M., and von Boehmer, H.: Expression of T-cell antigen receptor genes during fetal development in the thymus. Nature 315:232, 1985.

309. Haars, R., Kronenberg, M., Gallatin, W. M., Weissman, I. L., Owen, F. L., and Hood, L.: Rearrangement and expression of T cell antigen receptor and γ genes during thymic development. J. Exp. Med. 164:1, 1986.

310. Chien, Y. -H., Iwashima, M., Wettstein, D. A., Kaplan, K. B., Elliott, J. F., Born, W., and Davis, M. M.: T-cell receptor δ gene rearrangements in early thymocytes. Nature 330:722, 1987.

311. Pardoll, D. M., Fowlkes, B. J., Lechler, R. I., Germain, R. N., and Schwartz, R. H.: Early genetic events in T cell development analyzed by in situ hybridization. J. Exp. Med. 165:1624, 1987.

312. Born, W., Rathbun, G., Tucker, P., Marrack, P., and Kappler, J.: Synchronized rearrangement of T-cell γ and β chain genes in fetal thymocyte development. Science 234:479, 1986.

313. Havran, W. L., and Allison, J. P.: Developmentally ordered appearance of thymocytes expressing different T-cell antigen receptors. Nature 335:443, 1988.

314. Houlden, B. A., Cron, R. Q., Coligan, J. E., and Bluestone, J. A.: Systematic development of distinct T cell receptor-γδ T cell subsets during fetal ontogeny. J. Immunol. 141:3753, 1988.

315. Winoto, A., and Baltimore, D.: Separate lineages of T cells expressing and αβ and γδ receptors. Nature 338:430, 1989.

316. Takeshita, S., Toda, M., and Yamagishi, H.: Excision products of the T cell receptor gene support a progressive rearrangement model of the α/δ locus. EMBO J. 8:3261, 1989.

317. Bonneville, M., Janeway, C. A., Jr., Ito, K., Haser, W., Ishida, I., Nakanishi, N., and Tonegawa, S.: Intestinal intraepithelial lymphocytes are a distinct set of γδ T cells. Nature 336:479, 1988.

318. Ishida, I., Verbeek, S., Bonneville, M., Itohara, S., Berns, A., and Tonegawa, S.: T-cell receptor γδ and γ transgenic mice suggest a role of a γ gene silencer in the generation of αβ T cells. Proc. Natl. Acad. Sci. U.S.A. 87:3067, 1990.

319. Winoto, A., and Baltimore, D.: αβ lineage–specific expression of the α T cell receptor gene by nearby silencers. Cell 59:649, 1989.

320. Haynes, B. F.: The human thymic microenvironment. Adv. Immunol. 36:87, 1984.

321. Fowlkes, B. J., and Pardoll, D. M.: Molecular and cellular events of T cell development. Adv. Immunol. 44:207, 1989.

322. Haynes, B. F., Martin, M. E., Kay, H. H., and Kurtzberg, J.: Early events in human T cell ontogeny: Phenotypic characterization and immunologic localization of T cell precursors in early human fetal tissues. J. Exp. Med. 168:1061, 1988.

323. Deugnier, M. A., Imhof, B. A., Bauvois, B., Dunon, D., Denoyelle, M., and Thiery, J. -P.: Characterization of rat T cell precursors sorted by chemotactic migration toward thymotaxin. Cell 56:1073, 1989.

324. Reinherz, E. L., Kung, P. C., Goldstein, G., and Schlossman, S. F.: A monoclonal antibody with selective reactivity with functionally mature human thymocytes and all peripheral human T cells. J. Immunol. 123:1312, 1979.

325. Boyd, R. L., and Hugo, P.: Toward and integrated view of thymopoiesis. Immunol. Today 12:71, 1991.

326. Nikolic-Zugic, J.: Phenotypic and functional stages in the intrathymic development of αβ T cells. Immunol. Today 12:65, 1991.

327. Sprent, J., Lo, D., Gao, K. -K., and Ron, Y.: T cell selection in the thymus. Immunol. Rev. 101:173, 1988.

328. Zacharchuk, C. M., Mercep, M., Chakraborti, P. K., Simons, S. S., Jr., and Ashwell, J. D.: Programmed T lymphocyte death: Cell activation and steroid-induced pathways are mutually antagonistic. J. Immunol. 145:4037, 1990.

329. Mueller, D. L., Jenkins, M. K., and Schwartz, R. H.: Clonal expansion versus functional inactivation: A costimulatory signaling pathway determines the outcome of T cell antigen receptor occupancy. Annu. Rev. Immunol. 7:445, 1989.

329a. Harding, F. A., McArthur, J. B., Gross, J. A., Raulet, D. H., and Allison, J. P.: CD28-mediated signalling co-stimulates murine T cells and prevents induction of anergy in T-cell clones. Nature 356:607, 1992.

330. Kincade, P. W.: Formation of B lymphocytes in fetal and adult life. Adv. Immunol. 31:177, 1981.

331. Kincade, P. W., Lee, G., Pietrangeli, C. E., Hayashi, S. -I., and Gimble, J. M.: Cells and molecules that regulate B lymphopoiesis in bone marrow. Annu. Rev. Immunol. 7:111, 1989.

332. Namen, A. E., Lupton, S., Njerrild, K., Wignall, J., Mochizuki, D. Y., Schmierer, A., Mosley, B., March, C. J., Urdal, D., Gillis, S., Cosman, D., and Goodwin, R. G.: Stimulation of B cell precursors by cloned murine interleukin 7. Nature 333:571, 1988.

333. Takeda, S., Gillis, S., and Palacio, S.: In vitro effects of recombinant interleukin 7 on growth and differentiation of bone marrow pro-B and pro-T lymphocyte clones and fetal thymocyte clones. Proc. Natl. Acad. Sci. U.S.A. 86:1634, 1989.

334. Kocks, C., and Rojewsky, K.: Stable expression and somatic hyper-mutation of antibody V regions in B cell development pathways. Annu. Rev. Immunol. 7:537, 1989.

335. Gu, H., Tarlinton, D., Muller, W., Rajewsky, K., and Forster, I.: Most peripheral B cells in mice are ligand selected. J. Exp. Med. 173:1357, 1991.

336. Goodnow, C. C., Adelstein, S., and Basten, A.: The need for central and peripheral tolerance in the B cell repertoire. Science 248:1373, 1990.

337. Erikson, J., Radic, M. Z., Camper, S. A., Hardy, R. R., Carmack, C., and Weigert, M.: Expression of anti-DNA immunoglobulin trans genes in non-autoimmune mice. Nature 349:331, 1991.

338. Nemazee, D. A., and Burki, K.: Clonal deletion of B lymphocytes in a transgenic mouse bearing anti-MHC class I antibody genes. Nature 337:562, 1989.

339. Lanier, L. L., Yu, G., and Phillips, J. H.: Co-association of CD3ζ with a receptor (CD16) for IgG Fc on human natural killer cells. Nature 342:803, 1989.

340. Anderson, P., Caligiuri, M., and Ritz, J.: CD3-negative natural killer cells express ζ TCR as part of a novel molecular complex. Nature 341:159, 1989.

341. Kuster, H., Thompson, H., and Kinet, J. -P.: Characterization and expression of the gene for the human Fc receptor γ subunit. J. Biol. Chem. 265:6448, 1990.

342. Yin, Y. -J., Clayton, L. K., and Howard, F. D.: Molecular cloning of the CD3η subunit identifies a CD3ζ-related product in thymus-derived cells. Proc. Natl. Acad. Sci. U.S.A. 87:3319, 1990.

343. Bauer, A., McConkey, D. J. M., and Howard, F. D.: Differential signal transduction via T-cell receptor CD3ζ$_2$, CD3ζ-η, and CD3η$_2$ isoforms. Proc. Natl. Acad. Sci. U.S.A. 88:3842, 1991.

343a. Wegener, A.-M., Letourneur, F., Hoeveler, A., Brocker, T., Luton, F., and Mulissen, B.: The T cell receptor/CD3 complex is composed of at least two autonomous transduction modules. Cell 68:83, 1992.

344. Janeway, C. A., Rojo, J., and Saizawa, K.: The co-receptor function of murine CD4. Immunol. Rev. 109:77, 1989.

345. Rudd, C. E.: CD4, CD8, and the TCR-CD3 complex: A novel class of protein tyrosine kinase receptor. Immunol. Today 11:400, 1990.

346. Bjorkman, P. J., Saper, M. A., and Samraouri, B.: Structure of the human class I histocompatibility antigen, HLA-A2. Nature 329:506, 1987.

347. Bjorkman, P. J., Saper, M. A., and Samraouri, B.: The foreign antigen binding site and T cell recognition regions of class I histocompatibility antigens. Nature 329:512, 1987.

348. Brown, J. H., Jardetzky, T., and Saper, M. A.: A hypothetical model of the foreign antigen binding site of class II histocompatibility molecules. Nature 332:845, 1988.

349. Marrack, P., and Kappler, J.: The staphylococcal enterotoxins and their relatives. Science 248:705, 1990.

350. June, C. H., Fletcher, M. C., and Ledbetter, J. A.: Increases in tyrosine phosphorylation are detectable before phospholipase C activation after T cell receptor stimulation. J. Immunol. 144:1591, 1990.

351. Stanley, J. B., Gorczynski, R., and Huang, C. -K.: Tyrosine phosphorylation is an obligatory event in IL2 secretion. J. Immunol. 145:2189, 1990.

352. June, C. H., Fletcher, M. C., and Ledbetter, J. A.: Inhibition of tyrosine phosphorylation prevents T-cell receptor–mediated signal transduction. Proc. Natl. Acad. Sci. U.S.A. 87:7722, 1990.

353. Mustelin, T., Coggeshall, K. M., and Isakov, N.: T cell antigen receptor–mediated activation of phospholipase C requires tyrosine phosphorylation. Science 247:1584, 1990.

354. Abraham, N., Micelli, M. C., and Parnes, J. R.: Enhancement of T-cell responsiveness by the lymphocyte-specific tyrosine kinase p56^{lck}. Nature 350:62, 1991.

355. Samelson, L. E., Phillips, A. F., and Luong, E. T.: Association of the fyn-protein-tyrosine kinase with the T-cell antigen receptor. Proc. Natl. Acad. Sci. U.S.A. 87:4358, 1990.

356. Tonks, N. K., Diltz, C. D., and Fischer, E. H.: CD45, an integral membrane protein tyrosine phosphatase. J. Biol. Chem. 265:10674, 1990.

357. Clark, E. A., and Ledbetter, J. A.: Leukocyte cell surface enzymology; CD45 (LCA, T200) is a protein tyrosine phosphatase. Immunol. Today 10:225, 1989.

358. Pingel, J. T., and Thomas, M. L.: Evidence that the leukocyte common antigen is required for antigen induced T lymphocyte proliferation. Cell 58:1055, 1989.

359. Ostergaard, H. L., Shackelford, D. A., and Hurley, T. R.: Expression of CD45 alters phosphorylation of the lck-encoded tyrosine protein kinase in murine lymphoma T cell lines. Proc. Natl. Acad. Sci. U.S.A. 86:8959, 1989.

360. Mustelin, T., Coggeshall, K. M., and Altman, A.: Rapid activation of the T-cell tyrosine protein kinase p56^{lck} by the CD45 phosphotyrosine phosphatase. Proc. Natl. Acad. Sci. U.S.A. 86:6302, 1989.

361. Volarevic, S., Burns, C. M., and Sussman, J. J.: Intimate association of thy-1 and the T-cell antigen receptor with the CD45 tyrosine phosphatase. Proc. Natl. Acad. Sci. U.S.A. 87:7085, 1990.

362. Schraven, B., Samstag, Y., and Altevogt, P.: Association of CD2 and CD45 on human T lymphocytes. Nature 345:71, 1990.

363. Park, D. J., Rho, H. W., and Rhee, S. G.: CD3 stimulation causes phosphorylation of phospholipase C-γ1 on serine and tyrosine residues in a human T-cell line. Proc. Natl. Acad. Sci. U.S.A. 88:5453, 1991.

364. Trevellyan, J. M., Lu, Y., and Atluru, D.: Differential inhibition of T cell receptor signal transduction and early activation events by a

selective inhibitor of protein tyrosine kinase. J. Immunol. 145:3223, 1990.

365. Weiss, A., Imboden, J., and Hardy, K.: The role of the T3/antigen receptor complex in T-cell activation. Annu. Rev. Immunol. 4:593, 1986.

366. Beals, C. R., Wilson, C. B., and Perlmutter, R. M.: A small multigene family encodes G₁ signal-transduction proteins. Proc. Natl. Acad. Sci. U.S.A. 84:7886, 1987.

367. Graves, J. D., and Cantrell, D. A.: An analysis of the role of guanine nucleotide binding proteins in antigen receptor/CD3 antigen coupling to phospholipase C. J. Immunol. 146:2102, 1991.

368. Imboden, J. B., and Weiss, A.: The T-cell antigen receptor regulates sustained increases in cytoplasmic free Ca²⁺ through extracellular Ca²⁺ influx and ongoing intracellular Ca²⁺ mobilization. Biochem. J. 247:695, 1987.

369. Gelfand, E. W., Cheung, R. K., and Mills, G. B.: Uptake of extracellular Ca²⁺ and not recruitment from internal stores is essential for T lymphocyte proliferation. Eur. J. Immunol. 18:917, 1988.

370. Gardner, P.: Patch clamp studies of lymphocyte activation. Annu. Rev. Immunol. 8:231, 1990.

371. Davis, L. S., and Lipsky, P. E.: T cell activation induced by anti-CD3 antibodies requires prolonged stimulation of protein kinase C. Cell Immunol. 118:208, 1989.

372. Kumagai, N., Benedict, S. H., and Mills, G. B.: Induction of competence and progression signals in human T lymphocytes by phorbol esters and calcium ionophores. J. Cell Physiol. 137:329, 1988.

373. Patel, H. R., and Miller, R. A.: Analysis of protein phosphorylation patterns reveals unanticipated complexity in T lymphocyte activation pathways. J Immunol. 146:3332, 1991.

374. Chatila, T. A., and Geha, R. S.: Phosphorylation of T cell membrane proteins by activators of protein kinase C. J. Immunol. 140:4308, 1988.

375. Kammer, G. M.: The adenylate cyclase–cAMP–protein kinase A pathway and regulation of the immune response. Immunol. Today 9:222, 1988.

376. Monostori, E., Desai, D., and Brown, M. H.: Activation of human T lymphocytes via the CD2 antigen results in tyrosine phosphorylation of T cell antigen receptor ζ chains. J. Immunol. 144:1010, 1990.

377. June, C. H., Ledbetter, J. A., and Linsley, P. S.: Role of the CD28 receptor in T-cell activation. Immunol. Today 11:211, 1990.

377a. Vanderberghe, P., Freeman, G. J., Nodler, L. M., Fletcher, M. C., Kamoun, M., Turka, L. A., Ledbetter, J. A., Thompson, C. B., and June, C. H.: Antibody and B7/BB1–mediated ligation of CD28 receptor induces tyrosine phosphory lation in human T cells. J. Exp. Med. 175:951, 1992.

378. Lindsten, T., June, C. H., and Ledbetter, J. A.: Regulation of lymphokine messenger RNA stability by a surface-mediated T cell activation pathway. Science 244:339, 1990.

379. Fraser, J. D., Irving, B. A., and Crabtree, G. R.: Regulation of interleukin-2 gene enhancer activity by the T cell accessory molecule CD28. Science 251:331, 1991.

379a. Vanderberghe, P., Freeman, G. J., Nadler, L. M., Fletcher, M. C., Kamoun, M., Turka, L. A., Ledbetter, J. A., Thompson, C. B., and June, C. H.: Antibody and B7/BB1–mediated ligation of CD28 receptor induces tyrosine phosphorylation in human T cells. J. Exp. Med. 175:951, 1992.

380. Mentzer, S. J., Remold-O'Donnell, E., and Crimmins, M. A. V.: Sialophorin, a surface sialoglycoprotein defective in the Wiskott-Aldrich syndrome, is involved in human T lymphocyte proliferation. J. Exp. Med. 165:1383, 1987.

380a. Rosenstein, Y., Park, J. K., Hahn, W. C., Rosen, F. S., Bierer, B. E., and Burakoff, S. J.: CD43, a molecule defective in Wiskott-Aldrich syndrome, binds ICAM-1. Nature 354:233, 1991.

381. Jung, L. K. L., Fu, S. M., and Hara, T.: Defective expression of T cell–associated glycoprotein in severe combined immunodeficiency. J. Clin. Invest. 77:940, 1986.

382. Crabtree, G. R.: Contingent genetic regulatory events in T lymphocyte activation. Science 243:355, 1989.

383. Schuermann, M., Neuberg, M., and Hunter, J. B.: The leucine repeat motif in fos protein mediates complex formation with jun/AP-1 and is required for transformation. Cell 56:507.

384. Ullman, K. S., Northrop, J. P., and Verweif, C. L.: Transmission of signals from the T lymphocyte antigen receptor to the genes responsible for cell proliferation and immune function: The missing link. Annu. Rev. Immunol. 8:421, 1990.

385. Smith, K. A.: Interleukin-2: Inception, impact, and implications. Science 240:1169, 1988.

386. Mills, G. B., Cheun, R. K., and Grinstein, S.: Interleukin-2–induced lymphocyte proliferation is independent of increases in cytosolic-free calcium concentrations. J. Immunol. 134:2431, 1985.

387. Mills, G. B., Stewart, D. J., and Mellors, A.: Interleukin-2 does not induce phosphatidylinositol hydrolysis in activated T cells. J. Immunol. 136:3019, 1986.

388. Mills, G. B., Girarad, P., and Grinstein, S.: Interleukin-2 induces proliferation of T lymphocyte mutants lacking protein kinase C. Cell 55:91, 1988.

389. Mills, G. B., Cragoe, E. J., and Gelfand, E. W.: Interleukin-2 induces a rapid increase in intracellular pH through activation of a Na⁺/H⁺ antiport. Cytoplasmic alkalinization is not required for lymphocyte proliferation. J. Biol. Chem. 260:12500, 1985.

390. Merida, I., and Gaulton, G. N.: Protein tyrosine phosphorylation associated with activation of the interleukin 2 receptor. J. Biol. Chem. 265:5690, 1990.

391. Saltzman, E. M., White, K., and Casnellie, J. E.: Stimulation of the antigen and interleukin-2 receptors on T lymphocytes activates distinct tyrosine kinases. J. Biol. Chem. 265:10138, 1990.

392. Mills, G. B., May, C., and McGill, M.: Interleukin 2–induced tyrosine phosphorylation. J. Biol. Chem. 265:3561, 1989.

393. Shaw, A. C., Mitchell, N., and Weaver, Y. K.: Mutations of immunoglobulin transmembrane and cytoplasmic domains: Effects on intracellular signaling and antigen presentation. Cell 63:381, 1990.

394. Yamanashi, Y., Kakiuchi, T., and Mizuguchi, J.: Association of B cell antigen receptor with protein tyrosine kinase lyn. Science 251:192, 1991.

395. Quintrell, N., Lebo, R., and Varmus, H.: Identification of a human gene (hck) that encodes a protein-tyrosine kinase and is expressed in hemopoietic cells. Mol. Cell Biol. 7:2267, 1987.

396. Dymecki, S. M., Niederhuber, J. E., and Desiderio, S. V.: Specific expression of a tyrosine kinase gene, blk, in B lymphoid cells. Science 247:332, 1990.

397. Brunswick, M., Samelson, L. E., and Mond, J. J.: Surface immunoglobulin crosslinking activates a tyrosine kinase pathway in B cells that is independent of protein kinase C. Proc. Natl. Acad. Sci. U.S.A. 88:1311, 1991.

398. Roifman, C. M., Chin, K., and Gazit, A.: Tyrosine phosphorylation is an essential event in the stimulation of B lymphocytes by Staphylococcus aureus Cowan I. J. Immunol. 146:2965, 1991.

399. Gold, M. R., Matsuuchi, L., and Kelly, R. B.: Tyrosine phosphorylation of components of the B-cell antigen receptors following receptor crosslinking. Proc. Natl. Acad. Sci. U.S.A. 88:3436, 1991.

400. Carter, R. H., Park, D. J., and Rhee, S. G.: Tyrosine phosphorylation of phospholipase C induced by membrane immunoglobulin in B lymphocytes. Proc. Natl. Acad. Sci. U.S.A. 88:2745, 1991.

401. Lane, P. J., Ledbetter, J. A., and McConnell, F. M.: The role of tyrosine phosphorylation is signal transduction through surface Ig in human B cells. Inhibition of tyrosine phosphorylation prevents intracellular calcium release. J. Immunol. 146:715, 1991.

402. Padeh, S., Levitzki, A., and Gazit, A.: Activation of phospholipase C in human B cells is dependent on tyrosine phosphorylation. J. Clin. Invest. 87:1114, 1991.

403. Campbell, K. S., Justement, L. B., and Cambier, J. C.: Murine B-cell antigen receptor-mediated signal transduction. In Ligands, Receptors, and Signal Transduction in Regulation of Lymphocyte Function. Washington, D.C., American Society of Microbiology, 1990.

404. Lane, P. J. L., McConnell, F. M., and Schieven, G. L.: The role of class II molecules in human B cell activation: Association with phorphatidyl inositol turnover, protein tyrosine phosphorylation and proliferation. J. Immunol. 144:3684, 1990.

405. Cambier, J. C., Morrison, D. C., and Chein, M. M.: Modeling of T cell contact–dependent B cell activation: IL-4 and antigen receptor ligation primes quiescent B cell to mobilize calcium in response to Ia cross-linking. J. Immunol. 146:2075, 1991.

406. Mooney, N. A., Gullot-Courvalin, C., and Hivroz, C.: Early biochemical events after MHC class-II–mediated signaling on human B lymphocytes. J. Immunol. 145:2070, 1990.

407. Tohma, S., Hirohata, S., and Lipsky, P. E.: The role of CD11a/CD18-CD54 interactions in human T cell–dependent B cell activation. J. Immunol. 146:492, 1991.

408. Subbarao, B., and Mosier, D. E.: Induction of B lymphocyte proliferation by monoclonal anti-Lyb 2 antibody. J. Immunol. 130:2033, 1983.

409. Wacholtz, M. C., Patel, S. S., and Lipsky, P. E.: Leukocyte function-associated antigen 1 is an activation molecule for human T cells. J. Exp. Med. 170:431, 1989.

410. Duijvestin, A., and Hamann, A.: Mechanisms and regulation of lymphocyte migration. Immunol. Today 10:23, 1989.

411. Butcher, E. C.: The regulation of lymphocyte traffic. Curr. Top. Micro. Immunol. 128:85, 1986.

412. Mackay, C. R.: T cell memory: The connection between function, phenotype, and migration pathways. Immunol. Today 12:189, 1991.

413. Jalkanen, S., Steere, A. C., and Fox, R. I.: A distinct endothelial cell recognition system that controls lymphocyte traffic into inflamed synovium. Science 233:557, 1986.

414. Oppenheimer-Marks, N., and Ziff, M.: Binding of normal human mononuclear cells to blood vessel in rheumatoid arthritis synovial membrane. Arthritis Rheum. 29:789, 1986.

415. Manolios, N., Geczy, C., and Schrieber, L.: Lymphocyte migration in health and inflammatory rheumatic disease. Semin. Arthritis Rheum. 20:339, 1991.

416. Munro, J. M., Pober, J. S., and Cotran, R. S.: Tumor necrosis factor and interferon-γ induce distinct patterns of endothelial activation and

associated leukocyte accumulation in skin of *Papio anubis*. Am. J. Pathol. 135:121, 1989.

417. Butcher, E. C.: Cellular and molecular mechanisms that direct leukocyte traffic. Am. J. Pathol. 136:3, 1990.

418. Oppenheimer-Marks, N., Davis, L. S., and Lipsky, P. E.: Human T lymphocyte adhesion to endothelial cells and transendothelial migration: Alteration of receptor use relates to the activation status of both the T cell and the endothelial cell. J. Immunol. 145:140, 1990.

419. Pober, J. S., Gimbrone, M. A., and Lapiere, L. A.: Overlapping patterns of activation of human endothelial cells by interleukin 1, tumor necrosis factor, and immune interferon. J. Immunol. 137:1893, 1986.

420. Dustin, M. L., Rothlein, R., and Bhan, A. K.: Induction by IL1 and interferon-γ: Tissue distribution, biochemistry, and function of a natural adherence molecule (ICAM-1). J. Immunol. 137:245, 1986.

421. Hamann, A., Jablonski-Westrich, D., and Duijvestyn, A.: Evidence for an accessory role of LFA-1 in lymphocyte-high endothelium interaction during homing. J. Immunol. 140:693, 1988.

422. Pals, S. T., Den Otter, A., and Miedema, F.: Evidence that leukocyte function-associated antigen-1 is involved in recirculation and homing of human lymphocytes via high endothelial venules. J. Immunol. 140:1851, 1988.

423. Bevilacqua, M. P., Pober, J. S., and Menduck, D. L.: Identification of an inducible endothelial-leukocyte adhesion molecule. Proc. Natl. Acad. Sci. U.S.A. 84:9238, 1987.

424. Osborn, L., Hession, C., and Tizaid, R.: Direct cloning of vascular cell adhesion molecule 1, a cytokine-induced endothelial protein that binds to lymphocytes. Cell 59:1203, 1988.

425. Shimizu, Y., Shaw, S., and Graber, H.: Activation-independent binding of human memory T cells to adhesion molecule ELAM-1. Nature 349:799, 1991.

426. Picker, L. J., Kishimoto, T. K., and Smith, C. W.: ELAM-1 is an adhesion molecule for skin homing T cells. Nature 349:796, 1991.

427. Mantovani, A., and Dijana, E.: Cytokines as communication signals between leukocytes and endothelial cells. Immunol. Today 10:370, 1989.

428. Bacon, K. B., Westwick, J., and Camp, R. D. R.: Potent and specific inhibition of IL8, IL1-α, and IL1-β induced in vitro human lymphocyte migration by calcium channel antagonists. Biochem. Biophys. Res. Commun. 165:349, 1989.

429. Larsen, C. G., Anderson, A. O., and Appella, E.: The neutrophil-activating protein (NAP-1) is also chemotactic for T lymphocytes. Science 243:1464, 1989.

430. Schall, T. J., Bacon, K., and Toy, K. J.: Selective attraction of monocytes and T lymphocytes of the memory phenotype by cytokine RANTES. Nature 347:669, 1990.

431. Hodes, R. J., and Singer, A.: MHC restriction in T cell/B cell interactions: Role of B cell subpopulations and B cell activation. Annu. Immunol. 135:91, 1984.

432. Noelle, R. J., and Snow, E. C.: Cognate interactions between helper T cells and B cells. Immunol. Today 11:361, 1990.

433. Geppert, T. D., and Lipsky, P. E.: Antigen presentation at the inflammatory site. C.R.C. Crit. Rev. Immunol. 9:313, 1989.

434. Jelinek, D. F., and Lipsky, P. E.: The role of B cell proliferation in the generation of immunoglobulin secreting cells in man. J. Immunol. 130:2597, 1983.

435. Calame, K.: Mechanisms that regulate immunoglobulin gene expression. Annu. Rev. Immunol. 3:159, 1985.

436. Nakagawa, T., Hirano, T., Nakagawa, N., Yoshizaki, K., and Kishimoto, T.: Effect of recombinant IL-2 and γ-IFN on proliferation and differentiation of human B cells. J. Immunol. 134:959, 1985.

437. Romagnani, S., Guidizi, G., Almerigogna, F., Biagiotti, R., Alessi, A., Mingari, C., Liang, C., Moretta, I., and Ricci, M.: Analysis of the role of interferon-gamma, interleukin 2 and a third factor distinct from interferon-gamma and interleukin 2 in human B cell proliferation: Evidence that they can act at different times after B cell activation. Eur. J. Immunol. 16:623, 1986.

438. Jelinek, D., Splawski, J., and Lipsky, P.: The roles of interleukin 2 and interferon-gamma in human B cell activation, growth and differentiation. Eur. J. Immunol. 16:925, 1986.

439. Splawski, J., Jelinek, D., and Lipsky, P.: Immunomodulatory role of interleukin 4 on the secretion of immunoglobulin by human B cells. J. Immunol. 142:1569, 1989.

440. Paul, W., and Ohara, J.: B cell stimulatory factor-1/interleukin 4. Annu. Rev. Immunol. 5:429, 1987.

441. Snapper, C., Finkelman, F., and Paul, W.: Regulation of IgG1 and IgE production by interleukin 4. Immunol. Rev. 102:51, 1988.

442. Defrance, T., Vanbervliet, B., Aubry, J., Takebe, Y., Arai, N., Miyajima, A., Yokota, T., Lee, F., Arai, K., De Vries, J., and Banchereau, J.: B cell growth-promoting activity of recombinant human interleukin 4. J. Immunol. 139:1135, 1987.

443. Jelinek, D. F., and Lipsky, P. E.: Inhibitory influence of IL-4 on human B cell responsiveness. J. Immunol. 141:164, 1988.

444. Snapper, C., and Paul, W.: Interferon-gamma and B cell stimulatory factor-1 reciprocally regulate Ig isotype production. Science 236:944, 1987.

445. Lebman, D., and Coffman, R.: Interleukin 4 causes isotype switching to IgE in T cell–stimulated clonal B cell cultures. J. Exp. Med. 168:853, 1988.

446. Kepron, M., Chen, Y., Uhr, J., and Vitetta, E.: IL-4 induces the specific rearrangement of γ1 genes on the expressed and unexpressed chromosomes of lipopolysaccharide-activated normal murine B cells. J. Immunol. 143:334, 1989.

447. Pene, J., Rousset, F., Briere, F., Chretien, I., Bonnefoy, J., Spits, H., Yokota, T., Arai, N., Arai, K., and Banchereau, J.: IgE production by normal human lymphocytes is induced by interleukin 4 and suppressed by interferon γ and α and prostaglandin E₂. Proc. Natl. Acad. Sci. U.S.A. 85:6880, 1988.

448. Vercelli, D., Jabara, H., Arai, K., and Geha, R.: Induction of human IgE synthesis requires interleukin 4 and T/B cell interactions involving the T cell receptor/CD3 complex and MHC class II antigens. J. Exp. Med. 169:1295, 1989.

449. Lundgren, M., Persson, U., Larrson, P., Magnusson, C., Smith, C. I., Hammarstrom, L., and Severinson, E.: Interleukin 4 induces synthesis of IgE and IgG4 in human B cells. Eur. J. Immunol. 19:1311, 1989.

450. Muraguchi, A., Hirano, T., Tang, B., Matsuda, T., Horii, Y., Nakajima, K., and Kishimoto, T.: The essential role of B cell stimulatory factor 2 (BSF-2/IL-6) for the terminal differentiation of B cells. J. Exp. Med. 167:332, 1988.

451. Yamazaki, K., Taga, T., Hirata, Y., Kawanishi, Y., Seed, B., Taniguchi, T., Hirano, T., and Kishimoto, T.: Cloning and expression of the human interleukin-6 (BSF-2/INF-beta2) receptor. Science 241:825, 1988.

452. Splawski, J. B., McAnally, L. M., and Lipsky, P. E.: IL-2 dependence of the promotion of human B cell differentiation by IL-6 (BSF-2). J. Immunol. 144:562, 1990.

453. Horii, Y., Muraguchi, A., Suematsu, S., Matsuda, T., Yoshizaki, K., Hirano, T., and Kishimoto, T.: Regulation of BSF-2/IL-6 production by human mononuclear cells. J. Immunol. 141:1529, 1988.

454. Mito, S., Tominaga, A., Hitoshi, Y., Sakamoto, K., Honjo, T., Akagi, M., Kikuchi, T., Yamaguchi, N., and Takatsu, K.: Characterization of the high-affinity receptors for interleukin 5 on interleukin 5–dependent cell lines. Proc. Natl. Acad. Sci. U.S.A. 86:2311, 1989.

455. Clutterbuck, E., Shields, J., Gordon, J., Smith, S., Boyd, A., Callard, R., Campbell, H., Young, I., and Sanderson, C.: Recombinant human interleukin 5 is an eosinophil differentiation factor but has no activity in standard human B cell growth factor assays. Eur. J. Immunol. 17:1743, 1987.

456. Coffman, R., Shrader, B., Carty, J., Mosmann, T., and Bond, M.: A mouse T cell product that preferentially enhances IgA production: I. Biological characterization. J. Immunol. 139:3685, 1987.

457. Lebman, D., and Coffman, R.: The effects of IL-4 and IL-5 on the IgA response by murine Peyer's patch B cell subpopulations. J. Immunol. 141:2050, 1988.

458. Beagley, K., Elderidge, J., Kiyono, H., Everson, M., Koopman, W., Honjo, T., and McGhee, J.: Recombinant murine IL-5 induces high rate IgA synthesis in cycling IgA positive Peyer's patch B cells. J. Immunol. 141:2035, 1988.

459. Yokota, T., Arai, N., DeVries, J., Spits, H., Banchereau, J., Zlotnik, A., Rennick, D., Howard, M., Takabe, Y., Miyatake, S., Lee, F., and Arai, K.: Molecular biology of interleukin 4 and interleukin 5 genes and biology of their products that stimulate B cells, T cells and hemopoietic cells. Immunol. Rev. 102:157, 1988.

460. Sharma, S., Mehta, S., Morgan, J., and Maizel, A.: Molecular cloning and expression of a human B-cell growth factor gene in *Escherichia coli*. Science 235:1489, 1987.

461. Kehrl, J. H., Roberts, A. B., Wakefield, L. M., Jakowiew, S., Sporn, M. B., and Fauci, A. S.: Transforming growth factor β is an important immunomodulatory protein for human B lymphocytes. J. Immunol. 137:3855, 1986.

462. Petit-Koskas, E., Genot, E., Lawrence, D., and Kolb, J.: Inhibition of the proliferative response of human B lymphocytes to B cell growth factor by transforming growth factor-beta. Eur. J. Immunol. 18:111, 1988.

463. Coffman, R. L., Lebman, D. A., and Schrader, B.: Transforming growth factor β specifically enhances IgA production by lipopolysaccharide-stimulated murine B lymphocytes. J. Exp. Med. 170:1039, 1989.

464. vanVlasselaer, P., Punnonen, J., and deVries, J.: Transforming growth factor-β directs IgA switching in human B cells. J. Immunol 148:2062, 1992.

Chapter 8   Dennis A. Carson

Rheumatoid Factor

INTRODUCTION

Rheumatoid factors are autoantibodies directed against antigenic determinants on the Fc (for cystallizable) fragment of immunoglobulin G (IgG) molecules (Fig. 8–1). They have been found among the IgM, IgA, IgG, and IgE classes of Ig.[1-6] Most methods developed for the measurement of antibodies against exogenous antigens have also been applied to the assay of rheumatoid factor. These include agglutination, precipitation, complement fixation, and immunofluorescence assays.[7-10] Technical problems have arisen because the IgG antigens with which rheumatoid factors react are present in high concentration in serum and may interfere with a particular detection system. The development of radioimmunoassay (RIA) and enzyme-linked immunosorbent assay (ELISA) methods has facilitated the more precise quantification of IgM, IgG, and IgA rheumatoid factors.[11-17]

IgM rheumatoid factors are multivalent and, hence, are efficient agglutinators of antigen-coated particles. Commercially available sources of the latter include latex beads or bentonite particles that have been passively coated with human IgG. Cross-linking of the IgG-coupled latex or bentonite by IgM rheumatoid factor in serum produces a visible flocculus (Fig. 8–2). The quantity of IgM rheumatoid factor is then expressed as the highest dilution of serum yielding detectable agglutination.

Red blood cells coated with human or rabbit IgG are likewise agglutinated by IgM rheumatoid factors. Human red blood cells sensitized with certain incomplete IgG anti-Rh antibodies are well suited for the detection of IgM rheumatoid factors, particularly those with anti-Gm specificities.[18-21] Sheep red blood cells coated with rabbit IgG antibody are cross-linked by rheumatoid factor in the classic Rose-Waaler reaction. This test can be modified for the detection of complement-fixing rheumatoid factors.[9]

A positive Rose-Waaler test may be more specific for rheumatoid arthritis than the bentonite or latex flocculation assays, because the latter detect antiallotypic antibodies resulting from transplacental immunization or transfusion, as well as true autoantibodies.[21] However, because only a minor proportion of the anti-IgG antibodies in rheumatoid sera cross-react with rabbit IgG, titers in the Rose-Waaler test are usually lower than in those systems that employ human IgG as antigen. Furthermore, antisheep heterophile antibodies may give a false-positive reaction unless the sera are preabsorbed with sheep red blood cells.

Serum IgG will compete with IgG-coated particles for reaction with IgM rheumatoid factor. Through multivalent interactions, nonspecifically aggregated IgG in improperly treated sera or specific immune complexes will inhibit rheumatoid factor binding to a marked degree. Such "hidden rheumatoid factors" can be revealed by separation of the IgM and IgG fractions under dissociating conditions prior to performing the rheumatoid factor assays.[22] The C1q component of complement will agglutinate IgG-coated particles, particularly in plasma anticoagulated with calcium chelators.[23] Unlike IgM, however, the C1q molecule is denatured by heating serum at 56°C for 30 minutes.

Sensitive RIA and ELISA methods have been developed for the detection of IgM rheumatoid factors.[11-14, 16, 17] In a typical assay, plastic tubes or microtiter plates are coated with IgG. IgM rheumatoid factors in serum or synovial fluid specifically bind to the IgG fixed to the plates. After washing, the amount of IgM rheumatoid factor bound is quantitatively determined with an anti-IgM antibody that has been radioiodinated or linked to an enzyme such as alkaline phosphatase. In the latter instance, the amount of enzyme-linked antibody bound to the solid phase is determined by adding an appropriate substrate and then assaying product formation in a spectrophotometer.

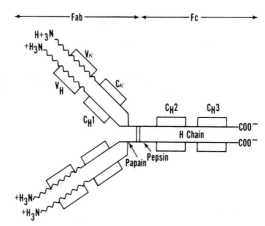

Figure 8–1. Structure of an IgG molecule of the G1 subclass containing kappa light chains. The antigens reacting with rheumatoid factor are in the Fc region.

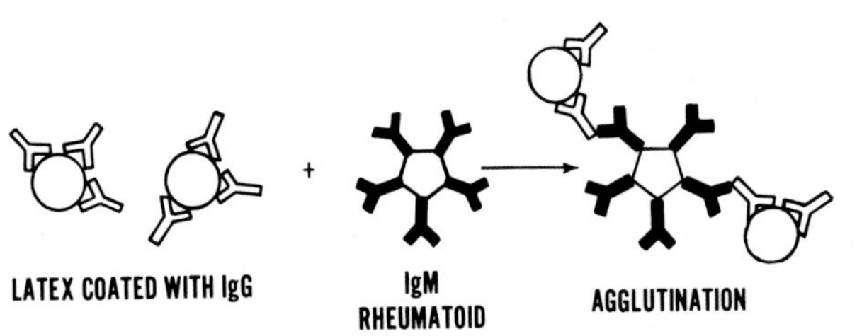

LATEX COATED WITH IgG   IgM RHEUMATOID FACTOR   AGGLUTINATION

Figure 8–2. Latex fixation reaction. Multivalent IgM rheumatoid factor cross-links IgG-coated latex particles to produce a visible flocculus.

One significant advantage of and ELISA methods is that they readily detect IgM rheumatoid factors in rheumatoid sera diluted 1000- to 100,000-fold. At such high dilutions, serum IgG and immune complexes infrequently compromise the accurate determination of IgM rheumatoid factor levels.

IgG rheumatoid factors are abundant in the sera, and particularly the synovial fluids, of many patients with severe rheumatoid arthritis.[12, 13, 16, 24–26] Unfortunately, the routine assay of IgG rheumatoid factors presents several difficulties (Table 8–1). All assays for IgM rheumatoid factor take advantage of the markedly increased avidity of pentavalent IgM rheumatoid factors for aggregated IgG as compared with monomeric IgG. With IgG rheumatoid factor, this phenomenon is not nearly as marked. For the same reason, IgG rheumatoid factors are inefficient agglutinators of IgG-coated particles or red blood cells. High concentrations of IgG in serum, and the tendency of IgG rheumatoid factors to self-associate rather than bind aggregated IgG, further make the assay of this antibody difficult. On occasion, IgG rheumatoid factor complexes precipitate in the cold or when serum is diluted 1:15 with water. This type of Ig rheumatoid factor is frequently monoclonal and is more commonly found in hypergammaglobulinemic purpura, cryoglobulinemia, and Sjögren's syndrome than in typical rheumatoid arthritis.[27–30]

IgG rheumatoid factors in rheumatoid arthritis are most definitely detected by their characteristic sedimentation profile as intermediate complexes in the analytic ultracentrifuge.[31, 32] Other assays for IgG rheumatoid factor require the prior removal of multivalent IgM rheumatoid factor by gel filtration, ion exchange chromatography, or digestion with the proteolytic enzyme pepsin. The last technique has the additional advantage of destroying the Fc portion of IgG, thereby releasing IgG rheumatoid factors trapped in self-associating complexes.[33] Care must be taken, however, to prevent further proteolysis of the IgG molecule with subsequent loss of antigen-binding activity.

Both ELISA and RIA methods have been developed for the detection of IgG rheumatoid factor.[12, 13, 16, 34, 35] They are performed analogously to the IgM rheumatoid factor assay, except that anti-IgG antibody is substituted for anti-IgM in the final step. Nonetheless, IgM rheumatoid factor must still be removed or destroyed prior to the IgG rheumatoid factor assay to avoid false-positive results.

The quantitative assay of IgG rheumatoid factor in serum is occasionally helpful in confirming a diagnosis of rheumatoid arthritis[12, 13, 16] or hypergammaglobulinemic purpura.[30] In patients with rheumatoid vasculitis or the hyperviscosity syndrome, IgG rheumatoid factor levels may assist in monitoring the response to therapy.[35] However, indications for the routine clinical assay of IgG rheumatoid factor have not been well defined.

Rheumatoid factors of the IgA class have been measured in rheumatoid serum by immunoelectrophoresis, quantitative immunoabsorption, and RIA and ELISA methods using class-specific anti-Ig reagents to distinguish them from the more abundant IgM rheumatoid factors.[6, 15, 36]

IgA rheumatoid factors are also found in the saliva of patients with rheumatoid arthritis and those with Sjögren's syndrome. Most salivary IgA, and presumably IgA rheumatoid factor, is produced locally.[36] The role of IgA rheumatoid factors in chronic inflammation of the exocrine glands is not known.

INCIDENCE OF RHEUMATOID FACTOR

Rheumatoid factors are not specific for rheumatoid arthritis. Rather, they are found in the sera of a variable portion of patients with acute and chronic inflammatory diseases and of some apparently normal people.[37–40] The exact incidence of rheumatoid factor in a population depends on the assay system

Table 8–1. COMPARISON OF RHEUMATOID FACTORS OF THE IgM AND IgG CLASSES

Property	IgM Rheumatoid Factor	IgG Rheumatoid Factor
Valence for IgG	5	2
Intrinsic affinity for antigen (liters/mole)	1×10^4–5×10^5	1×10^4–5×10^5
Agglutination of IgG-coated latex particles	Strong	Weak
Enhanced binding to aggregated IgG	Marked	Moderate
Usual sedimentation constants in ultracentrifuge	19S–22S	10S–18S
Self-association	No	Yes
Binding to IgG after treatment with		
Reducing agents	Decreased	Unchanged
Pepsin	Decreased	Unchanged or increased

Table 8–2. DISEASES COMMONLY ASSOCIATED WITH RHEUMATOID FACTOR

Category	Diseases
Rheumatic diseases	Rheumatoid arthritis, systemic lupus erythematosus, scleroderma, mixed connective tissue diseases, Sjögren's syndrome
Viral infections	AIDS, mononucleosis, hepatitis, influenza, and many others; after vaccination (may yield falsely elevated titers of antiviral antibodies)
Parasitic infections	Trypanosomiasis, kala-azar, malaria, schistosomiasis, filariasis, and others
Chronic bacterial infections	Tuberculosis, leprosy, yaws, syphilis, brucellosis, subacute bacterial endocarditis, salmonellosis
Neoplasms	After irradiation or chemotherapy
Other hyperglobulinemic states	Hypergammaglobulinemic purpura, cryoglobulinemia, chronic liver disease, sarcoid, other chronic pulmonary diseases

and the titer chosen to separate positive and negative reactors.

The titer of rheumatoid factor in a population, whether measured by the sensitized sheep cell agglutination test or by latex fixation, usually behaves as a continuous variable but differs among various ethnic groups.[41–43] With increasing age, both the percentage of persons with a particular titer and the mean titer of a population as a whole increase.[40, 41] In most populations, the distribution of titers among men and women is similar. Some studies have shown that the prevalence of rheumatoid factors and other autoantibodies in the general population tends to decline beyond the age of 70 to 80 years.[42] This decrease may be related to an increased mortality among autoantibody-positive people.

Diseases other than rheumatoid arthritis in which positive rheumatoid factor test results are frequent include rheumatic diseases, viral infections, chronic inflammatory diseases, and neoplasms after chemotherapy or radiotherapy.[37–41, 43] Many of these conditions are also associated with either hypergammaglobulinemia, indicative of polyclonal B lymphocyte activation, or circulating immune complexes. Table 8–2 is a partial list of diseases in which an increased incidence of rheumatoid factor has been reported.

In most but not all nonrheumatic conditions, titers of rheumatoid factor are lower than in rheumatoid arthritis. Thus, the specificity of the rheumatoid factor reaction for rheumatoid arthritis increases with serum titer.[40, 43] At a dilution of serum that excludes 95 percent of the normal population, at least 70 percent of patients with rheumatoid arthritis, as diagnosed by other criteria, will be positive by latex agglutination. The remaining patients are considered seronegative, i.e., having rheumatoid factor titers falling in the normal range. Some of the latter sera, particularly from patients with juvenile rheumatoid arthritis, may contain hidden IgM rheumatoid factors.[24, 44–47] A few patients have IgG rheumatoid factors in the absence of IgM. Some seronegative patients, on repeated testing, convert to seropositive. In general, the specificity of rheumatoid factor for rheumatoid arthritis is increased by positivity on two or more consecutive occasions, high titer, reactivity with both human and rabbit IgG, and distribution among the IgM, IgG, and IgA classes.

A variable percentage of adult rheumatoid patients, which in the author's experience represent not more than 10 percent of the total, remain seronegative by the usual criteria. These patients usually have milder synovitis than the seropositive patients, and they seldom develop extra-articular rheumatoid disease.[46, 47]

ETIOLOGY OF RHEUMATOID FACTOR

Genetic Control. Through genetic recombination and somatic mutation, the human immune system can generate millions of different antibodies. Although inherited factors therefore exert but a modest influence on the absolute ability to make IgM rheumatoid factor, they almost certainly influence the structure and specificity of the particular autoantibodies produced. Insight concerning such possible genetic regulation of rheumatoid factor has come mainly from structural studies of monoclonal proteins with rheumatoid factor activity.

Nearly 10 percent of monoclonal IgM from unrelated patients with mixed cryoglobulinemia or Waldenström's macroglobulinemia have anti-IgG autoantibody activity.[27, 48] A similar proportion of chronic lymphocytic leukemia cells have rheumatoid factor on the cell surface, although the autoantibody is not secreted.[49] Structural similarities among the monoclonal rheumatoid factors have been determined by serologic analysis with anti-idiotypic antibodies, by amino acid sequencing, and by gene cloning.[49–56] Anti-idiotypic antibodies recognize antigens in the variable regions of Ig light and heavy chains that differ from one antibody molecule to another. As early as 1973, Kunkel and colleagues[49] prepared an anti-idiotypic antibody that reacted with at least 60 percent of IgM rheumatoid factor cryoglobulins from unrelated persons. Gene cloning studies proved that the monoclonal IgM rheumatoid factors found in Waldenström's macroglobulinemia and mixed cryoglobulinemia are encoded by a small number of Ig light and heavy chain variable region genes,[56, 57] which are prevalent in all ethnic groups. However, several polymorphisms in the heavy chain genes encoding rheumatoid factors have been identified.[57] The anti-idiotypic antibodies to rheumatoid factors accurately identify the light and heavy chain polypeptide products of these genes. The anti-idiotypic antibodies have been used to study rheumatoid factor gene expression during the normal development of the immune system and in autoimmune diseases.[58-61]

Immunofluorescence analyses have revealed that B lymphocytes with presumed rheumatoid factor on the cell surface are remarkably common in the lymphoid tissues of normal people, despite the absence of rheumatoid factor in the circulation.[59, 61] Genes encoding rheumatoid factor rearrange early in development.[59] A remarkably high percentage of B lymphocytes in fetal spleen, for example, express rheumatoid factor. The rheumatoid factor B cells in normal adults are found mainly in the mantle zone regions of lymph nodes and tonsils.[61] These autoreactive B cells do not normally secrete rheumatoid factor. Instead, the rheumatoid factor B cells in the mantle zone probably are a specialized type of antigen-presenting cell that binds and processes antigens trapped in circulating immune complexes. This normal immune function of rheumatoid factor B cells is entirely independent of antibody synthesis.

Environmental Factors. At least three types of environmental stimuli potentially can trigger active rheumatoid factor synthesis in normal adults. They are (1) immunization with antigen-antibody complexes during anamnestic immune responses,[62-65] (2) polyclonal B cell activation,[66-67] and (3) bacterial superantigens.

Adoptive transfer experiments have elucidated the cellular requirements for the induction of rheumatoid factor synthesis during murine secondary immune responses.[63, 68] Optimal rheumatoid factor production requires the presence of T cells sensitized to the specific antigen being administered, as well as antibodies against the antigen. The rheumatoid factor precursor B cells can come from unimmunized or T cell–deficient mice. Importantly, the rheumatoid factor that is elicited during secondary immune responses is directed against the IgG isotype that is dominant in the antigen-antibody complex.

These results are explainable by the ability of activated B lymphocytes, as well as monocytes, to present antigen to helper T lymphocytes.[69] During secondary immune responses, antigen-antibody complexes are taken up and processed by rheumatoid factor precursor B lymphocytes, as well as by antigen-specific B cells.[70] Subsequently, peptides derived from the antigens appear on the cell surface in association with class II histocompatibility molecules. Unlike antibodies, T cell receptors for antigens recognize small linear peptides on the cell surface. When rheumatoid factor B cells present antigenic peptides derived from immune complexes, the antigen-reactive T lymphocytes can trigger rheumatoid factor production. This phenomenon is a form of linked recognition insofar as the helper T cell and the rheumatoid factor B cell recognize different antigens. The frequency of rheumatoid factor precursor cells in mouse spleen is remarkably high and may approach the frequency of cells producing specific antibody.[65]

Rheumatoid factors in human beings develop during the course of many acute and chronic inflammatory diseases.[71, 72] Although IgM rheumatoid factors predominate in most of these conditions, IgG rheumatoid factors are occasionally produced. As in the experimental models, sustained rheumatoid factor production usually depends on the continual presence of the immunologic stimuli. A well-studied example is subacute bacterial endocarditis, in which elimination of bacteria by antibiotics leads to the subsequent decline in rheumatoid factor titers.[71, 72]

With few exceptions, the nonrheumatic diseases and the animal models associated with rheumatoid factor induction are characterized by elevated levels of nonrheumatoid factor containing immune complexes or a diffuse elevation of serum Igs, or both, indicating polyclonal B lymphocyte activation.

The potential importance of polyclonal B lymphocyte activation in inducing rheumatoid factor production in humans has been emphasized.[66, 67] Polyclonal B lymphocyte activators are mitogens that stimulate lymphocytes to secrete Igs in the absence of specific antigenic stimulation. They are widespread in nature and include bacterial proteins and lipopolysaccharides,[73] mycoplasma components,[74] and certain viruses such as the Epstein-Barr virus.[75]

Lymphocytes from many normal adult humans will release low-affinity IgM rheumatoid factors after mitogenic stimulation by polyclonal B lymphocyte activators, such as the Epstein-Barr virus.[66] The rheumatoid factors that are induced by in vitro Epstein-Barr virus infection commonly express the major cross-reactive idiotypes that are found on Waldenström's macroglobulins with anti-IgG autoantibody activity. They may also derive from the minor subset of B lymphocytes that express the CD5 surface antigen.[76] Murine CD5 cells are commonly found in the peritoneal cavity, whereas human CD5 cells are enriched in the marginal zone regions of the lymphoid tissues. The CD5 B cells secrete IgM antibodies against bacterial polysaccharides, as well as certain autoantibodies.[77] However, they are resistant to T cell–dependent triggering to IgG synthesis and seldom undergo somatic mutation.

Bacterial "superantigens" are T cell mitogens that bind to particular T cell receptor subclasses and also to nonpolymorphic portions of HLA class II molecules. In this manner, the superantigens can link T cells nonspecifically with the abundant rheumatoid factor precursors in the blood and lymphoid tissues. As a result of such T-B cross-linking, rheumatoid factor is secreted in quantity. Hence, it is possible that the rheumatoid factors in endocarditis and other infections are induced not only by immune complexes but also by superantigens.[78]

IMMUNOCHEMICAL PROPERTIES OF RHEUMATOID FACTOR

Antigenic Specificity. Polyclonal IgM rheumatoid factors from the sera of patients with rheumatoid arthritis react with a diverse array of antigenic determinants localized to the Fc portion of the IgG molecule in both the C_H2 and C_H3 domains[79–80] (see Fig. 8–1). Recombinant DNA techniques have generated chimeric IgG molecules that express one or more of these determinants.[80] They include (1) cross-reactive antigens shared by human and animal IgG; (2) species-specific antigens found in human but not animal IgG; (3) subclass-specific antigens found on one or more but not all of the four subclasses of human IgG; (4) genetically defined alloantigens of the Gm type, which are autosomally inherited and differ from person to person, depending on their inheritance (each human IgG subclass has its own set of Gm antigen)[19–21]; and (5) neoantigens better expressed on aggregated, denatured, or enzymatically digested IgG than on monomeric native IgG.

Experiments have also identified IgM and IgG antibodies in rheumatoid sera reactive with antigens on the Fab region of intact, native IgG.[81] Strictly speaking, such anti-Fab antibodies are not true rheumatoid factors. They may be representative of the anti-idiotypic antibodies that regulate interactions among lymphocytes in an "immune network."[82]

The many specificities of IgM rheumatoid factors have been used by immunologists to unravel the genetic control of human IgG synthesis. However, no one antigenic determinant on the IgG molecule, with the possible exception of the Ga antigen,[78] has yet been shown to be of unique importance in rheumatoid arthritis. The important point to remember is that IgM rheumatoid factors in rheumatoid sera react with multiple antigenic determinants on autologous IgG. Although a proportion of rheumatoid factors do react better with Gm alloantigens, with animal IgG, or with denatured IgG than with native, autologous IgG, the difference is never absolute. Indeed, the varied array of antigenic determinants reacting with IgM rheumatoid factors in the sera of patients with rheumatoid arthritis reflects the polyclonality of the antibody molecules themselves.

Kinetics of Interaction of Rheumatoid Factor with IgG. The affinity of rheumatoid factors for IgG has been determined by analytic ultracentrifugation and equilibrium molecular sieving.[83–85] Typical association constants for both IgM and IgG rheumatoid factors average from 1×10^4 to 5×10^5 liters per mole. These values are from 10- to 100-fold less than the affinities of common heteroantibodies produced after exogenous immunization. A proportion of rheumatoid factors produced by plasma cells in vitro or eluted from synovium may have higher affinity.[86] These rheumatoid factors may not be detected in serum because of prior reaction with IgG and clearance by the reticuloendothelial system.

In spite of their intrinsically low affinity for antigen, rheumatoid factors can produce stable complexes with IgG under appropriate conditions. For multivalent IgM rheumatoid factor, this occurs when the IgG antigen is aggregated (Fig. 8–3). Although each individual antigen-antibody bond in such an

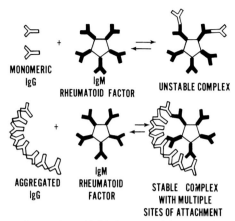

Figure 8–3. Interaction of IgM rheumatoid factor with monomeric and aggregated IgG.

IgM-IgG aggregate probably is, individually, of insufficient energy to yield a long-lived complex, the sum total of multiple interactions produces a stable structure.[83] From a biologic standpoint, the potentiating effect of multivalency is probably greater for those IgM rheumatoid factors of low affinity, because high-affinity antibodies, by definition, bind antigens securely even at low concentrations.

IgG rheumatoid factors have unique kinetic properties that distinguish them from all other autoantibodies and heteroantibodies, in that the antigens with which they react reside on the antibody molecule itself. Hence, IgG rheumatoid factors can self-associate and form immune complexes in the absence of exogenous antigen.[87–89] This self-associating ability favors the formation of immune complexes by anti-Ig antibodies of lower affinity than would be required to produce a similar reaction in a heterologous antigen-antibody system. By analogy with other systems, the ability of IgG rheumatoid factor to form high-molecular-weight complexes probably depends on the concentration and affinity of the autoantibody and the ratio of IgG rheumatoid factor to normal IgG. IgG3 rheumatoid factors are particularly likely to form large aggregates, because of the poor solubility of IgG3 molecules compared with other IgG subclasses.[90] IgM rheumatoid factor may, in addition, enhance the formation of IgG rheumatoid factor–containing complexes by cross-linking the reversibly aggregated IgG.

Physiologic Role of Rheumatoid Factors. As discussed earlier, the majority of the rheumatoid factor B lymphocytes in normal lymphoid tissues appear to be in the mantle zone regions.[61, 91] In experimental animals, antigen-antibody complexes that reach lymphoid tissues via the afferent lymphatic vessels often localize to the mantle and marginal zones.[92] The rheumatoid factor B cells in this region may bind and internalize immune complexes and subsequently present processed peptides to T lymphocytes in the context of HLA molecules.[70]

The physical interaction of an antigen-presenting

B lymphocyte with an antigen-specific T lymphocyte can lead either to lymphocyte activation or to anergy. The outcome may depend on the relative states of B and T cell activation, the type and density of surface adhesion molecules, and the patterns of secreted cytokines.[93, 94] As noted earlier, the remarkable abundance, physical location, and peculiar properties of rheumatoid factor B lymphocytes suggest that they play a significant role in antigen presentation and seldom differentiate into plasma cells. Antigen presentation by rheumatoid factor B cells may be important for the maintenance of peripheral tolerance and for the regulation of antigen-specific activation of T cells.[61]

The common appearance of IgM rheumatoid factors during acute infections also suggests that the secreted autoantibodies have an important physiologic function. The rheumatoid factors that are produced by polyclonal B lymphocyte activation can potentially amplify the early response of the humoral immune system to bacterial or parasitic exposure.[95] IgM rheumatoid factors have the ability to cross-link low-affinity IgG antibodies aligned on a surface of a viral or bacterial particle (see Fig. 8–3).[96] The net result is the formation of a relatively stable, multivalent, and multispecific complex.

When bound to aggregated IgG, rheumatoid factors of the IgM class activate complement remarkably efficiently.[97, 98] If the IgG is bound to a bacterium or parasite, the end result probably is either the lysis of the invading organism or its clearance from the circulation via the abundant complement receptors of the reticuloendothelial system. For this reason, IgM rheumatoid factor synthesis may represent an essential component of an effective polyclonal antibody response.

Under certain conditions, complexes of IgG and antigen potently inhibit immune responses.[99] The immune complexes can bind to the Fc-gamma-2 (Fcγ2) class of membrane receptors for the Fc fragment of IgG, which are expressed by most B lymphocytes. This interaction inhibits B lymphocyte activation by antigen and thereby impedes antibody production. Because IgM rheumatoid factors prevent immune complexes from binding to Fc receptors, they can substantially amplify IgG antibody responses.[100]

The physiologic functions of IgM-RF are summarized in Table 8–3.

ROLE OF RHEUMATOID FACTOR IN DISEASE

In patients with rheumatoid arthritis, Sjögren's syndrome, and mixed cryoglobulinemia, rheumatoid factors persist in the circulation in the absence of any known exogenous antigenic stimulus. Understanding the regulation of rheumatoid factor production may therefore yield clues concerning the immune pathogenesis of these diseases.

The rheumatoid factors produced in lymphoproliferative and autoimmune diseases are structurally dissimilar (Table 8–4). In lymphoproliferative disease, such as chronic lymphocytic leukemia, Waldenström's macroglobulinemia, mixed cryoglobulinemia, as well as in some cases of Sjögren's syndrome, the rheumatoid factors are monoclonal or oligoclonal and display cross-reactive idiotypic antigens.[54–61, 101, 102] The restricted nature of these rheumatoid factors is uncommon for antigen-driven immune responses, which typically undergo time-dependent diversification. The accumulation of somatic mutations, Ig class switching, and the recruitment of new antibody-secreting clones all contribute to antibody heterogeneity. These processes are controlled by helper T cells. In contrast, rheumatoid factor synthesis in lymphoproliferative diseases may result from unrestrained proliferation of immature B lymphocyte clones. In this regard, clinical studies have shown that a significant fraction of patients with mixed cryoglobulinemia eventually develop overt lymphoma.[101] Neoplastic transformation of B lymphocytes is an established complication of Sjögren's syndrome.[103]

In marked contrast, the rheumatoid factors in the sera of patients with rheumatoid arthritis are heterogeneous.[60, 102] The autoantibodies contain light and heavy chains distributed among all the variable region subgroups and among the IgM, IgG, and IgA classes. Sequence analyses indicate that these rheumatoid factors are the products of multiple B cell clones, whose Ig genes contain many somatic mutations.[104] Altogether, the results suggest that the production of rheumatoid factors in rheumatoid arthritis is driven by helper T lymphocytes.

Table 8–3. PHYSIOLOGIC FUNCTIONS OF IgM RHEUMATOID FACTOR

Factor	Function
Cell-associated rheumatoid factor	Antigen processing and presentation; maintenance of nonresponsiveness to autoantigens
Secreted rheumatoid factor	Stabilization of low-affinity IgG antigen complexes Immune complex clearance Enhancement of opsonization

Table 8–4. COMPARISON OF RHEUMATOID FACTORS IN LYMPHOPROLIFERATIVE AND AUTOIMMUNE DISEASES

Type of Disease	Characteristics
Lymphoproliferative	Restricted genes, cross-reactive idiotypes Limited or no somatic mutations Low affinity Mainly IgM
Autoimmune	Many genes, private idiotypes Multiple somatic mutations Higher affinity All Ig classes

Rheumatoid arthritis is an extravascular immune complex disease predominantly affecting synovial tissues.[105] The synovial fluids of rheumatoid arthritis patients, unlike their sera, frequently have markedly depressed complement levels and contain high-molecular-weight IgG aggregates as detected in the analytic ultracentrifuge or by cryoprecipitation.[25, 26] Partial isolation and characterization of the immune complexes from rheumatoid synovial fluids and tissues have yielded IgG rheumatoid factors, sometimes complexed with IgM rheumatoid factors, in the absence of other known antigens.[26] Thus, rheumatoid factors are likely to be of prime importance in the pathogenesis of the extravascular immune complex disease that produces rheumatoid synovitis.

In established rheumatoid arthritis, the synovium may convert to lymphoid granulation tissue. B lymphocytes with rheumatoid factor specificity are abundant in the rheumatoid synovium.[105–109] However, the specificities of the T lymphocytes that drive rheumatoid factor production in the inflamed synovium are not known. There is no evidence to indicate that the T cells recognize the IgG molecule itself. It must be remembered that activated rheumatoid factor B cells can present to T cells a variety of exogenous antigens complexed to IgG antibodies.[60] Hence, in the rheumatoid synovium, normal T lymphocytes reactive with exogenous antigens may be sufficient to sustain rheumatoid factor synthesis. As efficient antigen-presenting cells, rheumatoid factor B lymphocytes may also increase the chance of T cell autosensitization to self-components that are released from necrotic joint tissues, such as collagen, proteoglycans, and heat shock proteins. In this way, the abnormal conglomeration of activated rheumatoid factor B cells at synovial sites would create a vicious cycle that promotes T cell–dependent joint inflammation through a variety of mechanisms.

References

1. Waaler, E.: On the occurrence of a factor in human serum activating the specific agglutination of sheep blood corpuscles. Acta Pathol. Microbiol. Scand. 17:172, 1940.
2. Rose, H. M., Ragan, C., Pearce, E., and Lipman, M. O.: Differential agglutination of normal and sensitized sheep erythrocytes by sera of patients with rheumatoid arthritis. Proc. Soc. Exp. Biol. Med. 68:1, 1949.
3. Franklin, E. C., Holman, H. R. Muller-Eberhard, H. J., and Kunkel, H. G.: An unusual protein of high molecular weight in the serum of certain patients with rheumatoid arthritis. J. Exp. Med. 105:425, 1957.
4. Kunkel, H. G. Muller-Eberhard, H. J., Fudenberg, H. H., and Tomasi, T. B.: Gamma globulin complexes in rheumatoid arthritis and certain other conditions. J. Clin. Invest. 40:117, 1961.
5. Heimer, R., and Levin, F. M.: On the distribution of rheumatoid factors among the immunoglobulins. Immunochemistry 3:1, 1966.
6. Zuraw, B. L., O'Hair, C. H., Vaughan, J. H., Mathison, D. A., Curd, J. G., and Katz, D. H.: Immunoglobulin E–rheumatoid factor in the serum of patients with rheumatoid arthritis, asthma and other diseases. J. Clin. Invest. 68:1610, 1981.
7. Singer, J. M., and Plotz, C. M.: The latex fixation test: I. Application to the serologic diagnosis of rheumatoid arthritis. Am. J. Med. 21:888, 1956.
8. Epstein, W., Johnson, A., and Ragan, C.: Observations on a precipitin reaction between serum of patients with rheumatoid arthritis and a preparation (Cohn, fraction II) of human gamma globulin. Proc. Soc. Exp. Biol. Med. 91:235, 1956.
9. Tanimoto, K., Cooper, N. R., Johnson, J. S., and Vaughan, J. H.: Complement fixation by rheumatoid factor. J. Clin. Invest. 55:437, 1975.
10. McCormick, J. N.: An immunofluorescence study of rheumatoid factor. Ann. Rheum. Dis. 22:1, 1963.
11. Franchimont, P., and Suteneau, S.: Radioimmunoassay of rheumatoid factor. Arthritis Rheum. 12:483, 1969.
12. Carson, D. A., Lawrance, S., Catalano, M. A., Vaughan, J. H., and Abraham, G.: Radioimmunoassay of IgG and IgM rheumatoid factors reacting with human IgG. J. Immunol. 119:295, 1977.
13. Hay, C., Nineham, L. J., and Roitt, I. M.: Routine assay for detection of IgG and IgM anti globulins in seronegative and seropositive rheumatoid arthritis. Br. Med. J. 3:203, 1975.
14. Koopman, W. J., and Schrohenloher, R. E.: Sensitive radioimmunoassay for quantification of IgM rheumatoid factor. Arthritis Rheum. 34:302, 1980.
15. Dunne, J. V., Carson, D. A., Spiegelberg, H. L., Alspaugh, M. A., and Vaughan, J. H.: IgA rheumatoid factor in the sera and saliva of patients with rheumatoid arthritis and Sjögren's syndrome. Ann. Rheum. Dis. 38:161, 1979.
16. Pope, R. M., and McDuffy, S. J.: IgG rheumatoid factor: Relationship to seropositive rheumatoid arthritis and absence in seronegative disorders. Arthritis Rheum. 22:988, 1979.
17. Gripenberg, M., Wafis, F., Isomaki, H., and Lindes, E.: A simple enzyme immunoassay for the demonstration of rheumatoid factor. J. Immunol. Methods 31:109, 1979.
18. Waller, M. V., and Vaughan, J. H.: Use of anti-Rh sera for demonstrating agglutination activating factors in rheumatoid arthritis. Proc. Soc. Exp. Biol. Med. 92:198, 1956.
19. Grubb, R., and Laurell, A. B.: Hereditary serological human serum groups. Acta Pathol. Microbiol. Scand. 39:390, 1956.
20. Natvig, J. B., and Kunkel, H. B.: Detection of genetic antigens utilizing gamma globulins coupled to red blood cells. Nature 215:68, 1967.
21. Steinberg, A. C., and Wilson, J. A.: Hereditary globulin factors and immune tolerance in man. Science 140:303, 1963.
22. Allen, J. C., and Kunkel, H. G.: Hidden rheumatoid factors with specificity for native γ globulin. Arthritis Rheum. 9:758, 1966.
23. Ewald, R. W., and Schubart, A. F.: Agglutinating activity of the complement component C1q in the F-II latex fixation test. J. Immunol. 97:100, 1966.
24. Winchester, R. J., Kunkel, H. G., and Agnello, V.: Occurrence of γ-globulin complexes in serum and joint fluid of rheumatoid arthritis patients: Use of monoclonal rheumatoid factors as reagents for their demonstration. J. Exp. Med. 134:2865, 1971.
25. Hannestad, K.: Presence of aggregated γ-globulin in certain rheumatoid synovial effusions. Clin. Exp. Immunol. 2:511, 1967.
26. Winchester, R. J., Agnello, V., and Kunkel, H. G.: Gamma globulin complexes in synovial fluids of patients with rheumatoid arthritis: Partial characterization and relationship to lowered complement levels. Clin. Exp. Immunol. 6:689, 1970.
27. Meltzer, M., Franklin, E. C., Elias, K., McCluskey, K. J., and Cooper, N.: Cryoglobulinemia—a clinical and laboratory study: II. Cryoglobulins with rheumatoid factor activity. Am. J. Med. 40:837, 1966.
28. Theofilopoulos, A. N., Burtonboy, G., LoSpalutto, J. J., and Ziff, M.: IgM rheumatoid factor and low molecular weight IgM: An association with vasculitis. Arthritis Rheum. 17:272, 1974.
29. Grey, H. M., Kohler, P. F., Terry, W. D., and Franklin, E. C.: Human monoclonal γ-G cryoglobulins with anti-γ-globulin activity. J. Clin. Invest. 47: 1875, 1968.
30. Capra, J. D., Winchester, R. J., and Kunkel, H. G.: Hypergammaglobulinemic purpura: Studies on the unusual anti-γ-globulins characteristic of the sera of these patients. Medicine 50:125, 1971.
31. Chodirker, W. B., and Tomasi, T. B.: Low molecular weight rheumatoid factor. J. Clin. Invest. 42:876, 1963.
32. Schrohenloher, R. E.: Characterization of the γ-globulin complexes present in certain sera having high titers of anti-γ-globulin activity. J. Clin. Invest. 45:501, 1961.
33. Munthe, E., and Natvig, J. B.: Complement fixing intracellular complexes of IgG rheumatoid factor in rheumatoid plasma cells. Scand. J. Immunol. 1:217, 1972.
34. Pope, R. N., and McDuffy, S. J.: IgG rheumatoid factor: Analysis of various species of IgG for detection by radioimmunoassay. J. Lab. Clin. Med. 97:842, 1981.
35. Scott, D. G. I., Bacon, T. A., Allen, C., Elson, C. J., and Wallington, T.: IgG rheumatoid factor, complement and immune complexes in rheumatoid synovitis and vasculitis: Comparative and serial studies during cytotoxic therapy. Clin. Exp. Immunol. 43:54, 1981.
36. Elkow, K. B., Delacroix, D. L., Gharevi, A., Vauman, J. P., and Hughes, G. R.: Immunoglobulin A and polymeric IgA rheumatoid factors in systemic sicca syndrome: Partial characterization. J. Immunol. 129:577, 1982.
37. Dresner, E., and Trombly, P.: The latex-fixation reaction in nonrheumatic diseases. N. Engl. J. Med. 261:981, 1959.
38. Howell, D. S., Malcolm, J. M. and Pike, H.: The FII agglutinating

factors in the serum of patients with nonrheumatic diseases. Am. J. Med. 29:662, 1960.

39. Kunkel, H. G., Simon, H. J., and Fudenberg, H.: Observations concerning positive serologic reactions for rheumatoid factor in certain patients with sarcoidosis and other hyperglobulinemic states. Arthritis Rheum. 1:289, 1958.

40. Bennett, P. H., and Wood, P. H. N. (eds.): Population Studies of the Rheumatic Diseases. Amsterdam, Excerpta Medica, 1968.

41. Mikkelson, W. M., Dodge, H. J., Duff, I. V., and Kato, H.: Estimates of the prevalence of rheumatic disease in the population of Tecumseh, Michigan, 1950–60. J. Chron. Dis. 20:351, 1967.

42. Hooper, B., Whittingham, S., Mathews, J. D., Mackay, I. R., and Curnow, D. H.: Autoimmunity in a rural community. Clin. Exp. Immunol. 12:79, 1972.

43. Lawrence, J. S.: Rheumatism in Populations. London, William Heinemann, 1977.

44. Moore, T. L. Donner, R. W., Weiss, T. D., Baldassare, A. R., and Zuckner, J.: Hidden 19S rheumatoid factor in juvenile rheumatoid arthritis. Pediatr. Res. 14:1135, 1980.

45. Moore, T. L., Donner, R. W., Weiss, T. D., Baldassare, A. R., and Zuckner, J.: Specifity of hidden 19S 19M rheumatoid factor in patients with juvenile rheumatoid arthritis. Arthritis Rheum. 24:1283, 1981.

46. Masi, A. T., Maldonado-Cocco, J. A., Kaplan, S. B., Feigenbaum, S. L., and Chandler, R. W.: Prospective study of the early course of rheumatoid arthritis in young adults. Sem. Arthritis Rheum. 5:299, 1976.

47. Milzaao, S. C.: Seronegative peripheral arthritis. Clin. Rheum. Dis. 3:345, 1977.

48. Crowley, J. J., Goldfien, R. D. Schrohenloher, R. E., Spiegelberg, H. L., Silverman, G. J., Mageed, R. A., Jefferis, R., Koopman, W. J., Carson, D. A., and Fong, S.: Incidence of three cross-reactive idiotypes on human rheumatoid factor paraproteins. J. Immunol. 140:3411, 1988.

49. Kunkel, H. G. Agnello, V., Joslin, F. G., Winchester, R. J., and Capra, J. D.: Cross idiotypic specificity among monoclonal IgM proteins with anti-γ-globulin activity. J. Exp. Med. 137:331, 1973.

49a. Kipps, T. J., Robbins, B. A., Kuster, P., and Carson, R. A.: Autoantibody-associated cross-reactive idiotypes expressed at high frequency in chronic lymphocytic leukemia relative to B cell lymphomas of follicular center cell origin. Blood 72:422, 1988.

50. Capra, J. D., and Kehoe, J. M.: Structure of antibodies with shared idiotypy: The complete sequence of the heavy chain variable regions of two immunoglobulin M anti-gamma globulins. Proc. Natl. Acad. Sci. U.S.A. 71:4032, 1974.

51. Ledford, D. K., Goni, F., Pizzolato, M., Franklin, E. C., Solomon, A., and Frangione, B.: Preferential association of kappa-IIIb light chains with monoclonal human IgM-kappa autoantibodies. J. Immunol. 131:1322, 1983.

52. Carson, D. A., and Fong, S.: A common idiotype on human rheumatoid factors identified by a hybridoma antibody. Molec. Immunol. 20:1081, 1983.

53. Chen, P. P., Goni, F., Houghten, R. A., Fong, S., Goldfien, R., Vaughan, J. H., Frangione, B., and Carson, D. A.: Characterization of human rheumatoid factors with seven antiidiotypes induced by synthetic hypervariable region peptides. J. Exp. Med. 162:487, 1985.

54. Chen, P. P., Fong, S., Goni, F., Houghten, R. A., Frangione, B., Liu, F.-T., and Carson, D. A.: Analyses of human rheumatoid factors with antiidiotypes induced by synthetic peptides. Monogr. Allergy 22:12, 1987.

55. Chen, P. P., Liu, M.-F., Glass, C. A., Sinha, S., Kipps, T. J., and Carson, D. A.: Characterization of two immunoglobulin VH genes that are homologous to human rheumatoid factors. Arthritis Rheum. 32:72, 1989.

56. Liu, M.-F., Robbins, D. L., Crowley, J. J., Sinha, S., Kozin, F., Kipps, T. J., Carson, D. A., and Chen, P. P.: Characterization of four homologous L chain variable region genes that are related to 6B6.6 idiotype positive human rheumatoid factor L chains. J. Immunol. 142:688, 1989.

57. Olee, T., Yang, P. M., Siminovitch, K. A., Olsen, N. J., Hillson, J., Wu, J., Kozin, F., Carson, D. A., and Chen, P. P.: Molecular basis of autoantibody-associated restriction fragment length polymorphism that confers susceptibility to autoimmune diseases. J. Clin. Invest. 88:193, 1991.

58. Kipps, T. J., Tomhave, E., Chen, P. P., and Fox, R. I.: Molecular characterization of a major autoantibody-associated cross-reactive idiotype in Sjögren's syndrome. J. Immunol. 142:4261, 1989.

59. Kipps, T. J., Robbins, B. A., and Carson, D. A.: Uniform high frequency expression of autoantibody-associated cross-reactive idiotypes in the primary B cell follicles of human fetal spleen. J. Exp. Med. 171:189, 1990.

60. Koopman, W. J., Schrohenloher, R. E., and Carson, D. A.: Dissociation of expression of two rheumatoid factor cross-reactive κ L chain idiotypes in rheumatoid arthritis. J. Immunol. 144:3468, 1990.

61. Carson, D. A., Chen, P. P., and Kipps, T. J.: New roles for rheumatoid factor. J. Clin. Invest. 87:379, 1991.

62. Welch, M. J., Fong, S., Vaughan, J., and Carson, D.: Increased frequency of rheumatoid factor precursor B lymphocytes after immunization of normal adults with tetanus toxoid. Clin. Exp. Immunol. 51:299, 1983.

63. Nemazee, D. A., and Sato, V. L.: Induction of rheumatoid antibodies in the mouse: Regulated production of autoantibody in the secondary humoral response. J. Exp. Med. 158:529, 1983.

64. Fong, S., Vaughan, J. H., Tsoukas, C. D., and Carson, D. A.: Selective induction of autoantibody secretion in human bone marrow by Epstein-Barr virus. J. Immunol. 129:1941, 1982.

65. Van Snick, J., and Coulie, P.: Rheumatoid factors and secondary immune responses in the mouse: I. Frequent occurrence of hybridomas secreting IgM anti-IgG autoantibodies after immunization with protein antigens. Eur. J. Immunol. 13:890, 1983.

66. Slaughter, L., Carson, D. A., Jensen, F. C., Holbrook, T. L., and Vaughan, J. H.: In vitro effects of Epstein-Barr virus on peripheral blood mononuclear cells from patients with rheumatoid arthritis and normal subjects. J. Exp. Med. 148:1429, 1978.

67. Izui, S., Eisenberg, R. A., and Dixon, F. J.: IgM rheumatoid factors in mice injected with bacterial lipopolysaccharide. J. Immunol. 122:2096, 1979.

68. Coulie, P. G., and Van Snick, J.: Rheumatoid factor (RF) production during anamnestic immune responses in the mouse: III. Activation of RF precursor cells is induced by their interaction with immune complexes and carrier-specific helper T cells. J. Exp. Med. 161:88, 1985.

69. Lanzavecchia, A.: Antigen specific interaction between T and B cells. Nature 314:537, 1985.

70. Roosnek, E., and Lanzavecchia, A.: Efficient and selective presentation of antigen-antibody complexes by rheumatoid factor B cells. J. Exp. Med. 175:487, 1991.

71. Williams, R. C., and Kunkel, H. G.: Rheumatoid factor, complement and conglutinin aberrations in patients with subacute bacterial endocarditis. J. Clin. Invest. 41:666, 1962.

72. Carson, D. A., Bayer, A. S., Eisenberg, R. A., Lawrence S., and Theofilopoulos, A.: IgG rheumatoid factor in subacute bacterial endocarditis: Relationship to IgM rheumatoid factor and circulating immune complexes. Clin. Exp. Immunol. 31:100, 1978.

73. Banck, G., and Forsgren, A.: Many bacterial species are mitogenic for human blood B lymphocytes. Scand. J. Immunol. 8:347, 1978.

74. Biberfield, G.: Activation of human lymphocyte subpopulations by Mycoplasma pneumoniae. Scand. J. Immunol. 6:1145, 1977.

75. Rosen, A., Gergely, P., Jondal, M., Klein, G., and Britton, S.: Polyclonal Ig production after Epstein-Barr virus infection of human lymphocytes in vitro. Nature 267:52, 1977.

76. Casali, P., and Notkins, A. L.: CD5⁺ lymphocytes, polyreactive antibodies and the human B cell repertoire. Immunol. Today 10:364, 1989.

77. Kipps, T. J.: The CD5 B cell. Adv. Immunol. 47:117, 1989.

78. He, X. W., Goronzy, J., and Weyand, C.: Selective induction of rheumatoid factors by superantigens and human helper T cells. J. Clin. Invest. 89:673, 1992.

79. Natvig, J. B., Gaardner, P. I., and Turner, M. W.: IgG antigens of the Cγ2 and Cγ3 homology regions interacting with rheumatoid factors. Clin. Exp. Immunol. 12:177, 1972.

80. Shin, S. U., and Morrison, S. L.: Production and properties of chimeric antibody molecules. Methods Enzymol. 178:459, 1989.

81. Nasu, H., Chia, D. S., Knutson, D. W., and Barrett, E. V.: Naturally occurring human antibodies to the F(ab')₂ portion of IgG. Clin. Exp. Immunol. 42:378, 1980.

82. Jerne, N. K.: Towards a network theory of the immune system. Ann. Immunol. (Inst. Pasteur) 125c:374, 1974.

83. Eisenberg, R.: The specificity and polyvalency of binding of a monoclonal rheumatoid factor. Immunochemistry 13:355, 1976.

84. Lyet, J. P., and Normansell, D. E.: Low molecular weight rheumatoid factors in rheumatoid arthritis sera. Immunochemistry 11:417, 1974.

85. Wager, O., and Teppo, A.-M.: Binding affinity of human autoantibodies: Studies of cryoglobulin IgM rheumatoid factors and IgG autoantibodies to albumin. Scand. J. Immunol. 7:503, 1978.

86. Robbins, D. L., Morre, T. L., Carson, D. A., and Vaughan, J. H.: Relative reactivities of rheumatoid factors in serum and cells. Arthritis Rheum. 21:820, 1978.

87. Nardella, F. A., Teller, D. C., and Mannik, M.: Studies on the antigenic determinants in the self-association of IgG rheumatoid factor. J. Exp. Med. 154:112, 1981.

88. Pope, R. M., Teller, D. C., and Mannik, M.: The molecular basis of self-association of antibodies to IgG (rheumatoid factors) in rheumatoid arthritis. Proc. Natl. Acad. Sci. U.S.A. 71:517, 1974.

89. Pope, R. M., Mannik, M., Gilliland, B. C., and Teller, D. C.: The hyperviscosity syndrome in rheumatoid arthritis due to intermediate complexes formed by self-association of IgG-rheumatoid factors. Arthritis Rheum. 18:97, 1975.

90. Berney, T., Fulpius, T., Shibata, T., Reininger, L., Van Snick, J., Shan, H., Weisert, M., Marshak-Rothstein, A., and Izui, S.: Selective pathogenicity of murine rheumatoid factors of the cryoprecipitable IgG3 subclass. Int. Immunol. 4:93, 1992.

91. Axelrod, O., Silverman, G. J., Dev, V., Kyle, R., Carson, D. A., Kipps, T. J.: Idiotypic cross-reactivity of immunoglobulins expressed in Waldenstrom's macroglobulinemia, chronic lymphocytic leukemia, and mantle zone lymphocytes of secondary B-cell follicles. Blood 77:1484, 1991.

92. Kumararatne, D. S., Bazin, H., and MacLennon, I. C. M.: Marginal zones: The major B cell compartment of rat spleens. Eur. J. Immunol. 11:858, 1981.

93. Jenkins, M. K. Burrel, E., and Ashwell, J. D.: Antigen presentation of resting B cells. J. Immunol. 144:1585, 1990.

94. Noelle, R. J., and Snow, E. C. Cognate interactions between helper T cells and B cells. Immunol. Today 11:361, 1990.

95. Clagett, J. A., and Engel, D.: Polyclonal activation: A form of primitive immunity and its possible role in pathogenesis of inflammatory diseases. Dev. Comp. Immunol. 2:235, 1978.

96. Schmid, F. R., Roitt, I. M., and Rochas, M. J.: Complement fixation by a two component antibody system: Immunoglobulin G and immunoglobulin M antiglobulin (rheumatoid factor). J. Exp. Med. 132:673, 1970.

97. Zvaifler, N. J., and Schur, P. H.: Reaction of aggregated mercaptoethanol treated gamma globulin with rheumatoid factor–precipitin and complement fixation studies. Arthritis Rheum. 11:523, 1968.

98. Sabharwal, U. K., Vaughan, J. H., Fong, S., Bennett, P. H., Carson, D. A., and Curd, J. G.: Activation of the classical pathway of complement by rheumatoid factors. Arthritis Rheum. 25:161, 1982.

99. Rigley, K. P., Harnett, M. M., and Klaus, G. G. B.: Cross-linking of surface immunoglobulin Fcγ receptors on B lymphocytes uncomples the antigen receptors from the associated G protein. Eur. J. Immunol. 19:481, 1989.

100. Panoskaltis, A., and St. Clair, N. R.: Rheumatoid factor blocks regulator Fc signals. Cell Immunol. 123:177, 1989.

101. Brouet, J. C., Clauvel, J. P., Danon, F., Klein, M., and Seligman, M.: Biological and clinical significance of cryoglobulins: A report of 86 cases. Am. J. Med. 57:775, 1974.

102. Fong, S., Chen, P. P., Gilbertson, T. A., Weber, J. R., Fox, R. I., and Carson, D. A.: Expression of three cross reactive idiotypes on rheumatoid factor autoantibodies from patients with autoimmune diseases and seropositive adults. J. Immunol. 137:122, 1986.

103. Talal, N., and Bunim, J.: The development of malignant lymphoma in Sjögren's syndrome. Am. J. Med. 36:529, 1964.

104. Soto-Gil, R. W., Olee, T., Klink, B. K., Kenny, T. P., Robbins, D. L., Carson, D. A., and Chen, P. P.: A systematic approach to define the germline gene counterparts of a mutated autoantibody from a rheumatoid arthritis patient. Arthritis Rheum. 35:356, 1992.

105. Zvaifler, N. J.: The immunopathology of joint inflammation in rheumatoid arthritis. Adv. Immunol. 13:265, 1973.

106. Tighe, H., Silverman, G. J., Kozin, F., Tucker, R., Gulizila, R., Peebles, C., Lotz, M., Rhodes, G., Machold, K., Mosier, D. E., Carson, D. A.: Autoantibody production by severe combined immunodeficient mice reconstituted with synovial cells from rheumatoid patients. Eur. J. Immunol. 20:1843, 1990.

107. Hedberg, H.: Studies on the depressed hemolytic complement activity of synovial fluid in adult rheumatoid arthritis. Acta Rheumatol. Scand. 9:165, 1963.

108. Munthe, E., and Natvig, J. B.: Characterization of IgG complexes in eluates from rheumatoid tissue. Clin. Exp. Immunol. 8:249, 1971.

109. Petersen, J., Heilmann, C., Bjerium, O. J., Ingemann-Hansen, T., and Halkjair-Kristensen, J.: IgG rheumatoid factor secreting lymphocytes in rheumatoid arthritis: Evaluation of a haemolytic plaque forming cell technique. Scand. J. Immunol 17:471, 1983.

Chapter 9

Joe Craft
John A. Hardin

Antinuclear Antibodies

INTRODUCTION

Antinuclear antibodies (ANAs) are found in many different individuals, including healthy blood donors and patients with a variety of infectious, inflammatory, and neoplastic diseases. They are especially prominent in disorders such as systemic lupus erythematosus (SLE), scleroderma, mixed connective tissue disease (MCTD), and Sjögren's syndrome. In addition, patients with idiopathic adult dermatomyositis and polymyositis are characterized by the presence of antibodies to cytoplasmic nucleoproteins. Since mechanisms that account for these latter antibodies are likely to be closely related to those that account for autoimmune responses to nuclear components, it seems reasonable to refer to all antibodies to nucleic acids and nucleoproteins at any cellular location as ANAs.

We have come to refer to those diseases in which ANAs are a dominant laboratory feature as the ANA diseases (Table 9–1). These illnesses are distinguished by a tendency to occur more often in females, to produce systemic inflammation, to exhibit hereditary features, and to have some association with certain alleles of the class II major histocompatibility genes. Most notably, this group of diseases is distinguished by the presence of ANAs in high titers, in contrast with the relatively low levels usually associated with other conditions. This concept of a group of ANA diseases is helpful because it emphasizes the central role of autoimmunity to nucleoproteins in such patients, and it centers attention on ANAs as diagnostic tools.

The study of these autoantibodies is an important part of patient care and research into the rheumatic diseases for several reasons. It is now apparent that individual ANA specificities correlate with each of the different diseases previously mentioned, and

some ANAs help identify subsets of patients in each category. Moreover, some ANAs, such as those directed against deoxyribonucleic acid (DNA) and perhaps anti-Ro and anti-La antibodies, participate in the production of inflammation and tissue injury. Finally, ANAs are now being used widely as probes for a broad variety of intracellular structures to which animal antisera are not available. These latter studies, in turn, are providing new information about the structure and biologic function of their corresponding antigens. This information promises to provide insights into the pathogenesis of a range of autoimmune diseases.

This chapter describes the various ANAs, methods for their detection, and their clinical uses. In addition, the structure and function of many of the corresponding autoantigens that are targeted by ANAs will be described. As part of the source material for this chapter, the authors relied in part upon several reviews, particularly the chapter by Reichlin in the Third Edition of this text,[1] reviews of ANAs by Tan[2] and by Hardin,[3] and the history of research on ANAs by Lerner and Lerner.[4]

HISTORY

The study of ANAs began in 1948 with the work of Hargraves and colleagues,[5] who demonstrated that the concentrated bone marrow of patients with SLE contained "L.E." cells. This finding was followed by that of Haserick and Bortz,[6] who made the discovery that SLE plasma could produce these cells after mixing with normal bone marrow. The LE cell phenomenon soon became an important diagnostic test for SLE. Nearly a decade was to pass, however, before Holman and Kunkel[7] demonstrated that the basis for this phenomenon was antibodies to deoxyribonucleoprotein (more properly histones complexed with DNA), which acted as opsonins for directed phagocytosis by polymorphonuclear leukocytes of antibody-sensitized nuclei. This work, together with the discovery of autoantibodies to native DNA, initiated the era of discovery of many new ANA specificities that continues to the present time. The LE cell test, which yielded positive findings in about one half of patients with SLE, in most patients with drug-induced LE, and in small numbers of patients with Sjögren's syndrome and rheumatoid arthritis,[8] was a widely used diagnostic tool until the

Table 9–1. THE ANTINUCLEAR ANTIBODY DISEASES

Disease	Percentage (%) of Patients with ANAs*
SLE	99 (115)
Drug-induced lupus	100 (316)
Scleroderma	97 (40)
MCTD	93 (317)
Polymyositis/dermatomyositis	78 (226)
Sjögren's syndrome	~90 (311)

*References in parentheses.

164

middle of the 1970s when its use began to be supplanted by more specific tests for individual ANAs.

The second major turning point in the study of ANAs occurred when Friou[9] applied the new technique of indirect immunofluorescence to the study of ANAs. It soon became clear that this technique was much more sensitive than the LE cell test and yielded positive results in the majority of patients with SLE. Moreover, it could detect ANAs in a broad variety of other diseases as well. Thus, it became the method of choice for initial screening purposes.

The third crucial development was discovery that immunodiffusion could be used to demonstrate autoantibodies to soluble components of whole cells.[10] This technique permitted identification of a number of new ANA specificities such as the Sm[11] and nuclear ribonucleoprotein (nRNP) specificities[12] (it was subsequently shown that preparation of extractable nuclear antigens contained targets for both these specificities[13–16]) and the Ro/SS-A and La/SS-B specificities[17–19] (for simplicity, shortened in this chapter to Ro and La, respectively). In terms of present understanding and nomenclature, it is important to keep in mind that the relationships between ANA specificity and connective tissue disease or disease subset were defined largely through the use of this technique. For example, ANAs of the Sm specificity were shown to be highly diagnostic for SLE.[11, 20] In contrast, autoantibodies to nRNP were often found as a sole specificity in high titer in patients with overlap syndromes[14, 21] but were also present in some patients with other connective tissue diseases, most commonly SLE.[12, 13] It is not yet certain that the same strong diagnostic significance will hold up as these antibodies are defined by more sensitive assay systems.

Finally, in 1979 it became possible to apply the techniques of molecular biology to the analysis of ANAs and their antigens.[22] These studies initially demonstrated that the nRNP (hereafter referred to as U_1 RNP, as described later) and Sm autoantigens reside on discrete RNP particles, and they opened the door to the discovery that certain of these particles mediate splicing of premessenger ribonucleic acid (RNA) (for review, see reference 23).

Thus, as summarized in Table 9–2, our understanding of ANAs evolved from an initial period when an increasing array of ANA specificities and their clinical correlation were being recognized to the present time, in which much of the work focuses on gaining information about the structure and function of the various autoantigens. It appears that much of the future challenge will be to understand why selected cellular components are specifically targeted for autoimmune responses in individual connective tissue diseases.

SPECTRUM OF ANAS

The ANAs that have been identified in patients with various rheumatic diseases are listed in Table

Table 9–2. MILESTONES IN RESEARCH ON ANTINUCLEAR ANTIBODIES

Year	Discovery	Reference
1948	LE cells	Hargraves et al.[5]
1957	Antibodies to "deoxyribonucleoprotein"	Holman and Kunkel[7]
1957	Antibodies to DNA	Robbins et al.[74] Seligmann and Milgrom[75]
1959	Antibodies to soluble cell components	Deicher et al.[10]
1966	The Sm antigen	Tan and Kunkel[11]
1969	The Ro antigen	Clark et al.[17]
1971	The nRNP antigen	Mattioli and Reichlin[12]
1974	The La antigen	Mattioli and Reichlin[18]
1979	Identification of snRNPs as major autoantigens	Lerner and Steitz[22]

9–3. These autoantibodies have been categorized according to whether they bind components of chromatin, nuclear or cytoplasmic RNP particles, components of the nucleolus, or other cellular elements. Chromatin consists of DNA and the many different proteins, such as histones, that are bound to DNA. It serves as a reservoir for the genetic information and is found in a permanently densely packaged form that is genetically inactive (known as heterochromatin) and a more open form that contains transcriptionally active genes (known as euchromatin). Chromatin is insoluble in physiologic buffers, as discussed later under immunodiffusion. In contrast, RNP particles consist of one or more small RNA molecules and one or more associated polypeptides. These particles are found within both the nucleus and the cytoplasm, where they carry out enzymatic functions. Ribonucleoprotein particles are usually soluble in physiologic buffers.

The names of some specificities, such as Sm, are based on the prototype patient's name (i.e., Smith).[11] Others, such as Scl-70, are based on the associated disease (i.e., scleroderma)[24]; the cell organelle that bears the target antigen, such as NOR-90 (for an approximately 90-kD) protein of the chromosomal nucleolar organizing region)[25]; or the name of the antigen itself (i.e., RNA polymerase I)[26] (see Table 9–3).

Among the specificities listed in Table 9–3, individual specificities stand out because they are found most frequently, occur in high titer, and often have strong correlations with specific disease syndromes, as will be described in detail in this chapter. For example, one or more U_1 RNP, Sm, Ro, and La specificities are found in most patients with SLE, and as much as 20 percent of the patient's total IgG may be directed against one of the antigens corresponding to these specificities.[27] It has been estimated that individual patients with SLE have an average of three autoantibodies, usually including one or more of these specificities along with antibodies to DNA, histones, or both.[20, 28] Many other antibodies listed here, such as NOR-90, are quite rare, and their detection may require surveys of large groups of

Table 9–3. THE SPECTRUM OF ANAs

Chromatin
Anti–native DNA
Anti–single-stranded DNA
Anti–Z DNA
Anti-centromere
Anti-Ku
Anti-HMG proteins
Anti–topoisomerase I (Scl-70 antigen)
Anti–topoisomerase II
Anti-PBC 95K
Anti-lamins

Nucleolar Components
Anti-RNA polymerase I
Anti-Th
Anti-U_3 (fibrillarin)
Anti-Pm/Scl
Anti–NOR-90

Other Cellular Components
Anti-nuclear pore complexes
Anti-centrosomes
Anti-midbody
Anti-spindle
Anti-Mi
Anti-Su

Nuclear Ribonucleoproteins
Anti–U_1 RNP
Anti-Sm
Anti-Ro
Anti-La
Anti–U_2 RNP
Anti–U_4 U_6 RNP
Anti–U_5 RNP
Anti-5S rRNA[protein]

Cytoplasmic Components
Anti–Jo-1 (tRNA[histidyl synthetase])
Anti-tRNA[alanyl synthetase]
Anti-tRNA[threonyl synthetase]
Anti-tRNA[glycyl synthetase]
Anti–signal recognition particle (SRP)
Anti-ribosomes

patients.[25, 29] Certain ANAs tend to occur in sets in which individual antibody specificities appear to evolve in an ordered hierarchical manner.[3, 30] For example, anti–U_1 RNP antibodies may occur alone but almost always accompany anti-Sm antibodies (i.e., the latter rarely occur alone).[31, 32] Similarly, anti-La antibodies tend to occur in conjunction with anti-Ro antibodies, whereas the Ro specificity often occurs alone.[2, 33] As discussed in more detail later, such linked sets of antibodies tend to be directed against various epitopes on individual macromolecular structures, such as U_1 RNP particles. For example, the latter particle is the target for both anti–U_1 RNP and anti-Sm antibodies[32, 34] (reviewed in refs.[2, 3, 30, 35]).

DETECTION OF ANAS

Immunofluorescence. Most laboratories rely on indirect immunofluorescence as the initial screening test for ANAs. This method is highly sensitive and is capable of detecting all ANA specificities whose target antigens reside in sufficient quantities within substrate cells. Traditionally, frozen sections of mouse liver (or other rodent organs) or peripheral blood granulocytes were used as substrates. More recently, proliferating cell lines such as Hep-2 cells (derived from a human epithelial tumor cell line) have come into widespread use because cells that are rapidly growing and dividing contain a broader array and higher concentration of important nuclear and cytoplasmic antigens.

In the performance of the indirect immunofluorescence assay for ANAs (FANA), dilutions of the fluorescein-tagged anti-human immunoglobulin are chosen so that tests performed with panels of undiluted normal sera give positive results in about one third of the test sera. Thus, when diluted 1:10 to 1:40 for the assay, almost all of the normal test panel sera will be negative. When such conditions are met and large numbers of sera are tested, weakly positive nuclear staining will be found in about 5 percent of normal sera, and about 95 percent to 100 percent of SLE sera will be positive.[36]

Several factors should be considered in the interpretation of FANA assays. As implied earlier, about 5 percent of otherwise normal individuals will have weakly positive results. In such cases, titers are usually equal to or less than 1:320, and the nuclear staining pattern is most often homogeneous. The incidence of this finding is higher among women and older individuals. Conversely, rare SLE patients have negative FANAs. These individuals often have anti-Ro antibodies in the absence of other specificities,[1] an observation explained by the finding that the Ro antigen exists in cells in very low concentrations, particularly in rat or mouse tissues.[37] Thus, antibodies to the Ro antigen appear to be relatively difficult to detect in the FANA assay. This problem is minimized when proliferating cells are used as substrates. Additional patients with negative FANAs include those with antibodies to exclusively single-stranded DNA[1] or cytoplasmic RNPs such as the Jo-1 antigen[38] (now known to be histidyl transfer RNA (tRNA) synthetase[39]), which will produce cytoplasmic immunofluorescence. Finally, it should be noted that considerable variability is found when individual sera are tested in different laboratories. Factors involved include the subjective nature of the test, the quality of the reagents and microscope used for its performance, and the use of different types of substrates (proliferating cells versus organ tissues).

Limited but clinically useful information is often obtained in the FANA test from the pattern of nuclear fluorescence (Table 9–4); a corollary to this statement is that individual ANAs have different intracellular targets. Most commonly, staining is observed to occur in a homogeneous, speckled, nuclear rim, or nucleolar distribution. Nucleolar staining has been subdivided further into homogeneous, speckled, and clump patterns.[40] Certain sera from patients with scleroderma contain antibodies to chromosomal centromeres that produce nuclear staining in discrete speckles[41–43] or to topoisomerase I (Scl-70) that pro-

Table 9–4. CORRELATIONS OF ANAs AND DISEASES

FANA Pattern	Associated ANA	Disease Correlation
Homogeneous	Anti-histone	SLE, drug-induced LE, other diseases, "false-positive ANA"*
Rim	Anti-DNA, anti-lamin†	SLE
Fine-speckled	Anti-U₁ RNP	SLE, MCTD
	Anti-Sm	SLE
	Anti-La	SLE, Sjögren's syndrome
	Anti-Ro†	SLE, Sjögren's syndrome
	Anti-Ku	SLE, scleroderma/myositis
	Anti-PCNA/cyclin	SLE
	Anti-topoisomerase I	Scleroderma
Discrete speckled	Anti-centromere	CREST
	Anti-PBC 95K†	PBC
Nucleolar	anti-Th, anti-U₃ RNP, anti-RNA polymerase I, Pm-Scl	Scleroderma
	Ribosomes†	SLE
Cytoplasmic	tRNA synthetases	Polymyositis
	Ribosomes†	SLE
	Mitochondria†	PBC

SLE, systemic lupus erythematosus; MCTD, mixed connective tissue disease; CREST, syndrome of calcinosis, Raynaud's phenomenon, esophageal disorder, sclerodactyly, telangiectasias (scleroderma with limited skin involvement); PBC, primary biliary cirrhosis.

*Many ANAs will produce homogeneous fluorescence if assayed at low serum dilutions; anti-DNA antibodies may also produce homogeneous fluorescence.

†Anti-lamin antibodies are found rarely in SLE[318]; anti-La antibodies often give perinuclear staining in addition to nuclear speckling owing to leak during cell fixation; anti-Ro antibodies may not produce any staining (so-called "ANA-negative" patients); anti-topoisomerase I antibodies typically stain the nucleus in a grainy speckled manner[40]; anti-PBC 95K antibodies are found in approximately one third of patients with primary biliary cirrhosis and produce fewer speckles than anti-centromere antibodies[319]; anti-ribosomal antibodies may produce nucleolar and cytoplasmic fluorescence. (See text for details.)

duce grainy speckling throughout the nucleus.[40] Finally, as previously noted, autoantibodies from patients with idiopathic adult polymyositis and dermatomyositis tend to bind cytoplasmic antigens, such as the RNA proteins involved in protein synthesis, leading to a fluorescent staining pattern of the cytoplasm, with sparing of the nucleus unless other specificities are present. It should be noted, however, that these staining patterns may vary as sera are diluted. For example, sera containing antibodies to histones and small nRNP (snRNP) particles may typically produce the homogeneous pattern at lower dilutions and the fine-speckled pattern at higher dilutions. Nuclear staining patterns reported from various laboratories may be particularly inconsistent because of this additional variable caused by the the extent of serum dilution. Examples of some common staining patterns are shown in Figure 9–1.

Finally, from a clinical point of view, the presence of ANAs raises several additional considerations. In individual patients, their absence argues strongly against the presence of one of the connective tissue diseases, whereas high titers suggest but do not prove that the diagnosis resides in this category of disorders. On rare occasions, certain individuals, including family members of patients with connective tissue diseases, may have high titers of ANAs without manifestations of disease.

Immunodiffusion. The technique of double immunodiffusion is a simple and straightforward method for the detection of a variety of antibodies in patient sera, particularly those directed against various RNP particles (Fig. 9–2). For example, the most common anti-RNP antibodies (anti-Sm,[11] anti–U₁ RNP,[12] anti-Ro,[17, 19] and anti-La,[18, 19] as well as anti-Jo-1[38]) were first identified with this method, and the currently accepted clinical associations of these antibodies with various diseases are based largely on data developed with immunodiffusion. Certain anti-RNP antibodies that arise less frequently, such as anti–U₂ RNP, also can be detected with this technique.[44, 45] Thus, immunodiffusion remains an important diagnostic method.

Despite the relative insolubility of chromatin, antibodies to certain chromatin components that dissociate from DNA in saline buffer can also can be measured by immunodiffusion, including those that bind topoisomerase I (also called Scl-70),[24, 41] proliferating cell nuclear antigen (PCNA),[46] and the Ku proteins.[47] Additionally, antibodies to the nucleolar protein complex, PM-Scl (also called PM-1), can be measured in this way.[48] In contrast, autoantibodies that bind less abundant or less stable RNPs, such as the nucleolar Th and U₃ RNPs, or that bind relatively insoluble chromatin components, such as DNA and histones, are not routinely detectable in immunodif-

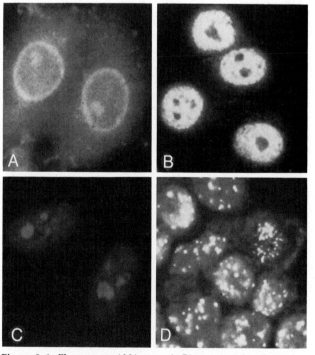

Figure 9–1. Fluorescent ANA test. *A,* Rim or peripheral staining pattern. *B,* Fine-speckled pattern. *C,* Nucleolar pattern; Hep-2 cells used as substrates. *D,* Centromere staining pattern, produced using human lymphoid cells. (*D* reprinted from the Clinical Slide Collection on the Rheumatic Diseases, copyright 1991. Used by permission of the American College of Rheumatology.)

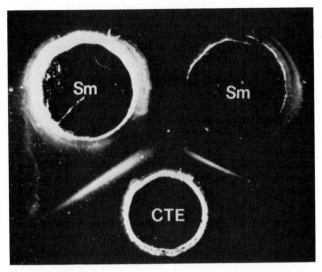

Figure 9–2. Double immunodiffusion assay. A soluble suspension of calf thymus extract (CTE) has been placed in the center well, and two sera with anti-Sm antibodies have been placed in the opposing wells (labeled Sm). Precipitin lines formed with 24 hours. (From Craft, J.: Antibodies to snRNPs in SLE. Rheum. Dis. Clin. North Am. 18:320, 1992, used by permission.)

fusion assays. As discussed later, such specificities must be identified through application of more sophisticated methods.

For its performance, this method requires only a prototype standard serum, tissue extract, and an agarose plate. Typically, tissue (e.g., rabbit or calf thymus) is disrupted with sonication in a saline buffer. The soluble phase is collected with centrifugation and is referred to as extractable nuclear antigens(s) (ENA). This material typically contains a wide variety of RNPs, including snRNPs and free proteins, but very little DNA and a paucity of proteins normally associated with DNA because of the insolubility of chromatin. As shown in Figure 9–2, a rosette of wells is cut into the agarose medium. Patient sera, either undiluted or diluted up to 1:8 or so, are placed in peripheral wells adjacent to sera of known specificity; the tissue extract is placed in the center well. The plate is incubated in a moist environment at room temperature. As the antibodies and antigens diffuse outward from the wells, collisions occur, and as antibodies bind their epitopes an insoluble lattice structure develops that can be observed as a precipitin band. If the antigen-antibody interaction of the test serum is the same as that for the prototype serum, the two precipitin lines will fuse to form a line of identity. Otherwise, they will spur across each other. Such precipitin lines require relatively large amounts of specific antibody (about 0.1 mg of IgG) and antigen, and the two components should be present in roughly equal amounts.

The sensitivity of immunodiffusion can be enhanced with the technique of counterimmunoelectrophoresis[49] (reviewed in reference 1). Negatively charged antigens such as DNA are moved electrophoretically in agarose against positively charged antibodies, producing the same type of lattice formation described earlier with about an order of magnitude more sensitivity. This method has mainly been applicable for the detection of antibodies to nucleic acids, and to the RNP/Sm and Ro/La systems.

ELISA (Enzyme-Linked Immunosorbent Assays). In these assays, a highly pure antigen is allowed to adhere to the surface of wells in a plastic tray and is followed with a protein-blocking solution so that all sites for nonspecific attachment of antibodies are occupied. Thus, when dilute patient serum is added, antibodies that recognize the antigen become selectively bound to the wells. The latter are detected with a second antibody conjugated to an enzyme such as alkaline phosphatase. Addition of a substrate that changes color when cleaved with the specifically bound enzyme permits quantification of bound patient antibody.

In comparison to immunodiffusion, the principal advantages of ELISA assays for the detection of autoantibodies are their relative speed (results are available within several hours, versus 24 to 48 hours for immunodiffusion) and sensitivity (approximates that of radioimmunoassays). They are also easier and safer to perform than are most radioimmunoassays. Their major limitations are the requirement for a pure antigen to serve as substrate and a relatively high rate of false-positive results.

ELISAs for ANAs were originally based on using immunoaffinity or biochemically purified antigen substrates. Since such purification methods are relatively laborious and yield small quantities of antigens, such assays have been established primarily for research purposes. It should be noted that the common autoantigens, including Ro,[50–53] La,[54] Sm,[55–59] U_1 RNP,[60–64] Jo-1,[65] and topoisomerase I (Scl-70),[66] have now been cloned and therefore potentially can be overproduced as recombinant proteins in *Escherichia coli*. Thus, recombinant DNA technology has begun to address the need for ready sources of highly pure antigens for commercial ELISA systems.

Immunoprecipitation Assays. Radioimmunoprecipitation provides a powerful method for detection of autoantibodies or autoantigens. One of the earliest radioimmunoprecipitation assays was the Farr assay for the detection of antibodies to native DNA.[67] This assay is carried out with radiolabeled DNA that is incubated with diluted patient sera. Ammonium sulfate, which insolubilizes immunoglobulin but not DNA, is then added. Thus, the radiolabeled DNA appears in the precipitates only if bound by antibodies in the patient serum. Usually, the results are recorded as the percentage of added DNA that is incorporated into the immunoprecipitate. Under these conditions, normal sera bind a small fraction of the added DNA (usually less than 20 percent), whereas SLE sera often bind considerably more (up to 100 percent).[68] Provided that the laboratory is careful to use only double-stranded DNA as the antigen, this assay is a precise method for detecting antibodies to native DNA and should

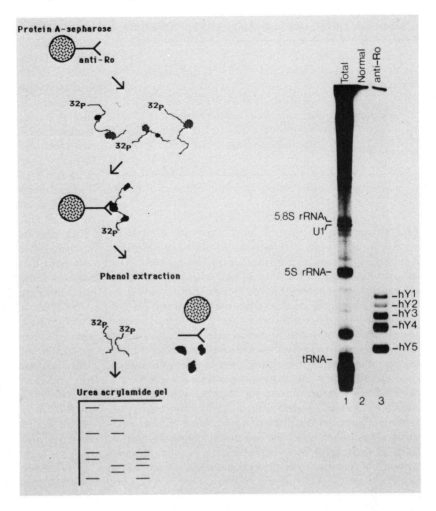

Figure 9–3. RNA immunoprecipitation assay. As shown in the left side of the figure, antibodies from a patient with SLE (in this case anti-Ro antibodies) are bound to sepharose beads coated with protein A; the latter binds the Fc portion of immunoglobulin of the IgG class. Antibody-coated beads are then mixed with a soluble cell extract, previously labeled in vivo with ^{32}phosphorus (^{32}P), which tags nucleic acids. Radiolabeled RNAs (as part of an RNP particle) can then be immunoprecipitated via their antigenic proteins, phenol-extracted to remove proteins (Ro proteins and immunoglobulins), and fractionated by gel electrophoresis. The right side of the figure contains the radiolabeled RNAs found in a total human (HeLa) cell extract (lane 1), and those immunoprecipitated by a normal control serum (lane 2) and a serum containing anti-Ro antibodies (lane 3). As shown, the Ro RNP contains four small RNAs (in human cells), the so-called hY RNAs (hY2 is a breakdown product of hY1).

be regarded as the gold standard for analysis of these antibodies.

In more recent years, radioimmunoprecipitation assays have been applied to the detection of a broad range of antibodies that recognize specific nucleoprotein particles such as snRNP and small cytoplasmic RNP (scRNP) particles, respectively.[69] It is largely through application of these assays that a large number of autoantigens have been identified. In these assays, cultured cells typically are labeled in vivo either with ^{32}P orthophosphate to label nucleic acids (Fig. 9–3) or with a radiolabeled amino acid such as ^{35}S-methionine to label proteins.[70] The cells are disrupted with sonication in a saline buffer so that all of their soluble components can be recovered. The resulting cell extract is incubated with patient antibodies attached to an insoluble carrier, such as sepharose beads coated with protein A; the latter protein binds to the Fc portion of immunoglobulins, particularly those of the IgG isotype (see Fig. 9–3). The antigen-antibody complexes that form are easily recovered, and the bound antigens are analyzed electrophoretically. In interpreting the results of the latter, it should be noted that immunoprecipitates may contain relatively intact nucleoprotein particles, and the entire array of constituent polypeptides or nucleic acids may be visualized, depending on the labeling procedure used.

Immunoprecipitation assays have a number of specific advantages, including a high level of sensitivity and specificity, because the radiolabeled antigen can be detected in minute quantity and because the antigen itself can be visualized directly. In comparison to immunodiffusion, they have much greater ability to detect antibodies against minor cellular components such as the Ro particle, and are somewhat more sensitive for the detection of antibodies against abundant antigens, such as the U_1 snRNP.[71] Although no formal comparisons of the sensitivity of ELISA versus that of immunoprecipitation have been made, we have found a number of sera that give positive results for anti-Ro and anti-La antibodies in the former but are negative in the latter assay.[71] In these cases, we cannot be sure that a specific anti-Ro or anti-La antibody is being detected in the ELISA. The principal disadvantages of immunoprecipitation assays are that they may require use of radioactivity and are more laborious compared to ELISA or immunodiffusion.

Immunoblots (Western Blots). In these assays, a source of antigens (cell extracts, or more purified proteins) is fractionated electrophoretically, followed

Table 9–5. DETECTION OF ANTIBODIES TO dsDNA

Detection Method	Percentage (%) of Positive Results
Precipitation in agar gel[77, 78]	7–33
Counterimmunoelectrophoresis[77]	37
Passive hemagglutination[79]	60
Complement fixation[74, 75, 78]	48–68
Radioimmunoassay[20, 67, 68]	50–75
IFA by the *Crithidia* technique[80–82]	58–95
ELISA[83–88]	70–92

dsDNA, double-stranded DNA.

by transfer to nitrocellulose and subsequent probing with patient serum.[72] Bound antibodies can then be detected with an antihuman antibody tagged with an enzyme or radioactive label. As with immunoprecipitations, a principal advantage of immunoblots is their specificity, since the antigenic protein targets of ANAs are visualized directly. An advantage of immunoblots over immunoprecipitation assays is that the former method provides information about which polypeptide carries the specific epitope that is being recognized, since the antigens are probed with antisera after electrophoretic separation, whereas immunoprecipitations demonstrate only the total protein or RNA composition of the bound antigen. In general, immunoblots are somewhat less sensitive than ELISAs, and their performance is more laborious. For certain autoantibodies, such as anti-Ro, which often target conformational epitopes that are disrupted by gel electrophoresis,[73] immunoblots may be ineffective. At present, the principal use of both immunoblots and immunoprecipitation assays is in the evaluation of ANAs at a research level and, on special occasions, to confirm results of immunodiffusion or ELISA.

Tests for Anti-DNA Antibodies. DNA was the first specific autoantigen to be identified in SLE.[74–76] While first detected in only a minority of patients with relatively insensitive immunodiffusion assays,[10] it soon became apparent that antibodies able to bind DNA could be detected in many patients when more sensitive assays were applied (Table 9–5). These antibodies are rarely found in diseases other than SLE,[68] their titers often fluctuate in accord with changes in disease activity,[78, 90] and the presence of immune complexes containing anti-DNA antibodies in eluates of nephritic kidneys indicated that they are a mechanism for tissue injury in SLE.[90–93] Thus, analysis of anti-DNA antibodies has become an important laboratory tool for the evaluation of patients with SLE. There is also evidence that anti-DNA antibodies "cross-react" with renal antigens and, by binding directly to glomeruli, may contribute to nephritis.[94]

A number of specific autoantigenic epitopes have been identified on DNA. From a clinical perspective, the most important specificity is represented by antibodies that bind the deoxyribose phosphate back-bone of DNA. These antibodies recognize native, double-stranded DNA. They are present in patients with SLE and, when found in high titer, are highly specific for this disorder. Another group of anti-DNA antibodies are specific for denatured DNA. These antibodies bind free purine and pyrimidine base sequences and thus bind only denatured DNA or segments within native DNA that have become single-stranded. Anti–single-stranded DNA antibodies are found in a number of different diseases, including SLE, drug-induced lupus, chronic active hepatitis, infectious mononucleosis, and rheumatoid arthritis.[79, 95] A third class of anti-DNA antibodies are represented by those that recognize specific DNA conformations. While the exact epitopes have not been defined, it has been shown that these antibodies can distinguish between DNA in either the most common right-handed helical, or B, form or the less common left handed-helical, or Z, form (a conformation thought to be associated with DNA segments involved with active gene expression).[96–98] Such conformation-dependent anti-DNA antibodies are relatively rare and are restricted to patients with SLE. Finally, while DNA is generally not immunogenic when injected into experimental animals, it has been possible to induce anti-DNA antibodies readily in mice inoculated with bacterial DNA.[99, 100] The resulting antibodies are specific for bacterial DNA. The specific feature(s) of the bacterial DNA that is being recognized in this system remains to be identified.

A number of assay systems are currently in widespread use for detection of anti-DNA antibodies (see Table 9–5). The earliest assays were based on immunodiffusion (positive in a minority of patients because of lack of sensitivity and capable of producing false-positive results because DNA immunoprecipitates with serum components other than specific antibody). Subsequent assays based on counterimmunoelectrophoresis, complement fixation, or passive hemagglutination improved sensitivity somewhat but were relatively cumbersome to perform. Radioimmunoassays based on Farr's technique or on the ability of Millipore (micropore) filters to bind immunoglobulin but not native DNA provided even better sensitivity but necessitated the use of radiolabeled DNA.

Several methods have been devised for ensuring that the DNA substrate is truly in nondenatured form. One of the most reliable is digestion with S1 nuclease, which removes overhanging single-stranded DNA ends, resulting in blunt-ended double-stranded DNA molecules. Alternative methods involve chromatography of the DNA on hydroxyapatite columns, which separates DNA molecules containing large single-stranded segments from double-stranded DNA. Native DNA can be difficult to maintain, since spontaneous denaturation tends to occur. The production of single-stranded segments as native DNA binds to plastic plates may be a particular problem for certain ELISAs. This latter concern may account for the relative lack of specificity for SLE

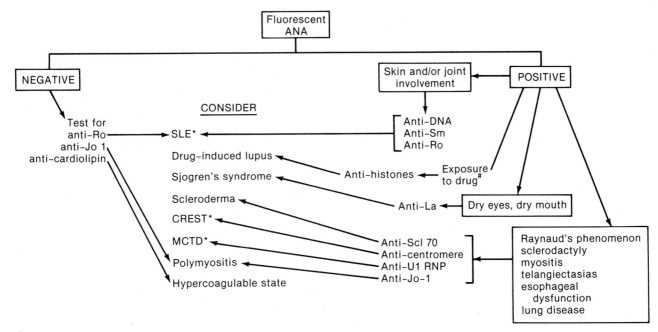

hydralazine, procainamide, quinidine, other drugs
. SLE = systemic lupus erythematosus; CREST = calcinosis, Raynaud's phenomenon, esophageal motility
disorder, sclerodactyly, and telangiectasias (scleroderma with limited skin involvement);
MCTD = mixed connective tissue disease.

Figure 9–4. Algorithm for the use of ANAs in the diagnosis of connective tissue disorders.

observed with some of the current assays for antibodies to native DNA.

EVALUATION OF PATIENTS FOR ANAS

The approach to the evaluation of a patient for ANAs is schematically described in the algorithm in Figure 9–4. A negative FANA generally indicates the absence of ANAs and argues against the diagnosis of SLE, or one of the ANA diseases. Thus, it is rarely profitable to order specialized tests for individual nuclear autoantigens such as DNA. However, if the clinical picture strongly suggests connective tissue disease, it is reasonable to consider specific assays for antibodies to antigens such as Ro and Jo-1, which test negative in FANA assays. On the other hand, since specific ANAs can have diagnostic significance, it is often useful to proceed to specialized assays when a positive FANA is obtained (see Fig. 9–4). For example, if SLE is suspected, the serum might be tested for anti-DNA, anti-Sm, anti–U_1 RNP, and anti-Ro antibodies. Similarly, if MCTD is suspected, the serum should be tested for anti–U_1 RNP antibodies; in the case of Sjögren's syndrome, the presence of anti-Ro and anti-La antibodies; in scleroderma, for antibodies to Scl-70 (topoisomerase I), chromosomal centromeres, or nucleoli; or in adult polymyositis or dermatomyositis, for antibodies to tRNA synthetases. It must be emphasized, however, that positive results in these more specialized assays alone do not signify specific diseases, rather they add weight to

diagnoses that should rely heavily on the clinical picture.

AUTOANTIBODY-AUTOANTIGEN SYSTEMS ASSOCIATED WITH RHEUMATIC DISEASES

Systemic Lupus Erythematosus

DNA. Antibodies to both native DNA and single-stranded DNA have clinical significance in SLE (reviewed in reference 101). Antibodies to native DNA are virtually diagnostic of SLE.[68, 79] Relatively low titers of this specificity are found occasionally in patients with Sjögren's syndrome and rheumatoid arthritis, and these patients are likely to have clinical features that overlap with SLE[68] (Table 9–6). Thus, the presence of anti-native DNA antibodies is one of the most helpful markers for diagnosing SLE. Patients with drug-induced lupus do not have antibodies to native DNA but may have antibodies to single-

Table 9–6. ANTI-NATIVE DNA

	Total No. Tested	No. Testing Positive (%)
SLE	44	32 (73)
Sjögren's syndrome	24	6 (25)
Other diseases	57	3 (5)
Normal subjects	84	2 (2)

Adapted and reprinted with permission from Pincus, T., Schur, P. H., et al.: Measurements of serum DNA-binding activity in SLE. The New England Journal of Medicine 281:701–705, 1969.

stranded DNA.[79] Such antibodies also occur in a wide variety of disorders, including SLE, chronic active hepatitis, infectious mononucleosis, and rheumatoid arthritis.[82, 95] Thus, they have poor diagnostic specificity for SLE. However, their importance in the immunopathogenesis of lupus is emphasized by their nearly universal occurrence in this disorder and their apparent presence in immune complexes that deposit in renal glomeruli.[102–104] In some patients, they appear to drive renal injury in the absence of anti-native DNA.[105] The specificity of antibodies to native DNA for SLE may be impaired if complete reliance is placed on ELISA technology, most probably because of the tendency of the latter assays to detect the relatively ubiquitous presence of antibodies to single-stranded DNA.

The presence of high levels of anti-native DNA antibodies along with hypocomplementemia is a risk factor for nephritis.[106–109] Some patients develop nephritis in the absence of these antibodies, however, whereas others have high levels for prolonged periods without exhibiting renal injury. One of the principal determinants of pathogenicity of the anti-DNA antibodies is their ability to fix complement.[78, 79] Thus, it is often wise to determine in individual patients how well these antibodies parallel disease activity. From that point onward, they may be considered as potentially useful for detecting early flare ups of disease. In patients who conform to this pattern, measurement of anti-DNA at 1- to 3-month intervals is often a reasonable plan.

A number of observations have contributed to the concept that anti-native DNA antibodies play a central role in the pathogenesis of SLE. First, they are one of the most common autoantibodies found in patients with this disease. When measured with radioimmunoprecipitation, they are found in the majority of patients with active disease. Additionally, with successful treatment, anti-DNA titers tend to fall and often become undetectable during periods of sustained remission. In some patients with worsening disease, anti-DNA titers have been observed to fall as levels of circulating free DNA (presumably released from injured tissues) rise, suggesting immune complex formation.[110] Finally, acid eluates of kidney tissue from patients with lupus nephritis have been found to contain enriched levels of anti-DNA antibodies (to both single- and double-stranded DNA), compared with the immunoglobulins in the circulation, thus providing good evidence for the deposition of DNA–anti-DNA immune complexes.[103, 104]

These observations imply that the DNA antigen is released from its intracellular compartment within the nucleus and exists within the circulation. DNA is a relatively stable molecule, and it can be isolated from plasma. Especially high levels are found in patients with ongoing tissue injury.[110a] Free DNA within the circulation is not completely heterogeneous. Rather it exists in discrete sizes that roughly approximate multiples of about 150 nucleotides, a size that corresponds to nucleosomal DNA segments.[110b] Similar lengths of DNA are released from cells undergoing programmed cell death (a process known as apoptosis). Presumably, this latter process accounts for at least some of the circulating DNA in patients with SLE. It seems likely that this DNA has both double- and single-stranded regions, and it is likely to be recognized by antibodies to both forms.

RNA. Antibodies able to bind deproteinized RNA were initially thought to be rare and of questionable diagnostic significance. More recently, it has become clear that autoantibodies to specific forms of naked RNA molecules are common. For example, antibodies to the small nuclear U_1 RNA[111] occur in approximately one third of patients with anti–U_1 RNP antibodies.[112] As with the latter specificity, anti–U_1 RNA antibodies appear to be restricted to patients with SLE and SLE/overlap syndromes,[112] but it is not clear whether the presence of such antibodies aids in the diagnosis of lupus or in estimating the prognosis of these patients. Antibodies to ribosomal RNAs have also been demonstrated in patients with SLE,[113] and it seems probable that additional autoantibody specificities for selected RNA molecules will found. At present, measurement of antibodies to specific RNA forms is largely a research tool.

Sm and U_1 RNP. Antibodies to the RNP antigen Sm were first identified by Tan and Kunkel in 1966[11] and are specific for the diagnosis of systemic lupus[20] (reviewed in references 2 and 114). When assayed by immunodiffusion, these antibodies are found in approximately 25 percent of all patients with SLE,[20] and their presence has been included as part of the revised criteria for the diagnosis of this disorder.[115] ELISAs for the detection of anti-Sm are more sensitive than immunodiffusion,[116–119] without sacrificing the specificity of the clinical correlation of these antibodies with SLE.[117, 119] Anti-Sm antibodies occur more frequently in peoples of Asian or African origin, in comparison with those of European origin[118, 119] and are approximately twice as common in black compared with white Americans with lupus.[118] For instance, these antibodies are found in approximately 30 to 40 percent of Japanese patients and patients of African ancestry with lupus, compared with some 10 to 20 percent of white patients.[117–120] Anti-Sm antibody titers sometimes vary over time,[121–123] although it is unusual for them to disappear when measured by sensitive immunoprecipitation assays.[122] They may, however, become undetectable by standard immunodiffusion tests.[121]

Several investigators have addressed the possible association of anti-Sm antibodies with disease flare ups in SLE and with disease subsets. Initial investigations using immunodiffusion assays suggested that patients with these antibodies had milder renal disease and less central nervous system involvement than those with anti-DNA antibodies,[124] although rising titers could predict disease flare ups[121] or more active disease.[28] However, a more recent study based on the sensitive ELISA for anti-Sm detection suggested that these antibodies did not correlate with particular disease manifestations.[119] Another study of more than 100 Japanese patients revealed that anti-Sm, when detected by ELISA, defined a group of patients with a low frequency of progression to end-stage renal disease (and thus with milder disease), despite a high prevalence of late-onset proteinuria, and despite a poorer prognosis overall than that of patients without anti-Sm.[117] These observations were supported by those involving a group of American patients with lupus that suggested that these antibodies, when detected by ELISA, were associated with renal disease, the progression of which was not defined.[123]

Overall, anti-Sm antibodies are very helpful in making the diagnosis of SLE. While the role of these antibodies in predicting or following the course of the illness is much less clearly drawn, in certain populations it is possible that these antibodies may identify a group of patients with a likelihood of developing certain disease manifestations.

Anti-U_1 RNP antibodies occur in up to 40 percent of patients with SLE[20, 28, 118, 125] (reviewed in references 2 and 114), often in conjunction with anti-Sm antibodies. These antibodies are sometimes found alone in SLE; however, the converse finding, patients with anti-Sm who lack anti-RNP, is unusual.[30–32, 116] Anti-RNP antibodies also are found in MCTD, typically alone and in high titer, and this entity is defined by the presence of this specificity.[14, 21, 116, 126] Anti-RNP antibodies also may rarely occur in patients with rheumatoid arthritis, Sjögren's syndrome, scleroderma, or polymyositis.[20, 116, 126] These antibodies are more common in black than in white individuals,[118] and antibody titers may vary over time.[123, 125, 127–129]

The molecular structure of the Sm and RNP antigens has now been well defined, and a working knowledge of this structure is helpful for interpretation of new diagnostic assays, including ELISAs for ANAs, and for understanding the immunologic abnormalities that characterize SLE. Structurally, the RNP and Sm antigenic determinants were first shown to be physically associated by Mattioli and Reichlin,[31] using double immunodiffusion. Subsequent investigations by Lerner and Steitz[22] demonstrated that both antigens are located on the U_1 snRNP particle, a complex of the U_1 RNA and nine associated polypeptides (reviewed in reference 130) (Fig. 9–5). As noted previously, anti-Sm and anti-RNP antibodies are commonly found together. This co-occurrence, or linkage, of these autoantibodies could potentially be explained if the U_1 snRNP, containing both antigenic determinants, per se, served as a self-immunogen in SLE, a concept for which indirect evidence is now available.[3]

The U_1 snRNP is one of an abundant group of U snRNPs, comprised of uridine-rich RNAs (U for uridine-rich) and proteins, all involved in processing of messenger RNA within the nucleus (reviewed in reference 23). The fine-speckled nuclear staining patterns of anti-Sm and anti-RNP antibodies in indirect

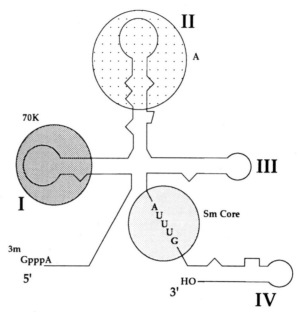

Figure 9–5. A schematic example of the U_1 snRNP, the intracellular target of anti-Sm and anti–U_1 RNP (formerly anti-nRNP) antibodies. Shown are the U_1 RNA and associated proteins of the U_1 snRNP. The 70K protein binds the first stem-loop of the U_1 RNA, the A protein the second stem-loop, and the so-called Sm core proteins, B', B, and D-G, bind a single-stranded region ($AU_{>3}G$) between the third and fourth stem-loops. The binding site of the C protein is not precisely known at present. (Adapted from Lutz-Freyermuth, C., and Keene, J. D.: The U1 RNA-binding site of the U1 small nuclear ribonucleoprotein (snRNP)-associated A protein suggests a similarity with U2 snRNPs. Mol. Cell. Biol. 9:2975–2982, 1989; and Query, C. C., Bentley, R. C., and Keene, J. D.: A specific 31-nucleotide domain of U1 RNA directly interacts with the 70K small nuclear ribonucleoprotein component. Mol. Cell. Biol. 9:4872–4881, 1989.)

immunofluorescence can be attributed to the fact that these snRNP particles are spread throughout the nucleus at sites of active gene transcription where messenger RNA is processed. Three of the nine proteins of the U_1 snRNP, 70K, A, and C, are the targets of anti–U_1 RNP antibodies[32] (appropriately called anti–U_1 RNP antibodies, rather than their original moniker, anti-nRNP antibodies, because these proteins are part of the U_1 snRNP.[22] Since these three polypeptides do not share known cross-reactive epitopes, the anti–U_1 RNP response is composed of at least three separate antibodies, anti-70K, anti-A, and anti-C, that may occur together or singly in a given patient[32, 34] (i.e., all three antibodies contribute to the anti–U_1 RNP response). ELISA assays based on measurement of antibodies to the individual proteins have now been established. Such assays are more sensitive than immunodiffusion; for example, more patients (an additional several percentage points) with anti-70K antibodies are detected using an ELISA.[125]

Anti-70K antibodies are found in nearly all patients with MCTD, when preselected for the presence of anti–U_1 RNP as measured by immunodiffusion or as determined by counterimmunoelectrophoresis.[128, 131, 132] In comparison, certain patients with SLE who have anti–U_1 RNP antibodies will also have anti-70K antibodies, from as few as 8 to 21 percent up to approximately 50 percent of such individuals.[123, 128, 131, 132] It should be noted, however, that one study using an ELISA based on recombinant 70K fusion proteins produced in *E. coli* indicated that as many as 85 percent of patients with SLE, who have anti–U_1 RNP antibodies detectable by immunodiffusion, will have anti-70K antibodies.[125]

These data show that the presence of anti-70K antibodies does not necessarily distinguish patients with MCTD from those with SLE. Yet, when these patients are grouped together, anti-70K antibodies are associated with myositis, esophageal hypomotility, Raynaud's phenomenon, and lack of nephritis,[123, 132] and when individuals with SLE are analyzed, these antibodies are associated with the latter two manifestations.[132] Thus, it does appear that anti-70K antibodies can perhaps be used as a marker for MCTD or for SLE with specific clinical features. The concept that these antibodies may be associated with specific disease subsets is strengthened by the finding that they are associated with HLA-DR4.[133] Although levels of anti-70K antibodies may vary over time, it is unclear whether these variations are associated with disease activity.[123, 125, 127–129] As for anti–U_1 RNP antibodies, anti-70K antibodies may be found in a small number of patients with rheumatoid arthritis, polymyositis, and scleroderma.[125]

Antibodies that bind the A protein are also found in the majority of patients who have anti–U_1 RNP antibodies.[32] However, in SLE, anti-A antibodies are approximately twice as frequent as anti-70K antibodies,[128, 134], occurring in as many as 75 percent of patients with anti–U_1 RNP by immunodiffusion,[123] or in around one quarter of all patients with SLE.[134] Uncertainty exists as to whether titers of anti-A antibodies rise in the setting of disease flare ups or whether these antibodies are markers for certain disease manifestations.[123, 129] Anti-C antibodies are also found in patients with anti–U_1 RNP antibodies,[32] but specific clinical associations of these antibodies have not been described.

Overall, antibodies to the 70K, A, and C proteins contribute to the anti–U_1 RNP response as detected by immunodiffusion or by other assays that measure antibodies to this entire RNP particle. Antibodies to the individual proteins may contribute to a greater or lesser degree to the overall anti–U_1 RNP response, depending on clinical manifestations.

The Sm antigen is made up of epitopes found on the B', B, and D proteins of the U_1 snRNP (and related U snRNPs) (see Fig. 9–5). Anti-Sm antibodies typically bind all three of these proteins; thus, a cross-reactive determinant is shared among these polypeptides, and any of them could be used as substrates in ELISA or other solid-phase assays. The B polypeptide is also weakly bound by anti–U_1 RNP antibodies, however, indicating that anti-D antibodies may be a more specific indicator of the anti-Sm response.[117]

The other abundant U snRNP particles contain specific proteins, in a fashion analogous to the three specific proteins (70K, A, and C) of the U_1 snRNP (reviewed in reference 114); however, these antibodies occur quite rarely and are of uncertain diagnostic significance. An exception to this statement are autoantibodies that bind the two specific proteins of the U_2 RNP, the so-called A' and B" proteins, which appear to occur in patients with overlap syndromes, particularly those associated with myositis.[34, 44, 45, 128, 135]

The 70K and A-E proteins of the U_1 snRNP have been cloned.[55–64, 136] Current investigations focus around which regions, or epitopes, of these proteins are bound by patient sera, and whether antibodies to a particular portion of a polypeptide have clinical significance. Knowledge of the precise structure of these proteins may provide clues as to why they become autoimmunogens in SLE and related diseases.

Ro/SS-A and La/SS-B. Anti–Ro/SS-A and anti–La/SS-B antibodies are a prominent feature of the humoral autoimmune response in patients with SLE and with Sjögren's syndrome (see references 137 and 138 for review). The Ro and La antigens were originally defined by immunodiffusion using sera from patients with SLE (and a few patients with Sjögren's syndrome),[17, 18] whereas the SS-A and SS-B antigens were separately defined using sera from patients with Sjögren's syndrome.[19, 139] Subsequently Ro and La were shown to be identical to SS-A and SS-B, respectively[140]; the latter is also the same as the Ha antigen.[141, 142] For convenience, the terms anti–Ro/SS-A and anti–La/SS-B (or anti–La/SS-B/Ha) will be shortened in this discussion to anti-Ro and anti-La, respectively.

Anti-Ro antibodies are found in approximately 25 to 50 percent of patients with SLE when sera from these patients are tested in counterimmunoelectrophoresis or double immunodiffusion,[17, 137, 138, 143–148] whereas anti-La occurs in about 10 to 15 percent of such patients,[146, 147] principally in those individuals who have SLE plus the sicca complex.[142, 147] ELISAs for the detection of both anti-Ro and anti-La are more sensitive than immunodiffusion or counterimmunoelectrophoresis.[146, 149] For example, an additional 5 to 10 percent or more of patients with lupus will have either or both of these antibodies when their sera are tested in ELISA in comparison with the latter assays,[146, 147, 150] although ELISA assays may not be as specific.[146] In patients with SLE, anti-Ro antibodies are associated with positive test results for rheumatoid factor (about 75 percent of patients) and hypergammaglobulinemia.[17, 143–145, 151] Anti-Ro antibodies may also occur in patients with other rheumatic syndromes, including as many as 18 percent of individuals with polymyositis, around 5 percent of patients with scleroderma, and approximately 5 percent of those with rheumatoid arthritis.[143, 146] In the latter group, these antibodies are associated with positive ANAs and more severe extra-articular disease.[152] Anti-La antibodies are more restricted in their disease expression, that is, to patients with SLE (generally with the sicca complex[142]) and Sjögren's syndrome, although they may be found in a small percentage of individuals with polymyositis.[146] Both anti-Ro and anti-La antibodies may also be found in small number of normal sera (a few percentage points) when assayed by ELISA, but antibody titers are lower than in patients with lupus or Sjögren's syndrome.[147, 153, 154] Titers of both specificities may also vary over time,[144, 150] but it is unclear whether these changes predict or reflect disease activity.

Anti-Ro antibodies often occur alone in SLE and in Sjögren's syndrome; however, the converse finding of isolated anti-La antibodies is unusual.[18, 146, 150, 153, 155] In this sense, the anti-Ro and anti-La antibody systems mimic that of anti–U_1 RNP and anti-Sm, where the latter antibody specificity rarely occurs alone. Patients with lupus with anti-Ro alone tend to have lower titers of these antibodies, in contrast with those individuals who also have anti-La.[147] Patients in the former group also have a greater frequency of renal disease,[143, 147, 155, 156] as well as having up to 20 to 30 percent of asymptomatic family members (first- and second-degree relatives) with anti-Ro,[157] whereas those in the latter group are older at disease onset and, as noted earlier, have a greater frequency of sicca complex.[147] HLA genes may exert effects on the expression of anti-Ro and anti-La, since individuals who are HLA-DR2/DR3 heterozygotes have a greater frequency of anti-Ro, and heterozygotes (with SLE or with primary Sjögren's syndrome) for HLA-DQ1/DQ2 have higher levels of these antibodies.[147, 158–160] Anti-Ro antibodies are also found in nearly all individuals with homozygous C2 deficiency who have a clinical picture of SLE; these patients are also commonly HLA-DR2 positive.[197] The notion that the frequency of these antibodies has a genetic basis is supported by the observation that they are more common in Japanese patients with SLE than in patients from the United States.[1]

Anti-Ro antibodies are associated with several subsets of SLE.[1] For example, about two thirds of patients with so-called "ANA-negative lupus" have anti-Ro antibodies detectable by immunodiffusion, with the bulk of the remainder having antibodies to single-stranded DNA.[143, 161] These individuals tend to have a high incidence of photosensitive dermatitis and a lower frequency of nephritis and neurologic disease, but many of them will have multisystem involvement. It should be noted, however, that when this group of patients was first described, ANAs were typically performed using organ tissues as substrates, which, as discussed earlier, are not as sensitive for detection of anti-Ro antibodies as rapidly dividing tumor cells. Moreover, the Ro antigen is less abundant in rodent tissues[162, 163] or less antigenic in these tissues,[163–165] which were often used as ANA substrates. Nevertheless, even when using Hep-2 cells as substrates for ANAs, a small percentage of patients with lupus will be ANA negative, and if the clinical suspicion of disease is high, these individuals should have tests for anti-Ro antibodies.

Anti-Ro antibodies are also found in about two thirds of patients with subacute cutaneous lupus, a disease subset characterized by a nonscarring and often photosensitive dermatitis.[166, 167] These individuals have mild systemic disease, similar to those individuals with ANA-negative lupus noted earlier[1, 143] and are often HLA-DR3 positive. Anti-Ro antibodies are also associated with photosensitivity in SLE.[143, 168] In patients with photosensitive skin disease and circulating anti-Ro, the antibodies themselves may be pathogenic, binding to Ro antigen expressed on the surface of keratinocytes, perhaps after ultraviolet light exposure.[169–172]

Another clinical syndrome associated with the presence of anti-Ro and anti-La antibodies is neonatal lupus. This syndrome is secondary to the transport of maternal IgG autoantibodies across the placenta after the first trimester, resulting in complete heart block that is typically irreversible, as well as transient skin rash, liver disease, and hematologic abnormalities in the neonate.[173] Such infants have IgG staining of the myocardium,[174, 175] as well as more focal deposition of immunoglobulin and complement around the fetal conduction system.[176] Initial studies revealed that as many as 85 percent of mothers of such infants had anti-Ro antibodies, as measured by immunodiffusion.[177–179] Subsequent studies using immunoblotting or ELISA assays have confirmed the association of maternal anti-Ro with congenital heart block, with mothers of virtually all these children having anti-Ro.[180, 181] Anti-Ro antibodies circulate in the serum of such infants for up 6 months following delivery and disappear coincident with the disappearance of skin rash, although the heart block is typically irreversible. The pathogenesis of the heart block is believed to be damage to the conducting system after it matures after approximately 16 weeks of gestation. In addition to the neonatal lupus syndrome, the presence of maternal anti-Ro antibodies also appears to be associated with the early onset of SLE in offspring as well its development in male children.[182]

As many as 90 percent of these mothers also have anti-La antibodies as measured by immunoblots or ELISA. Indeed, when lupus pregnancies that did not result in heart block were examined, anti-Ro was more frequent than anti-La, suggesting that the latter antibody system may be a better marker for heart block than anti-Ro.[180, 181] Although anti-Ro and anti-La antibodies are almost universally associated with neonatal lupus, it also should be noted that significantly less than 5 percent of mothers with such antibodies have children with this syndrome.[183, 184] Moreover, while such mothers may have connective tissue disease, including SLE, Sjögren's syndrome, or rheumatoid arthritis, it is not uncommon for them to be asymptomatic. Of interest as well is the report of mothers of two children with neonatal lupus, without congenital heart block, who had anti–U_1 RNP antibodies without anti-Ro.[185]

Like the Sm and U_1 RNP antigens, the molecular structure of the Ro and La antigens has now been well defined. The Ro antigen is a small RNP particle that consists of a 60-kD Ro polypeptide that binds four small RNAs, called Ro RNAs, in human cells.[186] Although the cellular location of the Ro protein is somewhat controversial, evidence suggests that it is nuclear in location,[154, 162] although its biologic function remains unknown.

New evidence also indicates that a 52-kD polypeptide is part of the Ro RNPs,[187] although its precise association with the Ro RNAs is not clear at present. While patients with SLE and Sjögren's syndrome make antibodies to both the 60-kD and the 52-kD forms of Ro, the isolated presence of antibodies to the 60-kD form (as determined by immunoblotting) appears to be restricted to patients with SLE, and the isolated occurrence of antibodies to the 52-kD component is restricted to patients with Sjögren's syndrome.[148] Unfortunately, the presence of these two types of antibodies cannot be distinguished by immunodiffusion assays; however, newer ELISAs for the detection of both forms of anti-Ro antibodies will soon be available. In certain tissues, other immunologic forms of the Ro polypeptides exist, including another 60-kD protein found in erythrocytes and a 54-kD protein found in erythrocytes and platelets[188–190]; the clinical significance of antibodies to these forms is unclear at present. Finally, another 60-kD Ro protein has also been identified that is homologous to a ubiquitous calcium-binding protein called calreticulin; hence this Ro protein is also called Ro-calreticulin.[191, 192] A more recent report hypothesizes that the Ro-calreticulin polypeptide may not be associated with the Ro RNAs and perhaps is not a true Ro protein.[193]

The Ro RNAs are transcribed by one of three cellular RNA polymerases, RNA polymerase III. These transcription products are transiently associated with the nuclear La polypeptide (accounting for the nuclear staining of anti-La antibodies in indirect immunofluorescence); that is, the La protein is found on the Ro RNAs and thus is physically associated with at least the originally defined 60-kD Ro polypeptide.[194–196] The physical association of these proteins provides a potential explanation for the frequent co-occurrence of anti-Ro and anti-La antibodies, if this RNP particle per se served as a self-immunogen in SLE, a concept for which indirect evidence is now available.[3]

The 60-kD and 52-kD Ro proteins and the La polypeptide have now been cloned.[50–54] Current investigations focus on which regions, or epitopes, of these proteins are bound by patient sera, and whether antibodies to a particular portion of a polypeptide have clinical significance. Knowledge of the precise structure of these proteins may provide clues as to why they become autoimmunogens in SLE and related diseases.

Proliferating Cell Nuclear Antigen (PCNA). Antibodies to PCNA, first identified in double immunodiffusion, occur in approximately 3 to 4 percent of patients with SLE.[197a] Patients with these antibodies do not have clinical features that distinguish them from other patients with lupus.[2] It was noted in early studies that anti-PCNA antibodies stained only dividing cells in indirect immunofluorescence. For example, when Hep-2 cells are used as substrates, nuclei of about 50 percent of cells are stained in a speckled pattern.[197a] Studies on synchronized cells showed that these antibodies recognized an antigen that had the bulk of its expression during late G and early S phase of the cell cycle just before DNA synthesis[198, 199]; hence the name proliferating cell nuclear antigen.[2] Parallel studies revealed that PCNA was homologous to another cell-cycle–specific protein called cyclin, and thus the name of this protein was changed to PCNA/cyclin.[200] Other work has shown that PCNA/cyclin is identical to the auxiliary protein for DNA polymerase-delta (δ) a nuclear particle required for DNA replication.[201, 202] Human anti-PCNA/cyclin antibodies have proved useful in helping to sort out the function of PCNA/cyclin in DNA replication[2] as well as in identifying those regions of the protein that are autoantigenic.[203]

Ribosomes. Approximately 5 to 10 percent of United States patients with SLE make antibodies to ribosomal proteins.[204] These sera typically produce cytoplasmic staining on immunofluorescence, with a portion also staining the nucleolus; recall that ribosomal assembly begins in the nucleolus followed by transport of these structures to the cytoplasm, where fully assembled ribosomes function in protein translation. In addition to binding specific regions of ribosomal RNAs[113] (see earlier under anti-RNA antibodies), anti-ribosomal antibodies bind only a few of the approximately 80 proteins in these complex structures.[204, 205] Antibodies to the P0, P1, P2, and S10 ribosomal protein components are the most frequently targeted.[204–206] Only about two thirds of these antibodies are detected by counterimmunoelectrophoresis or with cytoplasmic staining in immunofluorescence[207]; immunoblotting assays or ELISA (or radioimmunoassays) using synthetic ribosomal P peptides are more sensitive for their detection.[207, 208] Antibody levels may vary over time, and the presence and titer of antibodies to the P polypeptide components may be predictors of psychosis in SLE.[207, 208] These antibodies appear to be more common in Japanese patients, being present in as many as 40 percent of patients with active disease.[206]

Histones. Histones are the most ubiquitous proteins found in the nucleus of eukaryotic cells. Their function is to provide for orderly packaging of the many centimeters of DNA that must be contained in the tiny confines of each cell nucleus. The histones are highly conserved small proteins that are rich in very basic amino acids such as arginine and lysine. The resulting overall strong positive charge favors interaction with negatively charged DNA. There are five main types of histones, known as H1, H3, H2A, H2B, and H4. Within chromatin, the different histones occur in equimolar quantities, with the exception that histone H1 is present in amounts half those of the others.

A great deal of information has been learned about how histones relate to the architecture of chromatin through biochemical analysis, electron microscopy, and, most important, x-ray crystallography. Histones H3 and H4 spontaneously associate to form a tetramer composed of two copies of each molecule. Similarly, histones H2A and H2B associate to form dimers. Two H2A-H2B dimers bind to opposite sides of an H3-H4 tetramer to form a central spool for a segment of double-stranded DNA that is 146 nucleotides in length and that surrounds it in nearly two complete turns. This structure is know as the nucleosomal core particle. Individual core particles are connected through an intervening 40– to 60– base pair segment of DNA to which a single histone H1 molecule is attached. When viewed with electron microscopy the chromatin strand has the appearance of beads on a string, with the string representing the DNA strand (10 angstroms) [Å] and the beads (100 Å) corresponding to the nucleosomes. In conditions of higher salt concentrations, this fiber spontaneously forms a higher-order coil of approximately 300 Å mediated largely through interactions of adjacent H1 molecules. At this point, the DNA strand has been compacted approximately 40 fold.[209, 210]

Autoantibodies directed against histones occur in a number of diseases, including SLE,[211, 212] drug-induced lupus,[213–216] juvenile rheumatoid arthritis,[217, 218] and rheumatoid arthritis[219] as well as other conditions.[220] These antibodies typically produce a smooth, homogeneous staining of the nucleus. Because of the ubiquitous nature of antihistone antibodies, it is reasonable to suspect that the low titers of nuclear staining often referred to as "false-positive" ANAs in otherwise normal individuals is produced by the presence of anti-histone antibodies. In SLE, antibodies to histones are found in about two thirds of patients with active disease,[212] and in these patients the LE cell phenomenon is likely to be caused by such antibodies.[221] All the individual histones are recognized, but a predominant focus is directed against histones H1 and H2B.[212] The latter molecule may be particularly important in the induction of these responses because a major autoantigenic epitope resides at its extreme amino terminal.[222] In addition to antibodies that recognize individual histones, additional antibodies directed against histone complexes have been identified.[223]

High titers of anti-histone antibodies are especially characteristic of patients with drug-induced lupus. These antibodies are found in the majority of individuals who ingest procainamide or hydralazine and probably less frequently in patients taking quinidine, isoniazid, Dilantin (phenytoin), and a long list of other agents. Only a small portion of patients who develop these antibodies express clinical evidence of arthritis, serositis, fever, or other manifestations of drug-induced lupus.[224] The nature of the circulating anti-histone antibodies also distinguishes patients with active disease from those who are asymptomatic. Sera from symptomatic individuals with pro-

cainamide-induced and quinidine-induced lupus have been shown to bind to the H2A-H2B complex (associated with DNA).[225] In contrast, asymptomatic individuals with positive ANAs induced by procainamide are more likely to lack a specific pattern of histone binding, and persons with positive ANAs induced by chlorpromazine and hydralazine are more likely to bind free histones.[225] The role that these antibodies play in the pathogenesis of this syndrome remains unclear. Thus, measurement of antibodies to the H2A-H2B complex can distinguish patients with a drug-induced ANA versus individuals with the drug-induced lupus syndrome. The major limitation of measurements of anti-histone antibodies is the technical difficulty encountered in the assays. Methods that distinguish antibodies to histone complexes are currently limited to research laboratories.

Polymyositis

Approximately 85 percent of patients with polymyositis and adult dermatomyositis (PM/DM) have autoantibodies that produce cytoplasmic and/or nuclear (or nucleolar) staining in indirect immunofluorescence using Hep-2 cells, and 60 percent will produce precipitins in immunodiffusion.[226] These autoantibodies are especially notable for binding cytoplasmic RNPs. Among these, the most characteristic target group are tRNA synthetases, which are cytoplasmic enzymes responsible for catalysis of the attachment of amino acids to their tRNA during protein synthesis. Antibodies to these structures are found in approximately 30 to 40 percent of patients with polymyositis and in about 5 percent of patients with adult dermatomyositis.[227–230] Such autoantibodies are relatively specific for the diagnosis of these conditions, since they are not found in patients with SLE, Sjögren's syndrome, or scleroderma. Additionally, patients with polymyositis with antibodies to tRNA synthetases have a predilection for interstitial lung disease, which may be quite severe, in comparison to patients with PM/DM, who lack these specific autoantibodies.[231–235] It should also be noted that about 10 percent of patients with PM/DM also have an antibody specificity called Mi-2 that produces homogeneous nuclear fluorescence when tested for FANAs. These antibodies, which are detectable in double immunodiffusion, appear to be more specific for dermatomyositis than for polymyositis.[268]

The most common anti–tRNA synthetase autoantibody in PM/DM is anti–Jo-1.[236] When measured by immunodiffusion, these antibodies occur in approximately 20 to 30 percent of patients with polymyositis and much less commonly in patients with dermatomyositis or in patients with polymyositis-scleroderma overlap syndromes.[38, 226, 229, 230, 236–238] When ELISAs are used for detection of anti-Jo-1, as many as 35 percent of patients with polymyositis exhibit this specificity.[229, 235] The Jo-1 antigen is the synthetase responsible for linkage of the amino acid histidine to its tRNA, histidyl tRNA[synthease].[237, 239] Since the synthetase enzyme is associated with a tRNA during this process, the Jo-1 antigen is an RNP. In addition to interstitial lung disease, which occurs in approximately two thirds of patients with anti–Jo-1 (versus about 20 percent of patients with polymyositis without anti–Jo-1 antibodies),[231–235] this group of patients with polymyositis also has a high incidence of inflammatory arthritis (about 50 to 60 percent of patients with anti–Jo-1) and Raynaud's phenomenon.[228, 231, 235, 240] Patients with these antibodies may also have a higher prevalence of periarticular calcification.[240]

The production of anti–Jo-1 antibodies appears to be genetically restricted, occurring in patients who carry the HLA-DR3 and DRw52 haplotypes[238, 241]; other anti-tRNA synthetase antibodies, discussed later, also appear to be associated with the presence of HLA-DRw52.[241] Like other anti-RNP antibodies, including anti-Sm/RNP and anti-Ro/La, anti–Jo-1 antibodies appear to be driven by the target antigen; that is, it appears that the histidyl tRNA synthetase per se is involved in stimulating the production of these antibodies.[242, 243]

Autoantibodies to other tRNA synthetases also occur in PM/DM. The most common of these include antibodies to threonyl tRNA[synthetase],[244–246] and alanyl tRNA[synthetase],[247, 248] which occur in about 5 percent and 3 percent of PM/DM patients, respectively. These antibodies are also more common in patients with PM/DM with interstitial lung disease and arthritis.[244, 246–248] In addition, rare patients with PM/DM have been noted to have antibodies to glycyl and isoleucyl syntheses.[249] These rarer antibodies bind the protein component of the synthetase-tRNA complex; however, a portion of sera from patients with anti–alanyl tRNA[synthetase] antibodies also binds the naked alanyl tRNA directly; that is, these sera also contain anti-RNA antibodies.[247, 250] Indirect evidence suggests that these latter antibodies may arise through the idiotype–anti-idiotype network.[250]

Occasionally, patients with polymyositis may have autoantibodies to other components of the cell's protein translation and production apparatus,[251–254] including the signal recognition particle (SRP), a cytoplasmic RNP responsible for transfer of newly synthesized proteins to the endoplasmic reticulum. In contrast with anti-tRNA synthetase, anti-SRP antibodies appear to be a marker for polymyositis patients with a lower frequency of interstitial lung disease and arthritis,[254] although the myositis may be relatively steroid resistant.[255]

The PM-Scl (originally called PM-1[38, 256, 257]) and Ku antigens are also targeted by autoantibodies from patients with polymyositis, particularly those individuals who also have overlap features of scleroderma, or patients with scleroderma alone.[2, 256–259] PM-Scl is a nucleolar complex[260, 261] of 11 to 16 proteins that are not known to be associated with nucleic acids[261]; anti–PM-Scl antibodies are routinely detected by immunodiffusion. Two of these proteins,

one of 110 kD molecular weight, and another of 39 kD in size (which migrates aberrantly in gel electrophoresis at 75 kD), appear to be recognized by most anti-PM-Scl sera.[262, 263] Sera from approximately 8 percent of patients with polymyositis, and 3 percent of patients with scleroderma, contain anti–PM-Scl antibodies, and thus the nucleolus is stained in indirect immunofluorescence. Indeed, about 15 percent of all scleroderma patients whose sera stain the nucleolus in indirect immunofluorescence have anti–PM-Scl antibodies.[259] Anti–PM-Scl antibodies appear to be restricted to patients with these diseases.

Anti-Ku antibodies, named after the prototype patient, were first described in Japanese patients with scleroderma-polymyositis overlap syndromes.[264] Subsequently, these antibodies were also found in patients from the United States with SLE, scleroderma, and MCTD.[265] The antigenic target of anti-Ku antibodies is a 70-kD and 80-kD protein heterodimer (thus these antibodies are also called anti-p70/-p80[265–267] that binds DNA. These proteins are found throughout the nucleus and, during portions of the cell cycle, in the nucleolus. Generally, these antibodies produce fine-speckled staining of the nucleus in indirect immunofluorescence[265, 266] and, when present in high titer, nucleolar staining.[265] As noted previously, these antibodies can be detected in immunodiffusion assays.[264]

Scleroderma

When Hep-2 cells are used as substrates, virtually every patient with scleroderma (approximately 95 to 97 percent) will have a positive test result for ANAs in indirect immunofluorescence.[40, 41, 269] Patterns of nuclear staining include diffuse nuclear speckling, the larger speckles of anti-centromere antibodies, and nucleolar staining. It should be noted that both anti-centromere and anti-nucleolar antibodies may go undetected when organ tissues are used as substrates for immunofluorescence, rather than Hep-2 cells or other tissue culture cell lines.[40] Nucleolar immunofluorescence should at least suggest the diagnostic possibility of scleroderma, since antibodies that target this region of the cell are unusual in the other connective tissue diseases (anti-ribosomal antibodies may stain this portion of the cell, often in conjunction with cytoplasmic fluorescence, as noted previously). Sera from a small proportion of patients with isolated polymyositis will stain the nucleolus, however, via binding of the PM-Scl antigen, and rarely sera from patients with SLE will also stain the nucleolus via recognition of a nucleolar phosphoprotein, B23. This latter group of patients appear to have a high frequency of anti-cardiolipin antibodies.[270]

The two most common specificities in scleroderma are anti–Scl-70 and anti-centromere antibodies,[40–43, 269, 272] both of which produce nuclear fluorescence. These specificities are found rarely in patients with other connective tissue diseases and are good markers for the diagnosis of scleroderma.[40, 43, 269, 272] As noted earlier, anti-centromere antibodies produce a quite distinctive immunofluorescence pattern of discrete large speckles. While these antibodies are detectable by immunoblots or by ELISA,[273–275] they are not identifiable using immunodiffusion; however, an immunofluorescence staining pattern of discrete nuclear speckles is essentially diagnostic of this specificity. Anti–Scl 70 antibodies stain the nucleus in a grainy speckled pattern,[40] and typically their presence should be confirmed by the use of either immunodiffusion or more sophisticated assays.

The gene for the Scl-70 antigen has now been cloned and identified as topoisomerase I, an approximately 100-kD protein that catalyzes breaks in a single DNA strand that allow DNA to undergo topologic conversion.[276] This protein has proteolytic fragments, including one of 70 kD, hence the name Scl-70.[276, 277] Anti–Scl-70 antibodies are now more appropriately called anti-topoisomerase I (often shortened to anti-topo I). Autoantigenic centromere proteins have also been characterized, and the targets of anti-centromere antibodies appear to be three polypeptides of approximately 17, 80, and 140 kD called CENP-A, B, and C, respectively, with antibodies to CENP-B the most common and found in the highest titer among anti-centromere antibodies.[273, 274] This protein has also been cloned,[278, 279] and the availability of recombinant CENP-B and topoisomerase I will aid in the establishment of a new generation of ELISA assays.[275, 280, 281] Careful characterization of these proteins and their regions bound by anti–topoisomerase I and anti-centromere antibodies has also already provided pathogenetic clues to the etiology of the immune response in scleroderma.[280, 282, 283]

In general, anti–topoisomerase I antibodies are a marker for diffuse scleroderma, as compared with the more limited CREST form of the illness, with about two thirds of all scleroderma patients with these antibodies having diffuse disease.[284] Despite this high prevalence, the majority of patients with diffuse disease lack anti–topoisomerase I, with 20 to 33 percent of such patients in large series having these antibodies as measured by immunodiffusion,[284, 285] a proportion of that can be increased by a few percentage points when immunoblots or ELISAs are used for detection.[281, 285, 286] It should be noted, however, that in smaller series of European patients with scleroderma with diffuse disease, as many as 70 percent will have anti–topoisomerase I antibodies.[281, 286, 287] Additionally, from 4 to 18 percent of patients with limited scleroderma (CREST syndrome) will have anti–topoisomerase I antibodies detectable by immunodiffusion.[284, 285] These individuals tend to have more severe distal skin involvement and a higher percentage of lung involvement than do those patients with limited disease who lack anti–topoisomerase I antibodies, perhaps suggesting that anti–topoisomerase I may also be a marker for a form of diffuse disease whose progression has slowed or stopped.[284] About 5 percent of patients with isolated

Raynaud's syndrome will also have these antibodies,[285] and their presence in this group may have prognostic significance[288] for progression to scleroderma.[289] Among patients with the diffuse disease subset, individuals with anti–topoisomerase I antibodies have a higher frequency of pulmonary fibrosis, as well as digital pitting scars, and tend to have a higher incidence of cardiac involvement compared with those patients who lack these antibodies.[269, 284, 285] Although patients with diffuse disease have a poorer survival in terms of years from first symptom than that of patients with limited disease, anti–topoisomerase I antibodies in the former subset are not a predictive marker of limited survival.[284]

Anti-centromere antibodies, as defined by indirect immunofluorescence, are usually found in patients with the CREST variant of scleroderma. These antibodies have been reported to occur in as many as 96 percent of patients with CREST,[43] although in other, larger, series, they are found in approximately 50 percent of such patients.[40, 269, 284, 285, 290] Anti-centromere antibodies appear to be a good marker for limited disease, since they are found in only a relatively small percentage of patients with diffuse scleroderma.[40, 284, 285, 291] In individuals with proximal scleroderma, the presence of these antibodies also is indicative of less severe skin involvement.[284] About 15 to 30 percent of patients with primary Raynaud's syndrome will also have anti-centromere antibodies.[43, 285, 292] These latter individuals have more digital telangiectasias and abnormal nailfold capillaries as well as diminished digital blood compared with patients negative for anti-centromere antibodies, suggesting that among patients with primary Raynaud's syndrome, these antibodies are a marker for a transition to CREST.[289, 292] As noted earlier, patients with limited disease have a longer survival from the time of the first symptom compared with patients with diffuse disease, although anti-centromere antibodies in the former subset are not a predictor of better survival.[284] Despite the fact that certain patients with limited diseases may have anti–topoisomerase I antibodies, and some patients with diffuse disease may have anti-centromere antibodies, these specificities rarely coexist in the same patient.[284, 285, 293, 294]

As noted, sera from patients with scleroderma are also notable for staining the nucleolus in indirect immunofluorescence assays, with approximately 40 percent of such patients having such staining when Hep-2 cells are used as substrates, sometimes in conjunction with nuclear staining.[40, 41, 294] When carefully examined, scleroderma sera stain nucleoli in different patterns, including speckled, clumpy, and homogeneous[41]; such staining patterns reflect the location of the different components of the nucleolus being recognized. For example, antibodies to the PM-Scl complex, discussed earlier under the section on polymyositis, typically stain the nucleolus in a homogeneous manner.

A number of nucleolar autoantigens have now been defined. The nucleolar components most commonly recognized by sera from patients with scleroderma include the U_3[259] and Th snoRNPs[294-296] (*sno* stands for small nucleolar) and RNA polymerase I.[259, 294] Less commonly, the NOR-90 protein (a 90-kD polypeptide found within the nucleolar organizing region of the chromosomal satellites) serves as a target in this disease.[297] As a group these autoantibodies are all associated with scleroderma, and individually they may serve as markers for different disease manifestations. As already discussed, the nucleolar Ku and PM-Scl antigens are also bound by sera from patients with scleroderma, with a high prevalence of polymyositis.

The U_3 snoRNP consists of the U_3 small RNA (another uridine-rich RNA like the U_1 RNA of the U_1 snRNP) and several proteins,[298, 299] including one of 34 kD called fibrillarin that is probably the most abundant one in this particle, and the one that is recognized by anti-U_3 antibodies.[298] Sera that bind the U_3 particle via recognition of fibrillarin stain the nucleolus in a clumpy manner.[259] Functionally, the U_3 snoRNP is involved in processing of ribosomal RNA within the nucleolus.[300] Of patients with scleroderma anti-nucleolar antibodies, as many as one half may have anti–U_3 RNP (also called anti-fibrillarin) antibodies; these antibodies may also identify a group of patients with scleroderma who tend to have less joint involvement and who may include a higher proportion of men.[259]

The Th snoRNP particle, which is probably involved in nucleolar RNA processing events,[301] also consists of a small RNA and several associated polypeptides.[302] This snoRNP is also called the To particle[303, 304]; both the Th and the To identifiers are derived from prototype patients with this antibody specificity. Like anti–U_3 RNP antibodies, anti-Th antibodies stain the nucleolus in a clumpy manner.[305] Sera that contain these antibodies also faintly stain the nucleus in a fine-speckled manner[305]; this latter staining pattern is probably due to the fact that the Th particle appears to share an antigenic polypeptide with a nuclear RNP particle called RNase P.[301, 306] Patients with anti-Th antibodies tend to have more limited forms of scleroderma,[294-296] although certain patients with these antibodies may have diffuse disease.[296] As noted earlier, antibodies to the U_3 and Th snoRNPs cannot be detected by immunodiffusion, so the presence of these antibodies can be inferred only by nucleolar staining in indirect immunofluorescence, particularly in a clumpy pattern. Both these specificities can easily be detected by the more sensitive immunoprecipitation assay on a research basis.

RNA polymerase I is a protein complex that transcribes ribosomal RNA genes to produce their RNA products in the nucleolus prior to export to the cytoplasm. Anti-RNA pol I antibodies (anti–Pol I) occur in about 15 percent of patients with scleroderma whose sera stain the nucleolus in indirect immunofluorescence.[259, 294, 307] Like antibodies to the U_3 and Th snoRNPs, anti–polymerase I antibodies can be easily detected in immunoprecipitation assays[259, 294, 307] but are not found in immunodiffusion. However, these antibodies stain the nucleolus in a distinctive speckled manner, and such an appearance in indirect immunofluorescence should suggest the presence of this specificity.[259] Other autoantibodies (such as anti–NOR-90) may have a similar staining pattern, but these specificities are much less common than antibodies to RNA polymerase I.[294] It appears that antibodies to RNA polymerase I are associated with diffuse scleroderma of short duration with a frequent occurrence of internal organ involvement.[259, 294, 307]

Several other polypeptides, at present poorly characterized, are bound by sera from patients with scleroderma.[294] These specificities, which have been detected by sensitive immunoprecipitation assays, appear to be relatively rare and of ill-defined clinical importance at present. Finally, it should also be noted that as many as 50 percent of patients with morphea will have positive ANAs, typically with homogeneous or speckled nuclear staining.[308]

Sjögren's Syndrome

Antibodies to the Ro and La antigens predominate in sera from patients with Sjögren's syndrome. In retrospect, it now seems fairly certain that these specificities correspond respectively to the SjD and SjT precipitins originally described by Anderson and colleagues.[309] When tested by immunodiffusion, anti-Ro and anti-La antibodies are found in about 50 percent of sera from these patients.[310] More recent studies based on ELISA methods have demonstrated anti-Ro antibodies in 95 percent and anti-La antibodies in 87 percent of such patients.[311] The incidence of these antibodies appears to be approximately the same in patients with primary Sjögren's syndrome and in Sjögren's syndrome associated with SLE.

ANAs in Sjögren's syndrome have several clinical correlations. Because of its specificity, the anti-La antibody is a useful diagnostic marker that helps solidify the diagnosis in selected patients. As indicated earlier, this antibody is detectable in nearly all patients with Sjögren's syndrome when assays of high sensitivity are applied. In addition, it is rarely found in diseases other than Sjögren's syndrome and SLE, typically with the sicca complex. A group of patients with Sjögren's syndrome, cutaneous features of SLE, and anti-Ro antibodies have been described.[312] These individuals appear to constitute a specific clinical group associated with the HLA phenotype B8, DR-3, DRw52.[313] Among patients with Sjögren's syndrome, high titers of anti-Ro and anti-La antibodies (detectable by immunodiffusion) have been found to correlate with extraglandular manifestations such as neurologic involvement and with vasculitis.[314] The condition associated with human immunodeficiency virus (HIV) infection that resembles Sjögren's syndrome does not appear to include the presence of anti-Ro and anti-La antibodies.[315]

References

1. Reichlin, M.: Antinuclear antibodies. *In* Kelley, W. N., Harris, E. D., Ruddy, S., and Sledge, C. (eds.): Textbook of Rheumatology. 3rd ed. Philadelphia, W. B. Saunders Company, 1989, pp. 208–225.
2. Tan, E.: Antinuclear antibodies: Diagnostic markers for autoimmune diseases and probes for cell biology. Adv. Immunol. 44:93, 1989.
3. Hardin, J. A.: The lupus autoantigens and the pathogenesis of systemic lupus erythematosus. Arthritis Rheum. 29:457, 1986.
4. Lerner, E. A., and Lerner, M. R.: Whither the ANA? Arch. Dermatol. 123:358, 1987.
5. Hargraves, M. M., Richmond, H., and Morton, R.: Presentation of two bone marrow elements: The "tart" cell and "L. E. cell." Proc. Staff Meet. Mayo Clin. 23:25, 1948.
6. Haserick, J. R., and Bortz, D. W.: Normal bone marrow inclusion phenomena induced by lupus erythematosus plasma. J. Invest. Dermatol. 13:47, 1949.
7. Holman, H. R., and Kunkel, H. G.: Affinity between the lupus erythematosus serum factor and cell nuclei and nucleoprotein. Science 126:162, 1957.
8. Beck, J.: Antinuclear antibodies: Methods of detection and significance. Mayo Clin. Proc. 44:600, 1960.
9. Friou, G. J.: Clinical application of lupus serum nucleoprotein reaction using fluorescent antibody technique. J. Clin. Invest. 36:890, 1957.
10. Deicher, H. R. G., Holman, H. R., and Kunkel, H. G.: The precipitin reaction between DNA and a serum factor in systemic lupus erythematosus. J. Exp. Med. 109:97, 1959.
11. Tan, E. M., and Kunkel, H. G.: Characteristics of a soluble nuclear antigen precipitating with sera of patients with systemic lupus erythematosus. J. Immunol. 96:464, 1966.
12. Mattioli, M., and Reichlin, M.: Characterization of a soluble nuclear ribonucleoprotein antigen reactive with SLE sera. J. Immunol. 107:1281, 1971.
13. Reichlin, M., and Mattioli, M.: Correlation of a precipitating reaction to an RNA protein antigen and a low prevalence of nephritis in patients with systemic lupus. N. Engl. J. Med. 286:908, 1972.
14. Sharp, G. C., Irvin, W. S., Tan, E. M., Gould, R. G., and Holman, H. R.: Mixed connective tissue disease—an apparently distinct rheumatic disease syndrome associated with a specific antibody to an extractable nuclear antigen (ENA). Am. J. Med. 52:148, 1972.
15. Sharp, G. C., Irvin, W. S., Northway, J. D., et al.: Specificity of antibodies to extractable nuclear antigens (ENA) in mixed connective tissue disease (MCTD) and systemic lupus erythematosus (SLE). Arthritis Rheum. 15:125, 1972.
16. Northway, J. D., and Tan, E. M.: Differentiation of antinuclear antibodies giving speckled staining patterns in immunofluorescence. Clin. Immunol. Immunopathol. 1:140, 1972.
17. Clark, G., Reichlin, M., and Tomasi, T. B.: Characterization of a soluble cytoplasmic antigen reactive with sera from patients with systemic lupus erythematosus. J. Immunol. 102:117, 1969.
18. Mattioli, M., and Reichlin, M.: Heterogeneity of RNA protein antigens reactive with sera of patients with systemic lupus erythematosus. Description of a cytoplasmic nonribosomal antigen. Arthritis Rheum. 17:421, 1974.
19. Alspaugh, M. A., and Tan, E. M.: Antibodies to cellular antigens in Sjögren's syndrome. J. Clin. Invest. 55:1067, 1975.
20. Notman, D. D., Kurata, N., and Tan, E. M.: Profiles of antinuclear antibodies in systemic rheumatic diseases. Ann. Intern. Med. 83:464, 1975.
21. Sharp, G. C., Irvin, W. S., May, C. M., Holman, H. R., McDuffie, F. C., Hess, E. V., and Schmid, F. R.: Association of antibodies to ribonucleoprotein and Sm antigens with mixed connective-tissue disease, systemic lupus erythematosus, and other rheumatic diseases. N. Engl. J. Med. 295:1149, 1976.
22. Lerner, M. R., and Steitz, J. A.: Antibodies to small nuclear RNAs complexed with proteins are produced by patients with systemic lupus erythematosus. Proc. Natl. Acad. Sci. U.S.A. 76:5495, 1979.
23. Steitz, J. A., Black, D. L., Gerke, V., Parker, K. A., Kramer, A., Frendewey, D., and Keller, W.: Functions of the abundant U-snRNPs. *In* Birnstiel, M. L. (ed.): Structure and Function of Major and Minor Small Nuclear Ribonuclear Ribonucleoprotein Particles. Heidelberg, Springer-Verlag, 1988, pp. 115–154.
24. Douvas, A., Achten, M., and Tan, E. M.: Identification of a nuclear protein (Scl-70) as a unique target of human antinuclear antibodies in scleroderma. J. Biol. Chem. 254:10514, 1979.
25. Rodriguez, J. L., Gelpi, C., Juarez, C., and Hardin, J. A.: Anti–NOR-90: a new autoantibody in scleroderma that recognizes a 90-kDa component of the nucleolus-organizing region of chromatin. J. Immunol. 139:2579, 1987.
26. Reimer, G., Rose, K. M., Scheer, U., and Tan, E. M.: Autoantibody to RNA polymerase I in scleroderma sera. J. Clin. Invest. 79:65, 1987.
27. Maddison, P. J., and Reichlin, M.: Quantitation of precipitating anti-

28. Boey, M. L., Peebles, C. L., Tsay, G., Feng, P. H., and Tan, E. M.: Clinical and autoantibody correlations in Orientals with systemic lupus erythematosus. Ann. Rheum. Dis. 47:918, 1988.
29. Kipnis, R. J., Craft, J., and Hardin, J.: The analysis of antinuclear and antinucleolar autoantibodies of scleroderma by radioimmunoprecipitation assays. Arthritis Rheum. 33:1431, 1990.
30. Craft, J. E., and Hardin, J. A.: Linked sets of antinuclear antibodies: What do they mean? J. Rheumatol. (Suppl.) 14:106, 1987.
31. Mattioli, M., and Reichlin, M.: Physical association of two nuclear antigens and mutual occurrence of their antibodies: the relationship of the Sm and RNA protein (Mo) systems in SLE sera. J. Immunol. 110:1318, 1973.
32. Pettersson, I., Hinterberger, M., Mimori, T., Gottlieb, E., and Steitz, J. A.: The structure of mammalian small nuclear ribonucleoproteins. J. Biol. Chem. 259:5907, 1984.
33. Hendrick, J. P., Wolin, S. L., Rinke, J., Lerner, M. R., and Steitz, J. A.: Ro scRNPs are a subclass of La RNPs: further characterization of the Ro and La small ribonucleoproteins from uninfected mammalian cells. Mol. Cell. Biol. 1:1138, 1981.
34. Habets, W. J., Hoet, M., Bringmann, P., Lührmann, R., and van Venrooij, W.: Autoantibodies to ribonucleoprotein particles containing U2 small nuclear RNA. EMBO J. 4:1545, 1985.
35. Tan, E. M.: Interactions between autoimmunity and molecular and cell biology. J. Clin. Invest. 84:1, 1989.
36. Friou, G. F., Finch, S. C., and Detre, K. D.: Interaction of nucleic and globulin from lupus erythematosus serum demonstrated with fluorescent antibody. J. Immunol. 80:324, 1958.
37. Harmon, C. E., Deng, J.-S., Peebles, C. L., and Tan, E. M.: The importance of tissue substrate in the SS-A/Ro antigen-antibody system. Arthritis Rheum. 27:166, 1984.
38. Nishikai, M., and Reichlin, M.: Heterogeneity of precipitating antibodies in polymyositis and dermatomyositis. Characterization of the Jo-1 antibody system. Arthritis Rheum. 23:881, 1980.
39. Rosa, M. D., Hendrick, J. P., Jr., Lerner, M. R., Reichlin, M., and Steitz, J. A.: A mammalian tRNA^{his}-containing antigen is recognized by the polymyositis-specific antibody anti–Jo-1. Nucleic Acids Res. 11:853, 1983.
40. Bernstein, R. M., Steigerwald, J. C., and Tan, E. M.: Association of antinuclear and antinucleolar antibodies in progressive systemic sclerosis. Clin. Exp. Immunol. 48:43, 1982.
41. Tan, E. M., Rodan, G. P., Garcia, I., Moroi, Y., Fritzler, M. J., and Peebles, C.: Diversity of antinuclear antibodies in progressive systemic sclerosis. Anti-centromere antibody and its relationship to CREST syndrome. Arthritis Rheum. 23:617, 1980.
42. Moroi, Y., Peebles, C., Fritzler, M., Steigerwald, J., and Tan, E. M.: Autoantibody to centromere (kinetochore) in scleroderma sera. Proc. Natl. Acad. Sci. U.S.A. 77:1627, 1980.
43. Fritzler, J. J., Kinsella, T. D., and Garbutt, E.: The CREST syndrome: A distinct serologic entity with anticentromere antibodies. Am. J. Med. 69:520, 1980.
44. Mimori, T., Hinterberger, M., Pettersson, I., and Steitz, J. A.: Autoantibodies to the U2 small nuclear ribonucleoprotein in a patient with scleroderma-polymyositis overlap syndrome. J. Biol. Chem. 259:560, 1984.
45. Craft, J., Mimori, T., Olsen, T. L., and Hardin, J. A.: The U2 small nuclear ribonucleoprotein particle as an autoantigen: Analysis with sera from patients with overlap syndrome. J. Clin. Invest. 8:1716, 1988.
46. Miyachi, K., Fritzler, M. J., and Tan, E. M.: Autoantibody to a nuclear antigen in proliferating cells. J. Immunol. 121:2228, 1978.
47. Mimori, T., Akizuki, M., Yamagata, H., Inada, S., Yoshida, S., and Homma, M.: Characterization of a high molecular weight acidic nuclear protein recognized by autoantibodies in sera from patients with polymyositis-scleroderma overlap. J. Clin. Invest. 68:611, 1981.
48. Reichlin, M., Maddison, P. J., Targoff, I. N., Bunch, T., Arnett, F. C., Sharp, G., Treadwell, E., and Tan, E. M.: Antibodies to a nuclear/nucleolar antigen in patients with polymyositis-overlap syndrome. J. Clin. Immunol. 4:40, 1984.
49. Schur, P. H., DeAngelis, D., and Jackson, J. M.: Immunological detection of nucleic acid and antibodies to nucleic acids and nucleic antigens by counterimmunoelectrophoresis. Clin. Exp. Immunol. 17:209, 1974.
50. Deutscher, S. L., Harley, J. B., and Keene, J. D.: Molecular analysis of the 60-kDa human Ro ribonucleoprotein. Proc. Natl. Acad. Sci. U.S.A. 85:9479, 1988.
51. Ben-Chetrit, E., Gandy, B. J., Tan, E. M., and Sullivan, K. F.: Isolation and characterization of a cDNA clone encoding the 60-kD component of the human SS-A/Ro ribonucleoprotein autoantigen. J. Clin. Invest. 83:1284, 1989.
52. Chan, E. K., Hamel, J. C., Buyon, J. P., and Tan, E. M.: Molecular definition and sequence motifs of the 52-kD component of human SS-A/Ro autoantigen. J. Clin. Invest. 87:6876, 1991.

bodies to certain soluble nuclear antigens in SLE. Arthritis Rheum. 20:819, 1977.

53. Itoh, K., Itoh, Y., and Frank, M. B.: Protein heterogeneity in the human Ro/SSA ribonucleoproteins. The 52- and 60 kD Ro/SSA autoantigens are encoded by separate genes. J. Clin. Invest. 87:177, 1991.
54. Chambers, J. C., and Keene, J. D.: Isolation and analysis of cDNA clones expressing human lupus La antigen. Proc. Natl. Acad. Sci. U.S.A. 82:2115, 1985.
55. Rokeach, L., Haselby, J., and Hoch, S.: Molecular cloning of a cDNA encoding the human Sm-D autoantigen. Proc. Natl. Acad. Sci. U.S.A. 85:4832, 1988.
56. Rokeach, L. A., Jannatipour, M., Haselby, J. A., and Hoch, S. O.: Primary structure of a human small nuclear ribonucleoprotein polypeptide as deduced by cDNA analysis. J. Biol. Chem. 264:5024, 1989.
57. Ohosone, Y., Mimori, T., Griffith, A., Akizuki, M., Homma, M., Craft, J., and Hardin, J. A.: Molecular cloning of cDNA encoding Sm autoantigen: derivation of a cDNA for a B polypeptide of the U series of small nuclear ribonucleoprotein particles. Proc. Natl. Acad. Sci. U.S.A. 86:4249, 1989.
58. Ohosone, Y., Mimori, T., Griffith, A., Akizuki, M., Homma, M., Craft, J., and Hardin, J. A.: Molecular cloning of cDNA encoding Sm autoantigen: derivation of a cDNA for a B polypeptide of the U series of small nuclear ribonucleoprotein particles (correction). Proc. Natl. Acad. Sci. U.S.A. 86:8982, 1989.
59. van Dam, A., Winkel, I., Zijlstra-Baalbergen, J., Smeenk, R., and Cuypers, H. T.: Cloned human snRNP proteins B and B' differ only in their carboxy-terminal part. EMBO J. 8:3853, 1989.
60. Theissen, H., Etzerodt, M., Reuter, R., Schneider, C., Lottspeich, F., Argos, P., Lührmann, R., and Philipson, L.: Cloning of the human cDNA for the U1 RNA–associated 70K protein. EMBO J. 5:3209, 1986.
61. Spritz, R. A., Strunk, K., Surowy, C. S., Hoch, S. O., Barton, D. E., and Francke, U.: The human U1-70K protein: cDNA cloning, chromosomal localization, expression, alternative splicing and RNA-binding. Nucleic Acids Res. 15:10373, 1987.
62. Sillekens, P. T. G., Habets, W. J., Beijer, R. P., and Van Venrooij, W. J.: cDNA cloning of the human U1 snRNP–associated A protein: extensive homology between U1 and U2 snRNP-specific proteins. EMBO J. 6:3841, 1987.
63. Sillekens, P. T. G., Beijer, R. P., Habets, W. J., and Van Venrooij, W. J.: Human U1 snRNP-specific C protein: complete cDNA and protein sequence and identification of a multigene family in mammals. Nucleic Acids Res. 16:8307, 1988.
64. Yamamoto, K., Miura, H., Moroi, Y., Yoshinoya, M., Goto, M., Nishioka, K., and Miyamoto, T.: Isolation and characterization of a complementary DNA expressing human U1 small nuclear ribonucleoprotein C polypeptide. J. Immunol. 140:311, 1988.
65. Ramsden, D., Chen, J., Miller, F., Misener, V., Bernstein, R., Siminovitch, K., and Tsui, F. W. L.: Epitope mapping of the cloned human autoantigen, histidyl-tRNA synthetase: analysis of the myositis-associated anti-Jo-1 autoimmune response. J. Immunol. 143:2267, 1989.
66. D'Arpa, P., Machlin, P., Ratrie, H., Rothfield, N. F., Cleveland, D. W., and Earnshaw, W. C.: cDNA cloning of the human DNA topoisomerase I: Catalytic activity of a 67.7-kDa carboxyl-terminal fragment. Proc. Natl. Acad. Sci. U.S.A. 85:2543, 1988.
67. Wold, R. T., Young, F. E., Tan, E. M., and Farr, R. S.: Deoxyribonucleic acid antibody: A method to detect its primary interaction with deoxyribonucleic acid. Science 161:806, 1968.
68. Pincus, T., Schur, P. H., Rosa, J. A., Decker, J. L., and Talal, N.: Measurements of serum DNA-binding activity in SLE. N. Engl. J. Med. 281:701, 1969.
69. Lerner, M. L., and Steitz, J. A.: Snurps and scryps. Cell 25:298, 1981.
70. Craft, J., and Hardin, J. A.: Immunoprecipitation assays for the detection of soluble nuclear and cytoplasmic nucleoproteins. In Rose, N., Friedman, H., and Fahey, J. (eds.): Manual of Clinical Laboratory Immunology. 4th ed. Washington, D. C., American Society of Microbiology, 1992, pp. 747–754.
71. Evans, J., Arguelles, E., Harley, J., Reichlin, M., and Craft, J.: Antibodies to ribonucleoproteins in SLE (abstract). Arthritis Rheum. 31: S54, 1988.
72. Towbin, H., Staehlin, T., and Gordon, J.: Electrophoretic transfer of proteins from polyacrylamide gels to nitrocellulose sheets: procedure and some applications. Proc. Natl. Acad. Sci. U.S.A. 76:4350, 1979.
73. Boire, G., Lopez-Longo, F.-J., Lapointe, S., and Ménard, H.-A.: Sera from patients with autoimmune disease recognize conformational determinants on the 60-kd Ro/SS-A protein. Arthritis Rheum. 34:722, 1991.
74. Robbins, W. C., Holman, H. R., Deicher, H., and Kunkel, H. G.: Complement fixation with cell nuclei and DNA in lupus erythematosus. Proc. Soc. Exp. Biol. Med. 96:575, 1957.
75. Seligmann, M., and Milgrom, F.: Mise en evidence par la fixation du emplement de la reaction extre acid desoxyribonucleique et serum de malades atteints de lupus erythemateux dissemine. G. R. Acad. Sci. 245:1472, 1957.
76. Ceppallini, R., Polli, E., and Celada, F.: A DNA-reacting factor in serum of a patient with lupus erythematosus diffuse. Proc. Soc. Exp. Biol. Med. 96:572, 1957.

77. Davis, J. S., and Winfield, J. B.: Serum antibodies to DNA by counterimmunoelectrophoresis (EIC). Clin. Immunol. Immunopathol. 2:510, 1968.
78. Schur, P. H., and Sandson, J.: Immunological factors and clinical activity in systemic lupus erythematosus. N. Engl. J. Med. 278:533, 1968.
79. Koffler, D., Carr, R., Agnello, V., Feizi, T., and Kunkel, H. G.: Antibodies to polynucleotides: Distribution in human serum. Science 166:1648, 1969.
80. Davis, P., Christian, B., and Russell, A. S.: Immunofluorescent technique for the detection of antibodies to nDNA: Comparison with radioimmunoassay. J. Rheumatol. 4:15, 1977.
81. Sontheimer, R. D., and Gilliam, J. N.: An immunofluorescence assay for double-stranded DNA antibodies using Crithidia luciliae kinetoplast as a double-stranded DNA substrate. J. Lab. Clin. Med. 91:550, 1978.
82. Ballou, S. P., and Kushner, I.: Anti-native DNA detection by the Crithidia luciliae method: An improved guide to the diagnosis and clinical management of systemic lupus erythematosus. Arthritis Rheum. 22:321, 1979.
83. Isenberg, D. A., Dudeney, C., Williams, W., Addison, I., Charles, S., Clarke, J., and Todd, P. A.: Measurement of anti-DNA antibodies: a reappraisal using five different methods. Ann. Rheum. Dis. 46:448, 1987.
84. Tzioufas, A. G., Terzoglou, C., Stavropoulos, E. D., Athanasiadou, S., and Moutsopoulos, H. M.: Determination of anti-ds-DNA antibodies by three different methods: comparison of sensitivity, specificity, and correlation with lupus activity index (LAI). Clin Rheumatol. 9:186, 1990.
85. Smeenk, R., Brinkman, K., van den Brink, H., Termaat, R. M., Berden, J., Nossent, H., and Swaak, T.: Antibodies to DNA in patients with systemic lupus erythematosus. Their role in the diagnosis, the follow-up and the pathogenesis of the disease. Clin. Rheumatol. 9:100, 1990.
86. McMillan, S. A., and Fay, A. C.: Evaluation of five commercial kits to detect dsDNA antibodies. J. Clin. Pathol. 41:1223, 1988.
87. Emlen, W., Jarusiripipat, P., and Burdick, G.: A new ELISA for the detection of double-stranded DNA antibodies. J. Immunol. Methods. 132:91, 1990.
88. Tipping, P. G., Buchanan, R. C., Riglar, A. G., Dimech, W. J., Littlejohn, G. O., and Holdsworth, S. R.: Measurement of anti-DNA antibodies by ELISA: a comparative study with Crithidia and a Farr assay. Pathology 23:21, 1991.
89. Ginsberg, G., and Keiser, H.: A millipore filter assay for antibodies to native DNA in sera of patients with systemic lupus erythematosus. Arthritis Rheum. 16:199, 1973.
90. Koffler, D., Agnello, V., Moburn, R., and Kunkel, H. G.: Systemic lupus erythematosus: Prototype and immune complex nephritis in man. J. Exp. Med. 134:109, 1971.
91. Tan, E. M., Carr, R. I., Schur, P. H., and Kunkel, H. G.: Deoxyribonucleic acid (DNA) and antibodies to DNA in the serum of patients with systemic lupus erythematosus. J. Clin. Invest. 45:1732, 1966.
92. Koffler, D., Schur, P. H., and Kunkel, H. G.: Immunological studies concerning the nephritis of systemic lupus erythematosus. J. Exp. Med. 126:607, 1967.
93. Cochrane, C. G., and Koffler, D.: Immune complex disease in experimental animals and man. Adv. Immunol. 16:185, 1973.
94. Raz, E., Brezis, M., Rosenmann, E., and Eilat, D.: Anti-DNA antibodies bind directly to renal antigens and induce kidney dysfunction in the isolated perfused rat kidney. J. Immunol. 142:3076, 1989.
95. Koffler, D., Carr, R. I., Agnello, V., Thoburn, R., and Kunkel, H. G.: Antibodies to polynucleotides in human sera: Antigenic specificity and relationship to disease. J. Exp. Med. 134:294, 1971.
96. Carson, D. A.: The specificity of anti-DNA antibodies in systemic lupus erythematosus. J. Immunol. 146:1, 1991.
97. Thomas, T. J., Neryhew, N. L., and Messner, R. P.: DNA sequence and conformation specificity of lupus autoantibodies. Preferential binding to the left-handed Z-DNA form of synthetic polynucleotides. Arthritis Rheum. 31:367, 1988.
98. Stollar, B. D.: Immunochemistry of DNA. Int. Rev. Immunol. 5:1, 1989.
99. Karounos, D. G., Grudier, J. P., and Pisetsky, D. S.: Spontaneous expression of antibodies to DNA of various species origin in sera of normal subjects and patients with systemic lupus erythematosus. J. Immunol. 140:451, 1988.
100. Pisetsky, D. S., and Grudier, J. P.: Polyspecific binding of Escherichia coli beta-galactosidase by murine antibodies to DNA. J. Immunol. 143:3609, 1989.
101. Stollar, B. D.: Antibodies to DNA. CRC Crit. Rev. Biochem. 20:1, 1986.
102. Winfield, J. B., Koffler, D., and Kunkel, H. G.: Specific concentration of polynucleotide immune complexes in the cryoprecipitation of patients with systemic lupus erythematosus J. Clin. Invest. 56:563, 1975.
103. Andres, G. A., Accini, G. A., Beiser, S. M., Christian, C. L., Cinotti, G. A., Erlanger, B. F., Hsu, K. C., and Seegal, B. C.: Localization of fluorescein-labelled anti-nucleoside antibodies in glomeruli of patients with systemic lupus erythematosus nephritis. J. Clin. Invest. 49:2106, 1971.

104. Koffler, D., Agnello, V., and Kunkel, H. G.: Polynucleotide immune complexes in serum and glomeruli of patients with systemic lupus erythematosus. Am J. Pathol. 74:109, 1974.

105. Stollar, B. D.: The origin and pathogenic role of anti-DNA autoantibodies. Curr. Opin. Immunol. 2:607, 1989.

106. Miniter, M. F., Stollar, B. D., and Agnello, V.: Reassessment of the clinical significance of native DNA antibodies in systemic lupus erythematosus. Arthritis Rheum. 22:959, 1979.

107. Pillemer, S. R., Austin, H., Tsokos, G. C., and Balow, J. E.: Lupus nephritis: association between serology and renal biopsy measures. J. Rheumatol. 15:284, 1988.

108. Ebling, F. M., and Hahn, B. H.: Pathogenic subsets of antibodies to DNA. Int. Rev. Immunol. 5:79, 1989.

109. Beulieu, A., Quismorio, F. P., Friou, G. J., Vayuvegula, B., and Mirick, B.: IgG antibodies to double-stranded DNA in systemic lupus erythematosus sera: Independent variation of complement-fixing activity and total antibody content. Arthritis Rheum. 22:565, 1979.

110. Swaak, A. J. G., Aarden, L. A., Statius van Eps, L. W. S., and Feltkamp, T. E.: Anti-dsDNA and complement profiles as prognostic guides in sytemic lupus erythematosus. Arthritis Rheum. 22:226, 1979.

110a. Sano, H., and Morimoto, C.: Isolation of DNA from DNA/anti-DNA antibody immune complexes in systemic lupus erythematosus. J. Immunol. 126: 538, 1981.

110b. Ikebe, K., Gupta, C., and Tan, E. M.: Characterization of DNA in polyethylene glycol precipitated immune complexes from sera of patients with systemic lupus erythematosus. Clin. Exp. Immunol. 53:169, 1983.

111. Wilusz, J., and Keene, J. D.: Autoantibodies specific for U1 RNA and initiator methionine tRNA. J. Biol. Chem. 261:5467, 1986.

112. Van Venrooij, W. J., Hoet, R., Castrop, J., Hageman, B., Mattaj, I. W., and Van de Putte, L. B.: Anti–(U1) small nuclear RNA antibodies in anti–small nuclear ribonucleoprotein sera from patients with connective tissue diseases. J. Clin. Invest. 86:2154, 1990.

113. Chu, J.-L., Brot, N., Weissbach, H., and Elkon, K.: Lupus antiribosomal P antisera contain antibodies to a small fragment of 28S rRNA located in the proposed ribosomal GTPase center. J. Exp. Med. 174:507, 1991.

114. Craft, J.: Antibodies to snRNPs in SLE. Rheum. Dis. Clin. 18:311, 1992.

115. Tan, E. M., Cohen, A. S., Fries, J. F., Mase, A. T., McShane, D. J., Rothfield, N. F., Schaller, J. G., Talal, N., and Winchester, R. J.: The 1982 revised criteria for the classification of systemic lupus erythematosus. Arthritis Rheum. 25: 1271, 1982.

116. Reeves, W. H., Fisher, D. E., Lahita, R. G., and Kunkel, H. G.: Autoimmune sera reactive with Sm antigen contain high levels of RNP-like antibodies. J. Clin. Invest. 75:580, 1985.

117. Homma, M., Mimori, T., Takeda, Y., Akama, H., Yoshida, T., Ogasawara, T., and Akizuki, M.: Autoantibodies to the Sm antigen: immunological approach to clinical aspects of systemic lupus erythematosus. J. Rheumatol. 14(Suppl. 13):188, 1987.

118. Arnett, F. C., Hamilton, R. G., Roebber, M. G., Harley, J. B., and Reichlin, M.: Increased frequencies of Sm and nRNP autoantibodies in American blacks compared to whites with systemic lupus erythematosus. J. Rheumatol. 15:1773, 1988.

119. Field, M., Williams, D. G., Charles, P., and Maini, R. N.: Specificity of anti-Sm antibodies by ELISA for systemic lupus erythematosus: increased sensitivity of detection using purified peptide antigens. Ann. Rheum. Dis. 47:820, 1988.

120. Abuaf, N., Johanet, C., Chretien, P,. Absalon, B. I., Homberg, J. C., and Buri, J. F.: Detection of autoantibodies to Sm antigen in systemic lupus erythematosus by immunodiffusion, ELISA and immunoblotting: variability of incidence related to assays and ethnic origin of patients. Eur. J. Clin. Invest. 20:354, 1990.

121. Barada, F. A., Jr., Andrews, B. S., Davis, J. S., IV, and Taylor, R. P.: Antibodies to Sm in patients with systemic lupus erythematosus. Arthritis Rheum. 24:1236, 1981.

122. Fisher, D. E., Reeves, W. H., Wisniewolski, R., Lahita, R. G., and Chiorazzi, N.: Temporal shifts from Sm to ribonucleoprotein reactivity in systemic lupus erythematosus. Arthritis Rheum. 28:1348, 1985.

123. Takeda, Y., Wang, G. S., Wang, R. J., Anderson, S. K., Pettersson, I., Amaki, S., and Sharp, G. C.: Enzyme-linked immunosorbent assay using isolated (U) small nuclear ribonucleoprotein polypeptides as antigens to investigate the clinical significance of autoantibodies to these polypeptides. Clin. Immunol. Immunopath. 50:213, 1989.

124. Winn, D. M., Wolfe, J. F., Lindberg, D. A., Fristoe, F. A., Kingland, L., and Sharp, G. C.: Identification of a clinical subset of systemic lupus erythematosus by antibodies to the Sm antigen. Arthritis Rheum. 22:1334, 1979.

125. St. Clair, E. W., Query, C. C., Bentley, R., Keene, J. D., Polisson, R. P., Allen, N. B., Caldwell, D. S., Rice, J. R., Cox, C., and Pisetsky, D. S.: Expression of autoantibodies to recombinant (U1) RNP-associated 70K antigen in systemic lupus erythematosus. Clin. Immunol. Immunopathol. 54:266, 1990.

126. Sharp, G. C., Irvin, W. S., Laroque, R. L., Velez, C., Daly, V., Kaiser,

A. D., and Holman, H. R.: Association of autoantibodies to different nuclear antigens with clinical patterns of rheumatic disease and responsiveness to therapy. J. Clin. Invest. 50:350, 1971.

127. Houtman, P. M., Kallenberg, C. G. M., Limburg, P. C., van Leeuwen, M. A., van Rijswijk, M. H., and The, T. H.: Fluctuations in anti-nRNP levels in patients with mixed connective disease are related to disease activity as part of a polyclonal B cell response. Ann. Rheum. Dis. 45:800, 1986.

128. Pettersson, I., Wang, G., Smith, E. I., Wigzell, H., Hedfors, E., Horn, J., and Sharp, G. C.: The use of immunoblotting and immunoprecipitation of (U) small nuclear ribonucleoproteins in the analysis of sera of patients with mixed connective tissue disease and systemic lupus erythematosus. Arthritis Rheum. 29:986, 1986.

129. de Rooij, D. J., Habets, W. J., van de Putte, L. B., Hoet, M. H., Verbeek, A. L., and van Venrooij, W. J.: Use of recombinant RNP peptides 70K and A in an ELISA for measurement of antibodies in mixed connective tissue disease: a longitudinal follow-up of 18 patients. Ann. Rheum. Dis. 49:391, 1990.

130. Lührmann, R.: snRNP proteins. In Birnstiel, M. L. (ed.): Structure and Function of Major and Minor Small Nuclear Ribonuclear Ribonucleoprotein Particles. Heidelberg, Springer-Verlag, 1988, pp. 71–99.

131. Habets, W. J., de Rooij, D. J., Salden, M. H., Verhagen, A. P., van Eekelen, C. A. G., van de Putte, L. B., and van Venrooij, W. J.: Antibodies against distinct nuclear matrix proteins are characteristic for mixed connective tissue disease. Clin. Exp. Immunol. 54:265, 1983.

132. Reichlin, M., and van Venrooij, W. J.: Autoantibodies to the URNP particles: relationship to clinical diagnosis and nephritis. Clin. Exp. Immunol. 83:286, 1991.

133. Hoffman, R. W., Rettenmaier, L. J., Takeda, Y., Hewett, J. E., Pettersson, I., Nyman, U., Luger, A. M., and Sharp, G. C.: Human autoantibodies against the 70-kd polypeptide of U1 small nuclear RNP are associated with HLA-DR4 among connective tissue disease patients. Arthritis Rheum. 33:666, 1990.

134. Ehrfeld, H., Renz, M., Seelig, H. P., Hartung, K., Deicher, H., and Coldewey, R.: Antibodies to recombinant U1-70K and U1-A protein in systemic lupus erythematosus (SLE). Mol. Biol. Rep. 15:190, 1991.

135. Reeves, W. H., Fisher, D. E., Wisniewolski, R., Gottlieb, A. B., and Chiorazzi, N.: Psoriasis and Raynaud's phenomenon associated with autoantibodies to U1 and U2 small nuclear ribonucleoproteins. N. Engl. J. Med. 315:105, 1986.

136. Stanford, D. R., Kehl, M., Perry, C. A., Holicky, E., Harvey, S. E., Rohleder, A. M., Rehder, K., Lührmann, R., and Wieben, E. D.: The complete primary structure of the human snRNP E protein. Nucleic Acids Res. 16:10593, 1988.

137. Reichlin, M.: Significance of the Ro antigen system. J. Clin. Immunol. 6:339, 1986.

138. Reichlin, M., and Harley, J. B.: Antibodies to Ro(SSA) and the heterogeneity of systemic lupus erythematosus. J. Rheumatol. 14(Suppl. 13): 112, 1987.

139. Alspaugh, M. A., Talal, N., and Tan, E. M.: Differentiation and characterization of autoantibodies and their antigens in Sjögren's syndrome. Arthritis Rheum. 19:216, 1976.

140. Alspaugh, M. A., and Maddison, P.: Resolution of the identity of certain antigen-antibody systems in systemic lupus erythematosus and Sjögren's syndrome: An interlaboratory collaboration. Arthritis Rheum. 22: 796, 1979.

141. Akizuki, M., Powers, R., and Holman, H. R.: A soluble acidic protein of the cell nucleus which reacts with serum from patients with systemic lupus erythematosus and Sjögren's syndrome. J.Clin. Invest. 59:264, 1977.

142. Akizuki, M., Boehm-Truitt, M. J., Kassan, S. S., Steinberg, A. D., and Chused, T. M.: Purification of an acidic nuclear protein antigen and demonstration of its antibodies in subsets of patients with sicca syndrome. J. Immunol. 119:932, 1977.

143. Maddison, P. J., Mogavero, H., Provost, T. T., and Reichlin, M.: The clinical significance of autoantibodies to a soluble cytoplasmic antigen in systemic lupus erythematosus and other connective tissue diseases. J. Rheumatol. 6:189, 1979.

144. Scopelitis, E., Biundo, J. J., and Alspaugh, M. A.: Anti–SS-A antibody and other antinuclear antibodies in systemic lupus erythematosus. Arthritis Rheum. 23:287, 1980.

145. Bell, D. A., Komar, R., Chodirker, W. B., Block, J., and Cairns, E.: A comparison of serologic reactivity among SLE patients with or without anti-Ro (SS-A) antibodies. J. Rheumatol. 11:315, 1984.

146. Maddison, P. J., Skinner, R. P., Vlachoyiannopoulos, P., Brennand, D. M., and Hough, D.: Antibodies to nRNP, Sm, Ro(SSA) and La(SSB) detected by ELISA: their specificity and inter-relations in connective tissue disease sera. Clin. Exp. Immunol. 62:337, 1985.

147. Hamilton, R. G., Harley, J. B., Bias, W. B., Roebber, M., Reichlin, M., Hochberg, M. C., and Arnett, F. C.: Two Ro (SS-A) autoantibody responses in systemic lupus erythematosus. Correlation of HLA-DR/DQ specificities with quantitative expression of Ro (SS-A) autoantibody. Arthritis Rheum. 31:496, 1988.

148. Ben-Chetrit, E., Fox, R. I., and Tan, E. M.: Dissociation of immune

responses to the SS-A (Ro) 52-kd and 60-kd polypeptides in systemic lupus erythematosus and Sjögren's syndrome. Arthritis Rheum. 33:349, 1990.

149. Yamagata, H., Harley, H. B., and Reichlin, M.: Molecular properties of the Ro/SSA antigen and enzyme-linked immunosorbent assay for quantitation of antibody. J. Clin. Invest. 74:625, 1984.

150. Reichlin, M., and Harley, J. B.: Detection by ELISA of antibodies to small RNA protein particles in systemic lupus erythematosus patients whose sera lack precipitins. Trans. Assoc. Am. Physicians 99:161, 1986.

151. Maddison, P. J., Mogavero, H., Provost, T. T., and Reichlin, M.: The clinical significance of autoantibodies to a soluble cytoplasmic antigen in systemic lupus erythematosus and other connective tissue diseases. J. Rheumatol. 6:189, 1979.

152. Boire, G., and Menard, H. A.: Clinical significance of anti-Ro(SSA) antibody in rheumatoid arthritis. J. Rheumatol. 15:391, 1988.

153. Harley, J. B., Yamagata, H., and Reichlin, M.: Anti-La/SSB antibody is present in some normal sera and is coincident with anti-Ro/SSA precipitins in systemic lupus erythematosus. J. Rheumatol. 11:309, 1984.

154. Gaither, K. K., Fox, O. F., Yamagata, H., Mamula, M. J., Reichlin, M., and Harley, J. B.: Implications of anti-Ro/Sjögren's syndrome A antigen autoantibody in normal sera for autoimmunity. J. Clin. Invest. 79:841, 1987.

155. Wasicek, C. A., and Reichlin, M.: Clinical and serological differences between systemic lupus erythematosus patients with antibodies to Ro versus patients with antibodies to Ro and La. J. Clin. Invest. 69:835, 1982.

156. Maddison, P. J., and Reichlin, M.: Deposition of antibodies to a soluble cytoplasmic antigen in the kidneys of patients with systemic lupus erythematosus. Arthritis Rheum. 22:858, 1979.

157. Arnett, F. C., Hamilton, R. G., Reveille, J. D., Bias, W. B., Harley, J. B., and Reichlin, M.: Genetic studies of Ro (SS-A) and La (SS-B) autoantibodies in families with systemic lupus erythematosus and primary Sjögren's syndrome. Arthritis Rheum. 32:413, 1989.

158. Harley, J. B., Reichlin, M., Arnett, F. C., Alexander, E. L., Bias, W. B. and Provost, T. T.: Gene interaction at HLA-DQ enhances autoantibody production in primary Sjögren's syndrome. Science (Washington) 232:1145, 1986.

159. Harley, J. B., Sestak, A. L., Willis, L. G., Fu, S. M., Hansen, J. A., and Reichlin, M.: A model for disease heterogeneity in systemic lupus erythematosus. Relationships between histocompatibility antigens, autoantibodies, and lymphopenia or renal disease. Arthritis Rheum. 32:826, 1989.

160. Fujisaku, A., Frank, M. B., Neas B., Reichlin, M., and Harley, J. B.: HLA-DQ gene complementation and other histocompatibility relationships in man with the anti-Ro/SSA autoantibody response of systemic lupus erythematosus. J. Clin. Invest. 86:606, 1990.

161. Maddison, P. J., Provost, T. T., and Reichlin, M.: ANA-negative systemic lupus erythematosus: Serological analysis. Medicine (Baltimore) 60:87, 1981.

162. Harmon, C. E., Deng, J. S., Pebbles, C. L., and Tan, E. M.: The importance of tissue substrate in the SS-A/Ro antigen-antibody system. Arthritis Rheum. 27:166, 1984.

163. Boire, G., and Craft, J.: Biochemical and immunological heterogeneity of the Ro ribonucleoprotein particles: analysis with sera specific for the Ro^{hY5} particle. J. Clin. Invest. 84:270, 1989.

164. Reichlin, M., Rader, M., and Harley, J. B.: Autoimmune response to the Ro/SSA particle is directed to the human antigen. Clin. Exp. Immunol. 76:373, 1989.

165. Reichlin, M., and Reichlin, M. W.: Autoantibodies to the Ro/SS-A particle react preferentially with the human antigen. J. Autoimmun. 2:359, 1989.

166. Sontheimer, R. D., Maddison, P. J., Reichlin, M., Jordan, R. E., Stasthy, P., and Gilliam, J. N.: Serologic and HLA associations in subacute cutaneous lupus erythematosus, a clinical subset of lupus erythematosus. Ann. Intern. Med. 97:664, 1982.

167. Callen, J. P., and Klein, J.: Subacute cutaneous lupus erythematosus. Arthritis Rheum. 31:1007, 1988.

168. Mond, C. B., Peterson, M. G. E., and Rothfield, N. F.: Correlation of anti-Ro antibody with photosensitivity rash in systemic lupus erythematosus. Arthritis Rheum. 32:202, 1989.

169. LeFeber, W. P., Norris, D. A., Ryan, S. R., Huff, J. C., Lee, L. A., Kubo, M., Boyce, S. T., Kotzin, B. L., and Weston, W. L.: Ultraviolet light induces binding of antibodies to selected nuclear antigens on cultured human keratinocytes. J. Clin. Invest. 74:1545, 1984.

170. Lee, L. A., Weston, W. L., Krueger, G. G., Emam, M., Reichlin, M., Stevens, J. O., Surbrugg, S. K., Vasil, A., and Norris, D. A.: An animal model of antibody binding in cutaneous lupus. Arthritis Rheum. 29:782, 1986.

171. Lee, L. A., Gaither, K. K., Coulter, S. N., Norris, D. A., and Harley, J. B.: Pattern of cutaneous immunoglobulin G deposition in subacute cutaneous lupus erythematosus is reproduced by infusing purified anti-Ro (SSA) autoantibodies into human skin-grafted mice. J. Clin. Invest. 83:1556, 1989.

172. Furukawa, F., Kashihara-Sawami, M., Lyons, M. B., and Norris, D. A.: Binding of antibodies of the extractable nuclear antigens SS-A/Ro and SS-B/La is induced on the surface of human keratinocytes by ultraviolet light (UVL): Implications for the pathogenesis of photosensitive cutaneous lupus. J. Invest. Dermatol. 94:77, 1990.

173. Buyon, J. P., and Winchester, R.: Congenital complete heart block. A human model of passively acquired autoimmune injury. Arthritis Rheum. 33:609, 1990.

174. Litsey, S. E., Noonan, J. A., O'Connor, W. N., Cottrill, C. M., and Mitchell, B.: Maternal connective tissue disease and congenital heart block: demonstration of immunoglobulin in cardiac tissue. N. Engl. J. Med. 312:98, 1985.

175. Taylor, P. V., Scott, J. S., Gerlis, L. M., Esscher, E., and Scott, O.: Maternal antibodies against fetal cardiac antigens in congenital complete heart block. N. Engl. J. Med. 315:667, 1986.

176. Lee, L. A., Coulter, S., Erner, S., and Chu, H.: Cardiac immunoglobulin deposition in congenital complete heart block associated with maternal anti-Ro autoantibodies. Am. J. Med. 52:148, 1987.

177. Scott, J. S., Maddison, P. J., Taylor, P. V., Esscher, E., Scott, O., and Skinner, R. P.: Connective-tissue disease, antibodies to ribonucleoprotein, and congenital heart block. N. Engl. J. Med. 309:209, 1983.

178. Reed, B. R., Lee, L. A., Harmon, C., Wolfe, R., Wiggins, J., Peebles, C., and Weston, W. L.: Autoantibodies to SS-A/Ro in infants with congenital heart block. J. Pediatr. 103:889, 1983.

179. Watson, R. M., Lane, A. T., Barnett, N. K., Bias, W. B., Arnett, F. C., and Provost, T. T.: Neonatal lupus erythematosus: a clinical, serological and immunogenetic study with review of the literature. Medicine (Baltimore) 63:362, 1984.

180. Buyon, J. P., Ben-Chetrit, E., Karp, S., Roubey, R. A., Pompeo, L., Reeves, W. H., Tan, E. M., and Winchester, R.: Acquired congenital heart block. Pattern of maternal antibody response to biochemically defined antigens of the SSA/Ro-SSB/La system in neonatal lupus. J. Clin. Invest. 84:627, 1989.

181. Silverman, E., Mamula, M., Hardin, J., and Laxer, R.: Importance of the immune response to the Ro/La particle in the development of congenital heart block and neonatal lupus erythematosus. J. Rheumatol. 18:120, 1991.

182. Lehman, T. J., Reichlin, M., Santner, T. J., Silverman, E., Petty, R. E., Spencer, C. H., and Harley, J. B.: Maternal antibodies to Ro (SS-A) are associated with both early onset of disease and male sex among children with systemic lupus erythematosus. Arthritis Rheum. 32:1414, 1989.

183. Provost, T. T., Watson, R., Gaither, K., and Harley, J. B.: The neonatal lupus erythematosus syndrome. J. Rheumatol. 14 (Suppl. 13):199, 1987.

184. Ramsey-Goldman, R., Hom, D., Deng, J. S., et al.: Anti-SSA antibodies and fetal outcome in maternal systemic lupus erythematosus. Arthritis Rheum. 29:1269, 1986.

185. Provost, T. T., Watson, R., Gammon, W. R., Radowsky, M., Harley, J. B., and Reichlin, M.: The neonatal lupus syndrome associated with U1 RNP (nRNP) antibodies. N. Engl. J. Med. 316:1135, 1987.

186. Wolin, S. L., and Steitz, J. A.: The Ro small cytoplasmic ribonucleoproteins: identification of the antigenic protein and its binding site on the Ro RNAs. Proc. Natl. Acad. Sci. U.S.A. 81:1996, 1984.

187. Ben-Chetrit, E., Chan, E. K. L., Sullivan, K. F., and Tan, E. M.: A 52-kD protein is a novel component of the SS-A/Ro antigenic particle. J. Exp. Med. 167:1560, 1988.

188. Rader, M. D., O'Brien, C., Liu, Y. S., Harley, J. B., and Reichlin, M.: Heterogeneity of the Ro/SSA antigen. Different molecular forms in lymphocytes and red blood cells. J. Clin. Invest. 83:1293, 1989.

189. Itoh, Y., Rader, M. D., and Reichlin, M.: Heterogeneity of the Ro/SSA antigen and autoanti-Ro/SSA response: evidence of the four antigenically distinct forms. Clin. Exp. Immunol. 81:45, 1990.

190. Itoh, Y., and Reichlin, M.: Ro/SS-A antigen in human platelets. Arthritis Rheum. 34:888, 1991.

191. McCauliffe, D. P., Lux, F. A., Lieu, T. S., Sanz, I., Hanke, J., Newkirk, M. M., Bachinski, L. L., Itoh, Y., Siciliano, M. J., Reichlin, M., et al.: Molecular cloning, expression, and chromosome 19 localization of a human Ro/SS-A autoantigen. J. Clin. Invest. 85:1379, 1990.

192. McCauliffe, D. P., Zappi, E., Lieu, T. S., Michalak, M., Sontheimer, R. D., and Capra, J. D.: A human Ro/SS-A autoantigen is the homologue of calreticulin and is highly homologous with onchocercal RAL-1 antigen and an aplysia "memory molecule." J. Clin. Invest. 86:332, 1990.

193. Rokeach, L., Haselby, J. A., Meilof, J. F., Smeenk, R. J. T., Unnasch, T. R., Greene, B. M., and Hoch, S. O.: Characterization of the autoantigen calreticulin. J. Immunol. 147:3031, 1991.

194. Hendrick, J. P., Wolin, S. L., Rinke, J., Lerner, M. R., and Steitz, J. A.: Ro small cytoplasmic ribonucleoproteins are a subclass of La ribonucleoproteins: further characterization of the Ro and La small ribonucleoproteins from uninfected mammalian cells. Mol. Cell. Biol. 1:1138, 1981.

195. Eisenberg, R. A.: Association between the Ro and La antigenic determinants: immunodiffusion analysis of human spleen extract. J. Immunol. 135:1707, 1985.

196. Boire, G., and Craft, J.: Human Ro ribonucleoprotein particles: Characterization of native structure and stable association with the La polypeptide. J. Clin. Invest. 85:1182, 1990.
197. Provost, T. T., Arnett, F. C., and Reichlin, M.: Homozygous C2 deficiency, lupus erythematosus, and anti-Ro (SSA) antibodies. Arthritis Rheum. 26:1279, 1983.
197a. Miyachi, K., Fritzler, M. J., and Tan, E. M.: Autoantibody to a nuclear antigen in proliferating cells. J. Immunol. 121:2228, 1978.
198. Takasaki, Y., Deng, J. S., and Tan, E. M.: A nuclear antigen associated with cell proliferation and blast transformation: Its distribution in synchronized cells. J. Exp. Med. 154:1899, 1981.
199. Takasaki, Y., Fishwild, D., and Tan, E. M.: Characterization of proliferating cell nuclear antigen recognized by autoantibodies in lupus sera. J. Exp. Med. 159:981, 1984.
200. Mathews, M. B., Berstein, R. M., Franze, B. R., Jr., and Garrels, J. I.: Identity of the proliferating cell nuclear antigen and cyclin. Nature 309:374, 1984.
201. Bravo, R., Frank, R., Blundell, P. A., and Macdonald-Bravo, H.: Cyclin/PCNA is the auxiliary protein of DNA polymerase-δ. Nature 326:515, 1987.
202. Prelich, G., Tan, C. K., Kostura, M., Mathews, M. B., So, A. G., Downey, K. M., and Stillman, B.: Functional identity of proliferating cell nuclear antigen and a DNA plymerase-δ auxiliary protein. Nature 326:517, 1987.
203. Huff, J. P., Roos, G., Peebles, C. L., Houghten, R., Sullivan, K. F., and Tan, E. M.: Insights into native epitopes of proliferating cell nuclear antigen using recombinant DNA protein products. J. Exp. Med. 172:419, 1990.
204. Elkon, K. B., Parnassa, A. P., and Foster, C. L.: Lupus autoantibodies target ribosomal P proteins. J. Exp. Med. 162:459, 1985.
205. Bonfa, E., Parnassa, A. P., Rhoades, D. D., Roufa, D. J., Wool, I. G., and Elkon, K. B.: Antiribosomal S10 antibodies in humans and MRL/lpr mice with systemic lupus erythematosus. Arthritis Rheum. 32:1252, 1989.
206. Sato, T., Uchiumi, T., Ozawa, T., Kikuchi, M., Nakano, M., Kominami, R., and Arakawa, M.: Autoantibodies against ribosomal proteins found with high frequency in patients with systemic lupus erythematosus with active disease. J. Rheumatol. 18:1681, 1991.
207. Bonfa, E., and Elkon, K. B.: Clinical and serologic associations of the antiribosomal P protein antibody. Arthritis Rheum. 29:981, 1986.
208. Bonfa, E., Golombek, S. J., Kaufman, L. D., Skelly, S., Weissbach, H., Brot, N., and Elkon, K. B.: Association between lupus psychosis and anti-ribosomal P protein antibodies. N. Engl. J. Med. 317:265, 1987.
209. Burlingame, R. W., Lowe, W. E., Wang, B. C., and Moudrianakis, E. N.: Crystallographic studies of the octameric histone core of the nucleosome at a resolution of 3.3 angstroms. Science 228:546, 1985.
210. Klug, A., Finch, J. T., and Richmond, T. J.: Crystallographic structure of the octamer histone core of the nucleosome. Science 229:1109, 1985.
211. Rekvig, O. P., and Hannestad, K.: Human antibodies that react with both cell nuclei and plasma membranes display specificity for the octamer of histones H2A, H2B, H3, and H4 in high salt. J. Exp. Med. 152:1720, 1980.
212. Hardin, J. A., and Thomas, J. O.: Antibodies to histones in systemic lupus erythematosus: Localization of prominent autoantigens on histones H1 and H2B. Proc. Natl. Acad. Sci. U.S.A. 80:7410, 1983.
213. Craft, J. E., Radding, J. A., Harding, M. W., Bernstein, R. M., and Hardin, J. A.: Autoantigenic histone epitopes: a comparison between procainamide- and hydralazine-induced lupus. Arthritis Rheum. 30:689, 1987.
214. Portanova, J. P., Arndt, R. E., Tan, E. M., and Kotzin, B. L.: Anti-histone antibodies in idiopathic and drug-induced lupus recognize distinct intrahistone regions. J. Immunol. 138:446, 1987.
215. Gohill, J., Cary, P. D., Couppez, M., and Fritzler, M. J.: Antibodies from patients with drug-induced and idiopathic lupus erythematosus react with epitopes restricted to the amino and carboxyl termini of histone. J. Immunol. 135:3116, 1985.
216. Gohill, J., and Fritzler, M. J.: Antibodies in procainamide-induced and systemic lupus erythematosus bind the C-terminus of histone 1 (H1). Mol. Immunol. 24:275, 1987.
217. Malleson, P., Petty, R. E., Fung, M., and Candido, E. P.: Reactivity of antinuclear antibodies with histones and other antigens in juvenile rheumatoid arthritis. Arthritis Rheum. 32:919, 1989.
218. Monestier, M., Losman, J. A., Fasy, T. M., Debbas, M. E., Massa, M., Albani, S., Bohm, L., and Martini, A.: Antihistone antibodies in antinuclear antibody–positive juvenile arthritis. Arthritis Rheum. 33:1836, 1990.
219. Aitcheson, C. T., Peebles, C., Joslin, F., and Tan, E. M.: Characteristics of antinuclear antibodies in rheumatoid arthritis. Arthritis Rheum. 23:528, 1980.
220. Molden, D. P., Klipple, G. L., Peebles, C. L., Rubin, R. L., Nakamura, R. M., and Tan, E. M.: IgM anti-histone H3 antibodies associated with undifferentiated rheumatic disease syndromes. Arthritis Rheum. 29:39, 1986.

221. Tan, E. M.: An immunologic precipitin system between soluble nucleoprotein and serum antibody in systemic lupus erythematosus. J. Clin. Invest. 46:735, 1987.
222. Thomas, J. O., Wilson, C. M., and Hardin, J. A.: The major core histone antigenic determinants in systemic lupus erythematosus are in the trypsin-sensitive regions. FEBS Lett. 169:90, 1984.
223. Totoritis, M. C., Tan, E. M., McNally, E. M., and Rubin, R. L.: Association of antibody to histone complex H2A-H2B with symptomatic procainamide-induced lupus. N. Engl. J. Med. 318:1431, 1988.
224. Rubin, R. L.: Autoimmune reactions induced by procainamide and hydralazine. In Kammuller, M., Bloksama, M., and Siemen, W. (eds): Autoimmunity and Toxicology. Immune Disregulation Induced by Drugs and Chemicals. Amsterdam, Elsevier, 1988.
225. Burlingame, R. W., and Rubin, R. L.: Drug-induced anti-histone autoantibodies display two patterns of reactivity with substructures of chromatin. J. Clin. Invest. 88:680, 1991.
226. Reichlin, M., and Arnett, F. C.: Multiplicity of antibodies in myositis sera. Arthritis Rheum. 27:1150, 1984.
227. Bernstein, R. M., Bunn, C. C., Hughes, G. R. V., Francoeur, A. M., and Mathews, M. B.: Cellular protein and RNA antigens in autoimmune disease. Mol. Biol. Med. 2:105, 1984.
228. Bernstein, R. M., and Mathews, M. B.: Jo-1 and other myositis autoantibodies. In Brooks, P. M., and York, J. R. (eds.): Rheumatology-85, Excerpta Medica International Congress Series. New York, Elsevier Science Publishers, 1985, pp. 273–278.
229. Targoff, I. N., and Reichlin, M.: Measurement of antibody to Jo-1 by ELISA and comparison to enzyme inhibitory activity. J. Immunol. 138:2874, 1987.
230. Targoff, I. N.: Laboratory manifestations of polymyositis/dermatomyositis. Clin. Dermatol. 6:76, 1988.
231. Yoshida, S., Akizuk, M., Mimori, T., Yamagata, H., Inada, S., and Homma, M.: The precipitating antibody to an acidic nuclear protein antigen, the Jo-1, in connective tissue disease. A marker for a subset of polymyositis with interstitial pulmonary fibrosis. Arthritis Rheum. 1826:604, 1983.
232. Bernstein, R. M., Morgan, S. H., and Chapman, J.: Anti–Jo-1 antibody: a marker for myositis with interstitial lung disease. Br. Med. J. 289:151, 1984.
233. Hochberg, M. C., Feldman, D., Stevens, M. B., Arnett, F. C., and Reichlin, M.: Antibody to Jo-1 in polymyositis/dermatomyositis: association with interstitial pulmonary fibrosis. J. Rheumatol. 11:663, 1984.
234. Wasicek, C. A., Reichlin, M., Montes, M., and Raghu, G.: Polymyositis and interstitial lung disease in patient with anti–Jo-1 prototype. Am. J. Med. 76:538, 1984.
235. Biswas, T., Miller, F. W., Takagaki, Y., and Plotz, P. H.: An enzyme-linked immunosorbent assay for the detection and quantitation of anti–Jo-1 antibody in human serum. J. Immunol. Methods 98:243, 1987.
236. Nishikai, M., and Reichlin, M.: Heterogeneity of precipitating antibodies in polymyositis and dermatomyositis. Characterization of the Jo-1 antibody system. Arthritis Rheum. 23:881, 1980.
237. Mathews, M. B., and Bernstein, R. M.: Myositis autoantibody inhibits histidyl tRNA synthetase: A model for autoimmunity. Nature 304:177, 1983.
238. Arnett, F. C., Hirsch, T. J., Bias, W. B., Nishikai, M., and Reichlin, M.: The Jo-1 antibody system in myositis: relationships to clinical features and HLA. J. Rheumatol. 8:925, 1981.
239. Rosa, M. D., Hendrick, J. P., Jr., Lerner, M. R., Reichlin, M., and Steitz, J. A.: A mammalian tRNA^{his}-containing antigen is recognized by the polymyositis-specific antibody anti–Jo-1. Nucleic Acids Res. 11:853, 1983.
240. Oddis, C. V., Medsger, T. A., and Cooperstein, L. A.: A subluxing arthropathy associated with the anti–Jo-1 antibody in polymyositis/dermatomyositis. Arthritis Rheum. 33:1640, 1990.
241. Goldstein, R., Duvic, M., Targoff, I., Reichlin, M., McMenemy, A. M., Reveille, J. D., Warner, N. B., Pollack, M. S., and Arnett, F. C.: HLA-D region genes associated with autoantibody responses to histidyl-transfer RNA synthetase (Jo-1) and other translation-related factors in myositis. Arthritis Rheum. 33:1240, 1990.
242. Miller, F. W., Twitty, S. A., Biswas, T., and Plotz, P.: Origin and regulation of a disease-specific autoantibody response. J. Clin. Invest. 85:468, 1990.
243. Miller, F. W., Waite, K. A., Biswas, T., and Plotz, P.: The role of an autoantigen, histidyl-tRNA synthetase, in the induction and maintenance of autoimmunity. Proc. Natl. Acad. Sci. U.S.A. 87:9933, 1990.
244. Mathews, M. B., Reichlin, M., Hughes, G. R. V., and Bernstein, R. M.: Anti-threonyl tRNA synthetase, a second myositis-related autoantibody. J. Exp. Med. 160:420, 1984.
245. Okada, N., Mukai, R., Harada, F., Kabashima, T., Nakao, Y., Yamane, K., Ohshima, Y., Sakamoto, K., Kashiwagi, H., and Hamaguchi, H.: Isolation of a novel antibody which precipitates ribonucleoprotein complex containing threonine tRNA from a patient with polymyositis. Eur. J. Biochem. 139:425, 1984.
246. Targoff, I. N., Arnett, F. C., and Reichlin, M.: Antibody to threonyl-transfer RNA synthetase in myositis sera. Arthritis Rheum. 31:515, 1988.

247. Bunn, C. C., Bernstein, R. M., and Mathews, M. B.: Autoantibodies against alanyl tRNA synthetase and tRNA^ala coexist and are associated with myositis. J. Exp. Med. 163:1281, 1986.
248. Targoff, I. N., and Arnett, F. C.: Clinical manifestations in patients with antibody to PL-12 antigen (alanyl-tRNA synthetase). Am. J. Med. 88:241, 1990.
249. Targoff, I. N.: Autoantibodies to aminoacyl-transfer RNA synthetases for isoleucine and glycine. J. Immunol. 144:1737, 1990.
250. Bunn, C. C., and Mathews, M.: Autoreactive epitope defined as the anticodon region of alanine transfer RNA. Science 238:1116, 1987.
251. Targoff, I. N., Arnett, F. C., Berman, L., O'Brien, C., Reichlin, M.: Anti-KJ: a new antibody associated with the syndrome of polymyositis and interstitial lung disease. J. Clin. Invest. 84:162, 1989.
252. Reeves, W. H., Nigam, S. K., and Blobel, G.: Human autoantibodies reactive with signal-recognition particle. Proc. Natl. Acad. Sci. U.S.A. 83:9507, 1986.
253. Okada, N., Mimori, T., Mukai, R., Kashiwagi, H., and Hardin, J.: Characterization of human autoantibodies that selectively precipitate the 7SL RNA component of the signal recognition particle. J. Immunol. 138:3219, 1987.
254. Targoff, I. N., Johnson, A. E., and Miller, F. W.: Antibody to signal recognition particle in polymyositis. Arthritis Rheum. 33:1361, 1990.
255. Hirakata, M., Mimori, T., Akizuki, M., Craft, J., Hardin, J., and Homma, M.: Autoantibodies to small nuclear and cytoplasmic ribonucleoproteins in Japanese patients with inflammatory muscle disease. Arthritis Rheum. 35:449, 1992.
256. Wolfe, J. F., Adelstein, E., and Sharp, G. C.: Antinuclear antibody with distinct specificity for polymyositis. J. Clin. Invest. 59:176, 1977.
257. Treadwell, E. L., Alspaugh, M. A., Wolfe, J. F., and Sharp, G. C.: Clinical relevance of PM-1 antibody and physiochemical characterization of PM-1 antigen. J. Rheumatol. 11:658, 1984.
258. Genth, E., Mierau, R., Genetzky, P., von Mühlen, C. A., Kaufman, S., von Wilmowsky, H., Meurer, M., Krieg, T., Pollman, H.-J., and Hartl, P. W.: Immunogenetic associations of scleroderma-related antinuclear antibodies. Arthritis Rheum. 33:657, 1990.
259. Reimer, G., Steen, V. D., Penning, C. A., Medsger, T. A., Jr., and Tan, E. M.: Correlates between autoantibodies to nucleolar antigens and clinical features in patients with systemic sclerosis (scleroderma). Arthritis Rheum. 31:525, 1988.
260. Targoff, I. N., and Reichlin, M.: Nucleolar localization of the PM-Scl antigen. Arthritis Rheum. 28:226, 1985.
261. Reimer, G., Scheer, U., Peters, J. M., and Tan, E. M.: Immunolocalization and partial characterization of a nucleolar autoantigen (PM-Scl) associated with polymyositis/scleroderma overlap syndromes. J. Immunol. 137:3802, 1986.
262. Gelpi, C., Alguero, A., Angeles Martinez, M., Vidal, S., Juarez, C., and Rodriguez-Sanchez, J. L.: Identification of protein components reactive with anti-PM/Scl autoantibodies. Clin. Exp. Immunol. 81:59, 1990.
263. Alderuccio, F., Chan, E. K. L., and Tan, E. M.: Molecular characterization of an autoantigen of PM-Scl in the polymyositis/scleroderma overlap syndrome: a unique and complete human cDNA encoding an apparent 75-kD acidic protein of the nucleolar complex. J. Exp. Med. 173:941, 1991.
264. Mimori, T., Akizuki, M., Yamagata, H., Inada, S., Yoshida, S., and Homma, M.: Characterization of a high molecular weight acidic nuclear protein recognized by autoantibodies in sera from patients with polymyositis-scleroderma overlap. J. Clin. Invest. 68:611, 1981.
265. Reeves, W. H.: Use of monoclonal antibodies for the characterization of novel DNA-binding protein recognized by human autoimmune sera. J. Exp. Med. 161:18, 1985.
266. Mimori, T., Hardin, J. A., and Steitz, J. A.: Characterization of the DNA-binding protein antigen Ku recognized by autoantibodies from patients with rheumatic disorders. J. Biol. Chem. 261:2274, 1986.
267. Mimori, T., and Hardin, J. A.: Mechanism of interaction between Ku protein and DNA. J. Biol. Chem. 261:10375, 1986.
268. Targoff, I. N., and Reichlin, M.: The association between Mi2 antibodies and dermatomyositis. Arthritis Rheum. 28:796, 1985.
269. Catoggio, L. J., Bernstein, R. M., Black, C. M., Hughes, G. V., and Maddison, P. J.: Serological markers in progressive systemic sclerosis: clinical correlations. Ann. Rheum. Dis. 42:23, 1983.
270. Li, X., McNeilage, L. J., and Whittingham, S.: Autoantibodies to the major nucleolar phosphoprotein B23 define a novel subset of patients with anticardiolipin antibodies. Arthritis Rheum. 32:1165, 1989.
271. Douvas, A., Achten, M., and Tan, E. M.: Identification of a nuclear protein (Scl-70) as a unique target of human antinuclear antibodies in scleroderma. J. Biol. Chem. 254:10514, 1979.
272. Wade, J. P., Sack, B., and Schur, P.: Anticentromere antibodies—clinical correlates. J. Rheumatol. 15:1759, 1988.
273. Earnshaw, W. C., and Rothfield, N.: Identification of a family of human centromere proteins using autoimmune sera from patients with scleroderma. Chromosoma (Berl.) 91:313, 1985.
274. Earnshaw, W. C., Bordwell, B. J., Marino, C., and Rothfield, N.: Three human chromosomal autoantigens are recognized by sera from patients with anti-centromere antibodies. J. Clin. Invest. 77:426, 1986.
275. Rothfield, N., Whitaker, D., Bordwell, B., Weiner, E., Senecal, J.-L., and Earnshaw, W.: Detection of anti-centromere antibodies using cloned autoantigen CENP-B. Arthritis Rheum. 30:1416, 1987.
276. Shero, J. H., Bordwell, B., Rothfield, N., and Earnshaw, W. C.: High titers of autoantibodies to topoisomerase I (Scl-70) in sera from scleroderma patients. Science 231:737, 1986.
277. Van Venrooij, W. J., Stapel, S. O., Houben, H., Habets, W. J., Kallenberg, C. G. M., Penner, E., and Van de Putte, L. B.: Scl-86, a marker antigen for diffuse scleroderma. J. Clin. Invest. 75:1053, 1985.
278. Earnshaw, W. C., Sullivan, K. F., Machlin, P. S., Cooke, C. A., Kaiser, D. A., Pollard, T. D., Rothfield, N. F., and Cleveland, D. W.: Molecular cloning of cDNA for CENP-B, the major human centromere autoantigen. J. Cell. Biol. 104:817, 1987.
279. McNeilage, L. J., Whittingham, S., McHugh, N., and Barnett, A. J.: A highly conserved 72,000-dalton centromeric antigen reactive with autoantibodies from patients with progressive systemic sclerosis. J. Immunol. 137:2541, 1986.
280. D'Arpa, P., White-Cooper, H., Cleveland, D. W., Rothfield, N. F., and Earnshaw, W. C.: Use of molecular cloning methods to map the distribution of epitopes on topoisomerase I (Scl-70) recognized by sera of scleroderma patients. Arthritis Rheum. 33:1501, 1990.
281. Verheijen, R., Van den Hoogen, F., Beijer, R., Richter, A., Penner, E., Habets, W. J., and van Venrooij, W. J.: A recombinant topoisomerase I used for autoantibody detection in sera from patients with systemic sclerosis. Clin. Exp. Immunol. 80:38, 1990.
282. Earnshaw, W. C., Machlin, P. S., Bordwell, B. S., Rothfield, N. F., and Cleveland, D. W.: Analysis of anticentromere autoantibodies using cloned autoantigen CENP-B. Proc. Natl. Acad. Sci. U.S.A. 84:4979, 1987.
283. Maul, G. G., Jimenez, S. A., Riggs, E., and Ziemnicka-Kotula, D.: Determination of an epitope of the diffuse systemic sclerosis marker antigen DNA topoisomerase I: Sequence similarity with retroviral p30^gag protein suggests a possible cause for autoimmunity in systemic sclerosis. Proc. Natl. Acad. Sci. U.S.A. 86:8492, 1989.
284. Steen, V. D., Powell, D. L., and Medsger, T. A., Jr.: Clinical correlations and prognosis based on serum autoantibodies in patients with systemic sclerosis. Arthritis Rheum. 31:196, 1988.
285. Weiner, E. S., Earnshaw, W. C., Senecal, J. L., Bordwell, B., Johnson, P., and Rothfield, N. F.: Clinical associations of anticentromere antibodies and antibodies to topoisomerase I. Arthritis Rheum. 31:378, 1988.
286. Kumar, V., Kowalewski, C., Koelle, M., Qutaishat, S., Chorzelski, T., Beutner, E. H., Jarzabek-Chorzelska, M., Kolacinska, Z., and Jablonska, S.: Scl-70 antigen stability and its effect on antibody detection in scleroderma. J. Rheumatol. 15:1499, 1988.
287. Jarzabek-Chorzelska, M., Blaszczyk, M., Jablonska, S., Chorzelski, T., Kumar, V., and Beutner, E. H.: Scl-70 antibody—a specific marker of systemic sclerosis. Br. J. Dermatol. 115:393, 1986.
288. Weiner, E., Hildebrandt, S., Senecal, J.-L., Daniels, L., Noell, S., Joyal, F., Roussin, A., Earnshaw, W. C., and Rothfield, N.: Prognostic significance of anticentromere antibodies and anti-topoisomerase I antibodies in Raynaud's disease: A prospective study. Arthritis Rheum. 34:68, 1991.
289. Kallenberg, C. G. M., Wouda, A. A., Hoet, M. H., and van Venrooij, W. J.: Development of connective tissue disease in patients presenting with Raynaud's phenomenon: a six-year follow-up with emphasis on the predictive value of antinuclear antibodies as detected by immunoblotting. Ann. Rheum. Dis. 47:634, 1988.
290. Steen, V. D., Ziegler, G. L., Rodnan, G. P., and Medsger, T. A., Jr.: Clinical and laboratory associations of anticentromere antibody in patients with progressive systemic sclerosis. Arthritis Rheum. 27:125, 1984.
291. McCarty, G. A., Rice, J. R., Bembe, M. L., and Barada, F. A.: Anticentromere antibody—clinical correlations and association with favorable prognosis in patients with scleroderma variants. Arthritis Rheum. 26:1, 1983.
292. Sarkozi, J., Bookman, A. A. M., Lee, P., Keystone, E. C., and Fritzler, M. J.: Significance of anticentromere antibody in idiopathic Raynaud's syndrome. Am. J. Med. 83:893, 1987.
293. Ruffatti, A., Calligaro, A., Ferri, C., Bombardieri, S., Gambari, P. F., and Todesco, C.: Association of anticentromere and anti–Scl-70 antibodies in scleroderma: report of two cases. J. Clin. Lab. Immunol. 16:227, 1985.
294. Kipnis, R. J., Craft, J., and Hardin, J.: The analysis of antinuclear and antinucleolar autoantibodies of scleroderma by radioimmunoprecipitation assays. Arthritis Rheum. 33:1431, 1990.
295. Craft, J., and Gold, H.: The Th ribonucleoprotein particle: association with the RNA processing enzymes RNase MRP and RNase P. Mol. Biol. Rep. 14:109, 1990.
296. Okano, Y., and Medsger, T.: Autoantibody to Th ribonucleoprotein (nucleolar 7–2 RNA protein particle) in patients with systemic sclerosis. Arthritis Rheum. 33:1822, 1990.
297. Rodriguez, J. L., Gelpi, C., Juarez, C., and Hardin, J. A.: Anti–NOR-90: a new autoantibody in scleroderma that recognizes a 90-kDa

component of the nucleolus-organizing region of chromatin. J. Immunol. 139:2579, 1987.

298. Lischwe, M. A., Ochs, R. L., Reddy, R., Cook, R. G., Yeoman, L. C., Tan, E. M., Reichlin, M., and Busch, H.: Purification and partial characterization of a nucleolar scleroderma antigen (M_r = 34,000; pl, 8.5) rich in N^GN^G dimethylarginine. J. Biol. Chem. 260:14304, 1985.

299. Parker, K. A., and Steitz, J. A.: Structural analyses of the human U3 ribonucleoprotein particle reveal a conserved sequence available for base pairing with pre-rRNA. Mol. Cell Biol. 7:2899, 1987.

300. Kass, S., Tyc, K., Steitz, J. A., and Sollner-Webb, B.: The U3 small nucleolar ribonucleoprotein functions in the first step of preribosomal RNA processing. Cell 60:897, 1990.

301. Gold, H. A., Topper, J., Clayton, D., and Craft, J.: The human RNA processing enzyme RNase MRP is identical to the Th ribonucleoprotein autoantigen and related to RNase P. Science 245:1377, 1989.

302. Craft, J., and Gold, H.: New RNPs in higher eukaryotes. Mol. Biol. Rep. 14:97, 1990.

303. Hashimoto, C., and Steitz, J. A.: Sequential association of nucleolar 7–2 RNA with two different autoantigens. J. Biol. Chem. 258:1379, 1983.

304. Reddy, R., Tan, E. M., Henning, D., Nohga, K., and Busch, H.: Detection of a nucleolar 7–2 ribonucleoprotein and a cytoplasmic 8–2 ribonucleoprotein with autoantibodies from patients with scleroderma. J. Biol. Chem. 258:1383, 1983.

305. Craft, J.: Unpublished observation.

306. Gold, H. A., Craft, J., Hardin, J. A., Bartkiewicz, M., and Altman, S.: Antibodies in human sera that precipitate ribonuclease P. Proc. Natl. Acad. Sci. U.S.A. 85:5483, 1988.

307. Reimer, G., Rose, K. M., Scheer, U., and Tan, E. M.: Autoantibody to RNA polymerase I in scleroderma sera. J. Clin. Invest. 79:65, 1987.

308. Falanga, V., Medsger, T. J., and Reichlin, M.: Antinuclear and anti–single-stranded DNA antibodies in morphea and generalized morphea. Arch. Dermatol. 123(3):350, 1987.

309. Anderson, J. R., Grey, K. G., Beck, J., and Kinnear, W. F.: Precipitating autoantibodies in Sjögren's disease. Lancet 2:456, 1961.

310. Alexander, E. L., Hirsch, J. J., Arnett, F. C., Provost, T. T., and Stevens, M. B.: Ro (SSA) and La (SSB) antibodies in the clinical spectrum of Sjögren's syndrome. J. Rheumatol. 9:239, 1982.

311. Harley, J. B., Alexander, E. L., Bias, W. B., Fox, O. F., Provost, T. T., Reichlin, M., Yamagata, H., and Arnett, F. C.: Anti-Ro/SSA and anti–La/SSB in patients with Sjögren's syndrome. Arthritis Rheum. 29:196, 1986.

312. Provost, T. T., Talal, N., Harley, J. B., Reichlin, M., and Alexander, E.: The relationship between anti-Ro (SS-A) antibody–positive Sjögren's syndrome and anti-Ro (SS-A) antibody–positive lupus erythematosus. Arch. Dermatol. 124:63, 1988.

313. Provost, T. T., Talal, N., Bias, W., Harley, J. B., Reichlin, M., and Alexander, E. L.: Ro(SS-A)-positive Sjögren's/lupus erythematosus (SC/LE) overlap patients are associated with the HLA-DR3 and/or DRw6 phenotypes. J. Invest. Dermatol. 91:369, 1988.

314. Molina, R., Provost, T. T., and Alexander, E. L.: Two types of inflammatory vascular disease in Sjögren's syndrome: Differential association with seroreactivity to rheumatoid factor and antibodies to Ro/SSA and with hypocomplementemia. Arthritis Rheum. 28:1251, 1985.

315. Itescu, S., Brancato, L. J., Buxbaum, J., Gregersen, P. K., Rix, C. C., Croxson, T. S., Solomon, G. E., and Winchester, R.: A diffuse infiltrative CD8 lymphocytosis syndrome in human immunodeficiency virus (HIV) infection: A host immune response associated with HLA-DR5. Ann. Intern. Med. 112:3, 1990.

316. Blomgren, S. E., Condemi, J. J., and Vaughan, J. H.: Procainamide-induced lupus erythematosus. Clinical and laboratory observations. Am. J. Med. 52:338, 1972.

317. Kasukawa, R., Tojo, T., Miyawaki, S., Yoshida, H., Tanimoto, K., Nobunaga, M., Suzuki, T., Takasaki, Y., and Tamura, T.: Preliminary diagnostic criteria for classification of mixed connective tissue disease. In Kasukawa, R., and Sharp, G. C. (eds.): Mixed Connective Tissue Disease and Anti-nuclear Antibodies. Excerpta Medica International Congress Series 719. New York, Elsevier Science Publishers, 1987, pp. 41–54.

318. Reeves, W. H., and Ali, S. A.: Preferential use of lambda L chain in lamin B autoantibodies. J. Immunol. 143:3614, 1989.

319. Evans, J., Reuben, A., and Craft, J.: PBC-95K: A 95-kilodalton nuclear autoantigen in primary biliary cirrhosis. Arthritis Rheum. 34:731, 1991.

320. Lutz-Freyermuth, C., and Keene, J. D.: The U1 RNA-binding site of the U1 small nuclear ribonucleoprotein (snRNP)-associated A protein suggests a similarity with U2 snRNPs. Mol. Cell. Biol. 9:2975, 1989.

321. Query, C. C., Bentley, R. C., and Keene, J. D.: A specific 31-nucleotide domain of U1 RNA directly interacts with the 70K small nuclear ribonucleoprotein component. Mol. Cell. Biol. 9:4872, 1989.

Chapter 10

Immune Complexes and Complement

George Moxley
Shaun Ruddy

INTRODUCTION

The binding of antibodies to antigens to form immune complexes links the recognition of exogenous agents to protective biologic consequences. The combination of a viral protein with an antibody, for example, influences the immune response to that protein[1, 2] and activates the complement cascade. Portions of the C1q, C4, and C3 complement components modify the structure of the immune complex, inhibiting precipitation in tissues or solubilizing already deposited complexes. Complement fragments bound to the immune complex direct interaction with complement receptors on various cell surfaces, modifying the processing of immune complexes and enhancing their delivery to phagocytic cells.[3] Important interactions of immune complexes also occur by binding to cell surface receptors for the Fc portions of immunoglobulins.

The venerated concept that immune complexes cause disease began with the observations of von Pirquet on serum sickness. Eight to twelve days after an initial injection of horse serum, patients developed urticaria, fever, edema, and arthralgias; the reaction to a second injection was more rapid and more severe. Von Pirquet suggested that the interaction of immunogens with antibodies formed by the host produced toxic substances resulting in clinically apparent illness.[4] This proposed mechanism was later supported by Germuth[5] and Dixon and colleagues,[6] who used an animal model of serum sickness to show that the cardiovascular and renal manifestations due to tissue deposition of immune complexes were temporally correlated with the presence of both antigen and specific antibody in the circulation. They proposed that the antigen and antibody had interacted in the circulation, deposited locally, and resulted in anaphylactic and inflammatory responses. The notion that immune complexes cause disease has been central to the view of rheumatoid arthritis (RA), systemic lupus erythematosus (SLE), and other illnesses as autoimmune diseases. It also helps explain such diverse diseases as glomerulonephritis

and vasculitis as well as certain manifestations of subacute bacterial endocarditis and other infectious diseases.[1, 2] Chapters on immune complexes in previous editions of *Textbook of Rheumatology* have analyzed evidence regarding pathogenetic mechanisms in immune complex diseases. In some conditions, immune complexes form in the circulation and then localize in various tissues to cause inflammation; a prime example is serum sickness. In others, immune complexes form in interstitial fluids and cause local inflammation; a classic example is the Arthus reaction, in which antigens injected intradermally combine with antibody found in the interstitial fluid to trigger inflammation at the site of injection.

Not all immune complexes are alike in their capacity to induce tissue damage. Antigens differ in size, charge, and ability to bind to macromolecules, and antibodies differ in isotype, valence, affinity, relative charge, and ability to activate complement. The proportions of antigen and antibody contained in the complex vary, and, depending on the isotype of antibody, complement is activated and rheumatoid factors (RFs) bind. Other important pathogenetic factors in immune complex disease include local blood flow patterns, changes in vascular permeability, altered phagocytic function, and the effects of released complement fragments. In addition, the complement fragments bound to the immune complexes play a dominant role in the modification of immune complexes and their routing to complement receptors on cell surfaces for further modification and ultimate disposition.[3] Large complexes (favored by antibody excess) activate complement well and are rapidly cleared through binding to cell surface receptors. Small complexes (favored by antigen excess), which do not activate complement as well, are not very inflammatory. Complexes of intermediate size, which escape clearance mechanisms and activate complement well, are the most effective in inducing tissue damage. In any patient, at the moment when the circulation is sampled for immune complex levels, there is likely to be a variety of sizes and compositions of immune complexes.

METHODS FOR DEMONSTRATING IMMUNE COMPLEXES

Immune complexes are identified in tissues by indirect immunofluorescent methods detecting gran-

Supported by NIH Grant Numbers AR38478, AR07079-15, AI28532-03, and AI 13049-15, and a Virginia Commonwealth University Grant-in-Aid. This is publication number 250 from the Charles W. Thomas Fund.

188

Table 10–1. COMMONLY USED ANTIGEN-NONSPECIFIC ASSAYS FOR CIRCULATING IMMUNE COMPLEXES

Assay	Properties Allowing Detection	Complex Size Bias*/ Isotypes Detected	Confounding Factors
Fluid-phase C1q-binding[83]	1. Binding of radiolabeled C1q to complex 2. Insolubility in 2.5% PEG	Large IgG1, IgG2, IgG3, pentameric IgM	Heparin, C-reactive protein, rheumatoid factor (RF)
Solid-phase C1q-binding[84]	1. Binding of complex to C1q absorbed on microtiter well 2. Detection by radiolabeled antibody	Can detect monomeric IgG1, IgG2, IgG3, monomeric and pentameric IgM	RF
Raji cell[85]	1. Display of C3bi or C3dg on complex 2. Binding to CR2 on Raji cell 3. Detection by radiolabeled anti-IgG	Large IgG, IgM	EDTA, heat inactivation, RF, antilymphocyte antibody
Monoclonal rheumatoid factor[86]	1. Competition with IgG immunosorbent for binding to radiolabeled RF, or 2. Competition with radiolabeled aggregated γ-globulin for binding to solid-phase RF	Large IgG1, IgG2, IgG4	DNA, RF
Staphylococcal-binding[87]	1. Binding to protein A of *Staphylococcus aureus* 2. Removal of monomeric IgG by competition with rabbit IgG 3. Detection by radiolabeled antihuman IgG	Minimal bias IgG1–4, IgA1, IgM	RF, endotoxin, heparin
Conglutinin[88]	1. Display of C3bi on complex 2. Binding via C3bi on conglutinin coated on microtiter well 3. Developed with labeled anti-IgG or staphylococcal protein A	Large IgG, IgM	Endotoxin, heparin, EDTA, heat inactivation
Anti-C3[89]	1. Display of C3 on complex 2. Binding to C3-specific monoclonal antibody coated on microtiter well 3. Detection by labeled antihuman immunoglobulin	Not addressed[7]	Not addressed[7]

*Findings from McDougal, J.S., Hubbard, M., et al.[7]
EDTA, ethylenediamine tetra-acetic acid; PEG, polyethylene glycol.

ular deposits of immunoglobulin and complement. In biologic fluids, one can easily detect immune complexes if the antigen is known; for example, a virus or viral product in a complex may be precipitated with antibodies directed toward immunoglobulin or complement, or it is sedimented rapidly together with immunoglobulin in the ultracentrifuge. For the majority of disorders, including many rheumatic diseases, in which the antigens are unknown, nonspecific methods detect materials with attributes of immune complexes, such as bound complement fragments or high molecular weight. There are more than 40 different antigen-nonspecific methods, of which seven of the most commonly used are described in Table 10–1. Most methods detect aggregated gamma globulin (γ-globulin) as well as immune complexes and, therefore, are subject to interference by heating of sera or freeze-thaw effects. Some methods bear substantial biases in the kinds of immune complexes detected, such as the skewing toward detection of large immune complexes, a relative lack of reactivity toward materials between the size of monomeric IgG and pentameric IgM (200 to 900 kD),[7] and the detection of only certain isotypes of immu-

noglobulins. There are, in addition, substantial problems with variability both within and between assays, ranging up to 57 percent interassay variation and most marked for the Raji cell assay.[7] In part, this has to do with the crude nature of the standards used, heat-aggregated γ-globulin. In one collaborative survey, the range of values obtained by the various laboratories for an unknown, namely tetanus-antitetanus at 40 μg per ml, was 35 to 1420.[8] Because of this variation among laboratories, international standards for immune complexes have been proposed,[8] but this idea has not gained wide acceptance. Therefore, the technical characteristics of the assays do not favor uniform detection of all sizes and kinds of immune complexes or following levels except in serially obtained specimens compared in the same assay.

USE OF IMMUNE COMPLEX ASSAYS IN RHEUMATIC DISEASES

Patients with certain rheumatic diseases may be distinguished from normal subjects by the various

Table 10–2. PREDICTIVE VALUE OF IMMUNE COMPLEX ASSAYS IN DISTINGUISHING DISEASED INDIVIDUALS FROM NORMAL SUBJECTS*

Assay	Positive Predictive Value			Negative Predictive Value		
	RA	SLE	Vasculitis	RA	SLE	Vasculitis
Fluid-phase C1q-binding	88	91	67	81	50	76
Solid-phase C1q-binding	82	95	70	73	64	73
Raji cell	96	97	74	57	56	87
Monoclonal rheumatoid factor	92	85	90	54	66	58
Staphylococcal-binding	98	99	92	63	42	90
Conglutinin-binding	86	94	71	51	50	87

*This table represents accuracy in comparison between each clinical group and normal individuals. The figures reflect the mean, weighted for number of subjects, of all studies identified by use of Grateful Med with search terms for disease and prognosis or activity and antigen-antibody complex or immune complex disease and with patient and control groups numbering more than 20 subjects.

immune complex assays. The accuracy of such assays in RA, SLE, or vasculitis is illustrated in Table 10–2. Even with the use of the same published method for determining immune complexes, there is a wide range of values among the individual studies, such as the fluid-phase C1q-binding assay for SLE. Despite the variation among studies, one can derive from the positive and negative predictive values some indications about the empirical usefulness of this group of tests in distinguishing diseased from normal individuals. The most useful positive test for distinguishing a person with RA from a normal subject is the staphylococcal-binding assay, followed closely by the Raji cell assay; the most useful negative test in excluding RA is the fluid-phase C1q-binding assay. For distinguishing a person with SLE from a normal individual, the most useful test if positive is the staphylococcal-binding test, followed closely by the Raji cell assay; the diagnostic accuracy of the Raji cell assay for SLE is related partly to antilymphocyte antibody. In contrast, the most useful test in excluding SLE if negative is the monoclonal RF assay, followed by the solid-phase C1q-binding assay. For the diseases characterized by vasculitis, the most useful positive tests are the monoclonal RF and staphylococcal-binding assays, and the most useful negative tests are the Raji cell and the staphylococcal-binding assays.

Antigen-nonspecific immune complex assays may be positive in any of the diseases listed in Table 10–3. Although positive immune complex assays are of no differential diagnostic value, they are often

Table 10–3. DISEASES ASSOCIATED WITH POSITIVE TESTS FOR IMMUNE COMPLEXES

Rheumatic Diseases
  Rheumatoid arthritis and Felty's syndrome
  Primary Sjögren's syndrome
  Juvenile rheumatoid arthritis
  Systemic lupus erythematosus
  Scleroderma
  Mixed connective tissue disease
  Seronegative spondyloarthropathies: Reiter's syndrome, ankylosing spondylitis, psoriasis, Behçet's sydrome, idiopathic inflammatory bowel disease
  Vasculitis: mixed cryoglobulinemia, polyarteritis nodosa, Wegener's granulomatosis, serum sickness, Henoch-Schönlein purpura, hypocomplementemic cutaneous vasculitis
  Infectious arthritides: Lyme disease, viral arthritides
  Sarcoidosis

Neoplastic Disease
  Including but not limited to solid tumors such as melanoma and lymphoproliferative disorders

Glomerulonephritides

Bacterial Infections
  Including but not limited to endocarditis, meningococcal infection, and gonococcemia, streptococcal infections, syphilis, chronic infections such as in patients with underlying cystic fibrosis, recurrent infections in children, otitis media

Viral Infections
  Cytomegalovirus, hepatitis B, infectious mononucleosis, acquired immunodeficiency syndrome (AIDS), and AIDS-related complex,[90] and others

Various Parasitic Infections
  Such as toxoplasmosis and quartan malaria

Many Others
  Including inflammatory bowel disease, myocardial infarcts, sickle-cell anemia, atopic conditions, as well as other less common diseases

Data from Williams[1] and Theofilapoulos and Dixon,[2] in which a more complete listing can be found.

reflective of certain clinical subsets of disease. When compared with the levels of immune complexes in patients with RA restricted to the joints, levels from patients with extra-articular forms of RA (e.g., rheumatoid nodules and Sjögren's syndrome) were substantially higher in several studies.[9, 9a] Patients with rheumatoid vasculitis also have positive test results more frequently[10] and typically have higher levels.[11] Overall, the levels of immune complexes are higher in the more complicated forms of RA, but the difference in frequency of positivity is not enough to allow reliable identification of the clinical subset.

In SLE, no particular clinical manifestations correlate with the presence of antigen-nonspecific immune complexes as detected by the solid-phase C1q-binding assay, but patients with facial erythema or discoid lesions alone do not have a positive immune complex test.[12] This is similar to the direct demonstration of tissue-associated immunoglobulin and complement in clinically normal skin by the lupus band test: in discoid lupus, the test result is negative, whereas in SLE about 50 percent of patients have a positive test result.[13] In a study of patients with lupus nephritis, the levels of reactivity detected by the solid-phase C1q-binding were twice as high in diffuse proliferative as those in membranous lupus glomerulonephritis, and this was due to material the size of monomeric IgG.[14] One study of patients with SLE using the Raji cell assay showed a positive correlation with the numbers of organ systems involved,[15] and a second demonstrated a correlation with central nervous system involvement.[16]

In patients with cutaneous vasculitis of either the necrotizing or the lymphocytic type, the presence of fluid-phase C1q-binding activity was found to a far greater extent in the group with necrotizing vasculitis.[17] In one study of patients with scleroderma, those with positive Raji cell test results more frequently had diffuse disease, tendon friction rubs, and positive test results for antinuclear antibodies, and those with positive fluid-phase C1q-binding assays had more pulmonary involvement and positive RFs.[18] In a second study of patients with scleroderma, the fluid-phase C1q-binding, solid-phase C1q-binding, and conglutinin-binding assays were only infrequently positive.[19]

Immune complex assays have sometimes been used as indices of disease activity. In patients with RA, various measures of inflammatory joint disease or systemic inflammatory disease have been devised, typically including joint activity, morning stiffness, fatigue, analgesic use, and erythrocyte sedimentation rate [ESR] [systemic index]. Early studies of RA indicated a correlation of fluid-phase C1q-binding assay with systemic index and joint index (r = +0.695),[20] and higher levels of immune complexes occurred in individuals with high ESR and morning stiffness.[21] A carefully conducted prospective clinical study showed that the correlation of a systemic index with fluid-phase C1q-binding was significant but weak (r = +0.24–0.29); the correlation of the ESR

with clinical indices was stronger (r = +0.52–0.64).[9] In a similar prospective study comparing the value of single with serial determinations, the correlation value of tests on single samples with swollen joints or joint index was weak (r = +0.29–0.47 and +0.21–0.44, respectively). In specimens serially obtained from individual patients, the correlation with swollen joints or joint index was stronger than at a single point (r = +0.51 and +0.76, respectively).[22] Following serial levels in individual patients can, therefore, be of more value than attempting to correlate disease activity in a single specimen. These observations of weak or no correlation of various immune complex assays with systemic or joint index of RA have been affirmed many times with various assays.[9, 10, 21, 23] On the other hand, the fluid-phase C1q-binding assay is more useful in individual patients with RA followed serially.[22] Of special note is that in some studies the disease activity correlated better with tests other than immune complex assays, such as C3dg[20] or ESR.[9] With some therapies, such as cryofiltration,[24] slowly acting antirheumatic agents, doses of corticosteroids greater than 20 mg of prednisolone per day,[25] and lymphoplasmapheresis,[26] the improvement in clinical state was paralleled by a decline in the materials reacting in the various immune complex assays. For other therapies, such as total lymphoid irradiation, the clinical disease improved but the immune complexes did not decline.[27] There is no evidence for the utility of immune complex measurement in predicting RA activity; neither the fluid-phase nor the solid-phase C1q binding is predictive of disease activity or outcome.[23]

In SLE, comparison among the many studies is hampered by heterogeneity in the various disease manifestations in the patients included in the individual studies and the myriad ways of estimating disease activity. There has been considerable disagreement about whether there is little correlation of SLE activity with fluid-phase C1q-binding assay[28] results or strong correlation.[29] Just as extrarenal disease in one study correlated with Raji cell assay results, but renal disease did not,[15] and renal or pleural/pericardial SLE correlated best with results of fluid-phase C1q-binding assay in another study,[30] the differences in manifestations represented in the study subjects possibly influenced the degree of correlation with fluid-phase C1q-binding results. Solid-phase C1q-binding assay results have generally correlated strongly with various measures of lupus disease activity, including arthritis and nephritis, with the exception that skin disease alone was not associated with a positive test result.[12] The ability to discern the disease severity by means of the solid-phase C1q-binding assay has been confirmed,[31] and positive test results were found in most flare-ups of lupus.[32] The apparent conflict between mixed results for correlations with fluid-phase C1q binding and generally positive correlations with solid-phase C1q binding may be related mostly to monomeric IgG that binds to C1q, which is an effective index of disease activity.[14] Recent studies have demonstrated similar anti-C1q IgG in other disease states, such as hypocomplementemic urticarial vasculitis and rheumatoid vasculitis.[33, 34] In one SLE study, ESR and platelet count distinguished active disease as well as did solid-phase C1q binding.[31] Raji cell assay results have correlated with the numbers of organ systems involved but not with changes in renal function.[15] The conglutinin-binding assay showed a modest correlation with disease activity.[35]

The question of whether immune complexes predict future disease activity of SLE has conflicting answers. One group of investigators in a retrospective study of cycles of disease activity found that an elevation in fluid-phase C1q binding as well as depressed levels of C4 and results of the total serum hemolytic complement (CH$_{50}$) assay occurred prior to active nephritis episodes.[36] In addition, Abrass and coworkers[12] found in a carefully done prospective study that a change in the solid-phase C1q binding predicted a change in disease activity, requiring hospitalization or a change in medication 82 percent of the time; changes in fluid-phase C1q, anti-DNA antibody, and C3 were not predictive. It is important to note, however, that one subsequent study has not found a predictive value for solid-phase C1q binding.[32] Using the Raji cell assay, high levels of immune complexes prior to glucocorticoid therapy predicted the later development of lupus nephritis.[37] A recent study utilizing a modified anti-C3 assay showed higher levels in patients with higher SLE activity.[38]

There have been very few studies examining the extent to which immune complex assays parallel the activity of vasculitis. In patients with necrotizing vasculitis, results of the fluid-phase C1q-binding and monoclonal RF assays paralleled disease activity.[17] In a study of 28 patients with polyarteritis nodosa and 15 patients with Wegener's granulomatosis, effective therapy substantially diminished the frequency of positivity for the Raji cell assay, but not fluid-phase C1q binding.[39] In patients with polymyalgia rheumatica or temporal arteritis, there are higher Raji cell assay values with active disease.[40]

Correlations of activity of mixed connective tissue disease with results of the fluid-phase C1q-binding and Raji cell assays,[41] and of eosinophilic fascitis with Raji cell assay[42] results, have been described. In ankylosing spondylitis, there have been noted declining levels of immune complexes detected by solid-phase C1q-binding assay during the first year in association with major improvement in disease activity.[43] In patients with primary Sjögren's syndrome, the levels of immune complexes detected by fluid-phase C1q-binding or Raji cell assay did not correlate with disease activity or the development of lymphoid infiltrates in organs other than lymph nodes or spleen (pseudolymphoma).[44]

Summary of Clinical Uses. Immune complex assays may be useful in *categorization*, that is, when a disease state typically characterized by immune complexes, such as early RA, might be distinguished from a condition in which there are typically no immune complexes, such as arthralgia.[45] Preliminary indications are that a positive result would be likely to indicate RA with a nearly 75 percent accuracy, and a negative result would be likely to indicate arthralgia with an accuracy of slightly over 80 percent[45]; this has yet to be confirmed by other published reports. One may be able to sharpen this distinction by the judicious repetition of the assay; if the test result is again positive, it is more probable that the true underlying cause of the joint pain is related to a disease associated with immune complexes. The optimal clinical use of these assays requires careful consideration of the likelihood of disease prior to obtaining the study. The second clinical setting is the assessment of *disease activity*. However, it should be noted that there are other tests for disease activity that are not only more reflective of the actual clinical state but also considerably less expensive, such as the Westergren ESR for RA or temporal arteritis. For SLE, however, there may continue to be a role for the use of some immune complex assays, such as the solid-phase C1q-binding assay, in conjunction with anti-DNA antibodies and levels of C3 and C4 for the assessment and prediction of disease activity. In order to avoid the considerable assay-to-assay variation, side-by-side comparison of serially obtained specimens should be done.

COMPLEMENT ACTIVATION

The complement system includes 14 plasma proteins that interact in a cascade sequence to mediate a variety of inflammatory effects in addition to bacteriolysis, as well as six plasma proteins and five integral membrane proteins that regulate this cascade (Table 10–4).[46–49] Recognition of activating agents by either of two proteolytic pathways (Fig. 10–1) leads to a final common sequence that assembles the membrane attack complex (Fig. 10–2). The classic activation pathway—so called because it was discovered first—is triggered primarily by immune complexes formed from the union of IgG or IgM antibodies with their antigens. The alternative pathway—phylogenetically the more primitive—is activated principally by repeating polysaccharides and similar polymeric structures. Activation by either pathway generates enzymes with identical specificity: both pathways cleave the third complement component, C3, releasing the 8-kD activation peptide C3a and generating metastable C3b, which has a thioester bond capable of forming covalent bonds with the activating agent or adjacent cell membranes.[50, 50a] Both pathways also lead to cleavage of C5 and assembly of the membrane attack complex from the terminal sequence (C5b-9).

Classic Activation Pathway. C1 exists in serum as a calcium-dependent complex of one molecule of C1q with two molecules of C1r and C1s. The C1q molecule bears six globular heads that are recognition units for sites on the Fc portions of immunoglobulins

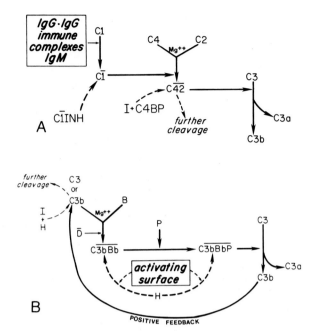

Figure 10–1. Pathways for complement activation. *A*, Classical pathway. *B*, Alternative pathway.

and probably for other activators of the classic pathway, including lipopolysaccharide and porins from gram-negative bacteria as well as ligand-bound C-reactive protein.[51] The binding of two or more recognition heads of C1q to an activator induces a rearrangement in C1r, converting it to an active protease that cleaves both itself and C1s. The natural substrates of the active $\overline{C1s}$ protease are C4 and C2. Both are cleaved, releasing activation peptides, with the major fragments being incorporated into a magnesium-dependent enzyme complex, $C\overline{4b2b}$, the classic pathway C3 convertase. Like C3, C4 also contains a labile thioester bond; C4b is metastable and capable of forming covalent amide or ester bonds with cell surface proteins or carbohydrates. Normal serum contains an α_2-neuraminoglycoprotein member of the SERPIN family, the C1 inhibitor, that complexes with both $\overline{C1s}$ and $\overline{C1r}$, irreversibly blocking the activities

of these proteases, thereby preventing the activation of C1s or the cleavage of C4 and C2. Formation of the classic pathway convertase is also inhibited by proteins that bind to C4b and inhibit the binding of C2b. These include C4 binding protein (C4BP), complement receptor 1 (CR1), and decay-accelerating factor (DAF).[52] C4BP and CR1 also act as cofactors for factor I, which further cleaves C4b into two inactive fragments, C4c and C4d.

Alternative Activation Pathway. Activation of this pathway does not require antibody and is triggered by polysaccharides such as those found in the coats of yeasts, pneumococci, and many gram-negative bacteria. This leads to cleavage of C3 and assembly of the membrane attack complex (MAC) by a mechanism that is independent of the classic pathway.[53] In a reaction that is strikingly similar to that of the classic pathway, four factors participate in the formation of the alternative pathway convertase.[54] Factor $\overline{D}$, C3, and factor B are the homologous proteins for C1s, C4, and C2, respectively. An extra protein, properdin,[54a] serves to stabilize the magnesium-dependent complex enzyme C3 convertase, $C\overline{3bBb}$, which is identical to $C\overline{4b2b}$ in its capacity to cleave C3 and C5 and to initiate the terminal sequence. Just as cleavage of C4 to C4b reveals a site for interaction with C2, cleavage of C3 to C3b permits its participation in a complex with factor B. Cleavage of C3b-bound B by $\overline{D}$ yields $C\overline{3bBb}$. Unlike C1, factor $\overline{D}$ already exists in plasma in its active form. Control of proteolysis is limited by the availability of substrate: $\overline{D}$ acts only on B that has complexed with C3b and not on free or unbound B. A positive feedback, or amplification, loop is built into the alternative pathway. C3b, the product of the cleavage reaction catalyzed by $C\overline{3bBb}$, is itself capable of complexing with additional B, rendering it susceptible to cleavage by $\overline{D}$, thereby producing additional $C\overline{3bBb}$. Uncontrolled cycling of this loop is prevented by the following reactions: (1) CR1, DAF, and factor H dissociate the $C\overline{3bBb}$ complex, rendering it inactive,[55–57] and (2) factor I further degrades C3b in the presence of CR1, methyl-accepting chemotaxis protein (MCP), or factor H, yielding C3c and C3dg.[58] Agents that trigger the alternative pathway do so by protecting newly formed $C\overline{3bBb}$ from dissociation and degradation by the control proteins. These agents increase the formation of the alternative pathway convertase by transforming an inefficient fluid-phase reaction into fruitful solid-state assembly of the enzyme complex. In the fluid phase, a small amount of C3 is continuously being hydrolyzed at its internal thioester bond, inducing a conformational change in C3 permitting B to complex with it and become susceptible to cleavage by $\overline{D}$. This reaction generates small amounts of C3 convertase and produces small amounts of C3b equivalents.[59] If C3b binds to the surface of host cells, regulatory mechanisms involving factor H, CR1, and MCP prevent further activation. Binding of C3b to foreign activators provides a haven on which the small amount of C3b produced by the fluid-phase

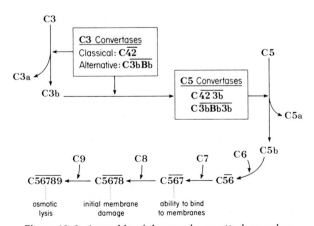

Figure 10–2. Assembly of the membrane attack complex.

Table 10–4. PROTEINS OF THE COMPLEMENT SYSTEM

Complement System and Components	Mol. Wt. (kD)	Mean Serum Conc. (μg/ml)	Cleavage Fragments
Classic activation pathway			
C1q	410	70	
C1r	83	35	
C1s	83	35	
C4	209	430	C4a, C4b, C4c, C4d
C2	110	25	C2a, C2b
Alternative activation pathway			
Properdin	220	25	
D	23	2	
B	93	250	Bb, Ba
C3	195	1300	C3a, C3b, C3c, C3d, C3g
Terminal sequence			
C5	190	75	C5a, C5b
C6	128	60	
C7	121	55	
C8	153	80	
C9	79	160	
Plasma control proteins			
C1 inhibitor	105	200	
C4 binding protein	550	250	
Factor H	150	360	
Factor I	88	35	
Anaphylatoxin inactivator	310	40	
S-protein (vitronectin)	83	500	
Membrane control proteins			
Complement receptor 1 (CD35)	190–280		
Membrane cofactor protein (MCP)	45–70		
Decay-accelerating factor (DAF)	70		
Homologous restriction factor	65		
Membrane inhibitor of reactive lysis (CD59)	18		

reactions can be deposited and protected from the action of control proteins, thereby shifting the slow fluid-phase reaction to an accelerated solid-state cleavage.

Terminal Sequence. The terminal sequence leads to formation of the MAC and damage to cell membranes.[60, 61] Binding of C3b to C$\overline{4b2b}$ forms a trimolecular complex that efficiently cleaves C5; binding of a second C3b molecule to C$\overline{3bBb}$ has the same effect. The products of cleavage of C5 by either the classic or the alternative pathway convertases are the 11-kilodalton (kD) activation peptide, C5a, and the remainder of the molecule, C5b. Activated C5b has a specific metastable binding site for C6 and combines with it to form C$\overline{5b6}$, which reacts with C7. Binding of the nascent complex of C$\overline{5b67}$ to cell membranes is the first step in assembling the MAC. The complex formed by components up through C8, C5b-8, is capable of membrane damage, but formation of a stable transmembrane channel requires the binding of multiple molecules of C9 that polymerize to form the mature MAC. The C5b-C9 complex is inserted through the lipid bilayer of the cell membrane, with hydrophobic residues on the exterior in contact with the lipid bilayer, leading to osmotic lysis of the cell. The precise mechanism by which the MAC mediates cytotoxicity remains unresolved.[62, 63] C9 is homologous in both amino acid sequence and function to perforin, the pore-forming protein of cytotoxic T lymphocytes. Action of the MAC is regulated by the glycolipid-anchored membrane proteins homologous restriction factor and membrane inhibitor of reactive lysis (CD59).[64] Both of these proteins function most efficiently on MACs formed from plasma proteins of the same species as the cells on which they are located, and protect host cells from lysis as innocent bystanders during complement activation. Vitronectin, or S-protein, which prevents the insertion of the C$\overline{5b67}$ complex into the lipid bilayer of cell membranes, probably also protects host cells from lysis.

BIOLOGIC CONSEQUENCES OF COMPLEMENT ACTIVATION

Although assembly of the C5b-9 complex and membrane damage is the most notorious effect of complement activation, a variety of other inflammatory events also ensue (Table 10–5). They include changes in vascular permeability that have been associated with the cleavage of C4 and C2 by C1 and may explain the pathogenesis of the angioedema associated with C1 inhibitor (INH) deficiency in hereditary angioedema.[49] The active enzyme C$\overline{3bBb}$ is chemotactic for polymorphonuclear neutrophils. The Bb fragment of factor B induces peritoneal macrophages to spread and increase their surface area. The activation peptides C3a and C5a are anaphylatoxins

Table 10–5. BIOLOGIC ACTIVITIES OF COMPLEMENT ACTIVATION

Product	Activity
C4, C2 kinin	Increase in vascular permeability; putative mediator of edema in hereditary angioedema
C3bBb	Chemotaxis of polymorphonuclear leukocytes
Bb	Spreading of monocytes
C3a	Anaphylatoxin: releases histamine from basophils and mast cells, serotonin from platelets; contracts smooth muscle
C5a	Anaphylatoxin: same activities as C3a on mast cells; marked chemotactic effect for monocytes and polymorphonuclear leukocytes
C5b-C9	Membrane attack complex: forms transmembrane channels leading to cytolysis

capable of inducing the secretion of histamine by mast cells and basophils. The degranulating effects on skin mast cells are observable at concentrations of 10^{-12} and 10^{-15} mol per L for C3a and C5a, respectively.[65] Both peptides also possess smooth muscle contractile activity that is independent of histamine release. The anaphylatoxic activities are blocked by scission of the terminal arginine from either C3a or C5a by carboxypeptidase N, a magnesium-dependent enzyme, that also has been termed the anaphylatoxin inactivator. C5a is responsible for most of the chemotactic activity in plasma after activation of the complement system. It attracts neutrophils, eosinophils, and monocytes and also releases lysosomal enzymes from polymorphonuclear neutrophils into phagocytic vacuoles or the surrounding medium. C3a does not appear to have chemotactic activity, but C3e, a polypeptide derived from the α-chain of C3, produces an initial leukopenia followed by a leukocytosis. C3e also causes release of leukocytes from the perfused rat femur and has been termed leukocyte-mobilizing factor.

The biologic activities of C3b and its degradation products iC3b and C3dg are governed by the types of cells bearing the receptors to which they bind (Table 10–6).[47] In addition to its function as a regulator of complement activation mentioned earlier, CR1 on the membranes of erythrocytes promotes the clearance of immune complexes by binding and transporting them to the liver and spleen, where they are removed from the circulation.[49, 66] CR1 on polymorphonuclear neutrophils and monocytes enhances the phagocytosis of C3b-coated particles by these cells. Recombinant soluble CR1, lacking transmembrane and cytoplasmic domains, inhibits both alternative and classic pathway activation and reduces tissue injury in the rat model of reperfusion injury to ischemic myocardium.[67, 67a] CR2, the receptor for C3d and C3dg, is present on B lymphocytes in a membrane complex that also contains CD19, a member of the immunoglobulin superfamily, as well as three other proteins of 130, 50, and 20 kD. Interaction of this complex with polymeric C3dg results in transmembrane signaling and priming of the cells for proliferation induced by anti-IgM.[68] The Epstein-Barr virus binds to the same domains of CR2 as do C3d and C3dg and achieves infection of cells via this route.[69] CR3, a member of the integrin family of adhesion molecules, specifically binds iC3b to polymorphonuclear neutrophils and monocytes and promotes the phagocytosis of iC3b-coated particles by these cells.[70] CR3 also promotes the attachment of polymorphonuclear neutrophils and monocytes to endothelium via direct interaction that does not involve complement proteins.

COMPLEMENT SYNTHESIS AND METABOLISM

Although in vitro culture studies have detected synthesis of many complement proteins by monocytes and macrophages,[71] the liver is the primary source of synthesis in vivo. Patients with severe hepatic failure have marked depressions in the levels of C4 and C3 in serum, and impaired synthesis of

Table 10–6. C3/C4 RECEPTORS

Receptor	Molecular Structure	Ligand	Cell Type	Function
CR1 (CD35)	190–280 kD Variable number of tandem short consensus repeats (SCR)	C3b C4b iC3b	Erythrocyte Neutrophils Monocytes B lymphocytes T lymphocytes Follicular dendritic cells	Immune complex clearance Enhanced phagocytosis Immune complex binding Antigen localization
CR2 (CD21)	145 kD, 15 SCR	iC3b (C3dg, C3d) EB virus	B lymphocytes Follicular dendritic cells	B cell activation (part of CD 19 complex) Antigen localization, lymphocyte memory Mediates viral infection
CR3 (CD11b/CD18)	α:150 β:95 Member of integrin family	iC3b	Neutrophils Monocytes	Enhanced phagocytosis Adhesion to endothelium

C3 has been measured directly in metabolic turnover studies.

Measurements of the fractional catabolic rates of C4, C3, C5, and factor B indicate that complement proteins are among the most rapidly metabolized of all plasma proteins.[72] The mean fractional catabolic rates in normal individuals are in the range of 50 percent of the plasma pool per 24 hours. Synthetic rates are significantly correlated with levels in serum, indicating that in normal individuals, the rate of synthesis is the major determinant of concentration in plasma. Levels in plasma reflect the balance between catabolism and synthesis. Increased synthetic rates induced by an inflammatory condition may produce elevated levels of complement proteins. When the disease progresses to a state in which increased utilization of complement proteins is occurring, levels may then fall into the normal range. For this reason, serial determinations of levels in an individual patient are often much more informative than measurements at isolated times.

With the exception of properdin, which is X linked, the synthesis of complement proteins is encoded by genes inherited in an autosomal codominant fashion (see Chapter 77).[73] Congenital deficiency is the consequence of inheritance of a null gene, which codes for nonsynthesis of the protein and is allelic with the normal structural gene. Inheritance of C4 is complicated by the existence of two adjacent loci, C4A and C4B,[74] which are separated by about 10 kilobases of DNA. At both of these loci, null (Q0) alleles are common, and levels in serum roughly correspond to the number of expressed C4 genes. Individuals homozygous for null alleles in both loci (C4AQ0,BQ0/C4AQ0,BQ0) are rare, but those with one, two, or three null alleles and levels in serum equal to three fourths, one half, or one fourth of the normal mean occur more frequently. The C4 genes are located on the sixth chromosome, in the region of the major histocompatibility complex, between the HLA-D/DR and HLA-B loci. The genes are about 30 kilobases downstream from the genes for C2 and factor B, the homologous proteins of the classic and alternative pathways, which are separated from each other by less than 2 kilobases.[75, 76]

The relatively high frequency of null alleles coding for nonsynthesis of complement proteins leads to wide variations in "normal" levels. Individuals who inherit a null allele at one of the two C4 loci, and who therefore have approximately 75 percent of the normal mean, are indistinguishable from those who have four fully functional genes. Even those who are heterozygous null at both loci and would be expected to have a level in plasma that was 50 percent of normal are often difficult to identify. The result is a very broad range of normal in the population. For most complement proteins the normal range is approximately ±50 percent of the normal mean. The very large normal range probably also reflects the fact that most complement proteins are "acute phase reactants," members of a class of proteins whose synthesis is increased in response to interleukin-1 (IL-1), IL-6, and tumor necrosis factor.

COMPLEMENT MEASUREMENT

Hemolytic Complement Assays. The total hemolytic complement assay (CH_{50} assay) is the traditional method for the determination of complement in serum or other body fluid.[77] It measures the ability of the test sample to lyse 50 percent of a standard suspension of sheep erythrocytes (E) coated with optimal amounts of rabbit antibody in a reaction that includes the entire classic activation pathway as well as the terminal sequence. The CH_{50} is a useful screening procedure for detecting homozygous deficiency of a complement protein but does not reliably detect heterozygous deficiency states. Specific hemolytic assays for each of the classic and alternative pathways and the terminal sequence are available, but their difficulty of performance has restricted them to the research laboratory. Because complement activity is heat labile, considerable care is required in proper collection and handling of specimens to preserve this activity. The inability to provide such care in many clinical situations limits the usefulness of complement activity measurements.

Immunoassays. Antibodies specific for each of the complement proteins are available, so that the concentrations of individual components may be measured by radial immunodiffusion or nephelometry. The most widely available clinically are assays for C4 and C3. Immunoassays measure the complement protein as antigen, without regard to whether or not it is active, so that special handling or processing of plasma samples is not required. Excepting certain kindreds with hereditary angioedema, in which the synthesis of nonfunctional but antigenically intact C1 inhibitor is inherited, the difference between the results of functional and immunochemical determinations in plasma is not clinically important. Functionally inactive products of the component sequence are cleared very rapidly from the plasma, so that participation of a component in an in vivo reaction is usually reflected by depressed levels in serum as measured by either functional or antigenic assays. In the case of closed body spaces such as the synovial, pleural, pericardial, and subarachnoid spaces, clearance of spent complement protein proceeds at a much slower rate, so that considerable divergence between the results of functional assays and immunoassays may be observed.

Detection of Activation or Cleavage Products. The limited proteolytic reactions of the complement system give rise to a number of activation peptides or degradation fragments. For example, the anaphylatoxins C4a, C3a, and C5a are N-terminal peptides liberated from C4, C3, and C5. In the alternative pathway, the fragment Ba is released from factor B when it is cleaved by factor D. Degradation of C4b by factor I in the presence of C4BP produces C4c and

C4d. Similarly, degradation of C3b by factor I in the presence of factor H, CR1, or MCP yields C3c and C3dg. Detection of such reaction products, whose concentrations in plasma or interstitial fluids are normally close to zero, often provides a more sensitive index of complement activation during disease than a fall in the concentration of a particular component in plasma.[78]

Sensitive and reproducible methods for the detection of nanogram quantities of the anaphylatoxin peptides (C3a, C4a, and C5a) have been developed. The plasma of patients undergoing extracorporeal circulation transiently contains elevated levels of C5a, which are temporally associated with the leukopenia and depressed partial pressure of oxygen (PO_2) observed during the initiation of this procedure.[79] Synovial fluid samples from patients with RA or gout have markedly increased levels of C3a, whereas the level of C5a is within normal limits.[80] Measurement of C3a is a more sensitive index of in vivo complement activation than is C5a because the latter peptide is avidly bound to receptors on leukocytes and is thereby rapidly cleared from the circulation.

Antibodies to neoantigens that arise during the formation of the MAC have been used to measure concentrations of C5b-9 (or more correctly SC5b-9, since the S-protein is present in the spent serum complex) in plasma and other biologic fluids. Patients with clinically active SLE have elevated plasma levels of C5b-9.[80a] Levels are increased in synovial fluid from patients with RA.[81] Cerebrospinal levels of SC5b-9 are increased in autoimmune neurologic diseases, such as multiple sclerosis and lupus cerebritis. Considering that increased levels of activation or cleavage products are indicative of complement activation during a disease, they are unlikely to be specific for any particular disease.

CLINICAL SIGNIFICANCE

Increases in Complement Levels. Elevations in complement levels occur frequently. They are due to increased synthesis and occur as part of the acute-phase response.[82] Characteristic changes are also observed in the levels of other plasma proteins, most notably increases in C-reactive protein, serum amyloid A protein, α_1-acid glycoprotein, and haptoglobin and decreases in transferrin and albumin levels. Elevations in levels of total hemolytic activity, C3, and C4 in plasma occur regularly in the active phase of virtually all rheumatic diseases, including RA, SLE, dermatopolymyositis, scleroderma, rheumatic fever, ankylosing spondylitis, and temporal arthritis. In these diseases, elevated levels are frequent, so that a level at the lower limit of normal may be inappropriate and indicate in vivo complement activation. Other conditions in which elevated levels have been observed include acute viral hepatitis, myocardial infarction, cancer, diabetes, pregnancy, sarcoidosis, amyloidosis, thyroiditis, inflammatory

Table 10–7. HYPOCOMPLEMENTEMIC STATES

Hyposynthesis
  Congenital deficiencies (see Chapter 75)
  Severe hepatic failure
  Severe malnutrition
  Glomerulonephritis*
  Systemic lupus erythematosus*

Hypercatabolism
  Deficiency of control proteins
    C1 inhibitor deficiency: hereditary angioedema
    C3b inactivator deficiency
    Factor H deficiency
  Rheumatic diseases with immune complexes
    Systemic lupus erythematosus
    Rheumatoid arthritis (with extra-articular disease)
    Systemic vasculitis
    Essential mixed cryoglobulinemia
  Infectious diseases
    Subacute bacterial endocarditis
    Infected atrioventricular shunts
    Pneumococcal sepsis
    Gram-negative sepsis
    Viremias, e.g., hepatitis B surface antigenemia, measles, dengue
    Parasitemias, e.g., trypanosomiasis, malaria, babesiosis
  Glomerulonephritis
    Post-streptococcal
    Membranoproliferative
    Idiopathic proliferative or focal sclerosing

*Usually associated with simultaneous and marked hypercatabolism.

bowel disease, typhoid fever, and pneumococcal pneumonia. The magnitude of the increase in the level of complement protein rarely exceeds twofold, compared with increases as high as 100- to 1000-fold with C-reactive protein.

Decreased Concentrations due to Hypercatabolism. Any disease associated with circulating immune complexes is likely to lead to acquired hypocomplementemia (Table 10–7), including SLE, RA, subacute bacterial endocarditis, hepatitis B surface antigenemia, pneumococcal infection, gram-negative sepsis, viremias such as measles, or recurrent parasitemias such as malaria. Essential mixed cryoglobulinemia, a disease characterized by arthritis or arthralgias, cutaneous vasculitis, and nephritis, is invariably accompanied by profound hypocomplementemia owing to classic pathway activation by the immune complexes that occur in this disease.

Systemic Lupus Erythematosus. Total hemolytic complement levels are depressed at some time in most patients with SLE,[36] whereas levels are generally normal in patients with discoid lupus. As a rule, depressions of complement levels are associated with increased severity of disease, especially renal disease. Component analyses have demonstrated low levels of C1, C4, C2, and C3. Serial observations often reveal decreased levels preceding clinical exacerbations; reductions in C4 occur before reductions of C3, other components, and total hemolytic complement activity. As attacks subside, levels return toward normal in the reverse order, with levels of C4 tending to remain depressed longer, even when the patient appears to be doing well clinically. The clinical usefulness of monitoring complement levels in patients with systemic lupus is controversial. Opinions range from those recommending complement measurements enthusiastically to those who find no value in these tests. Authors of studies with more detailed clinical characterizations of patients and longer follow-ups tend to conclude that complement determinations are useful adjuncts in the management of patients with known SLE and that they are useful tools in the diagnosis of this disease. The hemolytic activity of C4 in cerebrospinal fluid is labile, and measurements are not helpful in the diagnosis of central nervous system lupus unless base-line levels, determined while the patient has no central nervous system involvement, are available. Levels of complement in synovial fluid are usually profoundly depressed in patients with SLE.

Rheumatoid Arthritis. Levels of total hemolytic complement activity, C3, and C4 in serum are usually normal or elevated in patients with RA. Depressed levels are associated with extra-articular manifestations of the disease, particularly vasculitis. Such patients usually also have a high titer of RF in their serum, circulating immune complexes that are detectable by C1q-binding assays, and often small amounts of antinuclear antibody. Levels of complement in synovial fluid are low in patients with RA when the levels are measured by activity determination, and depression of the level of total hemolytic complement activity, C4, or C2 is most frequently found in patients with positive test results for RF. Levels of complement component protein measured in synovial fluid by radial immunodiffusion are usually normal, owing to the presence of antigenically intact but functionally inactive complement fragments that have not been cleared from the joint space. Cleavage fragments of C3 in synovial fluid include C3c and C3d, high proportions of C3d in relation to total C3, electrophoretically converted forms of C3, and increased C3a, Bb, and C5b-9 by radioimmunoassay. The clinical significance of complement measurements in synovial fluid is marginal. The only functional assay widely available is the assay for total hemolytic complement activity, and it is by no means uniformly subnormal in cases of RA, nor is the finding of a depressed level unique to RA. The abundant evidence for intra-articular activation of the complement system in RA is helpful in understanding the pathogenesis of the disease process, but it is rarely of value as a discriminating diagnostic test.

References

1. Williams, R. C. J.: Immune Complexes in Clinical and Experimental Medicine. Cambridge, Harvard University Press, 1980.
2. Theofilopoulos, A. N., and Dixon, F. J.: The biology and detection of immune complexes. Adv. Immunol. 28:89, 1979.
3. Schifferli, J. A., Ng, Y. C., and Peters, D. K.: The role of complement and its receptor in the elimination of immune complexes. N. Engl. J. Med. 315:488, 1986.
4. Von Pirquet, C. E.: Allergy. Arch. Intern. Med. 7:259, 1911.
5. Germuth,, F. G. J.: A comparative histologic and immunologic study in rabbits of induced hypersensitivity of the serum sickness type. J. Exp. Med. 97:257, 1953.
6. Dixon, F. J., Vazquez, J. J., Weigle, W. O., and Cochrane, C. G.: Pathogenesis of serum sickness. A. M. A. Arch. Pathol. 65:18, 1958.
7. McDougal, J. S., Hubbard, M., Strobel, P. L., and McDuffie, F. C.: Comparison of five assays for immune complexes in the rheumatic diseases: Performance characteristics of the assays. J. Lab. Clin. Med. 100:705, 1982.
8. Nydegger, U. E., and Svehag, S. E.: Improved standardization in the quantitative estimation of soluble immune complexes making use of an international reference preparation. Results of a collaborative multi-centre study. Clin. Exp. Immunol. 58:502, 1984.
9. McDougal, J. S., Hubbard, M., McDuffie, F. C., et al.: Comparison of five assays for immune complexes in the rheumatic diseases: An assessment of their validity for rheumatoid arthritis. Arthritis Rheum. 25:1156, 1982.
9a. McDougal, J. S., and McDuffie, F. C.: Immune complexes in man: detection and clinical significance. Adv. Clin. Chem. 25:1, 1991.
10. Reynolds, W. J., Yoon, S. J., Emin, M., Chapman, K. R., and Klein, M. H.: Circulating immune complexes in rheumatoid arthritis: A prospective study using five immunoassays. J. Rheumatol. 13:700, 1986.
11. Roberts-Thomson, R. J., Neoh, S. H., Bradley, J., and Milazzo, S. C.: Circulating and intra-articular immune complexes in rheumatoid arthritis: A comparative study of the C1q binding and monoclonal rheumatoid factor assays. Ann. Rheum. Dis. 39:438, 1980.
12. Abrass, C. K., Nies, K. M., Louie, J. S., Border, W. A., and Glassock, R. J.: Correlation and predictive accuracy of circulating immune complexes with disease activity in patients with systemic lupus erythematosus. Arthritis Rheum. 23:273, 1980.
13. Valenzuela, R., Bergfeld, W. F., and Deodhar, S. D.: Interpretation of Immunofluorescent Patterns in Skin Diseases. Chicago, American Society of Clinical Pathologists Press, 1984, p. 66.
14. Wener, M. H., Mannik, M., Schwartz, M. M., and Lewis, E. J.: Relationship between renal pathology and the size of circulating immune complexes in patients with systemic lupus erythematosus. Medicine 66:85, 1987.
15. Huston, K. A., Gupta, R. C., Donadio, J. V. J., McDuffie, F. C., and Ilstrup, D. M.: Circulating immune complexes in systemic lupus erythematosus: Association with other immunologic abnormalities but not with changes in renal function. J. Rheumatol. 5:423, 1978.
16. Andrews, B. S., Ascher, M. S., Barada, F. A. J., and Davis, J. S.: The Raji cell radioimmunoassay in patients with systemic lupus erythematosus: Clinical significance and relationships to other serologic variables assessed by discriminant analysis. J. Rheumatol. 12:718, 1985.
17. Mackel, S. E., Tappeiner, G., Brumfield, H., and Jordon, R. E.: Circulating immune complexes in cutaneous vasculitis: Detection with C1q and monoclonal rheumatoid factor. J. Clin. Invest. 64:1652, 1979.
18. Seibold, J. R., Medsger, J. A. J., Winkelstein, A., Kelly, R. H., and Rodnan, G. P.: Immune complexes in progressive systemic sclerosis (scleroderma). Arthritis Rheum. 25:1167, 1982.
19. Siminovitch, K., Klein, M., Pruzanski, W., et al.: Circulating immune complexes in patients with progressive systemic sclerosis. Arthritis Rheum. 25:1174, 1982.
20. Nydegger, U. E., Zubler, R. H., Gabay, R., et al.: Circulating complement breakdown products in patients with rheumatoid arthritis: Correlation between plasma C3d, circulating immune complexes, and clinical activity. J. Clin. Invest. 59:862, 1977.
21. Halla, J. T., Volonakis, J. E., and Schroenloher, R. E.: Immune complexes in rheumatoid arthritis sera and synovial fluids. Arthritis Rheum. 22:440, 1979.
22. Westedt, M. L., Daha, M. R., Baldwin, W. M. I., Stijnen, T., and Cats, A.: Serum immune complexes containing IgA appear to predict erosive arthritis in a longitudinal study in rheumatoid arthritis. Ann. Rheum. Dis. 45:809, 1986.
23. Reeback, J. S., Silman, A. J., Holborrow, E. J., Maini, R. N., and Hay, F. C.: Circulating immune complexes and rheumatoid arthritis: A comparison of different assay methods and their early predictive value for disease activity and outcome. Ann. Rheum. Dis. 44:79, 1985.
24. Krakauer, R. S., Wynsenbeek, A. J., Wallace, D. J., et al.: Therapeutic trial of cryofiltration in patients with rheumatoid arthritis. Am. J. Med. 74:951, 1983.
25. Forster, P. J., and McConkey, B.: The effect of antirheumatic drugs on circulating immune complexes in rheumatoid arthritis. Q. J. Med. 58(225):29, 1986.
26. Wallace, D., Goldfinger, D., Lowe, C., et al.: A double-blind, controlled study of lymphoplasmapheresis versus sham apheresis in rheumatoid arthritis. N. Engl. J. Med. 306:1406, 1982.
27. Nusslein, H. G., Herbst, M., Manger, B. J., et al.: Total lymphoid irradiation in patients with refractory rheumatoid arthritis. Arthritis Rheum. 28:1205, 1985.
28. Inman, R. D., Fong, J. K. K., Pussell, B. A., Ryan, P. J., and Hughes, G. R. V.: The C1q binding assay in systemic lupus erythematosus. Arthritis Rheum. 23:1282, 1980.

29. Hamburger, M. J., Lawley, T. J., Kimberly, R. P., Plotz, P. H., and Frank, M. M.: A serial study of splenic reticuloendothelial system Fc receptor functional activity in systemic lupus erythematosus. Arthritis Rheum. 25:48, 1982.

30. Valentijn, R. M., Van Overhagen, H., Hazevoet, H. M., et al.: The value of complement and immune complex determinations in monitoring disease activity in patients with systemic lupus erythematosus. Arthritis Rheum. 28:904, 1985.

31. Morrow, W. J. W., Isenberg, D. A., Todd-Pokropek, A., Parry, H. F., and Snaith, M. L.: Useful laboratory measurements in the management of systemic lupus erythematosus. Q. J. Med. 51:125, 1982.

32. Sturfelt, G., Johnson, U., and Sjoholm, A. G.: Sequential studies of complement activation in systemic lupus erythematosus. Scand. J. Rheumatol. 14:184, 1985.

33. Wisnieski, J. J., and Naff, G. B.: Serum IgG antibodies to C1q in hypocomplementemic urticarial vasculitis syndrome. Arthritis Rheum. 32:1119, 1989.

34. Siegert, C. E. H., Daha, M. R., van der Voort, E. A. M., and Breedvelt, F. C.: IgG and IgA antibodies to the collagen-like region of C1q in rheumatoid vasculitis. Arthritis Rheum. 33:1646, 1990.

35. Pussell, B. A., Lockwood, C. M., Scott, D. M., Pinching, A. J., and Peters, D. K.: Value of immune-complex assays in diagnosis and management. Lancet 2:359, 1978.

36. Lloyd, W., and Schur, P. H.: Immune complexes, complement, and anti-DNA in exacerbations of systemic lupus erythematosus (SLE). Medicine 60:208, 1981.

37. Boyd, R. D., Birchmore, D. A., Kaiser, D. L., Young, A. C., and Davis, J. S. I.: Acute effects of steroids on immune complex profile of patients with systemic lupus erythematosus. Arthritis Rheum. 26:637, 1983.

38. Huber, C., Ruger, A., Herrmann, M., Krapf, F., and Kalden, J. R.: C3-containing serum immune complexes in patients with systemic lupus erythematosus: correlation to disease activity and comparison with other rheumatic diseases. Rheumatol. Int. 9:59, 1989.

39. Ronco, P., Verroust, P., Mignon, F., et al.: Immunopathological studies of polyarteritis nodosa and Wegener's granulomatosis: A report of 43 patients with 51 renal biopsies. Q. J. Med. 52:212, 1983.

40. Papaioannou, C. C., Gupta, R. C., Hunder, G. G., and McDuffie, F. C.: Circulating immune complexes in giant cell arteritis and polymyalgia rheumatica. Arthritis Rheum. 23:1021, 1982.

41. Halla, J. T., Volanakis, J. E., and Schrohenloher, R. E.: Circulating immune complexes in mixed connective tissue disease. Arthritis Rheum. 22:484, 1979.

42. Seibold, J. R., Rodnan, G. P., Medsger, T. A. J., and Winkelstein, A.: Circulating immune complexes in eosinophilic fasciitis. Arthritis Rheum. 25:1180, 1982.

43. Espinoza, L. R., Gaylord, S. W., Bocanegra, T. S., Vasey, F. B., and Germain, B. F.: Circulating immune complexes in the seronegative spondyloarthropathies. Clin. Immunol. Immunopathol. 22:384, 1982.

44. Lawley, T. J., Moutsopoulos, H. M., Katz, S. I., Theofilopoulos, A. N., Chused, T. M., and Frank, M. M.: Demonstration of circulating immune complexes in Sjögren's syndrome. J. Immunol. 123:1382, 1979.

45. Jones, V. E., Jacoby, R. K., Wallington, T., and Holt, P.: Immune complexes in early arthritis. I. Detection of immune complexes before rheumatoid arthritis is definite. Clin. Exp. Immunol. 44:512, 1981.

46. Kinoshita, T.: Biology of complement: the overture. Immunol. Today 12:291, 1991.

47. Ross, G. D.: Complement and complement receptors. Curr. Opin. Immunol. 2:50, 1989.

48. Müller-Eberhard, H. J.: Molecular organization and function of the complement system. Annu. Rev. Biochem. 57:321, 1988.

49. Frank, M. M.: Complement in the pathophysiology of human disease. N. Engl. J. Med. 316:1525, 1987.

50. Law, S. K., and Levine, R. P.: Interaction between the third complement protein and cell surface macromolecules. Proc. Natl. Acad. Sci. U.S.A. 74:2701, 1977.

50a. Kim, Y. U., Carroll, M. C., Isenman, D. E., et al.: Covalent binding of C3b to C4b within the classical complement pathway C5 convertase. Determination of amino acid residues involved in ester linkage formation. J. Biol. Chem. 267:4171, 1992.

51. Sim, R. B., and Reid, K. B. M.: C1: molecular interactions with activating systems. Immunol. Today 12:307, 1991.

52. Farries, T. C., and Atkinson, J.: Evolution of the complement system. Immunol. Today 12:295, 1991.

53. Pillemer, L., Blum, L., Lepow, I. H., Ross, D. A., Todd, E. W., and Wardlaw, A. C.: The properdin system and immunity: I. Demonstration and isolation of a new serum protein, properdin, and its role in immune phenomena. Science 120:279, 1954.

54. Pangburn, M. K., and Muller-Eberhard, H. J.: The alternative pathway of complement. Springer Semin. Immunopathol. 7:163, 1984.

54a. Tuszynski, G. P., Rothman, V. L., Deutch, A. H., Hamilton, B. K., and Eyal, J.: Biological activities of peptides and peptide analogues derived from common sequences present in thrombospondin, properdin, and malarial proteins. J. Cell Biol. 116:209, 1992.

55. Nicholson-Weller, A., Burge, J., Fearon, D. T., Weller, P. F., and Austen, K. F.: Isolation of a human erythrocyte membrane glycoprotein with decay-accelerating activity for C3 convertases of the complement system. J. Immunol. 129:184, 1982.

56. Fearon, D. T.: Regulation of the amplification C3 convertase of human complement by an inhibitory protein isolated from human erythrocyte membrane. Proc. Natl. Acad. Sci. U.S.A. 76:5867, 1979.

57. Whaley, K., and Ruddy, S.: Modulation of C3b hemolytic activity by a plasma protein distinct from C3b inactivator. Science 193:1011, 1976.

58. Ruddy, S., and Austen, K. F.: C3b inactivator of man. II. Fragments produced by C3b inactivator cleavage of cell-bound or fluid phase C3b. J. Immunol. 107:742, 1971.

59. Lachmann, P. J., and Nicol, P.: Reaction mechanism of the alternate pathway of complement fixation. Lancet 3:465, 1973.

60. Muller-Eberhard, H. J.: The membrane attack complex of complement. Annu. Rev. Immunol. 4:503, 1986.

61. Podack, E. R.: Molecular mechanisms of cytolysis by complement and by cytolytic lymphocytes. J. Cell. Biochem. 30:133, 1986.

62. Bhakdi, S., and Tranum-Jensen, J.: Complement lysis: a hole is a hole. Immunol. Today 12:318, 1991.

63. Esser, A. F.: Big MAC attack: complement proteins cause leaky patches. Immunol. Today 12:316, 1991.

64. Lachmann, P. J.: The control of homologous lysis. Immunol. Today 12:312, 1991.

65. Hugli, T. E.: Structure and function of C3a anaphylatoxin. Curr. Top. Microbiol. Immunol. 153:181, 1989.

66. Frank, M. M., and Fries, L. F.: The role of complement in inflammation and phagocytosis. Immunol. Today 12:322, 1991.

67. Weisman, H. F., Bartow, T., Leppo, M. K., et al.: Soluble human complement receptor type 1: in vivo inhibitor of complement suppressing post-ischemic myocardial inflammation and necrosis. Science 249:146, 1990.

67a. Kalli, K. R., Hsu, P. H., Bartow, T. J., et al.: Mapping of the C3b-binding site of Cr1 and construction of a (Cr1)2-F(ab')2 chimeric complement inhibitor. J. Exp. Med. 174:1451, 1991.

68. Matsumoto, A. K., Kopicky-Burd, J., Carter, R. H., Tuveson, D. A., Tedder, T. F., and Fearon, D. T.: Intersection of the complement and immune systems: a signal transduction complex of the B lymphocyte–containing complement receptor type 2 and CD19. J. Exp. Med. 173:55, 1991.

69. Cooper, N. R.: Complement evasion strategies of microorganisms. Immunol. Today 12:327, 1991.

70. Corbi, A. L., Kishimoto, T. K., Miller, L. J., and Springer, T. A.: The human leukocyte adhesion glycoprotein Mac-1 (complement receptor type 3, CD11b) alpha subunit. Cloning, primary structure, and relation to the integrins, von Willebrand factor and factor B. J. Biol. Chem. 263:12403, 1988.

71. Lappin, D., Hamilton, A. D., Morrison, L., Aref, M., and Whaley, K.: Synthesis of complement components (C3, C2, B, and C1-inhibitor) and lysozyme by human monocytes and macrophages. J. Clin. Lab. Immunol. 20:101, 1986.

72. Ruddy, S., Carpenter, C. B., Chin, K. W., et al.: Human complement metabolism: An analysis of 144 studies. Medicine 54:165, 1975.

73. Perlmutter, D. H., and Colten, H. R.: Molecular basis of complement deficiencies. Immunodefic. Rev. 1:105, 1989.

74. Carroll, M. C.: Molecular genetics of the fourth component of human complement. Fed. Proc. 46:2457, 1987.

75. Porter, R. R.: The complement components coded in the major histocompatibility complexes and their biological activities. Immunol. Rev. 87:7, 1985.

76. Awdeh, Z. L., and Yunis, E. J.: Complotypes, extended haplotypes, male segregation distortion, and disease markers. Hum. Immunol. 15:366, 1986.

77. Schur, P. H.: Complement studies of sera and other biologic fluids. Hum. Pathol. 14:338, 1983.

78. Abramson, S. B., and Weissmann, G.: Complement split products and the pathogenesis of SLE. Hosp. Pract. 23:45, 1988.

79. Chenoweth, D. E., Cooper, S. W., Hugli, T. E., Stewart, R. W., Blackstone, E. H., and Kirklin, J. W.: Complement activation during cardiopulmonary bypass: evidence for generation of C3a and C5a anaphylatoxins. N. Engl. J. Med. 304:497, 1981.

80. Moxley, G. F., and Ruddy, S.: Elevated C3 anaphylatoxin levels in synovial fluids from patients with rheumatoid arthritis. Arthritis Rheum. 28:1089, 1985.

80a. Buyon, J. P., Tamerius, J., Ordorica, S., Young, B., and Abramson, S. B.: Activation of the alternative complement pathway accompanies disease flares in systemic lupus erythematosus during pregnancy. Arthritis Rheum. 35:55, 1992.

81. Brodeur, J. P., Ruddy, S., Schwartz, L. B., and Moxley, G. F.: Synovial fluid levels of complement SC5b-9 and fragment Bb are elevated in patients with rheumatoid arthritis. Arthritis Rheum. 34:1531, 1991.

82. Kushner, I.: C-reactive protein and the acute-phase response. Hosp. Pract. (Off.) 25:13, 16, 21, 1990.

83. Nydegger, U. E., Lambert, P. H., Gerber, H., and Miescher, P. A.: Circulating immune complexes in the serum in systemic lupus erythe-

matosus and in carriers of hepatitis B antigen: quantitation by binding to radiolabeled C1q. J. Clin. Invest. 54:297, 1974.

84. Hay, F. C., Nineham, L. J., and Roitt, I. M.: Routine assay for the detection of immune complexes of known immunoglobulin class using solid phase C1q. Clin. Exp. Immunol. 24:396, 1976.

85. Theofilopoulos, A. N., Wilson, C. B., and Dixon, F. J.: The Raji cell radioimmune assay for detecting immune complexes in human sera. J. Clin. Invest. 57:169, 1976.

86. Luthra, H. S., McDuffie, F. C., Hunder, G. G., and Samayoa, E. A.: Immune complexes in sera and synovial fluids of patients with rheumatoid arthritis: Radioimmunoassay with monoclonal rheumatoid factor. J. Clin. Invest. 56:458, 1975.

87. McDougal, J. S., Redecha, P. B., Inman, R. D., and Christian, C. L.:

Binding of immunoglobulin G aggregates and immune complexes in human sera to staphylococci containing protein A. J. Clin. Invest. 63:627, 1979.

88. Eisenberg, R. A., Theofilopoulos, A. N., Argyrios, N., and Dixon, F. J.: Use of bovine conglutinin for the assay of immune complexes. J. Immunol. 118:1428, 1977.

89. Aguado, M. T., Lambris, J. D., Tsokos, G. C., et al.: Monoclonal antibodies against complement 3 neoantigens for detection of immune complexes and complement activation. J. Clin. Invest. 76:1418, 1985.

90. Procaccia, S., Lazzarin, A., Colucci, A., et al.: IgM, IgG and IgA rheumatoid factors and circulating immune complexes in patients with AIDS and AIDS-related complex with serological abnormalities. Clin. Exp. Immunol. 67:236, 1987.

Chapter 11

Robert B. Zurier

Prostaglandins, Leukotrienes, and Related Compounds

INTRODUCTION

The oxygenation of unesterified arachidonic acid (C20:4 ω-6) and other polyunsaturated fatty acids by nearly all human cell types results in formation of several classes of bioactive products termed eicosanoids (eicosa-20). These include prostaglandins (PGs)—including prostacyclin—thromboxanes (TXs), leukotrienes (LTs), and lipoxins (LXs), which play critical roles in the regulation of immunity and inflammation, among other physiologic and pathologic processes.[1, 2] Although eicosanoids are derived from C20 polyunsaturated fatty acids, only a small percentage of these polyenoic acids, namely, dihomo-gamma (γ)-linolenic acid (DGLA), arachidonic acid (AA), and eicosapentaenoic acid (EPA), form the eicosanoids (Fig. 11–1).

Two groups of fatty acids are essential to the body: the omega-6 (ω-6) series derived from linoleic acid (18:2ω-6) and the ω-3 series derived from alpha (α)-linolenic acid (18:3ω-3). Using this notation, 18 refers to the number of carbon atoms in the fatty acid. The degree of saturation (the number of double carbon-carbon bonds) follows the number of carbon atoms. The ω refers to the number of carbon atoms from the methyl (omega) end of the fatty acid chain to the first double bond. Fatty acids are metabolized by an alternating sequence of desaturation (removal of two hydrogens) and elongation (addition of two carbons). Membrane phospholipids are the main storage site for polyunsaturated fatty acids and are particularly rich in eicosanoid precursors, which are located at the sn-2 position (Fig. 11–2). Phospholipase A_2 (PLA$_2$), in lysosomes or bound to cell membranes, catalyzes the break of the sn-2 bond, thus facilitating release of arachidonate or other polyunsaturates. The enzyme is crucial to eicosanoid synthesis regulation, since it is in the nonesterified state that the polyunsaturated precursors enter into the cascades leading to eicosanoid formation. Only a scant amount of oxidation at carbon 15 of arachidonic acid occurs catalytically when the fatty acid is still covalently bound as part of a phospholipid.[3] Furthermore, lysophospholipids "left over" after the action of PLA$_2$

are direct precursors of platelet-activating factor (PAF), a potent mediator of inflammation that is generated by acylation in the open sn-2 position of the lysophospholipid. In addition, PLC cleaves the head group (e.g., choline, inositol) from phospholipids, generating diacylglycerol from which arachidonic acid is released by a diacylglycerol lipase.

The tetraenoic precursor (arachidonic acid) is the most abundant of the three precursor fatty acids in cells of people who eat usual diets in Western culture. Metabolites of arachidonate constitute the "2" series (dienoic) prostaglandins (2 double bonds in the molecule), and the metabolic pathway has acquired the familiar name "arachidonic acid cascade." Figures 11–3 and 11–4 respectively illustrate the cyclooxygenase and 5-lipoxygenase pathways of the cascade.

CYCLOOXYGENASE PATHWAY

The first step in the pathway is a double dioxygenase or cyclooxygenase reaction combining two oxygen molecules on the polyunsaturated precursor. The cyclooxygenase from sheep vesicular glands has been cloned from a 2.7 kilobase messenger ribonucleic acid (mRNA) that codes for a 576 amino acid sequence corresponding to a molecular weight of 66,621 daltons (d)[4]; it does not have homology with any known protein. To form the characteristic five-carbon ring structure, the precursor fatty acids must have double bonds at carbons 8, 11, and 14 (numbering from the carboxyl group). When a molecule of oxygen is inserted across carbons 9 and 11, ring closure takes place enzymatically across C8 and C12, creating the unstable PG endoperoxides PGG and PGH and forming the cyclopentane ring. PGH serves as the common precursor for prostaglandins, prostacyclin, and TXs. Thus, in addition to the activity of PLs, regulation of PG synthesis also occurs at the level of PG endoperoxide synthase (PES) gene expression. PES levels are increased by interleukin-1 (IL-1), platelet-derived growth factor, and epidermal growth factor, agents that increase PG synthesis.[5]

Cell membranes constitute both the source of

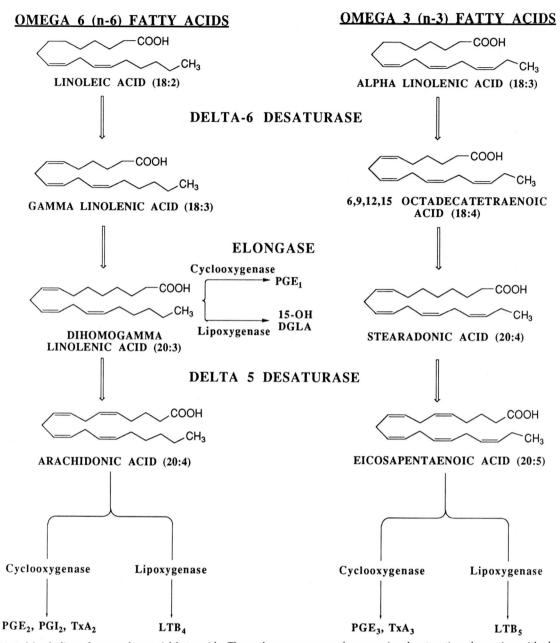

Figure 11–1. Metabolic pathways of essential fatty acids. The pathways are ones of progressive desaturation alternating with elongation. Eicosanoid precursors include dihomo-γ-linolenic acid, arachidonic acid, and eicosapentaenoic acid.

substrate arachidonate and the site of action of eicosanoid-forming enzymes. However, PG synthesis can also form at lipid bodies, non–membrane-bound lipid-rich cytoplasmic inclusions that develop in cells associated with inflammation. Lipid bodies isolated from human monocytes express PGH synthase activity.[6] Thus, lipid bodies, which are reservoirs of arachidonyl phospholipids, can function as domains of PG synthesis during an inflammatory reaction.

Prostaglandins

The basic structure of all PGs is a "prostanoic acid" skeleton, a 20-carbon fatty acid with a five-

membered ring at C8 through C12 (Fig. 11–3, inset). The term "prostaglandins" is employed widely but should be used to describe only those oxygenation products that contain the five-membered carbon ring. A family of acidic lipids found first in human seminal fluid, they were misnamed because it was thought they were produced in the prostate gland, rather than the seminal vesicles.[7–9]

The alphabetical PG nomenclature (PGE, PGF, PGD) relates to the chemical architecture of the cyclopentane ring. Thus, for example, PGE and PGF differ only in the presence of a ketone or hydroxyl function at C9 (see Fig. 11–3). These compounds are made by a variety of cells (PGE$_2$ by an isomerase, PGF$_{2\alpha}$ by a reductase), whereas PGD$_2$ appears to be

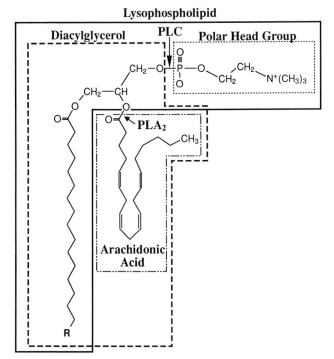

Figure 11–2. Arachidonic acid release from phospholipid. Shown here is phosphatidylcholine, the major membrane storage site for polyunsaturated fatty acids. PLA$_2$, phospholipase A$_2$; PLC, phospholipase C.

generated by an isomerase mainly in mast cells. In the nomenclature, a subscript numeral after the letters indicates the degree of unsaturation in the alkyl and carboxylic acid side chains. The numeral 1 indicates the presence of a double bond at C13-C14 (PGE$_1$), 2 marks the presence of an additional double bond at C5-C6 (PGE$_2$), and 3 denotes a third double bond at C17-C18 (PGE$_3$).

Prostaglandins are produced on demand and appear to exert their effects on the cell of origin or nearby structures. Thus, they have been termed local hormones. Although the precise role of the eicosanoids in inflammation is not clear, abundant experimental evidence supports the view that PGs participate in the development of the inflammatory response. Experimental evidence indicates that PGs are probably better at potentiating the effects of other mediators of inflammation than they are at inducing inflammation directly.[10] In addition, PGE compounds and intermediate hydroperoxides of arachidonic acid increase pain sensitivity to bradykinin and histamine. The effects of PGE are cumulative, depending on the concentration, time of exposure, or both. Therefore, even very small amounts of PGs, if allowed to persist at the site of injury, may in time cause pain. No precise pattern of prostaglandin effects on chemotaxis and chemokinesis of neutrophils has been defined. However, evidence has been presented that PGE$_2$, but not PGE$_1$, enhances markedly the chemotactic responsiveness of human monocytes to complement-activated human serum. None of the

PGs is directly chemotactic for monocytes. Mast cells, often overlooked as important in inflammatory responses, are seen in large numbers in synovium from patients early in the course of rheumatoid arthritis (RA); PGD$_2$ is the major PG formed by mast cells. There is also evidence that PGD$_2$ can mediate histamine release from mast cells exposed to anti-IgE antibody.

PGE$_2$ is the most potent stimulator of bone resorption among the PGs.[11] Its 13,14-dihydro derivative is nearly as potent, which is of interest because derivatives of the biologically active PGs are usually assumed not to be of functional significance. Addition of serum to the culture medium stimulates bone resorption, a process that is complement dependent and prostaglandin mediated. The mechanism may help explain bone erosion in joints of patients with RA, where complement is activated and PGE$_2$ concentrations are high.

Most of the effects of IL-1 on cells are associated with stimulation of PG production and inflammation.[12] The ILs belong to a group of proteins, including interferons and tumor necrosis factor (TNF), that mediates important regulatory functions among leukocytes in the immune system. The list of these "cytokines" is growing, and it is becoming increasingly evident that these proteins interact in a complex manner with eicosanoids. For example, TNF, in addition to its cytolytic and metabolic activities, stimulates a variety of cellular responses that maintain inflammation. TNF also induces production of PGE$_2$ in macrophages.[13]

Attempts to modify PG synthesis have been directed mainly at inhibition of cyclooxygenase activity by aspirin and other nonsteroidal anti-inflammatory drugs (NSAIDs). The cellular mechanisms by which glucocorticoids inhibit eicosanoid production both in vivo and in vitro are unclear. It has been reported that dexamethasone induces lipocortin I, a protein thought to inhibit phospholipase activity, resulting in a decrease in available arachidonate and subsequent eicosanoid production. However, other reports indicate that lipocortin does not inhibit cellular phospholipase activity, nor do glucocorticoids induce mRNA for lipocortin I in cells known to respond to dexamethasone. However, steroids do suppress cyclooxygenase mRNA levels and PG synthesis in cultured endothelial cells and studies in vitro and in vivo indicate that dexamethasone reduces induction of cyclooxygenase mass via production of new protein.[14]

Prostacyclin

Prostacyclin, discovered in 1976,[15] is a major member of the family of prostaglandins produced by endothelial cells. It is generated from PGH$_2$ by a distinct prostacyclin synthase, distribution of which appears to be more restrictive than the PG endoperoxide isomerases and reductases. Production of pros-

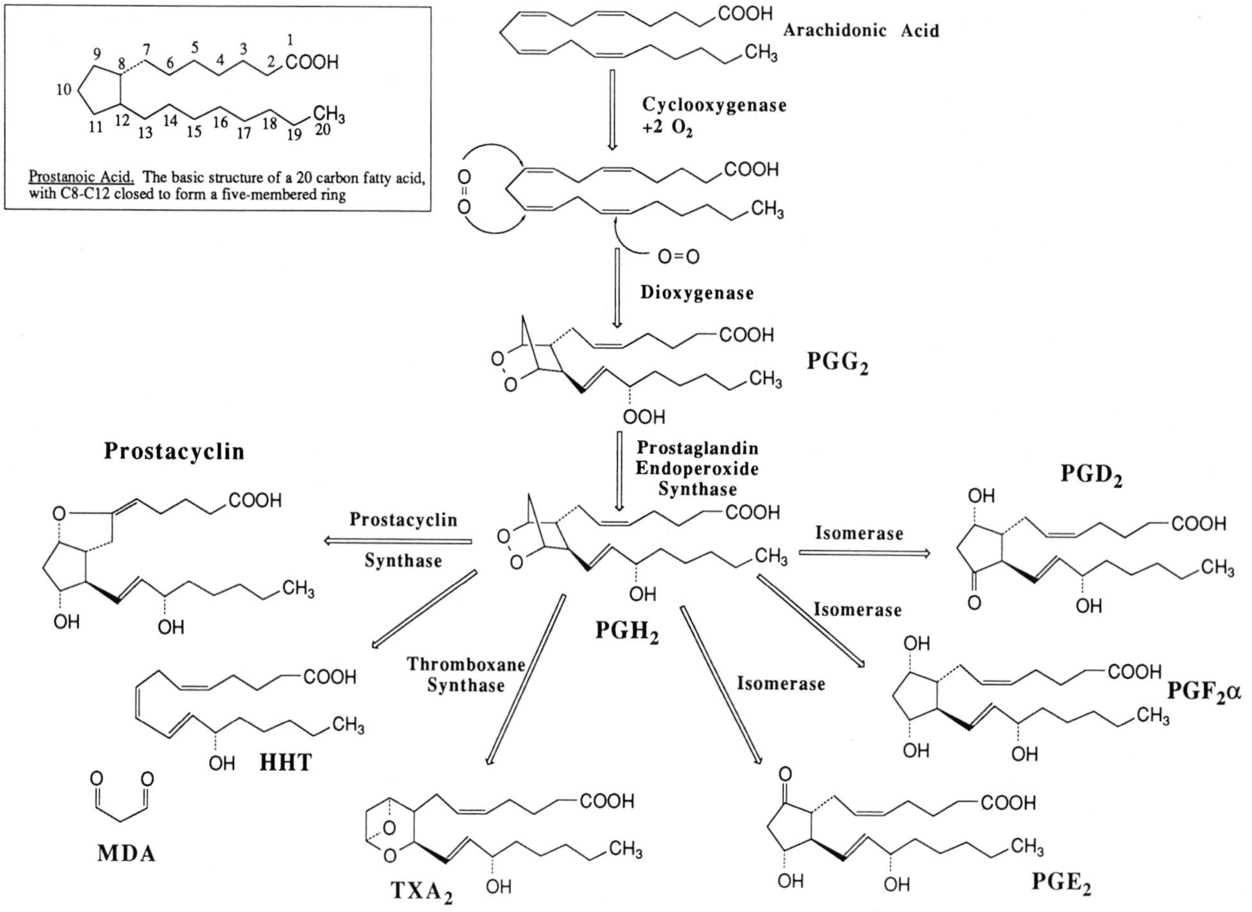

Figure 11–3. Cyclooxygenase pathway of arachidonic acid metabolism.

tacyclin can be stimulated by thrombin or generated by transfer of PGH₂ from platelets ("the endoperoxide steal"), contact with activated leukocytes, or stretching of the arterial wall. It is a powerful vasodilator and inhibits platelet aggregation through activation of adenylate cyclase, which leads to an increase in intracellular cyclic adenosine monophosphate (cAMP). It is metabolized rapidly (half-life in plasma is less than one circulation time) to the more stable, less biologically active 6-ketoprostaglandin $F_{1\alpha}$. The enzymatic products of its conversion (2,3-dinor-6-keto-$PGF_{1\alpha}$ and 6,15-diketo-2,3-dinor-$PGF_{1\alpha}$) are also chemically stable and have very little biologic activity. They are the major metabolites of prostacyclin excreted in urine, in which they can be assayed as indicators of prostacyclin generation.[16]

Prostacyclin generated in the vessel wall has antiplatelet and vasodilator actions, whereas thromboxane A_2, generated by platelets from the same precursors, induces platelet aggregation and vasoconstriction.[17] Thus, these two eicosanoids represent biologically opposite poles of a mechanism for regulating the interaction between platelets and the vessel wall and, therefore, formation of hemostatic plugs and intra-arterial thrombi. Given the central role of platelets in inflammatory reactions,[18] it is clear that an appropriate prostacyclin-thromboxane balance is

important to regulation of inflammation. The balance may be altered in patients with the antiphospholipid antibody syndrome. For example, serum and its IgG component from patients with the "lupus anticoagulant" inhibits prostacyclin production by aortic sections in tissue culture.

Endotoxin-mediated lung injury depends on neutrophil and platelet activation as well as activation of the clotting system and fibrin deposition. Prevention of lung tissue injury by prostacyclin infusion is associated with increased numbers of circulating platelets and a decrease in fibrin degradation products. Intravascular infusion of prostacyclin also reduces some of the clinical changes associated with pulmonary embolism. The instability of prostacyclin makes it cumbersome to administer therapeutically. Nonetheless, it has been used with limited success to treat peripheral vascular disease, including Raynaud's phenomenon. Infusions of stable analogues of PGI_2 are being studied, and orally active analogues are nearing clinical use.[16]

Thromboxanes

The endoperoxide PGH₂ can also be converted into TXs following the action of the enzyme TX synthase, which is quite active in the platelet. This microsomal enzyme has been purified from bovine and human platelets[19]; it converts PGH_2 into equal amounts of TXA_2 and 12-L-hydroxy-5,8,10-heptadecatrienoic acid (HHT). TXA_2 stimulates platelet activation, contributes to intravascular aggregation of platelets, and contracts arteriolar and bronchiolar smooth muscles. It is hydrolyzed rapidly (half-life = 30 sec) to the inactive product, TXB_2; thus, its actions are limited to the microenvironment of its release.

The extraordinary rapidity with which platelets adhere to damaged tissue, aggregate, and release potent biologically active materials suggests that the platelet is well suited to be a cellular trigger for the inflammatory process.[18] Thus, efforts directed at suppression of TX synthesis and platelet aggregation may result in limitation of inflammatory responses. Inhibition of platelet aggregation may be important to the anti-inflammatory effects of aspirin and other NSAIDs. Long-term administration of low doses of aspirin (40 mg per day)—the lowest dose predicted to cause total inhibition of TX formation in serum, according to mathematical modeling—has inhibitory effects on platelet function ex vivo that are indistinguishable from those caused by giving 325 mg per day of aspirin. Even low-dose aspirin, however, has some depressive effect on prostacyclin synthesis. Important in this regard is that recovery of vascular prostacyclin production may be more difficult to attain in elderly patients.[20]

Selective inhibition of TX synthase represents an approach that might be effected without depressing prostacyclin formation. The endoperoxide steal appears to function in vivo after administration of a TX synthase inhibitor. Antagonists of the receptors shared by endoperoxide and TXA_2 have been developed, and preliminary studies indicate these agents inhibit platelet aggregation in patients recalcitrant to TX synthase inhibition.[20]

LIPOXYGENASE PATHWAYS

In contrast with the cyclooxygenase pathway, where stable products have 3 atoms of oxygen covalently attached to arachidonic acid from 2 mol of molecular oxygen, lipoxygenases insert a single oxygen atom into the molecular structure of arachidonic acid. Separate lipoxygenases exist in certain cells and have strict structural requirements for their substrates; three major mammalian lipoxygenases exist that insert their oxygen atoms into the 5, 12, or 15 position of arachidonic acid with formation of a new double bond and hydroperoxy group. The hydroperoxy fatty acids (HPETE) can be reduced by peroxidases in the cell to yield the corresponding hydroxy fatty acids (HETE). For example, the exclusive lipoxygenase product of the human platelet is 12(S) hydroperoxyeicosatetraenoic acid (12-HPETE), which on reduction of the hydroperoxy group yields 12 hydroxyeicosatetraenoic acid (12-HETE). In contrast,

the human neutrophil makes predominantly 5-HPETE, but when high concentrations of arachidonate are added, 15-lipoxygenase can be demonstrated. Lipoxygenases that act on arachidonic acid are found in the cytosol fraction of cells. The human 5-lipoxygenase gene has been isolated and characterized.[21] In myeloid cells the 5-lipoxygenase pathway leads to formation of the biologically active leukotrienes (Fig. 11–4). As noted, the unstable HPETE is the initial metabolite of each lipoxygenase pathway. HPETE either is reduced to the more stable HETE or is converted by 5-lipoxygenase to LTA_4. LTA_4 can then be converted to LTB_4 (as in neutrophils and macrophages) or conjugated with reduced glutathione to form LTC_4 (as in eosinophils, mast cells, endothelial cells, and macrophages). Unlike 5-lipoxygenase, which is distributed mainly in myeloid cells, LTA_4 hydrolase, which converts LTA_4 to LTB_4, is widely distributed. A nearly full-length cDNA has been isolated that encodes for LTA_4 hydrolase and corresponds to a primary sequence of a 610 amino acid residue with a molecular weight of 69,153d.[22] From the cDNA sequence it was suggested that mRNA for LTA_4 may have a short half-life, which could account for the interesting properties of extremely rapid production and shut-down of LTB_4—and other eicosanoid—biosynthesis. It is clear that as mechanisms of eicosanoid production and activity are understood at a molecular level, the chances will increase of developing therapy that will influence the oxygenation pathways in a manner beneficial to the host.

LTA_4 can be exported from the cell of origin and converted in other cells by LTA_4 hydrolase to LTB_4. This variation on the "endoperoxide steal"—perhaps better called "transcellular metabolism"—also applies to conversion of LTA_4 to LTC_4 by LTC_4 synthase, a glutathione-S-transferase.[23] Thus, although human endothelial cells do not produce terminal products of the 5-lipoxygenase system, they do generate LTC_4 from LTA_4 provided by neutrophils. LTC_4 and its products LTD_4 and LTE_4 make up the biologic mixture previously known as slow-reacting substance of anaphylaxis.[24] LTD_4 and LTE_4 arise from LTC_4 following sequential removal of gamma (γ)-glutamic acid and glycine from LTC_4. The enzyme γ-glutamyl transpeptidase is present in many cells as part of a complex enzymatic system involved in glutathione biosynthesis and amino acid transport. Thus, in many systems the major sulfidopeptide LT has been reported to be LTD_4 rather than the precursor LTC_4. Removal of glycine from LTD_4 results in LTE_4 with concomitant loss of a significant amount of biologic activity.

The metabolic fate of LTs is not understood completely. LTB_4 is metabolized—via the cytochrome P450 oxidase system—by omega(ω)-oxidation to 20-hydroxy-LTB_4, which can be further oxidized to 20-carboxyl-LTB_4. Omega-oxidation of the C20 terminus of LTE_4 followed by beta (β)-oxidation results in novel metabolites. In addition, LTs are susceptible to oxidative degradation by chemical means, including attack by hypochlorous acid in neutrophils.[24]

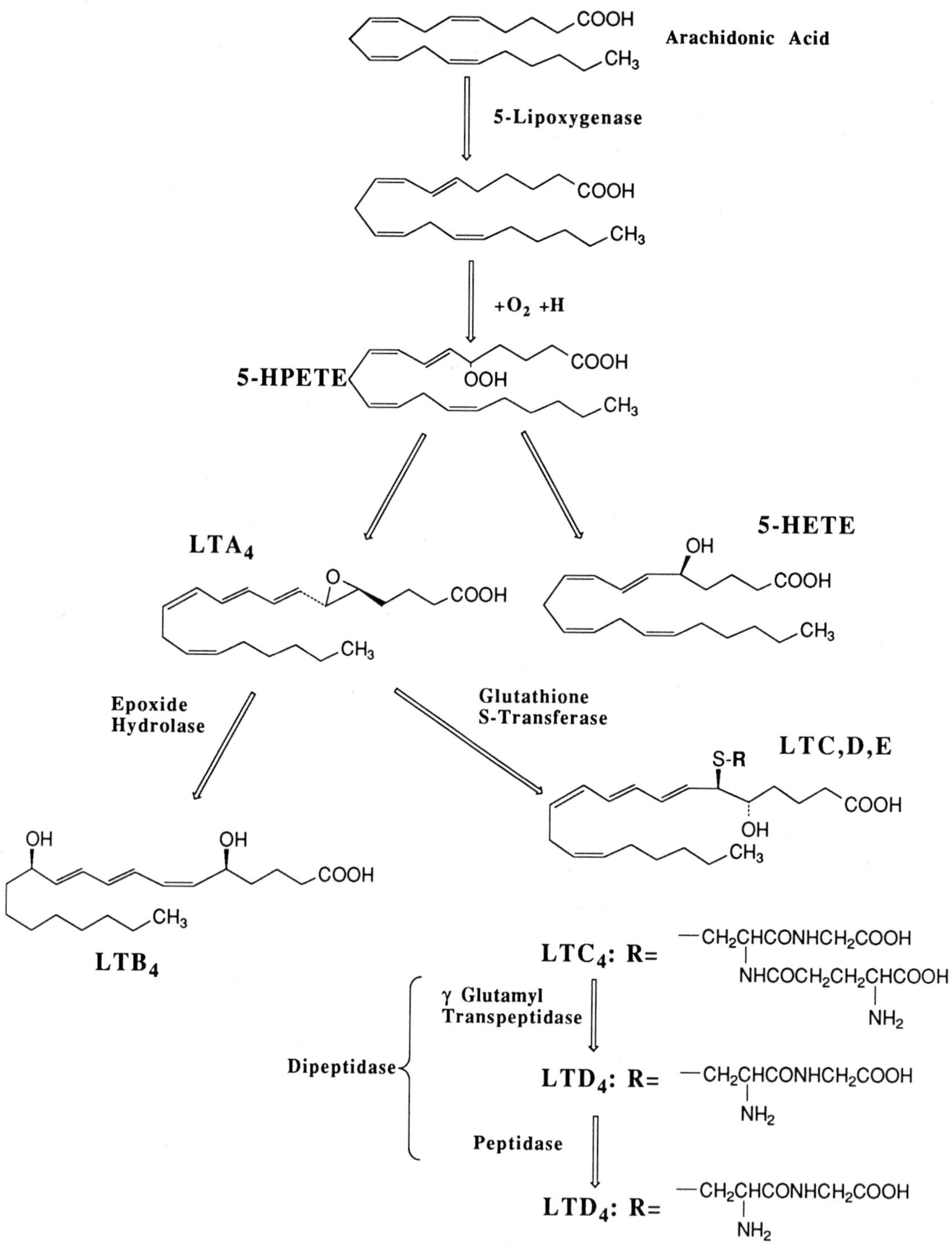

Figure 11–4. 5-Lipoxygenase pathway of arachidonic acid metabolism.

The biologic effects of compounds produced in the lipoxygenase pathway indicate their importance in inflammatory diseases. They have displaced the products of the cyclooxygenase pathway as candidates for the major mediators of inflammation formed by the oxygenation of arachidonic acid and are implicated as key mediators in several diseases, including inflammatory bowel disease, psoriasis, bronchial asthma, and RA.

5-HETE and 5-HPETE stimulate the generation of superoxide in human neutrophils. These compounds also augment intracellular calcium levels facilitating protein kinase C–dependent activation of a superoxide-generating system of neutrophils.[25] LTB_4 increases adherence of leukocytes to endothelial cells, a first step in the inflammatory response. LTB_4 does not appear to have a direct vascular contractile action, since it is inactive in the hamster cheek pouch preparation and several other microvasculature systems. In rabbit skin, administration of LTB_4 with a vasodilator PG induces plasma exudation, suggesting that LTB$_4$ may play a facilitating role in enhanced vascular permeability. Increased venule permeability does not occur in response to LTC$_4$, LTD$_4$, and LTE$_4$. LTB$_4$ is a potent chemotactic factor for neutrophils and is weakly chemotactic for eosinophils. LTB$_4$, and to a lesser extent 5-HETE, enhance migration of T lymphocytes in vitro.[23] Synovial cells produce 5-HETE but do not appear to produce significant amounts of LTB$_4$. However, macrophages that invade the synovium in patients with RA generate substantial quantities of 15- and 5-lipoxygenation products, including LTB$_4$. In addition to the local signs of inflammation induced by products of the lipoxygenase pathway, these compounds may contribute to the pain, tenderness, and aching so common in patients with RA.[26]

Synovial cell and endothelial cell proliferation are central to propagation of the rheumatoid joint lesion. Both LTB$_4$ and the cysteinyl LTs act as growth or differentiation factors for a number of cell types in vitro. For example, LTC$_4$ and LTD$_4$ promote proliferation of human glomerular epithelial cells in vitro. These compounds also increase proliferation of fibroblasts when PG synthesis is inhibited,[27] findings that emphasize the importance of interactions between the cyclooxygenase and lipoxygenase pathways.

LTB$_4$ also appears to serve an immunoregulatory function.[28] For example, it stimulates differentiation of competent CD8 T lymphocytes from precursors lacking the CD8 marker. In addition, LTB$_4$ stimulates interferon-γ and IL-2 production by T cells and biosynthesis of IL-1 by monocytes.

Modification of the Lipoxygenase Pathway

Strategies for inhibiting production or antagonizing the actions of LTs include development of selective LT receptor antagonists and inhibition of the production of all LT by blocking the action of 5-lipoxygenase. Early clinical trials with an LTD$_4$ receptor antagonist indicate that intravenous administration is well tolerated and attenuates LTD$_4$ and antigen-induced bronchoconstriction in patients with asthma.[29]

Several observations suggest that 5-lipoxygenase requires an activation step involving its translocation from cytosol to cell membrane before LT synthesis occurs. One new LT synthesis inhibitor prevents translocation to the membrane of 5-lipoxygenase. The inhibitor appears to bind with high affinity to a 5-lipoxygenase activating protein. This concept of inhibition engenders broad interest because other proteins, such as protein kinase C (and perhaps phospholipase C) translocate to the membrane.[30]

Molecular cloning studies have shown that a mRNA of 2.8 kilobases codes for 5-lipoxygenase.[31] Homology between lipoxygenases is strongest at the carboxyl-terminal end, suggesting that this is the region containing the active site. Definite identification of the active site and subsequent determination of its three-dimensional structure will be important to the development of 5-lipoxygenase inhibitors. The strategy can be applied of course to other enzymes in the arachidonic acid cascade.

Lipoxins

Another large family of arachidonic acid metabolites arises from the sequential action of 5- and 15-lipoxygenases. Addition of 15-HPETE and 15-HETE to human leukocytes results in the formation of a pair of oxygenated products containing a unique conjugated tetraene. One compound (lipoxin A$_4$) was identified as 5,6,15-L-trihydroxy-7,9,11,13-eicosatetraenoic acid, and the other proved to be its positional isomer 5-D-14,15-trihydroxy-6,8,10,12-eicosatetraenoic acid (Fig. 11–5). Since both of these compounds can arise via an interaction between lipoxygenase pathways, the trivial name lipoxins (LX) (lipoxygenase interaction products) was introduced. Platelet 12-lipoxygenase can transform neutrophil LTA$_4$ to LXs. The complete stereochemistry and multiple routes of biosynthesis for the biologically active lipoxin A$_4$ (LXA$_4$) and lipoxin B$_4$ (LXB$_4$) have been determined.[32]

That macrophages of rainbow trout generate LX rather than LT or PG as their major products of arachidonate metabolism indicate that LXs have a long evolutionary history.[33] The biologic actions of LXA$_4$ and LXB$_4$ are distinct from those of other eicosanoids. At submicromolar concentrations, LXA$_4$ induces rapid arteriolar dilation in the hamster cheek pouch and the rat kidney. LXA$_4$ antagonizes LTD$_4$-induced vasoconstriction in vivo and blocks binding of LTD$_4$ to its receptors on mesangial cells.[34] LXA$_4$ also suppresses LTB$_4$-induced inflammation in the hamster cheek pouch by blocking plasma leakage and leukocyte migration.

Unlike LTs, LXA$_4$ contracts guinea pig lung strips but not ileum smooth muscle preparations, which suggests a degree of organ specificity at the receptor level. Contractions induced by LXA$_4$ are characteristically slow in onset and are not blocked by either cyclooxygenase or lipoxygenase inhibitors. LXA$_4$ stimulates TX production in lung strips, and LXA$_4$ and LXB$_4$ stimulate prostacyclin formation by and release from cultured human endothelial cells. LXA$_4$ also blocks LTB$_4$-induced neutrophil inositol triphosphate generation and calcium mobilization, but not superoxide anion generation. Conversely, LXA$_4$ activates protein kinase C (PKC) and is more potent in this regard than diacylglycerol and arachidonic acid.[35] LXA$_4$ appears to be specific for the γ-subspecies of PKC. These results indicate that LXs may regulate the actions of vasoconstrictor LTs and suggest that LXA$_4$ may be an important modulator of intracellular signal transduction.

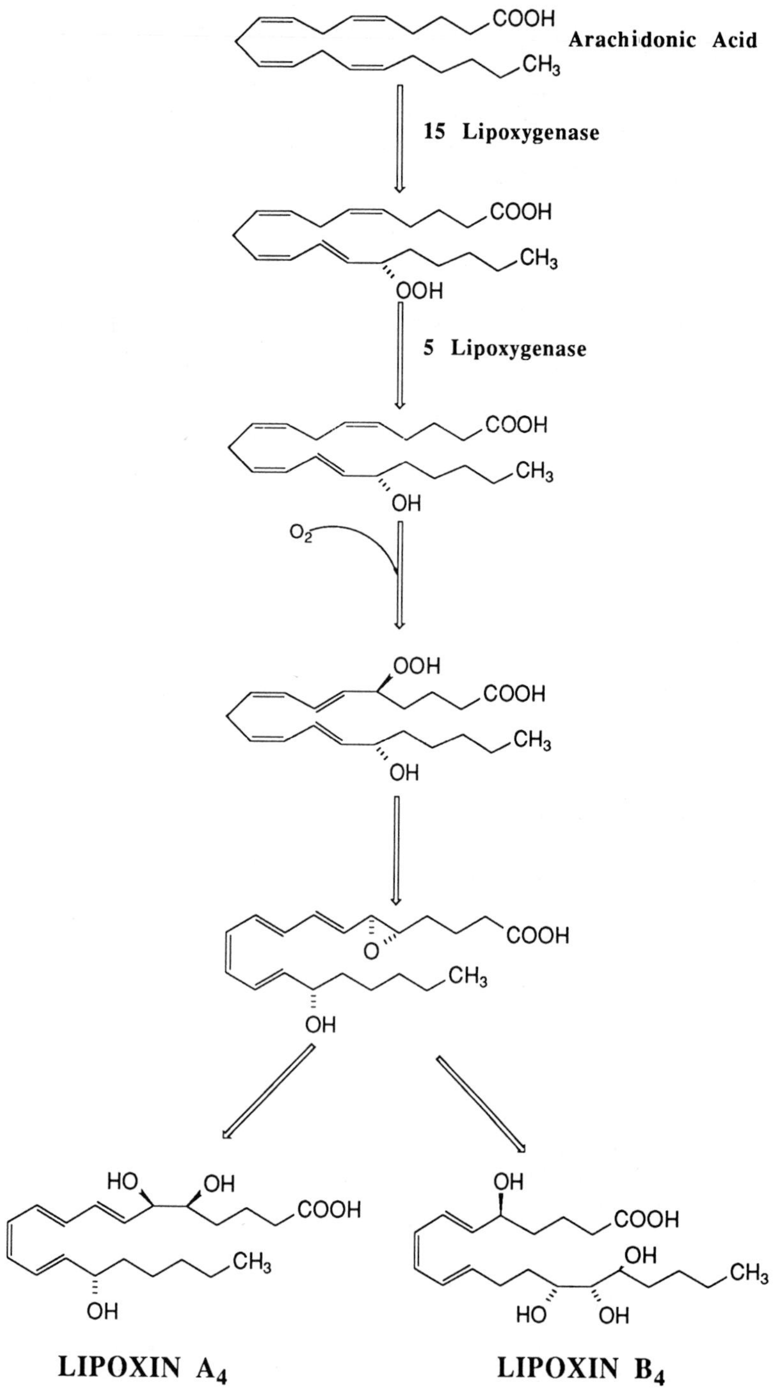

Figure 11–5. Lipoxin biosynthesis.

MONOOXYGENASE PATHWAY

Cytochrome P450, a ubiquitous monooxygenase, mediates metabolism of arachidonic acid to generate a series of products that possess potent pharmacologic activities,[36] including inhibition of calcium ion mobilization, platelet aggregation, and Na^2,K ATPase. The pathway involves insertion of oxygen into one of the four double bonds of arachidonate to form four epoxyeicosatetraenoic acids, which have been found in human urine. In addition, cytochrome P450 may be important in terminating the action of PGs and LTs.[24]

PROSTAGLANDINS AS REGULATORS OF INFLAMMATION AND IMMUNE RESPONSES

The role of PGs in the inflammatory process is not as well defined as once was supposed because the stable PGs PGE and PGI_2 have anti-inflammatory as well as inflammatory effects.[37] The observation that PGE_1 inhibits platelet aggregation led to the notion that cyclooxygenase products of arachidonic acid metabolism might have anti-inflammatory activity. (The potential anti-inflammatory effects of prostacyclin are noted in the section on prostacyclin.) As it becomes clearer that NSAIDs have anti-inflammatory effects other than interference with cyclooxygenase production and subsequent PG inhibition,[38] the potential protective effects of PGs are being considered.

Evidence from both in vitro and in vivo experiments indicates that PGs, notably PGE compounds, can suppress diverse effector systems of inflammation.[37] In addition, PGE can both enhance and diminish cellular and humoral immune responses, observations that reinforce a view of these compounds as *regulators* of cell function. A regulatory effect of PGE is not a new concept. For example, PGE inhibits the release of norepinephrine from the spleen in response to sympathetic nerve stimulation, and PGE is released from the spleen when it contracts in response to sympathetic nerve stimulation. Thus, by a feedback mechanism the contracting smooth muscle can reduce the stimulus leading to its contraction. PGE release may therefore be a defense mechanism aimed at minimizing potential injury.

Several studies in vitro have demonstrated the ability of PGE and PGI_2 to suppress functional responses of a variety of inflammatory cells besides platelets.[37] The ability of PGE to suppress production of LTB_4 by neutrophils[39] and IL-1 release by macrophages[13] in vitro may also help explain the potential anti-inflammatory effects of PGE. Eicosanoids interact with cytokines in a complex manner. Although PGE_2 suppresses release of IL-1 from stimulated macrophages, it has no effect on IL-1α or IL-1β mRNA accumulation. In contrast, 5×10^{-7} M PGE_2 causes a 70 percent reduction in TNF mRNA.[13] Thus, synthesis of TNF appears to be regulated by PGE at least at the level of transcription, whereas synthesis of IL-1α and IL-1β is regulated post-transcriptionally. The capacity of PGE and PGI_2 to suppress function of inflammatory cells appears to reside, in large part, in their capacity to influence cellular cyclic nucleotides and signal transduction pathways.

Additional studies in neutrophils, platelets, and monocytes suggest that PGs may also alter the functional characteristics of specific receptors, including Fc receptors, on cell membranes.[37] PGE also inhibits superoxide anion generation by human neutrophils activated in vitro.[40] In addition, neutrophils isolated from rats treated systemically with 15-S-15-methyl-PGE_1 (15-$MPGE_1$, a stable analogue of PGE_1) exhibit decreased superoxide anion production and lysosomal enzyme secretion after stimulation in vitro.[37]

That PGE compounds in vitro reduce release of other mediators of inflammation, including LTB_4, suggests that PGE might suppress inflammation in

vivo. PGE_1 does in fact prevent progression of adjuvant-induced arthritis and cartilage destruction in rats. 15-$MPGE_1$ resists degradation and is active even when given by mouth at 1/50th the parenteral dose. Oral administration of 15-$MPGE_1$ inhibits progression of adjuvant-induced arthritis; suppresses immune complex–induced vasculitis in skin of rats; prevents increases in vascular permeability induced by chemical mediators of inflammation, including histamine, serotonin, bradykinin, and C5a[37]; and reduces acute inflammation induced in a subcutaneous air pouch model by a chemotactic peptide, monosodium urate crystals, and LTB_4.[41]

In 15-$MPGE_1$–treated animals, hypersensitivity granulomas are suppressed dramatically, even when treatment begins after granulomas have developed. Characteristic increases in splenic B cells and in Ia antigen–positive granuloma macrophages are reduced markedly by treatment with 15-$MPGE_1$.[37] $PGF_{2\alpha}$ has no effect. The observations indicate that PGE can arrest ongoing cell-mediated immune reactions.

Much information about the effect of PGE on immune responses derives from studies of immune complex–induced nephritis.[42] A striking protective effect in murine lupus is associated with expression of the characteristically suppressed cell-mediated immune responses, reversal of abnormal development of prethymic cells, and enhanced functional maturity of thymocytes. Reduction by PGE of immune complex–induced renal injury and of proteinuria may be related to the ability of PGE to reduce vasoactive mediator–induced vascular permeability. Systemic treatment (subcutaneous or oral administration) of rats with PGE_1 or 15-$MPGE_1$ markedly attenuates vasopermeability induced by intradermal injection of histamine, serotonin, and bradykinin. PGE_2 and $PGF_{2\alpha}$ fail to reduce permeability. Electron microscopy studies indicate that treatment with PGE_1 preserves tight junctions of endothelial cells and prevents the endothelial cell gap formation that usually follows injection of a vasopermeability mediator.

Immune complex–induced vasculitis appears to be an early event at sites of inflammation (i.e., skin, kidney) in systemic lupus erythematosus patients and in subsynovial vessels in patients with RA. Formation of immune complexes in vessel walls leads to activation of complement and local generation of C5-derived chemotactic peptides. Treatment of an experimental model of vasculitis in rats with PGE_1 or 15-$MPGE_1$ inhibits increased vascular permeability, egress of leukocytes from blood vessels, and tissue injury even though vascular and perivascular deposition of antigens and complement is not prevented. The protection against tissue injury by orally administered PGE that was demonstrated in this model appears to be due in part to interference with directed motion of neutrophils and degranulation of these cells, as seen in studies done in vitro. Similarly, intravenous administration of PGE_1 in patients with peripheral vascular disease results in suppressed responses (chemotaxis, lysosomal enzyme release) of neutrophils harvested from peripheral blood.[42]

Intravenous infusion of PGE_1 can be used for short-term therapeutic effects, as shown by its capacity to improve renal function in patients with lupus nephritis.[43] PGE_1 administered intravenously also has the capacity to reduce levels of circulating immune complexes (CIC) in patients with autoimmune diseases.[44] The relatively long-term effects on CIC observed after intravenous infusion (up to several months) may help explain the long-term benefits of PGE_1 (the plasma half-life of which is measured in minutes) observed[45] in some patients with Raynaud's phenomenon and with vasculitis.

The availability of PGE_1 analogues that can be given by mouth paves the way for studies in diseases such as RA and SLE. When administered by itself in doses approved for human use, the PGE_1 analogue misoprostol does not exhibit immunosuppressive activity.[46] However, misoprostol improves renal function and reduces the incidence of acute rejection in renal-transplant recipients treated concurrently with cyclosporine and prednisone.[47] Synergy between PGE_1 and other immunosuppressive agents has also been observed in animals. Since NSAIDs and PGE share some of the same effects on cell function (e.g., reduction of neutrophil superoxide anion generation),[38] it is possible that they could be used together to suppress inflammation. This potential therapeutic strategy is demonstrated by in vitro studies in which macrophages pretreated with indomethacin exhibit an increased sensitivity to PGE_2–induced suppression of TNF mRNA and bioactivity.[48]

Because activated T lymphocytes appear to have a central role in the pathogenesis of many autoimmune and inflammatory diseases, the effects of PGE on T cell proliferation have been studied extensively in vitro.[49, 50] The agent induces a profound inhibition of T lymphocyte activation and proliferation in mitogen-stimulated cells. The phenomenon is associated with interference of early signal transduction mechanisms. Other studies indicate that PGE compounds are also capable of suppressing the IL-2–driven proliferative phase of preactivated long-term T cell cultures.

PGE and cAMP do not simply *suppress* cell function; transient increases in cellular cAMP, which may be induced by PGE and PGI_2—as well as by chemoattractant agents—can activate lymphocytes. For example, both a cyclooxygenase-dependent increase and a subsequent decrease (burst) of cAMP are necessary for initiation of proliferation by lymphocytes exposed to concanavalin A. Artificial maintenance of cAMP concentrations (by addition of theophylline or high-dose PGE) prevents cell proliferation. In addition, a population of low-density T lymphocytes exhibit enhanced blastogenic responses to phytohemagglutinin when treated in vitro with PGE. Moreover, the ability of T lymphocytes to adhere to virus-infected cells is enhanced by addition of PGE in vitro and by oral administration of PGE to humans.[42]

Further evidence of an immune response *regulatory* role for PGE is supplied by results of studies that document selective effects of physiologically relevant concentrations of PGE_2 on human B cell responses.[51] Thus, PGE_2 suppresses B cell DNA synthesis and proliferation stimulated by *Staphylococcus aureus* but has a minimal effect on pokeweed mitogen–stimuated B cell DNA synthesis. Further, PGE_2 causes a concentration-dependent inhibition of immunoglobulin generation by B cells stimulated with *Staphyloccocus aureus*. PGE can also modulate rheumatoid factor synthesis.

MODULATION OF EICOSANOID SYNTHESIS BY ADMINISTRATION OF PRECURSOR FATTY ACIDS

Attempts to modulate eicosanoid production have been directed at providing fatty acids other than arachidonate as substrates for oxygenation enzymes in an effort to generate a unique eicosanoid profile with different biologic effects.[52] Since eicosanoids derive from essential fatty acids, dietary manipulation or direct administration of precursor fatty acids has been used to alter the eicosanoid profile. Although the main reason for manipulation of eicosanoid precursor fatty acids has been to alter eicosanoid synthesis, it has become increasingly clear that the precursor fatty acids themselves may modulate immune reponses.[50] Animal and human studies have shown that changes in essential fatty acid intake can alter the fatty acid composition of cell membranes.

Fish oil lipids, rich in ω-3 fatty acids, inhibit formation of cyclooxygenase products and LTB_4 derived from arachidonate and reduce generation of cytokines by monocytes. Fish oil supplements have therefore been used in attempts to suppress inflammation in experimental models and in patients with RA.[53] Therapeutic benefits have been modest but encouraging. Evidence that fish oil supplements enhance collagen-induced arthritis in rats and exacerbate vasculitis in autoimmune mice dictates caution in premature uncontrolled use of therapies involving fish oils in inflammatory diseases.[54]

Certain plant seed oils contain relatively large amounts of γ-linolenic acid (GLA: 18:3 ω-6). GLA can be converted to dihomo-γ-linolenic acid (DGLA: 20:3 ω-6), the fatty acid precursor of the monoenoic (e.g., PGE_1) PGs (see Fig. 11–1). In humans, the Δ^5-desaturase that converts DGLA to arachidonic acid is sluggish. Thus, although administered GLA is readily converted to DGLA, concentrations of arachidonate do not increase appreciably. DGLA competes with arachidonate for oxidative enzymes, thereby reducing production of cyclooxygenase products derived from arachidonate. In addition, DGLA cannot be converted to inflammatory leukotrienes by 5-lipoxygenase. GLA enrichment of diet has suppressed acute and chronic inflammation and joint tissue injury in several experimental animal models.[54]

Controlled trials in which GLA was used to treat atopic eczema showed sufficient clinical benefit to warrant approval of GLA therapy by the National Health Service in England.[55] Administration of 1.1 g per day of GLA to volunteers and patients with RA (in an uncontrolled manner) for 12 weeks resulted in enrichment of leukocytes with DGLA, significant reductions in monocyte PGE_2, LTB_4, and LTC_4, and reduced synovitis in 6 of 7 patients.[56] Other studies show that GLA administration leads to increased PGE_1 production by monocytes.[54] PGE_1 is anti-inflammatory in many systems. The extremely short half-life of natural PGs has a purpose: it allows moment-to-moment regulation of cell function in response to external stimuli and internal messengers. Enrichment of cells with DGLA might enable PGE_1 concentrations to be altered as needed without overriding the physiologic controls that modulate rapid changes in its synthesis and degradation.

References

1. Needleman, P. Turk, J., Jakschik, B. A., Morrison, A. R., and Lefkowith, J. B.: Arachidonic acid metabolism. Annu. Rev. Biochem. 55:69, 1986.
2. Samuelsson, B., and Claesson, H. E.: Leukotriene B_4: Biosynthesis and role in lymphocytes. Adv. Prostaglandin Thromboxane Leukotriene Res. 20:1, 1990.
3. Brash, A. R.: Specific lipoxygenase attack on arachidonate and linoleate esterified in phosphatidylcholine: Precedent for an alternative mechanism in activation of eicosanoid biosynthesis. Adv. Prostaglandin Thromboxane Leukotriene Res. 15:197, 1985.
4. DeWitt, D. L., and Smith, W. L.: Primary structure of prostaglandin G/H synthase from sheep vesicular gland determined from the complementary DNA sequence. Proc. Natl. Acad. Sci. U.S.A. 85:1412, 1988.
5. Simonson, M. S., Wolfe, J. A., and Dunn, M. J.: Regulation of prostaglandin endoperoxide synthase. Adv. Prostaglandin Thromboxane Leukotriene Res. 21:69, 1990.
6. Weller, P. F., and Ryeom, S. W.: Cytoplasmic lipid bodies: nonmembrane sites for prostaglandin formation (submitted for publication).
7. Kurzrock, R., and Lieb, C. C.: Biochemical studies of human semen. II. The action of semen on the human uterus. Proc. Soc. Exp. Biol. Med. 28:268, 1930.
8. von Euler, U. S.: On the specific vasodilating and plain muscle stimulating substances from accessory genital glands in man and certain animals (prostaglandin and vesiglandin). J. Physiol. (Lond.) 88:213, 1936.
9. Bergström, S., Ryhage, R., and Samuelsson, B.: The structure of prostaglandins E_1, F_1, and F_2. Acta Chem. Scand. 16:501, 1962.
10. Ferreira, S. H.: Prostaglandins, aspirin-like drugs and analgesia. Nature (New Biol.) 240:200, 1972.
11. Raisz, L. G.: Recent advances in bone cell biology: interactions of vitamin D with other local and systemic factors. Bone Miner. 9:191, 1990.
12. Martin, M., and Resch, K.: Interleukin-1: More than a mediator between leukocytes. Trends Pharmacol. Sci. 9:171, 1988.
13. Scales, W. E., Chensue, S. W., Otterness, I., and Kunkel, S.L.: Regulation of monokine gene expression: Prostaglandin E_2 suppresses tumor necrosis factor but not interleukin-$I\alpha$ or β mRNA and cell-associated activity. J. Leukoc. Biol. 45:416, 1989.
14. Seibert, K., Masferrer, J. L., Jiyi, F., Honda, A., Raz, A., and Needleman, P.: The biochemical and pharmacological manipulation of cellular cyclooxygenase activity. Adv. Prostaglandin Thromboxane Leukotriene Res. 21:45, 1990.
15. Moncada, S., Gryglewski, R., Bunting, S., and Vane, J. R.: An enzyme isolated from arteries transforms prostaglandin endoperoxides to an unstable substance that inhibits platelet aggregation. Nature 263:663, 1976.
16. Vane, J. R., Anggard, E. E., and Botting, R. M.: Regulatory functions of the vascular endothelium. N. Engl. J. Med. 323:27, 1990.
17. Hamberg, M., Svensson, J., and Samuelsson, B.: Thromboxanes: a new group of biologically active compounds derived from prostaglandin endoperoxides. Proc. Natl. Acad. Sci. U.S.A. 72:2994, 1975.
18. Willis, A. L.: Platelet aggregation mechanisms and their implications in

haemostasis and inflammatory disese. In Ferreira, S. H., and Vane, J.R. (eds.): Inflammation, Handbook of Experimental Pharmacology. Berlin, Springer-Verlag, 1978, p. 138.
19. Yoshimoto, T., and Yamamoto, S.: Partial purification and assay of thromboxane A synthase from bovine platelets. Methods Enzymol. 86:109, 1982.
20. Oates, J. A., FitzGerald, G., Branch, R. A., Jackson, E. K., Knapp, H. R., and Roberts, L. J.: Clinical implications of prostaglandin and thromboxane A_2 formation. N. Engl. J. Med. 219:761, 1988.
21. Funk, C. D., Hoshiko, S., Matsumoto, T., Radmark, O., and Samuelsson, B.: Characterization of the human 5-lipoxygenase gene. Proc. Natl. Acad. Sci. U.S.A. 86:2587, 1989.
22. Minami, M., Ohno, S., Kawasaki, H., Radmark, O., Samuelsson, B., Jornvall, H., Shimizu, T., Seyama, Y., and Suzuki, K.: Molecular cloning of a cDNA coding for human leukotriene A_4 hydrolase. J. Biol. Chem. 262:13873, 1987.
23. Lewis, R. A., Austen, K. F., and Soberman, R. J.: Leukotrienes and other products of the 5-lipoxygenase pathway. N. Engl. J. Med. 323:645, 1990.
24. Murphy, R. C.: Biosynthesis and metabolism of eicosanoids. In Watkins, W. D., Peterson, M. B., and Fletcher, J. R. (eds.): Prostaglandins in Clininal Practice. New York, Raven Press, 1989, p. 1.
25. Heyworth, P. G., Karnovsky, M. L., and Badwey, J. A.: Protein phosphorylation associated with synergistic stimulation of neutrophils. J. Biol. Chem. 2674:14935, 1989.
26. Levine, J. D., and Goetzl, E. J.: Hyperalgesic properties of 15-lipoxygenase products of arachidonic acid. Proc. Natl. Acad. Sci. U.S.A. 83:5331, 1986.
27. Baud, L., Perez, J., Denis, M., and Ardaillou, R.: Modulation of fibroblast proliferation by sulfidopeptide leukotrienes: effect of indomethacin. J. Immunol. 138:1190, 1987.
28. Rola-Pleszczynski, M., Chavaillaz, P. A., and Lemaire, J.: Stimulation of interleukin-2 and interferon-gamma production by leukotriene B_4 in human lymphocyte cultures. Prostaglandins Leukotrienes Med. 23:207, 1986.
29. Ford-Hutchinson, A. W.: Regulation of the production and action of leukotrienes. Adv. Prostaglandin Thromboxane Leukotriene Res. 21:9, 1990.
30. Rouzer, C. A., Ford-Hutchinson, A. W., Morton, H. E., and Gillard, J. W.: MK886, a potent and specific leukotriene biosynthesis inhibitor blocks and reverses the membrane association of 5-lipoxygenase in ionophore-challenged leukocytes. J. Biol. Chem. 265:1436, 1990.
31. Dixon, R. A., Jones, R. E., Diehl, R. E., Bennett, C. D., Kargman, S., and Rouzer, C. A.: Cloning of the cDNA for human 5-lipoxygenase. Proc. Natl. Acad. Sci. U.S.A. 85:416, 1988.
32. Samuelsson, B., Dahlen, S. E., Lindgren, J. A., and Rouzer, C. A.: Leukotrienes and lipoxins: Structures, biosynthesis and biological effects. Science 237:1171, 1987.
33. Pettit, T. R., Rowley, A. F., and Secombes, C. J.: Lipoxins are major lipoxygenase products of rainbow trout macrophages. FEBS Lett. 259:168, 1989.
34. Badr, K. F., DeBoer, D. K., Schwartzberg, M, and Serhan, C. N.: Lipoxin A_4 antagonizes cellular and in vivo actions of leukotriene D_4 in rat glomerular mesangial cells: Evidence for competition at a common receptor. Proc. Natl. Acad. Sci. U.S.A. 86:3438, 1989.
35. Grandordy, B. M., Lacroix, H., Movoungu, E., Krilis, S., Crea, A. E. G., Spur, B. W., and Lee T. H.: Lipoxin A_4 inhibits phosphoinositide hydrolysis in human neutrophils. Biochem. Biophys. Res. Commun. 167:1022, 1990.
36. Oli, W. E. H., Guengenrich, F. P., and Oates, J. A.: Oxygenation of arachidonic acid by hepatic monooxygenases. J. Biol. Chem. 257:3771, 1982.
37. Fantone, J. C., Kunkel, S. L., and Zurier, R. B.: Effects of prostaglandins on in vivo immune and inflammatory reactions. In Goodwin, J. S. (ed.): Prostaglandins and Immunity. Boston, Martinus Nijhoff Publishing, 1985, p. 123.
38. Abramson, S. B., and Weissmann, G.: The mechanisms of action of nonsteroidal anti-inflammatory drugs. Arthritis Rheum. 32:1, 1989.
39. Ham, E. A., Soderman, D. D., Zanetti, M. E., and Kuehl, F. A., Jr.: Inhibition by prostaglandins of leukotriene B_4 release from activated neutrophils. Proc. Natl. Acad. Sci. U. S. A. 80:4349, 1983.
40. Sedgwick, J. B., Berube, M. L., and Zurier, R. B.: Stimulus-dependent inhibition of superoxide generation by prostaglandins. Clin. Immunol. Immunopathol. 34:205, 1985.
41. Tate, G., Mandell, B. F., Schumacher, H. R., and Zurier, R. B.: Suppression of acute inflammation by 15-methyl prostaglandin E_1. Lab. Invest. 59:192, 1988.
42. Zurier, R. B.: Inflammatory Diseases. In Watkins, W. D., Peterson, M. B., Fletcher, J. R. (eds.): Prostaglandins in Clinical Practice. New York, Raven Press, 1989, p. 79.
43. Nagayama, Y., Namura, Y., Tamura, T., and Muso, R.: Beneficial effect of prostaglandin E_1 in three cases of lupus nephritis with nephrotic syndrome. Ann. Allergy 61:289, 1988.
44. Yoshikawa, T., Suzuki, H., Kato, H., and Yano, S.: Effects of prosta-

glandin E₁ on collagen disease with high levels of circulating immune complexes. J Rheumatol. 17:1513, 1990.

45. Roberts, W. N., Hauptman, H. W., and Ruddy, S.: Reversal of the vasospastic component of lupus vasculopathy by prostaglandin E₁ infusion (abstr.). Arthritis Rheum. 32:S74, 1989.

46. Goodwin, J. S., and Clay, G. A.: Effect of chronic ingestion of a prostaglandin E₁ analog on immunologic function in healthy elderly subjects. Int. J. Immunopharmacol. 8:867, 1986.

47. Moran, M., Mozes, M. F., Maddux, M. S., Veremis, S., Bartkus, C., Ketel, B., Pollak, R., Wallenmark, K. C., and Jonasson, O.: Prevention of acute graft rejection by the prostaglandin E₁ analog misoprostol in renal-transplant recipients treated with cyclosporine and prednisone. N. Engl. J. Med. 322:1183, 1990.

48. Spengler, R. N., Spengler, M. L., Strieter, R. M., Remick, D. G., Larrick, J. W., and Kunkel, S. L.: Modulation of tumor necrosis factor-α gene expression. Desensitization of prostaglandin E₂–induced suppression. J. Immunol. 142:4346, 1989.

49. Chouaib, S., Welte, K., Mertelsmann, R., and Dupont, B.: Analysis of prostaglandin E₂ effect on T lymphocyte activation: abrogation of prostaglandin E₂ inhibitory effect by the tumor promoter 12-O-tetradecanoyl phorbol 13-acetate. J. Clin. Invest. 80:333, 1987.

50. Santoli, D., Phillips, P. D., Colt, T. L., and Zurier, R. B.: Suppression of interleukin 2–dependent human T cell growth in vitro by prostaglandins E and their precursor fatty acids. Evidence for a PGE-independent mechanism of inhibition by the fatty acids. J. Clin. Invest. 85:424, 1990.

51. Alvarellos, A., Lipsky, P. E., and Jasin, H. E.: PGE₂ modulation of rheumatoid factor synthesis. Arthritis Rheum. 31:1473, 1988.

52. Willis, A. L.: Nutritional and pharmacological factors in eicosanoid biology. Nutr. Rev. 39:289, 1981.

53. Kremer, J. M., Lawrence, D. A., Jubiz, W., DiGiacomo, R., Rynes, R., Bartholomew, L., and Sherman, M.: Dietary fish oil and olive oil supplementation in patients with rheumatoid arthritis. Clinical and immunological effects. Arthritis Rheum. 33:810, 1990.

54. Callegari, P., and Zurier, R.B.: Botanical lipids. Potential role in modulation of immunological responses and inflammatory reactions. Rheum. Dis. Clin. North Am. 17:415, 1991.

55. Burton, L.: Dietary fatty acids and inflammatory skin disease. Lancet 1:27, 1989.

56. Pullman-Mooar, S., Laposata, M., Lem, D., Holman, R. T., Leventhal, L. J., DeMarco, D., and Zurier, R.B.: Alteration of the cellular fatty acid profile and the production of eicosanoids in human monocytes by gammalinolenic acid. Arthritis Rheum. 33:1526, 1990.

Chapter 12

M. Amin Arnaout

Cell Adhesion Molecules

INTRODUCTION

In multicellular organisms, interactions of cells with each other and with extracellular matrix are critical to the normal development of the organism, to the maintenance of tissue architecture and integrity, and to the ability of the organism to respond effectively to infectious or immunologic stimuli. These cell-cell and cell-matrix interactions are vital to such well-recognized cellular processes as segregation, migration, differentiation, and target-killing and are mediated by families of cell surface glycoproteins, collectively referred to as cell adhesion molecules (CAMs). Knowledge of CAMs and an elucidation of their mechanisms of action and regulation are applicable not only to understanding the basic processes underlying morphogenesis, neuronal development, inflammation, and thrombogenesis but also to the design of chemotherapeutic agents that may either suppress adhesion-mediated events injurious to the host or enhance others that are beneficial. This chapter will review the structure and function of CAMs and how this emerging knowledge is beginning to modify our understanding of the pathogenesis of disease and our approaches to therapy for immune and inflammatory disorders, vascular occlusion, metastasis of tumors, and healing of damaged or severed tissues.

CELL ADHESION MOLECULE FAMILIES

A role for cell adhesion in differential binding and sorting of cells in multicellular organisms was first discovered in sponges. Wilson[1] found that when mechanically dissociated cells from two different species of marine sponge are mixed together, cells specifically sorted themselves out to produce the two types of the organism. That specific and tightly regulated cell recognition events underlie these and similar processes occurring during embryonic and neural development was later proposed by Moscona[2] and developed by Sperry[3] and Edelman.[4] It soon became evident that very similar processes are utilized in the immune system for antigen recognition,[5] immune surveillance,[6] and fighting infections[7] and in

The author's research was supported by NIH grants from NIAID and a grant from the March of Dimes.

the coagulation system in forming the hemostatic plug.[8]

A large number of molecules mediate cell adhesion in vertebrates. CAMs appear to segregate into at least five structurally distinct families (Fig. 12–1).

Cadherins

The cadherins are critical for establishing and maintaining the initial intercellular adhesive events required for formation of embryonic tissues and their stability. Members of this family are detected in blastomeres of mouse embryos at the one-cell stage and play an indispensable part in their compaction and implantation as well as in the subsequent processes leading to morphogenesis.[9] The addition to embryonic tissues of antibodies to cadherins leads to severe distortion in tissue architecture secondary to disruption of cell-cell adhesion.[10] Cadherins are also important in maintaining tight gap junctions and in control of intercellular spacing in adult tissues, since monoclonal antibodies (mAbs) also block re-formation of occluding junctions in epithelial and endothelial cells in vitro.[11]

Adhesion through cadherins is temperature dependent and requires Ca^{++}, which also protects these receptors from rapid proteolysis. Cadherins are homophilic receptors; that is, identical types of cadherins on homotypic or heterotypic cells bind to each other to establish cell-cell contact. This characteristic can be demonstrated in transfection studies in vitro. When singly dispersed L cells expressing one cadherin type are mixed with those expressing a different type, they adhere preferentially to those expressing the identical cadherin type. More than one cadherin may be expressed on a certain cell. Differential expression of cadherins during morphogenesis permits development of different spatiotemporal patterns in embryos.

At least a dozen cadherins are known to date: E (epithelial; uvomorulin)-, N (neural; A-CAM)-, and P (placental)-cadherins have been studied in detail. Their tissue distribution varies among different species. E-cadherin is usually expressed in the epithelial cells of various tissues, such as liver and kidney. N-cadherin is expressed in brain and cardiac muscle but may also be expressed in bovine endothelium. P-cadherin is prevalent in placenta in mice but not humans.

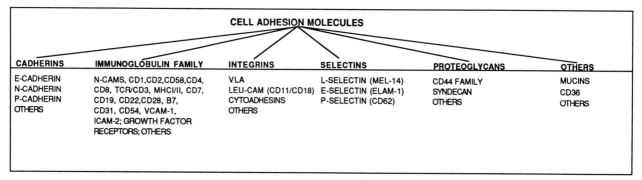

Figure 12–1. Families of cell adhesion molecules.

Cadherins, monomeric surface glycoproteins (Fig. 12–2) each consisting of 723 to 748 amino acids, are highly conserved with an overall homology of 43 to 58 percent.[12, 13] Each receptor has a single transmembrane domain, a highly conserved short C-terminal cytoplasmic tail subject to post-translational modifications, a large extracellular region with three internal repeats, presumptive sites for Ca^{++} binding, and a 113 amino-terminal region that determines the binding specificities. Interaction of the cytoplasmic tail with the cytoskeleton appears to be important in the localization of cadherins to tight junctions and for the overall function of these molecules.[14]

Immunoglobulin Supergene Family

The immunoglobulin (Ig) supergene family includes a large number of proteins with diverse functions and tissue distribution.[5] Members include the antigen-specific recognition proteins the Igs, T cell receptor (TCR), and HLA class I and II receptors. The unifying structural element in this family is a domain consisting of approximately 60 to 100 amino acids between two cysteine residues, arranged in a sandwich of two β-sheets of antiparallel strands forming the Ig fold and stabilized by a hydrophobic interior and the characteristic disulfide bond. The number of antiparallel strands in each sheet varies from three to four, giving rise to the V-set, C1-set, and C2-set folding patterns. The ellipsoidal (4 × 2.5 nm) Ig domain (revealed by crystallographic studies)[15] (see Fig. 12–2) is usually encoded by one exon. In some cases, however, an intron is present that roughly separates the coding regions of the two β-sheets, suggesting that the Ig domain may have arisen by a duplication of a primordial half-domain structure. The selective advantages for preserving the Ig domain throughout evolution despite the great diversity of sequence among the Ig-related molecules is not readily apparent. It has been hypothesized

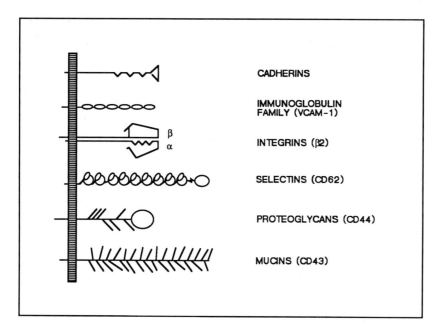

Figure 12–2. Schematic diagram of the structures of representative members of the various CAM families drawn roughly to scale. The three internal repeats in cadherins are indicated. The pattern of folding of cadherins is not yet determined. The immunoglobulin (Ig) domain, the characteristic structure of the Ig family, is depicted here as ellipsoidal with dimensions of 4 × 2.5 nm. Integrins are drawn following the head and tail morphology revealed by electron microscopic studies. A single disulfide bridge links the N-terminus of the β-chain to the middle portion of the molecule. The position of the metal-binding sites in the α-subunit is indicated (wavy line). The dimensions of the combined head and each tail, revealed by the electron microscopic studies, are 8 × 10 nm and 15 nm, respectively. The structure of CD62, a selectin, consists of 9 SCR (each 4.1 nm), assuming a rod-shaped structure (based on homology with complement short consensus repeats [SCRs]), the short EGF-like region (~2.3 nm),[135] and the globular lectin domain.[136] CD44 is depicted as an extended structure with chondroitin sulfate sites (not shown) and seven O-linked glycosylation sites in the middle portion and an N-terminal globular head representing the link-protein–like domain. CD43, a membrane mucin, is shown as a rod structure with mucin-like regions and arbitrarily positioned polysaccharide branches.

that one such advantage might be the known resistance of the Ig fold to proteolysis, an important factor in a stable extracellular recognition event. It also appears probable that adoption of the Ig fold in cell recognition and adhesion (e.g., as a guiding mechanism for axonal extension in the developing nervous system) antedated its adaptation in the immune system for antigen recognition.[5, 16]

Members of the Ig family contain one (e.g., Po and Thy1, CD1α) or more Ig domains and are expressed on the cell surface as monomers, dimers, or heterodimers. Serum Igs and α1 Bgp are secreted. The membrane-bound members are most often linked to the plasma membrane through a single hydrophobic region in their coding sequence. Some are anchored to the plasma membrane by linkage to glycolipid (GPI) and some exist in either form (e.g., CD58, N-CAM). GPI-linked or membrane-spanning forms have equivalent functional activities (e.g., CD58, N-CAM). Other members are associated with an integral membrane protein (e.g., β$_2$-microglobulin). Although mixing of segments from different protein families is not uncommon (e.g., selectins and complement proteins), this is unusual in the extracellular portion of the Ig family. The cytoplasmic portions of the Ig family are least related to each other, vary in length from three amino acids (e.g., IgM) to several hundreds, and may have domains integrated from other protein families (e.g., tyrosine kinases in platelet-derived growth factor [PDGF] receptor).

The major function of the Ig family is cell-to-cell recognition and antigen binding. The biologic processes mediated by the Ig family are vast and vital. They range from morphogenesis[17] to neuronal development,[18] antigen-dependent and antigen-independent immune reactions, and growth and differentiation.[5-7, 19] Cell-cell interaction may occur through Ca^{++}-independent homophilic (e.g., N-CAMs) or heterophilic (e.g., CD58 binding to CD2) interactions between members of the Ig family, or interactions between the Ig and other protein families, such as integrins (e.g., CD54 binding to CD11a/CD18 or V-CAM-1 binding to the α4β1 integrin). Some members of the Ig family also serve as viral receptors (e.g., CD4, CD54, and the poliovirus receptor).[20] Others display enzymatic activities (e.g., ecto-ATPase activity found in rat liver membrane-bound ATPase[21]).

Integrins

The integrins are heterodimeric surface membrane receptors mediating divalent-cation–dependent cell-cell and cell-matrix interactions.[22-25] Each integrin consists of a single α-subunit noncovalently associated with a single β-subunit (see Fig. 12–2). This association is required for cell-surface expression.[7] The sizes of the eight known α-subunits range from 140 to 200 kilodaltons (kD), as determined by electrophoresis on polyacrylamide gels under non-reducing conditions.[22–26b] Each α-subunit consists of a short C-terminal cytoplasmic region, a single membrane-spanning region, and a large extracellular region constituting the bulk of the protein. The extracellular region consists of seven tandem repeats each approximately 60 amino acids long, which could have arisen by a series of duplication events. In one group of α-subunits (CD11a, b, c, α1, and α2)[23, 24, 26] an additional peptide of 200 amino acids called the A-domain (or I-domain) is present between the second and third repeats. The extracellular region of the α-subunits of all other integrins undergoes a posttranslational cleavage near the C-terminal end, resulting in two disulfide-linked fragments. Members of the A-domain–containing group are more homologous to each other and have three metal-binding consensus sequences, whereas each member of the cleaved-α group, with one exception (α4), has four metal-binding sites.[23] The A-domain is present in several additional adhesion proteins. These include cartilage matrix protein, von Willebrand factor, collagen types VI, XII, XIV, and complement factors B and C2.[24, 27] The lack of other common features among these proteins suggests that the A-domain might have been the product of a primordial gene inserted into several proteins to enhance certain adhesion functions.

The β-subunits are smaller than the α-subunits (with the exception of β4) and are more homologous (40 to 48 percent). Each β-subunit consists of a large N-terminal extracellular region containing in its C-terminal half a characteristic cysteine-rich motif repeated four times. Each β-subunit spans the membrane once and has a short cytoplasmic tail containing potential phosphorylation sites. The large cytoplasmic tail of β4 may contribute to the unique localization of this subunit to hemidesmosomes.

Electron microscopy (EM) of several integrin heterodimers (α1β1, α2β1, α5β1, IIb/IIIa)[8, 28, 29] revealed a mushroom-like head comprising the two N-terminal halves of the α- and β-subunits (see Fig. 12–2) and two flexible tails, each comprising the remaining C-terminus of each subunit. The presence or absence of the A-domain does not therefore appear to affect the overall protein structure as revealed by EM.

Integrins can be divided into several subfamilies based on the nature of their associated β-subunit (Fig. 12–3). The largest group is the β1 integrins (also known as VLA, *very late activation* antigens). These are matrix receptors mediating interactions between cells and one or more components of the extracellular matrix (see Fig. 12–3), leading to cell attachment to matrix and modulation of specific cellular functions, such as growth and maturation, migration, proliferation, cytotoxicity, and phagocytosis.[22-24] β1 integrins can also facilitate entry of certain viruses, such as foot-and-mouth virus and human immunodeficiency virus (HIV) type I as well as certain bacteria into mammalian cells.[30-32] In addition to mediating cell-matrix adhesion, certain members of the β1 subfamily can also mediate cell-cell adhesion. For example,

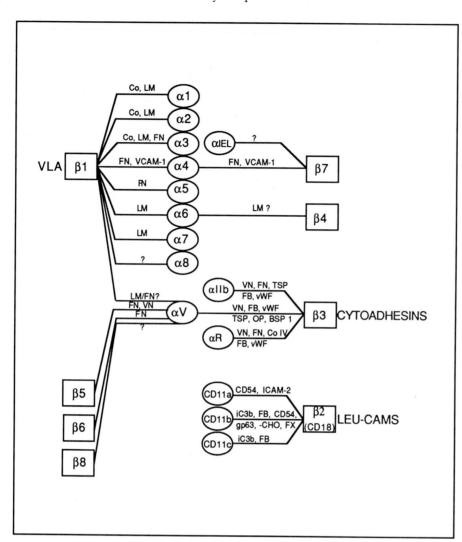

Figure 12–3. The integrin family (see text for details). ? indicates that ligand is unknown or that specificity is controversial. Compiled from references 22 to 26b, 45, 45a, and 45b.

α4β1 also mediates homotypic lymphocyte aggregation, B cell–T cell and T cell–endothelial cell adhesion,[33, 34] and α3β1 is also involved in homotypic aggregation of keratinocytes.[35]

β1 integrins are expressed on a variety of hematopoietic and nonhematopoietic cells (Table 12–1), and their expression is regulated by differentiation and by inflammatory stimuli. The critical functions mediated by β1 integrins are underscored by the fact that mutations in the β1-subunit homologue in *Drosophila* (called PS3 subunit) lead to the lethal myospheroid mutation, in which mutant embryos complete gastrulation and early morphogenesis and then die as a result of the failure to maintain muscle attachment sites once muscle cells begin to contract.[36] In addition, the deficiency of platelet α2β1 (Ia/IIa glycoprotein) in humans results in a bleeding tendency secondary to the complete inability of platelets to respond to collagen.[8] Finally, patients with β2 integrin deficiency (Leu-CAM deficiency) have nearly normal lymphocyte functions in vivo presumably owing in part to usage of several β1 integrins to normalize cytotoxic thymus-dependent lymphocyte (CTL) and natural killer cell (NK)–mediated killing and proliferative responses.[7]

Three members constitute the β2 integrins (also known as Leu-CAM or CD11/CD18).[24] β2 integrins generally mediate homotypic and heterotypic cell-cell interactions. Expression of this subfamily is restricted to leukocytes, with expression of certain members (CD11b and CD11c) limited normally to granulocytes, NKs, and monocytes. CD11a/CD18 has two ligands, CD54 and ICAM-2, both members of the Ig family. CD11b/CD18, the most abundant integrin in neutrophils, can interact with several ligands, such as iC3b, the major C3 opsonin in vivo, and CD54 as well as with clotting factors fibrinogen (FB) and factor X. This receptor also mediates binding of macrophages to a variety of parasites, such as *Leishmania* (through the parasite protein gp63) and *Histoplasma* sp.[24] In granulocytes and monocytes (phagocytes), the majority of CD11b/CD18 and CD11c/CD18 are stored in intracellular granules and are readily brought to the cell surface upon cell activation. β2 integrins play major roles in leukocyte function. In vitro, anti-CD11/CD18 mAbs inhibit chemotaxis of phagocytes, adhesion to various substrates, phagocytosis of C3-opsonized bacteria and fungi, adhesion to cytokine-activated endothelium, proliferation of lymphocytes and NKs, and cell-me-

Table 12–1. DISTRIBUTION OF INTEGRINS

Integrin	PMN	B Cell	T Cell R*	T Cell A*	Mo	Thy	Platelets	Epi	Endo	Neural	Fib/Myo/Mel
α1B1	NA	±	±	+++	+	±	−	−	−	+	+/NA/+
α2β1	−	+	±	+++	++	+	++	+	+	NA	+/+/+
α3β1	−	+	+	+++	+	±	+	+	+	NA	+/+/+
α4β1	−	+++	+++	+++	++	+++	−	−	−	+	+/+/+
α5β1	±	±	++	+++	++	±	±	+	+	+	+/+/−
α6β1	−	±	+++	++	+++	++	+	−	−	−	NA/−/+
α7β1	−	−	−	−	−	−	−	−	−	NA	−/+/+
α8β1	−	−	−	−	−	−	−	−	−	++	±/±/NA
αVβ1	NA	NA	NA	NA	NA	NA	NA	NA	NA	+	+/NA/+
CD11a (αL) β2	++	+	++	+++	++	+	−	−	−	−	−
CD11b (αM) β2	+++	−	−	−	++	−	−	−	−	−	−
CD11c (αX) β2	+	−	−	±	++	−	−	−	−	−	−
αIIbβ3	−	−	−	−	−	−	+++	−	−	−	−
αRβ3	+	−	−	−	+	−	−	−	−	−	−
αVβ3	NA	+	−	+	+	NA	±	−	+	+	−/+/+
α6(αE) β4	−	−	−	−	−	−	−	+	−	−	−
αVβ5(βX)	NA	−	−	−	+	NA	−	+	NA	NA	+/NA/NA
αVβ6(βS)	−	−	−	−	−	−	−	+	+	−	+/NA/NA
α4β7	−	+	+	++	±	NA	−	−	−	−	−
αIELβ7	−	+	+	NA	+	NA	NA	−	−	−	−
αVβ8	−	−	−	−	−	−	−	+	NA	+	NA/−/NA

*R, Resting; A, activated; bracketed subunits refer to old or not commonly used nomenclature.

Minus (−), not detected; ±, trace; ++, moderate; +++, abundant; −/+, presence or absence, respectively, of antigen in tissues; NA, not available. Endo, endothelial; Epi, epithelial; Fib, fibroblasts; Mel, melanocytes; Mo, monocytes; Myo, myoblasts; PMN, neutrophils; Thy, thymocytes. Compiled from references 22 to 26b, 45a, 45b, and 45c.

diated killing of targets. In vivo, β2 integrins are critical to the extravasation of phagocytes (but not of lymphocytes) to inflamed tissues and to the ability of phagocytes to ingest serum opsonized particles. No other adhesion pathways are able to compensate for these functions in phagocytic cells, especially neutrophils, as shown in patients with Leu-CAM deficiency. Inherited absence of lymphocyte β2 integrins is inconsequential in vivo, perhaps because of the compensatory function of other CAM families, such as β1 integrins,[7, 23] CD2/CD58,[19] CD44,[37] and CD43.[38]

Integrins sharing the β3-subunit are the platelet IIb/IIIa (αIIbβ3) and the vitronectin receptor (αVβ3). In addition, a third receptor, leukocyte response integrin, which promotes phagocytosis in monocytes and perhaps in neutrophils, appears to share the β3-subunit.[39] It may be identical to a recently defined integrin on murine lymphocytes mediating CD11a- and CD2-independent killer-target cell adhesion.[39a] The presumably distinct α-subunit of this receptor (here referred to as αR) has not been cloned.

β3 integrins mediate homotypic adhesion (e.g., platelet aggregation) as well as adhesion to matrix components. In platelets, IIb/IIIa accounts for 1 to 2 percent of the total platelet protein.[8] The importance of IIb/IIIa in vivo is reflected by the fact that inherited deficiency of this integrin results in a bleeding disorder (Glanzmann's thrombasthenia) secondary to failure of platelets to aggregate in response to activation.[8] Although their cell distribution is rather restricted to one or two cell types (Table 12–1), β3

integrins are highly promiscuous receptors, binding to a large number of matrix proteins (see Fig. 12–3).

One or two members have been identified so far in the remaining newly described five β subfamilies[40–45] (see Fig. 12–3). Expression of α4β6 is restricted to epithelial cells (see Table 12–1). β7 associates with an α4-subunit to form the lymphocyte homing receptor for Peyer's patches, or with αIEL to form the αIELβ7 receptor predominantly expressed on intraepithelial cells and may be critical in mucosal immunity. β5, β6, and β8 share αV, the most promiscuous of the α-subunits being also shared by β1 and β3.

Several integrins can bind to a single ligand. For example, α3β1, α4β1, α5β1, and αVβ1 bind to fibronectin; α1β1, α2β1, and α3β1 bind to collagen; α1β1, α2β1, and α6β1 bind to laminin.[23, 46, 47] Despite this apparent redundancy, binding of different receptors to the same ligand is usually mediated by one or more distinct sites in the ligand. For example, whereas α5β1 binds to fibronectin through its arginine–glycine–aspartic acid(RGD)–containing region, α4β1 binding to fibronectin occurs in an RGD-independent manner through the alternatively spliced CS1 site[48] within the III connecting segment region. α4β1 also binds to a second site near the heparin II domain.[49] In addition, some receptors can bind, through separate regions in the receptor, to two or more distinct sites in the same ligand. Thus, three binding sites in fibronectin (two RGD sites in the α-chain and a non-RGD site in the γ-chain) bind to three separate sites in αIIbβ3.[8, 50, 51] This characteristic probably permits different signals to be transmitted by the same matrix component through one or more integrin receptors.

The complex interactions between integrins and their ligands are regulated at several levels. Differentiation or activation signals modulate expression of these heterodimers on a variety of cells. Differentiation of myeloid cell lines, such as U937 or HL60, is accompanied by expression of the β2 integrins CD11b and CD11c and several members of the β1 subfamily.[23, 24] Activation of lymphocytes leads to increased expression of CD11a/CD18 as well as several members of the β1 family, whereas the levels of α6β1 decrease (see Table 12–1). Nearly all β1, β2, and β3 integrins are up-regulated by transforming growth factor-β (TGF-β).[52] In certain subfamilies (e.g., β2 integrins CD11b and CD11c and the β3 integrin IIb/IIIa), marked increases in surface expression occur more rapidly (within minutes), secondary to recruitment of already synthesized receptors stored within intracellular granules to the cell surface.[8, 23, 24]

While the function of some receptors appears to be constitutive (e.g., platelet αVβ3, T lymphocyte α1β1, α2β1, and α3β1[8, 53]), that of others is manifested only in activated cells (e.g., platelet IIb/IIa and T lymphocyte α4β1, α5β1, and α6β1)[53, 54] and reflects conformational changes in the receptors.[55] In the same integrin, certain functions are constitutive, whereas others may require receptor activation. Some of the activation-dependent changes may also be mediated by rapid and reversible stimulus-induced phosphorylation of the cytoplasmic portion of integrins.[24]

Integrins can also be differentially regulated by divalent-cations and alternative splicing events. The RGD-independent binding of α2β1 to collagen,[56] α3β1 to fibronectin,[57] and α6β1 to laminin[58] are inhibited by Ca++ but increased by Mg++, suggesting that similar alterations in Ca++ versus Mg++ levels in vivo may modify usage of various integrins, even those expressed on the same cell. Whether this is one mechanism by which cells regulate integrin specificity remains to be determined. Alternative splicing of the β1-,[58a] β3-,[59] β4-,[40] α3-,[59a] and α6-subunits[42a] has been described and probably reflects the potential for transmitting different signals through modified interaction with the cytoskeleton.

Integrin function is also regulated by the cell type and by the type and distribution of various ligands. Thus, platelet α2β1 binds only to collagen, but in other cells it also binds to laminin and fibronectin.[60] Certain ligands dramatically increase expression of a respective receptor; for example, expression of α3β1 is dramatically increased in cell lines allowed to adhere to fibronectin.[61] Several integrins can bind to a single ligand. Alternative splicing of the CS1 site in fibronectin, a major α4β1 binding site, determines the type of interacting receptor.[48, 62] While many ligands are constitutively expressed, some are expressed only as a result of target cell activation. For example, expression of V-CAM-1, an α4β1 ligand on endothelial cells, occurs only as a result of activation of these cells with tumor necrosis factor (TNF), IL-1 and other inflammatory mediators.[63] Similarly, expression of iC3b, FB or factor X, and various ligands for CD11b/CD18 occurs on activation of the complement or clotting systems, respectively.[24]

Not only do integrins provide a link between the extracellular matrix and cytoskeleton, but also they transmit direct signals that modify the activities of other integrins and other metabolic activities within cells. Fibronectin and, to a lesser extent, collagens synergize with anti-CD3 antibodies in eliciting T cell proliferation.[64] Ligation of α5β1 on macrophages can activate the β2 integrin CD11b/CD18 to mediate phagocytosis.[65] Ligand binding also induces clustering of integrins on the cell surface.[66, 67] Cross-linking of CD11a/CD18 results in phosphoinositide turnover and a rise in intracellular Ca++.[68] Cross-linking of CD11b on mouse macrophages produces an activation profile similar to that induced by interferon-γ (INF-γ).[69] Ligand binding to IIb/IIIa increases tyrosine-specific protein phosphorylation[70] and Na+-H+ exchange in epinephrine-activated platelets.[71] Perturbations of integrins can also directly lead to alterations in gene expression. Ligation of α5β1 in synovial fibroblasts or lymphocytes, for example, leads, respectively, to induction of the matrix-degrading metalloproteinases collagenase and stromelysin and to IL-2 transcription.[72, 72a]

Selectins

Selectins (or LEC-CAMs) are a family of monomeric cell surface adhesion receptors that play a role in lymphocyte recirculation and in recruitment of leukocytes to inflammatory sites.[73] Each selectin consists of a short cytoplasmic tail, a single membrane-spanning region, and an extracellular region characterized by a single N-terminal lectin-like domain, an adjacent epidermal growth factor (EGF)–like domain followed by a variable number of short consensus repeats (SCRs) present in several complement regulatory proteins, thus giving rise to the acronym LEC (*Lectin*, *EGF*, *Complement*) (see Fig. 12–2). Three members have been described so far in this family, MEL-14, ELAM-1, and CD62.[74-77] The MEL-14 (L-selectin, LEC-CAM-1, gp90MEL, LAM-1, Leu-8, Ly-22) is constitutively expressed on a majority of leukocytes and contains 2 SCRs. Expression of ELAM-1 (E-selectin, LEC-CAM-2) is restricted to vascular endothelium, occurs in a transient manner in response to IL-1 or TNF, and contains 6 SCRs. Peak expression of ELAM-1 occurs within 4 hours and usually disappears from the cell surface after 24 hours despite the continuous presence of the stimulus. CD62 (P-selectin GMP140, PADGEM, LEC-CAM-3) is the largest of the three molecules, with 9 SCRs. Alternatively spliced forms of CD62 containing 8 SCRs and/or lacking the transmembrane portion were also described. CD62 is normally stored in α granules of platelets and Weibel-Palade bodies of endothelial cells and is rapidly mobilized, within minutes, to the cell surface following degranulation of these cells. Both MEL-14 and CD62 map to the same region on chromosome 1, bands 23–25, suggesting that this family may be encoded by a cluster of loci.[77]

All three selectins are involved in cell-cell interactions involving leukocytes and endothelial cells. Binding through selectins requires Ca^{++} but not metabolic energy, since it can occur at 4°C or by cells fixed with paraformaldehyde.

MEL-14 is a lymphocyte-homing receptor mediating normal lymphocyte binding to peripheral lymph node (PN) endothelium.[78] Lymphocyte homing to other lymphoid tissues such as Peyer's patches, lung-associated endothelium, or chronically inflamed synovium is not mediated by MEL-14. Anti–MEL-14 mAbs prevent accumulation of circulating lymphocytes within PN in vivo, markedly reducing, for example, the size of the intrinsically enlarged PN in MRL-lpr/lpr mice.[79] These antibodies also reduce significantly neutrophil accumulation in inflamed tissues in vivo and adhesion of neutrophils to inflamed endothelium in vitro.[80]

The activation-dependent endothelial glycoprotein ELAM-1 also mediates the binding of phagocytes (but not other leukocytes) to cytokine-activated endothelium. At 37° C, approximately 20 to 30 percent of the binding of neutrophils to endothelium treated for 4 hours with IL-1 is inhibited by anti–ELAM-1, with the balance being CD11/CD18-dependent.[81]

The endothelium–platelet glycoprotein CD62 facilitates adherence of phagocytes (but not lymphocytes) to activated platelets and endothelial cells. Binding of resting neutrophils to purified CD62 is not inhibited by anti-CD11/CD18 mAbs. On the other hand, binding of TNF-α–activated neutrophils to endothelium or to plastic, a CD11b/CD18-mediated function, is inhibited by CD62.[82] These data suggest that an activated form of CD11b/CD18 may interact with CD62 or that the two adhesion pathways may be utilized sequentially by the neutrophil (see later).

The ligands for two of the three selectins have been characterized.[83–88] Based on their lectin-like structure and the ability of simple sugars to inhibit selectin-mediated adhesion, it was anticipated that the ligands may be carbohydrate in nature. The sialyl Lewis X oligosaccharide NeuNAcα2-3Galβ1-4(Fucα1-3)GlcNAc is a ligand for ELAM-1. Antibodies specific for this sialylated fucosylated lactoseaminoglycan inhibit ELAM-1–dependent adhesion. Both the sialic acid and the fucose residues are essential for recognition by ELAM-1. The sialylated Lewis X oligosaccharide is also rich in tumor cells (e.g., colonic carcinoma cell lines), explaining why adhesion of these cells to vascular endothelium is ELAM-1 mediated. CD62 recognizes the lacto-*N*-fucopentaose III (LNFIII) structure Galβ1-4(Fucα1-3)GlcNAcβ1-3Galβ1-4Glc, a pentasaccharide containing the non-sialylated form of the Lewis X epitope. This epitope is identical with CD15, an epitope previously defined by mAbs raised against the neutrophil surface. The

fucose residue in the nonsialyl Lewis X (CD15) epitope is essential for CD62 binding. LNF III isolated from human milk inhibits adhesion of myeloid cells to COS cells transfected with CD62 complementary DNA (cDNA). Several glycoproteins or glycolipids containing one or more of the lactoseamine unit (Galβ1,4 GlcNAcβ1) may be subject to sialylation and/or fucosylation mediated, respectively, by α-(2,3)-sialyltransferase or α-(1,3)-fucosyltransferases, resulting in the respective ligands for CD62 and ELAM-1. This has been shown directly by transfecting cDNA encoding for a (1,3)-fucosyltransferase into nonmyeloid cells, leading to expression of the ELAM-1 ligand.

Although the exact structure recognized by MEL-14 is not yet determined, it is also an oligosaccharide with sialic acid and fucose components.[87] Fucoidin (an algal polysaccharide consisting mainly of mannose, sialic acid, and fucose-4-sulfate) as well as the negatively charged phosphomannose PPME both inhibit MEL-14–mediated adhesion.

The full spectrum of the protein or lipid backbone molecules that display the various oligosaccharide ligands for selectins remains to be determined. It is probable that these specific molecules may express additional peptides, carbohydrate, or other negatively charged residues that enhance binding of selectins to their physiologic ligands. This may explain, for example, the ability of fucoidin and heparin to interact with CD62. The role of the EGF-like domain and the SCR in the function of selectins is unknown, since neither appears to be required for ligand binding. The EGF-like domain may facilitate adherence to the ligand, as in some other proteins with a similar domain. The SCR repeats may either provide an appropriate distance from the cell surface for optimal binding to the carbohydrate ligand or play a role in preventing amplification of the complement cascade at or near the cell surface, as in other complement SCR-containing proteins.

Selectins may play an important role in the initial adhesion of neutrophils and monocytes to cytokine-activated endothelium. This contact helps anchor the neutrophil to endothelium and leads through yet poorly understood events to the integrin-mediated chemotaxis and transendothelial migration. Phenotypic alterations in leukocytes and endothelium may be important intermediary events. The local activation of phagocytes by inflammatory mediators leads to rapid loss of MEL-14 and the ELAM-1 ligand from the cell surface of activated neutrophils,[89, 90] presumably secondary to proteolytic cleavage. This physical or functional inactivation of these receptors/ligands may then permit integrin-dependent adhesion and transmigration, processes that are facilitated by expression of inducible molecules such as CD54 on the endothelium. The pivotal role of the integrin-mediated component is underscored by the lack of neutrophil extravasation to inflammatory sites in inherited Leu-CAM deficiency.

The physiologic role of some selectins (CD62) in

the binding of platelets to neutrophils and to monocytes is unclear, although it may be important in wound healing and atherosclerosis. Neutrophils in contact with activated platelets were reported to induce a marked decrease in platelet activity.[91] Other studies, however, found increased platelet activity in the presence of neutrophils, suggesting that different in vitro models may be measuring different physiologic components of neutrophil-platelet interactions.

Proteoglycans

Proteoglycans constitute a large protein family with one common feature, the presence of one or more glycosaminoglycan side chains. These side chains are utilized in conjunction with the core protein to mediate interactions with many substrates, including matrix proteins and growth factors. Two cell surface proteoglycans used as CAMs are described here. Many others probably exist or await characterization.

CD44 is a lymphocyte-homing receptor mediating specific adhesion of lymphocytes to mucosal high endothelial venules (HEVs).[92-94] CD44 is identical to several independently identified cell surface glycoproteins known as gp90[Hermes], Pgp1, ECM III, and Ina and Inb blood group antigen.[37] CD44 has a wide cell distribution, being expressed in brain, medullary thymocytes, mature T cells, B cells, monocytes, granulocytes, erythrocytes, fibroblasts, keratinocytes, and carcinoma cell lines. CD44 is expressed in large amounts on macrophages and granulocytes ($\sim 10^6$ receptors per cell).[37]

Human CD44 consists of a 341 amino acid core with a single membrane-spanning region. The cytoplasmic portion is 72 amino acids long with several serine residues that can serve as substrates for Ser/Threo kinases. A second form with a cytoplasmic tail of only three amino acids is produced by a minor mRNA species, presumably by alternative splicing.[94] The C-terminal region of the extracellular portion of the protein contains several O-linked and N-linked carbohydrates as well as four serine-glycine dipeptides serving as potential chondroitin sulfate attachment sites, thus accounting for the cell-specific variable electrophoretic patterns of the mature protein, which ranges in size from approximately 90 to 200 kilodaltons (kD). The extracellular N-terminal region contains a single 98 amino acid domain that is repeated two or more times in members of the hyaluronate-binding proteins as link protein where this globular domain stabilizes binding of proteoglycans to hyaluronate by linking both structures.

CD44 is the major cell surface hyaluronate receptor.[95] It also recognizes a mucosal addressin expressed on mucosal HEVs.[92] CD44 recognizes a hexasaccharide element of the basic disaccharide repeat motif of hyaluronic acid. It is also involved in several cell-cell and cell-matrix interactions. CD44 enhances homotypic adhesion (aggregation) of fibroblasts and their binding to collagens I and VI and to fibronectin (hence the name ECM III receptor).[96] It also enhances homotypic adhesion and migration of macrophages.[97] Several heterotypic interactions, such as adhesion of T cells to sheep erythrocytes or to monocytes, CD2- or CD3-induced T cell proliferation,[37] and interaction between hematopoietic and stromal bone marrow cells,[98] are facilitated by CD44. Its up-regulation on carcinoma cell lines and on certain lymphomas may reflect its expression on actively proliferating normal cells and may be important in tumor spreading and metastasis.

CD44 appears to have distinct binding sites for mucosal HEVs and for hyaluronate. Anti-CD44 mAbs that inhibit hyaluronate binding are localized to the link-protein segment, whereas those that inhibit homing are directed to the proteoglycan portion of the molecule.[94] Recombinant CD44-Ig hybrids bind only weakly to HEVs but much more strongly to the underlying hyaluronate-rich matrix,[95] reflecting perhaps differences in the glycosylation profiles of the native and recombinant receptor. The coordinate expression and function of CD44 with other homing receptors (e.g., MEL-14 on B cells, β1 and β2 integrins on memory or activated T cells and CD2/CD58) may explain the enhanced affinity of these cells to their respective targets.[37]

Syndecan, a cell surface proteoglycan matrix receptor,[99] consists of a core protein of 311 amino acids, spans the membrane once, and has a short cytoplasmic tail that can interact with the cytoskeleton. The extracellular domain contains two potential glycosaminoglycan attachment sites containing heparan sulfate and chondroitin sulfate. In simple epithelia, syndecan is located basolaterally and is lost when cells become terminally differentiated. Syndecan is predominantly expressed by mature epithelia but is also found on cells of the B cell lineage and in embryonic and nondifferentiated cells. Syndecan binds epithelial cells through its heparan sulfate moiety to collagens I, III, and V, fibronectin, and thrombospondin.[99] Syndecan may normally function by stabilizing epithelial cell layers through high-affinity binding to underlying matrix and may serve as a depot for growth factors known to bind to other heparan sulfate proteoglycans.[100]

Others

Several additional proteins with demonstrable or suggestive roles in cell-cell and cell-matrix interactions have been identified. One of these molecules is CD36 (known as GP IV on platelets), an 88-kD monomeric cell surface protease-resistant glycoprotein also expressed by monocytes, endothelial cells, nucleated erythroid cells, and a number of tumor cell lines, including melanomas and fibrosarcomas.[101] It is a heavily glycosylated, 438-residue protein with a central extracellular cysteine-rich domain and two potential hydrophobic membrane-spanning regions.[102] CD36 mediates platelet binding to thrombospondin and to collagen type I.[103, 104] It also mediates cytoadherence of *Plasmodium falciparum*–parasitized erythrocytes to CD36+ endothelial or melanoma cells, and of monocytes to thrombin-activated platelets. Interaction with various ligands may involve more than one binding site in CD36, since COS cells expressing recombinant CD36 express some adhesive functions but not others.[102]

The dumbbell-shaped GP Ib-IX complex is the major mucin of platelets contributing to its net negative surface charge.[8, 105] GP Ib consists of two disulfide-linked subunits, each spanning the membrane once. The extracellular portion of the larger α-subunit (145 kD) consists of a globular N-terminal region, containing seven leucine-rich glycoprotein[106, 107] (LRG) repeats of unknown function and a thrombin-binding site, and an elongated portion, close to the plasma membrane, containing the von Willebrand factor (vWF)–binding site.[108] The smaller β-subunit (24 kD) contains a single LRG repeat and is noncovalently bound to the highly homologous GP IX, a 17-kD single-LRG–containing transmembrane protein. Palmitoylation through thioester linkages to the cytoplasmic and intramembranous cysteine residues of GP Ibβ and GP IX might account for the tight association leading to the larger globular domain of the complex.[109] The GP Ib–GP IX complex mediates the initial binding of resting platelets to subendothelium through its interaction with immobilized (but not soluble) vWF and also mediates binding to thrombin.[8] GP Ib is also responsible for the discoid shape of the resting platelet through the association of its 100 amino acid cytoplasmic tail with actin-binding protein 280 (ABP-280).[110] Activation of platelets results in proteolytic cleavage of ABP-280, thus disrupting its association with GP Ib and altering cell shape. Inherited deficiency of GP Ib/IX in humans (Bernard-Soulier syndrome) leads to a bleeding disorder secondary to failure of platelets to adhere to immobilized vWF. These cells also appear large and polymorphic, perhaps as a result of loss of membrane-cytoskeletal associations.[8]

CD43 (leukosialin) is a major membrane mucin of leukocytes. It consists of an extracellular 235 amino acid region, a 23aa membrane-spanning domain, and a 135-residue cytoplasmic C-terminal tail.[111] The extracellular region consists of 80 to 90 mucin-type O-linked polysaccharides consisting of sialylated *N*-acetylgalactoseamine and is relatively resistant to proteolysis. CD43 is expressed on all leukocytes and platelets and shows two major cell-specific glycosylation patterns, a 115-kD form on mononuclear cells and a 135-kD form on platelets and granulocytes.[38] Evidence suggesting a role for CD43 as an adhesion molecule is indirect at present. Monoclonal Abs to CD43 induce monocyte-dependent proliferation of human peripheral blood T cells in a time course and a quantity similar to that observed using anti-CD3 mAbs. These antibodies also induce monocyte aggregation.[112] The physiologic role of CD43 is reflected by the fact that defective CD43 is associated with accelerated platelet destruction and impaired T cell proliferative responses seen in patients with Wiskott-Aldrich syndrome.

RELEVANCE OF CAMS TO COMMON DISORDERS

The important biologic role played by various CAMs is emphasized by the rare congenital defects identified, to date, affecting certain CAMs and resulting in lethal mutations, life-threatening infections, or bleeding disorders. Much more common pathologic disorders, however, ranging from vascular occlusion to ischemia-reperfusion injury, acute and chronic inflammatory disorders, and tumor metastasis, are initiated or propagated by CAMs. This Jekyll-Hyde role of CAMs, as important players in host survival and in host injury, suggests that intervention measures aimed at enhancing or suppressing CAM functions may be beneficial. Following are some important examples.

Immunologic Tissue Injury

A critical component of the inflammatory response is extravasation of inflammatory cells to injured or infected tissues. While vital to host defense against infections, infiltration of leukocytes into damaged tissues can exacerbate the pathologic sequelae of myocardial infarction, hemorrhagic shock, burns, frost bite, transplant rejection, limb reimplantation, and rheumatoid arthritis. Increased tissue damage in these instances is caused by influx of neutrophils into tissues injured by ischemia or immune reactions, driven by increased blood flow and activated by tissue-released chemoattractants. Activated neutrophils then cause further tissue injury secondary to release of proteolytic enzymes and oxygen-free radicals.[7] Prevention or suppression of phagocyte extravasation under these conditions may have desirable consequences. The first indication for the validity of such an approach came from elucidation of the molecular basis of Leu-CAM deficiency, in which deficient β2 integrin expression on neutrophils resulted in lack of extravasation of these cells at acute inflammatory sites.[7] In several animal models of acute inflammation, induction of an acquired form of Leu-CAM deficiency (through use of anti-CD11 or anti-CD18 mAbs) was remarkably effective in reducing neutrophil infiltration into inflamed tissues, such as skin, meninges, lung, gastrointestinal tract, and myocardium.[89] Monoclonal Abs against CD54 were also effective in reducing emigration of neutrophils into rabbit lung in response to phorbol myristate acetate or allergenic stimuli.[113] More recently, anti-CD54 Abs were found as effective as anti-CD3 mAbs in treating acute rejection of transplanted organs.[114] Although the ability of the host to fight infection and to repair tissues is compromised, the temporary need for such therapy, expectantly in acute clinical situations, may make these associated side effects acceptable.

Monoclonal Abs directed against various selectins[81, 90, 115, 116] have also been shown to inhibit neutrophil binding to endothelium. In addition, anti–MEL-14 mAbs as well as the recombinant receptor have been shown to be effective in limiting neutrophil emigration into inflamed tissues in experimental animals.[116] Most of the effect, however, is seen in the first 2 hours of acute inflammation, consistent with the role of selectins in the early events of the inflammatory response.[116] The more persistent inhibitory effects seen with anti–β2 integrin therapy are perhaps a reflection of the rapid down-regulation of selectins and/or their ligands as well as the additional role of β2 integrin in the transmigration and phagocytic activities of migrating cells.[7]

Little information is available on the potential role of anti-adhesive therapy in chronic inflammatory disorders. Under these conditions, mononuclear cells usually predominate. Inherited Leu-CAM deficiency does not impair the ability of lymphocytes to migrate to inflamed tissues,[7] suggesting that anti–β2 integrin therapy may not be as effective in non–phagocyte-mediated inflammatory disorders. The recent demonstration that V-CAM-1/α4β1[63, 117] and perhaps other adhesive pathways (as discussed previously) mediate mononuclear cell–endothelial cell interactions suggests that interventions targeting such systems may prove useful therapeutically.

Since some CAMs such as CD54 and the poliovirus receptor serve as viral receptors, attempts are being made to prevent cell infectivity using modified forms of the receptors.[118–121] These viruses tend to mutate frequently, thus circumventing development of effective immunity. It was presumed that mutations abrogating the ability of the virus to bind to its respective receptor do not arise, since they will be lethal. Thus, inhibition of viral entry by using blockers for the single conserved viral component (receptor-binding site) could prove effective therapeutically. In vitro studies have shown the ability of the respective recombinant soluble receptor to block infectivity. The validity of this approach as a future definitive therapy remains to be established, however, since viral mutants resistant to neutralization with soluble cellular polio receptors have been isolated.[122]

Thrombogenesis

The inability of platelets genetically deficient in IIb-IIIa to aggregate in response to many agonists also suggested that anti-IIb-IIIa mAb therapy might be useful in a variety of life-threatening thrombotic complications.[123] Blocking of IIb-IIIa–mediated platelet aggregation with mAbs has been effective in preventing thrombosis in the coronary and carotid arteries in vivo. Inhibition of IIb-IIIa could also be effected by using peptides recognized by this receptor (e.g., the RGD peptide). Cyclization of certain RGD-derived peptides has increased their affinities to IIb-IIIa by several orders of magnitude compared with the linear peptide, with a concurrent decrease in binding to other integrins, suggesting that they could prove useful and specific in vivo.[124] A class of highly effective and naturally occurring RGD-containing sequences has also been found in snake venom toxins.[125] Although nonspecific in their natural form, modified forms of these peptides (so-called disintegrins) could also prove valuable therapeutically. The mainstay of anti-platelet therapy is currently aspirin, which prevents thromboxane generation. In vitro, however, this inhibitory effect is easily overcome by slightly increasing the concentration of the agonist. Novel reagents that interfere with the aggregation response irrespective of the agonists used (such as IIb-IIIa–directed therapy) may therefore be complementary and highly effective anti-thrombotic reagents.

Tissue Repair

In tissue repair as in tissue formation during embryogenesis, a coordinate spatiotemporal expression of several classes of CAMs (e.g., cadherins, several Ig members such as N-CAM, Ng-CAM, growth factor receptors, integrins) and their cognate ligands (e.g., proteoglycans, laminins, tenascin) may be required to provide the defined migratory pathways, differentiation and growth signals, and patterned migration of various groups of cells to re-establish tissue integrity. Preliminary data are beginning to accumulate elucidating the nature of the changes occurring during the reparative response. Keratinocytes from injured but not normal tissue express certain β1 integrins that these cells use for migration.[126] Since the reparative process is significantly influenced by availability of matrix components, attempts have been made to promote healing in defined experimental conditions by providing matrix elements with encouraging results. Thus, exogenous application of fibronectin was found to facilitate healing of corneal ulcers.[126] Repair of tissues in which intricate cellular networks are needed to re-establish normal function (e.g., when the spinal cord is severed) may be a more formidable task. In this system, however, it is probable that the lack of regenerative ability of neuronal tissue may be secondary, in part, to the absence of critical matrix components (e.g., various forms of laminin) and growth factors needed to provide the physical and biochemical guidance signals required for restoring normal connections. Preliminary data are now available that suggest that laminins can facilitate restoration of normal neuronal connections in damaged tissue.[127]

Tumor Metastasis

For solid tumors to metastasize, they have to be released from the restrictions of their immediate extracellular environment, migrate across matrix networks into the blood stream, re-establish binding to and transmigration across endothelial cells in selected organs, and grow in their new environment unhindered. These complex processes must involve increased expression of CAMs at certain stages of tumor development and their down-regulation at others. Loss of certain CAMs may result in leukemic transition of some lymphomas and dissemination to other organs, guided in part by the nature of homing receptors expressed on their cell surface.[128] Abnormalities in a CAM (a product of the DCC gene) are present in 70 percent of colorectal cancers, suggesting that alterations in the normal cell adhesion phenotype may predispose to or promote metastasis.[129] We are only beginning to understand the complexity of some of these CAM-dependent processes. One interesting phenotype of tumor cells, at least in vitro, is that they intrinsically synthesize less matrix compared with normal cells,[130] permitting tumor cells the freedom of motion. This can be reversed to a certain degree experimentally by overexpressing the down-regulated integrin (e.g., $\alpha5\beta1$ receptor in tumorigenic Chinese hamster ovary cells). Such transfected cells now show reduced ability to form tumors in nude mice.[131] On the other hand, migration of tumor cells requires increased expression of certain CAMs. In metastatic but not benign melanomas, for example, $\beta3$ integrins and CD54 are strongly expressed.[132, 133] RGD-containing peptides can inhibit migration of melanomas in vitro and reduce the number of metastatic pulmonary nodules in mice injected with B16F10 melanoma cell line.[134] Although these studies suggest that modulation of tumor metastasis may be feasible, they also highlight the complexity of this process and the need for further investigations.

CONCLUSIONS AND FUTURE DIRECTIONS

Overwhelming evidence has now established that cell-cell and cell-matrix adhesion—far from being a mere gluing phenomenon—is a basic and highly regulated process that permeates every discipline in biology from morphogenesis to immune recognition and tissue regeneration. Several families, those mentioned here and undoubtedly others to be discovered, contribute to the complexity and diversity of this process. The profound impact that this area of investigation has had so far on the understanding of the molecular basis of common clinical disorders and on providing possible novel avenues of therapy is unfolding. Ultimate success will directly depend on a more thorough comprehension of the regulatory and signal-transducing pathways that control patterns of cell movement and provide the growth control and direction necessary for the programmed development of form, tissue repair, and immune recognition.

ACKNOWLEDGMENT

I wish to thank Ms. Elena Fiamma for secretarial assistance.

References

1. Wilson, H. V.: On some phenomena of coalescence and regeneration in sponges. J. Exp. Zool. 5:245, 1907.
2. Moscona, A. A.: Cell suspensions from organ rudiments of chick embryos. Exp. Cell Res. 3:536, 1952.
3. Sperry, R. W.: Chemoaffinity in the orderly growth of nerve fiber patterns and connections. Proc. Natl. Acad. Sci. U.S.A. 50:703, 1963.
4. Edelman, G. M.: Cell adhesion and morphogenesis: the regulator hypothesis. Proc. Natl. Acad. Sci. U.S.A. 81:1460, 1984.
5. Williams, A. F., and Barclay, A. N.: The immunoglobulin superfamily—domains for cell surface recognition. Annu. Rev. Immunol. 6:381, 1988.
6. Stoolman, L. M.: Adhesion molecules controlling lymphocyte migration. Cell 56:907, 1989.
7. Arnaout, M. A.: Leukocyte adhesion molecules deficiency: Its structural basis, pathophysiology, and implications for modulating the inflammatory response. Immunol. Rev. 114:145, 1990.
8. Kieffer, N., and Phillips, D. R.: Platelet membrane glycoproteins: Functions in cellular interactions. Annu. Rev. Cell Biol. 6:329, 1990.
9. Takeichi, M.: The cadherins: cell-cell adhesion molecules controlling animal morphogenesis. Development 102:639, 1988.
10. Takeichi, M.: Cadherins: A molecular family important in selective cell-cell adhesion. Annu. Rev. Biochem. 59:237, 1990.
11. Gumbiner, B., and Simons, K.: A functional assay for proteins involved in establishing an epithelilial occluding barrier: Identification of a uvomorulin-like peptide. J. Cell Biol. 102:457, 1986.
12. Heimark, R. L., Degner, M., and Schwartz, S. M.: Identification of a Ca^{2+}-dependent cell-cell adhesion molecule in endothelial cells. J. Cell Biol. 110:1745, 1990.
13. Liaw, C. W., Cannon, C., Power, M. D., Kiboneka, P. K., and Rubin, L. L.: Identification and cloning of two species of cadherins in bovine endothelial cells. EMBO J. 9:2701, 1990.
14. McCrea, P. D., Turck, C. W., and Gumbiner, B.: A homolog of the *armadillo* protein in *Drosophila* (plakoglobin) associated with E-cadherin. Science 254:1359, 1991.
15. Bjorkman, P. J., Saper, M. A., Samraoui, B., Bennet, W. S., Strominger, J. L., and Wiley, D. C.: Structure of the human class I histocompatibility antigen HLA-A2. Nature (Lond.) 329:512, 1987.
16. Edelman, G. M.: Morphoregulatory molecules. Biochemistry 27:3533, 1988.
17. Edelman, G. M.: Cell adhesion molecules in the regulation of animal form and tissue pattern. Annu. Rev. Cell Biol. 2:81, 1986.
18. Dodd, J., and Jessell, T. M.: Axon guidance and the patterning of neuronal projections in vertebrates. Science 242:692, 1988.
19. Makgoba, M. W., Sanders, M. E., and Shaw, S.: The CD2–LFA-3 and LFA-1–ICAM pathways: relevance to T-cell recognition. Immunol. Today 10:417, 1989.
20. White, J. M., and Littman, D. R.: Viral receptors of the immunoglobulin superfamily. Cell 56:725, 1989.
21. Lin, S.-H., and Guidotti, G.: Cloning and expression of a cDNA coding for a rat liver plasma membrane ecto-ATPase. J. Biol. Chem. 264:14408, 1989.
22. Hynes, R. O.: Integrins: a family of cell surface receptors. Cell 48:549, 1987.
23. Hemler, M. E.: VLA proteins in the integrin family: structures, functions, and their role on leukocytes. Annu. Rev. Immunol. 8:365, 1990.
24. Arnaout, M. A.: Structure and function of the leukocyte adhesion molecules CD11/CD18. Blood 75:1037, 1990.
25. Ruoslahti, E., and Pierschbacher, M. D.: New perspectives in cell adhesion: RGD and integrins. Science (Wash.) 238:491, 1987.
25a. Sonnenberg, A., Calafat, J., Janssen, H., Daams, H., van der Raaij Helmer, L. M., Falcioni, R., Kennel, S. J., Aplin, J. D., Baker, J., Loizidou, M., and Garrod, D.: Integrin $\alpha6/\beta4$ complex is located in hemidesmosomes, suggesting a major role in epidermal cell–basement membrane adhesion. J. Cell Biol. 113:907, 1991.
26. Ignatius, M. J., Large, T. H., Houde, M., Tawil, J. W., Burton, A., Esch, F., Carbonetto, S., and Reichardt, L. F.: Molecular cloning of

the rat integrin α1-subunit: a receptor for laminin and collagen. J. Cell Biol. 111:709, 1990.

26a. Kramer, R. H., Vu, M. P., Cheng, Y. F., Ramos, D. M., Timpl, R., and Waleh, N.: Laminin-binding integrin α7β1: functional characterization and expression in normal and malignant melanocytes. Cell Regul. 2:805, 1991.

26b. Bossy, B., Bossy-Wetzel, E., and Reichardt, L. F.: Characterization of the integrin α8 subunit: a new integrin β1–associated subunit, which is prominently expressed on axons and on cells in contact with basal laminae in chick embryos. EMBO J. 10:2375, 1991.

27. Bonaldo, P., Russo, V., Bucciotti, F., Bressan, G. M., and Colombatti, A.: Alpha-1 chain of chick type VI collagen. J. Biol. Chem. 264:5575, 1989.

28. Kelly, T., Molony, L., and Burridge, K.: Purification of two smooth muscle glycoproteins related to integrin. J. Biol. Chem. 262:17189, 1987.

29. Nermut, M. V., Green, N. M., Eason, P., Yamada, S. S., and Yamad, K. M.: Electron microscopy and structural model of human fibronectin receptor. EMBO J. 7:4093, 1988.

30. Fox, G., Parry, N. R., Barnett, P. V., McGinn, B., Rowlands, D. J., and Brown, F.: The cell attachment site on foot-and-mouth disease virus includes the amino acid sequence RGD (arginine-glycine-aspartic acid). J. Gen. Virol. 70:625, 1989.

31. Brake, D. A., Debouck, C., and Biesecker, G.: Identification of an Arg-Gly-Asp (RGD) cell adhesion site in human immunodeficiency virus type I transactivating protein, tat. J. Cell Biol. 111:1275, 1990.

32. Isberg, R. R., and Leong, J. M.: Multiple β1 chain integrins are receptors for invasin, a protein that promotes bacterial penetration into mammalian cells. Cell 60:861, 1990.

33. Takada, Y., Elices, M. J., Crouse, C., and Hemler, M. E.: The primary structure of the α4 subunit of VLA4: Homology to other integrins and a possible cell-cell adhesion function. EMBO J. 8:1361, 1989.

34. Elices, M. J., Osborn, L., Takada, Y., Crouse, C., Luhowskyj, S., Hemier, M. E., and Lobb, R. R.: VCAM-1 on activated endothelium interacts with the leukocyte integrin VLA-4 at a site distinct from the VLA-4/fibronectin binding site. Cell 60:577, 1990.

35. Carter, W. G., Wayner, E. A., Bouchard, T. S., and Kaur, P.: The role of integrins α2β1 and α3β1 in cell-cell and cell-substrate adhesion of human epidermal cells. J. Cell Biol. 110:1387, 1990.

36. MacKrell, A. J., Blumberg, B., Haynes, S. R., and Fessler, J. H.: The lethal myospheroid gene of Drosophila encodes a membrane protein homologous to vertebrate integrin β subunits. Proc. Natl. Acad. Sci. U.S.A. 85:2633, 1988.

37. Haynes, B. F., Telen, M. J., Hale, L. P., and Denning, S. M.: CD44—a molecule involved in leukocyte adherence and T-cell activation. Immunol. Today 10:423, 1989.

38. Bierer, B. E., Peterson, A., Park, J., Remold-O'Donnell, E., Rosen, F. S., Seed, B., and Burakoff, S. J.: T cell activation: The T cell erythrocyte receptor (CD2) and sialophorin (CD43). Therp. Adv. Clin. Immunol. 8:51, 1988.

39. Gresham, H. D., Goodwin, J. L., Allen, P. M., Anderson, D. C., and Brown, E. J.: A novel member of the integrin receptor family mediates Arg-Gly-Asp–stimulated neutrophil phagocytosis. J. Cell. Biol. 108:1935, 1989.

39a. Takahashi, T., Nakamura, T., Koyanagi, M., Kato, K., Hashimoto, Y., Yagita, H., and Okumura, K.: A murine very late activation antigen–like extracellular matrix receptor involved in CD2- and lymphocyte function-associated antigen–1–independent killer-target cell interaction. J. Immunol. 145:4371, 1990.

40. Suzuki, S., and Naitoh, Y.: Amino acid sequence of a novel integrin β4 subunit and primary expression of the mRNA in epithelial cells. EMBO J. 9:757, 1990.

41. Sheppard, D., Rozzo, C., Starr, L., Quaranta, V., Erle, D. J., and Pytela, R.: Complete amino acid sequence of a novel integrin β subunit (β6) identified in epithelial cells using the polymerase chain reaction. J. Biol. Chem. 265:11502, 1990.

42. Kajiji, S., Tamura, R. N., and Quaranta, V.: A novel integrin (αE-β4) from human epithelial cells suggests a fourth family of integrin adhesion receptors. EMBO J. 8:673, 1989.

42a. Hogervorst, F., Kuikman, I., van Kessel, A. G., and Sonnenberg, A.: Molecular cloning of the human α6 integrin subunit. Alternative splicing of α6 mRNA and chromosomal localization of the α6 and β5 genes. Eur. J. Biochem. 199:425, 1991.

43. Holtzmann, B., and Weissman, I. L.: Peyer's patch–specific lymphocyte homing receptors consist of a VLA-4–like α chain associated with either of two integrin β chains, one of which is novel. EMBO J. 8:1735, 1989.

44. Ramaswamy, H., and Hemler, M. E.: Cloning, primary structure and properties of a novel human integrin β subunit. EMBO J. 9:1561, 1990.

45. Erle, D. J., Ruegg, C., Sheppard, D., and Pytela, R.: Complete amino acid sequence of an integrin beta subunit (β7) identified in leukocytes. J. Biol. Chem. 266:11009, 1991.

45a. Moyle, M., Napier, M. A., and McLean, J. W.: Cloning and expression of a divergent integrin subunit β8. J. Biol. Chem. 266:19650, 1991.

45b. Dedhar, S., Robertson, K., and Gray, V.: Induction of expression of the αvβ1 and αvβ3 integrin heterodimers during retinoic acid–induced

neurol differentiation of murine embryonal carcinoma cells. J. Biol. Chem. 266:21846, 1991.

45c. Parker, C. M., Cepek, K., Russell, G. J., Shaw, S. K., Posnett, D., Schwarting, R., and Brenner, M. B.: A family of B7 integrins on human mucosal lymphocytes. Proc. Natl. Acad. Sci. 89:1924, 1992.

46. Bodary, S. C., and Mclean, J. W.: The integrin β1 subunit associates with the vitronectin receptor αV subunit to form a novel vitronectin receptor in human embryonic kidney cell line. J. Biol. Chem. 265:5938, 1990.

47. Vogel, B. E., Tarone, G., Giancotti, F. G., Gailit, J., and Ruoslahti, E.: A novel fibronectin receptor with an unexpected subunit composition (αvβ1). J. Biol. Chem. 265:5934, 1990.

48. Humphries, M. J., Akiyama, S. K., Komoriya, A., Olden, K., and Yamada, K. M.: Identification of an alternatively spliced site in human plasma fibronectin that mediates cell-type–specific adhesion. J. Cell Biol. 103:2637, 1986.

49. Wayner, E. A., and Carter, W. G.: Identification of multiple cell adhesion receptor for collagen and fibronectin in human fibrosarcoma cells possessing unique α and β subunits. J. Cell Biol. 105:1873, 1987.

50. D'Souza, S. E., Ginsberg, M. H., Burke, T. A., Lam, S. C., and Plow, E. F.: Localization of an Arg-Gly-Asp recognition site within an integrin adhesion receptor. Science (Wash.) 242:91, 1988.

51. D'Souza, S. E., Ginsberg, M. H., Burke, T. A., and Plow, E. F.: The ligand-binding site of the platelet integrin receptor GP IIb-IIIa is proximal to the second calcium-binding domain of its α-subunit. J. Biol. Chem. 265:3440, 1990.

52. Ignotz, R. A., Heino, J., and Massagué, J.: Regulation of cell adhesion receptors by transforming growth factor-β. J. Biol. Chem. 264:92, 1989.

53. Arencibia, I., and Sundqvist, K.-G.: Collagen receptor on T lymphocytes and the control of lymphocyte motility. Eur. J. Immunol. 19:929, 1989.

54. Shimizu, Y., van Seventer, G. A., Horgan, K. J., and Shaw, S.: Regulated expression and binding of three VLA (β1) integrin receptors on T cells. Nature (Lond.) 345:250, 1990.

55. Coller, B. S.: A new murine monoclonal antibody reports an activation-dependent change in the conformation and/or microenvironment of the platelet glycoprotein IIb/IIIa complex. J. Clin. Invest. 76:101, 1985.

56. Staatz, W. D., Rajpara, S. M., Wayner, E. A., Carter, W. G., and Santoro, S. A.: The membrane glycoprotein Ia-IIa (VLA-2) complex mediates the Mg++-dependent adhesion of platelets to collagen. J. Cell Biol. 108:1917, 1989.

57. Elices, M. J., Urry, L. A., and Hemler, M. E.: Receptor functions for the integrin VLA-3: Fibronectin, collagen, and laminin binding are differentially influenced by ARG-GLY-ASP peptide and by divalent cations. J. Biol. Chem. 112:169, 1991.

58. Sonnenberg, A., Modderman, P. W., and Hogervorst, F.: Laminin receptor on platelets is the integrin VLA-6. Nature (Lond.) 360:487, 1988.

58a. Altruda, F., Cervella, P., Tarone, G., Botta, C., Balzac, F., Stefanuto, G., and Silengo, L.: A human integrin β1 subunit with a unique cytoplasmic domain generated by alternative mRNA processing. Gene 95:261, 1990.

59. van Kuppevelt, T. H., Languino, L. R., Gailit, J. O., Suzuki, S., and Ruoslahti, E.: An alternative cytoplasmic domain of the integrin β3-subunit. Proc. Natl. Acad. Sci. U.S.A. 86:5415, 1989.

59a. Tamura, R. N., Cooper, H. M., Collo, G., and Quaranta, V.: Cell type–specific integrin variants with alternative α-chain cytoplasmic domains. Proc. Natl. Acad. Sci. U.S.A. 88:10183, 1991.

60. Kirchhofer, D., Languino, L. R., Ruoslahti, E., and Pierschbacher, M. D.: α2β1 integrins from different cell types show different binding specificities. J. Biol. Chem. 265:615, 1990.

61. Rettig, W. J., Murty, V. V., Mattes, M. J., Chaganti, R. S., and Old, L. J.: Extracellular matrix–modulated expression of human cell surface glycoproteins A42 and J143: intrinsic and extrinsic signals determine antigenic phenotype. J. Exp. Med. 164:1581, 1986.

62. Hynes, R. O.: Fibronectins. New York, Springer-Verlag, 1990.

63. Osborn, L., Hession, C., Tizard, R., Vassallo, C., Luhowskyj, S., Chi-Rosso, G., and Lobb, R.: Direct expression cloning of vascular cell adhesion molecule-1, a cytokine-induced endothelial protein that binds to lymphocytes. Cell 59:1203, 1989.

64. Matsuyama, T., Yamada, A., Kay, J., Yamada, K. M., Akiyama, S. K., Schlossman, S. F., and Morimoto, C.: Activation of CD4 cells by fibronectin and anti-CD3 antibody: A synergistic effect mediated by the VLA-5 fibronectin receptor complex. J. Exp. Med. 170:1133, 1989.

65. Wright, S. D., Craigmyle, L. S., and Silverstein, S. C.: Fibronectin and serum amyloid-P component stimulate C3b- and C3bi-mediated phagocytosis in cultured human monocytes. J. Exp. Med. 158:1338, 1983.

66. Detmers, P. A., Wright, S. D., Olsen, E., Kimball, B., and Cohn, Z. A.: Aggregation of complement receptors on human neutrophils in the absence of ligand. J. Cell Biol. 105:1137, 1987.

67. Isenberg, W. M., McEver, R. P., Philips, D. R., Shuman, M. A., and Bainton, D. F.: The platelet fibrinogen receptor: An immunogold surface replica study of agonist-induced ligand binding and receptor clustering. J. Cell Biol. 104:1655, 1987.

68. Pardi, R., Bender, J. R., Dettori, C., Gianazza, E., and Engleman, E.

G.: Heterogeneous distribution and transmembrane signalling properties of lymphocyte-function–associated antigen (LFA-1) in human lymphocyte subsets. J. Immunol. 143:3157, 1989.

69. Ding, A., Wright, S. W., and Nathan, C.: Activation of mouse peritoneal macrophages by monoclonal antibodies to MAC-1 (complement receptor type 3). J. Exp. Med. 165:733, 1987.

70. Ferrell, J. E., and Martin, G. S.: Tyrosine-specific protein phosphorylation is regulated by glycoprotein IIb/IIIa in platelets. Proc. Natl. Acad. Sci. U.S.A. 86:2234, 1989.

71. Banga, H. S., Simons, E. R., Brass, L. F., and Rittenhouse, S. E.: Activation of phospholipase A and C in human platelets exposed to epinephrine: Role of glycoproteins IIb/IIIa and dual role of epinephrine. Proc. Natl. Acad. Sci. U.S.A. 83:9197, 1989.

72. Werb, Z., Tremble, P. M., Behrendtsen, E., Crowley, E., and Damsky, C. H.: Signal transduction through the fibronectin receptor induces collagenase and stromelysin gene expression. J. Cell Biol. 109:877, 1989.

72a. Yamada, A., Nikaido, T., Nojima, Y., Schlossman, S. F., and Morimoto, C.: Activation of human CD4 T lymphocytes. Interaction of fibronectin with VLA-A receptor on CD4 cells induces the AP-1 transcription factor. J. Immunol. 146:53, 1991.

73. Brandley, B. K., Swiedler, S. J., and Robbins, P. W.: Carbohydrate ligands of the LEC cell adhesion molecules. Cell 63:861, 1990.

74. Bevilacqua, M. P., Stengalin, M. P., Gimbrone, M. A., and Seed, B.: Endothelial leukocyte adhesion molecule 1: An inducible receptor for neutrophils related to complement regulatory proteins and lectins. Science 243:1160, 1989.

75. Johnston, G. I., Cook, R. G., and McEver, R. P.: Cloning of GMP-140, a granule membrane protein of platelets and endothelium: Sequence similarity to proteins involved in cell adhesion and inflammation. Cell 56:1033, 1989.

76. Lasky, L. A., Singer, M. S., Yednock, T. A., Dowbenko, D., Fennie, C., Rodriguez, H., Nguyen, T., Stachel, H., and Rosen, S. D.: Cloning of a lymphocyte homing receptor reveals a lectin domain. Cell 56:1045, 1989.

77. Tedder, T. F., Isaacs, C. M., Ernst, T. J., Demetri, G. D., Adler, D. A., and Disteche, C. M.: Isolation and chromosomal localization of cDNA's encoding a novel human lymphocyte surface molecule LAM-1. Homology of the mouse lymphocyte homing receptor and other human adhesion proteins. J. Exp. Med. 170:123, 1989.

78. Gallatin, W. M., Weisman, I. L., and Butcher, E. C.: Cell-surface molecule involved in organ-specific homing of lymphocytes. Nature (Lond.) 304:30, 1983.

79. Mountz, J. D., Gause, W. C., Finkleman, F. D., and Steinberg, A. D.: Prevention of lymphadenopathy in MRL-lpr/lpr mice by blocking peripheral lymph node homing with MEL-14 in vivo. J. Immunol. 140:2943, 1988.

80. Jutila, M. A., Rott, L., Berg, E. L., and Butcher, E. C.: Function and regulation of the neutrophil MEL-14 antigen in vivo: comparison with LFA-1 and MAC-1. J. Immunol. 143:3318, 1989.

81. Luscinskas, F. W., Brock, A. F., Arnaout, M. A., and Gimbrone, M. A.: Endothelial-leukocyte adhesion molecule-1 (ELAM-1)–dependent and leukocyte (CD11/18)-dependent mechanisms contribute to polymorphonuclear leukocyte adhesion to cytokine-activated human vascular endothelium. J. Immunol. 142:2257, 1989.

82. Gamble, J. R., Skinner, M. P., Brendt, M. C., and Vadas, M. A.: Prevention of activated neutrophil adhesion to endothelium by soluble adhesion protein GMP 140. Science (Wash.) 249:414, 1990.

83. Larsen, E., Palabrica, T., Sajer, S., Gilbert, G. E., Wagner, D. D., Furie, B. C., and Furie, B.: PADGEM-dependent adhesion of platelets to monocytes and neutrophils is mediated by a lineage-specific carbohydrate, LNF III (CD15). Cell 63:467, 1990.

84. Lowe, J. B., Stoolman, L. M., Nair, R. P., Larsen, R. D., Behrend, T. L., and Marks, R. M.: ELAM-1–dependent cell adhesion to vascular endothelium determined by a transfected human fucosyltransferase cDNA. Cell 63:475, 1990.

85. Philips, M. L., Nudelman, E., Gaeta, F. C. A., Perez, M., Singhal, A. K., Hakomori, S., and Paulson, J. C.: ELAM-1 mediates cell adhesion by recognition of a carbohydrate ligand, sialyl-Lex. Science (Wash.) 250:1130, 1990.

86. Tiemeyer, M., Sweidler, S. J., Ishihara, M., Moreland, M., Schweingruber, H., Hirtzer, P., and Brandley, B. K.: Carbohydrate ligands for endothelial-leukocyte adhesion molecule 1. Proc. Natl. Acad. Sci. U.S.A. 88:1138, 1991.

87. True, D. D., Singer, M. S., Lasky, L. A., and Rosen, S. D.: Requirement for sialic acid on the endothelial ligand of a lymphocyte homing receptor. J. Cell Biol. 111:2757, 1990.

88. Walz, G., Aruffo, A., Kolanus, W., Bevilacqua, M., and Seed, B.: Recognition by ELAM-1 of the sialyl-Lex determinant on myeloid and tumor cells. Science (Wash.) 250:1132, 1990.

89. Carlos, T. M., and Haraln, J. M.: Membrane proteins involved in phagocyte adherence to endothelium. Immunol. Rev. 114:5, 1990.

90. Kishimoto, T. K., Jutila, M. A., Berg, E. L., and Butcher, E. C.: Neutrophil Mac-1 and Mel-14 adhesion proteins are inversely regulated by chemotactic factors. Science (Wash.) 245:1238, 1989.

91. Marcus, A. J.: Thrombosis and inflammation as multicellular processes: Pathophysiologic significance of transcellular metabolism. Blood 76:1903, 1990.

92. Streeter, P. R., Berg, E. L., Rouse, B. T. N., Bargatz, R. F., and Butcher, E. C.: A tissue-specific endothelial cell molecule involved in lymphocyte homing. Nature (Lond.) 331:41, 1988.

93. Stamenkovic, I., Amiot, M., Pesando, J. M., and Seed, B.: A lymphocyte molecule implicated in lymph node homing is a member of the cartilage link protein family. Cell 56:1057, 1989.

94. Goldstein, L. A., Zhou, D. F. H., Picker, L. J., Minty, C. N., Bargatze, R. F., Ding, J. F., and Butcher, E. C.: A human lymphocyte homing receptor, the hermes antigen, is related to cartilage proteoglycan core and link proteins. Cell 56:1063, 1989.

95. Aruffo, A., Stamenkovic, I., Melnick, M., Underhill, C. B., and Seed, B.: CD44 is the principal cell surface receptor for hyaluronate. Cell 61:1303, 1990.

96. Carter, W. G., and Wayner, E. A.: Characterization of the class III collagen receptor, a phosphorylated transmembrane glycoprotein expressed in nucleated human cells. J. Biol. Chem. 263:4193, 1988.

97. Green, S. J., Tarone, G., and Underhill, C. B.: Aggregation of macrophages and fibroblasts is inhibited by a monoclonal antibody to the hyaluronate receptor. Exp. Cell Res. 178:224, 1988.

98. Miyake, K., Medina, K. L., Hayashi, S. I., Ono, S., Hamaoka, T., and Kincaide, P. W.: Monoclonal antibodies to Pgp-1/CD44 block lymphohempoiesis in long-term bone marrow cultures. 171:477, 1990.

99. Saunders, S., Jalkanen, M., O'Farrell, S., and Bernfield, M.: Molecular cloning of syndecan, an integral membrane proteogylcan. J. Cell Biol. 108:1547, 1989.

100. Saksela, O., Moscatelli, D., Sommer, A., and Rifkin, D. B.: Endothelial cell–derived heparan sulphate binds basic fibroblast growth factor and protects it from proteolytic degradation. J. Cell Biol. 107:743, 1988.

101. Bernstein, I. D., Andrews, R. G., Cohen, S. F., and McMaster, B. E.: Normal and malignant human myelocytic and monocytic cells identified by monoclonal antibodies. J. Immunol. 128:876, 1982.

102. Oquendo, P., Hundt, E., Lawler, J., and Seed, B.: CD36 directly mediates cytoadherence of Plasmodium falciparum–parasitized erythrocytes. Cell 58:95, 1989.

103. Asch, A. S., Barnwell, J., Silverstein, R. L., and Nachman, R. L.: Isolation of the thrombospondin membrane receptor. J. Clin. Invest. 79:1054, 1987.

104. Tandon, N., Kralisc, U., and Jamieson, G. A.: Identification of glycoprotein IV (CD36) as a primary receptor for platelet collagen adhesion. J. Biol. Chem. 264:7576, 1989.

105. Fox, J. E. B., Aggerbeck, L. A., and Berndt, M. C.: Structure of the glycoprotein Ib-IX complex from platelet membranes. J. Biol. Chem. 263:1525, 1988.

106. Takahashi, N., Takahashi, Y., and Putman, F. W.: Periodicity of leucine and tandem repetition of a 24 amino acid segment in the primary structure of leucine-rich α_2-glycoprotein of human serum. Proc. Natl. Acad. Sci. U.S.A. 82:1906, 1985.

107. Heingard, D., and Oldberg, A.: Structure and biology of cartilage and bone matrix noncollagenous macromolecules. FASEB J. 3:2042, 1989.

108. Lopez, J. A., Chung, D. W., Fujikawa, K., Hagen, F. S., Papayannopoulou, T., and Roth, G. J.: Cloning of the α chain of human platelet glycoprotein Ib: α transmembrane protein with homology to leucine-rich α_2-glycoprotein. Proc. Natl. Acad. Sci. U.S.A. 84:5615, 1987.

109. Muszbeck, L., and Laposata, M.: Glycoprotein Ib and glycoprotein IX in human platelets are acylated with palmitic acid through thioester linkage. J. Biol. Chem. 264:9716, 1989.

110. Fox, J. E. B., Boyles, J. K., Berndt, M. C., Steffen, P. K., and Anderson, L. K.: Identification of a membrane skeleton in platelets. J. Cell Biol. 106:1525, 1988.

111. Shelley, C. S., Remold-O'Donnell, E., Davis, A. E., III, Bruns, G. A. P., Rosen, F. S., Carroll, M. C., and Whitehead, A. S.: Molecular characterization of sialophorin (CD43), the lymphocyte surface sialoglycoprotein defective in Wiskott-Aldrich syndrome. Proc. Natl. Acad. Sci. U.S.A. 86:2819, 1989.

112. Nong, Y.-H., Remold-O'Donnell, E., LeBien, T. W., and Remold, H. G.: A monoclonal antibody to sialophorin (CD43) induces homotypic adhesion and activation of human monocytes. J. Exp. Med. 170:259, 1989.

113. Barton, R. W., Rothlein, R., Ksiazek, J., and Kennedy, C.: The effect of anti-intercellular adhesion molecule on phorbol ester–induced rabbit lung inflammation. J. Immunol. 143:1278, 1989.

114. Cosimi, A. B., Conti, D., Delmonico, F. L., Preffer, F. I., Wee, S.-L., Rothlein, R., Faanes, R., and Colvin, R. B.: In vivo effects of mAb to ICAM-1 (CD54) in non-human primates with renal allografts. J. Immunol. 144:4604, 1990.

115. Geng, J.-G., Bevilacqua, M. P., Moore, K. L., McIntyre, T. M., Prescott, S. M., Kim, J. M., Bliss, G. A., Zimmerman, G. A., and McEver, R. P.: Rapid neutrophil adhesion to activated endothelium mediated by GMP-140. Nature 343:757, 1990.

116. Watson, S. R., Fennie, C., and Lasky, L. A.: Neutrophil influx into an inflammatory site inhibited by a soluble homing receptor-IgG chimaera. Nature 349:164, 1991.

117. Osborn, L.: Leukocyte adhesion to endothelium in inflammation. Cell 62:3, 1990.
118. Dalgleish, A. G., Beverley, P. C., Clapham, P. R., Crawford, D. H., Greaves, M. F., and Weiss, R. A.: The CD4 (T4) antigen is an essential component of the receptor for the AIDS retrovirus. Nature (Lond.) 312:763, 1984.
119. Klatzmann, D., Champagne, E., Chamaret, S., Gruest, J., Guetard, D., Hercend, T., Gluckman, J. C., and Montagnier, L.: T-lymphocyte T4 molecule behaves as the receptor for human retrovirus LAV. Nature (Lond.) 312:767, 1984.
120. Greve, J. M., Davis, G., Meyer, A. M., Forte, C. P., Yost, S. C., Marlor, C. W., Kamarck, M. E., and McClelland, A.: The major human rhinovirus receptor is ICAM-1. Cell 56:839, 1989.
121. Mendelsohn, C. L., Wimmer, E., and Racaniello, V. R.: Cellular receptor for poliovirus: Molecular cloning, nucleotide sequence, and expression of a new member of the immunoglobulin superfamily. Cell 56:855, 1989.
122. Kaplan, G., Peters, D., and Racaniello, V. R.: Poliovirus mutants resistant to neutralization with soluble cell receptors. Microbiology 250:1596, 1990.
123. Coller, B. S.: Platelets and thrombolytic therapy. N. Engl. J. Med. 322:33, 1990.
124. Kirchhofer, D., Gailit, J., Ruoslahti, E., Grzesiak, J., and Pierschbacher, M. D.: Cation-dependent modulation of GPIIb/IIIa ligand specificity. J. Biol. Chem. 265:18525, 1990.
125. Cook, J. J., Huang, T. F., Rucinski, B., Strzyzewski, M., Tuma, R. F., Williams, J. A., and Niewiarowski, S.: Inhibition of platelet hemostatic plug formation by trigramin. Am. J. Physiol. 256:H1038, 1989.
126. Clark, R. A.: Fibronectin matrix deposition and fibronectin receptor expression in healing and normal skin. J. Invest. Dermatol. 94:128S, 1990.
127. Davis, G. E., Blaker, S. N., Engvall, E., Varon, S., Manthorpe, M., and Gage, F. H.: Human amnion membrane serves as a substratum for growing axons in vitro and in vivo. Science (Wash.) 236:1106, 1987.
128. Jalkanen, S., Wu, N., Bargatze, R. F., and Butcher, E. C.: Human lymphocytes and lymphoma homing receptors. Annu. Rev. Med. 38:467, 1987.
129. Fearon, E. R., Cho, K. R., Nigro, J. M., Kern, S. E., Simons, J. W., and Ruppert, J. M.: Identification of a chromosome 18q gene that is altered in colorectal cancers. Science 247:49, 1990.
130. Ruoslahti, E.: Integrins. J. Clin. Invest. 87:1, 1991.
131. Giancotti, F. G., and Ruoslahti, E.: Elevated levels of $\alpha5\beta1$ fibronectin receptor suppress the transformed phenotype of Chinese hamster ovary cells. Cell 60:849, 1990.
132. McGregor, B. C., McGregor, J. L., Weiss, L. M., Wood, G. S., Hu, C. H., Boukerche, H., and Warnke, R. A.: Presence of cytoadhesins (IIb/IIIa-like glycoproteins) on human metastatic melanomas but not on benign melanocytes. Am. J. Clin. Pathol. 92:495, 1989.
133. Natali, P., Nicotra, M. R., Calabro, A., Bigotti, A., Romano, G., Temponi, M., and Ferrone, S.: Differential expression of intercellular adhesion molecule-1 (ICAM-1) in primary and metastatic melanoma lesions. Cancer Res. 50:1271, 1990.
134. Humphries, M. J., Yamada, K. M., and Olden, K.: Investigation of the biologic effects of anti–cell adhesion synthetic peptides that inhibit experimental metastasis of B16-F10 melanoma cells. J. Clin. Invest. 81:782, 1988.
135. Taylor, H. C., Lightner, V. A., Beyer, W. F., Jr., McCaslin, D., Briscoe, G., and Erickson, H. P.: Biochemical and structural studies of tenascin/hexabrachion proteins. J. Cell. Biochem. 41:71, 1989.
136. Drickamer, K.: Two distinct classes of carbohydrate-recognition domains in animal lectins. J. Biol. Chem. 263:9557, 1988.

Chapter 13

William P. Arend
Jean-Michel Dayer

Cytokines and Growth Factors

INTRODUCTION

An important advancement in basic science over the past 10 to 20 years has been a greater understanding of how cells communicate with each other. During embryogenesis as well as in normal functioning of the mature organism, soluble molecules transmit information between cells. These mediators are released by cells of origin in response to specific signals and influence the response and function of target cells largely through exerting a positive or negative influence on gene expression. In addition to playing an important role in normal physiology, unregulated or excess effects of these soluble polypeptides are thought to be involved in mediating pathophysiologic events in many human autoimmune or inflammatory diseases.

These molecules of cell communication are known as interleukins (ILs), interferons (INFs), growth factors, and colony-stimulating factors.[1] *Cytokines* is a generic term referring to factors released by cells, *lymphokines* implying an origin from lymphocytes, and *monokines*, a derivation from monocytes. Cytokines are involved in the growth and differentiation of normal cells, primarily of the hematopoietic system or of mesenchymal origin. An important general principle is that each cytokine exhibits multiple effects, opposing and antagonizing, or supplementing and synergizing with other cytokines. Thus, a biologic response observed in cell culture in vitro or in a tissue in vivo represents the net effects of multiple factors.

Cytokines are particularly important as local mediators of intercellular communication in normal or diseased tissues.[2] These factors may act on the same cell that produced them in an *autocrine* fashion or on adjacent cells in a *paracrine* fashion (Fig. 13–1). Autocrine stimulation can occur in two ways: either a released cytokine interacting with cell surface receptors, or an intracellular factor binding with internal receptors without ever being secreted. Cytokines may also function in an *endocrine* fashion through exerting effects at a distance from the tissue of origin. In addition, some cytokines may remain associated with the cell surface and act through direct cell contact. By all mechanisms, cytokines bind to specific receptors on target cells and induce intracellular

signal transduction pathways. The resultant biologic responses to soluble or membrane-bound cytokines are determined by changes in gene transcription, mRNA translation, and protein synthesis and secretion.

This chapter summarizes recent information on those cytokines that have particular effects on cells of the immune or inflammatory systems. It should be emphasized that the research field of cytokine biology is progressing rapidly. Knowledge concerning the possible role of cytokines in specific rheumatic disease processes is in its infancy and should greatly expand over the next decade.

INTERLEUKIN-1

History. During the past 50 years, investigators working in different areas have been convinced that phagocytic cells such as monocyte-macrophages or polymorphonuclear cells release polypeptides that are highly relevant to inflammation and immunity. At an early descriptive stage, it was considered that endogenous pyrogens (EPs) originated from neutrophils and immunologic peptides (lymphokines) from

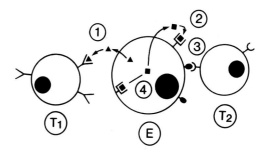

Figure 13–1. Different mechanisms of intercellular communication mediated by cytokines. In a paracrine manner (1), a cytokine-producing effector cell (E) releases a cytokine molecule (solid triangle) that interacts with a nearby target cell (T₁). An autocrine pathway (2) results when an effector cell (E) secretes a cytokine molecule (solid squares) that interacts with its receptor on the surface of the same cell. Direct cell-cell communication (3) occurs when a membrane-bound cytokine on the effector cell interacts with an appropriate receptor on a contiguous target cell (T₂). Lastly, a modified autocrine pathway (4) may exist when an intracellular cytokine (squares) interacts with its receptor on the inside of the cell. (From Kelley, J.: Cytokines of the lung. Am. Rev. Respir. Dis. 141:765, 1990. Used by permission.)

227

lymphocytes (reviewed in references 3 and 4). The notion of monokines was first introduced as lymphocyte-activating factor (LAF) in 1972. EP from human monocytes was purified to homogeneity at the same time as human mononuclear cell factor (MCF), which stimulates the production of collagenase and prostaglandin E_2 in human synovial cells. It was established subsequently that MCF was identical to LAF, the latter being purified to homogeneity. The term *interleukin-1* was coined at the Second International Lymphokine Workshop held in Ermatingen, Switzerland, in 1979. By that time it was clear that different individual biologic activities found within the culture medium of stimulated monocyte-macrophages were probably manifestations of a single molecule or a family of very closely related peptides. This was formally established in 1984 to 1985 by the cloning of two different genes that code for two distinct proteins: (IL-1α) and (IL-1β).[5]

Protein Chemistry and Gene Structure of Interleukin-1. There are two mature forms of IL-1 (reviewed in references 3 and 5). IL-1α is composed of 159 amino acids (17.5 kD, pI 5) and is mainly cell associated (95 percent), although the degree varies with the cells and the stimuli. IL-1β consists of 153 amino acids (17.3 kD, pI 7) and is mainly released into the extracellular environment after stimulation. IL-1β has a three-dimensional structure of a stable globular protein formed by six pairs of antiparallel β strands. The mature forms of human IL-1α and IL-1β share only 26 percent amino acid sequence homology. The two forms of IL-1 are initially synthesized as 31-kD precursor polypeptides, 271 amino acids for IL-1α and 269 for IL-1β. Only the precursor forms of IL-1 exist inside the cell, and they are present in the cytosolic fraction. Neither form contains a hydrophobic signal peptide sequence that could mediate secretion; the mechanisms of IL-1 egress remain unclear. The precursor form of IL-1α is biologically active, whereas the 31-kD form of IL-1β is inactive. Cleavage of the carboxy-terminal portion of the 31-kD peptides by nonspecific proteases (e.g., elastase, plasmin) or by specific proteases such as IL-1β convertase[6] in the cell microenvironment produces mature 17-kD IL-1. Membrane-bound IL-1α probably originates from endogenous movement of the precursor molecule to the cell surface, although some investigators favor the concept of exogenous binding of released IL-1α to receptors.

Both IL-1α and IL-1β genes are located on the second human chromosome comprising 12 and 9.7 kilobase (kb) of DNA, respectively, and both genes contain seven exons. The promoter region of the IL-1β genomic DNA contains tissue-specific regulatory sequences as well as consensus sequences responsive to stimulation by lipopolysaccharide (LPS) and phorbol esters. In response to specific agents, IL-1β mRNA accumulates 10- to 500-fold more than IL-1α mRNA, but both are short lived. The translated protein products are detectable 15 to 30 minutes after stimulation.

Regulation of Interleukin-1 Production. Almost any cell perturbation can induce IL-1 gene expression, particularly in monocytes. These stimuli can be manifold and include direct cell contact, extracellular matrix elements, soluble factors, certain forms of soluble immune complexes, complement fragments, crystals, bacteria, and viruses. The relative importance of some of these inducing agents is still difficult to assess because minute amounts (ng to pg) of contaminating LPS can trigger IL-1 production. Among the cytokines known to stimulate IL-1 production, tumor necrosis factor-α (TNF-α) appears to be important,[7] but IL-1 can also induce its own production in an autocrine or paracrine fashion. The leukotriene B_4 (LTB$_4$) appears to stimulate IL-1 production, whereas prostaglandin E_2 has the opposite effect.

Cellular Sources of Interleukin-1. Activated monocytes are a major source of IL-1 (100 ng per 10^6 cells per 48 hours for IL-1β, and ten times less for IL-1α). With the exception of red blood cells and platelets, however, almost all cells can produce IL-1 to some extent. Monocytes and macrophages are the primary cells responsible for producing large amounts of IL-1. Activated T cells contain IL-1α, which may be membrane associated, possibly playing a role in the initiation of the immune response. Among other cells relevant to the inflammatory response that can produce IL-1 are endothelial cells, B cells (Epstein-Barr virus–transformed B cells), and occasionally dermal or synovial fibroblasts. Finally, microglial cells in the central nervous system produce IL-1, and it is known that IL-1 can induce slow-wave sleep, fever, decreased appetite, and hormones controlled by the hypothalamus.[3]

Signal Transduction Mediated by Interleukin-1 and Receptors. High-affinity cell membrane receptors for IL-1 have been characterized and two distinct receptors (types I and II) have been cloned (reviewed in references 8 through 10). Both IL-1α and IL-1β appear to bind to both IL-1 receptors but not with equivalent avidity. Type I IL-1 receptors are approximately 80 kD and are present on T cells, endothelial cells, epithelial cells, and chondrocytes. Type II IL-1 receptors are approximately 56 kD and can be found on B cells, neutrophils, and macrophages. Both receptors are sparsely present, i.e., approximately 100 to 2000 receptors per cell. The mechanisms of IL-1–induced signal transduction remain unclear and may vary with the target cell.[11, 12] IL-1 induces phosphorylation of 27-, 44-, and 65-kD intracellular proteins; the former is a heat-shock protein (HSP 27). Depending on the cells examined and their relative degree of differentiation, IL-1 can activate phospholipase A or C activity, induce Ca^{2+} influx, stimulate cyclic AMP (cAMP) production, enhance phosphoinositol metabolism, or induce ornithine decarboxylase activity. IL-1 can also induce the oncogenes c-*jun*, c-*fos*, or c-*myc*. The importance of IL-1 as an activator of cells depends on the state of differentiation of specific target cells and on the coupling of signal transduction

Table 13–1. BIOLOGIC EFFECTS OF IL-1 THAT MAY
OCCUR IN RA

Systemic
  Fever
  Decreased appetite
  Muscle breakdown
  Synthesis of acute-phase proteins
  Increased GM-CSF production
Local
  Prostaglandin E$_2$, collagenase, and neutral protease production
    by fibroblasts and chondrocytes
  Chemotaxis of polymorphonuclear leukocytes, lymphocytes,
    and monocytes
  Adherence of white blood cells to endothelial cells
  Fibroblast proliferation
  Increased production of collagen and an inhibitor of neutral
    proteases
  Stimulation of T and B lymphocytes

mechanisms to activation of particular genes in each target cell.

Systemic and Local Effects of Interleukin-1 on Immune and Inflammatory Diseases. The systemic effects of IL-1, which include the induction of metabolic changes, extend to the central nervous system, bone marrow, blood vessel walls, the liver, and other tissues[3-5] (Table 13–1). The metabolic effects of IL-1 include an increase in adrenocorticotropic hormone, corticosteroids, and hepatic proteins (C-reactive protein, serum amyloid A, and complement components), and a decrease in plasma zinc, iron, albumin, and transferrin. The induction of the acute-phase proteins, however, is mainly mediated by IL-6, the principal hepatocyte-stimulating factor. Together with TNF-α, IL-1 may contribute to the anemia observed in many inflammatory diseases such as rheumatoid arthritis (RA). This effect is probably due to the marked suppression by these cytokines of colony formation by erythroid progenitor cells.

The local effects of IL-1 on both immune and inflammatory cells may be more important to inflammatory joint diseases, such as RA.[13-15] These effects of IL-1 include enhancement in T and B lymphocyte function; chemotaxis of neutrophils, lymphocytes, and monocytes; and increased expression of adhesion molecules on endothelial cells. IL-1 may further enhance chemotaxis indirectly by inducing the release of other chemoattractant cytokines. IL-1 may be involved in early events in rheumatoid synovitis by assisting in the migration of other cells and by stimulating a variety of responses in endothelial cells. Probably the most important aspect of IL-1 at the local level is its effect on tissue destruction: IL-1 stimulates the production of collagenase and other neutral proteinases, and of prostaglandin E$_2$ by synovial cells, chondrocytes, and bone-derived cells.

On the other hand, IL-1 may contribute to joint scarring and fibrosis through other mechanisms[15] including stimulation of fibroblast proliferation either directly or indirectly through inducing platelet-derived growth factor (PDGF) production. IL-1 may also induce the fibroblast production of fibronectin,

type I collagen, proteoglycans, and an inhibitor of collagenase and other neutral proteases. In addition, IL-1 alters collagen production in chondrocytes, reducing production of type II collagen and enhancing synthesis of types I and III collagen. Because type II collagen is the predominant form in articular cartilage, this effect of IL-1 may result in a further weakening of the joint. Furthermore, collagen types II, III, and IX may stimulate IL-1 production. Finally, IL-1 has complex effects on proteoglycans in cartilage, inhibiting synthesis and enhancing degradation.[16]

The effects of IL-1 on synovial fibroblasts and chondrocytes represent an example of agonist and antagonist influences occurring simultaneously.[15] Collagenase and its inhibitor may be produced at the same time by the same cells; the relative amounts of induction of each may vary according to the cell stimulus. In addition, both collagenase and collagen may be synthesized simultaneously, although the collagen type that is produced may lead to fibrosis instead of adequate tissue repair. Thus, the degree and distribution of destruction in the rheumatoid joint may depend partly on the relative production of collagenase, enzyme inhibitors, and collagen by chondrocytes and synovial fibroblasts. However, it has not been determined in humans whether all of these in vitro effects of IL-1 on cell functions also occur in vivo.

There is now strong evidence for the presence and role of IL-1 in inflammatory joint diseases.[15] In these diseases, IL-1 may be more important as a local mediator of cell-cell communication than as a systemic mediator.

Interleukin-1 in Experimental Synovitis in Vivo. Observations in experimental animal models of arthritis support the hypothesis that IL-1 may be an important mediator of tissue destruction. Intra-articular injection of IL-1 in rabbits induces a transient infiltration of neutrophils into the joint space followed by mononuclear cells, although few cells are observed in the synovium.[17] Loss of proteoglycan from the mid-zone of the articular cartilage also follows IL-1 injection into the joint, a response that appears to be separate from the cellular infiltration. Repeated injection of IL-1 into ankles of normal rats results in a chronic synovitis with mononuclear cells and fibrosis but without cartilage and bone destruction.[18] However, in joints previously injected with a streptococcal cell wall peptidoglycan-polysaccharide complex, subsequent injection of IL-1 markedly accentuates the inflammatory response with pannus formation and cartilage destruction.[18] Collagen-induced arthritis in mice, an animal model of inflammatory arthritis, is accelerated by the subcutaneous infusion of IL-1.[19] All of these studies suggest that IL-1 is capable of mediating tissue destruction. However, in rats with antigen-induced arthritis, IL-1 injection into knee joints leads to a reduction in inflammation and joint destruction.[20] This ameliorative effect was observed when IL-1 was administered

Table 13–2. EVIDENCE SUGGESTING THE PRESENCE OF IL-1 IN RA

Synovial Fluid
  Levels of IL-1 bioactivity variable
  Elevated levels of IL-1α and IL-1β proteins
  Cells may not spontaneously produce IL-1
Synovial Tissue
  Spontaneous in vitro production of IL-1α and IL-1β
  High levels of IL-1α and IL-1β mRNA
Blood
  IL-1β present, and levels correlate with disease activity
Other
  Disease-modifying drugs may alter IL-1 production or effects
    on target cells

either before or after induction of arthritis. Further studies are necessary to establish whether this phenomenon might be due, in part, to desensitization to IL-1 or to the induction of IL-1 inhibitors.[21]

A study on antigen-induced arthritis in rabbits suggests the presence of substances that may inhibit IL-1 effects, biologically active IL-1 being detected in synovial fluids only from early arthritic joints.[22] In contrast, IL-1 inhibitor activity was present in control synovial fluids and in increased amounts in chronic arthritis synovial fluids. After induction of arthritis initially, no IL-1 activity could be detected in synovial fluids, but later markedly increased IL-1 production by synovial explants was observed. These observations imply that IL-1 levels in joint fluids may not be an accurate reflection of what is occurring in the synovial tissues, mainly because of the presence of IL-1 inhibitors in these fluids. Thus, in animal models of synovitis, IL-1 may accelerate tissue destruction, induce primarily reparative responses, or be accompanied by the production of IL-1 inhibitors, again emphasizing the dual nature of IL-1–induced biologic effects.

Interleukin-1 in Rheumatoid Arthritis. Much evidence exists to suggest that IL-1 may play a role in rheumatoid synovitis[13–15, 23] (Table 13–2; see Chapter 51). Attempts to measure IL-1 activity in human synovial fluids using bioassays have yielded variable results, probably because of the ubiquitous presence of IL-1 and IL-2 inhibitors in these fluids. Enzyme-linked immunosorbant assay or radioimmunoassay for IL-1α and IL-1β proteins variably demonstrate the presence of increased levels in synovial fluids from both active RA patients and from non-RA patients.[24] However, these assays may be influenced by the viscosity of synovial fluids and by the presence of rheumatoid factors.

Studies on IL-1 production by RA synovial fluid or tissue macrophages also have yielded conflicting results. Although synovial fluid cells may not produce high levels of IL-1,[25] rheumatoid synovial tissue obtained at arthroscopy synthesizes large amounts of both IL-1α and IL-1β in vitro.[26] This high IL-1 production was not observed with non-RA synovial tissue and in the rheumatoids correlated with arthroscopic and radiologic evidence of destructive arthri-

tis. Thus, IL-1 in synovial fluids of both RA and non-RA patients may be derived primarily from cells in the inflamed synovium. In support of this conclusion is the finding of high levels of IL-1α and IL-1β mRNAs in rheumatoid synovial membrane.[27–29]

Additional studies offer further evidence that IL-1 may be an important mediator of tissue destruction in RA. Levels of circulating IL-1β in RA patients correlate with clinical disease activity.[30] Circulating monocytes from recently active RA patients spontaneously secrete IL-1 in vitro,[31] probably reflecting monocytopoiesis as immature cells secrete more IL-1. Finally, although suggestive evidence exists, further studies are necessary to establish whether disease-modifying drugs used in RA may inhibit the production or biologic effects of IL-1.

INTERLEUKIN-1 INHIBITORS

In recent years, many studies have revealed the existence of inhibitory activities toward IL-1 that could modulate the local effects of IL-1 in the rheumatoid joint. Several such activities have been described in cell supernatants and in human urine and have been termed *IL-1 inhibitors*. However, these factors may be acting at different levels and in different ways, in a specific or a nonspecific manner. Their possible mechanisms include reducing IL-1 production, binding to IL-1 and preventing its action, degrading IL-1, modulating IL-1 receptor expression, blocking IL-1 receptors, or interfering with IL-1 activity at the postreceptor level. Many of the biologic activities reported as "IL-1 inhibitors" have not been purified nor their mechanisms of action characterized (reviewed in refs. 32–34).

Inhibition at the Levels of Induction and Production. Because LPS induces IL-1 to a considerable extent, agents that block LPS effects could be considered inhibitors of IL-1 production. Some of these agents combine with the LPS molecule, preventing the triggering signal at the membrane level; an example is the antibiotic polymyxin, which affects only some types of LPS (LPS from *Escherichia coli* but not from *Neisseria gonorrhoeae*). Membrane glycolipids such as sialogangliosides (but not asialogangliosides) prevent LPS induction of IL-1 production. Serum lipoproteins such as high-density lipoprotein (HDL) decrease LPS-induced IL-1 production.[35] Inhibition of the proteolytic cleavage of IL-1β may be another mechanism of preventing production of 17-kD extracellular IL-1β. An increase in cellular cAMP or a decrease in available Ca^{2+} may also reduce IL-1 production by stimulated monocytes.

Other cytokines such as IL-4, IL-6, and IFN-α may decrease the production of IL-1 in some cells under particular conditions. However, these cytokines do not affect IL-1 exclusively but also reduce TNF-α and other monocyte-macrophage products.

Interleukin-1 Binding Proteins or Antagonistic Factors. Several molecules may bind to IL-1, potentially blocking its biologic activity. These molecules include the 85-kD uromodulin from urine, later identified as the Tamm Horsefall glycoprotein,[36] and more recently an IL-1β–binding protein in human plasma.[37] These binding proteins may be important carrier molecules, but it is not certain that they inhibit IL-1 biologic activities. For example, the "F"α₂-macroglobulin binds to IL-1β without affecting its biologic activity.[38]

Other possible mechanisms of blocking IL-1 effects include specific autoantibodies, soluble receptors, and opposing cytokines. Recently, several groups have identified autoantibodies to cytokines, most being directed against IL-1α or TNF-α and primarily of the immunoglobin G4 (IgG4) subclass.[39] These antibodies may also function as carrier molecules, and their role as potential inhibitors of cytokine effects in vitro or in vivo has not been established. Soluble receptors to IL-1 have recently been described in the supernatants of cultured cells.[40, 41] However, it is not yet known whether soluble IL-1 receptors are found in human plasma or urine, as is the case for receptors for TNF-α, IL-6, INF-γ (IFN-γ), and other cytokines. A soluble form of the IL-1 receptor, produced by recombinant DNA technology, has been shown to block some effects of IL-1 in vivo.[42, 43] Finally, other cytokines may oppose the effects of IL-1 and function as apparent inhibitors. For example, transforming growth factor-β (TGF-β) antagonizes many effects of IL-1 on target cells, in part through decreasing the expression of IL-1 receptors.

Interleukin-1 Receptor Antagonist. A specific inhibitor of IL-1 that binds to the IL-1 receptor but fails to stimulate target cells was originally described by two laboratories (reviewed in references 44 and 44a). A 22-kD IL-1 inhibitor was found in the urine of patients with fever or with monocytic leukemia.[45] A similar activity was discovered in the supernatants of human monocytes cultured on a substrate of immune complexes or adherent IgG.[46] Both laboratories demonstrated that this native IL-1 inhibitor bound to IL-1 receptors on thymoma cells, synovial fibroblasts, and chondrocytes but failed to stimulate detectable biologic responses in these cells. Thus, this molecule functioned as a specific receptor antagonist of IL-1, the first known human protein with such a mechanism of action.

The human IL-1 receptor antagonist [IL-1ra] has been purified from supernatants of either monocytes cultured on adherent IgG[47] or the human myelomonocytic leukemia cell line U937.[48] The molecular and biochemical characteristics of IL-1ra are summarized in Table 13–3. The native IL-1ra exists in two forms, each having an identical 152–amino acid sequence: a 22- to 25-kD form with varying degrees of glycosylation, and a nonglycosylated 17-kD form. Complementary DNAs for the human IL-1ra have been cloned and expressed in *E. coli* with production of nonglycosylated 17-kD recombinant IL-1ra.[49] The recombinant IL-1ra exhibits identical biologic properties to either native form of the molecule; thus, glycosylation is not required for receptor binding.

Table 13–3. MOLECULAR AND BIOCHEMICAL CHARACTERISTICS OF IL-1RA

Synthesized as a 177–amino acid propeptide with a 25–amino acid leader sequence

Mature protein 152 amino acids with an N-linked glycosylation site

Natural molecule has two primary forms: 22–25-kD molecules with varying degrees of glycosylation and nonglycosylated 17-kD form

Sequence homology 30 percent with IL-1β and 19 percent with IL-1α

Exhibits no immunologic cross-reactivity with either IL-1α or IL-1β

Produced by monocytes, macrophages, neutrophils, keratinocytes, and other epithelial cells

Binds to type I IL-1 receptors on target cells with the same avidity as IL-1 but fails to elicit biologic responses

Biologic Properties of Interleukin-1 Receptor Antagonist. The biologic properties of the recombinant IL-1ra have been examined in recent studies and are summarized in Table 13–4. This molecule binds to type I IL-1 receptors on murine T cells and human fibroblasts with an avidity equal to that of IL-1. The inhibition of IL-1–induced biologic responses in T cells, fibroblasts, and chondrocytes in vitro requires 10- to 100-fold excess amounts of IL-1ra.[50] This observation probably results from the fact that target cells are exquisitely sensitive to tiny amounts of IL-1, requiring only 2 to 5 percent of available receptors to be occupied before a complete biologic response is seen. Because excess IL-1 receptors are present on all target cells, large amounts of IL-1ra are necessary to block IL-1 binding to a small number

Table 13–4. BIOLOGIC EFFECTS OF IL-1RA

Effects on Cartilage and Bone
Inhibition of IL-1 induced collagenase and prostaglandin E₂ production in synovial cells and chondrocytes
Inhibition of IL-1–induced Ca²⁺ release
Inhibition of hyaluronic acid synthesis in synovial cells
Reversal of the IL-1–induced inhibition of glycosaminoglycan synthesis in chondrocytes
Effects on Other Tissues
Inhibition of IL-1–induced adherence of neutrophils and eosinophils to endothelial cells
Inhibition of IL-1–induced proliferation of murine thymocytes
Reversal of the IL-1–induced inhibition of insulin content and secretion in pancreatic β cells
Effects on Systemic Functions (in vivo)
Reduction of mortality in endotoxic shock (rabbits)
Inhibition of IL-1–induced corticosterone production (mice)
Inhibition of IL-1–induced hypotension and induction of acute-phase proteins (rabbits)
Inhibition of collagen-induced but not of antigen-induced arthritis (mice)
Inhibition of immune complex–induced ulcerative colitis (rabbits)

of these receptors. The relevance of this observation to the possible in vivo role of IL-1ra in normal physiology or in pathophysiologic conditions remains to be established.

IL-1ra is produced primarily by monocytes with enhanced production by in vitro–derived or tissue macrophages, particularly under the differentiating influence of granulocyte-macrophage colony-stimulating factor (GM-CSF).[51] In addition, synovial macrophages from patients with RA and alveolar macrophages from patients with interstitial lung disease produce large amounts of IL-1ra.[52, 53] These observations are of particular interest because IL-1β production is down-regulated as monocytes differentiate into macrophages in vitro or in vivo. Thus, both IL-1β and IL-1ra are produced in nearly equal amounts by peripheral monocytes, but greatly excessive amounts of IL-1ra are produced by macrophages. An alternative form of IL-1ra is synthesized by keratinocytes and other epithelial cells in vitro and in vivo. This form of IL-1ra lacks a full leader peptide; thus, this molecule is not secreted but remains inside the cell.[54] The biologic role of this intracellular variant of IL-1ra in normal and diseased human skin remains to be established.

In Vivo Effects of Interleukin-1 Receptor Antagonist. The availability of recombinant IL-1ra has permitted the performance of in vivo studies examining the consequences of blocking IL-1 effects in various experimental animal models of disease. These initial published studies are summarized in Table 13–4 and indicate that IL-1ra has potent in vivo biologic effects in a variety of acute and chronic animal diseases. The only human studies performed to date indicate that elevated IL-1ra levels are present in the serum and urine of patients with juvenile RA[55] and in the synovial fluid of patients with RA.[56]

The current belief that IL-1 has an important role in the pathophysiology of RA and other autoimmune and inflammatory diseases has led to the concept that interruption of in vivo IL-1 effects would be desirable. However, IL-1 has numerous potentially important normal functions. Carefully performed clinical trials are necessary to evaluate whether IL-1–binding proteins or receptor antagonists are not only safe but efficacious in human disease.

TUMOR NECROSIS FACTOR-α

History. TNF-α was originally described as a monocyte product that induced tumor lysis in experimental animals and cachexia in mice (hence the name *cachectin*) (reviewed in references 57 and 58). In 1984, the TNF-α gene was cloned and expressed, and other properties, probably more important, were discovered. TNF-α possesses a wide range of cell regulatory, immune, and inflammatory properties that overlap with other members of the cytokine network, such as IL-1 and IFN-γ. TNF-α interacts with these and other cytokines and enhances or inhibits their action.

Protein Chemistry and Gene Structure. The biologically active TNF-α molecule exists in solution as a trimer with approximately 17-kD subunits.[59, 60] TNF-α is produced in the cell as a 26-kD propeptide and also is present (approximately 1 to 2 percent) within the cell membrane, where it is biologically active. The structure of TNF-α resembles other transmembrane proteins with hydrophobic and hydrophilic regions; the membrane form is cleaved to yield the 17-kD extracellular molecule of 157 amino acids. In contrast, lymphotoxin (LT), or TNF-β, does not appear to exist as a transmembrane protein. TNF-α and TNF-β are antigenically distinct but possess 30 percent amino acid sequence homology and share the same cell surface receptor. TNF-α and TNF-β genes are present within the major histocompatibility complex (MHC) region on the short arm of chromosome 6 in humans. The 3′ untranslated region of TNF-α DNA contains a 33-nucleotide sequence composed entirely of A and T residues (TTATTTAT). Other cytokine genes (LT, GM-CSF, IL-1, IFN-γ) have similar sequences that appear to regulate mRNA stability. The corresponding (UA)-rich domain in the 3′ untranslated portion of the TNF-α mRNA regulates translation of the protein. TNF-α mRNA pre-exists in resting macrophages, but translation is strongly suppressed. On activation by LPS, however, TNF-α translation is specifically activated, leading to efficient protein production. The UA-rich domain itself may be an important substrate for the regulatory effects of glucocorticoid. Dexamethasone may prevent translational activation through a mechanism involving this UA-rich element in the 3′ untranslated region of cytokine mRNAs.

Regulation and Sources of Tumor Necrosis Factor-α Production. Production of TNF-α and LT is induced not only by LPS but also by a variety of other stimuli, including tumor promoters, viruses, and mitogens. TNF-α and LT also can be stimulated by other cytokines, notably IFN-γ, IL-1, and the CSFs. IL-1 and TNF-α are usually synthesized and secreted simultaneously, although their production appears to be regulated separately and controlled by different mechanisms.

Initially, it was thought that only monocytes and macrophages produced TNF-α and that T lymphocytes produced TNF-β. However, there is evidence that lymphocytes and transformed cell lines of hematopoietic and nonhematopoietic origin can produce TNF-α. As monocytes mature into macrophages, their ability to produce IL-1 decreases dramatically, but TNF-α production appears to be maintained at a high level.

Signal Transduction Mediated by Tumor Necrosis Factor-α and Receptors. TNF-α exerts its biologic activity by interacting with specific cell surface receptors. These receptors exist on a variety of normal and malignant cells in numbers ranging from 10^3 to 10^4 receptors per cell. At present, two distinct receptors

Table 13–5. NATURAL INHIBITORS OF TNF

Levels of Action	Mechanisms	Substances
Induction of synthesis	TNF-α steady-state mRNA levels (transcriptional and post-transcriptional action)	Prostaglandin E_2 (high concentrations)
		Glucocorticoids
	Inhibition of phospholipase A_2 and lipoxygenase	Bromophenacylbromide
		Quinacrine
	Increase in cAMP	Theophylline
		Cholera toxin
Processing	26-kD propeptide to mature protein	Proteases (?)
Binding to mature protein	Binding proteins (soluble fragments of TNF-α receptors)	TNF-α–binding protein I
		TNF-α–binding protein II
Postreceptor binding	Dephosphorylation	Phosphatases
	Protein kinase C	Inhibitors of protein kinase C
	G protein	Pertussis toxin
	Phospholipase A_2	Glucocorticoids
Target cell metabolism	Lysosomal enzymes	Chloroquine
	Free oxygen radicals	Free oxygen radical scavengers, catalase, glutathione peroxidase

for TNF-α are known.[61, 62] One TNF-α receptor, of 55 kD (415 amino acids), possesses leader, extracellular, transmembrane, and intracellular domains that exhibit a high degree of sequence homology to the extracellular domain of the nerve growth factor receptor. The second TNF-α receptor, of 75 kD (461 amino acids), is also a transmembranous molecule. The extracellular fragments of both TNF-α receptors can be shed and possess inhibitory properties toward TNF-α biologic activities (see later). The existence of two TNF-α receptors contributes to TNF-α binding to target cells to varying degrees; the receptors are not equally distributed on various cell types.

One of the ways in which cytokines interact and influence each other's action is by transmodulation of receptor expression. TNF-α receptor mRNA and cell surface expression can be up-regulated by IFN-α, IFN-β, and IFN-γ.

Systemic and Local Effects of Tumor Necrosis Factor-α in Immune and Inflammatory Diseases. The main pathologic role of TNF-α appears to be mediation of septic shock and acute respiratory distress syndrome.[63, 64] Many effects of TNF-α on cells overlap with those of IL-1. Thus, at the local level, TNF-α stimulates collagenase and prostaglandin E_2 production by synovial or other fibroblasts, and it may play a role in synovial inflammation. TNF-α also acts in synergism with other cytokines (e.g., IFN-γ in inducing c-*myc*, and IL-1 in inducing collagenase). In some conditions, TNF-α induces IL-1 production.

TNF-α gene alleles exist in NZW mice and are correlated with reduced serum TNF-α levels. It has been hypothesized that the decreased TNF-α levels predispose to the systemic lupus erythematosus (SLE)–like autoimmune disease seen in these mice. In fact, the administration of TNF-α reduces the severity of autoimmune diabetes in BB rats.[65] In contrast, patients with SLE exhibit normal levels of TNF-α in the circulation and display a normal increase in TNF-α levels with infection. Interestingly, the cachexia of chronic congestive heart failure is accompanied by high circulating levels of TNF-α.[66]

Intra-articular injection of TNF-α into rabbit knees induces less cellular influx and no loss in cartilage proteoglycan in comparison with IL-1. However, injection of both TNF-α and IL-1 produces a greater inflammatory response than is observed with either cytokine alone.[67] Thus, TNF-α may augment the tissue-damaging potential of IL-1 in experimental synovitis. TNF-α protein can be detected in more than half of rheumatoid synovial fluids, particularly those from patients producing rheumatoid factors or patients with active disease (reviewed in reference 15). In addition, TNF-α protein is synthesized by rheumatoid synovial tissue in vitro. Immunoperoxidase staining reveals TNF-α protein in 50 percent of rheumatoid synovial tissue specimens, primarily in synovial lining cells and interstitial macrophages.

INHIBITORS OF TUMOR NECROSIS FACTOR

Because TNF-α may be associated with various human diseases, it is important to understand potential mechanisms likely to block TNF-α either at the level of production or at the level of biologic activities (reviewed in reference 68). Potential natural inhibitors of TNF-α are summarized in Table 13–5.

Inhibition of Tumor Necrosis Factor-α Synthesis, Processing, and Release. Prostaglandin E_2 in high concentrations in vitro (100 nM) suppresses LPS-induced TNF-α mRNA accumulation by exerting effects at both transcriptional and post-transcriptional levels. TNF-α activates the cyclooxygenase pathway, and the resultant prostaglandin E_2 produced reciprocally down-regulates TNF-α production. Other agents causing an increase in cAMP also may reduce TNF-α production. In contrast, the lipoxygenase pathway appears to stimulate TNF-α production. Glucocorticoids markedly suppress the endotoxin-induced increase of TNF-α mRNA through both transcriptional and post-transcriptional mechanisms. Finally, inhibition of the protease that cleaves the 26-kD precursor propeptide of TNF-α into the fully active form represents another potential mechanism for regulation of TNF-α effects.

Inhibition of Tumor Necrosis Factor-α Effects by Binding Proteins. Originally discovered in the urine of febrile patients, TNF-α inhibitory activities have since been found in biologic fluids.[68, 69] Similar activities have been found in the plasma of cancer patients and, to a lesser extent, in normal urine. Purification to homogeneity of the TNF-α inhibitory material yielded a protein with a novel amino acid sequence. This protein binds to the ligand itself to form a stable complex, its affinity being higher for TNF-α than for TNF-β. The TNF-α inhibitor has been shown to be a soluble fragment of the TNF-α receptor itself. Because there are two different TNF-α receptors, of 55 and 75 kD, there are two different soluble fragments that originate from the two chains and are referred to as *TNF-α–binding proteins I and II*. Proteolytic cleavage of the two TNF-α receptor molecules probably represents an important mechanism for controlling the release of the two soluble receptor proteins that have been detected in the supernatants of alveolar macrophages and in synovial fluids. Whether these naturally occurring soluble TNF-α receptor molecules function as inhibitors or carriers of TNF-α in vivo remains to be established.[69a]

Inhibition at the Level of the Target Cells. Reversible phosphorylation of intracellular proteins controlled by various kinases may be one mechanism of TNF-α effects on target cells. Dephosphorylation of these proteins by activating specific phosphates might be a mechanism whereby the cell could resist TNF-α. The TNF-α transduction mechanism may also involve receptor coupling to guanosine triphosphate (GTP)–binding proteins, leading to an increase or decrease in cytoplasmic cAMP through modulation of adenylate cyclase activity. A pivotal role of a pertussis toxin–sensitive G protein in at least some biologic responses to TNF-α has been established. In addition, phospholipase A₂ is activated through a GTP-binding protein, and blocking this enzyme might be essential to regulation of TNF-α cytotoxicity.

There are two distinct mechanisms by which TNF-α destroys cells: an early mechanism that is dependent on new protein synthesis, and a later one that is independent of new protein synthesis. Both dexamethasone and indomethacin block TNF-α–induced cytotoxicity, suggesting that phospholipase A₂ may play a key role in cytotoxicity. In addition, the cytocidal action of TNF-α has been shown to involve lysosomal enzymes, and inhibition of enzyme activities might block TNF-α–induced cytotoxicity. Finally, scavengers of toxic oxygen metabolites decrease cytotoxicity of TNF-α. Therefore, enzymes such as catalase, glutathione peroxidase, or superoxide dismutase may be essential for resisting the cytotoxic effects of TNF-α.

Inhibition by Down-Regulation of the Tumor Necrosis Factor-α Receptor. TNF-α receptor function is down-regulated by IL-1 and mitogens in some cells, a phenomenon that is probably mediated by protein kinase C. This response is not due to enhanced internalization of the TNF-α receptor, nor to its shedding, but to an influence on the affinity of ligand binding. In contrast, stimulation of protein kinase A results in the enhancement of TNF-α receptor expression.

In summary, both TNF-α and IL-1 are ubiquitous factors that may play predominant roles in mediating events of tissue destruction in many human diseases. Regulation of the production or effects of these cytokines may have important beneficial consequences.[15, 44, 68]

INTERLEUKIN-6

IL-6 is a glycoprotein of 26 kD with 184 amino acids. The IL-6 gene is located on chromosome 7, and there appear to be three different alleles. IL-6 is produced by monocytes, T lymphocytes, and fibroblasts and was previously known as B cell stimulatory factor-2 or INF-β₂.[70, 71] IL-6 has multiple biologic effects, including modulation of growth and differentiation of T lymphocytes, synergism with IL-3 in hematopoietic colony formation, and enhancement of Ig production by B cells. However, IL-6 was previously known as hepatocyte stimulating factor, and its most important function appears to be the induction of synthesis of acute-phase proteins in the liver.[72] IL-6 is produced by various cell types and is induced by other inflammatory cytokines, such as IL-1, TNF-α, and PDGF, as well as by viruses and bacterial products such as endotoxins. Elevated circulating levels of IL-6 have been observed in some malignant diseases or disorders with autoimmune phenomena such as autoantibody and rheumatoid factor production. IL-6 is produced in large amounts by synovial cells stimulated with IL-1 or TNF-α. In addition, high levels of IL-6 are present in synovial fluids of various inflammatory and noninflammatory arthropathies. Immunohistologic staining of rheumatoid synovium, and in situ hybridization for presence of mRNA, reveals IL-6 to be present primarily in fibroblasts.

Although some of the biologic activities of IL-6 are similar to those of IL-1 and TNF-α, IL-6 fails to stimulate prostaglandin E₂ or collagenase production by fibroblasts and synovial cells.[73, 74] In vitro, IL-6 actually decreases IL-1–induced prostaglandin E₂ production by these cells. In addition, IL-6 induces synthesis of tissue inhibitor of metalloproteinases (TIMP), a specific inhibitor of collagenase. However, IL-6 is more potent in inducing hepatic synthesis of acute-phase proteins and in enhancing Ig production by B lymphocytes than is either IL-1 or TNF-α. Thus, in joint diseases, IL-6 may amplify some IL-1 and TNF-α effects but decrease other biologic consequences. An important feature of IL-6 is its ability to influence chondrocyte metabolism and, in synergy with TNF-β, to increase the proliferation of these cells.[74] In fact, IL-6 is involved in the proliferation

Table 13–6. INFLAMMATORY EFFECTS OF IL-6 AND IL-8

Cytokine	Sources	Properties
IL-6	Monocytes, endothelial cells, fibroblasts, T lymphocytes	Induces Ig production; stimulates hepatic production of acute-phase proteins
IL-8/NAP-1	Monocytes, endothelial cells, fibroblasts, epithelial cells	Chemotactic for neutrophils; induces many neutrophil responses

NAP-1, neutrophil-activating peptide-1.

and differentiation of various cell types, including osteoclasts, hepatocytes, smooth muscle cells, megakaryocytes, keratinocytes, and mesangial cells. Thus, IL-6 may be an important regulator of mesenchymal and epithelial tissue metabolism.

Interleukin-6 in Human Diseases. IL-6 may play an important role in a variety of human diseases characterized by polyclonal B cell activation.[75] The hypergammaglobulinemia of cardiac myxoma, RA, chronic human immunodeficiency virus infection, and alcoholic liver disease may be due in large part to excessive IL-6 production. In addition, IL-6 may be involved in the plasmacytosis seen in various malignancies. In fact, IL-6 may function as an autocrine growth factor for plasma cells in multiple myeloma, as well as in other lymphoid malignancies. Finally, mesangial proliferative glomerulonephritis may be characterized by IL-6 stimulation of mesangial cell growth in an autocrine fashion.

In summary, IL-6 may be primarily responsible for induction of synthesis of the acute-phase proteins in the liver as well as for the hypergammaglobulinemia that characterizes many chronic human autoimmune and inflammatory diseases (Table 13–6). A unique role for IL-6, however, may be the autocrine stimulation of plasma cells and lymphoid cells in human malignancies.

INTERLEUKIN-8/NEUTROPHIL-ACTIVATING PEPTIDE-1 AND RELATED MOLECULES

IL-8 is a member of a recently described family of related chemotactic peptides. IL-8 is also known as *neutrophil-activating peptide-1, neutrophil chemotactic factor,* and *monocyte-derived neutrophil chemotactic factor.* Because this factor is produced by cells other than monocytes and has effects on cells other than neutrophils, *IL-8* is the preferred terminology.[76, 77, 77a]

Interleukin-8. IL-8 is a 10-kD protein that is synthesized as a larger precursor.[76] Heterogeneity exists in the mature forms of IL-8, probably due to N-terminal proteolytic processing of the secreted molecule. IL-8 possesses four cysteine residues forming two intrachain disulfide bonds that are essential for biologic activity. IL-8 is related both in structure and biologic properties to a variety of other peptides, including platelet basic protein, connective tissue–activating peptide-III, platelet factor-4, and macrophage inflammatory protein-2. IL-8 binds to specific membrane receptors, distinct from those of other

chemotactic factors such as C5a, f-Met-Leu-Phe, LTB$_4$, or platelet-activating factor. However, the mechanism of signal transduction appears to be similar for all of those factors and involves GTP-binding proteins, a transient rise in cytosolic free Ca^{2+} and activation of protein kinase C.

IL-8 is produced by peripheral monocytes, tissue macrophages, endothelial cells, fibroblasts, and a variety of other tissue cells.[76] TNF-α and IL-1 are potent inducing agents for IL-8 production in all of these cells. In addition, LPS can stimulate IL-8 production in monocytes, macrophages, and endothelial cells. The mRNA for IL-8 remains at high levels for up to 24 to 36 hours in stimulated cells, in contrast to the transient appearance of mRNAs for other inflammatory cytokines. This cell response suggests that IL-8 protein may be produced for a more prolonged period.

IL-8 is a potent chemoattractant for neutrophils. In addition, IL-8 induces other responses in neutrophils, including increased expression of the adhesion molecules CD11b/CD18,[78] release of lysosomal enzymes, and generation of oxygen metabolites. In contrast to other chemotactic peptides, these IL-8 effects are not observed with monocytes or platelets, and IL-8 is only a weak stimulator of eosinophils and basophils. Chemotactic activity of IL-8 toward lymphocytes also may exist.[79]

IL-8 may be an important chemotactic agent for neutrophils in both inflammatory synovitis and crystal-induced arthritis and may facilitate migration of inflammatory cells through the synovial endothelium (see Chapter 51). IL-8 levels are high in the synovial fluids of RA patients.[80] Furthermore, IL-1 stimulates IL-8 release from cultured rheumatoid synovial cells. IL-8 levels are also elevated in the synovial fluids of patients with gout; either sodium urate or calcium pyrophosphate crystals will induce IL-8 release from monocytes in vitro.[81] In addition to inflammatory arthritis, IL-8 may be responsible for the influx of neutrophils into other tissues undergoing an acute inflammatory response, for example, the lung in adult respiratory distress syndrome.[82] IL-1 and TNF-α enhance neutrophil chemotaxis not only through stimulating IL-8 production by multiple cells but also through inducing expression of adhesion molecules on endothelial cells in postcapillary venules.

Monocyte Chemotactic Factors. Another series of proteins that appear to be related to the IL-8 family are monocyte chemotactic factor (MCF) and human monocyte chemoattractant protein-1 (MCF).[83] MCP-1 has 21 percent amino acid sequence homology to IL-8 and bears structural similarity. MCF is produced by monocytes, dermal fibroblasts, and endothelial cells, whereas MCP-1 is made by monocytes and T lymphocytes. These peptides are not only chemotactic for monocytes but also activate these cells to release lysosomal enzymes and generate oxygen metabolites. The roles of MCP-1 in acute or chronic inflammatory diseases remain to be investigated.

In summary, the multiple members of the IL-8 and related families may prove to be important chemotactic agents for white blood cells in many human diseases. Both IL-6 and IL-8 may play important roles as nonspecific mediators of acute and chronic inflammatory events (see Table 13-6).

LYMPHOKINES

Lymphocytes can release a variety of cytokines, depending on the stimulating conditions and the degree of cell activation. Lymphocyte-derived cytokines are known historically as *lymphokines*, although this term is a misnomer because most of these factors can be produced by other cells as well.[84] Those cytokines produced by lymphocytes and whose function is primarily exerted on the immune system will be discussed here, namely, IL-2, IL-4, IL-5, and IFN-γ. Other cytokines released by lymphocytes that will be briefly touched on include IL-3, IL-7, IL-9, IL-10, and IL-11. IL-1, IL-6, and GM-CSF may also be produced by T lymphocytes and are discussed elsewhere in this chapter.

Interleukin-2. IL-2 is a 15.5-kD glycoprotein that was originally called *T cell growth factor*. An apparent size heterogeneity of IL-2 is due to variable degrees of glycosylation and sialylation of a single protein.[85] The organization of the IL-2 gene is similar to the genes of IL-4 and GM-CSF, suggesting that these factors may have arisen from a common progenitor. IL-2 is produced by CD4$^+$ helper T cells after stimulation with a mitogen or an antigen presented in complex with a class II MHC molecule. IL-2 functions in an autocrine or paracrine fashion to augment T cell growth, enhance growth and differentiation of activated B cells, stimulate natural killer (NK) cell function, and activate macrophages. The prime function of IL-2 is to enhance clonal proliferation of T lymphocytes that have been stimulated with an antigen-MHC complex. Its effects on B cells and macrophages may be of secondary importance.

IL-2 stimulates target cells by binding to specific cell surface receptors present on multiple cell types. The current view is that the IL-2 receptor possesses two chains, p55 (the α-chain and Tac antigen), and p70-75 (the β-chain). Both chains separately bind IL-2 and may be expressed individually on some cells. However, both chains must be expressed together to produce a high-affinity IL-2 receptor and one that is capable of generating biologic responses.

Abnormalities of the IL-2–IL-2 receptor system

may be present in several autoimmune diseases.[86] Early studies suggested that IL-2 production may be deficient in patients with RA, SLE, or other autoimmune diseases. This conclusion was based primarily on the observation that peripheral T cells from patients with these diseases exhibited little IL-2 production in vitro after stimulation with mitogens. However, more recent studies indicate that these cells recover function after short periods of culture and that the IL-2–IL-2 receptor system in these diseases actually may be hyperactive in vivo. IL-2 may be produced in excessive amounts in vivo, and IL-2 receptor–bearing cells may hyper-respond to this lymphokine. The apparently paradoxic observations of decreased IL-2 production or responsiveness in vitro may be due to enhanced internalization of the IL-2–IL-2 receptor complex and a transient exhaustion of the capacity to produce IL-2. The probable importance of IL-2 in driving autoimmune processes is substantiated by the beneficial effects of monoclonal antibodies to the IL-2 receptor in murine lupus or collagen-induced arthritis in mice.

Soluble Interleukin-2 Receptors. Further evidence for the importance of IL-2 in chronic autoimmune or inflammatory diseases is the presence of IL-2 inhibitors in synovial fluids from patients with RA, psoriatic arthritis, or Reiter's syndrome.[87] These IL-2 inhibitors appear to be heterogeneous and have not been well characterized. However, in some instances, the IL-2 inhibitor may be a soluble form of the IL-2 receptor.[88] In fact, elevated levels of soluble IL-2 receptors have been described in the sera of patients with a variety of neoplastic, immune, or inflammatory diseases.[88] The circulating levels of soluble IL-2 receptors appear to correlate with the degree of clinical activity of the underlying disease, suggesting their release by activated cells. The clinical usefulness of measuring these levels appears to be greatest in non-Hodgkin's lymphoma, acquired immunodeficiency syndrome,[89] and possibly also in SLE.[90] The soluble IL-2 receptor binds IL-2 too weakly to interfere with IL-2 activation of target cells.[91] However, the soluble receptor has been hypothesized to function as a carrier molecule in vivo to deliver IL-2 from sites of production to target cells in other organs.

Interleukin-3. IL-3 is a 14- to 28-kD protein that is produced by T lymphocytes and that functions as a hematopoietic growth factor.[92] In addition to enhancing growth of early progenitor cells in the bone marrow, IL-3 stimulates monocyte cytotoxicity, promotes eosinophil survival, and induces eosinophil functions. IL-3 also may induce histamine release from basophils, stimulate class II MHC antigen expression on macrophages,[93] and synergize with LPS to enhance IL-1 production by macrophages.[94] The IL-3 gene is associated with the genes for GM-CSF and macrophage-CSF (M-CSF); further details on the growth-promoting properties of IL-3 are discussed under the section colony-stimulating factors.

Interleukin-4. Although IL-2 primarily stimulates growth of T cells, IL-4, IL-5, and IL-6 enhance proliferation and differentiation of B cells. IL-4 is a 19-kD protein that was originally called *B cell stimulatory factor-1* or *B cell growth factor-1*.[95] IL-4 is produced by a subclass of murine T helper cells, the T_H2 cells; human T cells may not exhibit this same classification scheme. In addition, both IL-3 and IL-4 are also produced by mast cells. The wide range of IL-4 effects on B cells includes promotion of growth, increased expression of class II MHC molecules, enhancement of IgG1 and IgE production, and induction of expression of Fc receptors for IgE. Thus, IL-4 acts on resting as well as activated B cells, again through a specific cell membrane receptor.

Since the original description of IL-4, this cytokine has been shown to have multiple effects on T lymphocytes, macrophages, and endothelial cells. IL-4 synergizes with IL-2 as a growth factor for T lymphocytes and thymocytes. IL-4 alone enhances proliferation of mitogen-stimulated CD8+ T cells as well as CD4− CD8− thymocytes (so-called double-negative cells). In addition, IL-4 appears to be necessary for the induction of cytotoxic T lymphocyte activity. Thus, IL-4 has potent effects on T cell growth and proliferation. Interestingly, IFN-γ blocks many of the effects of IL-4 on both B and T cells, as well as inhibits the generation of IL-4–producing cells.

IL-4 demonstrates both stimulatory and inhibitory effects on monocyte and macrophage function. IL-4 increases expression of class II MHC molecules on these cells, thus enhancing their capacity for antigen presentation.[96] IL-4 also induces fusion of macrophages to form multinucleated cells and, thus, may play a role in the formation of granulomata. In contrast, IL-4 inhibits many monocyte functions, such as Fc receptor expression[97]; superoxide production[98]; and the production of multiple cytokines, including IL-1, IL-6, and TNF-α.[99] The potent effects of IL-4 on inhibition of monocyte cytokine production appear to be mediated at the level of transcription. IL-4 also acts on endothelial cells and synergizes with IL-1β to enhance lymphocyte binding through increasing expression of vascular cell adhesion molecule-1 (VCAM-1).[100] In contrast, IL-4 inhibits endothelial cell expression of other adhesion molecules that are induced by IL-1, TNF-α, or IFN-γ and that mediate binding of neutrophils.[101] Thus, IL-4 may alter the quality of cells in an inflammatory infiltrate by promoting lymphocyte migration from blood but decreasing neutrophil egress.

Interleukin-5. IL-5 is another T cell–derived factor that acts primarily on B cells and eosinophils.[102] IL-5 is a 55-kD glycoprotein that was formerly known as *T cell–replacing factor* or *B cell growth factor-II*. IL-5 is involved in an antigen-stimulated immune response through enhancing IL-2 receptor expression on B and T cells as well as promoting Ig secretion by B cells. However, the most potent effects of IL-5 are on eosinophils, where this cytokine induces differentiation and growth. In addition, IL-5 is chemotactic for mature eosinophils and induces superoxide anion production in these cells. The effects of IL-5 on

enhancing antibody production by B cells are also seen with IL-6. However, IL-5 is more active than any other cytokine on eosinophils.

Interleukins 7, 9, 10, and 11. The remaining ILs not discussed elsewhere in this chapter are IL-7, IL-9, IL-10, and IL-11. These molecules have been more recently described and are not well characterized. IL-7 is a 25-kD protein produced by bone marrow stromal cells and is a potent growth factor for precursors of B lymphocytes.[103] In addition, IL-7 plays a role in T cell activation through inducing IL-2 production and IL-2 receptor expression in mitogen-stimulated T cells.[104] IL-9 is a 40-kD glycoprotein that is secreted by T lymphocytes and that induces proliferation of T cell clones, thymocytes, and mast cells.

IL-10, also known as *cytokine synthesis inhibitory factor*, is a 35-kD homodimeric protein produced by a subset of T lymphocytes, mast cells, and B lymphocytes.[105] IL-10 has multiple biologic effects, including inhibition of cytokine synthesis by subsets of T lymphocytes and monocytes,[105a] enhancement of mast cell survival, and induction of class II MHC expression on B lymphocytes. IL-10 synergizes with IL-4 for effects on mast cells and with both IL-2 and IL-4 for induction of thymocyte proliferation. Finally, IL-11 is a 20-kD protein produced by bone marrow stromal cells that possesses both lymphopoietic and hematopoietic properties.[106] IL-11 stimulates plasmacytoma proliferation and T cell helper function for B cells. IL-11 also synergizes with IL-3 in enhancing colony formation of murine megakaryocytes. Thus, along with other cytokines, IL-11 has potent growth factor properties and may also be an important regulator of mature T cell function.

Interferon-γ. INF-γ is an important immunoregulatory molecule that has no structural similarity and little functional overlap with the antiviral proteins IFN-α and IFN-β.[107] IFN-γ is a homodimer consisting of two identical 25-kD glycoproteins. Variable degrees of glycosylation account for the size heterogeneity in IFN-γ. This cytokine is secreted by activated T helper cells, CD8+ T cytotoxic cells, and NK cells. IFN-γ appears to be produced coordinately with IL-2 by antigen-stimulated cells.

A major effect of IFN-γ is to up-regulate the expression of class I and II MHC molecules on different cell types, including macrophages, endothelial cells, fibroblasts, chondrocytes, and many other tissue cells. This effect of IFN-γ may permit these cells to function efficiently in antigen presentation, thus further enhancing an ongoing immune response. IFN-γ also is a potent activator of macrophages, usually in association with LPS or other agents, leading to enhanced Fc receptor expression, phagocytosis, and bacterial killing. IFN-γ activates NK cells and cytotoxic T cells as well. IFN-γ stimulates IgG antibody production in B cells but, paradoxically, does not induce class II MHC expression on these cells. Furthermore, IFN-γ opposes many of the stimulatory effects of IL-4 on B cells, including class II MHC expression, proliferation, and the class

Table 13–7. LYMPHOKINES (PRODUCTS OF T LYMPHOCYTES)

Lymphokine	Properties
IL-2	Enhances clonal proliferation of T lymphocytes
	Enhances growth of B lymphocytes
	Stimulates NK cell function
	Activates macrophages
IL-3	Hematopoietic growth factor
	Stimulates monocyte and eosinophil functions
IL-4	Growth factor for B lymphocytes
	Enhances switch from IgG to IgE production
	Synergizes with IL-2 as a growth factor for T cells
	Stimulates monocyte expression of class II MHC molecules
	Inhibits monocyte production of IL-1, IL-6, and TNF-α
IL-5	Induces growth and differentiation of eosinophils
	Enhances IL-2 receptor expression on B and T cells
	Promotes Ig secretion by B cells
IL-7	Growth factor for B cell precursors
IL-9	Induces proliferation of T cells
IL-10	Inhibits cytokine synthesis by T cell subsets
IL-11	Lymphopoietic and hematopoietic growth factor
IFN-γ	Up-regulates class I and II MHC expression on multiple cells
	Activates many macrophage functions
	Opposes effects of IL-4 on B cells and of TGF-β on fibroblasts

switch from IgG to IgE production. These antagonistic effects of IL-4 and IFN-γ on B cells represent another example of the importance of multiple cytokines in regulation of cell function.

INFs have been implicated in autoimmune diseases, particularly in SLE.[107] The sera of SLE patients contain an unusual acid-labile form of IFN-α, the relevance of which remains unclear. SLE T lymphocytes may exhibit deficient production of and response to IFN-γ, possibly reflecting a basic abnormality in T cell function in this disease. Finally, IFN-γ antagonizes the stimulatory effects of TNF-α on rheumatoid synovial fibroblast functions, including HLA-DR expression, proliferation, collagenase production, and GM-CSF production.[108] Deficient IFN-γ production in the rheumatoid joint may permit these TNF-α effects to be manifested in an unopposed fashion.

In summary, T cell–derived cytokines or lymphokines are released after antigen stimulation and have important roles in enhancing proliferation and function of both T and B cells. In addition, some of these molecules are potent activators of macrophages. The effects of these molecules further illustrate the principle that cytokines work in a network, exhibiting both synergistic and opposing properties (Table 13–7).

TRANSFORMING GROWTH FACTOR-β

TGF-β is a member of a family of peptides that function primarily as mediators of growth and differentiation. TGF-β may play an important role in regulating the normal embryonic development of mesenchymal tissues. In autoimmune and inflammatory diseases, TGF-β effects may contribute to both tissue injury and repair.

TGFs were first identified by their ability to induce phenotypic transformation of cultured fibroblasts.[109] The TGF family is now known to contain multiple members, with TGF-α and TGF-β being structurally unrelated. TGF-α has a size of 5.6 kD, is similar in structure and properties to epidermal growth factor (EGF), and binds to the EGF receptor.[110] TGF-β is a larger protein of 25 kD that does not bind to the EGF receptor but shares with TGF-α and EGF the ability to affect growth of cells in culture. TGF-α is a homodimer or heterodimer of two covalently linked subunits of equal size.[111] There are at least five isoforms of TGF-β composed of dimers of varying subunit peptides. Other members of the TGF family include proteins called *inhibins* and *activins*.[112] These proteins exhibit more restricted functions than the pleiotropic effects of TGF-β.

Cells in a variety of tissues contain mRNA for TGF-β, but protein production is more restricted. The major cellular sources of TGF-β are platelets and macrophages. Both cells contain the major isoform TGF-β_1 in excess of TGF-β_2, whereas the latter predominates in bone. All TGF-β is released from cells in a latent form, bound to larger proteins that remain poorly characterized. This TGF-β complex can be activated in vitro by exposure to low or high pH as well as by denaturation with chaotropic ions. The mechanism of activation of latent TGF-β in vivo is not known, but proteases secreted by inflammatory cells may be responsible. Specific receptors for TGF-β are found on multiple cells throughout the body. The presence of active TGF-β may be regulated or limited at two primary levels: induction of protein synthesis and secretion in particular cells, and activation of latent TGF-β in the pericellular environment.

Biologic Properties of Transforming Growth Factor-β. The general properties of TGF-β include both positive and negative effects on growth and differentiation of mesenchymal cells. The net proliferative response observed may be influenced by the presence of other cytokines and by the conditions of culture. A major principle in understanding the possible role of TGF-β *in vivo* is the importance of a particular set or combination of cytokines. For example, TGF-β and PDGF together induce anchorage-independent growth of fibroblasts containing the *myc* oncogene, whereas the combination of TGF-β and EGF is inhibitory to growth of these cells. Overall, TGF-β is thought to diminish the growth rate of many cell types in vivo, possibly in an autocrine or paracrine fashion.

The effects of TGF-β on cell growth probably are mediated through PDGF.[113] Moreover, the concentration of TGF-β influences whether enhancement or inhibition of cell growth occurs. Recent studies have indicated that low concentrations of TGF-β induce proliferation of connective tissue cells through the autocrine stimulation of PDGF production. In contrast, high concentrations of TGF-β decrease cell proliferation through both the down-regulation of PDGF receptors and a direct inhibition of cell growth. TGF-β has been shown to inhibit the growth of synovial fibroblasts in vitro after stimulation with PDGF.

A potentially important function of TGF-β in inflammatory diseases is the recruitment of monocytes. TGF-β is the most potent known chemotactic agent for monocytes. Release of TGF-β by platelets in diseased tissues may induce the egress of monocytes from the blood. In addition, TGF-β may stimulate monocyte transcription of other proinflammatory cytokines such as IL-1 or TNF-α.[114] Paradoxically, TGF-β does not induce production of IL-1 and TNF proteins by human monocytes and actually inhibits at a post-transcriptional level LPS-induced cytokine production. It is not known whether TGF-β blocks the ability of other substances to stimulate IL-1 translation and protein secretion. TGF-β induces Fc receptor III expression on human monocytes, potentially enhancing the phagocytic potential of these cells.[115] In addition, TGF-β may deactivate macrophages for H_2O_2 production and down-regulate HLA-DR expression. However, as monocytes differentiate into macrophages, the cells down-regulate their TGF-β receptors and become less responsive to the stimulatory effects of TGF-β. Thus, although TGF-β may recruit monocytes into inflammatory sites, the net effect of this cytokine on macrophage function would appear to be inhibitory and anti-inflammatory.

Transforming Growth Factor-β–Induced Immunosuppression. TGF-β also has potent immunosuppressive effects on both B and T lymphocytes and on NK cells. Both B and T cells are capable of synthesizing and secreting TGF-β, but this cytokine may inhibit cell function in an autocrine or paracrine fashion. TGF-β inhibits B cell proliferation in vitro after IL-2 stimulation and blocks Ig secretion induced by IL-2 or IL-4. In addition, TGF-β inhibits IL-1–induced T cell proliferation in a similar fashion. TGF-β did not block IL-1–dependent production of IL-2 or IL-2 receptors in T lymphocytes in one study; thus, it may inhibit DNA synthesis at a later step.[116] However, another study reported that TGF-β inhibits growth and differentiation of hematopoietic and lymphoid cells by decreasing expression of IL-1 receptors.[117] In this study, TGF-β blocked IL-1–induced IL-2 production by murine thymoma cells. Thus, TGF-β may inhibit B and T lymphocyte function at two levels, by down-regulating IL-1 receptor expression and by blocking DNA synthesis distally. Finally, TGF-β inhibits both constitutive and IFN-γ–induced NK cell function. As discussed in the following section, TGF-β is present in various chronic disease tissues and may be responsible for the suppressed function of T cells from these lesions.

Another major effect of TGF-β on connective tissue is stimulation of repair and fibrosis. TGF-β induces production of type I collagen and fibronectin by fibroblasts through both transcriptional and post-transcriptional mechanisms. However, TGF-β–induced collagen production is reversed by IFN-γ.[118] This observation represents another example of the opposing or regulatory effects of one cytokine on another. TGF-β may further contribute to tissue fibrosis by decreasing production of neutral proteinases and by enhancing production of inhibitors of these enzymes in fibroblasts.[119] These effects are not observed with TGF-β alone but only in the presence of growth factors such as EGF, basic fibroblast growth factor (FGF), or PDGF. These combined cytokine effects lead to decreased synthesis and release of tissue-damaging enzymes such as collagenase and plasminogen activators. In contrast, production of TIMP and of plasminogen activator inhibitor (PAI) in fibroblasts is enhanced by TGF-β. These effects of TGF-β on fibroblast protein production are accompanied by comparable changes in steady-state mRNA levels. The net effect of TGF-β on fibroblasts is to enhance synthesis and inhibit degradation of fibrous tissue.

In summary, TGF-β exhibits varied effects on inflammatory, immune, and connective tissue cells in vitro (Table 13–8). The predicted result of TGF-β presence in vivo would be an influx of monocytes, inhibition of macrophage and lymphocyte function, and a stimulation of matrix formation. This overall effect would appear to dampen acute inflammatory events and enhance tissue repair and scarring. Studies in experimental animal models of disease and in human diseases substantiate this conclusion.

Transforming Growth Factor-β in Animal and Human Diseases. TGF-β is thought to play a role in many human diseases, including inflammatory joint diseases, scleroderma, glomerulonephritis, and pulmonary fibrosis. In these diseases, TGF-β may be released by platelets or macrophages and mediate effects on local cells such as fibroblasts.

Many chronic inflammatory diseases are characterized by deficient cellular immune responses. In streptococcal cell wall–induced arthritis in rats, a model resembling RA, TGF-β appears to be responsible for this immunosuppression.[120] In addition,

Table 13–8. BIOLOGIC PROPERTIES OF TGF-β

Target Cell	Properties
Monocytes-macrophages	Chemotaxis, activates or inhibits various functions
T and B lymphocytes	Inhibits functions by decreasing IL-1 receptor expression
Connective tissue cells	Enhances or inhibits growth (through PDGF)
	Induces production of type I collagen and fibronectin
	Decreases neutral proteinase production
	Enhances production of enzyme inhibitors

TGF-β may be involved in both acute and chronic inflammatory events in arthritis. Intra-articular injection of TGF-β in rats induces swelling, erythema, and an influx of mononuclear cells, followed by synovial fibroblast hyperplasia.[121] The latter response is thought to be due to TGF-β induction of growth factor production in monocytes. Latent TGF-β is present in rheumatoid synovial effusions, and rheumatoid synovial tissue cells contain TGF-β mRNA as well as produce TGF-β protein in vitro.[122] Finally, TGF-β protein is present in both the lining and sublining layers of rheumatoid synovium in vivo and stimulates collagen production by synovial fibroblasts in vitro.[123] All of these data suggest that TGF-β is an important mediator of both acute inflammation and fibrosis in the rheumatoid synovium.

Scleroderma is another disease in which TGF-β is thought to play a primary role in pathophysiology.[124] The extensive dermal and organ fibrosis in this disorder results from excessive collagen production by fibroblasts. TGF-β mRNA is present in infiltrating monocytes, perivascular areas of the dermis, and subcutaneous tissues of scleroderma skin.[125] Furthermore, adjacent fibroblasts contain TGF-β protein as well as type I procollagen mRNA. However, TGF-β also plays a role in normal skin function because this protein can be found in epithelial cells from normal as well as diseased skin.[126] In addition to stimulating fibroblast matrix synthesis, TGF-β may contribute to pathologic changes in scleroderma by inhibiting endothelial cell growth. However, the potentially injurious effects of TGF-β in scleroderma may be opposed by other cytokines. TGF-β induction of type I procollagen mRNA in human fibroblasts is antagonized by both TNF-α and IFN-γ.[127] These cytokines act through different mechanisms. TNF-α inhibits transcription of the type I procollagen gene, whereas IFN-γ destabilizes the mRNA. These observations have given rise to clinical trials examining the effects of IFN-γ in scleroderma patients.

TGF-β may also be involved in various forms of glomerulonephritis or fibrotic pulmonary diseases. TGF-β mRNA levels are elevated in the glomeruli of rats with experimental glomerulonephritis and correlate with increased tissue levels of proteoglycans and fibronectin.[128] Furthermore, antiserum to TGF-β markedly reduces both extracellular matrix formation and histologic progression of the glomerular disease in this animal model.[129] Finally, TGF-β has been incriminated in two different animal models of lung disease: bleomycin-induced pulmonary fibrosis in rats[130] and pulmonary hypertension in sheep.[131]

In summary, TGF-β may interact with other cytokines in mediating acute and chronic inflammatory events in many human diseases. Whether TGF-β plays a primary role in any of these disorders or has any potential for use in therapy remains to be proven.

OTHER GROWTH FACTORS

Additional growth factors besides TGF-β that may play roles in autoimmune and inflammatory diseases include PDGF, EGF, and FGF. These polypeptides are thought to regulate growth of normal cells as well as of transformed cells such as occur in neoplasms or in RA. Multiple growth factors appear to be present in most tissues and exert synergistic effects.

Platelet-Derived Growth Factor. In addition to platelets, PDGF is produced by endothelial cells, macrophages, and other cells.[132, 133] The structure of PDGF is analogous to that of TGF-β. PDGF is a 30-kD dimer of two polypeptide chains linked by disulfide bonds. The two chains, A and B, are approximately 60 percent similar, with the A chain existing as two structural variants. PDGF is a homodimer of A (PDGF-AA) or B (PDGF-BB) chains as well as a heterodimer (PDGF-AB). Each of these forms of PDGF may exhibit differences in biologic properties. The primary forms released by platelets are PDGF-AB and PDGF-BB. Two different PDGF receptors exist: the type A receptor binds all three isoforms of PDGF, whereas the type B receptor preferentially binds PDGF-BB. The PDGF receptor is a functional tyrosine kinase; thus, phosphorylation of selected substrates is a main mechanism of signal transduction after receptor binding. Therefore, whether a response to PDGF is observed will depend on the isoform of PDGF synthesized as well as on the type and density of PDGF receptors present.

Epidermal Growth Factor. EGF is partially homologous to TGF-α; both peptides bind to the same receptor and induce the same biologic responses.[134] EGF is a 6-kD molecule with three internal disulfide bonds. EGF is found in most body fluids, and the major producing cells in humans are the submandibular glands and Brunner's glands in the duodenum. The EGF receptor is present on most cells in the body, except those of the hematopoietic system. The cytoplasmic domain of the EGF receptor exhibits tyrosine kinase activity; ligand binding leads to phosphorylation of the receptor itself as well as of intracellular substrates. TGF-α and EGF are potent angiogenic factors capable of inducing new capillary growth. In addition, these peptides stimulate proliferation and differentiation of many epithelial and mesenchymal cells. Interestingly, the growth-promoting effects of TGF-α and EGF on many cells are opposed by TGF-β. Thus, the balance between these factors influences the resultant effect on cell growth.

Fibroblast Growth Factors. Two types of FGF have been described: acidic (aFGF) and basic (bFGF).[136] Both are 15- to 18-kD single polypeptide chains and are synthesized by a variety of cells, including macrophages, fibroblasts, endothelial cells, and epithelial cells. Two FGF receptors have been described, with both forms of FGF binding to both receptors, although in a differential fashion.

Growth Factors in Rheumatoid Synovitis. Growth factors derived from macrophages appear to be responsible for the intense proliferation of fibroblast-like cells in the rheumatoid synovium.[136a] This fibroblast growth assumes some of the characteristics of transformed cells with a "tumor-like" nature to

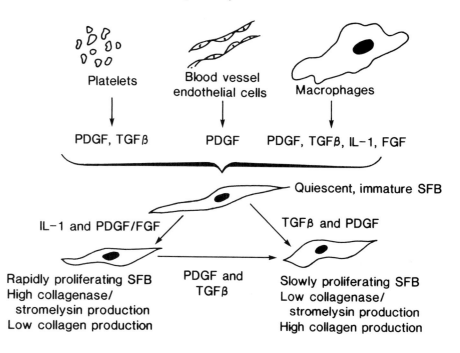

Figure 13–2. A hypothetical model of paracrine control of rheumatoid synovial fibroblast-like cells by TGF-β and other growth factors, such as PDGF, FGF, and IL-1. The diagram depicts paracrine factors such as PDGF, FGF, and IL-1 (derived from platelets, endothelial cells, macrophages, etc.) stimulating quiescent, immature synovial fibroblast-like cells to adapt a highly proliferative and invasive phenotype. TGF-β, on the other hand, appears to inhibit the invasive, tumor-like phenotype. (From Wilder, R. L., Lafayatis, R., Roberts, A. B., et al.: Transforming growth factor-β in rheumatoid arthritis. Ann. N.Y. Acad. Sci. 593:197, 1990. Used by permission.)

the rheumatoid pannus (see Chapter 51). Rheumatoid synovial cells in vitro grow to high-saturation densities and under anchorage-independent conditions, thus resembling transformed cells.[136] These growth characteristics are dependent on the presence of serum, with PDGF the main involved factor. In support of the importance of growth factors in inducing growth and proliferation of rheumatoid synovial cells in vivo is the observation that PDGF is a potent stimulator of in vitro growth of these cells. EGF enhances while TGF-β inhibits the PDGF-dependent growth of rheumatoid synovial cells in vitro.[136] In addition, the ability of rheumatoid synovial fluid to promote growth of synoviocytes in vitro is inhibited 68 percent by neutralizing antibodies to PDGF.[137] Furthermore, rheumatoid synovial tissue contains both mRNA and protein for PDGF-BB, in association with a precursor form of aFGF.[138] These proteins are present primarily in infiltrating macrophages in the rheumatoid synovium.

FGFs also have been described in noninflammatory synovial fluids, and both FGF mRNA and protein are present in rheumatoid and osteoarthritic synovium.[139] In both noninflammatory and inflammatory joint diseases, FGFs may participate in induction of collagenase production and angiogenesis, as well as in stimulation of fibroblast growth.

Rheumatoid synovial cells exhibit complex responses to the combination of PDGF and IL-1.[140] IL-1 inhibits PDGF-induced fibroblast proliferation, probably through inducing the production of prostaglandin E_2. In addition, PDGF, EGF, and FGF all enhance IL-1 induction of prostaglandin E_2 production by rheumatoid synovial cells. As a contrasting response, PDGF inhibits IL-1 induction of collagenase production by these cells in vitro. However, the type

and degree of differentiation of fibroblasts markedly influence their responses to cytokines. As opposed to synovial cells, both IL-1 and PDGF stimulate collagenase gene transcription and protein production in dermal fibroblasts. In fact, PDGF enhances transcription of IL-1 receptors in murine dermal fibroblasts, producing an even greater cellular response in the presence of both factors. Thus, the combination of PDGF and IL-1 leads primarily to antagonistic effects on synovial cells, whereas synergistic responses occur in dermal fibroblasts.

In summary, in addition to TGF-β, other growth factors such as PDGF, EGF, and FGF may play important roles in the rheumatoid synovium, particularly in stimulating fibroblast proliferation (Fig. 13–2). These cytokines also may be involved in other human diseases characterized by tissue fibrosis.

COLONY-STIMULATING FACTORS

The CSFs were originally described as hematopoietic growth factors but are now known to exert multiple effects on mature neutrophils, monocytes, and lymphocytes.[141, 142] This group of glycoproteins includes GM-CSF, G-CSF, M-CSF, and IL-3 (previously known as multi-CSF). Erythropoietin, which has growth-promoting effects only on erythroid precursor cells, is another CSF that will not be discussed here.

The genes for GM-CSF, M-CSF, and IL-3 are all located in the same region of the long arm of chromosome 5. This genetic association suggests that these proteins may share some biologic properties. This is indeed true, because the effects of these factors on growth and differentiation of bone marrow precursor cells are overlapping and synergistic. GM-CSF and IL-3 are multipotential hematopoietic growth factors whose effects on early precursor cells are enhanced by other cytokines such as IL-1 and IL-6. In contrast, G-CSF and M-CSF are more lineage-specific growth factors that act later on cells already committed to the granulocytic or macrophage series. More restricted effects on growth of particular types of cells are observed with IL-3, specifically for basophils and mast cells.

The effects of CSFs on mature cells are specific for each CSF, vary with the level of cell differentiation, and are greatly influenced by the presence of other cytokines. G-CSF, approximately 20 kD in size, and M-CSF, 50 to 70 kD in size, are both produced by monocytes, fibroblasts, and endothelial cells. G-CSF enhances the growth and survival, as well as various functions, of neutrophils present in tissues. M-CSF, formerly called *CSF-1*, is a potent chemotactic factor for monocytes and enhances the differentiation of monocytes into macrophages. The effects of serum on macrophage differentiation in vitro is probably due primarily to the presence of M-CSF. Furthermore, M-CSF injected intravenously into mice increases the level of circulating monocytes and tissue macrophages, with these macrophages exhibiting a more differentiated phenotype. Thus, in rheumatic diseases, G-CSF and M-CSF may influence the accumulation and differentiation of phagocytic cells in tissues, possibly enhancing their protective or injurious potential.

Granulocyte-Macrophage Colony-Stimulating Factor. GM-CSF has a potentially great relevance to cell function in autoimmune and inflammatory diseases. GM-CSF is a 14- to 35-kD glycoprotein that exhibits heterogeneity in glycosylation and is produced by T cells, monocytes, fibroblasts, and endothelial cells.[143] GM-CSF exerts effects on mature granulocytes, eosinophils, basophils, and monocytes and primes neutrophils for a series of responses triggered by other agents. These responses include chemotaxis, immobilization in tissues, phagocytosis, and production of oxygen metabolites. In addition, GM-CSF stimulates neutrophil production of other cytokines, including IL-1, G-CSF, and M-CSF. Finally, GM-CSF enhances eosinophil cytotoxicity and leukotriene synthesis as well as stimulates histamine release from basophils. Thus, the priming or activating effect of GM-CSF on neutrophils, eosinophils, and basophils enhances the capacity of these cells to contribute to the inflammatory response.

It is on monocytes and macrophages, however, where GM-CSF may exert the most important influence. First, GM-CSF enhances monocyte migration into inflamed tissues by stimulating expression of the adhesion molecules CD18[144] and CD11b.[145] Once in the tissues, GM-CSF stimulates monocytes to synthesize more membrane-bound IL-1α[146] and to secrete prostaglandin E$_2$[147] and also primes these cells to secrete more TNF-α in response to LPS and IFN-γ.[147] GM-CSF also stimulates HLA-DR and DP expression on human monocytes. The enhanced expression of both membrane-bound IL-1α and of class II MHC molecules leads to greater accessory cell function in GM-CSF–stimulated monocytes. Monocytes pretreated with GM-CSF promote both mitogen- and antigen-induced lymphocyte proliferation. This last effect of GM-CSF might be important to rheumatic diseases where enhanced antigen presentation may lead to a more intense and prolonged immune response. Finally, GM-CSF influences differentiation of macrophages from monocytes and markedly enhances IL-1ra production by these cells.

The postulated role of CSFs in inflammatory arthritis has been substantiated by recent studies in patients with RA. Rheumatoid synovial fluid and tissue exhibit little evidence for the chronic production of the T cell products IL-2, IL-3, and IFN-γ.[148] In contrast, both protein and mRNA are abundant for M-CSF, GM-CSF, and a mast cell growth factor. This last observation is of particular interest because rheumatoid synovium contains increased numbers of mast cells, and these cells are thought to be involved in pathophysiologic events. TNF-α produced in the rheumatoid joint may enhance the effects of GM-CSF on induction and maintenance of class II MHC antigen expression on tissue macrophages.[149] RA is the only human disease where GM-CSF protein and mRNA have been found in the injured tissue,[150] although with further study other diseases may exhibit similar findings.

In summary, CSFs may be involved in rheumatic diseases at two levels: induction of growth and proliferation of hematopoietic progenitor cells in the bone marrow as well as activation of mature granulocytes and monocytes. The effects of CSFs on peripheral and tissue phagocytic cells enhance the ability of these cells to release other cytokines and inflammatory mediators. Furthermore, monocytes and macrophages may acquire a greater ability to present antigen to lymphocytes, thus driving both humoral and cellular immune responses. Activation of T cells leads to production of GM-CSF and IL-3, whereas monocyte production of GM-CSF and G-CSF results from stimulation by endotoxin or by other cytokines such as IL-1 and TNF-α. Fibroblasts and endothelial cells may constitutively produce M-CSF, but GM-CSF and G-CSF production is stimulated in these cells by IL-1 and TNF-α. Thus, local cytokine release stimulates further CSF production, which, in turn, leads to more cytokine production by fibroblasts and macrophages. This self-perpetuating cycle may lead to chronic inflammation and prolonged tissue destruction in diseases such as RA in the absence of an ongoing significant component of T cell activation (Fig. 13–3).

CONCLUSION

This chapter has summarized many aspects of the molecular biology, biochemistry, and biology of those cytokines whose effects are exerted primarily on cells of the immune and inflammatory systems.

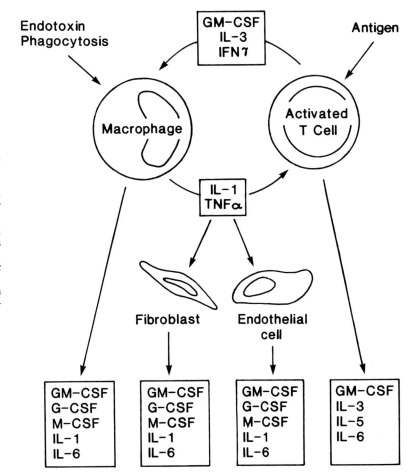

Figure 13–3. Regulation of production and cellular sources of colony-stimulating growth factors. Macrophages are stimulated by endotoxin, phagocytosis, or factors released by antigen-stimulated T cells. Both macrophages and activated T cells directly release growth factors. In addition, macrophages release IL-1 and TNF, which, in turn, stimulate cytokine production by fibroblasts and endothelial cells. (From Groopman, J. E., Molina, J.-M. and Scadden J.T.: Hematopoietic growth factors: Biology and clinical applications. N. Engl. J. Med. 321:1449, 1989. Reprinted with permission from *The New England Journal of Medicine*.)

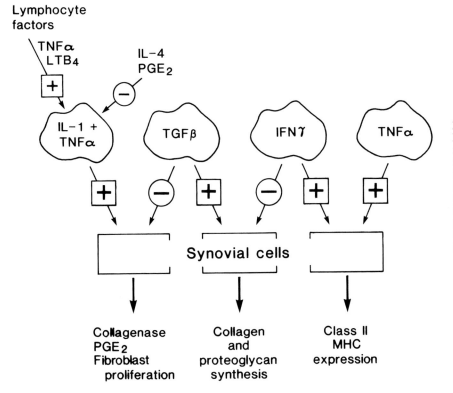

Figure 13–4. Contrasting effects of cytokines on synovial cell function in rheumatoid arthritis. Cytokine-producing cells respond to both positive and negative influences. In addition, different cytokines may affect synovial cells in a positive or negative fashion, depending on the cell function examined. TGF-β may oppose some of the stimulatory effects of IL-1 and TNF, whereas IFN-α may oppose some of the effects of TGF-β.

Cytokines may play an important role in the initiation and maintenance of autoimmune and inflammatory disease as mediators of cell-cell interactions. As an example, some of these effects of cytokines on synovial cell function in RA are summarized in Figure 13–4. Both agonist and antagonist effects of cytokines may be present at the same time in this disease process. The net biologic response at any point in time will depend on which cytokine(s) are present in excess. In addition, inhibitors of IL-1 and TNF-α may be present locally, limiting the biologic effects of these potent proinflammatory cytokines.

In normal physiology, cytokines regulate the growth and differentiation of hematopoietic and mesenchymal cells in both positive and negative fashions. However, cytokines have overlapping, redundant, and synergistic effects so that multiple factors are usually involved in any particular biologic response. Cytokines exhibit both enhancing and inhibitory effects on immune and inflammatory cells. It is important to note that the cytokine network is, in large part, self-regulating through the simultaneous presence of factors with opposing properties, feedback inhibition of production, and induction of specific cytokine-binding proteins or receptor antagonists.

The possibility exists that in some human autoimmune or inflammatory diseases, the normal cytokine balances may be disrupted. This abnormal state may occur through the unregulated production of proinflammatory factors or inadequate exertion of anti-inflammatory cytokines or mechanisms. This chapter has emphasized the importance of regulatory mechanisms in the cytokine network. Present goals of investigation include determining whether particular cytokines can be incriminated in specific disease processes and how these effects can be prevented or blocked.

Cytokines as therapeutic agents in human diseases are called *biologic response modifiers*. Whether interruption of the effects of a single cytokine will significantly alter the course of a human disease remains to be established. A more likely eventuality might be the therapeutic use of multiple cytokines in an effort to alter the diseased milieu. In any case, cytokine biology has brought a new dimension to the understanding of cellular events in rheumatic diseases and holds the promise of therapeutic potential.

References

1. Arai, K. I., Lee, F., Mijajima, A., et al.: Cytokines: Coordinators of immune and inflammatory responses. Annu. Rev. Biochem. 59:783, 1990.
2. Kelley, J.: Cytokines of the lung. Am. Rev. Respir. Dis. 141:765, 1990.
3. Dinarello, C. A.: Interleukin-1 and its biologically related cytokines. Adv. Immunol. 44:153, 1989.
4. di Giovine, F. S., and Duff, G. W.: Interleukin-1: The first interleukin. Immunol. Today 11:13, 1990.
5. Schmidt, J. A., and Tocci, M. J.: Interleukin 1. *In* Sporn, M. B., and Roberts, A. B. (eds): Peptide Growth Factors and Their Receptors. vol. 1. Berlin, Springer-Verlag, 1990, p. 473.
6. Kostura, M. J., Tocci, M. J., Limiuco, G., et al.: Identification of a monocyte specific pre-interleukin-1β convertase activity. Proc. Natl. Acad. Sci. U.S.A. 86:5227, 1989.
7. Brennan, F. M., Chantry, D., Jackson, A., et al.: Inhibitory effect of TNFα antibodies on synovial cell interleukin-1 production in rheumatoid arthritis. Lancet 2:244, 1989.
8. Rosoff, P. M.: IL-1 receptors: Structure and signals. Semin. Immunol. 2:129, 1990.
9. Dower, S. K., Qwarnstrom, E. E., et al.: Biology of the interleukin-1 receptor. J. Invest. Dermatol. 94:68S, 1990.
10. Dower, S. K., and Sims, J. E.: Molecular characterization of cytokine receptors. Ann. Rheum. Dis. 49:452, 1990.
11. Mizel, S. B.: Cyclic AMP and interleukin-1 signal transduction. Immunol. Today 11:390, 1990.
12. O'Neill, L. A. J., Bird, T. A., and Saklatvala, J.: Interleukin-1 signal transduction. Immunol. Today 11:392, 1990.
13. Dayer, J. M., and Demczuk, S.: Cytokines and other mediators in rheumatoid arthritis. Semin. Immunopathol. 7:387, 1984.
14. Zvaifler, N. J.: New perspectives on the pathogenesis of rheumatoid arthritis. Am. J. Med. 85A:12, 1988.
15. Arend, W. P., and Dayer, J.-M.: Cytokines and cytokine inhibitors or antagonists in rheumatoid arthritis. Arthritis Rheum. 33:305, 1990.
16. Arner, E. D., and Pratta, M. A.: Independent effects of interleukin-1 on proteoglycan breakdown, proteoglycan synthesis, and prostaglandin E₂ release from cartilage in organ culture. Arthritis Rheum. 32:288, 1989.
17. Pettipher, E. R., Higgs, G. A., and Henderson, B.: Interleukin 1 induces leukocyte infiltration and cartilage proteoglycan degradation in the synovial joint. Proc. Natl. Acad. Sci. U.S.A. 83:8749, 1986.
18. Stimpson, S. A., Dalldorf, F. G., Otterness, I.G., and Schwab, J. H.: Exacerbation of arthritis by IL-1 in rat joints previously injured by peptidoglycan-polysaccharide. J. Immunol. 140:2964, 1988.
19. Hom, J. T., Bendele, A. M., and Carlson, D. G.: *In vivo* administration with IL-1 accelerates the development of collagen-induced arthritis in mice. J. Immunol. 141:834, 1988.
20. Jacobs, C., Young, D., Tyler, S., et al.: *In vivo* treatment with IL-1 reduces the severity and duration of antigen-induced arthritis in rats. J. Immunol. 141:2967, 1988.
21. Wallach, D., Holtmann, H., Engelmann, H., and Nophar, Y.: Sensitization and desensitization to lethal effects of tumor necrosis factor and IL-1. J. Immunol. 140:2994, 1988.
22. Henderson, B., Rowe, F. M., Bird, C. R., and Gearing, A. J. H.: Production of interleukin 1 in the joint during the development of antigen-induced arthritis in the rabbit. Clin. Exp. Immunol. 74:371, 1988.
23. Duff, G.: Interleukin-1 in inflammatory joint disease. *In* Bomford, R., and Henderson, B. (eds.): Interleukin-1, Inflammation and Disease. Amsterdam, Elsevier Science Publishers, 1989, p. 243.
24. Hopkins, S. J., Humphreys, M., and Jayson, M. I. V.: Cytokines in synovial fluid: I. The presence of biologically active and immunoreactive IL-1. Clin. Exp. Immunol. 72:422, 1988.
25. Bhardwaj, N., Lau, L. L., Rivelis, M., and Steinman, R. M.: Interleukin-1 production by mononuclear cells from rheumatoid synovial effusions. Cell. Immunol. 114:405, 1988.
26. Miyasaka, N., Sato, K., Goto, M., et al.: Augmented interleukin-1 production and HLA-DR expression in the synovium of rheumatoid arthritis patients: Possible involvement in joint destruction. Arthritis Rheum. 31:480, 1988.
27. Buchan, G., Barrett, K., Turner, M., et al.: Interleukin-1 and tumour necrosis factor mRNA expression in rheumatoid arthritis: prolonged production of IL-1α. Clin. Exp. Immunol. 73:449, 1988.
28. Firestein, G. S., Alvaro-Garcia, J. M., and Maki, R.: Quantitative analysis of cytokine gene expression in rheumatoid arthritis. J. Immunol. 144:3347, 1990.
29. MacNaul, K. L., Hutchinson, N. I., Parsons, J. N., et al: Analysis of IL-1 and TNFα gene expression in human rheumatoid synoviocytes and normal monocytes by *in situ* hybridization. J. Immunol. 145:4154, 1990.
30. Eastgate, J. A., Symons, J. A., Wood, N. C., et al: Correlation of plasma interleukin 1 levels with disease activity in rheumatoid arthritis. Lancet 2:706, 1988.
31. Shore, A., Jaglal, S., and Keystone, E.C.: Enhanced interleukin 1 generation by monocytes *in vitro* is temporarily linked to an early event in the onset or exacerbation of rheumatoid arthritis. Clin. Exp. Immunol. 65:293, 1986.
32. Dayer, J.-M., and Seckinger, P.: Natural inhibitors and antagonists of interleukin 1. *In* Bomford, R., and Henderson, B. (eds.): Interleukin-1, Inflammation and Disease. Amsterdam, Elsevier Science Publishers, 1989, p. 283.
33. Arend, W. P., Joslin, F. G., Thompson, R. C., and Hannum, C. G.: An interleukin 1 inhibitor from human monocytes: Production and characterization of biological properties. J. Immunol. 143:1851, 1989.
34. Larrick, J. W.: Native interleukin 1 inhibitors. Immunol. Today 10:61, 1989.

35. Baumberger, C., Ulevitch, R. J., and Dayer, J.-M.: Modulation of endotoxic activity of lipopolysaccharides by high-density lipoprotein. Pathobiology 59:378, 1991.

36. Muchmore, A. V., and Decker, J. M.: Uromodulin. An immunosuppressant 85-kilodalton glycoprotein isolated from human pregnancy urine is a high affinity ligand for recombinant interleukin 1α. J. Biol. Chem. 261:13404, 1986.

37. Eastgate, J. A., Symons, J. A., and Duff, G. W.: Identification of an interleukin-1 beta binding protein in human plasma. FEBS Lett. 260:213, 1990.

38. Borth, W., Scheer, B., Urbansky, A., et al.: Binding of IL-1β to α-macroglobulins and release by thioredoxin. J. Immunol. 145:3747, 1990.

39. Bendtzen, K., Svenson, M., Jonsson, V., and Hippe, E.: Autoantibodies to cytokines: Friends or foes? Immunol. Today 11:167, 1990.

40. Giri, J. G., Newton, R. C., and Horuk, R.: Identification of soluble interleukin-1 binding protein in cell-free supernatants. J. Biol. Chem. 265:17416, 1990.

41. Symons, J. A., and Duff, G. W.: A soluble form of the interleukin-1 receptor produced by a human B cell line. FEBS Lett. 272:133, 1990.

42. Dower, S. K., Wignall, J. M., Schooley, K., et al.: Retention of ligand binding activity by the extracellular domain of the IL-1 receptor. J. Immunol. 142:4314, 1989.

43. Fanslow, W. C., Sims, J. E., Sassenfeld, H., et al.: Regulation of alloreactivity in vivo by a soluble form of the interleukin-1 receptor. Science 248:739, 1990.

44. Arend, W. P.: Interleukin-1 receptor antagonist: Discovery, structure, and properties. Prog. Growth Factor Res. 2:193, 1990.

44a. Arend, W. P.: Interleukin-1 receptor antagonist: A new member of the interleukin-1 family. J. Clin. Invest. 88:1445, 1991.

45. Balavoine, J. F., de Rochemonteix, B., Williamson, K., et al.: Prostaglandin E₂ and collagenase production by fibroblasts and synovial cells is regulated by urine-derived human interleukin 1 and inhibitor(s). J. Clin. Invest. 78:1120, 1986.

46. Arend, W. P., Joslin, F. G., and Massoni, R. J.: Effects of immune complexes on production by human monocytes of interleukin 1 or an interleukin 1 inhibitor. J. Immunol. 134:3868, 1985.

47. Hannum, C. H., Wilcox, C. J., Arend, W. P., et al.: Interleukin-1 receptor antagonist activity of a human interleukin-1 inhibitor. Nature 343:336, 1990.

48. Carter, D. B., Deibel, M. R., Jr., Dunn, C. J., et al.: Purification, cloning, expression and biological characterization of an interleukin-1 receptor antagonist protein. Nature 344:633, 1990.

49. Eisenberg, S. P., Evans, R. J., Arend, W. P., et al.: Primary structure and functional expression from complementary DNA of a human interleukin-1 receptor antagonist. Nature 343:341, 1990.

50. Arend, W. P., Welgus, H. G., Thompson, R. C., and Eisenberg, S. P.: Biological properties of recombinant human monocyte-derived interleukin 1 receptor antagonist. J. Clin. Invest. 85:1694, 1990.

51. Roux-Lombard, P., Modoux, C., Dayer, J.-M.: Production of interleukin-1 (IL-1) and a specific IL-1 inhibitor during human monocyte-macrophage differentiation: Influence of GM-CSF. Cytokine 1:45, 1989.

52. Roux-Lombard, P., Modoux, C., and Dayer, J.-M.: Inhibition of IL-1 and TNFα activities in synovial fluids and cultured synovial fluid cell supernatants. Calcif. Tissue Int. 42:S(A47), 1988.

53. Rochemonteix, B. G., Nicod, L. P., Junod, A. F., and Dayer, J.-M.: Characterization of a specific 20- to 25-kD interleukin-1 inhibitor from cultured human lung macrophages. Am. J. Respir. Cell Mol. Biol. 3:355, 1990.

54. Haskill, S., Martin, G., Van Le L., et al.: cDNA cloning of a novel intracellular form of the human interleukin-1 receptor antagonist associated with epithelium. Proc. Natl. Acad. Sci. U.S.A. 88:3631, 1991.

55. Prieur, A.-M., Kaufmann, M. T., Griscelli, C., and Dayer, J. M.: Specific interleukin-1 inhibitor in serum and urine of children with systemic juvenile chronic arthritis. Lancet 2:1240, 1987.

56. Malyak, M., Joslin, F. G., and Arend, W. P.: Synovial fluid IL-1ra levels as determined by a modified sandwich ELISA (Abstract). Arthritis Rheum. 33:S149, 1990.

57. Beutler, B., and Cerami, A.: The history, properties, and biological effects of cachectin. Biochemistry 27:7575, 1988.

58. Beutler, B.: Cachectin/tumor necrosis factor and lymphotoxin. In Sporn, M. B., Roberts, A. B. (eds.): Peptide Growth Factors and Their Receptors. vol. 2. Berlin, Springer-Verlag, 1990, p. 39.

59. Sherry, B., and Cerami, A.: Cachectin/tumor necrosis factor exerts endocrine, paracrine and autocrine control of inflammatory responses. J. Cell Biol. 107:1269, 1988.

60. Jones, E. Y., Stuart, D. I., and Walker, N. P. C.: Structure of tumour necrosis factor. Nature 338:225, 1989.

61. Gray, P. W., Barrett, K., Chantry, D., et al.: Cloning of human tumor necrosis factor (TNF) receptor cDNA and expression of recombinant soluble TNF-binding protein. Proc. Natl. Acad. Sci. U.S.A. 87:7380, 1990.

62. Kohno, T., Brewer, M. T., Baker, S. L., et al.: A second tumor necrosis factor gene product can shed a naturally occurring tumor necrosis factor inhibitor. Proc. Natl. Acad. Sci. U.S.A. 87:8331, 1990.

63. Le, J., and Vilcek, J.: Tumor necrosis factor and interleukin-1: Cytokines with multiple overlapping biological activities. Lab. Invest. 56:234, 1987.

64. Cerami, A., and Beutler, B.: The role of cachectin/TNF in endotoxic shock and cachexia. Immunol. Today 9:28, 1988.

65. Satoh, J., Seino, H., Shintani, S., et al.: Inhibition of type 1 diabetes in BB rats with recombinant human tumor necrosis factor-α. J. Immunol. 145:1395, 1990.

66. Levine, B., Kalman, J., Mayer, L., et al.: Elevated circulating levels of tumor necrosis factor in severe chronic heart failure. N. Engl. J. Med. 323:236, 1990.

67. Henderson, B., and Pettipher, E. R.: Arthritogenic actions of recombinant IL-1 and tumour necrosis factor α in the rabbit: Evidence for synergistic interactions between cytokines in vivo. Clin. Exp. Immunol. 75:306, 1989.

68. Seckinger, P., and Dayer, J.-M.: Natural inhibitors of tumor necrosis factor. In Aggarwal, B. B., and Vilcek, J. (eds.): Tumor Necrosis Factor: Structure, Function, and Mechanism of Action. New York, Marcel Dekker, 1992, p. 217.

69. Lantz, M., Gullberg, U., Nilsson, E., and Olsson, I.: Characterization in vitro of a human tumor necrosis factor-binding protein. A soluble form of a tumor necrosis factor receptor. J. Clin. Invest. 86:1396, 1990.

69a. Aderka, D., Engelmann, H., Maor, Y., Brakebusch, C., and Wallach, D.: Stabilization of the bioactivity of tumor necrosis factor by its soluble receptor. J. Exp. Med. 175:323, 1992.

70. Akira, S., Hirano, T., Taga, T., and Kishimoto, T.: Biology of multifunctional cytokines: IL 6 and related molecules (IL 1 and TNF). FASEB J. 4:2860, 1990.

71. Van Snick, J.: Interleukin-6: An overview. Annu. Rev. Immunol. 8:253, 1990.

72. Heinrich, P. C., Castell, J. V., and Andus, T.: Interleukin-6 and the acute phase response. Biochem. J. 265:621, 1990.

73. Seckinger, P., Yaron, I., Meyer, F. A., et al.: Modulation of the effects of interleukin-1 on glycosaminoglycan synthesis by the urine-derived interleukin-1 inhibitor, and not by interleukin 6. Arthritis Rheum. 33:1, 1990.

74. Guerne, P.-A., Vaughan, J.H., Carson, D. A., and Lotz, M.: Interleukin-6 (IL-6) and joint tissues. Ann. N. Y. Acad. Sci. 557:558, 1989.

75. Hirano, T., Akira, S., Taga, T., and Kishimoto, T.: Biological and clinical aspects of interleukin 6. Immunol. Today 11:443, 1990.

76. Baggiolini, M., Walz, A., and Kunkel, S. L.: Neutrophil-activating peptide-1/interleukin 8, a novel cytokine that activates neutrophils. J. Clin. Invest. 84:1045, 1989.

77. Matsushima, K., and Oppenheim, J. J.: Interleukin 8 and MCAF: Novel inflammatory cytokines inducible by IL 1 and TNF. Cytokine 1:2, 1989.

77a. Baggiolini, M., and Sorg, C. (eds.): Interleukin-8 (NAP-1) and Related Chemotactic Cytokines. Basel, S. Karger AG, 1992.

78. Detmers, P. A., Lo, S. K., Olsen-Egbert, E. O., et al.: Neutrophil-activating protein 1/interleukin 8 stimulates the binding activity of the leukocyte adhesion receptor CD11b/CD18 on human neutrophils. J. Exp. Med. 171:1155, 1990.

79. Larsen, C. G., Anderson, A. O., Appella, E., et al.: The neutrophil-activating protein (NAP-1) is also chemotactic for T lymphocytes. Science 243:1464, 1989.

80. Brennan, F. M., Zachariae, C. O. C., Chantry, D., et al.: Detection of interleukin 8 biological activity in synovial fluids from patients with rheumatoid arthritis and production of interleukin 8 mRNA by isolated synovial cells. Eur. J. Immunol. 20:2141, 1990.

81. Terkeltaub, R., Zachariae, C., Santoro, D., et al.: IL-8 as a potential mediator of crystal-induced synovitis (Abstract). Arthritis Rheum. 33:S20, 1990.

82. Cohen, A. B., MacArthur, C., Idell, S., et al.: A peptide from alveolar macrophages that releases neutrophil enzymes into the lungs in patients with the adult respiratory distress syndrome. Am. Rev. Respir. Dis. 137:1151, 1988.

83. Leonard, E.J., and Yoshimura, T.: Human monocyte chemoattractant protein-1 (MCP-1). Immunol. Today 11:97, 1990.

84. Vitetta, E. S., and Paul, W. E.: Role of lymphokines in the immune system. In Sporn, M. B., and Roberts, A. B. (eds.): Peptide Growth Factors and Their Receptors. vol. 2. Berlin, Springer-Verlag, 1990. p. 401.

85. Smith, K. A.: Interleukin-2: Inception, impact, and implications. Science 240:1169, 1988.

86. Kroemer, G., and Wick, G.: The role of interleukin 2 in autoimmunity. Immunol. Today 10:246, 1989.

87. Smith, M. D., and Roberts-Thomson, P. J.: Interleukin 2 and interleukin 2 inhibitors in human serum and synovial fluid: II. Mitogenic stimulation, interleukin 2 production and interleukin 2 receptor expression in rheumatoid arthritis, psoriatic arthritis and Reiter's syndrome. J. Rheum. 16:897, 1989.

88. Miossec, P., Elhamiani, M., Chichehian, B., et al.: Interleukin 2 (IL 2) inhibitor in rheumatoid synovial fluid: Correlation with prognosis and soluble IL 2 receptor levels. J. Clin. Immunol. 10:115, 1990.

89. Rubin, L. A., and Nelson, D. L.: The soluble interleukin-2 receptor: Biology, function and clinical application. Ann. Intern. Med. 113:619, 1990.

90. ter Borg, E. J., Horst, G., Limburg, P. C., and Kallenberg, C. G. M.: Changes in plasma levels of interleukin-2 receptor in relation to disease exacerbations and levels of anti-dsDNA and complement in systemic lupus erythematosus. Clin. Exp. Immunol. 82:21, 1990.

91. Miossec, P., Elhamiani, M., Edmonds-Alt, X., et al.: Functional studies of soluble low-affinity interleukin-2 receptors in rheumatoid synovial fluid. Arthritis Rheum. 33:1688, 1990.

92. Ihle, J. N.: interleukin 3. In Sporn, M. B., and Roberts, A. B. (eds.): Peptide Growth Factors and Their Receptors. vol. 1. Berlin, Springer-Verlag, 1990, p 541.

93. Frendl, G., and Beller, D. I.: Regulation of macrophage activation by IL-3: I. IL-3 functions as a macrophage-activating factor with unique properties, inducing Ia and lymphocyte function-associated antigen-1 but not cytotoxicity. J. Immunol. 144:3392, 1990.

94. Frendl, G., Fenton, M. J., and Beller, D. I.: Regulation of macrophage activation by IL-3: II. IL-3 and lipopolysaccharide act synergistically in the regulation of IL-1 expression. J. Immunol. 144:3400, 1990.

95. Yokota, T., Arai, N., Arai, K. I., and Zlotnick, A.: Interleukin 4. In Sporn, M. B., and Roberts, A. B. (eds.): Peptide Growth Factors and Their Receptors. vol. 1. Berlin, Springer-Verlag, 1990, p. 577.

96. Gerrard, T. L., Dyer, D. R., and Mostowski, H. S.: IL-4 and granulocyte-macrophage colony-stimulating factor selectively increase HLA-DR and HLA-DP antigens but not HLA-DQ antigens on human monocytes. J. Immunol. 144:4670, 1990.

97. te Velde, A. A., Huijbens, R. J. F., de Vries, J. E., and Figdor, C. G.: IL-4 decreases FcγR membrane expression and FcγR-mediated cytotoxic activity of human monocytes. J. Immunol. 144:3046, 1990.

98. Abramson, S. L., and Gallin, J. I.: IL-4 inhibits superoxide production by human mononuclear phagocytes. J. Immunol. 144:625, 1990.

99. te Velde, A. A., Huijbens, R. J. F., Heije, K., de Vries, J. E., and Figdor, C. G.: Interleukin-4 (IL-4) inhibits secretion of IL-1β, tumor necrosis factor α, and IL-6 by human monocytes. Blood 76:1392, 1990.

100. Masinovsky, B., Urdal, D., and Gallatin, W. M.: IL-4 acts synergistically with IL-1β to promote lymphocyte adhesion to microvascular endothelium by induction of vascular cell adhesion molecule-1. J. Immunol. 145:2886, 1990.

101. Thornhill, M. H., and Haskard, D. O.: IL-4 regulates endothelial cell activation by IL-1, tumor necrosis factor, or IFN-γ. J. Immunol. 145:865, 1990.

102. Nonjo, T., and Kishimoto, T.: Interleukin 5. In Sporn, M. B., and Roberts, A. B. (eds.): Peptide Growth Factors and Their Receptors. vol. 1. Berlin, Springer-Verlag, 1990, p. 609.

103. Namen, A. E., Lupton, S., Hjerrild, K., et al.: Stimulation of B-cell progenitors by cloned murine interleukin-7. Nature 333:571, 1988.

104. Morrissey, P. J., Goodwin, R. G., Nordan, R. P., et al.: Recombinant interleukin 7, pre-B cell growth factor, has costimulatory activity on purified mature T cells. J. Exp. Med. 169:707, 1989.

105. MacNeil, I. A., Suda, T., Moore, K. W., et al.: IL-10, a novel growth cofactor for mature and immature T cells. J. Immunol. 145:4167, 1990.

105a. deWaal Malefyt, R., Abrams, J., Bennett, B., Figdor, C. G., and deVries, J. A.: Interleukin-10 (IL-10) inhibits cytokine synthesis by human monocytes: An autoregulatory role of IL-10 produced by monocytes. J. Exp. Med. 174:1209, 1991.

106. Paul, S. R., Bennett, F., Calvetti, J. A., et al.: Molecular cloning of a cDNA encoding interleukin 11, a stromal cell-derived lymphopoietic and hematopoietic cytokine. Proc. Natl. Acad. Sci. U.S.A. 87:7512, 1990.

107. Vilček, J.: Interferons. In Sporn, M. B., and Roberts, A. B. (eds.): Peptide Growth Factors and Their Receptors. vol. 2. Berlin, Springer-Verlag, 1990, p. 3.

108. Alvaro-Gracia, J. M., Zvaifler, N. J., and Firestein, G. S.: Cytokines in chronic inflammatory arthritis: V. Mutual antagonism between interferon-gamma and tumor necrosis factor-alpha on HLA-DR expression, proliferation, collagenase production, and granulocyte macrophage colony-stimulating factor production by rheumatoid arthritis synoviocytes. J. Clin. Invest. 86:1790, 1990.

109. Sporn, M. B., Roberts, A. B., Wakefield, L. M., and de Crombrugghe, B.: Some recent advances in the chemistry and biology of transforming growth factor-beta. J. Cell. Biol. 105:1039, 1987.

110. Massagué, J.: Transforming growth factor-α: A model for membrane-anchored growth factors. J. Biol. Chem. 265:21393, 1990.

111. Sporn, M. B., and Roberts, A. B.: TGF-β: Problems and prospects. Cell. Reg. 1:875, 1990.

112. Roberts, A. B., and Sporn, M. B.: The transforming growth factor-βs. In Sporn, M. B., and Roberts, A. B. (eds.): Peptide Growth Factors and Their Receptors. vol. 1. Berlin, Springer-Verlag, 1990, p. 419.

113. Battegay, E. J., Raines, E. W., Seifert, R. A, et al.: TGF-β induces bimodal proliferation of connective tissue cells via complex control of an autocrine PDGF loop. Cell 63:515, 1990.

114. Chantry, D., Turner, M., Abney, E., and Feldmann, M.: Modulation of cytokine production by transforming growth factor-β. J. Immunol. 142:4295, 1989.

115. Welch, G. R., Wong, H. L., and Wahl, S. M.: Selective induction of FcγRIII on human monocytes by transforming growth factor-β. J. Immunol. 144:3444, 1990.

116. Wahl, S. M., Hunt, D. A., Wong, H. L., et al.: Transforming growth factor-β is a potent immunosuppressive agent that inhibits IL-1–dependent lymphocyte proliferation. J. Immunol. 140:3026, 1988.

117. Dubois, C. M., Ruscetti, F. W., Palaszynski, E. W., et al.: Transforming growth factor β is a potent inhibitor of interleukin 1 (IL-1) receptor expression: Proposed mechanism of inhibition of IL-1 action. J. Exp. Med. 172:737, 1990.

118. Narayanan, A. S., Page, R. C., Swanson, J., et al.: Collagen synthesis by human fibroblasts. Biochem. J. 260:463, 1989.

119. Overall, C. M., Wrana, J. L., and Sodek, J.: Independent regulation of collagenase, 72-kDa progelatinase, and metalloendoproteinase inhibitor expression in human fibroblasts by transforming growth factor-β. J. Biol. Chem. 264:1860, 1989.

120. Wahl, S. M., Hunt, D. A., Bansal, G., et al.: Bacterial cell wall-induced immunosuppression. J. Exp. Med. 168:1403, 1988.

121. Allen, J. B., Manthey, C.L., Hand, A. R., et al.: Rapid onset of synovial inflammation and hyperplasia induced by transforming growth factor β. J. Exp. Med. 171:231, 1990.

122. Wilder, R. L., Lafyatis, R., Roberts, A. B., et al.: Transforming growth factor-β in rheumatoid arthritis. Ann. N.Y. Acad. Sci. 593:197, 1990.

123. Lafyatis, R., Thompson, N. L., Remmers, E. F., et al.: Transforming growth factor-β production by synovial tissues from rheumatoid patients and streptococcal cell wall arthritic rats: Studies on secretion by synovial fibroblast-like cells and immunohistologic location. J. Immunol. 143:1142, 1989.

124. LeRoy, E. C., Smith, E. A., Kahaleh, M. B., et al.: A strategy for determining the pathogenesis of systemic sclerosis. Arthritis Rheum. 32:817, 1989.

125. Kulozik, M., Hogg, A., Lankat-Buttgereit, B., and Krieg, T.: Co-localization of transforming growth factor β2 with α1(I) procollagen mRNA in tissue sections of patients with systemic sclerosis. J. Clin. Invest. 86:917, 1990.

126. Gruschwitz, M., Müller, P. U., Sepp, N., et al.: Transcription and expression of transforming growth factor type beta in the skin of progressive systemic sclerosis: A mediator of fibrosis? J. Invest. Dermatol. 94:197, 1990.

127. Kähäri, V. M., Chen, Y. O., Su, M. W., et al.: Tumor necrosis factor-α and interferon-γ suppress the activation of human type I collagen gene expression by transforming growth factor-β1. J. Clin. Invest. 86:1489, 1990.

128. Okuda, S., Languino, L. R., Ruoslahti, E., and Border, W. A.: Elevated expression of transforming growth factor-β and proteoglycan production in experimental glomerulonephritis. J. Clin. Invest. 86:453, 1990.

129. Border, W. A., Okuda, S., Languino, L. R., et al.: Suppression of experimental glomerulonephritis by antiserum against transforming growth factor β1. Nature 346:371, 1990.

130. Khalil, N., Bereznay, O., Sporn, M., Greenberg, A. H.: Macrophage production of transforming growth factor β and fibroblast collagen synthesis in chronic pulmonary inflammation. J. Exp. Med. 170:727, 1989.

131. Perkett, E. A., Lyons, R. M., Moses, H. L., et al.: Transforming growth factor-β activity in sheep lung lymph during the development of pulmonary hypertension. J. Clin. Invest. 86:1459, 1990.

132. Raines, E. W., Bowen-Pope, D. F., and Ross, R.: Platelet-derived growth factors. In Sporn, M. B., and Roberts, A. B. (eds.): Peptide Growth Factors and Their Receptors. vol. 1. Berlin, Springer-Verlag, 1990, p. 173.

133. Heldin, C. H., and Westermark, B.: Platelet-derived growth factor: Mechanism of action and possible in vivo function. Cell. Reg. 1:555, 1990.

134. Carpenter, C., and Wahl, M. I.: The epidermal growth factor family. In Sporn, M. B., and Roberts, A. B. (eds.): Peptide Growth Factors and Their Receptors. vol. 1. Berlin, Springer-Verlag, 1990, p. 69.

135. Baird, A., and Pöhlen, P.: Fibroblast growth factors. In Sporn, M. B., and Roberts, A. B. (eds.): Peptide Growth Factors and Their Receptors. vol. 1. Berlin, Springer-Verlag, 1990, p. 369.

136. Lafyatis, R., Remmers, E. F., Roberts, A. B., et al.: Anchorage-independent growth of synoviocytes from arthritic and normal joints: Stimulation by exogenous platelet-derived growth factor and inhibition by transforming growth factor-beta and retinoids. J. Clin. Invest. 83:1267, 1989.

136a. Remmers, E. F., Sano, H., and Wilder, R. L.: Platelet-derived growth factors and heparin-binding (fibroblast) growth factors in the synovial tissue pathology of rheumatoid arthritis. Semin. Arthritis Rheum. 21:191, 1991.

137. Remmers, E. F., Lafyatis, R., Kumkumian, G. K., et al.: Cytokines and growth regulation of synoviocytes from patients with rheumatoid arthritis and rats with streptococcal cell wall arthritis. Growth Factors 2:179, 1990.

138. Remmers, E. F., Sano, H., Lafyatis, R., et al.: Production of platelet derived growth factor β chain (PDGF-B/c-sis) mRNA and immuno-

reactive PDGF B-like polypeptide by rheumatoid synovium: Coexpression with heparin binding acidic fibroblast growth factor-1. J. Rheumatol. 18:7, 1991.

139. Sano, H., Forough, R., Maier, J. A. M., et al.: Detection of high levels of heparin binding growth factor-1 (acidic fibroblast growth factor) in inflammatory arthritic joints. J. Cell. Biol. 110:1417, 1990.

140. Kumkumian, G. K., Lafyatis, R., and Remmers, E. F.: Platelet-derived growth factor and IL-1 interactions in rheumatoid arthritis: Regulation of synoviocyte proliferation, prostaglandin production, and collagenase transcription. J. Immunol. 143:833, 1989.

141. Groopman, J. E., Molina, J.-M., and Scadden, D. T.: Hematopoietic growth factors: Biology and clinical applications. N. Engl. J. Med. 321:1449, 1989.

142. Kelso, A., and Metcalf, D.: T lymphocyte–derived colony-stimulating factors. Adv. Immunol. 48:69, 1990.

143. Monroy, R. L., Davis, T. A., and MacVittie, T. J.: Granulocyte-macrophage colony-stimulating factor: More than a hemopoietin. Clin. Immunol. Immunopathol. 54:333, 1990.

144. Elliott, M. J., Vadas, M. A., Cleland, L. G., et al.: IL-3 and granulocyte-macrophage colony-stimulating factor stimulate two distinct phases of adhesion in human monocytes. J. Immunol. 145:167, 1990.

145. Griffin, J. D., Spertini, O., Ernst, T. J., et al.: Granulocyte-macrophage colony-stimulating factor and other cytokines regulate surface expression of the leukocyte adhesion molecule-1 on human neutrophils, monocytes, and their precursors. J. Immunol. 145:576, 1990.

146. Inamura, N., Sone, S., Okubo, A., et al.: Heterogeneity in responses of human blood monocytes to granulocyte-macrophage colony-stimulating factor. J. Leukocyte Biol. 47:528, 1990.

147. Heidenreich, S., Gong, J. H., Schmidt, A., et al.: Macrophage activation by granulocyte/macrophage colony-stimulating factor: Priming for enhanced release of tumor necrosis factor-α and prostaglandin E_2. J. Immunol. 143:1198, 1989.

148. Firestein, G. S., Xu, W. D., Townsend, K., et al.: Cytokines in chronic inflammatory arthritis: I. Failure to detect T cell lymphokines (interleukin 2 and interleukin 3) and presence of macrophage colony-stimulating factor (CSF-1) and a novel mast cell growth factor in rheumatoid synovitis. J. Exp. Med. 168:1573, 1988.

149. Alvaro-Garcia, J. M., Zvaifler, N. J., and Firestein, G. S.: Cytokines in chronic inflammatory arthritis: IV. Granulocyte/macrophage colony-stimulating factor-mediated induction of class II MHC antigen on human monocytes: A possible role in rheumatoid arthritis. J. Exp. Med. 170:865, 1989.

150. Xu, W. D., Firestein, G. S., Taetle, R., et al.: Cytokines in chronic inflammatory arthritis: II. Granulocyte-macrophage colony-stimulating factor in rheumatoid synovial effusions. J. Exp. Med. 83:876, 1989.

Zena Werb
Caroline M. Alexander

Chapter 14
Proteinases and Matrix Degradation

INTRODUCTION

One of the most striking aspects of the inflammatory process is the remodeling of the connective tissues. The influx of inflammatory cells results in increases in cell proliferation and synthesis and degradation of extracellular matrix (ECM) components. The net result of these processes is the destruction of normal tissue structures, replacement of these structures by inflammatory and fibrotic tissue, and, finally, loss of function. The degradation of ECM may be coupled to cell migration or to remodeling during growth and synthesis of connective components, or it may be purely destructive (Table 14–1). This chapter considers the proteolytic events responsible for inflammation and connective tissue remodeling and the cellular and molecular mechanisms controlling these processes.*

EXTRACELLULAR MATRIX-DEGRADING PROTEINASES

The enzymes that are most important in the degradation of the ECM macromolecules in connective tissues are *proteinases* or *endopeptidases* that cleave internal peptide bonds of proteins. They may be found intracellularly in lysosomes, where they act on proteins taken up by endocytosis, or extracellularly in the pericellular space and at a distance from the cells of origin. Numerous proteinases and peptidases are found not only intracellularly but also extracellularly in various tissue fluids and plasma.

There are four classes of proteinases that can be classified by catalytic mechanism: the *aspartic* and *cysteine* proteinases, which are mostly active at acid pH, and the *serine* and *metalloproteinases*, which are active at neutral and slightly alkaline pH.[1, 2] The proteinases most likely to play a role in ECM degradation are listed in Tables 14–2 and 14–3. Most of

these proteinases have been cloned and sequenced, although their biologic and pathologic roles are understood incompletely.

Aspartic Proteinases

Most intracellular protein digestion in mammalian cells occurs at acid pH in lysosomes. The most prominent lysosomal proteinase acting at acid pH is *cathepsin D*, an enzyme in the same multigene family as pepsin and renin.[1, 2] These enzymes require aspartic acid residues as part of their catalytic mechanism. Cathepsin D is a glycoprotein that is normally synthesized as a glycoprotein proenzyme of 42 kilodaltons (kD). It is then sorted to lysosomes and endosomes by recognition of phosphorylated mannose on the high-mannose N-linked oligosaccharides by mannose-6-phosphate receptors, where it is then slowly cleaved to the active enzyme by mechanisms that are poorly understood.

Cathepsin D is found in the lysosomes of most cells, including fibroblasts; however, its activity is higher in phagocytic cells, such as macrophages, and is increased by connective tissue activation. Under inflammatory conditions and during periods of rapid ECM destruction, cathepsin D is secreted extracellularly by macrophages and connective tissue cells, mostly as the proenzyme; however, at physiologic neutral pH, even the activated form of cathepsin D would be expected to have no proteolytic activity. It is possible, under the active metabolic conditions

Table 14–1. EXTRACELLULAR MATRIX REMODELING EVENTS INVOLVING PROTEOLYSIS

Emigration of inflammatory cells out of blood vessels, through the basement membrane and underlying loose connective tissue

Migration and proliferation of microvascular endothelial cells and fibroblasts during neovascularization

Editing of excess matrix components during rapid connective tissue synthesis and assembly

Removal of obsolete matrix components from migration, signaling, and assembly pathways

Breakdown of connective tissue components coupled to synthesis during tissue expansion and growth

Destruction of extracellular matrix during inflammation, activation of connective tissue cells, and fibrosis

---

*This chapter concentrates on the major general concepts in this area and on new developments since publication of the third edition in 1989. For a more comprehensive treatment of the older literature, please consult Reference 1.

Supported by a contract from the Office of Health and Environmental Research, U.S. Department of Energy (DE–AC03–76–SF01012), and by grants from the National Institutes of Health (HD 23539 and HD 26732).

Table 14–2. PROTEINASES OF CONNECTIVE TISSUES

Class	Examples	Location	pH range	Protein Inhibitors
Aspartic	Cathepsin D	L, E	3–6	α_2M
Cysteine	Cathepsin B	L, E	3–7	α_2M
	Cathepsin L	L, E		α-CPI
Serine	Plasmin	E	6–10	α_2M, PN-1,
	Kallikrein	E		α_2-antiplasmin
	Thrombin	E		PN-1
	uPA	E, S		PN-1, PAI-1, PAI-2
	tPA			PAI-1
	PMN elastase	G, E		α_1-Proteinase inhibitor
	Cathepsin G	G, E		α-CPI
	Mast cell chymase	G, E		α-CPI
	Mast cell tryptase	G, E		Aprotinin
	Granzymes	G, E		
Metallo	Collagenase	E	6–9	α_2M, TIMP-1, TIMP-2
	Stromelysin 1, 2	E		
	PMN collagenase	G, E		
	Macrophage elastase	E		
	Gelatinase (92 kD)	E, G		
	Gelatinase (72 kD)	E		
	Pump-1	E		None
	Membrane neutral endopeptidase 22.11	S		None known

E, extracellular; S, cell surface; L, lysosomal; G, granules; PN-1, protease nexin-1.

found in inflammatory foci and in granulation tissue, that the CO_2 and lactic acid production could create an environment of sufficiently low pH in the pericellular space to permit the proteolytic activity of cathepsin D.[3]

Cathepsin D degrades cartilage proteoglycans, with an optimum at pH 5, by cleaving the hyaluronic acid–binding region and by producing a few cleavages in the polysaccharide-rich regions.[1, 4, 5] Few peptide bonds in native collagens are susceptible to this enzyme.

There is little inhibitory activity for cathepsin D in mammalian tissues. Alpha$_2$-macroglobulin (α_2M) (Table 14–4) can bind the enzyme, but this inhibitor is unstable at acid pH. Pepstatin, a pentapeptide inhibitor from fungi, is a potent, specific inhibitor of aspartic proteinases that can be used experimentally to inhibit cathepsin D.[3]

Cysteine Proteinases

Cysteine proteinases have been associated with inflammatory reactions. *Cathepsin B* and *cathepsin L* are the best-known lysosomal cysteine proteinases. These enzymes are related to each other and, evolutionarily, to papain, and have catalytic sites that require cysteine and histidine residues.[6] Both cathepsin B and L are synthesized as proenzymes of M_r and sorted into lysosomes, where they are activated slowly, by limited proteolysis, to enzymes of 25 kD.[1] However, most of the cathepsin L of inflammatory macrophages and tumor cells is actively secreted in both proenzyme and active forms. The lysosomal cysteine proteinases are inhibited by α_2M and by protein inhibitors of the cystatin family, such as the plasma protein α_1-cysteine proteinase inhibitor.[7]

In human tissues, the cysteine proteinases with greatest activity against collagen and proteoglycan are cathepsins L and N.[8, 9] Like cathepsin B, cathepsin L is a lysosomal enzyme that is active at acid pH. Cathepsin B and L both cleave the N-terminal peptides of collagen that contain the covalent cross-links within and between molecules, but cathepsin L is very much the more active of the two.[9] Cathepsin B cleaves the hyaluronic acid–binding region from cartilage proteoglycan and degrades the glycosaminoglycan attachment region to rather small fragments.[1, 9]

Cathepsins B and L are inactivated by thiol-blocking reagents in general, but more selective inhibitors usable in biologic systems are leupeptin, E-64, and certain chloromethanes.[1] Leupeptin (propionyl-leucyl-leucyl-L-argininaldehyde) is a tight-binding, reversible inhibitor of cathepsin B. E-64 (L-*trans*-epoxysuccinyl-leucylamido(4-guanidino) butane) is an irreversible inhibitor of these enzymes.

Serine Proteinases

The family of endopeptidases, with a catalytically essential serine residue at their active site, is the largest class of mammalian proteinases. These enzymes are most active at about neutral pH. Their physiologic importance is reflected by the fact that serine proteinase inhibitors represent 10 percent of all plasma protein.[10] The serine proteinases include many of the proteins of the cascades of coagulation, fibrinolysis, complement, and kinins in the plasma, such as thrombin, plasmin, Cls, Clr, and kallikrein, as well as trypsin, chymotrypsin, and elastase from the exocrine pancreas. Plasmin and the plasminogen activators, plasma kallikrein, the tissue kallikreins,

Table 14–3. PROTEINASE SUSCEPTIBILITY OF EXTRACELLULAR MATRIX PROTEINS

Matrix Protein	Proteinases
Cartilage	
Cartilage proteoglycans	Stromelysin, Pump-1, plasmin, mast cell chymase, cathepsin G, PMN elastase, cathepsin B, cathepsin L
Collagen type II	Collagenase
IX	Stromelysin
X	Collagenase, 72-kD gelatinase
XI	92-kD gelatinase
Interstitial Connective Tissue	
Collagen type I	Collagenase, PMN collagenase, cathepsins B, L, N
III	Collagenase, plasmin
V	92-kD gelatinase, 72-kD gelatinase
VII	Collagenase, 92-kD gelatinase, 72-kD gelatinase
XII	Unknown
Fibronectin	Stromelysin, cathepsin G, uPA, plasmin, PMN elastase, macrophage elastase, stromelysin, cathepsin L, 72-kD gelatinase, 92-kD gelatinase
Elastin	PMN elastase, macrophage elastase, 72-kD gelatinase, stromelysin, cathepsin D
Basement Membrane	
Collagen type IV	Stromelysin, 72-kD gelatinase, 92-kD gelatinase, plasmin, PMN elastase, mast cell chymase
Heparan sulfate proteoglycans	Mast cell chymase, PMN elastase
Laminin	Plasmin, stromelysin, PMN elastase
Denatured collagen	92-kD gelatinase, 72-kD gelatinase, PMN elastase, cathepsin B, cathepsin L

and the serine proteinases from the granules of the polymorphonuclear leukocytes (PMN), T cells, and mast cells may play a role in ECM degradation.

Plasminogen Activators. Two distinct genes for plasminogen activators, the *tissue-type plasminogen activator* (tPA), made largely by endothelial cells, and the *urokinase-type plasminogen activator* (uPA), contribute to the activation of plasminogen, the zymogen of plasmin (reviewed in References 11 and 12). Activation of plasminogen can also occur through the action of the bacterial protein streptokinase. uPA is

a trypsin-like serine proteinase secreted as a proenzyme of 55 kD that must be cleaved into two chains of 20 kD and 34 kD connected by a single disulfide bridge for activity.[13] Although the physiologic activator of uPA has not been identified, kallikrein and plasmin are able to perform this activation cleavage. tPA is a serine proteinase of 72 kD that is activated by removal of an activation peptide. It can also be converted to a two-chain form by plasmin, but both the single- and two-chain tPA are equally effective in activating plasminogen.[13]

Plasminogen activators are secreted proteinases that are produced by macrophages, fibroblasts, synovial cells, endothelial cells, and PMN (reviewed in Reference 12). Both proenzyme and active forms of uPA bind tightly to the surface of macrophages and fibroblasts via a specific saturable receptor, which then focalizes the enzyme activity to the pericellular space and even the invasion front of moving cells[14, 15] and protects the enzyme from endogenous inhibitors.[13] The receptor is a phospholipid-anchored membrane protein that recognizes the N-terminal epidermal growth factor (EGF)-like domain.[16] uPA is inhibited by protease nexin-1, an inhibitor produced by fibroblasts that also inhibits plasmin and thrombin, and by plasminogen activator inhibitors (PAI)-1 and PAI-2 made by fibroblasts, macrophages, and endothelial cells.[11, 12] uPA is also inhibited by aprotinin, a 7-kD inhibitor from mast cells. tPA is inhibited by PAI-1 and PAI-2.[12]

tPA activates plasminogen efficiently in a trimolecular complex of fibrin, plasminogen, and tPA, and, because of this, activation is blocked by 6-aminohexanoic acid and related fibrinolytic compounds (reviewed in Reference 12). tPA has no other known protein substrates. uPA efficiently activates plasminogen in solution, as well as plasminogen that is substrate bound to fibrin or ECM. It also has limited proteolytic activity against cellular and matrix proteins, including fibronectin.[12]

Plasmin. The inactive precursor of plasmin, plasminogen, occurs in the plasma at a concentration of about 20 mg per deciliter and is activated by uPA and tPA. Plasmin preferentially cleaves on the carboxyl side of peptide bonds containing lysyl residues.

Table 14–4. POLYPEPTIDE INHIBITORS OF MATRIX-DEGRADING PROTEINASES

Inhibitor	Molecular Weight (kD)	Source	Specificity
α_2M	725	Plasma, macrophages	All classes
α-CPI		Plasma	Cysteine proteinases
α_1-Proteinase inhibitor	54	Plasma, macrophages	PMN elastase, other cysteine proteinases
Protease nexin-1		Fibroblasts	Trypsin-like serine proteinases
PAI-1		Fibroblasts, endothelial cells	tPA, uPA
PAI-2		Macrophages	tPA, uPA
α_1-Antichymotrypsin		Plasma	Chymotrypsin-like proteinases
Aprotinin	7	Mast cells	Serine proteinases
TIMP-1	28	Fibroblasts, endothelial cells, macrophages, bone	Metalloproteinases
TIMP-2	21	Endothelial cells, fibroblasts, cartilage	Metalloproteinases

Plasmin is very active in degrading fibrin, and plasminogen has a high affinity for fibrin, so that a fibrin clot has a built-in mechanism for its own dissolution.[11, 12] This sequestration of proenzymes on substrates may represent a common pattern for proteinases acting on insoluble proteins, because granulocyte elastase and collagenase also bind to their respective substrates. Plasmin also degrades cartilage proteoglycan.[17] Although it has little direct action on collagen, plasmin can activate procollagenase.[12, 18] The major plasma inhibitors of plasmin are the α_2-plasmin inhibitor and α_2-M.[12, 13] It is also inhibited by aprotinin. The major tissue inhibitor of plasmin is protease nexin-1, an inhibitor secreted by fibroblasts and other cells.[12]

Plasma Kallikrein. Plasma kallikrein is generated from the inactive precursor prokallikrein by the action of coagulation factor XII (Hageman factor) or kallikrein itself.[19] Plasma kallikrein acts on high-molecular-weight kininogen to yield bradykinin. Kallikrein also has the capacity to activate procollagenase and prostromelysin (reviewed in References 20 and 21), and although active kallikrein is normally present in rheumatoid synovial fluid only at very low concentrations, it may be a significant activator.

Polymorphonuclear Leukocyte Elastase. The PMN elastase is present in the azurophil granules of PMN and monocytes as a precursor containing two additional amino acid residues (GlyGlu) compared to the active form; this is true for cathepsin G as well.[22, 23] It is a protein of about 28 kD that acts on cartilage proteoglycan to remove the hyaluronic acid–binding region and then to fragment the glycosaminoglycan attachment region.[24] Elastin, the cross-linked structural protein important for the elastic strength of the arterial walls, lung, joint capsule, and skin, is highly resistant to proteolytic degradation, but it is degraded by PMN elastase.[1] Unlike the collagenases, the elastases are not specific for the substrate after which they are named but have very broad proteolytic activity. PMN elastase also actively degrades fibronectin and laminin,[25] making it a proteinase that is highly destructive to ECM.

PMN elastase degrades collagen fibers by first degrading the N-terminal peptides, with the elimination of the cross-links that play a crucial part in the stabilization of collagen fibers. The individual molecules then separate, and, if solubilized, denature in a few hours at 37°C and are degraded to small peptides and amino acids by further proteolytic activity. PMN elastase is several times more active against cartilage collagen (type II) than against type I collagen, whereas the reverse is true of the specific collagenases.[26] The enzyme also degrades the type IV collagen of basement membranes, which is resistant to interstitial collagenase.[27]

Extracellular activity of PMN elastase is controlled by α_1-proteinase inhibitor and α_2-M.[10, 28] Inhibitors of PMN elastase include not only diisopropyl fluorophosphate and phenylmethylsulfonylfluoride (general inhibitors of the serine proteinases) but also specific reagents such as methyl-N-succinyl-dialanyl-prolys-valyl-chloromethane, which can be used experimentally in vivo. Two drugs used clinically, gold sodium thiomalate and pentosan polysulfate, also inhibit leukocyte elastase.[1]

Cathepsin G. Cathepsin G, the "chymotrypsin-like" enzyme of PMN, is structurally and catalytically related to the pancreatic chymotrypsins and to the chymases of mast cell granules. Molecular cloning of cathepsin G revealed that it is synthesized as a proenzyme, although the propeptide is only two residues.[23] Like PMN elastase, cathepsin G occurs only in the azurophil granules of PMN[23] and of monocytes.[29]

The action of cathepsin G on cartilage proteoglycan is somewhat more restricted than that of PMN elastase, and the enzyme has little or no action on elastin or type I collagen.[24] Cathepsin G is effective in solubilizing collagen from cartilage and may generate physiologically active products from complement components.[24] Physiologic inhibitors of cathepsin G include the plasma proteins α_1-antichymotrypsin, α_1-proteinase inhibitor, and α_2M.[10, 28] Cathepsin G is an activator of metalloproteinases.[30]

Mast Cell Proteinases. Mast cells contain three major serine proteinases: (1) mast cell chymase (mast cell proteinase I) and (2) atypical mast cell chymase (mast cell proteinase II), both of which are homologous to cathepsin G[1, 23, 31]; and (3) tryptase, a trypsin that is found in a stoichiometric complex with tryptstatin, which is identical to aprotinin, a 7-kD proteinase inhibitor from pancreatic mast cells. Mast cell chymase is a broad-spectrum proteinase, actively degrading proteoglycans and type IV collagen.[32] The mast cell chymases are inhibited by α_1-antichymotrypsin and α_2M. The substrates of tryptase are poorly understood; however, this enzyme does not activate procollagenase but does activate stromelysin.[33]

Serine Esterases of Lymphocytes. Activated lymphocytes from peripheral blood and spleen, cytotoxic lymphocytes, natural killer cells, and lymphocytes engaged in antibody-dependent cell-mediated cytotoxicity have recently been shown to have granules containing abundant quantities of serine esterases, called *granzymes*, of both trypsin- and chymotrypsin-like specificity.[34, 35] Because these abundant enzymes are released on stimulation with calcium ionophores and interactions with target cells, and because of the similarity of several of these enzymes to cathepsin G and mast cell chymases, it is possible that they may be present in inflammatory sites and immune reactions and have a role in degrading ECM proteins.[35]

Metalloproteinases

The fourth class of proteinases contains the enzymes that are dependent on Zn^{2+} ions for activity, and they are additionally stabilized and perhaps

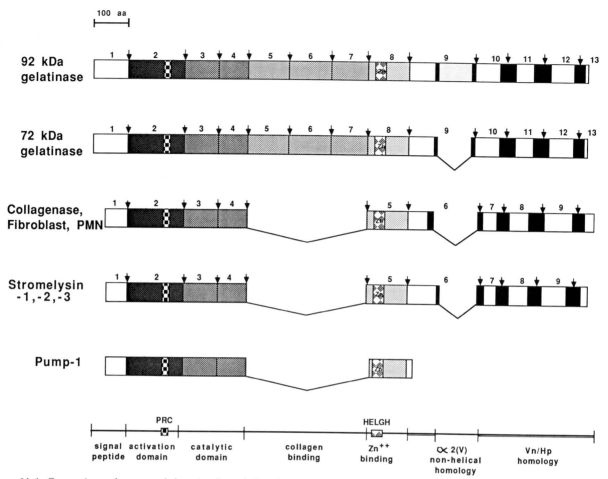

Figure 14–1. Comparison of conserved domains from deduced amino acid sequences for Pump-1, human collagenase, stromelysin-1, stromelysin-2, stromelysin-3, 72 kD and 92 kD gelatinases. Arrows indicate exon/intron boundaries, and numbers indicate the exons. The single letter code for amino acids is used. Vn/Hp indicates the vitronectin-hemopexin domain.

activated by Ca^{2+}. The metalloproteinase gene family (reviewed in References 36 through 38a) consists of eight well-characterized members in human tissues that have been cloned and show sequence conservation (Fig. 14–1).

Collagenase. The interstitial collagenases (also called *matrix metalloproteinase* [MMP]-1) are specific for collagen as substrate and cleave all three chains of the triple helix at one susceptible point, between residues 775 and 776 of the $\alpha_1(I)$ chain. The bonds cleaved are between residues of glycine and isoleucine of collagens of types I, II, and III.[1, 39] Similar bonds occur elsewhere in the collagen molecules, but it is not clear why this region of the helix is particularly sensitive to proteolysis. Mutations in this region in signal chain of the type I collagen triple helix render the molecule insensitive to proteolysis by collagenase.[40] Collagenase also cleaves collagens of types VII and VIII and makes two cleavages in collagen type X but does not degrade basement membrane collagen type IV, or types V or VI collagen.[41, 42]

The primary sequence of collagenase (Fig. 14–1) consists of activation, catalytic, zinc binding, and

hemopexin-vitronectin homology domains.[43, 44] Removal of the hemopexin domain gives a molecule that is no longer capable of degrading triple-helical collagen, but instead has stromelysin-like specificity.[45]

Rheumatoid synovial collagenase is about fivefold more active against type I collagen than the type II cartilage collagen when both are in solution.[46] Covalent cross-linking of the molecules in fibrils makes them more resistant to the action of collagenase than is soluble collagen, and cartilage collagen is particularly highly cross-linked. Collagenase has significant activity on denatured collagen; however, it prefers the native conformation of the collagen triple helix (reviewed in Reference 1).

About 95 percent of the inhibitory capacity of plasma for collagenase is due to $\alpha_2 M$, which reacts more slowly with the PMN collagenase than with interstitial collagenase from other cells.[47] The major tissue inhibitor is the tissue inhibitor of metalloproteinases (TIMP) of about 28 kD,[48] which can enter the interstitial spaces such as cartilage matrix, unlike $\alpha_2 M$.[49] A new member of the TIMP family, TIMP-2, also inhibits collagenase.[50–52] Collagenase and the other mammalian metalloproteinases are commonly found in culture and tissues in inactive proenzyme form. The procollagenases of 53 and 57 kD are activated by a multienzyme cascade described later. Collagenase is inhibited by zinc chelating agents such as 1,10-phenanthroline. Some thiol compounds, such as thiorphan and penicillamine, are effective inhibitors. Gold salts and phosphonamidates are also inhibitors (reviewed in Reference 13). Interstitial collagenase is produced by a wide variety of cells, including macrophages, fibroblasts, synovial cells, osteoblasts, chondrocytes, and endothelial cells.[1]

PMN Collagenase. There are two distinct human collagenases. PMNs have an enzyme that has a sequence different from that produced by cells of tissues such as the synovium, although sequence analysis indicates it is closely related to collagenase.[53] The PMN collagenase (also called *MMP-8*), of about 75 kD, is stored in the specific granules of PMN and secreted in response to appropriate stimuli.[54] PMN collagenase degrades type I collagens more readily than type III collagen and prefers collagen in solution to fibrillar collagen.[55] PMN collagenase occurs in much smaller amounts in the cells than do elastase and cathepsin G, and its significance in collagen degradation remains to be determined.[54]

Stromelysin. The major metalloproteinase, other than collagenase, found in cultures of fibroblasts, synovium, and other cells is stromelysin,[38, 43, 56, 57] which has also been called *proteoglycanase, MMP-3, transin,* and *neutral proteinase.* It is produced as a proenzyme of about 51 kD that is activated to forms of 41 kD and further degraded to active enzymes of 21 to 25 kD.[38, 43, 56, 58] Stromelysin has a wide variety of connective tissue and plasma protein substrates, including proteoglycans; collagen of types IV, V, VII, IX; denatured type I collagen; laminin; fibronectin; elastin; α_1-proteinase inhibitor; immunoglobulins; and substance P.[38, 42, 43, 56, 59, 60] In addition, it has a significant function in the multienzyme cascade involved in activating procollagenase.[33, 61, 61a]

Stromelysin is inhibited by α_2M and TIMP.[61] Stromelysin is produced by the same range of cells as collagenase. Although it is frequently synthesized and secreted coordinately with collagenase, it is clear in human fibroblasts, chondrocytes, and macrophages that collagenase and stromelysin may be regulated independently.[56, 62, 63] By site-directed mutagenesis, the importance of the three histidine residues in the region of the zinc-binding sequence VAAHELGH in stromelysin have been found to be essential for catalytic activity.[64] The sequence PRC containing the cysteine in the activation domain has also been shown to regulate autoactivation of stromelysin.[64]

Stromelysin-2. A second enzyme closely related to stromelysin, called *stromelysin-2* (also called *MMP-10, transin-2*), with sequence identity of nearly 80 percent, has been cloned and characterized.[36, 38, 65, 66] It has nearly identical substrate specificity with stromelysin but very distinct regulation.[66] Its role in inflammatory diseases is unknown.

Stromelysin-3. Recently, a new member of the metalloproteinase family has been cloned as a stromal gene induced in human breast carcinoma.[67] It is in the same size class and general domain structure of stromelysin and collagenase, although it is distantly related to both (about 40 percent sequence identity). It has been named stromelysin-3, although nothing is yet known about its substrates. Because it is also expressed in human embryonic fibroblasts after treatment with growth factors or phorbol esters, it may have significance in inflammatory diseases.

72-kD Gelatinase. A gelatin-degrading proteinase of 72 kD (also called *MMP-2, type IV collagenase, matrilysin*) that is secreted by many cells in culture, including fibroblasts and macrophages, has been characterized as an enzyme that degrades type IV collagen.[68–70] The 72 kD shows sequence homology with collagenase and stromelysin and even more so with the 92-kD gelatinase.[70, 71] The difference in size compared to collagenase is due to an additional domain homologous with the collagen-binding domain of fibronectin, inserted next to the zinc-binding pocket of the active site. It also requires proteolytic cleavage for activation and is inhibited by TIMP-1 and TIMP-2.[51, 70] The 72-kD gelatinase in proenzyme form binds one molecule of TIMP-2.[51] A second molecule is required to inhibit the activated enzyme. The TIMP-2 bound to the proenzyme may stabilize it against autoactivation. In addition to denatured collagen and type IV collagen, it has significant proteolytic activity against fibronectin and collagen types V, VII, and X but not against collagen types I and VI.[42, 70, 72]

92-kD Gelatinase. The 92-kD gelatinase (also called *type IV collagenase, type V collagenase, MMP-9, invasin*) is a major secretion product of stimulated PMN and macrophages.[71, 73] In PMN, this gelatinase is present in specific granules, although it was previously thought to be in a unique "C"-type granule because of release kinetics different from those of PMN collagenase and lactoferrin.[74, 75] It is related in sequence to the 72-kD gelatinase, characterized by a domain closely related to the binding sequence of fibronectin.[71] It also has a sequence related to the nonhelical C-terminal domain of α_2(V) collagen.

Like other metalloproteinases, the 92-kD gelatinase is a proenzyme that requires limited proteolytic cleavage for activation. However, the plasminogen activator–plasmin cascade does not activate this enzyme. In the PMN it is present in several higher-molecular-weight forms that revert to the 92-kD size on reduction.[73] The active forms of this gelatinase cleave denatured collagens, fibronectin, elastin, and collagens of types IV, V, VII, and XI.[71, 73] It is inhibited by TIMP-1 and, in parallel with 72-kD gelatinase and TIMP-2, the proenzyme form of the 92-kD enzyme binds one molecule of TIMP-1, requiring a second molecule for inhibition of the activated form. It does not cross-react immunologically with the 72-kD gelatinase. Which of the myriad "gelatinases" described in the literature are due to the 72 or 92 kD or other gelatinases remains to be determined.

Pump-1. Pump-1 (also known as *punctated metalloproteinase, small uterine metalloproteinase, MMP-7*) was initially described as a truncated cDNA with the proenzyme activation, catalytic, and zinc-binding sequences of metalloproteinases but lacking the hemopexin domain found in all other members of the family.[36, 65] It has now been shown to have a substrate specificity like that of stromelysin, degrading fibronectin, proteoglycans, and gelatin.[76] It also is a coactivator of collagenase. It is expressed in involuting uterus and certain tumors and is induced in fibroblasts by concanavalin A.[77]

Macrophage Elastase. Stimulated macrophages secrete a 21-kD metalloproteinase that degrades elastin, proteoglycan, type IV collagen, fibronectin, and also protein inhibitors of other proteinases, including α_1-proteinase inhibitor.[78] The proenzyme form of the elastase is about 50 kD and is related to stromelysin and collagenase.[78a] If this enzyme is produced by the macrophage-like cells of the synovial lining, it has the potential to contribute to tissue damage.

Other Metalloproteinases. In culture, many types of cells have been shown to produce proenzyme forms of metalloproteinases. Numerous proteinase bands, inhibitable by zinc chelators, are present in the medium of stimulated cells, and many of these have not been characterized.

ENDOGENOUS PROTEINASE INHIBITORS

The activities of proteinases *in vivo* are modulated by the naturally occurring inhibitors of the enzymes. The inhibitors likely to be important in the control of ECM degradation are those that are secreted by tissue cells or that derive from the plasma (see Table 14–4).

α_2-Macroglobulin

Most protein inhibitors of proteinases are classified as inhibitors of aspartic, cysteine, or serine proteinases or metalloproteinases, but α_2M inhibits enzymes from all four groups.[10] α_2M interacts stoichiometrically, usually binding 2 mol of proteinase per mol of α_2M. Only active endopeptidases interact with α_2M, forming essentially irreversible complexes. Saturation of an α_2M molecule with a proteinase prevents the subsequent binding of other proteinase molecules. The bound enzyme is inhibited against high-molecular-weight substrates and is protected from other high-molecular-weight inhibitors. α_2M-enzyme complexes are removed rapidly from tissue fluids by binding to specific α_2M receptors on macrophages or on other cells, followed by endocytosis. Limited reactivation of α_2M-collagenase complexes is unlikely to be the source of active enzyme in vivo because native α_2M is extremely resistant to proteolytic breakdown. Each of the four identical subunits of α_2M has near the center of its polypeptide chain a short sequence of amino acids that is highly sensitive to attack by most proteinases. When a proteinase cleaves this region, a conformational change in the α_2M molecule occurs such that the proteinase molecule is physically trapped within it. α_2M contains a thiol ester group, formed between side chains of neighboring cysteine and glutamic acid residues, that becomes chemically reactive after cleavage of the α_2M and forms covalent links to the trapped proteinase molecule or other molecules that may be in the vicinity.[10] The covalent-linking reaction of α_2M does not contribute to its inhibition of proteinases.

α_2M occurs in plasma at a concentration of about 250 mg per deciliter, but its M_r of 725,000 prevents it from escaping into the synovial fluid of a normal joint. α_2M is synthesized in liver but also locally by monocyte-macrophages[79] and, thus, could find its way into tissue spaces. During inflammation, rheumatoid synovial fluid has about the same concentration of α_2M as plasma.

Cysteine Proteinase Inhibitors

The major extracellular inhibitors of the cysteine proteinases are α_2M[10] and a specific plasma protein, *α-cysteine proteinase inhibitor* (α-CPI).[80] α-CPI occurs in several forms of 60 kD or more. It is a modular inhibitor, having domains that function as kininogen precursor,[81] as well as inhibitory domains. α-CPI enters tissue spaces, whereas the α_2M molecule is too large to do so.

In human cells, there are two cytoplasmic inhibitors of cysteine proteinases, called *cystatins*, both of M_r of approximately 13 kD, and inhibitory activity corresponding to these cystatins was extracted from human articular cartilage.[82]

Serpins

The primary inhibitors of serine proteinases in the joint are basically those derived from the plasma.[10] α_2M is an important inhibitor of plasmin, kallikrein, leukocyte elastase, cathepsin G, and the metalloproteinases; however, the most prominent and specific inhibitors are a multigene superfamily called the *serpins*.[83] The serpins are glycoproteins of 50 to 100 kD that include the plasma inhibitors *α₁-proteinase inhibitor*, which inhibits primarily PMN elastase and cathepsin G; *antithrombin III*, which inhibits thrombin; *C1-inhibitor*, which inhibits kallikrein; *α₂-antiplasmin*, which inhibits plasmin; and *α₁-antichymotrypsin*, which inhibits cathepsin G and the chymotrypsin-like enzymes of mast cells and cytotoxic lymphocytes. Tissue inhibitors of the serpin class include *protease nexin-1*, which inhibits uPA, plasmin, trypsin, and plasmin; *PAI-1* from endothelial cells and fibroblasts, which inhibits tPA and uPA; and *PAI-2* from macrophages.[12] α_1-Proteinase inhibitor can also be synthesized locally in tissues by

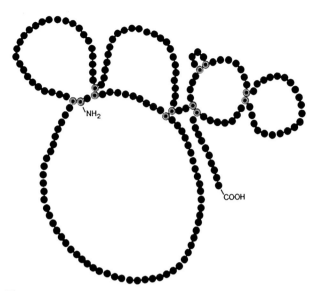

Figure 14–2. Diagrammatic representation of the TIMP molecule showing location of the disulfide bonds.

macrophages.[84] The inhibition of proteinase by serpins is tight and, in most instances, covalent.

Metalloproteinase Inhibitors

The major inhibitor of the collagenases and the other metalloproteinases in plasma and rheumatoid synovial fluid is α_2M.[10] Although plasma levels of metalloproteinase activity are probably controlled by α_2M, tissue levels are controlled by *TIMP*, which forms tight-binding complexes with all known members of the matrix metalloproteinase family, including collagenase and stromelysin, and is produced by virtually all mesenchymal tissues (reviewed in References 1, 36, and 38). TIMP cDNA has been cloned and sequenced[48]; the 20,685 dalton (D) protein is glycosylated and has 12 Cys residues that are disulfide bonded[85] to form a compact molecule (Fig. 14–2) resistant to boiling. The N-terminal domain of TIMP contains the inhibitory activity, TIMP may be coexpressed with metalloproteinases in several cell types, such as macrophages, endothelial cells, chondrocytes, and fibroblasts (reviewed in Reference 1); however, its regulation is distinct from that of the proteinases.[62, 86]

TIMP is but one member of a family of inhibitors of metalloproteinases. Several other inhibitors have been identified[87, 88] and found to be regulated independently of TIMP. A second form, TIMP-2, has been cloned.[50–52] Interestingly, TIMP-2 forms a 1:1 stoichiometric complex with the precursor form of the 72-kD gelatinase and is involved in regulating activation.[88a, b] A second mole of TIMP-2 is needed to inactivate the enzyme.[51] The physiologic function and inhibition profile of the TIMP family members have yet to be elucidated.

ENZYMATIC MECHANISMS FOR EXTRACELLULAR MATRIX DEGRADATION

The macromolecules of the ECM consist of complex fibrous proteins and glycoproteins that function as the major structural proteins of animals. In adult organisms, most intact connective tissues turn over slowly. However, the orderly degradation of interstitial ECM and basement membrane is one of the fundamental processes governing growth, development, morphogenesis, remodeling, and repair under both normal and pathologic conditions. The degradative mechanisms that operate under one set of conditions may not apply to other tissues or conditions. The differing primary structures of the genetically distinct collagen types, glycoproteins, and proteoglycans may require distinct enzymes. Various cells make different combinations of proteinases, proteinase inhibitors, and activators of zymogens. The extent and type of intermolecular cross-links, and the assembly of the collagen types and other connective tissue proteins into supramolecular structures, may also influence the susceptibility of the matrix to proteolysis. Degradation may take place at extracellular sites or in the lysosomal system within cells.

Degradation Related to Synthesis of Extracellular Matrix

It is widely recognized that newly synthesized collagen and proteoglycans are degraded more readily than molecules in mature matrix. For example, a significant proportion of collagen (about 30 percent) is degraded within minutes of its synthesis, probably intracellularly.[89] Intracellular processes may "edit" collagens so that abnormal molecules containing synthetic errors generated at the transcriptional, translational, or post-translational levels can be destroyed. Another possibility is regulation of the proper α_1(I):α_2(I) chain ratio during synthesis of type I collagen. The processing of procollagens to collagens by cleavage of the amino and carboxyl terminal extension peptides by specific procollagen peptidases is another example of a requirement for specialized enzymes to effect proteolysis during collagen synthesis and assembly. Degradative mechanisms may also control matrix assembly and the proportion of collagen types and proteoglycans secreted into interstitial spaces.

Degradation Related to Turnover of Extracellular Collagens and Other Matrix Macromolecules

Depolymerization of Cross-linked Collagen Fibers. The degradation of collagens becomes more complex once they are in place extracellularly. Polymeric collagen fibrils containing intermolecular cross-links are generally much more resistant to degradation than are soluble collagens (reviewed in Reference 1). It is not known whether the amino or carboxyl terminal cross-link regions of the collagen molecule must be cleaved before the helical portion of the molecules can be attacked; however, a number of enzymes, including PMN elastase[27, 90] and cathepsins B and L, cleave the terminal peptides of type I collagen in vitro and may have similar actions on collagens of types II, III, and IV. Specific collagenases can solubilize some peptides even from highly cross-linked collagen. Enzymes with depolymerase activity at neutral pH that could be present in vivo include granulocyte elastase, cathepsin G, and some less well characterized proteinases. Cysteine proteinases, such as cathepsins B, N, H, and L, that are active at acid pH and also cleave the nonhelical extension peptides of collagen types I and II, could depolymerize insoluble collagen fibers within lysosomes and in pericellular spaces where the local pH is acidified by metabolic products such as lactic acid.

Cleavage of the Helical Portion of Collagen. The triple helix of collagen endows the molecules with their property of resistance to proteolysis. One group of collagenolytic enzymes attacks the native collagen molecule, cleaving all three subunits at a specific locus characteristic of each enzyme. The collagenases have a high degree of substrate specificity and a strong preference for collagen in its native form; denatured collagen (gelatin) and peptides containing the cleaved sequence are poor substrates by comparison. The other proteinases that degrade the helical sequences, such as granulocyte elastase, may also degrade other proteins. The cleavage products of specific collagenases are resistant to further proteolysis unless they denature. Enzymes of a second group cleave the native collagen molecules at numerous sites. The collagenolytic cathepsins may degrade the collagen molecule sequentially inward from the ends. During rapid collagen breakdown, collagen fibrils are found within cells enclosed in membrane-bounded vesicles, presumably secondary lysosomes. The fibrils are probably cleaved from an intact fiber by the combined action of specific and nonspecific collagenolytic enzymes. Once within lysosomes, cathepsins B, N, H, and L may cleave the collagen fibrils.

Degradation of Denatured Collagens. Once the collagen fibril is attacked by collagenase or one of the other enzymes, making limited cleavage in the helical portion of molecule, fragments dissociate from the fibril and, at 37°C, immediately denature into gelatin. At sites of collagen degradation, numerous enzymes are present that may further degrade the gelatin to amino acids and oligopeptides. The 72- and 92-kD gelatinases are produced along with collagenase in a number of systems. Proteinases derived from plasma, such as plasmin, may also play an important role in the degradation to gelatin. There are also a number of other exopeptidases in extracellular fluids and within cells.[2] As an alternative to

Table 14–5. COLLAGEN-TYPE SPECIFICITY OF COLLAGENOLYTIC ENZYMES

Enzyme	Collagen-type Specificity
Collagenase (MMP-1)	I = III > II, VII, X
	IV, V, VI no reaction
PMN collagenase (MMP-5)	I > III
72-kD gelatinase (MMP-2, type IV collagenase, matrilysin)	IV, V, VII, X denatured collagen
	I, II, III, VI no reaction
92-kD gelatinase (MMP-9, type V collagenase, inradolysin)	V, IV, VII, X, XI, denatured collagen
	I, III no reaction
Stromelysin	IV, V, VII, IX
	I, VI no reaction
PMN elastase	III, IV
	II > I, V nonhelical peptides only
Mast cell proteinases	IV > I
Plasmin	III, IV, V
Collagenolytic cathepsins B, L, N	I, II, IV

extracellular degradation by neutral proteinases and peptidases, the large fragments derived from the primary collagenolytic event may be endocytosed and degraded by lysosomal enzymes within connective tissue and inflammatory cells.

Type-Specific Collagenolysis. There are more than 14 defined types of collagen. Of these collagens, only types I, II, III, VII, VIII, and X are susceptible to the classic interstitial collagenase (Table 14–5). In types I, II, and III collagens, a Gly-Ile bond is cleaved to give two fragments of ¾ and ¼ length,[39] whereas type X is cleaved at two sites.[41, 72] PMN collagenase cleaves types I and II collagens at the same rate, whereas type III collagen is relatively resistant[90]; skin fibroblast collagenase cleaves all three collagens at the same rate. PMN collagenase also cleaves type X collagen poorly.[72] Type III collagen is susceptible to a number of other proteinases, including plasmin and neutrophil elastase in a site near the collagenase cleavage site.[91] The structure of collagen fibers is complex. It may be necessary to cleave the fibril-associated collagens, such as type IX in cartilage and types XII and XIV in other interstitial matrices, to gain access to the fibrillar collagens.[92] Type IX collagen is cleaved by stromelysin.[59]

Type V collagen is a minor component of ECM and is found in basement membranes and in pericellular areas. The 92-kD gelatinase was first characterized as a metalloproteinase degrading the helical region of this collagen and has been isolated from macrophages and PMN.[71, 73] This enzyme is extremely effective at degrading denatured collagens and has activity on types IV, VII, and XI collagens.[71]

Type IV collagen is the major structural component of basement membrane. It has a distinctive structure and architecture, and the collagenous sequences are interrupted in several places by nonhelical domains. The study of the degradation of type IV collagen has been hampered by the lack of an acceptable substrate. Soluble type IV collagen from tumors, pepsin-solubilized collagen, and insoluble lens capsule have all been used. Two type IV–degrading metalloproteinases have been identified as the gelatinases of 72 and 92 kD that require activation.[70, 71] They cleave type IV collagen near the amino terminus and also cleave types V and VII collagens. Stromelysin degrades many of the components of ECM, including type IV collagen.[56, 57] Type IV collagen is also degraded by serine proteinases such as human neutrophil elastase[26] and mast cell chymase.[31]

The collagenolytic cathepsins, active at acid pH, degrade collagens of types I and II,[8, 9] but their specificity for other collagen types has not been determined. However, because their mechanism of action is more like that of the bacterial collagenases, it is probable that these enzymes are able to degrade the whole spectrum of collagen types.

Differential Susceptibility of Collagen Types to Cleavage. In addition to collagen-type specificity of collagenolytic enzymes, the various collagen types differ in their susceptibility to collagenolytic attack. Cartilage collagen (type II) in solution and in fibril form generally is more resistant to attack by a variety of specific collagenases than are types I and III. It is not clear whether the greater extent of glycosylation of type II collagen may be responsible for this difference. Collagen type III appears to be the most susceptible to attack by a large variety of nonspecific and specific collagenases that all hydrolyze peptide bonds near the cleavage site for specific collagenases. However, it is interesting to note that granulocyte elastase is able to cleave the nonhelical peptides of type II collagen much more rapidly than those of type I and degrades type IV collagen well.[27] Stromelysin cleaves types IV, VII, and IX collagen but not types I, V, and VI.[42, 56, 59] The 72-kD gelatinase is unable to cleave collagens of types I, II, and III but cleaves types IV, V, VII, and X collagens.[70, 72] Collagenase from human skin cleaves types, I, II, III, VII, VIII, and X but not types IV and V.[70, 72] The 92-kD gelatinase is unable to cleave collagens of types I and III but cleaves types IV, V, VII, and XI.[71] Thus, there is a marked difference in susceptibility of native substrates to a particular collagenase.

In tissues, collagens are assembled into complex fibrillar patterns containing more than one type of collagen. These mixtures of collagen types may produce constraints on the rate of degradation. Other components of the ECM, including fibronectins, proteoglycans, and elastin bundled together into complex connective tissue, may also play an important role in regulating the rate of collagen degradation in tissues. Glycoproteins may regulate the degradation of collagen and elastin. The rate of glycosaminoglycan degradation may be reduced in the presence of collagen.

Influence of Temperature on Collagen Degradation. Because peripheral tissues such as skin and joints have normal temperatures of 30°C to 33°C, and these temperatures are increased by inflammation, collagen's altered susceptibility to degradation by temperature may have important consequences. The rate of degradation of collagen fibrils of types I and II is influenced markedly by temperature. An increase of 2° in the range of 30°C to 37°C increases the rate of collagen degradation about four-fold.[93] At temperatures above 33°C, the cleavage fragments produced by the primary collagenolytic event denature. In the form of gelatin polypeptides, they become susceptible to many proteinases.

CELLULAR REGULATION OF PROTEINASE ACTIVITY

The first observations and subsequent isolation of collagenases and plasminogen activator from vertebrate tissues depended on the fact that these enzymes appear not to be stored for subsequent release but are synthesized de novo and are secreted from cells in culture in either an inactive or an active form. These observations have led to questions about how proteinase activity is regulated.

Cellular Origins of ECM-Degrading Proteinases

The specific proteinases, their activators, and their inhibitors originate from a number of different cells of mesenchymal, endothelial, and epithelial origin within connective tissues (Table 14–6). Fibro-

Table 14–6. CELLULAR SOURCES OF PROTEINASES AND PROTEINASE INHIBITORS IN THE JOINT

Cell Type	Proteinase	Proteinase Inhibitor
Synovial fibroblasts	Collagenase, stromelysin, Pump-1, 72-kD gelatinase, 92-kD gelatinase, uPA, cathepsin L, cathepsin D	TIMP-1, TIMP-2, PAI-1, protease nexin-1
Monocyte-macrophages	Collagenase, 92-kD gelatinase, stromelysin, elastase, uPA, cathepsin L, cathepsin D	α_1-Proteinase inhibitor, α_2M, TIMP-1, PAI-1
Chondrocytes	Collagenase, stromelysin, gelatinases, cathepsin D	TIMP-2, TIMP-1
Endothelial cells	Collagenase, stromelysin, tPA	TIMP-1, TIMP-2 PAI-1
PMN	PMN collagenase, PMN elastase, cathepsin G, uPA, 92-kD gelatinase	
Mast cells	Mast cell chymases, tryptase	Aprotinin
Osteoblasts-osteocytes	Collagenase, stromelysin	TIMP-1
Cytotoxic lymphocytes	Granzymes	

blasts and stromal cells from a variety of tissues, including synovium, cornea, skin, and gingiva, can, when appropriately triggered, produce prodigious amounts of collagenase, stromelysin, and gelatinases in proenzyme forms that require subsequent activation (reviewed in Reference 1). They also produce the metalloproteinase inhibitor TIMP. These cells also produce uPA and the uPA inhibitors PAI-1 and protease nexin-1. Macrophages have also been shown to produce collagenolytic activities and TIMP[94] when stimulated. Their secretion of the 92-kD gelatinase capable of specific cleavage of type V collagen is significant because type V collagen forms a major part of interstitial collagen fibrils yet is resistant to degradation by virtually all other collagenolytic enzymes. Monocytes contain PMN elastase and cathepsin G.[29] Macrophages can also be triggered to secrete uPA and PAI-2.[12] They also actively secrete the lysosomal proteinases cathepsins B, L, and D.[95] Chondrocytes can be stimulated to produce collagenolytic activity against types I and II collagens, stromelysin, and TIMP.[96, 97] Rheumatoid synovial cells, which are of mesenchymal origin, can produce large amounts of collagenase, stromelysin, gelatinases, TIMP, and uPA.[18, 46, 56, 62, 97] Endothelial cells produce collagenase, stromelysin, and gelatinases, as well as large amounts of TIMP-1, TIMP-2, and other inhibitors of metalloproteinases.[87, 96, 98] Endothelial cells also produce tPA and PAI-1.[98, 99]

PMN collagenase and 92-kD gelatinase are present in specific granules and degrade types I and V collagens.[54, 73, 74] The second collagenolytic system of PMN is the PMN elastase present in azurophil granules.[27] This serine proteinase degrades a wide variety of plasma and interstitial proteins, including collagens of types III and IV, and depolymerizes cross-linked fibrils of type I collagen, increasing their susceptibility to type I–specific collagenase. PMNs are not particularly effective in degrading type II collagen.

Thus, the spectrum of enzymes varies considerably with the cell types involved in an inflammatory reaction and with their states of activation.

Control of Metalloproteinase Gene Expression

Although a range of ECM-degrading potential is exhibited by a variety of cells, many cells secrete little if any metalloproteinase unless appropriately triggered. Factors involved in the stimulation or suppression of metalloproteinase activity in tissue or cell culture are well described and appear to act directly on the enzyme-producing cells (Table 14–7).

Collagenase is expressed by cells cultured from a variety of cells and tissues. Synovial fibroblasts can be induced in culture to express collagenase and stromelysin transcripts, each at a level of about 1 percent of the total mRNA of the cell,[100, 101] and collagenase and stromelysin mRNA and protein can be readily demonstrated in rheumatoid synovium by

Table 14–7. FACTORS AFFECTING PRODUCTION OF COLLAGENASE AND OTHER METALLOPROTEINASES

Stimulatory Factors	Inhibitory Factors
Cell-cell interactions	Glucocorticoids
Cell-matrix interactions via integrins	
Fibronectin fragments	
Soluble collagen	
Interleukin-1α and -1β	Retinoids
Tumor necrosis factor-α	Increased production of endogenous inhibitors
Growth factors (EGF, PDGF, FGF, TGF-α, NGF, relaxin)	Hormones (estrogens, progesterone)
β-Adrenergic hormones	
Proteinases	Indomethacin
Phagocytosis	Transforming growth factor-β
Formation of multinucleate giant cells	Autocrine inhibitory factor
Prostaglandin E	Interferon-γ
Phorbol diester tumor promoters	Transformation (E1a)
Protein phosphotyrosine phosphatase inhibitors	
Bacterial toxins	
Colchicine	
Serum amyloid A	
β₂-Microglobulin	
Heat shock	
Ultraviolet irradiation	
Cytochalasin B	
Calcium ionophores	
Iron	
Cell aging	
Transformation (src, ras, SV-40, other oncogenes)	

in situ methods.[102-105] The rather broad tissue specificity and potentially high expression levels of metalloproteinases, in contrast to the low or undetectable collagen turnover rates observed in the normal organism, suggest a complex control of metalloproteinase activity in vivo, which is partially achieved at the level of proteinase gene expression.

Numerous events, both physical and chemical, induce expression of metalloproteinases. An emerging body of knowledge points to a correlation between alteration of cell adhesion to ECM, cytoskeletal architecture, and the expression of metalloproteinase genes[101] (reviewed in Reference 38). Most of the inducing agents interact via cell surface receptors to alter the actin cytoskeleton. After a critical induction period, the cells may regain their normal cytoarchitecture but are committed to express the proteinase genes.[101] However, changes in cytoskeletal architecture may only parallel the inducing stimuli for expression of metalloproteinases because chondrocytes, which are already round, can be stimulated by interleukin-1 (IL-1) to secrete the ECM-degrading proteinases.[96] Rheumatoid synovial cells actively secreting metalloproteinases have an altered actin cytoskeleton and a stellate appearance.[18] Metalloproteinases may also have a role in changing the adhesion of cells during mitosis.[1]

Appropriate to the role of metalloproteinases in

inflammatory responses, collagenase and stromelysin are induced by the inflammatory mediator IL-1 in human fibroblasts, synovial cells, and chondrocytes.[62, 97, 106–109] Expression of collagenase is also induced by cachectin–tumor necrosis factor-α (TNF-α) in human synovial and dermal fibroblasts.[62, 108, 110] Lymphokines also induce collagenase in macrophages.[111] Expression of metalloproteinases is repressed by anti-inflammatory glucocorticoids.[18] Nucleotide sequences conferring inducibility by IL-1 and repression by glucocorticoids have been identified 5′ to the stromelysin gene.[112] In the collagenase gene, it is now clear that glucocorticoids exert their action through an interaction of the glucocorticoid receptor with activator protein 1 (AP-1) (Fos/Jun), which down-regulates transcription.[113]

Collagenase and stromelysin expression increase during fibroblast aging and in response to stress in culture,[114] and, with increasing age, stromelysin can be extracted from human cartilage.[115] Osteoarthritic cartilage contains degraded type II collagen around chondrocytes and fragments of cartilage link protein that can be attributed to stromelysin action.[116, 117] There is also immune modulation of metalloproteinase activity. Interferon-gamma (γ) suppresses the IL-1–induced expression of collagenase and stromelysin in fibroblasts, chondrocytes, and macrophages.[61a, 118] The action on stromelysin is at the mRNA level, whereas collagenase activity is decreased because of a decrease in stromelysin-dependent activation.

Production of plasminogen activator and type IV collagenase is stimulated in capillary endothelial cells by angiogenic preparations containing fibroblast growth factor (FGF).[98] Endothelial cells invade type I collagen or fibrin matrices and form tube-like structures when stimulated with phorbol esters or by transformation, in a process inhibited by transforming growth factor-beta-1 (TGF-β1) and uPA inhibitors.[119–121] A gradient of angiogenic stimulus may be required for stimulation of collagenase synthesis.[122] Angiogenesis factor–stimulated degradation of types IV and V collagen by an enzyme apparently bound to the membranes of endothelial cells has also been observed.[122]

Expression of collagenase synthesis can be obtained by stimulation of fibroblasts with platelet-derived growth factor (PDGF), FGF, EGF and TGF-α (reviewed in Reference 37). Relaxin also induces collagenase expression concomitantly with a decrease in collagen synthesis,[123] thus promoting a net degradative phenotype. Nerve growth factor (NGF) induces stromelysin in neuronal cells.[37] In addition, TGF-β decreases metalloproteinase expression[63] by inducing a protein that binds to a specific TGF-β inhibitor element in the metalloproteinase gene and inhibits transcription regulated by AP-1.[124] The action of cytokines and growth factors in regulating proteinase expression may be regulated negatively by ECM, which binds these factors and acts as a reservoir,[12] and by receptor competition. One of the best understood of these is the IL-1–like IL-1 receptor antagonist, which is made by the same cells as IL-1 and functions to compete with IL-1, decreasing its inductive effects.[109] Blockage of metalloproteinase mRNA induction by cycloheximide suggests that a newly synthesized inducer protein might also be involved.[93]

One intriguing mode of regulation is seen in the induction of collagenase and plasminogen activator synthesis and morphologic alteration by treatment of fibroblasts with proteinases, including plasmin. It may be predicted that active collagenase, stromelysin, or plasmin should induce synthesis of this set of gene products, a fine example of positive autoregulation that may be physiologically important. The fragments of fibronectin produced by plasmin and metalloproteinases may also amplify the induction by acting as agonistic ligands for the fibronectin receptor.[101] Phagocytosis of urate crystals, particles, and iron, and their storage within lysosomes, also induces secretion of collagenase by fibroblasts and macrophages.[125] The mechanism governing the secretion of collagenase after phagocytosis is not known, but prolonged lysosomal storage of materials appears to be necessary. Not all cells respond to the phagocytic stimulus alone, although the phagocytic stimulus coupled with an additional stimulant such as lymphocyte supernatants, proteinases, or pharmacologic agents appears to work in a two-stage manner to stimulate collagenase secretion. Fusion of fibroblasts into multinucleate giant cells, which are often found in sites of rapid collagen degradation, can also induce the production of collagenase.[126] Autocrine induction of collagenase after an initiating event by factors including serum amyloid A, β_2-microglobulin, and ultraviolet irradiation–induced factor[127–130] also may play a role in amplifying the stromal response.

Prostaglandins of the E series (PGE) are associated with the production of collagenase and uPA in rheumatoid synovial cells.[108] Under some conditions it appears that the micromolar concentrations of these prostaglandins that can be found in vivo and in tissue culture medium are able to induce the secretion of collagenase by macrophages and synovial cells. The response of cells to exogenous PGE, which is intimately connected with cellular concentrations of cyclic adenosine monophosphate (cAMP), may be variable because of the transient increases in cAMP. It is also possible that the response of cells to mononuclear factors, lymphokines, and possibly some of the other stimulating factors may be mediated indirectly by an increase in PGE concentration of cells.

Bacterial lipopolysaccharide endotoxin induces collagenase expression by macrophages.[94] Collagen in solution may induce collagenase production by fibroblasts, possibly by inducing IL-1 expression[131] or by direct action on integrin-type collagen receptors.[101] Although fibroblasts normally produce collagens of types I and III as part of their differentiated function, fibroblasts growing on insoluble collagen fibrils or ECM do not secrete collagenase until triggered by another factor such as a proteinase.

Fewer agents have been shown to repress metalloproteinase gene expression (Table 14–7). Synovial fibroblast–derived inhibitors of collagenase synthesis have also been described.[129] It is possible that these inhibitors are TGF-β, which may play a critical role in regulation of ECM.[132] TGF-β antagonizes the inducing effects of EGF and FGF for collagenase and stromelysin gene expression directly at the transcriptional level.[63, 124] Because of its function in increasing TIMP expression, it is doubly effective in reducing metalloproteinase function. Interferon-γ suppresses collagenase and stromelysin expression induced by IL-1.[61a, 118, 133] Glucocorticoids both prevent initiation of gene transcription and repress ongoing collagenase gene expression by direct interaction with AP-1 transcription factors.[112, 113] These compounds also decrease the secretion of PGE by cells; however, it appears that the major action of glucocorticoids on secretion of collagenase is direct. Indomethacin, a compound that inhibits PGE production directly, may decrease production of collagenase by macrophages and synovial cells in other situations. Retinoic acid and its derivatives also inhibit the secretion of collagenase.[134] The adenovirus E1A oncogene suppresses expression of metalloproteinases at the transcriptional level.[135]

Sequences upstream from the collagenase and stromelysin genes that mediate the regulatory effects of some of the inducers and repressors have been identified.[110, 112, 124, 135–138] A sequence (TRE) that mediates phorbol ester response by binding the activated DNA-binding protein AP-1, which is composed of Fos (or a related protein) and Jun (or a related protein) or two Jun molecules, has been identified in the collagenase and stromelysin genes. Consensus sequences for TGF-β1 responsive elements and glucocorticoid receptor–binding sequences have been identified in the stromelysin gene. The upstream sequences also specify cAMP responsiveness.[135–137] Thus far, the consensus sequences for the AP-1 binding sequences[137] appear to account for the variety of inducing agents for metalloproteinase gene expression. Collagenase, stromelysin, and stromelysin-2 genes have identical exon-intron organizations and are clustered on the long arm of human chromosome 11 (11q21–22), suggesting relatively recent gene duplication.[139, 140] Although all three genes have similar elements in their 5′ upstream promoters, they are regulated separately in most cells and tissues.

The genes for the 72- and 92-kD gelatinases are also closely linked on chromosome 16q21.[141, 142] The genes for these two enzymes are very similar with respect to exon-intron organization, except that the region with sequence similarity to $\alpha_2(V)$ is not encoded by a separate exon. The 5′ promoter sequences for these two genes are distinct and reflect their distinct tissue-specific expression and regulation. The promoter for the 92-kD gelatinase contains two AP-1 sites[142]; however, the sequences specifying expression in PMN and monocytes have not been identified. The 72-kD gelatinase promoter has both negative and positive regulatory elements.[143, 144] It has no AP-1 site and appears more like a housekeeping gene. The negative elements may produce tissue-specific extinction of expression.[143]

Table 14–8. FACTORS REGULATING EXPRESSION OF TIMP

Regulator	Effect
Interleukin-1	Stimulation
Interleukin-6	Stimulation
Lipopolysaccharide endotoxin	Stimulation
Phorbol esters	Stimulation
Retinoids	Stimulation
Transforming growth factor-β	Stimulation
Extracellular matrix interactions	Inhibition
Concanavalin A	Inhibition
Cytochalasins	Inhibition

Control of Expression of Metalloproteinase Inhibitors

The control of expression of TIMP and other metalloproteinase inhibitors effectively regulates expression of metalloproteinase activity.[38, 87, 96] TIMP and metalloproteinase genes are regulated independently (Tables 14–7 and 14–8). Stimulation of human macrophages with lipopolysaccharide concomitantly increases collagenase and TIMP synthesis.[94] TIMP is expressed constitutively by fibroblasts, and although TIMP expression is stimulated by phorbol esters and IL-1, which also stimulate metalloproteinases,[106] other inducers of collagenase and stromelysin, such as TNF-α, gel contraction, and cytochalasin B,[62, 145] do not increase TIMP expression. Interestingly, IL-6 enhances TIMP but not metalloproteinase expression.[86] Furthermore, TGF-β[63] and retinoids[146] increase TIMP expression while repressing metalloproteinase gene expression. TIMP is on the X chromosome. Its regulatory elements have been isolated, but except for an AP-1–like sequence, they have not been studied.[147]

Regulation of Expression of the Plasminogen Activator–Plasmin System

The plasminogen activator–plasmin system controls a variety of events requiring extracellular proteolysis (Table 14–9). Although uPA may have some direct proteolytic activity other than activation of plasminogen, tPA is known only to activate plasminogen (reviewed in Reference 12). Thus, the key player is plasmin, which directly degrades ECM glycoproteins and type III collagen and also acts as an amplifier by activating the metalloproteinases such as collagenase and stromelysin.[12, 18] Hence, the major control of this system lies in the production of active plasmin from its precursor. This is accomplished by regulating the expression of uPA and tPA

Table 14–9. PLASMINOGEN ACTIVATOR AND PLASMIN FUNCTIONS IN ECM DEGRADATION

Enzyme	Activity
uPA	Activation of plasminogen to plasmin
	Direct cleavage of fibronectin
tPA	Activation of plasminogen to plasmin
Plasmin	Degradation of fibrin, proteoglycans, laminin, fibronectin, type III collagen
	Activation of procollagenase, prostromelysin
	Inactivation of TIMP

genes and by regulating the expression of endogenous inhibitors of uPA, tPA, and plasmin (Table 14–10).

uPA gene expression is induced by phorbol esters, IL-1, and TNF-α and is repressed by glucocorticoids and TGF-β,[12, 144] which also regulate metalloproteinase gene expression in a similar manner (see Table 14–7). This related regulation of uPA and metalloproteinase genes strengthens the notion that the two systems work synergistically in ECM degradation. Interestingly, interferon-γ induces uPA[148] while repressing metalloproteinases.[118] tPA gene expression is also stimulated by phorbol esters but, unlike uPA, glucocorticoids are also stimulatory. However, the expression of tPA activity decreases with glucocorticoids because expression of genes for the endogenous inhibitors PAI-1 and PAI-2 is also markedly increased with glucocorticoids.[1, 12]

The expression of PAI-1 is also stimulated by phorbol esters, which also induce uPA or tPA expression, further refining the control of proteolysis by maintaining a fine balance between enzyme and inhibitor. TGF-β induces expression of PAI-1 and PAI-2 while repressing uPA expression and similarly represses metalloproteinase expression while stimulating TIMP production,[1, 12] making it a doubly effective molecule in preventing ECM destruction. Expression of protease nexin-1, the inhibitor of plasmin and uPA, is stimulated by phorbol esters and mitogens, further adding to a fine-tuning of the enzyme-inhibitor balance.

Receptors for Plasminogen Activator. Plasminogen activators are also regulated by cellular and matrix interactions. In the case of tPA, its high affinity for, and modulation of its activity by, binding to fibrin serves to localize the production of plasmin.[12]

There are two types of high-affinity interactions of cells for serine proteinases. One pathway by which uPA and plasmin, as well as other serine proteinases, specifically bind to fibroblasts involves the cell-secreted inhibitors, protease nexins. The secreted protease nexins bind active uPA or plasmin in a covalent complex involving the active site of enzyme, thus inactivating it. The protease nexin–proteinase complex then binds to specific receptors via the protease nexin portion, which are then rapidly internalized, and the complexes are degraded.[13] The second type of receptor binds the proteinases directly to the cell surface. There are distinct high-affinity binding sites for thrombin, elastase, and uPA.[12, 13] In this instance, the bound enzyme is not internalized by the cell. The uPA receptor has an affinity of about 10^{-10} M.[13] The uPA binds via a binding domain in the first 35 amino acid residues of the amino terminal end and, thus, retains catalytic activity.[13] The membrane-bound uPA described previously is, in fact, receptor-bound uPA. The proenzyme form of uPA binds the uPA receptor with an affinity close to that of active two-chain uPA. It is possible that the receptor is the cellular site for activation of pro-uPA to uPA, through the action of a specific proteinase of unknown characteristics.

There is an advantage of receptor-bound uPA. Specific inhibitors of uPA such as protease nexin-1, PAI-1, and PAI-2 do not affect the membrane-bound enzyme while completely blocking the secreted enzyme.[12, 13] This mechanism has the advantage of focalizing uPA actively to the cell surface.[14]

uPA receptors are also regulated. Phorbol esters increase the number of receptors by ten-fold in a monocyte-macrophage cell line.[12] On exposure to chemoattractants, uPA receptors become concentrated at the leading edge of macrophages.[14]

Expression of Lysosomal Proteinases. The lysosomal proteinases cathepsins D, B, and L are prominent in inflammatory disease, such as in the pannus-cartilage junction,[149, 150] and the major proteinases

Table 14–10. FACTORS REGULATING PLASMINOGEN ACTIVATORS IN INFLAMMATORY CELLS

Enzyme or Inhibition	Cell Type	Regulator	Regulation
uPA	Fibroblasts	Phorbol esters	Stimulation
		Interleukin-1	Stimulation
		Interferon-γ	Stimulation
		Glucocorticoids	Inhibition
		TGF-β	Inhibition
tPA	Endothelial cells	Phorbol esters	Stimulation
		Glucocorticoids	Stimulation
PAI-1	Fibroblasts, endothelial cells	Phorbol esters	Stimulation
		Glucocorticoids	Stimulation
		TGF-β	Stimulation
PAI-2		Glucocorticoids	Stimulation
Protease nexin-1	Fibroblasts	Phorbol esters	Stimulation
		Mitogens	Stimulation

extracted from cartilage are these lysosomal proteinases. These proteinases increase in amount in inflammatory cells and in osteoarthritic cartilage.[150] Yet, there are no data supporting a direct role for these lysosomal proteinases in ECM degradation.[151] Thus, it is possible either that stimulated lysosomal enzyme synthesis and release are secondary to endocytosis of ECM fragments released by enzymes acting at neutral pH or that these enzymes have other roles, such as activation of proenzymes or destruction of inhibitors.[152] In addition, the same cells and tissues, such as cartilage, that produce abundant lysosomal proteinases also contain or produce metalloproteinases.[97, 153]

Release of Proteinases from Granules of PMN, Mast Cells, Monocytes, and Lymphocytes

Most of the processes for expression of proteinases capable of degrading ECM components described earlier require a close coupling between expression of a gene and synthesis of a proenzyme, followed by its prompt secretion. PMN, monocytes, mast cells, and cytotoxic lymphocytes contain large amounts of proteinases stored in granules. Proteinases from the azurophil and specific granules of PMN and from azurophil granules of monocytes may be released extracellularly during phagocytosis of tissue debris and immune complexes.[1, 106, 154] Contact of PMN with surfaces coated with immune complexes or aggregated immunoglobulins leads to focal degranulation and matrix degradation.[154] The area of matrix destruction is highly impermeable to fluid-phase proteinase inhibitors, making this type of proteinase release particularly insidious. PMN are found in large numbers in synovial fluid, but it is unlikely that release of their proteinases into synovial fluid mediates ECM destruction because of the large amounts of inhibitors in synovial fluid.

Mast cells degranulate their proteinases in response to secretogues such as IgE immune complexes,[31] and lymphocytes release their serine esterases in response to specific receptor-mediated cell-cell interactions.[34, 35] Such reactions may well occur during the inflammatory and immune reactions of rheumatoid arthritis. However, a direct role for these cells and their proteinases in ECM degradation remains to be determined.

Oxidative Damage and the Degradation of Extracellular Matrix. Oxygen radicals are a prominent product of the phagocytosis of debris and response to chemotactic factors of PMN and macrophages. These reactive molecules contribute to ECM destruction in inflammatory sites by four different mechanisms. They denature proteins, making them more susceptible to degradation[155, 156]; they directly break peptide[155] and polysaccharide[157] bonds; they destroy inhibitors, such as α_1-proteinase inhibitor, that have active-site methionine residues[156, 158]; and they activate the proenzyme forms of PMN metalloproteinases, such as PMN collagenase.[159] There are direct data suggesting that hydrogen peroxide degrades human proteoglycan aggregate.[157] Taken together, this suggests that oxidative damage promotes ECM degradation.

Extracellular Regulation of Matrix Degradation

One of the key factors in our understanding of connective tissue catabolism is the regulation of the activity of proteinases. Degradation of collagen is likely to be rate limiting in most instances of ECM degradation. For collagens, one mechanism of regulation is the variation in susceptibility to collagenases by the genetic type of collagen in the tissue, as well as the degree of cross-linking of the collagen. Other proteinases may also be involved in the breakdown of collagen in vivo by removing proteoglycans and glycoproteins surrounding collagen fibrils and by breaking collagen cross-links before the action of collagenase and the further degradation of the products of the initial cleavage. A second mechanism involved in the local control of metalloproteinase activity is that of inhibitors and activators. Metalloproteinase inhibitors, as well as proenzyme forms and putative activators, have been found in association with connective tissue (Fig. 14–3).

Control of Metalloproteinase Activation

It has been appreciated for many years that collagenase activation occurs by multiple pathways because it can be achieved by proteolytic treatment with such enzymes as trypsin, plasmin, kallikrein, or cathepsin B,[18, 152] as well as by incubation with organomercurial agents, such as mersalyl[148, 152, 160–163] (Table 14–11). Only recently has the nature of the multienzyme cascade been elucidated in vitro,[160, 163] but there are few data on the actual activation mechanism in vivo.[18, 164] There is a pathway involving initial cleavage by trypsin between amino acid residues 81 and 82, followed by a concentration-inde-

Table 14–11. ACTIVATORS OF MATRIX METALLOPROTEINASES

Enzymes	Chemical Activators
PMN elastase	Oxygen radicals
Cathepsin G	4-Chloromercuribenzoate
Plasmin	4-Aminophenylmercuric acetate
Trypsin	Mersalyl
Kallikrein	3 M sodium iodide or sodium thiocyanate
Cathepsin B	
Stromelysin, collagenase, Pump-1	Sodium dodecyl sulfate
Endogenous serine proteinase	
Mast cell tryptase	
Mast cell chymase	
Dental plaque	

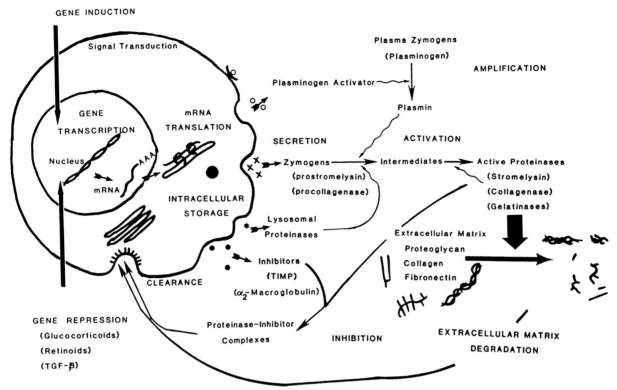

Figure 14–3. Diagrammatic representation of the factors regulating the extracellular expression of ECM-degrading proteinases.

pendent autocatalysis that can be achieved by organomercurial treatment alone.[163] Collagenase is activated in the absence of stromelysin; however, stromelysin-1 and -2, stromelysin-like Pump-1, or small forms of collagenase are required for the full activation of procollagenase by trypsin.[45, 58, 61a, 76, 163, 165] Stromelysin is activated by the proteinases that activate collagenase, as well as by mast cell tryptase,[32] PMN elastase, and cathepsin G.[30] Although activation of proenzymes has not generally been demonstrated as the rate-limiting step in collagenolysis, activation with mersalyl does enhance the penetration of endothelial cells through amniotic membranes, implying that activation steps are limiting. In vivo, the generation of plasmin by uPA or tPA is likely to be a significant activation mechanism for collagenase and stromelysin.[18] The mechanism of activation of the 72-kD and 92-kD gelatinases in vivo is unknown; however, plasmin does not activate these enzymes. Neutrophil serine proteinases cathepsin G and elastase can activate the 72-kD gelatinase.[30] The focalization of uPA to the cell surface by uPA receptors[12] may serve to confine the area of activation of metalloproteinases, thus permitting a local imbalance of TIMP:enzyme ratios with subsequent ECM degradation locally in the pericellular space. Other serine proteinases from mast cells and plasma may also be important.[33, 166]

Metalloproteinase activity is not expressed until the interaction of the cysteine in the activation prosequence (PRCGxPDV) with the catalytically active zinc is perturbed.[162] This is generally accompanied

by an autolytic reaction that removes approximately 8 kD of N-terminal sequence. Many disparate reagents can act as activators in the test tube, from caotropes (such as 4-aminophenylmercuric acetate) to the proteinases described earlier. The common feature of all these reagents is their ability to destabilize the propeptide-zinc interaction.[161] Activating proteinases chew into the propeptide sequence, promoting an autolytic cleavage seven residues beyond the cysteine-chelating zinc. The propeptide sequence is apparently critical to the stability of the proteinase: if the residues in the propeptide sequence R^{89} and C^{90} (numbered according to the sequence of rat stromelysin) are altered by site-directed mutagenesis, the enzyme is autolytic and is secreted as fragments. Mutation of surrounding residues enables the enzyme to sidestep the need for an activator, and it is secreted in autoactivated form.[64]

PMN are able to activate their metalloproteinases directly. Direct activation of PMN collagen by oxygen radicals during the respiratory burst[158] accompanying phagocytosis may be an important mechanism. Macrophages are also able to degrade ECM in the absence of any exogenous enzymes, such as plasmin, and active cysteine proteinases and metalloproteinase are present in their medium.[1] Experiments with calcium ionophores, which induce not only collagenase and stromelysin gene expression in fibroblasts but also show limited and focal activation of their proenzymes, have implicated lysosomal hydrolases (cathepsin B or L), a phosphoramidon-inhibitable endopeptidase, or a serine proteinase in the first step of activation, and a metalloproteinase (collagenase or stromelysin or both) in the second step. Thus, there are two pathways, one plasminogen dependent and the other plasminogen independent, for activation of the ECM-degrading metalloproteinases. Procollagenases also bind to collagen; thus, once secreted in an inactive form, collagenase may bind to collagen and remain in sites of potential collagenolysis until activated by a proteinase or thiol-binding compound.

Maintenance of the Proteinase-Inhibitor Balance. The degradation of ECM macromolecules is mediated by the availability of active proteolytic enzymes in the face of large amounts of proteinase inhibitors from plasma and local tissue sources. These inhibitors serve to control cascade activation reactions and limit proteolysis to areas where the enzyme-inhibitor balance is in favor of the enzyme. Tissues like cartilage that are resistant to degradation and invasion by synovial pannus and blood vessels are rich in inhibitors such as TIMP.[49] In inflammatory sites, several mechanisms change the balance in favor of enzyme by inactivation of inhibitors. The serpin inhibitors are particularly sensitive to inactivation.[10] PMN elastase proteolytically inactivates antithrombin III, α_2-antiplasmin, and C1 inactivator.[167, 168] Metalloproteinases, such as macrophage elastase, stromelysin, and PMN collagenase, and cysteine proteinases, such as cathepsin B, proteolytically inactivate α_1-proteinase inhibitor.[78, 169] Oxidation of the active methionine of α_1-proteinase inhibitor by oxygen radicals produced by the respiratory burst of PMN and monocytes also inactivates this inhibitor.[159] TIMP can also be destroyed through proteolysis by PMN elastase.[170] It is clear that altering the proteinase-inhibitor balance by increasing TIMP exogenously by injection inhibits cell invasion,[171] and decreasing TIMP endogenously with antisense TIMP increases cell invasiveness.[172]

Specific Localization of ECM-Degrading Enzymes. Several factors may influence the limiting of proteolytic enzymes to specific sites of ECM breakdown (Table 14–12). Receptors for enzymes such as uPA limit the activity of enzymes to the cell surface. Cell- and tissue-specific collagenolytic enzymes may help achieve selective functions. Human granulocytes contain both a distinct collagenase and an elastase within granules, and mast cells contain a granule-bound proteinase that activates metalloproteinases. Selective mobilization of these granule enzymes may be associated with localized collagenolysis. Through recruitment of specific cells by selective induction of collagenase secretion or by attraction of specific cells to sites of collagen degradation by chemoattractants, additional specificity may be achieved. Collagen peptides are chemotactic for fibroblasts and monocytes. To fulfill specific proteolytic functions, organelles and membranes may be equipped with their own collagenases and other proteinases. Matrix-degrading enzymes may also be associated with the cell surface,[14] which would restrict ECM degradation to areas of contact.

Table 14–12. FACTORS CONTROLLING THE RATE OF ECM PROTEOLYSIS IN VIVO

Recruitment of cells with proteolytic potential
Induction or repression of production of proteolytic enzymes
Limited tissue distribution and concentration of proteinases by sequestration in vesicles, by cell surface localization, and by rate of diffusion
Activation of enzymes by limited proteolysis by cellular and plasma zymogens
Control by tissue and interstitial inhibitors of ECM-degrading proteinases and of accessory proteinases
Specificity of susceptibility of ECM molecules to actions of specific proteinases
Sequestration of proenzymes on collagen fibers and ECM matrix
Alteration in rate of endocytosis of ECM fragments
Variation of tissue temperature during inflammation
Modulation of the susceptibility of collagen and other ECM macromolecules to degradation by mineralization, cross-linking (aging), and interaction with other connective tissue components

Locally, high concentrations of collagenolytic enzymes may be achieved by binding to collagen fibrils near sites of secretion. The rate of extracellular diffusion of molecules of M_r similar to that of collagenase is quite slow. Both in vivo and in vitro localized areas of connective tissue degradation can be seen around individual cells.[116, 164] Most tissue proteolytic enzymes are secreted concomitantly with inhibitors.[62, 63, 86] Proteolytic activity would then be limited to the immediate vicinity of secretion of an active enzyme or the site of activation of a proenzyme. Such mechanisms are involved in limiting the cascade systems of enzymes of complement and coagulation.

FUTURE PROSPECTS

Despite decades of research, the exact role of any proteinase in ECM degradation and the regulatory mechanisms that set the balance from homeostasis to connective tissue remodeling or destruction remain obscure. Knowledge at the molecular level has been progressing rapidly and should lead to new insights within the next decade. In particular, methodologies for deleting genes or overexpressing them show promise for enhancing our understanding.

Now that the major tissue proteinases have been isolated, a clearer understanding of the way that they may be involved in disease processes can be achieved. However, it is equally clear that a plethora of additional proteinases are present, and their roles in the remodeling processes need to be established.

It has become increasingly evident that the proteinase inhibitors and the proteinase-inhibitor balance may hold the key to the regulation of the degradative processes and, perhaps, ultimately to therapy. There are additional protein proteinase inhibitors to be discovered.

Important ECM-degrading enzymes may be cell associated or even integral membrane proteins. This area needs further exploration. Are there surface receptors for the metalloproteinases and their inhibitors?

Finally, ECM degradation is but one wing of the larger problem of tissue growth and remodeling. The data showing that growth regulatory peptide factors such as cytokines, TGF-β, and PDGF are important regulators of proteolytic enzyme and inhibitor expression, as well as of ECM synthesis, suggest that further analysis of growth factors and their control may be fruitful in understanding the whole problem of ECM synthesis and destruction in inflammatory and immunologically mediated disease processes.

References

1. Werb, Z.: Proteinases and matrix degradation. *In* Kelley, W. N., Harris, E. D., Jr., Ruddy, S. and Sledge, C. B. (eds.): Textbook of Rheumatology, 3rd ed. Philadelphia, W. B. Saunders, 1989, pp. 300–321.
2. Bond, J. S., and Butler, P. E.: Intracellular proteases. Annu. Rev. Biochem. 56:333, 1987.
3. Dingle, J. T., Barrett, A. J., Poole, A. R., and Stovin, P.: Inhibition by pepstatin of human cartilage degradation. Biochem. J. 127:443, 1972.
4. Morrison, R. I. G., Barrett, A. J., Dingle, J. T., and Prior, D.: Cathepsins B1 and D: Action on human cartilage proteoglycans. Biochim. Biophys. Acta 302:411, 1973.
5. Roughley, P. J., and Barrett, A. J.: The degradation of cartilage proteoglycans by tissue proteinases: Proteoglycan structure and its susceptibility to proteolysis. Biochem. J. 167:629, 1977.
6. Barrett, A. J., and Kirschke, H.: Cathepsin B, cathepsin H and cathepsin L. Methods Enzymol. 80:535, 1981.
7. Barrett, A. J., Rawlings, N. D., Davies, M. E., Machleidt, W., Salvesen, G., and Turk, V.: Cysteine proteinases of the cystatin superfamily. *In* Barrett, A. J., and Salvesen, G. (eds.): Proteinase Inhibitors. Amsterdam, Elsevier, 1986.
8. Maciewicz, R. A., Etherington, D. J., Kos, J., and Turk, V.: Collagenolytic cathepsins of rabbit spleen: A kinetic analysis of collagen degradation and inhibition by chicken cystatin. Coll. Rel. Res. 7:295, 1987.
9. Kirschke, H., Kembhavi, A. A., Bohley, P., and Barrett, A. J.: Action of rat liver cathepsin L on collagen and other substrates. Biochem. J. 201:367, 1982.
10. Travis, J., and Salvesen, G. S.: Plasma proteinase inhibitors. Annu. Rev. Biochem. 52:655, 1983.
11. Saksela, O.: Plasminogen activation and regulation of pericellular proteolysis. Biochim. Biophys. Acta 823:35, 1985.
12. Saksela, O., and Rifkin, D. B.: Cell-associated plasminogen activation: Regulation and physiological functions. Annu. Rev. Cell Biol. 4:93, 1988.
13. Blasi, F., Vassalli, J.-D. and Dano, K.: Urokinase-type plasminogen activator: Proenzyme, receptor, and inhibitors. J. Cell. Biol. 104:801, 1987.
14. Eistrecher, A., Muhlhauser, J., Carpentier, J. L., Orci, L., and Vassalli, J.-D.: The receptor for urokinase type plasminogen activator polarises expression of the protease to the leading edge of migrating monocytes and promotes degradation of enzyme inhibitor complexes. J. Cell Biol. 111:783, 1990.
15. Pollanen, J., Hedman, K., Nielsen, L. S., Cano, K., and Vaheri, A.: Ultrastructural localisation of plasma membrane-associated urokinase-type plasminogen activator at focal contacts. J. Cell Biol. 106:87, 1988.
16. Appella, E., Robinson, E. A., Ullrich, S. J., Stoppelli, M. P., Corti, A., Cassani, G., and Blasi, F.: The receptor-binding sequence of urokinase: A biological function for the growth factor module of proteases. J. Biol. Chem. 262:4427, 1987.
17. Lack, C. H., and Rogers, H. J.: Action of plasmin on cartilage. Nature 182:948, 1958.
18. Werb, Z., Mainardi, C. L., Vater, C. A., and Harris, E. D., Jr.: Endogenous activation of latent collagenase by rheumatoid synovial cells. N. Engl. J. Med. 296:1017, 1977.
19. Heimark, R. L., and Davie, E. W.: Bovine and human plasma prekallikrein. Methods Enzymol. 80:157, 1981.
20. Moscatelli, D., and Rifkin, D. B.: Membrane and matrix localisation of proteinases: A common theme in tumour cell invasion and angiogenesis. Biochim. Biophys. Acta 948:67, 1988.
21. Nagase, H., Cawston, T. E., DeSilva, M., and Barrett, A. J.: Identification of plasma kallikrein as an activator of latent collagenase in rheumatoid synovial fluid. Biochim. Biophys. Acta 702:133, 1982.
22. Sinha, S., Watorek, W., Karr, S., Giles, J., Bode, W., and Travis, J.: Primary structure of human neutrophil elastase. Proc. Natl. Acad. Sci. U.S.A. 84:2228, 1987.
23. Salveson, G. S., Farley, D., Shuman, J., Przybyla, A., Reilly, C., and Travis, J.: Molecular cloning of human cathepsin G: Structural similarity to mast cell and cytotoxic lymphocyte proteinases. Biochemistry 26:2289, 1987.
24. Keiser, H. Greenwald, R. A., Feinstein, G., and Janoff, A.: Degradation of cartilage proteoglycan by human leukocyte neutral proteases—a model of joint injury: II. Degradation of isolated bovine nasal cartilage proteoglycan. J. Clin. Invest. 57:625, 1976.
25. Campbell, E. J., Senior, R. M., McDonald, J. A., and Cox, D. L.: Proteolysis by neutrophils: Relative importance of cell-substrate contact and oxidative inactivation of proteinase inhibitors in vitro. J. Clin. Invest. 70:845, 1982.
26. Starkey, P. M., Barrett, A. J., and Burleigh, M. C.: The degradation of articular collagen by neutrophil proteinases. Biochim. Biophys. Acta 483:386, 1977.
27. Pipoly, D. J., and Crouch, E. C.: Degradation of native type IV procollagen by human neutrophil elastase: Implications for leucocyte-mediated degradation of basement membranes. Biochemistry 26:5748, 1987.
28. Ohlsson, K., and Ohlsson, L.: Neutral proteases of human granulocytes: III. Interaction between granulocyte elastase and plasma protease inhibitors. Scand. J. Clin. Lab. Invest. 34:349, 1974.
29. Welgus, H. G., Connolly, N. L., and Senior, R. M.: 12-O-Tetradecanoyl-phorbol-13-acetate–differentiated U937 cells express a macrophage-like profile of neutral proteinases: High levels of secreted collagenase and collagenase inhibitor accompany low levels of intracellular elastase and cathepsin G. J. Clin. Invest. 77:1675, 1986.
30. Okada, Y., and Nakanishi, I.: Activation of matrix metalloproteinase 3 (stromelysin) and matrix metalloproteinase 2 (gelatinase) by human neutrophil elastase and cathepsin G. FEBS Lett. 249:353, 1989.
31. Benfey, P. H., Yin, F. H., and Leder, P.: Cloning of the mast cell protease RMCP II: Evidence for cell specific expression and a multigene family. J. Biol. Chem. 262:5377, 1987.
32. Sage, H., Woodbury, R. G., and Bornstein, P.: Structural studies on human type IV collagen. J. Biol. Chem. 254:9893, 1979.
33. Gruber, B. L., Marchese, M. J., Suziki, K., Schwartz, L. B., Okada, Y., Nagase, H., and Ramamurthy, N. S.: Synovial procollagenase activation by human mast cell tryptase dependence upon matrix metalloproteinase 3 activation. J. Clin. Invest. 84:1657, 1989.
34. Masson, D., and Tscopp, J.: A family of serine esterases in lytic granules of cytolytic T lymphocytes. Cell 49:679, 1987.
35. Pasternak, M. S., Verret, C. R., Liu, M. A., and Eisen, H. N.: Serine esterase in cytotoxic T lymphocytes. Nature 322:740, 1986.
36. Matrisian, L. M.: Metalloproteinases and their inhibitors in matrix remodeling. Trends Genet. 6:121, 1990.
37. Matrisian, L. M., and Hogan, B. L. M.: Growth factor-regulated proteases and extracellular matrix remodelling during mammalian development. Curr. Top. Dev. Biol. 24:219, 1990.
38. Alexander, C. M., and Werb, Z.: Proteinases and extracellular matrix remodeling. Curr. Opin. Cell Biol. 1:974, 1989.
38a. Woessner, J. F., Jr.: Matrix metalloproteinases and their inhibitors in connective tissue remodeling. FASEB J. 5:2145, 1991.
39. Miller, E. J., Harris, E. D., Jr., Finch, F. E., Jr., Chung, E., McCroskery, P. A., and Butler, W. T.: Cleavage of type II and III collagens with mammalian collagenase: Site of cleavage and primary structure at the NH₂-terminal portion of the smaller fragment released from both collagens. Biochemistry 15:787, 1976.
40. Wu, H., Byrne, M. H., Stacey, A., Goldring, M. B., Birkhead, J. R., Jaenisch, R., and Krane, S. M.: Generation of collagenase-resistant collagen by site-directed mutagenesis of murine pro alpha1(I) collagen gene. Proc. Natl. Acad. Sci. U.S.A. 87:5888, 1990.
41. Schmid, T. M., Mayne, R., Jeffrey, J. J., and Linsenmayer, T. F.: Type X collagen contains two cleavage sites for a vertebrate collagenase. J. Biol. Chem. 261:4184, 1986.
42. Okada, Y., Naka, K., Minamoto, T., Ueda, Y., Oda, Y., Nakanishi, I., and Timpl, R.: Localization of type VI collagen in the living cell layer of normal and rheumatoid synovium. Lab. Invest. 63:647, 1990.
43. Whitham, S. E., Murphy, G., Angel, P., Rahmsdorf, H. J., Smith, B. J., Lyons, A., Harris, T. J. R., Reynolds, J. J., and Docherty, A. J. P.: Comparison of human stromelysin and collagenase by cloning and sequence analysis. Biochem. J. 240:913, 1986.
44. Goldberg, G. L., Wilhelm, S. M., Kronberger, A., Bauer, E. A., Grant, G. A., and Eisen, A. Z.: Human fibroblast collagenase: Complete primary structure and homology to an oncogene transformation-induced rat protein. J. Biol. Chem. 261:6600, 1986.
45. Clark, I. M., and Cawston, T. E.: Fragments of human fibroblast collagenase: Purification and characterisation. Biochem. J. 263:201, 1989.
46. Woolley, D. E., Lindberg, K. A., Glanville, R. W., and Evanson, J. M.: Action of rheumatoid synovial collagenase on cartilage collagen: Different susceptibilies of cartilage and tendon collagen to collagenase attack. Eur. J. Biochem. 50:437, 1975.

47. Werb, Z., Burleigh, M. C., Barrett, A. J., and Starkey, P. M.: The interaction of α₂-macroglobulin with proteinases: Binding and inhibition of mammalian collagenase and other metal proteinases. Biochem. J. 139:359, 1974.

48. Docherty, A. J. P., Lyons, A., Smith, B. J., Wright, E. M., Stephens, P. E., Harris, T. J. R., Murphy, G., and Reynolds, J. J.: Sequence of human tissue inhibitor of metalloproteinases and its identity to erythroid-potentiating activity. Nature 318:66, 1985.

49. Moses, M. A., Sudhalter, V., and Langer, R.: Identification of an inhibitor of neovascularization from cartilage. Science 248:1408, 1990.

50. Boone, T. C., Johnson, M. J., De Clerck, Y. A., and Langley, K. E.: cDNA cloning and expression of a metalloproteinase inhibitor related to tissue inhibitor of metalloproteinases. Proc. Natl. Acad. Sci. U.S.A. 87:2800, 1990.

51. Stetler-Stevenson, W. G., Krutzsch, H. C., and Liotta, L. A.: Tissue inhibitor of metalloproteinase (TIMP-2): A new member of the metalloproteinase inhibitor family. J. Biol. Chem. 264:17374, 1989.

52. Stetler-Stevenson, W. G., Brown, P. D., Onisto, M., Levy, A. T., and Liotta, L. A.: Tissue inhibitor of metalloproteinases-2 (TIMP-2) mRNA expression in tumour cell lines and human tumour tissues. J. Biol. Chem. 265:13933, 1990.

53. Hasty, K. A., Pourmotabbed, T. F., Goldberg, G. I., Thompson, J. P., Spinella, D. G., Stevens, R. M., and Mainardi, C. L.: Human neutrophil collagenase: A distinct gene with homology to other matrix metalloproteinases. J. Biol. Chem. 265:11421, 1990.

54. Hasty, K. A., Hibbs, M. S., Kang, A. H., and Mainardi, C. L.: Secreted forms of human neutrophil collagenase. J. Biol. Chem. 261:5645, 1986.

55. Horwitz, A. L., Hance, A. J., and Crystal, R. G.: Granulocyte collagenase: Selective digestion of type I relative to type III collagen. Proc. Natl. Acad. Sci. U.S.A. 74:897, 1977.

56. Chin, J. R., Murphy, G., and Werb, Z.: Stromelysin, a connective tissue-degrading metalloendopeptidase secreted by stimulated rabbit synovial cells in parallel with collagenase: Biosynthesis, isolation, characterization and substrates. J. Biol. Chem. 260:12367, 1985.

57. Wilhelm, S. M., Collier, I. E., Kronberger, A., Eisen, A. Z., Marmer, B. I., Grant, G. A., Bauer, E. A., and Goldberg, G. I.: Human skin fibroblast stromelysin: Structure, glycosylation, substrate specificity, and differential expression in normal and tumorigenic cells. Proc. Natl. Acad. Sci. U.S.A. 84:6725, 1987.

58. Nagase, H., Enghild, J. J., Suzuki, K., and Salvesen, G.: Stepwise activation mechanisms of the precursor of matrix metalloproteinase 3 (stromelysin) by proteinases and (4-aminophenyl) mercuric acetate. Biochemistry 29:5783, 1990.

59. Okada, Y., Konomi, H., Yada, T., Kimata, K., and Nagase, H.: Degradation of type IX collagen by matrix metalloproteinase 3 (stromelysin) from human rheumatoid synovial cells. FEBS Lett. 244:473, 1989.

60. Teahan, J., Harrison, R., Izquierdo, M., and Stein, R. L.: Substrate specificity of human fibroblast stromelysin: Hydrolysis of substance P and its analogues. Biochemistry 28:8497, 1989.

61. Murphy, G., Cockett, M. I., Stephens, P. E., Smith, B. J., and Docherty, A. J. P.: Stromelysin is an activator of procollagenase: A study with natural and recombinant enzymes. Biochem. J. 248:265, 1987.

61a. Unemori, E. N., Bair, M. J., Bauer, E. A., and Amento, E. P.: Stromelysin expression regulates collagenase activation in human fibroblasts. Dissociable control of two metalloproteinases by interferon gamma. J. Biol. Chem. 266:23477, 1991.

62. MacNaul, K. L., Chartrain, N., Lark, M., Tocci, M. J., and Hutchinson, N. I.: Discoordinate expression of stromelysin, collagenase, and tissue inhibitor of metalloproteinases-1 in rheumatoid synovial fibroblasts: Synergistic effects of interleukin-1 and tumor necrosis factor-α on stromelysin expression. J. Biol. Chem. 265:17238, 1990.

63. Edwards, D. R., Murphy, G., Reynolds, J. J., Whitham, S. E., Docherty, A. J. P., Angel, P., and Heath, J. K.: Transforming growth factor beta modulates the expression of collagenase and metalloproteinase inhibitor. EMBO J. 6:1899, 1987.

64. Sanchez-Lopez, R., Nicholson, R., Gesnel, M.-C., Matrisian, L. M., and Breathnach, R.: Structure-function relationships in the collagenase family member transin. J. Biol. Chem. 263:11892, 1988.

65. Muller, D., Quantin, B., Gesnel, M.-C., Millon-Collard, R., Abecassis, J., and Breathnach, R.: The collagenase gene family consists of at least four members. Biochem. J. 253:187, 1988.

66. Nicholson, R., Murphy, G., and Breathnach, R.: Human and rat malignant tumor-associated mRNAs encode stromelysin-like metalloproteinases. Biochemistry 28:5195, 1989.

67. Bassett, P., Bellocq, J. P., Wolf, C., Stoll, I., Hutin, P., Limacher, J. M., Podhajcer, O. L., Chenard, M. P., Rio, M. C., and Chambon, P.: A novel metalloproteinase gene specifically expressed in stromal cells of breast carcinomas. Nature 348:699, 1990.

68. Garbisa, S., Ballin, M., Daga-Gordini, D., Fastelli, G., Naturale, M., Negro, A., Semenzato, G., and Liotta, L. A.: Transient expression of type IV collagenolytic metalloproteinase by human mononuclear phagocytes. J. Biol. Chem. 261:2369, 1986.

69. Salo, T., Turpeenniemi-Hujanen, T., and Tryggvason, K.: Tumor-promoting phorbol esters and cell proliferation stimulate secretion of basement membrane (type IV) collagen-degrading metalloproteinase by human fibroblasts. J. Biol. Chem. 260:8526, 1985.

70. Collier, I. E., Wilhelm, S. M., Eisen, A. Z., Marmer, B. L., Grant, G. A., Seltzer, J. L., Kronberger, A., He, C., Bauer, E. A., and Goldberg, G. I.: H-ras transformed human bronchial epithelial cells (TBE-1) secrete a single metalloprotease capable of degrading basement membrane collagen. J. Biol. Chem. 263:6579, 1988.

71. Wilhelm, S. M., Collier, I. E., Marmer, B. L., Eisen, A. Z., Grant, G. A., and Goldberg, G. I.: SV-40 transformed human lung fibroblasts secrete a 92-kDa type IV collagenase which is identical to that secreted by normal human macrophages. J. Biol. Chem. 264:17213, 1989.

72. Welgus, H. G., Fliszar, C. J., Seltzer, J. L., Schmid, T. M., and Jeffrey, J. J.: Differential susceptibility of type X collagen to cleavage by two mammalian interstitial collagenases and 72-kDa type IV collagenase. J. Biol. Chem. 265:13521, 1990.

73. Hibbs, M. S., Hasty, K. A., Seyer, J. M., Kang, A. H., and Mainardi, C. L.: Biochemical and immunological characterization of the secreted forms of human neutrophil gelatinase. J. Biol. Chem. 260:2493, 1985.

74. Hibbs, M., and Bainton, D. F.: Human neutrophil gelatinase is a component of specific granules. J. Clin. Invest. 84:1395, 1989.

75. Dewald, B., RindlerLudwig, R., Bretz, U., and Baggiolini, M.: Subcellular localization and heterogeneity of neutral proteases in neutrophilic polymorphonuclear leucocytes. J. Exp. Med. 141:709, 1975.

76. Quantin, B., Murphy, G., and Breathnach, R.: Pump-1 cDNA codes for a protein with characteristics similar to those of classical collagenase family members. Biochemistry 28:5327, 1989.

77. Overall, C. M., and Sodek, J.: Concanavalin A produces a matrix-degradative phenotype in human fibroblasts: Induction and endogenous activation of collagenase, 72-kDa gelatinase and Pump-1 is accompanied by the suppression of the tissue inhibitor of matrix metalloproteinases. J. Biol. Chem. 265:21141, 1990.

78. Banda, M. J., and Werb, Z.: Limited proteolysis by macrophage elastase inactivates human α₁-proteinase inhibitor. J. Exp. Med. 152:1563, 1980.

78a. Shaprio, S. D., Griffin, G. L., Gilbert, D. J., and Jenkins, N. A.: Molecular cloning, chromosome localization, and bacterial expression of a murine macrophage metalloelastase. J. Biol. Chem. 267:4664, 1992.

79. Hovi, T., Mosher, D., and Vaheri, A.: Synthesis of α₂-macroglobulin by human monocyte-derived macrophages. J. Exp. Med. 145:1580, 1977.

80. Sasaki, M., Taniguichi, K., and Minakata, K.: Multimolecular forms of thiol proteinase inhibitor in human plasma. J. Biochem. 89:169, 1981.

81. Ohkubo, I., Kurachi, K., Takasawa, T., Shiokawa, H., and Sasaki, M.: Isolation of a human cDNA for α₂-thiolproteinase inhibitor and its identity with low molecular weight kininogen. Biochemistry 23:5691, 1984.

82. Killackey, J. J., Roughley, P. J., and Mort, J. S.: Proteinase inhibitors of human articular cartilage. Coll. Rel. Res. 3:419, 1983.

83. Carrell, R. W., and Boswell, D. R.: Serpins: The superfamily of plasma serine proteinase inhibitors. In Barrett, A. J., and Salvesen, G. (eds.): Proteinase Inhibitors. Amsterdam, Elsevier, 1986.

84. Mornex, J.-E., Chytil-Weir, A., Martinet, A., Courtney, M., LeCocq, J.-P., and Crystal, R. G.: Expression of α₁-proteinase inhibitor by human monocyte-derived macrophages. J. Clin. Invest. 77:1952, 1986.

85. Williamson, R. A., Marston, F. A., Angal, S., Koklitis, P., Panico, M., Morris, H. R., Carne, A. F., Smith, B. J., Harris, T. V., and Freedman, R. B.: Disulphide bond assignment in human tissue inhibitor of metalloproteinases. Biochem. J. 268:267, 1990.

85a. Murphy, G., Houbrechts, A., Cockett, M. I., Williamson, R. A., O'Shea, M., and Docherty, A. J.: The N-terminal domain of tissue inhibitor of metalloproteinases retains metalloproteinase inhibitory activity. Biochemistry 30:8097, 1991.

86. Sato, T., Ito, A., and Mori, Y.: Interleukin-6 enhances the production of tissue inhibitor of metalloproteinases (TIMP) but not that of matrix metalloproteinases by human fibroblasts. Biochem. Biophys. Res. Commun. 170:824, 1990.

87. Herron, G. S., Banda, M. J., Clark, E. J., Gavrilovic, J., and Werb, Z.: Secretion of metalloproteinases by stimulated capillary endothelial cells: II. Expression of collagenase and stromelysin activities is regulated by endogenous inhibitors. J. Biol. Chem. 261:2814, 1980.

88. Cawston, T. E., Curry, V. A., Clark, I. M., and Hazleman, B. L.: Identification of a new metalloproteinase inhibitor that forms tight-binding complexes with collagenase. Biochem. 269:183, 1990.

88a. Howard, E. W., and Banda, M. J.: Binding of tissue inhibitor of metalloproteinases 2 to two distinct sites on human 72-kDa gelatinase. Identification of a stabilization site. J. Biol. Chem. 266:17972, 1991.

88b. Howard, E. W., Bullen, E. C., and Banda, M. J.: Preferential inhibition of 72- and 92-kDa gelatinases by tissue inhibitor of metalloproteinases-2. J. Biol. Chem. 266:13070, 1991.

89. Berg, R. A., Schwartz, M. L., and Crystal, R. G.: Regulation of the production of secretory proteins: Intracellular degradation of newly synthesized "defective" collagen. Proc. Natl. Acad. Sci. U.S.A. 77:4746, 1980.

90. Hasty, K. A., Jeffrey, J. J., Hibbs, M. S., and Welgus, H. G.: The collagen substrate specificity of human neutrophil collagenase. J. Biol. Chem. 262:10048, 1987.

91. Mainardi, C. L., Hasty, D. L., Seyer, J. M., and Kang, A. H.: Specific cleavage of human type III collagen by human polymorphonuclear leukocyte elastase. J. Biol. Chem. 255:12006, 1980.

92. Gordon, M. K., Gerecke, D. R., Nishimura, I., Ninomiya, Y., and Olsen, B. R.: A new dimension in the extracellular matrix. Connect. Tiss. Res. 20:179, 1989.

93. Harris, E. D., Jr., and McCroskery, P. A.: The influence of temperature and fibril stability on degradation of cartilage collagen by rheumatoid synovial collagenase. N. Engl. J. Med. 290:1, 1974.

94. Welgus, H. G., Campbell, E. J., Cury, J. D., Eisen, A. Z., Senior, R. M., Wilhelm, S. M., and Goldberg, G. I.: Neutral metalloproteinases produced by human mononuclear phagocytes: Enzyme profile, regulation, and expression during cellular development. J. Clin. Invest. 86:1496, 1990.

95. Schorlemmer, H.-U., Davies, P., and Allison, A. C.: Ability of activated complement components to induce lysosomal enzyme release from macrophages. Nature 261:48, 1976.

96. Gavrilovic, J., Hembry, R. M., Reynolds, J. J., and Murphy, G.: Tissue inhibitor of metalloproteinases (TIMP) regulates extracellular type I collagen degradation by chondrocytes and endothelial cells. J. Cell. Sci. 87:357, 1987.

97. Murphy, G., McGuire, M. B., Russell, R. G. G., and Reynolds, J. J.: Characterization of collagenase, other metallo-proteinases and an inhibitor (TIMP) produced by human synovium and cartilage in culture. Clin. Sci. 61:711, 1981.

98. Moscatelli, D. A., Rifkin, D. B., and Jaffe, E. A.: Production of latent collagenase by human umbilical vein endothelial cells in response to angiogenic preparations. Exp. Cell. Res. 156:379, 1985.

99. Loskutoff, D. J., Ng, T., Sawdey, M., and Lawrence, D.: Fibrinolytic system of cultured endothelial cells: Regulation by plasminogen activator inhibitor. J. Cell. Biochem. 32:273, 1986.

100. Aggeler, J., Frisch, S. M., and Werb, Z.: Collagenase is a major gene product of induced rabbit synovial fibroblasts. J. Cell. Biol. 98:1656, 1984.

101. Werb, Z., Tremble, P., Behrendtsen, O., Crowley, E., and Damsky, C.: Signal transduction through the fibronectin receptor induces collagenase and stromelysin gene expression. J. Cell Biol. 109:877, 1989.

102. McCachren, S. S., Haynes, B. F., and Niedel, J. E.: Localisation of collagenase mRNA in rheumatoid arthritis synovium by in situ hybridisation histochemistry. J. Clin. Immunol. 10:19, 1990.

103. Sawai, T., Murakami, K., Ohtani, Y., Kurkinnen, M., Kyogoku, M., and Hayashi, M.: Stromelysin synthesizing cells in synovial tissues of rheumatoid arthritis demonstrated by in situ hybridization and immunohistochemical methods. Tohoku J. Exp. Med. 160:285, 1990.

104. Case, J. P., Sano, H., Lafyatis, R., Remmers, E. F., Kumkumian, G. K., and Wilder, R. L.: Transin/stromelysin expression in the synovium of rats with experimental erosive arthritis. J. Clin. Invest. 84:1731, 1989.

105. Woolley, D. E., Crossley, M. J., and Evanston, J. M.: Collagenase at sites of cartilage erosion in the rheumatoid joint. Arthritis Rheum. 20:1231, 1977.

106. Murphy, G., Reynolds, J. J., and Werb, Z.: Biosynthesis of tissue inhibitor of metalloproteinases by human fibroblasts in culture: stimulation by 12-O-tetradecanoyl-phorbol-13-acetate and interleukin 1 in parallel with collagenase. J. Biol. Chem. 260:3079, 1985.

107. Schnyder, J., Payne, T., and Dinarello, C. A.: Human monocyte or recombinant interleukin 1's are specific for the secretion of a metalloproteinase from chondrocytes. J. Immunol. 138:496, 1987.

108. Dayer, J.-M., Beutler, B., and Cerami, A.: Cachectin/tumor necrosis factor stimulates collagenase and prostaglandin E_2 production by human synovial cells and dermal fibroblasts. J. Exp. Med. 162:2163, 1985.

109. Smith, R. J., Chin, J. E., Sam, L. M., and Justen, J. M.: Biologic effects of an interleukin-1 receptor antagonist protein on interleukin-1-stimulated cartilage erosion and chondrocyte responsiveness. Arthritis Rheum. 34:78, 1991.

110. Brenner, D. A., O'Hara, M., Angel, P., Chojkier, M., and Karin, M.: Prolonged activation of jun and collagenase genes by tumour necrosis factor α. Nature 337:661, 1989.

111. Wahl, L. M., Wahl, S. M., Mergenhagen, S. E., and Martin, G. R.: Collagenase production lymphokine-activated macrophages. Science 187:261, 1975.

112. Frisch, S. M., and Ruley, H. E.: Transcription from the stromelysin promoter is induced by interleukin-1 and repressed by dexamethasone. J. Biol. Chem. 262:16300, 1987.

113. Jonat, C., Rahmsdorf, H. J., Park, K. K., Cato, A. C., Gebel, S., Ponta, H., and Herrlich, P.: Antitumor promotion and anti-inflammation: Down-modulation of AP-1 (Fos/Jun) activity by glucocorticoid hormone. Cell 62:1189, 1990.

114. Sottile, J., Mann, D. M., Diemer, V., and Millis, A. J. T.: Regulation of collagenase and collagenase mRNA production in early- and late-passage human diploid fibroblasts. J. Cell. Physiol. 138:281, 1989.

115. Gunja-Smith, Z., Nagase, H., and Woessner, J. F., Jr.: Purification of the neutral proteogycan-degrading metalloproteinase from human articular cartilage tissue and its identification as stromelysin/matrix metalloproteinase-3. Biochem. J. 258:115, 1989.

116. Dodge, G. R., and Poole, A. R.: Immunohistochemical detection and immunochemical analysis of articular cartilages and in explants of bovine articular cartilage cultured with interleukin-1. J. Clin. Invest. 83:647, 1989.

117. Ngugen, Q., Murphy, G., Roughley, P. G., and Mort, J. S.: Degradation of proteoglycan aggregate by cartilage metalloproteinases: Evidence for the involvement of stromelysin in the generation of link protein heterogeneity in situ. Biochem. J. 259:61, 1989.

118. Shapiro, S. D., Campbell, E. J., Kobayashi, D. K., and Welgus, H. G.: Immune modulation of metalloproteinase production in human macrophages: Selective pretranslational suppression of interstitial collagenase and stromelysin biosynthesis by interferon-γ. J. Clin. Invest. 86:1204, 1990.

119. Montesano, R., and Orci, L.: Tumor-promoting phorbol esters induce angiogenesis in vitro. Cell 42:469, 1985.

120. Montesano, R., Pepper, M. S., Mohle-Steinlein, U., Risau, W., Wagner, E. F., and Orci, L.: Increased proteolytic activity is responsible for the aberrant morphogenetic behaviour of endothelial cells expressing the middle T oncogene. Cell 62:435, 1990.

121. Pepper, M. S., Belin, D., Montesano, R., Orci, L., and Vassalli, J.-D.: Transforming growth factor-beta 1 modulates basic fibroblast growth factor-induced proteolytic and angiogenic properties of endothelial cells in vitro. J. Cell. Biol. 111:743, 1990.

122. Kalebic, T., Garbisa, S., Glaser, B., and Liotta, L. A.: Basement membrane collagen: Degradation by migrating endothelial cells. Science 221:281, 1983.

123. Unemori, E. N., and Amento, E. P.: Relaxin modulates synthesis and secretion of procollagenase and collagen by human dermal fibroblasts. J. Biol. Chem. 265:10681, 1990.

124. Kerr, L. D., Miller, D. B., and Matrisian, L. M.: TGF-B1 inhibition of transin/stromelysin gene expression is mediated through a fos binding sequence. Cell 61:267, 1990.

125. Brinckerhoff, C. E., Gross, R. H., Nagase, H., Sheldon, L. A., Jackson, R. C., and Harris, E. D., Jr.: Increased level of translatable collagenase mRNA in rabbit synovial cells treated with phorbol myristate acetate or crystals of monosodium urate monohydrate. Biochemistry 21:2674, 1982.

126. Brinckerhoff, C. E., and Harris, E. D., Jr.: Collagenase production by cultures containing multinucleated cells derived from synovial fibroblasts. Arthritis Rheum. 21:745, 1978.

127. Brinckerhoff, C. E., Benoit, M. C., and Culp, W. J.: Autoregulation of collagenase production by a protein synthesized and secreted by synovial fibroblasts: A cellular mechanism for control of collagen degradation. Proc. Natl. Acad. Sci. U.S.A. 82:1916, 1985.

128. Stein, B., Rahmsdorf, H. J., Steffen, A. Litfin, M., and Herrlich, P.: UV-induced damage is an intermediate step in UV-induced expression of human immunodeficiency virus type 1, collagenase, c-fos and metallothionein. Mol. Cell. Biol. 9:5169, 1989.

129. Vance, B. A., Kowalski, C. G., and Brinckerhoff, C. E.: Heat shock of rabbit synovial fibroblasts increases expression of mRNAs for two metalloproteinases, collagenase and stromelysin. J. Cell Biol. 108:2037, 1989.

130. Schorpp, M., Mallick, U., Rahmsdorf, H. J., and Herrlich, P.: UV-induced extracellular factor from fibroblasts communicates the UV response to nonirradiated cells. Cell 37:861, 1984.

131. Dayer, J.-M., Trentham, D. E., and Krane, S. M.: Collagens act as ligands to stimulate human monocytes to produce mononuclear cell factor (MCF) and prostaglandins (PGE2). Coll. Rel. Res. 2:523, 1982.

132. Roberts, A. B., Heine, U. I., Flanders, K. C., and Sporn, M. B.: Transforming growth factor-beta: Major role in regulation of extracellular matrix. Ann. N.Y. Acad. Sci. 580:225, 1990.

133. Andrews, H. J., Bunning, R. A., Plumpton, T. A., Clark, I. M., Russell, R. G., and Cawston, T. E.: Inhibition of interleukin-1-induced collagenase production in human articular chondrocytes in vitro by recombinant human interferon-γ. Arthritis Rheum. 33:1733, 1990.

134. Brinckerhoff, C. E., McMillan, R. M., Dayer, J.-M., and Harris, E. D.: Inhibition by retinoic acid of collagenase production by rheumatoid synovial cells. N. Engl. J. Med. 303:432, 1980.

135. van Dam, H., Offringa, R., Smits, A. M., Bos, J. L., Jones, N. C., and van der Eb, A. J.: The repression of the growth factor-inducible genes JE, c-myc and stromelysin by adenovirus E1A is mediated by conserved region 1. Oncogene 4:1207, 1989.

136. Gutman, A., and Wasylyk, B.: The collagenase gene promoter contains a TPA and oncogene-responsive unit encompassing the PEA3 and AP1 binding sites. EMBO J. 9:2241, 1990.

137. Angel, P., Baumann, I., Stein, B., Delius, H., Rahmsdorf, H. J., and Herrlich, P.: 12-O-tetradecanyol-phorbol-13-acetate (TPA) induction of the human collagenase gene is mediated by an inducible enhancer element located in the 5'-flanking region. Mol. Cell. Biol. 7:2256, 1987.

138. Kerr, L. D., Holt, J. T., and Matrisian, L. M.: Growth factors regulate

transin gene expression by c-fos-dependent and c-fos-independent pathways. Science 242:1424, 1988.

139. Spurr, N. K., Gough, A. C., Gosden, J., Rout, D., Porteous, D. J., Van Heyningen, V., and Docherty, A. J.: Restriction fragment length polymorphism analysis and assignment of the metalloproteinases stromelysin and collagenase to the long arm of chromosome 11. Genomics 2:119, 1988.

140. Jung, J. Y., Warter, S., and Rumpler, Y.: Localization of stromelysin 2 gene to the q22.3–23 region of chromosome 11 by in situ hybridization. Ann. Genet. 33:21, 1990.

141. Huhtala, P., Eddy, R. L., Fan, Y. S., Byers, M. G., Shows, T. B., and Tryggvason, K.: Completion of the primary structure of the human type IV collagenase preproenzyme and assignment of the gene (CLG4) to the q21 region of chromosome 16. Genomics 6:554, 1990.

142. Collier, I. E., Bruns, G. A. P., Goldberg, G. I., and Gerhard, D. S.: On the structure and chromosome localization of the 72-kDa and 92-kDa human type-IV collagenase genes. Genomics 9:429, 1991.

143. Frisch, S. M., and Morisaki, J. H.: Positive and negative transcriptional elements of the human type IV collagenase gene. Mol. Cell. Biol. 10:6524, 1990.

144. Huhtala, P., Chow, L. T., and Tryggvason, K.: Structure of the human type IV collagenase gene. J. Biol. Chem. 265:11077, 1990.

145. Unemori, E. N., and Werb, Z.: Reorganization of polymerized actin: A possible trigger for induction of procollagenase in fibroblasts cultured in and on collagen gels. J. Cell Biol. 103:1021, 1986.

146. Clark, S. D., Kobayashi, D. K., and Welgus, H. G.: Regulation of the expression of tissue inhibitor of metalloproteinases and collagenase by retinoids and glucocorticoids in human fibroblasts. J. Clin. Invest. 80:1280, 1987.

147. Flenniken, A. M., and Williams, B. R. G.: Developmental expression of the endogenous TIMP gene and a TIMP-lacZ fusion gene in transgenic mice. Genes Dev. 4:1094, 1990.

148. Collart, M. A., Belin, D., Vassalli, J.-D., de Kossodo, S., and Vassalli, P.: γ Interferon enhances macrophage transcription of the tumor necrosis factor/cachectin, interleukin 1, and urokinase genes, which are controlled by short-lived repressors. J. Exp. Med. 164:2113, 1986.

149. Poole, A. R., Hembry, R. M., and Dingle, J. T.: Cathepsin D in cartilage: The immunohistochemical demonstration of extracellular enzyme in normal and pathological conditions. J. Cell. Sci. 41:139, 197.

150. Bayliss, M. T., and Ali, S. Y.: Studies on cathepsin B in human articular cartilage. Biochem. J. 171:149, 1978.

151. Hembry, R. M., Knight, C. G., Dingle, J. T., and Barrett, A. J.: Evidence that cathepsin D is not responsible for the resorption of cartilage matrix in culture. Biochim. Biophys. Acta 714:307, 1982.

152. Eeckhout, Y., and Vaes, G.: Further studies on the activation of procollagenase, the latent precursor of bone collagenase: Effects of lysosomal cathepsin B, plasmin and kallikrein, and spontaneous activation. Biochem. J. 166:21, 1977.

153. Hasty, K. A., Reife, R. A., Kang, A. H., and Stuart, J. M.: The role of stromelysin in the cartilage destruction that accompanies inflammatory arthritis. Arthritis Rheum. 33:388, 1990.

154. Campbell, E. J., and Campbell, M. A.: Pericellular proteolysis by neutrophils in the presence of proteinase inhibitors: Effects of substrate opsonization. J. Cell Biol. 106:667, 1988.

155. Davies, K. J. A., Lin, S. W., and Pacifici, R. E.: Protein damage and degradation by oxygen radicals: IV. Degradation of denatured protein. J. Biol. Chem. 262:9914, 1987.

156. Johnson, D., and Travis, J.: The oxidative inactivation of human α_1-proteinase inhibitor. J. Biol. Chem. 254:4022, 1979.

157. Roberts, C. R., Roughley, P. J., and Mort, J. S.: Degradation of human proteoglycan aggregate induced by hydrogen peroxide: Protein fragmentation, amino acid modification and hyaluronic acid cleavage. Biochem. J. 259:805, 1989.

158. Ossanna, P. J., Test, S. T., Matheson, N. R., Regiani, S., and Weiss, S. J.: Oxidative regulation of neutrophil elastase-alpha-1-proteinase inhibitor interactions. J. Clin. Invest. 77:1939, 1986.

159. Weiss, S. J., Peppin, G., Ortiz, X., Ragsdale, C., and Test, S. T.: Oxidative autoactivation of latent collagenase by human neutrophils. Science 227:747, 1985.

160. Stetler-Stevenson, W. G., Krutzsch, H. C., Wacher, M. P., Margulies, I. M. K., and Liotta, L. A.: The activation of human type IV collagenase proenzyme: Sequence identification of the major conversion product following organomercurial activation. J. Biol. Chem. 264:1353, 1989.

161. Springman, E. B., Angleton, E. L., Birkedal-Hansen, H., and van Wart, H. E.: Multiple modes of activation of latent human fibroblast collagenase: Evidence for the role of a cys73 active-site zinc complex in latency and a "cysteine switch" mechanism for activation. Proc. Natl. Acad. Sci. U.S.A. 87:364, 1990.

162. van Wart, H. E., and Birkedal-Hansen, H.: The cysteine switch: A principle of regulation of metalloproteinase activity with potential applicability to the entire matrix metalloproteinase gene family. Proc. Natl. Acad. Sci. U.S.A. 87:5578, 1990.

163. Grant, G. A., Eisen, A. Z., Marmer, B. L., Roswitt, W. T., and Goldberg, G. I.: The activation of human skin fibroblast procollagenase: Sequence identification of the major conversion products. J. Biol. Chem. 262:5886, 1987.

164. Unemori, E. N., and Werb, Z.: Collagenase expression and endogenous activation in rabbit synovial fibroblasts stimulated by the calcium ionophore A23187. J. Biol. Chem. 263:16252, 1988.

165. Vater, C. A., Nagase, H., and Harris, E. D., Jr.: Proactivator-dependent activation of procollagenase induced by treatment with EGTA. Biochem. J. 237:853, 1986.

166. Birkedal-Hansen, H., Cobb, C. M., Taylor, R. E., and Fullmer, H. M.: Activation of fibroblast procollagenase by mast cell proteases. Biochim. Biophys. Acta 438:273, 1976.

167. Jordan, R. E., Kilpatrick, J., and Nelson, R. M.: Heparin promotes the inactivation of antithrombin by neutrophil elastase. Science 237:237, 1987.

168. Brower, M. S., and Harpel, P. C.: Proteolytic cleavage and inactivation of α_2-plasmin inhibitor and C1-inactivator by human polymorphonuclear leukocyte elastase. J. Biol. Chem. 257:9849, 1982.

169. Michaelis, J., Vissers, M. C., and Winterbourn, C. C.: Human neutrophil collagenase cleaves α1-antitrypsin. Biochem. J. 270:809, 1990.

170. Okada, Y., Watanabe, S., Nakanishi, I., Kishi, J.-I., Hayakawa, T., Watorek, W., Travis, J., and Nagase, H.: Inactivation of tissue inhibitor of metalloproteinases by neutrophil elastase and other serine proteinases. FEBS Lett. 229:157, 1988.

171. Schultz, R. M., Silberman, S., Persky, B., Bajkowski, A. S., and Carmichael, D. F.: Inhibition by human recombinant tissue inhibitor of metalloproteinases of human amnion invasion and lung colonization by murine B16-F10 melanoma cells. Cancer Res. 48:5539, 1988.

172. Khokha, R., Waterhouse, P., Yagel, S., Lala, P. K., Overall, C. M., Norton, G., and Denhardt, D. T.: Antisense RNA-induced reduction in murine TIMP confers oncogenicity on Swiss 3T3 cells. Science 243:947, 1989.

Chapter 15
Neutrophils and Eosinophils

Per Venge
Håkan Bergstrand
Lena Håkansson

INTRODUCTION

The vital importance of the neutrophil granulocyte in the defense against bacteria is easily demonstrated by the life-threatening infections experienced by patients who lack these cells in their peripheral blood or who have a major defect in the function of the cell.[1-4] It is assumed, and even probable, that the neutrophil plays a major pathophysiologic role in a number of different diseases, including rheumatic disorders, owing to the destructive power of this cell. On the other hand, although discovered more than 100 years ago, the physiologic role of the eosinophil granulocyte is still enigmatic. Currently, the most popular hypothesis is that it plays a role in the defense against invading parasites. Indeed, the eosinophil and eosinophil products are capable of killing various parasites in vitro. Eosinophils have been seen accumulating around invading parasites in tissue, but the few individuals who seem to lack eosinophils are surprisingly healthy. That the eosinophil has a role in disease, however, has become increasingly clear during the last decade. Thus, activated eosinophils are found in most inflammatory diseases, adjacent to sites of tissue destruction, and patients who have hypereosinophilia in their blood generally develop severe and often life-threatening symptoms directly related to the number of eosinophils present in tissues and in the peripheral blood.

THE NEUTROPHIL

The neutrophil granulocyte matures from a common stem cell for erythrocytes, thrombocytes, macrophages, eosinophils, basophils, and mast cells, that is, the hematopoietic stem cell.[2, 3] Thus, the neutrophil is remotely related to all other blood cells, with only one major exception—the lymphocytes. The first identifiable neutrophil precursor cell in the bone marrow in myelopoiesis is the myeloblast. This precursor further matures into the promyelocyte. These two precursor cells contain a rather homogeneous population of primary, or azurophil, granules. The next maturation stage is the myelocyte which contains another population of granules, that is, the specific, or secondary, granules. The mature neutro-

phil granulocyte has an abundance of small heterogeneous granules that may be separated into several different subpopulations based on their densities and their content of specific proteins (Table 15–1). The marrow transit time (the time it takes for a myeloblast to become a mature neutrophil) is about 14 days in normal healthy individuals. After this, the neutrophil survives for 2 more days, with a blood transit time (half-life) of about 6.7 hours. The graveyard of the neutrophil is mainly the spleen and liver, but a proportion will also die in the lungs and intestine. It has been estimated that the turnover of neutrophils is about 10^{11} cells per day. In various diseases, such as in acute and chronic inflammatory diseases, the turnover of neutrophils may be dramatically increased.

The principles that regulate myelopoiesis and differentiation to the mature neutrophil include a number of growth and differentiation factors collectively called cytokines (see later). With respect to myelopoiesis, the best known are the colony-stimulating factors granulocyte-macrophage colony-stimulating factor (GM-CSF) and G-CSF, which are now used clinically to stimulate myelopoiesis in neutropenic patients.

Biochemistry

Azurophil (Primary) Granules

The azurophil granules contain as their main constituents several proteolytic enzymes and a wide array of bactericidal proteins (see Table 15–1).

Proteases

Cathepsin G. Cathepsin G is one of the most basic proteins in the human organism, with an isoelectric point (pI) above pH 11.[1] It is a chymotrypsin-like protease with optimal activity at nearly neutral pH. Cathepsin G also has bactericidal activity that is independent of its enzymatic activity.[5] The proteolytic activity is neutralized by several plasma protease inhibitors, among which alpha$_1$ (α_1)-antichymotrypsin is the most specific. However, α_1-antitrypsin and α_2-macroglobulin are also efficient inhibitors of cathepsin G. The major biological activities of cathepsin

Table 15–1. NEUTROPHIL GRANULE POPULATIONS AND THEIR PROTEIN CONTENT

Primary (Azurophil) Granules	Secondary (Specific) Granules
Cathepsin G	Lactoferrin
Elastase	Lysozyme
Nonspecific collagenase, proteinase 3, proteinase 4, p29b, AGP7	Specific collagenase
	Plasminogen activator
	Vitamin B_{12}–binding protein
Myeloperoxidase (MPO)	C5a-cleaving enzyme
Lysozyme	Cytochrome b_{558}
Defensins	NADPH oxidase
Azurocidin, CAP37	40-kD protein
Bactericidal/permeability-increasing protein (BPI), CAP57	Gelatinase
	β_2-Microglobulin
Acid hydrolases	GTP-binding protein

G are probably related to its proteolytic activity and comprise the cleavage of a number of proteins, including complement factors, coagulation factors, angiotensin, bradykinin, and basement membrane laminin.[6–9] In many instances, these cleavages give rise to active products, but in other cases active products are inactivated. Examples of this are the generation of chemotactic products after cleavage of the complement factor C5 and the activation of latent neutrophil collagenase[10] or matrix metalloproteinases[11] and the inactivation of chemotactic peptides.

Elastase. Elastase is a basic serine protease, with a molecular weight (M_r) of about 30 kilodaltons (kD).[12] It is an elastolytic enzyme with a broad substrate specificity and will digest most proteins.[13] The major inhibitor of elastase in plasma is α_1-antitrypsin, but α_2-macroglobulin is also effective. In addition, elastase is inhibited by a locally produced inhibitor, the so-called secretory leukocyte-protease inhibitor (SLPI).[14] The proteolytic activity of elastase provides it with a role in tissue injury.[13, 15] Subjects deficient in the major elastase inhibitor, α_1-antitrypsin, have an increased propensity to develop emphysema. Other studies have suggested that elastase is involved in the glomerular injury[16] in glomerulonephritis. Digestion of several clotting factors[6, 17] by elastase released to the extracellular plasma environment may account for the coagulation abnormalities seen in patients with septicemia. Basement membrane structures such as laminin are also degraded by elastase, and endothelial cells are injured.[9] Degradation of fibronectin by elastase gives rise to several biologically active products, some of which have cell-adhesive properties, and others gelatin-binding properties.[18]

Nonspecific Collagenase, Proteinase 3, Proteinase 4, p29b, and AGP7 (Azurophil Granule Protein 7). All these names probably identify the same 29-kD serine protease.[19–23] Originally the enzyme was thought to be a collagenase, since it has the capacity to degrade collagen.[19] It was, however, also apparent that the enzyme has a broad serine esterase activity, which therefore prompted the name nonspecific collagenase. The amino acid sequence shows a high

degree of homology with the other serine proteases in the azurophil granules but also with azurocidin (see later). The enzyme specificity of p29b is very similar to that of elastase,[22] and, like elastase, proteinase 3 produces emphysema when given intratracheally to hamsters.[20] Autoantibodies specific for nonspecific collagenase are found in patients with Wegener's granulomatosis who have positive test results for antineutrophil cytoplasmic antibodies (ANCA) (see Chapter 64).

Antibiotic Proteins

Myeloperoxidase. Myeloperoxidase (MPO) is a basic heme-containing protein[24] that is made up of heavy (α) and light (β) chains of 57.5 and 14 kD, respectively. These subunits are arranged sometimes in a 2:2 relationship but probably more often in a 2:1 relationship.[25] MPO is present in blood monocytes but absent in macrophages. In tissues, therefore, the measurement of MPO has been used to quantitatively estimate neutrophil involvement.[26] MPO is a strong peroxidase and takes part in the production of short-lived and reactive oxygen-derived radicals, such as OCl^- (hypochlorite), and long-lived radicals, such as chloramines.[15] Biological activities related to this property of MPO include microbicidal activities, tumor cell killing, the inactivation of α_1-proteinase inhibitor and chemotactic peptides, induction of platelet release, transformation of prostaglandins, reduction of the opsonizing activity of IgG and complement factor C3b, down-regulation of the activity of natural killer cells against tumors, damage to fibronectin,[27, 28] and degradation of articular cartilage.[29, 30] In spite of these demonstrations, the precise role of MPO in vivo is still somewhat enigmatic. Thus, the deficiency of MPO,[31] which in certain areas is relatively common,[32] is rarely related to any specific problems of the individual. Immunoassays of MPO have been developed and used to measure MPO in blood[33–35] and in various tissue fluids.[36] Interestingly, MPO measurements in blood may be used to quantitatively estimate bone marrow activity in leukemic patients.[34] As for other azurophil granule proteins, antibodies against MPO may be found in blood in some inflammatory diseases, such as systemic vasculitis.[37]

Lysozyme. Lysozyme, located in both primary (azurophil) and secondary (specific) granules, is described in more detail later in the section on the secondary granule constituents.

Defensins. Defensins comprise a group of four peptides with molecular weights of less than 4 kD.[38, 39] The defensins are the most abundant of all granule proteins in the neutrophil, making up about 50 percent of all proteins in the granules. Defensins are active in killing both bacteria and viruses but are far less potent than other antibiotic proteins of the neutrophil.[39]

Azurocidin, or CAP37. Azurocidin, or CAP37 (cationic antimicrobial protein of M_r 37 kD) is an antibiotic protein that resembles serine proteases, with homologies to cathepsin G, elastase, and proteinase 3/p29b,[22, 39] but it has lost its protease activity as the result of an amino acid replacement in the catalytic site of the sequence. Apart from being an antibiotic protein, CAP37 was shown to be a potent chemotactic principle for monocytes.[40]

BPI. BPI (bactericidal/permeability-increasing protein)[41, 42] is probably the same protein as the more recently described protein CAP57 (cationic antimicrobial protein M_r 57 kD).[39] BPI/CAP57 is a potent killer of gram-negative bacteria, such as Escherichia coli. It also binds to lipopolysaccharides and may neutralize some of the effects of endotoxin on neutrophils, such as receptor up-regulation.[39]

Specific (Secondary) Granules

Most prominent among the components of the secondary granules are lactoferrin and lysozyme. Others include a vitamin B_{12}–binding protein, a newly identified 40-kD protein with unknown function, β_2-microglobulin, gelatinase,[43] a guanosine-5'-triphosphate (GTP)–binding protein,[44] and a specific collagenase.[45] Specific granules also function as reservoirs of components of the NADPH-oxidase[46] and of plasma membrane receptors.

Lactoferrin. Lactoferrin is an 80-kD iron-binding protein with a high degree of homology with transferrin.[47] Lactoferrin is also produced by exocrine glands, such as the mammary gland, and is believed to take part in the first-line defense against microorganisms by interfering with the iron metabolism of the microbe. The few children described with a lactoferrin deficiency all are highly susceptible to life-threatening infections.[48] Lactoferrin has been shown to take part in the feedback regulation of myelopoiesis[49] and also to promote adherence to endothelial cells.[50] Furthermore, lactoferrin, by virtue of its iron-binding capacity, may interfere with the oxygen-derived molecules produced by the neutrophil, although there is no real concensus as to the biological consequence of this interaction.[51] Immunoassay of lactoferrin in the circulation provides a sensitive and quantitative marker of the turnover and activity of neutrophils both in patients with leukemia[33, 34, 52] and in patients with inflammatory disease.[35, 53, 54]

Lysozyme. Lysozyme is a 15-kD protein found in both the specific and the azurophil granules of human neutrophils. As with lactoferrin, it is also produced by a number of other cells, including monocytes/macrophages and glandular cells. It is probable that lysozyme has a role as a first-line defense molecule, since it has some bactericidal properties and is ubiquitously distributed on all mucous membranes.[55] Lysozyme may be measured in the circulation as a marker of macrophage activity, since approximately 90 percent of all lysozyme in the circulation derives from the monocyte/macrophage pool of cells. Thus, the classic use of serum/plasma measurements of lysozyme is in the diagnosis of monocytic leukemia.[33, 55]

Signal Transduction

The biochemical processes that transduce a message initiated by stimulation of the neutrophil at the level of the cell membrane are very complex and, as yet, are not fully clarified. A highly schematic overview of the signal transduction pathways in the neutrophil is provided in Figure 15–1.

Binding of chemoattractants, such as formyl-methionyl-leucylphenylalanine (f-MLP), leukotriene B_4 (LTB$_4$), platelet-activating factor (PAF), and C5a, to specific membrane receptors results in the activation of receptor-associated, predominantly pertussis toxin–sensitive, GTP-binding protein(s). This, in turn, triggers a phosphatidylinositol-(4,5)-bisphosphate–specific phospholipase C (PLC), catalyzing the generation from the substrate of two second messengers, inositol-(1,4,5)-trisphosphate (IP$_3$) and diacylglycerol (DAG).[56–60] Recent work has also indicated important but less clearly defined roles in signal transduction for phospholipases of the A$_2$ and D types, generating arachidonic acid and phosphatidic acid as possible second messengers, respectively.

IP$_3$ releases calcium from intracellular stores—endoplasmic reticulum or, in neutrophils, calciosomes. Recent findings point to the importance of oscillations in calcium levels as a means of generating signals and to a complementary role for inositol-1,3,4,5-tetrabisphosphate (IP$_4$) in regulating cytosolic calcium levels either by inducing uptake in intracellular stores or by enhancing calcium influx.[56–58, 61]

Diacylglycerol activates protein kinase C (PKC) in a way that is mimicked by phorbol esters. The PKC family is composed of at least nine different isozymes that are differentially expressed in different cells and may be distinctly modulated; the PKC isozymes perhaps play specific roles in signal transduction pathways.[59, 60, 62]

Products of arachidonic acid metabolism, such as leukotrienes, prostaglandins, and epoxides, may influence neutrophil activity. Some of the effects of arachidonic acid may occur via direct activation of PKC,[62] others perhaps via inhibition of a GTPase-activating protein.[63] The arachidonic acid metabolites act mainly via membrane receptors coupled to G-proteins.

Stimuli such as insoluble immune complexes or serum-treated zymosan (STZ) interact with neutrophil receptors for C3b and C3bi and with IgG receptors of the Fc receptor II (FcRII) and FcRIII types; the signal transduction pathways thus initiated are also believed to involve the IP$_3$- and DAG-responsive receptors and the arachidonic acid system, but also other pathways are considered. Some stimuli trigger tyrosine kinase–mediated phosphorylation(s)[64]; inhibitor studies suggest a role in chemoattractant-

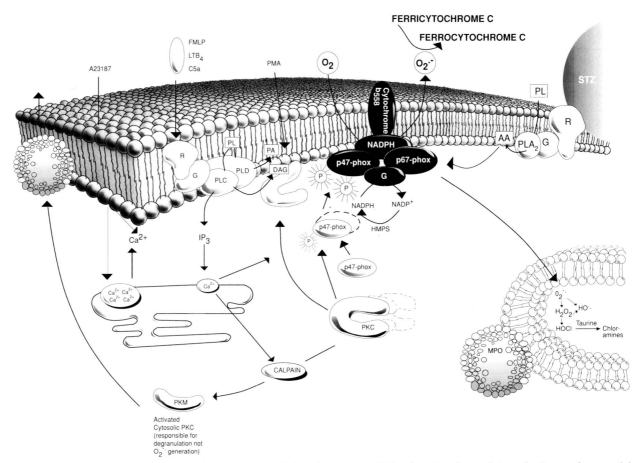

Figure 15–1. Schematic representation of the concepts of the phagocyte oxidative burst and signal transduction pathways. AA, arachidonic acid; C5a, complement factor 5a; DAG, diacylglycerol; f-MLP, formyl-methionyl-leucyl-phenylalanine; G, GTP-binding protein; IP_3, inositol 1,4,5-trisphosphate; LTB_4, leukotriene B_4; MPO, myeloperoxidase; NADPH in black balloon, NADPH-binding protein; PA, phosphatidic acid; PKC, protein kinase C; PKM (protein kinase C fragment); PL, phospholipid; PLA_2 phospholipase A_2; PLC, phospholipase C; PLD, phospholipase D; PMA, 4β-phorbol 12-myristate 13-acetate; R, receptor; STZ, serum-treated zymosan.

induced oxidative burst rather than in degranulation.[65]

Phosphorylation of specific target proteins by activated kinases change their conformation and thereby also their activity; such target proteins include constituents of the cytoskeleton as well as components of NADPH oxidase. Phosphorylations mediated by PKC lead mainly to activation of the neutrophil; however, PKC isozymes, apparently in a form of a so-called "cross-talk," may modulate the activity of other signal transduction pathways.[66] For example, one function of PKC in activated neutrophils is to reduce agonist-induced rises in cytosolic calcium. Phosphorylations of target proteins by cyclic nucleotide–dependent kinases, activated by hormones or drugs via specific membrane receptors, often lead to similar reductions in cellular response.[56, 67, 68]

Signal transduction pathways for degranulation and oxidative metabolism differ in certain aspects.[69, 70] For example, with phorbol myristate acetate (PMA) as a stimulus, the oxidative response can be induced in the virtual absence of gross degranulation, whereas f-MLP triggers granule exocytosis with little hydrogen peroxide generation. The latter response is possibly mediated by a proteolytically generated activated PKC fragment, that is, PKM.[69] Still, degranulation is possibly a step in the activation of the oxidative burst. Moreover, cytosolic proteins of the annexin family (including lipocortins), which bind membrane phospholipids in a calcium-dependent manner, promote aggregation of isolated specific granules; such proteins possibly mediate membrane-membrane contact during degranulation.[71] However, exocytosis of specific and azurophilic granules is differentially regulated, possibly by distinct subsets of low molecular weight G-proteins.[72]

To respond optimally to an appropriate challenge, granulocytes have to be adequately "primed." Such priming is often accomplished by treatment of the cells with low, nontriggering concentrations of secretagogues or with appropriate cytokines or lipopolysaccharide; the biochemical mechanisms for the priming are not unequivocally defined but may include changes in intracellular levels of calcium and/or diacylglycerol/phosphatidic acid but also other principles (see later).

Neutrophil Functions

Adherence

Adherence of neutrophils to vascular endothelial cells is the initial key event leading to the accumulation of neutrophils at an inflammatory site. The increased adherence of neutrophils to endothelial cells and the increased adhesiveness of endothelial cells, which is a part of the inflammatory response, are regulated by a series of events involving adhesion molecules expressed on neutrophils and endothelial cells. The control of adherence and the interaction with endothelial cells are discussed in Chapters 12 and 19, respectively.

Migration

Migration of neutrophils out into the tissue after adhesion to the endothelial cells is the second crucial mechanism behind the accumulation of neutrophils at an inflammatory focus. To accomplish the migration of neutrophils to an inflammatory site the cells are subjected to substances that regulate their direction and speed of migration.[73, 74]

Chemotactic and Chemokinetic Factors. Chemotactic agents govern the direction of cell migration. When exposed to a gradient of a chemotactic agent, neutrophils migrate toward the increasing concentration of the agent. Chemokinetic factors enhance the speed of directed as well as undirected migration. It is believed that chemotactic factors govern the final step of migration to the inflammatory foci, while chemokinetic factors, by enhancing the speed of migration, increase the possibility of the neutrophils' detecting the gradient of a chemotactic factor. The detection of the chemotactic factor gradient is a crucial event, since a gradient within a tissue structure is maintained only within a very short distance.

Neutrophils respond to a number of chemotactic factors in vitro (Table 15–2). The complement-derived C5a, the arachidonic acid metabolite LTB_4, PAF, and the tripeptide f-MLP are the most potent of these chemotactic factors, active at nanomolar concentrations.[74a, 74b] The complement component C5a is rapidly degraded in serum to C5a desarg, which is a chemotactic factor significantly less potent than C5a. Serum, however, also contains an anionic polypeptide called cochemotaxin that potentiates the chemotactic activity of C5a desarg. Further investigations indicate that cochemotaxin is identical to vitamin D–binding protein (group-specific component globulin, gc-globulin).[74c]

The Motile Apparatus of Neutrophils. Migration as well as phagocytosis and degranulation requires changes in the shape and consistency of the cell's

Table 15–2. CHEMOTACTIC AND CHEMOKINETIC FACTORS FOR NEUTROPHILS AND EOSINOPHILS

Chemotactic Factors
C5a (complement-derived)
f-MLP (formyl-methionylleucylphenylalanine) (bacterial origin)
LTB_4 (leukotriene B_4) (metabolite of arachidonic acid)
HETEs (metabolite of arachidonic acid)
PAF (platelet-activating factor, 1-O-alkyl-2-acetyl-sn-glycero-3-phosphocholine)
Thrombin
Collagen fragments
Kallikrein
Fibrinopeptides
IL-8 (interleukin-8)

Chemokinetic Factors
C3-related products
α_1-Antiproteinase inhibitor
α_2-Macroglobulin
Orosomucoid
Albumin (ethanol-treated)
PAF

peripheral cytoplasm and pseudopods, which are the regions involved in these movements. The extension of the cytoplasm is maintained by a network of actin microfilaments.[75] Actin exists in two forms, as a monomer called G-actin and as filaments named F-actin. Alterations of the actin filaments involve sequestration of filaments, nucleation of monomers, and filament assembly. The three-dimensional network formed by actin is based on actin-binding protein and α-actinin. Actin-binding protein is a cross-linking protein that forms the right angles of the network. α_1-Actinin, the other cross-linking agent, joins the actin filaments side to side as bundles. The length and maintenance of actin filaments are regulated by several proteins. Acumentin and gelsolin, by different actions, maintain a shortened filament length. Profilin, when in its high-affinity state, binds G-actin at a 1:1 molar ratio and thereby prevents formation of nuclei or incorporation into preformed actin filaments.

Strong evidence suggests that myosin is the protein that contracts the cytoplasm of the neutrophil. Myosin is regulated by calcium and magnesium. Activation of the Mg-ATPase activity of myosin results in contraction. One mechanism behind the interaction between the contractive effect of myosin and the extensive effect of actin filaments is probably that contraction moves actin from areas of high calcium concentrations to areas of low calcium concentrations. A few seconds after a chemotactic factor–receptor complex is formed, it becomes associated with the cytoskeleton, an association dependent on filamentous actin and regulated by a G-protein.[76]

Defects of Neutrophil Migration. Few primary defects of neutrophil migration have been described. Granulocytes from patients with leukocyte adhesion deficiency (LAD) also demonstrate defective migratory responses both in vitro and in vivo.[77, 78] A study of infection-prone children demonstrated defects of the neutrophil chemotactic response, primary or secondary, that was related to the severity of their infections.[79] A number of reports have described neutrophil migratory dysfunction due to chemotactic factor and chemokinetic factor defects as well as cell-directed inhibitors of migration.[73, 74] A few patients with C5 deficiency have been described. Sera from these patients show a reduced capacity to generate complement-derived chemotactic activity. These patients were subject to severe bacterial infections. An inhibitor of C5a-derived chemotactic activity has been demonstrated in sera from patients with systemic lupus erythematosus (SLE). The inhibitor, antigenically related to the fragment Bb of the complement factor B, binds to cochemotaxin and thereby interferes with the C5-derived chemotactic activity. Chemotactic factor inactivator (CFI) is a term for activities present in serum and bronchoalveolar lavage fluid (BAL) that decreases the chemotactic effect of C5a and other chemotactic substances. The mechanisms of the inhibitory effect of CFIs vary. One factor with protease activity has been described. Another CFI interacts with the vitamin D–binding protein (cochemotaxin). Whether the latter CFI is identical to the C5a inhibitor found in sera from patients with SLE is at present unknown. A chemokinetic inhibitory factor (CIF) has been demonstrated in sera of patients with chronic lymphocytic leukemia (CLL). Chemokinetic inhibitory factor is a lymphokine produced by B-CLL cells as well as normal blood and spleen B lymphocytes.[80] The presence of CIF in the sera of patients with CLL was related to an increased propensity to infection.

Phagocytosis

Phagocytosis is the process by which particles recognized by neutrophils are internalized. Recognition is dependent on the presence of opsonins, such as immunoglobulins and complement components (C3b), on the particles and is mediated by receptors for immunoglobulins and complement components on the surface membrane of neutrophils. Binding of opsonins to the cell surface receptor activates the motile apparatus of the cell via gelation and contraction of actin filaments, and pseudopods are formed around the particle, which is eventually engulfed.

Fc and C3b Receptors on the Surface Membrane of Neutrophils (Table 15–3). The receptors that recognize the Fc part of IgG and C3b/iC3b are the most important receptors involved in phagocytosis. Under normal conditions, the neutrophils express the low-affinity receptors FcγRII (CDw32) and FcγRIII (CD16).[81–84] FcγRII interacts with IgG complexes consisting of two or more IgG molecules and thereby induces phagocytosis, respiratory burst, and degranulation. The subclass specificity of FcγRII is IgG1 ≈ IgG3>>IgG2 = IgG4. FcγRIII interacts with dimeric complexes of IgG1 and IgG3 and is able to induce granule secretion but not phagocytosis or respiratory burst. The FcγRIII, however, possesses the unique

Table 15–3. Fc AND COMPLEMENT RECEPTORS ON NEUTROPHILS AND EOSINOPHILS

Receptor	Cells	Cellular Function
FcαR	Neutrophils Eosinophils	Phagocytosis Secretion Respiratory burst
FcγRI (CD64)	Cytokine-activated neutrophils	Phagocytosis Respiratory burst
FcγRII (CDw32)	Neutrophils Eosinophils	Phagocytosis Respiratory burst Secretion
FcγRIII (CD16)	Neutrophils	Secretion
FcεRII (CD23-rel)	Eosinophils	Secretion Respiratory burst
CR1 (CD35)	Neutrophils Eosinophils	Phagocytosis Secretion
CR3 (CD11b/ CD18)	Neutrophils Eosinophils	Phagocytosis Secretion

function of inducing opsonin-independent phagocytosis of bacteria that possess lectin-like substances on their surface. The FcγRIII is coupled to a phospholipase C–sensitive glycosyl-phosphatidylinositol (PIG) anchor. The expression of FcγRIII depends on upregulation and release of the receptor. FcγRIII is released upon stimulation of neutrophils with f-MLP and PMA. Expression of the high-affinity FcγRI is induced on neutrophils by interferon-gamma (γ). FcγRI mediates phagocytosis of monomeric IgG and IgG complexes with a subclass specificity of IgG1 ≈ IgG3>IgG4>>IgG2. Interaction of IgG with FcγRI mediates phagocytosis and superoxide generation.

Neutrophils express two kinds of C3b receptors, CR1, which interacts with C3b, and C4b and CR3, which interact with iC3b.[85–88] CR1 interacts with the actin filaments of the cytoskeleton of neutrophils. Expression of CR1 is increased by tumor necrosis factor (TNF) and f-MLP, probably by recruitment of receptors from an hitherto unidentified intracellular store. CR3 is present both in the plasma membrane and in the specific granule fraction. Tumor necrosis factor and f-MLP up-regulate CR3 by recruitment from the specific granule fraction. It has been known for a long time that coating of particles with both C3b and IgG enhances the rate of phagocytosis compared with that of particles coated with IgG only. The demonstration of an association between the CR3 receptor and the FcγRIII, by a subset of CD11b/CD18 receptors, is probably one explanation for the synergistic effect of C3b on IgG-mediated phagocytosis.[84]

Under normal conditions, the FcαRs on neutrophils exist in a low-affinity state, but activation of granulocytes with GM-CSF and G-CSF induces a change to a high-affinity state and an acquisition of IgA-mediated phagocytic capability.[89] The FcαR recognizes both IgA1 and IgA2.

Fc Receptor Deficiencies. Patients with paroxysmal nocturnal hemoglobinuria (PNH), a disorder characterized by a defect in the biosynthesis of a PIG anchor, show a varying deficiency in FcγRIII expression. The NA1/NA2 polymorphism of FcγRIII is involved in alloimmune and autoimmune neutropenias and blood transfusion reactions.[84] The few "NA null" individuals (meaning that they lack the NA antigen but not the PIG anchor) who have been detected were healthy and had no circulating immune complexes and no increased susceptibility to infections. A newborn baby to a "NA null" mother, however, developed transient immune neutropenia.

Secretion of Primary and Secondary Granule Constituents

The extracellular release of granule constituents may be brought about by active mobilization of the granule material to the exterior of the cell or passive diffusion out of the cell because of the loss of cellular integrity. The latter may take place at cell death but is also believed to take place during phagocytosis because of the imperfect closure of the phagocytic vacuole.[1, 90] Thus, when the neutrophil ingests a particle such as a bacterium, the granules are mobilized to the vacuolar membrane in order to release their material into the vacuole. At a very early stage of this process, part of the granule material is released into the vacuole before the ingestion phase is completed and the phagocytic vacuole is properly closed. This phenomenon is sometimes referred to as "regurgitation while feeding." Active secretion of granule material may take place during the chemotactic migration of the neutrophil. The actual meaning of this secretion is not well understood but may be of importance for the capacity of the neutrophil to penetrate certain tissue structures such as basal membranes during the migration from blood to tissue.

The kinetics of degranulation and secretion of primary granule constituents are very different from that of the secondary granules, which implies that the mechanisms that govern the degranulation of these two granule populations are fundamentally different. The primary granules, with their contents of very potent and potentially destructive material, primarily release their content into the phagocytic vacuole, whereas secondary granule constituents are mobilized to the plasma membrane and released to the exterior of the cell. Secretion of the constituents of both granules may be achieved with C5a, PMA, or other soluble stimuli but requires, in the case of primary granules, concentrations that are 10 to 100 times those required to induce secondary granule secretion. Even with these high concentrations, hardly more than 15 to 25 percent of the primary granule constituents is released, in contrast with the secondary granules, which release 50 to 70 percent of their material with the lower secretagogue concentrations.

Induction of neutrophil degranulation is brought about by a variety of soluble stimuli, such as the chemotactic agents C5a, IL-8,[91] LTB$_4$, f-MLP, the phorbol ester PMA, and Ca ionophores, or the exposure to particles opsonized with immunoglobulins and complement products, such as C3b. As shown in Table 15–3, secretion is induced by the interaction with either IgA or IgG, and the IgG signal for secretion is primarily mediated through the FcγRII and RIII receptors. Some cytokines, such as GM-CSF, enhance the secretion of primary and secondary granule proteins from human neutrophils,[92] partly by up-regulation of receptors in the plasma membrane (see Table 15–4) but probably also by changing intracellular Ca levels.[93]

Oxidative Metabolism

At appropriate triggering, neutrophils respond with a marked increase in oxygen consumption. This respiratory or oxidative burst, which is not inhibited by blockers of the mitochondrial respiration such as cyanide or azide, is due to the activation of an oxidase catalyzing the one-electron reduction of oxygen to superoxide radicals at the expense of NADPH generated in the hexose monophosphate shunt according to the reaction $2 O_2 + NADPH \rightarrow 2 O_2^- + NADP^+ + H^+$. The superoxide radicals formed are dismutated, mainly in phagocytic vacuoles, to hydrogen peroxide and are further converted, in reactions involving the primary granule constituent MPO, to hydroxyl radicals and other reactive products of oxygen such as hypohalides and chloramines. This respiratory burst is part of the phagocytes' armament for microbicidal purposes. However, if inappropriately released from the cell (e.g., at frustrated phagocytosis), the formed reactive oxygen species are potentially harmful to the tissue of the host.

The oxidative burst is not absolutely dependent on phagocytic events or associated with degranulation; rather, it seems to be a unique process that may be induced and modulated independent from other functions of the neutrophil.[69, 70, 94–98]

NADPH Oxidase. The NADPH oxidase is normally present in the cells in a dormant form. On priming and activation of the cells, some components of the oxidase are translocated from the cytosolic compartment to the membrane; others apparently initially reside in the membrane.

The evidence today favors participation in the oxidase catalyzed reaction of the following components (see Fig. 15–1): a membrane-associated cytochrome, a cytosolic 47-kD protein (p47-*phox* for phagocyte oxidase), a 67-kD protein (p67-*phox*) that is cytosolic and/or associated with the cytoskeleton,[99] possibly a 45-kD flavoprotein, and a NADPH-binding component that is not unequivocally identified but may be a 32-kD protein.[96, 99–101] A GTP-binding, *ras*-like protein, *rapl*, is linked to the cytochrome and may constitute a component of the NADPH oxidase.[102]

The *cytochrome* has a low redox potential, -245 mV, and an α band of light absorption at 558 nm. It is therefore referred to as cytochrome b$_{-245}$ or cytochrome b$_{558}$. It has been purified and shown to be composed of the heme and two protein subunits, an α chain of 22 kD (p22-*phox*) and a glycosylated β chain of molecular weight 76 to 93 kD (gp91-*phox*). The genes for both these chains have been cloned[95, 96]; the amino acid sequences show little resemblance to those of other mammalian cytochromes. The genes for the p47-*phox*[103] and p67-*phox*[104] have also recently been cloned; the p47-*phox* contains several potential phosphorylation sites. Apparently, p47-*phox* is needed for activation of the oxidase but perhaps not for the continued expression of its activity.[99]

Priming of Cells for an Oxidative Burst. Whereas for human macrophages, IFN-γ and somatotropin are necessary and sufficient as primers, other cytokines such as GM-CSF and TNF-α have been attributed priming properties for neutrophils.[105] The neutrophil is also reportedly primed for enhanced oxygen radical generation by lipopolysaccharide and by exposure to low concentrations of secretagogues, such as f-MLP, LTB$_4$, and PAF, which per se do not trigger a response.[106–108]

The mechanism(s) for the priming of the oxidative burst are not clarified; f-MLP does not prime cells according to pathways that trigger a response. Granulocytes primed with GM-CSF respond with a respiratory burst to increases in the level of cytosolic calcium; in cells harvested from blood such an event is, by itself, not sufficient to trigger the cells.[109] GM-CSF– and TNF-α–primed cells also express enhanced responses to G-protein triggering; such cells produce cell-associated PAF and/or phosphatidic acid (through a phospholipase D [PLD] pathway), which perhaps plays a second messenger role.[110, 111] PKC inhibitors augment GM-CSF–induced priming.[112] Interferon-γ, lipopolysaccharides and TNF treatment of CGD neutrophils leads to increased mRNA transcript levels of cytochrome b$_{-245}$,[108] indicating that priming may involve PKC activity as well as increased transcription of NADPH oxidase enzyme components.

Neutrophils in suspension respond to chemoattractant challenge with a transient burst of radical generation, whereas *adherent cells* respond according to a more protracted time course, suggesting differences in the control of the burst in these situations.[113, 114] For example, triggering of adherent neutrophils, but not cells in suspension, with STZ is accompanied by a change in cytosolic calcium.[115]

Triggering of the Oxidative Burst. Activation of the NADPH oxidase in vitro can be accomplished by triggering cells with various particulate stimuli, such as STZ, or soluble, receptor-associating stimuli such as f-MLP, LTB$_4$, C5a, and PAF. More artificial secretagogues, such as PMA or a calcium ionophore (e.g., A23187), are often utilized to trigger a vigorous burst in vitro.

The signal transduction pathways differ with the stimulus employed and the cell examined, but the final pathway results in stimulation of PKC activity and partial phosphorylation of the p47-*phox* cytosolic component,[116] which then becomes associated with the cytoskeleton. Phalloidin, which prevents actin depolymerization induced by f-MLP, also inhibits oxidase activation. However, an inhibitor (cytochalasin B) and an enhancer (tetracaine) of f-MLP–induced actin polymerization augment f-MLP–triggered oxidative responses. P47-*phox* is translocated to the cell membrane,[99, 116, 117] where it "docks" with the C-terminal tail of the 91-kD cytochrome b$_{558}$ subunit.[118] The protein then undergoes further phosphorylations. In fact, continuous phosphorylation of p47-*phox* occurs during the respiratory burst[116]; inhibition of a normally vigorous phosphatase activity may also lead to activation of the respiratory burst.[119] Translocation of the p47-*phox* mediates the assembly of the oxidase components on the membrane.[120]

Both chains of the cytochrome b$_{-245}$ are also phosphorylated during superoxide generation; these phosphorylations are kinetically not associated with activation of the NADPH oxidase but may rather be involved in cessation of the activity.[116]

Fluoride, f-MLP, and C5a, presumably acting through G-protein(s), trigger neutrophil oxidative responses that are independent of changes in intracellular calcium levels and/or DAG and PKC activation.[121] A possible second messenger in such situations is phosphatidic acid generated via a wortmannin-sensitive PLD pathway[116, 122]; DAG possibly *modulates* such responses. Another possible messenger is arachidonic acid, which can trigger the NADPH oxidase in subcellular systems (see later); superoxide generation induced by PMA is blocked by inhibitors of arachidonic acid–generating PLA$_2$.[123]

Triggering of an oxidative response by C3b and IgG (the FcRII) receptors or by concanavalin A (Con A) also utilizes pathways that do not appear to involve Ca^{2+} increase and PKC activation and seem to be different from those utilized by stimulation with f-MLP.[121, 124]

Activation of NADPH Oxidase in Subcellular Systems. Activation of the NADPH oxidase can be accomplished in suitably reconstituted subcellular systems by arachidonic acid or detergents such as SDS (sodium dodecyl sulfate). In this system, PKC activity does not seem to be involved, since phorbol esters express low activating efficacy and since activation can be accomplished in the virtual absence of ATP. Still, DAGs synergize with the anionic amphiphile in activation of superoxide generation as well as p47-*phox* phosphorylation in this system.[116] Triggering needs a membrane component and possibly four or even five different cytosolic components, one of which is a GTP-binding protein.[125]

Pharmacologic Modulation of the Oxidative Burst. Besides antioxidants, conceivably acting as scavengers of oxygen radicals rather than NADPH oxidase inhibitors, naturally occurring inhibitors of the oxidative burst have been identified[126]: adenosine, antiproteases, polyamines, streptococcal pneumolysin,[94] 1-*O*-alkyl-2-acyl-*sn*-glycerols, formed during stimulation of the cells, which may inhibit the oxidative burst as a result of PKC inhibition,[106] and a lipid thiobis ester from the neutrophil cytosol that apparently inhibits the NADPH oxidase reversibly.[127]

Of currently used clinical drugs, azelastine reduces, whereas xanthine derivatives differentially modulate in vitro phagocyte radical generation. These agents presumably act at the level of the secretagogue signal transduction. Agents that increase cyclic adenosine monophosphate (cAMP) often reduce receptor-mediated neutrophil oxidative responses, whereas agents that increase cyclic guanosine monophosphate (cGMP) may enhance such responses. Agents that elevate cAMP reduce f-MLP–induced superoxide generation in concert with inhibition of DAG production by PLD.[67, 128] Several reports fail to record substantial inhibition of phagocyte oxygen radical generation by glucocorticoid treatment either in vitro or in vivo.

Of other experimental agents, diphenyl iodonium and analogues, which block the activity of the flavin adenine dinucleotide (FAD)–binding protein of the NADPH oxidase, are more potent inhibitors of this oxidase than of the mitochondrial correspondent; these agents may be the most suitable probes available for inhibiting the NADPH oxidase in vitro.[126] Protein kinase inhibitors such as staurosporine and its more specific PKC inhibitor analogues,[129, 130] sphingosine analogues,[131] and certain amphiphilic drugs such as the naphthalene sulfonamide W-7 and the purported intracellular calcium antagonist TMB-8 also block neutrophil superoxide radical generation. Tyrosine kinase inhibitors such as erbstatin selectively block oxidative responses triggered by f-MLP and PAF receptor stimulation.[65]

Chronic Granulomatous Disease. A severe clinical syndrome, chronic granulomatous disease (CGD), which is characterized by serious recurrent bacterial and fungal infections often associated with massive granuloma formation, is due to lack of phagocyte NADPH oxidase activity following defects in one or more of the putative components of the enzyme.[95, 96, 100] Multiple genetically distinct forms of CGD exist.[100] Approximately 50 percent of all CGDs are due to X-linked defects in the heavy chain of the cytochrome, some one third are due to autosomal recessive defects in the p47-*phox*, whereas a few percent of CGDs lack functional p67-*phox*.

Patients with CGD of the X chromosome–linked category lack both chains of the cytochrome; the defect has been pinpointed to the gene coding for the β chain. Patients of the autosomal recessive category seem to express both chains normally; however, in these patients the p47-*phox* is not appropriately phosphorylated. Either it may be missing or the pertinent serine or threonine residue(s) may be displaced by mutation.

Tissue Injury Induced by the Oxidative Burst. Phorbol esters, which are highly potent and effective stimuli of the oxidative metabolism, are extremely effective inflammation-inducing agents in animals in vivo. Free radicals exacerbate ischemic tissue injury.

Numerous in vitro studies have shown adverse effects on biological material of reactive oxygen species.[15, 132, 133] All of these observations suggest an important role for the oxidative burst in inducing tissue damage at sites of inflammation.

Specifically, oxygen-derived species may contribute to the induction of acute lung injury as well as to neutrophil-induced tissue damage at vascular sites of immune complex deposition[94, 134] and to nonspecific bronchial hyper-reactivity in asthma.[135] In joints, the role of oxygen-derived reactive species may even be a more primary one; oxidant attactant on proteins may transform them to autoantigens and/or increase their susceptibility to degradation by proteolytic agents.[15, 136]

Priming

Priming denotes an increased responsiveness of cells to stimuli of, for instance, chemotactic responses, adherence, and secretory responses. Several interleukins are capable of priming the function of neutrophils (Table 15–4). Interleukin-4 (IL-4) facili-

Table 15–4. PRIMING OF NEUTROPHILS AND EOSINOPHILS BY CYTOKINES

Cytokine	Affected Cell	Effect On
IL-3	Neutrophil Eosinophil	Adherence CR3 expression Cytotoxicity
IL-4	Neutrophil	Phagocytosis
IL-5	Eosinophil	Adherence CR3 expression Cytotoxicity Secretion
IL-6	Neutrophil	Secretion
IL-8	Neutrophil	Adherence CR1,CR3 expression Chemotaxis Respiratory burst Secretion
GM-CSF	Neutrophil Eosinophil	Adherence CR1 and CR3 expression FcγRIII expression Cytotoxicity
IFN-γ	Neutrophil Eosinophil	FcγRII and RIII expression Cytotoxicity
IFN-α	Eosinophil	Cytotoxicity
IFN-β	Eosinophil	Cytotoxicity
TNF-α	Neutrophil Eosinophil	Adherence CR1 and CR3 expression Respiratory burst
EAF	Eosinophil	Respiratory burst CR3 expression Secretion Cytotoxicity
ECEF	Eosinophil	Cytotoxicity

IL, interleukin; GM-CSF, granulocyte-macrophage colony-stimulating factor; IFN, interferon; TNF, tumor necrosis factor; EAF, eosinophil-enhancing factor; ECEF, eosinophil cytotoxicity-enhancing factor.

tated the killing of opsonized bacteria by an increased phagocytosis, and IL-6 was shown to enhance the cytotoxicity of neutrophils.[137, 138] IL-8, also called neutrophil-activating peptide (NAP), is a potent primer of most aspects of a neutrophil's function, such as chemotaxis, respiratory burst, secretion, and cytotoxicity.[139] An increased expression of CD11b/CD18 (CR3) and CR1 might be one explanation behind its priming activity. GM-CSF, apart from its effect on neutrophil proliferation and differentiation, also affects the function of mature neutrophils, such as adherence, phagocytosis, and degranulation.[140] GM-CSF increases the expression of CR1 and CR3 (CD11b/CD18) by de novo synthesis, thereby enhancing the adherence of neutrophils to endothelium.[88, 140] GM-CSF also induces an increased FcγRIII expression owing to de novo protein synthesis. The GM-CSF receptors on neutrophils are coupled to G-proteins, which probably are involved in the priming mechanism. GM-CSF also increases the generation of DAG by neutrophils. TNF-α enhances neutrophil respiratory burst and adherence to endothelium probably as a result of induction of an increased expression of CR1 and CR3.[88, 140]

THE EOSINOPHIL

The human eosinophil granulocyte derives from a common hematopoietic stem cell and is remotely related to neutrophils, basophils, mast cells, and monocytes/macrophages. Important growth factors involved in eosinophil maturation are GM-CSF and IL-3 at an early stage, and IL-5 at a later stage.[141] The most immature and identifiable eosinophil precursor cell is the promyelocytic eosinophil, characterized by its content of large crystalloid-containing granules in which are found eosinophil specific proteins. These granules are also abundant in mature human eosinophil granulocytes and help identify these cells under the electron microscope. Normally only 1 to 4 percent

of all leukocytes in the blood are eosinophil granulocytes. It has been estimated, however, that the tissues contain 100 to 300 times as many eosinophils, which indicates that the eosinophil is to be regarded predominantly as a tissue cell. The half-life of the eosinophil in the blood is 4 to 5 hours, whereas the half-life in tissues is considerably longer, probably several days and perhaps even weeks. Like the neutrophil, the eosinophil expresses its activity by the production and extracellular release of the granule proteins and other newly formed mediators, such as oxygen-derived metabolites and some lipids (Fig. 15–2).[142, 143]

Biochemistry

Granules and Granule Proteins

The granules of human eosinophils are separated into two major populations: peroxidase-positive and peroxidase-negative. The peroxidase-positive granules contain as one feature characteristic crystalloids. These crystalloids contain the four major proteins of the human eosinophil, that is, major basic protein (MBP), eosinophil cationic protein (ECP), eosinophil peroxidase (EPO),[144] and eosinophil protein X,[145] or eosinophil-derived neurotoxin (EPX/EDN). All four proteins appear to be present in the heavy, peroxidase-positive granules, whereas only ECP and EPX/EDN are present in the other, lighter population. A fifth major protein of the eosinophil is the Charcot-Leyden crystal (CLC) protein, which presumably is a plasma membrane protein. This protein is shed from the eosinophil and forms typical extracellular needle-like crystals in tissues of heavy eosinophil infiltration. Both MBP and the CLC protein are also found in basophils, whereas ECP, EPO, and presumably EPX/EDN are specific to the eosinophil. These specificities have important implications when these proteins are used as specific markers of eosinophil

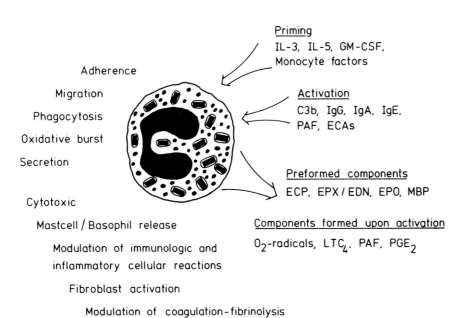

Figure 15–2. The human eosinophil.

activity in vivo. Characteristic of the four granule proteins are their high isoelectric points, the pI for ECP and EPO is above pH 11. They are also fairly small, ranging from about 14 kD, for MBP, to 67 kD, for EPO. All four proteins have been cloned, and their primary structures have revealed large contents of the basic amino acid arginine.[146-151] The amino acid sequences of ECP and EPX/EDN show a large degree of homology, about 70 percent, with each other. Also, a homology to pancreatic ribonuclease was shown, and both proteins have ribonuclease activities, with EPX/EDN being the most active.[152] The close relationship between ECP and EPX/EDN is also demonstrated by the monoclonal antibody EG2, which recognizes a common epitope on the two proteins.[153] The relative content of these four major proteins in normal human eosinophil granules is roughly equal, ranging from 10 to 15 μg per 10^6 eosinophils. The content in eosinophils obtained from patients with eosinophilia, however, may vary quite considerably.

Granule Proteins

Eosinophil Cationic Protein (ECP). ECP is a one-chain, zinc-containing protein with an M_r varying from 18 to 21 kD. The heterogeneity is due to differences in glycosylation of the protein molecule.[154] Besides being a ribonuclease, ECP is a potent cytotoxic molecule with the capacity to kill mammalian cells as well as nonmammalian cells, such as parasites. The noncytotoxic properties of ECP include the alteration of glycosaminoglycan production by human fibroblasts and stimulation of airway mucus secretion.[155] The former finding may point to a role in tissue repair processes and may have a bearing on the findings of the eosinophil presence in fibrotic processes.[156] The latter may be of great importance for the understanding of the role of the eosinophil in diseases such as asthma, since this disease is characterized by, among other things, hypersecretion of the airways. Another finding of potential interest is the capacity of ECP to inhibit T lymphocyte proliferation as a response to mitogens, but also in mixed leukocyte reactions. This effect is seen in vitro at very low concentrations, that is, less than 10^{-8} mol per L. Hence, by virtue of its granule proteins the eosinophil may be active in the regulation of T cell–mediated reactions. ECP also shortens the coagulation time of plasma by mechanisms related to the enhancement of the activity of factor XII. These findings may be of relevance in the hypereosinophilic syndrome, in which thromboembolic phenomena are very common,[142, 157] but also in allergic reactions in which activation of factor XII has been demonstrated concomitant to the activation of the eosinophil.[158] Another study showed an effect on fibrinolysis with preactivation of plasminogen, with consequent enhancement of plasminogen activator activation of plasminogen. It should be emphasized that most of the described effects of ECP in vitro take place at

concentrations that are comparable to those found in vivo, that is, 10^{-9} to 10^{-6} mol per L. Locally, these concentrations may even be exceeded. Thus, in sputum of asthmatic patients and in the synovial fluid of patients with rheumatoid arthritis,[159] concentrations as high as 10^{-5} mol per L have been found. One important question therefore is, how is the cytotoxic activity of these proteins regulated extracellularly? So far, two potential mechanisms have been described. Thus, by virtue of its acidic nature heparin will bind and neutralize the activity of ECP. No in vivo data exist however, to support this potential mechanism. Another potential mechanism is the binding of ECP to α_2-macroglobulin, probably at the site of the binding of proteolytic enzymes. The binding of ECP to α_2-macroglobulin in vivo is indicated by the existence of high molecular weight forms of ECP in the sera of patients with eosinophilia and who also have very high levels of ECP in sera.[160] This interaction with α_2-macroglobulin may be an important mechanism of neutralizing the actions of ECP, since it is the only obvious interaction of ECP with any plasma component.

Sensitive immunoassays for ECP serve as an indicator of eosinophil activation and turnover[160] not only in asthma and allergic diseases[161, 162] but also in inflammatory diseases of the gut, skin, joints, brain, and so forth.[36, 159, 163]

Eosinophil Protein X and Eosinophil-Derived Neurotoxin. EPX and EDN are the same protein.[143, 154] Since no agreement has been reached as to how to name this protein, the provisional name EPX/EDN is used in this chapter. EPX/EDN is slightly less basic than ECP but has a similar size, that is, an M_r of 18 kD.[145, 147, 149] EPX/EDN is a potent ribonuclease and about 100 times more active than ECP.[152] EPX/EDN also has some cytotoxic properties, as the name EDN implies. Thus, when injected into the brains of experimental animals, EPX/EDN produced damage to the tissues reminiscent of the so-called Gordon's phenomenon, with destruction of Purkinje's cells of the cerebellum and the development of ataxia. The neurotoxic activity of EPX/EDN, however, is not restricted to this protein, since ECP produces Gordon's phenomenon at concentrations about 100 times lower than those of EPX/EDN. In analogy with ECP, EPX/EDN inhibits T lymphocyte proliferation in a noncytotoxic fashion and at concentrations similar to those of ECP. EPX/EDN does not kill parasites as efficiently as ECP. The effect of EPX/EDN on parasites, such as the larvae of *Schistosoma mansoni*, is very characteristic and different from the effect of ECP. Thus, when the parasite is exposed to EPX/EDN, it is reversibly paralyzed. This phenomenon could be an important defense mechanism and facilitate the eradication of the parasite.

Eosinophil Peroxidase. EPO is a two-chain protein with a total M_r of 67 kD.[144] The main function of EPO is that of a peroxidase, and together with a halide and H_2O_2, EPO constitutes a potent cytotoxic mechanism. EPO damages nasal sinus mucosa,[164] and it also has a number of noncytotoxic effects on mammalian cells. Thus, EPO induces degranulation of mast cells and causes platelet aggregation.[165] In addition, EPO may be involved in the inactivation of lipid mediators, such as the leukotrienes.[166] EPO is taken up by the neutrophils via a specific and probably receptor-related mechanism.[167] This uptake could be an important regulatory mechanism, which actively neutralizes the toxic effects of EPO, but it also increases the adhesiveness of the neutrophil. EPO can be measured in several body fluids, including plasma, by sensitive immunoassays.[144]

Major Basic Protein. The name *major basic protein* derives from the fact that in guinea pig eosinophils this protein seems to be dominating, making up about 50 percent of the protein content of the granule proteins.[142, 143] As mentioned previously, MBP is stored in the granules in the peculiar and typical crystalloids. The M_r of MBP is 13.9 kD. MBP is not unique to the eosinophil but is also found in other cells, such as basophils and some placental cells. The major biological function of eosinophilic MBP is related to its cytotoxic activities and involves the killing and damage of parasites and mammalian cells, such as pneumocytes and nasal mucosal cells. In analogy with the other eosinophil granule proteins, MBP also has a number of noncytotoxic effects on various cells. These include degranulation of basophils and mast cells, platelet aggregation, induction of neutrophil superoxide production, contraction of airway smooth muscle, and inhibition of airway mucus production.[143, 155, 165, 168, 169] Interesting functions of MBP are the effects on respiratory epithelium,[168] which may partly explain the development of the hyper-responsiveness of the airways in asthmatic patients.[170] Control of MBP activity involves binding and neutralization by heparin[158]; mast cells also sequester MBP.[171] Measurement of MBP in serum or plasma is less suitable as a marker of eosinophil turnover and activity in the body than the aforementioned proteins, since very high levels of MBP are also found in conditions unrelated to eosinophil involvement, such as pregnancy.

Other Enzymatic Activities. In addition to the four major proteins, the human eosinophil contains in its granules several other enzymatic activities,[142, 172] including collagenolytic, histaminase, phospholipase, and arylsulfatase B activities. Even transforming growth factor-α and GM-CSF are expressed in human eosinophils.[172a] These activities may indicate a regulatory role of eosinophils in allergy, since the eosinophil acquires the potential to inactivate a number of the mediators of allergic inflammation, such as histamine, PAF, and leukotrienes.

Newly Formed Mediators

The eosinophil is a very capable producer of oxygen-derived toxic metabolites, such as O_2^-, H_2O_2, and OH· and is, in this respect in fact, fully comparable to the neutrophil.[142, 143, 161, 173] The eosinophil also produces a number of lipid mediators, including prostaglandins (PGE_2), leukotrienes (LTC_4), and PAF. Both LTC_4 and PAF are potent spasmogenic lipids. PAF is also a chemotactic signal for the eosinophils themselves, and it induces secretion of eosinophil granule proteins.[174]

Functions

Adherence

Eosinophils adhere to endothelium, although their adherence has not been extensively studied, probably because of the normally low number of eosinophils in the blood. However, accumulation of eosinophils in the lungs of asthmatic patients and nasal mucosa of rhinitis patients, tissues that under normal conditions do not contain eosinophils, suggests a recruitment of eosinophils from the blood stream, that initially involves the adherence of eosinophils to endothelial cells.[175]

Migration

Eosinophils are migratory cells, although their rate of migration is slower than that of neutrophils. Eosinophils respond to the chemotactic factors C5a, LTB_4, HETEs, PAF, and f-MLP (see table 15–2).[142] PAF is claimed to be the most potent chemotactic factor for eosinophils, while their response to f-MLP is weaker than that of neutrophils. Interleukin-5 also serves as a chemotactic factor for eosinophils. To explain the selective accumulation of eosinophils observed in allergic disorders, many investigators have been searching for chemotactic factors selective for eosinophils. Increased eosinophil chemotactic activity has been demonstrated in sera and BAL from allergic asthmatic patients after allergen inhalation challenge and during the pollen season.[161] The eosinophil chemotactic activity in sera and BAL was a sensitive marker of allergen exposure and was diminished by immunotherapy. Another possible mechanism behind eosinophil accumulation, an increased responsiveness of the cells, has also been described. Eosinophils from patients with asthma demonstrated enhanced chemotactic and chemokinetic responses compared with normal eosinophils.

Secretion

Secretion of granule proteins from eosinophils may be induced by a receptor-coupled mechanism. The receptors most commonly involved are probably IgG, IgA, IgE, and C3b receptors (see Table 15–3), but lipid mediators such as PAF may also induce eosinophil degranulation.[174] The actual mechanism of release of the individual granule proteins is not well understood, although release of peroxidase and MBP but not of ECP has been demonstrated after exposure to IgE complexes[176] in contrast with the release of ECP only, after exposure to IgG complexes. A commonly used method of studying secretion from human eosinophils is the use of C3b-coated particles.[177] This model has emphasized the importance of a large surface in addition to a specific ligand in order to induce degranulation of the eosinophil. This phenomenon is reminiscent of the putative mechanism of parasite killing. However, even in the presence of a surface not more than 15 to 20 percent of the total amount of granule proteins is released. It is therefore likely that other and more potent mechanisms are operative in vivo, since tissue eosinophils in many cases give the impression of an almost complete emptying of the eosinophil. One mechanism that may be involved in enhancing the degranulation from human eosinophils is related to various cytokines, such as GM-CSF, IL-3, and IL-5 (Carlson, Peterson, Venge, unpublished). Thus, we showed that prior exposure of eosinophils to IL-5 significantly enhanced secretion of ECP and other granule proteins. Still, however, not more than 20 to 30 percent of the granule protein content was released, which probably means that we have to look for still other mechanisms. One interesting group of eosinophil-enhancing factors are those produced by the monocyte.[178] These have been shown to enhance eosinophil cytotoxicity and production of oxygen radicals. Their effects on eosinophil degranulation, however, remain to be shown.

Priming (see Table 15–4)

Interleukin-5 is a potent primer of most aspects of eosinophil function.[141, 179] High-affinity receptors for IL-5 have been demonstrated in the plasma membrane of eosinophils. IL-5 increased the adherence of eosinophils to endothelial cells via the CD11/CD18 adhesion molecules by an up-regulation of the expression of CD11/CD18. The observed enhanced cytotoxicity induced by IL-5 is probably partly secondary to increased adherence. Interleukin-3 increased the cytotoxicity of eosinophils. GM-CSF induces an increased adherence via an increased expression of CD11/CD18 adhesion molecules.[142, 178, 180] The increased CD11/CD18 expression is due to both a mobilization from intracellular stores and de novo protein synthesis. Furthermore, GM-CSF also enhanced the cytotoxicity of eosinophils. Interferon-α, β, and γ all are inducers of increased eosinophil cytotoxicity, although IFN-γ is reported to be the most potent of all cytokines. The two cytokines called EAF and ECEF, derived from supernatants of cultured monocytes, and, in the case of ECEF, also from T lymphocytes, both induce increased cytotoxicity of eosinophils.[142] EAF and ECEF, which are now molecularly characterized, are distinct from all other hitherto described cytokines. ECEF, which shows molecular heterogeneity, may however include EAF.

Table 15–5. SOME CAUSES OF BLOOD EOSINOPHILIA

Allergic disease
Asthma
Parasite disease
Chronic inflammatory diseases (e.g., rheumatoid disorders, skin diseases)
Cancer (e.g., Hodgkin's disease, colon and urogenital cancer, lung cancer)
Postinfectious and post acute inflammation (e.g., after acute myocardial infarction)
Hematologic (e.g., chronic myeloid leukemia, eosinophil leukemia)
Hypereosinophilic syndrome
Others

Eosinophilia and the Hypereosinophilic Syndrome

Blood eosinophilia, a very common finding in humans, is generally defined as more than 400×10^6 eosinophils per L of blood. However, in nonatopic, healthy individuals, this number is very seldom above 250×10^6 per L. The most common causes of blood eosinophilia are given in Table 15–5 and can roughly be categorized into asthma and allergy, chronic inflammatory disease, postinfectious eosinophilia, parasite infestation, cancer, hematologic disease, and a group of unknown causes. It is wise to regard blood eosinophilia as a signal of disease until otherwise has been proved. In order to take full advantage of the blood eosinophil count, one has to make sure that the eosinophils are counted either in a chamber or in one of the modern machines. Calculation of eosinophils based on differential counts under the microscope is of little value. Although blood eosinophilia mostly is a signal of an underlying disease and generally disappears when the disease has been cured, sometimes blood eosinophilia by itself may give rise to disease. This is the

Table 15–6. SYMPTOMS FREQUENTLY FOUND IN PATIENTS WITH THE HYPEREOSINOPHILIC SYNDROME*

80 to 100 Percent
Retinal lesions
Endomyocardial disease
Thromboembolic disease

50 to 80 Percent
Skin involvement
Lymphatic and spleen involvement
Anorexia, weight loss
Fever, sweating
Central nervous system involvement

20 to 50 Percent
Lung involvement
Renal disease
Gastrointestinal involvement, including diarrhea
Joint disease

*The symptoms are ordered in the relative frequency of occurrence.
Adapted from Spry, C. J. F.: Eosinophils: A Comprehensive Review and Guide to the Scientific and Medical Literature. New York, Oxford University Press, 1988.

case in the hypereosinophilic syndrome of unknown cause and in tropical eosinophilia.[142, 157] In these diseases, most of the symptoms can be directly related to the activity of the eosinophils, and consequently the therapeutic strategy is the reduction of the number of eosinophils, for example, by glucocorticoids or, in severe cases, by cytostatics. The most common symptoms of patients with the hypereosinophilic syndrome, given in Table 15–6, very clearly reflect the potential of the eosinophil. The recognition and definition of the hypereosinophilic syndrome during the 1970s was another very important component in the recognition of the eosinophil as a pro-inflammatory and potentially harmful cell.

References

1. Olsson, I., and Venge, P.: The role of the human neutrophil in the inflammatory reaction. Allergy 35:1, 1980.
2. Klebanoff, S. J., and Clark, R. A.: The Neutrophil. Function and Clinical Disorders. New York, North-Holland, 1978.
3. Bainton, D. F.: Phagocytic cells: developmental biology of neutrophils and eosinophils. In Gallin, J. I., Goldstein, I. M., and Snyderman, R. (eds.): Inflammation. Basic Principles and Clinical Correlates. New York, Raven Press, 1988, pp. 265–280.
4. Gallin, J. I.: Phagocytic cells: disorders of function. In Gallin, J. I., Goldstein, I. M., and Snyderman, R. (eds.): Inflammation. Basic Principles and Clinical Correlates. New York, Raven Press, 1988, pp. 493–512.
5. Bangalore, N., Travis, J., Onunka, V. C., Pohl, J., and Shafer, W. M.: Identification of the primary antimicrobial domains in human neutrophil cathepsin G. J. Biol. Chem. 265:13584, 1990.
6. Schmidt, W., Egbring, R., and Havemann, K.: Effect of elastase-like and chymotrypsin-like neutral proteases from human granulocytes on isolated clotting factors. Thromb. Res. 6:315, 1975.
7. Tonnesen, M. G., Klempner, M. S., Austen, K. F., and Wintroub, B. U.: Identification of a human neutrophil angiotensin II–generating protease as cathepsin G. J. Clin. Invest. 69:25, 1982.
8. Reilly, C. F., Schechter, N. B., and Travis, J.: Inactivation of bradykinin and kallidin by cathepsin G and mast cell chymase. Biochem. Biophys. Res. Commun. 127:443, 1985.
9. Heck, L. W., Blackburn, W. D., Irwin, M. H., and Abrahamson, D. R.: Degradation of basement membrane laminin by human neutrophil elastase and cathepsin G. Am. J. Pathol. 136:1267, 1990.
10. Capodici, C., Muthukumaran, G., Amoruso, M. A., and Berg, R. A.: Activation of neutrophil collagenase by cathepsin G. Inflammation 13(3):245, 1989.
11. Okada, Y., and Nakanishi, I.: Activation of matrix metalloproteinase 3 (stromelysin) and matrix metalloproteinase 2 ("gelatinase") by human neutrophil elastase and cathepsin G. FEBS Lett. 249:353, 1989.
12. Ohlsson, K., and Olsson, I.: The neutral proteases of human granulocytes: Isolation and partial characterization of granulocyte elastases. Eur. J. Biochem. 42:519, 1974.
13. Janoff, A.: Human granulocyte elastase: Further delineation of its role in connective tissue damage. Am. J. Pathol. 68(3):579, 1972.
14. Ohlsson, K., Rosengren, M., Stetler, G., Brewer, M., Hale, K. K., and Thompson, R. C.: Structure, genomic organization, and tissue distribution of human secretory leukocyte-protease inhibitor (SLPI): A potent inhibitor of neutrophil elastase. In Taylor, J. C., and Mittman, C. (eds.): Pulmonary Emphysema and Proteolysis: 1986. Orlando, FL, Academic Press, 1987, pp. 307–324.
15. Weiss, S. J.: Tissue destruction by neutrophils. N. Engl. J. Med. 320:365, 1989.
16. Johnson, R. J., Couser, W. G., Alpers, C. E., Vissers, M., Schulze, M., and Klebanoff, S. J.: The human neutrophil serine proteinases, elastase and cathepsin G, can mediate glomerular injury in vivo. J. Exp. Med. 168:1169, 1988.
17. Hastka, J.: The importance of granulocyte elastase in haematological diagnosis. Blut 57:69, 1988.
18. McDonald, J. A., and Kelley, D. G.: Degradation of fibronectin by human leukocyte elastase: Release of biologically active fragments. J. Biol. Chem. 255:8848, 1980.
19. Ohlsson, K., and Olsson, I.: The neutral proteases of human granulocytes: Isolation and partial characterization of two granulocyte collagenases. Eur. J. Biochem. 36:473, 1973.
20. Kao, R. C., Wehner, N. G., Skubitz, K. M., Gray, B. H., and Hoidahl, J. R.: Proteinase 3: A distinct human polymorphonuclear leukocyte proteinase that produces emphysema in hamsters. J. Clin. Invest. 82:1963, 1988.
21. Ohlsson, K., Linder, C., and Rosengren, M.: Monoclonal antibodies specific for neutrophil proteinase 4. Production and use for isolation of the enzyme. Biol. Chem. Hoppe Seyler 371:549, 1990.
22. Campanelli, D., Detmers, P. A., Nathan, C. F., and Gabay, J. E.: Azurocidin and a homologous serine protease from neutrophils. Differential antimicrobial and proteolytic properties. J. Clin. Invest. 85:904, 1990.
23. Wilde, C. G., Snable, J. L., Griffith, J. E., and Scott, R. W.: Characterization of two azurophil granule proteases with active-site homology to neutrophil elastase. J. Biol. Chem. 265:2038, 1990.
24. Schultz, J.: Myeloperoxidase. In Sbarra, A. J., and Strauss, R. R. (eds.): The Reticuloendothelial System. A comprehensive Treatise. 2. Biochemistry and Metabolism. New York, Plenum Press, 1980, pp. 231–253.
25. Kinkade, J. M., Jr., Pember, S. O., Barnes, K. C., Shapira, R., Spitznagel, J. K., and Martin, L. E.: Differential distribution of distinct forms of myeloperoxidase in different azurophilic granule subpopulations from human neutrophils. Biochem. Biophys. Res. Commun. 114:296, 1983.
26. Schmekel, B., Karlsson, S. E., Linden, M., Sundström, C., Tegner, H., and Venge, P.: Myeloperoxidase in human lung lavage: I. A marker of local neutrophil activity. Inflammation 14:447, 1990.
27. Klebanoff, S. J.: Antimicrobial mechanisms in neutrophilic polymorphonuclear leukocytes. Semin. Hematol. 12(2):117, 1975.
28. Vissers, M. C. M., and Winterbourn, C. C.: Oxidative damage to fibronectin. I. The effects of the neutrophil myeloperoxidase system and HOCl. Arch. Biochem. Biophys. 285:53, 1991.
29. Katrantzis, M., Baker, M. S., Handley, C. J., and Lowther, D. A.: The oxidant hypochlorite (OCl$^-$), a product of the myeloperoxidase system, degrades articular cartilage proteoglycan aggregate. Free Radic. Biol. Med. 10:101, 1991.
30. Green, S. P., Baker, M. S., and Lowther, D. A.: Depolymerization of synovial fluid hyaluronic acid (HA) by the complete myeloperoxidase (MPO) system may involve the formation of a HA-MPO ionic complex. J. Rheumatol. 17:1670, 1990.
31. Salmon, S. E., Cline, M. J., Schultz, J., and Lehrer, R. I.: Myeloperoxidase deficiency: Immunologic study of a genetic leukocyte defect. N. Engl. J. Med. 282(5):250, 1970.
32. Cramer, R., Soranzo, M. R., Dri, P., Rottini, G. D., Bramezza, M., Ciricelli, S., and Patriarca, P.: Incidence of myeloperoxidase deficiency in an area of northern Italy: histochemical, biochemical, and functional studies. Br. J. Haematol. 51:81, 1982.
33. Öberg, G., Dahl, R., Ellegaard, J., Sundström, C., Vaeth, M., and Venge, P.: Diagnostic and prognostic significance of serum measurements of lactoferrin, lysozyme, and myeloperoxidase in acute myeloid leukemia (AML): recognition of a new variant, high-lactoferrin AML. Eur. J. Haematol. 38:148, 1987.
34. Öberg, G., Simonsson, B., Smedmyr, B., Tötterman, Th., and Venge, P.: Myeloid regeneration after bone-marrow transplantation monitored by serum measurements of myeloperoxidase, lysozyme, and lactoferrin. Eur. J. Haematol. 38:356, 1987.
35. Venge, P., Nilsson, L., Nyström, S.-O., and Åberg, T.: Serum and plasma measurements of neutrophil granule proteins during cardiopulmonary bypass. A model to estimate human turnover of lactoferrin and myeloperoxidase. Eur. J. Haematol. 39:339, 1987.
36. Hällgren, R., Colombel, J. F., Dahl, R., Fredens, K., Kruse, A., Jacobsen, S., Venge, P., and Rambaud, J. C.: Neutrophil and eosinophil involvement of the small bowel in patients with celiac disease and Crohn's disease. Studies on the secretion rate and immunohistochemical localization of the granulocyte granule constituents in jejunum. Am. J. Med. 86:56, 1989.
37. Lee, S. S., Adu, D., and Thompson, R. A.: Anti-myeloperoxidase antibodies in systemic vasculitis. Clin. Exp. Immunol. 79:41, 1990.
38. Lehrer, R. I., and Ganz, T.: Antimicrobial polypeptides of human neutrophils. Blood 76:2169, 1990.
39. Spitznagel, J. K.: Antibiotic proteins of human neutrophils. J. Clin. Invest. 86:1381, 1990.
40. Pereira, H. A., Shafer, W. M., Pohl, J., Martin, L. E., and Spitznagel, J. K.: CAP37, a human neutrophil-derived chemotactic factor with monocyte-specific activity. J. Clin. Invest. 85:1468, 1990.
41. Weiss, J., Elsbach, P., Olsson, I., and Odeberg, H.: Purification and partial characterization of a potent bactericidal and membrane-active protein from granules of human polymorphonuclear leukocytes. J. Biol. Chem. 253:2664, 1978.
42. Elsbach, P., and Weiss, J.: A reevaluation of the roles of the O_2-dependent and O_2-independent microbicidal systems of phagocytes. Rev. Infect. Dis. 5:843, 1983.
43. Hibbs, M. S., and Bainton, D. F.: Human neutrophil gelatinase is a component of specific granules. J. Clin. Invest. 84:1395, 1989.
44. Dexter, D., Rubins, J. B., Manning, E. C., Khachatrian, L., and Dickey, B. F.: Compartmentalization of low molecular mass GTP-binding

proteins among neutrophil secretory granules. J. Immunol. 145:1845, 1990.

45. Murphy, G., Bretz, U., Baggiolini, M., and Reynolds, J. J.: The latent collagenase and gelatinase of human polymorphonuclear neutrophil leucocytes. Biochem. J. 192:517, 1980.

46. Borregaard, N., Heiple, J. M., Simons, E. R., and Clark, R. A.: Subcellular localization of the b-cytochrome component of the human neutrophil microbicidal oxidase: Translocation during activation. J. Cell Biol. 97:52, 1983.

47. Reiter B.: The biological significance of lactoferrin. Int. J. Tiss. Reac. 5:87, 1983.

48. Lomax, K. J., Gallin, J. I., Rotrosen, D., Raphael, G. D., Kaliner, M. A., Benz, E. J., Boxer, L. A., and Malech, H. L.: Selective defect in myeloid cell lactoferrin gene expression in neutrophil specific granule deficiency. J. Clin. Invest. 83:514, 1989.

49. Broxmeyer, H. E., Smithyman, A., Eger, R. R., Meyers, P. A., and de Sousa, M.: Identification of lactoferrin as the granulocyte-derived inhibitor of colony-stimulating activity production. J. Exp. Med. 148:1052, 1978.

50. Boxer, L. A., Björksten, B., Björk, J., Yang, H.-H., Allen, J. M., and Baehner, R. L.: Neutropenia induced by systemic infusion of lactoferrin. J. Lab. Clin. Med. 99:866, 1982.

51. Klebanoff, S. J., and Waltersdorph, A. M.: Prooxidant activity of transferrin and lactoferrin. J. Exp. Med. 172:1293, 1990.

52. Birgens, H. S.: The biological significance of lactoferrin in haematology. Scand. J. Haematol. 33:225, 1984.

53. Hällgren, R., Venge, P., and Wikström, B.: Hemodialysis-induced increase in serum lactoferrin and serum eosinophil cationic protein as signs of local neutrophil and eosinophil degranulation. Nephron 29:233, 1981.

54. Lash, J. A., Coates, T. D., Lafuze, J., Baehner, R. L., and Boxer, L. A.: Plasma lactoferrin reflects granulocyte activation in vivo. Blood 61:885, 1983.

55. Osserman, E. F.: Lysozyme. N. Engl. J. Med. 292:424, 1975.

56. Sandborg, R. R., and Smolen, J. I.: Biology of disease. Early biochemical events in leukocyte activation. Lab. Invest. 59:300, 1988.

57. Berridge, M. J., and Irvine, R. F.: Inositol phosphates and cell signalling. Nature 341:197, 1989.

58. Downes, C. P., and MacPhee, C. H.: myo-Inositol metabolites as cellular signals. Eur. J. Biochem. 193:1, 1990.

59. Nishizuka, Y.: The role of protein kinase C in cell surface signal transduction and tumour promotion. Nature 308:693, 1984.

60. Bell, R., and Burns, D. J.: Minireview. Lipid activation of protein kinase C. J. Biol. Chem. 266:4661, 1991.

61. Tsien, R. W., and Tsien, R. Y.: Calcium channels, stores, and oscillations. Annu. Rev. Cell. Biol. 6:715, 1990.

62. Nishizuka, Y.: The molecular heterogeneity of protein kinase C and its implication for cellular regulation. Nature 334:661, 1988.

63. Han, J.-W., McCormick, F., and Macara, I. G.: Regulation of ras-GAP and the neurofibromatosis-1 gene product by eicosanoids. Science 252:576, 1991.

64. Berkow, R. L., and Dodson, R. W.: Alterations in tyrosine protein kinase activities upon activation of human neutrophils. J. Leukocyte Biol. 49:599, 1991.

65. Naccache, P. H., Gilbert, C., Caon, A. C., Gaudry, M., Huang, C.-K., Bonak, V. A., Umezawa, K., and McColl, S. R.: Selective inhibition of human neutrophil functional responsiveness by erbstatin, an inhibitor of tyrosine protein kinase. Blood 76:2098, 1990.

66. Houslay, M. D.: Review. "Cross-talk": a pivotal role for protein kinase C in modulating relationships between signal transduction pathways. Eur. J. Biochem. 195:9, 1991.

67. Huang, C.-K.: Protein kinases in neutrophils: a review. Membr. Biochem. 8:61, 1989.

68. Smolen, J. E., Stoehr, S. J., and Kuczynski, B.: Cyclic AMP inhibits secretion from electrophorated human neutrophils. J. Leukocyte Biol. 49:172, 1991.

69. Pontremoli, S., Melloni, E., Michetti, M., Sacco, O., Salamino, F., Sparatore, B., and Horecker, B. L.: Biochemical responses in activated human neutrophils mediated by protein kinase C and a Ca²⁺-requiring proteinase. J. Biol. Chem. 261:8309, 1986.

70. Huizinga, T. W. J., Dolman, K. M., Van Der Linden, N. J. M., Kleijer, M., Nuijens, J. H., Von Dem Borne, A. E. G. K., and Roos, D.: Phosphatidylinositol-linked FcRIII mediates exocytosis of neutrophil granule proteins but does not mediate initiation of the respiratory burst. J. Immunol. 144:1432, 1990.

71. Ernst, J. D., Hoye, E., Blackwood, R. A., and Jaye, D.: Purification and characterization of an abundant cytosolic protein from human neutrophils that promotes Ca²⁺-dependent aggregation of isolated specific granules. J. Clin. Invest. 85:1065, 1990.

72. Philips, M. R., Abramson, S. B., Kolasinski, S. L., Haines, K. A., Weissmann, G., and Rosenfeld, M. G.: Low molecular weight GTP-binding proteins in human neutrophil granule membranes. J. Biol. Chem. 266:1289, 1991.

73. Keller, H. U., Wilkinson, P. C., Abercombie, M., Becker, E. L., Hirsch,

G. J., Miller, M. E., Ramsey, W. S., and Zigmond, S. H.: A proposal for the definition of terms related to locomotion of leukocytes and other cells. Clin. Exp. Immunol. 27:377, 1977.

74. Snyderman, R., Phillips, J., and Mergenhagen, S. E.: Polymorphonuclear leukocyte chemotactic activity in rabbit serum and guinea pig serum treated with immune complexes. Infect. Immun. 1:521, 1970.

74a. Palmblad, J., Malmsten, C. L., Uden, A.-M., Rådmark, O., Engstedt, L., and Samuelsson, B.: Leukotriene B₄ is a potent and stereospecific stimulator of neutrophil chemotaxis and adherence. Blood 58:658, 1981.

74b. Valone, F. H., and Goetzl, E. J.: Specific binding by human polymorphonuclear leukocytes of the immunological mediator 1-O-hexadecyl/octadecyl-2-acetyl-sn-glycero-3-phosphorylcholine. Immunology 48:141, 1983.

74c. Perez, H. D., Kelly, E., Chenoweth, D., and Elfman, F.: Identification of the C5a des arg cochemotaxin. Homology with vitamin D–binding protein (group-specific component globulin). J. Clin. Invest. 82:360, 1988.

75. Stossel, T. P.: The mechanical responses of white blood cells. In Gallin, J. I., Goldstein, I. M., and Snyderman, R. (eds.): Inflammation. Basic Principles and Clinical Correlates. New York, Raven Press, 1988, pp. 325–343.

76. Bengtsson, T.: Correlation between chemotactic peptide-induced changes in chlorotetracycline fluorescence and F-actin content in human neutrophils: A role for membrane-associated calcium in the regulation of actin polymerization. Exp. Cell Res. 191:57, 1990.

77. Anderson, D. C., Schmalsteig, F. C., Finegold, M. J., Hughes, B. J., Rothlein, R., Miller, L. J., Kohl, S., Tosi, M. F., Jacobs, R. L., Waldrop, T. C., Goldman, A. S., Shearer, W. T., and Springer, T. A.: The severe and moderate phenotypes of heritable Mac-1, LFA-1 deficiency: Their quantitative definition and relation to leukocyte dysfunction and clinical features. J. Infect. Dis. 152:668, 1985.

78. Styrt, B.: History and implications of the neutrophil glycoprotein deficiencies. Am. J. Hematol. 31:288, 1989.

79. Bondestam, M., Håkansson, L., Foucard, T., and Venge, P.: Defects in polymorphonuclear neutrophil function and susceptibility to infection in children. Scand. J. Clin. Lab. Invest. 46:685, 1986.

80. Siegbahn, A., Simonsson, B., and Venge, P.: The chemokinetic inhibitory factor (CIF) in serum of CLL patients: Correlation with infection propensity and disease activity. Scand. J. Haematol. 35:80, 1985.

81. Huizinga, T. W., Roos, D., and von dem Borne, A. E.: Neutrophil Fc-γ receptors: A two-way bridge in the immune system. Blood 75:1211, 1990.

82. Unkeless, J. C.: Function and heterogeneity of human Fc receptors for immunoglobulin G. J. Clin. Invest. 83:355, 1989.

83. Anderson, C. L.: Human IgG Fc receptors. Clin. Immunol. Immunopathol. 53:S63, 1989.

84. Kimberley, R. P., Tappe, N. J., Merriam, L. T., Redecha, P. B., Edberg, J. C., Schwartzman, S., and Valinsky, J. E.: Carbohydrates on human Fcγ receptors. Interdependence of the classical IgG and nonclassical lectin-binding sites on human FcγRIII expressed on neutrophils. J. Immunol. 142:3923, 1989.

85. Albelda, S. M., and Buck, C. A.: Integrins and other cell adhesion molecules. FASEB J. 4:2868, 1990.

86. Arnaout, M. A.: Structure and function of the leukocyte adhesion molecules CD11/CD18. Blood 75:1037, 1990.

87. Yong, K., and Khwaja, A.: Leucocyte cellular adhesion molecules. Blood Rev. 4:211, 1990.

88. Pober, J. S., and Cotran, R. S.: The role of endothelial cells in inflammation. Transplantation 50:537, 1990.

89. Monteiro, R. C., Kubagawa, H., and Cooper, M. D.: Cellular distribution, regulation, and biochemical nature of an Fcα receptor in humans. J. Exp. Med. 171:597, 1990.

90. Henson, P. M., Henson, J. E., Fittschen, C., Kimani, G., Bratton, D. L., and Riches, D. W. H.: Phagocytic cells: Degranulation and secretion. In Gallin, J. I., Goldstein, I. M., and Snyderman, R. (eds.): Inflammation. Basic Principles and Clinical Correlates. New York, Raven Press, 1988, pp. 363–390.

91. Willems, J., Joniau, M., Clinque, S., and Van Damme, J.: Human granulocyte chemotactic peptide (IL-8) as a specific neutrophil degranulator: Comparison with other monokines. Immunology 67:540, 1989.

92. Devereux, S., Porter, J. B., Hoyes, K. P., Abeysinghe, R. D., Saib, R., and Linch, D. C.: Secretion of neutrophil secondary granules occurs during granulocyte-macrophage colony-stimulating factor–induced margination. Br. J. Haematol. 74:17, 1990.

93. Sha'afi, R. I., and Molski, F. P.: Role of ion movements in neutrophil activation. Annu. Rev. Physiol. 52:365, 1990.

94. Sbarra, A. J., and Strauss, R. R. (eds.): The respiratory burst and its physiological significance. New York, Plenum Press, 1988.

95. Orkin, S. H.: Molecular genetics of chronic granulomatous disease. Annu. Rev. Immunol. 7:277, 1989.

96. Segal, A. W.: The electron transport chain of the microbicidal oxidase of phagocytic cells and its involvement in the molecular pathology of chronic granulomatous disease. J. Clin. Invest. 83:1785, 1989.

97. Klebanoff, S. J.: Phagocytic cells: products of oxygen metabolism. *In* Gallin, J. I., Goldstein, I. M., and Snyderman, R. (eds.): Inflammation. Basic Principles and Clinical Correlates. New York, Raven Press, 1988, pp. 391–444.

98. Borregaard, N.: The respiratory burst. An overview. *In* Sbarra, A. J., and Strauss, R. R. (eds.): The Respiratory Burst and Its Physiological Significance. New York, Plenum Press, 1988, pp. 1–31.

99. Woodman, R. C., Ruedi, J. M., Jesaitis, A. J., Okamura, N., Quinn, M. T., Smith, R. M., Curnutte, J. T., and Babior, B. M.: Respiratory burst oxidase and three of four oxidase-related polypeptides are associated with the cytoskeleton of human neutrophils. J. Clin. Invest. 87:1345, 1991.

100. Smith, R. M., and Curnutte, J. T.: Review article: Molecular basis of chronic granulomatous disease. Blood 77:673, 1991.

101. Umei, T., Babior, B. M., Curnutte, J. T., and Smith, R. M.: Identification of the NADPH-binding subunit of the respiratory burst oxidase. J. Biol. Chem. 266:6019, 1991.

102. Quinn, M. T., Parkos, C. A., Walker, L., Orkin, S. H., Dinauer, M. C., and Jesaitis, A. J.: Association of a *ras*-related protein with cytochrome b of human neutrophils. Nature 342:198, 1989.

103. Volpp, B. D., Nauseef, W. M., Donelson, J. E., Moser, D. R., and Clark, R. A.: Cloning of the cDNA and functional expression of the 47-kilodalton cytosolic component of human neutrophil respiratory burst oxidase. Proc. Natl. Acad. Sci. U.S.A. 86:7195, 1989 (published erratum in Proc. Natl. Acad. Sci. U.S.A. 86:9563, 1989).

104. Leto, T. L., Lomax, K. J., Volpp, B. D., Nunoi, H., Sechler, J. M. G., Nauseef, W. M., Clark, R. A., Gallin J. I., and Malech, H. L.: Cloning of a 67-kD neutrophil oxidase factor with similarity to a noncatalytic region of p60^{c-src}. Science 248:727, 1990.

105. McColl, S. R., Beauseigle, D., Gilbert C., and Naccache, P. H.: Priming of the human neutrophil respiratory burst by granulocyte-macrophage colony-stimulating factor and tumor necrosis factor-α involves regulation at a post-cell surface receptor level. J. Immunol. 145:3047, 1990.

106. Bass D. A., McPhail, L. C., Schmitt, J. D., Morris-Natschke, S., McCall, C. E., and Wykle, R. L.: Selective priming of rate and duration of the respiratory burst of neutrophils by 1,2-diacyl and 1-O-alkyl-2-acyl diglycerides. Possible relation to effects on protein kinase C. J. Biol. Chem. 264:19610, 1989.

107. Koenderman, L., Yazdanbakhsh, M., Roos, D., and Verhoeven, A. J.: Dual mechanisms in priming of the chemoattractant-induced respiratory burst in human granulocytes. A Ca^{2+}-dependent and a Ca^{2+}-independent route. J. Immunol. 142:623, 1989.

108. Cassatella, M. A., Bazzoni, F., Flynn, R. M., Dusi, S., Trinchieri, G., and Rossi, F.: Molecular basis of interferon-gamma and lipopolysaccharide enhancement of phagocyte respiratory burst capacity. Studies on the gene expression of several NADPH oxidase components. J. Biol. Chem. 265:20241, 1990.

109. Sullivan, R., Fredette, J. P., Griffin, J. D., Leavitt, J. L., Simons, E. R., and Melnick, D. A.: An elevation in the concentration of free cytosolic calcium is sufficient to activate the oxidative burst by granulocytes primed with recombinant human granulocyte-macrophage colony-stimulating factor. J. Biol. Chem. 264:6302, 1989.

110. Bourgoin, S., Plante, E., Gaudry, M., Naccache, P. H., Borgeat, P., and Poubelle, P. E.: Involvement of a phospholipase D in the mechanism of action of granulocyte-macrophage colony-stimulating factor (GM-CSF): Priming of human neutrophils in vitro with GM-CSF is associated with accumulation of phosphatidic acid and diradylglycerol. J. Exp. Med. 172:767, 1990.

111. Bauldry, S. A., Bass, D. A., Cousart, S. L., and McCall, C. E.: Tumor necrosis factor-α priming of phospholipase D in human neutrophils. Correlation between phosphatidic acid production and superoxide generation. J. Biol. Chem. 266:4173, 1991.

112. Khwaja, A., Roberts, P. J., Jones, H. M., Yong, K., Jaswon, M. S., and Linch, D. C.: Isoquinoline sulfonamide protein kinase inhibitors H7 and H8 enhance the effects of granulocyte-macrophage colony-stimulating factor (GM-CSF) on neutrophil function and inhibit GM-CSF receptor internalization. Blood 76:996, 1990.

113. Nathan, C. F.: Respiratory burst in adherent human neutrophils: triggering by colony-stimulating factors CSF-GM and CSF-G. Blood 73:301, 1989.

114. Nathan, C. F.: Neutrophil activation on biological surfaces. Massive secretion of hydrogen peroxide in response to products of macrophages and lymphocytes. J. Clin. Invest. 80:1550, 1987.

115. Koenderman, L., Tool, A. T. J., Hooybrink, B., Roos, D., Hansen, C. A., Williamson, J. R., and Verhoeven, A. J.: Adherence of human neutrophils changes Ca^{2+} signaling during activation with opsonized particles. FEBS Lett. 270:49, 1990.

116. Heyworth, P. G., and Badwey, J. A.: Mini-review: Protein phosphorylation associated with the stimulation of neutrophils. Modulation of superoxide production by protein kinase C and calcium. J. Bioenerg. Biomembr. 22:1, 1990.

117. Nauseef, W. M., Volpp, B. D., McCormick, S., Leidal, K. G., and Clark, R. A.: Assembly of neutrophil respiratory burst oxidase. Protein kinase C promotes cytoskeletal and membrane association of cytosolic oxidase components. J. Biol. Chem. 266:5911, 1991.

118. Rotrosen, D., Kleinberg, M. E., Nunoi, H., Leto, T., Gallin, J. I., and Malech, H. L.: Evidence for a functional cytoplasmic domain of phagocyte oxidase cytochrome b$_{558}$. J. Biol. Chem. 265:8745, 1990.

119. Grinstein, S., Hill, M., and Furuya, W.: Activation of electropermeabilized neutrophils by adenosine 5′-[gamma-thio] triphosphate (ATP [S]). Role of phosphatases in stimulus-response coupling. Biochem. J. 261:755, 1989.

120. Heyworth, P. G., Curnutte, J. T., Nauseef, W. M., Volpp, B. D., Pearson, D. W., Rosen, H., and Clark, R. A.: Neutrophil nicotinamide adenine dinucleotide phosphate oxidase assembly. Translocation of p47-*phox* and p67-*phox* requires interaction between p47-*phox* and cytochrome b$_{558}$. J. Clin. Invest. 87:352, 1991.

121. Della Bianca, V., Grzeskowiak, M., and Rossi, F.: Studies on molecular regulation of phagocytosis and activation of the NADPH oxidase in neutrophils. IgG- and C3b-mediated ingestion and associated respiratory burst independent of phospholipid turnover and Ca^{2+} transients. J. Immunol. 144:1411, 1990.

122. Rossi, F., Grzeskowiak, M., Della Bianca, V., Calzetti, F., and Gandini, G.: Phosphatidic acid and not diacylglycerol generated by phospholipase D is functionally linked to the activation of the NADPH oxidase by FMLP in human neutrophils. Biochem. Biophys. Res. Commun. 168:320, 1990.

123. Henderson, L. M., Chappel, J. B., and Jones, O. T. G.: Superoxide generation is inhibited by phospholipase A$_2$ inhibitors. Role for phospholipase A$_2$ in the activation of the NADPH oxidase. Biochem. J. 264:249, 1989.

124. Walker, B. A. M., Hagenlocker, B. E., Stubbs, E. B., Jr., Sandborg, R. R., Agranoff, B. W., and Ward, P. A.: Signal transduction events and FcgammaR engagement in human neutrophils stimulated with immune complexes. J. Immunol. 146:735, 1991.

125. Gabig, T. G., Eklund, E. A., Potter, G. B., and Dykes, J. R., II: A neutrophil GTP-binding protein that regulates cell free NADPH oxidase activation is located in the cytosolic fraction. J. Immunol. 145:945, 1990.

126. Cross, A. R.: Inhibitors of the leukocyte superoxide generating oxidase: mechanisms of action and methods for their elucidation. Free Radic. Biol. Med. 8:71, 1990.

127. Eklund, E. A., and Gabig, T. G.: Purification and characterization of a lipid thiobis ester from human neutrophil cytosol that reversibly deactivates the O$_2^-$-generating oxidase. J. Biol. Chem. 265:8426, 1990.

128. Tygai, S. R., Olson, S. C., Burnham, D. N., and Lambeth, J. D.: Cyclic AMP–elevating agents block chemoattractant activation of diradylglycerol generation by inhibiting phospholipase D activation. J. Biol. Chem. 266:3498, 1991.

129. Robinson, J. M., Heyworth, P. G., and Badwey, J. A.: Utility of staurosporine in uncovering differences in signal transduction pathways for superoxide production in neutrophils. Biochim. Biophys. Acta 1055:55, 1990.

130. Twomey, B., Muid, R. E., Nixon, J. S., Sedgwick, A. D., Wilkinson, S., and Dale, M. M.: The effect of new potent selective inhibitors of protein kinase C on the neutrophil respiratory burst. Biochem. Biophys. Res. Commun. 171:1087, 1990.

131. Merrill, A. H., and Stevens, V. L.: Modulation of protein kinase C and diverse cell functions by sphingosine—a pharmacologically interesting compound linking sphingolipids and signal transduction. Biochim. Biophys. Acta 1010:131, 1989.

132. Halliwell, B.: Oxidants and human disease: some new concepts. FASEB J. 1:358, 1987.

133. Doelman, C. J. A., and Bast, A.: Oxygen radicals in lung pathology. Free Radic. Biol. Med. 9:381, 1990.

134. Warren, J. S., Yabroff, K. R., Mandel, D. M., Johnson, K. J., and Ward, P. A.: Role of O$_2^-$ in neutrophil recruitment into sites of dermal and pulmonary vasculitis. Free Radic. Biol. Med. 8:163, 1990.

135. Barnes, P. J.: Reactive oxygen species and airway inflammation. Free Radic. Biol. Med. 9:235, 1990.

136. Harris, E. D.: Rheumatoid arthritis: Pathophysiology and implications for therapy. N. Engl. J. Med. 322:1277, 1990.

137. Boey, H., Rosenbaum, R., Castracane, J., and Borish, L.: Interleukin-4 is a neutrophil activator. J. Allergy Clin. Immunol. 83:978, 1989.

138. Borish, L., Rosenbaum, R., Albury, L., and Clark, S.: Activation of neutrophils by recombinant interleukin-6. Cell. Immunol. 121:280, 1989.

139. Baggiolini, M., Walz, A., and Kunkel, S. L.: Neutrophil-activating peptide-1/interleukin-8, a novel cytokine that activates neutrophils. J. Clin. Invest. 84:1045, 1989.

140. Steinbeck, M. J., and Roth, J. A.: Neutrophil activation by recombinant cytokines. Rev. Infect. Dis. 11:549, 1989.

141. Clutterbuck, E. J., and Sanderson, C. J.: Regulation of human eosinophil precursor production by cytokines: A comparison of recombinant human interleukin-1 (rhIL-1), rhIL-3, rhIL-5, rhIL-6, and rh granulocyte-macrophage colony-stimulating factor. Blood 75:1774, 1990.

142. Spry, C. J. F.: Eosinophils: A Comprehensive Review and Guide to the Scientific and Medical Literature. New York, Oxford University Press, 1988.

143. Gleich, G. J., and Adolphson, C. R.: The eosinophil leukocyte: structure and function. Adv. Immunol. 39:177, 1986.
144. Carlson, M. G. Ch., Peterson, C. G. B., and Venge, P.: Human eosinophil peroxidase: purification and characterization. J. Immunol. 134:1875, 1985.
145. Peterson, C. G. B., and Venge, P.: Purification and characterization of a new cationic protein—eosinophil protein-X (EPX)—from granules of human eosinophils. Immunology 50:19, 1983.
146. Rosenberg, H. F., Ackerman, S. J., and Tenen, D. G.: Human eosinophil cationic protein. Molecular cloning of a cytotoxin and helminthotoxin with ribonuclease activity. J. Exp. Med. 170:163, 1989.
147. Rosenberg, H. F., Tenen, D. G., and Ackerman, S. J.: Molecular cloning of the human eosinophil-derived neurotoxin: A member of the ribonuclease gene family. Proc. Natl. Acad. Sci. U.S.A. 86:4460, 1989.
148. Barker, R. L., Loegering, D. A., Ten, R. M., Hamann, K. J., Pease, L. R., and Gleich, J. G.: Eosinophil cationic protein cDNA: Comparison with other toxic cationic proteins and ribonucleases. J. Immunol. 143:952, 1989.
149. Hamann, K. J., Barker, R. L., Loegering, D. A., Pease, L. R., and Gleich, J. G.: Sequence of human eosinophil-derived neurotoxin cDNA: Identity of deduced amino acid sequence with human nonsecretory ribonucleases. Gene 83:161, 1989.
150. Barker, R. L., Loegering, D. A., Arakawa, K. C., Pease, L. R., and Gleich, J. G.: Cloning and sequence analysis of the human gene encoding eosinophil major basic protein. Gene 86:285, 1990.
151. Ten, R. M., Pease, L. R., McKean, D. J., Bell, M. P., and Gleich, G. J.: Molecular cloning of the human eosinophil peroxidase: Evidence for the existence of a peroxidase multigene family. J. Exp. Med. 169:1757, 1989.
152. Gullberg, U., Widegren, B., Arnason, U., Egesten, A., and Olsson, I.: The cytotoxic eosinophil cationic protein (ECP) has ribonuclease activity. Biochem. Biophys. Res. Commun. 139:1239, 1986.
153. Tai, P.-C., Spry, C. J. F., Petterson, C., Venge, P., and Olsson, I.: Monoclonal antibodies distinguish between storage and secreted forms of eosinophil cationic protein. Nature 309:182, 1984.
154. Venge, P., and Peterson, C. G. B.: Eosinophil biochemistry and killing mechanisms. In Morley, J., and Coldite, I. (eds.): Eosinophils in Asthma. New York, Academic Press, 1989, pp. 163-N177.
155. Lundgren, J. D., Davey, R. T., Jr., Lundgren, B., Mullol, J., Marom, Z., Logun, C., Baraniuk, J., Kaliner, M. A., and Shelhamer, J. H.: Eosinophil cationic protein stimulates and major basic protein inhibits airway mucus secretion. J. Allergy Clin. Immunol. 87:689, 1991.
156. Rennard, S. I., Bitterman, P. B., and Crystal, R. G.: IV.: Mechanisms of fibrosis. Am. Rev. Respir. Dis. 130:492, 1984.
157. Liesveld, J. L., and Abboud, C. N.: State of the art: The hypereosinophilic syndromes. Blood Rev. 5:29, 1991.
158. Dahl, R., and Venge, P.: Activation of blood coagulation during inhalation challenge tests. Allergy 36:129, 1981.
159. Hällgren, R., Bjelle, A., and Venge, P.: Eosinophil cationic protein in inflammatory synovial effusions as evidence of eosinophil involvement. Ann. Rheum. Dis. 43:556, 1984.
160. Venge, P., Roxin, L.-E., and Olsson, I.: Radioimmunoassay of human eosinophil cationic protein. Br. J. Haematol. 37:331, 1977.
161. Venge, P., and Håkansson, L.: The eosinophil and asthma. In Kaliner, M., Barnes, P. J., and Persson, C. G. A. (eds.): Asthma: Its Pathology and Treatment. New York, Marcel Dekker, Inc., 1991, pp. 477–502.
162. Venge, P.: What is the role of the eosinophil? Thorax 45:161, 1990.
163. Hällgren, R., Feltelius, N., Svensson, K., and Venge, P.: Eosinophil involvement in rheumatoid arthritis as reflected by elevated serum levels of eosinophil cationic protein. Clin. Exp. Immunol. 59:539, 1985.
164. Hisamatsu, K., Ganbo, T., Nakazawa, T., Murakami, Y., Gleich, G. J., Makiyama, K., and Koyama, H.: Cytotoxicity of human eosinophil granule major basic protein to human nasal sinus mucosa in vitro. J. Allergy Clin. Immunol. 86:52, 1990.
165. Rohrbach, M. S., Wheatley, C. L., Slifman, N. R., and Gleich, G. J.: Activation of platelets by eosinophil granule proteins. J. Exp. Med. 172:1271, 1990.
166. Henderson, W. R., Jörg, A., and Klebanoff, S. J.: Eosinophil peroxidase-mediated inactivation of leukotrienes B_4, C_4, and D_4. J. Immunol. 128:2609, 1982.
167. Zabucchi, G., Menegazzi, R., Cramer, R., Nardon, E., and Patriarca, P.: Mutual influence between eosinophil peroxidase (EPO) and neutrophils: neutrophils reversibly inhibit EPO enzymatic activity and EPO increases neutrophil adhesiveness. Immunology 69:580, 1990.
168. White, S. R., Ohno, S., Munoz, N. M., Gleich, G. J., Abrahams, C., Solway, J., and Leff, A. R.: Epithelium-dependent contraction of airway smooth muscle caused by eosinophil MBP. Am. J. Physiol. Lung Cell. Mol. Physiol. 259:L294, 1990.
169. Moy, J. N., Gleich, G. J., and Thomas. L. L.: Noncytotoxic activation of neutrophils by eosinophil granule major basic protein: Effect on superoxide anion generation and lysosomal enzyme release. J. Immunol. 145:2626, 1990.
170. Gleich, G. J., Flavahan, N. A., Fujisawa, T., and Vanhoutte, P. M.: The eosinophil as a mediator of damage to respiratory epithelium: A model for bronchial hyperreactivity. J. Allergy Clin. Immunol. 81:776, 1988.
171. Butterfield, J. H., Weiler, D., Peterson, E. A., Gleich, G. J., and Leiferman, K. M.: Sequestration of eosinophil major basic protein in human mast cells. Lab. Invest. 62:77, 1990.
172. Weller, P. F.: The immunobiology of eosinophils. N. Engl. J. Med. 324:1110, 1991.
172a. Moqbel, R., Hamid, Q., Ying, S., Barkans, J., Hartnell, A., Tsicopoulos, A., Wardlaw, A. J., and Kay, A. B.: Expression of mRNA and immunoreactivity for the granulocyte/macrophage colony-stimulating factor in activated human eosinophils. J. Exp. Med. 174:749, 1991.
173. Barnes, P. J.: New concepts in the pathogenesis of bronchial hyperresponsiveness and asthma. J. Allergy Clin. Immunol. 83:1013, 1989.
174. Kroegel, C., Yukawa, T., Dent, G., Venge, P., Fan Chung, K., and Barnes, P. J.: Stimulation of degranulation from human eosinophils by platelet-activating factor. J. Immunol. 142:3518, 1989.
175. Dahl, R., Venge, P., and Fredens, K.: The eosinophil. In Barnes, P. J., Rodger, I., and Thomson, N. (eds.): Asthma: Basic Mechanisms and Clinical Management. London, Academic Press, 1988, pp. 115–130.
176. Capron, M., and Prin, L.: The IgE receptor of eosinophils. Springer Semin. Immunopathol. 12:327, 1990.
177. Winqvist, I., Olofsson, T., and Olsson, I.: Mechanisms for eosinophil degranulation; release of the eosinophil cationic protein. Immunology 51:1, 1984.
178. Silberstein, D. S., and David, J. R.: The regulation of human eosinophil function by cytokines. Immunol. Today 8:380, 1987.
179. Thorne, K. J. I., Richardson, B. A., Mazza, G., and Butterworth, A. E.: A new method for measuring eosinophil-activating factors, based on the increased expression of CR3α chain (CD11b) on the surface of activated eosinophils. J. Immunol. Methods 133:47, 1990.
180. Cannistra, S. A., and Griffin, J. D.: Regulation of the production and function of granulocytes and monocytes. Semin. Hematol. 25:173, 1988.

Chapter 16

Ranjeny Thomas
Peter E. Lipsky

Monocytes and Macrophages

Mononuclear phagocytes reside in every organ and tissue in the body and carry out a number of diverse functions that are essential for host defense and normal homeostasis. Members of this family of cells play a critical role in the induction and regulation of both humoral and cellular immune responses,[1] act as the main protection against a number of microorganisms,[2] and may help prevent the spread and development of neoplastic cells.[3] In addition, mononuclear phagocytes are involved in the removal of senescent, damaged, or dying cells from the circulation, bone remodeling and resorption,[4] and tissue repair and scar formation after injury.[5] Finally, mononuclear phagocytes play an important role as effector cells at sites of chronic inflammation.[6] Their migratory, pinocytic, phagocytic, intracellular digestive, and secretory activities, as well as the capacity to respond to a number of environmental stimuli, enable them to carry out these varied activities. Thus, the mononuclear phagocytes constitute a family of lineally related but diverse cells scattered throughout the body that can respond to environmental stimuli and differentiate to achieve their various functions.

HISTORICAL PERSPECTIVE

The idea that phagocytes played an important part in host defense was first suggested by the Russian biologist Elie Metchnikoff in 1883.[7] He described the function and distribution of phagocytes initially in invertebrates and then in the liver, spleen, lymph nodes, and central nervous system of vertebrates, including humans. To distinguish mononuclear phagocytes from the smaller leukocytes of the circulating blood, which he called *microphages*, Metchnikoff called them *macrophages*.

The macrophage system as defined by Metchnikoff was expanded by Aschoff, who introduced the term *reticuloendothelial system* (RES) to cover the entire range of cells that possessed the endocytic capacity to take up vital dyes. The cells constituting the system were thought to be involved in the formation of the reticulum of the lymph nodes and spleen, or to be those cells lining blood or lymph sinusoids. The concept of the RES has been largely abandoned because it defines a system of cells linked

only by their ability to take up vital dyes in vivo.[8] Certain cells such as blood monocytes, which do not take up vital dyes efficiently in vivo, are excluded inappropriately from this system. Moreover, the RES includes cells such as reticulum cells and endothelial cells that are not lineally related to other cells of the system.

Evolving knowledge indicated that macrophages were a family of cells with unique features, especially that of phagocytosis, derived from a common bone marrow precursor. This morphologically, functionally, and lineally related family of cells[9] is now known as the *mononuclear phagocyte system* (Table 16–1).

CHARACTERISTICS OF MATURE MONONUCLEAR PHAGOCYTES

Morphology of Peripheral Blood Monocytes

Peripheral blood monocytes and tissue and organ macrophages are mature mononuclear phagocytes. The peripheral blood monocyte is a large round cell with a diameter of 10 to 18 μm. It contains a well-developed Golgi apparatus, numerous lysosomal granules, and mitochondria evenly distributed throughout the cytoplasm. The nucleus is eccentric and kidney shaped, with moderately condensed

Table 16–1. MONONUCLEAR PHAGOCYTE SYSTEM

Cell Type	Location
Monoblast	Bone marrow
Promonocyte	Bone marrow
Monocyte	Bone marrow and peripheral blood
Macrophage	Tissue and organs
	Connective tissue (histiocytes)
	Liver (Kupffer cells)
	Lung (alveolar macrophages)
	Lymph nodes (free and fixed macrophages)
	Spleen (macrophages)
	Bone marrow (macrophages)
	Serous cavities (pleural and peritoneal macrophages)
	Bone (osteoclasts)
	Nervous system (microglial cells)
	Synovium (type A and C cells)
	Inflammatory sites (macrophages and epithelioid and giant cells)

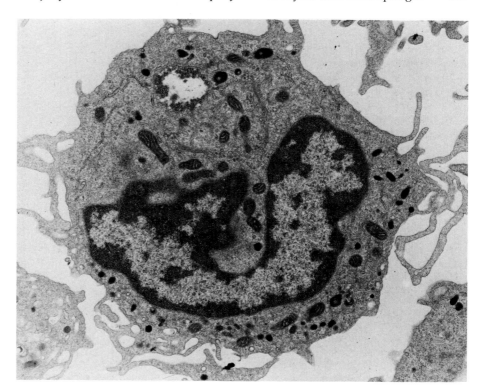

Figure 16–1. A human peripheral blood monocyte. The reniform nucleus, numerous mitochondria, and endocytic vacuoles are typical morphologic features of mononuclear phagocytes.

chromatin. Pseudopodia extend from the cell surface, and there is evidence of endocytic activity (Fig. 16–1).

Monocytes circulate in the peripheral blood with a half-life estimated at 8 to 71 hours in humans. They subsequently penetrate tissues in a random fashion independent of age[10] and in numbers proportional to the size of the organ. Once monocytes leave the circulation they do not return. The total blood monocyte pool is composed of circulating and marginated components. The marginated pool, which constitutes up to 75 percent of the total, consists of monocytes adhering to or rolling along the endothelial cells of blood vessels.

Entry of Peripheral Blood Monocytes into the Tissues

Monocytes that are adherent to the endothelial cells of all the postcapillary venules can migrate between them, through the basement membrane, and enter tissues.[11] Because monocytes leaving the circulation acquire the characteristics of macrophages within a few hours, vascular endothelium may be an important substrate with which monocytes must directly interact to differentiate further, as well as to emigrate. Several leukocyte cell surface glycoprotein families known as the integrins have been demonstrated to be involved in both monocyte and neutrophil–endothelial cell interactions.[12, 13]

The most important integrins involved in monocyte adhesion to endothelial cells are known as the leukocyte cell adhesion molecules (leu-CAMs) or CD18 family of adhesion molecules. These are glycoprotein heterodimers sharing a common beta subunit.[12] There are three adhesion receptors: leukocyte functional antigen-1 (LFA-1), also known as CD11a/CD18; Mac-1 (CD11b/CD18); and glycoprotein 150,95 (CD11c/CD18).[14] LFA-1 is found on all leukocytes; Mac-1 on monocytes, macrophages, granulocytes, natural killer (NK) cells, and some lymphocytes; and GP 150,95 on monocytes, granulocytes, and some cytotoxic lymphocytes. LFA-1 binds to two transmembrane glycoprotein counter-receptors, intercellular adhesion molecules 1 (CD54) and 2 (ICAM-1 and 2), both of which are members of the immunoglobulin supergene family.[15] Whereas ICAM-1 is an inducible molecule expressed on leukocytes and endothelial and epithelial cells in response to cytokines, endotoxin, and phorbol esters, ICAM-2 is constitutively expressed on endothelial cells and is not enhanced by inflammatory stimuli.[13] CD11b/CD18 has been identified as the receptor (CR3) for the complement component C3bi (CR3bi), but it also can recognize and bind to ICAM-1 expressed by endothelial cells.[12] GP 150,95 (CR4) also functions as an adhesion molecule, mediating the binding of monocytes to stimulated human umbilical vein endothelial cells independent of other receptor–ligand interactions.[16] Its ligand on endothelial cells has not been characterized.

Quantitative as well as qualitative changes occur in the CD11/CD18 receptors after cell activation. Chemoattractants or phorbol esters induce up-regulation of surface CD11b/CD18 and CD11c/CD18 by translocating receptors stored in intracellular vesicles to the cell surface.[17] Additional or alternative modifications of these receptors, such as conformational changes or phosphorylation, appear to be required for regulating adhesive interactions. Exposure of monocytes to the chemoattractant f-methionine-leucine-phenylalanine leads to phosphorylation of CD18 within seconds.[18] Indirect evidence suggests that this may alter the function of cytoskeletal elements, since cells from patients with leu-CAM deficiency cannot polymerize actin filaments in response to chemoattractants.

Several additional adhesion receptors used to bind various connective tissue molecules have also been shown to be expressed by monocytes, including receptors for hyaluronic acid (probably CD44), laminin, elastin, collagen, fibronectin, and proteoglycans. Adherence of monocytes to exposed vascular substratum, especially after injury, may be another mechanism of migration from blood vessels.

Finally, a group of lymphoid tissue homing receptors may be involved in monocyte and neutrophil migration into inflammatory sites. Leukocyte endothelial cell adhesion molecule (LECAM, L-selectin) is expressed by neutrophils and monocytes. Antibody to LECAM-1 blocks normal binding of neutrophils to lymphoid high endothelial venules. During inflammation, LECAM-1 is down-regulated or lost by neutrophils.[19] In contrast, the monocyte binds poorly to high endothelial venules in uninflamed lymph nodes. However, inflammation increases the binding of monocytes to high endothelial venule endothelium, and both LECAM-1 and CD11b/CD18 mediate this interaction.[19] Granulocytes and monocytes also express high levels of a homing cell adhesion molecule (HCAM), which binds a ligand on the high endothelial venules of mucosal lymphoid tissue known as the *mucosal addressin*.[20] The involvement of this receptor complex in monocyte migration is not yet known.

A rare, inherited deficiency of leu-CAM (CD11/CD18) expression has enhanced understanding of the role of these molecules in both normal and inflammatory settings.[17] These patients have abnormalities in the gene encoding CD18 and therefore express diminished amounts of all three members of the leu-CAM family. Phagocytes from these patients have marked defects in adhesion-related functions, including chemotaxis, aggregation, endothelial cell and complement (C3bi)-binding, and cell-mediated cytotoxicity (ADCC). The children develop recurrent and often fatal bacterial infections. Studies of these patients indicate that all three of the CD11/CD18 antigens are crucial in adhesion-dependent functions of monocytes and granulocytes.[17]

Besides the alteration of adhesion molecules after inflammatory stimuli, the accumulation of monocytes at inflammatory sites is governed in part by local elaboration of chemoattractants, which influence the direction and speed of their movement. Monocytes move in the direction of increasing concentrations of chemoattractant. A number of factors have been shown to be chemotactic for monocytes, including bacterial products such as N-formylated oligopeptides, cleavage products generated as a result of complement activation—primarily C5a, thrombin, and denatured albumin—and connective tissue components such as fibronectin fragments, elastin fragments, collagen, and collagenase-digested collagen.[21] In addition, several monocyte- and lymphocyte-derived cytokines and factors produced by erythrocytes,[21] tumor cells, and platelets, such as platelet-derived growth factor (PDGF) and transforming growth factor-β (TGF-β), are chemoattractants.

A family of chemoattractant cytokines has recently been characterized.[22] Monocyte chemoattractant protein-1 (MCP-1) is an 8.7-kD chemoattractant protein probably secreted by phytohemagglutinin- or lipopolysaccharide-stimulated monocytes.[23] Cytokine RANTES, secreted by T cells, is another potent attractor of blood monocytes.[24] Activated lymphocytes also produce a cytokine, migration inhibition factor (MIF), that inhibits macrophage migration and may contribute to the localization of recently arrived monocytes.[25] The control of monocyte migration into tissues under normal conditions has not been delineated. It is possible that some of these chemoattractants may control diapedesis under normal circumstances.

Besides stimulating directional cell movement, chemoattractants induce several additional functional responses, including random motility (chemokinesis), cell-to-substrate adhesiveness and cell-to-cell aggregation. Alternate cycles of hyperadherence (through enhanced expression of leukocyte adhesion molecules) and detachment from tissue substrates may be the basis of directional cell movement in response to chemoattractants. Higher concentrations of chemoattractants also induce exocytosis of lysosomal enzymes and production of reactive oxygen intermediates.

Cellular movement is initiated by a rapidly regulated remodeling of the branching network of actin filaments found in the macrophage cytoplasm. In human leukocytes, three actin-binding proteins appear to have major effects on the actin filament architecture. Actin-binding protein cross-links actin filaments into the cytoplasmic orthogonal actin network.[26] Gelsolin is a multifunctional actin-binding protein that severs actin filaments, nucleates actin filament assembly, and blocks the fast-exchanging end of actin filaments.[27] It is associated with the cytoplasmic side of intracellular membranes, including rough endoplasmic reticulum, cytoplasmic vesicles, mitochondria, and the plasma membrane of macrophages. Profilin is an actin monomer-binding protein whose affinity for actin is regulated by polyphosphoinositides in vitro.

Chemoattractants exert their concentration-dependent effects on mononuclear phagocytes through a series of membrane chemoattractant receptor–mediated biochemical and cellular events, leading to regulation of the cytoskeleton and cell movement. The occupied receptor interacts with a G protein, transmitting a signal to the enzyme phospholipase C by means of the G-α-GTP complex thus formed.[28] This enzyme splits phosphatidylinositol-4,5,-biphosphate (PIP$_2$) to diacyl glycerol and inositol-1,4,5-trisphosphate (IP$_3$). IP$_3$ acts as an internal ionophore, inducing the release of intracellular calcium ions from the endoplasmic reticulum. Diacyl glycerol activates the enzyme protein kinase C (PKC). An increase in intracellular calcium appears to be a sufficient signal for the release of granule contents, which can be the source of new membrane chemotactic receptors.[29] Furthermore, up-regulation of the complement receptor CR3 (Mac-1) is blocked by an inhibitor of release of intracellular calcium stores.[30] Micromolar concentrations of calcium activate gelsolin to bind and sever F-actin filaments and cap the filament ends. PIP and PIP$_2$ release gelsolin from the filament ends.[27] Without bound gelsolin, monomeric actin becomes available, and polymerization begins. This process is important for chemotactic force generation and subsequent monocyte motility.

Peripheral Blood Monocyte Differentiation into Tissue Macrophages

Once in the tissues, the monocyte matures into a functionally more active cell, the tissue macrophage. These cells vary in diameter from 10 to 80 μm. They contain one or more oval or indented, often eccentrically located, nuclei and may have prominent nucleoli. Their cytoplasm is more abundant than that of the monocyte and contains numerous dense granules, endocytic vacuoles, and mitochondria. The dense granules are lysosomes—membrane-bound structures that contain a variety of hydrolytic enzymes. A membrane-associated proton pump maintains an acid environment. The primary lysosomes bud from the Golgi apparatus and may fuse with phagocytic or autophagocytic vacuoles to form digestive bodies or secondary lysosomes. The cytoplasm also contains ribosomes, polyribososmes, microfilaments, microtubules, varying amounts of endoplasmic reticulum, and a variety of vacuoles that contain the remains of engulfed material. Many ruffles, pseudopodia, and flaps can be seen on their surface.[31]

Macrophages have a very long life span in the tissues, often surviving for months or even years. It has generally been held that tissue macrophages are the direct descendants of blood monocytes. Although this may be true for alveolar macrophages,[32] it has been suggested that some resident macrophage populations, such as Kupffer cells and peritoneal macrophages, may renew themselves by local proliferation.[33] In this case, an influx of monocytes may be important only during inflammation.[32] During an intense local inflammatory response, local proliferation of immature macrophages may be observed.

In chronic inflammation, macrophages may form tight clusters or granulomas. Under these conditions,

their endocytic activities become less prominent, and many mitochondria develop and take on the characteristics of epithelioid cells.[34] Epithelioid cells are large, macrophage-like cells with abundant cytoplasm and round or oval nuclei. They contain numerous mitochondria, lysosomes, and large vacuoles. In some cases, newly emigrated monocytes fuse to form multinucleated giant cells. The resulting syncytia have a life span of only a few days. The mechanism of fusion is unclear, but both interleukin-4 (IL-4) and interferon-gamma (IFNγ) may be involved. Many giant cells express class II MHC antigens and may function as antigen-presenting cells.[35] The proto-oncogene c-fms (the gene for macrophage colony-stimulating factor receptor, vide infra) is down-regulated in cultures of human monocytes that have been stimulated to form giant cells. It has been concluded that these cells represent highly stimulated cells of the mononuclear phagocytic lineage at a terminal stage of differentiation.[36]

Macrophages are found outlining blood vessels in the connective tissue and are particularly prominent in the lung, liver, spleen, and bone marrow (see Table 16–1). The synovial lining layer also contains cells of macrophage lineage. Primarily on the basis of light and electron microscopic studies, these cells have been classified as macrophage-like type A and C cells as distinct from fibroblast-like B cells.[37] The application of a panel of monoclonal antibodies specific for monocyte/macrophage-associated antigens, class II MHC antigens, and fibroblast-associated antigens has permitted further documentation of the lineage of synovial lining cells.[38] Thus, synovial lining type A cells are phagocytic, express monocyte/macrophage-associated antigens detected by a variety of monoclonal antibodies and receptors for the Fc region of the IgG molecule and the third component of complement (C3), and are likely to be bone marrow derived. The deeper type B cells react only with monoclonal antibodies that identify fibroblasts and are probably locally derived.[38] Finally, cells with dendritic morphology, abundant class II antigen, and some monocyte/macrophage-associated antigens have been identified in synovial tissue obtained from patients with rheumatoid arthritis.[38, 39]

Macrophage Heterogeneity

Macrophages are heterogeneous with respect to morphology and function, as might be expected from their widespread tissue distribution. Evidence of functional heterogeneity has been obtained from an examination of the capacity of various macrophage populations to function as antigen-presenting cells. Whereas inflammatory macrophages, alveolar macrophages, and Kupffer cells (the macrophages of the liver) are endocytically active and may express class II MHC antigens, only the inflammatory macrophages are fully competent antigen-presenting cells and stimulators of allogeneic T lymphocytes.[40–42] Besides variability in antigen-presenting cell function, there is considerable variability in the capacity of macrophages from various anatomic sites to mediate tumor-cell killing and to carry out other metabolic activities.[43]

Mononuclear phagocyte heterogeneity is thought to result from differences in their stage of differentiation, as well as from the modulating influences of the local environment during normal and altered homeostasis.[44, 45] For instance, regular tissue macrophages overall are a more functionally quiescent population of cells than are peripheral blood monocytes, presumably because of the influence of local regulatory factors.[44] In contrast, macrophages activated at inflammatory sites exhibit enhancement of phagocytosis, pinocytosis, and microbicidal and tumoricidal activities as a result of stimulation by a variety of products generated at inflammatory sites.[44, 45]

MATURATION OF THE MONONUCLEAR PHAGOCYTES IN THE BONE MARROW

The maturation of mononuclear phagocytes within the bone marrow involves a multistep process (Fig. 16–2). Partial definition of these events was made possible by the development of semisolid culture systems to support the clonal growth of hematopoietic colonies. The initial observation that hematopoietic precursors were unable to survive or proliferate in vitro led to the discovery of four regulatory glycoproteins, referred to as the colony-stimulatory factors (CSFs) (Table 16–2). Granulocyte macrophage CSF (GM-CSF) and multi-CSF (IL-3) can stimulate the formation of granulocytes and macrophages.[46] Granulocyte CSF (G-CSF) stimulates only granulocyte formation, and macrophage CSF (M-CSF) only monocyte formation. Restricted development of cells of monocyte or granulocyte lineage from the bipotential stem cell depends on the relative concentrations of these CSFs. Thus, low concentrations of GM-CSF produce few colonies, which are predominantly monocytic, whereas high concentrations result in predominant granulocyte colonies.[46]

IL-6 has since been shown to have colony-stim-

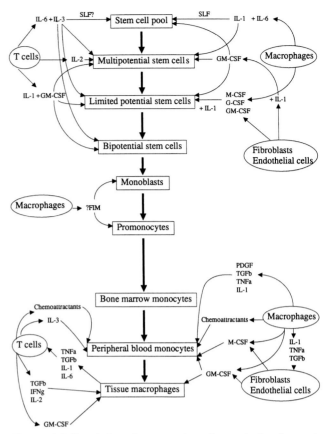

Figure 16–2. Regulation of mononuclear phagocyte development. Factors produced by mononuclear phagocytes as well as by other cell types, such as T cells, fibroblasts, and endothelial cells, control mononuclear phagocyte ontogeny and differentiation. SLF, Steel factor.

ulating activity. Its protein sequence shows a distinct similarity to that of G-CSF.[47] Recombinant human IL-6 synergizes with IL-3 in the proliferation of stem cell colonies but by itself does not induce colony formation later in myelopoiesis, that is, at the bipotential cell stage. However, IL-6 suppresses colony formation induced by G-CSF but not M-CSF.[48] This may occur by either competitive inhibition or down-regulation of G-CSF receptors by IL-6.

Recently, a new hemopoietic factor, called Steel factor, has been purified from the supernatants of liver and bone marrow stromal cell cultures.[49] Alone, it shows modest effects on pluripotent stem cell cultures, but it synergizes dramatically on stem cells with other factors such as erythropoietin, IL-1, IL-6, and IL-7.[50] The importance of Steel factor is evidenced by the severe deficiency of hematopoiesis in animals with defects in its production.

Unique membrane receptors exist for each CSF and are found on bipotential stem cells and their progenitors.[51] Most cells simultaneously exhibit receptors for more than one type of CSF. Progenitor cells can respond to any of the four CSFs. One CSF may modulate the capacity of myelomonocytic precursors to respond to other CSFs and thereby regulate their capacity to differentiate down specific path-

Table 16–2. COLONY-STIMULATING FACTORS (CSFs)

Human CSF	Other Names	Cellular Sources
Multi-CSF	IL-3	Activated T cells
GM-CSF	CSF-α	Activated T cells
	CSF2	Macrophages
	Pluriprotein-α	Endothelial cells
		Fibroblasts, stromal cells
G-CSF	CSF-β	Macrophages
	Pluriprotein	Endothelial cells
		Fibroblasts
M-CSF	CSF1	Macrophages
		Endothelial cells
		Fibroblasts

ways.[52] Thus, binding of GM-CSF to its receptor down-modulates receptors for G-CSF and M-CSF.[51, 52] In addition, receptor binding of G-CSF down-modulates receptors for M-CSF, whereas receptor binding of M-CSF down-modulates binding for GM-CSF. The M-CSF and Steel factor receptors have been identified as the proto-oncogene products c-*fms* and c-*kit*, respectively. These both contain intracellular tyrosine kinase domains.[49, 53]

There is marked synergy between CSFs and IL-1. IL-1 may regulate hematopoiesis by inducing alterations of progenitor responsiveness or by enhancing CSF production by auxiliary stromal cells (especially T cells but also monocytes, endothelial cells, and fibroblasts). IL-1 allows IL-3 to act on multipotent stem cells that are more primitive than those normally responsive to IL-3 alone.[54] This action is mediated in part by the enhancement of CSF receptors on primitive multipotent hematopoietic precursors. In cells of the hematopoietic stroma, IL-1 can increase translation of IL-6, GM-CSF, and G-CSF genes by stabilizing their messenger RNA (mRNA) transcripts.[55] Thus IL-1 provides another mechanism by which immature cells may be directed to the macrophage lineage.

Growth hormone may also influence myelopoiesis. Both growth hormone and somatomedin-C double the number of granulocyte colonies in the presence of GM-CSF, suggesting that bone marrow stromal cells respond to growth hormone by synthesizing somatomedin-C. Thus, the effect of growth hormone may be mediated in the bone marrow in a paracrine fashion, just as it is in other target tissues.[56]

Besides the proliferative actions of the CSFs, each is capable of maintaining functional membrane integrity, inducing cellular maturation, and stimulating the functional activity of mature cells.[46] The CSF receptors therefore mediate diverse biologic responses, depending on the differentiation status of the myeloid cell. M-CSF primes mature monocytes to secrete IL-1, tumor necrosis factor-α (TNF-α), and colony-stimulating activity, and it enhances tumoricidal activity and cell-mediated cytotoxicity. GM-CSF and IL-3 stimulate macrophage cytotoxicity. Although neither factor alone seems to stimulate monocyte toxicity, both GM-CSF– and IL-3–treated monocytes kill more effectively when exposed to a second activating signal provided by endotoxin.[57] It is likely that TNF-α secretion is responsible for these effects. Because both GM-CSF and IL-3 are secreted by activated T lymphocytes, these factors may serve to enhance endotoxin-induced macrophage killing in an area of local inflammation. GM-CSF also stimulates the expression of class II MHC molecules by monocytes, and thereby may allow them to be more effective antigen-presenting cells at sites of inflammation.[58]

Although it is not clear whether the factors produced by inflammatory tissue macrophages reach the bone marrow to stimulate the earliest monocyte/macrophage progenitors, it is likely that the ontogeny of mononuclear phagocytes is regulated by cells of the mononuclear phagocyte lineage as well as by other cell types (see Fig. 16–2). Resting peripheral monocytes have no detectable mRNA for G-CSF or M-CSF, but gene expression and protein secretion are inducible by activation with interferon-γ, GM-CSF, and IL-3.[59] GM-CSF and IL-3 appear to selectively induce monocyte M-CSF secretion, whereas endotoxin induces G-CSF. Both endothelial cells and fibroblasts produce M-CSF, G-CSF, and GM-CSF, although production of M-CSF by human endothelial cells requires activation by IL-1 and TNF-α.[57]

Recombinant DNA technology has enabled the production of sufficient amounts of CSFs for clinical use. Administration of recombinant GM-CSF leads to a significant increase in nadir white blood cell count with only mild side effects, including low-grade fever, bone discomfort, myalgia, and headache after cycles of chemotherapy.[60] In some patients with advanced malignancy, administration of GM-CSF has led to a decrease in tumor progression.[60] In vitro, continuous exposure of cells to GM-CSF is required to stimulate proliferation and functional activity.[46] Likewise, clinically, subcutaneous and continuous intravenous routes of administration are found to be more effective than intravenous pulse or bolus doses of GM-CSF. The future of these agents is promising, and further studies are underway to include larger patient groups and combinations of CSFs, and to evaluate their use in a variety of clinical situations associated with decreased numbers of myelomonocytic cells.

In mice and rabbits, a factor is secreted by macrophages at the site of inflammation and then transported to the bone marrow. This substance, called factor-inducing monocytopoiesis (FIM), is a thermolabile protein with a molecular weight of 18 to 25 kD. In the marrow, it stimulates monocyte production by increasing the proliferative activity of monoblasts and promonocytes and by enhancing the transit of monocytes from bone marrow to blood.[61] This may lead to the appearance in the circulation of immature monocytes normally retained in the bone marrow.

Monocyte maturation is accompanied by alterations in cellular morphology and histochemistry. The monoblast is a round cell with a diameter of 10 to 12 μm that contains the cytoplasmic enzymes characteristic of mononuclear phagocytes, including peroxidase, nonspecific esterase, and lysozyme.[62] The monoblast is pinocytically and phagocytically active and possesses receptors for both the Fc region of IgG and C3.[62] Promonocytes are 10 to 25 μm in diameter and constitute about 0.25 percent of all nucleated bone marrow cells.[10] They are adherent to glass and contain cytoplasmic esterase and peroxidase activity, but have few Fc receptors (FcRs) and C3 receptors.[10, 62] Although capable of endocytosis, these cells are poorly phagocytic compared with monocytes, which have better developed lysosomes and more FcRs and C3 receptors.[62]

Table 16–3. DIFFERENTIATION MARKERS OF MYELOID CELLS

Designation	Characteristics and Function of Molecule	Pluripotent Cell	Bipotential Cell	Blood Monocyte	Granulocyte
CD34	Glycoprotein (phosphorylated by protein kinase C)	+ +	+ +	−	−
CD33	Glycoprotein	+	+	+ +	+ +
CD13	Aminopeptidase N (a membrane anchored metalloprotease)	−	+	+ +	+ +
CD15	Lacto-N-fucopentanose III (LNF III X hapten) polysaccharide	−	−	+	+ +
CD14	Receptor for lipopolysaccharide-binding protein	−	−	+ +	+ +
M-CSF receptor	c-fms oncoprotein	−	+	+ +	−
CD31	30–410-kD glycoprotein	+	+	+ +	+ +

Adapted from Civin, C. I.: Human monomyeloid cell membrane antigens. Exp. Hematol. 18:461, 1990. Used by permission.

Table 16–3 depicts the differentiation markers of myeloid cells, demonstrating similarities and differences between the developing cells and their mature progeny. Table 16–4 shows the surface markers of mature cells, divided into functional groups. The function of some of these cell surface molecules is not known. Mature monocytes, macrophages, and activated macrophages bear different constellations of cell surface markers. For example, CD23 (low-avidity IgE receptor), CD25 (α-chain of the IL-2 receptor), and CD69 (activation-induced molecule) are found on activated macrophages. Furthermore, other functional subsets of macrophages can be defined by their expression of different cell surface markers.[63]

ACTIVITIES OF MATURE MONONUCLEAR PHAGOCYTES

The various activities of mononuclear phagocytes can be considered in terms of simple and complex functions (Table 16–5). A simple function is a single ability or activity, whereas a complex function involves the coordination of a variety of simple functions. For example, phagocytosis, pinocytosis, and intracellular digestion are simple functions that are part of microbial digestion, a complex function. Mononuclear phagocytes possess a number of physiologic characteristics that permit them to accomplish their varied functions. Among these features is the display of a variety of cell surface molecules. Mononuclear phagocytes express more than 30 distinct receptors that enable them to recognize and interact with various molecules in their external environment (see Table 16–4). Another feature is the capacity to synthesize and secrete some 100 defined substances that act both intracellularly and extracellularly.

Cell Surface Molecules

Immunoglobulin Fc Receptors

Mononuclear phagocytes possess surface receptors that specifically recognize the Fc region of the IgG and IgE antibody molecules.[64] The human Fc-γ receptors (FcγRs) can be divided into three classes on the basis of ligand affinity and reactivity with class-specific monoclonal antibodies. FcR I (CD64) has high affinity for monomeric IgG and is found only on cells of myeloid origin. FcR II (CDw32) binds aggregated or polyvalent IgG (IgG1 or IgG3) and is found on monocytes, lymphocytes, and granulocytes. FcR III (CD16) has a low affinity for aggregated IgG and is found mainly on granulocytes and NK cells, and to a lesser extent on monocytes and macrophages.[65]

The major biologic role for FcRs is the facilitation of phagocytosis. Although antibody is not an obligatory requirement for endocytosis of many particles, its presence greatly enhances this process. Whereas interaction with FcR initiates fairly weak binding of particles to mononuclear phagocytes, such interactions are potent stimulators of phagocytosis.[64] The FcR is also likely to play a central role in a number of other functions of macrophages, including cell-mediated cytotoxicity, "arming" in tumor immunity, and triggering of the secretion of biologically active molecules such as prostaglandins, lysosomal acid hydrolases, and reactive oxygen metabolites.[64] In addition, cytophilic antibody bound to FcRs can enhance the amount of foreign antigen taken up by a macrophage and subsequently presented to antigen-specific T cells.[66]

Complement Receptors

Mononuclear phagocytes bear at least three cell surface receptors that recognize activation fragments of the third component of complement (C3a, C3b, and C3bi) and one for an activation fragment of the fifth component of complement, anaphylotoxin (C5a).[67, 68] Two distinct C3 receptors (CR1 and CR3) appear to recognize different portions of the C3 molecule (C3 and C3bi, respectively).[67, 68] Whereas binding of particles is effectively induced by interaction with C3 receptors, such interactions are ineffective triggers of phagocytosis by resting

Table 16–4. SURFACE MARKERS ON MYELOID CELLS

Designation	Characteristics and Function of Molecule	Blood Monocyte	Granulocyte	Macrophage
Adhesion Molecules				
CD11a	LFA-1 α-chain p 180	+ +	+ +	+
CD11c	p150, 95 α-chain (CR4)	+ +	+ +	+
CD18	95-kD glycoprotein chain, linked to CD11a, b, and c	+ +	+ +	+ +
CDw49d	VLA α4-chain. Binds V-CAM and fibronectin	+ +	−	
CDw49f	VLA α6-chain. Laminin receptor	+ +	−	
CD29	Common β-chain of VLA protein family	+ +	+ +	+ +
CD44	Leukocyte endothelial cell adhesion molecule (LECAM-II)	+ +	+ +	+ +
CD58	LFA-3. Binds CD2 molecule on T cells	+ +	+ +	+ +
CD36	85-kD glycoprotein	−	−	+ +
Complement Receptors				
CD11b	α-subunit of complement receptor, or C3bi (CR3). Fibrinogen receptor	+ +	+ +	
CD35	CR1. Binds C3b, C3bi, C3c, C4b	+ +	+ +	−
Immunoglobulin Receptors				
CD64	FcγR I	+ +	+ +	+ +
CD32	FcγR II. Low-affinity IgG receptor	+ +	+ +	+ +
CD16	FcγR III	+ +	+ +	+ +
CD23	FcεR IIa and b. Low-affinity IgE receptor	−	+ +	−
Other Receptors				
CD74	Class II MHC molecule (DR), invariant chain complex	+ +	−	+ +
CD45	Transmembrane glycoprotein with 4 isoforms, resulting from	+ +	+ +	+ +
CD45RA	differential splicing	+ +	−	−
CD45RB		+ +	−	+ +
CD45RO		+ +	+ +	+ +
CD25	α-Chain of IL-2 receptor complex. Low-affinity IL-2 receptor	−	−	+ −
CD9	24-kD single-chain protein	+ +	−	−
CD46	Doublet glycoprotein of 56–66 kD Membrane cofactorprotein (MCP)	+ +	+ +	+ +
CD47	47–52-kD glycoprotein	+ +	+ +	+ +
CD48	41-kD PI-linked glycoprotein	+ +	+ +	+ +
CD43	95-kD highly sialated integral membrane protein	+ +	+ +	+ +
CD53	35-kD transmembrane glycoprotein	+ +	+ +	+ +
CD55	70-kD PI-linked membrane glycoprotein. Decay-accelerating factor	+ +	+ +	+ +
CD59	18–20-kD glycoprotein. Mediates inhibition of the membrane attack complex	+ +	+ +	+ +
CD63	53-kD glycoprotein	+ +	+ +	+ +
CD68	110-kD glycoprotein	+ +	−	+ +
CD71	Transferrin receptor	+ +	+ +	+ +
CDw17	Lactosyl ceramide	+ +	+ +	−
CDw50	?	+ +	+ +	+ +
CDw52	21–29-kD glycoprotein. Campath 1 antigen	+ +	+ +	+ +
CDw65	Fucoganglioside. Ceramide dodecasaccharide 4c	+	+ +	−

macrophages.[67, 69] There is marked synergy between C3 receptors and FcRs in facilitation of phagocytosis, the former mediating binding and the latter phagocytosis. Engagement of C3 receptors can also lead to prostaglandin release.[67, 69] The interaction of C5a with its macrophage receptor induces secretion of IL-1 and initiates chemotaxis.[70] Interferon-γ depresses binding of ligand by C3 receptors, and this is reversed by fibronectin.[71]

Fibronectin Receptors

Fibronectin and laminin are found in the substratum of blood vessels and in connective tissue. The fibronectin and laminin receptors are members of the VLA family of integrins, which share a common β1-subunit (CD 29). α1β1 (VLA-1, CD49a/CD29) and α2β1 (VLA-2, CD49b/CD29) bind collagen and α4β1 (VLA-4, CD49d/CD29); α5β1 (VLA-5, CD49e/CD29) and α$_v$β1 (CD51) bind fibronectin. The monocyte/macrophage fibronectin receptor is structurally and functionally similar to its fibroblast equivalent.[72] α3β1 (VLA-3, CD49c/CD29) acts as a receptor for collagen, laminin, and fibronectin, and α6β1 (VLA-6, CD49f/CD29) is a laminin receptor.[12] VLA-4 also mediates adhesion of leukocytes to an inducible endothelial cell surface protein, called VCAM-1.[73] The sites on VLA-4 involved in VCAM-1 binding are distinct from those involved in fibronectin binding.

Interaction of these matrix molecules with their

Table 16–5. PANOPLY OF MONONUCLEAR
PHAGOCYTE ACTIVITIES

Simple Functions	Complex Functions
Migration	Tissue remodeling
Pinocytosis	Senescent or dead cell removal
Phagocytosis	Antimicrobial activity
Intracellular digestion	Antiviral activity
	Antineoplastic activity
	Antibody-dependent cell-mediated cytotoxicity
	Immunoregulation
	Lipid and lipoprotein metabolism
	Wound healing

specific mononuclear phagocyte receptors may be involved in migration of macrophages to sites of exposed interstitium, as in damaged tissue. In addition, engagement of fibronectin receptors in vitro results in enhanced functional expression of Fc and C3 receptors and consequently augmented phagocytosis and secretion of neutral proteases. CD11b/CD18, fibronectin, vitronectin, and laminin receptors are stored in vesicles in monocytes and polymorphonuclear leukocytes (PMNs). At least in PMNs, activation of the cell leads to the expression of these molecules on the cell surface. Macrophages bind laminin after activation with interferon-γ or stimuli that activate PKC. PKC stimulation induces phosphorylation of the cytoplasmic domain of the α6 subunit, and this may induce anchorage of this subunit to the cytoskeleton after binding to a laminin substratum.[74]

Cytokine Receptors

Mononuclear phagocytes have receptors for many cytokines that modify their behavior. These include receptors for chemoattractants, CSFs,[46] IL-1, IL-2, IL-4, IL-6, interferon-α and γ,[75] TGF-β, and PDGF. TGF-β can up-regulate the expression of FcR III in monocytes, thus modulating phagocytosis, and can stimulate production of IL-1, TNF-α, and additional TGF-β by monocytes.

The IL-1 receptor on monocytes is immunologically distinct from that on T lymphocytes and is up-regulated in a synergistic fashion by dexamethasone and prostaglandin E$_2$.[76] Monocytes respond to IL-1 by up-regulating endogenous IL-1 production and by producing cyclooxygenase metabolites of arachidonic acid.[77] The IL-6 receptor appears to be conserved between monocytes, T cells, and B cells. IL-1 and IL-6 down-regulate IL-6 mRNA levels in monocytes.[78] Both low- and high-affinity IL-2 receptors are found on stimulated but not resting macrophages.[79] They are up-regulated by lipopolysaccharide and interferon-γ. IL-2 stimulation leads to a respiratory burst by activated macrophages.[79] IL-4 down-regulates the production of IL-1, TNF-α, and IL-6 by monocytes. It also reduces the capacity of monocytes to produce oxygen radicals in response to interferon-γ, and thus

it may play a role as a regulator of macrophage function at inflammatory sites.[80, 80a]

Hormone and Other Biologic Messenger Receptors

Mononuclear phagocytes express receptors for polypeptide hormones, bioactive lipids, and other biologically active substances.[75] Many of these have the capacity to regulate the function of mononuclear phagocytes. Insulin suppresses expression of FcRs. Glucocorticoids may exert their anti-inflammatory effects by inhibition of phospholipase A$_2$ activity and thus the synthesis of prostaglandins. In addition, they may inhibit IL-1 secretion, proteinase secretion, and the response to interferon-γ.[81] Calcitriol facilitates monocyte maturation. It thus exerts a paracrine effect on differentiated monocytes and macrophages, which are present at the sites of granulomata, where calcitriol is produced by macrophage 1α-hydroxylase activity. Phorbol esters augment many macrophage functions by directly activating PKC. Prostaglandins of the E series diminish phagocytic potential, decrease MHC class II expression, and decrease the secretion of IL-1 and TNF-α.[81, 82]

Many, if not most, of the secreted products of mononuclear phagocytes are released on interaction of particular cell surface receptors with their ligands. In addition to those already mentioned, these include secretion of neutral proteases when the receptor for acetylated proteins is engaged,[83] and secretion of lysosomal enzymes when the receptor for N-formylated peptides is engaged.

Secretory Products

Mononuclear phagocytes secrete a variety of substances either constitutively or after a specific stimulus, such as a cell surface receptor–ligand interaction. The array of products secreted by macrophages is determined by their stage of differentiation, local environmental influences, and state of activation. In addition to their influence on host defense and normal and altered homeostasis at many different levels, the secretory products of macrophages can directly or indirectly affect macrophage activities. Substances released by macrophages are shown in Table 16–6.[84] From the table, it is clear that macrophages produce diverse substances sometimes with different—opposing—effects and sometimes with similar—complementary—effects on the organism.

Enzymes

The lysosomal acid hydrolases of macrophages are involved primarily in intracellular digestion. However, macrophages may also be stimulated to release these enzymes selectively into the environmental milieu. Phagocytosis of some particles, such as latex particles or erythrocytes, induces the release

Table 16–6. SECRETORY PRODUCTS OF MACROPHAGES

Polypeptide Hormones
Interleukin-1α and β (IL-1)
Interleukin-6 (IL-6)
Tumor necrosis factor-α (TNF-α)
Interferon-α
Neutrophil-activating factor
Transforming growth factor-β (TGF-β)
Transforming growth factor-α
Platelet-derived growth factor (PDGF)
Fibroblast growth factors (FGF)
Fibroblast-activating factors
Plasmacytoma growth factor
Thymosin B4
Insulin-like growth factor-1 (somatomedin-C)
Somatotropin
Erythropoietin
Colony-stimulating factor for granulocytes and macrophages (GM-CSF)
Colony-stimulating factor for macrophages (M-CSF, CSF-1)
Colony-stimulating factor for granulocytes (G-CSF)
Factor-inducing monocytopoiesis (FIM)
Erythroid colony-potentiating factor/tissue inhibitor of metalloproteinases (TIMP)
Adrenocorticotropic hormone (ACTH)
β-Endorphin
Bombesin
Substance P
Complement (C) Components
Classical pathway: C1, C2, C3, C4, C5, C6, C7, C8, C9; active component fragments generated by macrophage proteinases: C3a, C3b, C5a, Bb
Alternative pathway: factor B, factor D, properdin
Inhibitors: factor I (of C3b), factor H (β-1H)
Coagulation Factors
Intrinsic pathway: IX, X, V, prothrombin
Extrinsic pathway: VII
Surface activities: tissue factor, prothrombinase
Antithrombolytic: plasminogen activator inhibitor-2, plasmin inhibitors
Proteolytic Enzymes
Metalloproteases; macrophage elastase, collagenase, stromelysin, 92- and 68-kD gelatinase, angiotensin convertase
Serine proteases: urokinase-type plasminogen activator (UPA), cytolytic proteinase
Aspartyl proteases: cathepsin D
Cysteine protease: cathepsin L, cathepsin B

Other Enzymes
Lipases: lipoprotein lipase, phospholipase
Glucosaminidase: lysozyme
Lysosomal acid hydrolases: proteases, lipases, (deoxy) ribonucleases, phosphatases, glycosidases, sulfatases (approximately 40)
Deaminase: arginase
Inhibitors of Enzymes
Protease inhibitors: α_2-macroglobulin, α_1-protease inhibitor (α_1-PI)/α_1-antitrypsin, plasminogen activator inhibitor-2 (PAI-2), plasmin inhibitors, TIMP/collagenase inhibitor
Phospholipase inhibitor: lipomodulin (macrocortin)
Proteins of Extracellular Matrix or Cell Adhesion
Fibronectin
Gelatin-binding protein/92-kD gelatinase
Thrombospondin
Chondroitin sulfate proteoglycans
Heparan sulfate proteoglycans
Other Binding Proteins
For metals: transferrin, acidic isoferrins
For vitamins: transcobalamin II
For lipids: apolipoprotein E, lipid transfer protein
For growth factors: α_2-macroglobulin, IL-1
For inhibitors: TGF-β–binding protein
For biotin: avidin
Bioactive Lipids
Cyclooxygenase products: prostaglandin E$_2$ (PGE$_2$),
Prostaglandin F$_{2\alpha}$, prostacyclin (PGI$_2$), thromboxane
Lipoxygenase products: monohydroxyeicosatetraenoic acids (HETE), leukotrienes (LT) B$_4$, C, D, E
Platelet-activating factors (PAF): 1-O alkyl-2-acetyl-*sn*-glyceryl-3-phosphorylcholine
Other Bioactive Low-Molecular-Weight Substances
Oligopeptides: glutathione
Steroid hormones: 1$_\alpha$, 25-dihydroxyvitamin D3
Purine and pyrimidine products: thymidine, uracil, uric acid, deoxycytidine, cAMP, neopterin
Reactive oxygen intermediates: superoxide, hydrogen peroxide, hydroxyl radical, singlet oxygen, hypohalous acids
Reactive nitrogen intermediates: nitrites, nitrates

From Rappolee, D. A., Werb, Z.: Secretory products of phagocytes. Curr. Opin. Immunol. 1:47, 1988. Used by permission.

of about 10 to 25 percent of the macrophage's lysosomal granules over a brief period. Other ingested particles, however, such as streptococcal cell walls, zymosan, or asbestos, induce the release of up to 80 percent of the lysosomal enzymes into the extracellular environment. Many of the particles that cause such release of lysosomal enzymes into the extracellular environment lead to chronic inflammation when injected into experimental animals. Lysosomal release may also be induced by interaction of macrophages with immune complexes or interferon-γ.[85]

Lysozyme represents the major secretory product of the macrophage. It is a cationic protein that hydrolyzes *N*-acetyl muramic β-1,4-N-acetyl glucosamine linkages in bacterial cell walls, leading to lysis

of susceptible organisms. The synthesis and secretion of a number of lysosomal neutral proteinases (see Table 16–6) are inducible in activated macrophages and are markedly stimulated by phagocytosis.[86] Up to 75 percent of the newly synthesized enzymes are secreted into the extracellular fluid. The exact mechanisms involved in the secretion of these enzymes have not yet been elucidated.

Enzyme and Cytokine Inhibitors

Cultured human monocytes secrete products that are inhibitory to enzymes and cytokines. These often play a role in autocrine regulation of other secreted products. Enzyme inhibitors include α_2-macroglobulin, a protease inhibitor of lysosomal hydro-lases, plasminogen activator, elastase, and collagen-ase. When α_2-macroglobulin–protease complexes bind to the α_2-macroglobulin receptor, secretion of neutral proteases is shut off.[83] The regulation of this reciprocal secretion of active enzymes and enzme inhibitors remains to be delineated. Activated human monocytes secrete an inhibitor of IL-1.[87] The kinetics and factors affecting secretion of the cytokine and its natural antagonist appear to differ. The IL-1 inhibitor has been purified and the gene encoding it cloned and sequenced. It is a 22-kD secreted protein with some homology to IL-1. It inhibits the action of IL-1 by competitively inhibiting its binding to the IL-1 receptor.[87] Thus, the IL-1 receptor antagonist may have utility as an anti-inflammatory agent. Two other macrophage products inhibit the effects of IL-1—TGFβ, which is inhibitory at a point distal to the interaction of IL-1 with its receptor,[88] and prostaglan-din E_2, which inhibits synthesis of IL-1 at a post-transcriptional stage.[82] Both IL-1 and TNF-α induce prostaglandin synthesis by macrophages and other cell types.[89]

Macrophages are capable of synthesizing the whole spectrum of lipoxygenase (leukotriene) and cyclooxygenase (prostaglandin) products. This differs from other cells, which tend to be more specialized. The specific spectrum synthesized by a macrophage population at any one time depends on the nature of the stimulus, the tissue of origin of the cells, and their stage of cellular activity.[90]

Simple Functions

Phagocytosis

Phagocytosis is an essential component of many complex functions, such as tissue remodeling, wound healing, microbial destruction, and clearance of senescent or dead cells, particulate debris, and biologically active molecules. The most critical step in phagocytosis is the cell's ability to discriminate between normal self and damaged self or foreign particles. This recognition and attachment process is mediated primarily through cell surface receptors. In the case of bacteria, opsonins function by binding specifically to bacterial surface molecules as well as to macrophage receptors. There are two types of opsonin—the C3b and C3bi fragments of C3, and antimicrobial IgG (and other immunoglobulins).[91] Re-ceptors for immunoglobulin, complement, and fibro-nectin bind particles complexed with these opsonins. Other receptors, such as those for mannose or fucose-terminal glycoproteins and acetylated proteins, bind ligands directly. Finally, a nonspecific particle recep-tor has been defined on the surface of macrophages. It binds such particles as glutaraldehyde-treated erythrocytes and latex particles.

There appears to be marked synergy between the two opsonins, in that particle-bound C3 can markedly reduce the amount of IgG necessary to induce phagocytosis. Although resting macrophages are unable to ingest C3-opsonized particles, inter-feron-γ–activated macrophages can ingest particles opsonized by C3 only.[69]

The normal consequence of binding of a particle to the macrophage membrane is the initiation of ingestion. The cytoplasm extends to form pseudo-podia, which spread to surround the particle. The pseudopodia fuse on the distal side of the particle, resulting in the formation of a phagocytic vesicle or phagosome. The lining of this vacuole is composed of inverted plasma membrane. The vesicle buds off from the cell periphery and migrates to the cyto-plasm. Initial binding of a particle to the macrophage surface, even after opsonization with IgG antibody, does not always trigger ingestion. Rather, for IgG-opsonized particles, a zipper-like mechanism seems to be involved. Phagocytosis of a particle requires initial attachment of the macrophage to the FcR, followed by sequential attachment of sites on the particle to adjacent macrophage FcRs. In this way, the macrophage membrane is guided around the particle. Phagocytosis of one particle does not trigger ingestion of other particles attached to the macro-phage surface.

Pinocytosis

If a material has no binding to the plasma mem-brane, it is taken up as a simple solute. This process is referred to as *fluid-phase pinocytosis*.[92] Compounds that bind to the plasma membrane are concentrated at this site and are thus interiorized to a greater extent. The clathrin-coated pit is the main port of entry of pinocytosed ligands.[92] Both occupied and unoccupied receptors are internalized by clathrin-coated pits. Very rapidly, the internalized vesicles lose their coats (referred to as *early endosomes*) and are capable of fusing with one another. Within min-utes, these are converted into a sorting endosome where the fate of receptors and ligands is decided. Some molecules recycle back to the surface in recy-cling endosomes, whereas others are directed to the lysosome in late endosomes. The late endosome fuses with the lysosome.[93] Fluid-phase pinocytosis and hormone-stimulated endocytosis can also occur in the absence of coated pits.

The uptake of soluble immune complexes pro-vides an example of such pinocytosis. These are bound by the macrophage FcR and thus interiorized at a markedly accentuated rate compared with that of soluble protein alone. Both these pinocytic proc-esses are means of antigen uptake by macrophages involved in immunoregulation, and of regulatory factor uptake by all macrophages during growth, differentiation, and execution of function.

Intracellular Digestion

The fusion of endocytic vacuoles, formed as a result of either phagocytosis or pinocytosis, with primary or secondary lysosomes initiates the process of intracellular digestion that results in the degradation of internalized microorganisms or other ingested materials. Intracellular vacuoles are able to exchange their contents by means of membrane fusion. This leads to a constant exchange of digestive enzymes and materials from the extracellular environment.

Intracellular digestion is an enzymatic process utilizing preformed lysosomal hydrolases. Acid hydrolases are synthesized in the endoplasmic reticulum and are stored within the cell in primary and secondary lysosomes. Endocytosis of a number of materials leads to an increase in the level of intracellular macrophage lysosomal hydrolases and other enzymes.[94]

Materials that are endocytosed by macrophages usually do not regain access to the external environment in an undigested form unless the macrophage is killed.[2] After uptake, nondigestible materials, such as colloidal gold or certain bacterial constituents, are stored within secondary lysosomes of the macrophages, where they remain for long periods. Similarly, when digestible proteins are taken up, less than 2 percent of the intracellular material is subsequently released in an undegraded form.

Complex Functions

Complex functions of mononuclear phagocytes include selective removal of senescent autologous cells, resistance to bacterial and viral infection, protection against the development and spread of neoplastic cells, and initiation and regulation of immune responses.

Selective Removal of Senescent Autologous Cells

Mononuclear phagocytes play a central role in the disposal of cell fragments and aging and dying cells, such as senescent erythrocytes. The mononuclear phagocytes of the liver, bone marrow, and spleen remove most of these cells. A number of possible mechanisms have been suggested to explain the ability of macrophages to distinguish normal from aged red blood cells (RBCs). Aged RBCs are less deformable and have a reduced membrane net negative charge in comparison with normal RBCs. In addition, phagocytosis of aged RBCs by macrophages appears to require participation of IgG molecules present in serum. Therefore, the turnover of senescent RBCs, like the clearance of infectious agents, may be regulated by IgG FcR-mediated phagocytosis.

Antimicrobial Function

Several lines of evidence suggest that one of the major antimicrobial mechanisms of mononuclear phagocytes is the production of oxygen metabolites.[95] The susceptibility of an organism to killing is directly related to its ability to trigger the secretion of oxygen metabolites during its ingestion and is inversely related to its level of antioxidant defense pathways. Oxygen metabolites mediate cell injury by disrupting the structure of proteins, lipids, and nucleic acids and by activating thiol groups in enzymes. Oxygen-independent antimicrobial mechanisms include growth inhibition by acidification of the phagosome; iron removal by iron-binding proteins; action of cationic proteins, interferon, and complement components; and digestion by lysozyme and lysosomal hydrolases.[95–97]

Tachyzoites of the parasite *Toxoplasma gondii* reside in macrophage vacuoles, which fail to fuse with acidifying lysosomes, and hence resist macrophage killing. To enter the cell, the tachyzoites bind macrophage VLA-6 by means of laminin adsorbed to their surface. This resistance to killing can be overcome by altering the trophozoite's mode of entry into the cell. Phagocytosis of antibody-coated trophozoites mediated by FcR results in vacuoles capable of fusion with lysosomes.[98] Phagocytosis and fusion appear to involve a domain of the FcR cytoplasmic tail.

Macrophage Activation

Monocytes or macrophages recruited in response to injury or infection are less mature than resident macrophages but are able to generate a respiratory burst, produce reactive oxygen intermedates, release secretory products, and exhibit enhancement in phagocytosis and microbicidal and tumoricidal activities.[99] This is as a result of activation by cytokines produced at the inflammatory site, and by microbial products such as lipopolysaccharide and muramyl dipeptide. The most important cytokine is interferon-γ, secreted by T cells. Other cytokines, including GM-CSF and TNF-α induce generation of reactive oxygen and nitrogen intermediates by macrophages. TNF-α and IL-4 independently synergize with interferon-γ for macrophage activation in parasitic killing.[100] Concomitant with the development of the activated state, other functions such as the ability to multiply may be lost. Some resident macrophages are selectively refractory to the actions of interferon-γ. Kupffer cells fail to generate a respiratory burst after interferon-γ, although class II antigen expression is enhanced.

Two macrophage inflammatory proteins (MIP-1 and MIP-2) are secreted by endotoxin-activated macrophages. Both can cause a localized inflammatory reaction, are chemotactic for and activate human neutrophils in vitro, and synergize with some hemopoietic factors to enhance GM-CSF formation. MIP-1 can act as an endogenous pyrogen.[22] It has become clear that MIP-1 and MIP-2 are members of two large families of cytokines secreted by activated T cells, activated fibroblasts, and macrophages. MIP-1 belongs to a family of cytokines that includes RANTES and the mouse fibroblast gene product JE (probably MCP-1).[23] MIP-2 is a member of the platelet factor 4 family. Platelet factor 4 is also chemotactic for neutrophils. These two families may have arisen from a common gene precursor.[22] IL-8 is another cytokine, produced by lipopolysaccharide-stimulated macrophages, that activates and is chemotactic for neutrophils.[101] Thus, these cytokines, secreted by stimulated macrophages and other cells at the site of inflammation, are important attractors of activated neutrophils to these sites.

As first described by Metchnikoff[7] and later defined by Mackaness, the term *macrophage activation* refers to the development by macrophages of enhanced microbicidal function. Although this phenomenon was found to be induced primarily by interferon-γ,[102] this cytokine can either up- or down-regulate many functional, metabolic, and morphologic properties of macrophages, only some of which are involved in enhanced antimicrobial function. Thus, some investigators have adopted a broader use of the term *macrophage activation* to encompass all the cellular effects of interferon-γ. The concept of macrophage activation is further complicated by the finding that factors other than interferon-γ, such as IL-2, IL-4, and GM-CSF, can mimic or enhance its action on macrophages. Consequently, there is no consensus on the definition of macrophage activation, except that it is a differentiation stage of heightened functional competence.

Antiviral Function

Mononuclear phagocytes have been demonstrated to be important in host defense against viral infection. Host susceptibility to a virus is related to its ability to replicate within the mononuclear phagocytes. For example, adult mice are resistant to infection with herpes simplex virus, whereas newborn mice are highly susceptible to this infection. Herpes simplex is able to replicate in the macrophages of newborn mice but not in adult macrophages. The ability to limit replication of this virus matures in the first 3 weeks of life. Newborn mice can be effectively protected against herpes simplex infection by adoptive transfer of adult macrophages.[103]

On the other hand, pathogens that resist intracellular killing can use macrophage FcRs and C3 receptors for opsonized particles to gain entry into the macrophage, then commence replication unchecked. In the presence of subneutralizing amounts of antiviral antibodies, this phenomenon is known as antibody-dependent enhancement of viral infectivity (ADE).[104] An important example is the entry of human immunodeficiency virus I into macrophages by means of human FcR III and FcR II.[105]

Antineoplastic Function

Macrophages are commonly found in neoplasms in proportions of up to 30 percent. The number can be influenced by the tumor containing them; that is,

some tumors produce chemotactic factors or CSFs, whereas others secrete chemotaxis-inhibiting factors, lymphokines, complement, or substances that prevent macrophage activation.[106]

It has been demonstrated that young mononuclear phagocytes, such as inflammatory macrophages, but not resident tissue macrophages, acquire competance to lyse neoplastic cells in a contact-dependent, nonphagocytic manner in a series of operationally defined stages. In the first stage, macrophages interact with interferon-γ and thereby gain responsiveness to a second signal, such as the lipid A component of bacterial endotoxin or maleylated proteins.[83] Interferon-γ renders macrophages capable of selectively binding tumor cells but not lysing them. Cytolytic competence is acquired only after full activation by the triggering stimuli.

Other factors, which may or may not be secreted by mononuclear phagocytes themselves, can prime the macrophage for cytolytic competence. Interferon-γ and TNF-α are synergistic in their induction of tumoricidal activity in macrophages. Prostaglandin E$_2$ stimulates tumoricidal activity in activated macrophages but depresses antitumor effects in resident macrophages.[107] Somatotropin is as effective as interferon-γ in priming macrophages for superoxide production. Finally, the macrophage products hydrogen peroxide[95] and the complement components[108] are important for tumoricidal killing.

Another antineoplastic mechanism involves antibody coating (arming) of tumor cells. Antibody-coated tumor cells then interact with FcRs on activated macrophages and thereby trigger the release of oxygen metabolites, hydrogen peroxide, and lysosomal enzymes that either kill tumor cells or limit their growth.[109]

Immunoregulation (Fig. 16–3)

Mononuclear phagocytes play a critical role in the induction, regulation, and expression of both cellular and humoral immune responses. Although macrophages are involved in the responses of lymphocytes, they differ from these cells in that they do not themselves possess immunologic specificity but rather act as nonspecific accessory cells.[1]

Antigen uptake is an important function of macrophages in the initiation of an immune response. Antigens may enter the macrophage by fluid–phase pinocytosis. Because antigen may be taken up by absorptive endocytosis after the interaction of antigen with receptors on the surface of the antigen-presenting cell, antigen uptake is augmented by IgG FcR binding in the presence of IgG.[110] Autologous, homologous, and heterologous proteins are taken up in a similar manner, indicating that foreignness per se is not recognized by the macrophage.[111] Such antigens are processed through the endosomes. The processing is sensitive to inhibitors of endosomal and lysosomal proteases. Determinants thus produced associate exclusively with class II MHC molecules in

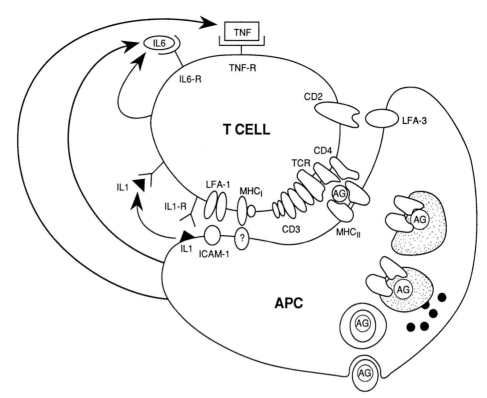

Figure 16–3. Mononuclear phagocytes as antigen-presenting cells (APC). Mononuclear phagocytes endocytose and then process foreign antigen (Ag), which associates with class II MHC molecules (MHC$_{II}$) in the endosome. T cell stimulation requires physical interaction between the class II-Ag complex and the T cell receptor (TCR). During this interaction, a variety of receptor ligand interactions transmit co-stimulatory signals that enhance T cell activation. In addition, cytokines produced by mononuclear phagocytes enhance T cell responses.

the endosome and are transported to the plasma membrane by the Golgi apparatus and its vesicles.[112] An alternative, cytosolic processing pathway exists for proteins that are endogenously synthesized or that penetrate plasma or endosomal membranes. Endogenous synthesis of viral proteins within the target cell and the fusion of a virus with cell membranes are examples of this. These determinants typically associate with class I MHC molecules.

Class I molecules consist of a highly polymorphic glycoprotein α-chain noncovalently bound to β$_2$-microglobulin. Class II molecules consist of two noncovalently bound membrane glycoproteins (α and β), at least one of which is polymorphic. Crystallographic analysis of the structure of the class I molecule reveals a groove at the surface of the molecule formed by the two amino terminal domains.[113] Functional studies strongly indicate that the groove is involved in antigen binding. Although the three-dimensional structure of the class II molecule is not yet available, a similar antigen-binding groove can be predicted.[114]

The class II MHC molecule, expressed by macrophages, can be up-regulated by interferon-γ as well as IL-4 and GM-CSF. In contrast, prostaglandins of the E series (which are secreted after interferon-γ, IL-1, or TNF-α stimulation of macrophages), interferon-α, IL-6, lipopolysaccharide, glucocorticoids, and maleylated proteins in the α$_2$-macroglobulin protease complex are known inhibitors of MHC class II expression.[115, 116] TNF-α down-regulates class II expression to a moderate degree, mostly by suppression of transcription. Not only does IL-4 increase MHC class II expression, it also increases expression

of the adhesion antigens CD11b/CD18 and CD11c/CD18,[117] both of which may be important accessory molecules in mediating T cells and antigen-presenting cells during antigen presentation. GM-CSF enhances MHC class II specifically by macrophages and also enhances a number of other functional activities of these cells that may make them more effective antigen-presenting cells.[58] Kupffer cells constitutively express class I and II MHC molecules and can function as antigen-presenting cells.[118] Microglial cells can also express class II and function as antigen-presenting cells after exposure to interferon-γ.[119] In contrast, alveolar macrophages have poor antigen-presenting ability.

T cell activation requires physical interaction between the T cell receptor and processed antigen presented by the MHC molecule of the antigen-presenting cell. Signals thus generated may be transduced to T cells by CD3—a molecular complex of at least five components that is noncovalently linked to the T cell receptor.[120] Macrophages are not unique in their capacity to act as antigen-presenting cells. Thus, Langerhans' cells of the skin, dendritic cells of the lymphoid organs and blood, and activated B cells can all function as antigen-presenting cells.[1, 121–123]

Among these accessory cells exist cells of both high accessory cell potency, such as dendritic cells and blood monocytes, and low potency, such as resident tissue macrophages. Both B cells and monocytes may develop dendritic morphology in culture,[124, 125] and cells with dendritic morphology and high accessory ability have been produced by culturing monocytes.[124] Cytokines derived from either monocytes or B cells may modify antigen-presenting capacity acquired during differentiation. Thus, IL-1, IL-6, and TNF-α can enhance responses of T cells stimulated by low-potency antigen-presenting cells.[126] Peripheral blood dendritic cells express CD13 and CD33 but not CD14, indicating that they are likely of myeloid origin. Their cell surface phenotype, potent APC capacity, and reduced capacity for phagocytosis and digestion indicate that dendritic cells are functionally distinct from monocytes.[126a]

Some resident tissue (e.g., lung and liver) macrophages that express class II antigens are, however, inadequate antigen-presenting cells for resting T cells.[40, 41] Thus, in addition to the interaction between the processed antigen–class II complex on the macrophage and the antigen receptor on the T cell, antigen-presenting macrophages may be required to deliver other activation signals to resting T cells. These appear to involve a variety of T cell surface molecules and their macrophage ligands, including CD2/LFA-3, CD4/class II, LFA-1/ICAM-1, and CD28, CD5, and MHC class I with undefined ligands.[127] Other molecules are almost certainly involved in this cosignaling process. It is therefore likely that poor antigen-presenting cells, such as lung and liver macrophages, do not express or secrete the ligands for one or more of these T cell surface molecules. Macrophages that possess all or even some of the properties of a complete antigen-presenting cell, however, have been shown to be capable of facilitating the function for such incomplete antigen-presenting cells.[42, 128] Thus, macrophages can also play an auxiliary role in antigen presentation to resting T cells.

Several secretory products of macrophages are involved in immunoregulation. IL-1 was the first example of a macrophage-derived cytokine involved in the initiation and propagation of immune responses.[129] IL-1 enhances IL-2 and interferon-γ production, induces IL-2 receptors on T cells, and augments cytotoxic T cell activity. TNF-α is another secretory product of macrophages that may augment T cell responsiveness to antigen directly[130] or by stimulation of other cytokines such as IL-6.[131] In addition, TNF-α may enhance or diminish the capacity of macrophages to initiate T cell responses by stimulating them to produce IL-1 as well as prostaglandin E_2.[89] Macrophages also produce substances that suppress T cell activation directly or indirectly. These include prostaglandin, hydrogen peroxide, arginase, oxygen metabolites,[95, 96, 132] and the IL-1 receptor inhibitor.[87]

CONCLUSION

The mononuclear phagocyte system is a dynamic collection of lineally related cells whose functions are extremely varied and critical to normal homeostasis and host defense. Mononuclear phagocytes participate in a variety of physiologic and pathologic events. This ability relies on their capacity to respond to environmental stimuli with an increase in maturation of effector cells, enhancement of tissue migration, and functional modulation of individual cells to meet the immediate needs of the organism.

References

1. Unanue, E. R., and Allen, P. M.: The basis for the immunoregulatory role of macrophages and other accessory cells. Science 236:551, 1987.
2. Andrews, P. W., Jackett, P. S., and Lowrie, D. B.: Killing and degradation of microorganisms by macrophages. In Dean, R. T., and Jessup, W. (eds.): Mononuclear Phagocytes: Physiology and Pathology. Amsterdam, Elsevier, 1985.
3. Varesio, L.: Induction and expression of tumoricidal activity by macrophages. In Dean, R. T., and Jessup, W. (eds.): Mononuclear Phagocytes: Physiology and Pathology. Amsterdam, Elsevier, 1985.
4. Stashenko, P., Dewhirst, F. E., Peros, W. J., Kent, R. L., and Ago, J. M.: Synergistic interactions between interleukin 1, tumor necrosis factor, and lymphotoxin in bone resorption. J. Immunol. 138:1464, 1987.
5. Dohlman, J. G., and Goetzl, W. J.: Determinants of generation and structural heterogeneity of fibroblast-activating principles of human mononuclear phagocytes. In van-Furth, R. (ed.): Mononuclear Phagocytes: Characteristics, Physiology and Function. Dordrecht, Martinus Nijhoff, 1985.
6. Larsen, G. L., and Henson, P. M.: Mediators of inflammation. Annu. Rev. Immunol. 1:335, 1983.
7. Metchnikoff, E.: Lectures on the comparative pathology of inflammation. In Starling, F. A., and Starling, E. H. (eds.): London, Kegan, Paul, Trench, Treubner and Company, 1883.
8. van-Furth, R., Langevoort, H. L., and Schaberg, A.: Mononuclear phagocytes in human pathology: Proposal for an approach to improved classification. In van-Furth, R. (ed.): Mononuclear Phagocytes in Immunity, Infection and Pathology. Oxford, Blackwell Scientific Publications, 1975.
9. van-Furth, R., Cohn, Z. A., Hirsch, J. G., Spector, W. G., and Langevoort, H. L.: The mononuclear phagocyte system: A new classification of macrophages, monocytes, and their precursor cells. Bull. WHO 46:845, 1972.
10. van-Furth, R.: Macrophage activity and clinical immunology: Origin and kinetics of mononuclear phagocytes. Ann. N.Y. Acad. Sci. 278:161, 1976.
11. Harlan, J. M.: Leukocyte-endothelial interactions. Blood 65:513, 1985.
12. Albelda, S. M., and Buck, C. A.: Integrins and other cell adhesion molecules. FASEB J. 4:2868, 1990.
13. Arnaout, M. A.: Structure and function of the leukocyte adhesion molecules CD11/CD18. Blood 75:1037, 1990.
14. Springer, T. A., Dustin, M. L., Kishimoto, T. K., and Marlin, S. D.: The lymphocyte function-associated LFA-1, CD2, and LFA-3 molecules: Cell adhesion receptors of the immune system. Annu. Rev. Immunol. 5:223, 1987.
15. Wawryk, S. O., Novotny, J. R., Wicks, I. P., Wilkinson, D., Maher, D., Salvaris, E., Welch, K., Fecondo, J., and Boyd, A. W.: The role of the LFA-1/ICAM-1 interaction in human leukocyte homing and adhesion. Immunol. Rev. 108:135, 1989.
16. Stacker, S. A., and Springer, T. A.: Leukocyte integrin p150,95 (CD11c/CD18) functions as an adhesion molecule binding to a counter-receptor on stimulated endothelium. J. Immunol. 146:648, 1991.
17. Dana, N., and Arnaout, M. A.: Leukocyte adhesion molecular (CD11/CD18) deficiency. In Kazatchine, M. (ed.): Balliere's Clinical Immunology and Allergy. Philadelphia, W.B. Saunders Company, 1988.
18. Chatila, T. A., Geha, R. S., and Arnaout, M. A.: Constitutive and stimulus-induced phosphorylation of CD11/CD18 leukocyte adhesion molecules. J. Cell Biol. 109:3435, 1989.
19. Kishimoto, T. K., Jutila, M. A., Berg, E. L., and Butcher, E. C.: Neutrophil Mac-1 and MEL-14 adhesion proteins inversely regulated by chemotactic factors. Science 245:1238, 1989.
20. Streeter, P. R., Berg, E. L., Rouse, B. T., Bargatze, R. F., and Butcher, E. C.: A tissue-specific endothelial cell molecule involved in lymphocyte homing. Nature 331:41, 1988.
21. Wilkinson, P. C.: Cellular and molecular aspects of chemotaxis of macrophages and monocytes. In Nelson, D. S. (ed.): Immunobiology of the Macrophage. New York, Academic Press, 1976.
22. Wolpe, S. D., and Cerami, A.: Macrophage inflammatory proteins 1 and 2: members of a novel superfamily of cytokines. FASEB J. 3:2565, 1989.
23. Yoshimura, T., and Leonard, E. J.: Production by human fibroblasts of monocyte chemoattractant protein-1, the product of gene JE. J. Immunol. 144:2377, 1990.
24. Schall, T. J., Bacon, K., Toy, K. J., and Goeddel, D. V.: Selective

attraction of monocytes and T lymphocytes of the memory phenotype by cytokine RANTES. Nature 347:669, 1990.

25. Weiser, W. Y., Temple, P. A., Witek-Giannotti, J. S., Clark, S. C., and David, J. R.: Molecular cloning of a cDNA encoding a human macrophage migration inhibitory factor. Proc. Natl. Acad. Sci. U.S.A. 86:7522, 1989.

26. Hartwig, J. H., Chambers, K. A., and Stossel, T. P.: Association of gelsolin with actin filaments and cell membranes of macrophages and platelets. J. Cell Biol. 108:467, 1989.

27. Yin, H. L.: Gelsolin: calcium- and polyphosphoinositide-regulated actin-modulating protein. Bioessays 7:176, 1987.

28. Lad, P. M., Olson, C. V., Grewal, I. S., and Scott, S. J.: A pertussis toxin-sensitive GTP-binding protein in the human neutrophil regulates multiple receptors, calcium mobilization, and lectin-induced capping. Proc. Natl. Acad. Sci. U.S.A. 82:8643, 1985.

29. Allen, R. A., Traynor, A. E., Omann, G. M., and Jesaitis, A. J.: The chemotactic peptide receptor. Hematol. Oncol. Clin. North Am. 2:33, 1988.

30. Berger, M., Birx, D. L., Wetzler, E. M., OShea, J. J., Brown, E. J., and Cross, A. S.: Calcium requirements for increased complement receptor expression during neutrophil activation. J. Immunol. 135:1342, 1985.

31. Fedorko, M. E., and Hirsch, J. G.: Structure of monocytes and macrophages. Semin. Hematol. 7:109, 1970.

32. van-Furth, R., Diesselhoff-Den Dulk, M. M. C., Sluiter, W., and van-Dissel, J. T.: New perspectives on the kinetics of mononuclear phagocytes. In van-Furth, R. (ed.): Mononuclear Phagocytes: Characteristics, Physiology and Funtion. Dordrecht, Martinus Nijhoff, 1985.

33. Bouwens, L., Baekeland, M., and Wisse, E.: A balanced view on the origin of Kupffer cells. In Kirn, A., Knook, D. L., and Wisse, E. (eds.): Cells of the Hepatic Sinusoid. Vol 1. Rijswijk, The Netherlands, Kupffer Cell Foundation, 1986.

34. Papadimitriou, J. M., and Spector, W. G.: The origin, properties and fate of epithelioid cells. J. Pathol. 105:187, 1971.

35. Papadimitriou, J. M., and van Bruggen, I.: Evidence that multi-nucleate giant cells are examples of mononuclear phagocytic differentiation. J. Pathol. 148:149, 1986.

36. Kreipe, H., Radzun, H. J., Rudolph, P., Barth, J., Hansmann, M. L., Heidorn, K., and Parwaresch, M. R.: Multinucleated giant cells generated in vitro: Terminally differentiated macrophages with down-regulated c-fms expression. Am. J. Pathol. 130:232, 1988.

37. Kinsella, T. D., Baum, J., and Ziff, M.: Studies of isolated synovial lining cells of rheumatoid and non-rheumatoid synovial membranes. Arthritis Rheum. 13:734, 1970.

38. Burmester, G. R., Dimitriu-Bona, A., Waters, S. J., and Winchester, R. J.: Identification of three major synovial cell lining populations by monoclonal antibodies directed to Ia antigens and antigens associated with monocytes/macrophages and fibroblasts. Scand. J. Immunol. 17:69, 1983.

39. Tsai, V., Bergroth, V., and Zvaifler, N. J.: Synovial dendritic cells and T cells in rheumatoid arthritis. Scand. J. Rheumatol. 74:79, 1988.

40. Mayernik, D. G., Ul-Haq, A., and Rinehart, J. J.: Differentiation-associated alteration in human monocyte-macrophage accessory cell function. J. Immunol. S130:21, 1983.

41. Toews, G. B., Vial, W. C., Dunn, M. M., Guzzetta, P., Nunez, G., Stastny, P., and Lipscomb, M. F.: The accessory cell function of human alveolar macrophages in specific T cell proliferation. J. Immunol. 132:181, 1984.

42. Rubinstein, D., Roska, A. K., and Lipsky, P. E.: Antigen presentation by liver sinusoidal lining cells after antigen exposure in vivo. J. Immunol. 138:1377, 1987.

43. Vicenzi, E., Biondi, A., Bordignon, C., Rambaldi, A., Donati, M. B., and Mantovani, A.: Human mononuclear phagocytes from different anatomical sites differ in their capacity to metabolize arachidonic acid. Clin. Exp. Immunol. 57:385, 1984.

44. Dougherty, G. J., and McBride, W. H.: Macrophage heterogeneity. J. Clin. Lab. Immunol. 14:1, 1984.

45. Todd, R. F., and Schlossman, S.: Utilization of monoclonal antibodies in the characterization of monocyte–macrophage differentiation antigens. In Bellanti, J. A., and Herscowitz, H. B. (eds.): Immunology of the Reticuloendothelial System: A Comprehensive Treatise. New York, Plenum Press, 1984.

46. Metcalf, D.: The molecular control of cell division, differentiation commitment and maturation in hemopoietic cells. Nature 339:27, 1989.

47. Ikebuchi, K., Wong, G. G., Clark, S. C., Ihle, J. N., Hirai, Y., and Ogawa, M.: Interleukin-6 enhancement of interleukin 3-dependent proliferation of multipotential hemopoietic precursors. Proc. Natl. Acad. Sci. U.S.A. 84:9035, 1987.

48. Katayama, K., Koizumi, S., Ueno, Y., Ohno, I., Ichihara, T., Horita, S., Miyawaki, T., and Taniguchi, N.: Antagonistic effects of interleukin 6 and G-CSF in the later stage of human granulopoiesis in vitro. Exp. Hematol. 18:390, 1990.

49. Zsebo, K. M., Williams, D. A., Geissler, E. N., Broudy, V. C., Martin, F. H., Atkins, H. L., Hsu, R. Y., Birkett, N. C., Okino, K. H., and Murdock, D. C.: Stem cell factor is encoded at the SI locus of the mouse and is the ligand for the c-kit tyrosine kinase receptor. Cell 63:213, 1990.

50. Martin, F. H., Suggs, S. V., Langley, K. E., Lu, H. S., Ting, J., Okino, K. H., Morris, C. F., McNiece, I. K., Jacobsen, F. W., and Mendiaz, E. A.: Primary structure and functional expression of rat and human stem cell factor DNAs. Cell 63:203, 1990.

51. Nicola, N. A.: Why do hemopoietic growth factors interact with each other? Immunol. Today 8:134, 1987.

52. Walker, F., Nicola, N. A., Metcalf, D., and Burgess, A. W.: Hierarchical down-modulation of hemopoietic growth factor receptors. Cell 43:269, 1985.

53. Sherr, C. J., Rettenmier, C. W., Sacca, R., Roussel, M. F., Look, A. T., and Stanley, E. R: The c-fms proto-oncogene product is related to the receptor for the mononuclear phagocyte growth factor, CSF-1. Cell 41:665, 1985.

54. Stanley, E. R.: Action of the colony-stimulating factor, CSF-1. In Evered, D., Nugent, J., and O'Connor, M. (eds.): Biochemistry of Macrophages. London, Pitman, 1986.

55. Bagby, G. C., Shaw, G., and Segal, G. M.: Human vascular endothelial cells, granulopoiesis, and the inflammatory response. J. Invest. Dermatol. 93:48S, 1989.

56. Kelley, K. W.: The role of growth hormone in modulation of the immune response. Ann. N.Y. Acad. Sci. 594:95, 1990.

57. Cannistra, S. A., and Griffin, J. D.: Regulation of the production and function of granulocytes and monocytes. Semin. Hematol. 15:173, 1988.

58. Alvaro-Gracia, J. M., Zvaifler, N. J., and Firestein, G. S.: Cytokines in chronic inflammatory arthritis IV. Granulocyte/macrophage colony-stimulating factor–mediated induction of class II MHC antigen on human monocytes: a possible role in rheumatoid arthritis. J. Exp. Med. 170:865, 1989.

59. Horiguchi, J., Warren, M. K., and Kufe, D.: Expression of the macrophage-specific colony-stimulating factor in human monocytes treated with granulocyte-macrophage colony-stimulating factor. Blood 69:1259, 1987.

60. Lieschke, G. J., Maher, D., Cebon, J., O'Connor, M., Green, M., Sheridan, W., Boyd, A., Rallings, M., Bonnem, E., Metcalf, D., et al.: Effects of bacterially synthesized recombinant human granulocyte-macrophage colony-stimulating factor in patients with advanced malignancy. Ann. Intern. Med 110:357, 1989.

61. Sluiter, W., Hulsig-Hesselink, E., and van-Furth, R.: Synthesis and release of factor inducing monocytopoiesis (FIM) by macrophages. In Rossi, F., and Patriarca, P. (eds.): Biochemistry and Function of Phagocytes. New York, Plenum Press, 1982.

62. Tomida, M.: Regulation of differentiation of normal and leukemic precursors, In Dean, R. T., and Jessup, W. (eds.): Mononuclear Phagocytes: Physiology and Pathology. Amsterdam, Elsevier, 1985.

63. Thiele, D. L., and Lipsky, P. E.: Mononuclear phagocytes: Phenotype and function. Surv. Immunol. Res. 3:142, 1984.

64. Unkeless, J. C., Fleit, H., and Mellman, I. S.: Structural aspects and heterogeneity of immunoglobulin Fc receptors. Adv. Immunol. 31:247, 1981.

65. Mellman, I. S.: Relationships between structure and function in the Fc receptor family. Curr. Opin. Immunol. 1:16, 1988.

66. Grey, H. M., and Chesnut, R.: Antigen processing and presentation to T cells. Immunol. Today 6:101, 1985.

67. Bodmer, J. L.: Membrane receptors for particles and opsonins. In Dean, R. T., and Jessup, W. (eds.): Mononuclear Phagocytes: Physiology and Pathology. Amsterdam, Elsevier, 1985.

68. Dierich, M. P.: Complement-dependent ligand receptor interactions in inflammatory responses. In Russo, F., Mencia-Huerta, M. J. M., and Chignard, M. (eds.): Advances in Inflammation Research. Vol 10. New York, Raven Press, 1986.

69. Griffin, F. M., Jr.: Activation of macrophage complement receptors for phagocytosis. Contemp. Top. Immunobiol. 13:57, 1984.

70. Snyderman, R., Phillips, J. K., and Mergenhagen, S. E.: Biological activity of complement in vivo: Role of C5 in the accumulation of polymorphonuclear leukocytes in inflammatory exudates. J. Exp. Med. 134:1131, 1971.

71. Wright, S. D., Detmers, P. A., Jong, M. T., and Meyer, B. C.: Interferon-gamma depresses binding of ligand by C3b and C3bi receptors on cultured human monocytes, an effect reversed by fibronectin. J. Exp. Med. 163:1245, 1986.

72. Brown, D. L., Phillips, D. R., Damsky, C. H., and Charo, I. F.: Synthesis and expression of the fibroblast fibronectin receptor in human monocytes. J. Clin. Invest. 84:366, 1989.

73. Elices, M. J., Osborn, L., Takada, Y., Crouse, C., Luhowskyj, S., Hemler, M. E., and Lobb, R. R.: VCAM-1 on activated endothelium interacts with the leukocyte integrin VLA-4 at a site distinct from the VLA-4/fibronectin binding site. Cell 60:577, 1990.

74. Shaw, L. M., Messier, J. M., and Mercurio, A., M.: The activation dependent adhesion of macrophages to laminin involves cytoskeletal anchoring and phosphorylation of the alpha 6 beta 1 integrin. J. Cell. Biol. 110:2167, 1990.

75. Adams, D. O., and Hamilton, T. A.: Phagocytic cells: Cytotoxic activities of macrophages. *In* Gallin, J. I., Goldstein, R., and Snyderman, R. (eds.): Inflammation: Basic Principles and Clinical Correlates. New York, Raven Press, 1988.

76. Spriggs, M. K., Lioubin, P. J., Slack, J., Dower, S. K., Jonas, U., Cosman, D., Sims, J. E., and Bauer, J.: Induction of an interleukin-1 receptor (IL-1R) on monocytic cells: Evidence that the receptor is not encoded by a T cell-type IL-1R mRNA. J. Biol. Chem. 265:22499, 1990.

77. Kammer, G. M.: The adenylate cyclase-cAMP-protein kinase A pathway and regulation of the immune response. Immunol. Today 9:222, 1988.

78. Bauer, J., Bauer, T. M., Kalb, T., Taga, T., Lengyel, G., Hirano, T., Kishimoto, T., Acs, G., Mayer, L., and Gerok, W.: Regulation of interleukin 6 receptor expression in human monocytes and monocyte-derived macrophages: Comparison with the expression in human hepatocytes. J. Exp. Med. 170(5):1537, 1989.

79. Holter, W., Goldman, C. K., Casabo, L., Nelson, D. L., Greene, W. C., and Waldmann, T. A.: Expression of functional IL-2 receptors by lipopolysaccharide and interferon-gamma stimulated human monocytes. J. Immunol. 138:2917, 1987.

80. Abramson, S. L., and Gallin, J. I.: IL-4 inhibits superoxide formation by human mononuclear phagocytes. J. Immunol. 144:625, 1990.

80a. Wong, H. L., Lotze, M. T., Wahl, L. M., and Wahl, S. M.: Administration of recombinant IL-4 to humans regulates gene expression, phenotype, and function in circulating monocytes. J. Immunol. 148:2118, 1992.

81. Snyder, D. S., Beller, D. I., and Unanue, E. R.: Prostaglandins modulate macrophage Ia expression. Nature 299:163, 1982.

82. Knudsen, P. J., Dinarello, C. A., and Strom, T. B.: Prostaglandins posttranscriptionally inhibit monocyte expression of interleukin 1 activity by increasing intracellular cyclic adenosine monophosphate. J. Immunol. 137:3189, 1986.

83. Johnson, W. J., Pizzo, S. V., Imber, M. J., and Adams, D. O.: Receptors for maleylated proteins regulate secretion of neutral proteases by murine macrophages. Science 218:574, 1982.

84. Rappolee, D. A., and Werb, Z.: Secretory products of phagocytes. Curr. Opin. Immunol. 1:47, 1988.

85. Pantalone, R. M., and Page, R. C.: Lymphokine-induced production and release of lysosomal enzymes by macrophages. Proc. Natl. Acad. Sci. U.S.A. 72:2091, 1975.

86. Gordon, S.: Regulation of enzyme secretion by mononuclear phagocytes: Studies with macrophage plasminogen activator and lysozyme. Fed. Proc. 37:2754, 1978.

87. Arend, W. P., Joslin, F. G., and Massoni, R. J.: Effects of immune complexes on production by human monocytes of interleukin 1 or an interleukin 1 inhibitor. J. Immunol. 134:3868, 1985.

88. Wahl, S. M., Hunt, D. A., Wong, H. L., Dougherty, S., McCartney-Francis, N., Wahl, L. M., Ellingsworth, L., Schmidt, J. A., Hall, G., Roberts, A. B., et al.: Transforming growth factor-beta is a potent immunosuppressive agent that inhibits IL-1-dependent lymphocyte proliferation. J. Immunol. 140:3026, 1988.

89. Bachwich, P. R., Chensue, S. W., Larrick, J. W., and Kunkel, S. L.: Tumor necrosis factor stimulates interleukin-1 and prostaglandin E2 production in resting macrophages. Biochem. Biophys. Res. Commun. 136:94, 1986.

90. Schade, U. F., Burmeister, I., Elekes, E., Engel, R., and Wolter, D. T.: Mononuclear phagocytes and eicosanoids: Aspects of their synthesis and biological activities. Blut 59:475, 1989.

91. Ofek, I., and Sharon, N.: Lectinophagocytosis: a molecular mechanism of recognition between cell surface sugars and lectins in the phagocytosis of bacteria. Infect. Immun. 56:539, 1988.

92. Duncan, R., and Pratten, M. K.: Pinocytosis: Mechanism and regulation. *In* Dean, R. T., and Jessup, W. (eds.): Mononuclear Phagocytes: Physiology and Pathology. Amsterdam, Elsevier, 1985.

93. Kaplan, J., and Ward, D. M.: Movement of receptors and ligands through the endocytic apparatus in alveolar macrophages. Am. J. Physiol. 258:L263, 1990.

94. Axline, S. G.: Functional biochemistry of the macrophage. Semin. Hematol. 7:142, 1970.

95. Nathan, C. F.: Secretion of toxic oxygen products by macrophages: Regulatory cytokines and their effect on the oxidase. *In* Evered, D., Nugent, J., and O'Connor, M. (eds.): Biochemistry of Macrophages. London, Pitman, 1986.

96. Nathan, C. F.: Secretion of oxygen intermediates: role in effector functions of activated macrophages. Fed. Proc. 41:2206, 1982.

97. Rothermel, C. D., Rubin, B. Y., Jaffe, E. A., and Murray, H. W.: Oxygen-independent inhibition of intracellular *Chlamydia psittaci* growth by human monocytes and interferon-gamma–activated macrophages. J. Immunol. 137:689, 1986.

98. Joiner, K. A., Fuhrman, S. A., Miettinen, H. M., Kasper, L. H., and Mellman, I. S.: *Toxoplasma gondii*: Fusion competence of parasitophorous vacuoles in Fc receptor–transfected fibroblasts. Science 249:641, 1990.

99. Nathan, C. F.: Mechanisms of macrophage antimicrobial activity. Trans. R. Soc. Trop. Med. Hyg. 77:620, 1983.

100. Bogdan, C., Mol, H., Solbach, W., and Rollinghoff, M.: Tumor necrosis factor-alpha in combination with interferon-gamma, but not with interleukin-4 activates murine macrophages for elimination of *Leishmania* major amastigotes. Eur. J. Immunol 20:1131, 1990.

101. Djeu, J. T., Matsushima, K., Oppenheim, J. J., Shiotsuki, K., and Blanchard, D. K.: Functional activation of human neutrophils by recombinant monocyte–derived neutrophil chemotactic factor/IL-8. J. Immunol. 144:2205, 1990.

102. Nathan, C. F.: Interferon-gamma and macrophage activation in cell-mediated immunity. *In* Steinman, R. M., and North, R. J. (eds.): Mechanisms of Host Resistance to Infectious Agents, Tumors and Allografts. New York, Rockefeller University Press, 1986.

103. Hirsch, M. S., Zisman, B., and Allison, A. C.: Macrophages and age-dependent resistance to herpes simplex virus in mice. J. Immunol. 104:1160, 1970.

104. Kauffmann, S. H., and Reddehase, M. J.: Infection of phagocytic cells. Curr. Opin. Immunol. 2:43, 1989.

105. Homsy, J., Meyer, M., Tateno, M., Clarkson, S., and Levy, J. A.: The Fc and not CD4 receptor mediates antibody enhancement of HIV infection in human cells. Science 244:1357, 1989.

106. Lipton, J. H., and Sachs, L.: Characterization of macrophage- and granulocyte-inducing proteins for normal and leukemic myeloid cells produced by the Krebs ascites tumor. Biochim. Biophys. Acta 673:552, 1981.

107. Taffet, S. M., and Russell, S. W.: Macrophage-mediated tumor cell killing: Regulation of expression of cytolytic activity by prostaglandin E$_2$. J. Immunol. 126:424, 1981.

108. Pettersen, H. B., Johnson, E., and Hetland, G.: Human alveolar macrophages synthesize active complement components C6, C7, and C8 in vitro. Scand. J. Immunol. 25:567, 1987.

109. Adams, D. O., Johnson, W. J., Fiorito, E., and Nathan, C. F.: Hydrogen peroxide and cytolytic factor can interact synergistically in effecting cytolysis of neoplastic targets. J. Immunol. 127:1973, 1981.

110. Cohn, Z. A.: Biochemistry of macrophages: The first line of defence—Chairman's introduction. Ciba Found. Symp. 118:1, 1986.

111. Babbitt, B. P., Matsueda, G., Haber, E., Unanue, E. R., and Allen, P. M.: Antigenic competition at the level of peptide-Ia binding. Proc. Natl. Acad. Sci. U.S.A. 83:4509, 1986.

112. Yewdell, J. W., and Bennink, J. R.: The binary logic of antigen processing and presentation to T cells. Cell 62:203, 1990.

113. Bjorkman, P. J., Saper, M. A., Samraoui, B., Bennett, W. S., Strominger, J. L., and Wiley, D. C.: The foreign antigen binding site and T cell recognition regions of class I histocompatibility antigens. Nature 329:512, 1987.

114. Brown, J. H., Jardetzky, T., Saper, M. A., Samraoui, B., Bjorkman, P. J., and Wiley, D. C.: A hypothetical model of the foreign antigen binding site of class II histocompatibility molecules. Nature 332:845, 1988.

115. Fertsch, D., Schoenberg, D. R., Germain, R. N., Tou, J. Y., and Vogel, S. N.: Induction of macrophage Ia antigen expression by rIFN-gamma and down-regulation by IFN-alpha/beta and dexamethasone are mediated by changes in steady-state levels of Ia mRNA. J. Immunol. 139:244, 1987.

116. Stuart, P. M., Zlotnik, A., and Woodward, J. G.: Induction of class I and class II MHC antigen expression on murine bone marrow-derived macrophages by IL-4 (B cell stimulatory factor 1). J. Immunol. 140:1542, 1988.

117. te-Velde, A. A., Klomp, J. P., Yard, B. A., de-Vries, J. E., and Figdor, C. G.: Modulation of phenotypic and functional properties of human peripheral blood monocytes by IL-4. J. Immunol. 140:1548, 1988.

118. Rogoff, T. M., and Lipsky, P. E.: Role of the Kupffer cells in local and systemic immune responses. Gastroenterology 80:854, 1981.

119. Frei, K., Siepl, C., Groscurth, P., Bodmer, S., and Fontana, A.: Immunobiology of microglial cells. Ann. N.Y. Acad. Sci. 540:218, 1988.

120. Brenner, M. B., Trowbridge, I. S., and Strominger, J. L.: Cross-linking of human T cell receptor proteins: Association between the T cell idiotype beta subunit and the T3 glycoprotein heavy subunit. Cell 40:183, 1985.

121. Bjercke, S., Elg, J., Braathen, L., and Thorsby, E.: Enriched epidermal Langerhans cells are potent antigen-presenting cells for T cells. J. Invest. Dermatol. 83:286, 1984.

122. Klinkert, W. E., LaBadie, J. H., and Bowers, W. E.: Accessory and stimulating properties of dendritic cells and macrophages isolated from various rat tissues. J. Exp. Med. 156:1, 1982.

123. Ashwell, J. D., DeFranco, A. L., Paul, W. E., and Schwartz, R. H.: Antigen presentation by resting B cells: Radiosensitivity of the antigen-presentation function and two distinct pathways of T cell activation. J. Exp. Med. 159:881, 1984.

124. Najar, H. M., Bru-Capdeville, A. C., and Gieseler, R. H.: Differentiation of human monocytes into accessory cells at serum-free conditions. Eur. J. Cell Biol. 51:339, 1990.

125. Corradi, M. P., Jelinek, D. F., Ramberg, J. E., and Lipsky, P. E.: Development of a cell with dendritic morphology from a precursor of B lymphocyte lineage. J. Immunol. 138:2075, 1987.

126. Ruppert, J., and Peters, J. H.: IL-6 and IL-1 enhance the accessory activity of human blood monocytes during differentiation to macrophages. J. Immunol. 146:144, 1991.

126a. Thomas, R., Davis, L. S., and Lipsky, P. E.: Evidence for the myeloid lineage of human peripheral blood dendritic cells. FASEB J. 6:1973, 1992.

127. Geppert, T. D., and Lipsky, P. E.: Antigen presentation at the inflammatory site. Crit. Rev. Immunol. 9:313, 1989.

128. Roska, A. K., and Lipsky, P. E.: Dissection of the functions of antigen-presenting cells in the induction of T cell activation. J. Immunol. 135:2953, 1985.

129. Oppenheim, J. J., Kovacs, E. J., Matsushima, K., and Durum, S. K.: There is more than one interleukin-1. Immunol. Today 1986.

130. Yokota, S., Geppert, T. D., and Lipsky, P. E.: Enhancement of antigen- and mitogen-induced human T lymphocyte proliferation by tumor necrosis factor-alpha. J. Immunol. 140:531, 1988.

131. Lotz, M., Jirik, F., Kabouridis, P., Tsoukas, C., Hirano, T., Kishimoto, T., and Carson, D. A.: B cell stimulating factor 2/interleukin 6 is a costimulant for human thymocytes and T lymphocytes. J. Exp. Med. 167:1253, 1988.

132. Denham, S., and Rowland, I. J.: Inhibition of the reactive proliferation of lymphocytes by activated macrophages: the role of nitric oxide. Clin. Exp. Immunol. 87:157, 1992.

Chapter 17

The Mast Cell

Immediate-type hypersensitivity reactions (type I) typically begin in tissues with the activation of mast cells, which often leads to the recruitment and activation of basophils, eosinophils, and other cell types. Mediators of mast cells stored preformed inside secretory granules (Table 17–1) are released with cell activation. Other mediators not present in a preformed state are synthesized (Tables 17–2 and 17–3) and secreted directly. In humans, preformed mediators include histamine, proteoglycans (heparin, chondroitin sulfates), and neutral proteases (tryptase, chymase, cathepsin G–like protease, and carboxypeptidase), along with modest amounts of ubiquitous acid hydrolases. Newly generated mediators include lipids, principally the arachidonic acid metabolites, prostaglandin D_2 (PGD_2) and leukotriene C_4 (LTC_4), and smaller amounts of LTB_4. In addition, cytokines such as interleukin-4 (IL-4) and tumor necrosis factor alpha (TNF-α) are produced by activated mast cells (see Table 17–3). Together, these products of mast cells account for much of the host response.

Mast cells are positioned in tissues at potential portals of entry of noxious substances. Normally residing in the circulation, basophils enter tissues at sites of inflammation, particularly during the late phase of allergic reactions and during the early phase of delayed-type hypersensitivity reactions. The selected participation of basophils and different types of mast cells in various clinical conditions—as well as the duration, intensity, and tissue distribution of a particular response—depend on various characteristics of the agonist, immunologic sensitivity of the host, the target tissue involved, and any underlying abnormality.

Two types of mast cells have been observed in human tissues. The distinctive tissue distributions and mediator compositions of each mast cell type suggest a purposeful presence for each and a higher level of complexity concerning the pathobiologic mechanisms and pharmacologic control of mast cell–mediated reactions than previously appreciated. This chapter focuses on the different types of human mast cells and on human basophils because of their obvious relevance to human disease.

DIFFERENT TYPES OF MAST CELLS

Histochemistry, Composition, Distribution, and Morphology

Two distinct types of human mast cells have been described based on different protease compo-

Table 17–1. PREFORMED MEDIATORS OF MAST CELLS AND BASOPHILS

Cell Type	Biogenic Amine	Neutral Protease	Proteoglycan
Human Mast Cells			
MC$_T$ (mucosal)	Histamine	Tryptase	Heparin, chondroitin sulfate E
MC$_{TC}$ (connective tissue)	Histamine Chymase Carboxypeptidase Cathepsin G-like	Tryptase	Heparin, chondroitin sulfate E
Human Basophils	Histamine		Chondroitin sulfate A
Rat Mast Cells			
Mucosal (RBL-1)	Histamine	Chymase II (RMCPII)	Chondroitin sulfate di-B
Connective tissue	Histamine Serotonin	Chymase I (RMCPI) Carboxypeptidase A Tryptase–trypstatin	Heparin
Mouse Mast Cells			
Mucosal	Histamine	Chymases MMCP-1, 2, 4	Chondroitin sulfate E
Connective tissue	Histamine Serotonin	Chymases MMCP-4, 5 Tryptase MMCP-6 Carboxypeptidase	Heparin
Bone marrow derived IL-3 dependent	Histamine Serotonin	Tryptase MMCP-6 mRNA Carboxypeptidase A mRNA	Chondroitin sulfate E
Dog Mast Cells	Histamine	Chymase Tryptase	Heparin Chondroitin disulfate

Table 17–2. NEWLY GENERATED METABOLITES OF ARACHIDONIC ACID FROM MAST CELLS AND BASOPHILS

Cell Type	Lipoxygenase		Cyclooxygenase PGD$_2$
	LTC$_4$	LTB$_4$	
Human Mast Cells			
MC$_T$	+ +	+	+ +
MC$_{TC}$	+ +	+	+ +
Human Basophils	+ +		−
Rat Mast Cells			
Bone marrow derived IL-3 dependent	+ +		+
Connective tissue	+	+	+ +
Mouse Mast Cells			
Bone marrow derived IL-3 dependent	+ +	+	−
Connective tissue	+	+ +	

+ + = more than 10 ng/10^6 cells; + = 1 to 10 ng/10^6 cells; − = none detected.

sitions of the secretory granules. MC$_{TC}$ cells contain chymase, carboxypeptidase, cathepsin G–like protease, and tryptase; MC$_T$ cells contain only tryptase (Fig. 17–1; see color section at the front of this volume).[1] These proteases are the most discriminating markers of different mast cell types in humans and rodents. Human mast cell types cannot be precisely distinguished from one another by the histochemical staining, perhaps because heparin proteoglycan is present in all.

In histologically normal tissues (Table 17–4), mast cell concentrations are particularly high in the human alveolar wall, bowel mucosa, dermis, nasal and conjunctival mucosa, and around blood vessels, consistent with the clinical alterations known to occur in allergic diseases at these sites. Only modest numbers of mast cells reside in normal human synovium. MC$_T$ cells are the predominant, but not exclusive, type of mast cell found in the lung, particularly

alveoli, and in the small intestinal mucosa, whereas MC$_{TC}$ cells are the predominant type found in the skin, the gastrointestinal submucosa,[2] and the normal synovium. The relative abundance of MC$_{TC}$ and MC$_T$ cells may change with tissue inflammation or fibrosis, making it impossible to base a subtype designation on location alone.

Mature mast cells of all types have a nucleus without deeply divided lobes, numerous cytoplasmic granules, and thin elongated folds of their plasma membrane.[3] Human basophils are polymorphonuclear, contain larger and less numerous granules, and exhibit a comparatively smooth plasma membrane contour. Among MC$_{TC}$ and MC$_T$ cells, differences in granule morphology correspond to differences in protease composition[4, 5]; MC$_T$ granules often are scroll-rich, whereas MC$_{TC}$ granules often have gratings and lattices and are scroll-poor. All granules in both cell types contain tryptase and heparin; all granules in MC$_{TC}$ cells also contain chymase.

Functional and Pharmacologic Differences

Degranulation of human mast cells in response to various agents and inhibition of degranulation by antiallergic drugs have been studied in dispersed preparations of mast cells obtained from various anatomic sites. Such preparations often contain a mixture of MC$_T$ and MC$_{TC}$ cells, depending on the site examined, the pathologic condition of the donor organ and the method of dispersion and purification. In addition, differences in the secretory response between mast cells isolated from different tissues may relate to microenvironmental influences rather than to lineage.

Mast cells derived from human foreskin (MC$_{TC}$ type) release histamine in response to immunologic (antigen and anti-IgE) and a variety of nonimmunologic agents, such as the calcium ionophore A23187,

Table 17–3. CYTOKINES PRODUCED BY MAST CELLS AND BASOPHILS

Cell Type	Cytokines	
	mRNA	*Protein*
Human		
Mast cells	TNF-α	TNF-α, IL-4
Basophils		TNF-α, IL-4
Rodent mast cells	TNF-α	TNF-α
	GM-CSF	
	TGF-β	
	IF-γ	
	MIP-1α	
	MIP-1β	
	MCAF	
	IL-1	IL-1
	IL-2	
	IL-3	IL-3
	IL-4	IL-4
	IL-5	IL-6
	IL-6	
	IL-10	

Table 17–4. CHARACTERISTICS OF HUMAN MC$_{TC}$ AND MC$_T$ CELL TYPES

Characteristic	MC$_{TC}$ Cell	MC$_T$ Cell
Normal tissue distribution		
Skin	+ +	−
Intestinal submucosa	+ +	+
Intestinal mucosa	+	+ +
Alveolar wall	−	+ +
Bronchi and bronchioles	+	+ +
Nasal mucosa	+ +	+ +
Conjunctiva	+ +	+
Synovium	+ +	+
Protease content	Tryptase, chymase, cathepsin G–like, and carboxypeptidase	Tryptase
T lymphocyte dependency	No	Yes
Granule morphology	Grating or lattice Completely scroll-poor	Completely scroll-rich

+ + = abundant; + = present; − = negligible.

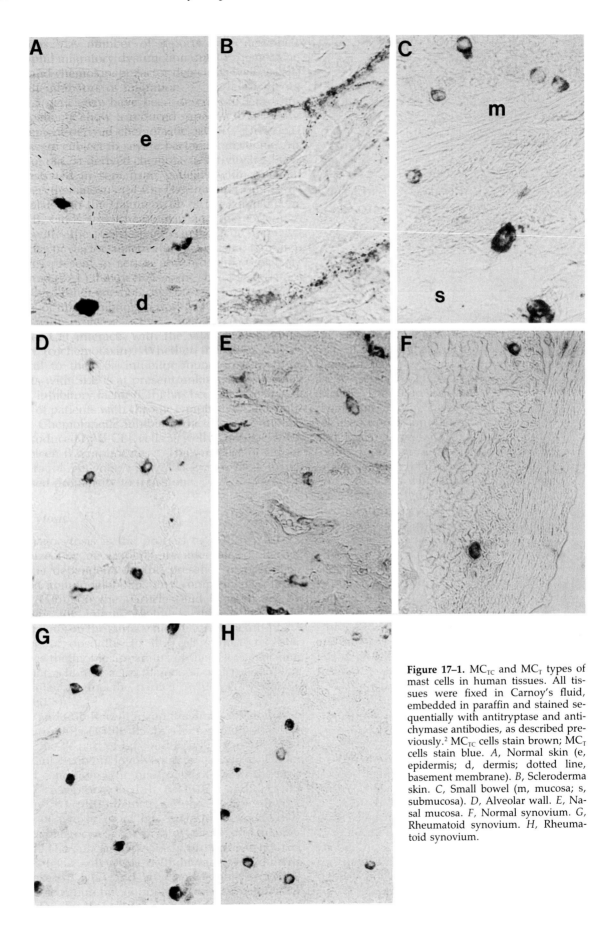

Figure 17–1. MC_TC and MC_T types of mast cells in human tissues. All tissues were fixed in Carnoy's fluid, embedded in paraffin and stained sequentially with antitryptase and antichymase antibodies, as described previously.[2] MC_TC cells stain brown; MC_T cells stain blue. *A*, Normal skin (e, epidermis; d, dermis; dotted line, basement membrane). *B*, Scleroderma skin. *C*, Small bowel (m, mucosa; s, submucosa). *D*, Alveolar wall. *E*, Nasal mucosa. *F*, Normal synovium. *G*, Rheumatoid synovium. *H*, Rheumatoid synovium.

compound 48/80, morphine sulfate, substance P, and the anaphylatoxin C5a. In contrast, mast cells isolated from lung (90 percent MC_T) are activated by anti-IgE and calcium ionophore A23187, but not by the other agents listed.[6] Mast cells isolated from human colonic mucosa (mast cell type varies) are activated by anti-IgE and the calcium ionophore A23187, but not by compound 48/80, morphine sulfate, or f-met peptide.[7] Compound 48/80 and the anaphylatoxins C3a and C5a also are ineffective in activating dispersed human adenoidal mast cells.[8] Analysis of the distribution of MC_T and MC_{TC} cells in the different preparations of dispersed human mast cells would help to clarify whether functional differences relate to the MC_{TC}/MC_T classification or to microenvironmental influences.

Disodium cromoglycate is widely used for the treatment of allergic asthma, rhinitis, and conjunctivitis, but experimental support for inhibition of mast cell degranulation as its mechanism of action is weak.[9] For example, no effect on skin-derived MC_{TC} cells has been observed.[10] Beta (β)-adrenergic receptor agonists produce 10 to 50 percent inhibition of IgE-dependent histamine release from dispersed human lung mast cells,[11, 12] whereas generation of LTC_4 and PGD_2 is inhibited to a greater extent.[13] In vivo, local instillation of nasal glucocorticoids diminished mediator release during the immediate response to nasal allergen challenge,[14] perhaps because of the capacity for local steroids to diminish mast cell concentrations as demonstrated in the synovium,[15] skin,[16] and rectal mucosa,[17] or to prevent the superficial migration of mast cells that apparently occurs in atopic subjects during the allergy season.[18]

Mast Cell Types and Human Disease

Several studies have begun to address the presence of distinct mast cell types in human diseases not typically associated with atopy. For example, mast cell hyperplasia has been noted in rheumatoid synovium near sites of cartilage erosion.[19] MC_{TC} cells appear to be associated with areas of dense fibrosis, whereas variable ratios of both MC_T and MC_{TC} cells were found at sites of active inflammation.[20] Increased mast cell numbers also have been documented in persons with scleroderma.[21] A possible role for mast cells in the tissue destruction and fibrosis that occurs with rheumatoid arthritis and scleroderma has been suggested. The ability of purified tryptase to activate latent collagenase derived from rheumatoid synovium[22] may be relevant to these observations. Characterization of mast cell types by the presence of specific markers has provided a means with which to begin to delineate mast cell involvement in disease processes. These findings are likely to have important pathogenetic, diagnostic, and therapeutic outcomes.

Growth and Differentiation of Mast Cells

A current working model for the lineage of human mast cells and basophils is shown in Figure 17–2. MC_T and MC_{TC} cells arise from a common nonmyeloid progenitor; basophils arise from myeloid precursors. Mast cell progenitors are kit^+, $IL-3R^-$, whereas basophil progenitors appear to be kit^-, $IL-3R^+$. IL-3 is a growth factor for human basophils in vitro[23, 24] but not for human mast cells. Consistent with this observation is the presence of IL-3 binding sites on basophils[25] but not mast cells.[26] Progenitors committed to a mast cell lineage are released from the marrow into the circulation, then enter their tissue sites of residence and mature along MC_{TC} or MC_T pathways. Basophils complete their maturation in the bone marrow and enter the circulation as mature granulated cells. The presence of receptors for laminin on the surface of rodent mast cells,[27, 28] though not yet shown in humans, may facilitate the tissue localization of mast cells.

Whether the predominance of a particular type of mast cell in different tissues is due to local influences on the development of committed mast cell progenitors to a particular mast cell type or is due to the selective recruitment of mast cells already directed toward a particular type is unclear. However, two experiments suggest that these mast cell types develop along distinct pathways. First, in humans with inherited combined immunodeficiency disease and in those with acquired immunodeficiency syndrome, marked and selective decreases in MC_T cell concentrations occur in the bowel, whereas the concentration and distribution of MC_{TC} cells are unaffected.[29] This finding suggests that the appearance in tissues of MC_T cells is dependent on functional T lymphocytes and that MC_{TC} cell development proceeds independently. Second, immature MC_T cells contain granules with complete scrolls and tryptase alone, whereas MC_{TC} cells have granules with electron-dense cores surrounded by a less electron-dense matrix and tryptase together with chymase.[30] Thus, commitment to a particular mast cell type occurs by the time granules begin to form. T lymphocyte–associated activity appears to be important in the development of MC_T cells, whereas fibroblast-derived factors, particularly stem cell factor (SCF), the ligand for kit, appear to be important in the development of both mast cell types. Co-cultures of cord blood mononuclear cells[31] and fetal liver cells[32] with murine 3T3 fibroblasts routinely yield mast cells in excess of basophils. A great portion of fibroblast-derived activity may be duplicated by human SCF, which by itself promotes the growth of mast cells from cord blood and fetal liver.[32a] The particular level of T lymphocyte involvement and the maturational stage at which certain capabilities are acquired or lost, such as proliferation, dedifferentiation, interconversion, and activation and secretion, also need to be clarified.

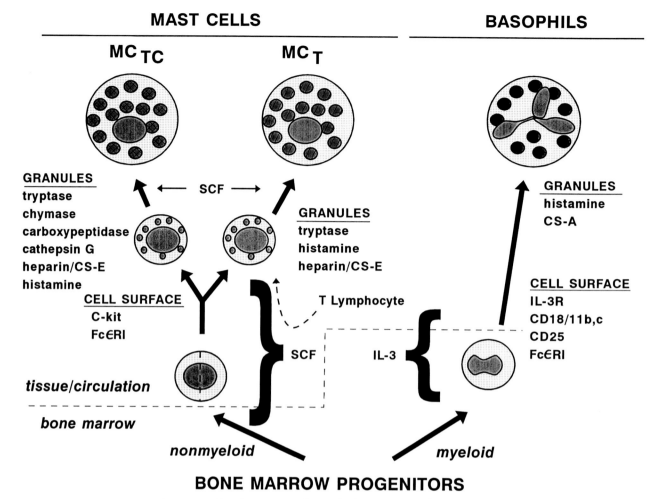

Figure 17–2. Developmental pathways for human mast cells and basophils.

MEDIATORS OF MAST CELLS AND BASOPHILS

Preformed Granule–Associated Mediators
(see Tables 17–1 and 17–5)

Biogenic Amines

Histamine, derived from histidine, is the sole biogenic amine in human mast cells and basophils.

Table 17–5. CELLULAR LEVELS OF PREFORMED MEDIATORS IN HUMAN MAST CELLS AND BASOPHILS

	Level (pg/cell)		
Mediator	MC_{TC} Cell	MC_T Cell	Basophil
Histamine	1–3	1–2	1–2
Tryptase	35	10	0.04
Chymase	5	<0.04	<0.04
Cathepsin G–like	+ +	<0.04	<0.04
Carboxypeptidase	5–20	<0.04	<0.04
Heparin	3–8	3–8	−
Chondroitin sulfate			
Type E	+	+	−
Type A	+	+	+

+ = present; − = not detected.

Histamine (β-imidazolylethylamine) is formed from histidine[33] by histidine decarboxylase (Fig. 17–3).[34, 35] Histamine is then stored in secretory granules where, at the acidic pH of the unstimulated cell, it is associated with carboxyl groups of proteoglycans or proteins. Histamine is the only preformed mediator of human mast cells with direct potent vasoactive and smooth muscle spasmogenic effects. With degranulation, histamine is released and dissociates from the proteoglycan–protein complex. Extracellular histamine is metabolized within minutes of release, suggesting that it is destined to act locally. Histamine levels of 1 to 3 pg per human mast cell or basophil have been reported. Histamine concentrations of about 0.1 mol per L are estimated to exist inside secretory granules, whereas concentrations of about 2 nmol per L exist in plasma. Intermediate levels in samples obtained from other sites reflect rates of local production and removal. Elevated levels of histamine in plasma or urine are detected after anaphylactic reactions to allergens or radiocontrast dyes and in a portion of subjects with mastocytosis, consistent with mast cell involvement. However, in patients in septic shock and in those with hereditary angioneurotic edema during attacks, histamine levels

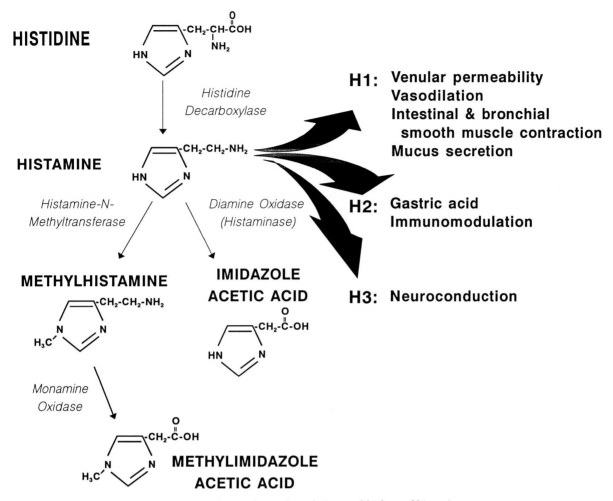

Figure 17–3. The synthesis, degradation, and biology of histamine.

are not elevated, which is consistent with a lack of mast cell involvement.

Histamine exerts its biologic and pathobiologic effects through its interaction with cell-specific receptors designated H1, H2, and H3,[36-38] which initially were defined with the recognition of specific agonists and antagonists. H1 receptors are blocked by chlorpheniramine, H2 receptors are blocked by cimetidine, and H3 receptors are blocked by thioperamide. Because many of the previously described H2 effects were based on using burimamide or impromidine, which show H3 cross-antagonism, some of the recognized H2-mediated activities may require re-evaluation, particularly those that affect inflammation and immunoregulation. Examples of receptor-specific agonists include 2-methylhistamine at H1 receptors, dimaprit at H2 receptors, and α-methylhistamine at H3 receptors.

Effects of histamine (see Fig. 17–3) mediated by H1 receptors include enhanced vasopermeability between venular endothelial cells, vasodilation, contraction of bronchial and gastrointestinal smooth muscle, and increased mucus secretion at various sites. Increased vasopermeability facilitates the tissue deposition of factors from plasma that may be im-

portant for tissue growth and repair and of foreign material or immune complexes that result in tissue inflammation. H2 receptor agonists stimulate gastric acid secretion by parietal cells. H2 agonists also inhibit secretion by cytotoxic lymphocytes and granulocytes, augment suppression by T lymphocytes,[39] enhance epithelial permeability across human airways,[40] stimulate chemokinesis of neutrophils and eosinophils and expression of eosinophil C3b receptors, and activate endothelial cells to release a potent inhibitor of platelet aggregation, PGI_2 (prostacyclin). Stimulation of H3 receptors affects neurotransmitter release and histamine formation in the central and peripheral nervous system.[41] Bronchial hyperreactivity to irritant stimuli in atopic patients with asthma may in part be mediated by histamine-mediated cholinergic hyperexcitability.

The combined effects of H1 and H2 receptor–mediated activities of histamine are required for the full expression of vasoactivity. For example, the triple response caused by an intradermal injection of histamine—namely, central erythema (histamine arteriolar vasodilation), circumferential erythema (axon reflex vasodilation mediated by neuropeptides), and a central weal (histamine vasopermeability, edema)—

is mostly blocked by H1 receptor antagonists but is completely blocked only with a combination of H1 and H2 receptor antagonists.[42] Analogous results have been observed for the tachycardia, widened pulse pressure, diastolic hypotension, flushing, and headaches that result from intravenous infusion of histamine.[43]

Neutral Proteases

Neutral proteases are enzymes that catalyze the cleavage of peptide bonds and perform best near neutral pH. Such enzymes are the dominant protein components of secretory granules in human and rodent mast cells.[44] In addition, such enzymes serve as selective markers that distinguish mast cells from other cell types, including basophils, and different mast cell subpopulations from one another.

Tryptase is the principal enzyme accounting for the trypsin-like activity first detected in human mast cells by histochemical techniques.[45, 46] Substantial amounts of tryptase are present in MC_{TC} cells derived from foreskin (35 pg per cell) and in MC_T cells derived from lung (10 pg per cell), where it is located in secretory granules and is released in parallel with histamine during degranulation.[47] Negligible amounts have been measured in human basophils (0.04 pg per cell). Other cell types have no detectable tryptase. Thus, the enzyme is a discriminating marker of human mast cells.

Tryptase is a tetrameric serine endoprotease of 134,000 daltons with subunits of 31,000 to 34,000 daltons, each with an active enzymatic site[45] and common antigenic sites.[48] At least two highly homologous tryptase cDNA molecules have been cloned,[49–51] and the two corresponding genes are present in the normal haploid genome on chromosome 16.

Tryptase activity is measured by hydrolysis of synthetic trypsin-like substrates, whereas the absence of inhibition by the biologic inhibitors of serine esterases present in plasma, lung, and urine clearly distinguishes tryptase from pancreatic trypsin and from most other serine esterases. Tryptase, like all other mast cell proteases examined thus far, resides in secretory granules fully active, apparently bound to proteoglycan molecules distinct from those to which chymase and carboxypeptidase are bound.[51a] The enzyme is uniquely stabilized in its active tetrameric form by heparin,[52] to which it is ionically bound under physiologic conditions. When free in solution, tryptase subunits rapidly dissociate from one another into inactive monomers, without any evidence for autodegradation.[53]

Several tryptase-mediated activities of potential biologic interest have been examined in vitro (Table 17–6). For example, tryptase rapidly inactivates fibrinogen as a coagulable substrate for thrombin[54]; the lack of fibrin deposition and the rapid resolution of urticaria and angioedema reactions may, in part, reflect this same activity in vivo. Although chroma-

Table 17–6. POTENTIAL BIOLOGIC PROPERTIES OF TRYPTASE AND CHYMASE

Protease	Property
Tryptase	Fibrinogenolysis*
	High-molecular-weight kininogen destruction*
	Prostromelysin activation*
	Fibroblast proliferation†
	Pulmonary smooth muscle hyperreactivity to histamine†
	Neuropeptide degradation†
Chymase	Generation of angiotensin II*
	Basement membrane degradation*
	Glandular mucus secretion†
	Neuropeptide degradation†

*Human.
†Dog.

tographically purified tryptase generated anaphylatoxin C3a from C3,[55] affinity purified tryptase is inactive against C3 and C5. Finally, tryptase activates latent collagenase derived from rheumatoid synovial cells, apparently by first activating prostromelysin (metalloproteinase III),[22] which in turn activates latent collagenase. The increased numbers of mast cells found in rheumatoid synovium[15] and in inflammatory cutaneous lesions of scleroderma,[21] together with the increased tissue turnover that occurs in each condition, suggest a related role for tryptase. Also of interest are the observations that dog tryptase potentiates histamine-mediated contraction of guinea pig pulmonary smooth muscle[56] and proliferation of fibroblasts.[44]

Chymase is the principal enzyme accounting for the chymotrypsin-like activity present in human cutaneous mast cells. The enzyme was purified from human skin,[57] and the corresponding gene cloned and localized to human chromosome 14.[58] Chymase was selectively localized to a subpopulation of mast cells by enzymatic and immunohistochemical techniques.[2] Dispersed MC_{TC} cells obtained from skin contain 4.5 pg of chymase per mast cell.

Human chymase is a monomer of 30,000 daltons with endopeptidase activity that cleaves on the C-terminal side of aromatic resides, such as Phe. Inhibition of chymase by diisopropylfluorophosphate (DFP) and tosyl-L-phenylalanine chloromethylketone classifies it as a serine esterase. Like tryptase, chymase is stored fully active in mast cell secretory granules, presumably bound to heparin or chondroitin sulfate E. Unlike tryptase, chymase stability is not substantially affected by heparin,[59] and its activity is inhibited by classic biologic inhibitors of serine proteinases, such as α_1-antichymotrypsin, α_1-proteinase inhibitor, and α_2-macroglobulin.[60] No chymotrypsin-like enzymatic activity has been detected in MC_T cells.

Potential biologic activities of chymase, like those of tryptase, are based on in vitro observations (see Table 17–6). Of potential interest are findings that chymase converts angiotensin I to II about four times as efficiently as angiotensin-converting enzyme,[61] inactivates bradykinin,[62] and attacks the lamina lucida of the basement membrane at the dermal–epidermal junction of human skin.[63] Dog chymase has been shown to stimulate mucus production from glandular cells in vitro,[64] suggesting a similar role in asthma and allergic rhinitis, where release of chymase in proximity to glandular tissue might be involved in the state of hypersecretion.

Human mast cell cathepsin G is a neutral protease found in neutrophils and monocytes. The presence of a cathepsin G–like protein in MC_{TC} cells has been demonstrated with immunohistochemical, Western blot, and enzymatic techniques.[65] Western blot analysis showed a stained band at 30,000 daltons. This co-migrated with chymase and a minor species of cathepsin G present in neutrophils. The major form of neutrophil cathepsin G migrates at 28,000 daltons. Based on enzymatic activity, substantial levels of this cathepsin G–like protease are present in MC_{TC} cells.

Human mast cell carboxypeptidase was detected and localized to secretory granules in MC_{TC} cells by immunohistochemical techniques[66] and by the IgE-mediated release of an activity from human mast cells that cleaves the carboxyterminal His^9–Leu^{10} bond of angiotensin I and behaves like a zinc metalloexopeptidase.[67] Human mast cells dispersed from skin contain 5 to 16 pg of carboxypeptidase per cell.[68] Human mast cell carboxypeptidase is a monomeric enzyme with a molecular weight of 34,500 daltons.[68] Based on analysis of the complementary DNA–derived amino acid sequence and gene structure,[69] the human enzyme is more homologous to human pancreatic carboxypeptidase B than A, but the catalytic site is more homologous to human pancreatic carboxypeptidase A, as are its substrate specificities for carboxyterminal Phe and Leu residues.

Proteoglycans

The presence of highly sulfated proteoglycans in secretory granules of mast cells and basophils results in metachromasia when these cells are stained with basic dyes. Proteoglycans are composed of glycosaminoglycan side chains (repeating unbranched disaccharide units of a uronic acid and hexosamine moieties that are variably sulfated) covalently linked to a single-chain protein core by means of a specific trisaccharide–protein linkage region consisting of Gal-Gal-Xyl-Ser. Although proteoglycans are most abundant as components of extracellular matrix, this review concerns only the intracellular proteoglycans. Two proteoglycans, *heparin* and *chondroitin sulfate E,* have been associated with purified human mast cells,[70, 71] whereas *chondroitin sulfate A* is the predominant type in human basophils.[72] Heparin is selectively concentrated only in mast cells; chondroitin sulfates A and E are also found in other cell types.

The characteristic disaccharide units of heparin, chondroitin sulfate E and chondroitin sulfate A, are shown in Figure 17–4. The average number of sulfate

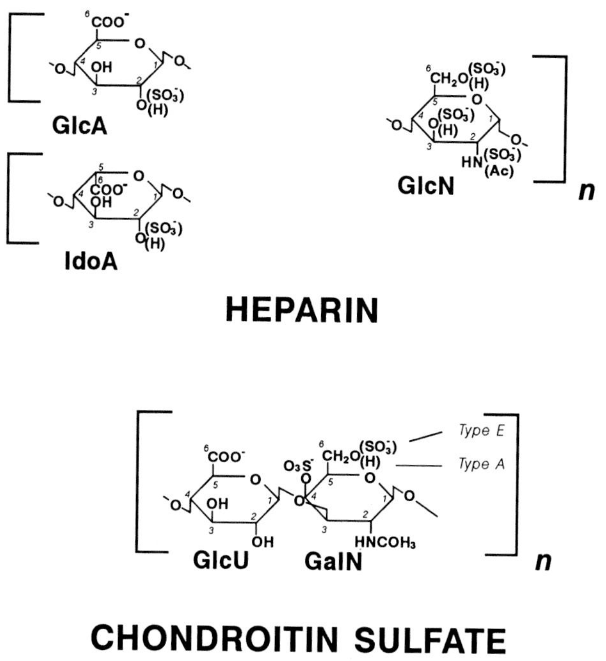

HEPARIN

CHONDROITIN SULFATE

Figure 17–4. Structural characteristics of mast cell and basophil proteoglycans.

residues per respective disaccharide is 2.5, 1.5, and 1.0. The characteristic susceptibility of heparin to nitrous acid is due to attack at the *N*-sulfate residue; chondroitin sulfates lack this residue and are resistant to nitrous acid.

The same peptide core is associated with heparin and chondroitin sulfate proteoglycans, and both proteoglycan types may reside in the same cell, even on the same peptide core. In humans, the core protein is 17,600 daltons and contains a glycosaminoglycan-attachment region of 18 amino acids,[73] where two or three glycosaminoglycans of about 20,000 daltons are attached.[74, 75] The attachment region is rich in alternating Ser and Gly residues, and the gene is located on chromosome 10.

The biologic functions of endogenous mast cell proteoglycans are somewhat speculative. These proteoglycans bind to histamine, neutral proteases, and acid hydrolases at the acidic pH inside mast cell secretory granules and may facilitate uptake and packaging of these mediators into the secretory granules. Mast cell proteoglycans may regulate the stability and activities of many of the enzymes present. After release from mast cells, the proteoglycans may continue to affect those substances that remain associated, particularly the neutral proteases. The stabilizing effect of heparin and, to a lesser degree, chondroitin sulfate E, on human tryptase activity[52, 53] may be crucial for the full expression of mast cell–mediated events. Heparin and chondroitin sulfate E (to a lesser extent) express anticoagulant, anticomplement, antikallikrein, and Hageman factor autoactivation activities. Heparin neutralizes the ability of eosinophil-derived major basic protein to kill schistosomula and enhances the binding of fibronectin to

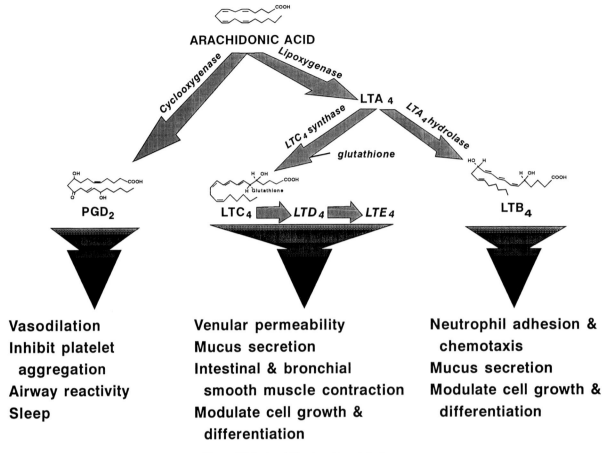

Figure 17–5. Arachidonic acid metabolism.

collagen. Heparin may sequester or protect growth factors such as fibroblast growth factor in the extracellular matrix and may modulate the cell adhesion properties of matrix proteins such as vitronectin, fibronectin, and laminin. The anticoagulant activities of human and commercial porcine heparin are similar and depend on a specific pentasaccharide sequence.[76] When heparin is saturated with tryptase, however, as in the mast cell, many of these activities may be attenuated.

Newly Generated Lipid Mediators

Liberation of the 20-carbon polyunsaturated fatty acid called *arachidonic acid* from cellular lipid stores occurs with mast cell activation, at which time it is either reincorporated into lipids or oxidatively metabolized. Unstimulated human mast cells derived from lung incorporate exogenous arachidonic acid into neutral lipids and phospholipids in a ratio of about 7:2,[77] and store these lipids in membranes and cytoplasmic lipid bodies.[78] Arachidonate released by hydrolysis of these lipids is then metabolized along either the cyclooxygenase pathway to prostaglandins (PGs) and thromboxanes (TXs), or the 5-, 12-, or 15-

lipoxygenase pathway to monohydroxyl fatty acids, lipoxins, and leukotrienes (LTs) that include both LTB$_4$ and the sulfidopeptides LTC$_4$, LTD$_4$, and LTE$_4$ (slow-reacting substances of anaphylaxis [SRS-A]). Platelet-activating factor, a phospholipid-derived mediator, has not been shown to be a secretory product of human mast cells and basophils. Synthesis of selected products by different cell types is governed by the repertoire of metabolic enzymes present in each cell; the major eicosanoid products of mast cells and selected properties are shown in Figure 17–5.

On activation, dispersed and purified preparations of human mast cells obtained from lung, skin, and intestine produce PGD$_2$ and LTC$_4$ in weight ratios of approximately 5:1.[79] Smaller amounts of LTB$_4$ isomers are also produced. There is no evidence that lipid products can be used to distinguish MC$_T$ from MC$_{TC}$ cell activation. In contrast, peripheral blood basophils obtained from normal human subjects synthesize LTC$_4$ but not PGD$_2$.[80] Detection of LTC$_4$ and histamine, but not PGD$_2$, in biologic fluids is used as one criterion of basophil activation. However, to conclude that the absence of PGD$_2$ in the presence of LTC$_4$ and histamine in biologic fluids proves activation of basophils is hazardous, because basophils obtained from subjects with chronic myelogenous leukemia apparently produce substantial amounts of PGD$_2$.[81] Also, cells other than mast cells and basophils produce PGD$_2$ and LTC$_4$. Thus, when these products are detected in a complex biologic milieu, their cell source is ambiguous.

The biologic importance of mast cell–derived products of arachidonic acid is difficult to ascertain. A metabolite of PGD$_2$ has been detected in the urine of patients with active systemic mastocytosis, but not in normal subjects.[82] The importance of PGD$_2$ production in the subgroup of these patients with recurrent hypotensive episodes was suggested when administration of aspirin inhibited generation of the PGD$_2$ metabolite and led to clinical improvement. Sulfidopeptide leukotrienes derived from allergen-activated mast cells are suggested to play an important role in asthma.

Cytokines (see Table 17–3)

Compelling evidence that rodent mast cells, when activated, produce cytokines emerged in 1987 when expression of IL-4 messenger RNA[83] and a cytolytic factor appearing to be TNF-α[84] was reported. Rodent mast cells in culture constitutively transcribe cytokines TNF-α and IL-6; corresponding biologic activities also are present. Activated mast cells also transcribe macrophage inflammatory protein-1α (MIP-1α), MIP-1β, monocyte chemotactic and inflammatory factor (MCAF), IL-1, IL-2, IL-3, IL-4, IL-5, IL-10, granulocyte-macrophage colony-stimulating factor (GM-CSF), TGF-β, and gamma (γ) interferon, biologic activities having been detected for IL-1, IL-3, and IL-4. Particularly interesting is the capacity of non-T, non-B murine spleen cells to generate IL-4 when stimulated by FcεRI. Both immature mast cells (kit$^+$) and immature basophils (kit$^-$) apparently are responsible for producing this IL-4. The capacity of rodent mast cells to produce their own growth factors—namely, IL-3, IL-4, and possibly IL-10—implicates an autocrine function of these cytokines. Preliminary reports suggest an analogous situation for human mast cells. Cytokine production may occur hours after mast cells are activated, in marked variance to the unloading of granule mediators that begins within minutes and the generation of arachidonic acid metabolites that begins within minutes and lasts up to about 30 minutes. In humans, production of TNF-α has been demonstrated in human skin mast cells and in basophils.[85, 86] Possibly relevant to the late cellular phase of immediate hypersensitivity reactions is the finding that the increased levels of ELAM-1 on endothelial cells are induced by TNF-α from stimulated cutaneous mast cells.[87]

ACTIVATION AND REGULATED SECRETION

Immunologic activation of mast cells and basophils typically begins by cross-linkage of IgE bound to the high-affinity FcεRI receptor (Ka = 10^9 M^{-1}) with multivalent allergen (Fig. 17–6). In vivo, auto-antibodies against IgE have been detected in patients with idiopathic urticaria[88] and immune complex–mediated diseases,[89] implicating the potential for mast cell activation to play a role in the pathogenesis of these disorders. The FcεRI receptor is composed of four subunits,[90] αβγ$_2$, shown schematically in Figure 17–6. The α-chain contains the IgE-binding domain. The β-chain and the two disulfide-linked γ-chains are not accessible on the surface and may be involved with signal transduction. The γ-chains also are present in the CD16 and FcγRIII receptors of natural killer cells and may substitute for the T cell receptor (TCR) ζ-chain.

Regulated secretion by mast cells and basophils also may be induced by nonimmunologic agonists. Multivalent lectins, like bivalent concanavalin A,[91] cross-link membrane FcεRI or IgE. Calcium ionophores activate by translocating calcium.[92] Basic biomolecules such as compound 48/80, C3a, C5a, morphine, mellitin, eosinophil-derived major basic protein, and various neuropeptides such as substance P[93, 94] directly perturb the plasma membrane of human mast cells derived from skin but are inactive against mast cells derived from lung. The peptide f-Met-Leu-Phe activates human basophils but not mast cells. Various histamine-releasing factors derived from monocytes, lymphocytes, platelets, and neutrophils also have been described that are of potential clinical significance. Dexamethasone in vitro inhibits activation–secretion by human basophils[95] but not by human lung–derived mast cells.[96]

The earliest biochemical events involved in signal transduction after FcεRI aggregation are likely to be mediated by a network of heterotrimeric guanidine triphosphate–GTP-binding proteins and tyrosine and serine–threonine kinases and phosphatases, which in turn activate adenyl cyclase, phospholipase C, phospholipase A2, and various ion channels. Cyclic adenosine monophosphate (cAMP) may be an important second messenger in the coupled activation–secretion process, and transmembrane activation of adenyl cyclase appears to be linked to FcεRI-mediated activation.[97] However, evidence was not found for an early rise in cAMP after activation of human mast cells.[98, 99] Adenosine added to antigen- or calcium ionophore–stimulated human mast cells at low concentrations augments ongoing release of both histamine and LTC$_4$, but it has no effect on mediator release from unstimulated mast cells.[100] In contrast, release of these mediators from human basophils is inhibited.

Metabolism of phospholipids, which reside mostly in secretory granules,[101] occurs early during the secretory response, is necessary for the later secretion of lipid mediators, and may be important for regulated secretion to ensue. Levels of inosine triphosphate (IP$_3$) and diacylglycerol increase early after FcεRI receptor aggregation in rodent mast cells[102–104] and human basophils,[105] and should lead to activation of PKC.

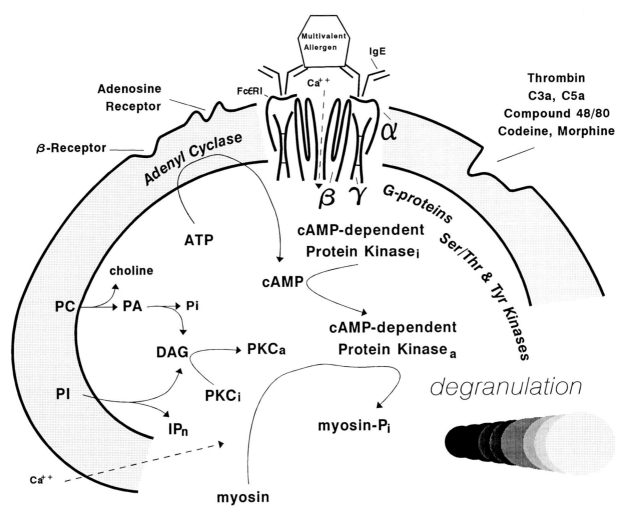

Figure 17–6. Early biochemical steps involved in the activation of mast cells.

BIOLOGY AND PATHOBIOLOGY OF HUMAN MAST CELLS

The two major barriers to the assessment of mast cell involvement in clinical events have been the localization of this cell type in tissue rather than the circulation and the lack of a marker, detectable in biologic fluids, with sufficient sensitivity and specificity to indicate activation of mast cells occurring in tissues. In the case of basophils, numbers in the circulation are small, making quantitation difficult, and have not been shown to correlate with basophil participation in immediate hypersensitivity or inflammatory events. Several mediators of mast cells have been considered as potentially useful indicators of mast cell or basophil activation. Mast cell neutral proteases have the greatest potential utility because of their abundant presence in and selective localization to mast cell secretory granules. A specific immunoassay for tryptase was developed to quantify total amounts of the enzyme in complex biologic fluids.[106] In serum, tryptase levels in normal persons are undetectable (less than 1 ng per ml) but are elevated in systemic mast cell disorders, such as anaphylaxis and mastocytosis.[47, 107] Basophil involvement is more difficult to assess. Histamine levels, when elevated in the absence of detectable tryptase or PGD_2, suggest basophil involvement. But proof requires demonstration of basophils at the site of inflammation, as preformed in the skin[108, 109] and nose.[110] Unfortunately, no one mediator has been found that can serve as a specific indicator of basophil activation. Analysis of levels of tryptase, PGD_2, and histamine has been used to suggest that mast cell degranulation occurs only during the early phase of immediate hypersensitivity reactions, whereas basophil activation occurs during the late phase in skin, lung, and nasal tissues.

Arthritis

Possible roles for mast cell involvement in arthritis are well documented.[111] Increased concentrations and depth of mast cells in synovial tissue are found in patients with rheumatoid arthritis.[112, 113]

Increased numbers of the MC_{TC} type of mast cell are seen in association with mononuclear infiltrates, increased MC_{TC} cells with fibrosis.[20] Mast cells free in synovial fluid are occasionally observed.[114] Suppression of mast cell hyperplasia occurs after intrasynovial injection of glucocorticoid but not after treatment with low-dose methotrexate.[15] IgE rheumatoid factors have been observed in synovial fluid capable of activating mast cells in vitro.[115] A recent study, however, found no effect of astemizole on the clinical course of rheumatoid arthritis, suggesting that if mast cells are involved, released histamine has little impact on the disease.[116] Released tryptase may affect cartilage and bone turnover and synovial fibrosis. In synovial fluid taken from subjects with various arthritides, including osteoarthritis, rheumatoid arthritis, and acute gout, levels of tryptase did not correlate with a particular pathogenic etiology or with the degree of complement activation, although lower levels of tryptase were found more often in fluids with higher levels of C3a.[117] Whether tryptase levels in synovial fluid accurately reflect levels of mast cell activation in synovial tissue is not clear. Larger volumes of synovial fluid, faster rates of exchange of soluble proteins across vascular surfaces, and higher turnover rates in inflamed tissue may obscure higher production rates of tryptase at such sites. Thus, a better understanding of the mechanism of mast cell involvement in synovial inflammation is needed.

Scleroderma and Fibrosis

Involvement of mast cells in fibrotic disorders has been suggested, based on the observation of increased numbers of mast cells in various conditions characterized by fibrosis, such as scleroderma,[21, 118] fibrotic lung diseases,[119, 120] and keloids.[121] Although mostly Mc_{TC} cells are defected in scleroderma skin, MC_T cells are also found, and both mast cell types often appear fragmented.[121a] Increased numbers and fragmentation of mast cells have been observed by electron microscopy in the skin of a single patient with rapidly progressive scleroderma.[122] In a murine model of chronic graft-versus-host disease in which dermal fibrosis occurs, "phantom" mast cells have been described.[123] This term refers to putative mast cells that have no granules (and consequently unstainable by basic dyes) but that exhibit surface staining for high-affinity IgE receptors. These phantom mast cells appear in the skin of persons with scleroderma before fibrosis.[124] Whether such cells represent immature precursor mast cells infiltrating the skin, an enhanced activation state, or the dedifferentiation of resident mast cells is not clear.

Experimentally, bidirectional effects have been noted between mast cells and fibroblasts. Mouse skin–derived 3T3 fibroblasts prolong the survival of human lung mast cells[125] in vitro and mature rodent mast cells. The maturational effect is consistent with previous findings in mice,[126] suggesting that mast

cell differentiation from noncommitted cells depends on factors secreted by T lymphocytes, whereas maturation of granules depends on fibroblast factors. As discussed earlier, the production of stem cell factor by fibroblasts accounts for a substantial portion of the fibroblast effect on mast cell growth and differentiation. Also, cultured rat embryonic skin fibroblasts phagocytose granules released from co-cultured rat mast cells,[127] increased levels of collagenase and β-hexosaminidase being found in the culture media. Degranulation of lymph-node–derived murine mast cells co-cultured with murine embryonic skin fibroblasts resulted in structural alterations in the fibroblast monolayer.[128] Mouse 3T3 fibroblasts co-cultured with mouse bone marrow–derived mast cells lose their contact inhibition.[129] Canine tryptase enhances proliferation of rat- and hamster-derived fibroblasts, but contact inhibition is maintained.[44] These interactions between mast cells and fibroblasts suggest potential pathways for mast cell involvement in the development of tissue fibrosis in humans.

References

1. Irani, A. A., and Schwartz, L. B.: Neutral proteases as indicators of human mast cell heterogeneity. In Schwartz, L. B. (ed.): Neutral Proteases of Mast Cells. Basel, Karger, 1990.
2. Irani, A. A., Schechter, N. M., Craig, S. S., et al.: Two types of human mast cells that have distinct neutral protease compositions. Proc. Natl. Acad. Sci. U.S.A. 83:4464, 1986.
3. Dvorak, A. M.: The fine structure of human basophils and mast cells. In Holgate, S. T. (ed.): Mast Cells, Mediators and Disease. London, Kluwer Academic Publishers, 1988.
4. Craig, S. S., Schechter, N. M., and Schwartz, L. B.: Ultrastructural analysis of human T and TC mast cells identified by immunoelectron microscopy. Lab. Invest. 58:682, 1988.
5. Craig, S. S., and Schwartz, L. B.: Human MC_{TC} type of mast cell granule: The uncommon occurrence of discrete scrolls associated with focal absence of chymase. Lab. Invest. 63:581, 1990.
6. Church, M. K., Pao, G. J. K., and Holgate, S. T.: Characterization of histamine secretion from mechanically dispersed human lung mast cells: Effects of anti-IgE, calcium ionophore A 23187, compound 48/80, and basic polypeptides. J. Immunol. 129:2116, 1982.
7. Fox, C. C., Dvorak, A. M., Peters, S. P., et al.: Isolation and characterization of human intestinal mucosal mast cells. J. Immunol. 135:483, 1985.
8. Schmutzler, W., Delmich, K., Eichelberg, D., et al.: The human adenoidal mast cell: Susceptibility to different secretagogues and secretion inhibitors. Int. Arch. Allergy Appl. Immunol. 77:177, 1985.
9. Flint, K. C., Leung, K. B. P., Pearce, F. L., et al.: Human mast cells recovered by bronchoalveolar lavage: Their morphology, histamine release and the effects of sodium cromoglycate. Clin. Sci. 68:427, 1985.
10. Ting, S., Zweiman, B., and Lavker, R. M.: Cromolyn does not modulate human allergic skin reactions in vivo. J. Allergy Clin. Immunol. 71:12, 1983.
11. Church, M. K., and Hiroi, J.: Inhibition of IgE-dependent histamine release from human dispersed lung mast cells by anti-allergic drugs and salbutamol. Br. J. Pharmacol. 90:421, 1987.
12. Peters, S. P., Schulman, E. S., Schleimer, R. P., et al.: Dispersed human lung mast cells: Pharmacologic aspects and comparison with human lung tissue fragments. Am. Rev. Respir. Dis. 126:1034, 1982.
13. Undem, B. J., Peachell, P. T., and Lichtenstein, L. M.: Isoproterenol-induced inhibition of immunoglobulin E–mediated release of histamine and arachidonic acid metabolites from the human lung mast cell. J. Pharmacol. Exp. Ther. 247:209, 1988.
14. Pipkorn, U., Proud, D., Lichtenstein, L. M., et al.: Inhibition of mediator release in allergic rhinitis by pretreatment with topical glucocorticosteroids. N. Engl. J. Med. 316:1506, 1987.
15. Malone, D. G., Wilder, R. L., Saavedra-Delgado, A. M., et al.: Mast cell numbers in rheumatoid synovial tissues: Correlations with quantitative measures of lymphotic infiltration and modulation by anti-inflammatory therapy. Arthritis Rheum. 30:130, 1987.

16. Lavker, R. M., and Schechter, N. M.: Cutaneous mast cell depletion results from topical corticosteroid usage. J. Immunol. 135:2368, 1985.

17. Goldsmith, P., McGarity, B., Walls, A. F., et al.: Corticosteroid treatment reduces mast cell numbers in inflammatory bowel disease. Dig. Dis. Sci. 35:1409, 1990.

18. Enerback, L., Pipkorn, U., and Granerus, G.: Intraepithelial migration of nasal mucosal mast cells in hay fever. Int. Arch. Allergy Appl. Immunol. 80:44, 1986.

19. Wasserman, S. I.: The mast cell and synovial inflammation: Or, what's a nice cell like you doing in a joint like this? Arthritis Rheum. 27:841, 1984.

20. Irani, A. A., Golzar, N., DeBlois, G., et al.: Distribution of mast cell subsets in rheumatoid arthritis and osteoarthritis synovia. (Abstract.) Arthritis Rheum. 30:66, 1987.

21. Hawkins, R. A., Claman, H. N., Clark, R. A., et al.: Increased dermal mast cell populations in progressive systemic sclerosis: A link in chronic fibrosis. Ann. Intern. Med. 102:182, 1985.

22. Gruber, B. L., Marchese, M. J., Suzuki, K., et al.: Synovial procollagenase activation by human mast cell tryptase dependence upon matrix metalloproteinase 3 activation. J. Clin. Invest. 84:1657, 1989.

23. Valent, P., Schmidt, G., Besemer, J., et al.: Interleukin-3 is a differentiation factor for human basophils. Blood 73:1763, 1989.

24. Dvorak, A. M., Saito, H., Estrella, P., et al.: Ultrastructure of eosinophils and basophils stimulated to develop in human cord blood mononuclear cell cultures containing recombinant human interleukin-5 or interleukin-3. Lab. Invest. 61:116, 1989.

25. Valent, P., Besemer, J., Muhm, M., et al.: Interleukin 3 activates human blood basophils via high-affinity binding sites. Proc. Natl. Acad. Sci. U.S.A. 86:5542, 1989.

26. Valent, P., Besemer, J., Sillaber, C., et al.: Failure to detect IL-3–binding sites on human mast cells. J. Immunol. 145:3432, 1990.

27. Thompson, H. L., Burbelo, P. D., and Metcalfe, D. D.: Regulation of adhesion of mouse bone marrow–derived mast cells to laminin. J. Immunol. 145:3425, 1990.

28. Thompson, H. L., Burbelo, P. D., Yamada, Y., et al.: Identification of an amino acid sequence in the laminin A chain mediating mast cell attachment and spreading. Immunology 72:144, 1991.

29. Irani, A. M., Craig, S. S., DeBlois, G., et al.: Deficiency of the tryptase-positive, chymase-negative mast cell type in gastrointestinal mucosa of patients with defective T lymphocyte function. J. Immunol. 138:4381, 1987.

30. Craig, S. S., Schechter, N. M., and Schwartz, L. B.: Ultrastructural analysis of maturing human T and TC mast cells in situ. Lab. Invest. 60:147, 1989.

31. Furitsu, T., Saito, H., Dvorak, A., et al.: Development of human mast cells in vitro. Proc. Natl. Acad. Sci. U.S.A. 86:10039, 1989.

32. Irani, A. A., Craig, S. S., Nilsson, G., et al.: Characterization of human mast cells developed in vitro from fetal liver cells cocultured with murine 3T3 fibroblasts. Immunology 1992 (in press).

32a. Schwartz, L. B., Irani, A. A., Nilsson, G., and Ishizaka, T.: Recombinant human stem cell factor is a major growth factor for human mast cells. Clin. Res. 40:343A, 1992.

33. Bauza, M. T., and Lagunoff, D.: Histidine transport by isolated rat peritoneal mast cells. Biochem. Pharmacol. 30:1271, 1981.

34. Schayer, R. W.: Histidine decarboxylase in mast cells. Ann. N.Y. Acad. Sci. 103:164, 1963.

35. Yamauchi, K., Sato, R., Tanno, Y., et al.: Nucleotide sequence of the cDNA encoding L-histidine decarboxylase derived from human basophilic leukemia cell line, KU-812-F. Nucleic Acids Res. 18:5891, 1990.

36. Polk, R. E., Healy, D. P., Schwartz, L. B., et al.: Vancomycin and the red-man syndrome: Pharmacodynamics of histamine release. J. Infect. Dis. 157:502, 1988.

37. Arrang, J. M., Garbarg, M., Lancelot, J. C., et al.: Highly potent and selective ligands for histamine H3-receptors. Nature 327:117, 1987.

38. Black, J. W., Duncan, W. A. M., Durant, C. J., et al.: Definition and antagonism of histamine H2-receptors. Nature 236:385, 1972.

39. Melmon, K. L., Rocklin, R. E., and Rosenkranz, R. P.: Autacoids as modulators of the inflammatory and immune response. Am. J. Med. 71:100, 1981.

40. Braude, S., Coe, C., Royston, D., et al.: Histamine increases lung permeability by an H2-receptor mechanism. Lancet 2:372, 1984.

41. Arrang, J. M., Devaux, B., Chodkiewicz, J. P., et al.: H3-receptors control histamine release in human brain. J. Neurochem. 51:105, 1988.

42. Robertson, I., and Greaves, M. W.: Responses of human skin blood vessels to synthetic histamine analogues. Br. J. Clin. Pharmacol. 5:319, 1978.

43. Kaliner, M., Shelhamer, J. H., and Ottesen, E. A.: Effects of infused histamine: Correlation of plasma histamine levels and symptoms. J. Allergy Clin. Immunol. 69:283, 1982.

44. Ruoss, S. J., Hartmann, T., and Caughey, G. H.: Mast cell tryptase is a mitogen for cultured fibroblasts. J. Clin. Invest. 88:493, 1991.

45. Schwartz, L. B., Lewis, R. A., and Austen, K. F.: Tryptase from human pulmonary mast cells: Purification and characterization. J. Biol. Chem. 256:11939, 1981.

46. Hopsu, V. K., and Glenner, G. G.: A histochemical enzyme kinetic system applied to the trypsin-like amidase and esterase activity in human mast cells. J. Cell Biol. 17:503, 1963.

47. Schwartz, L. B., Lewis, R. A., Seldin, D., et al.: Acid hydrolases and tryptase from secretory granules of dispersed human lung mast cells. J. Immunol. 126:1290, 1981.

48. Schwartz, L. B.: Monoclonal antibodies against human mast cell tryptase demonstrate shared antigenic sites on subunits of tryptase and selective localization of the enzyme to mast cells. J. Immunol. 134:526, 1985.

49. Miller, J. S., Westin, E. H., and Schwartz, L. B.: Cloning and characterization of complementary DNA for human tryptase. J. Clin. Invest. 84:1188, 1989.

50. Vanderslice, P., Ballinger, S. M., Tam, E. K., et al.: Human mast cell tryptase: Multiple cDNAs and genes reveal a multigene serine protease family. Proc. Natl. Acad. Sci. U.S.A. 87:3811, 1990.

51. Miller, J. S., Moxley, G., and Schwartz, L. B.: Cloning and characterization of a second complementary DNA for human tryptase. J. Clin. Invest. 86:864, 1990.

51a. Goldstein, S. M., Leung, J., Schwartz, L. B., et al.: The protease composition of human skin mast cell protease-proteoglycan complexes. Tryptase resides in a complex distinct from chymase and carboxypeptidase. J. Immunol. 1992 (in press).

52. Schwartz, L. B., and Bradford, T. R.: Regulation of tryptase from human lung mast cells by heparin: Stabilization of the active tetramer. J. Biol. Chem. 261:7372, 1986.

53. Alter, S. C., Metcalfe, D. D., Bradford, T. R., et al.: Regulation of human mast cell tryptase: Effects of enzyme concentration, ionic strength and the structure and negative charge density of polysaccharides. Biochem. J. 248:821, 1987.

54. Schwartz, L. B., Bradford, T. R., Littman, B. H., et al.: The fibrogenolytic activity of purified tryptase from human lung mast cells. J. Immunol. 135:2762, 1985.

55. Schwartz, L. B., Kawahara, M. S., Hugli, T. E., et al.: Generation of C3a anaphylatoxin from human C3 by human mast cell tryptase. J. Immunol. 130:1891, 1983.

56. Sekizawa, K., Caughey, G. H., Lazarus, S. C., et al.: Mast cell tryptase causes airway smooth muscle hyperresponsiveness in dogs. J. Clin. Invest. 83:175, 1989.

57. Schechter, N. M., Fraki, J. E., Geesin, J. C., et al.: Human skin chymotryptic protease: Isolation and relation to cathepsin G and rat mast cell proteinase I. J. Biol. Chem. 258:2973, 1983.

58. Caughey, G. H., Zerweck, E. H., and Vanderslice, P.: Structure, chromosomal assignment, and deduced amino acid sequence of a human gene for mast cell chymase. J. Biol. Chem. 266:12956, 1991.

59. Sayama, S., Iozzo, R. V., Lazarus, G. S., et al.: Human skin chymotrypsin-like proteinase chymase: Subcellular localization to mast cell granules and interaction with heparin and other glycosaminoglycans. J. Biol. Chem. 262:6808, 1987.

60. Schechter, N. M., Sprows, J. L., Schoenberger, O. L., et al.: Reaction of human skin chymotrypsin-like proteinase chymase with plasma proteinase inhibitors. J. Biol. Chem. 264:21308, 1989.

61. Wintroub, B. U., Schechter, N. B., Lazarus, G. S., et al.: Angiotensin I conversion by human and rat chymotryptic proteinases. J. Invest. Dermatol. 83:336, 1984.

62. Reilly, C. F., Tewksbury, D. A., Schechter, N. M., et al.: Rapid conversion of angiotensin I to angiotensin II by neutrophil and mast cell proteinases. J. Biol. Chem. 257:8619, 1982.

63. Briggaman, R. A., Schechter, N. M., Fraki, J., et al.: Degradation of the epidermal–dermal junction by a proteolytic enzyme from human skin and human polymorphonuclear leukocytes. J. Exp. Med. 160:1027, 1984.

64. Sommerhoff, C. P., Caughey, G. H., Finkbeiner, W. E., et al.: Mast cell chymase: A potent secretagogue for airway gland serous cells. J. Immunol. 142:2450, 1989.

65. Schechter, N. M., Irani, A.-M. A., Sprows, J. L., et al.: Identification of a cathepsin G–like proteinase in the MC$_{TC}$ type of human mast cell. J. Immunol. 145:2652, 1990.

66. Irani, A.-M. A., Goldstein, S. M., Wintroub, B. U., et al.: Human mast cell carboxypeptidase: Selective localization to MC$_{TC}$ cells. J. Immunol. 147:247, 1991.

67. Goldstein, S. M., Kaempfer, C. E., Proud, D., et al.: Detection and partial characterization of a human mast cell carboxypeptidase. J. Immunol. 139:2724, 1987.

68. Goldstein, S. M., Kaempfer, C. E., Kealey, J. T., et al.: Human mast cell carboxypeptidase: Purification and characterization. J. Clin. Invest. 83:1630, 1989.

69. Reynolds, D. S., Gurley, D. S., Stevens, R. L., et al.: Cloning of cDNAs that encode human mast cell carboxypeptidase A, and comparison of the protein with mouse mast cell carboxypeptidase A and rat pancreatic carboxypeptidases. Proc. Natl. Acad. Sci. U.S.A. 86:9480, 1989.

70. Thompson, H. L., Schulman, E. S., and Metcalfe, D. D.: Identification of chondroitin sulfate E in human lung mast cells. J. Immunol. 140:2708, 1988.

71. Stevens, R. L., Fox, C. C., Lichtenstein, L. M., et al.: Identification of chondroitin sulfate E proteoglycans and heparin proteoglycans in the secretory granules of human lung mast cells. Proc. Natl. Acad. Sci. U.S.A. 85:2284, 1988.

72. Metcalfe, D. D., Bland, C. E., and Wasserman, S. I.: Biochemical and functional characterization of proteoglycans isolated from basophils of patients with chronic myelogenous leukemia. J. Immunol. 132:1943, 1984.

73. Stevens, R. L., Avraham, S., Gartner, M. C., et al.: Isolation and characterization of a cDNA that encodes the peptide core of the secretory granule proteoglycan of human promyelocytic leukemia HL-60 cells. J. Biol. Chem. 263:7287, 1988.

74. Metcalfe, D. D., Soter, N. A., Wasserman, S. I., et al.: Identification of sulfated mucopolysaccharides including heparin in the lesional skin of a patient with mastocytosis. J. Invest. Dermatol. 74:210, 1980.

75. Metcalfe, D. D., Lewis, R. A., Silbert, J. E., et al.: Isolation and characterization of heparin from human lung. J. Clin. Invest. 64:1537, 1979.

76. Oscarsson, L. G., Pejler, G., and Lindahl, U.: Location of the anti-thrombin-binding sequence in the heparin chain. J. Biol. Chem. 264:296, 1989.

77. Peters, S. P., MacGlashan, D. W., Schulman, E. S., et al: Arachidonic acid metabolism in purified human lung mast cells. J. Immunol. 132:1972, 1984.

78. Dvorak, A. M., Dvorak, H. F., Peters, S. P., et al.: Lipid bodies: Cytoplasmic organelles important to arachidonate metabolism in macrophages and basophils. J. Immunol. 131:2965, 1983.

79. Robinson, C.: Mast cells and newly-generated lipid mediators. In Holgate, S. T. (ed.): Immunology and Medicine: Mast Cells, Mediators and Disease. London, Kluwer Academic Publishers, 1988.

80. MacGlashan, D. W., Jr., Peters, S. P., Warner, J., et al.: Characteristics of human basophil sulfidopeptide leukotriene release: Releasability defined as the ability of basophils to respond to dimeric cross-links. J. Immunol. 136:2231, 1986.

81. Rothenberg, M. E., Caulfield, J. P., Austen, K. F., et al.: Biochemical and morphological characterization of basophilic leukocytes from two patients with myelogenous leukemia. J. Immunol. 138:2616, 1987.

82. Roberts, L. J., II, Sweetman, B. J., Lewis, R. A., et al.: Increased production of prostaglandin D2 in patients with systemic mastocytosis. N. Engl. J. Med. 303:1400, 1980.

83. Brown, M. A., Pierce, J. H., Watson, C. J., et al.: B Cell stimulatory factor-1/interleukin-4 mRNA is expressed by normal and transformed mast cells. Cell 50:809, 1987.

84. Young, J. D.-E., Liu, C.-C., Butler, G., et al.: Identification, purification, and characterization of a mast cell–associated cytolytic factor related to tumor necrosis factor. Proc. Natl. Acad. Sci. U.S.A. 84:9175, 1987.

85. Steffen, M., Abboud, M., Potter, G. K., et al.: Presence of tumour necrosis factor or a related factor in human basophil/mast cells. Immunology 66:445, 1989.

86. Klein, L. M., Lavker, R. M., Matis, W. L., et al.: Degranulation of human mast cells induces an endothelial antigen central to leukocyte adhesion. Proc. Natl. Acad. Sci. U.S.A. 86:8972, 1989.

87. Walsh, L. J., Trinchieri, G., Waldorf, H. A., et al.: Human dermal mast cells contain and release tumor necrosis factor α, which induces endothelial leukocyte adhesion molecule 1. Proc. Natl. Acad. Sci. U.S.A. 88:4220, 1991.

88. Gruber, B. L., Baeza, M. L., Marchese, M. J., et al.: Prevalence and functional role of anti-IgE autoantibodies in urticarial syndromes. J. Invest. Dermatol. 90:213, 1988.

89. Gruber, B. L., Kaufman, L. D., Marchese, M. J., et al.: Anti-IgE autoantibodies in systemic lupus erythematosus: Prevalence and biologic activity. Arthritis Rheum. 31:1000, 1988.

90. Metzger, H., Alcarez, G., Hohman, R., et al.: The receptor with high affinity for immunoglobulin E. Annu. Rev. Immunol. 4:419, 1986.

91. Becker, E. L., and Austen, K. F.: Mechanisms of immunologic injury of rat peritoneal mast cells: I. The effect of phosphonate inhibitors on the homocytotropic antibody–mediated histamine release and the first component of rat complement. J. Exp. Med. 124:379, 1966.

92. Foreman, J. C., Mongar, B. D., and Gomperts, B. D.: Calcium ionophores and movement of calcium ions following the physiological stimulus to a secretory process. Nature (Lond.) 245:249, 1973.

93. Hagermark, O., Hokfelt, T., and Pernow, B.: Flare and itch induced by substance P in human skin. J. Invest. Dermatol. 71:233, 1978.

94. Church, M. K., Lowman, M. A., Rees, P. H., et al.: Plenary lecture: Mast cells, neuropeptides and inflammation. Agents Actions 27:8, 1989.

95. Schleimer, R. P., Lichtenstein, L. M., and Gillespie, E.: Inhibition of basophil histamine release by anti-inflammatory steroids. Nature (Lond.) 292:454, 1981.

96. Schleimer, R. P., Schulman, E. S., MacGlash, D. W., et al.: Effects of dexamethasone on mediator release from human lung fragments and purified human lung mast cells. J. Clin. Invest. 71:1830, 1983.

97. Holgate, S. T., Lewis, R. A., and Austen, K. F.: Role of adenylate cyclase in the immunologic release of mediators from rat mast cells: Agonist and antagonist effects of purine- and ribose-modified adenosine analogs. Proc. Natl. Acad. Sci. U.S.A. 77:6800, 1980.

98. Peachell, P. T., MacGlashan, D. W., Jr., Lichtenstein, L. M., et al.: Regulation of human basophil and lung mast cell function by cyclic adenosine monophosphate. J. Immunol. 140:571, 1988.

99. Peachell, P. T., Columbo, M., Kagey-Sobotka, A., et al.: Adenosine potentiates mediator release from human lung mast cells. Am. Rev. Respir. Dis. 138:1143, 1988.

100. Peachell, P. T., Lichtenstein L. M., and Schleimer, R. P.: Differential regulation of human basophil and lung mast cell function by adenosine. J. Pharmacol. Exp. Ther. 256:717, 1991.

101. Chock, S. P., and Schmauder-Chock, E. A.: Phospholipid storage in the secretory granule of the mast cell. J. Biol. Chem. 264:2862, 1989.

102. Beaven, M. A., Moore, J. P., Smith, G., et al.: The calcium signal and phosphatidyl-inositol turnover in 2H3 cells. J. Biol. Chem. 259:7137, 1984.

103. Ishizaka, T., Conrad, D. H., Schulman, E. S., et al.: Biochemical analysis of initial triggering events of IgE-mediated histamine release from human lung mast cells. J. Immunol. 130:2357, 1983.

104. White, J. R., Plaznik, D. H., and Ishizaka, T.: Antigen-induced increase in protein kinase C activity in plasma membranes of mast cells. Proc. Natl. Acad. Sci. U.S.A. 82:8193, 1985.

105. Ishizaka, T., Conrad, D. H., Huff, T. F., et al.: Unique features of human basophilic granulocytes developed in in vitro culture. Int. Arch. Allergy Appl. Immunol. 77:137, 1985.

106. Wenzel, S., Irani, A. M., Sanders, J. M., et al.: Immunoassay of tryptase from human mast cells. J. Immunol. Methods 86:139, 1986.

107. Schwartz, L. B., Metcalfe, D. D., Miller, J. S., et al.: Tryptase levels as an indicator of mast-cell activation in systemic anaphylaxis and mastocytosis. N. Engl. J. Med. 316:1622, 1987.

108. Shalit, M., Schwartz, L. B., Golzar, N., et al.: Release of histamine and tryptase in vivo after prolonged cutaneous challenge with allergen in humans. J. Immunol. 141:821, 1988.

109. Charlesworth, E. N., Hood, A. F., Soter, N. A., et al.: Cutaneous late-phase response to allergen: Mediator release and inflammatory cell infiltration. J. Clin. Invest. 83:1519, 1989.

110. Walden, S. M., Proud, D., Bascom, R., et al.: Experimentally induced nasal allergic responses. J. Allergy Clin. Immunol. 81:940, 1988.

111. Mican, J. M., and Metcalfe, D. D.: Arthritis and mast cell activation. J. Allergy Clin. Immunol. 86(Suppl.):677, 1990.

112. Crisp, A. J., Chapman, C. M., Kirkham, S. E., et al.: Articular mastocytosis in rheumatoid arthritis. Arthritis Rheum. 27:845, 1984.

113. Godfrey, H. P., Ilardi, C., Engber, W., et al.: Quantitation of human synovial mast cells in rheumatoid arthritis and other rheumatic diseases. Arthritis Rheum. 27:852, 1984.

114. Malone, D. G., Irani, A. M., Schwartz, L. B., et al.: Mast cell numbers and histamine levels in synovial fluids from patients with arthritides of various etiologies. Arthritis Rheum. 29:956, 1986.

115. Gruber, B., Ballan, D., and Gorevic, P. D.: IgE rheumatoid factors: Quantification in synovial fluid and ability to induce synovial mast cell histamine release. Clin. Exp. Immunol. 71:289, 1988.

116. Chard, M. D., and Crisp, A. J.: Astemizole, an H₁ antagonist, has no additional therapeutic effect in rheumatoid arthritis. J. Rheumatol. 18:203, 1991.

117. Brodeur, J. P., Ruddy, S., Schwartz, L. B., et al.: Synovial fluid levels of complement SC5b-9 and fragment Bb are elevated in patients with rheumatoid arthritis. Arthritis Rheum. 34:1531, 1991.

118. Nishioka, K., Kobayashi, Y., Katayama, I., et al.: Mast cell numbers in diffuse scleroderma. Arch. Dermatol. 123:205, 1987.

119. Kawanami, O., Ferrans, V., Fulmer, J. D., et al.: Ultrastructure of pulmonary mast cells in patients with fibrotic lung disorders. Lab. Invest. 40:717, 1979.

120. Goto, T., Befus, D., Low, R., et al.: Mast cell heterogeneity and hyperplasia in bleomycin-induced pulmonary fibrosis in rats. Am. Rev. Respir. Dis. 130:797, 1984.

121. Smith, C. J., Smith, J. C., and Finn, M. C.: The possible role of mast cells (allergy) in the production of keloid and hypertrophic scarring. J. Burn Care Rehab. 8:126, 1987.

121a. Irani, A. A., Gruber, B. L., Kaufman, L. D., et al.: Mast cell changes in scleroderma: Presence of MC_T cells in the skin and evidence of mast cell activation. Arthritis Rheum. 1992 (in press).

122. Claman, H. N.: Mast cell changes in a case of rapidly progressive scleroderma: Ultrastructural analysis. J. Invest. Dermatol. 92:290, 1989.

123. Choi, K. L., Giorna, R., and Claman, H. N.: Cutaneous mast cell depletion and recovery in murine graft-vs-host disease. J. Immunol. 138:4093, 1987.

124. Seibold, J. R., Giorno, R. C., and Claman, H. N.: Dermal mast cell degranulation in systemic sclerosis. Arthritis Rheum. 33:1702, 1990.

125. Levi-Schaffer, F., Austen, K. F., Caulfield, J. P., et al.: Co-culture of human lung-derived mast cells with mouse 3T3 fibroblasts: Morphology and IgE-mediated release of histamine, prostaglandin D2, and leukotrienes. J. Immunol. 139:494, 1987.

126. Davidson, S. M. A., Mansour, A., Gallily, R., et al.: Mast cell differentiation depends on T cells and granule synthesis on fibroblasts. Immunology 48:439, 1983.

127. Subba Rao, P. V., Friedman, M. M., Atkins, F. M., et al.: Phagocytosis of mast cell granules by cultured fibroblasts. J. Immunol. 130:341, 1983.

128. Ginsburg, H., Amira, M., Padawer, J., et al.: Structural alterations in fibroblast monolayers caused by mast cell degranulation. J. Leukocyte Biol. 45:491, 1989.

129. Dayton, E. T., Caulfield, J. P., Hein, A., et al.: Regulation of the growth rate of mouse fibroblasts by IL-3–activated mouse bone marrow–derived mast cells. J. Immunol. 142:4307, 1989.

Chapter 18

Frank H. Valone

Platelets

INTRODUCTION

Platelets evolved from primitive cells that had both hemostatic and phagocytic capabilities.[1] The primary function of platelets is to respond to tissue injury by maintaining vascular integrity and initiating tissue repair.[2, 3] Platelets retain many immunologic capabilities and may contribute to host defense.[4, 5] Inappropriate platelet activation, however, may lead to vascular disruption, development of inflammatory diseases, and ultimately, tissue fibrosis through the action of platelet-derived growth factors (PDGF). Platelets are anucleate, discoid, cytoplasmic fragments that are approximately 2 μm in diameter. They form a heterogeneous population that can be subdivided by density centrifugation or flow cytometry into subpopulations that differ in content and function.[6, 7] Platelets derive from specific cytoplasmic projections of megakaryocytes in the bone marrow and have a circulating half-life of 7 to 11 days.[8] Because platelets lack nuclei, they are incapable of protein synthesis. Platelets contain, however, most of the subcellular organelles found in other cells, including mitochondria, microtubules, glycogen granules, Golgi cisternae, and ribosomes.[9] The most prominent organelles, which comprise 20 percent of the platelet volume, are secretory granules, i.e., dense granules (or dense bodies) and alpha (α) granules. These granules contain a rich array of biologically active factors that, in conjunction with newly formed lipid mediators, may contribute to host defense, tissue repair, or development of immunologic diseases.

MECHANISMS OF PLATELET ACTIVATION

The process of platelet activation after vascular disruption is characterized by numerous amplifying and inhibitory pathways. The pathways interact to form a hemostatic plug initially to prevent further blood loss. Platelets then promote healing through recruitment of other cells and release of growth factors. Platelets are activated after vascular injury by two general mechanisms: adhesion to disrupted vascular surfaces, and direct activation by soluble factors (Table 18–1). Under conditions of low flow

rates and low shear force, platelets adhere to components of the subendothelial matrix such as collagen and microfibrils as well as the adhesive proteins, fibronectin, vitronectin, and laminin.[10] Platelets adhere to interstitial collagen types I and III and to basement membrane collagen type IV. Under conditions of high shear forces, such as those found in arteries and the microvasculature, von Willebrand factor is required for optimal platelet adhesion to the subendothelium.[11] Von Willebrand factor, which is derived mainly from platelets and endothelial cells, promotes adhesion by interacting with subendothelial matrix components, including collagen and heparin-like glycosaminoglycans, and with the platelet receptor, glycoprotein IIb/IIIa.[12, 13] Adherent platelets form a layer over the subendothelial surface. Additional platelets are then recruited by fluid-phase mediators to stick specifically to the adherent platelets through a process termed *platelet aggregation*. Fibrinogen is an essential cofactor for aggregation.[14] The fluid-phase factors that mediate aggregation include thrombin[15] and platelet products such as ADP,[16] endoperoxides prostaglandin G_2 (PGG_2) and

Table 18–1. ACTIVATORS OF PLATELETS DURING HEMOTASTASIS AND INFLAMMATORY REACTIONS

Mechanism	Activator
Adhesion	Collagen
	Microfilaments
	Fibronectin
	Laminin
	Vitronectin
	Urate crystals
Fluid phase	
Nonimmunologic	
Hemostatic	Thrombin
	Collagen
	ADP
	Epinephrine
	Arachidonic acid metabolites (e.g., PGG_2, PGH_2, thromboxane A_2)
Other	Serotonin
	Vasopressin
	Double-stranded DNA
Immunologic	PAF
	Immune complexes
	Antibodies to drugs
	Micro-organisms
	Substance P
Enhancers of activation	Complement
	Single-stranded DNA
	Lipopolysaccharides (endotoxin)

Supported by the Veterans Administration and American Cancer Society grant IM522.

319

PGH$_2$, and thromboxanes.[17, 18] Potent platelet activators, including thrombin, platelet-activating factor (PAF),[19] collagen,[20] endoperoxides, and thromboxanes, stimulate platelets to release the contents of their granules, a process that is termed the *release reaction*. Granule contents that enhance further platelet aggregation include serotonin, ADP, von Willebrand factor, fibrinogen, and thrombospondin. Fibrinogen, thrombospondin, fibronectin, vitronectin, and von Willebrand factor share a critical amino acid sequence, Arg-Gly-Asp. The receptor for these molecules, glycoprotein IIb/IIIa, is a member of a superfamily of heterodimeric adhesion receptors.

Structurally related receptors mediate intercellular adhesion by a variety of cells and are termed *integrins* or *cytoadhesions*.[21, 22] The integrin family has numerous members, including the beta (β)-2 subfamily (LFA-1, MAC-1) and the β-1 subfamily (receptors for fibronectin, laminin, and collagen). The capacity of activated platelets to recruit other platelets through release of activating factors creates a positive feedback loop that promotes formation of a hemostatic plug. Factors that limit this process include the endothelial products prostacyclin[23] and endothelium-derived relaxing factor, which may be nitric oxide.[24] Platelet activation is also inhibited by PGD$_2$[25] and 12-hydroxyeicosatetraenoic acid (12-HETE).[26] Immunologic and nonimmunologic factors that stimulate platelet aggregation in the absence of vascular disruption are described in a later section.

Aspirin and other nonsteroidal anti-inflammatory drugs inhibit platelet activation. The common mechanism of action for these agents is inhibition of platelet cyclooxygenase. This enzyme is a critical element in the pathway that metabolizes the fatty acid arachidonic acid to the endoperoxides PGG$_2$ and PGH$_2$ and thromboxanes A$_2$ and B$_2$, which are potent platelet stimuli.[27, 28] Aspirin irreversibly acetylates cyclooxygenase, whereas the other drugs typically inhibit the enzyme reversibly. Platelets are incapable of protein synthesis, so a single aspirin tablet inhibits the cyclooxygenase of circulating platelets until they are replaced by new, unaffected platelets. Not all stimuli require cyclooxygenase for platelet activation. Aspirin effectively inhibits platelet activation by ADP, immune complexes, and small amounts of collagen[29, 30] but has little or no effect on platelet activation by thrombin and PAF.[31, 32]

PLATELET-DERIVED MEDIATORS OF INFLAMMATION

The processes of platelet adhesion, aggregation, and release reaction promote hemostasis and wound repair. The same processes can contribute to rheumatic diseases when inappropriate or uncontrolled platelet activation occurs. Platelet activation may result from hemostatic pathways after vascular disruption by local inflammation or from effects of immunologically generated fluid-phase platelet activators (see Table 18–1). Platelets release a host of lipid, peptide, and protein mediators that may contribute to tissue damage and fibrosis (Table 18–2). Multiple

Table 18–2. PLATELET-DERIVED MEDIATORS OF INFLAMMATION

Class	Mediator	Actions
Lipid		
Cyclooxygenase-dependent	Thromboxane A$_2$	Vasoconstrictor; proaggregant; increases neutrophil adherence
	Thromboxane B$_2$	More stable thromboxane A$_2$ derivative
	Prostaglandins D$_2$, E$_2$, F$_2$	Vasoactive; modulates hemostasis and leukocyte function
	HHT	Chemotactic
Lipoxygenase-dependent	12-HPETE	Vasoconstrictor; cyclooxygenase inhibitor; stimulates leukocyte LTB$_4$ synthesis
	12-HETE	Chemotactic
Phospholipid	PAF	Proaggregant; increases vascular permeability; neutrophil and monocyte activation
Protein/Peptide		
Dense body	Serotonin	Vasoconstrictor; increases vascular permeability; fibrogenic
Alpha granule	PDGF	Chemotactic
	PF4	Proaggregant; chemotactic; induces basophil histamine release
	TG-β	Neutrophil and monocyte activation
"Granule" contents	IL-1β	Pyrogen; tissue inflammation
	Cationic permeability factor	Stimulates mast cell histamine; chemotactic
	Elastase	Neutral proteinase
	Collagenase	Neutral proteinase
	α$_1$-Antitrypsin	Protease inhibitor
	α$_2$-Macroglobulin	Protease inhibitor
	α$_2$-Antiplasmin	Primary plasmin inhibitor
	Plasminogen activator inhibitor-1	Inhibits plasminogen activators

Table 18–3. GROWTH FACTORS RELEASED BY
PLATELETS

Mediator	Action
PDGF	Connective tissue mitogen; cell-transforming factor
Transforming growth factor beta (TGF-β)	Modulates cell proliferation; stimulates matrix synthesis; fibrogenic
β-TG (CTAP III)	Fibroblast proliferation
IL-1	Modulates fibroblast proliferation
Endothelial cell growth factor	Endothelial proliferation
Epidermal growth factor	Epidermal and epithelial proliferation

pathophysiologic processes may occur, including (1) promoting cell aggregation, altering blood flow, and increasing vascular permeability; (2) recruiting inflammatory cells; (3) directly damaging tissues; and (4) stimulating cell proliferation and fibrosis. Platelets also release protease inhibitors that serve to limit tissue damage during inflammatory reactions. Some of these factors that affect inflammation such as platelet factor-4 (PF4) are unique to platelets, whereas most are found in a variety of cells.

Serotonin is a weak stimulus of platelet activation but is a potent vasoconstrictor and interacts with thromboxane A_2 to increase vascular permeability and promote collagen synthesis.[33] Platelets metabolize arachidonic acid via a cyclooxygenase pathway to yield the cyclic endoperoxides PGG_2 and PGH_2, which are converted by thromboxane synthetase to thromboxane A_2 and its more stable product, thromboxane B_2.[17, 18, 34] The endoperoxides and thromboxanes are potent platelet stimuli and vasoconstrictors. Minor cyclooxygenase products of platelets include PGE_2, PGD_2, and 12-L-hydroxy-5, 8, 10-heptadecatrienoic acid (HHT). The former products have diverse effects on cell function, whereas HHT is primarily chemotactic. Arachidonic acid is also oxygenated by a platelet 12-lipoxygenase to the 12-monohydroperoxy and 12-monohydroxy fatty acids 12-hydroxyperoxyeicosatetraenoic (12-HPETE) and 12-HETE. These products inhibit platelet cyclooxygenase and platelet activation,[35] but they also stimulate neutrophil function.[36] Neutrophils and platelets exchange arachidonic acid metabolites to produce lipoxygenase products that neither cell can produce alone. Nonsteroidal anti-inflammatory drugs are potent inhibitors of platelet cyclooxygenase but have no effect on platelet lipoxygenase.

Activated platelets have interleukin-1β (IL-1β) on their surfaces.[37] Expression of IL-1β does not require release of platelet granules, suggesting that IL-1β is sequestered in membranes rather than being a granule constituent that is released during platelet activation. IL-1β has complex effects.[37a] IL-1β and PDGF stimulate synoviocyte proliferation in the presence of cyclooxygenase inhibitors, whereas IL-1β inhibits proliferation in the absence of the inhibi-

tors.[38] IL-1β also stimulates PGE_2 and collagenase production by rheumatoid synoviocytes and dermal fibroblasts, which may result in bone resorption and cartilage destruction.[39]

PF4 is a 29-Kilodalton (kD) basic protein that is found only in platelets. PF4 affects diverse processes, including vascular permeability,[40] chemotaxis of neutrophils and monocytes,[41] and stimulation of elastase and calcium mobilization from bone.[42] PF4 forms complexes with glycosaminoglycans, and this interaction may be important for its biologic effects. Platelets contain proteases that may promote tissue damage and protease inhibitors that limit tissue damage and prevent clot dissolution.

GROWTH FACTORS RELEASED BY PLATELETS

Activated platelets release several proteins and glycoproteins that stimulate cell proliferation and extracellular matrix deposition (Table 18–3). PDGF is a 30 to 35 kd protein that stimulates migration and proliferation of fibroblasts and stimulates proliferation of smooth muscle and glial cells.[43, 44, 44a] Despite its name, PDGF is found in numerous cells. PDGF is composed of A and B chains, and the B chain is nearly identical to the human *cis* oncogene.[44] This observation suggests that PDGF may have a fundamental role in autocrine regulation of cell proliferation. Exploration of PDGF's actions has offered important insights into the biologic and pathologic roles of oncogenes. Thromboglobulin-β (TG-β) is an 8.8-kD protein that exists as a tetramer and whose amino acid sequence is approximately 50 percent homologous with PF4. TG-β, connective tissue–activating peptide (CTAP) III, PF4, and low-affinity PF4 are antigenically related and may derive from a single precursor molecule termed *platelet basic protein.*[45] TG-β and CTAP III stimulate synovial cells and fibroblasts, although stimulation may require cofactors including IL-1.[46] CTAP III stimulates DNA and glycosaminoglycan synthesis in cells derived from connective tissue and has been identified in synovial fluids and tissues.[47, 48] Transforming growth factor (TGF)-β is a 25-kD protein that has complex effects on cell growth and differentiation, depending on the target cell.[49] TGF-β induces loss of contact inhibition of cells in culture and, in the presence of cofactors such as PDGF, induces colony formation. TGF-β stimulates early bone growth, suggesting that it may be important to bone repair after injury.[50] In contrast, TGF-β may inhibit growth of synoviocytes stimulated by PDGF.[51] Injection of TGF-β into animals induces fibrosis and angiogenesis.[52]

PLATELET ACTIVATION BY MEDIATORS OF INFLAMMATION

Platelets may be activated during inflammatory processes by typical hemostatic pathways if the vasculature has been disrupted by ongoing tissue inflammation or injury. Alternatively, platelets may be activated by factors unique to tissue inflammation that may be soluble (e.g., PAF) or particulate (e.g., urate crystals). Several of these factors, including PAF, immune complexes, complement components, and urate cystals, have been identified in inflamed synovial tissues and fluids.

Platelet-Activating Factor. PAF is a low-molecular-weight phospholipid that is produced after immunologic and nonimmunologic activation of a variety of cells, including neutrophils, monocytes, endothelial cells, and platelets.[53] PAF has a wide range of target cells, including platelets, neutrophils, monocytes, eosinophils, T and B lymphocytes, and endothelial cells.[54, 55, 55a] PAF stimulates neutrophil adherence, chemotaxis, and release of inflammatory products. Similarly, PAF stimulates monocyte chemotaxis, cytotoxicity, and release of inflammatory cytokines, including IL-1 and tumor necrosis factor (TNF). Despite having a short half-life in vivo, PAF induces prolonged tissue inflammation that is characterized by infiltration of eosinophils, neutrophils, or mononuclear leukocytes, depending on target tissue and time after administration.[56] This effect probably results from release of secondary mediators, including leukotrienes, IL-1, and TNF.[57] These cytokines have potent proinflammatory effects[58] and have been shown to contribute to joint injury and bone resorption.[59, 60] PAF participates in several positive feedback loops that serve to prolong tissue injury. PAF induces synthesis of IL-1 and TNF by monocytes-macrophages,[57] and these cytokines induce PAF synthesis by the same cells.[61] PAF also induces its own synthesis by cells such as neutrophils and monocytes, which, in turn, are activated by PAF.

Immune Complexes and Complement. Platelets have a 40-kD receptor for the Fc portion of immunoglobulins (FcR), which is apparently identical to FcR III found on other cells, including neutrophils.[62] Immunoglobulin bound to surfaces, antigen-antibody complexes, and IgG aggregates all effectively bind to FcR. Cross-linking of FcR induces platelet aggregation and release of inflammatory mediators. There is apparently some specificity for platelet aggregation by small IgG aggregates found in rheumatoid synovial fluid compared with larger complexes, which are cleared more rapidly.[63] Platelet activation by soluble immune complexes may contribute to vasculitis and nephritis of serum sickness[64, 65] and may result in thrombocytopenia due to platelet sequestration and increased rate of clearance. Similarly, drug-induced thrombocytopenia may result from platelet sequestration or lysis, or both, by circulating drug-antibody complexes. Quinidine-induced purpura is one of the best studied of the drug-induced thrombocytopenias[66]; the pathogenesis of this disorder is complex and involves immunologic and nonspecific drug-antibody binding to platelets. Heparin-induced thrombocytopenia occurs in up to 5 percent of patients who receive this drug and may

be complicated by acute arterial thrombosis; this disorder results from binding of heparin-antiheparin immune complexes to platelet FcR, resulting in platelet activation and rapid clearance from the circulation.[67] Gold-induced thrombocytopenia occurs in 1 to 5 percent of patients regardless of the gold preparation used[68]; this complication occurs early in therapy, usually before patients receive 1 g of gold. Thrombocytopenia may result from marrow aplasia but more typically results from immune destruction with shortened platelet survival.[69] Platelet-associated IgG is increased during episodes of thrombocytopenia, and thrombocytopenia responds to immunologic therapy such as administration of corticosteroids or gamma globulin. HLA-DR3 is associated with development of toxic reactions to gold. More than 85 percent of patients with gold-induced thrombocytopenia are HLA-DR3 positive compared with 30 percent of patients with rheumatoid arthritis.[68]

Human platelet activation via FcR does not require complement activation, whereas complement facilitates platelet activation by immune complexes in some species.[70] Complement components may enhance human platelet activation by thrombin and other stimuli. In contrast, Clq inhibits platelet activation by collagen.[71] This effect is primarily on aggregation rather than platelet adhesion to collagen. Complement may contribute to platelet lysis by antiplatelet antibodies. Platelets are activated directly by assembly of C5b-9 on platelet membranes via either the classic or alternative complement pathways.[72] C5b-9 increases platelet binding of coagulation factors Va and Xa and increases platelet prothrombinase activity. Platelets may also facilitate complement activation by cleavage of C5 by membrane-bound thrombin.[73]

DNA. Free DNA has been described in plasma in conditions associated with tissue injury, including vasculitis and systemic lupus erythematosus (SLE). Both native, double-stranded DNA and single-stranded DNA bind to platelets. Native DNA activates platelets directly, whereas single-stranded DNA enhances platelet activation by other agonists.[74–76] Circulating immune complexes of DNA–anti-DNA contribute to immune thrombocytopenia in SLE.

Microorganisms. Platelets bind bacteria directly via a unique receptor-ligand mechanism.[77] Bacterial binding induces platelet aggregation and release reaction via an antibody-FcR–dependent pathway. Platelet-bacteria interactions may contribute to vegetation formation during endocarditis but may also limit growth of bacteria through the effects of platelet bactericidal factors. Platelets also contribute to host resistance to parasites, including *Schistosoma mansoni* and filarial parasites.[78] Platelets have low-affinity receptors for IgE that are similar to IgE receptors on macrophages and eosinophils. Specific IgE antiparasite antibodies facilitate platelet binding and killing of parasites. The specific cytotoxic mechanisms may involve oxygen radicals and cytotoxic proteins released by platelets.

Table 18–4. PLATELET-NEUTROPHIL INTERACTIONS
DURING INFLAMMATION

Increased synthesis of inflammatory mediators
  PAF
  Leukotrienes
Increased neutrophil activation
  Adherence
  Cytotoxicity
  Release of oxygen radicals
  Release of granule constituents
  Phagocytosis
Increased platelet activation
Impaired cell activation
  Release of oxygen radicals
  Platelet aggregation

Urate Crystals. Monosodium urate crystals, the causative agent of gout, can potentially interact with platelets in both extravascular and intravascular sites. Urate crystals form a surface that activates platelets by interacting with specific platelet membrane proteins, including glycoprotein IIb/IIIa.[79] Platelet activation by urate crystals is novel because urate induces selective secretion of dense body constituents followed by platelet lysis.

PLATELET-NEUTROPHIL INTERACTIONS

Activated platelets release numerous factors, including PF4, 12-HETE, and HHT, which are chemotactic for neutrophils. Subsequent interactions of these cells are enhanced by PADGEM, which is a platelet surface protein similar to the adhesion proteins ELAM-1 and MEL-14.[80, 80a] Interactions between platelets and neutrophils may either promote or limit inflammation[81] (Table 18–4). Platelets and neutrophils cooperate to synthesize PAF synergistically.[82] Platelets release the inactive precursor lyso-PAF, which is then converted to PAF by the neutrophils. A similar exchange occurs for intermediate products of arachidonic acid metabolism.[83] Neutrophils and platelets cooperate to synthesize leukotrienes and novel arachidonic acid metabolites that neither cell can produce alone. Platelet-derived adenine nucleotides have complex effects on release of oxygen radicals by neutrophils. ADP and ATP enhance release, whereas AMP and adenosine inhibit release.[84] Platelets scavenge oxygen radicals by a glutathione-dependent pathway that may limit the toxic effects of these radicals.[85] Similarly, PDGF reduces the neutrophil oxidative burst while enhancing phagocytosis.[86] Superoxide, hydrogen peroxide, and cathepsin G released by activated neutophils stimulate release of platelet constituents.[87, 88] This effect is balanced by a nitric oxide–like factor produced by activated neutrophils that inhibits platelet aggregation.[89]

MEASURING PLATELET ACTIVATION AND LOCALIZATION IN INFLAMMATION AND FIBROSIS

It has been technically difficult to determine the contribution of platelets to animal models of inflammatory disease and fibrosis because of limited sensitivity of available tests. Platelet aggregation may be reversible; therefore, transient aggregates formed during inflammation may be missed in pathologic studies. Degranulated and partially digested platelets have unremarkable ultrastructural features and may be difficult to identify by microscopy. More successful approaches involve radiolabeling platelets with indium or chromium and measuring local accumulation of radioactivity. Alternatively, local accumulation of platelet-specific proteins can be measured. A final approach is to determine the effects of selective depletion of platelets.

Measuring platelet activation in human disease would serve two purposes. First, it would implicate platelets in the pathogenesis of the disease. Second, it may offer a means to measure disease activity and the effects of therapy. One approach to this problem is to measure platelet turnover. This is a cumbersome test that does not measure activation, per se, but rather measures the changes in half-life that may result from activation. Levels of platelet stimuli, such as PAF and immune complexes, can also be measured, but such studies do not indicate if platelets are activated. Local or systemic release of platelet products, including PF4 and TG-β, are frequently used as indicators of platelet activation. These are useful research tools but are difficult to measure, especially in blood, and are unlikely to be useful for routine clinical purposes. Monoclonal antibodies that only bind to activated platelets have recently been developed, and these may be useful, specific measures of platelet activation.[90, 90a]

ANIMAL MODELS

Numerous studies have examined the contribution of platelets to immunologic reactions in animal models. Platelet deposition at sites of tissue injury has been demonstrated by accumulation of ^{51}Cr-labeled platelets or by microscopic techniques during sponge implantation,[91] Arthus reaction in the skin,[92, 93] and IgE-mediated anaphylaxis.[94] Platelets are required for the active Arthus reaction[93] and generalized Shwartzman reaction[95] because platelet depletion blocks these reactions. Platelets contribute to immune complex deposition, local inflammation, and cellular proliferation during acute serum sickness[96] and immune complex nephritis.[97] Platelet depletion diminishes these processes but does not eliminate tissue damage. Similarly, platelet depletion does not block IgE-mediated anaphylaxis completely. The failure of platelet depletion fully to abrogate these complex processes most likely results from the redundancy of immunologic pathways that contribute to tissue inflammation. Animal and human platelets differ significantly in their immunologic responses. For example, rat platelets do not respond to PAF. Thus, delineation of the platelet contribution to inflammation and fibrosis requires studies in humans.

RHEUMATOID ARTHRITIS

Several types of studies indicate that platelets may contribute to tissue damage in rheumatoid arthritis. Thrombocytosis is frequently observed in patients with rheumatoid arthritis, and higher platelet counts may correlate with more active disease.[98] Whether the thrombocytosis is simply reactive or contributes to disease pathogenesis is unknown. Despite the elevated platelet counts, platelets from patients with rheumatoid arthritis frequently have modestly shortened half-lives.[99] Platelet half-life does not correlate with levels of circulating immune complexes or with clinical and laboratory measures of disease activity. Circulating antibodies that stimulate platelet secretion are found frequently in patients with rheumatoid arthritis.[100] Platelet activation by these antibodies may account for the decreased granular constituents of circulating platelets and their shortened half-lives. Local platelet consumption in inflamed joints may also contribute to shorten platelet life spans because indium-labeled platelets tend to localize selectively to inflamed joints.[101] Increased numbers of platelets are recovered from synovial fluids of patients with rheumatoid arthritis compared to patients with osteoarthritis, with mean levels of 14,988 per mm^3 and 1592 per mm^3, respectively.[102] These levels are 1 to 10 percent of platelet levels in blood. Synovial fluid platelet counts correlate well with laboratory and clinical measures of disease activity. Analysis of the contents of platelets recovered from rheumatoid synovial fluid indicates that the platelets have released their granular constituents.[103] This observation supports a number of studies that demonstrate platelet products, including PF4 and TG-β in rheumatoid synovial fluid.

SCLERODERMA AND RAYNAUD'S PHENOMENON

Sclerodema is a connective tissue disorder characterized by cellular proliferation and fibrosis in the vasculature and tissues of the skin, musculoskeletal system, and internal organs.[104] Platelet activation by subendothelium exposed by immune injury to the endothelium may contribute to the pathogenesis of this disorder. Activated platelets release growth factors including PDGF, endothelial cell growth factor, IL-1, and TG-β, which may contribute to intimal proliferation and tissue fibrosis. Platelets from patients with sclerodema have increased adherence to collagen.[105] Increased numbers of circulating platelet aggregates and platelet products such as TG-β are found frequently.[106] Serotonin and other platelet factors may contribute to the episodic vasoconstriction that is characteristic of Raynaud's phenomenon. The platelets of these patients are abnormally sensitive to activation by low concentrations of ADP and serotonin.[107] Calcium channel blockers are effective for treating Raynaud's phenomenon,[108] and this effect parallels the drugs' capacity to inhibit platelet activation. Recent studies, however, suggest that platelet activation occurs mainly in patients with vascular disruption due to scleroderma and does not contribute to episodes of vasoconstriction.[109, 110]

SYSTEMIC LUPUS ERYTHEMATOSUS AND GLOMERULONEPHRITIS

Patients with SLE have circulating single- and double-stranded DNA and circulating immune complexes, some of which are DNA–anti-DNA complexes. Platelet-associated DNA is increased in SLE with DNA bound to specific platelet receptors and incorporated in immune complexes.[76] Single-stranded DNA enhances platelet activation by IgG complexes without activating platelets directly. In contrast, double-stranded DNA activates platelets in vitro directly. Platelet-associated IgG is also increased in SLE. A portion of the IgG is bound to the platelet FcR in the form of immune complexes. In addition, patients frequently have antiplatelet antibody.[111] Antiplatelet antibodies in SLE and chronic idiopathic immune thrombocytopenia are often directed toward glycoprotein IIb/IIIa. Increased platelet-associated IgG correlates with other serologic markers of disease activity but not with activity of glomerulonephritis.[112] Platelet activation by circulating immune complexes and antiplatelet antibodies contributes to platelet dysfunction and thrombocytopenia. Platelets of patients with SLE have decreased content of serotonin, and plasma has increased levels of platelet constituents, suggesting platelets are activated in vivo. The lupus anticoagulant may contribute to platelet activation in SLE by inhibiting endothelial cell synthesis of the platelet inhibitor prostacyclin.[113] Several studies indicate that platelet activation contributes to the pathogenesis of glomerulonephritis in SLE. Increased platelet cationic proteins are bound to the glomerular basement membrane, and increased PDGF is found in capillary walls.[114, 115] Cationic proteins can neutralize the basement membrane's negative charge, thereby increasing protein loss. PDGF can enhance cellular proliferation and the resulting renal dysfunction.

The author gratefully acknowledges the expert secretarial assistance of Ms. Junetta Garrard.

References

1. Hirsh, J., Buchanan, M. R., Ofosu, F. A., and Weitz, J.: Evolution of thrombosis. Ann. N. Y. Acad. Sci. 516:362, 1987.
2. Siess, W.: Molecular mechanisms of platelet activation. Physiol. Rev. 69:58, 1989.

3. Steen, V. M., and Holmsen, H.: Current aspects on human platelet activation and responses. Eur. J. Haematol. 38:383, 1987.

4. Oxholm, P., and Winther, K.: Thrombocyte involvement in immune inflammatory reactions. Allergy 41:1, 1986.

5. Page, C. P.: Platelets as inflammatory cells. Immunopharmacology 17:51, 1989.

6. Corash, L., Costa, J. L., et al.: Heterogeneity of human whole blood platelet subpopulations: III. Density-dependent differences in subcellular constituents. Blood 64:185, 1984.

7. Davis, T., Drotts, D., Weil, G., et al.: Flow cytometric measurements of cytoplasmic calcium changes in human platelets. Cytometry 9:138, 1988.

8. Shulman, N. R., and Jordan, J. V.: Platelet kinetics. In Colman, R. W., et al. (eds.): Hemostasis and Thrombosis: Basic Principles and Clinical Practice. Philadelphia, J. B. Lippincott, 1988, pp. 431–451.

9. Zucker-Franklin, D.: Platelet morphology and function. In Williams, W. J., Beutler, E., Erslev A. J., and Rechtman, M. A. (eds.): Hematology. New York, McGraw-Hill, 1990, 1172–1181.

10. Baumgartner, H. R., Turitto, V., and Weiss, H. J.: Effect of shear rate on platelet interaction with subendothelium in citrated and native blood: II. Relationships among platelet adhesion, thrombus dimensions, and fibrin formation. J. Lab. Clin. 95:208, 1980.

11. Baumgartner, H. R., Tscopp, T. B., and Meyer, D.: Shear rate dependent inhibition of platelet adhesion and aggregation on collagenous surfaces by antibodies to factor VIII/von Willebrand factor. Br. J. Haematol. 44:127, 1980.

12. Stel, H. V. Sakariassen, K. S., De Groot, P. G., et al.: von Willebrand factor in the vessel wall mediates platelet adherence. Blood 65:85, 1985.

13. Ruggeri, Z. M., and Zimmerman, T. S.: von Willebrand factor and von Willebrand disease. Blood 70:895, 1987.

14. McLean, J. R. Maxwell, R. E., and Hertler, D.: Fibrinogen and adenosine diphosphate-induced aggregation of platelets. Nature 202:605, 1964.

15. Berndt, M. C. Gregory, C., Dowden, G., et al.: Thrombin interactions with platelet membrane proteins. Ann. N. Y. Acad. Sci. 485:374, 1986.

16. Garder, A., Jonsen, J., LaLand, S., et al.: Adenosine diphosphate in red cells as a factor in the adhesiveness of human blood platelets. Nature 192:531, 1961.

17. Hamburg, M., and Samuelsson, B.: Prostaglandin endoperoxides, novel transformations of arachidonic acid in human platelets. Proc. Natl. Acad. Sci. U.S.A. 71:3400, 1974.

18. Brass, L. F.: The biochemistry of platelet activation. In Hoffman, R., et al. (eds.): Hematology: Basic Principles and Practice. New York, Churchill Livingstone, 1991, pp. 1176–1197.

19. Braquet, P., Touqui, L., Shen, T. Y., et al.: Perspectives in platelet activating factor research. Pharmacol. Rev. 39:97, 1987.

20. Charo, I. F., Feinman, R. D., and Detwiler, T. C.: Interrelations of platelet aggregation and secretion. J. Clin. Invest. 60:866, 1977.

21. Hynes, R. O.: Integrins: A family of cell surface receptors. Cell 48:549, 1987.

22. Springer, T. A.: Adhesion receptors of the immune system. Nature 346:425, 1990.

23. Weksler, B. B.: Prostacyclin. Prog. Hemost. Thromb. 6:113, 1982.

24. Palmer, R. M., Ferrige, A. G., and Moncada, S.: Nitric oxide release accounts for the biological activity of endothelium-derived relaxing factor. Nature 327:524, 1987.

25. Oelz, O., Oelz, R., Knapp, H. R., et al.: Biosynthesis of prostaglandin D₂: I. Formation of prostaglandin D₂ by human platelets. Prostaglandins 13:225, 1977.

26. Aharony, D., Smith, J.B., and Silver, M. J.: Regulation of arachidonate-induced platelet aggregation by the lipoxygenase product, 12-hydroperoxyeicosatetraenoic acid. Biochim. Biophys. Acta 718:193, 1982.

27. Vane. J. R.: Inhibition of prostaglandin synthesis as a mechanism of action for aspirin-like drugs. Nature 231:232, 1971.

28. Vane, J., and Botting, R.: Inflammation and the mechanism of action of anti-inflammatory drugs. FASEB J. 1:89, 1987.

29. Kinlough-Rathbone, R. L., Packhamn, M. A., Reimers, H. J., et al.: Mechanisms of platelet shape change, aggregation, and release induced by collagen, thrombin, or A23, 187. J. Lab. Med. 90:707, 1977.

30. Valone, F. H.: Synergistic platelet activation by IgG and the phospholipid platelet-activating factor 1-0-alkyl-2-acetyl-sn-glycero-3-phosphorylcholine. J. Clin. Immunol. 6:57, 1986.

31. Hoak, J. C., Czervionke, R. L., Fry, G. L., et al.: Interaction of thrombin and platelets with the vascular endothelium. Fed. Proc. 39:2606, 1980.

32. Lauri, D., Cerletti, C., and De Gaetano, G.: Amplification of primary response of human platelets to platelet-activating factor: Aspirin-sensitive and aspirin-insensitive pathways. J. Lab. Clin. Med. 105:653, 1985.

33. DeClerck, F., Somers, Y., and Van Gorp, L.: Platelet-vessel wall interactions in hemostasis: Implications of 5-hydroxytryptamine. Agents Actions 15:627, 1984.

34. Hammarstrom, S., and Falaradeau, P.: Resolution of prostaglandin endoperoxide synthase and thromboxane synthase of human platelets. Proc. Natl. Acad. Sci. U.S.A. 74:3691, 1977.

35. Aharony, D., Smith, J. B., and Silver, M. J.: Regulation of arachidonate-induced platelet aggregation by the lipoxygenase product, 12-hydroperoxyeicosatetraenoic acid. Biochim. Biophys. Acta 718:193, 1982.

36. Goetzl, E. J., Woods, J. M., and Gorman, R. R. : Stimulation of human eosinophil and neutrophil polymorphonuclear leukocyte chemotaxis and random migration by 12-L-hydroxy-5,8,10,14-eicosatetraenoic acid. J. Clin. Invest. 59:179, 1977.

37. Hawrylowicz, C. M., Santoro, S. A., Platt, F. M., et al.: Activated platelets express IL-1 activity. J. Immunol. 143:4015, 1989.

37a. Kirkham, E.: Interleukin-1, immune activation pathways, and different mechanisms in osteoarthritis and rheumatoid arthritis. Ann. Rheum. Dis. 50:395, 1991.

38. Kumkumain, G. K., Lafyatis, R., Remmers, E. F., et al.: Regulation of synoviocyte proliferation, prostaglandin production, and collagenase transcription. J. Immunol. 143:833, 1989.

39. Dayer, J. M. de Rochemonteix, B., Burrus, B., et al.: Human recombinant interleukin-1 stimulates collagenase and prostaglandin E₂ production by human synovial cells and dermal fibroblasts. J. Clin. Invest. 77:645, 1986.

40. Goldberg, I. D., Stemerman, M. B., and Handin, R. I.: Vascular permeation of platelet factor 4 after endothelial injury. Science 209:611, 1980.

41. Deuel, T. F., Senior, R. M., Hang, D. C., et al.: Platelet factor-4 is chemotactic for neutrophils and monocytes. Proc. Natl. Acad. Sci. U.S.A. 78:4584, 1981.

42. Horton, J. E., Harper, J., and Harper, E.: Platelet factor 4 regulates osteoclastic bone resorption in vitro. Biochim. Biophys. Acta 630:459, 1980.

43. Williams, L. T., Antoniades, H. N., and Goetzl, E. J.: Platelet-derived growth factor stimulates mouse 3T3 cell mitogenesis and leukocyte chemotaxis through different structural determinants. J. Clin. Invest. 72:1759, 1983.

44. Ross, R., Raines, E. W., and Bowen-Pope, P. F.: The biology of platelet-derived growth factor. Cell 46:155, 1986.

44a. Cromack, D. T., et al.: TGF-beta and PDGF mediated tissue repair: identifying mechanisms of action using impaired and normal models of wound healing. Prog. Clin. Biol. Res. 365:359, 1991.

45. Harrison, P., Savidge, G. F., and Cramer, E. M.: The origin and physiological relevance of alpha granule adhesive proteins. Br. J. Haematol. 74:125, 1990.

46. Brandt, E., Ernst, M., Loppnow, H., and Flad, H. D.: Characterization of a platelet derived factor modulating phagocyte functions and co-operating with interleukin I. Lymphokine Res. 8:281, 1989.

47. Sloan, T. B., Weiss, J. J., Anderson, B., et al.: Connective tissue activation. XVI. Detection of a human platelet derived connective tissue activating peptide (CTAP-III) in human sera and plasma and in synovial fluids and tissues. Proc. Soc. Exp. Biol. Med. 164:267, 1980.

48. Castor, C. W., Bignall, M. C., Hossler, P. A., et al.: Connective tissue activation. XXI. Regulation of glycosaminoglycan metabolism by lymphocyte (CTAP-I) and platelet (CTAP-III) growth factors. In Vitro 17:777, 1981.

49. Assoian, R. K., and Sporn, M. B.: Type beta transforming growth factor in human platelets: Release during platelet degranulation and action on vascular smooth muscle cells. J. Cell Biol. 102:1217, 1986.

50. Centrella, M., Massague, J., and Canalis, E.: Human platelet-derived transforming growth factor-beta stimulates parameters of bone growth in fetal rat calvariae. Endocrinology 119:2306, 1986.

51. Lafyatis, R., Remmers, E. F., Roberts, A. B., et al.: Anchorage-independent growth of synoviocytes from arthritic and normal joints: Stimulation by exogenous platelet-derived growth factor and inhibition by transforming growth factor-beta and retinoids. J. Clin. Invest. 83:1267, 1989.

52. Sporn, M. B., Roberts, A. B., Wakefield, I. M., et al.: Transforming growth factor-B: Biological function and chemical structure. Science 233:532, 1986.

53. Prescott, S. M., Zimmerman, G. A., and McIntyre, T. M.: Platelet-activating factor. J. Biol. Chem. 265:17381, 1990.

54. Winslow, C. M., and Lee, M. L.: New Horizons in Platelet-Activating Factor Research. New York, John Wiley and Sons, 1987.

55. Snyder, F.: Platelet-Activating Factor and Related Lipid Mediators. New York, Plenum Publishing, 1987.

55a. Baumann, W. J.: Third International Conference on Platelet-Activating Factor and Structurally Related Alkyl Ether Lipids. Lipids 26:965, 1991.

56. Archer, C. B., Page, C. P., Morley, J., et al.: Accumulation of inflammatory cells in response to intracutaneous platelet activating factor (Paf-acether) in man. J. Dermatol. 112:285, 1985.

57. Valone, F. H., Barthelson, R., and Ruis, N. M.: Mechanisms for biphasic or persistent immunological reactions induced by platelet-activating factor. In Tauber, A. I., Wintroub, B. U., and Simon, A. S. (eds.): Biochemistry of the Acute Allergic Reaction, Fifth International Symposium. New York, Alan R. Liss, 1988.

58. Le, J., and Vilcek, J.: Tumor necrosis factor and interleukin 1: Cytokines with multiple overlapping biological activities. Lab. Invest. 56:234, 1987.

59. Dayer, J. M., Beutler, B., and Cerami, N.: Cachectin/tumor necrosis factor stimulates collagenase and prostaglandin E_2 production by human synovial cells and dermal fibroblasts. J. Exp. Med. 162:2163, 1985.

60. Mizel, S. B., Dayer, J. M., Krane, S. M., et al.: Stimulation of rheumatoid synovial cell collagenase and prostaglandin production by partially purified lymphocyte activating factor (interleukin 1). Proc. Natl. Acad. Sci. U.S.A. 78:2474, 1981.

61. Valone, F. H., and Epstein, L. B.: Biphasic platelet-activating factor synthesis by human monocytes stimulated with interleukin 1 beta, tumor necrosis factor or gamma interferon. J. Immunol. 141:3945, 1988.

62. Gosselin, E. I., Brown, M. E., Anderson, C. L., et al.: The monoclonal antibody 41H16 detects the leu 4 responder form of human Fc gamma RIII. J. Immunol. 144:1871, 1990.

63. Slapleigh, C., Valone, F. H., Schur, P. G., et al.: Platelet-activating activity in synovial fluids of patients with rheumatoid arthritis, juvenile rheumatoid arthritis, gout and non-flammatory arthropathies. Arthritis Rheum. 23:800, 1980.

64. Lawley, T. J., Bielory, L., Gascon, P., et al.: A prospective and immunologic analysis of patients with serum sickness. N. Engl. J. Med. 311:1407, 1984.

65. Donald, J. V., Anderson, C. F., Mitchell, J. C., et al.: A prospective clinical trial of platelet-inhibitor therapy. N. Engl. J. Med. 310:1421, 1984.

66. Lerner, W., Caruso, R., Faig, D., et al.: Drug-dependent and non–drug-dependent anti-platelet antibody in drug-induced immunologic thrombocytopenic purpura. Blood 66:306, 1985.

67. Kelton, J. G., Sheridan, D., Santos, A., et al.: Heparin-induced thrombocytopenia: Laboratory studies. Blood 72:925, 1988.

68. Adachi, J. D., Bensen, W. G., Kassam, Y., et al.: Gold induced thrombocytopenia: 12 cases and a review of the literature. Semin. Arthritis Rheum. 16:287, 1987.

69. Walker, D. J., Saunders, P., and Griffiths, I. D.: Gold induced thrombocytopenia. J. Rheumatol. 13:225, 1986.

70. Pfueller, S. L., and Luscher, E. F.: The effects of aggregated immunoglobulins on human blood platelets in relation to their complement-fixing abilities. J. Immunol. 109:517, 1972.

71. Peerschke, E. I. B., and Ghebrehiwet, B.: Modulation of platelet responses to collagen by C1q receptors. J. Immunol. 144:221, 1990.

72. Wiedmer, T., Esmon, C. T., and Sims, P. J.: On the mechanism by which complement proteins C5b-9 increase platelet prothrombinase activity. J. Biol. Chem. 257:11256, 1986.

73. Polley, M. J., and Nachman, R. L.: The human complement system in thrombin-mediated platelet function. In Gordon, J.L. (ed.): Platelets in Biology and Pathology. Amsterdam, Elsevier/North-Holland, 1981.

74. Dorsch, C. A., and Killmayer, J.: The effect of native and single stranded DNA on the platelet release reaction. Arthritis Rheum. 26:179, 1983.

75. Fidel, B. A., Schoenberger, J. S., and Gewurz, H.: Modulation of platelet activation by native DNA. J. Immunol. 123:2479, 1979.

76. Frampton, G., Perl, S., Bennett, A., et al.: Platelet-associated DNA and anti-DNA antibody in systemic lupus erythematosus with nephritis. Clin. Exp. Immunol. 63:621, 1986.

77. Sullam, P., Payan, D., Dazin, P. F., et al.: Quantitation of S. salvarius binding to human platelets in vitro. Infect. Immun. 58:3802, 1990.

78. Capron, A., Joseph, M., Ameisen, J.C., et al.: Platelets as effectors in immune and hypersensitivity reactions. Int. Arch. Allergy Appl. Immunol. 82:307, 1987.

79. Jaques, B. C., and Ginsberg, M. H.: The role of cell surface proteins in platelet stimulation by monosodium urate cytstals. Arthritis Rheum. 25:508, 1982.

80. Larsen, E., Celi, A., Gilbert, G. E., et al.: PADGEM protein: A receptor that mediates the interaction of activated platelets with neutrophils and monocytes. Cell 59:305, 1989.

80a. Celi, A., et al.: PADGEM: an adhesion receptor for leukocytes on stimulated platelets and endothelial cells. Proc. Soc. Exp. Biol. Med. 198:703, 1991.

81. Henson, P. M.: Interactions between neutrophils and platelets. Lab. Invest. 62:391, 1990.

82. Coeffier, E., Delautier, D., Le Couedic, J. P. et al.:Cooperation between platelets and neutrophils for PAF-acether (platelet-activating factor) formation. J. Leukoc. Biol. 47:234, 1990.

83. Marcus, A. J., Safier, L. B., Ullman, H. L., et al.: Cell-cell interactions in the eicosanoid pathway. Ann. N. Y. Acad. Sci. 516:407, 1987.

84. Ward, P. A., Cunningham, T. W., McCulloch, K. K., et al.: Platelet enhancement of 0^-_2 responses in stimulated human neutrophils. Lab. Invest. 58:37, 1988.

85. Franco, D., Ballestrero, A., Ottonello, L., et al.: Platelets as scavengers of neutrophil-derived oxidants: A possible defense mechanism at sites of vascular injury. Thromb. Haemost. 61:415, 1989.

86. Wilson, E., Laster, S. M., Gooding, L. R., et al.: Platelet-derived growth factor stimulates phagocytosis and blocks agonist-induced activation of the neutrophil oxidative burst: A possible cellular mechanism to protect against oxygen radical damage. Proc. Natl. Acad. Sci. U.S.A. 84:2213, 1987.

87. Clark, R. A., and Klebanoff, S. J.: Neutrophil-platelet intraction mediated by myeloperoxidase and hydrogen peroxide. J. Immunol. 124:399, 1980.

88. Renesto, P., Ferrer-Lopez, P., and Chignard, M.: Interference of recombinant eglin C, a proteinase inhibitor extracted from leeches, with neutrophil-mediated platelet activation. Lab. Invest. 62:409, 1990.

89. Salvemini, D., De Nucci, G., Gryglewski, R. J., et al.: Human neutrophils and mononuclear cells inhibit platelet aggregation by releasing a nitric oxide-like factor. Proc. Natl. Acad. Sci. U.S.A. 86:6328, 1989.

90. Abrams, C. S., Ellison, N., Budzynski, A. Z., et al.: Direct detection of activated platelets and platelet-derived microparticles in humans. Blood 75:128, 1990.

90a. Abrams, C., and Shattil, S. J.: Immunological detection of activated platelets in clinical disorders. Thromb. Haemost. 6:467, 1991.

91. Bolam, J. P., and Smith, M. J.: Accumulation of platelets at acute inflammatory sites. Br. J. Pharmacol. 61:158, 1977.

92. Kravis, T. C., and Henson, P. M.: Accumulation of platelets at sites of antigen-antibody mediated injury. J. Immunol. 118:1569, 1977.

93. Margaretten, W., and McKay, D. G.: The requirement for platelets in the active arthus reaction. Am. J. Pathol. 64:257, 1971.

94. Pinckard, R. N., Halonen, M., Palmer, J., et al.: Intravascular aggregation and pulmonary sequestration of platelets during IgE-induced systemic anaphylaxis in the rabbit. J. Immunol. 119:2185, 1977.

95. Margaretten, W., and McKay, D.: The role of the platelet in the generalized Shwartzman reaction. J. Exp. Med. 129:585, 1969.

96. Henson, P.M., and Cochrane, C. G.: Acute immune complex disease in rabbits. J. Exp. Med. 133:554, 1971.

97. Johnson, R. J., Garcia, R. L., Pritzl, P., et al.: Platelets mediate glomerular cell proliferation in immune complex nephritis induced by anti-mesangial cell antibodies in the rat. Am. J. Pathol. 136:369, 1990.

98. Hutchinson, R. M., Davis, P., and Jayson, M. I. V.: Thrombocytosis in rheumatoid arthritis. Ann. Rheum. Dis. 35:138, 1976.

99. Vollertsen, R. S., Fuster, V., Con, D. L., et al: In vivo platelet survival in rheumatoid arthritis. Mayo Clin. Proc. 57:620, 1982.

100. Weissbarth, E., Baruth, B., Mielke, H., et al.: Platelets as target cells in rheumatoid arthritis and systemic lupus eythematosus: A platelet specific immunoglobulin inducing the release reaction. Rheumatol. Int. 2:67, 1982.

101. Farr, M., Scott, D. L., Constable, J. J., et al.: Thrombocytosis of active rheumatoid disease. Ann. Rheum. Dis. 42:545, 1983.

102. Farr, M., Wainwright, A., Salmon, M., et al.: Platelets in the synovial fluid of patients with rheumatoid arthritis. Rheumatol. Int. 4:13, 1984.

103. Endresen, G. K. M.: Evidence for activation of platelets in the synovial fluid from patients with rheumatoid arthritis. Rheumatol. Int. 9:19, 1989.

104. Medsger, T. A., Jr.: Systemic sclerosis (scleroderma), eosinophil fasciitis, and calcinosis. In McCarthy, D. (ed.): Arthritis and Allied Conditions. Philadelphia, Lea & Febiger, 1985, pp. 994–1036.

105. Kahaleh, M. B., Scharstein, K. K., and LeRoy, E. C.: Enhanced platelet adhesion to collagen in scleroderma. Effect of scleroderma plasma and scleroderma platelets. J. Rheumatol. 12:3, 1985.

106. Kahaleh, M. D., Osborn, I., and LeRoy, E. C.: Elevated levels of circulating platelet aggregates and beta-thromboglobulin in scleroderma. Ann. Inter. Med. 96:610, 1982.

107. Biondi, M. L., and Marasini, B.: Abnormal platelet aggregation in patients with Raynaud's phenomenon. J. Clin. Pathol. 42:716, 1989.

108. Rodeheffer, R. I., Rommer, J. A., Wigley, F. M., et al.: Controlled double-blind trial of nifedipine in the treatment of Raynaud's phenomenon. N. Engl. J. Med. 308:880, 1983.

109. Seibold, J. R., and Harris, J. N.: Plasma B-thromboglobulin in the differential diagnosis of Raynaud's phenomenon. J. Rheumatol. 12:99, 1985.

110. Wigley, F. M., Wise, R. A., Malamet, R., et al.: Dissociation of platelet-activation from vasospasm. Arthritis Rheum. 30:281, 1987.

111. Berchtold, P., Harris, J. P., Tani, P., et al.: Autoantibodies to platelet glycoproteins in patients with disease-related immune thrombocytopenia. Br. J. Haematol. 73:365, 1989.

112. Bennett, A., Frampton, G., and Cameron, J. S.: Platelet-associated IgG in idiopathic glomerulonephritis and the nephritis of systemic lupus erythematosus. Br. J. Haematol. 62:695, 1986.

113. Schorer, A. E., Wickham, N. W. R., and Watson, K. V.: Lupus anticoagulant induces a selective defect in thrombin-mediated endothelial prostacyclin release and platelet aggregation. Br. J. Haematol. 71:399, 1989.

114. Camussi, G., Tetta, C., Mazzucco, G., et al.: Platelet cationic proteins are present in glomeruli of lupus nephritis patients. Kidney Int. 30:555, 1986.

115. Frampton, G., Hildreth, G., Hartley, B., et al.: Could platelet-derived growth factor have a role in the pathogenesis of lupus nephritis? Lancet 1:343, 1988.

Chapter 19

Ramzi S. Cotran

Endothelial Cells

INTRODUCTION

Endothelial cells line the lumina of all blood vessels and, in this unique position, form the interface between the blood and tissues. In the past decade, it has become clear that endothelial cells perform a wide variety of critical physiologic functions and interact in an active way with cellular and soluble components of the blood and with other cells in the vascular wall.[1, 2] In addition, the roles of endothelial cells in inflammation have been expanded: they respond to various stimuli, not simply as targets for injury, but by undergoing alterations in function and structure that directly influence the evolution and outcome of the inflammatory response. Some of these alterations are increases and decreases in normal constitutive functions, and others are due to induction of new functions and new molecules. This chapter briefly reviews the recent studies that ascribe an active role for the endothelium in inflammation and immune injury and that may be particularly relevant to inflammatory rheumatic diseases.

Endothelial cells contribute to all phases of acute and chronic inflammation, from the initial vascular events characterized by vasodilatation and increased vascular permeability; to the acute cellular events manifested by leukocyte adhesion, transmigration, and activation; to the chronic cellular response, dominated by lymphocytic infiltration; and finally to the healing and fibrotic reactions highlighted by neovascularization (angiogenesis) and fibroplasia.

Definitions

Before the role of endothelium in these events is considered, certain terms that are being used increasingly to define these endothelial responses operationally should be introduced (Table 19–1).

Necrosis and *lysis* are endothelial reactions that have long been appreciated from ultrastructural studies and that have been ascribed to direct effects of exogenous injurious agents, such as burns, chemicals, or bacterial toxins[3] but that could also be potentially caused by endogenous chemical mediators, such as oxygen-derived free radicals released from leukocytes. This type of injury results in increased vascular permeability and frequently in local thrombus formation. It often results in *desquamation* of the

endothelium, but desquamation can in principle occur without the endothelial cells' necessarily undergoing necrosis or lysis. It is possible, for example, that activation of certain proteolytic enzymes in the subendothelial space may cause a disruption of the cell-matrix adhesive proteins, followed by endothelial detachment.[4] Such an event may also cause increased vascular permeability.

Endothelial stimulation is a term defined operationally here to denote a rapid (minutes), reversible response of the endothelium that is independent of new protein synthesis.[2] The best example of endothelial stimulation is the endothelial cell contraction that occurs immediately after injection of histamine, serotonin, and other vasoactive mediators, and that results in the formation of the classical intracellular gaps in venules.[5] Another is the rapid redistribution of the adhesive glycoprotein granule-membrane protein 140 (GMP-140, P selectin, or CD62)[6, 7] when endothelial cells are stimulated with thrombin or histamine[6] (see later discussion).

In contrast to stimulation, *endothelial activation* is a response that requires hours or even days to occur, is dependent on new or altered protein synthesis, and is most commonly induced by inflammatory cytokines, such as interleukin-1 (IL-1), tumor necrosis factor (TNF), and interferon-gamma (γ).[1, 2] The classical example of endothelial activation is the induction of the endothelial adhesion molecule ELAM-1 (E-selectin) by IL-1[8] and class II MHC molecules by interferon-γ.[9]

Endothelial dysfunction is a relatively nonspecific term, first used in the context of the role of endothelial injury in atherogenesis, to describe endothelial cells undergoing potentially irreversible alterations in functional state without losing their structural integrity.[10] Increased pinocytosis, changes in membrane fluidity, and altered growth characteristics are examples of such dysfunction. Although such sublethal injury to the endothelium may be of importance, most of the examples initially described as

Table 19–1. ENDOTHELIAL RESPONSES IN INFLAMMATION

Endothelial necrosis, lysis, and desquamation
Endothelial stimulation
Endothelial activation
Endothelial dysfunction
Endothelial regeneration and neovascularization

representing endothelial dysfunction are now known to be examples of either endothelial activation, or what was defined earlier as endothelial stimulation.

Finally, *neovascularization, or angiogenesis,* is a process that represents an integrated series of endothelial responses—endothelial migration, proliferation, and maturation— that is characteristic of the healing phase of inflammation and chronic inflammatory responses.[11]

A great deal of overlap exists among these responses in terms of mediators and mechanisms involved, as well as of final effects. For example, cytokines that are classic inducers of endothelial activation, such as TNF, render endothelial cells more susceptible to endothelial lysis by leukocyte products[12] and may also cause angiogenesis.[13] Indeed, the many shared molecular mechanisms between activation and proliferation have made the distinction between traditional growth factors and cytokines difficult to uphold.

ROLE OF ENDOTHELIUM IN THE VASCULAR EVENTS OF ACUTE INFLAMMATION

The first hallmark of acute inflammation is local *vasodilatation.* Vasodilatation serves to enhance the subsequent increases in vascular permeability and neutrophil exudation that characterize the inflammatory response. Although vasodilatory mediators may potentially originate from plasma or circulating blood cells, vascular endothelium can contribute to the vasodilatation by elaborating at least three potential vasodilators—prostacyclin (PGI_2), nitric oxide/endothelial-derived growth factor (NO/EDGF), and platelet-activating factor (PAF).[14] Agonists such as thrombin, histamine, and leukotriene C_4 stimulate endothelial production of these vasodilators in vitro, and the stimulation is mediated by rises in concentration of cytosolic calcium.[15] The molecular mechanisms underlying these reactions are detailed elsewhere in this book. The net amounts of vasodilators produced are highly variable, and the precise role that vascular (rather than extravascular) mediators play is unclear. For example, the net quantities of prostacyclin synthesized by endothelium depends on the endothelial cell levels of phospholipase A_2, the dose of the agonists, and the levels of endothelial cell prostacyclin synthetase activities. The last, in particular, is subject to regulation by certain cytokines, such as IL-1 and TNF.[16] Thus, IL-1 and TNF markedly enhance the production of prostacyclin by endothelial cells. With regard to NO/EDRF, evidence strongly suggests that the endothelial moiety is critical in the induction of vasodilatation in vivo.[17]

Much more is known of the role of endothelium in the *increased vascular permeability* characteristic of acute inflammation. The ultrastructural studies of the 1960s and more recent studies in vitro and in vivo have established several fundamental types of endothelial responses that result in increased vascular permeability. Although certain stimuli specifically cause only one type of response, most natural inflammatory reactions are associated with combinations of such events.

Endothelial Contraction

In most experimental models of inflammation studied—from the simple injection of vasoactive amines, such as histamine or serotonin, to the complex permeability changes induced by physical, chemical, thermal, toxic, or immunogenic injury— the principal morphologic basis for vascular leakage is the formation of intercellular gaps in the endothelium that allow the passage of plasma across the vascular wall.[18] Except in some experimental models, this histamine type of vascular injury occurs almost exclusively in small and medium-sized venules.[19] Persuasive evidence suggests that the gaps form as a result of contraction of endothelial cells mediated by the vasoactive agents, a classical example of *endothelial stimulation.* This sort of mediated injury is relatively short-lived and is seen with all the permeability-increasing chemical mediators thus far studied, including histamine, serotonin, bradykinin, C3a, C5a, PAF, and the vasoactive leukotrienes.[20] Although the precise cause of the venular localization of such increased permeability is still uncertain, Simionescu and colleagues found a greater density of surface histamine receptors in venular endothelium than in capillary endothelium.[21] Recent in vitro studies have confirmed that histamine causes endothelial cell contraction, and that the process is mediated by an intracellular pathway involving calmodulin and myosin light-chain kinase.[22]

Cytoskeletal and Junctional Reorganization: Endothelial Retraction

An apparently different mechanism of reversible endothelial intercellular leakage has been reported in endothelial cell monolayers in vitro. When exposed to cytokines such as IL-1, TNF, and interferon-γ for 4 to 6 hours, endothelial cells in confluent monolayers begin to undergo a structural reorganization of their cytoskeletons such that they retract from one another at the junctions, causing intercellular discontinuities that lead to long-lived (24 hours or more) increases in permeability.[23, 24] The retraction is reversible and requires protein synthesis. The TNF effect is sensitive to pertussis toxin and thus may involve a G-protein mediator.[24] Its genesis is thus altogether different from that of endothelial contraction induced by histamine and is an example of cytokine-induced endothelial activation. Whether there are in vivo correlates to this type of increased permeability is unclear, but cytokine-induced retraction is an attractive explanation for so-called delayed–prolonged vascular leakage caused by stimuli such as X-irradiation or ultraviolet irradiation, immunologically mediated delayed hypersensitivity, certain bacterial toxins, and mild to moderate thermal injury.[25] The pathogenesis of such delayed–prolonged leakage remains poorly understood. Although some studies have suggested that this is a type of *direct*, albeit delayed, injury by the exogenous agent,[26] the contribution of cytokine-induced retraction to such responses deserves further study.

Direct Endothelial Injury

Originally described after necrotizing thermal and chemical injury, direct endothelial injury is a type of vascular leakage characterized ultrastructurally by degenerative changes in the endothelium with vacuolization, fragmentation, membrane blebbing, and frequently outright denudation with local thrombus formation. The injury involves capillaries, venules, and arterioles, and results in immediate and sustained increases in local vascular permeability.[3]

Leukocyte-Mediated Vascular Leakage

A variety of in vitro and in vivo studies indicate that leukocytes, in the process of adhesion and transmigration across the vascular wall, may injure endothelial cells, leading to increased vascular permeability. The mechanism of such injury involves oxygen-derived free radicals and proteolytic enzymes[27]; it is detailed elsewhere in this book. The occurrence and severity of the endothelial injury that accompanies leukocyte–endothelial interactions vary and appear to depend on the state of activation of neutrophils. For example, in a model of neutrophil emigration induced by serum in the rat, closed junctions are maintained during the process of neutrophil extravasation, and no vascular leakage occurs.[28] In contrast, the leukocytic exudation that accompanies immune complex–mediated injury or injections of chemotactic complement fragments, which also cause leukocyte activation, results in considerable increases in vascular permeability and ultrastructural evidence of endothelial injury and denudation. The process has been studied most extensively in pulmonary-induced inflammation in which increases in vascular permeability can be measured. In some of these models, interventions that prevent leukocyte adhesion[29] or protect against toxic oxygen leukocyte products[30] inhibit edema formation.

Regeneration of Endothelium

The final mechanism of leakage accounts for the increased permeability of new regenerating capillaries in healing inflammation during the process of endothelial proliferation. Leakage in this setting occurs as a result of open intercellular junctions and is enhanced by the relatively incomplete basement membranes in immature endothelial cells.[31] In addition, a recent study by Joris and colleagues suggests that proliferation of endothelium in the microcirculation may cause endothelial regeneration without the formation of new blood vessels but with the occurrence of distinct increases in vascular permeability that involve mostly capillaries.[32] Such seems to be the cause of leakage induced experimentally by placing pieces of infarcted tissue in a vascular bed[32] and, by analogy, in the vicinity of necrotic or infarcted tissue.

Role of Endothelium in Leukocyte Adhesion and Transmigration

Adhesion of blood leukocytes to vascular endothelium is one of the earliest events in acute immunogenic and nonimmunogenic inflammation, and it is the prelude to the process of leukocyte emigration. In the past few years, there has been an explosion in research on the mechanisms by which such adhesion is stimulated and of the molecular mediators of leukocyte–endothelial interactions. These studies have shown that a variety of mediators, such as chemotactic peptides, complement components, leukotriene B$_4$, and cytokines, affect adhesion by modulating the surface expression of complementary adhesion molecules present on the leukocytes and endothelial cells. In addition, these molecules affect not only the adhesive process but also the initial transient binding of leukocytes to endothelium, called rolling, and the subsequent transmigration across the venular wall. The molecular characteristics of adhesion molecules in general are detailed in Chapter 12. Here, only those endothelial molecules relevant to leukocyte–endothelial interactions in inflammation and, in particular, their demonstrated biologic roles are considered.

The adhesion receptors involved in leukocyte–endothelial interactions belong to three molecular families—the selectins, the immunoglobulins, and the integrins[33] (see Chapter 12).

Selectins

Selectins are characterized by an extracellular N-terminal domain related to mammalian C-type lectins, an epidermal growth factor–like domain, and two to nine domains related to the short consensus repeats of complement regulatory proteins.[33, 34] Selectins include E-selectin (ELAM-1), P-selectin (GMP-140, PADGEM, CD62), and L-selectin (LAM-1, Mel-14 antigen, or LECCAM-1).

ELAM-1 was the first specific endothelial adhesion molecule identified.[35] Cultured endothelial cells do not basally express ELAM-1, but within 1 hour of exposure to IL-1 or TNF, endothelial cells begin to synthesize ELAM-1 and express it on their surface. Expression of ELAM-1 is maximal 4 to 6 hours after cytokine treatment and then declines, even in the presence of the cytokine. In culture, ELAM-1 has been shown to promote the adhesion of neutrophils and, to a somewhat lesser extent, eosinophils, basophils, monocytes, and a subpopulation of memory

T cells.[36, 37] The major ligand for ELAM-1 on leukocytes is a sialylated form of the Lewis X glycan, which is covalently attached to various cell surface glycoproteins.[34, 38, 39]

There is substantial evidence for a role of ELAM-1 in leukocyte, principally neutrophil, adhesion in vivo. First, ELAM-1 can be induced in the skin of baboons after intradermal injections of TNF and LPS.[40, 41] Within 2 hours after injections of TNF or LPS, ELAM-1 begins to be expressed, and this is correlated with neutrophil adhesion and extravasation. Second, ELAM-1 can be induced by antigen in vivo and in skin organ cultures in the late-phase reactions of immediate hypersensitivity in human skin.[42] In this model, ELAM-1 is largely confined to postcapillary venular endothelium, the anatomic site of leukocyte adhesion and extravasation, and its appearance is associated with inflammatory influx. Finally, antibodies to ELAM-1 have been shown to inhibit neutrophil adhesion in a model of pulmonary inflammation induced by immune complexes and, at the same time, to markedly reduce the pulmonary edema that occurs in these animals.[29] Antibodies to ELAM-1 also abrogated antigen-induced acute airway neutrophil infiltration and late-phase airway obstruction in a primate model of extrinsic asthma.[43]

The second endothelial adhesive selectin is P-selectin or GMP-140 (also called PADGEM). This molecule was originally described in the α granule of platelets, being rapidly redistributed to the plasma membrane of platelets on stimulation with thrombin or histamine.[7] In endothelium, GMP-140 is present constitutively on the membrane of Weibel-Palade granules and can also be rapidly translocated to the plasma membrane on exposure of endothelium to thrombin or histamine.[6] GMP-140 also functions as a lectin, binding to Lewis X or sialylated Lewis X moieties attached to macromolecules on the surface of neutrophils and monocytes.[44] In vitro GMP-140 mediates adhesion of neutrophils and monocytes to cultured endothelium.[45] The process of initiating the translocation of GMP-140 to the cell surface, such that the endothelium becomes more adhesive, is rapid and does not require protein synthesis; it is thus an example of endothelial stimulation in contrast to IL-1 and TNF induction of ELAM-1 expression. The process can be mimicked by calcium ionophores and is thought to depend on increased concentrations of cytosolic calcium.

The precise role of GMP-140 in leukocyte–endothelial adhesion is beginning to be explored. Because of its rapid up-regulation by relatively acute mediators (e.g., histamine, thrombin), it is thought to be particularly important in early phases of adhesion. Recent studies of leukocyte interaction with artificial lipid bilayers containing purified GMP-140 have shown that this molecule may be a mediator of the initial rolling of leukocytes, a prelude to their firm adhesion.[46] Other studies have shown an important relation between the expression of GMP-140 and the stimulation of the production of PAF by endothelial cells. Endothelial cells are normally devoid of PAF but are rapidly stimulated by the same agonists that cause GMP-140 redistribution (histamine, thrombin, calcium ionophores) to synthesize PAF, a portion of which is expressed on the endothelial surface.[47] Such PAF then mediates further adhesion of neutrophils by a mechanism in which the PAF first recognizes a receptor for PAF on neutrophils and then induces functional up-regulation of the CD11/CD18 adhesive glycoprotein on neutrophils.[48] Under appropriate flow conditions then, both GMP-140 and PAF (by the CD11a/CD18 mechanism) act to mediate maximal neutrophil adherence in early inflammation. Finally, recent studies suggest that oxygen free radicals induce the prolonged expression of GMP-140 on endothelial cell surfaces, resulting in prolonged and enhanced neutrophil adhesions.[49] However, none of these postulated contributions of GMP-140, derived from in vitro studies, have yet been shown to occur in vivo.

The third adhesive selectin is L-selectin (LAM-1, LECCAM-1, Mel-14 antigen). Originally identified in mice by antibody Mel-14, and in humans by monoclonal antibody Leu-8, this selectin is present on lymphocytes, where it serves as the peripheral lymph node homing receptor (see Chapter 12), and on neutrophils, where it mediates neutrophil–endothelial adhesion. The endothelial ligand for L-selectin has not been unequivocally identified. In neutrophils, L-selectin appears to be associated with sialylated Lewis X moieties that may bind to ELAM-1.[50]

Antibodies to L-selectin inhibit neutrophil rolling,[51, 52] and like P-selectin, it is thought to mediate early adhesive events. The role of L-selectin in lymphocyte trafficking is discussed later.

Immunoglobulin and Integrin Adhesive Proteins

The endothelial adhesive glycoproteins belonging to the immunoglobulin gene superfamily are ICAM-1 and VCAM-1, and both interact with glycoproteins of the integrin gene superfamily on leukocytes. ICAM-1 is expressed basally on endothelial cells, but its expression is markedly increased in vitro by LPS, IL-1, TNF, and to a lesser extent by γ-interferon.[53] The time sequence of ICAM-1 induction differs from that of ELAM-1, in that increased expression is not maximally reached for 24 hours or even longer.[1] ICAM-1 mediates both neutrophil and lymphocyte adhesion to cytokine-activated endothelial cells in vitro.[54, 55] The leukocyte receptors for ICAM-1 are LFA-1 and MAC-1 integrins (CD11a/CD18 and CD11b/CD8).[55, 56] Neutrophils need to be activated with chemotactic agents (e.g., C5a) or previous ELAM-1 binding[57] to be induced to bind to ICAM-1. This increased adhesivity is mediated by increased avidity of binding, rather than by increased total surface expression of integrin molecules.[58] Recent in vitro studies using endothelial cultures exposed to varying flow conditions suggest that the ICAM-1/integrin interaction is critical to the adhesion

Table 19–2. LEUKOCYTE–ENDOTHELIAL ADHESION MOLECULES IN INFLAMMATION

Endothelial Molecule	Leukocyte Ligand	Main Function
E-selectin (ELAM-1)	Sialylated Lewis X Others	Cytokine-induced neutrophil, eosinophil, basophil, macrophage, and memory T cell adhesion
P selectin (GMP-140, CD62)	Sialylated Lewis X	Neutrophil rolling/early adhesion Monocyte adhesion
L-selectin ligand	L-selectin (LECCAM-1)	Neutrophil rolling/early adhesion Lymphocyte homing
ICAM-1 (CD54)	LFA-1; Mac-1	Neutrophil and lymphocyte adhesion and transmigration
VCAM-1 (INCAM-110)	VLA-4	Lymphocyte, monocyte, eosinophil, and basophil adhesion

strengthening that follows the initial rolling of neutrophils on a selectin,[46] and it also enhances neutrophil *transmigration.*[54] The importance of this interaction in vivo is evidenced by the marked inhibition of neutrophil exudation in patients with leukocyte adhesion deficiency, who have mutations in the common β subunit of the CD11/CD18 complex.[59] ICAM-1 expression can also be induced in baboon skin in vivo with TNF, with a time sequence consistent with its expression in vitro (i.e., expression commencing between 9 and 12 hours, and reaching a maximum by 24 to 48 hours).[40]

The second endothelial adhesive glycoprotein of the immunoglobulin superfamily is VCAM-1 (also called INCAM-110).[60, 61] VCAM-1 is present constitutively on normal unstimulated cells, but its expression is markedly enhanced in IL-1– and TNF-activated endothelial cells.[60] In cultured endothelium, VCAM-1 is induced slowly, reaching peak expression in about 24 hours of cytokine stimulation. An important difference between VCAM-1, ELAM-1, and ICAM-1 is that VCAM-1 can also be induced by the cytokine IL-4.[62, 63] There is also synergism between IL-4 and TNF in the induction of VCAM-1 in vitro.[63] The leukocyte receptor for VCAM-1 is the β1-integrin protein VLA-4.[64] Antibodies to VCAM-1 inhibit lymphocyte adhesion in vitro.[60] In vivo, VCAM-1 is present in sites of lymphocyte infiltration in inflammation,[65] and its induction in baboon skin by cytokines (TNF, IL-4) correlates with the occurrence of significant CD3+ lymphocyte infiltrates.[66] It is thus thought that VCAM-1 is an important lymphocyte adhesion molecule. It does not, however, seem to mediate T cell transmigration, at least in vitro.[67]

Table 19–2 is a summary of the endothelial–leukocyte adhesion molecules involved in inflammation. The precise roles of these adhesion molecules is being dissected in numerous in vitro and in vivo models, but several points should be made with regard to their possible contribution in inflammation.

First, a number of factors influence leukocyte adhesion and transmigration in various assays in vitro. Hemodynamic conditions, such as altered shear stress, clearly influence both adhesion and transmigration. For example, the CD11a/CD18/ICAM-1–dependent component of adhesion of neutrophils to endothelium, which is evident under static conditions in adhesion assays, is lost at shear stresses below the physiologic range. At wall shear stress

estimated to exist in postcapillary venules, the selectin GMP-140 mediates neutrophil binding, but ICAM-1 does not, even when the ICAM-1–integrin mechanism is activated by stimulating neutrophils with PMA. In contrast, under static conditions, there is only minimal and reversible adhesion of neutrophils to GMP-140, but strong adhesion of PMA-stimulated neutrophils, and these attachments are highly resistant to increased shear stress.[46] LAM-1 (L-selectin) and its putative endothelial ligand mediate endothelial attachment in rotating but not static cultures.[68]

The second important factor in these in vitro studies is the state of activation of the leukocyte itself. Resting neutrophils (and also probably memory T cells; see later discussion) readily adhere to cytokine-activated endothelial cells bearing ELAM-1 and VCAM-1, but not ICAM-1. Activated neutrophils shed LAM-1 (L-selectin) and therefore do not adhere to the putative LAM-1 ligand on endothelium.[69] In addition, activated neutrophils are less adhesive to ELAM-1, but there is no unequivocal evidence that the ELAM-1 ligand, sialylated Lewis X, is shed from the surface of leukocytes on activation. Activated neutrophils, however, are much more adhesive to ICAM-1, this being dependent on the increased avidity of the CD11/CD18 integrin. The loss of LAM-1– and ELAM-1–dependent binding that is associated with neutrophil activation, coupled with the increased avidity for ICAM-1, favors transmigration, a process dependent on the CD11/CD18 interactions with ICAM-1.

A third influence on leukocyte adhesion and transmigration is the potential role of *endogenous* endothelial mediators—induced *pari passu* with the initial stimulant or activator of endothelium—on *subsequent* leukocyte–endothelial interactions. One such example has already been mentioned—the role of PAF, stimulated in endothelium by histamine and thrombin, in affecting subsequent CD11/CD18–dependent adhesion.[48] Activated endothelial cells are known to synthesize and secrete a variety of endogenous cytokines with potential biologic activities (Table 19–3).[1] These include IL-1[70]; IL-8,[71] a neutrophil and T cell chemotactic factor; MCP-1, an activator of monocyte chemokinesis[72]; GM-CSF,[1] an activator of neutrophil and monocyte chemotaxis; and IL-6, a T and B cell activator. The role of these endogenous cytokines in the evolution of the cellular events is unclear, and with certain cytokines, it is a matter of

Table 19–3. ENDOTHELIAL-DERIVED CYTOKINES

Interleukin-1
Interleukin-6
Interleukin-8
MCP-1
GM-CSF
G-CSF
TGB-β
Endothelial cell–derived growth factor

current confusion. For example, intradermal injections of IL-8 in vivo are clearly chemotactic, causing significant neutrophil accumulation in the skin,[73] whereas systemically administered IL-8 inhibits inflammatory leukocyte accumulation. In vitro, IL-8 renders neutrophils less adherent for ELAM-1, inhibits leukocyte adhesion in some in vitro assays[75] but enhances endothelial transmigration in others.[76] Whether endothelial-derived IL-8 in vivo serves to inhibit leukocyte adhesion to and detachment from adherent cells, or, in contrast, to induce neutrophil migration and thus leukocyte accumulation is still open to question.

These considerations have led to a number of models for neutrophil–endothelial recognition and the contribution of adhesion molecules in inflammation.[2, 77] These models postulate an initial, primary, rapid, and relatively loose adhesion pathway that involves mainly L- and P-selectins and, in cytokine-activated endothelium, the E-selectin ELAM-1. In the presence of chemoattractants or leukocyte-activating factors (produced by endothelium or other cells, or stimulated by an initial ELAM-1 leukocyte adhesion[57]), loosely adherent leukocytes increase their ability to bind stably to endothelium, largely through the integrin/ICAM-1 pathway, and to undergo transmigration. It has been speculated that the existence of a number of receptor pairs and the requirement of several sequential events provide mechanisms for the diversity and specificity of endothelial–leukocyte adhesion, not only for neutrophils but for other leukocytes as well.[77]

Persuasive evidence about the relevance of adhesion molecules in vivo is accumulating from two types of studies. The first involves the immunohistochemical demonstration of adhesion molecules in experimentally induced reactions or natural disease processes, and the second uses antibodies to adhesion molecules to inhibit leukocyte adhesion or extravasation in experimental models of inflammation. Immunocytochemical methods were the first to document that ELAM-1 (E-selectin), a molecule initially induced only in culture, can be elaborated in vivo, in an elicited delayed hypersensitivity in human skin.[78] ELAM-1, ICAM-1, and VCAM-1 have since been localized in a variety of human pathologic processes, including the late-phase reaction of immediate hypersensitivity,[42] septic shock,[79] the vasculature of tumors characterized by excessive cytokine production (T cell lymphoma, Hodgkin's disease,

and Kaposi's sarcoma[80]), allograft rejection,[81] and other inflammatory–immune conditions of the skin and viscera.[81, 82] However, although reflecting a state of endothelial activation, the expression of these inducible endothelial cell adhesion molecules is not sufficient evidence that they are involved in leukocyte adhesion when present.[83] Indeed, under some of the conditions, correlation between the presence of the adhesion molecule and the existence of intravascular or perivascular leukocytes is poor. The reasons for these discrepancies have been detailed elsewhere,[83] and include the following: (1) the molecule observed by antibody staining may not be on the cell surface or may be present in an inactivated form that is not recognized by the leukocyte receptor; (2) the state of the leukocyte is such that it does not bear the leukocyte receptor in a sufficiently interactive form on its surface; (3) other physiologic conditions necessary for binding are absent (e.g., the appropriate hemodynamic changes such as shear stress); and (4) additional molecules required for adhesion or transmigration of leukocytes may be absent. Such may be the case in septic shock, in which ELAM-1 expression is widespread but in which neutrophil adhesion is confined to certain organs, such as lung, capillaries, and venules.[79]

Immunohistochemical studies in animal models after injection of cytokines or lipopolysaccharide have provided some more interpretable correlations between the presence of adhesion molecules and leukocyte infiltrates. In studies in baboons, it was shown that TNF causes rapid rises in ELAM-1, beginning 2 hours after TNF injection, that correlate with neutrophil adhesion and extravasation, and it later causes rises in ICAM-1 and VCAM-1.[40, 41] Further, IL-4, as it does in vitro, enhances VCAM-1 expression induced by TNF.[66]

More convincing studies are those that have used antibodies to adhesion molecules to inhibit leukocyte accumulation and, in certain instances, its functional consequences. For example, antibodies to or soluble forms of the leukocyte CD11/CD18 complex,[84] L-selectin,[69, 85] and ICAM-1 have been shown to reduce leukocyte influx in models of acute inflammation. In particular, antibodies to ELAM-1 inhibit neutrophil infiltration and pulmonary edema in immune complex pulmonary injury in the rat[29] and both neutrophil influx and airway obstruction in a model of late phase airway reaction induced by antigen in the primate.[44]

Role of Endothelium in Chronic and Immunologic Inflammation

We conclude this chapter by briefly examining the role of endothelial cells in chronic inflammatory and immunologic reactions, since these may be particularly relevant to chronic inflammatory arthritis. Recent studies, reviewed in detail elsewhere,[1, 86] have shown important interactions among cytokines, endothelial proteins, and lymphocytes in lymphocyte homing, infiltration, and proliferation.

As for the neutrophil, lymphocyte homing to peripheral lymph nodes, gut-associated lymphoid tissue (e.g., Peyer's patches), and inflamed endothelium is governed by complementary adhesion molecules on lymphocytes and endothelial cells.[86] Because there is a certain degree of specificity in the actual tissues to which various lymphocyte populations home, the endothelial ligands for the homing receptors are called *addressins*.[87] It is also clear that circulating naive T cells, activated T cells, memory T cells, and B cells, may use different sets of molecules in their journey through the vascular system. The best studied of the homing receptors is L-selectin, initially described as the Mel-14 antigen of mouse lymphocytes (HEV), which recognizes ligands in the high endothelial venules of peripheral lymph nodes.[88] L-selectin is abundant on the surface of naive T cells, which have low levels of LFA-1 and of other adhesion molecules (such as VLA-4, CD29, and CD44), and accounts for homing of T cells derived from resting lymph nodes to HEVs. The specific addressin in peripheral lymph node HEVs that reacts with L-selectin is unknown; in the mouse, however, the monoclonal antibody MECA-79 blocks such homing and reacts preferentially with the high endothelial venules in peripheral lymph nodes. Similarly, the endothelial addressin in Peyer's patches, recognized by the monoclonal antibody MECA-367, preferentially stains only high endothelial venules in Peyer's patches.[87] The chemical nature of this molecule and its receptor on the lymphocytes are currently unknown.

All three cytokine-induced endothelial adhesion molecules described here—ELAM-1, ICAM-1, and VCAM-1—recognize certain lymphocyte subsets. ELAM-1 binds to a subset of memory T lymphocytes[36] through a sialylated carbohydrate that may be a form of sialylated Lewis X.[90] This ELAM-1 binding ligand is present on some 80 to 90 percent of T lymphocytes in human skin in chronic inflammatory infiltrates, and it has thus been suggested that ELAM-1 may indeed be a skin endothelial addressin for memory T cells.[89] Memory T cells are also characterized by the expression of low-molecular-weight isoform of CD45 (CD45RO), and high levels of LFA-1[90] and VLA-4.[65] They can thus bind to cytokine-activated endothelial cells by using ELAM-1, LFA-1/ICAM-1, and the VCAM-1/VLA-4 recognition mechanisms. When activated by antigen, T cells become even more adhesive to endothelium by increasing the avidity of their LFA-1 and VLA-4 for the endothelial ligands.[91] Further, activated T cells are more susceptible to transmigration in vitro, particularly when the endothelium is activated by cytokines.[64a, 64b, 67, 68]

In addition to IL-1 and TNF, which increase lymphocyte binding to endothelium, interferon-γ and IL-4 also have profound effects on lymphocyte–endothelial interactions. Interferon-γ induces the expression of ICAM-1, up-regulates the expression of both ELAM-1 and VCAM-1 when combined with TNF,[92] and markedly up-regulates the endothelial expression of class I and II MHC antigens.[86, 87] IL-4 induces increases in VCAM-1 expression and synergizes with TNF or IL-1 in this activity.[60–63] It does not induce ELAM-1 or ICAM-1, and, indeed, it may inhibit the expression of these two molecules. Interferon-γ and IL-4 treatment increase T cell adhesion to cultured endothelium without inducing neutrophil adhesion. All these effects of cytokines serve to amplify lymphocyte recruitment. Indeed, it has been shown in baboons that injections of IL-4 and TNF induce marked increases in the expression of VCAM-1 and ICAM-1, and in the infiltration by CD3+ T lymphocytes in vivo.[66]

These considerations may explain the preponderance of memory T cells in chronic inflammatory infiltrates, including the infiltrates of rheumatoid arthritis.[93] The CD45RO+ memory T cells are characterized by increased expression of a number of adhesive molecules, including VLA-4, LFA-1, ICAM-1, and also CD2 and LFA-3, and the complementary endothelial adhesion molecules are induced by the leukocyte-derived cytokines. There is also evidence, however, that memory cells are more selectively retained at inflammatory sites.[93]

In addition to its role in lymphocyte recruitment, the endothelium responds to its interaction with lymphocytes, particularly activated T cells in a number of other ways. As stated earlier, interferon-γ, produced by activated T cells, increases class II MHC expression. The phenomenon clearly occurs in vivo and has been shown in the endothelium of mouse skin allografts,[94] guinea pig experimental allergic encephalomyelitis,[95] and allograft coronary arteries after transplantation.[96] The precise role of increased class II MHC expression is unknown. Current evidence, detailed elsewhere[86] suggests that endothelial cells can act as antigen-presenting cells in vitro, although whether they do so in vivo is still unproved. Endothelial cells can also be induced by their interactions with lymphocytes to stimulate T cells, probably by their ability to enhance IL-2 production by such T cells.[97] Some of this so-called co-stimulator activity of endothelial cells depends on cell contact and involves, in part, interactions between endothelial cell LFA-3 (CD59) and T cell CD2.[98]

Finally, activated endothelial cells, as previously described, elaborate a variety of cytokines, some of which can act as co-stimulators of T cell proliferation, (e.g., IL-1 and, in particular, IL-6).[100] IL-6 has pleiotropic effects relevant in immune reactions and may account for the augmented B cell responses ascribed to endothelial cells.[101] Other endothelial-derived cytokines that may be involved in the various phases of chronic inflammation include IL-8, MCP-1, GM-CSF, G-CSF, TGF-β, and EDGF. These may contribute to mononuclear cell accumulation, fibroplasia, and angiogenesis, which characterize chronic inflammation.

SUMMARY

Endothelial cells contribute to all phases of acute and chronic inflammation by undergoing specific alterations in structure and function, and by elaborating adhesion molecules, cytokines, growth factors, and other mediators. Endothelial responses can be rapid, not requiring protein synthesis (endothelial stimulation) or can be slow and long-lived, depending on the synthesis of new proteins (endothelial activation).

Endothelial cells participate in the acute vascular events of inflammation by producing vasodilatory mediators, including prostacyclin and NO/EDRF. Increased vascular permeability results from direct endothelial injury; from endothelial contraction induced by vasoactive mediators and resulting in widening of intercellular junctions; from endothelial retraction, induced by cytokines and dependent on cytoskeletal reorganization; from injury induced by leukocytes in the process of adhesion and emigration; or from endothelial regeneration.

Endothelial cells are central to the process of leukocyte adhesion and transmigration. Leukocyte–endothelial attachments are governed by complementary adhesion molecules on the surface of leukocytes and endothelium. The surface expression, avidity, and contribution of adhesion receptor pairs in these interactions depend on the state of activation of the leukocytes and of endothelium and also on rheologic factors, such as shear stress. The most well-studied receptor pair is the P-selectin/sialylated Lewis X, which appears to mediate early adhesive events (rolling) under conditions of flow; L-selectin and its putative endothelial ligand, also involved in rolling; ELAM-1/sialylated Lewis X, which mediates adhesion of neutrophils and other leukocytes to cytokine-activated endothelium; integrin/ICAM-1, which mediates firm adhesion and transmigration of activated leukocytes; and VCAM-1/VLA-4, involved in lymphocyte and monocyte adhesion in immune cytokine–activated endothelium. The presence of a number of adhesion receptor pairs and the requirement for sequential steps in rolling, firm adhesion, and transmigration may account for the diversity and specificity of leukocyte–endothelial interactions. These adhesion molecules are expressed in vivo in a variety of inflammatory–immune conditions, and there is increasing evidence that inhibition of the activity of these molecules may abrogate leukocyte accumulation and the resultant tissue injury in some experimental models.

Finally, interactions between cytokines, endothelium, and lymphocytes mediated by means of similar complementary adhesion molecules accounts for the recruitment of lymphocytes in chronic immune reactions, and can explain the preponderance of memory T cells in chronic inflammatory reactions. Endothelial cells also contribute to chronic inflammation by the elaboration of cytokines and growth factors that may participate in T cell proliferation, mononuclear cell infiltration, fibroplasia, and angiogenesis.

References

1. Pober, J. S., and Cotran, R. S.: Cytokines and endothelial cell biology. Physiol. Rev. 70:427, 1990.
2. Pober, J. S., and Cotran, R. S.: Overview: The role of endothelial cells in inflammation. Transplant 50:537, 1990.
3. Cotran, R. S., and Majno, G.: A light and electron microscopic analysis of vascular injury. Ann. N.Y. Acad. Sci. 116:750, 1964.
4. Weiss, S. J.: Tissue destruction by neutrophils. N. Engl. J. Med. 320:365, 1989.
5. Majno, G., Shea, S. M., and Leventhal, M.: Endothelial contraction induced by histamine-type mediators: An electron microscopic study. J. Cell Biol. 42:647, 1969.
6. McEver, R. P., Beckstead, J. H., Moore, K. L., Marshall-Carson, L., and Bainton, D. F.: GMP-140, a platelet gamma-granule membrane protein, is also synthesized by vascular endothelial cells and is localized in Wiebel-Palade bodies. J. Clin. Invest. 84:92, 1989.
7. Hattori, R., Hamilton K. K., Fugate, R. D., McEver, R. P., and Sims, P. J.: Stimulated secretion of endothelial von Willebrand factor is accompanied by rapid redistribution to the cell surface of the intracellular granule membrane protein GMP-140. J. Biol. Chem. 264:7768, 1989.
8. Bevilacqua, M. P., Pober, J. S., Mendrick, D. L., Cotran, R. S., and Gimbrone, M. A., Jr.: Identification of an inducible endothelial leukocyte adhesion molecule, ELAM-1. Proc. Natl. Acad. Sci. U.S.A. 84:9238, 1987.
9. Pober, J. S., Gimbrone, M. A., Jr., Cotran, R. S., Reiss, L. S., and Burakoff, S. I.: Ia expression by vascular endothelium is inducible by activated T cells and by human gamma-interferon. J. Exp. Med. 157:1339, 1983.
10. Gimbrone, M. A., Jr.: Endothelial dysfunction and the pathogenesis of atherosclerosis. In Gotto, A. M., Jr., and Smith, L. C. (eds.): Atherosclerosis. Vol. 5. New York, Springer-Verlag, 1980, pp. 415–425.
11. Folkman, J., and Klagsburn, M.: Angiogenic factors. Science 235:442, 1987.
12. Varani, J., Bendelow, M. J., Sealey, D. E., et al.: Tumor necrosis factor enhances susceptibility of vascular endothelial cells to neutrophil-mediated killing. Lab. Invest. 59:292, 1988.
13. Leibovich, S. J., Polverini, P. J., Shepard, H. M., Wiseman, D. M., Shively, V., and Nuseir, N.: Macrophage-induced angiogenesis is mediated by tumour necrosis factor-α. Nature [Lond.] 329:630, 1987.
14. Brenner, B. M., Troy, J. L., and Baltermann, B. J.: Endothelium-dependent vascular responses: Mediators and mechanisms. J. Clin. Invest. 84:1373, 1989.
15. Jaffe, E. A., Grulich, J., Weksler, B. B., Hampel, G., and Watanabe, K.: Correlation between thrombin-induced prostacyclin production and inositol trisphosphate and cytosolic free calcium levels in cultured human endothelial cells. J. Biol. Chem. 262:8557, 1987.
16. Zavoico, G. B., Ewenstein, B. M., Schafer, A. I., and Pober, J. S.: Interleukin-1 and related cytokines enhance thrombin-stimulated PGI$_2$ production in cultured endothelial cells without affecting thrombin-stimulated von Willebrand factor secretion or platelet activator factor biosynthesis. J. Immunol. 142:3993, 1989.
17. Moncada, S., Palmer, R. J., and Higgs, E. A.: Nitric oxide: Physiology, pathophysiology and pharmacology. Pharmacol. Rev. 43:109, 1991.
18. Cotran, R. S.: Endothelial cells. In Kelley, W. N., Harris, E. D., Jr., Ruddy, S., and Sledge, C. B. (eds.): Textbook of Rheumatology. Philadelphia, W. B. Saunders Company, 1989, pp. 389–415.
19. Majno, G., Palade, G. E., and Schoefl, G. I.: Studies on inflammation, II. The site of action of histamine and serotonin along the vascular tree: A topographic study. J. Biophys. Biochem. Cytol. 11:607, 1961.
20. Joris, I., Majno, G., Corey, E. J., and Lewis, R. A.: The mechanism of vascular leakage induced by leukotriene E4: Endothelial contraction. Am. J. Pathol. 126:19, 1987.
21. Simionescu, N., Heltianu, C., Autohe, F., and Simionescu, M.: Endothelial cell receptors for histamine. Ann. N.Y. Acad. Sci. 401:132, 1982.
22. Wysolmerski, R. B., and Lagunoff, D.: Involvement of myosin light chain kinase in endothelial cell retraction. Proc. Natl. Acad. Sci. U.S.A. 87:16, 1990.
23. Stolpen, A. H., Guinan, E. C., Fiers, W., Pober, J. S.: Recombinant tumor necrosis factor and immune interferon act singly and in combination to reorganize human vascular endothelial cell monolayers. Am. J. Pathol. 123:16, 1986.
24. Brett, J., Gerlach, H., Nawroth, P., Steinberg, S., Godman, G., and Stern, D.: Tumor necrosis factor/cachectin increases permeability of

endothelial cell monolayers by a mechanism involving regulatory G proteins. J. Exp. Med. 169:1977, 1989.

25. Cotran, R. S.: The delayed and prolonged vascular leakage in inflammation, II. An electron microscopic study of the vascular response after thermal injury. Am. J. Pathol. 46:589, 1965.

26. Gabbiani, G., Badonnel, M. C., Mathewson, S. M., and Ryan, G. B.: Acute cadmium intoxication: Early selective lesion of endothelial clefts. Lab. Invest. 30:686, 1974.

27. Varani, J., Ginsburg, I., Schuger, L., et al.: Endothelial cell killing by neutrophils: Synergistic interaction of oxygen products and proteases. Am. J. Pathol. 135:435, 1989.

28. Hurley, J. V.: Acute Inflammation. Baltimore, Williams & Wilkins, 1972.

29. Mulligan, M. S., Varani, J., Dame, M. K., Lane, C. L., Smith, W. C., Anderson, D. C., and Ward, P.: Role of ELAM-1 in neutrophil-mediated lung injury. J. Clin. Invest. 88:38, 1991.

30. Johnson, K. J., and Ward, P. A.: Role of oxygen metabolites in immune complex injury of the lung. J. Immunol. 126:2365, 1981.

31. Schoefl, G.: Studies on inflammation, III. Growing capillaries: Their structure and permeability. Virchows Arch. A337:97, 1963.

32. Joris, I., Cuenand, H. F., Doern, G. V., Underwood, J. M., and Majno, G.: Capillary leakage in inflammation. A study by vascular labeling. Am. J. Pathol. 137:1353, 1990.

33. Springer, T. A.: Adhesion receptors of the immune system. Nature 346:425, 1990.

34. Bevilacqua, M. P., Corless, C., and Lo, S. K.: Endothelial–leukocyte adhesion molecule-1 (ELAM-1): A vascular selection that regulates inflammation. In Cochrane, C., and Gimbrone, M. A., Jr. (eds.): Cellular and Molecular Mechanisms of Inflammation: Vascular Adhesion Molecules. San Diego, Academic Press, 1991, pp. 1–13.

35. Bevilacqua, M. P., Pober, J. S., Mendrick, D. L., Cotran, R. S., and Gimbrone, M. A., Jr.: Identification of an inducible endothelial–leukocyte adhesion molecule. Proc. Natl. Acad. Sci. U.S.A. 84:9238, 1987.

36. Bochner, B. S., Luscinskas, F. W., Gimbrone, M. A., Jr., Newman, W., Sterbinsky, S. A., Derse-Anthony, C. P., Klunk, D., and Schleimer, R. P.: Adhesion of human basophils, eosinophils, and neutrophils to interleukin 1–activated human vascular endothelial cells: Contributions of endothelial cell adhesive molecules. J. Exp. Med. 173:1553, 1991.

37. Shimizu, Y. S., Shaw, S., Graber, N., Gopal, T. V., Horgan, K. J., van Seventer, G. A., and Newman, W.: Activation-independent binding of human memory T cells to adhesion molecule ELAM-1. Nature 349:799, 1991.

38. Lowe, J. B., Shoolman, L. M., Nair, R. P., Larsen, R. D., Bertrend, T. L., and Marks, B. M.: ELAM-1–dependent cell adhesion to vascular endothelium determined by a transfected human fucosyltransferase cDNA. Cell 63:475, 1990.

39. Walz, G., Aruffo, A., Kolanus, W., Bevilacqua, M., and Seed, B.: Recognition by ELAM-1 of the sialyl-Le^x determinant on myeloid and tumor cells. Science 250:1132, 1990.

40. Munro, J. M., Pober, J. S., and Cotran, R. S.: Tumor necrosis factors and interferon-gamma induce distinct patterns of endothelial activation and associated leukocyte accumulation in skin of Papis anubis. Am. J. Pathol. 135:121, 1989.

41. Munro, J. M., Pober, J. S., and Cotran, R. S.: Recruitment of neutrophils in the local endotoxin response: Association with de novo endothelial expression of the adhesion molecule ELAM-1. Lab. Invest. 64:295, 1991.

42. Lueng, D. C., Pober, J. S., and Cotran, R. S.: Expression of endothelial–leukocyte adhesion molecule-1 in elicited late phase reactions. J. Clin. Invest. 87:1805, 1991.

43. Gundel, R. H., Wagner, C. D., Torcellini, C. A., Clarke, C. C., Haynes, N., Rothlein, R., Smith, C. W., and Letts, L. G.: Endothelial–leukocyte adhesion molecule-1 mediates antigen-induced acute airway inflammation and late-phase airway obstruction in monkeys. J. Clin. Invest. 88:1407, 1991.

44. Polley, M. J., Phillips, M. L., Wayner, E., Nudelman, E., Singhal, A. K., Hakamore, S.-I., and Paulson, J. C.: CD62 and endothelial cell–leukocyte adhesion molecule 1 (ELAM-1) recognize the same carbohydrate ligand, sialyl-Lewis X. Proc. Natl. Acad. Sci. U.S.A. 88:6224, 1991.

45. Geng, J. G., Bevilacqua, M. P., Moore, K. L., et al.: Rapid neutrophil adhesion to activated endothelium mediated by GMP-140. Nature 343:757, 1990.

46. Lawrence, M. B., and Springer, T. A.: Leukocytes role on a selection at physiologic flow rates: Distinction from and prerequisite for adhesion through integrins. Cell 65:1, 1991.

47. Zimmerman, G. A., McIntyre, T. M., Mehra, M., and Prescott, S. M.: Endothelial cell–associated platelet-activating factor: A novel mechanism for signalling intracellular adhesion. J. Cell Biol. 110:529, 1990.

48. Lorant, D. E., Patel, K. D., McIntyre, T. M., McEver, R. P., Prescott, S. M., and Zimmerman, G. A.: Coexpression of GMP-140 and PAF by endothelium stimulated with histamine or thrombin: a juxtacrine system for adhesion and activation of neutrophils. J. Cell Biol. 115:223, 1991.

49. Patel K. O., Zimmerman, G. A., Prescott, S. M., McEver, R. P., and McIntyre, T. M.: Oxygen radicals induce human endothelial cells to express GMP-140 and bind neutrophils. J. Cell. Biol. 112:749, 1991.

50. Picker, L. J., Warnock, R. A., Buras, A. R., Doerschuk, C. M., Berg, E. L., and Butcher, E. C.: The neutrophil selection LECAM-1 presents carbohydrate ligands to the vascular selections ELAM-1 and GMP-140. Cell 66:921, 1991.

51. Von Adrian, V. H., Chambers, V. H., McEvoy, L., Bargaze, R. F., Arfors, K. E., and Butcher, E. C.: A two-step model of leukocyte-endothelial interactions: distinct roles of LECAM-1 and the leukocyte β2 integrins in vivo. Proc. Natl. Acad. Sci. U.S.A. 88:538, 1991.

52. Ley, K., Gaehtgens, P., Fennie, C., Singer, M. S., Lasky, L. A., and Rosen, S. D.: Lectin-like cell adhesion molecule 1 mediates leukocyte rolling in mesenteric venules in vivo. Blood 77:2553, 1991.

53. Pober, J. S., Gimbrone, M. A., Jr., Lapierre, L. A., Mendrick, D. L., Fiers, W., Rothlien, R., and Springer, T. A.: Overlapping patterns of activation of human endothelial cells by interleukin 1, tumor necrosis factor, and immune interferon. J. Immunol. 137:1893, 1986.

54. Smith, C. W., Rothlein, R., Hughes, B. J., et al.: Recognition of an endothelial determinant for CD18-dependent human neutrophil adherence and transendothelial migration. J. Clin. Invest. 82:1746, 1988.

55. Dustin, M. L., and Springer, T. A.: Lymphocyte function–associated antigen-1 (LFA-1) interaction with intercellular adhesion molecule-1 (ICAM-1) is one of at least three mechanisms for lymphocyte adhesion to cultured endothelial cells. J. Cell Biol. 107:321, 1988.

56. Diamond, M. S., Staunton, D. E., de Fougerolles, A. R., Stacker, S. A., Garcia-Aguilar, J., Hibbs, M. L., and Springer, T. A.: ICAM-1 (CD54): a counter-receptor for Mac-1 (CD11b/CD18). J. Cell Biol. 111:3129, 1991.

57. Lo, S. K., Lee, S., Ramos, R. A., Lobb, R., Rosa, M., Chi-Russo, G., and Wright, S. D.: Endothelial–leukocyte adhesion molecule 1 stimulates the adhesive activity of leukocyte integrin CR3 (CD11b/CD18, Mac-1, alpha m beta 2) on human neutrophils. J. Exp. Med. 173:1493, 1991.

58. Lo, S. K., Deturers, P. A., Levin, S. M., and Wright, S. P.: Transient adhesion of neutrophils to endothelium. J. Exp. Med. 169:1779, 1989.

59. Anderson, R., and Springer, T.: Leukocyte adhesion deficiency. Annu. Rev. Med. 38:175, 1978.

60. Rice, G. E., Munro, J. M., Bevilacqua, M. P.: Inducible cell adhesion molecule 110 (INCAM-110) is an endothelial receptor for lymphocytes: A CD11/CD18-independent adhesion mechanism. J. Exp. Med. 171:1369, 1990.

61. Osborn, L., Hession, C., Tizard, R., Vassallo, S., Luhowskyj, G., ChiRosso, G., and Lobb, R.: Direct expression cloning of vascular cell adhesion molecule 1, a cytokine-induced endothelial protein that binds to lymphocytes. Cell 59:1203, 1989.

62. Thornhill, M. H., and Haskard D. O.: IL-4 regulates endothelial cell activation by IL-1, tumor necrosis factor, or IFN-gamma. J. Immunol. 145:865, 1990.

63. Thornhill, M. H., Kyan-Aung, V., and Haskard, D. O.: IL-4 increases human endothelial cell adhesiveness for T cells but not for neutrophils. J. Immunol. 144:3060, 1990.

64. Elices, M. J., Osborn, L., Takada, Y., Crouse, C., Luhowskyj, S., Hemler, M. E., and Lobb, R. R.: VCAM-1 on activated endothelium interacts with the leukocyte integrin VLA-4 at a site distinct from the VLA-4/fibronectin binding site. Cell 60:577, 1990.

65. Rice, G. E., Munro, M., Corless, C., and Bevilacqua, M. P.: Vascular and non-vascular expression of ICAM-110. Am. J. Pathol. 138:385, 1991.

66. Briscoe, D. M., Pober, J. S., and Cotran, R. S.: Interleukin-4 (IL-4) modulates the effect of tumor necrosis factor (TNF) on endothelial cell adhesion molecule induction in vivo. J. Am. Soc. Nephrol. 2:534, 1991.

67. Oppenheimer-Marks, N., Davis, L. S., Boque, D. T., Ramberg, J., and Lipsky, P. E.: Differential utilization of ICAM-1 and VCAM-1 during the adhesion and transendothelial migration of human T lymphocytes. J. Immunol. 147:2913, 1991.

68. Spertini, O., Luscinskas, F. W., Kansas, G. S., Munro, J. M., Griffin, J. D., Gimbrone, M. A., Jr., and Tedder, T. F.: Leukocyte adhesion molecule-1 (LAM-1) interacts with an inducible endothelial cell ligand to support leukocyte adhesion. J. Immunol. 147:2565, 1991.

69. Jutila, M. A., Berg, E. L., Kishimoto, T. K., Picker, L. J., Bargatze, R. F., Bishop, D. K., Orosz, C. G., Wu, N. W., and Butcher, E. C.: Inflammation-induced endothelial cell adhesion to lymphocytes, neutrophils and monocytes. Transplant 48:727, 1989.

70. Kurt-Jones, E. A., Fiers, W., and Pober, J. S.: Membrane IL-1 induction on human endothelial cells and dermal fibroblasts. J. Immunol. 139:2317, 1987.

71. Streiter, R. M., Kunkel, S. L., Showell, H. J., Remick, D. G., Phan, S. H., Ward, P. A., and Marks, R. M.: Endothelial cell gene expression of a neutrophil chemotactic factor by TNF-γ, LPS and IL-β. Science 243:1467, 1989.

72. Rollins, B. J., and Pober, J. S.: IL-4 induces the synthesis and secretion of MCP-1/JE by human endothelial cells. Am. J. Pathol. 138:1315, 1991.

73. Matsushima, K., and Oppenheim, J. J.: Review article: Interleukin 8

and MCAF: Novel inflammatory cytokines inducible by IL-1 and TNF. Cytokine 1:2, 1989.

74. Hechtman, D. H., Cybulsky, M. I., Fuchs, H. J., Baker, J. B., and Gimbrone, M. A., Jr.: Inhibitor of polymorphonuclear leukocyte accumulation at sites of acute inflammation. J. Immunol. 147:83, 1991.

75. Gimbrone, M. A., Jr., Obin, M. S., Brock, A. F., et al.: Endothelial interleukin-8: A novel inhibitor of leukocyte–endothelial interactions. Science 246:1601, 1989.

76. Huber, A. R., Kunkel, S. L., Todd, R. F., and Weiss, S. J.: Regulation of transendothelial neutrophil migration by endogenous interleukin-8. Science 254:99, 1991.

77. Butcher, E. C.: Leukocyte–endothelial cell recognition: Three or more steps to diversity and sensitivity. Cell 67:1033, 1991.

78. Cotran, R. S., Gimbrone, M. A., Jr., Bevilacqua, M. P., Mendrick, D. L., Pober, J. S.: Induction and detection of a human endothelial activation antigen in vivo. J. Exp. Med. 164:661, 1986.

79. Redl, H., Dinges, H. P., Buurman, W. A., van der Linden, C. J., Pober, J. S., Schlag, G., Cotran, R. S.: Expression of endothelial leukocyte adhesion molecule-1 (ELAM-1) in septic but not traumatic/hypovolemic shock in the baboon. Am. J. Pathol. 139:461, 1991.

80. Cotran, R. S., and Pober, J. S.: Endothelial activation: Its role in inflammatory and immune reactions. In Simionescu, N., and Simionescu, M. (eds.): Endothelial Cell Biology. New York, Plenum Publishing Corp., 1988, pp. 335–347.

81. Briscoe, D. M., Schoen, F. J., Rice, G. E., Bevilacqua, M. P., Ganz, P., and Pober, J. S.: Induced expression of endothelial–leukocyte adhesion molecules in human cardiac allografts. Transplantation 51:537, 1991.

82. Goerdt, S., Zwadlo, G., Schlegel, R., Hagemier, H., Sorg, C.: Characterization and expression kinetics of an endothelial activation antigen present in acute inflammatory tissues. Exp. Cell. Biol. 55:117, 1987.

83. Pober, J. S., and Cotran, R. S.:What can be learned from the expression of endothelial adhesion molecules in tissues? (Editorial.) Lab. Invest. 64:301, 1991.

84. Rothlein, R., Barton, R. W., and Wingquist, R.: The role of intercellular adhesion molecule-1 (ICAM-1) in the inflammatory response. In Cochrane, C., and Gimbrone, M. A., Jr. (eds.): Cellular and Molecular Mechanisms of Inflammation: Vascular Adhesion Molecules. San Diego, Academic Press, 1991, pp. 171–180.

85. Watson, S. R., Fennie, C., and Lasky, L. A.: Neutrophil influx into an inflammatory site is inhibited by a soluble homing receptor—IgG chimera. Nature 349:164, 1991.

86. Pober, J. S., and Cotran, R. S.: Immunologic interaction of T lymphocytes with vascular endothelium. Adv. Immunol. 50:261, 1991.

87. Butcher, E. C.: Cellular and molecular mechanisms that direct leukocyte trafficking. Am. J. Pathol. 136:3, 1990.

88. Gallatin, W. M., Weissman, I. L., and Butcher, E. C.: A cell surface molecule involved in organ-specific homing of lymphocytes. Nature 303:30, 1983.

89. Berg, E. L., Yoshino, T., Rott, L. S., Robinson, M. K., Warnock, R.

A., Kishimoto, K., Picker, L. J., and Butcher, E. C.: The cutaneous lymphocyte antigen is a skin homing receptor for the vascular lectin endothelial cell–leukocyte adhesion molecule 1. J. Exp. Med. 174:1461, 1991.

90. Sanders, M. E., Makgoba, M. W., Sharrow, S. O., Stephany, D., Springer, T. A., Young, H. A., and Shaw, S: Human memory T lymphocytes express increased levels of three cell adhesion molecules (LFA-3, CD-2, and LFA-1) and three other molecules (UCHL1, CDw29, and Pgp-1) and have enhanced IFN-gamma production. Immunology 140:1401, 1988.

91. Van Epps, D. E., Potter, J., Vachula, M., Smith, C. W., and Dudason, D. C.: Suppression of human lymphocyte chemotatis and migration by anti-LFA-1 antibodies. J. Immunol. 143:3207, 1989.

92. Hughes, C. C. W., Savage, L. O. S., and Pober, J. S.: The endothelial cell as a regulation of T cell function. Immunol. Rev. 117:88, 1990.

93. Ziff, M.: Role of the endothelium in chronic inflammatory synovitis. Arthritis Rheum. 34:1345, 1991.

94. de Waal, R. M. W., Bogman, M. J. J., Maass, C. N., Cornelissen, L. M. H., Tax, W. J. M., and Koene, R. A. P.: Variable expression of Ia antigens on the vascular endothelium of mouse skin allografts. Nature 303:426, 1983.

95. Sobel, R. A., Blanchette, B. W., Bhan, A. K., and Colvin, R. B.: The immunopathology of experimental allergic encephalomyelitis, II. Endothelial cell Ia increases prior to inflammatory cell infiltration. J. Immunol. 132:2402, 1984.

96. Salomon, R. N., Hughes, C. C. W., Schoen, F. J., Payne, D. D., Pober, J. S., and Libby, P. Human coronary transplantation-associated arteriosclerosis: Evidence for a chronic immune reaction to activated graft endothelial cells. Am. J. Pathol. 138:791, 1991.

97. Guinan, E. C., Smith, B. R., Doukas, J. T., Miller, R. A., and Pober, J. S.: Vascular endothelial cells enhance T cell responses by markedly augmenting IL-2 concentrations. Cell. Immunol. 118:166, 1989.

98. Savage, C. O. S., Hughes, C. C. W., Pepinsky, R. S., Wallner, B. P., Freedman, A. S., and Pober, J. S.: Endothelial cell lymphocyte function–associated antigen-3 and an unidentified ligand act in concert to provide costimulation to human peripheral blood CD4 + T cells. Cell. Immunol. 137:150, 1991.

99. Jirik, F. R., Podor, T. J., Hirano, T., Kishimoto, T., Loskutoff, D. J., Carson, D. A., and Lotz, M.: Bacterial lipopolysaccharide and inflammatory mediators augment IL-6 secretion by human endothelial cells. J. Immunol. 142:144, 1989.

100. Leeuwenberg, J. F. M., von Asmuth, E. J. V., Jeunhomme, T. M. A. A., and Buurman, W. A.: IFN-gamma regulates the expression of the adhesion molecules ELAM-1 and IL-6 production by human endothelial cells in vitro. J. Immunol. 145:2110, 1990.

101. Teitel, J. M., Shore, A., McBarron, J., Leary, P. L., and Schiavone, A. Endothelial cells modulate both T-cell–dependent and T-cell–independent plaque-forming cell generation in vitro. Int. Arch. Allergy Appl. Immunol. 91:66, 1990.

Fibroblast Function and Fibrosis

INTRODUCTION

The fibroblast is an omnipresent cell that functions primarily in the deposition and degradation of the extracellular matrix. It is ubiquitously distributed in the soft connective tissues of the musculoskeletal system and parenchymal organs. The fibroblast plays a central role in the normal processes of tissue remodeling and wound healing and is believed to be equally important in the pathogenesis of diseases characterized by fibrosis, including progressive systemic sclerosis (PSS), pulmonary fibrosis, and hepatic cirrhosis. The prevalence of fibrosing diseases has generated a great deal of investigative interest in the study of this cell, and our knowledge of fibroblast biology has greatly increased in the past decade. In this chapter, the biology of the fibroblast is reviewed. To establish an orientation and a relationship of fibroblast function to disease processes, the mechanisms of the pathogenesis of fibrosis are reviewed first.

MECHANISMS OF PATHOGENESIS OF FIBROSIS

In studying the pathogenetic mechanisms of tissue fibrosis, one is constrained by the difficulty of conducting biochemical experiments on human material. Therefore, much of our insight into this subject is derived from morphologic observations of human diseases, biochemical studies of autopsy material, and careful experimentations on a spectrum of animal models with varying relevance to human diseases. In addition, much insight has been gained from *in vitro* studies of fibroblast cultures. Most of the specific diseases characterized by tissue fibrosis share certain clinical and morphologic features with each other as well as with many pertinent animal models.

Morphologically, the end-stage of these disorders is characterized by a disruption of normal architecture with proliferation of connective tissue. In parenchymal organs such as liver and lung, this fibroproliferative process results in an abnormal cellular arrangement that generally is associated with clinically recognizable organ dysfunction. In other conditions, such as retroperitoneal fibrosis, where the process takes place in a nonvital locale (i.e., retroperitoneal fat), the normal tissue is again replaced by dense connective tissue, but the clinical consequences are not as apparent in the earlier stages.

Although there may be one or two exceptions, the fibrotic reaction is generally associated with an inflammatory response, and evidence indicates that the deposition of connective elements occurs in the wake of this inflammation. This implies that some injurious event occurs in the target tissue that results in an inflammatory response that, in turn, leads to a fibrotic response.

Thus, one can generalize about fibrosis and identify three distinct but interrelated phases of the process: the phase of tissue injury, the inflammatory phase, and the reparative phase. It is quite likely that these three phases are represented to some degree in all fibrosing disorders and that the apparent clinical differences can be correlated with the predominance of one or another component at a given stage of the process. Morphologic observations would support the concept of three phases, although there is significant overlap, and evidence of all three phases can be found in a given tissue section.

Wound Healing—A Model of Tissue Fibrosis. Before reviewing the factors that are influential in each of these phases, a brief discussion of normal wound healing is in order. The healing process in mammals is in contrast to the regenerative response of lower vertebrates (amphibians) in which the amputation of a limb results in the growth of a new limb. Without the process of wound healing, our species would probably not have survived.

Schilling has divided the wound healing process into four phases: (1) wounding, (2) the inflammatory phase, (3) the proliferative phase, and (4) the remodeling phase.[1] This classification is similar to the one proposed earlier for the phases of tissue fibrosis, and the parallels between wound repair and tissue fibrosis have been previously emphasized.[2] The immediate response to a wound is the activation of the coagulation system. The inflammatory phase rapidly follows and is characterized by the migration of neutrophils, eosinophils, and mononuclear cells to the wound. Neutrophils are the first to appear and are the predominant cell in the first 24 to 48 hours, followed by macrophages (days 2 to 4).[3] These inflammatory cells are presumably attracted to the site by specific chemoattractants. The role of these cells appears to be complex and important to the process (see Chapter 15). Neutrophils are believed to function primarily in the prevention of infection. It has been shown that, in the absence of infection, wound healing proceeded normally in guinea pigs rendered neutropenic by antineutrophil serum.[4] In subsequent studies by the same investigators, it was demonstrated that the presence of macrophage-monocytes in the wound was essential for effective healing.[5-6] This is most likely related to the elaboration of cytokines by macrophages (see later discussion).

The next stage of wound healing is the reparative phase. This includes the processes of neovascularization and fibroblast activation and occurs in the wake of the inflammatory reaction. Both these processes are probably initiated in response to signals generated during the inflammatory phase. There is evidence that would implicate both the clotting system[7] (see Chapter 18) and the macrophage[8, 9] (see Chapter 16). Fibroblasts are attracted into the wound and are probably stimulated to proliferate and to synthesize collagen and other connective tissue elements. The timing of this phenomenon is somewhat controversial. Studies from different investigators have reported conflicting results indicating that the rate of collagen synthesis reaches maximum levels several days to 2 weeks postwounding.[10-12] A recent study has demonstrated that collagen production was several hundred times higher on day 7 of a healing human wound than on day 2.[13]

The deposition of new connective tissue in the wound forms granulation tissue that, to form a mature scar, must be contracted and remodeled. *In vitro* observations would indicate that wound contraction is a process that requires active participation by the fibroblast and is associated with a phenotypic change in this cell.[14] The process of wound remodeling occurs in association with wound contraction. Collagenase, gelatinase, and other hydrolytic enzymes are secreted by wound fibroblasts, and new matrix proteins are deposited, resulting in a healed wound. Wound contraction and remodeling result in the realignment of fibrous elements along tension lines. Remodeling is carefully controlled by factors that cause the release, activation, and inhibition of proteolytic enzymes, the action of which is balanced by the synthesis and processing of matrix proteins (see Chapter 14). In this phase, cross-linking of collagen occurs, and this process is essential to the formation of an effective wound. If this process is inhibited by a lathyrogen, the resulting wound is weak and the collagen is more easily extractable.[15] In addition to being less easy to solubilize, cross-linked collagen is relatively resistant to degradation by collagenase.[16]

This process of wound healing is summarized in Table 20–1. It has been the subject of investigation for several decades, and this model, as briefly described earlier, is supported by an abundance of

Table 20–1. EVENTS IN WOUND HEALING

Event	Approximate Time After Injury (days)
Injury	
Coagulation	0–2
Inflammation	
PMNs	1–4
Monocytes	2–6
Repair	
Fibroblast migration	3–7
Neovascularization	6–10
Collagen synthesis (biochemical)	2–21
Collagen deposition (morphologic)	7–21
Contraction, remodeling, and cross-linking	7 and later

PMN, polymorphonuclear leukocyte.

clinical and basic research. The pathogenesis of the fibrotic disorders is not as well defined, but evidence would support the concept that tissue injury, inflammation, and tissue repair are involved to some degree in most, if not all, of these conditions. In these disorders, the phases overlap considerably; specifically, the inflammatory component persists into the reparative phase.

Phases of Fibrosis. It is appropriate to expand on these three phases (injury, inflammation, and repair), with specific focus on how they relate to the pathogenesis of fibrosis.

Tissue Injury. Regardless of the nature of the fibrotic condition, it is almost certain that a specific insult initiates the process by inciting an inflammatory response. The nature of this insult is quite variable and includes infectious agents, immunologic reactions, environmental factors, drugs and toxins, tissue ischemia, and trauma. In some diseases, such as alcoholic cirrhosis, postnecrotic cirrhosis, silicosis, and radiation fibrosis, the identity of the initiating agent is obvious. Unfortunately, many others of these conditions are idiopathic and the inciting agent(s) are not known.

Pharmacologic agents can induce fibrotic conditions. It is quite likely that these agents induce fibrosis by injuring the target tissue. This is especially likely in the case of retroperitoneal fibrosis associated with ergot alkaloids. Methysergide is a vasoactive substance and may induce an inflammatory response by this mechanism.

In its early states, retroperitoneal fibrosis is associated with an inflammatory infiltrate. The fibrotic conditions associated with the carcinoid syndrome are likely to share pathogenetic features with ergot-induced diseases considering the structural similarities between these ergot alkaloids and serotonin. An association has been made between tissue fibrosis and certain β-adrenergic blockers.[17-19]

The Inflammatory Response. In the wound healing model, the inflammatory response is immediate. In contrast, fibrosing conditions are not as acute, usually progressing over a period of weeks to years. In addition, immunologic mechanisms are not operative in wound healing but are probably central in the pathogenesis of certain fibrotic disorders.

Linking of the inflammatory response and the immune response to fibrosis is an area in which our knowledge has grown rapidly in the past few years. It is clear that soluble mediators, including cytokines and growth factors generated during the inflammatory phase as well as cell-cell interactions, influence the reparative phase and probably represent a bridge between these two phases. It is well known by clinical observations, however, that tissue injury and inflammation do not always progress to scarring. For example, only a minority of alcoholics progress to cirrhosis, and certain bacterial infections resolve without residual fibrosis despite intense inflammation. The scientific basis for these observations is not known and may be the most compelling question to be answered in the study of these processes. It is very likely that host factors play a role. A familial occurrence has been observed in certain of these syndromes (Dupuytren's diathesis, retroperitoneal fibrosis)[20, 21], and keloids are more frequently seen in blacks. It is also probable that the intensity of the tissue destruction mediated by proteinases, oxidative products, prostaglandins, and other factors released during this phase is a determining factor in the degree to which normal architecture is disrupted by the healing phase. Furthermore, the development of delayed-type hypersensitivity and the local generation of specific modulators of fibroblast function are believed to be important in certain conditions.

The Reparative Phase. As mentioned earlier, scar formation occurs in the wake of inflammation in wound healing. Similarly, tissue fibrosis occurs in the wake of the inflammatory reaction. The transition to the reparative phase is generally not sharply demarcated in these diseases, and the two processes overlap considerably. Morphologic observations would support this in that inflammatory infiltration and fibrosis are often seen in the same biopsy specimen.

Although it is likely that events in all three phases are critical in the fibrotic process, the relative role of each step is unknown. It is becoming clear that the reparative process is extremely important in determining the ultimate lesion in response to a given stimulus. In one provocative study, it was shown that hamsters developed interstitial pulmonary fibrosis in response to cadmium chloride but developed bullous emphysema in response to the identical agent if the animals were rendered lathyritic by the administration of β-aminopropionitrile, a compound that inhibits cross-linking of collagen.[22] This observation strongly suggests that regulation of the repair process is key in the development of fibrosis, at least in the lung.

The cell that is central in the reparative phase is the fibroblast. In the last decade, the complexities of this cell have been the subject of investigation of researchers of many disciplines. In the past decade, the techniques of cell biology and molecular genetics

have permitted the passage of this study to a more precise science with highly characterized mediators and fibroblast functions.

FIBROBLAST FUNCTION

The fibroblast is a multifaceted cell, and and the functions of this cell can be influenced by a variety of stimuli. Specifically, the fibroblast functions that are most relevant to tissue repair include (1) chemotactic migration; (2) proliferation; (3) adherence to extracellular matrix and to other cells; (4) biosynthesis, processing, and deposition of the major connective tissue elements (collagen, glycosaminoglycans, elastin, and fibronectin); and (5) tissue remodeling (which involves all the above in addition to the synthesis, release, and activation of proteinases that degrade these matrix proteins.)

Migration and Chemoattraction of Fibroblasts. Early in the reparative phase of wound healing, local fibroblasts migrate into the site of tissue injury[23] in response to specific signals related to the inflammatory phase. Similarly, it is likely that fibroblast attraction to sites of inflammation is crucial in the pathogenesis of fibrotic diseases. It should be pointed out that unlike other cells that respond to certain substances by migration toward them (neutrophils and monocytes), the fibroblast is not a cell that circulates in the blood stream. Therefore, the chemotaxis of fibroblasts results in the recruitment of local cells. Growth factors then stimulate the proliferation of these cells, resulting in an increase in the number of fibroblasts at the site. This is in contrast to the chemotaxis of circulating blood cells in which large numbers of these cells are attracted to the site of inflammation but do not proliferate locally.

Both promoters and inhibitors of fibroblast migration and chemotaxis have been described and are summarized in Table 20–2. It is apparent that this process can be linked to the inflammatory phase through the coagulation system, the complement system, neutrophils, and macrophages and by the degradation products of certain connective tissue proteins.[6, 24-29] Inflammatory mediators, including cytokines, growth factors, and eicosanoids, have been shown to be chemotactic for fibroblasts. Transforming growth factor (TGF)-β and platelet-derived growth factor (PDGF) are potent growth factors for fibroblasts as well as potent chemoattractants and adherence promoters (see following) and, therefore, have multiple effects on the cell that would act in concert to promote healing and fibrosis (see Chapter 13). In the case of PDGF, the BB homodimer and AB heterodimer are potent chemoattractants, whereas the AA homodimer is inactive and inhibits the chemoattraction induced by the other PDGF isoforms.[41] Tumor necrosis factor (TNF) has been recently shown to be chemotactic for fibroblasts; the activity has been shown to reside in a peptide corresponding to residues 31 to 68 of the protein.[33] The eicosanoids 5(S)-

Table 20–2. MEDIATORS OF FIBROBLAST MIGRATION

Factor	Sources	Characteristics	Reference No.
Promoters of Migration			
Platelet-derived growth factor	Platelets Macrophages	Disulfide-bonded dimer of approximately 35,000 M_r	30
Transforming growth factor-β	Platelets, other cells	Disulfide-bonded dimer (116 amino acids/chain)	31
Brain-derived growth factor	Brain tissue	17,000 M_r protein similar to acidic FGF	32
Tumor necrosis factor	Macrophages, other cells	Residues 31–68 is active peptide	33
Peptides derived from matrix proteins			
Collagen	Matrix		28
Fibronectin	Matrix macrophages	140-kD cell attachment region	26, 34
Elastin	Matrix	VGVAPG sequence	27, 35
Serum-derived chemotactic factor for fibroblasts	Complement (C5)	80,000 M_r protein	24
LTB₄, 5(S)-HETE, and 12(S)-HETE	Leukocytes, other cells	Arachidonate metabolites	36
Inhibitors of Migration			
Interferon-γ and -α	Various cells	Family of proteins	37
Serum inhibitor of fibroblast migration	Serum	230,000 M_r protein	38
Retinoids			39
Neutrophil factor	Neutrophil	16,000 M_r protein	40

hydroxyeicosatetraenoic acid (HETE), LTB₄, and 12(S)-HETE have also been shown to be chemoattractants for fibroblasts.[36] The attraction of fibroblasts to peptides generated by the degradation of collagen, elastin, and fibronectin would seem to be an important physiologic mechanism linking the repair process to normal enzymatic wound debridement.

In view of the work of Leibovich and Ross,[5] the macrophage plays a central role in the process of dermal wound healing and probably plays a role in inflammation-related fibrosis. This is strengthened by several observations. First, the macrophage is a source of PDGF and TGF-β,[42, 43] two peptides that promote fibroblast activation. In addition, this cell produces fibronectin, which is a fibroblast chemoattractant.[26, 34] Furthermore, macrophages secrete specific connective tissue–degrading proteinases into the extracellular space.[44] The products released by these proteinases attract fibroblasts to deposit new matrix. Thus, the macrophage can recruit fibroblasts into the area of inflammation by several mechanisms.

Fibroblast Proliferation and Growth Factors. In both wound healing and tissue fibrosis, the local proliferation of fibroblasts is believed to be important in the resulting scar formation. In recent years, investigators have identified several regulatory mechanisms governing fibroblast growth that have greatly increased our understanding of the process. It has been well known for decades that cultured fibroblasts proliferate in serum-containing medium but not in unsupplemented culture medium. It is now clear that polypeptide growth factors are responsible for the mitogenic effect of fetal calf serum. Furthermore, it is now clear that certain of these growth factors are produced by a variety of cells, including fibroblasts, and they can act as autocrine as well as paracrine factors. The rapidly expanding body of growth factor literature has also documented the multiple effects these growth factors have on

fibroblast function, suggesting a central role for them in the process of wound healing and fibrosis.

Platelet-Derived Growth Factor. PDGF is a protein that is a major growth factor for fibroblasts and is responsible for much of the mitogenic activity of whole serum. PDGF is a disulfide-bonded dimer with a molecular weight (M_r) of approximately 35 kilodaltons (kD). Two distinct gene products (A and B chains) combine in all possible combinations to make up the mature protein, thereby forming both heterodimer forms (AB) and homodimer forms (AA and BB). There is considerable homology between these chains, and the B chain is the product of the c-*sis* oncogene. It is released from the alpha (α) granules of platelets during activation. It is also synthesized by a variety of normal, neoplastic, and transformed cells as well as by inflammatory cells, including macrophages. PDGF can act as a paracrine or an autocrine growth factor.[45–48]

Cells that respond to PDGF include fibroblasts and smooth muscle cells but not epithelial cells, endothelial cells, or lymphocytes, which are devoid of receptors for this protein.[49, 50] The molecular structure of the PDGF receptor has been recently elucidated, and it is of interest that its structure mirrors that of its ligand.[51] The model for this receptor is that it consists of two subunits, each a distinct gene product designated α and β. The mature receptor can consist of two α subunits, two β subunits, or one of each. These subunits have been well characterized and are strikingly homologous. Each is a polypeptide of approximately 100,000 daltons (d) with a disulfide-rich extracellular binding domain, a transmembrane segment, and an intracellular tyrosine kinase domain. Ligand binding depends on the two-subunit structure, and specificity is determined by the subunit structure. The α subunit binds both A and B chains with high affinity, whereas the β subunit binds only B chains. Thus, the α = α subunit structure can bind all three forms of PDGF, the $\alpha = \beta$ receptor binds the AB and BB dimers, and the $\beta = \beta$ receptor binds only the BB homodimeric form of PDGF. Some studies have demonstrated differential effects of the various forms of PDGF as well as differential expression of the receptor subunits.[41] Fibroblasts appear preferentially to express the β subunit, and this subunit has been found to be increased in inflammatory states and in atherosclerotic lesions.[52, 53] Thus, considering the relatively ubiquitous distribution of PDGF, its activity is likely to be governed by both quantity and quality of receptor expression.

Binding of PDGF to its receptor initiates a series of events that results in mitosis. The receptor associates with protein kinase C, and a series of intracellular events occur including phosphorylation of proteins, turnover of phosphoinositides, and mobilization of calcium.[45, 54] Signal transduction occurs with internalization of the receptor ligand complex and down-regulation of receptors. These result in the expression of genes associated with early events in mitosis such as c-fos.[55]

PDGF has been shown to have other effects on fibroblasts. It has been shown to be chemotactic[30, 41] and to induce collagenase secretion.[56] PDGF has been shown to induce the contraction of collagen gels by fibroblasts. This process is mediated by a β-1 integrin and is a response to the AB and BB isoforms but not the AA form.[57, 58] Cells transfected with the c-sis oncogene overexpress the B chain of PDGF and were found to produce excess fibronectin but not collagen.[59] Studies have indicated that the interactions and relationships between PDGF and other growth factors and cytokines are complex. PDGF has been shown to induce the expression of the interleukin-1 (IL-1) receptor gene[60] and can induce the phosphorylation of the epidermal growth factor (EGF) receptor inhibiting high-affinity binding of EGF.[61] Being an autocrine factor, the effects of other cytokines have been found to be attributable to endogenous PDGF. The mitogenic effect of IL-1 has been shown to be due to the induction of PDGF.[62] TNF has been shown to induce the AA isoform of PDGF,[63] and a similar mechanism has been proposed for TGF-β.[64]

PDGF has been shown to promote wound healing in vivo. Its expression by epithelial cells and fibroblasts in fresh wounds has been documented,[65] and the application of PDGF has been shown to promote wound healing.[66, 67] A comparison of the effect of PDGF with that of TGF-β revealed that the latter compound promoted the deposition of collagen bundles, whereas PDGF induced the production of glycosaminoglycan and appeared to promote the influx of macrophages.[68] It has also been shown that PDGF induces the fibroblast production of a chemoattractant for monocytes.[69]

Transforming Growth Factor-α–Epidermal Growth Factor. This is a family of growth factors that bind to a common receptor, the EGF receptor,

which is expressed on the surface of a variety of cell types. The original EGF that was isolated from mouse submaxillary gland was characterized as a small (approximately 6 kD) protein with a characteristic primary structure containing six half-cystines.[70–72] The cloning of the cDNA of this protein has revealed that the precursor protein is much larger than 6 kD having approximately 1200 amino acid residues and that the basic EGF unit was found in eight repeats. Near the carboxy-terminus is a typical transmembrane sequence, and it is now known that EGF can exist as a membrane protein. This basic structure of a membrane-bound growth factor with EGF-like domains and the ability to bind to the EGF receptor is shared by several other proteins, and it is now clear that this is a family of related growth factors that includes TGF-α, vaccinia growth factor, and amphiregulin. The first TGF-α, is abundant in human tissues and has been identified in the macrophages of healing wounds.[73] This protein has been characterized as a membrane-bound protein with a single EGF-like domain and can be cleaved from the cell surface to yield free growth factor. Both the free and membrane-bound form can interact with the EGF receptor, and this protein can therefore act as a paracrine growth factor and as a growth factor that acts through cell-cell contact, a phenomenon called *juxtacrine stimulation.*[74]

The EGF receptor is a protein that shares some of the characteristics of the PDGF receptor in that it contains a large extracellular domain that binds the ligand, a small transmembrane domain, and a large intracellular domain that is a tyrosine kinase. The interaction of ligand with the receptor initiates a series of events that leads to the expression of early genes of mitosis. The activation of these proteins leads to phosphoinositide turnover, diacyl glycerol generation, and calcium mobilization. The complex of receptor and ligand is internalized and probably degraded.[75, 76] Although at least two different signaling pathways for growth factors have been suggested on the basis of pertussis toxin sensitivity,[77] the hydrolysis of phosphoinositides appears to be common to both systems. Thus, subtle differences do exist in the effects of different growth factors, but it is likely that specific receptor expression is the key factor determining the response of a cell to a given growth factor.

Fibroblast Growth Factor. One of the earliest growth factors described, the term *fibroblast growth factor* (FGF) refers to a family of growth factors, primarily two proteins that share about 50 percent homology and are named *acidic FGF* and *basic FGF* according to their relative charge.[78] These are proteins of approximately 18 kD in molecular size and bind to the same receptor. FGFs have two binding domains, one that mediates receptor binding and one that mediates heparin binding.[79] They are mitogenic for a variety of cells and are potent angiogenic factors. The affinity for heparin may be related to these proteins being found in extracellular matrix of cultured endothelial cells complexed with heparin sulfate.[78, 80] FGF's presence in extracellular matrix as an active growth promoter raises an interesting and novel concept in cell-matrix interaction. *In vivo*, FGF has been shown to promote wound healing and, specifically to promote the formation of granulation tissue.[81, 82] This is consistent with the broad mitogenic effect and the angiogenesis ascribed to this factor (see Chapter 51).

Other factors that are mitogenic for fibroblasts include insulin, insulin-like growth factor, somatomedin A and C, IL-1, thrombin, and thrombospondin. It has become clear that certain of these factors work through the induction of an autocrine growth factor, such as PDGF, as in the case of IL-1, TNF, and thrombin.[62, 63, 83] Others (insulin, insulin-like growth factor, etc.) have been called *progression factors* because they act in synergy with other growth factors known as competence factors (e.g., PDGF). As the molecular and cellular mechanisms of mitogenesis are dissected, this distinction has become less clear. Bleomycin is a pharmacologic agent that has been shown to be mitogenic for fibroblasts.[84]

A major antagonist of fibroblast proliferation is interferon-gamma (γ). This is a cytokine that appears to be a general antagonist of the elements of the fibrotic process and is further discussed later. It has been shown to inhibit the mitogenic activity of PDGF, EGF, and FGF.[85] Retinoids have also been shown to inhibit fibroblast proliferation.[86]

Fibroblast Adherence. The anchoring of fibroblasts to their surrounding extracellular matrix is believed to be important in the synthesis and organization of the extracellular matrix and is probably essential in the processes of wound healing and tissue fibrosis. The adhesion of fibroblasts to other cells, including inflammatory phagocytes, probably plays a major role in the cell-cell communications characteristic of the inflammatory reaction. Several families of cell surface proteins or cell adhesion molecules (CAMs) have been defined, which mediate the adherence of cells to matrix and to other cells.

The first major family of cell adhesion proteins is the integrins.[87–89] These are heterodimers consisting of two noncovalently associated subunits, α and β. Each chain is a transmembrane protein consisting of a large amino-terminal extracellular domain, a hydrophobic transmembrane domain, and a carboxy-terminal cytoplasmic domain that associates with the cytoskeletal components talin and vinculin. The β subunits are similar to one another with remarkable homology and are conserved throughout the phylogenetic tree. To date, six different β subunits and eleven different α subunits have been characterized. The individual integrins have been classified on the basis of the β chains and are defined as $\alpha_x\beta_y$. The major integrins identified in humans are of the β-1 to 3 families and are listed in Table 20–3.

The β-1 integrins are the very late activation antigens of T lymphocytes integrins (VLA). These integrins are widely distributed among cells and are

Table 20–3. INTEGRINS

α Subunit	Ligands	Other Names
β-1 Integrins		
1	Laminin, collagens I, IV	
2	Collagens I, IV, VI, V	
3	Laminin, fibronectin, collagens I, IV	
4	Fibronectin	
5	Fibronectin	Fibronectin receptor
6	Laminin	
V	Fibronectin	
β-2 Integrins		
L	ICAM-1, 2	LFA-1
M	C3bi, fibrinogen ICAM-1, factor X	MAC-1
X	C3bi	Glycoprotein 150,95
β-3 Integrins		
II$_b$	Fibrinogen, von Willebrand factor, fibronectin, vitronectin	Glycoprotein IIb/IIIa
V	Vitronectin	Vitronectin receptor

largely matrix receptors. The classic fibronectin receptor, $\alpha_5\beta_1$, is one of seven distinct integrins of this subfamily, which are defined by their α-chain and ligand specificity. The other members of this family bind laminin or the various collagen types, or both. The binding of integrins to their ligands is divalent cation dependent, and the ligand specificity is probably determined by the α-chain. The specificity of ligand binding can be reduced to specific peptide sequences. The classic example of this is the Arg-Gly-Asp (RGD) specificity of the fibronectin receptor. Although RGD-specific binding is shared by other integrins, some integrin-matrix interactions are not dependent on the presence of RGD sequences.

The β-2 integrin family consists of leukocyte adhesion molecules and are also called *LEU-CAMs*.[87–89] These include several well-characterized surface proteins. LFA-1, which is $\alpha_L\beta_2$, is present on leukocytes; its ligand is ICAM-1, a cell adhesion molecule that is expressed by fibroblasts and endothelial cells. This LFA-1/ICAM-1 interaction is believed to play a major role in the adherence of inflammatory phagocytes to other cells in inflammatory situations, including fibroblasts.[90] MAC-1 (CD11b/CD18, Mo-1, CR-3) also binds to ICAM-1 as well as other proteins and may also play a role in inflammation.

The β-3 family of integrins includes the well-characterized fibrinogen receptor of platelets, glycoprotein IIb/IIIa ($\alpha_{IIb}\beta_3$), which also may mediate the binding of platelets to fibronectin and von Willebrand factor. The other β-3 integrin is the vitronectin receptor, which has multiple ligands. Other families of integrins are likely to emerge with the discovery of new β-chains. A body of evidence is accumulating that would indicate that cellular expression of specific integrins is essential in a variety of biologic phenomena. Cell migration is closely linked to cell adhesion and, therefore, integrin expression may govern the specificity of this process. Thus, integrin expression is believed to play a regulatory role in embryogenesis, tissue repair, tumor invasion, among many other processes. Integrin-mediated adhesion in wound healing and fibrosis is believed to play a regulatory role in the migration of fibroblasts into the wound as well as the re-epithelialization process.[89] Wound contraction *in vitro* is also associated with integrin expression.[91]

In addition to the integrins, other cell surface proteins have been identified as receptors for extracellular matrix proteins. The best characterized of these is the family of 67-kD proteins that bind laminin, collagen, and elastin.[92] Binding to these receptors does not appear to be RGD sensitive but has been found to be mediated by specific sequences in the ligands: YIGSR for the laminin receptor and VGVAPG for the elastin receptor.[93] An 85-kD protein has been described as a hyaluronate-binding protein.[94] Cell surface proteoglycans rich in heparin sulfate have been found to be involved in both cell-cell and cell-matrix adhesion.[95, 96]

The other major category of CAMs comprise those proteins that primarily mediate cell-cell interactions. These include homophilic (act as both receptor and ligand) and heterophilic (receptor and ligand are different molecules) CAMs. Although there are numerous different proteins in this category, the one that is of interest to the subject of this chapter is ICAM-1. This is a 76- to 114-kD protein of the immunoglobulin superfamily. It is expressed on endothelial cells, fibroblasts, and other cells, and its expression can be induced. It is the ligand for LFA-1 and mediates the adhesion of leukocytes to fibroblasts,[90, 97] thus playing a major role in local inflammatory reactions.

Biosynthesis, Processing, and Deposition of Collagen. Having migrated to the sites of inflammation and anchored to the surrounding tissue, the fibroblast then engages in the essence of the healing process and deposits matrix components in the extracellular space. This process is very complex and involves much more than the expression of the gene coding for the matrix protein. The biosynthesis of collagen, for example, requires several post-translational processing steps to deposit native triple-helical molecules that can be incorporated into mature fibrils (see Chapter 2). This process requires the presence of several enzymes, which are also expressed by fibroblasts, and the presence of certain cofactors. In addition, the fibroblast synthesizes the other matrix components (proteoglycans, fibronectin, etc.) and assembles these molecules into a functional matrix. The production of collagen will be discussed as a marker for matrix synthesis because the production of fibronectin and proteoglycans generally parallels collagen deposition.

As discussed in detail later, the production of collagen by fibroblasts *in vitro* is readily manipulated by a variety of substances. However, it is logical to ask whether the rate of production of collagen (or other matrix elements) is critical in the development of fibrosis. If fibroblasts migrate into a tissue that is relatively devoid of these cells and subsequently proliferate, connective tissue matrix should accumulate even if the rate of collagen synthesis per cell is normal. Certain observations would indicate that the fibroblast synthesizes collagen at an enhanced rate in the process of fibrosis. First, in certain models of pulmonary fibrosis (bleomycin, ozone), cultured lung explants exhibit an increased rate of collagen synthesis[98, 99] as do fibroblasts derived from the lungs of bleomycin-treated rats. Immunochemical examination of human lung tissue from patients with fibrotic diseases exhibited fibroblasts in situ with an increased expression of type I collagen.[100] Furthermore, it has been well established that scleroderma skin fibroblasts also have an enhanced rate of collagen synthesis and collagen mRNA synthesis and that this "scleroderma phenotype" persists in culture after passage[101] (see Chapter 66).

It may seem logical that the connective tissue deposited in fibrotic states simply represents a difference in the quantity of qualitatively normal interstitium. This is not necessarily the case. In common fibrotic diseases such as idiopathic pulmonary fibrosis, cirrhosis, and keloids, the fibrotic matrix contains an increase in type I collagen reflected by an increase in the type I:III ratio.[102, 103] In progressive systemic sclerosis, fibrotic lung contains types I and III collagen in normal ratios but increased collagen overall.[104] In Dupuytren's contracture, the thickened fascia contains a substantial amount of type III collagen that is not present in normal palmar fascia.[105]

The formation of a functional extracellular matrix requires the coordinated expression of a number of related and unrelated genes, including those coding for matrix proteins (collagen, core protein of GAGs) as well as regulatory enzymes (e.g., procollagen proteinases, hydroxylases, cross-linking enzymes). In the past, studies have used collagen gene expression as a marker for the process and measured the amount of procollagen secreted in a cell culture system, usually fibroblast monolayer cultures. These methods do not assess the processing of procollagen into fibrils, a process that is essential to the formation of scar tissue. Since the isolation of the genes encoding for this protein, the focus of these studies is on transcriptional regulation of the collagen gene by measuring mRNA levels and by using various DNA constructs to assess the role of DNA regulatory elements and *trans*-acting factors. (The regulatory elements in the collagen gene are discussed in Chapter 2.)

Various substances have been reported to influence collagen production by fibroblasts, and they are listed in Table 20–4. A simple classification of these agents is not obvious, but certain agents probably play a role in the physiologic regulation of matrix deposition. A mechanism of feedback inhibition was suggested when it was observed that the amino-

Table 20–4. MODULATORS OF COLLAGEN
SYNTHESIS

Promoters of Collagen Production

Transforming growth factor-β
Interleukin-1
Interleukin-4
Hepatic fibrogenic factor
Ascorbate
Bradykinin
Insulin
Bleomycin
γ-aminobutyric acid

Inhibitors of Collagen Production

Procollagen propeptides (NH$_2$ and COOH extensions)
γ-Interferon
Tumor necrosis factor
Factors that increase cAMP (prostaglandin E$_2$, β-adrenergic
  agonists)
Glucocorticoids
Parathyroid hormone
Retinoids

terminal extension propeptides of the α_1(I)- and
α_1(III)-chains were found to inhibit the synthesis of
collagen by fibroblasts.[106] Further studies have demonstrated that a synthetic peptide constructed from
a highly conserved portion of the carboxy-terminal
extension of the α_2(I)-chain inhibited the synthesis of
collagen and fibronectin.[107] These extension peptides
are cleaved from the molecule in the extracellular
space during normal processing of collagen and appear to be stable, being detected in tissues and body
fluids.[108]

Ascorbate has two distinct effects on the production of collagen by fibroblasts. It has been known
for many years that it served as a cofactor in the
post-translational hydroxylation of proline and lysine
residues. More recently, it has been found specifically
to increase collagen synthesis in a manner independent of its role in hydroxylation.[109]

The inflammatory response provides many distinct signals that modulate collagen synthesis, and
these are believed to be key factors in the fibrotic
process.

Transforming Growth Factor-β. It is now known
that TGF-β represents a family of at least five gene
products with significant sequence homology that
are potent promoters of the fibrotic response. It is
found in platelets and is produced in one or another
isoform by essentially all cells. The prototype of the
family is TGF-β1, which is a disulfide-bonded dimer
of identical 12-kD polypeptide chains.[110] It is released
from cells in a latent form and can be converted to
its active form by transient acidification. TGF-β is a
pleiotropic cytokine with multifaceted biologic effects. It induces anchorage-independent growth of
fibroblasts while inhibiting the proliferation of other,
more differentiated cells such as keratinocytes and
epidermal cells.[111, 112] Its fibrogenic property is believed to be related to its effect on the expression of
connective tissue genes. It has been shown to stim-

ulate collagen, fibronectin, and proteoglycan synthesis.[113–115] The expression of metalloproteinases is
inhibited, whereas the expression of proteinase inhibitors (tissue inhibitor of metalloproteinases [TIMP],
platelet-activating inhibitor) is stimulated,[116–118] resulting in a negative influence on matrix degradation.
TGF-β also affects cell-matrix adhesion and cell-cell
interactions by regulating the expression of certain
integrins. It up-regulates the expression of the matrix
receptors of the β-1 integrin subfamily ($\alpha_{1, 2, 3, 5}/\beta_1$)
and the β-3 integrin ($\alpha_V\beta_3$), which is the vitronectin
receptor. This up-regulation of matrix receptors may
influence the migration of fibroblasts and the process
of wound contraction. TGF-β also up-regulates the
expression of the β-2 integrin LFA-1, thereby influencing the adhesion of fibroblasts to inflammatory
phagocytes, which is likely to promote the retention
of macrophages and neutrophils in sites of fibrosis
and wound healing.[119, 120]

The action of TGF-β is initiated by the binding
of the cytokine to specific cell surface receptors.
Binding sites for TGF-β have been found on virtually
all cells tested. Although the receptor structure is not
as well characterized as the other growth factor
receptors, the TGF-β receptor appears to be a large
glycosylated protein. It does not appear to possess
certain properties of these other receptors in that it
is not a phosphoprotein, and ligand binding does
not induce down-regulation or receptor clustering.[121]
Little is known of the mechanisms involved in signal
transduction of this cytokine. However, evidence
would suggest that the activation of the α_2(I) collagen
gene by TGF-β involves a nuclear factor-1 binding
site in the 5' flanking region of the gene.[122]

Other cytokines have been shown to modulate
the production of collagen *in vitro*. IL-1 stimulates
the production of collagen by cells cultured in serum-
free medium. In serum-containing medium, it has
little effect and may even down-regulate collagen
production. This down-regulation may represent an
antagonism of IL-1 for the effect of other cytokines
present in the serum (e.g., TGF-β) or may be due to
the down-regulation of collagen production by prostaglandin E$_2$.[123, 124] IL-4 has been shown to stimulate
collagen production.[125] TNF and interferon-γ down-
regulate collagen production.[124, 126] A fibrogenic factor
that stimulated types I, III, and V collagen synthesis
has been identified in fibrotic liver and appears to be
a complex phospholipid-polypeptide.[124, 125] Other
substances that have been reported to stimulate
collagen production include bradykinin and insulin.[123, 127]

There is ample evidence that would indicate that
10 to 40 percent of newly synthesized collagen can
be wasted by intracellular degradation. This event
may be related to lysosomal function, and this may
be the site of intracellular degradation. It has been
speculated that this process may provide a mechanism for the cell to dispose of structurally imperfect
collagen chains. There is a relationship between
collagen production and agents that elevate intracel-

lular cyclic AMP (cAMP). Thus, dibutyryl-cAMP and β-adrenergic agents, such as isoproterenol, cause a significant suppression of collagen secretion by fibroblasts. This effect is linked to the rate of intracellular wastage of collagen, which may be the major mechanism of this effect. The suppression of collagen production is type selective in that it occurs at the expense of type I collagen.[128] Alterations of collagen deposition mediated by this pathway may be one way in which the qualitative abnormalities of fibrosis-related collagen may be affected.

Glucocorticoids have a profound effect on the production of collagen by fibroblasts. These agents have been shown to inhibit collagen production *in vitro* in fibroblasts as well as in a cell-free systems.[129] It has also been shown that cortisol caused a decrease in the translatable type I procollagen mRNA in the developing chick embryo calvarium.[130] A similar effect has been described with parathyroid hormone.[131]

In view of the central role of collagen deposition in fibrotic diseases, the quest for pharmacologic agents that may inhibit this process has proceeded. There has been recent interest in retinoids, which inhibit collagen production by normal skin fibroblasts and keloid fibroblasts. This effect appears to be at the level of gene transcription because levels of mRNA are reduced.[132] Ethyl-2,3-dihydroxybenzoate, an analog of α-keto glutarate and ascorbate, has been shown to reduce collagen production by fibroblasts by inhibition of prolyl hydroxylase.[133] Another group of compounds that modulate collagen production are the proline analogues. These include *cis*-hydroxyproline, azetidinecarboxylic acid, and 3,4-dehydroproline. These agents are incorporated into the nascent collagen chains and prevent triple-helix formation. These imperfect molecules are presumably degraded intracellularly, and the net result is a decrease in the secretion of normal procollagen. There have been reports indicating that this class of compounds has a beneficial effect on experimental animal models of fibrosis.[134]

Contraction of Collagen Gels by Fibroblasts— A Model for Wound Contraction. Most of the *in vitro* studies of fibroblasts have been performed on monolayers of these cells that have been allowed to attach and proliferate on a plastic surface. Although the study of cultured cells was a technical advance two decades ago, it is a departure from the physiologic situation in which the fibroblast is in three-dimensional contact with the extracellular matrix. When fibroblasts are cultured in a three-dimensional gel of type I collagen, the cells actively contract the collagen gel to approximately 10 percent of its original volume.[135] This process has been studied as a model for wound contraction. The process requires cytoskeletal integrity and is mediated by a β-1 integrin.[57, 58] The morphologic and physiologic changes that occur are striking. Cells become elongated and bipolar; adhesion plaques are lost; and the cytoskeletal elements are rearranged. Collagen production is decreased during the process and reaches 10 percent of control

values. During the process of gel contraction, collagenase gene expression is up-regulated up to 30-fold, active collagenase is found in the supernatant, and collagen is degraded.[14] Although the trigger for this process is not clear, it is an attractive model for wound contraction.

The Expression of Matrix-Degrading Proteolytic Enzymes by Fibroblasts. In maintaining the homeostasis of the extracellular matrix, the fibroblast must degrade the existing matrix proteins in precise balance with the synthesis and deposition of new matrix proteins. It is clear that this process involves the enzymes of the matrix metalloproteinase family (see Chapter 14). This family includes at least six gene products, of which at least four are expressed by fibroblasts, collagenase, stromelysin, 70-kD gelatinase, and 92-kD gelatinase, the aggregate action of which is capable of degrading the extracellular matrix. These enzymes share significant sequence homology, and certain regions of the proteins are highly conserved. The regulation of the activity of these enzymes occurs at several levels. Gene expression and synthesis of each of these enzymes are subject to a variety of factors. Once secreted, the latent enzyme must be converted to an active form. Finally, naturally occurring inhibitors are produced by the same cells and can modulate enzyme activity.

Collagenase, stromelysin, and 70-kD gelatinase are secreted constitutively by fibroblasts. The former two are generally up-regulated and down-regulated by the same substances, whereas the gelatinase is independently regulated. The 92-kD gelatinase is generally not expressed by fibroblasts, but gene expression can be induced by phorbol myristate acetate and TNF.[136] The modulation of metalloproteinase expression is accomplished by some of the same agents discussed earlier. However, the production of these enzymes is independent of the production of collagen and the proliferation of fibroblasts. IL-1 and TNF are both potent inducers of collagenase expression,[137, 138] and these agents have divergent effects on collagen production, IL-1–inducing collagen production in serum-free conditions, and TNF down-regulating collagen production.[124] TGF-β stimulates collagen synthesis while down-regulating collagenase production and inducing TIMP production.[118] PDGF and EGF are mitogens, and both induce metalloproteinase production.[56, 139] IL-6 induces TIMP production, but collagenase production is not affected.[140] Thus, although the expression of metalloproteinases has been associated with an invasive phenotype, it is not clearly linked to collagen production or to cellular proliferation. It is of interest that the binding of fibroblasts to fibronectin through the integrin fibronectin receptor has been shown to induce collagenase production.[141] Thus, the collagenolytic activity associated with collagen gel contraction may be mediated through this mechanism, and cell migration that is mediated through integrin receptors may be associated with collagen breakdown.

Certain pharmacologic agents also affect the release of these enzymes from fibroblasts and other cells. Glucocorticoids in pharmacologic concentrations inhibit collagenase release as well as collagen production.[142] Retinoids have also been shown to inhibit the synthesis of collagenase and gelatinase.[143] Tetracycline has been shown to inhibit collagenase activity *in vitro* and *in vivo*.[144]

A SYNTHESIS

It is apparent from a multitude of studies that the fibroblast is a target cell of a variety of growth factors and cytokines. Most of our knowledge is based on precise methods of cell culture and molecular biology. One must be careful not to focus entirely on the parts but to maintain the whole picture in mind. Many of the observations made on the effect of growth factors on fibroblasts have been examined in the more complex models of wound healing. Virtually all of the growth factors discussed earlier have been shown to promote wound healing *in vivo*, and most have been identified *in situ* in wound healing models. Some subtle but interesting differences have been observed. The subcutaneous infusion of TNF induces a proliferative response resembling granulation tissue, whereas high concentrations induce massive tissue necrosis.[145] The comparison of the effects of PDGF and TGF-β have led to interesting observations. PDGF appears to induce not only the migration of inflammatory cells and fibroblasts into the wound but also the production of TGF-β, which seems to have a more profound effect on the stimulation of mature collagen fibers and matrix production.[146, 147] The observations that the fibroblast is capable of producing many of these mediators, that they act as both paracrine and autocrine factors, and that one factor can either induce the production of another or modulate a cellular response to another have led to the development of the concept of a cytokine network (see Chapter 13). The environment of the healing joint or the localized fibrotic response is rife with peptide and nonpeptide mediators, and the cell is exposed to this mixture of compounds with varied effect. What, then, determines the net response of the fibroblast? The answer to this question is not clear. It is possible that the net response is related to the balance between agonists and antagonists in the environment. However, it is more likely that the expression of specific receptors and adhesion proteins on the fibroblast should play a major role in the response. The latter mechanism could lead to the clonal expansion of phenotypically similar fibroblasts, a concept for which there is experimental support. It is likely that in the next several years further light will be shed on this complex issue.

References

1. Schilling, J. A.: Wound healing. Surg. Clin. North Am. 56:859, 1976.
2. Shoshan, S.: Wound healing. Int. Rev. Conn. Tiss. Res. 9:1, 1981.
3. Ross, R., and Benditt, E. P.: Wound healing and collagen formation. I. Sequential changes in components of guinea pig skin wounds observed in the electron microscope. J. Biophys. Biochem. Cytol. 11:677, 1961.
4. Simpson, D. M., and Ross, R.: The neutrophilic leukocyte in wound repair: A study with antineutrophil serum. J. Clin. Invest. 51:2009, 1972.
5. Leibovich, S. J., and Ross, R.: The role of the macrophage in wound repair: A study with hydrocortisone and antimacrophage serum. Am. J. Pathol. 78:71, 1975.
6. Diegelmann, R. F., Cohen, I. K., and Kaplan, A. M.: The role of macrophages in wound repair: A review. Plast. Reconstr. Surg. 68:107, 1981.
7. Knighton, D. R., Hunt, T. K., Thakral, K. K., and Goodson, W. H.: Role of platelets and fibrin in wound healing: An *in vivo* study of angiogenesis and collagen synthesis. Ann. Surg. 196:379, 1982.
8. Thakral, K. K., Goodson, W. H., and Hunt, T. K.: Stimulation of wound blood vessel growth by wound macrophages. J. Surg. Res. 26:430, 1979.
9. Polverini, P. J., Cotran, R. Z., Gimbrone, M. A., and Unanue, E. R.: Activated macrophages induce vascular proliferation. Nature 269:804, 1977.
10. Madden, J. W., and Peacock, E. E., Jr.: Studies on the biology of collagen during wound healing. I. Rate of collagen synthesis and deposition in cutaneous wounds of the rat. Surgery 64:288, 1968.
11. Mussini, E., Hutton, J. J., and Udenfriend, S.: Collagen proline hydroxylase in wound healing, granuloma formation, scurvy, and growth. Science 157:927, 1967.
12. Stein, H. D., and Keiser, H. R.: Collagen metabolism in granulating wounds. J. Surg. Res. 11:277, 1971.
13. Hanipuro, K., Melkko, J., Ristelli, L., Kairaluoma, M., and Ristelli, J.: Synthesis of type I collagen in healing wounds in humans. Ann. Surg. 213:75, 1991.
14. Mauch, C., and Krieg, T.: Fibroblast-matrix interactions and their role in the pathogenesis of fibrosis. Rheum. Dis. Clin. North Am. 16:93, 1990.
15. Arem, A. J., Misiorowski, R., and Chvapil, M.: Effect of low-dose bAPN on wound healing. J. Surg. Res. 27:228, 1979.
16. Vater, C. A., Harris, E. D., Jr., and Siegel, R. C.: Native cross-links in collagen fibrils induce resistance to human synovial collagenase. Biochem. J. 181:639, 1979.
17. Pierce, J. R., Jr., Trostle, D. C., and Warner, J. J.: Propranolol and retroperitoneal fibrosis. Ann. Intern. Med. 95:244, 1981.
18. Marshall, A. J., Bradley, H., Davies, J. D., Lee, R. F. J., Low-Beer, J. S., and Read, A. E.: A study of practolol periotonitis. J. Med. 46:135, 1977.
19. Wallis, A. A., Bell, R., and Sutherland, P. W.: Propranolol and Peyronie's disease. Lancet 2:980, 1977.
20. Early, P. F.: Population studies in Dupuytren's contracture. J. Bone Joint Surg. 43B:602, 1962.
21. Comings, D. E., Skubi, K. B., Van Eyes, J., and Motulsky, A.: Familial multifocal fibrosclerosis. Ann. Intern. Med. 66:884, 1967.
22. Niewoehner, D. E., and Hoidal, J. R.: Lung fibrosis and emphysema: Divergent responses to a common injury? Science 217:359, 1982.
23. Baum, J. L.: Source of the fibroblast in central corneal wound healing. Arch. Ophthalmol. 85:473, 1971.
24. Postlethwaite, A. E., Snyderman, R., and Kang, A. H.: Generation of a fibroblast chemotactic factor from serum by the activation of complement. J. Clin. Invest. 64:1379, 1979.
25. Postlethwaite, A. E., Snyderman, R., and Kang, A. H.: The chemotactic attraction of human fibroblasts to a lymphocyte-derived factor. J. Exp. Med. 144:1188, 1976.
26. Postlethwaite, A. E., Keski-Oja, G., Balian, G., and Kang, A. H.: Induction of fibroblast chemotaxis by fibronectin: localization of the chemotactic region to a 140,000-molecular weight non–gelatin-binding fragment. J. Exp. Med. 153:494, 1981.
27. Senior, R. A., Griffin, G. L., and Mecham, R. P.: Chemotactic responses of fibroblasts to tropoelastin and elastin-derived peptides. J. Clin. Invest. 70:614, 1982.
28. Postlethwaite, A. E., Seyer, J. M., and Kang, A. E.: Chemotactic attraction of human fibroblasts to type I, II, and III collagens and collagen-derived peptides. Proc. Natl. Acad. Sci. U.S.A. 75:871, 1978.
29. Gauss-Muller, V., Kleinman, H. K., Martin, G. R., and Schiffman, E.: Role of attachment and attractants in fibroblast chemotaxis. J. Lab. Clin. Med. 96: 1076, 1980.
30. Seppa, H., Grotendorst, G., Seppe, S., et al.: Platelet-derived growth factor is chemotactic for fibroblasts. J. Cell Biol. 921:584, 1982.
31. Postlethwaite, A. E., Keski-Oja, J., Moses, H. L., and Kang, A. H.: Stimulation of the chemotactic migration of human fibroblasts by transforming growth factor-β. J. Exp. Med. 165:251, 1987.
32. Senior, R. M., Huang, S. S., Griffin, G. L., and Huang, J. S.: Brain-derived growth factor is a chemoattractant for fibroblasts and astroglial cells. Biochem. Biophys. Res. Comm. 141:67, 1986.
33. Postlethwaite, A. E., and Seyer, J. M.: Stimulation of fibroblast che-

motaxis by human recombinant tumor necrosis factor α (TNF-α) and a synthetic TNF-α 31–68 peptide. J. Exp. Med. 172:1749, 1990.

34. Rennard, S. I., Hunninghake, G. W., Bitterman, P. B., and Crystal, R. G.: Production of fibronectin by the human alveolar macrophage. Mechanisms for the recruitment of fibroblasts to sites of tissue injury in interstitial lung disease. Proc. Natl. Acad. Sci. U.S.A. 78:7147, 1981.

35. Senior, R. M., Griffin, G. L., Mecham, R. P., Wrenn, D. S., Prasad, K. U., and Urry, D. W.: Val-Gly-Val-Ala-Pro-Gly, a repeating peptide in elastin, is chemotactic for fibroblasts and monocytes. J. Cell Biol. 99:870, 1984.

36. Rieger, G. M., Hein, R., Adelmann-Grill, B. C., Ruzicka, T., and Krieg, T.: Influence of eicosanoids on fibroblast chemotaxis and protein synthesis in vitro. J. Dermatol. Sci. 1:347, 1990.

37. Adelmann-Grill, B. C., Hein, R., Wach, F., and Krieg, T.: Inhibition of fibroblast chemotaxis by recombinant human interferon-γ and interferon-α. J. Cell. Physiol. 130:270, 1987.

38. Ochs, M. E., Postlethwaite, A. E., and Kang, A. H.: Identification of a protein in serum that inhibits fibroblast chemotactic and random migration in vitro. J. Invest. Dermatol. 88:183, 1987.

39. Hein, R., Mensing, H., Muller, P. K., Braun-Falco, O., and Krieg, T.: Effect of vitamin A and its derivatives on collagen production and chemotactic response of fibroblasts. Br. J. Dermatol. 111:37, 1984.

40. Mensing, H., and Czarnetzki, B. M.: Generation and characterization of a neutrophil-derived inhibitor of fibroblast chemotaxis. Arch. Dermatol. Res. 278:184, 1986.

41. Siegbahn, A., Hammacher, A., Westermark, B., and Heldin, C. H.: Differential effects of the various isoforms of platelet-derived growth factor on chemotaxis of fibroblasts, monocytes, and granulocytes. J. Clin. Invest. 85:916, 1990.

42. Sporn, M. B., and Roberts, A. B.: Peptide growth factors and inflammation, tissue repair, and cancer. J. Clin. Invest. 78:29, 1986.

43. Martinet, Y., Bitterman, P. B., Mornex, J. F., Grotendorst, G. R., Martin, G. R., and Crystal, R. G.: Activated human monocytes express the c-sis proto-oncogene and release a mediator showing PDGF-like activity. Nature 319:158, 1986.

44. Shapiro, S. D., Campbell, E. J., Kobayashi, D. K., and Welgus, H. G.: Immune modulation of metalloproteinase production in human macrophages. Selective pretranslational suppression of interstitial collagenase and stromelysin biosynthesis by interferon-γ. J. Clin. Invest. 86:1204, 1990.

45. Ross, R., Raines, E. W., and Bowen-Pope, D. F.: The biology of platelet-derived growth factor. Cell 46:155, 1986.

46. Doolittle, R. F., Hunkapiller, M. W., Hood, L. E., Devare, S. G., Robbins, K. C., Aaronson, S. A., and Antoniades, H. N.: Simian sarcoma virus onc gene, v-sis is derived from the gene (or genes) encoding a platelet-derived growth factor. Science 221:521, 1983.

47. Waterfield, M. D., Scrace, G. T., Whittle, N., Stroobant, P., Johnsson, A., Wasteson, A., Westermark, B., Heldin, C.-H., Huang, J. S., and Duell, T. F.: Platelet-derived growth factor is structurally related to the putative transforming protein p28sis of simian sarcoma virus. Nature 304:35, 1983.

48. Heldin, C.-H., Betsholtz, C., Johnsson, A., Nister, M., Ek, B., Ronnstrand, L., Wasteson, A., and Westermark, B.: Platelet-derived growth factor. Mechanism of action and relationship to oncogenes. J. Cell. Sci. [Suppl.] 3:65, 1985.

49. Heldin, C.-H., Westermark, B., and Wasteson, A.: Specific receptors for platelet-derived growth factor on cells derived from connective tissue and glia. Proc. Natl. Acad. Sci. U.S.A. 78:3364, 1981.

50. Singh, J. P., Chaikan, M. A., and Stiles, C. D.: Phylogenetic analysis of platelet-derived growth factor by radio-receptor assay. J. Cell Biol. 95:667, 1982.

51. Hart, C. E., and Bowen-Pope, D.: Platelet-derived growth factor receptor: Current views of the two subunit model. J. Invest. Dermatol. 94: 53s, 1990.

52. Seifert, R. A., Hart, C. E., Phillips, P. E., Forstrom, J. W., Ross, R., Murray, M. J., and Bowen-Pope, D. F.: Two different subunits associate to create isoform-specific platelet-derived growth factor receptors. J. Biol. Chem. 264:8771, 1988.

53. Rubin, K., Tingstrom, A., Hansson, G. K., Larsson, L., Ronnstrand, L., Klareskog, L., Claesson-Welsh, L., Heldin, C. H., Fellström, B., and Terracio, L.: Induction of B-type receptors for platelet-derived growth factor in vascular inflammation: Possible implications for development of vascular proliferative lesions. Lancet 1:1353, 1988.

54. Kumijian, D. A., Wahl, M. I., Rhee, S. G., and Daniel, T. O.: Platelet-derived growth factor (PDGF) binding promotes physical association of PDGF receptor with phospholipase C. Proc. Natl. Acad. Sci. U.S.A. 86:8232, 1989.

55. Kruijer, W., Cooper, J. A., Hunter, T., and Verma, I. M.: Platelet-derived growth factor induces rapid but transient expression of the c-fos gene and protein. Nature 312:711, 1984.

56. Bauer, E. A., Cooper, T. W., Huang, J. S., Altman, J., and Duell, T. F.: Stimulation of in vitro human skin collagenase expression by platelet-derived growth factor. Proc. Natl. Acad. Sci. U.S.A. 82:4132, 1985.

57. Gullberg, D., Tingstrom, A., Thuresson, A. C., Olsson, L., Terracio, L., Borg, T. K., and Rubin, K.: Beta 1 integrin-mediated collagen gel contraction is stimulated by PDGF. Exp. Cell Res. 186:264, 1990.

58. Clark, R. A., Folkvord, J. M., Hart, C. E., Murray, J., and McPherson, J. M.: Platelet isoforms of platelet-derived growth factor stimulate fibroblasts to contract collagen matrices. J. Clin. Invest. 84:1036, 1989.

59. Allen-Hoffmann, B. L., Schlosser, S. J., Brondyk, W. H., and Fahl, W. E.: Fibronectin levels are enhanced in human fibroblasts overexpressing the c-sis protooncogene. J. Biol. Chem. 265:5219, 1990.

60. Chiou, W. J., Bonin, P. D., Harris, P. K., Carter, D. B., and Singh, J. P.: Platelet-derived growth factor induces interleukin-1 receptor gene expression in Balb/c 3T3 fibroblasts. J. Biol. Chem. 264:21442, 1989.

61. Decker, S. J., Harris, P.: Effects of platelet-derived growth factor on phosphorylation of the epidermal growth factor receptor in human skin fibroblasts. J. Biol. Chem. 264:9204, 1989.

62. Raines, E. W., Dower, S. K., and Ross, R.: Interleukin-1 mitogenic activity for fibroblasts and smooth muscle cells is due to PDGF-AA. Science 243:393, 1989.

63. Paulsson, Y., Austgulen, R., Hofsli, E., Heldin, C. H., Westermark, B., Nissen-Meyer, J.: Tumor necrosis factor-induced expression of platelet-derived growth factor A-chain messenger RNA in fibroblasts. Exp. Cell Res. 180:490, 1989.

64. Soma, Y and Grotendorst, G. R.: TGF-β stimulates primary skin fibroblast DNA synthesis via an autocrine production of PDGF-related peptides. J. Cell. Physiol. 140:246, 1989.

65. Antoniades, H. N., Galanopoulos, T., Neville-Golden, J., Kiritsy, C. P., and Lynch, S. E.: Injury induces in vivo expression of platelet-derived growth factor (PDGF) and PDGF receptor mRNAs in skin epithelial cells and PDGF mRNA in connective tissue fibroblasts. Proc. Natl. Acad. Sci. U.S.A. 88:565, 1991.

66. Mustoe, T. A., Purdy, J., Gramates, P., Deuel, T. F., Thomason, A., and Pierce, G. F.: Reversal of impaired wound healing in irradiated rats by platelet-derived growth factor-BB. Am. J. Surg. 158:345, 1989.

67. Pierce, G. F., Mustoe, T. A., Senior, R. M., Reed, J., Griffin, G. L., Thomason, A., and Deuel, T. F.: In vivo incisional wound healing augmented by platelet-derived growth factor and recombinant c-sis gene homodimeric proteins. J. Exp. Med. 167:974, 1988.

68. Pierce, G. F., Vande Berg, J., Rudolph, R., Tarpley, J., and Mustoe, T. A.: Platelet-derived growth factor-BB and transforming growth factor-β 1 selectively modulate glycosaminoglycans, collagen, and myofibroblasts in excisional wounds. Am. J. Pathol. 138:629, 1991.

69. Yoshimura, T., and Leonard, E. J.: Secretion by human fibroblasts of monocyte chemoattractant protein-1, the product of gene JE. J. Immunol. 144:2377, 1991.

70. Cohen, S.: Isolation of a mouse submaxillary gland protein accelerating incisor eruption and eyelid opening in the new-born animal. J. Biol. Chem. 237:1555, 1962.

71. Savage, C. R., Jr., Inagami, T., and Cohen, S.: The primary structure of epidermal growth factor. J. Biol. Chem. 247:7612, 1972.

72. Carpenter, G, and Cohen, S.: Epidermal growth factor. J. Biol. Chem. 265:7709, 1990.

73. Rappolee, D. A., Mark, D., Banda, M. J., and Werb, Z.: Wound macrophages express TGF-α and other growth factors in vivo: Analysis by mRNA phenotyping. Science 241:708, 1988.

74. Massague, J.: Transforming growth factor-α: A model for membrane-anchored growth factors. J. Biol. Chem. 265:21393, 1990.

75. Stoscheck, C. M., and Carpenter, G: Down regulation of epidermal growth factor receptors: Direct demonstration of receptor degradation in human fibroblasts. J. Cell. Biol. 98:1048, 1984.

76. King, L. E., Gates, R. E., Stoscheck, C. M., and Nanney, L. B.: The EGF/TGF-α receptor in skin. J. Invest. Dermatol. 94:164s, 1990.

77. Chambard, J. C., Paris, S., Lallemain, G., and Pouyssegur, J.: Two growth factor signalling pathways in fibroblasts distinguished by pertussis toxin. Nature 326:800, 1987.

78. Gospodarowicz, D.: Fibroblast growth factors: Chemical structure and biologic function. Clin. Orthop. Rel. Res. 257:231, 1990.

79. Baird, A., Schubert, D., Ling, N., and Guillemin, R.: Receptor- and heparin-binding domains of basic fibroblast growth factor. Proc. Natl. Acad. Sci. U.S.A. 85:2324, 1988.

80. Vlodavsky, I., Folkman, J., Sullivan, R., Fridman, R., Ishai-Miochaeli, R., Sasse, J., and Klagsbrun, M.: Endothelial cell-derived basic fibroblast growth factor: Synthesis and deposition into subendothelial extracellular matrix. Proc. Natl. Acad. Sci. U.S.A. 84:2292, 1987.

81. Buntrock, P., Buntrock, M., Marx, I., Kranz, D., Jentsch, K. D., and Heder, G.: Stimulation of wound healing using brain extract with fibroblast growth factor (FGF) activity. Exp. Pathol. 26:247, 1984.

82. Davidson, J., Buckley, A., Woodward, S. J., McGee, G., and Demetrious, A.: Mechanism of accelerated wound repair using EGF and bFGF. In Hunt, T. K., et al. (eds.): Growth Factors and Other Aspects of Wound Healing. New York, Alan R. Liss, 1988, p. 63.

83. Daniel, T. O., Gibbs, V. C., Milfay, D. F., Garovoy, M. R., and Williams, L. T.: Thrombin stimulates c-sis gene expression in microvascular endothelial cells. J. Biol. Chem. 261:9579, 1986.

84. Moseley, P. L., Hemken, C., and Hunninghake, G. W.: Augmentation of fibroblast proliferation by bleomycin. J. Clin. Invest. 78:1150, 1986.

85. Oleszak, E.: Inhibition of mitogenic activity of PDGF, EGF, and FGF by interferon-γ. Exp. Cell Res. 179:575, 1988.

86. Daly, T. J., and Weston, W. L.: Retinoid effects on fibroblast proliferation and collagen synthesis in vitro and on fibrotic disease in vivo. J. Am. Acad. Dermatol. 15:900, 1986.

87. McDonald, J. A.: Receptors for extracellular marix components. Am. J. Physiol. 257:L331, 1989.

88. Albelda, S. M., and Buck, C.: Integrins and other cell adhesion molecules. FASEB J. 4:2868, 1990.

89. Rouslahti, E.: Integrins. J. Clin. Invest. 87:1, 1991.

90. Piela, T. H., and Korn, J. H.: ICAM-1-dependent fibroblast-lymphocyte adhesion: Discordance between surface expression and function of ICAM-1. Cell. Immunol. 129:125, 1990.

91. Gullberg, D,. Tingstrom, A., Thuresson, A. C., Olsson, L., Terracio, L., Borg, T. K., and Rubin, K.: Beta 1 integrin-mediated collagen gel contraction is stimulated by PDGF. Exp. Cell. Res. 186:264, 1990.

92. Liotta, L. A., Wewer, U. M., Rao, C. N., and Bryant, G.: Laminin receptor. In Edelman, G. M., and Thiery, J.-P. (eds.): The Cell in Contact. New York, John Wiley, 1985, pp. 333–344.

93. Meachem, R. P., Hinek, A., Griffin, G. L., Senior, R. M., and Liotta, L. A.: The elastin receptor shows structural and functional similarities to the 67-kDa tumor cell laminin receptor. J. Biol. Chem. 264:16652, 1989.

94. Underhill, C. B., Thurn, A. L., and Lacy, B. E.: Characterization and identification of the hyaluronate binding site from membranes of SV-3T3 cells. J. Biol. Chem. 260:8128, 1985.

95. LeBaron, R. G., Esko, J. D., Woods, A., Johansson, S., and Hook, M.: Adhesion of glycosaminoglycan-deficient Chinese hamster ovary cell-mutants to fibronectin substrata. J. Cell Biol. 106:945, 1988.

96. Saunders, S., Halkanen, M., O'Farrell, S., and Bernfield, M.: Molecular cloning of syndecan, an integral membrane proteoglycan. J. Cell. Biol. 108:1547, 1989.

97. Wawryk, S. O., Novotny, J. R., Wicks, I. P., Wilkinson, D., Maher, D., Salvaris, E., Welch, K., Fecondo, J., and Boyd, A. W.: The role of the LFA-1/ICAM-1 interaction in human leukocyte homing and adhesion. Immunol. Rev. 108:135, 1989.

98. Collins, J. F., McCullough, B., Coalson, J. J., and Johanson, W. G., Jr.: Bleomycin-induced pulmonary fibrosis in babboons. II. Further studies on connective tissue changes. Am. Rev. Respir. Dis. 125:305, 1981.

99. Last, J. A., Greenberg, D. B., and Castleman, W. L.: Ozone-induced alterations in collagen metabolism of rat lungs. Toxicol. Appl. Pharmacol. 51:241, 1979.

100. McDonald, J. A., Broekelmann, T. J., Matheke, M. L., Crouch, E., Koo, M., and Kuhn, C. III: A monoclonal antibody to the carboxyterminal domain of procollagen type I visualizes collagen-synthesizing fibroblasts. Detection of an altered fibroblast phenotype in lungs of patients with pulmonary fibrosis. J. Clin. Invest. 78:1237, 1986.

101. Buckingham, R. B., Prince, R. K., Rodnan, G. P, and Taylor, F.: Increased collagen accumulation in dermal fibroblast cultures from patients with progressive systemic sclerosis. J. Lab. Clin. Med. 92:5, 1978.

102. Seyer, J. M., Hutcheson, E. T., and Kang, A. H.: Collagen polymorphism in idiopathic chronic pulmonary fibrosis. J. Clin. Invest. 57:1498, 1976.

103. Seyer, J. M., Hutcheson, E. T., and Kang, A. H.: Collagen polymorphism in normal and cirrhotic human liver. J. Clin. Invest. 59:241, 1977.

104. Seyer, J. M., Kang, A. H., and Rodnan, G.: Investigation of type I and type III collagens of the lung in progressive systemic sclerosis. Arthritis Rheum. 24:625, 1981.

105. Brickley-Parsons, D., Climcher, M. J., Smith, R., Albin, R., and Adams, J. P.: Biochemical changes in the collagen of the palmar fascia in patients with Dupuytren's disease. J. Bone Joint Surg. 63A:787, 1981.

106. Wiestner, M., Krieg, T., Horlein, D., Glanville, RW., Fietzek, P., and Muller, P. K.: Inhibiting effect of procollagen peptides on collagen biosynthesis in fibroblast culture. J. Biol. Chem. 254:7016, 1979.

107. Aycock, R. S., Raghow, R., Stricklin, G. P., Seyer, J. M., and Kang, A. H.: Post-transcriptional inhibition of collagen and fibronectin synthesis by a synthetic homolog of a portion of the carboxyl-terminal propetide of human type I collagen. J. Biol. Chem. 261: 14355, 1986.

108. Ristelli, L., and Ristelli, J.: Radioimmunoassay for monitoring connective tissue metabolism. Rheumatology 10:216, 1986.

109. Pinnell, S. R.: Regulation of collagen synthesis. J. Invest. Dermatol. 79:73s, 1982.

110. Frolik, C. A., Dart, L. L., Meyers, C. A., Smith, D. M., and Sporn, M. B.: Purification and initial characterization of a type β transforming growth factor from human platelets. Proc. Natl. Acad. Sci. U.S.A. 80:3676, 1983.

111. DeLarco, J. E., and Todaro, G. J.: Growth factors from murine sarcoma virus–transformed cells. Proc. Natl. Acad. Sci. U.S.A. 75:4001, 1978.

112. Tucker, R. F., Shipley, G. D., Moses, H. L., and Holley, R. W.: Growth inhibitor from BSC-1 cells closely related to platelet type β transforming growth factor. Science 226:705, 1984.

113. Roberts, A. B., Sporn, M. B., Assoian, R. K., Smith, J. M., Roche, N. S., Wakefield, L. M., Heine, U. I., Liotta, L. A., Falanga, V., Kehrl, J. H., and Fauci, A. S.: Transforming growth factor type-β: Rapid induction of fibrosis and angiogenesis in vivo and stimulation of collagen formation in vitro. Proc. Natl. Acad. Sci. U.S.A. 83:4167, 1986.

114. Ignotz, R. A., Endo, T., and Massague, J.: Regulation of fibronectin and type I collagen mRNA levels by transforming growth factor-b. J. Biol. Chem. 262:6443, 1987.

115. Raghow, R., Postlethwaite, A. E., Keski-Oja, J., Moses, H. L., and Kang, A. H.: Transforming growth factor-b increases state levels of type I procollagen messenger RNAs posttranscriptionally in cultured human dermal fibroblasts. J. Clin. Invest. 79:1285, 1987.

116. Bassols, A., and Massague, J.: Transforming growth factor-β regulates the expression and structure of extracellular matrix chondroitin/dermatan proteoglycans. J. Biol. Chem. 263:3039, 1988.

117. Keski-Oja, J., Raghow, R., Sawdey, M., Loskutoff, D. J., Postlewaite, A. E., Kang, A. J., et al.: Regulation of mRNAs for type I plasminogen activator inhibitor, fibronectin, and type I procollagen by transforming growth factor. J. Biol. Chem. 263:311, 1988.

118. Edwards, D. R., Murphy, G., Reynolds, J. J., Whitlam, S. E., Docherty, A. J. P., Angel, P., et al.: Transforming growth factor-β modulates the expression of collagenase and metalloproteinase inhibitor. EMBO J. 6:1899, 1987.

119. Heino, J., Ignotz, R. A., Hemler, M. E., Crouse, C., and Massague, J.: Regulation of cell adhesion receptors by transforming growth factor-β: Concomitant regulation of integrins that share a common β1 subunit. J. Biol. Chem. 264:380, 1989.

120. Ignotz, R. A., Heino, J., and Massague, J.: Regulation of cell adhesion receptors by transforming growth factor-β: Regulation of vitronectin receptor and LFA-1. J. Biol. Chem. 264:388, 1989.

121. Wakefield, L. M., Smith, D. M., Flanders, K. C., and Sporn, M. B.: Distribution and modulation of the cellular receptor for transforming growth factor-β. J. Cell Biol. 105:965, 1987.

122. DeCrombrugghe, B., Karsenty, G., Maity, S., Vuorio, T., Rossi, P., Ruteshouser, E. C., McKinney, S. H., and Lozano, G.: Transcriptional mechanisms of types I and III collagen genes. Ann. N.Y. Acad. Sci. 580:88, 1990.

123. Goldstein, R. H., and Polgar, P.: The effect and interaction of bradykinin and prostaglandins on protein and collagen production by lung fibroblasts. J. Biol. Chem. 257:8630, 1982.

124. Elias, J. A., Freundlich, B., Adams, S., and Rosenbloom, J.: Regulation of human lung fibroblast collagen production by recombinant interleukin-1, tumor necrosis factor, and interferon-γ. Ann. N.Y. Acad. Sci. 580:233, 1990.

125. Postlethwaite, A. E., Katai, H., and Raghow, R.: Stimulation of extracellular matrix biosynthesis in fibroblasts by interleukin 4. Arthritis Rheum. 32 (Suppl.):B167, 1989.

126. Amento, E. P., Bhan, A. K., McCullagh, K. G., and Krane, S. M.: Influences of γ-interferon on synovial fibroblast-like cells. Ia induction and inhibition of collagen synthesis. J. Clin. Invest. 76:8378, 1985.

127. Fine, A., Poliks, C. F., Donahye, L. P., Smith, B. D., and Goldstein, R. H.: The differential effect of prostaglandin E2 on transforming growth factor-β and insulin-induced collagen formation in lung fibroblasts. J. Biol. Chem. 264:16988, 1989.

128. Rennard, S. I., Stier, L. E., and Crystal, R. G.: Intracellular degradation of newly synthesized collagen. J. Invest. Dermatol. 79:77s, 1982.

129. Roskowski, R. J., Sheehy, J., and Cutroneo, K. R.: Glucocorticoid-mediated selective reduction of functioning collagen messenger ribonucleic acid. Arch. Biochem. Biophys. 210:74, 1981.

130. Oikarinen, J., and Ryhanen, L.: Cortisol decreases the concentration of translatable type-I procollagen mRNA species in the developing chick-embryo calvaria. Biochem. J. 198:519, 1981.

131. Kream, B. E., Rowe, D. W., Gworek, S. C., and Raisz, L. G.: Parathyroid hormone alters collagen synthesis and procollagen mRNA levels in fetal rat calvaria. Proc. Natl. Acad. Sci. U.S.A. 77:5654, 1980.

132. Oikarinen, H., Oikarinen, A. I., Tan, E. M., Abergel, R. P., Meeker, C. A., Chu, M. L., Prockop, D. J., and Uitto, J.: Modulation of procollagen gene expression by retinoids. Inhibition of collagen production by retinoic acid accompanied by reduced type I procollagen messenger ribonucleic acid levels in human skin fibroblast cultures. J. Clin. Invest. 75:1545, 1985.

133. Sasaki, T., Majamaa, K., and Uitto, J.: Reduction of collagen production in keloid fibroblast cultures by ethyl-3, 4-dihydroxybenzoite: Inhibition of prolyl hydroxylase activity as a mechanism of action. J. Biol. Chem. 262:9397, 1987.

134. Riley, D. J., Kerr, J. S., Berg, R. A., Ianni, B. D., Pietra, G. G., Edelman, N. H., and Prockop, D. H.: Prevention of bleomycin-induced pulmonary fibrosis in the hamster by cis-4-hydroxy-L-proline. Am. Rev. Respir. Dis. 123:388, 1981.

135. Bell, E., Ivarsson, B., and Merrill, C.: Production of tissue-like structure by contraction of collagen lattices by human fibroblasts of different proliferative potential. Proc. Natl. Acad. Sci. U.S.A. 76:1274, 1979.

136. Okada, Y., Tsuchiya, H., Shimizu, H., Tomita, K., Nakanishi, I., Sato, H., Seiki, M., Yamashita, K., and Hayakawa, T.: Induction and

stimulation of 92-kDa gelatinase/type IV collagenase production in osteosarcoma and fibrosarcoma cell lines by tumor necrosis factor-α. Biochem. Biophys. Res. Commun. 171:610, 1990.

137. Conca, W., Kaplan, P. B., and Krane, S. M.: Increases in levels of procollagenase messenger RNA in cultured fibroblasts induced by human recombinant interleukin 1B or serum follow c-*jun* expression and are dependent on new protein synthesis. J. Clin. Invest. 83:1753, 1989.

138. Dayer, J.-M., Beutler, B., and Cerami, A.: Cachectin/tumor necrosis factor stimulates collagenase and prostaglandin E_2 production by human synovial cells and dermal fibroblasts. J. Exp. Med. 162:2163, 1985.

139. McDonnell, S. E., Kerr, L. D., and Matrisian, L. M.: Epidermal growth factor stimulation of stromelysin mRNA in rat fibroblasts requires induction of proto-oncogenes c-*fos* and c-*jun* and activation of protein kinase C. Mol. Cell. Biol. 10:4284, 1990.

140. Lotz, M., and Guerne, P. A.: Interleukin-6 induces the synthesis of tissue inhibitor of metalloproteinases-1/erythroid potentiating activity (TIMP-1/EPA). J. Biol. Chem. 266:2017, 1991.

141. Werb, Z., Tremble, P. M., Behrendtsen, O., Crowley, E., and Damsky, C. H.: Signal transduction through the fibronectin receptor induces collagenase and stromelysin gene expression. J. Cell Biol. 109:877, 1989.

142. Werb, Z.: Biochemical actions of glucocorticoids on macrophages in culture. J. Exp. Med. 147:1695, 1978.

143. Bauer, E. A., Seltzer, J. L., and Eisen, A. Z.: Retinoic acid inhibition of collagenase and gelatinase expression in human skin fibroblast cultures. Evidence for a dual mechanism. J. Invest. Dermatol. 81:162, 1983.

144. Greenwald, R. A., Golub, L. M., Lavietes, B., Ramamurthy, N. S., Gruber, B., Laskin, R. S., and McNamara, R. F.: Tetracyclines inhibit human synovial collagenase *in vivo* and *in vitro*. J. Rheumatol. 14:28, 1987.

145. Piguet, P. F., Grau, G. E., and Vassali, P.: Subcutaneous perfusion of tumor necrosis factor induces local proliferation of fibroblasts, capillaries and epidermal cells, or massive tissue necrosis. Am. J. Pathol. 136:103, 1990.

146. Lynch, S. E., Colvin, R. B., and Antoniades, H. N.: Growth factors in wound healing: Single and synergistic effects on partial thickness porcine skin wounds. J. Clin. Invest. 84:640, 1989.

147. Pierce, G. F., Mustoe, T. A., Lingellbach, J., Masakowski, V. U., Griffin, G. L., Senior, R. M., and Duel, T. F.: Platelet-derived growth factor and transforming growth factor-β enhance tissue repair activities by unique mechanisms. J. Cell. Biol. 109:429, 1990.

148. Goldring, S. R., Stephenson, M. L., Downie, E., Krane, S. M., and Korn, J. H.: Heterogeneity in hormone responses and patterns of collagen synthesis in cloned dermal fibroblasts. J. Clin. Invest. 85:798, 1990.

Section III
General Evaluation of the Patient

Chapter 21

Clement J. Michet
Gene G. Hunder

Examination of the Joints

HISTORY IN THE PATIENT WITH MUSCULOSKELETAL DISEASE

A detailed description of symptoms related to the musculoskeletal system provides much of the information necessary to making a diagnosis. The goal of the interview is to understand precisely what the patient means by what is said about the symptoms. In obtaining a history of the patient's illness, the physician must probe for details of the sequence and severity of symptoms and patterns of progression, exacerbation, or remission. The effects of the previous therapy, associated diseases, and stress must be elucidated. The functional impact of the disease on the patient must be defined.

The effects of current or previous therapy on the course of the illness are important. Frequently, these are not volunteered by the patient. Assessment of compliance is extremely important; even an ideal therapeutic regimen will fail if the patient does not comply with the outlined program.

The patient's behavior usually provides clues to the nature of the illness and the patient's response to it. It is important to determine whether the patient is reacting appropriately to an illness or is overly concerned or has ignored the joint symptoms. The patient's understanding of the illness affects the response to it.

Pain

Pain is the complaint that most commonly brings the patient with musculoskeletal disease to the physician. Pain is a complex, subjective sensation that is often difficult to define, explain, or measure. It has different meanings to different people and even to the same person at different times. Response to pain is affected by the patient's current emotional status as well as previous experiences, including observations of others in pain.

Pain must be localized anatomically. If the pain is in a joint, an articular disorder is likely to be present. Pain between joints may suggest bone or muscle disease or referred pain. Pain in bursal areas, fascial planes, or along tendons, ligaments, or nerve distributions suggests disease in these structures. Pain arising from deeper structures is often less focal than pain originating from superficial tissues. Pain in small joints of the hands or feet tends to be more accurately localized than pain in larger, more proximal joints such as the shoulder, hip, or spine. Pain from the hip joint, for example, may be felt in the groin, buttock, or over the greater trochanter or referred to the anterior portion of the thigh or knee. When pain is diffuse, variable, poorly described, or unrelated to anatomic structures, a psychological problem or fibromyalgia may be suspected.

Although variable from one patient to another, the character of the pain often helps in understanding the patient's illness. For example, "aching" in a joint area suggests an arthritic disorder, whereas "burning" or "prickling" in an extremity may indicate a neuropathy. An "intolerable" or "excruciating" pain in a patient who otherwise is able to carry out normal activities suggests that emotional factors may be amplifying symptoms.

Presence or absence of pain at rest usually helps the evaluation. Joint pain present both at rest and with movement is more suggestive of an inflammatory process, whereas pain mainly or only during motion often indicates a mechanical disorder such as degenerative arthritis or traumatic arthritis. However, many patients with more advanced degenerative joint disease also have pain at night.

Swelling

An important finding in rheumatic diseases is swelling. Patients vary in their perception of swelling and ability to describe it. The interviewer needs to determine where and when the swelling occurs; it is helpful to learn whether the swelling is visible to others. Description of the exact location of the swelling helps in understanding whether the swelling conforms to an anatomically discrete area such as a particular joint, bursa, or other specific extra-articular areas. An obese person may interpret normal collections of adipose tissue over the medial aspects of the elbow or knee and lateral aspect of the ankle as swellings.

Information about the onset, persistence, and influencing factors helps define the nature of the swelling. Discomfort with use of the swollen part may indicate synovitis or bursitis because of tension on these tissues during motion of a joint. However, when inflamed tissues are not put under stress during joint movement, pain is minimal; for example, movement of the knee is generally painless in cases of prepatellar bursitis. Swelling in a confined area such as a synovial sac or bursa is most painful when it has developed acutely. In such instances, even light palpation may be intolerable. In chronic swelling when the synovial sac has stretched or when the distention has developed gradually, pain is generally less severe.

Limitation of Motion

Patients with rheumatic disorders frequently complain of limitation of motion. Determination of the extent of disability resulting from lack of motion is important. The length of time restrictions of motion have been present can be helpful in predicting reversibility of the disability. It is helpful also to know whether the limitation of motion began abruptly, as with a tendon rupture or onset of a psychogenic episode, or gradually, as in slowly progressive inflammatory disease.

Stiffness

Stiffness is a word that has different meanings to different patients. Some equate it with pain or fatigue; others equate it with soreness, weakness, or restrictions of movement; and still others use the term without being able to tell clearly what they feel. Most rheumatologists define stiffness as discomfort perceived by the patient attempting to move joints after a period of inactivity. When it occurs, stiffness or "gelling" usually develops after inactivity of one or more hours. Mild stiffness may resolve within a few minutes. When severe, as in rheumatoid arthritis or polymyalgia rheumatica, the stiffness may improve only over one to several hours.

Morning stiffness can be a prodromal symptom of arthritis, and it is a criterion of the American Rheumatism Association for the diagnosis of rheumatoid arthritis (see Chapter 53). It should be differentiated from the discomfort associated with movement of a mechanically damaged joint. Morning stiffness associated with noninflammatory joint diseases is almost always of short duration, usually less than one-half hour, and of less severity than stiffness of inflammatory joint disease. In addition, in mechanical, degenerative, or other destructive joint disease, the degree of stiffness is related to the extent of overuse of the damaged joint and responds usually within a few days to adequate limitation of the use of the affected joint. In degenerative joint disease, stiffness may be more noticeable during the day after resting an hour or more than it is in the morning.

The absence of stiffness does not exclude the possibility of the presence of systemic inflammatory rheumatic diseases such as rheumatoid arthritis, but its absence is uncommon. Stiffness from neurologic disorders of the Parkinsonism type, without a recognized inflammatory basis, also occurs and sometimes is conspicuous, although the "limbering up" component is lacking.

Weakness

When present, a loss of motor power or muscular strength is nearly always objectively demonstrated during the examination, at least in relation to what a patient was formerly able to do. True weakness can be noted only when muscles are actively being used. In musculoskeletal disorders, weakness is usually persistent rather than intermittent. Muscle weakness as a result of inflammatory myopathies occurs typically in proximal portions of the extremities, whereas weakness caused by most neuropathies is found in distal or peripheral parts.

Fatigue

A common and important complaint of many patients with musculoskeletal disease, *fatigue* is, nonetheless, an imprecise term. It can be defined as an inclination to rest even though pain and weakness are not limiting factors. It implies exhaustion and depletion of energy. Fatigue is a normal phenomenon after variable degrees of activity but resolves after rest. In rheumatic diseases, fatigue may be prominent even when the patient has not been active physically. If the arthritis improves, fatigue tends to lessen. In the absence of organic disease, anxiety and muscular tension or related emotional states are prominent factors in producing chronic fatigue. Patients with an inflammatory arthritis may complain of weakness when they are experiencing stiffness. The differentiation of fatigue from stiffness and weakness may be facilitated by remembering that stiffness is a discomfort during movement and weakness is an inability to move normally against resistance. Fatigue may be sensed when the patient is resting and is an aversion to activity.

SYSTEMATIC METHOD OF EXAMINATION

As with the general physical examination, a systematic method of examining joints is the quickest and easiest way of obtaining a thorough assessment of the status of the joint. Many rheumatologists begin with the joints of the upper extremities and proceed to the joints of the trunk and lower extremity, but each examiner should establish his or her own routine.[1, 2] Gentle handling of tender and painful joints will enhance cooperation by the patient and allow an accurate evaluation of the joints.

Important Physical Signs of Arthritis

The general aim of the examination of the joints is to detect abnormalities in structure and function. Some of the more common signs of articular disease are swelling, tenderness, limitation of motion, and instability.

Swelling. Swelling about a joint may be caused by intra-articular effusion; synovial thickening; periarticular soft tissue inflammation, such as bursitis or tendinitis; bony enlargement; or extra-articular fat pads. All these causes need to be differentiated from each other. Familiarity with the anatomic configuration of the synovial membrane in various joints aids in differentiating soft tissue swelling due to synovitis (articular effusion or synovial thickening) from swelling of periarticular tissues. The presence of an effusion of a joint is often visible or palpable as bulging of the joint capsule. The presence of palpable fluid in a joint in the absence of immediately preceding trauma usually indicates synovitis. The normal synovial membrane is too thin to palpate, whereas the thickened synovial membrane in rheumatoid arthritis may have a "doughy" or "boggy" consistency. In some joints the extent of the synovial cavity can be delineated on physical examination by compressing the fluid into one of the extreme limits of synovial reflection. The edge of the resulting bulge may thus be palpated more easily. If this palpable edge is within the anatomic confines of the synovial membrane and disappears on release of the compression, the distention may be regarded as representing synovial effusion; if it persists, it is an indication of a thickened synovial membrane. Reliable differentiation between synovial membrane thickening and effusion is not always possible by physical examination. Occasional intrasynovial loose bodies or fibrin clots may be palpated.

Localization of tenderness by palpation should help determine whether the reaction is intra-articular or in a periarticular structure such as a fat pad, tendon attachments, ligaments, bursae, muscles, or skin. It is also useful to palpate noninvolved structures to help assess the significance of tenderness.

Limitation of Motion. Because limitation of motion is a common manifestation of articular disease, it is important to know the normal type and range of motion of each joint to detect restriction resulting from abnormalities of the joint or adjacent structures. Comparison of an unaffected joint of the opposite extremity helps evaluate individual variations. In patients with joint disease, passive range of motion is often greater than active motion, providing the patient is relaxed during the examination. This may be due to pain, weakness, or the state of the articular or periarticular structures. Stressing passive joint motion at the extremes of flexion and extension is an alternative method for determining joint tenderness.

Crepitation. A palpable or audible grating or crunching sensation produced by motion, crepitation may or may not be accompanied by discomfort. Crepitation occurs when roughened articular or extra-articular surfaces are rubbed together either by active motion or by manual compression. Fine crepitation is often palpable over joints involved by chronic inflammatory arthritis and usually indicates roughening of the opposing cartilage surfaces as a result of erosion or the presence of granulation tissue. Coarse crepitation is also due to irregularity of the cartilage surfaces caused by either inflammatory or noninflammatory arthritis. Bone-on-bone crepitus produces a higher-frequency palpable and audible "squeak." Crepitation from within the joints should be differentiated from cracking sounds caused by the slipping of ligaments or tendons over bony surfaces during motion. The latter are usually less significant to the diagnosis of joint disease and may be heard over many normal joints. In scleroderma, a peculiar coarse, creaking, leathery crepitation may be palpable or audible about various joints and tendon sheaths.

Deformity. Deformity is malalignment of the joint and may occur as a bony enlargement, articular subluxation, contracture, or ankylosis in abnormal positions. Deformed joints do not function normally, usually restrict activities, and may be associated with pain when put under stressful use.

Instability. Joint instability is present when the joint has greater than normal movement in any plane. *Subluxation* is defined as a partial displacement of the articular surfaces with some persistent joint surface-to-surface contact, whereas a dislocated joint has lost all cartilage surface contact. Instability is best determined by supporting the joint between the examiner's two hands and stressing the adjacent bones in directions in which the normal joint does not move.

Other Aspects of Examination

Muscle testing is discussed in Chapter 24. Examination of the cervical spine and low back is discussed in Chapters 25 and 27, respectively.

Recording the Joint Examination

A permanent record of examination of the joints is important in determining the status and following

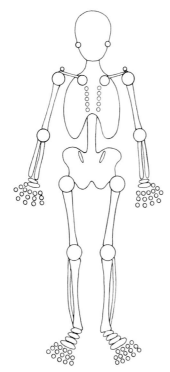

Figure 21–1. Skeleton diagram for recording joint examination findings. (From Polley, H. F., and Hunder, G. G.: Rheumatologic Interviewing and Physical Examination of the Joints. Philadelphia, W. B. Saunders Company, 1978.)

the progress of arthritic diseases. A variety of recording methods have been described. To avoid a cumbersome chart, suitable abbreviations for joints can be used, such as *TM* for temporomandibular or *SC* for sternoclavicular. In recording the degree of swelling (S), tenderness (T), and limitation of motion (L) of a joint, a quantitative estimate of gradation based on a system of grades from 0 (normal) to 4 (highly abnormal) is convenient. The abbreviation *S* refers to synovial effusion, thickening, or a combination of these. *T*, tenderness of structures other than joints, should be specifically described. In the case of limitation of motion, *L*, grade 1 may be used to indicate about 25 percent loss of motion; grade 2, about 50 percent loss; grade 3, about 75 percent loss; and grade 4, 100 percent loss, or ankylosis. In most instances, when more accuracy is desired, it is preferable to record degrees of motion in one or more joints using a goniometer. A table can be constructed with a column for each S, T, and L and the findings recorded for each joint.

A still more abbreviated, narrative form of recording the joint examination may be used, especially when a limited number of joints are involved. An example is as follows: Lt Sh S_0, T_2, L_1; Rt Wr S_2, T_2, L_1; Lt-MCP$_{2 \text{ through } 5}$ S_1, T_0, L_1; Rt Knee S_1 (bulge), T_0, L_1 (lacks 10 degrees of extension).

Alternative methods include the use of a schematic skeleton with marked articulations that may be used to record the status of individual joints (Fig. 21–1); determination of the total number of tender or swollen joints, or both, and the use of this number as a joint count or joint index; measurement of the size of joints by use of a tape measure or jeweler's rings; determination of the degree of warmth by use of thermography; and measurement of the amount of tenderness by use of a dolorimeter. Grip strength can be measured by asking a patient to squeeze a partially inflated (20 mm Hg) sphygmomanometer cuff. The use of joints can be assessed by determining the speed and the ability to perform other specified coordinated functions.

There is an inherent tendency toward variability in making any of these clinical assessments. For observations such as joint tenderness or grip strength, interobserver variation is often greater than intraobserver differences.[3, 4] However, there may also be significant intraobserver variation in observing the same patient, even over a short interval. Furthermore, biologic factors also contribute to variability, such as circadian changes in joint size and grip strength among rheumatoid patients observed over a 24-hour interval.[5] Not all physical findings in examination of one joint are equally reliable, and there may be considerable interobserver variation. For instance, assessment of bony swelling and tenderness of the tibiofemoral joint has less observer variation than do signs of patellofemoral pathology during examination of osteoarthritic knees.[6]

EXAMINATION OF SPECIFIC JOINTS

Temporomandibular Joint

The temporomandibular joint is formed by the condyle of the mandible and the fossa of the temporal bone just anterior to the external auditory canal. It is uncommon for this joint to be visibly swollen. The joint is palpated by placing a finger just anterior to the external auditory canal and asking the patient to open and close the mouth and to move the mandible from side to side. Because of normal differences in soft tissue thickness, the presence of synovial thickness or swelling of minimal or moderate degree can be detected most easily if the synovitis is unilateral or asymmetric. Vertical movement of the temporomandibular joint can be measured by determining the space between the upper and lower incisor teeth with the patient's mouth open maximally. This distance is normally 3 to 6 cm. Lateral movement can be determined by using incisor teeth as landmarks.

Many forms of arthritis affect the temporomandibular joints. Juvenile rheumatoid arthritis commonly affects these joints and may produce arrest of bone growth of the mandible with resultant micrognathia. Audible or palpable crepitus or clicking occur frequently in those patients without evidence of severe arthritis.

Cricoarytenoid Joint

The paired cricoarytenoid joints are formed by the articulation of the base of the small pyramidal arytenoid cartilage and the upper posterolateral border of the cricoid cartilage. The vocal ligaments (cords) are attached to the arytenoid cartilages. The cricoarytenoid joints are normally very mobile diarthrodial joints that move both medially and laterally and rotate during opening and closing of the vocal cords.

Examination of these joints is performed by direct or indirect laryngoscopy. Erythema, swelling, and lack of mobility during phonation may result from inflammation of the joints.

The cricoarytenoid joints may be affected in rheumatoid arthritis, trauma, and infection. Involvement in rheumatoid arthritis is more common than clinically apparent. Early symptoms include a sense of fullness or discomfort in the throat that is worse on speaking or swallowing. Hoarseness may occur, and significant airway obstruction has been reported.

Sternoclavicular, Manubriosternal, and Sternocostal Joints

The medial ends of the clavicles articulate on each side of the sternum at its upper end to form the sternoclavicular joints. The articulations of the first ribs and the sternum (sternocostal joints) are immediately caudad. The articulation of the manubrium and body of the sternum is at the level of the attachment of the second costal cartilage to the sternum. The third through seventh sternocostal joints articulate distally along the lateral borders of the sternum. The sternoclavicular joints are the only articulations in this group that are always diarthrodial in form. The others may be amphiarthroses or synchondroses. The sternoclavicular joints are the only true points of articulation of the shoulder girdle with the trunk. These joints lie beneath the skin; therefore, any synovitis is visible and easily palpated. Movement of these joints is slight and cannot be measured accurately.

Involvement of the sternoclavicular joints is common in ankylosing spondylitis, rheumatoid arthritis, and degenerative arthritis but is frequently overlooked. The sternoclavicular joint also may be the site of septic arthritis, especially in drug abusers. Tenderness of the manubriosternal or costosternal joints is much more frequent than actual swelling. Many older patients with no systemic rheumatic disorder may be found to have tender sternocostal joints or costal cartilages (costochondritis). Actual swelling of the upper costal cartilages or areas of the costochondral junctions (Tietze's syndrome) is uncommon.

Acromioclavicular Joint

The acromioclavicular joint is formed by the lateral end of the clavicle and medial margin of the acromion process of the scapula. Bony enlargement of this joint is often seen in middle-aged or older persons, but soft tissue swelling is not usually visible or palpable. Local tenderness, or pain with adduction of the arm across the front of the chest, helps pinpoint the involvement in this joint. Arthritis of the acromioclavicular joint is usually secondary to trauma leading to degenerative disease. It is not usually severely affected in rheumatoid arthritis. Movement occurs at this joint during shoulder motion, but actual measurements need not be made in the routine joint examination.

Shoulder

See Chapter 26.

Elbow

The elbow joint (see also Chapter 105) is composed of three bony articulations. The principal one is the humeroulnar joint, which is a hinge joint. The radiohumeral and proximal radioulnar articulations allow rotation of the forearm.

To examine the elbow joint, the examiner's thumb is placed between the lateral epicondyle and the olecranon process in the lateral paraolecranon groove, and one or two fingers are placed in the corresponding groove medial to the olecranon (Fig. 21–2). The elbow should be relaxed and moved passively through flexion, extension, and rotation.

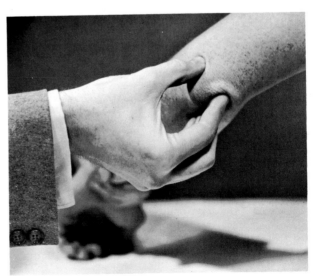

Figure 21–2. Palpation of the paraolecranon grooves of the elbow joint. (From Polley, H. F., and Hunder, G. G.: Rheumatologic Interviewing and Physical Examination of the Joints. Philadelphia, W. B. Saunders Company, 1978.)

Limitation of motion and crepitus may thus be noted. Synovial swelling is most easily palpated as it bulges under the examiner's thumb when the elbow is passively extended fully. Synovial membrane can sometimes be palpated over the posterior aspect of the joint between the olecranon process and distal humerus. Synovitis is commonly associated with limitation of extension of the joint.

The olecranon bursa overlies the olecranon process of the ulna. Olecranon bursitis is common after repeated or chronic local trauma or occurs in rheumatic diseases such as rheumatoid arthritis and tophaceous gout.

The medial and lateral epicondyles of the humerus and tendinous attachments are common sites of tenderness (tennis or golfer's elbow, lateral or medial epicondylitis, respectively).

Muscle function of the elbow can be assessed by testing flexion and extension. The prime movers of flexion are the biceps brachii (C5 and 6), brachialis (C5 and 6), and brachioradialis (C5 and 6) muscles.* The prime mover of extension is the triceps brachii muscle (C7 and 8).

Wrist and Carpal Joints

The wrist is a complex joint (see also Chapter 104). The true wrist, or radiocarpal articulation, is formed proximally by the distal end of the radius and the articular disc and distally by a row of three of the carpal bones, the scaphoid, the lunate, and the triangular. The distal radioulnar joint is usually separated from the wrist joint. The mid-carpal joints are formed by the junction of the proximal and distal rows of the carpal bones, which are, from the radial to the ulnar side, the trapezium, trapezoid, capitate, and hamate. The mid-carpal and carpometacarpal articular cavities often communicate.

The long flexor tendons of the muscles of the forearm cross the front of the wrist and are enclosed in a flexor tendon sheath under the flexor retinaculum (transverse carpal ligament). The flexor retinaculum and the underlying carpal bones form the carpal tunnel. The median nerve also runs through the carpal tunnel superficial to the flexor tendons. The extensor tendons of the forearm pass under the extensor retinaculum (dorsal carpal ligament) enclosed in a synovial sheath.

The palmar aponeurosis (fascia) spreads out into the palm from the flexor retinaculum. In Dupuytren's contracture, the palmar aponeurosis becomes thickened and contracted, drawing one or more fingers into flexion at the metacarpophalangeal joint. The fourth finger is usually affected earliest, then the fifth and the third. The first two digits are rarely involved. The skin frequently feels adherent to the palmar fascia.

---

*Level of spinal cord innervation of specific muscles is shown in parentheses following each muscle discussed throughout the chapter.

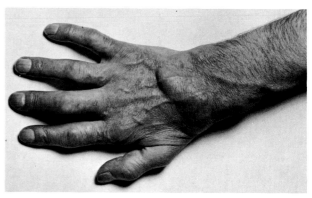

Figure 21–3. Localized swelling of the dorsal wrist tenosynovium in a patient with rheumatoid arthritis. (From Polley, H. F., and Hunder, G. G.: Rheumatologic Interviewing and Physical Examination of the Joints. Philadelphia, W. B. Saunders Company, 1978.)

A ganglion is a cystic enlargement arising from a joint capsule; it characteristically occurs on the dorsum of the wrist between the tendons of the common extensors of the digits and the radial extensors at the base of the second metacarpal bone.

Subluxation of the ulna occurs secondary to chronic inflammatory arthritis. The subluxed ulna appears as a prominence on the dorsolateral wrist and presses against the extensor digitorum communis tendons, especially those of the fourth and fifth digits. Attrition may result in rupture of these tendons. The long extensor tendon of the thumb is also particularly vulnerable to wear and fraying as a result of its course over bony prominences.

Swelling of the wrist may be due to involvement of the sheaths of the tendons crossing the wrist or the wrist joint itself, or both. When swelling is due to tenosynovitis, the outpouching tends to be more localized and is altered by flexing and extending the fingers (Fig. 21–3). Articular swelling is more diffuse and protrudes anteriorly and posteriorly from under the tendons.

Synovitis of the wrist joint is detected most reliably by palpating over the dorsal surface (Fig. 21–4). Because of structures overlying both the dorsal and the palmar aspects of the wrist, accurate localization of the margins of the synovial membrane may be difficult. To examine the wrist, the physician should palpate or pinch this joint gently between the thumbs and fingers to detect abnormalities of bony and soft tissue structures. Swelling in hypertrophic osteoarthropathy, if present, extends proximal to the wrist and does not have the typical consistency of either synovial fluid swelling or pitting edema. In addition, clubbing may be present.

Tenosynovitis and trigger finger can be detected by palpating crepitus or nodules along the tendons in the palm while the patient slowly flexes and extends the fingers. Tendon nodules causing triggering usually occur at the level of the metacarpal heads, where a thickening of the deep fascia forms the

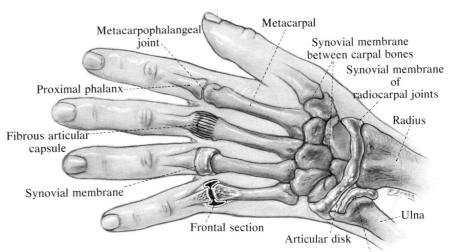

Figure 21–4. Illustration of the relationship of the synovial membranes of the wrist and carpal and metacarpal joints to the surrounding bony structures. (From Polley, H. F., and Hunder, G. G.: Rheumatologic Interviewing and Physical Examination of the Joints. Philadelphia, W. B. Saunders Company, 1978.)

proximal annular ligament in the sheath of the flexor tendons (proximal pulley).

Movements of the wrist include palmar flexion (flexion), dorsiflexion (extension), radial deviation, ulnar deviation, and circumduction. Pronation and supination of the hand and forearm occur primarily at the proximal and distal radioulnar joints. The only carpometacarpal joint that moves to any degree is the carpometacarpal joint of the thumb, which possesses the movements of a sellar joint. Crepitus at this joint is common in degenerative arthritis.

The wrist can normally be extended to about 70 degrees and flexed to 80 or 90 degrees. Ulnar deviation averages 50 degrees and radial deviation 20 to 30 degrees. Loss of dorsiflexion is the most incapacitating functional impairment of wrist motion.

Stenosing tenosynovitis at the radial styloid process (de Quervain's tenosynovitis) characteristically involves the long abductor and short extensor tendons of the thumb. Tenderness near the radial styloid process can be localized to these tendons by having the patient make a fist with the thumb in the palm of his or her hand. The examiner then moves the patient's wrist into ulnar deviation. The development of severe pain over the radial styloid is a positive Finkelstein's test and is caused by stretching the thumb tendons in the stenosed sheath.

Carpal tunnel syndrome results from pressure on the median nerve in the carpal tunnel and is discussed in detail in Chapter 101.

Muscle function of the wrist can be measured by testing flexion and extension as well as supination and pronation of the forearm. Prime movers in wrist flexion are the flexor carpi radialis (C6 and 7) and flexor carpi ulnaris (C8 and T1) muscles. Each of these two muscles can be tested separately. This can be accomplished if the examiner provides resistance to flexion at the base of the second metacarpal bone in the direction of extension and ulnar deviation in the case of the flexor carpi radialis and resistance at the base of the fifth metacarpal in the direction of

extension and radial deviation in the case of the flexor carpi ulnaris. The prime extensions of the wrist are the extensor carpi radialis longus (C6 and 7), extensor carpi radialis brevis (C6 and 7), and extensor carpi ulnaris (C7 and 8) muscles. The radial and ulnar extensor muscles can also be tested separately. Prime movers in supination of the forearm are the biceps brachii (C5 and 6) and supinator (C6). Prime movers in pronation are the pronator teres (C6 and 7) and pronator quadratus (C8 and T1).

Metacarpophalangeal, Proximal, and Distal Interphalangeal Joints

The metacarpophalangeal joints are hinge joints. Lateral collateral ligaments that are loose in extension tighten in flexion, thereby preventing lateral movement of the digits. The extensor tendons that cross the dorsum of each joint strengthen the articular capsule. When the extensor tendon of the digit reaches the distal end of the metacarpal head, it is joined by fibers of the interossei and lumbricales and expands over the entire dorsum of the metacarpophalangeal joint and onto the dorsum of the adjacent phalanx. This expansion of the extensor mechanism is known as the extensor hood.

The proximal and distal interphalangeal joints are also hinge joints. The ligaments of the interphalangeal joints resemble those of the metacarpophalangeal joints. When the fingers are flexed, the bases of the proximal phalanges slide toward the palmar side of the heads of the metacarpal bones. The metacarpal heads form the rounded prominences of the knuckle, with the metacarpal joint spaces lying about 1 cm distal to the apices of the prominences.

The skin on the palmar surface of the hand is relatively thick and covers a fat pad between it and the metacarpophalangeal joint. This makes palpation of the palmar surface of the joint more difficult than the dorsal surfaces.

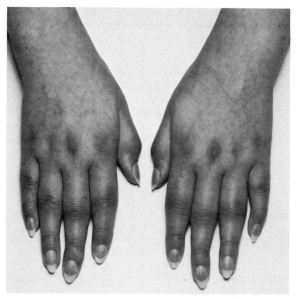

Figure 21–5. Symmetric proximal interphalangeal joint swelling in a patient with systemic lupus erythematosus.

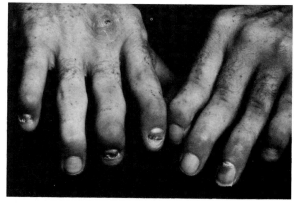

Figure 21–6. Swan-neck deformities in a patient with chronic Reiter's syndrome.

Swelling of the fingers may result from articular or periarticular causes. Synovial swelling produces (1) symmetric enlargement of a joint itself, whereas extra-articular swelling may be diffuse, extending beyond the joints, or (2) asymmetric enlargement, involving only one side of the digit or joint (Fig. 21–5). Chronic swelling and distension of the metacarpophalangeal joints tend to produce stretching and laxity of the articular capsule and ligaments. This laxity, combined with muscle imbalance and other forces, results in the extensor tendons of the digits slipping off the metacarpal heads to the ulnar sides of the joints. The abnormal pull of the displaced tendons is one of the factors that causes ulnar deviation of the fingers in chronic inflammatory arthritis.

"Swan-neck" deformity describes the appearance of a finger in which there is a flexion contracture of the metacarpophalangeal joint, hyperextension of the proximal interphalangeal joint, and flexion of the distal interphalangeal joint. These changes are produced by contraction of the interossei and other muscles that flex the metacarpophalangeal joints and extend the proximal interphalangeal joints. This deformity is characteristic of rheumatoid arthritis but may be seen in other chronic arthritides such as lupus erythematosus (Fig. 21–6).

The term *boutonnière deformity* is used to describe a finger with a flexion contracture of the proximal interphalangeal joint associated with hyperextension of the distal interphalangeal joint. The deformity is relatively common in rheumatoid arthritis and results when the central slip of the extensor tendon of the proximal interphalangeal joint becomes detached from the base of the middle phalanx, allowing palmar dislocation of the lateral bands. The dislocated bands cross the fulcrum of the joint and then act as flexors instead of extensors of the joint.

Another abnormality is "telescoping" or shortening of the digits produced by resorption of the ends of the phalanges secondary to destructive arthropathy. Shortening of the fingers is associated with wrinkling of the skin over involved joints and also is called *opera-glass hand* or *la main en lorgnette*. Bony hypertrophic or osteophytic articular nodules on the distal interphalangeal joints are called *Heberden's nodes*, and when they are located on the proximal interphalangeal joints are called *Bouchard's nodes*.

The metacarpophalangeal joints are palpated on the dorsal aspect of the metacarpal heads on each side of the extensor tendons (Fig. 21–7), with the proximal phalanges flexed 20 to 30 degrees. Small amounts of swelling in one or more joints can best be detected by comparing the joints in question with others. Synovitis of metacarpophalangeal joints is

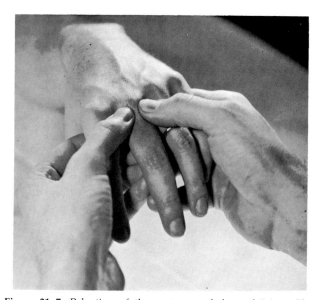

Figure 21–7. Palpation of the metacarpophalangeal joints. The examiner's thumbs palpate the dorsal aspect of the joint while the index fingers palpate the volar aspect of the metacarpal head. (From Polley, H. F., and Hunder, G. G.: Rheumatologic Interviewing and Physical Examination of the Joints. Philadelphia, W. B. Saunders Company, 1978.)

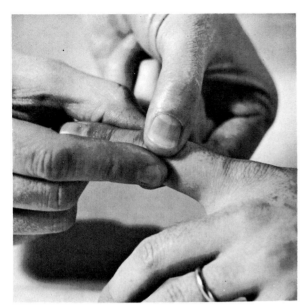

Figure 21–8. Palpation of the proximal interphalangeal joint. Anteroposterior compression of the joint by the examiner's thumb and index finger while the other thumb and index finger palpate for medial and lateral synovial distention. (From Polley, H. F., and Hunder, G. G.: Rheumatologic Interviewing and Physical Examination of the Joints. Philadelphia, W. B. Saunders Company, 1978.)

often associated with lateral compression tenderness, which can be elicited by gently squeezing the patient's hand at the level of the joints.

The proximal and distal interphalangeal joints are best examined by palpating gently over the lateral and medial aspects of the joint where the flexor and extensor tendons do not interfere with assessment of the synovial membrane. Alternatively, the joint can be compressed anteroposteriorly by the thumb and index finger of one of the examiner's hands while the other thumb and index finger palpate for synovial distention medially and laterally (Fig. 21–8).

The presence of clubbing of the fingernails can be detected by repeated gentle palpation of the distal nail edge with one hand while using the other hand to palpate the proximal edge of the nail for elevation from the nail bed. Alternatively, the examiner can palpate the proximal edge of the patient's nail with the tip of one or more fingers or thumbs pointing distally (same direction as the patient's fingers). When clubbing is present, the proximal edge of the nail "floats" in its bed.

A general assessment of the strength of the hands can be made when the patient makes a tight fist by gripping two or more of the examiner's fingers. A more accurate measure, which can be used in comparative studies, is obtained having the patient squeeze a partially inflated sphygmomanometer (at 20 mm Hg).

It is often helpful to test strength of the fingers separately. The prime movers of flexion of the second through fifth metacarpophalangeal joints are the dor-

sal and palmar interosseus muscles (C8 and T1). The lumbrical muscles (C6, 7, and 8) flex the metacarpophalangeal joints when the proximal phalangeal joints are extended. The flexors of the proximal interphalangeal joints are the flexor digitorum superficialis muscles (C7 and 8, T1), and the flexor of the distal interphalangeal joints is the flexor digitorum profundus muscle (C7 and 8, T1).

The prime extensors of the metacarpophalangeal joints and interphalangeal joints of the second through fifth fingers are the extensor digitorum communis (C6, 7, and 8), the extensor indicis proprius (C6, 7, and 8), and the extensor digiti minimi (C7) muscles. The interossei and lumbrical muscles simultaneously flex the metacarpophalangeal joints and extend the interphalangeal joints. The dorsal interosseus muscles (C8 and T1) and abductor digiti minimi (C8) abduct the fingers, whereas the palmar interosseus muscles adduct the fingers.

The thumb is moved by a number of muscles. Prime flexor of the first metacarpophalangeal joint is the flexor pollicus brevis muscle (C6, 7, and 8, T1). The prime flexor of the interphalangeal joint is the flexor pollicus longus muscle (C8 and T1). The metacarpophalangeal joint of the thumb is extended by the extensor pollicus brevis muscle, and the prime extensor of the interphalangeal joint is the extensor pollicus longus muscle (C6, 7, 8, and 9).

The prime abductors of the thumb are the abductor pollicis longus (C6 and 7) and the abductor pollicis brevis (C6 and 7) muscles. Motion takes place primarily at the carpometacarpal joint. The prime mover in thumb adduction is the adductor pollicis muscle (C8 and T1). Motion takes place primarily at the carpophalangeal joint. The prime movers in opposition of the thumb and fifth fingers are the opponens pollicis muscles (C6 and 7) and opponens digiti minimi muscle (C8 and T1).

Hip

The hip joint is a spheroidal or ball-and-socket joint consisting of the rounded head of the femur and the cup-shaped acetabulum (see also Chapter 108). Stability of the joint is ensured by the fibrocartilaginous rim of the glenoid labrum and the dense articular capsule and surrounding ligaments, including the iliofemoral, pubofemoral, and ischiocapsular ligaments that reinforce the capsule. The hip joint is also surrounded by powerful muscle groups. The primary hip flexor is the iliopsoas muscle assisted by the sartorius and the rectus femoris muscles. Hip adduction is accomplished by the three adductors, the longus, brevis, and magnus, plus the gracilis and pectineus muscles. The gluteus medius is the major hip abductor, whereas the gluteus maximus and hamstrings extend the hip. There are several clinically important bursae about the hip joint. Anteriorly, the iliopsoas bursa lies between the psoas muscle and the joint surface. The trochanteric bursa lies between the gluteus maximus muscle and the posterolateral greater trochanter, and the ischiogluteal bursa overlies the ischial tuberosity.

Examination of the hip begins by observing the patient's stance and gait. The patient should stand in front of the examiner so that the anterior iliac spines are visible. If pelvic tilt or obliquity is present, it may be related to a structural scoliosis, anatomic leg-length discrepancy, or hip disease. Hip contractures may result in abduction or adduction deformities. To compensate for an adduction contracture, the pelvis is tilted upward on the side of the contracture. This allows the legs to be parallel during walking and weight bearing. With a fixed abduction deformity, the pelvis becomes elevated on the normal side during standing or walking. This causes an apparent shortening of the normal leg and forces the patient to stand or walk on the toes of the normal side or to flex the knee on the abnormal leg.

Viewed from the rear, with the legs parallel, the patient with hip disease and an adducted hip contracture may have asymmetric gluteal folds due to pelvic tilt, with the diseased side elevated. In this situation, the patient is unable to stand with the foot of the involved leg flat on the floor. In abduction contracture, the findings are reversed; with both legs extended and parallel, the uninvolved side is elevated.

A hip flexion deformity commonly occurs in diseases of the hip but is often overlooked. Unilateral flexion of the hip in the standing position reduces weight bearing on the involved side and relaxes the joint capsule, causing less pain. This posture may be noted when observing the patient from the side. There is a hyperlordotic curve of the lumbar spine to compensate for lack of full hip extension.

The patient with possible hip disease should be observed walking. With a normal gait, the abductors of the weight-bearing leg contract to hold the pelvis level or elevate the non–weight-bearing side slightly. Two abnormalities of gait may be observed in hip disease. With a painful hip, the most common abnormality is the antalgic gait. In this gait, the person leans over the diseased hip during the phase of weight bearing on that hip, placing the body weight directly over the joint to avoid painful contraction of the hip abductors. Alternatively, a Trendelenburg gait may develop. Here, with weight bearing on the affected side, the pelvis drops and the trunk shifts to the normal side. Although the antalgic gait is said to be seen with painful hips and the Trendelenburg gait in conditions with weak hip abductors, neither gait is specific and either accompanies a painful hip. A mild Trendelenburg gait is seen commonly in normal persons.

The Trendelenburg test is a measure of the gluteus medius hip abductor weakness. The patient is asked to stand bearing weight only on the involved side. Normally, the abductors will hold the pelvis level or the nonsupported side slightly elevated. If the non–weight-bearing side drops, the test is positive for weakness of the weight-bearing gluteus medius. This test is nonspecific and may be observed in primary neurologic or muscle disorders or in a variety of hip diseases, leading to weakness of the abductors, including coxa vara, congenital dislocation, slipped capital femoral epiphysis, or femoral neck fracture.

In the supine position, the presence of a hip flexion contracture is suggested by persistence of lumbar lordosis and pelvic tilt masking the contracture by allowing the involved leg to remain in contact with the examination table. The Thomas test demonstrates the flexion contracture. In this test, the opposite hip is fully flexed to flatten the lumbar lordosis and fix the pelvis. The involved leg should then be extended toward the table as far as possible. The diseased hip's flexion contracture will become more obvious and can be estimated in degrees from full extension. While the patient is supine, measurement for leg length discrepancy is performed with the legs fully extended. To detect true leg length discrepancy, each leg is measured from the anterior superior iliac spine to the medial malleolus. A difference of 1 cm or less is unlikely to cause any abnormality of gait. An apparent leg-length discrepancy may result from pelvic tilt or abduction or adduction contractures of the hip.

The hip joint range of motion includes flexion, extension, abduction, adduction, internal and external rotation, and circumduction. The degree of flexion permitted varies with the manner in which it is assessed. When the knee is held flexed 90 degrees, the hip normally flexes to an angle of 120 degrees between the thigh and long axis of the body. If the knee is held in extension, the hamstrings limit the hip flexion to about 90 degrees. Abduction is measured with the patient still supine with the leg in an extended position perpendicular to the pelvis. Pelvic stabilization is achieved by placing one arm across the pelvis with the hand on the opposite anterior iliac spine. With the other hand, the examiner grasps the patient's ankle and abducts the leg until the pelvis is noted to begin moving. Normally, abduction is to approximately 45 degrees. The maneuver is repeated on the other side. The examiner may also stand at the foot of the table, grasp both ankles, and simultaneously abduct the legs. Differences between the two hips can be appreciated, and the intermalleolar distance is measured. Abduction is commonly limited in hip joint disease. Adduction is tested by grasping the ankle and raising the leg off the examination table by flexing the hip enough to allow the tested leg to cross over the opposite leg. Normal adduction is to about 20 to 30 degrees. Hip rotation may be tested with both hip and knee flexed to 90 degrees or with the leg extended.

Normal hip external rotation is to 45 degrees, and internal rotation is to 40 degrees. These figures vary somewhat in normal persons. There is also a difference in rotation between the flexed and extended hip. Owing to the increased stabilization of the joint by the surrounding ligaments in the extended position, rotation decreases with extension. To test hip rotation, the extended leg is grasped above the ankle and rotated externally and internally from the neutral position. Limitation of internal rotation of the hip is a sensitive indicator of hip joint disease.

Extension is tested with the patient in the prone position. Estimating actual hip joint extension can be difficult, because some of the apparent motion arises from hyperextension of the lumbar spine, pelvis rotation, motion of the buttock soft tissue, and flexion of the opposite hip. The pelvis and lumbar spine are partially immobilized by placing one arm across the posterior iliac crest and lower lumbar spine. The examiner places the other hand under the thigh with the knee flexed and hyperextends the thigh. Normal extension ranges up to 10 to 20 degrees. Limitation of extension is most often secondary to a hip flexion contracture.

The iliotibial band is a part of the fascia lata extending from the iliac crest, sacrum, and ischium over the greater trochanter to the lateral femoral condyle, tibial condyle, and fibular head and along the lateral intermuscular system, separating the hamstrings from the vastus lateralis. The tensor fascia lata may cause an audible snap as it slips over the greater trochanter if the weight-bearing leg moves from hip flexion and adduction to a neutral position, as in climbing stairs. Most commonly observed in young women, the "snapping" hip usually does not cause any significant degree of pain.

In patients complaining of lateral hip pain, the soft tissues over the greater trochanter should be palpated for tenderness. The lateral surface of the trochanter is tender in cases of trochanteric bursitis. Swelling occasionally may be palpable and helps to differentiate actual bursitis from gluteus tendinitis or attachment tenderness in which there is posterolateral trochanteric tenderness without swelling. If lateral tenderness without swelling is present, differentiation between the two conditions can be difficult. The pain of trochanteric bursitis is aggravated by actively resisted abduction of the hip.

Patients complaining of anterior hip or groin pain should be examined for iliopsoas bursitis. Swelling and tenderness may be noted in the middle one third of the inguinal ligament lateral to the femoral pulse. The pain is aggravated by hip extension and reduced by flexion. The bursitis may be a localized problem or represent extension of hip synovitis to the bursa, because there is communication between the two structures in approximately 15 percent of cases. In the latter instance, the bursitis actually represents a synovial cyst. It is impossible to differentiate a bursitis from a cyst on examination. If the patient is tender in the region of the iliopsoas bursa but no swelling is palpable, it is not possible to differentiate this condition from an overlying tendonitis of the iliopsoas muscle. The inguinal region should be carefully palpated for other abnormalities

such as hernias, femoral aneurysms, adenopathy, tumor, and psoas abscess masses.

Muscle strength testing should include the hip flexors, extensors, abductors, and adductors. The primary hip flexor is the iliopsoas muscle (L2 and 3). Flexion may be tested with the patient sitting at the end of the table. The pelvis is stabilized by placing one hand on the ipsilateral iliac crest while the patient actively flexes the hip. The examiner uses the other hand to exert downward pressure against the thigh proximal to the knee. A second approach is to have the patient assume the supine position and hold the leg to be tested in 90 degrees of flexion at the hip while the examiner attempts to straighten the hip. Hip extension is tested with the patient lying prone. The primary hip extensor is the gluteus maximus muscle (L5 and S1). With the knee flexed to remove hamstring action, the patient is instructed to extend the hip and thigh off the surface of the table as the examiner places one forearm across the posterior iliac crest to stabilize the pelvis by placing one hand downward against the iliac crest to prevent the lateral trunk muscles from elevating the pelvis and leg off the table. The patient is instructed to abduct the thigh and leg while the examiner places downward pressure with his or her other hand against the distal lateral thigh. The leg nearest the table is then tested for hip adduction. The primary adductor is the adductor longus (L3 and 4). The examiner holds the upper leg in slight abduction while the patient adducts the lower leg off the table against the resistance of the examiner's other hand proximal to the knee.

An alternative method for testing abduction and adduction enables the examiner to compare the two legs simultaneously. The patient lies supine with the legs fully extended and the hips moderately abducted. To test abduction, the patient actively pushes out against the examiner's resistance against the lateral malleoli. Adduction is tested by movement against resistance at the medial malleoli.

Knee

The knee is a compound condylar joint with three articulations: the patellofemoral and the lateral and medial tibial femoral condyles with their fibrocartilaginous menisci. The joint is stabilized by the articular capsule, the ligamentum patellae, and the medial and lateral collateral and anterior and posterior cruciate ligaments. The collateral ligaments provide medial and lateral stability, whereas the cruciates provide anteroposterior support and rotatory stability. Normal knee motion is a combination of flexion or extension and rotation. With flexion, the tibia internally rotates, and with extension, it externally rotates on the femur. The surrounding synovial membrane is the largest of any of the body's joints; it extends up to 6 cm proximal to the joint as the suprapatellar pouch beneath the quadriceps femoris muscle. There are several clinically significant bursae

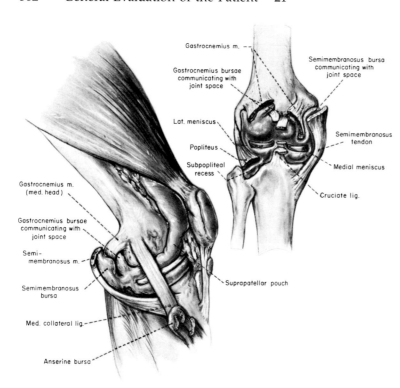

Gastrocnemius m.

Gastrocnemius bursae
communicating with
joint space

Lat. meniscus

Popliteus

Subpopliteal
recess

Semimembranosus bursa
communicating with
joint space

Semimembranosus
tendon

Medial meniscus

Cruciate lig.

Gastrocnemius m.
(med. head)

Gastrocnemius bursae
communicating with
joint space

Semi-
membranosus m.

Semimembranosus
bursa

Med. collateral lig.

Anserine bursa

Suprapatellar pouch

Figure 21–9. Medial and posterior aspects of the knee with important muscle attachments and bursae illustrated. (From Polley, H. F., and Hunder, G. G.: Rheumatologic Interviewing and Physical Examination of the Joints. Philadelphia, W. B. Saunders Company, 1978.)

about the knee, including the superficial prepatellar bursa, the superficial and deep infrapatellar bursae, the anserine bursa distal to the medial tibial plateau, and the posterior medial semimembranous and posterolateral gastrocnemius bursae (Fig. 21–9). Knee extension is provided for primarily by the quadriceps femoris muscle and flexion by the hamstrings. The biceps femoris externally rotates over the lower leg on the femur, whereas the popliteus and semitendinous muscles supply internal rotation. The knee flexes to a maximum of 135 degrees in most persons. Excessive extension beyond 0 degrees is observed in some people in the form of genu recurvatum.

Examination of the knees should always include observation of the standing patient. Weight bearing places deforming stress on the knees. Genu varum, or lateral deviation of the knee joint (with medial deviation of the lower leg); genu valgum, or medial deviation of the knee (and lateral deviation of the lower leg); and genu recurvatum, or posterior bowing, are often more easily appreciated in the standing patient. Limp, flexion contracture, locking, or giving way should be noted. Locking is the sudden loss of ability to extend the knee; it is painful and may be associated with an audible noise such as a click, pop, or snap.

Asymmetry from swelling or muscle atrophy may be noted on initial inspection. Patellar malalignment should be noted, including high-riding or laterally displaced patellae. The examiner should inspect the knee from the rear to identify popliteal swelling due to a popliteal or Baker's cyst, which is most commonly a medial semimembranous bursal swelling. If the calves appear asymmetric, measure-

ment of calf circumference should be performed when the patient is lying on the examination table. Popliteal cysts may dissect down into the calf muscles, producing enlargement and palpable fullness. Edema may be present if the cyst causes secondary venous or lymphatic obstruction. Acute dissection or rupture of a popliteal cyst can mimic thrombophlebitis, the so-called pseudothrombophlebitis syndrome, with local pain, heat, redness, and swelling.

In the supine position, inability to extend the knee fully may be related to a flexion contracture or a large synovial effusion. Suprapatellar swelling with fullness of the distal anterior thigh that obliterates the normal depressed contours along the side of the patella usually indicates a knee joint effusion or synovitis. Localized swelling over the surface of the patella is generally secondary to prepatellar bursitis, whereas localized anterolateral or medial swelling along the joint line may represent cystic swelling of menisci.

Quadriceps femoris muscle atrophy usually develops in chronic arthritis of the knee. Atrophy of the vastus medialis is the earliest change and may be appreciated by comparing the two thighs for medial asymmetry and circumference. Usually measurement of the thigh circumference is performed at approximately 15 cm above the joint to avoid spurious results due to suprapatellar effusions.

For adequate palpation of the knee, the joint must be relaxed. This is usually best accomplished with the patient supine and the knees as fully extended as possible and not touching. Palpation should begin over the anterior thigh approximately 10 cm above the patella. To identify the superior margin of the suprapatellar pouch, which is an extension of the knee joint cavity, the examiner should palpate the tissues moving distally toward the knee. Swelling, warmth, thickness, nodules, loose bodies, and tenderness should be noted. A thickened synovial membrane has a boggy, doughy consistency different from the surrounding soft tissue and muscle. It is usually palpated earlier over the medial aspect of the suprapatellar pouch and medial tibiofemoral joint. To enhance detection of knee fluid, any fluid in the suprapatellar pouch is compressed with the palm of one hand placed just proximal to the patella. The synovial fluid forced into the inferior distal articular cavity is then palpated with the opposite thumb and index finger laterally and medially to the patella. If the examiner alternates compression and release of the suprapatellar pouch, the synovial thickening can be differentiated from a synovial effusion, because the effusion will intermittently distend the joint capsule under the thumb and index finger of the opposite hand, whereas the synovial thickening will not. The examiner should be cautious not to compress the suprapatellar pouch too firmly or push the tissues distally because the patella or normal soft tissue, including the fat pads, will fill the palpated space and be misinterpreted as synovitis or joint swelling. With a large effusion, the patella can be ballotted by pushing it posteriorly against the femur with the right forefinger while maintaining suprapatellar compression with the left hand.

At the other extreme, effusions as small as 4 to 8 ml can be detected by eliciting the bulge sign. This test is performed with the knee extended and relaxed. The examiner strokes or compresses the medial aspect of the knee proximally and laterally with the palm of one hand to move the fluid from the area. The lateral aspect of the knee is then tapped or stroked, and a fluid wave or bulge is noted to appear medially (Fig. 21–10). If the maneuver is not positive with the first attempt, it should be repeated with the pressure applied to the other areas of the lateral side of the knee.

The medial and lateral tibiofemoral joint margins are palpated for tenderness and bony lipping or exostosis, as seen in osteoarthritis. Palpating the joint margins can be done easily with the hip flexed to 45 degrees, the knee flexed to 90 degrees, and the foot resting on the examining table. Tenderness over joint margins may represent articular cartilage disease, involvement of the medial meniscus or anterior cruciate ligament, or lateral involvement of the collateral ligament, iliotibial band, or fibial head.

Bursitis can be differentiated from articular synovitis by palpation of localized tenderness and swelling. The anserine bursa is located at the medial tibial plateau between the medial collateral ligament and the tendons of the sartorius, gracilis, and semitendinous muscles. The prepatellar bursa, if quite swollen, can be mistakenly interpreted as knee joint synovitis unless the bursal margins are carefully outlined by palpation. Infrapatellar bursitis is pal-

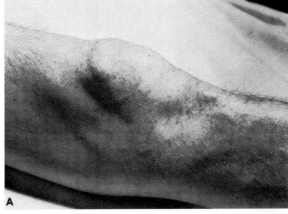

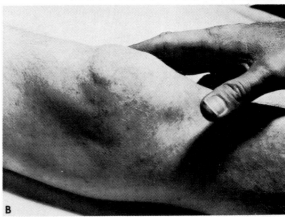

Figure 21–10. Demonstration of the bulge sign for a small synovial knee effusion. The medial aspect of the knee has been shaded to move the synovial fluid from this area (shaded depressed area in *A*). *B* shows bulge in previously shaded area after lateral aspect of the knee has been tapped. (From Polley, H. F., and Hunder, G. G.: Rheumatologic Interviewing and Physical Examination of the Joints. Philadelphia, W. B. Saunders Company, 1978.)

pated either overlying the infrapatellar tendon at the level of the tibia (superficial) or lying beneath the tendon (deep). The infrapatellar fat pad beneath the tendon at the level of the joint line may also be tender.

Determination of the cause of patellofemoral pain is clinically difficult. A number of physical signs have been described.[7] Patellar palpation is best performed with the knee extended and relaxed. The patella is compressed and moved so that its entire articular surface will come into contact with the underlying femur. Slight crepitation may be observed in many normally functioning knees. Pain with crepitation may suggest patellofemoral degenerative arthritis or chondromalacia patellae. Retropatellar pain occurring with active knee flexion and extension and secondary to patellofemoral disease may be differentiated from tibiofemoral articular pain. To test this, the examiner should attempt to lift the patella away from the knee while passively moving the knee through range of motion. Painless motion during this maneuver indicates that the patellofemoral joint is the source of the difficulty. In addition, the patellar inhibition test also helps to clarify the presence of patellofemoral arthritis. In this test, the examiner compresses the patella distally away from the femoral condyles while instructing the patient to isometrically contract the quadriceps. Sudden patellar pain and quadriceps relaxation are interpreted as a positive test for chondromalacia, but frequency of false-positive results is high.

The patella should be checked for stability in patients suspected of having recurrent patellar dislocation. With the knee in 30-degree flexion, the patella is pushed laterally with the patient supine and the knee passively extended and while relaxed. A distressed reaction from the patient is considered a positive apprehension test. Subluxation of the patella can also be appreciated while moving the knee through range of motion from 0 to 90 degrees of flexion or back to full extension.

Another cause of joint snapping and symptoms suggesting an internal derangement is the plica syndrome caused by bands of synovial tissue.[8] In cases of mediopatella plica syndrome, a tender band-like structure may be palpated parallel to the medial border of the patella. During flexion and extension, a palpable or audible snap is appreciated. Patellar crepitance may also be noted.

Ligamentous instability is tested by applying valgus and varus stress to the knee and by using the drawer test. The knee should be extended and relaxed. The abduction or valgus test is performed by stabilizing the lower femur while placing a valgus stress on the knee by abducting the lower leg with the other hand placed proximal to the ankle. A medial joint line separation with the knee fully extended indicates a tear of the medial compartment ligaments plus the posterior cruciate ligament. The test is then performed with the knee in 30 degrees of flexion. If the test is negative at 0 degrees but positive at 30 degrees, the instability represents a tear of the medial compartment ligaments with the posterior cruciate ligament remaining intact. The adduction or varus test is then performed at 0 degrees. Separation of the lateral joint line indicates a lateral compartment ligament tear with an associated tear of the posterior cruciate ligament.

The degree of ligamentous laxity observed during testing should be graded on a scale of 1 to 3.[9] A mild grade 1 instability indicates that the joint surfaces separate 5 mm or less; moderate grade 2 represents a separation of 5 to 10 mm. A severe instability, grade 3, is a separation greater than 10 mm. In cases of trauma, opening of the joint space indicates ligamentous instability secondary to rupture or stretching of the ligaments. However, in cases of chronic arthritis of the tibiofemoral compartment, there may be apparent medial or lateral separation due to the "pseudolaxity" created by loss of cartilage and bone. If the ligaments are intact, the resulting degree of valgus or varus displacement with stressing will not be any greater than in the normal knee.

The drawer test is performed with the hip flexed to 45 degrees and the knee to 90 degrees. To stabilize the knee, the examiner either sits on the foot while grasping the posterior calf with both hands or supports the lower leg between his or her lateral chest wall and forearm. The anterior drawer test is performed by pulling the tibia forward. This maneuver has been said to test whether the anterior cruciate ligament is intact. However, anterior subluxation may actually represent more complex instability. Rotatory instability of the knee may also exist. With the tibia in neutral, a positive anterior drawer test in which the lateral tibial plateau subluxes forward while the medial stays in normal position represents anterolateral rotatory instability. If both plateaus sublux, tears of the middle one third of the medial lateral capsular ligaments are present. If the subluxation is not present with the tibia internally rotated, the posterior cruciate ligament is intact. A positive anterior drawer test with the leg in external rotation represents a tear of the medial capsular ligament. The Lackman test, a modification of the anterior drawer sign, and the pivot shift test are more reliable in the evaluation of acute anterior cruciate ligament injuries.[10, 11] A posterior drawer test in a chronically unstable knee suggests that damage has occurred to the posterior cruciate ligament.

The jerk test measures anterolateral instability. With the hip flexed to 45 degrees and the knee to 90 degrees, the tibia is internally rotated while valgus stress is applied to the knee. The leg is extended and at approximately 30 degrees of flexion subluxation of the lateral femorotibial articulation relocates. The change in acceleration rate of the two joint surfaces (during the maneuver) is felt as a sudden jerk.

Meniscal injury should also be tested for during the survey for joint instability. Symptoms that suggest a meniscal tear include locking during extension, joint clicking or popping during motion, and localized line tenderness along the joint. To examine the medial meniscus, the medial tibiofemoral joint line should be palpated with the lower leg internally rotated and the knee flexed to 90 degrees. Localized tenderness suggests involvement of the medial meniscus. With the knee flexed to 90 degrees, the lateral joint line is palpated for localized tenderness that would indicate lateral meniscal injury. The McMurray test is performed to elicit evidence of a posterior meniscal tear. In this procedure, the patient's knee is placed in full extension and the examiner places one hand over the knee with the fingers along the side of the knee along one joint line and the thumb along the other side. The other hand holds the leg at the ankle and is used to flex, extend, and rotate the lower leg. With the knee flexed and the lower leg externally rotated 15 degrees, a palpable or audible snap occurring when the knee is extended from full to 90 degrees of flexion is a positive test and suggests a tear of the medial meniscus. A lateral snap or click occurring with the knee internally rotated 30 degrees and moved into extension suggests a lateral meniscal tear. In addition, a positive lateral test may represent a tear of the popliteus tendon, which can accompany a lateral meniscal tear. The Apley maneuver also tests for a torn meniscus. With the patient lying prone and the knee flexed to 90 degrees, the examiner places downward compression on the foot while rotating the tibia on the femur. Pain elicited during this maneuver suggests a meniscal tear. The distraction test is then performed by the examiner placing his or her knee on the patient's posterior thigh to stabilize the leg while applying an upward distractive force on the foot. Pain from rotating the tibia suggests ligament damage. When verified by arthroscopy, physical signs of meniscal tears are not always reliable. Tenderness along the joint line is most sensitive but not as specific as manipulative tests such as the Mc-Murray test or a newly suggested maneuver, the "medial-lateral grind" test.[12]

Range of motion of the knee in flexion and extension should be from full extension (0 degrees), to full flexion of 120 to 150 degrees. Some normal persons may be able to hyperextend to up to 15 degrees. Loss of full extension due to a flexion contracture is a common finding that accompanies chronic arthritis of the knee. In advanced arthritis, such as seen in some cases of rheumatoid arthritis, a posterior subluxation of the tibia on the femur may be observed.

Muscle strength testing includes testing flexion supplied by the hamstrings, i.e., the biceps femoris, semitendinosus, and semimembranosus (L5 to S3) and extension supplied by the quadriceps femori (L2, 3, and 4). The hamstrings are tested best with the patient prone and attempting to flex the knee from 90 degrees to beyond.

The ankle should be kept in neutral position or dorsiflexed to remove gastrocnemius action. With the leg externally rotated, the biceps femoris, which inserts on the fibula and lateral tibia, is primarily tested, whereas flexion with internal rotation tests the semitendinosus and semimembranosus muscles, which insert on the medial side of the tibia. Extension is tested with the patient sitting upright with the knee fully extended. The examiner stabilizes the thigh with downward pressure just proximal to the knee and places downward pressure at the ankle to test the knee extensors.

Ankle

The ankle is a hinged joint, and movement is limited to plantar flexion and dorsiflexion. It is formed by the distal ends of the tibia and fibula and proximal aspect of the body of the talus. The tibia forms the weight-bearing portion of the ankle joint; the fibula articulates on the side of the tibia. The malleoli of the tibia and fibula extend downward beyond the weight-bearing part of the joint and articulate with the sides of the talus. Malleoli provide

lateral stablity by enveloping the talus in a mortise-like fashion.

The articular capsule of the ankle is lax on the anterior and posterior aspects of the joint, allowing extension and flexion, but is tightly bound bilaterally by ligaments. The synovial membrane of the ankle on the inside of the capsule usually does not communicate with any other joints, bursae, or tendon sheaths in the region of the ankle or foot.

Strong medial and lateral ligaments of the ankle contribute to the lateral stability of the joint. The medial or deltoid ligament, the only ligament on the medial side of the ankle, is a triangle-shaped fibrous band that tends to resist eversion of the foot. It may be torn in eversion sprains of the ankles. The lateral ligaments of the foot consist of three distinct bands forming the posterior talofibular, the calcaneofibular, and the anterior talofibular ligaments. These ligaments may be torn in inversion sprains of the ankle. All tendons crossing the ankle joint lie superficial to the articular capsule and are enclosed in synovial sheaths (8 cm in length) for part of their course across the ankle. On the anterior aspect of the ankle, the tendons and synovial tendon sheaths of the tibialis anterior, extensor digitorum longus, peroneus tertius, and extensor hallucis longus overlie the articular capsule and synovial membrane. On the medial side of the ankle posteriorly and inferiorly to the medial malleolus lie the flexor tendons and tendon sheaths of the tibialis posterior, flexor digitorum longus, and flexor hallucis longus (Fig. 21–11). All three of these muscles plantar flex and supinate the foot. The tendon of the flexor hallucis longus is located more posteriorly than the other flexor tendons and lies beneath the Achilles tendon for part of its course. The tendon calcaneus (Achilles tendon) is a common tendon of the gastrocnemius and soleus muscles and inserts into the posterior surface of the calcaneus, where it is subject to external trauma, various inflammatory reactions, and irritations from bony spurs beneath it. On the lateral aspect of the ankle, posteriorly and inferiorly to the lateral malleolus, a synovial sheath encloses the tendons of the peroneus longus and peroneus brevis. These muscles extend the ankle (plantar flex) and evert (pronate) the foot. Each of the tendons adjacent to the ankle may be involved separately in traumatic or disease processes.

There are three sets of fibrous bands or retinacula that hold down the tendons that cross the ankle in their passage to the foot. The extensor retinaculum consists of a superior part (transverse crural ligament) in the anterior and inferior portions of the leg and an inferior part in the proximal portion of the dorsum of the foot. The flexor retinaculum is a thickened fibrous band on the medial side of the ankle. On the lateral side of the ankle, the peroneal retinaculum forms a superior and an inferior fibrous band. These bands bind down tendons of the peroneus longus and peroneus brevis as they cross the lateral aspect of the ankle.

Synovial swelling of the ankle joint is most likely

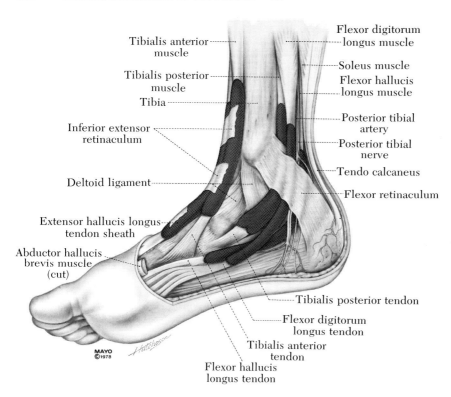

Tibialis anterior muscle

Tibialis posterior muscle

Tibia

Inferior extensor retinaculum

Deltoid ligament

Extensor hallucis longus tendon sheath

Abductor hallucis brevis muscle (cut)

Flexor digitorum longus muscle

Soleus muscle

Flexor hallucis longus muscle

Posterior tibial artery

Posterior tibial nerve

Tendo calcaneus

Flexor retinaculum

Tibialis posterior tendon

Flexor digitorum longus tendon

Tibialis anterior tendon

Flexor hallucis longus tendon

MAYO ©1978

Figure 21–11. Medial aspect of the ankle demonstrating the relationships between the tendons, ligaments, and posterior tibial artery and nerve. (From Polley, H. F., and Hunder, G. G.: Rheumatologic Interviewing and Physical Examination of the Joints. Philadelphia, W. B. Saunders Company, 1978. © Mayo Clinic, 1978. By permission of Mayo Foundation.)

to cause fullness over the anterior or anterolateral aspect of the joint, because the capsule is more lax in this area. Mild swelling of the joint may not be apparent on inspection because of the many structures that cross the joint superficially to the synovial membrane. Efforts should be made to differentiate between superficial linear swelling localized to the distribution of the tendon sheaths from more diffuse fullness and swelling due to involvement of the ankle joint. Similarly, it is difficult to observe synovitis of the intertarsal joints. Intertarsal joint synovitis may produce an erythematous puffiness or fullness over the dorsum of the foot.

From the normal position of rest in which there is a right angle between the leg and foot, labeled 0 degrees, the ankle normally allows about 20 degrees of dorsiflexion and about 45 degrees of plantar flexion. Inversion and eversion of the foot occur mainly at the subtalar and other intertarsal joints. From the normal position of the foot, the subtalar joint normally permits about 20 degrees of eversion and 30 degrees of inversion. To test the subtalar joint, the examiner grasps the calcaneus with one hand and attempts to invert and evert it, holding the ankle motionless.

A general assessment of muscular strength of the ankle can be obtained by asking the patient to lift the weight of the body on the toes and heels. If the patient can walk on toes and heels, the muscle strength of the flexors and extensors of the ankle can be considered normal. In many instances, however, joint pains may prevent the patient from walking, or it is desired to test muscles individually.

Prime movers in plantar flexion of the ankle are the gastrocnemius (S1 and 2) and the soleus (S1 and 2) muscles. The prime mover in dorsiflexion and inversion of the foot is the tibialis anterior muscle (L4 and 5, S1). The examiner applies graded resistance on the medial and dorsal aspect of the foot when testing the tibialis anterior muscle. The prime mover in inversion is the tibialis posterior muscle (L5 and S1). To test the tibialis posterior muscle, the foot should be in plantar flexion. The examiner applies graded resistance on the medial border of the forefoot while the patient attempts to invert the foot. The prime movers in eversion of the foot are the peroneus longus (L4 and 5, S1) and peroneus brevis (L4 and 5, S1) muscles.

Foot

See Chapter 28.

References

1. Polley, H. F., and Hunder, G. G.: Rheumatologic Interviewing and Physical Examination of the Joints. 2nd ed. Philadelphia, W.B. Saunders Company, 1978.
2. Hoppenfeld, S.: Physical Examination of the Spine and Extremities. Englewood Cliffs, NJ, Appleton-Century-Crofts, 1976.
3. Ritchie, D. M., Boyle, J. A., McInnes, J. M., Jasani, M. K., Dalakos, T. G., Grieveson, P., and Buchanan, W. W.: Clinical studies with an articular index for the assessment of joint tenderness in patients with rheumatoid arthritis. Q. J. Med. 147:393, 1968.
4. Lee, P., Baxter, A., Dick, W. C., and Webb, J.: An assessment of grip strength measurement in rheumatoid arthritis. Scand. J. Rheumatol. 3:17, 1974.

5. Boardman, P. L., and Hart, F. D.: Clinical measurement of the anti-inflammatory effects of salicylates in rheumatoid arthritis. Br. Med. J. 4:264, 1967.
6. Cushnaghan, J., Cooper, C., Dieppe, P., Kirwan, J., McAlindon, T., and McCrae, F.: Clinical assessment of osteoarthritis of the knee. Ann. Rheum. Dis. 49:768, 1990.
7. Carson, W. G., James, S. L., Larson, R. L., Singer, K. M., and Winternitz, W. W.: Patellofemoral disorder: Physical and radiographic evaluation. Clin. Orthop. Rel. Res. 185:165, 1984.
8. Hardaker, W. T., Whipple, T. L., and Bassett, F. H.: Diagnosis and treatment of the plica syndrome of the knee. J. Bone Joint Surg. 62A:221, 1980.
9. Hughston, J. C., Andrews, J. R., Cross, M. J., and Moschi, A.: Classification of knee ligament instabilities: I. The medial compartment and cruciate ligaments. J. Bone Joint Surg. 58A:159, 1976.
10. Katz, J. W., and Fingeroth, R. J.: The diagnostic accuracy of ruptures of the anterior cruciate ligament comparing the Lachman test, the anterior drawer sign, and the pivot shift test in acute and chronic knee injuries. Am. J. Sports Med. 14:88, 1986.
11. Jonsson, T., Althoff, B., Peterson, L., and Renstrom, P.: Clinical diagnosis of ruptures of the anterior cruciate ligament. Am. J. Sports Med. 10:100, 1982.
12. Anderson, A. F., and Lipscomb, A. B.: Clinical diagnosis of meniscal tears: Description of a new manipulative test. Am. J. Sports Med. 14:291, 1986.

Chapter 22

Monarticular Arthritis

W. Joseph McCune

INTRODUCTION

With rare exceptions, any joint disorder is capable of presenting initially as monarthritis. Monarthritis, therefore, presents a diagnostic challenge to even the most experienced clinician. In fact, frequently it remains incompletely understood after initial evaluation. Nonetheless, it is almost always possible to identify those patients who require vigorous evaluation and treatment to prevent rapid disease progression. One can then proceed in a measured and systematic manner with the remainder of patients, in whom the short-term clinical course and response to simple therapeutic measures may provide additional useful information. This chapter is intended to aid the clinician in distinguishing true arthritis from syndromes that also present with pain in the surrounding structures of joints, in narrowing the list of diagnostic possibilities based on the clinical presentation, and in effectively using diagnostic tests. Special attention is given to common entities presenting as acute inflammatory arthritis suggesting joint sepsis.

DIFFERENTIAL DIAGNOSIS

Confronted with a patient complaining of pain or swelling in the region of a single joint, the physician must first attempt to localize the anatomic site of the abnormality. "Joint pain" can be the result of abnormalities in the joint itself, adjacent bone, surrounding ligaments, tendons, bursae, or soft tissues.

Arthritis involving a diarthroidal joint causes stiffness, reduced range of motion, and pain during normal use. With few exceptions (e.g., the patello-femoral joint in chondromalacia[1]) joint abnormalities can be detected during both passive and active range of motion. Stiffness of the joint may be particularly noticeable in the morning (morning stiffness) or after a period of cessation of activity (gelling). It is important to compare the abnormalities noted with findings in the contralateral, presumably unaffected, joint. Every effort should be made to identify effusions on physical examination. Effusions almost always result from intra-articular pathology, although they occasionally may accompany adjacent pathology, such as osteomyelitis, fractures, or tumors.[2] Small effusions may be demonstrable only by arthrocentesis, particularly in the knee. The presence of

excess synovial fluid does not specifically indicate joint inflammation unless the white blood cell count is elevated. The range of disorders causing monarthritis is listed in Table 22–1.

The conditions discussed in the following sections may be confused with arthritis (Table 22–2).

Internal Derangements (Particularly of the Knee or Shoulder). Torn menisci or ligaments, or loose bodies, may episodically wedge into the joint, producing clicking, locking, or giving away. These conditions may precede or accompany degenerative arthritis and may be a consequence of inflammatory arthritis. In inflammatory disorders, similar symptoms may also be produced by fronds of proliferative synovium that become lodged within the joint. Symptoms are frequently intermittent, occurring at irregular intervals. They may often be elicited on physical examination by repeatedly flexing and extending the joint in various degrees of internal and external rotation.[3]

Bone Pain. Pain in bone usually results from involvement by a disease process of either the periosteum or the marrow space, because sensory nerves are located in these areas. Bone pain is commonly caused by fractures, osteomyelitis, hemoglobinopathies, hematologic malignancy,[4] primary or metastatic bone tumors, and occasionally by infiltrative processes such as Paget's disease. Characteristically, it is accompanied by tenderness to pressure over involved periosteum or pain on weight bearing. Involvement of subchondral bone may also be associated with effusions and abnormalities of the joint on examination. There may be surprisingly little discomfort during passive range of motion unless the articular surface is involved. When symptoms are long-standing, radiographs are characteristically positive. The importance of identifying such lesions makes radiographs an essential part of the evaluation of both children and adults with monarticular disease. Paget's disease may be associated with both bone pain and arthritic symptoms owing to expansion and deformity of subchondral bone and cartilage, particularly in the hips and knees.[5]

Tendinitis or Bursitis. Findings are usually localized to one side of the joint.[6] There is local tenderness and often more pain with active motion, which stresses the involved structures, than with passive motion of the joint. An exception to this rule is supraspinatus tendinitis of the shoulder. Because of the intimate relationship of the supraspinatus tendon to the internal structures of the shoulder,

Table 22–1. DIFFERENTIAL DIAGNOSIS OF MONARTICULAR ARTHRITIS

Usually Monarticular	Often Polyarticular
Common	
Septic arthritis	Rheumatoid arthritis
Bacterial	Osteoarthritis
Tuberculous	Psoriatic arthritis
Fungal	Reiter's syndrome
Lyme disease	Calcium pyrophosphate
Gout	deposition disease
Internal derangement	Chronic articular hemorrhage
Ischemic necrosis	Most JRA and juvenile
Hemarthrosis	spondylitis
Coagulopathy	Erythema nodosum/sarcoid
Warfarin (Coumadin)	Serum sickness
Trauma/overuse	Acute hepatitis B
Pauciarticular JRA	Rubella
Neuropathic	Henoch-Schönlein
Congenital hip dysplasia	Systemic lupus erythematosus
Osteochondritis dissecans	Lyme disease
Reflex sympathetic dystrophy	Parvovirus
Hydroxyapatite deposition	Dialysis arthropathy
Hemoglobinopathies	Other crystal-induced
Loose body	arthropathies
"Palindromic rheumatism"	
Paget's disease involving joint	
Stress fracture	
Osteomyelitis	
Osteogenic sarcoma	
Metastatic tumor	
Synovial osteochondromatosis	
Rare	
Pigmented villonodular	Undifferentiated connective
synovitis	tissue disease
Plant thorn synovitis	Relapsing polychondritis
Familial Mediterranean fever	Enteropathic disease
Synovioma	Ulcerative colitis
Synovial metastasis	Regional enteritis
Intermittent hydrarthrosis	Bypass arthritis
Pancreatic fat necrosis	Whipple's disease
Gaucher's disease	Chronic sarcoidosis
Behçet's disease	Hyperlipidemias types II and
Regional migratory	IV
osteoporosis	Still's disease
Giant cell arteritis/polymyalgia	Pyoderma gangrenosum
rheumatica	Pulmonary hypertrophic
Sea urchin spine	osteoarthropathy
Amyloidosis (myeloma)	Chondrocalcinosis-like
	syndromes due to
	ochronosis,
	hemochromatosis, Wilson's
	disease
	Rheumatic fever
	Paraneoplastic syndromes

passive and active motion may produce similar pain, and there may be no localized tenderness. Clinical findings can usually be reduced or eliminated by local instillation of lidocaine. The presence of a puncture site,[7] prior glucocorticoid injection, an adjacent source of infection such as an ulcerated rheumatoid nodule,[8] or severe inflammation may signify infectious bursitis. The usual agents are gram-positive organisms that are easily identified on Gram stain and culture.[7, 9] Isolated tendinitis is less commonly due to hematogenous spread of infection except in disseminated gonococcal disease, which commonly presents with dorsal tenosynovitis of the wrists,[10, 11] and brucellosis. Identification of septic bursitis or tendinitis is particularly important when arthrocentesis of a joint underlying the infected area is contemplated, so that introduction of micro-organisms into a sterile joint space may be avoided. The infected olecranon or prepatellar bursae commonly mimic septic arthritis. On careful physical examination, the range of motion of the joint is usually more than would be expected in a patient with septic arthritis who has a similar degree of soft tissue swelling.

Neuropathic Pain. Compression or irritation of peripheral nerves may produce pain referred to the region of joints, such as pain radiating from the wrist to the palmar surface of the first four digits in carpal tunnel syndrome,[12] hip region pain in lumbosacral radiculopathies, or shoulder pain with brachial plexopathies. Such symptoms are usually in the distribution of a peripheral nerve(s) and tend to follow an irregular time course, with sudden exacerbations, particularly at night. Maneuvers that compress the affected nerve at the site of injury, such as straight leg raising or percussion of the median nerve at the waist,[13] are helpful when they exactly reproduce the patient's pain in the distribution of a peripheral nerve. In difficult cases, nerve conduction studies may be useful. Diffuse polyneuropathies may produce pain that is poorly localized and superficially resembles joint pain in a stocking-glove distribution. Pain that localizes exactly to a joint in the setting of a polyneuropathy may be related to neuropathic joint disease of reflex sympathetic dystrophy or may have an unrelated cause.[14]

Soft Tissue Infections. These infections may simulate arthritis, particularly when occurring in the region of deeply buried joints that are difficult to examine. "Hip pain" may result from cellulitis, pyomyositis, psoas or retroperitoneal abscesses, or intrapelvic pathology such as diverticulitis. Fever and the acute onset of hip pain and stiffness with normal radiographs and synovial fluid findings suggest soft tissue or bone infection. Pain referred to the sacroiliac joint may result from similar conditions and perirectal abscesses. Infectious processes in these locations present with unremitting, severe pain, marked elevation of the erythrocyte sedimentation rate, and variably severe systemic toxicity.[15–17] Physical examination may reveal muscular rigidity and guarding, local tenderness, increased girth of the affected limb, or draining sinuses. Imaging studies may be essential in identifying deep infections. Occasionally, bubbles are identified in soft tissue using plain radiographs, but the usual approach includes radionuclide scanning using gallium or indium compounds combined with computed tomography (CT) or ultrasound. Magnetic resonance (MR) imaging has recently been shown to provide superior imaging of pathologic conditions in muscle and may be an important adjunct to ultrasound or CT for identifying deep infection. However, technical considerations make needle-directed aspirations, which are often indi-

Table 22–2. REGIONAL PERIARTICULAR SYNDROMES

Region	Periarticular Syndrome	Nonarticular Syndrome
Jaw	Temporomandibular joint dysfunction	Temporal arteritis Molar dental problems Parotid swelling Preauricular lymphadenitis
Shoulder	Subacromial bursitis Long head bicipital tendinitis Rotator cuff tear	Pancoast's tumor Brachial plexopathy Cervical nerve root injury
Elbow	Olecranon bursitis Epicondylitis	Ulnar nerve entrapment
Wrist	Extensor tendinitis (including de Quervain's tenosynovitis) Gonococcal tenosynovitis	Carpal tunnel syndrome
Hand	Palmar fasciitis (Dupuytren's contracture) Ligamentous/capsular injury	
Hip	Greater trochanteric bursitis Adductor syndrome Ischial bursitis Fascia lata syndrome	Meralgia paresthetica Deep infection Paget's disease Neoplasm
Knee	Anserine bursitis Prepatellar bursitis Meniscal injury Ligamentous tear-laxity Baker's cyst	Neoplasm Osteomyelitis
Ankle	Peroneal tendinitis Achilles bursitis Calcaneal fasciitis Sprain Erythema nodosum	Tarsal tunnel syndrome
Foot	Plantar fasciitis	Morton's neuroma Vascular insufficiency Cellulitis

cated in such situations, much more effectively performed with CT or ultrasound guidance.

Compartment Syndromes. Compartment syndromes may result from trauma, infection, or hemorrhage, particularly in the hand, forearm, and lower leg. Immediate diagnosis is essential, and operative decompression may be necessary.

Psychiatric Disorders. These disorders are less frequently associated with truly localized complaints than with generalized malaise and arthralgias unless they are work related.

IMPORTANT HISTORICAL FEATURES OF MONARTICULAR ARTHRITIS

Is the arthritis acute or chronic? Extremely rapid onset of pain (over seconds or minutes) suggests an internal derangement, fracture, trauma, or loose body.

Acute onset over several hours to 1 week is typical of most forms of inflammatory arthritis, particularly bacterial infection and crystal-induced synovitis. In normal persons, a history of more protracted onset of symptoms is less suggestive of bacterial infection and may suggest the possibility of tuberculous or fungal arthritis (although these forms of arthritis sometimes present acutely), an inflammatory

arthritis, or structural disease. When a careful history reveals long-standing symptoms in a joint, it is important to distinguish exacerbations of pre-existing disease, such as worsening of degenerative joint disease with excessive use, from a second superimposed process, such as infection.[18]

Is the underlying process mechanical or inflammatory? This question is most reliably answered by the synovial fluid white blood cell count (Table 22–3). In addition, when the joint disease has been present long enough for fluctuations in severity to be observed (usually more than a week), it is useful to consider the historical features that help to distinguish these forms of joint disease. Waxing and waning of disease activity unrelated to patterns of use, including fluctuations of pain and swelling, protracted morning stiffness, and gelling, suggest inflammation. Pain that occurs only after use, improves with rest, and involves weight-bearing joints suggests mechanical disease. In the author's experience, the response to pharmacologic agents frequently is less helpful in distinguishing inflammatory versus structural arthritis than is commonly believed. Not all patients with inflammatory arthritis are significantly helped by nonsteroidal anti-inflammatory drugs. Conversely, patients with early osteoarthritis frequently do better when they ingest the equivalent of three aspirin tablets before or after activity. Com-

Table 22–3. SYNOVIAL FLUID AND ASSOCIATED LABORATORY FINDINGS IN MONARTICULAR ARTHRITIS

Synovial Fluid White Blood Cell Count	Predominant Cell	Appearance	Viscosity	Micro-organisms	Crystals	RBC	Glucose	Protein	Complement	Cartilage Debris	Other
0–200 Normal	M	Clear	↑	–	–	–	90%	1.5–2	–	–	Small amount not demonstrable on physical examination
0–2000 Osteoarthritis	M	Clear	↑	–	+/– Occasional CPPD	–	–	–/↑	–	+	Radiographs positive in advanced disease; synovial fluid findings variable
Structural Internal derangement	M	Clear	↑	–	–	+/– +/–	–	–/↑		+	MR scan, arthrogram (knee) arthroscopy
Neuropathic						+++/–					Marked radiographic changes
Osteochondritis dissecans							–				MR scan, CT scan
Ischemic necrosis							–				MR scan, bone scan, radiograph in advanced cases
Traumatic	RBC	Cloudy Bloody	↑	–	–	+++	–	↑/↑↑↑			Radiograph
2000–10,000 Pigmented villonodular synovitis	RBC	Brown Bloody	↓	–	–	++	↓	↑↑		–	Synovial biopsy
Amyloid	M	Slightly turbid		–	–						Congo red: synovial fluid Monoclonal gammopathy
Enteropathic arthritis	M/P	Slightly turbid		–	–	–					Positive stool occult blood LE cells
Systemic lupus erythematosus	M	Slightly turbid	↑	–	–	–			↓		Serum autoantibodies
5000–50,000 Juvenile rheumatoid arthritis	P	Slightly turbid	↓	–	–	–	↓	↑/↑↑	–/↓	–	Synovial fluid leukocytes may be ≥ 100,000 Serum: + ANA (50%) + rheumatoid factor (< 20%)
Sarcoidosis		Slightly turbid	↓	–	–	–					Chest radiographs, slit lamp examination
Reiter's syndrome	P	Slightly turbid	↓	–	–	–	↓	↑/↑↑	↑	–	
Psoriatic arthritis	P	Slightly turbid	↓	–	–	–	↓				Negative rheumatoid factor, ANA positive sign
Rheumatoid arthritis	P	Turbid	↓↓	–	–	–	↓↓	↑/↑↑↑	↓		Serum (+) rheumatoid factor (50–80%) + ANA
Tuberculous arthritis	M	Turbid	↓↓	+/–	–	–	↓↓↓	↑↑/↑↑↑			PPD usually positive unless anergic Synovial biopsy essential

Table continued on following page

Table 22–3. SYNOVIAL FLUID AND ASSOCIATED LABORATORY FINDINGS IN
MONARTICULAR ARTHRITIS *Continued*

Synovial Fluid White Blood Cell Count	Predominant Cell	Appearance	Viscosity	Micro-orga-nisms	Crystals	RBC	Glucose	Protein	Com-ple-ment	Cartilage Debris	Other
10,000–150,000											
CPPD-pseu-dogout	P	Turbid	↑↓	–	CPPD (approximately 60%)	–	↓	↑↑	+/–		Repeated crystal examinations Radiographs: chondrocalci-nosis
Gout	P	Turbid	↑	–	Monosodium urate (>90%)	–	↓	↑↑			Serum uric acid unreliable
Gonococcal infection	P	Turbid to pus	↓↓	+/–		–	↓↓	↑↑↑			Synovial fluid culture 20–50% positive Culture portals of entry Urogenital Gram stain
Nongono-coccal bacte-rial	P	Turbid to pus	↓↓↓	+		–	↓↓↓	↑↑↑			Gram stain—gram-positive organisms Synovial fluid, blood cultures

M, mononuclear; P, polynuclear; RBC, red blood cell; ANA, antinuclear antibodies; CPPD, calcium pyrophosphate dihydrate; LE, lupus erythematosus.

plete abrogation of long-standing symptoms after intra-articular glucocorticoids for a period of weeks suggests either resolution of inflammation or a placebo effect. Constitutional signs of illness in the otherwise well patient are not a feature of structural arthritis.

Is the arthritis truly monarticular? Careful inquiry may elicit evidence of antecedent or coincident involvement of additional joints. A history of inflammatory symptoms in multiple joints for more than a month suggests a chronic inflammatory condition that is not infectious. Multiple arthralgias of shorter duration may accompany the onset of many illnesses. Truly migratory disease, in which there is only one inflamed joint but a clear-cut history of recent inflammatory arthritis of other joints occurring sequentially, suggests gonococcal arthritis or rheumatic fever.

Coexistent Involvement of the Axial Spine. Evidence of enthesopathies or spondylitis should be sought. The patient should be specifically questioned about recurrent pain or morning stiffness in the low back. Symmetric sacroiliitis with uniformly distributed radiographic changes involving the lumbosacral spine suggests ankylosing spondylitis, whereas asymmetric or patchy disease in a man or woman suggests Reiter's disease[19] or psoriatic[20] or entero-pathic[21] spondylitis. These latter findings should prompt evaluation for iritis, urethritis, and gastrointestinal blood loss, abnormalities that may not be initially reported by the patient. The combination of spondylitis with transient, painful, inflammatory arthritis of large joints is characteristic of ankylosing spondylitis and inflammatory bowel disease, whereas spondylitis and radiographic evidence of chronic peripheral large or small joint disease with erosions, periosteal proliferation, or "ray" involvement suggests Reiter's disease or psoriatic arthritis.

Patchy spondylitis and inflammatory arthritis of a distal interphalangeal joint is virtually diagnostic of these latter two conditions. Spondylitis is usually clinically apparent before the development of associated structural disease in the hip or shoulder. Diffuse spinal ligamentous calcification may also be clinically or radiographically evident in diffuse skeletal hyperostosis with a peripheral arthropathy or enthesopathy. Brucellosis can present with infectious spondylitis, tendinitis, arthritis, and fever.[22]

Focal spinal involvement associated with monarticular disease occurs in tuberculosis, myeloma with amyloid, steroid osteopenia with associated ischemic necrosis, metastatic cancer, and infection. The author has also noted the coexistence of transient low back pain and stiffness with flares of the arthropathy of relapsing polychondritis. As these conditions are relatively uncommon, it should be remembered that patients with degenerative disease not infrequently report back pain and peripheral joint pain at the same time.

The diagnostic approach to monarthritis is shown in Figure 22–1. Associated systemic features are listed in Table 22–4.

APPROACH TO THE PATIENT WITH ACUTE INFLAMMATORY MONARTHRITIS

The evaluation of acute inflammatory monarthritis deserves special emphasis because immediate benefit may result from identification and treatment of the underlying disease. In most instances, the physician must make a working diagnosis of infection, crystal-induced arthritis, or the onset of a potentially chronic inflammatory arthropathy. Following diagnosis, one can institute either definitive

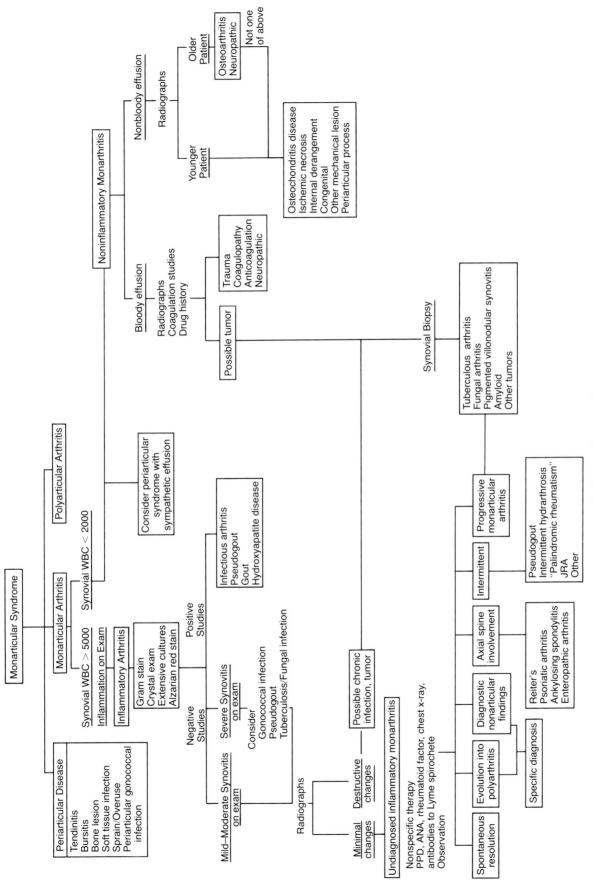

Figure 22–1. The diagnostic approach to monarthritis.

Table 22-4. SYSTEMIC FEATURES OF
MONARTICULAR ARTHRITIS

System	Diagnosis
Skin	Febrile-onset juvenile rheumatoid arthritis
	Psoriatic arthritis
	Reiter's syndrome
	Enteropathic arthritis
	Sarcoid arthritis
	Familial Mediterranean fever
	Septic arthritis (especially *Neisseria gonorrhoeae* and *meningitidis*)
	Hyperlipoproteinemia
	Hemachromatosis
	Fat necrosis due to pancreatic disease
	Amyloidosis
	Lyme arthritis
	Systemic lupus erythematosus
	Serum sickness
	Sporotrichosis
Nasopharynx and ear	Reiter's syndrome
	Gout
	Relapsing polychondritis
Eye	Juvenile rheumatoid arthritis
	Reiter's syndrome
	Relapsing polychondritis
	Sarcoidosis
Gastrointestinal tract	Crohn's disease
	Whipple's disease
	Hemachromatosis
	Fat necrosis due to pancreatic disease
	Ulcerative colitis
	Bypass arthritis
	Ulcerative colitis
Heart and circulation	Amyloidosis
	Reiter's syndrome
	Relapsing polychondritis
	Endocarditis
	Lyme arthritis
	Ankylosing spondylitis
	Systemic lupus erythematosus
Respiratory tract	Sarcoidosis
	Relapsing polychondritis
	Whipple's disease
	Tuberculosis
Nervous system	Meningococcal arthritis
	Neuropathic arthropathy
	Lyme arthritis
	Systemic lupus erythematosus
Genitourinary system	Systemic lupus erythematosus
	Amyloidosis
	Gout
Hematologic	Coagulopathies
	Gaucher's disease
	Hemachromatosis
	Myeloma/amyloid
	Leukemia

therapy or measures to provide symptomatic relief. Each of these disorders is capable of presenting with the explosive onset of inflammation over a few hours, but the "hyperacute" presentation is most typical of infection or gout. As a rule, the diagnosis of gout can be made immediately in almost all affected patients. Infectious arthritis can be diagnosed by Gram stain in some patients and proved by culture in most within 48 hours. The diagnosis of pseudogout is often uncertain until repeated aspirations are performed and cultures are negative. The presence of other conditions may be suggested by extra-articular disease features, but often laboratory testing and continued observation are needed before the diagnosis is certain. The following observations are intended to aid in the differential diagnosis of these entities.

Infectious Arthritis

In evaluating an acutely inflamed joint, one must first ask, "Is the likelihood of septic arthritis sufficient to hospitalize the patient?" Joint sepsis produces dramatic inflammation followed quickly by irreversible destruction of cartilage and bone. It may also be the initial sign of life-threatening systemic infection. In healthy adults, the signs are usually obvious. The patient complains of intense local pain and resists attempts to examine the affected joint. Superficial joints are swollen, warm, tender, sometimes red, and have markedly restricted range of motion. As a general rule, large joints are more frequently affected than small ones in the absence of local trauma or peripheral vascular disease.[9, 10, 23-26] The severity of constitutional symptoms varies with the organism and the host: fever, rigors, and leukocytosis are usually present in staphylococcal arthritis and frequently absent in gonococcal arthritis. Unfortunately, persons at highest risk for joint sepsis are those in whom confounding factors obscure symptoms or blunt the inflammatory response. Infection should be strongly suspected in less acutely "sick" appearing patients when both systemic risk factors, such as glucocorticoid therapy, immunodeficiency or immunosuppression, diabetes, intravenous drug abuse, or a remote focus of infection (e.g., pulmonary, cardiac, or genitourinary), *and* local pathology, such as inflammatory arthritis, effusions, penetrating trauma, previous injection of glucocorticoids, or a prosthetic joint, are present. Patients who have difficulty communicating, such as the very old and very young, may have occult infection of deep joints such as the hip for days or weeks that can remain undetected even in a hospital setting. In these patients, when a careful physical examination yields equivocal results, radionuclide scans may help identify joints that should be aspirated.

Although the clinical picture is never diagnostic of a particular infectious agent, certain presentations are characteristic. Gonococcal infection rarely escapes attention, because it tends to present as an inordinately painful monarticular or polyarticular arthritis or painful, hot, diffuse tenosynovitis in an otherwise vigorous person. However, there is frequent difficulty in establishing the diagnosis. This may result from failure to perform cultures on appropriate media or failure to carefully examine Gram stains from cervical or urethral discharges. In addition, tenosynovitis may be mistaken for a "sprain." We periodically admit patients to the hospital who are wearing elastic bandages obtained at other clinics for presumed trauma to the wrist. Although truly "migratory" arthritis is characteristic of gonococcal infection, the illness frequently presents in monarticular or additive forms. Skin lesions ranging from macules to pustules and vesicles are well described[27] but, in the author's experience, are usually quite subtle and most easily identified in retrospect when they disappear during treatment. Appropriate culture techniques are described later in the chapter. In suspected gonococcal infection, a dramatic response to penicillin alone within 24 hours may occur if treatment is instituted early and virtually always occurs within 72 hours if the organism is sensitive.[28]

Meningococcal arthritis occasionally presents with clinical and Gram stain findings identical to those of gonococcal disease. At initial presentation, some patients do not appear to be severely ill. Such patients may be misdiagnosed as having gonococcal arthritis[23] and obviously would not fare well on low-dose penicillin or outpatient regimens that have been proposed for treatment of presumed gonococcal infection.

Gram-negative infections should be suspected in the very young, very old, and intravenous drug abusers. Pain and swelling in the symphysis pubis, sacroiliac joints, or sternoclavicular joints in an intravenous drug abuser suggests gram-negative infection and should prompt aggressive diagnostic procedures.[29–34] Inflammation of diarthrodial joints in these patients is compatible with endocarditis or another source of hematogenously spread infection or immune complex disease related to acute or chronic hepatitis B infection.

Lyme arthritis presents as a true inflammatory arthritis weeks to months after initial exposure and after development of the early syndrome of fevers, arthralgias, lymphadenopathy, and rash. This curable infection should be suspected in patients with compatible symptoms, a history of travel to endemic areas, or coexistent neurologic or cardiac abnormalities. If infection is suspected, serum antibodies to *Borrelia burgdorferi* should be obtained.[35–38]

Viral illness, including hepatitis B, infectious mononucleosis, rubella, and rubella vaccination, may present with a serum sickness–like syndrome that can be manifested exclusively by inflammatory arthritis. It is usually nondestructive and self-limited.[23]

Crystal-Induced Arthritis

Crystal-induced arthritis commonly presents as acute monarticular arthritis. It is particularly likely when there is a history of recurrent, self-limited attacks of self-limited inflammation of the same joint. Fortunately, the most fulminant arthropathy, gout, is also the most easily and reliably diagnosed: mono-

sodium urate crystals can be identified in at least 95 percent of acute joint effusions by polarized microscopy and even in some asymptomatic joints.[39] Calcium pyrophosphate crystals, on the other hand, are often not identified initially in patients who are later diagnosed as having pseudogout.[40] Hydroxyapatite crystals present a particular problem in diagnosis, because they are reliably identified only by electron microscopy or Alzarian red stain.[41] As a general rule, identification of crystals in joint fluid does not prove the absence of coexistent infection. Crystal-induced arthropathies are particularly common and difficult to manage in patients who are uremic or undergoing dialysis.

Gouty arthritis is said to be definitely present when intracellular urate crystals are identified in synovial fluid and probably present if the crystals are extracellular. The most characteristic clinical features are extremely rapid onset of severe pain and inflammation and extension of the inflammatory process into the surrounding tissues, producing the appearance of cellulitis. Desquamation of overlying skin may occur as the attack progresses. In the ankle, the initial phases visually resemble the periarthritis of erythema nodosum, but the pain is much more severe.[42, 43] Podagra is characteristic but not pathognomonic of gout,[44] and first attacks of gout can occur in other large joints. It should be stressed that hyperuricemia does not establish the diagnosis of gouty arthritis, nor does normouricemia rule it out. Low-grade fever, associated with gout since it was first described by Thomas Sydenham in 1788, is more common in polyarticular than in monarticular gout. Although response to intravenous colchicine is not pathognomonic of gout, complete abolition of the inflammatory process by this intervention in appropriately selected patients is highly suggestive.

Calcium pyrophosphate dihydrate deposition is associated with acute or chronic inflammatory arthritis and may be superimposed on osteoarthritis.[40] Pseudogout, if untreated, tends to run a more prolonged time course than gout, reaching maximum severity after 1 to 3 days and resolving in 1 week or longer. A most taxing clinical problem commonly encountered is the combination of severe inflammation, often of a knee or wrist, and an initial joint aspiration containing 5000 or more leukocytes but no crystals in a patient who is elderly and may be obtunded or have coexistent risk factors for joint infection. Interpretation of subsequent arthrocentesis must address the issue of possible "strip mining" of crystals embedded in cartilage by an unrelated inflammatory process. If there is no history of recurrent similar attacks in the same joint, it may be most prudent to hospitalize and observe such patients until cultures are completed. The decision to administer antibiotics empirically in the interim is made on an individual basis.

Hemarthroses may result from trauma, hemangiomas, or other vascular malformations, excessive anticoagulation, or inherited coagulopathies.[45–47] Persistent bloody effusions should lead to consideration of a tumor, particularly pigmented villonodular synovitis.[48, 49]

Other Causes of Acute Inflammatory Arthritis

If a patient does not have one of the aforementioned disorders, there is a significant likelihood that the cause will remain elusive for a time and that the physician will be obliged to make a practical decision about how aggressively to pursue a diagnosis. Often it is possible to observe a patient with tolerable symptoms using nonspecific agents for symptomatic relief until the disorder either goes away or develops into polyarticular disease or until there are systemic findings that clarify the diagnosis. Therefore, the initial workup under these circumstances should be as focused as possible so that a satisfactory result can be achieved with the greatest possible economy of patient discomfort and medical resources.

It is useful to separate such patients according to whether or not they appear "sick" and have constitutional signs of illness. In general, if patients are suffering exclusively from a disorder that primarily causes arthritis, it is unusual for them to appear particularly toxic if there is only one symptomatic joint. Some systemic diseases also rarely cause constitutional signs. In these patients, the following disorders should be specifically considered.

Juvenile Rheumatoid Arthritis. Although the majority of children with juvenile rheumatoid arthritis (JRA) presenting as monarticular disease will eventually develop involvement of additional joints, about 25 percent will have isolated monarthritis that may recur intermittently into adulthood. Such patients tend to have persistent or recurrent nondestructive synovitis with no or minimal radiographic evidence of joint destruction. Antinuclear antibodies are more frequent than is rheumatoid factor; both monarticular disease and antinuclear antibodies correlate with the development of iritis.[50, 51]

Palindromic Rheumatism Versus Early Rheumatoid Arthritis. Episodic inflammation with total resolution of symptoms is often a prelude to rheumatoid arthritis,[52] particularly in patients who are rheumatoid factor positive.

Rheumatoid Arthritis. This disorder may present with acute or insidious onset on monarthritis. Often a detailed history will reveal gradual onset of fatigue or arthralgias. Physical examination may reveal unsuspected involvement of other joints, particularly the metatarsophalangeal joints.

Seronegative Arthropathies. Involvement of distal joints suggests Reiter's disease or psoriatric arthritis, as does the presence of fusiform swelling or "ray" involvement (inflammation of two or more adjacent joints on the same digit, often with swelling that appears to bridge involved joints). It should be remembered that up to 25 percent of patients with psoriatic arthritis have been reported to develop arthritis before psoriatic skin or nail changes.[53, 54] Careful examination of the scalp, eyebrows, unbilicus, and anal crease for psoriatic plaques and a search for pitting of the nail beds may yield evidence of unsuspected psoriasis. Urethritis, iritis, circinate balinitis, and keratoderma blennorrhagicum as well as previously mentioned evidence of axial involvement are consistent with Reiter's disease. Patients should be questioned about prior diarrhea or urethritis.[55-58] Lyme disease has been reported to present as a seronegative arthropathy.[59]

Arthropathies Associated with Systemic Illness. In patients who show significant signs of systemic illness, one should consider the following diagnoses.

Enteropathic Arthritis. Whipple's disease, which is quite rare, is well known to present frequently with arthritis at a time when the bowel disease is not evident. It may remain undiagnosed for years unless the diagnosis is carefully considered. Regional enteritis and ulcerative colitis are more likely to be symptomatic when arthritis develops.[60-62] Mild to moderately severe large joint arthritis in a seronegative patient with iron deficiency anemia or occult blood in the stool suggests these diagnoses.

Systemic Autoimmune Disease. Systemic lupus erythematosus occasionally presents with monarticular arthritis, although polyarthritis is more common.[63] Monarticular or large joint pain in a steroid-treated lupus patient suggests avascular necrosis[64] or infection. Sarcoidosis often presents as arthritis of the ankles, wrists, or knees, usually bilateral, which may be associated with erythema nodosum or hilar adenopathy.[65] Henoch-Schönlein purpura,[66] Takayasu's disease,[67] overlap syndromes,[68, 69] polymyalgia rheumatica,[70] or giant cell arteritis[71] can present with monarticular or polyarticular arthritis, although in many of these disorders, polyarthritis is the rule.

Familial Mediterranean fever typically causes exquisitely painful monarthritis with moderately impressive physical findings.[72, 73] The combination of fever and an evanescent rash suggests Still's disease[74] or rheumatic fever.[75] The combination of polyarthritis with ocular, nasal, or tracheal inflammation suggests Wegener's syndrome or relapsing polychondritis.[76]

CHRONIC INFLAMMATORY MONARTICULAR ARTHRITIS

Chronic Monarticular Inflammation. Many disorders that can present as acute monarticular inflammation will progress to polyarticular involvement, remit and relapse, or spontaneously resolve. Persistent monarticular inflammation raises special concern that a more narrow spectrum of disorders is present, particularly chronic infections or tumors. Synovial biopsy and arthroscopy may be useful in identifying the etiology of chronic monarthritis (see Chapter 36).

Chronic infections result from slow-growing organisms or the presence of foreign bodies in the joint. Typically, there are persistent signs of inflammation, including stiffness, pain, and warmth, and characteristically there is synovial thickening whether or not an effusion is present. Although symptoms need not be dramatic, they tend to be progressive and unremitting over a period of weeks to months, eventually resulting in significant distortion of the normal contours of the affected extremity and radiographic evidence of cartilage and bone destruction.

Tuberculosis, which is currently enjoying a resurgence in the United States, almost always affects a single diarthroidial joint.[77] A positive tuberculin test may be the only clue,[78-80] or there may be radiographic evidence of old and recent pulmonary involvement, vertebral osteomyelitis, or genitourinary or soft tissue infection. The infection may originate from a focus of subchondral bone, and radiographic evidence of osteomyelitis may be evident. Infection with atypical mycobacteria or *Candida*, coccidioidomycosis, or blastomycosis can produce similar syndromes.[79] Adequate tissue for all necessary stains and cultures can be reliably obtained by open biopsy, but arthrocentesis alone is clearly inadequate. Closed needle biopsy of the knee can yield diagnostic material, but it is the author's opinion that if stains are not diagnostic after closed needle biopsy, there should be little delay in obtaining a larger specimen.

Chronic infections may also result from penetrating wounds or the introduction of foreign bodies. Superficially located joints on the hands and the feet are most likely to be penetrated during normal activity, often without awareness on the part of the person. Sporotrichosis should be suspected in a gardener with involvement of a hand joint, especially if there is surrounding soft tissue reaction.[81]

Tumors should always be suspected when there is chronic monarticular inflammation, particularly pigmented villonodular synovitis.[82, 83] Metastases to synovium from solid tumors[84, 85] or joint involvement by hematologic malignancies are rare; however, as has been previously noted, tumors involving periarticular structures can mimic arthritis.

NONINFLAMMATORY MONARTICULAR ARTHRITIS

Structural joint disease can be said to be present when there is little synovial inflammation in proportion to the degree of destruction of bone and cartilage and the synovial fluid white blood cell count is less than 2000. Truly noninflammatory fluid, however, contains less than 200 cells per mm. Osteoarthritis may present as monarthritis, particularly in the knee, hip, shoulder, first radiocarpal joint, or first metatarsophalangeal joint (hallux rigidus). In addition, osteoarthritis may produce inflammatory changes in individual distal interphalangeal joints. In particular, inflammation associated with malalignment frequently occurs in the fifth distal interphalangeal joint. Although a history of gradual onset is usual, early symptoms may be ignored until overuse, entrapment

of a loose body, or some other mechanical event triggers obvious symptoms. Elderly patients with osteoarthritis may actually have inflammatory joint effusions containing calcium pyrophosphate crystals.[44] In monarticular disease, a predisposing factor, such as congenital dysplasia of the hip, trauma to or prior surgical removal of ligaments or fibrocartilage from the knee, prior inflammatory arthritis or infections, occupational stress, or extreme obesity, should be sought. Unless subjected to repeated physical stress, a patient with osteoarthritis will not present with isolated involvement of the elbows and wrists. Well-established symptoms are almost always associated with radiographic findings.

Osteoarthritis is much less likely to be present under the following circumstances.

Young Patient. Hip symptoms suggest congenital dysplasia of the hip or a slipped femoral capital epiphysis.[86, 87] Spontaneous osteonecrosis may occur in the hip (Legg-Calvé-Perthes disease), metatarsal bones (Freiberg's disease), capitellum of the humerus, or carpal lunate. Osteochondritis dissecans should be suspected in a child or teenager who, after minor trauma, develops relatively sudden onset of knee pain followed by mechanical dysfunction.[88]

Sudden Onset of Symptoms. Rapid development of "osteoarthritis" should lead to consideration of the possibility of a fracture related to osteopenia, an adjacent destructive process such as metastatic tumor, or avascular necrosis.

Osteonecrosis is a common cause of monarthritis of the hip, shoulders, and knees in young people with systemic diseases requiring glucocorticoid therapy. It occurs in a variety of other conditions such as alcoholism, barotrauma, hemoglobinopathies, diabetes, hyperlipidemia, hyperuricemia, and systemic lupus erythematosus. Patients may have minimal or negative radiographic findings, particularly during the early stages of the process when surgical core decompression or careful joint protection may offer some hope of favorably altering the clinical course. Clinical judgment is therefore required to select those patients for whom sensitive but expensive diagnostic procedures, such as MR or radionuclide bone scanning, are indicated.

DIAGNOSTIC STUDIES

Synovial Fluid Analysis

The primary purpose of synovial fluid analysis is to answer the following questions: is the effusion inflammatory? is it infected? does it contain intracellular or extracellular crystals? Decisions about how to handle joint fluid are aided by the clinical setting but also should reflect the gross appearance of the fluid at the time of aspiration. The more the specimen resembles pus, the more vigorously infection and crystal disease should be sought and the more persistently attempts should be made to obtain as much fluid as possible. If fluid is scarce, much valuable information can be obtained by sending a single drop for culture and placing a drop on a slide and immediately performing polarized microscopy and a Gram stain. If there is sufficient fluid also to obtain a cell count and differential white blood cell count, then most of the important information will have been obtained. Typical findings in monarticular arthritis are shown in Table 22–3.[89, 90] Synovial fluid analysis is discussed in detail in Chapter 36.

Cultures

If septic arthritis is a possibility, blood, synovial fluid, and urine cultures are indicated. As previously noted, gonococcal cultures are indicated in almost all patients; cervical-urethral, rectal, and pharyngeal cultures should be placed on Thayer-Martin medium. Cultures from normally sterile sites, including the synovial cavity, tenosynovial space, and intracutaneous lesions, should be placed on chocolate agar without added preservative. Occasionally, cultures of synovium yield bacteria, even though simultaneous fluid cultures are sterile (see Chapter 86).

Radiography

Plain radiographs of the affected and contralateral joints should almost always be obtained. In most patients with arthritis of less than 1 week's duration, no intra-articular pathology will be revealed, but the initial films may be important as a baseline for determining the extent of disease progression at follow-up. In those with no prior joint complaints, soft tissue calcification or evidence of intra-articular pathology not known to the patient, such as osteoarthritis, chondrocalcinosis, or loose bodies, is a frequent finding. An unsuspected bony lesion such as a fracture, evidence of osseous or hematologic malignancy, osteomyelitis, or Paget's disease may be detected. Care should be taken to include enough surrounding bone in the radiograph to identify such lesions.

In chronic monarthritis, useful information is usually present in the radiographs. Absence of pathology in inflammatory disease is most typical of pauciarticular JRA but is noted in many forms of inflammatory synovitis. These findings may also be noted in lupus, although alignment changes and osteopenia are more typical. Most chronic infectious processes will be associated with significant destruction. Marginal erosions and osteopenia suggest rheumatoid arthritis, whereas marginal erosions and normal or increased bone density suggest seronegative arthritis or chondrocalcinosis. Although symptoms are well known to precede radiographic changes in some patients with early osteoarthritis, the absence of radiographic changes in a patient with severe chronic joint pain suggests another diagnosis (see Chapter 37).

Nuclear Medicine

Radionuclide scans are useful primarily because of their sensitivity. They are employed when it is important to search for a site of infection that cannot be detected or localized by other means, e.g., in deeply buried joints that are difficult to examine, fibrocartilaginous joints in which range of motion is poorly tested, and the spine.

Technetium polyphosphate is used because of its safety, sensitivity, and convenience; however, it lacks specificity and localizes at virtually every site of intra-articular pathology of any kind, including osteoarthritis. Indium and gallium scans are more cumbersome than technetium scans and are more specific for infection, but these studies may be positive in periarticular soft tissue infections as well as osseous lesions. It has been said that the combination of a positive bone scan and a positive gallium scan is virtually diagnostic of musculoskeletal infection,[91] although these tests are infrequently employed together. In general, the decision to obtain a radionuclide scan implies the intent to obtain synovial fluid or a synovial biopsy if the scan is positive (see Chapter 37).

Magnetic Resonance Scanning

MR imaging has been shown to be superior to other imaging modalities in the diagnosis of ischemic necrosis of bone[92–94] and possibly also Legg-Calvé-Perthes disease,[95] particularly in early cases. Often a patient with clinical evidence of unilateral osteonecrosis will be found by MR imaging to have evidence of early changes on the opposite side. MR imaging continues to have increasing applications in evaluation of articular and periarticular disease. In the knee, it provides a more accurate and noninvasive alternative to arthrography for detection of meniscal and cruciate ligament injuries.[96, 97] MR can identify fractures that are occult on plain radiographs. Because of its superior definition of soft tissue pathology, MR is useful in investigating deep infections about the hip, such as psoas abscesses, which may mimic arthritis.[98] MR is also useful in detecting disorders of alignment, mass lesions, and cord abnormalities in the spine.[91] Recent studies indicate that MR with gadolinium can also be useful in identifying the extent of rheumatoid synovitis.[99, 100] Although superior in most cases to CT scanning in detecting subchondral bone and marrow involvement by tumor or osteomyelitis, it does not provide the ability to survey the entire body that is characteristic of radionuclide scans. Trabecular bone pathology, such as osteonecrosis, osteomyelitis, solid tumors, hematologic malignancies, and infarctions in hemoglobinopathies, are well demonstrated. Although not infallible, MR imaging is the modality of choice in evaluation of possible osteonecrosis and is more likely than radionucleotide scanning to identify bilateral disease. Periarticular pathology, including tendon ruptures, ligamentous tears, soft tissue tumors, and infections, can be demonstrated (see Chapter 37).

Synovial and Bone Biopsy

Synovial biopsy plays a major role in the diagnosis of chronic unexplained monarticular arthritis.[101] Tuberculous or fungal synovitis is more frequently identified by staining and culture of open biopsy material than by similar studies of synovial fluid. It is the author's opinion that in the knee, closed-needle biopsy should be performed initially, rather than open biopsy. Arthroscopic or open biopsy should follow promptly if histologic studies do not yield a diagnosis. In other joints, however, arthroscopic or open biopsy is usually the procedure of choice in most adults. In acute inflammatory arthritis, surgical biopsy is indicated in the diagnosis of infection of fibrocartilaginous joints, such as the sacroiliac and sternoclavicular joints, and probably the symphysis pubis if an initial attempt at aspiration is not diagnostic.[102-104] General anesthesia is often required for pain control (see Chapter 36).

If osteomyelitis is suspected, immediate consideration should be given to obtaining a bone biopsy prior to initiating antibiotic therapy.[105]

References

1. Radin, E. L.: Chondromalacia of the patella. Bull. Rheum. Dis. 34:1, 1984.
2. Lagier, R.: Synovial reaction caused by adjacent malignant tumors: Anatomicopathological study of three cases. J. Rheumatol. 4:65, 1977.
3. Feagin, J. A. Jr.: The office diagnosis and documentation of common knee problems. Clin. Sports Med. 8:453, 1989.
4. Isenberg, D. A., and Schoenfield, Y.: The rheumatologic complications of hematologic disorders. Semin. Arthritis Rheum. 12:348, 1983.
5. Altman, R. D.: Paget's disease of bone (osteitis deformans). Bull. Rheum. Dis. 34:1, 1984.
6. Larsson, L. G., and Baum, J.: The syndromes of bursitis. Bull. Rheum. Dis. 34:1, 1984.
7. Ho, G., Jr., Tice, A. D., and Kaplan, S. R.: Septic bursitis in the prepatellar and olecranon bursae. Ann. Intern. Med. 89:21, 1978.
8. Viggiano, D. A., Garrett, J. C., and Clayton, M. L.: Septic arthritis presenting as olecranon bursitis in patients with rheumatoid arthritis. J. Bone Joint Surg. 62A:1011, 1980.
9. Ho, G., Jr., and Su, E. Y.: Antibiotic therapy of septic bursitis. Arthritis Rheum. 24:905, 1981.
10. Brogadir, S. P., Schimmer, B. M., and Myers, A. R.: Spectrum of the gonococcal arthritis-dermatitis syndrome. Semin. Arthritis Rheum. 8:177, 1979.
11. McCord, W. C., Nies, K. M., and Louie, J. S.: Acute venereal arthritis. Arch. Intern. Med. 137:858, 1977.
12. Dorwart, B. B.: Carpal tunnel syndrome: A review. Semin. Arthritis Rheum. 14:134, 1984.
13. Spinner, R. J., Bachman, J. W., and Amadio, P. C.: The many faces of carpal tunnel syndrome. Mayo Clin. Proc. 64:829, 1989.
14. Putten, J.: Neurological Differential Diagnosis. New York, Springer Verlag, 1980.
15. Gibson, R. K., Rosenthal, S. J., and Lukert, B. P.: Pyomyositis. Am. J. Med. 11:421, 1982.
16. Chedozi, L. C.: Pyomyositis. Am. J. Surg. 137:255, 1979.
17. Kallen, P. S., Louie J. S., Nies, K. M., and Bayer, A. S.: Infectious myositis and related syndromes. Am. J. Med. 11:421, 1982.
18. Goldenberg, D. L.: Infectious arthritis complicating rheumatoid arthritis and other chronic rheumatic disorders. Arthritis Rheum. 32:496, 1989.
19. Resnick, D., and Niwayana, G.: Reiter's disease. In Resnick, D., and Niwayana, G. (eds.): Diagnosis of Bone and Joint Disorders. 2nd ed. Philadelphia, W. B. Saunders Company, 1988, pp. 1171–1199.
20. Resnick, D., and Niwayana, G.: Psoriatic arthritis. In Resnick, D., and Niwayana, G. (eds.): Diagnosis of Bone and Joint Disorders. 2nd ed. Philadelphia, W. B. Saunders Company, 1988, pp. 1218–1251.
21. Resnick, D.: Enteropathic arthritis. In Resnick, D., and Niwayana, G. (eds.): Diagnosis of Bone and Joint Disorders. Philadelphia, W. B. Saunders Company, 1981.
22. Gotuzzo, E., Alarcon, G. S., Bocanegra, T. S. Carrillio, C., Guerra, J. C., Rolands, I., and Espinoza, L. R.: Articular involvement in human brucellosis: A retrospective analysis of 304 cases. Semin. Arthritis Rheum. 12:245, 1982.
23. Goldenberg, D. L., and Reed, J. I.: Bacterial arthritis. N. Engl. J. Med. 312:764, 1985.
24. Sharp, J. T., Lidsky, M. D., Duffy, J., and Duncan, M. W.: Infectious arthritis. Arch. Intern. Med. 139:1125, 1979.
25. Goldenberg, D. L., and Cohen, A. S.: Acute infectious arthritis. Am. J. Med. 60:369, 1976.
26. Rosenthal, J., Bole, G. G., and Robinson, W. D.: Acute nongonococcal infectious arthritis. Arthritis Rheum. 23:889, 1980.
27. Abu-Nassar, H., Hill, N., Fred, H. I., and Yow, E. M.: Cutaneous manifestations of gonoccocemia. Arch. Intern. Med. 112:145, 1963.
28. Seifert, M. H., Warin, A. P., and Miller, A.: Articular and cutaneous manifestations of gonorrhoea: Review of sixteen cases. Ann. Rheum. Dis. 33:140, 1974.
29. Miskew, M. D., Block, R. A., and Witt, P. F.: Aspiration of infected sacroiliac joints. J. Bone Joint Surg. 61A:1071, 1979.
30. Gordon, G., and Kabins, S. A.: Pyogenic sacroiliitis. Am. J. Med. 69:50, 1980.
31. Bayer, A. S., Chow, A. W., Louie, J. S., and Guze, L. B.: Sternoarticular pyoarthrosis due to gram-negative bacilli. Arch. Intern. Med. 137:1036, 1977.
32. Bayer, A. S., Chow, A. W., Louie, J. S., Nies, K. M., and Guze, L. B.: Gram-negative bacillary septic arthritis: Clinical, radiographic, therapeutic, and prognostic features. Semin. Arthritis Rheum. 7:123, 1977.
33. Lewkonia, R. M., and Kinsella, T. D.: Pyogenic sacroiliitis: Diagnosis and significance. J. Rheumatol. 8:153, 1981.
34. Goldin, R. H., Chow, A. W., Edwards, J. E., Jr., Louie, J. S., and Guze, L. B.: Sternoarticular septic arthritis in heroin users. N. Engl. J. Med. 289:616, 1973.
35. Steere, A. C., Malawista, S. E., Hardin, J. A., Ruddy, S., Askenase, P. W., and Andiman, W. A.: Erythema chronicum migrans and Lyme arthritis. Ann. Intern. Med. 86:685, 1977.
36. Steere, A. C., Malawista, S. E., Newman, J. H., Spieler, P. N., and Bartenhagen, N. H.: Antibiotic therapy in Lyme disease. Ann. Intern. Med. 93:1, 1980.
37. Shrestha, M., Grodzicki, R. L., and Steere, A. C.: Diagnosing early Lyme disease. Am. J. Med. 78:235, 1985.
38. Steere, A. C.: Lyme disease. N. Engl. J. Med. 321:586, 1989.
39. Bomalaski, J. S., Lluberas, G., and Schumacher, H. R., Jr.: Monosodium urate crystals in the knee joints of patients with asymptomatic nontophaceous gout. Arthritis Rheum. 29:1480, 1986.
40. Masuda, I., and Ishikawa, K.: Clinical features of pseudogout attack: A review of fifty cases. Clin. Orthop. Rel. Res. 229:123, 1988.
41. Gatter, R. A.: A Practical Handbook of Joint Fluid Analysis. Philadelphia, Lea & Febiger, 1984.
42. Yu, T.: Diversity of clinical features in gouty arthritis. Semin. Arthritis Rheum. 13:360, 1984.
43. Grahame, R., and Scott, J. T.: Clinical survey of 354 patients with gout. Ann. Rheum. Dis. 29:461, 1970.
44. McCarty, D. J.: Calcium pyrophosphate dihydrate crystal deposition disease—1975. Arthritis Rheum. 19:275, 1976.
45. Ahlberg, A., and Silwer, J.: Arthropathy in von Willebrand's disease. Acta Med. Scand. 41:539, 1970.
46. Wild, J. H., and Zvaifler, N. J.: Hemarthrosis associated with sodium warfarin therapy. Arthritis Rheum. 19:98, 1976.
47. McLaughlin, G. E., McCarty, D. J., Jr., and Segal, B. L.: Hemarthrosis complicating anticoagulant therapy. J.A.M.A. 196:202, 1966.
48. Calabro, J. J.: Cancer and arthritis. Arthritis Rheum. 10:553, 1967.
49. Myers, B. W., and Masi, A. T.: Pigmented villonodular synovitis and tenosynovitis: A clinical epidemiologic study of 166 cases and literature review. Medicine 59:223, 1980.
50. Chylack, L. T., Jr.: The ocular manifestations of juvenile rheumatoid arthritis. Arthritis Rheum. 20(Suppl.):224, 1976.
51. Cassidy, J. T., Sullivan, D. B., and Petty, R. E.: Clinical patterns of chronic iridocyclitis in children with juvenile rheumatoid arthritis. Arthritis Rheum. 20(Suppl.):224, 1976.
52. Schumacher, H. R.: Palindromic onset of rheumatoid arthritis. Arthritis Rheum. 25:361, 1982.
53. Wright, V.: Psoriasis and arthritis. Ann. Rheum. Dis. 15:348, 1956.

54. Sherman, M. S.: Psoriatic arthritis. J. Bone Joint Surg. 34:831, 1952.
55. Good, A. E.: Reiter's disease: A review with special attention to cardiovascular and neurologic sequelae. Semin. Arthritis Rheum. 3:252, 1974.
56. Calin, A., and Fries, J.: An "experimental" epidemic of Reiter's syndrome revisited: Follow-up evidence on genetic and environmental factors. Ann. Intern. Med. 84:564, 1976.
57. McEwen, C., DiTata, D., Lingg, C., Porini, A., Good, A., and Rankin T.: Ankylosing spondylitis and spondylitis accompanying ulcerative colitis, regional enteritis, psoriasis, and Reiter's disease: A comparative study. Arthritis Rheum. 14:291, 1971.
58. Calin, A.: Reiter's syndrome. Med. Clin. North Am. 61:365, 1977.
59. Weyand, C., and Goronzy, I.: Immune response to *Borrelia burgdorferi* in patients with reactive arthritis. Arthritis Rheum. 32:1057, 1989.
60. LeVine, M. E., and Dobbins, W. O., III: Joint changes in Whipples disease. Semin. Arthritis Rheum. 3:79, 1973.
61. Weiner, S. R., and Utsinger, P.: Whipple disease. Semin. Arthritis Rheum. 15:157, 1986.
62. Kelley, J. J., III, and Weisiger, B. B.: The arthritis of Whipple's disease. Arthritis Rheum. 6:615, 1963.
63. Ropes, M. W.: Systemic lupus erythematosus. Cambridge, Harvard University Press, 1976.
64. Zizic, T. M., Hungerford, D. S., and Stevens, M. B.: Ischemic bone necrosis in systemic lupus erythematosus. Medicine 59:134, 1980.
65. Spilberg, I., Siltzbach, L. E., and McEwen, C.: The arthritis of sarcoidosis. Arthritis Rheum. 12:126, 1969.
66. Cream, J. J., Gumpel, J. M., and Peachey, R. D. G.: Schönlein-Henoch purpura in the adult. Q. J. Med. 39:461, 1970.
67. Hall, S., Barr, W., Lie, J. T., Stanson, A. W., Kazmier, F. J., and Hunder, G. G.: Takayasu arthritis. Medicine 64:89, 1985.
68. Bennett, R. M., and O'Connell, D. J.: Mixed connective tissue disease: A clinicopathologic study of 20 cases. Semin. Arthritis Rheum. 10:25, 1980.
69. Nimelstein, S. H., Brody, S., McShane, D., and Holman, H. R.: Mixed connective tissue disease: A subsequent evaluation of the original 25 patients. Medicine 59:239, 1980.
70. Healey, L.: Long-term follow-up of polymyalgia rheumatica: Evidence for synovitis. Semin. Arthritis Rheum. 23:322, 1984.
71. Ginsburg, W. W., Cohen, M. D., Hall, S. B., Vollertsen, R. S., and Hunder, G. G.: Seronegative polyarthritis in giant cell arthritis. Arthritis Rheum. 28:1362, 1985.
72. Meyerhoff, J.: Familial Mediterranean fever: Report of a large family, review of the literature, and discussion of the frequency of amyloidosis. Medicine 59:66, 1980.
73. Sohar, E., Pras, M., and Gafni, J.: Familial Mediterranean fever and its articular manifestations. Clin. Rheum. Dis. 1:195, 1975.
74. Larson, E. B.: Adult Still's disease. Medicine 63:82, 1984.
75. Ben-Dov, I., and Berry, E.: Acute rheumatic fever in adults over the age of 45 years: An analysis of 23 patients together with a review of the literature. Semin. Arthritis Rheum. 10:100, 1980.
76. Michet, C. J., Jr., McKenna, C. H., Luthra, H. S., and O'Fallon, W. M.: Relapsing polychondritis. Ann. Intern. Med. 104:74, 1986.
77. Nathanson, L., and Cohen, W.: A statistical and roentgen analysis of two hundred cases of bone and joint tuberculosis. Radiology 36:550, 1940.
78. Berney, S., Goldstein, M., and Bishko, F.: Clinical and diagnostic features of tuberculosis arthritis. Am. J. Med. 53:36, 1972.
79. Goldenberg, D. L., and Cohen, A. S.: Arthritis due to tuberculous and fungal microorganisms. Clin. Rheum. Dis. 4:211, 1978.
80. Alvarez, S., and McCabe, W. R.: Extrapulmonary tuberculosis revisited: A review of experience at Boston City and other hospitals. Medicine 63:25, 1984.
81. Wilson, D. E., Mann, J. J., Bennett, J. E., and Utz, P.: Clinical features of extracutaneous sporotrichosis. Medicine 63:25, 1984.
82. Byers, P. D., Cotton, R. E., Deacon, W. W., Lowy, M., Newman, P. H., Sissons, H. A., and Thompson, A. D.: The diagnosis and treatment of pigmented villonodular synovitis. J. Bone Joint Surg. 50:290, 1968.
83. Docken, W. P.: Pigmented villonodular synovitis. Semin. Arthritis Rheum. 9:1, 1979.
84. Goldenberg, D. L., Kelley, W., and Gibbons, R. B.: Metastatic adenocarcinoma of synovium presenting as an acute arthritis. Arthritis Rheum. 18:107, 1975.
85. Cadman, N. L., Soule, E. H., and Kelly, P. J.: Synovial sarcoma. Cancer 18:613, 1965.
86. Wilson, P. D., Jacobs, B., and Schecter, L.: Slipped capital femoral epiphysis. J. Bone Joint Surg. 14:549, 1967.
87. Ponseti, I. V., and McClintock, R.: The pathology of slipping of the upper femoral epiphysis. J. Bone Joint Surg. 38A:71, 1956.
88. Pappas, A. M.: The osteochondroses. Pediatr. Clin. North Am. 14:549, 1967.
89. Hollander, J. L., Reginato, A., and Torralba, T. P.: Examination of synovial fluid as a diagnostic aid in arthritis. Med. Clin. North Am. 50:1280, 1966.
90. Cohen, A. S., and Goldenberg, D.: Synovial Fluid in Laboratory Diagnostic Procedures in the Rheumatic Diseases. New York, Grune & Stratton, 1984.
91. Modic, M. T., Feiglin, D. H., Piraino, D. W., Boumphrey, F., Weinstein, M. A., Duchesneau, P. M., and Rehm, S.: Vertebral osteomyelitis: Assessment using MR radiology. B.R.S. Inform. Tech. 157:157, 1985.
92. Thickman, D., Axel, L., Kresel, H. Y., Steinberg, M., Chen H., Velchick, M., Fallon, M., and Dalinka, M.: Magnetic resonance imaging of avascular necrosis of the femoral head. Skeletal Radiol. 15:133, 1986.
93. Totty, W. G., Murphy, W. A., Ganz, W. I., Kumar, B., Daum, W. J., and Siegel, B. A.: Magnetic resonance imaging of the normal and ischemic femoral head. A.J.R. 143:1273, 1984.
94. Mitchell, M. D., Kundel, H. L., Steinberg, M. E., Kressel, H. Y., Alavi, A., and Axel, L.: Avascular necrosis of the hip: Comparison of MR, CT, and scintigraphy. A.J.R. 147:67, 1986.
95. Scoles, P. V., Yoon, Y. S., Makley, J. T., and Kalamchi, A.: Nuclear magnetic resonance imaging in Legg-Calve-Perthes disease. J. Bone Joint Surg. 66:1357, 1984.
96. Turner, D. A., Prodromos, C. C., Petasnick, J. P., and Clark, J. W.: Acute injury of the ligaments of the knee: Magnetic resonance evaluation. Radiology 154:717, 1985.
97. Reicher, M. A., Hartzman, S., Duckwiler, G. R., Bassett, L. W., Anderson, L. J., and Gold, R. H.: Meniscal injuries: Detection using MR imaging. Radiology 159:753, 1986.
98. Weintraub, J. C., Cohen, J. M., and Maravilla, K. R.: Iliopsoas muscles: MR study of normal anatomy and disease. Radiology 156:435, 1985.
99. Bjorkengren, A. G., Geborek, P., Rydholm, U., and Petterson, H.: MR imaging of the knee in acute rheumatoid arthritis: Synovial uptake of godolinium-DOTA. A.J.R. 155:329, 1990.
100. Kursunoglu-Brahme, S., Riccio, T., Weisman, M. H., Resnick, D., Zvaifler, N., Sanders, M. E., and Fix, C.: Rheumatoid knee: Role of gadopentetate-enhanced MR imaging. Radiology 176:831, 1990.
101. Schumacher, H. R.: Joint pathology in infectious arthritis. Clin. Rheum. Dis. 4:33, 1978.
102. Sequeira, W., Jones, E., Siegel, M. E., Lorenz, M., and Kallick, C.: Pyogenic infections of the public symphysis. Ann. Intern. Med. 96:604, 1982.
103. Roca, R. P., and Yoshikawa, T. T.: Primary skeletal infections in heroin users: A clinical characterization, diagnosis, and therapy. Clin. Orthop. Rel. Res. 144:238, 1979.
104. Gordon, G., and Kabins, S. A.: Pyogenic sacroiliitis. Am. J. Med. 69:50, 1980.
105. Evarts, C. M.: Diagnostic techniques: Closed biopsy of bone. Clin. Orthop. Rel. Res. 107:100, 1975.

Polyarticular Arthritis

INTRODUCTION

Chronic polyarticular pain is the most common symptom complex bringing patients to a rheumatologist. In a review of my own office and hospital consultations, 58 percent of patients were seen because of chronic pain in multiple joints. This is in accordance with the experience of others.[1]

Not only is the evaluation of chronic polyarthritis the most common intellectual exercise facing the rheumatologist, but also it is one of the most rewarding. In most of the conditions to be discussed, it is the skilled, experienced physician, using the "tools" of history and physical examination, who can formulate a correct diagnosis and treatment plan. Although radiographs and certain laboratory tests are helpful, they are used primarily as adjuncts, and their findings are virtually never diagnostic by themselves. There are few areas left in medicine where the bedside skills of the physician are so important, and few areas that share the excitement of physicians being able to use their experience and intellectual abilities to the benefit of patients.

It is the goal of this chapter to present a logical methodology for dealing with individuals presenting with chronic polyarticular pain.

DIFFERENTIAL DIAGNOSIS

Arthritis versus Arthralgia. In the minds of most patients, "arthritis" is usually thought of as a *disease*, one whose manifestation is joint pain. Most people regard all joint pains as related, so that the first problem facing the clinician is to determine whether arthritis is, in fact, present, and then, if it is, which of the patient's complaints are related to the arthritis. Because of the tendency to lump together all musculoskeletal pain, considerable skill in history-taking is required, along with considerable patience and tact.

As is apparent, the first problem one faces in evaluating a patient with polyarticular complaints is establishing the *type* of problem present. In some cases, this is relatively easy, whereas other cases will challenge all of the physician's skills. Table 23–1 lists the major considerations in patients with chronic polyarticular pain.

Tendinitis and Related Disorders. These include painful shoulder syndromes, tennis elbow (lateral epicondylitis), golfer's elbow (medial epicondylitis), trochanteric bursitis, prepatellar bursitis, Achilles tendinitis, and tendinitis along the radial aspect of the wrist (de Quervain's disease). Whereas nearly all of these are overuse syndromes, the activity involved need not be particularly strenuous. Repetitive light activities (e.g., secretarial work) are frequently the culprits. In these syndromes, pain is often maximal at the beginning of an activity and then starts to subside as the activity is continued. Although these conditions often present as monarticular pain (e.g., tennis elbow), a surprisingly large number of patients have polyarticular pain. A thorough history, including a description of job and sports activities, is essential. In many cases, physical examination reveals areas of local tenderness near, but distinct from, the joint. Pain may be exacerbated by movement of the affected structures against resistance. For example, a useful test for lateral epicondylitis is to ask the patient to attempt wrist extension against resistance, which produces pain over the lateral epicondyle and along the extensor surface of the proximal forearm. Swelling, if present at all, is usually minimal and limited to tendon sheaths and bursae, rather than joints.

Muscle Disorders. This group includes inflammatory muscle diseases (polymyositis), metabolic disorders, postinfectious syndromes, and dystrophies. Although weakness predominates in most of these conditions, and arthritis therefore is not a serious consideration, an occasional patient will present with periarticular pain as a primary complaint. This pain is usually maximal with fatigue (as at the end of the day), and night cramps may also be present. Careful examination will reveal muscle weakness, although considerable skill and experience are necessary to determine whether weakness is "real" or apparent, that is, the sudden relaxation of muscles induced by pain. Refer to Chapter 69 for a detailed discussion of muscle diseases.

Table 23–1. DIFFERENTIAL DIAGNOSIS OF POLYARTICULAR PAIN

Polyarthritis	Neuropathies
Tendinitis	Diseases of the spine
Muscle disorders	Primary bone diseases
Polymyalgia rheumatica	Periostitis
Vasculitis	Fibrositis
Vaso-occlusive disease	Malingering

Polymyalgia Rheumatica. This disorder of the elderly is associated with severe proximal muscle pain and minimal objective findings. Since many of these patients have pre-existing polyarticular disorders, such as osteoarthritis and tendinitis, it requires some skill and experience to differentiate among these problems. In this condition, a careful history is by far the most important part of the examination; it will be dominated by severe pain and stiffness that the patient will almost always localize to muscle (see Chapter 65). Several authors[2, 3, 3a] have pointed out the difficulty in distinguishing polymyalgia rheumatica from older-onset rheumatoid arthritis and have stressed that in the early stages it may be impossible to tell them apart.

Vasculitis. Although frank *arthritis* is an uncommon manifestation of vasculitis, joint or muscle pain, often severe, is present in the majority of patients. The pain is often described as deep, aching, and constant. Most patients, of course, are systemically ill, with fever, weight loss, and a variety of nonarticular problems (see Chapter 64).

Vaso-occlusive Diseases. These include atherosclerosis, cholesterol emboli, diabetes, Raynaud's disease, and Buerger's disease. If the disease is in small vessels, pain may be prominent in the digits, and there will usually be overlying skin changes, including pallor, cyanosis, and purpura. The pain, in this case, is usually burning or aching and is often severe at night. If proximal vessels are involved, a more typical pattern of claudication will be present. Patients with aortoiliac disease, presenting as claudication in the buttocks and thighs, often appear in the rheumatologist's office. The syndrome of widespread cholesterol embolization can be particularly difficult for the rheumatologist to diagnose, since these patients may have polyarthralgias, myalgias, renal disease, elevated erythrocyte sedimentation rates, eosinophilia, and positive test results for rheumatoid factor and antinuclear antibody.[4]

Neurologic Diseases. These include peripheral neuropathies, compression neuropathies such as the carpal tunnel syndrome, and infiltrative diseases including amyloidosis and Waldenström's macroglobulinemia. Pain is usually associated with paresthesias and is usually worse at night. Although patients may localize pain to joints, it is more typically diffuse, and examination will reveal no objective joint abnormalities. However, since these conditions are more frequent in the elderly, who may have pre-existing joint disease, a careful history and physical examination are often necessary to differentiate between neuropathies and polyarthritis.

Diseases of the Spine. A variety of diseases of the spine, including spinal stenosis (congenital or acquired), spondylolisthesis, and tumors of the lower cord and cauda equina, may present in a similar fashion. The pain is usually primarily in the buttocks and is worse with certain postures or activities. In spinal stenosis, for example, pain is typically that of *neurogenic claudication*, with aching in the buttocks and thighs brought on by certain activities—often worse *going down hills* or steps. In elderly patients, many with pre-existing hip disease, one must be especially careful in evaluating these complaints. It is especially unfortunate to see patients who, following bilateral total hip replacement, continue to complain of their original pain. (Thorough approaches to diagnoses of back and neck pain are detailed in Chapters 25 and 27.)

Primary Bone Diseases. Metastatic tumors and myeloproliferative disorders may masquerade as polyarticular arthritis. In childhood, leukemia is especially apt to present as widespread joint pain, and any large series of patients with the initial diagnosis of juvenile rheumatoid arthritis will contain a small percentage who ultimately are found to have leukemia.[5, 6] In adults, myeloma and a variety of widely metastatic cancers present as bone (and joint) pain. In childhood leukemia, joint effusions, warmth, and tenderness may be present (see Chapter 70). These objective findings are rare in adults.

Other widespread bone diseases, especially osteonecrosis (see Chapter 97), may occasionally resemble polyarticular arthritis. When osteonecrosis involves peripheral joints, such as the knee and ankle, swelling and tenderness may be impressive,[7] and only a high index of suspicion will lead the physician to the correct diagnosis. Finally, in these days of vigorous sports participation by middle-aged and older individuals, it is not uncommon to see multiple stress fractures mimicking polyarthritis in the feet.

Periostitis. Periostitis, especially as part of the syndrome of *hypertrophic pulmonary osteoarthropathy*, may cause severe widespread joint pain, tenderness, and warmth. Careful examination will reveal tenderness not only around joint structures but also along the shaft of the bone (see Chapter 93).

Fibrositis and Psychogenic Pain Syndromes. Although these are not the same, the problem for the physician is similar, in that patients complain of a variety of musculoskeletal pains, yet objective examination reveals nothing other than areas of tenderness, usually in typical "trigger points" (see Chapter 29).

Malingering. These people are similar to those with psychogenic pain syndromes, but they have a clear-cut objective—that of achieving some sort of compensation for an injury or disease.

Polyarticular Arthritis. The term *arthritis* implies primary joint disease, so that patients must have had either historical or (preferably) physical evidence of joint disease. Interestingly, joint swelling, one of the most important physical findings, is not very valuable historically, because patients are usually unable to evaluate swelling unless it is severe. In addition to the subjective tightness that many painful joints manifest, a history of joint swelling may be used to describe conditions ranging from edema to urticaria.

Once the diagnosis is believed to be polyarticular arthritis, and not one of the other conditions listed in Table 23–1, a number of features must be sought in an attempt to differentiate the large numbers of diseases that can cause polyarticular arthritis.

HISTORY, PHYSICAL EXAMINATION, AND LABORATORY TESTS

History

As Mackenzie and others have pointed out, the clinical history is "by far the most important diagnostic tool"[8] in the evaluation of polyarticular disorders. A number of items deserve special attention.

Onset. One should direct attention early to the nature of the first symptoms. This is not always easy, especially if months or years have passed, because most patients prefer to talk about their current symptoms. It is also difficult because most patients think of "arthritis" as a disease, rather than a symptom or finding, and in their histories they may discuss all the joint problems of a lifetime, even obviously traumatic ones. It is sometimes frustrating to listen to individuals reciting irrelevant incidents of joint pain, but a little patience by the physician at this point usually is rewarded by real insight into the disease process.

Course. Once the true onset of disease has been defined, the physician must determine what has occurred since, and at what rate. Chronic arthritis may be relentlessly progressive from the onset, or it may be intermittent, with periods of partial or complete remission. In addition, as individual joints become involved, the process may be migratory or additive. The term "migratory polyarthritis" implies that previously involved joints become asymptomatic as new joints become inflamed, that is, the disease appears to "migrate" from joint to joint.

Specific Joint Symptoms. These include features such as locking, giving way without warning, palpable or audible crepitation, warmth, and swelling (may be unreliable historically—see preceding).

Systemic Symptoms. Patients seeing a doctor because of joint pain will often not see, unless asked, any relationship between their joint pain and such symptoms as fever, night sweats, weight loss, and generalized morning stiffness. These should be specifically sought and, when possible, quantified.

Rheumatic Disease Systems Review. In addition to systemic symptoms, the patient with arthritis must be specifically asked about conditions associated with various forms of arthritis, including rash (photosensitive? psoriatic? purpuric? petechial?), alopecia, Raynaud's phenomenon, sicca syndrome, uveitis, scleritis, oral or genital ulcers, urethritis or cervicitis, symptoms of inflammatory bowel disease, and pleurisy.

Past History. One should inquire about prior similar episodes, rheumatic fever and other unusual childhood diseases, and previous hospitalizations. It must be noted that previous diagnoses are not always correct. Therefore, a childhood history of rheumatic fever, for example, needs to be explored, since a number of children who have been labeled as having rheumatic fever in fact had juvenile rheumatoid arthritis, and vice versa. Special importance should be given to events of the immediate weeks or months preceding the joint disease. Many of these will not be associated in the patient's mind with the joint complaints and must therefore be specifically sought by the physician. These include, among others, prior sore throats, febrile illnesses, venereal disease, sexual contacts, diarrhea, rashes, and uveitis.

Family History. In addition to any type of arthritis, one should inquire about a family history of any associated condition such as psoriasis, uveitis, and inflammatory bowel disease. In patients suspected of ankylosing spondylitis, it may be important to obtain the history of any family members with chronic back pain and then attempt to determine the nature of that condition.

Physical Examination

With the large number of diseases presenting as polyarthritis, it is apparent that nothing short of a complete physical examination will suffice. Special consideration must be given to searching for certain features, such as small patches of psoriasis, psoriatic nails, oral and genital ulcers, funduscopic changes, murmurs, rubs, bruits, and peripheral pulses as well as a careful neurologic examination.

The examination of the musculoskeletal system, of course, must be systematic and thorough. Each joint should be examined for warmth, synovial thickening, effusions, crepitation, deformity, and tenderness. Both active and passive range of motion should be tested. The spine examination should include the range of motion of the cervical and lumbar spine, chest expansion, tenderness of the spinous processes and sacroiliac joints, abnormal curves, and muscle spasm.

Laboratory Tests

Nonspecific tests of inflammation include hematocrit, erythrocyte sedimentation rate, C-reactive protein, and white blood cell count. Tests sometimes helpful in specific diseases include rheumatoid factor, uric acid, protein electrophoresis, anti-streptolysin O, anti-*Borrelia* antibodies, and, rarely, HLA-B27 antigen.[9]

If obtainable, *synovial fluid* should be examined for viscosity (and/or mucin clot), white blood cell count, and glucose. If appropriate, further available tests might include polarized light examination for crystals; synovial fluid culture; Gram stain; occasionally, synovial fluid protein; and, rarely, examination of synovial fluid for complement levels or specific antibodies, such as rheumatoid factor.

Radiographic Features

Important radiographic features that may help in the evaluation include cartilage loss, erosions, periarticular osteoporosis, osteophytes, periostitis, and soft tissue changes. In many cases, properly chosen radiographs may be virtually diagnostic or may eliminate certain diseases from further consideration.

APPROACH TO THE PATIENT WITH POLYARTHRITIS

Once polyarthritis is established as the cause of joint pain, a logical, stepwise approach can lead to the correct diagnosis in nearly all cases (Table 23–2). The first problem is usually to determine whether or not the arthritis is *inflammatory*.

Historical features supporting inflammation include prolonged morning stiffness, fever, weight loss, and spontaneous joint swelling. Physical examination often reveals local warmth and synovial thickening as well as effusions. Laboratory findings of inflammation include anemia, an elevated sedimentation rate, and often more specific tests, such as rheumatoid factor or antinuclear antibody, may be helpful. Radiographs of affected joints may show uniform cartilage loss, periarticular osteoporosis, or erosions of subchondral bone. If synovial fluid is present, evaluation is most helpful, with reduced viscosity and an elevated white cell count being present in most inflammatory conditions.

If an *inflammatory polyarthritis* is present, there are a number of classification schemes that are useful. Often the most helpful first step is to ascertain the presence or absence of early *axial* involvement.

Table 23–2. CLASSIFICATION OF POLYARTHRITIS

Inflammatory
Peripheral, with Axial Involvement
　　Ankylosing spondylitis (especially juvenile onset), Reiter's
　　　syndrome, enteropathic arthritis, psoriatic arthritis
Peripheral Pauciarticular
　　Psoriatic arthritis, Reiter's syndrome, rheumatic fever,
　　　polyarticular gout, enteropathic arthritis, Behçet's disease,
　　　bacterial endocarditis
Peripheral Polyarticular
　　Rheumatoid arthritis, systemic lupus erythematosus, AIDS

Noninflammatory (Osteoarthritis)
Hereditary
　　Osteoarthritis of the hands, primary generalized
　　　osteoarthritis
Traumatic Osteoarthritis
　　Osteoarthritis following local injury, osteoarthritis of the
　　　knees in obese people, chondromalacia following
　　　aggressive exercise programs, osteoarthritis in the elderly
Metabolic Diseases (may have an unusual pattern)
　　Hemochromatosis, ochronosis, acromegaly
Idiopathic

Inflammatory Polyarthritis with Axial Involvement

Ankylosing spondylitis is the prototype of this group of diseases. Peripheral arthritis is common early in juveniles and young adults with ankylosing spondylitis, and in teenage boys it is often the only finding. The arthritis involves predominantly the lower extremities and includes knees, ankles, and feet in the majority of patients.[9] Enthesopathy, or pain at the sites of tendon and ligament attachment to bone, may be the dominant early feature, especially when the heels and feet are involved.

Reiter's syndrome usually causes a similar inflammatory polyarthritis involving primarily joints of the lower extremities but having a greater predilection for involvement of the feet, especially the metatarsophalangeal joints and heels. The axial disease may be limited to the sacroiliac joints or may be a prominent feature, with involvement of most of the lumbar spine. Although only one quarter to one third of patients with Reiter's syndrome have overt back disease on presentation, the majority develop either unilateral or bilateral sacroiliitis and spine disease during the course of the disease.[11] The extra-articular features of Reiter's syndrome, including conjunctivitis, urethritis, and mucocutaneous changes, are often not present at the same time as the arthritis and therefore must be sought historically (see Chapter 57).

Enteropathic arthritis,[12] or the arthritis of inflammatory bowel disease, may present as either axial or peripheral arthritis, or the two may coexist. The axial arthritis is identical to ankylosing spondylitis and is strongly associated with HLA-B27. Once present, the spondylitis runs a progressive course regardless of the activity of the bowel disease. Spondylitis typically develops at approximately the same time as does the bowel disease but may precede it by many years or, in some cases, may even follow the onset of the bowel disease. The peripheral arthritis, on the other hand, usually waxes and wanes with the activity of the bowel disease. The arthritis typically involves four or fewer joints at a given time, most prominently the large joints of the lower extremity. The arthritis is associated occasionally with erythema nodosum and, rarely, with pyoderma gangrenosum (see Chapter 59).

Psoriatic arthritis (see later) may cause both an axial and a peripheral arthritis, but the axial disease is infrequently an important presenting manifestation (see Chapter 58).

Whipple's disease typically causes a polyarthritis similar to Reiter's syndrome, with sacroiliitis plus a peripheral arthritis usually involving only a few joints at a time.

If axial arthritis includes prominent cervical spine involvement, especially early in the course, one must also consider various forms of *juvenile chronic polyarthritis*, including adult-onset Still's disease (see Chapter 70). Finally, in rare cases, typical adult rheumatoid arthritis may involve the spine, especially the cervical region, in the early stages.

Polyarthritis Limited to Peripheral Joints

Many classification systems can be used to differentiate these diseases, but one of the most helpful is to separate patients according to the number of involved joints. In this context, the term *pauciarticular* is generally used to describe disease affecting four or fewer joints, although certain latitude may be taken, such as counting the midfoot or wrist as a single joint. In addition, these arbitrary terms are usually used to describe the early stages only, since most of these diseases become polyarticular late in the course.

Pauciarticular Peripheral Arthritis

Psoriatic arthritis, which may precede skin disease in a minority of patients, usually begins as an asymmetric pauciarticular disease, often including distal interphalangeal joints or entire digits, producing the "sausage digit" appearance. The arthritis is typically asymmetric, with occasional patients showing severe damage of one group of joints, such as one hand, with no involvement of the contralateral side. There is a good correlation between psoriatic nail involvement and psoriatic arthritis, especially the pauciarticular form, but the overall correlation with the amount of psoriasis is not as strong. Occasionally, patients have extensive joint destruction owing to psoriatic arthritis, with only a few patches of skin and nail disease (see Chapter 58). Although most cases of psoriatic arthritis begin insidiously, the disease may, on occasion, present as an acute monarticular or oligoarticular disease resembling gout and may be precipitated by local trauma.[13]

Reiter's syndrome (see earlier) may spare the entire axial skeleton and may present in a manner very similar to that of psoriatic arthritis, but with a greater predilection for lower extremity disease (see Chapter 57).

Adult rheumatic fever, which seems to be increasing in frequency, often causes a very painful pauciarticular disease, most prominent in the larger joints of the lower extremities. The typical *migratory* pattern of childhood rheumatic fever is uncommon in adults,[14] and the response to aspirin less dramatic. Finally, although some fever is usually present, carditis is uncommon, and other features, such as chorea, rash, and subcutaneous nodules, are rare. In addition, the presentation in adults may be less "acute," with a more insidious arthritis developing over several days or 1 to 2 weeks (see Chapter 71).

Unfortunately, *gout* all too often presents to the rheumatologist as undiagnosed chronic polyarthritis. These are virtually always patients whose initial presentation was misdiagnosed, and in later stages chronic polyarticular gout can resemble rheumatoid arthritis. Particularly confusing, at times, is the syndrome of acute and chronic gouty arthritis superimposed on osteoarthritis of the finger joints.[15] A careful history of the disease onset is essential, and examination of synovial fluid will yield the diagnosis (see Chapter 76). Rarely, chronic *pseudogout* may present as polyarticular arthritis.

Behçet's disease, uncommon in the United States, almost invariably causes chronic polyarthritis limited to a few joints. The disease is characterized by very painful acute flare ups, often associated with oral, genital, and ophthalmologic manifestations.

Acquired immunodeficiency syndrome (AIDS) is being seen more and more by rheumatologists. Reiter's syndrome, psoriatic arthritis, and a painful polyarthritis possibly specific for human immunodeficiency virus (HIV) all have been described, frequently as the presenting manifestation of HIV infection.[16] Another presentation of HIV infection resembles systemic lupus erythematosus, with fever, rash, polyarthritis, proteinuria, and hematologic abnormalities.[17] Of course, many forms of septic polyarthritis may complicate HIV infection (see Chapter 73).

Enteropathic arthritis (see earlier) may present with only peripheral pauciarticular arthritis, usually strongly associated with the activity of the bowel disease. It characteristically involves larger joints of the lower extremities (see Chapter 59).

Relapsing polychondritis usually causes severe inflammation of the ears, nose, and sclera, associated with a pauciarticular arthritis. The joint disease often begins abruptly, may last several weeks, and is nondestructive. The most commonly involved joints are the knees and wrists, although generalized polyarthralgias are frequent. Low back pain, due to sacroiliitis, occurs in a minority of patients (see Chapter 81).

Sarcoidosis causes a number of articular problems. The most frequent is arthritis in association with the syndrome of erythema nodosum and bilateral hilar adenopathy. In these patients, the ankles are almost invariably involved, with knees being the next most frequent. Occasionally, in patients with long-standing sarcoidosis, a chronic, destructive polyarthritis resembling rheumatoid arthritis may develop (see Chapter 83).

The arthritis of *Lyme disease* is usually monarticular or oligoarticular, but a chronic symmetric polyarthritis has also been described.[18]

The arthritis of *bacterial endocarditis* is also typically monarticular or oligoarticular. However, polyarthralgias are common, and the frequent association of a positive rheumatoid factor test can add to the diagnostic difficulties.[22]

Amyloid arthropathy may include virtually all joints, but pauciarticular involvement of the upper extremities is most frequent. Bilateral shoulder disease may cause joint enlargement known as the shoulder pad sign. This finding, especially in association with carpal tunnel syndrome and purpura in skin folds, should always make one suspect primary amyloidosis. The amyloidosis caused by beta$_2$ (β_2)-microglobulin deposition in chronic dialysis patients is particularly prone to synovial and periarticular deposition and may present with an impressive destructive arthritis of large joints, especially the knees, shoulders, and hips[19] (see Chapter 82).

Finally, as mentioned earlier, ankylosing spondylitis may present without axial involvement, especially in juveniles.

Polyarticular Peripheral Arthritis

Rheumatoid arthritis, of course, is the prototype of this group of diseases (see Chapter 53). Indeed, because of its frequency, the differential diagnosis in patients with inflammatory polyarthritis is often thought of as "rheumatoid arthritis versus everything else." Rheumatoid arthritis accounts for about one fourth of all patients referred to rheumatologists.[1] However, if anything, more errors are made by overdiagnosis rather than by failure to recognize the disease, and rheumatologists frequently see patients with osteoarthritis, gout, and other conditions who are receiving therapy for rheumatoid arthritis. Typically beginning in multiple small joints in a symmetric fashion, rheumatoid arthritis has many variations, even including months or years of recurrent monarthritis, "palindromic rheumatism,"[20] before a typical pattern evolves. The symmetry of rheumatoid arthritis is sometimes overemphasized, and it should be stressed that this is a general, rough symmetry. It is quite rare to see rheumatoid arthritis cause extensive damage to one hand, for example, and completely spare the other. However, a specific joint, such as a particular metacarpophalangeal joint, need not be equally involved bilaterally.

The arthritis of rheumatoid arthritis is typically additive, with sequential involvement of groups of joints. Early in the course, especially, there may be impressive fluctuation in symptoms, but most joints will remain more or less symptomatic as new joints are involved. The earliest joints involved are usually small joints of the hands (Fig. 23–1; see also color section at the front of this volume) and feet, but the distal interphalangeal joints are spared until late in the course.

Systemic lupus erythematosus (see Chapter 61) often presents as chronic polyarthritis, and confusion with rheumatoid arthritis occurs frequently in such patients. The arthritis is typically intermittent, may be extremely painful, and is nondestructive. Mixed connective tissue disease may cause an identical arthritis.

Scleroderma often begins as painful swollen hands, with early contractures as a prominent feature. Indeed, the patient with puffy hands and Raynaud's phenomenon is often termed "undifferentiated connective tissue disease" in recognition of the fact that the condition of such patients may evolve into systemic lupus, scleroderma, mixed connective tissue disease, or rheumatoid arthritis. Some may remain "undifferentiated" for many years.

Psoriatic arthritis, although typically pauciarticular at onset, may evolve into a polyarticular disease resembling rheumatoid arthritis (see Chapter 58). This presents particular diagnostic problems in children, whose disease may resemble pauciarticular juvenile rheumatoid arthritis at onset and then evolve into a pattern resembling polyarticular juvenile or adult rheumatoid arthritis.[21]

Gonococcal arthritis, unlike the monoarthritis typical of most septic joint disease, usually presents with fever, widespread tenosynovitis, and papular or pustular skin lesions. As it evolves over several days, it may gradually involve one or more joints in a frankly purulent arthritis.

Noninflammatory Polyarthritis (Osteoarthritis)

Many of the features supporting the diagnosis of noninflammatory polyarthritis are simply the absence of features suggesting inflammation. However, there are a number of specific findings that are helpful in establishing a diagnosis of osteoarthritis.

Historically, the patient will usually describe pain primarily during and following use of the affected joints, with minimal pain at rest. Morning stiffness and gelling after periods of rest are likely to be brief, lasting no more than a few minutes. Swelling also is usually brought on by activity, often by a sudden increase in the level of activity. In some forms of osteoarthritis, notably nodal osteoarthritis of the hands, a careful family history is very important.

Physical examination often reveals coarse crepitation, and loose bodies and other debris may be palpable while the joint is carried through a range of motion. Bony osteophytes may be palpable, especially in the fingers.

Routine tests of inflammation will be normal unless another disease is present. Since osteoarthritis increases in frequency with advancing age, it should be stressed that positive tests for rheumatoid factor become less valuable in older people. The frequency of positive tests in healthy individuals is a function of age. Synovial fluid examination is very useful in establishing a diagnosis of osteoarthritis, with findings of a normal or only a slightly reduced viscosity, a low white blood cell count (usually fewer than 3000 cells per mm^3), and often bits of collagen and other debris.

The ultimate diagnostic test for osteoarthritis is the radiograph. There are a number of important biochemical changes in cartilage that precede radiographic changes, but for all practical purposes symptomatic osteoarthritis is always accompanied by radiographic changes.

Osteoarthritis of the hands (see Chapter 79), a hereditary disease much more prevalent in women, typically develops within a few years of the meno-

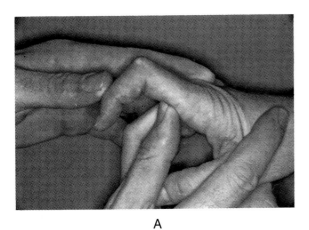
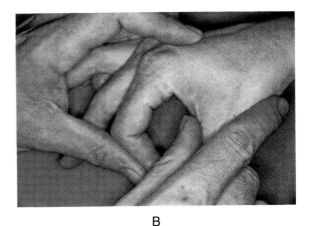

A   B

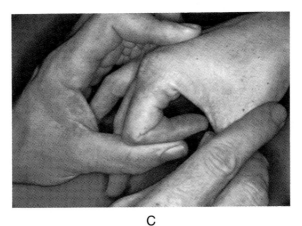

C

Figure 23–1. Bunnell's sign. This sign is used to distinguish synovitis of the proximal interphalangeal joint from spasm of the intrinsic muscles due to metacarpophalangeal synovitis as the cause of decreased motion of the proximal interphalangeal joint. *A,* With the metacarpophalangeal joint extended, decreased flexion of the proximal interphalangeal joint is noted. If normal flexion is noted (i.e., the tip of the finger can touch the volar pad), then involvement of all three joints (metacarpophalangeal, proximal interphalangeal, and distal intraphalangeal) is excluded. *B,* With the metacarpophalangeal joint flexed, the contracted intrinsic muscles are relaxed. Restricted motion with the metacarpophalangeals flexed therefore is indicative of proximal interphalangeal involvement. *C,* Normal proximal interphalangeal motion when the metacarpophalangeal joints are flexed indicates that the prior proximal interphalangeal restriction was due to intrinsic muscle contracture, presumably caused by metacarpophalangeal synovitis.

pause and is often associated with mild inflammation for the first year or two that a particular joint is involved. The joints may intermittently be warm and tender, but joint aspiration usually shows very thick fluid with low white blood cell counts. After 1 or 2 years, the evidence of inflammation, if any, gradually subsides, and the typical osteophytes of Heberden's and Bouchard's nodes develop. The disease is strikingly symmetric, although the degree of involvement may vary somewhat. This condition spares the metacarpophalangeal joints and the wrists, except for the first carpometacarpal joint. The other joints all may be involved, or the disease may limit itself to a few proximal or distal interphalangeal joints, almost always in a symmetric fashion. Although most people have disease limited to the hands, there is a modest increased risk of developing osteoarthritis elsewhere, especially the hips and knees. When the hips are involved in association with the hands, the disease may affect primarily the medial aspect of the joint,

rather than the more common superior margin of the joint.

Primary generalized osteoarthritis is a rare, hereditary disease with a high frequency of osteoarthritis of multiple joints. The disease usually begins in middle age and involves "typical" joints early, such as the hips, knees, and hands. However, eventually the disease may involve other joints, such as the shoulders and ankles. Although calcium pyrophosphate deposition disease has been associated with some of these families, in the majority a metabolic error has not yet been discovered. Recently, however, a specific genetic defect was identified in three such families.[22a]

Osteoarthritis secondary to metabolic diseases is being increasingly recognized, as particular patterns of osteoarthritis have been described in association with several disorders. In fact, a number of diseases have patterns of osteoarthritis that are characteristic enough to suggest the underlying disorder.

Hemochromatosis, an underdiagnosed but relatively common disorder,[23] presents with arthritis in more than half the patients at the time of diagnosis, and arthritis is often the initial symptom. Although the arthritis may eventually become quite extensive, the earliest involvement is usually in weight-bearing joints, especially the hips, and in the hands. The hand involvement is quite characteristic, with osteoarthritis involving the metacarpophalangeal joints, especially the second and third. It is typically associated with the development of large, hook-like osteophytes on the metacarpal heads. The diagnosis is confirmed by serum iron and ferritin studies and by the demonstration of tissue iron overload, especially in the liver.

Calcium pyrophosphate deposition disease has many patterns and may present only as recurrent monarthritis (pseudogout). However, it may be widespread and may be associated with generalized osteoarthritis, including severe involvement of unusual joints, such as the wrist and patellofemoral joint. Hyperparathyroidism is found in approximately 10 percent of all cases of generalized calcium pyrophosphate deposition disease.

Hypothyroidism is associated with symmetric, noninflammatory, highly viscous effusions, frequently in joints with pre-existing osteoarthritis. The hands, feet, and knees are most frequently involved. The fluid characteristically contains calcium pyrophosphate crystals but little or no evidence of inflammation.

Ochronosis may cause a widespread form of osteoarthritis, especially involving the hips and spine. In the spine, it usually is associated with widespread disc calcification.

Acromegaly usually causes severe polyarthritis owing to bone and cartilage overgrowth, with the most severe involvement being in the hips and spine. In the lumbar spine, it may cause spinal stenosis as a result of bony hypertrophy. In the hands and feet, a characteristic pattern includes enlarged ends of bones, with increased joint spaces due to cartilage overgrowth.

Post-traumatic osteoarthritis includes several polyarticular syndromes. *Chondromalacia* of the patella has multiple etiologies, but as a clinical presentation it usually is seen in physically active young and middle-aged women. A typical pattern is bilateral knee pain in a woman who has recently taken up jogging or aerobics. The pain is primarily activity related, but prolonged sitting with bent knees also often is painful. Physical findings may include small effusions, laxity of the patellar ligaments, and patellofemoral crepitation.

Charcot's arthropathy is the term used to describe the severe joint destruction and disorganization seen in a variety of neurologic diseases. Although tabes dorsalis with severe knee involvement was originally described, the most common form of Charcot's arthropathy seen today is ankle and foot involvement secondary to diabetic neuropathy.

Hemophilia causes a severe destructive arthritis following repeated episodes of intra-articular hemorrhage (see Chapter 90). Clinical and radiographic features of both inflammation and osteoarthritis may coexist. The late stage resembles osteoarthritis but has certain characteristic radiographic features, such as widening of the intercondylar notch of the femur.

Obesity causes a number of joint problems, with the most characteristic being bilateral osteoarthritis of the knees, especially in women.[24] Various *developmental defects*, such as congenitally shallow acetabula, are often asymptomatic until osteoarthritis develops later in life.

References

1. Hooker, R. S., and Brown, J. B.: Rheumatology referral patterns. HMO Practice 4:61, 1990.
2. Healey, L. A.: Late-onset rheumatoid arthritis vs. polymyalgia rheumatica: making the diagnosis. Geriatrics 43:65, 1988.
3. Deal, C. L., Meenan, R. F., Goldenberg, D. L., et al.: The clinical features of elderly-onset rheumatoid arthritis. Arthritis Rheum. 28:987, 1985.
3a. Healy, L. A.: Polymyalgia rheumatica and seronegative RA may be the same entity. J. Rheumatol. 19:270, 1991.
4. Cappiello, R. A., Espinoza, L. R., Adelman, H., et al.: Cholesterol embolism: a pseudovasculitic syndrome. Semin. Arthritis Rheum. 18:240, 1989.
5. Kunnamo, I., Kallio, P., Pelkonen, P., et al.: Clinical signs and laboratory tests in the differential diagnosis of arthritis in children. Am. J. Dis. Child. 141:34, 1987.
6. Brewer, E. J.: Pitfalls in the diagnosis of juvenile rheumatoid arthritis. Pediatr. Clin. North Am. 33:1015, 1986.
7. Lotke, P. A., and Steinberg, M. E.: Osteonecrosis of the hip and knee. Bull. Rheum. Dis. 35(2):1, 1985.
8. Mackenzie, A. H.: Differential diagnosis of rheumatoid arthritis. Am. J. Med. 85(Suppl. 4):2, 1985.
9. Khan, M. A.: Editorial comment. J. Rheumatol. 16:634, 1989.
10. Burgos-Vargas, R., and Clark, P.: Axial involvement in the seronegative enteropathy and arthropathy syndrome and its progression to ankylosing spondylitis. J. Rheumatol. 16:192, 1989.
11. Lionarons, R. J., van Zoeren, M., Verhagen, J. N., et al.: HLA-B27–associated reactive spondyloarthropathies in a Dutch military hospital. Ann. Rheum. Dis. 45:141, 1986.
12. Gravallese, E. M., and Kantrowitz, F. G.: Arthritic manifestations of inflammatory bowel disease. Am. J. Gastroenterol. 83:703, 1987.
13. Langevitz, P., Buskila, D., and Gladman, D. D.: Psoriatic arthritis precipitated by physical trauma. J. Rheumatol. 17:695, 1990.
14. Wallace, M. R., Garst, P. D., Papadimos, T. J., et al.: The return of acute rheumatic fever in young adults. JAMA 262:2557, 1989.
15. Lally, E. V., Zimmerman, B., Ho, G., Jr., et al.: Urate-mediated inflammation in nodal osteoarthritis: clinical and roentgenographic correlations. Arthritis Rheum. 32:86, 1989.
16. Winchester, R.: AIDS and the rheumatic diseases. Bull. Rheum. Dis. 39(5):1, 1990.
17. Kopelman, R. H., and Zolla-Pazner, S.: Association of human immunodeficiency virus infection and autoimmune phenomenon. Am. J. Med. 84:82, 1988.
18. Steere, A. C., Schoen, R. T., and Taylor, E.: The clinical evolution of Lyme arthritis. Ann. Intern. Med. 107:725, 1987.
19. Alfrey, A. C.: Beta$_2$-microglobulin amyloidosis. Nephrology Letter 6:27, 1989.
20. Hannonen, P., Mottonen, T., and Oka, M.: Palindromic rheumatism. A clinical survey of sixty patients. Scand. J. Rheum. 16:413, 1987.
21. Southwood, T. R., Petty, R. E., Malleson, P. N., et al.: Psoriatic arthritis in children. Arthritis Rheum. 32:1007, 1989.
22. Churchill, M. A., Geraci, J. E., and Hunder, G. G.: Musculoskeletal manifestations of bacterial endocarditis. Ann. Intern. Med. 87:754, 1977.
22a. Ala-Kokko, L., Baldwin, C. T., Moskowitz, R. W., Prockop, D. J.: Single base mutation in the Type II procollagen gene (COL2A1) as a cause of primary osteoarthritis associated with a mild chondrodysplasia. Proc. Natl. Acad. Sci. U.S.A. 87:6565, 1990.
23. Edwards, C. Q., Griffen, L. M., Goldgar, D., et al.: Prevalence of hemochromatosis among 11,065 presumably healthy blood donors. N. Engl. J. Med. 318:1355, 1988.
24. Felson, D. T., Anderson, J. J., Naimark, A., et al.: Obesity and knee osteoarthritis. The Framingham study. Ann. Intern. Med. 109:18, 1988.

Chapter 24
Weakness

Marc L. Miller

Weakness is a common complaint of patients with a variety of medical problems. Patients with such diverse conditions as congestive heart failure, polymyositis, depression, myasthenia gravis, and hypothyroidism may all come to medical attention complaining of weakness. When tested, some of these patients have true muscle weakness, whereas others may complain of weakness but actually have normal muscle strength. Therefore, the first step in evaluating the patient complaining of weakness is to determine whether true muscle weakness is present. The next steps are to determine where the problem lies in the neuromuscular system and then to find the cause (Fig. 24–1). A practical approach to the evaluation of the patient complaining of weakness is presented; however, a comprehensive discussion of the neuromuscular disorders causing weakness is beyond the scope of this chapter. For such a discussion, the reader is referred to standard textbooks.[1–5]

DIFFERENTIAL DIAGNOSIS OF TRUE MUSCLE WEAKNESS

The wide variety and great number of disorders of the neuromuscular system that can produce muscle weakness make a systematic approach to differential diagnosis necessary. One useful approach is to place the various lesions into categories determined by the organization of the neuromuscular system, beginning with the motor cortex and proceeding through the corticospinal tracts, anterior horn cells, spinal nerve roots, peripheral nerves, neuromuscular junction, and, finally, to muscle. Once the anatomic site has been identified, the disorders at each site can be categorized as genetic, inflammatory and immunologic, infectious, neoplastic, toxic, or metabolic in origin (Table 24–1).

Lesions of upper motor neurons presenting with weakness range from the common acute stroke syndromes, space-occupying lesions, such as brain tumors, and spinal cord lesions related to trauma, infection, tumor, or hypertrophic degenerative skeletal changes to the less common demyelinating diseases and congenital leukodystrophies.

At the anterior horn cell level, one must consider amyotrophic lateral sclerosis, a paraneoplastic syndrome, or a familial spinal muscular atrophy as the cause of weakness. Poliomyelitis, as an acute cause of anterior horn cell disease, is much less common today but is still a threat in unimmunized persons.

Lesions of the peripheral nervous system present most commonly in one of two patterns. The first pattern is a polyneuropathy with weakness associated with sensory symptoms caused by heavy metal exposures or drug toxicity or by an autoimmune reaction (e.g., Guillain-Barré syndrome). The second pattern is sometimes associated with diabetes mellitus or various vasculitic syndromes and presents as a mononeuropathy or mononeuritis multiplex. Inherited progressive degeneration of peripheral nerves (e.g., Charcot-Marie-Tooth disease) can result in a specific pattern of weakness. Demyelinating diseases may also affect the peripheral nerves.

The neuromuscular junction may be affected by antiacetylcholinesterase receptor antibodies (e.g., myasthenia gravis or drug-induced myasthenia) or by inhibition of acetylcholinesterase by organophosphate exposure.

Finally, weakness is the most common presentation of muscle disease and usually presents as a painless proximal process. The major categories of muscle disease are inflammatory myopathy occurring alone as polymyositis or dermatomyositis or in combination with another connective tissue disease; drug-induced myopathy; endocrine myopathy associated with thyroid disease, Cushing's syndrome, or hyperparathyroidism; muscular dystrophies; infectious myopathy due to toxoplasmosis or human immunodeficiency virus (HIV); and a variety of diffuse clinical syndromes affecting glycogen, lipid metabolism, or mitochondrial function. These categories are reviewed in detail in Chapter 69.

History of Present Illness

Patients with anemia, cardiopulmonary disease, musculoskeletal pain, depression, or anxiety as well as those who are malingering may present with complaints of weakness without objective findings of weakness. Cachexia due to poor nutrition, malignancy, chronic infections, and inflammatory diseases, or patients with deconditioning due to inactivity may have similar symptoms. These patients describe many functional difficulties with walking, climbing stairs, or household and workplace tasks. It is usually the patients with milder disease rather than those with advanced disease (e.g., obvious

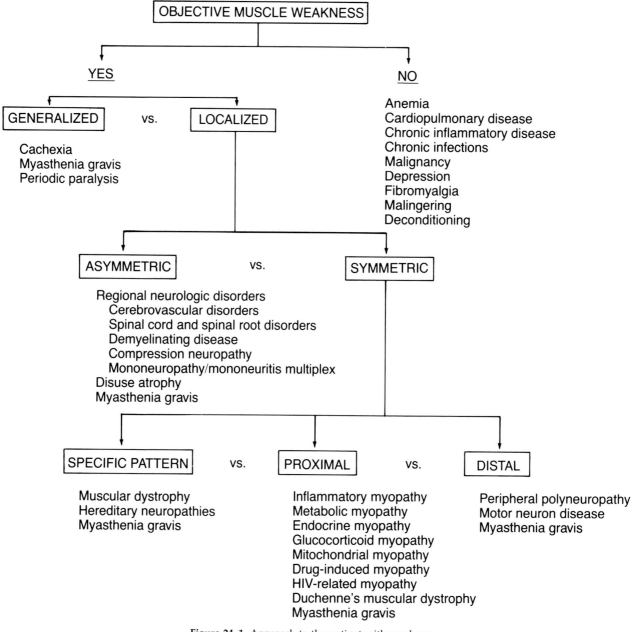

Figure 24–1. Approach to the patient with weakness.

Table 24–1. DIFFERENTIAL DIAGNOSIS OF WEAKNESS

	Site of Lesion				
Diagnostic Category	*Upper Motor Neuron*	*Anterior Horn Cell*	*Peripheral Nerve*	*Neuromuscular Junction*	*Muscle*
Genetic	Leukodystrophies	Spinal muscular atrophies	Peroneal muscular atrophy	Myasthenia gravis	Muscular dystrophies
Inflammatory/ immunologic	Vasculitis (stroke syndrome)	Amyotrophic lateral sclerosis	Guillain-Barré syndrome	Myasthenia gravis	Polymyositis
Infectious	Brain abscess	Poliomyelitis	Leprosy	Botulism	Human immunodeficiency virus
Neoplastic	Brain or brainstem tumor	Paraneoplastic syndrome	Myeloma-associated amyloidosis	Eaton-Lambert syndrome	Malignancy-associated myositis
Toxic/drug	Radiation	Lead	Lead	Penicillamine	Glucocorticoids
Metabolic/ endocrine	Vitamin B_{12} deficiency	? Hypoglycemia	Diabetic polyneuropathy	—	Hypothyroidism

congestive heart failure) who pose diagnostic dilemmas.

Careful, guided questioning of the patient will show that activity is limited by shortness of breath, pain, fatigue, or malaise rather than true weakness. Vegetative symptoms of depression, symptoms of congestive failure or chronic respiratory insufficiency, and constitutional symptoms suggestive of malignancy or chronic infection should be sought. Morning stiffness implies inflammatory joint disease. Proximal muscle stiffness and aching, sometimes with headache, visual symptoms, and jaw claudication, suggest polymyalgia rheumatica or giant cell arteritis. Painful muscle cramps, muscle strain, and localized and diffuse pain syndromes can interfere with motor function. Patients with fibromyalgia may complain of weakness and also fatigue and pain. A psychosocial history is important in considering the diagnosis of malingering or depression.

Patients with true muscle weakness may use a wide variety of words to express symptoms, such as "heaviness," "stiffness" of the limbs, or "lack of energy." Other patients may describe a functional deficit in terms of difficulty with walking a distance, climbing stairs, getting in or out of a car, brushing their hair, or opening jars. Still others may describe their problem specifically as weakness, which is confirmed after more detailed questioning (Table 24–2).

Onset and Duration

The duration of symptoms before medical attention is sought depends on the lifestyle of the person as well as on the underlying disorder. Patients with muscle weakness will see a physician when the weakness interferes with function. Physically active, conditioned people, such as laborers or athletes, will often notice very early, mild decrements in strength, whereas more sedentary, poorly conditioned persons may have long-standing advanced weakness before coming to medical attention.

The pattern of onset and progression can provide a clue to diagnosis. The muscular dystrophies, inflammatory myopathy, motor neuron disease, and myasthenia gravis typically have a gradual onset. Patients present with a history of gradual decline in strength and function. In contrast, sudden onset of weakness, beginning peripherally and moving proximally, suggests Guillain-Barré syndrome. Myasthenia gravis, inflammatory myopathies, infections such as poliomyelitis, or the periodic paralyses can have a sudden onset.

Weakness gradually and steadily worsens in most cases of inflammatory myopathy, the muscular dystrophies, and motor neuron disease. An intermittent course with sudden flares and periods of remission of weakness can characterize early myasthenia gravis, the metabolic myopathies due to abnormal glycogen and lipid metabolism, and the periodic paralyses. Weakness may develop suddenly during or immediately after exercise in some of the metabolic myopathies.

Distribution

The distribution of weakness is a guide to diagnosis (see Fig. 24–1). Is the weakness generalized or localized? If generalized, chronic wasting states, such as advanced metastatic malignancies, or chronic inflammatory disorders, such as untreated or unremitting rheumatoid arthritis, should be considered. These patients are cachectic and have diffuse muscle atrophy. If the weakness is localized, the next step is to determine if the weakness is symmetric or asymmetric. Does it involve only one extremity, suggestive of nerve root entrapment or peripheral nerve lesion? Does it involve part of one hand, as in compression neuropathy seen in carpal tunnel syndrome? If the history suggests a symmetric pattern, are predominantly proximal or distal muscle groups involved?

Proximal Weakness. Patients with proximal weakness of the lower extremities will complain of difficulty rising from chairs—the lower the chair, the greater the difficulty. Likewise, ascending stairs or climbing into a bus may pose problems. Patients with proximal weakness of the upper extremities will complain of difficulty performing tasks over their head, such as reaching for objects on a high shelf, and may have trouble brushing their hair or teeth, which may be described as a heaviness in their arms.

Distal Weakness. Distal weakness is manifested as a decrease in grip strength and may cause problems with manual tasks such as opening jars or using hand tools. If there is lower extremity distal weakness (e.g., foot drop), the patient may report tripping repeatedly over rugs or rough surfaces.

Isolated Functional Deficit. Patients should be questioned about difficulty with specific localized functions, which can be signs of neuromuscular disease. Unilateral foot drop is often seen in neuropathy associated with vasculitis. Shortness of breath can develop from involvement of respiratory muscles in the inflammatory myopathies or muscular dystrophies. Diplopia can be an early sign of myasthenia gravis. Dysphagia, dysphonia, or regurgitation into the nasopharynx can occur with bulbar lesions, in motor neuron disease, or in inflammatory myopathy involving the pharyngeal and upper esophageal muscles.

Table 24–2. THE HISTORY IN EVALUATION OF WEAKNESS

Pattern of onset and course
Distribution of weakness
Associated pain and sensory symptoms
Past medical history
Sex, family history, age at onset
Medication, dietary, and exposure history
Review of systems for systemic disease

Pain and Sensory Symptoms

The presence or absence of associated pain and sensory symptoms should be noted. Disorders of anterior horn cells, the motor segments of spinal roots, or the neuromuscular junction are rarely painful. Inflammatory myopathy is typically painless except in severe cases. The metabolic myopathies are characteristically associated with pain after exercise. Infectious myopathies, such as trichinosis and viral myositis, and vasculitis affecting arteries in muscle are usually painful. Pain at rest, paresthesias, or numbness associated with weakness suggest a peripheral neuropathy, dorsal nerve root compression, or spinal cord lesion. Joint disease may cause localized weakness and pain. (All of Section III may be relevant reading.) Joint swelling and erythema, morning stiffness, and gelling phenomenon suggest arthritis as the cause of weakness. The presence of bone pain may be a clue that the weakness is due to the myopathy associated with osteomalacia.

Past Medical History

A complete past medical history may provide important diagnostic information. A history of chronic renal failure or diabetes mellitus could explain a peripheral polyneuropathy or proximal leg weakness. Medication history is crucial; long-term phenytoin therapy for a seizure disorder can interfere with vitamin D metabolism, leading to osteomalacia-related myopathy. Patients taking lovastatin for hypercholesterolemia may develop an insidious myositis. Persons with a remote history of poliomyelitis may present many years after their recovery from the acute illness with a "post-polio" syndrome of new muscular weakness.[6]

The neuromuscular manifestations of HIV infection have been described in recent years. These include peripheral neuropathies, an inflammatory myopathy indistinguishable from polymyositis that may be the consequence either of the HIV infection itself or of treatment with zidovudine, a noninflammatory atrophic muscle wasting syndrome, and possibly motor neuron disease.[7, 8] A history of HIV infection or of risk factors for HIV infection should therefore be sought in patients with unexplained inflammatory myopathy, cachexia, or weakness. Patients with known HIV infection who develop weakness should be evaluated for HIV- or zidovudine-related myopathy or neuropathy.

Sex, Family History, and Age

The sex of the patient, family history, and age at onset of weakness must be considered. The patient's sex is important in considering the X-linked recessive muscular dystrophies: Duchenne, Becker, and some cases of scapuloperoneal muscular atrophy.

A family history of neuromuscular disease suggests a genetic basis,[9] and in such instances a family tree should be constructed to define the mode of inheritance. Mild cases may be overlooked unless the family members are formally examined and appropriate screening tests are performed. The muscular dystrophies have characteristic inheritance patterns. These disorders can be X-linked recessive (Duchenne and Becker), autosomal dominant (fascioscapulohumeral), or autosomal recessive (limb-girdle). Primary hypokalemic and hyperkalemic periodic paralyses are autosomal dominant disorders. The glycogen and lipid storage diseases are autosomal recessive disorders. Some disorders of peripheral nerves are genetically determined. Peroneal muscular atrophy (Charcot-Marie-Tooth disease) is inherited in some kindreds as an autosomal dominant trait and in others as an autosomal recessive trait.

Age at onset of weakness may provide clues to diagnosis and clinical associations. The mitochondrial myopathies have characteristic ages of onset[10] as do the muscular dystrophies. Primary hypokalemic and hyperkalemic periodic paralyses typically present in childhood, whereas the secondary forms of these disorders are not age related. Myasthenic syndromes presenting in the elderly suggest an underlying malignancy.

Medication, Dietary, and Exposure History

Many medications have been implicated as causes of peripheral neuropathy,[11] myopathy,[12] or disorders of neuromuscular transmission.[13] In most instances, these are rare toxic effects of the drug. Glucocorticoid myopathy is by far the most commonly encountered drug-induced cause of weakness. This condition is dose related and usually develops in patients taking the equivalent of prednisone 20 mg or more per day.

Dietary history is important when considering the diagnosis of trichinosis. Undercooked pork or ground beef (contaminated in the grinding process by raw pork) may lead to *Trichinella* infection. Alcohol use should be determined because myopathy is a common complication of chronic alcohol abuse.[14]

Exposure to organophosphate compounds widely used in pesticides may result in acute cholinergic crisis with paralysis and cholinergic signs or in a delayed-onset polyneuropathy with distal weakness.[15] Cases of organophosphate poisoning have occurred sporadically in accidents or suicide attempts or in major outbreaks due to contamination of beverages or cooking oil. A third organophosphate poisoning syndrome has been described, with intermediate onset and severe weakness of proximal limb muscles, neck flexors, and respiratory muscles.[16]

Heavy metals, including lead, thallium, and gold, can produce peripheral neuropathies. Exposure is usually due to accidental or suicidal intoxication, except with gold, in which the neuropathy has been reported rarely in patients treated with gold salts for rheumatoid arthritis.[17]

Review of Systems

A complete review of systems should be obtained to look for underlying conditions. Weakness from an inflammatory myopathy, vasculitis, or joint disease or disuse can accompany systemic lupus erythematosus, rheumatoid arthritis, progressive systemic sclerosis, or Sjögren's syndrome. Symptoms of thyroid disease and Cushing's syndrome should be elicited when appropriate. A history of dark urine suggests myoglobinuria, which may result from one of the metabolic myopathies, acute alcoholic myopathy, or severe polymyositis.

PHYSICAL EXAMINATION

Table 24–3 lists key features of the physical examination in the evaluation of weakness.

General Examination

Signs of anemia, congestive heart failure, or malignancy are clues that the patient may have substituted a complaint of dyspnea, fatigue, or malaise for true muscle weakness. Patients with chronic illnesses or malignancy may have marked generalized muscular atrophy without obvious weakness, a helpful sign that primary neuromuscular disease is not present.

The skin should be examined for signs of vasculitis, rashes characteristic of systemic lupus erythematosus and dermatomyositis, and changes characteristic of scleroderma. Premature baldness may be a sign of myotonic dystrophy, as may be premature cataracts. In true myotonia, the patient may have difficulty relaxing a handshake or other muscle contractions. Physical signs of thyroid disease and Cushing's syndrome suggest an endocrine myopathy.

Table 24–3. PHYSICAL EXAMINATION IN EVALUATION OF WEAKNESS

Examination	Features
General physical	Signs of anemia, cardiopulmonary disease, malignancy, chronic inflammatory or infectious disease, depression, associated connective tissue disease, endocrine disorders, nonmuscular manifestations of muscle disease
Joint	Synovitis, contractures, deformity
Muscle	Assessment of muscle bulk, tone, tenderness; documentation of objective weakness; distribution of weakness; signs of noncooperation
Neurologic	Deep tendon reflexes, sensory examination

Joint examination may reveal synovitis suggestive of rheumatoid arthritis or other connective tissue disease. Joint inflammation, pain, deformity, or contracture may interfere with a patient's effort on formal strength testing and therefore render the evaluation of muscle strength uninterpretable. Hip joint disease, particularly in children, may produce a waddling gait that can be confused with hip girdle weakness seen in muscular dystrophy. Children with hip joint disease have decreased hip motion, pain on motion, and flexion contractures but no weakness, wasting, or reflex changes.

Muscle Examination

Muscle examination (reviewed in detail in Chapters 5, 21, and 69) should be performed with the patient undressed. Muscle bulk should be assessed—atrophy suggests a long-standing problem. Patients with inflammatory myopathy typically have normal muscle bulk at the time of profound muscle weakness. The progression to diffuse atrophy in untreated or unresponsive patients occurs over a period of months. Patients with Duchenne's dystrophy develop hypertrophy of the calf muscles early in the course of disease, followed by pseudohypertrophy due to fatty replacement of normal muscle and, in the late stages, atrophy. The distribution of atrophy provides objective confirmation of the location of weakness. Patients with primarily distal involvement, as in motor neuron disease, have wasting of the intrinsic muscles of the hands and feet with preservation of deltoid and quadriceps bulk. The converse is true of patients with polymyositis and other proximal myopathies. Asymmetric atrophy usually suggests a regional neurologic problem.

Fasciculations are a valuable clue to the diagnosis of motor neuron disease, although benign fasciculations may be seen in normal persons. Muscle tenderness is seen in infectious myopathies, such as trichinosis or viral myositis, and in conditions not associated with true weakness, such as fibromyalgia, muscle strain, or muscle spasm. Myoedema can be demonstrated by tapping the muscle with a reflex hammer and then observing a sustained ridge in the muscle. Myoedema may occur in hypothyroid myopathy or in cachectic patients with malignancy or malnutrition. Muscle tone should be assessed, because spasticity seen in demyelinating disease may be misinterpreted as weakness by the patient. Quantification of muscle strength by grading systems is discussed in detail in Chapter 69.

Assessment of Distribution of Weakness

Systematic testing of all muscle groups allows the examiner to determine the distribution of involved muscles (see Fig. 24–1). Disuse atrophy from prolonged bedrest, advanced muscle wasting from malignancy, long-standing periodic paralysis, and some cases of myasthenia gravis produce generalized weakness. If the weakness is localized, is it asymmetric or symmetric? If asymmetric, does the distribution suggest a motor cortex or spinal cord lesion or a spinal nerve root or peripheral nerve lesion? If symmetric, is the weakness predominantly proximal or distal?

Proximal muscle weakness involves the axial muscle groups, deltoids, and hip flexors. Patients with proximal weakness may have difficulty flexing or extending the neck against resistance. Flexion is most easily tested. The patient rests the chin on the chest while the examiner places his or her hand on the patient's forehead. The patient then resists as the examiner gradually exerts increasing force to extend the head. Proximal weakness may be assessed by observing the patient sit up from the supine position. If neck flexor weakness is present, the head will lag behind as the patient sits up. Sitting up may be difficult or even impossible in patients with more severe proximal weakness and sometimes may be the only detectable evidence of weakness. The patient with quadriceps weakness may be unable to rise from a seated position without the use of the hands and arms or may be unable to perform a deep knee bend. These persons may suddenly drop into the chair when trying to sit down slowly. Patients with proximal leg weakness may rise from sitting on the floor by "climbing up their legs with their hands." This action is called *Gower's sign* and is characteristic of, but not specific for, Duchenne's muscular dystrophy.

Distal weakness is characterized by decreased grip strength or weakness of wrist flexion or extension. Distal lower extremity weakness may produce foot drop or decreased plantar flexion strength. More subtle degrees may be demonstrated by the patient's inability to toe- or heel-walk.

The inflammatory, metabolic and endocrine, and glucocorticoid myopathies and some forms of muscular dystrophy generally produce proximal weakness, whereas peripheral neuropathies and motor neuron disease are associated predominantly with distal weakness.

Facial expression should be observed for facial asymmetry and ptosis. Fasciculations and furrowing of the tongue may be signs of motor neuron disease.

Fatigability

Fatigability, or progressive weakness with continued use, is characteristic of myasthenia gravis and can be demonstrated by exercising one side and then comparing its strength with the rested side. In Eaton-Lambert syndrome associated with malignancy, muscle strength paradoxically increases with repetition.

Malingering

An often difficult aspect of the evaluation of complaints of weakness is the identification of the hysterical or malingering patient. Assessment of muscle strength depends on the cooperation and full effort of the patient. The malingerer may show inconsistencies, such as inability to lift a leg when directed to do so against the examiner's resisting hand while being able to rise easily from a seated position when distracted. Similarly, patients may be able to walk on their heels but unable actively to dorsiflex the ankles when asked to resist the examiner's pull on their feet. "Give" weakness, in which there is momentary muscle contraction followed by a sudden give in resistance, is not seen with true weakness in the absence of pain and is a good indication of malingering. The failure of synergistic muscle groups to contract (e.g., quadriceps and contralateral hip extensors) or the simultaneous contraction of agonist and antagonist groups (e.g., ipsilateral quadriceps and hamstrings) also suggests inappropriate effort.

Neurologic Examination

The examiner should have a good appreciation of neuroanatomy and be able to identify lesions of the peripheral and central nervous systems. The Medical Research Council guide to the examination of the peripheral nerves is an excellent reference.[18] Asymmetry of the deep tendon reflexes may indicate a localized central or peripheral nervous system lesion. Reflexes are generally maintained in inflammatory myopathy and myasthenia gravis but are lost or diminished in the muscular dystrophies in parallel with the extent of weakness as well as in the Eaton-Lambert myasthenic syndrome. Hyperthyroidism and hypothyroidism may cause brisk or diminished responses with slow relaxation phase, respectively. Pathologic plantar responses suggest an upper motor neuron lesion.

Sensory modalities should also be tested. Peripheral nerve entrapments, such as carpal tunnel syndrome, often produce diminished light touch or pinprick sensation or abnormal two-point discrimination. Later, muscle atrophy and weakness develop. Spinal nerve root impingement and peripheral neuropathies may produce sensory abnormalities. Sensation may be markedly compromised in a peripheral, symmetric pattern in the Guillain-Barré syndrome; in polyarteritis, segmental hypesthesias are found in the distribution of certain peripheral nerves.

LABORATORY TESTING

After a thorough history and review of systems and a careful physical examination, the explanation for the patient's weakness is often obvious or the number of alternatives are greatly reduced; however, the diagnosis sometimes remains elusive. In addition to confirming a diagnosis already suspected follow-

Table 24–4. LABORATORY SCREENING IN
EVALUATION OF WEAKNESS

Screening tests
  Complete blood count with differential
  Erythrocyte sedimentation rate
  C-reactive protein
  Serum muscle enzymes

Specific tests
  Serologic tests
    Antinuclear antibodies
    Rheumatoid factor
    Complement
    Cryoglobulins
    Hepatitis B surface antigen
  Thyroid function tests, parathyroid hormone
  Antiacetylcholine receptor antibody
  Electromyography and nerve conduction tests
  Muscle biopsy

ing the history and physical examination, laboratory testing can help distinguish among various possibilities when the diagnosis is not clear (Table 24–4).

Screening Tests

The patient with a complaint of weakness but without objective weakness on examination should be further evaluated with a complete blood count, sedimentation rate or C-reactive protein, liver function tests, electrolytes, and renal function tests to exclude anemia, chronic hepatic or renal disease, malignancy, and chronic inflammatory or infectious processes. A sedimentation rate greater than 100 mm per hour in a patient with normal renal function is invariably caused by malignancy, infection, or vasculitis. Chest radiograph and arterial blood gas measurement may demonstrate chronic pulmonary disease with hypoxemia or congestive heart failure. Measurements of muscle enzymes and thyroid function are indicated when myopathy or thyroid disease is still suspected despite normal or equivocal physical findings.

Patients with objective weakness require further investigation to establish a diagnosis. Eosinophilia may be a sign of myopathy due to the hypereosinophilic syndrome[19] or to a parasitic infestation. Elevation of serum muscle enzymes, including creatine kinase (CK), aldolase, lactic dehydrogenase, and aspartate aminotransferase, helps confirm the presence of myopathy and is suggestive of inflammatory myopathy or muscular dystrophy. Serial measurements of muscle enzymes are useful in assessing the response to treatment in inflammatory myopathy; however, muscle enzyme elevations are not specific for inflammatory myopathy and muscular dystrophy. Motor neuron disease, metabolic myopathies, hypokalemic periodic paralysis, parasitic infestations, drug-induced myopathies such as those caused by clofibrate or lovastatin, and alcoholic myopathy may also be associated with increased enzyme levels.

Other causes of increased CK include intramuscular injections, crush injuries, myocardial infarction, and strenuous exercise.[20]

Specific Laboratory Tests

Once the presence of true weakness is established and nonspecific screening laboratory tests indicate a systemic illness but no definitive diagnosis, a number of more specific tests are indicated.

Serologic tests, including antinuclear antibodies and complement levels, should be obtained in patients with inflammatory myopathy to screen for associated connective tissue disease. Cryoglobulins and hepatitis B surface antigen should be obtained in patients with suspected vasculitis.

Thyroid function tests should be obtained in patients with diffuse weakness. Both hypothyroidism and hyperthyroidism can produce a proximal myopathy. Hypothyroidism may be associated with an increased level of CK in patients both with and without objective weakness. The presence of increased CK in a patient with hypothyroidism and muscle weakness does not indicate the coincidental presence of an inflammatory myopathy.[21]

Elevated parathyroid hormone indicates that weakness is secondary to osteomalacia[22] or hyperparathyroidism.[23] Antiacetylcholine receptor antibodies are usually elevated in myasthenia gravis.[24]

Specific tests after exercise are described in detail in Chapter 69, as are the electromyogram and techniques for a proper muscle biopsy.

WEAKNESS AND RHEUMATIC DISEASES

Of particular concern to physicians caring for patients with rheumatic diseases is the new onset or exacerbation of weakness in the patient with an already established rheumatic disease. In this setting, the task facing the physician is to determine whether the weakness is a manifestation of the underlying disease, a complication of the treatment of the underlying disease, or the result of a second disorder.

There are several causes of weakness in rheumatoid arthritis (see Chapter 52). Chronic synovitis and joint contractures and deformities can lead to disuse atrophy, localized weakness, and peripheral nerve entrapment. Patients with severe rheumatoid disease may develop generalized weakness from muscle wasting and disuse. Rheumatoid vasculitis involving the vasa nervorum of peripheral nerves may result in either the symmetric pattern of a polyneuropathy or the asymmetric pattern of mononeuritis multiplex.[25] Chronic glucocorticoid treatment commonly causes proximal muscle weakness. Antimalarials can produce a myopathy characterized by proximal weakness and the presence of muscle fiber vacuolization on light microscopy and curvilinear bodies on electron microscopy.[26] Toxic effects of D-penicillamine include the development of myasthenia gravis[27] and polymyositis.[28] Finally, an inflammatory myopathy may develop in a patient with established rheumatoid arthritis in which the clinical features of polymyositis and rheumatoid arthritis overlap.

The new onset of weakness in patients with systemic lupus erythematosus can be due to steroid myopathy or vasculitis or the development of an inflammatory myopathy (see Chapter 61). Similarly, myositis with weakness may occur with progressive systemic sclerosis (see Chapter 65) or Sjögren's syndrome (see Chapter 55), although myositis is often asymptomatic in these conditions.

A not uncommon clinical dilemma in rheumatology is distinguishing weakness due to undertreated or progressive polymyositis from weakness due to glucocorticoid myopathy (see Chapter 69). The temporal relationship of the weakness to steroid administration and dose, serum muscle enzymes, electromyography, and muscle biopsy may all be helpful in making this distinction, but this differential diagnosis can often be difficult.[29]

The new onset of weakness in a patient with gout treated with chronic colchicine maintenance raises the possibility of colchicine neuromyopathy, which may be misdiagnosed as inflammatory myopathy.[30]

CONCLUSION

The complaint or finding of weakness can present an enormous challenge in both diagnosis and treatment to the conscientious physician. An approach informed by a sound knowledge of the wide spectrum of conditions causing weakness and based on a thorough medical history, physical examination, and appropriate laboratory testing is most likely to be rewarding to the patient and physician alike.

References

1. Walton, J. (ed.): Disorders of Voluntary Muscle. 5th ed. Edinburgh, Churchill Livingstone, 1988.
2. Kakulas, B. A., and Adams, R. D.: Diseases of Muscle. 4th ed. Philadelphia, Harper and Row, 1985.
3. Engel, A. G., and Banker, B. Q. (eds.): Myology. New York, McGraw-Hill, 1986.
4. Dyck, P. J., Thomas, P. K., Lambert, E. H., and Bunge, R. (eds.): Peripheral Neuropathy. 2nd ed. Philadelphia, W.B. Saunders, 1984.
5. Adams, R. D. and Victor, M.: Principles of Neurology. 4th ed. New York, McGraw-Hill, 1989.
6. Dalakos, M. C., Elder, G., Hallett, M., Ravits, J., Baker, M., Papadopoulos, N., Albrecht, P., and Sever, J.: A long-term follow-up study of patients with post-poliomyelitis neuromuscular symptoms. N. Engl. J. Med. 314:959, 1986.
7. Dalakos, M. C., and Pezeshkpour, G. H.: Neuromuscular diseases associated with human immunodeficiency virus infection. Ann. Neurol. 23(Suppl.):S38, 1988.
8. Dalakos, M. C., Illa, I., Pezeshkpour, G. H., Laukaitis, J. P., Cohen, B., and Griffin, J. L.: Mitochondrial myopathy caused by long-term zidovudine therapy. N. Engl. J. Med. 322:1098, 1990.
9. Emery, A. E. H.: Genetic aspects of neuromuscular disease. In Walton, J. (ed.): Disorders of Voluntary Muscle. 5th ed. Edinburgh, Churchill Livingstone, 1988, pp. 869–890.
10. DiMauro, S., Bonilla, E., Zeviani, M., Nakagawa, M., and DeVivo, D. C.: Mitochondrial myopathies. Ann. Neurol. 17:521, 1985.
11. Dyck, P. J., Low, P. A., and Stevens, J. C.: Diseases of peripheral nerves. In Clinical Neurology. Vol. 4. Philadelphia, Harper and Row, 1990, pp 1–126.
12. Zuckner, J.: Drug-induced myopathies. Semin. Arthritis Rheum. 19:259, 1990.
13. Argov, Z., and Mastaglia, F. L.: Disorders of neuromuscular transmission caused by drugs. N. Engl. J. Med. 301:409, 1979.
14. Urbano-Marquez, A., Estruch, R., Navarro-Lopez, F., Grau, J. M., Mont, L., and Rubin, E.: The effects of alcoholism on skeletal and cardiac muscle. N. Engl. J. Med. 320:409, 1989.
15. Lotti, M., Becker, C. E., and Aminoff, M. J.: Organophosphate polyneuropathy: Pathogenesis and prevention. Neurology 34:658, 1984.
16. Senanayake, N., and Karalliedde, L.: Neurotoxic effects of organophosphorous pesticides: An intermediate syndrome. N. Engl. J. Med. 316:761, 1987.
17. Katrak, S. M., Pollock, M., O'Brien, C. P., Nukada, H., Allpress, S., Calder, C., Palmer, D. G., Grennan, D. M., McCormack, P. L., and Laurent, M. P.: Clinical and morphologic features of gold neuropathy. Brain 103:671, 1980.
18. Medical Research Council: Aids to the Examination of the Peripheral Nervous System. Memorandum No. 45. London, Her Majesty's Stationery Office, 1981.
19. Chusid, M. J., Dale, D. C., West, B. C., and Wolff, S. M.: The hypereosinophilic syndrome. Medicine 54:1, 1975.
20. Ross, J. H., Attwood, E. C., Atkin, G. E., and Villar, R. N.: A study on the effects of severe repetitive exercise on serum myoglobin, creatine kinase, transaminases and lactate dehydrogenase. Q. J. Med. 206:268, 1983.
21. Mastaglia, F. L., Ojeda, V. J., Sarnat, H. B., and Kakulas, B. A.: Myopathies associated with hypothyroidism. Aust. N. Z. J. Med. 18:799, 1988.
22. Schott, G. D., and Wills, M. R.: Muscle weakness in osteomalacia. Lancet 1:626, 1976.
23. Patten, B. M., Bilezikian, J. P., Mallette, L. E., Prince, A., Engel, W. K., and Aurbach, G. D.: Neuromuscular disease in primary hyperparathyroidism. Ann. Intern. Med. 80:182, 1974.
24. Lindstrom, J. M., Seybold, M. E., Lennon, V. A., Whittingham, S., and Duane, D. D.: Antibody to acetylcholine receptor in myasthenia gravis: Prevalence, clinical correlates and diagnostic value. Neurology 26:1054, 1976.
25. Conn, D. L., and Dyck, P. J.: Angiopathic neuropathy in connective tissue diseases. In Dyck, P. J., Thomas, P. K., Lambert, E. H., and Bunge, R. (eds.): Peripheral Neuropathy. 2nd ed. Philadelphia, W.B. Saunders, 1984, pp. 2027–2043.
26. Estes, M. L., Ewing-Wilson, D., Chou, S. M., Mitsumoto, H., Hanson, M., Shirey, E., and Ratliff, N. B.: Chloroquine neuromyotoxicity. Am. J. Med. 82:447, 1987.
27. Gordon, R. A., and Burnside, J. W.: D-Penicillamine–induced myasthenia gravis in rheumatoid arthritis. Ann. Intern. Med. 84:578, 1977.
28. Cucher, B. G., and Goldman, A. L.: D-Penicillamine–induced polymyositis in rheumatoid arthritis. Ann. Intern. Med. 85:615, 1976.
29. Askari, A., Vignos, R. J., and Moskowitz, R. W.: Steroid myopathy in connective tissue disease. Am. J. Med. 61:485, 1976.
30. Kuncl, R. W., Duncan, G., Watson, D., Alderson, K., Rogawski, M. A., and Peper, M.: Colchicine myopathy and neuropathy. N. Engl. J. Med. 316:1562, 1987.

Chapter 25
Kenneth K. Nakano

Neck Pain

INTRODUCTION

Pain localized to the neck may either herald a specific cervical spine disorder or produce a confusing diagnostic problem. Neck pain can originate from the involved cervical anatomic structures, or it may be so perceived but be due to referral from another site[1] (Table 25–1). Musculoskeletal conditions involve neurologic anatomy, and the converse appears equally true.

Patients complain of neck pain less frequently than they complain of low back pain in clinical practice; a major difference between the complaints is that neck pain becomes far less disabling, seldom compromising work capacity.[2] Neck stiffness is a common disorder; 25 to 30 percent of people aged 25 to 29 years in the working population report one or more attacks of stiff neck.[3] For the working population over 45 years of age, the reports increase to 50 percent. Episodes of "simple" stiff neck last 1 to 4 days and seldom require medical care. Brachial neuralgia (pain radiating to the shoulder and arm) occurs later in life than stiff neck, with a frequency of 5 to 10 percent in the 25- to 29-year age group that subsequently increases to 25 to 40 percent after age 45 years. Overall, 45 percent of working men experience at least one attack of stiff neck, 23 percent report at least one episode of brachial neuralgia, and 51 percent suffer both these symptoms. The frequency of brachial neuralgia is approximately three times higher in those who complain of stiff neck, suggesting common factors in the pathogenesis.

Table 25–1. STRUCTURES CAUSING NECK PAIN

Acromioclavicular joint
Heart and coronary artery disease
Apex of lung, Pancoast's tumor, bronchogenic cancer (C3, C4, C5 nerve roots in common)
Diaphragm muscle (C3, C4, C5 innervation)
Gallbladder
Spinal cord tumor
Temporomandibular joint
Fibrositis and fibromyositis syndromes (upper thoracic spine, proximal arm and shoulder)
Aorta
Pancreas
Disorders of any somatic or visceral structure (produces cervical nerve root irritation)
Peripheral nerves
Central nervous system (posterior fossa lesions)
Hiatus hernia (C3, C4, C5)
Gastric ulcer

Pain in the neck exists in all occupational groups; stiff neck appears first, followed by headache and shoulder-arm pain.[3] Studies have reported that, at any time, as many as 12 percent of women and 9 percent of men experience pain in the neck with or without associated arm pain, and 35 percent of the population can recall an episode of neck pain.[2] A history of stiff neck and arm pain was elicited in 80 percent of a population of male industrial and forest workers.[2] In a series of male workers in a broad spectrum of jobs, the number was modified to 51 percent, but only 5.4 percent had experienced any work loss as a consequence of the pain.[2]

The pain-sensitive structures of the neck include the ligaments, nerve roots, articular facets and capsules, muscles, and dura. Pain in the neck region can originate from many tissue sites and results from a number of mechanisms (Table 25–2).

Normal function of the cervical spine requires physiologic movements of the joints, bones, spinal cord, nerve roots (through the intervertebral foramina), muscles, ligaments, tendons, fascia, sympathetic nervous system, and the vascular supply to all these structures. Because most structures in the neck potentially become pain sensitive, a knowledge of the dermatome pattern of pain distribution becomes necessary in clinical diagnosis.

ANATOMY AND BIOMECHANICS

The most complicated articular system in the body and the most mobile segment of the spine is the neck. Through a cylinder connecting the head to the thorax pass structures requiring the greatest protection and possessing the least: the carotid and vertebral arteries, the spinal cord, and the spinal nerve roots. The head, weighing 6 to 8 lb, balances on the seven cervical vertebrae in a flexible chain held together by 14 apophyseal joints, 5 intervertebral discs, 12 joints of Luschka, and a system of ligaments (anterior longitudinal, posterior longitudinal, ligamentum flavum, interspinous and ligamentum nuchae), and muscles (14 paired anterior, lateral, and posterior; Figs. 25–1 and 25–2). Thirty-seven separate joints carry out the myriad movements of the head and neck in relation to the trunk and serve specialized sense organs.

The shape and mode of articulation of the joints influence the axes and ranges of movement of the

Table 25–2. CERVICAL SPINE SYNDROMES

Localized Neck Disorders
Osteoarthritis (apophyseal joints, C1-C2-C3 levels most often)
Rheumatoid arthritis (atlantoaxial)
Juvenile rheumatoid arthritis
Sternocleidomastoid tendinitis
Acute posterior cervical strain
Pharyngeal infections
Cervical lymphadenitis
Osteomyelitis (staphylococcal, tuberculosis)
Meningitis
Ankylosing spondylitis
Paget's disease
Torticollis (congenital, spasmodic, drug-involved, hysterical)
Neoplasms (primary or metastatic)
Occipital neuralgia (greater and lesser occipital nerves)
Diffuse idiopathic skeletal hyperostosis
Rheumatic fever (infrequently)
Gout (infrequently)

Lesions Producing Neck and Shoulder Pain
Postural disorders
Rheumatoid arthritis
Fibrositis syndromes
Musculoligamentous injuries to neck and shoulder
Osteoarthritis (apophyseal and Luschka)
Cervical spondylosis
Intervertebral osteoarthritis
Thoracic outlet syndrome
Nerve injuries (serratus anterior, C3–C4 nerve root, long thoracic nerve)

Lesions Producing Predominantly Shoulder Pain
Rotator cuff tears and tendinitis
Calcareous tendinitis
Subacromial bursitis
Bicipital tendinitis
Adhesive capsulitis
Reflex sympathetic dystrophy
Frozen shoulder syndromes
Acromioclavicular secondary osteoarthritis
Glenohumeral arthritis
Septic arthritis
Tumors of the shoulder

Lesions Producing Neck and Head Pain with Radiation
Cervical spondylosis
Rheumatoid arthritis
Intervertebral disc protrusion
Osteoarthritis (apophyseal and Luschka joints; intervertebral disc; osteoarthritis)
Spinal cord tumors
Cervical neurovascular syndromes
    Cervical rib
    Scalene muscle
    Hyperabduction syndrome
    Rib-clavicle compression

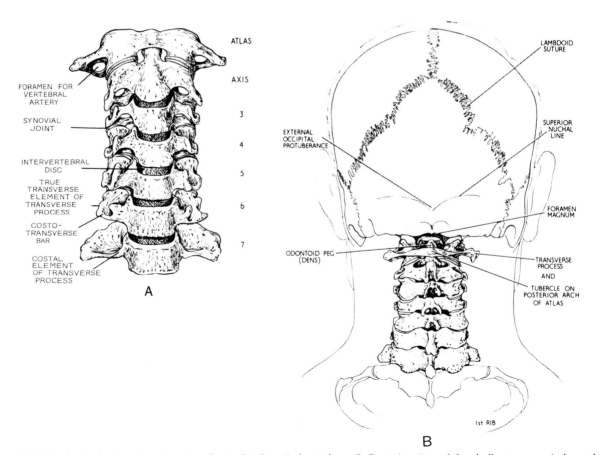

Figure 25–1. *A,* Cervical spine. Anterior view of articulated cervical vertebrae. *B,* Posterior view of the skull, seven cervical vertebrae, and first thoracic vertebra.

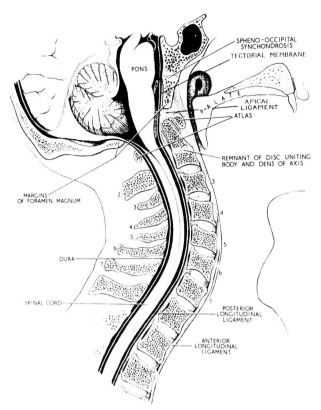

Figure 25–2. Sagittal view of the lower head and neck to show the relationship of the spinal cord and brainstem to the bones, ligaments, and joints between the bodies of the cervical vertebrae. The cervical lordosis can be seen as well as the relationship of the anterior and posterior longitudinal ligaments to intervertebral discs and the ligaments at the craniovertebral junction.

neck. The neck normally moves more than 600 times each hour, whether one is awake or asleep. The cervical spine is subject to stress and strain with daily activities such as sitting, lying down, speaking, rising, walking, turning, gesturing, and so forth. The articular surfaces of the vertebral bodies are covered by plates of avascular hyaline cartilage and united by intervertebral discs. The intervertebral discs increase in area from below the axis (C2) downward, and cervical lordosis results from their wedge shape (see Figs. 25–1 and 25–2). The thickness of the discs varies; the two deepest discs lie below the sixth and fifth vertebra, respectively. Each intervertebral disc consists of fibrocartilage and contains a nucleus pulposus, which changes in shape but cannot be compressed.[4]

Anterior and posterior longitudinal ligaments extend upward to the occipital bone and downward into the sacrum, joining the vertebral bodies. The anterior lonitudinal ligament attaches to the bodies and becomes tightly fixed at the discs (Fig. 25–2); a sudden extending force may rupture it and lead to severe hyperextension associated with damage to the spinal cord. The posterior ligament attaches to the discs and adjacent bones but not to the center.

The specialized atlanto-occipital and atlantoaxial joints are controlled by intersegmental muscles. The

head and atlas move together around the odontoid peg and the upper articular facets of the axis (Fig. 25–1B), the long transverse processes of the atlas providing the levers used in rotation. The odontoid's anterior surface articulates with the posterior surface of the anterior arch of the atlas. The total excursion of the head can be measured in flexion, extension, rotation, and lateral flexion (Table 25–3). The overall range of movement in the sagittal plane (flexion and extension) approximates 90 degrees, with about three-fourths due to extension.[5] Approximately 10 degrees of flexion and 25 degrees of extension occur at the atlanto-occipital joints.[6] In this range of movement, the ligaments help protect the spinal cord from damage by the normal, fractured, or dislocated odontoid process. The lower parts of the cervical spine contribute to the remainder of full range in this plane.[7] The maximum range of movement between individual vertebrae occurs at the level of the joints between the fourth and fifth vertebrae in young children and between the fifth and sixth vertebrae in teenagers and adults. The total range of rotation of the head and neck encompasses 80 to 90 degrees. Approximately 35 to 45 degrees occurs at the atlantoaxial joint and is associated with a screwing movement of the upper vertebra on the lower vertebra, a movement that reduces the cross-sectional area of the spinal canal. Lateral flexion does not occur in isolation but accompanies some rotation. Usually there is about 30 degrees of lateral mobility on both sides in the lower cervical spine.[6] The spinal canal shortens on the side of the concavity of the spine and lengthens on the side of the convexity.

With age, the nucleus pulposus becomes vulnerable to acute and chronic trauma.[8] With loss of disc substance, the annulus fibrosus may bulge into the spinal canal, and because of its eccentric position, the nucleus tends to prolapse backward if any tear develops in the annulus. The commonest sites for both types of herniation are the most mobile regions (i.e., at C5–6 and C6–7). With degenerative changes, the disc space narrows and the spinal column shortens.[9] The intervertebral foramina become narrowed, movements become restricted, and unusual mechanical strains on the synovial joints result. These changes may be confined to a localized area or may become widespread in generalized degenerative disease. The formation of osteophytes leads to encroachement on the spinal canal and intervertebral foramina.[9] The canal may also be further narrowed by bulging of the ligamenta flava. Changes in the

Table 25–3. AGE AND THE NORMAL CERVICAL SPINE MOTION

Age in Years	Flexion Extension (degrees)	Lateral Rotation (degrees)	Lateral Flexion (degrees)
<30	90	90	45
31–50	70	90	45
>50	60	90	30

caliber of the vertebral arteries can result because of degenerative changes in the joints of the cervical spine. Arterial branches supplying joints and nervous tissue can be distorted at rest and further obstructed with movement. With severe vertebral artery stenosis, syncope results occasionally from rotation of the head.

Mere bony changes do not necessarily correspond with the segmental level of neurologic damage. Two reasons exist for this: (1) there is the disproportionate growth of the spinal cord and column—the first thoracic segment of the spinal cord lies opposite the seventh cervical vertebra (see Fig. 25–2), and the upper rootlets of the lower cervical and first thoracic nerves cross over two intervertebral discs, whereas the lower rootlets of these two nerves normally cross only one disc (Fig. 25–3); and (2) severe degeneration of the discs may shorten the vertebral canal to such an extent that the spinal cord, which remains unaltered in length, drops down relative to the bones—the spinal nerve roots may then become acutely folded as they travel toward the intervertebral foramina, the lowest roots becoming the most severely affected.

Familiarity with the distribution of sensory, motor, and autonomic components in segmental nerves becomes necessary for localization of neurologic segments in the clinical examination (Fig. 25–4 and Table 25–4). For practical purposes, the lower fibers of the cervical plexus supply the top of the shoulder; C5 and C6 nerve roots supply the lateral side of the arm and forearm; C6, C7, and C8 nerve roots innervate the hand; and C8 extends into the forearm. The T1 segment innervates the medial side of the arm and forearm. Visceral pain can be referred in some in-

stances to well-defined segmental areas (Fig. 25–5); for example, pain of the point of the shoulder (C3–4) may be associated with acute cholecystitis. The segmental supplies of individual muscles are listed in Table 25–4.

Nerve Root Compression. A radicular nerve normally occupies 20 to 25 percent of the intervertebral foramen. There may be considerable variation in the anatomy of the lower cervical nerves and their root pouches, and as age advances, they become relatively fixed and vulnerable to damage.[10] Two types of disc lesions cause pressure on the radicular nerves or nerve roots: (1) a dorsolateral protrusion that does not invade the intervertebral foramen but compresses the intrameningeal nerve roots against the vertebral laminae; and (2) an intraforaminal protrusion from the uncinate part of the disc that compresses the radicular nerve against the articular process. The extent of root compression depends on the angulation of the radicular nerve and its location in the foramen, as well as the size and position of the protrusion. Marginal lipping of the vertebrae and narrowing of the discs lead to secondary osteophyte formation of the articular processes and consequent posterolateral narrowing of the foramen.

Blood Supply. Variations in the pattern of blood vessels in the cervical spinal cord exist, but the main blood supply comes through a few major articular arteries.[11] The anterior and posterior spinal arteries act more as connecting links than as main channels of blood. The blood supply to the spinal cord can be impaired in patients with cervical spondylosis when one or more radicular arteries become compressed. The resultant ischemia may be either continuous or intermittent, and sometimes the maximum impair-

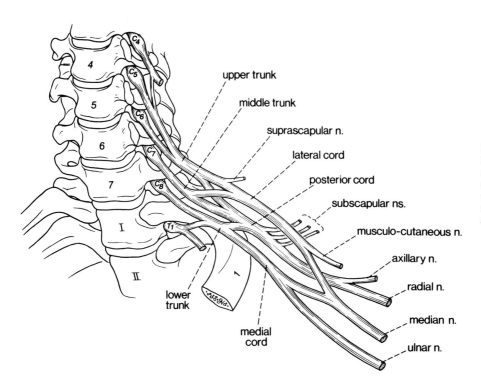

Figure 25–3. Brachial plexus and lower cervical spine. Note nerve roots, trunk, cords, and the peripheral nerves. The brachial plexus goes under the clavicle and over the first rib, accompanied by the subclavian artery and vein.

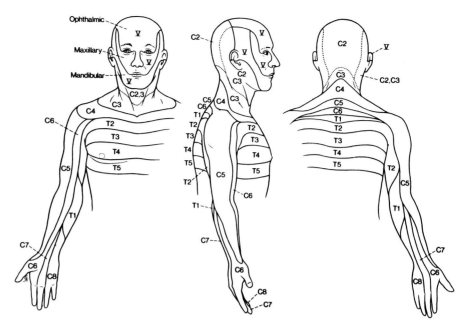

Figure 25–4. Dermatome distribution of nerve fibers from C1 through T5 carrying senses of pain, heat, cold, vibration, and touch to the head, neck, arm, hand, and thoracic area. The sclerotomes and myotomes are similar but with some overlap. Pain arising from structures deep to the deep fascia (myotome and sclerotome) do not precisely follow the dermatome distribution.

ment occurs only when the head is in a certain position (usually extension).

The vertebral arteries vary in size, and one (usually the left) may be larger than the other. The vertebral arteries lie within the vertebral canal, on their medial aspect closely related to the neurocentral joint, and pass immediately anterior to the emerging cervical nerve roots. Each nerve root receives a small arterial branch. Spondylotic changes of the cervical vertebrae may displace the artery laterally and, in

severe cases, posteriorly as well. The degree of displacement depends on the size and position of the body prominence that arises as a result of spondylosis. Atheroma of the vertebral artery also may be important in the production of symptoms. Cerebellar infarction may result from a critical reduction of blood flow to the vertebral artery in the neck. When the blockage occurs in the cervical part of the vertebral artery, the cerebellar infarcts tend to be bilateral, approximately symmetric, and in the territory of the

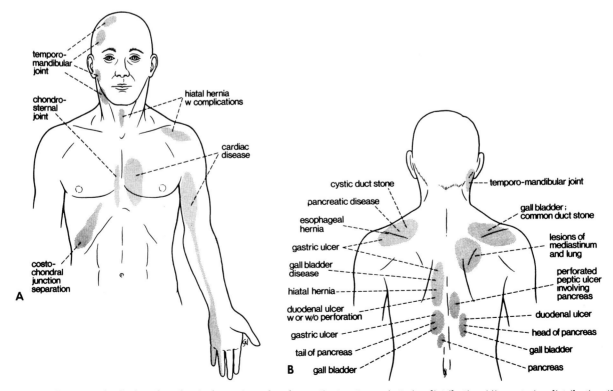

Figure 25–5. Patterns of reflexly referred pain from visceral and somatic structures. Anterior distribution (*A*); posterior distribution (*B*).

Table 25–4. NERVES AND TESTS OF PRINCIPAL MUSCLES

Nerve	Nerve Roots	Muscle	Test
Accessory	Spinal	Trapezius	Elevation of shoulders Abduction of scapula
	Spinal	Sternocleidomastoid	Tilting of head to same side with rotation to opposite side
Brachial plexus		Pectoralis major	
	C5,C6	Clavicular part	Adduction of arm
	C7,C8,T1	Sternocostal part	Adduction, forward depression of arm
	C5,C6,C7	Serratus anterior	Fixation of scapula during forward thrusting of the arm
	C4,C5	Rhomboid	Elevation and fixation of scapula
	C4,C5,C6	Supraspinatus	Initiate abduction arm
	(C4),C5,C6	Infraspinatus	External rotation arm
	C6,C7,C8	Latissimus dorsi	Adduction of horizontal, externally rotated arm, coughing
Axillary	C5,C6	Deltoid	Lateral and forward elevation of arm to horizontal
Musculocutaneous	C5,C6	Biceps Brachialis	Flexion to supinated forearm
Radial	C6,C7,C8	Triceps	Extension of forearm
	C5,C6	Brachioradialis	Flexion of semiprone forearm
	C6,C7	Extensor carpi radialis longus	Extension of wrist to radial side
Posterior interosseous	C5,C6	Supinator	Supination of extended forearm
	C7,C8	Extensor digitorum	Extension of proximal phalanges
	C7,C8	Extensor carpi ulnaris	Extension of wrist to ulnar side
	C7,C8	Extensor indicis	Extension of proximal phalanx of index finger
	C7,C8	Abductor pollicis longus	Abduction of first metacarpal in plane at right angle to palm
	C7,C8	Extensor pollicis longus	Extension of first interphalangeal joint
	C7,C8	Extensor pollicis brevis	Extension of first metacarpophalangeal joint
Median	C6,C7	Pronator teres	Pronation of extended forearm
	C6,C7	Flexor carpi radialis	Flexion of wrist to radial side
	C7,C8,T1	Flexor digitorum superficialis	Flexion of middle phalanges
	C8,T1	Flexor digitorum profundus (lateral part)	Flexion of terminal phalanges, index and middle fingers
	C8,T1	Flexor pollicis longus (anterior interosseous nerve)	Flexion of distal phalanx, thumb
	C8,T1	Abductor pollicis brevis	Abduction of first metacarpal in plane at right angle to palm
	C8,T1	Flexor pollicis brevis	Flexion of proximal phalanx, thumb
	C8,T1	Opponens pollicis	Opposition of thumb against 5th finger
	C8,T1	1st and 2nd lumbricals	Extension of middle phalanges while proximal phalanges are fixed in extension
Ulnar	C7,C8	Flexor carpi ulnaris	Observe tendons while testing abductor digiti minimi
	C8,T1	Flexor digitorum profundus (medial part)	Flexion of distal phalanges of ring and little fingers
	C8,T1	Hypothenar muscles	Abduction and opposition of little finger
	C8,T1	3rd and 4th lumbricals	Extension of middle phalanges while proximal phalanges are fixed in extension
	C8,T1	Adductor pollicis	Adduction of thumb against palmar surface of index finger
	C8,T1	Flexor pollicis brevis	Flexion of proximal phalanx, thumb
	C8,T1	Interossei	Abduction and adduction of fingers

superior cerebellar artery. Most often the obstruction is incomplete, and blood flow may be reduced only when the patient turns or extends the head. Rotation and extension of the head to one side can obstruct the contralateral vertebral artery, and in patients with atherosclerosis, rotation and extension of the head can produce posterior circulation abnormalities such as nystagmus, vertigo, weakness, dysarthria, drop attacks, and a Babinski response. An anterior spinal artery–spinal cord syndrome results from either compromise of the anterior spinal artery or compression of one of the main radicular arteries by osteophytes or adhesions associated with nerve root-sleeve fibro-sis. In diseases involving the major blood vessels (e.g., arteriosclerosis, diabetes, syphilis), the blood supply of the spinal cord may be impaired, especially if the condition is associated with spondylosis.

CLINICAL EVALUATION

The essential means in the diagnosis and management of cervical pain include elicitation of the history and the physical examination. Radiologic and electrodiagnostic procedures assist in confirming the clinical formulation.

History and Symptoms

Pain. The most common symptom of cervical spine disorders is pain (Fig. 25–6). Clinically, the approach to pain is to define it in terms of type of onset, distribution, frequency, constancy versus intermittency, duration, quality, association with neurologic symptoms and signs, localization, and various associated features. Cervical nerve root irritation causes a well-localized area of pain (see Fig. 25–4), whereas poorly defined areas of pain arise from deep connective tissue structures, muscle, joint, bone, or disc. The patient's ability to describe the pain provides the examiner with essential clues to diagnosis. Retro-orbital, temporal, and occipital pain reflects a referral pattern from the atlas, axis, C3, and their surrounding structures. In cervical spine disorders, pain may appear in the back, sides, or front of the neck and may radiate to the upper thoracic spine, shoulders, or scapular regions or into one or both upper limbs. Additionally, this pain may be produced, relieved, or exaggerated by various normal movements of the cervical spine. The areas of pain designation may be tender (i.e., transverse process, spinous process, apophyseal joints, or anterior vertebral bodies).

Stiffness with consequent limitation of motion of the neck, shoulder, elbow, wrist, and even fingers

may occur subsequent to injury response, articular involvement, nerve root irritation, or reflex sympathetic dystrophy.

Tenosynovitis and tendinitis often accompany syndromes of the cervical spine and may involve the rotator cuff, tendons about the wrist or hand with stenosis or fibrosis of tendon sheaths, and palmar fascia.

Paresthesias. Numbness and tingling follow the segmental distribution of the nerve roots (see Fig. 25–4) in cervical spine disorders; however, these symptoms often occur without demonstrable sensory change. The symptoms appear on one side or bilaterally on awakening and frequently abate with a change in the position of the neck and upper limbs. Paresthesias involving the face, head, or tongue suggest involvement of the upper three nerve roots of the cervical plexus, whereas numbness of the neck, shoulders, arm, forearms, and fingers indicate involvement of the C5 to T1 nerve roots (see Fig. 25–4).

Weakness. Muscular weakness, hypotonia, and fasciculation indicate a lower motor neuron disorder secondary to an anterior radiculopathy (Table 25–4). More than one root innervates a given muscle, and the appearance of muscle weakness and atrophy suggests dysfunction of several roots. Pain and guarding produce functional weakness. On the other hand, a motor deficit may elicit sensory symptoms, i.e., a feeling of "heaviness" of the limbs.

Headache and Occipital Neuralgia. Head pain appears commonly and is characteristic of cervical spine disorders; it results from nerve root or sympathetic nerve compression, vertebral artery pressure, autonomic dysfunction, and posterior occipital muscle spasm, as well as osteoarthritic changes of the apophyseal joints of the upper three cervical vertebrae.[12] Occipital headache occurs commonly in the age group in which spondylosis appears and becomes associated with pain in the neck and upper limbs. The pain may, in turn, spread to the eye region, become dull rather than pulsating, and is aggravated by strain, sneeze, and cough as well as by movements of the head and neck. Furthermore, the headache begins on arising and worsens as the day progresses.

Pseudoangina Pectoris. A lesion at C6 and C7 may produce neurologic or myalgic pain with tenderness in the precordium or scapular region, raising confusion with angina pectoris. Pain from C6 and C7 may become compressive, increase with exercise, refer down the arm, or be aggravated by neck movement or associated with torticollis or muscle spasm in the neck. Differentiation between heart disease and radiculopathy can be made in the presence of other neurologic signs of C6 and C7 dysfunction (e.g., muscle weakness, fasiculation, sensory changes). However, difficulty will arise in clinical situations where true and pseudoangina coexist.

Eye Symptoms. "Blurring" of vision relieved by changing neck position, increased tearing, pain in

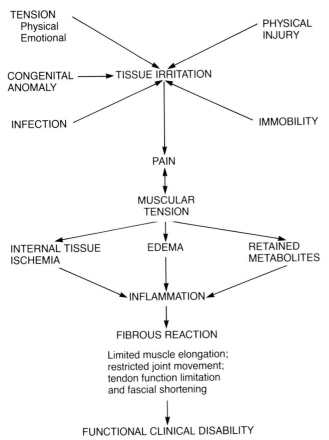

Figure 25–6. Mechanisms producing neck pain and disability.

one or both eyes, retro-orbital pain, and descriptions of the eyes being "pulled backward or pushed forward" may be reported by the patient with a cervical spine disorder. These symptoms result from irritation of the cervical sympathetic nerve supply to eye structures via the plexuses surrounding the vertebral and internal carotid arteries and their branches.

Ear Symptoms. Changes in equilibrium develop with irritation of surrounding sympathetic plexuses or vertebral artery vascular insufficiency, or both. Gait disturbances associated with or without tinnitus and altered auditory acuity result from vascular insufficiency secondary to vasospasm or compression of the vertebral arteries by cervical structures.

Throat Symptoms. Dysphagia results from muscle spasm, anterior osteophyte compression of pharynx and esophagus, or abnormalities of cervical cranial nerve and sympathetic communications.

Miscellaneous Symptoms. Occasionally, bizarre symptoms appear in patients with cervical spine disorders. Dyspnea ("can't get a deep breath or enough air") results from a C3 to C5 deficit (innervation of the respiratory muscles). Cardiac palpitations and tachycardia associated with unusual positions or hyperextension of neck appear with irritation of the C4 nerve root, which innervates the diaphragm and pericardium, or of the cardiac sympathetic nerve supply. Nausea and emesis, ill-defined pain, and paresthesias may accompany spinal cord compression. Drop attacks with abrupt loss of proprioception and collapse without loss of consciousness may suggest posterior circulation insufficiency.

A complex variety of symptoms and signs results from cervical nerve root dysfunction, sympathetic nervous system involvement, cervical spinal cord compression, posterior circulation insufficiency, as well as diseases and injury of cervical bone, muscles, and joints. The clinician must consider all of these factors in evaluating patients with neck pain before attributing the symptoms as "functional" or psychoneurotic.

CLINICAL EXAMINATION

A general physical and neurologic examination yields objective information from the precise identification of the pain-sensitive structure as well as the mechanism of pain production. Systematic examination of patients with cervical spine syndromes includes head, neck, upper thoracic spine, shoulders, arms, forearms, wrists, and hands with the patient fully undressed. The clinician observes the patient's posture, movements, facial expression, gait, and various positions (e.g., sitting, standing, supine). As the patient walks into the office, the clinician observes the patient's head position and how naturally and rhythmically the head and neck move with body movement.

The neck should be inspected for normal anatomic position of the hyoid bone, thyroid cartilage,

thyroid gland, the normal cervical lordosis, as well as scars or pigmentation. Palpation of bony structures in the neck should be done with the patient supine to relax the overlying muscles. In palpating the anterior neck, the examiner stands at the patient's side and supports the neck from behind with one hand, palpating with the other, relaxing the spine as much as possible. The horseshoe-shaped hyoid bone lies above the thyroid cartilage and is at the level of the C3 vertebra. With the index finger and thumb (pincer like), the examiner feels the stem of the horseshoe, and as the patient swallows, the hyoid bone moves up and then down. The thyroid cartilage possesses a superior notch and a flaring upper portion (sits at the C4 level), whereas the lower border lies at the C5 level. Below the lower border of the thyroid cartilage, the examiner palpates the first cricoid ring (opposite the C6 vertebra); this is the upper border of the trachea and is just superior to the site of emergency tracheostomy. The cricoid ring moves with swallowing. About 2 to 3 cm lateral to the first cricoid ring, the carotid tubercle, the anterior tubercle of the transverse process of C6, can be felt. The carotid arteries lie adjacent to the tubercle, and their pulsation can be appreciated. Palpation of both carotid tubercles simultaneously results in restriction of carotid arterial flow causing a carotid reflex. The carotid tubercle proves useful as a landmark in stellate sympathetic ganglion injections. The transverse process of C1 lies between the angle of the jaw and the styloid process of the skull. Because it is the broadest transverse process of the cervical spine, palpation is facilitated. Normal anatomic movements of the atlanto-occipital and atlantoaxial joints and bony structures can be appreciated by a lateral sliding movement, holding the atlas between the thumb and index finger by the transverse processes.

The posterior landmarks of the cervical spine include the occiput, inion, superior nuchal line, mastoid process, spinous processes of each vertebra, and apophyseal joints. Initially, the examiner palpates the occiput, then the inion, marking the center point of the superior nuchal line (the line feels like a transverse ridge extending outward on both sides of the inion). The round mastoid process sits at the lateral edge of the superior nuchal line (see Fig. 25–1B). The spinous process of the axis (C2) can be palpated below the indented area immediately under the occiput. As each spinous process from C2 to T1 is palpated, the examiner notes the cervical lordosis. Occasionally, the bifid spinous processes of C3 to C6 can be appreciated. The C7 (vertebra prominens) and T1 spinous processes are larger than the others. Alignment of the spinous processes should be noted. The apophyseal joints can be felt as small, rounded domes deep to the trapezius muscles about 1 in lateral to the spinous processes. To palpate these joints, the patient must be relaxed because spasm and tension preclude access on examination. The joint involved can be determined by lining up with the hyoid bone at C3, the thyroid cartilage at C4 and

C5, and the first cricoid ring at C6. These joints often become tender with osteoarthritis, especially in the upper cervical spine, whereas the C5–6, C6–7 level will be most often involved in cervical spondylosis.

Examination of soft tissues in the neck should be divided into two anatomical areas: anterior and posterior. The anterior portion is bordered laterally by the two sternocleidomastoid muscles, superiorly by the mandible, and inferiorly by the suprasternal notch (an upside-down triangle). The posterior aspect includes the entire area posterior to the lateral border of the sternocleidomastoid muscle. The supine position appears optimal in the examination. The sternocleidomastoid muscle can be examined anteriorly by asking the patient to turn the head to the opposite side; the muscle then stands out and can be palpated from origin to insertion. The opposite muscle can be compared for any discrepancies in size, bulges, or strength. Hyperextension injuries overstretch the muscle with resultant hemorrhage into the tissue. Localized swelling may be due to hematomas. In torticollis, the sternocleidomastoid muscles will be involved. The lymph node chain resides along the medial border of the sternocleidomastoid muscle and normally cannot be palpated. Small, tender lymph nodes can be palpated if enlarged secondary to infections (throat, ear), metastases, or tumor. Enlarged lymph nodes may, in turn, produce torticollis. The thyroid gland overlies the thyroid cartilage in an "H" pattern, the bar being the isthmus with the two lobes situated laterally. Normally, the thyroid gland is smooth and palpable without enlargement. Diffuse enlargement of the thyroid gland, cysts, or nodules or tenderness from thyroiditis should be noted. The carotid arteries, best felt near the carotid tubercle on C6, should be examined separately owing to the carotid reflex secondary to simultaneous palpation. Carotid pulsation normally should be symmetric.

The parotid gland overlies part of the sharp angle of the mandible, usually indistinct to palpation; but when enlarged, the usually sharp and bony angle of the mandible feels soft and boggy owing to overlying glandular tissue (e.g., mumps, Sjögren's syndrome, and endocrine disorders). The supraclavicular fossa above the clavicle should be examined for lymph nodes, unusual excursion with respiration, swelling, fat accumulation, and asymmetry with the opposite side. The platysma muscle crosses the supraclavicular fossa but is too thin to alter its contour. Observation during voluntary platysma contracture may reveal lumps or asymmetry. The apex and dome of the lung extend upward into the supraclavicular fossa. Cervical ribs can sometimes be palpated.

Posteriorly, with the patient sitting, the clinician examines the trapezius muscle, lymph nodes, greater occipital nerves, and superior nuchal ligament. The trapezius muscle origin extends from the inion to the spinous process of T12 and inserts laterally in a continuous arc into the clavicle, the acromion, and the spine of the scapula. The trapezius should be felt from origin to insertion, beginning high on the neck. Flexion injuries may traumatize the trapezius, and hematomas in the muscle occur frequently. Furthermore, the trapezius is the site of focal points of pain and tenderness in fibrositis syndromes. The two trapezius muscles should be palpated bilaterally and simultaneously while looking for tenderness, lumps, swelling, or asymmetry of the two muscles. Embryologically, the trapezius and sternocleidomastoid muscles form as one muscle, later splitting, but they retain a common attachment along the base of the skull to the mastoid process while their nerve supply, the spinal accessory nerve (ninth cranial nerve), remains the same. The lymph node chain lies at the anterolateral border of the trapezius and normally cannot be palpated. The greater occipital nerves sit laterally to the inion, extending upward in the scalp, and can be easily palpated when tender and inflamed. A flexion-extension injury of the spine commonly produces traumatic inflammation and swelling of the occipital nerves with resultant painful occipital neuralgia, a frequent cause of headache. The superior nuchal ligament arises from the inion and extends to the C7 and T1 spinous processes. It is under the examining finger when the spinous processes are felt and may become tender, irregular, and lumpy if overstretched or injured.

Range of Motion. The cervical spine has a large range of motion (see Table 25–3), which, in turn, provides a wide scope of vision and remains essential to the sense of balance. The basic movements of the neck include flexion, extension, lateral flexion to the right and left, and rotation to the right and left. About half of the total flexion and extension of the neck occurs at the occiput-C1 level, the other half being equally distributed among the other six cervical vertebrae, with a slight increase at the C5–6 level. Approximately half of rotation occurs at the atlantoaxial joint (odontoid); the other half distributes equally among the other five vertebrae. All vertebrae share in lateral flexion. A decrease in specific motion may occur with blocking at a joint, pain, fibrous contractures, bony ankylosis, muscle spasm, mechanical alteration in joint and skeletal structures, or a tense and uncooperative patient. Other causes of muscle spasm include injury to muscles, involuntary splinting over painful joints or skeletal structures, and irritation or compression of cervical nerve roots of the spinal cord.

All range of cervical spine motion should be performed in the following manner: (1) actively and to the extreme of motion (to assess muscle function and strength), as observed by the examiner; (2) passively (to assess nonmobile structures, ligaments, capsules, and fascia), as the examiner moves the relaxed cervical spine through all its motions; and (3) against resistance (to study origin and insertions of tendon and ligaments and assess motor strength), with each motion maximally attempted against force of the examiner's hand.

Flexion and Extension. The patient nods the head forward and touches chin to sternum. If the examiner's finger can be placed between the patient's chin and sternum, there is 10 degrees limitation of flexion, whereas 30 degrees of limitation exists if three fingers can be inserted within the above area. Observation of the cervical spine curve should be done as the examiner instructs the patient to look from floor to ceiling. The arc of neck motion normally remains smooth and not halting or irregular. In full hyperextension, the base of the occiput normally touches the spinous process of T1.

Lateral Flexion. The patient attempts to touch his or her ear to the shoulder without rotation or shoulder shrugging. Clinically normal people can laterally flex 45 degrees in either direction.

Rotation. The patient rotates the head maximally, usually being able to bring his or her chin into alignment with the shoulder. Normally, the motion remains smooth, whereas torticollis restricts motion.

Passive Range of Motion. The examiner asks for complete relaxation and takes the patient's head firmly in his or her hands, putting the spine through maximal flexion, extension, lateral flexion, and rotation. Passive motion may be more extensive than active motion if muscles remain stiff and painful or possess involuntary spasm. In cases of head or cervical spine injury, passive range of motion should not be done because of the risk of neurologic trauma to an unstable spine.

Motion against Resistance. All ranges of neck motion can be done with the examiner offering firm resistance to each movement. The anchorage of muscle, tendon insertion and origin, muscle strength, and muscular function should be assessed. This phase of the examination should be done with the patient seated. The primary (sternocleidomastoid muscles) and secondary (three scalenes and small prevertebral muscles) flexors of the neck can be assessed by the examiner placing his or her left hand flat on the patient's upper sternum and right (resisting) hand with the palm cupped on the patient's forehead; the patient then flexes his or her neck, slowly increasing the power to maximal pressure. The primary (paravertebral extensor mass, splenius and semipinalis capitis, and trapezius) and secondary (small intrinsic neck) extensor muscles should be assessed by the examiner placing his or her left hand over the patient's upper posterior chest and scapular area, with the examiner's right palm cupped over the patient's occiput; the patient then gradually increases neck extension to his or her maximum. Lateral flexor muscles (three scalenes and the small intrinsic neck) can be examined by placing the examiner's left hand on the patient's shoulder (for stability) and with right palm (fingers extended) against the side of his or her head; the patient then laterally flexes against the examiner's resistance. The rotators of the neck (sternocleidomastoid and intrinsic neck muscles) can be tested to right lateral rotation by placing the stabilizing left hand of the examiner on the patient's left shoulder and the examiner's right hand along the right side of the patient's mandible, while the patient rotates against resistance. Left rotation is tested in the reverse fashion. Either sternocleidomastoid muscle functioning alone provides the main pull to the side being tested.

SPECIAL CLINICAL TESTS OF THE CERVICAL SPINE

Head Compression Test. With narrowing of the intervertebral foramina, pressure and shearing forces on the apophyseal joint surfaces, intervertebral disc compression, or pressure on stiff ligamentous and muscle structures, there is pain on compression of the head onto the cervical spine. If radicular pain or paresthesias with referral to the upper limb occur with the head compression test, nerve root irritation is strongly suggested. On the other hand, if the pain remains in the neck, soft connective tissues or joints appear as the pain-sensitive structures involved. The test should be performed with the patient sitting; the examiner places one hand across the other on the top of the patient's head with gradually increased downward pressure; the patient then reports any pain or paresthesias and its distribution. Application of pressure may also be down with the head tilted to either side, backward, or forward.

Head Distraction Test. This test should be done with the patient seated; the open palm of the examiner's hand should be placed under the patient's chin while the examiner's other hand goes under the patient's occiput; gradually the force of lifting the patient's head increases, removing the weight of the skull and distracting the foramina, discs, and joints. Nerve root compression may be relieved with disappearance of symptoms with opening of the intervertebral foramina or extension of the disc spaces. Additionally, pressure on joint capsules of apophyseal joints diminishes with head distraction.

Valsalva Maneuver. Holding one's breath against a closed glottis raises intrathecal pressure. If an intraspinal tumor or a herniated disc exists, this test produces pain that radiates in a dermatome distribution. Vigorous cough or sneeze, likewise, elicits pain in the above situations.

Dysphagia Test. Soft tissue swelling, hematoma, vertebral subluxation, or cervical osteophytic projections produce pain or restriction to swallowing.

Ophthalmologic Tests. Pupillary signs may differ from one side to the other or vary from one time to another in certain patients with cervical spine disorders, thereby indicating irritability of sympathetic nerve supply in the neck controlling the pupillary muscles. This should not be confused with Horner's syndrome, which follows complete interruption or paralysis of the sympathetic fibers resulting in miosis, vasomotor and sweating changes, and ptosis on the affected side.

Table 25–5. CLINICAL FEATURES DIFFERENTIATING UPPER AND LOWER MOTOR NEURON WEAKNESS

Clinical Feature	Upper Motor Neuron Weakness	Lower Motor Neuron Weakness
Weakness	Greater in extensors of upper limbs and in flexors of lower limbs (pyramidal distribution); usually involves one side of body but may also produce paraparesis, quadriparesis, or (rarely) monoparesis; usually does not produce weakness in one muscle group or bilateral cranial weakness	Nonpyramidal distribution; may be present in one muscle group; paraparesis, quadriparesis, and bilateral cranial nerve weakness also seen
Deep tendon reflexes	Usually increased, but acutely may be decreased; also may be decreased with parietal and cerebellar lesions	Decreased
Tone to passive motion	Increased; may be decreased with cerebellar and parietal lesions	Decreased
Pathologic reflexes associated	Babinski and others Defect of cortical association areas; frontal-release signs; defect of sensation; cerebellar defects; cranial nerve defects	Absent Cranial nerve signs; sensory sign

Adson Test. The Adson test examines the subclavian artery when it may be compressed by a cervical rib, the scalene muscles, or other thoracic outlet abnormalities. The examiner palpates the patient's radial pulse in abduction, extension, and external rotation of the arm. The patient then takes a deep inspiration while rotating the head maximally toward the side being tested. With subclavian artery compression, a marked decrease in volume or absence of the radial pulse on the affected side results.

Shoulder Depression Test. This test indirectly determines if there is irritation on compression of nerve root, dural root sleeve fibrosis or adhesions, foraminal encroachment, or adjacent joint capsule thickening and adhesions. The examiner stands beside the patient, who tilts the head to one side. With one of the examiner's hands on the patient's shoulder and the other hand on the patient's head, the examiner exerts downward pressure on the patient's shoulder and lateral flexion pressure on the patient's head in the opposite direction. This test places a tug on the nerve roots; with root sleeve fibrosis, foraminal osteophytes, or adhesions, radicular pain or paresthesias often result.

Muscle Weakness and Atrophy. Weakness of the muscles may be difficult to assess because innervation of shoulder girdle, arm, forearm, and muscles occurs by two or more roots (see Table 25–4).

Muscular weakness has many possible causes; to narrow the choice down to one or a few, one must ascertain the anatomic localization of the patient's complaints. Tables 25–5 and 25–6 provide guidelines and offer differential clinical features separating upper and lower motor neuron weakness. Atrophy may follow weakness owing to disuse or pain. Interossei hand muscle atrophy can appear with cervical spine disease.

Reflexes. Reflexes indicate the state of the nervous system and its afferent pathways (Table 25–7). Certain abnormal reflexes appear only with spasticity and paralysis; these indicate injury to the corticospinal tract. The primary deep tendon reflexes (Tables 25–8 and 25–9), abdominal reflexes, and plantar responses should be routinely examined; bulbocavernosus and anal reflexes should be tested in all suspected lower spinal cord (conus or cauda equina) lesions and in cases of sphincter disturbances.

In eliciting the deep tendon reflexes, adequate relaxation of the patient and a mild degree of passive tension on the muscle become essential, especially in the radial (supinator) and ankle jerks. The examiner varies the tension on the muscle by manipulating the joint, and reinforcement procedures enable the patient to relax completely, as by pulling one of his or her hands with the other (Jendrassik maneuver). When the examiner elicits the triceps jerk, the small contraction of the triceps muscle should be disregarded because most muscles contract if directly percussed.

The tendon jerk normally occurs in only a part of each muscle, and in a myopathy, the reflex jerk

Table 25–6. DIFFERENTIATING SYMPTOMS OF LOWER MOTOR NEURON WEAKNESS

Signs and Symptoms	Neuropathy	Myopathy*	Motor Neuron or Anterior Horn Cell Dysfunction	Neuromuscular Junction Dysfunction
Weakness	Mainly distal or nerve distribution	Proximal	May be distal or proximal and involve midline muscles (neck flexor weak)	Mainly bulbar respiratory, and proximal
Deep tendon reflexes	Decreased	Decreased	Increased	Normal
Myotactic reflexes	Increased	Decreased	Increased	Normal
Sensory loss paresthesias	Usually present	Absent	Absent	Absent
Fasciculations	May be present	Absent	Present	Absent
Fatigue	Mild	Mild	Mild	Severe
Tenderness	May have dysesthesias	May be present	Cramps	Absent

*Myoglobinuria or myotonia may differentiate certain myopathies.

Table 25–7. RELATION OF REFLEXES TO PERIPHERAL NERVES AND SPINAL CORD SEGMENTS

Reflex	Site and Mode of Elicitation	Response	Muscle(s)	Peripheral Nerve(s)	Cord Segment
Scapulohumeral reflex	Tap on lower end of medial border of scapula	Adduction and lateral rotation of dependent arm	Infraspinatus and teres minor	Suprascapular (axillary)	C4 to C6
Biceps jerk	Tap on tendon of biceps brachii	Flexion at elbow	Biceps brachii	Musculocutaneous	C5 and C6
Supinator jerk (also called radial reflex)	Tap on distal end of radius	Flexion at elbow	Brachioradialis (and biceps brachii and brachialis)	Radial (musculo-cutaneous)	C5 and C6
Triceps jerk	Tap on tendon of triceps brachii above olecranon, with elbow flexed	Extension at elbow	Triceps brachii	Radial	C7 and C8
Thumb reflex	Tap on tendon of flexor pollicis longus in distal third of forearm	Flexion of terminal phalanx of thumb	Flexor pollicis longus	Median	C6 to C8
Extensor finger and hand jerk	Tap on posterior aspect of wrist just proximal to radiocarpal joint	Extension of hand and fingers (inconstant)	Extensors of hand and fingers	Radial	C6 to C8
Flexor finger jerk	Tap on examiner's thumb placed on palm of hand; sharp tap on tips of flexed fingers (Trömner's sign)	Flexion of fingers	Flexor digitorum superficialis (and profundus)	Median	C7 and C8 (T1)
Epigastric reflex (exteroceptive)	Brisk stroking of skin downward from nipple in mammillary line	Retraction of epigastrium	Transversus abdominis	Intercostal	T5 and T6
Abdominal skin reflex (exteroceptive)	Brisk stroking of skin or abdominal wall in lateromedial direction	Shift of skin of abdomen and displacement of umbilicus	Muscles of abdominal wall	Intercostal, hypogastric, and ilioinguinal	T6 and T12
Cremasteric reflex (exteroceptive)	Stroking skin on medial aspect of thigh (pinching adductor muscles)	Elevation of testis	Cremaster	Genital branch of genitofemoral	L2 and L3 (L1)
Adductor reflex	Tap on medial condyle of femur	Adduction of leg	Adductors of thigh	Obturator	L2, L3, and L4
Knee jerk	Tap on tendon of quadriceps femoris below patella	Extension at knee	Quadriceps femoris	Femoral	(L2), L3, and L4
Gluteal reflex (exteroceptive)	Stroking skin over gluteal region	Tightening of buttock (inconstant)	Gluteus medius and gluteus maximus	Superior and inferior gluteal	L4, L5, and S1
Posterior tibial reflex	Tap on tendon of tibialis posterior behind medial malleolus	Supination of foot (inconstant)	Tibialis posterior	Tibial	L5
Semimembranosus and semi-tendinosus reflex	Tap on medial hamstring tendons (patient prone and knee slightly flexed)	Contraction of semimembranosus and semitendinosus muscles	Semimembran-osus and semitendinosus	Sciatic	S1
Biceps femoris reflex	Tap on lateral hamstring tendon (patient prone and knee slightly flexed)	Contraction of biceps femoris	Biceps femoris	Sciatic	S1 and S2
Ankle jerk	Tap on tendon calcaneus	Plantar flexion of foot	Triceps surae and other flexors of foot	Tibial	S1 and S2
Bulbocavernosus reflex (exteroceptive)	Gentle squeezing of glans penis or pinching of skin of dorsum of penis	Contraction of bulbocavernosus muscle, palpable at root of penis	Bulbocavernosus	Pudendal	S3 and S4
Anal reflex (exteroceptive)	Scratch or prick of perianal skin (patient lying on side)	Visible contractcion of anus	Sphincter ani externus	Pudendal	S5

Table 25–8. THE SIX PRIMARY REFLEXES

Reflex	Nerve Roots Necessary for Reflex	Muscle Carrying Out the Reflex
Ankle jerk	S1	Gastrocnemius
Posterior tibial	L5	Posterior tibial
Knee	L2–L4	Quadriceps
Biceps	C5, C6	Biceps
Radial	C5, C6	Brachioradialis
Triceps	(C6), C7, C8	Triceps

may be lost in the quadriceps through wasting in the vastus internus, although the power of contraction of the remainder persists to a fair degree. Some clinically normal people show reduced reflexes, and before the examiner completes the assessment, he or she should ascertain whether other evidence of peripheral nerve (sensory loss, atrophy, etc.) or muscle disease exists.

Examination of Related Area. Shoulder lesions may closely mimic cervical spine disease, and a complete shoulder examination becomes necessary in these situations. The shoulder syndromes usually demonstrate little or no neurologic component. Rotator cuff tendinitis, calcareous deposits in tendons, and capsulitis often coexist with cervical spine disease. Reflex sympathetic dystrophy may occur, with the initial triggering pain mechanism arising in the spine. Similar changes may occur at the elbow, wrist, and fingers. Finger motion may be limited because of swelling secondary to circulatory reflex ischemic changes from sympathetic nerve irritation. Fibrous nodules and contracture of palmar fascia occur following cervical spine disease or injury.

The temporomandibular joint, teeth, lower jaw, or scalp infections may refer pain to the temporomandibular joint area and to the neck. The jaw reflex (mediated by the fifth cranial nerve and involving the masseter and temporalis muscles) can be examined by placing the index finger on the mental area of the chin with the patient's mouth in rest position (slightly open); a reflex hammer then taps the fingers and the jaw reflexly closes. An absent or decreased jaw jerk suggests abnormality in the course of the trigeminal nerve, whereas a brisk reflex suggests an upper motor neuron lesion. The jaw jerk proves useful in separating cervical spine disease from primary trigeminal nerve dysfunction.

Table 25–9. FOUR-POINT GRADING SCALE FOR REFLEXES

Grade	State of Reflexes
0	Absent despite full relaxation and reinforcement maneuvers
1	Reduced but not absent
2	Normal physiologic reflexes
3	Increased response but no reduplication or excessive spread
4	Marked increase with reduplication, clonus, and spread

RADIOGRAPHIC EXAMINATION

Radiographs are essential in the evaluation of the patient with a cervical spine disorder. Clinicians should assess both the clinical and radiographic studies of their patients and not depend solely on the radiologist. Clinical correlation is necessary because gross radiologic signs and abnormalities may be associated with minimal or no clinical disturbance, whereas the reverse situation (minimal radiographic change and yet the patient demonstrates neurologic signs) may also occur.

Routine radiographic views include (1) anteroposterior of the atlas and axis through the open mouth; (2) anteroposterior of the lower five vertebrae; (3) lateral views in flexion, neutral, and extension; and (4) both right and left oblique.

Conventional radiographic diagnosis of intraspinal disease depends on the use of plain radiographs, myelography, and computed tomography (CT).[13] Magnetic resonance imaging (MRI) combines the best features of these conventional techniques; it can display vertebrae, intervertebral discs, the thecal space, neural elements, blood vessels, and paraspinal structures without the use of radiographic or intravenous or intrathecal contrast agents, or both (Figs. 25–7 to 25–9).[14–26] Patients undergoing spinal MRI should be evaluated with at least two pulse sequences, a combination of a T_1-weighted and a T_2-weighted technique. Sagittal images are preferred, occasionally supplemented with axial slices through the level of clinical interest. MRI is the preferred modality for most congenital anomalies (particularly Chiari malformations), syringomyelia, cord neoplasms, multiple sclerosis, and early disc degeneration. Children are particularly good candidates for MRI spinal evaluation because the general anesthesia associated with myelography is obviated and the examination is painless and without ionizing radiation. CT and MRI are approximately equivalent for evaluation of extrameduallary tumors, trauma, and moderate to large protruded intervertebral discs. Certain acutely traumatized patients must be excluded from MRI owing to accompanying life support apparatus (see Chapter 37).

ELECTRODIAGNOSTIC STUDIES

Various electromyography (EMG), nerve conduction velocity (NCV), and somatosensory evoked response (SER) patterns help differentiate normal conditions from a diffuse polyneuropathy, focal entrapment neuropathy, radiculopathy, myopathy, disorder of the neuromuscular junction (e.g., myasthenia gravis), and anterior horn cell disease (e.g., amyotrophic lateral sclerosis) (Table 25–10). No single feature of the EMG provides a diagnosis (except in true myotonia); rather, it requires the summated information of needle EMG coupled with NCV and SER as well as the clinical examination as performed

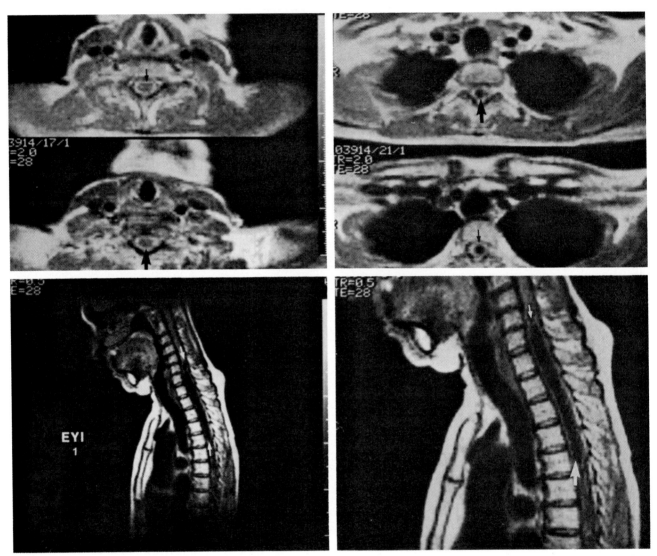

Figure 25–7. MRI scan demonstrating a cervical-thoracic (C6–7 to T5–6) syrinx. (From Nakano, K. K.: J. Neurol. Orthopaed. Med. Surg. 6:113, 1985. Used by permission.)

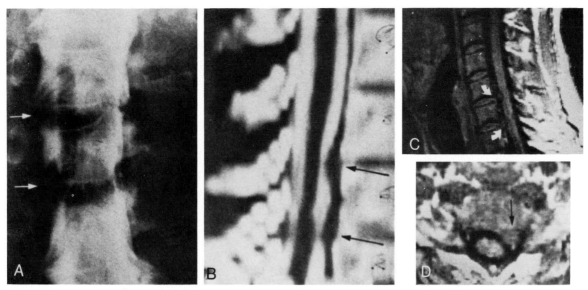

Figure 25–8. Operatively verified disc herniation at the fifth and sixth disc level. *A,* Oblique myelogram showing typical filling defects (*arrows*). *B,* Reconstructed CT image after myelography showing disc protrusions (*arrows*). *C,* Sagittal T1-weighted MR image shows possible herniated disc material emerging behind intervertebral spaces and vertebral bodies (*arrows*). *D,* Axial T1-weighted images confirmed herniated discs. Left-sided herniation at fifth disc level (*arrow*). (From Nakstad, P. H., Hald, J. K., Bakke, S. T., et al.: MRI in cervical disk herniation. Neuroradiology 31[5]:383, 1989. Used by permission.)

by a clinician. EMG studies should be done with disposable, sterile monopolar or concentric needles.

Clinicians often confront the problem of evaluating a patient with weakness. Weakness, in turn, may be secondary to disease within the muscle, nerve, neuromuscular junction, or upper motor neuron (spinal cord, brainstem, or cerebrum; see Tables 25–5 and 25–6). The specific need for definitive therapy, including surgery, can be established only when the physician becomes aware of the cause, extent, and prognosis of the weakness. Evaluation of the electrical activity of muscle tissue and of muscle

response to nerve stimulation solves many of these problems.

LABORATORY TESTS

The clinical laboratory offers some help in diagnosis and management of neck pain in specific diseases (e.g., rheumatoid arthritis, hyperparathyroidism, multiple myeloma, ankylosing spondylitis, human immunodeficiency virus, or metastatic malignant cancer). Cerebrospinal fluid (CSF) evaluation

Figure 25–9. *A,* Prolapsed disc. T2-weighted sagittal image of lumbar spine shows small protrusion of disc material of high signal intensity at L5–S1 level (*arrow*). Protruded disc material is bounded by outer annulus fibrosus and posterior longitudinal ligament of low signal intensity posteriorly. *B,* Extruded disc. T2-weighted sagittal image of lumbar spine shows large extradural mass contiguous with nucleus pulposus in disc. Inferior outer annulus fibrosus is disrupted (*arrow*). (From Murayama, S., Numaguchi, Y., and Robinson, A. E.: The diagnosis of herniated intervertebral disks with MR imaging: A comparison of gradient-refocused-echo and spin-echo pulse sequences. A.J.N.R. 11:18, 1990. Copyright © by American Society of Neuroradiology.)

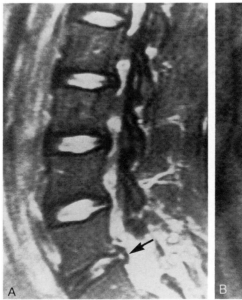
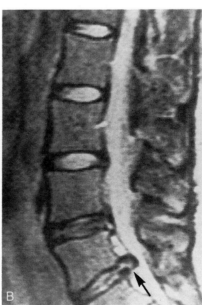

Table 25–10. SUMMARY OF EMG, NCV, AND SER FINDINGS BY LOCATION IN DISEASE IN THE MOTOR UNIT

	Location						
	Spinal Cord		Nerve Root				
Study	ANTERIOR HORN CELL	ANTERIOR MOTOR	DORSAL PRE-	GANGLION POST-	Peripheral Nerve	Neuromuscular Junction	Muscle
Motor NCV	N	N	N	N	+	N	N
Sensory NCV	N	N	N	±	+	N	N
EMG	+	+	N	N	+	±	+
Repetitive stimulation	±	±	N	N	±	+	N
F wave	+	+	N	N	+	N	N
H reflex	+	+	+	+	+	N	N
SER	±	±	+	+	+	N	N

N = Normal
+ = Abnormal
± = Occasional abnormality

should be done in patients with neck pain suspected of having infection (meningitis, meningismus) or subarachnoid hemorrhage. In the latter conditions, the CSF is diagnostic.

DIFFERENTIAL DIAGNOSIS IN PATIENTS WITH NECK PAIN

Many clinical conditions arising outside the cervical spine but perceived in or about the neck area (see Fig. 25–5) mimic cervical nerve root irritation, muscle spasm, ligament strain, bone disease, or joint disorders. Although Table 25–1 lists multiple structures potentially causing neck pain, clinical evaluation usually differentiates between the entities. Table 25–11 summarizes various cervical spine syndromes and the associated pathogenetic process.

Disorders of somatic or visceral structures having cervical nerve root innervation (same embryologic origin) cause pain felt in the neck. Because these areas constitute reflexly referred pain along the segmental distribution of the nerve roots, such areas of referral are not tender on deep palpation. Areas of superficial peripheral tenderness develop due to reflex or direct sympathetic irritation secondary to vasomotor changes. Referred painful areas do not have muscle spasm and often are described as a burning or cramping sensation. Nausea, emesis, and pallor may accompany this type of pain.

Peripheral neuropathy may produce pain both proximal as well as distal to the irritative site. With peripheral neuropathy, however, muscle spasm is not associated. Spinal cord tumor produces a poorly localized and ill defined neck pain, hyperreflexia, and spasticity; immobilization does not relieve the pain, and deep tenderness and local muscle spasms are absent. Furthermore, in spinal cord lesions paralysis or weakness exists below the cord level (not dermatome) associated with sensory changes and Babinski signs. Cerebral or subarachnoid hemorrhage, meningitis, head and neck trauma, or a central tumor produce cervical spine pain, mimicking cervical spine syndromes producing nerve root irrita-

tion. In these instances, the clinical examination, MRI and CT scans, CSF tests, and angiographic studies differentiate between the various conditions.

An important point to remember in the differential diagnosis of neck pain is that compression or irritation of cervical nerve roots with radiation of pain associates with deep tenderness at the site of pain. Segmental areas of deep tenderness, not painful until palpated, indicate nerve root involvement. Lidocaine 1 percent injection in the painful area results in transient reproduction of the radicular pain followed by relief from pain for days or weeks in patients with nerve root irritation. If local anesthetic injection fails to reproduce (and relieve) the pain, one then looks at potential visceral or somatic structures having the same segmental nerve supply.

Table 25–11. CERVICAL SPINE SYNDROMES AND THEIR PATHOGENESIS

Clinical Condition	Pathogenetic Process
Neck sprain/strain	Trauma; psychophysiologic
Radiculopathy	Nerve root compression; osteoarthritis
Cervical myelopathy	Trauma; spondylosis; other
C1–C2, C1–occipital dislocation	Trauma; infection; inflammation
Osteoporosis	Metabolic bone disease
Ankylosing spondylitis	Hyperostosis
Gout	Urate crystal deposits
Paget's disease	Unknown; possibly viral
Fibrous dysplasia of bone	Genetic
Ossification of posterior longitudinal ligament	Hypertrophy and calcification
Ligamentum flavum calcification	Calcific deposits
Osteomyelitis	Infection
Neoplastic disease	Neoplastic primary or metastasis
Occipital neuralgia	Neuritis of C2 nerve root
Vertebral artery syndromes	Atherosclerosis; trauma; osteoarthritis; RA
Thoracic outlet syndromes	Neurogenic/vascular
Double crush syndromes	Cervical radiculopathy and peripheral entrapments
Esophageal syndromes	Osteoarthritis, RA, trauma
Psychiatric diseases	Mental illness (conversion)

RA, rheumatoid arthritis.

Neck pain occurs in malingerers, depressed persons, patients seeking compensation, hysterical and psychoneurotic patients, and automobile accident victims.[27] If these patients possess no concomitant nerve root irritation, they will derive no relief from local anesthesia injected in the painful area(s). Absence of muscle spasm, an antalgic position, and feigning limitation of motion should arouse the examiner's suspicion.

Skilled clinical elicitation of historical data and physical examination constitute the principal and most reproducible means of differential diagnosis[11, 28] (Fig. 25–10). In evaluating the patient with neck pain, the examiner soon realizes that there may be a syndrome of neck pain alone, head and neck pain, neck and shoulder pain, shoulder pain alone, shoul-

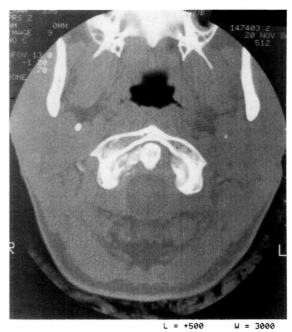

Figure 25–11. High-resolution odontoid C1–2 and foramen magnum CT of a patient with the "crowned dens syndrome" demonstrating the calcification between the odontoid and the right lateral mass of C1.

der and arm pain, or just arm, forearm, hand, or finger pain. Symptoms of altered sensation and vascular insufficiency often accompany the complaint of neck pain. Symptoms or signs arising in the head and upper cervical spine arise only from structures at the C1 to C4 level. An unusual example of this fact is the "crowned dens syndrome"[29, 30] in which the patient experiences acute neck pain followed by headache that is associated with calcification surrounding the odontoid process (Fig. 25–11). Rarely, canal stenosis at the level of the atlas can present with muscular weakness and wasting of the upper limbs and spastic paresis of the lower limbs.[31] Symptoms in the lower neck, shoulder, and arm arise from structures at the C4 to T1 levels. When the examiner observes muscle weakness in the patient with neck pain, he or she must differentiate between nerve root compromise,[32] myelopathy,[33–36] peripheral neuropathy, or a primary muscle disease (see Table 25–6). Infrequently, a synovial cyst of the cervical spine presents as an extradural lesion with radicular pain or pain localized in the involved level of the spine.[37]

TREATMENT

Medical Regimen

Opinions differ as to the best treatment of neck pain and the various cervical spine syndromes discussed in this chapter. Cautious clinical, electrodiagnostic, radiographic, CT, and MRI assessment must precede the planning of treatment, and other causes of pain in the neck and upper limbs must be

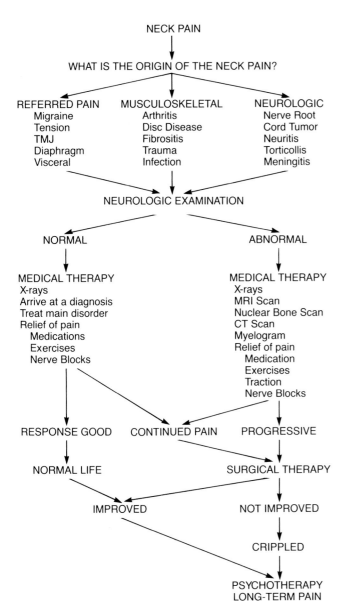

Figure 25–10. Algorithm in the clinical evaluation of patients with neck pain.

excluded before treatment commences. In any treatment regimen, the clinician must consider (1) the severity of the symptoms; (2) the presence or absence of neurologic findings; and (3) the severity of the condition as seen by electrodiagnostic evaluation and radiographic procedures (which may necessitate CT, MRI, and myelography).

Medical therapy aims at the relief of pain and stiffness in the neck and arms. Early mobilization exercises in patients with acute sprains often improves outcome.[38] Bedrest should be reserved for severe acute cases, chronic cases with an acute exacerbation of symptoms, or patients in whom ambulatory treatment fails. The patient lies flat in bed with one pillow and with the head in the most comfortable position. For the relief of pain, adequate analgesics should be prescribed. Salicylates and anti-inflammatory and analgesic medications usually suffice; however, if severe pain develops, codeine, meperidine, or morphine may become necessary. Muscle relaxants, hypnotics, or diazepam may be used concomitantly. With complete bedrest and sufficient analgesic, anti-inflammatory, and muscle relaxant medications, acute neck pain usually subsides within 7 to 10 days. When the acute pain subsides, the patient commences active exercises.

In cervical spondylosis and other musculoskeletal-type syndromes, limitation of neck movement benefits the patient, and cervical collars can be used to achieve this end. The several types of cervical collars range from those that immobilize the cervical spine to those intended merely to provide temporary support and limit excessive movement. Patients with nerve root pain often find relief of their symptoms after wearing a collar. Generally, patients with generalized spondylosis do less well than those with focal spondylosis. Before prescribing a cervical collar, it becomes essential to assess the degree of disability, and the type of collar selected should depend on the degree of immobilization desired. Felt, foam, and rubber collars restrict gross movement, whereas plastic and plaster collars give more secure immobilization. Any collar must fit well and maintain the neck in the most comfortable position. Most people dislike wearing collars; however, some patients seem to become dependent on wearing a collar and cannot be persuaded easily to remove it. In general, the patient should leave the collar off after about 2 months to prevent weakness and wasting of the neck muscles. After the acute, painful stage abates, active exercise in conjunction with collar use should be encouraged.

Traction. Traction, either continuous or intermittent, should be considered when bedrest fails. Continuous traction should be reserved for more severe cases with symptoms of nerve root compression. Many patients cannot tolerate traction, and a few become worse with it. Analgesics and muscle relaxants can be used in doses sufficient to prevent restlessness. Sometimes it becomes necessary to set up a traction apparatus using a weight of only 5 lb to keep the patient immobile in bed and avoid the unpleasant effects of heavier traction. Some difference in opinion exists about the correct direction of pull in traction. Some authors believe that the most comfortable position should be found and traction exerted in this direction; others recommend that the head be in extension, whereas other authorities consider slight flexion as the best position. A weight of 10 lb should be attached to a pulley at the head of the bed, which should be raised to increase the pull and prevent the trunk from sliding up. The weight may be increased to 20 lb according to muscular development or may be varied during the day; some authorities recommend 10 to 12 lb during the day and 5 to 8 lb at night.[39] Intermittent traction may be applied manually or mechanically by pulley and weight with the head halter. The direction of pull should be in the most comfortable position. A weight between 15 and 25 lb and traction applied for 15 to 20 minutes generally suffices. Treatment should be repeated daily if necessary. Occasionally, side effects of traction occur, and rarely, hemianopic visual field defects develop. Traction appears unsuitable for patients with gross radiographic-visible changes of the cervical spine, because of the danger of spinal cord compression or pressure on the vertebral arteries.

Exercises. Active exercises should be used in most regimens of treatment. The exercises can be grouped into (1) anterior neck–mobilizing exercises; (2) shoulder-raising exercises; and (3) muscle-strengthening exercises. Shoulder exercises, aimed at elevating the shoulder girdle and relieving drag on the nerve roots, can be combined with the use of a cervical collar.

Head positioning may be employed to relieve symptoms, because placing the head in certain positions relieves pain. The head should be carried at all times in its optimum position of slight flexion with the chin drawn in.

Other Measures. Massage may be useful in patients with painful muscle spasms; however, in most instances, massage is not prescribed in cervical spine disorders. Injection of local anesthetics or steroids into painful areas may provide relief of pain and spasm with subsequent improvement in cervical movement. Ice applied to painful areas in acute situations often helps, whereas heat in the form of ultrasound or infrared radiation helps subsequently to relieve muscle spasm.

Sometimes catastrophes, with severe neurologic complications and even death, have occurred with neck manipulation as a treatment of neck pain.[40] These complications usually result from vascular disturbances of the vertebral arteries, which appear to be particularly vulnerable at the C1, where they enter the skull. Rotation and hyperextension can become dangerous movements.

Surgery

Two groups of patients appear appropriate for surgical consideration.[41] In the first group, symptoms relate principally to the nerve roots emerging from the cervical spine, and the condition presents itself with either neck or arm pain. In the second group, a slowly progressive spinal cord syndrome involves the legs first and then the arms.

One of the primary factors in the pathogenesis of radiculopathy and myelopathy is compression. Treatment is aimed at the elimination of this pressure. The most clear-cut indication for surgery is the presence of a neurologic deficit related to compression that is unrelieved by medical treatment. Radicular symptoms respond readily to surgical treatment. In the past the initial surgical approach was from the posterior midline, but recently many surgeons have advocated an anterior approach. In the anterior approach, the disc space may or may not be fused. In patients with defined neurologic deficits, results have been excellent in 80 to 90 percent of cases, irrespective of surgical approach. This appears especially so with a centrally herniated disc.[42, 43] In cases of myelopathy, the surgical approach may be either anterior or posterior. However, surgical repair of cervical myelopathies is less effective than in cases of acute radiculopathy, with approximately 60 to 70 percent of treated patients remaining stable or improving. In patients with cervical bone canal diameter of 11 mm or less at several levels, a long posterior decompression may be necessary. In cases with a diffuse bulging disc or an osteophytic ridge, and where the bony elements are normal (or slightly small), the site of compression and approach may be anterior (several levels may be operated on at the same time). In patients with a large, centrally herniated cervical disc with a total myelographic block, the surgeon may have difficulty deciding on the appropriate approach, and it should be stressed that opinions differ as to the optimal surgical technique in these cases.[44–46]

Careful clinical investigation supplemented by EMG, NCV, and SER to exclude peripheral nerve disease becomes essential in patients with radicular symptoms.

Patient Education

Finally, an important aspect in the treatment of patients with neck pain entails patient education. The clinician should define the problem, instruct the patient in the rationale of the treatment, and teach the patient how to care for his or her neck in standing, sitting, driving, and other activities of daily living.

SUMMARY

Many medical conditions produce neck pain both locally and in its referred aspect. Confirming the source of dysfunction in the neck, understanding the mechanism by which the symptoms occur, and recognizing the tissues capable of eliciting clinical signs assume importance. A careful, thorough his-

tory and complete physical and neurologic examination usually reveal the problem clearly. When clinicians recognize which symptoms can be reproduced and which movements and positions reproduce them, they will arrive at a diagnosis and direct effective therapy. Following the principles established on that basis reaffirms the fact that a diagnosis need not be a diagnosis of exclusion.

References

1. Smythe, H.: The "repetitive strain injury syndrome" is referred pain from the neck. J. Rheumatol. 15:1604, 1988.
2. Hult, L.: The Munkfors investigation. Acta Orthop. Scand. 16(Suppl.):1, 1954.
3. Holt, L.: Frequency of symptoms for different age groups and professions. In Hirsch, C., and Zotterman, Y. (eds.): Cervical Pain. New York, Pergamon Press, 1971, pp. 17–20.
4. Cassidy, J. J., Hiltner, A., and Baer, E.: Hierarchical structure of the intervertebral disc. Clin. Rheumatol. 8:282, 1989.
5. Waltz, T. A.: Physical factors in the production of the myelopathy of cervical spondylosis. Brain 90:395, 1967.
6. Penning, L.: Functional Pathology of the Cervical Spine. Amsterdam, Excerpta Medica, 1968.
7. Lind, G., Sihlbom, H., Nordwall, A., et al.: Normal range of motion of the cervical spine. Arch. Phys. Med. Rehabil. 70:692, 1989.
8. Schmorl, G., and Junghans, H.: The Human Spine in Health and Disease. New York, Grune and Stratton, 1959.
9. Hayashi, H., Ohada, K., Hamada, H., et al.: Etiological factors in myelopathy: A radiological evaluation of the aging changes in the cervical spine. Clin. Orthop. Rel. Res. 214:200, 1987.
10. Brain, W. R.: Some unsolved problems in cervical spondylosis. Br. Med. J. 1:771, 1963.
11. Nakano, K. K.: Neurology of Musculoskeletal and Rheumatic Disorders. Boston, Houghton-Mifflin, 1979.
12. Emeads, J.: The cervical spine and headache. Neurology 38:1874, 1988.
13. Nepper-Rasmussen, J.: CT of dens axis fractures. Neuroradiology 31:104, 1989.
14. Han, J. S., Kaufman, B., El Yousef, S. J., et al.: NMR imaging of the spine. A.J.R. 141:1137, 1983.
15. Modic, M. T., Weinstein, M. A., Pavlicek, W., et al.: MRI of the cervical spine. A.J.N.R. 5:15, 1983.
16. Modic, M. T., Weinstein, M. A., Pavlicek, W., et al.: MRI imaging of the spine. Radiology 148:757, 1983.
17. Bradley, W. G., Waluch, V., Yadley, R. A., et al.: Comparison of CT and NMR in 400 patients with suspected disease of the brain and spinal cord. Radiology 152:695, 1984.
18. Kucharczyk, W.: CNS tumors in children: Detection by MRI. Radiology 155:131, 1985.
19. Nakstad, P. H., Hald, J. K., Bakke, S. J., et al.: MRI in cervical disc herniation. Neuroradiology 31:382, 1989.
20. Tsuruda, J. S., Norman, D., Dillon, W., et al.: Three-dimensional gradient-recalled MR imaging as a screening tool for the diagnosis of cervical radiculopathy. A.J.N.R. 10:1263, 1989.
21. Murayama, S., Numaguchi, Y., and Robinson, A. E.: The diagnosis of herniated intervertebral disks with MR imaging: A comparison of gradient-refocused-echo and spin-echo pulse sequences. A.J.N.R. 11:17, 1990.
22. Castillo, M., Malko, J. A., and Hoffman, J. C., Jr.: The bright intervertebral disk: An indirect sign of abnormal spinal bone marrow on T1-weighted MR images. A.J.N.R. 11:23, 1990.
23. VanDyke, C., Ross, J. S., Tkach, J., et al.: Gradient-echo MR imaging of the cervical spine: Evaluation of extradural disease. A.J.R. 153:393, 1989.
24. Quint, D. J., Patel, S. C., and Sanders, W. P.: Importance of absence of CSF pulsation artifacts in the MR detection of significant myelographic block at 1.5T. A.J.N.R. 10:1089, 1989.
25. Ross, J. S., Modic, M. T., and Masaryk, T. J.: Tears of the anulus fibrosus: Assessment with Gd-DTPA-enhanced MR imaging. A.J.N.R. 10:1251, 1989.
26. Breger, R. K., Williams, A. L., Daniels, D. L., et al.: Contrast enhancement in spinal MR imaging. A.J.R. 153:387, 1989.
27. Newman, P. K.: Whiplash injury. Br. Med. J. 301:6749, 1990.
28. Hoppenfeld, S.: Orthopaedic Neurology. Philadelphia, J. B. Lippincott, 1977.
29. Nakano, K. K., and Newbill, D. C.: An unusual source of acute neck pain: Calcifications surrounding the odontoid process. Straub Proc. 52 (April):13, 1987.
30. Bouvet, P., LeParc, J. M., Michalski, B., et al.: Acute neck pain due to

calcifications surrounding the odontoid process: The crowned dens syndrome. Arthritis Rheum. 12:1417, 1985.

31. Sawada, H., Akiguchi, I., Fukuyama, H., et al.: Marked spinal stenosis at the level of the atlas. Neuroradiology 31:346, 1989.

32. Laban, M. M., Braker, A. M., and Meerschaert, J. R.: Airport induced "cervical traction" radiculopathy: The OJ syndrome. Arch. Phys. Med. Rehabil. 70:845, 1989.

33. Johnston, R. A.: Management of old people with neck trauma. Br. Med. J. 299:633, 1989.

34. Crawford, P. M., and Shepherd, D. I.: Hyperextension injuries to the cervical cord in the elderly. Br. Med. J. 299:669, 1989.

35. Yablon, I. G., Ordia, J., Mortara, R., et al.: Acute ascending myelopathy of the spine. Spine 14:1084, 1989.

36. Wen, D. U., Bergman, T. A., and Haines, S. J.: Acute cervical myelopathy from hereditary multiple exostoses: Case report. Neurosurgery 25:472, 1989.

37. Patel, S. C., and Sanders, W. P.: Synovial cyst of the cervical spine: Case report and review of the literature. A.J.N.R. 9:602, 1988.

38. McKinney, L. A.: Early mobilisation and outcome in acute sprains of the neck. Br. Med. J. 299:1006, 1989.

39. Cyriax, J.: Textbook of Orthopedic Medicine. Vol. 2. London, Cassell, 1965.

40. Miller, R. G., and Burton, R.: Stroke following chiropractic manipulation of the spine. J.A.M.A. 229:189, 1974.

41. Dunsker, S. B.: Cervical Spondylosis: Seminars in Neurological Surgery. New York, Raven Press, 1981.

42. Simeone, F. A., and Rothman, R. H.: Cervical disc disease. In Simeone, F. A., and Rothman, R. H. (eds.): The Spine. Philadelphia, W. B. Saunders Company, 1982, pp. 440–499.

43. Lunsford, L. N., Bissonette, D. J., Jannetta, P. J., et al.: Anterior surgery for cervical disc disease. J. Neurosurg. 53:1, 1980.

44. Murphy, K. P., Opitz, J. L., Cabanela, M. E., et al.: Cervical fractures and spinal cord injury: Outcome of surgical and nonsurgical management. Mayo Clin. Proc. 65:949, 1990.

45. Snyder, G. M., and Bernhardt, M.: Anterior cervical fractional interspace decompression for treatment of cervical radiculopathy: A review of the first 66 cases. Clin. Orthop. Rel. Res. 246:92, 1989.

46. Vassilouthis, J., Kalovithouris, A., Papandreou, A., et al.: The symptomatic incompetent cervical intervertebral disc. Neurosurgery 25:232, 1989.

Shoulder Pain

Shoulder pain is one of the most common musculoskeletal problems seen in an outpatient setting. The clinician must differentiate between pain from a local shoulder problem and that referred from another source. Owing to its role as the link between the thorax and the upper extremity and the close proximity of major neurovascular structures, the shoulder is frequently painful as an early manifestation of systemic disease. Left shoulder pain may be the initial presentation of coronary artery disease. Hepatic or splenic disease may initially present as shoulder pain. The purpose of this chapter is to provide the reader with practical guidelines for the diagnosis and treatment of painful shoulder disorders seen in a rheumatology practice. Improvements in diagnostic tests such as magnetic resonance imaging (MRI), arthrography–computed tomography (arthro-CT), sonography, and electromyography (EMG) have facilitated early diagnosis of shoulder pain. Moreover, these improved techniques have led to a better understanding of rotator cuff diseases, impingement, instability patterns, and a variety of other disorders about the shoulder.

A detailed analysis of shoulder problems and the treatment of major trauma are beyond the scope of this chapter and have been covered by other authors.[1-5] The conditions to be discussed are divided, albeit artificially, into disorders of the periarticular structures, disorders of the glenohumeral joint, and regional disorders (Table 26–1).

DIAGNOSTIC AIDS

Anatomy

An understanding of the structural and functional anatomy is a requisite for the clinician treating shoulder pain. One must visualize the three-dimensional relationships, muscular functions, ligamentous and tendinous attachments, and routing of neurovascular structures. Figure 26–1 shows the musculoskeletal and topographic localization of pain in association with common shoulder disorders. Figure 26–2 shows the relationship of the posterior musculature coursing anteriorly underneath the acromion to insert on the greater tuberosity. These muscles, combined with the subscapularis inserting on the lesser tuberosity, form the functionally important rotator cuff. By understanding the relationship between the rotator cuff and the subacromial region bounded inferiorly by the humeral head and superiorly by the undersurface of the acromion, the clinician not only can visualize the problems of an impingement syndrome but also can accurately aspirate and inject this space. Knowledge of the route of the tendon of the long head of the biceps through the bicipital groove and onto the superior aspect of the glenoid helps in an understanding of bicipital tendinitis. Before attempting to diagnose and treat shoulder pain, the reader should review in some detail one of the many sources describing the structural and functional relationships of the shoulder girdle.[2, 3]

The use of arthroscopy for both diagnosis and treatment of shoulder problems has led to an increased understanding of the arthroscopic anatomy of the capsular region. Figure 26–3 shows the glenohumeral ligaments, which are important in maintaining the stability of the shoulder joint. Anterior stability is predominantly conferred by the inferior

Table 26–1. COMMON CAUSES OF SHOULDER PAIN

Periarticular Disorders
Rotator cuff tendinitis/impingement syndrome
Calcific tendinitis
Rotator cuff tear
Bicipital tendinitis
Acromioclavicular arthritis
Glenohumeral Disorders
Inflammatory arthritis
Osteoarthritis
Osteonecrosis
Cuff arthropathy
Septic arthritis
Glenoid labrum tears
Adhesive capsulitis
Glenohumeral instability
Regional Disorders
Cervical radiculopathy
Brachial neuritis
Nerve entrapment syndromes
Sternoclavicular arthritis
Reflex sympathetic dystrophy
Fibrositis
Neoplasms
Miscellaneous
   Gallbladder disease
   Splenic trauma
   Subphrenic abscess
   Myocardial infarction
   Thyroid disease
   Diabetes mellitus
   Renal osteodystrophy

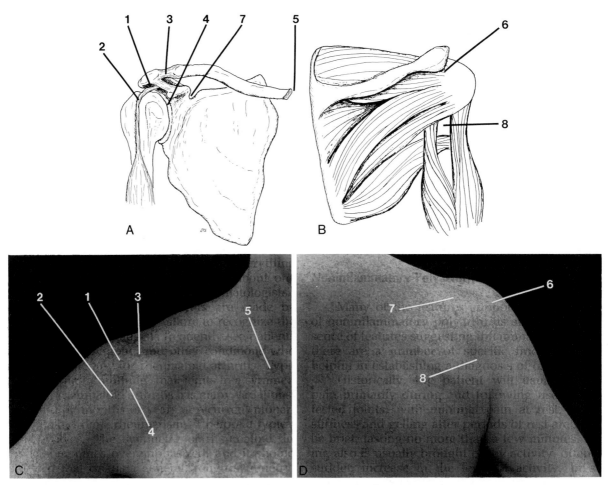

Figure 26–1. Musculoskeletal (*A* and *B*) and topographical (*C* and *D*) areas localizing pain and tenderness associated with specific shoulder problems. *1*, Subacromial space (rotator cuff tendinitis/impingement syndrome, calcific tendinitis, rotator cuff tear). *2*, Bicipital groove (bicipital tendinitis, biceps tendon subluxation and tear). *3*, Acromioclavicular joint. *4*, Anterior glenohumeral joint (glenohumeral arthritis, osteonecrosis, glenoid labrum tears, adhesive capsulitis). *5*, Sternoclavicular joint. *6*, Posterior edge of acromion (rotator cuff tendinitis, calcific tendinitis, rotator cuff tear). *7*, Suprascapular notch (suprascapular nerve entrapment). *8*, Quadrilateral space (axillary nerve entrapment). These areas of pain and tenderness frequently overlap.

glenohumeral ligament. The labrum serves to enlarge the contact area of the articular surface as well as to confer stability to the joint. Lesions of the labrum indicate certain instability patterns and may be a source of pain from internal derangement of the shoulder.

History

Most shoulder problems can be diagnosed by taking a detailed history. The association with trauma, rapidity of onset, and character and localization of the pain frequently lead the clinician to the proper diagnosis. For instance, anterior dislocations of the glenohumeral joint are usually associated with a force directed to the arm with the shoulder in an abducted and externally rotated position, whereas dislocations of the acromioclavicular (AC) joint are usually due to direct trauma to the shoulder region. The gradual onset of pain in the subacromial region

that is increased with forward elevation of the shoulder is characteristic of rotator cuff tendinitis with impingement. The presence of a snap or click on forward elevation combined with weakness frequently indicates a rotator cuff tear associated with impingement. The burning quality and characteristic radiation of pain are indicative of a neuropathic process.

Physical Examination

A comprehensive physical and neurologic examination with particular attention to the involved extremity is essential. Careful recording of range of motion should include both active and passive forward flexion, abduction, internal and external rotation in a neutral position and at 90 degrees of abduction, and forward elevation. Forward elevation is defined as the functional arc between forward flexion and abduction and represents the most im-

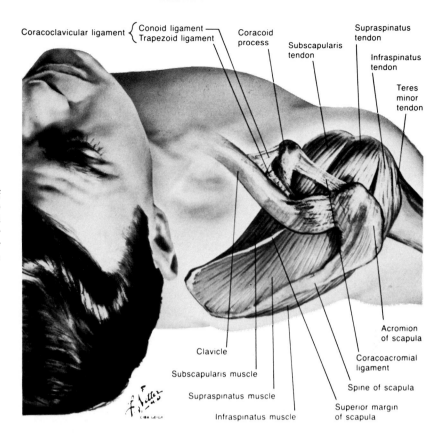

Figure 26–2. Superior view of the rotator cuff musculature as it courses anteriorly underneath the coracoacromial arch to insert upon the greater tuberosity. (Reproduced by permission of Ciba-Geigy. From The Ciba Collection of Medical Illustrations, Volume 8, Part I.)

Labels: Coracoclavicular ligament { Conoid ligament / Trapezoid ligament }; Coracoid process; Subscapularis tendon; Supraspinatus tendon; Infraspinatus tendon; Teres minor tendon; Clavicle; Subscapularis muscle; Supraspinatus muscle; Infraspinatus muscle; Acromion of scapula; Coracoacromial ligament; Spine of scapula; Superior margin of scapula

portant motion in terms of placing the hand in a functional position. Abduction should be divided into that which occurs at the glenohumeral joint and that which occurs at the scapulothoracic articulation. Careful recording of these values on serial examinations aid in measuring response to therapy.

The localization of tenderness can help differentiate common entities such as glenoid labrum tears, rotator cuff tendinitis, and bicipital tendinitis. Although all three are associated with tenderness in the anterior aspect of the shoulder, the tenderness of rotator cuff tendinitis is generally subacromial and that of bicipital tendinitis migrates laterally and superiorly as the shoulder is abducted and externally rotated. Tenderness in the quadrilateral space or suprascapular notch is frequently associated with nerve entrapment syndromes. Neurologic examination should include sensory testing of the upper extremity with particular reference to the area innervated by the axillary nerve. Results of evaluation of all muscle systems should be graded and recorded and the presence of atrophy or fasciculations noted. Examination of the ipsilateral elbow, wrist, and hand is important not only in planning therapy but also in determining functional expectations.

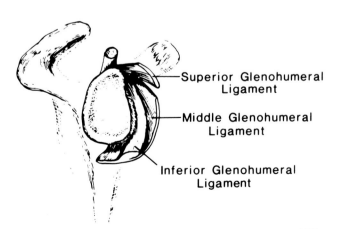

Figure 26–3. Schematic representation of the superior, middle, and inferior glenohumeral ligaments as visualized arthroscopically.

Labels: Superior Glenohumeral Ligament; Middle Glenohumeral Ligament; Inferior Glenohumeral Ligament

Plain Radiographs

For most nontraumatic painful shoulder syndromes, the use of an anteroposterior or glenohumeral view of the involved shoulder in internal and external rotation suffices. In cases of injury to the shoulder girdle, a "trauma series," involving an anteroposterior view, scapular Y view, and axillary view, has become standard protocol. The axillary view is particularly helpful in assessing posterior or anterior subluxation of the humeral head. It has been recognized that impingement-induced rotator cuff tendinitis can be caused by or, if already present, increased by anterior subluxation. In such cases, an axillary view or even fluoroscopy can be helpful in demonstrating the subluxation.[6, 7] In cases of suspected AC joint injury, an anteroposterior view of the shoulder with a weight held in the ipsilateral hand frequently demonstrates subluxation at the AC joint. Several special shoulder radiographs are available for the evaluation of specific lesions such as Bankart's lesion of the anterior inferior glenoid rim (West Point view) or a Hill-Sachs lesion (Didiee view, Hermodsson view).

Scintigraphy

Technetium methyldiphosphonate (99mTc-MDP) or gallium may be of diagnostic help in evaluating skeletal lesions about the shoulder joint. Bone scans are generally not helpful in the diagnosis of non-neoplastic or noninfectious shoulder disease.

Scintigraphy may have a role in differentiating those patients with complete rotator cuff tears that proceed to cuff tear arthropathy. As is discussed later in this chapter, this is an important distinction because patients with complete rotator cuff tears may do well, whereas those who develop progressive changes of cuff tear arthropathy have progressive arthritis, pain, and significant functional impairment. The presence of synovitis or calcium pyrophosphate deposition disease (CPPD) may be an important factor in the pathogenesis of cuff tear arthropathy. In such cases, scintigraphy may demonstrate the increased blood flow and blood pooling associated with the chronic synovitis.

Arthrography

Single-contrast arthrography, double-contrast arthrography, and double-contrast arthrotomography (DCAT) are valuable tools in evaluating problems of the rotator cuff, glenoid labrum, biceps tendon, and shoulder capsule.[8-11] Figure 26–4 shows a normal double-contrast arthrogram of the shoulder. Rotator cuff tears can be demonstrated by both single-contrast and double-contrast studies. The proponents of double-contrast arthrography believe that the extent of the tear, the preferred surgical approach, and the quality of the rotator cuff tissue are best determined by double-contrast studies.[9-11] Figure 26–5 demonstrates extravasation of contrast material into the subacromial space from a rotator cuff tear. Arthrography can be misleading by underestimating the extent of a rotator cuff tear. Tears of the glenoid labrum without shoulder dislocation are now being recognized as sources of anterior shoulder pain in athletes.

Glenoid labrum tears (Fig. 26–6) with or without associated glenohumeral subluxation can frequently be identified by DCAT.[11, 12] Kneisl et al.[13] reported on 55 patients who underwent DCAT followed by a diagnostic shoulder arthroscopy. DCAT predicted

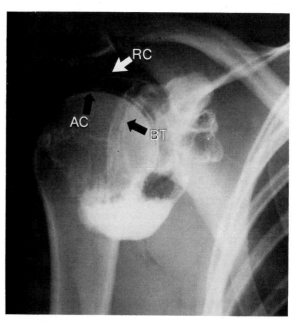

Figure 26–4. Normal double-contrast arthrogram showing the inferior edge of the rotator cuff *(RC)* as it courses through the subacromial space to the greater tuberosity; the tendon of the long head of the biceps *(BT)*; and the articular cartilage of the humeral head *(AC)*.

the arthroscopic findings in 76 percent of anterior labra and 96 percent of posterior labra. This test was 100 percent sensitive and 94 percent specific in diagnosing complete rotator cuff tears. Partial rotator

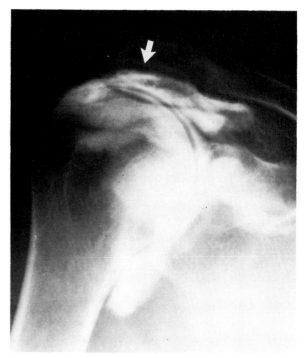

Figure 26–5. Single-contrast arthrogram demonstrating a massive rotator cuff tear with extravasation of contrast into the subacromial space *(arrow)*.

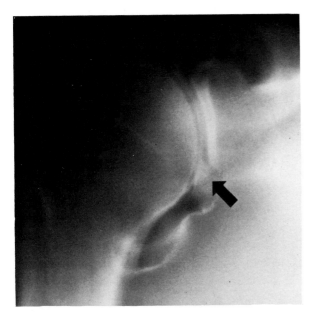

Figure 26–6. A double-contrast arthrotomogram demonstrating a tear of the anteroinferior portion of the glenoid labrum *(arrow)*.

cuff tears identified at arthroscopy were missed in 83 percent of patients undergoing DCAT. The authors believed DCAT was better in diagnosing interarticular and cuff pathology in the presence of instability than if pain alone was a presenting diagnosis.[13]

Shoulder arthrography can confirm a diagnosis of adhesive capsulitis by showing a contracted capsule with an obliterated axillary recess (Fig. 26–7).

The use of subacromial bursography has been reported to be beneficial in visualizing the outer surface of the rotator cuff and the subacromial space in cases of impingement.[14, 15] Fukuda et al.[16] reported

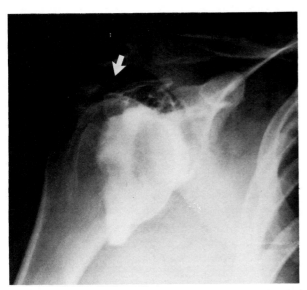

Figure 26–7. Double-contrast arthrogram in patient with calcific tendinitis *(arrow)* and adhesive capsulitis. Note the contracted capsule with diminution of the synovial space and obliteration of the axillary recess.

a small series of younger patients (average age 41.8 years) who underwent subacromial bursography following a negative glenohumeral arthrogram. These patients demonstrated pooling of contrast medium on a bursal side of a tear, which was confirmed at the time of surgery. At the time of surgical exploration, these patients underwent wedge resection and primary repair of these partial tears. It is unclear whether patients undergoing open or arthroscopic decompression for impingement require resection or repair of such partial lesions.[16] Subacromial bursography is not routinely used diagnostically and in the author's opinion is of little value in planning surgical procedures.

Computed Tomography

CT is helpful in evaluating the musculoskeletal system, and CT combined with contrast arthrography (arthro-CT) has become a major diagnostic tool for the evaluation of glenoid labrum tears, loose bodies, and chondral lesions (Fig. 26–8). Rafii et al.[17] reported on the use of arthro-CT in the evaluation of shoulder derangement. In this study, there was a 95 percent accuracy of arthro-CT in investigating lesions of the labrum and articular surface.[17] Moreover, arthro-CT may still be the best test for determining full-thickness rotator cuff tears when a decision about surgical repair must be made.

Ultrasonography

The technologic improvement of sonographic equipment has allowed improved ultrasonographic study of the rotator cuff. The technique is noninvasive and rapid and involves no radiation exposure.[12–15] The cuff is examined in both horizontal and transverse planes with the arm in different positions to visualize various areas of the cuff. These techniques generally provide visualization of the distal cuff, where most rotator cuff tears are located.[12–15] Figure 26–9 shows normal and abnormal ultrasound images of the rotator cuff in both longitudinal and transverse planes.

Several studies report a high sensitivity and specificity for the ultrasonographic diagnosis of a rotator cuff tear.[12, 15–17] The specificity and sensitivity of the procedure are reported to be greater than 90 percent as determined by both arthrographic and surgical correlation.[15, 17] This technique has also been used for the postoperative evaluation of a rotator cuff repair and for evaluation of abnormalities of the biceps tendon.[18, 19]

Ultrasonography (US) of the rotator cuff requires an ultrasonographer experienced not only in performing the technique but also in interpreting the images. Abnormalities in the rotator cuff can be seen as hyperechoic areas, hypoechoic areas, or discontinuities in the cuff. Ultrasound scans of associated

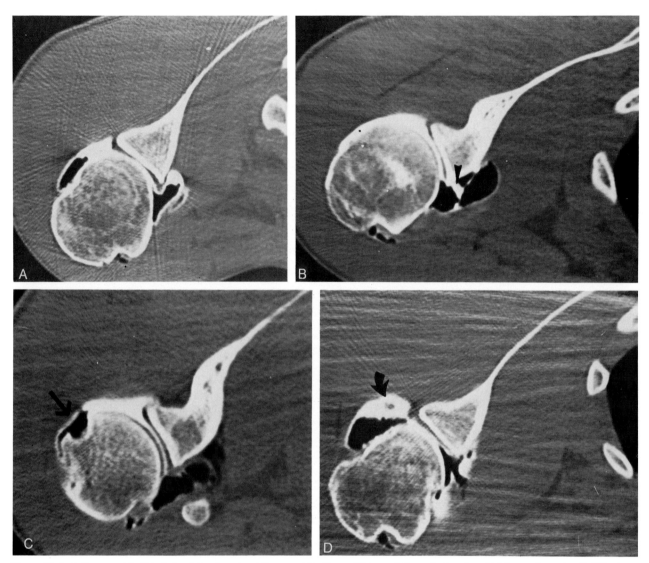

Figure 26–8. Arthrographic CT of shoulder showing *(A)* normal findings; *(B)* tear of the anterior glenoid labrum *(arrowhead)*; *(C)* a large defect of the articular surface of the posterior portion of the humeral head (Hill-Sachs lesion) *(arrow)*; and *(D)* loose body in the posterior recess *(arrow)*.

lesions, such as calcific tendinitis or subluxation of the humeral head, and even the normal biceps tendon can be misinterpreted as a rotator cuff lesion.[20] Small echogenic areas within an injured rotator cuff may, at times, be confused with partial rotator cuff lesions. Further experience with this procedure and correlation with arthrography, arthroscopy, and open surgery should further delineate its role in the evaluation of the painful shoulder.

Gardelin and Perin[27] reported US to be 96 percent sensitive in determining rotator cuff and biceps tendon pathology. Mack et al.[28] found US even to be valuable in evaluating the postoperative patient with recurrent shoulder symptoms. In a prospective study, Hodler et al.[29] compared US with MRI and arthrography in evaluating rotator cuff lesions in 24 shoulders. US identified 14 of 15 torn cuffs, MRI 10 of 15, and arthrography 15 of 15.[29] US identified

seven of nine intact rotator cuffs, whereas MRI was accurate in eight of nine intact cuffs.[29] Vestring et al.[30] found US to be as accurate as MRI in the diagnosis of humeral head defects and joint effusions but inferior to MRI in the diagnosis of labrum lesions, rotator cuff lesions, subacromial spurs, and synovial inflammatory disease. US has also been reported to be valuable in identifying dislocation of the biceps tendon, particularly when it is associated with a full-thickness rotator cuff tear.

In the author's opinion, US has been helpful in the evaluation of an acutely injured shoulder if a rotator cuff tear is suspected. In the hands of an experienced sonographer, US may be the most cost-effective test for initial evaluation of a rotator cuff injury, but most surgeons would require arthro-CT or MRI confirmation before surgical exploration.[27–31]

US has been helpful in the evaluation of an

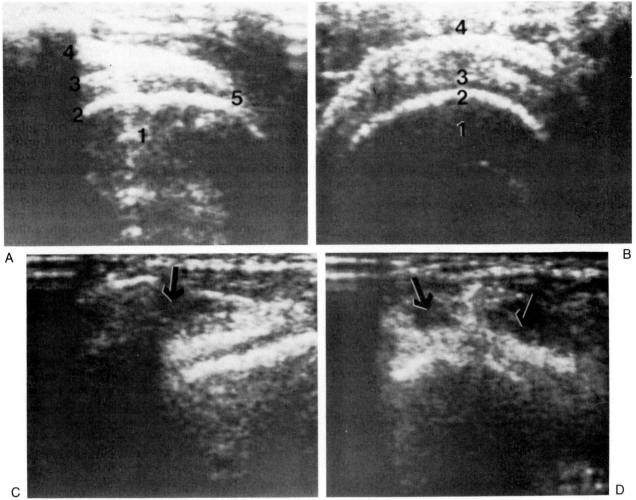

Figure 26–9. *A,* Normal longitudinal view of rotator cuff by ultrasound showing *(1)* humeral head, *(2)* the superior articular surface, *(3)* the rotator cuff, *(4)* the deltoid tendon, and *(5)* the tapering of the cuff to its insertion on the greater tuberosity. *B,* Transverse view of a normal intact rotator cuff covering the humeral head. *C,* Rotator cuff tear showing hypoechoic area *(arrow)* on a longitudinal view. *D,* Rotator cuff tear demonstrating hypoechoic area *(arrows)* on transverse view.

acutely injured shoulder if a rotator cuff tear is suspected. In most centers, arthrographic or MRI confirmation of a complete rotator cuff tear would be obtained before surgical exploration.

Arthroscopy

Diagnostic arthroscopy and arthroscopic surgery have greatly aided in the diagnosis and treatment of knee injuries (see Chapter 38). These arthroscopic techniques have proved to be of value in the diagnosis and treatment of glenohumeral and subacromial disorders. They have been recommended for evaluating glenohumeral synovitis, articular cartilage damage, loose bodies, and particularly for diagnosing labrum tears. In combination with physical examination, history, and examination under anesthesia, arthroscopy has been helpful in the diagnosis of chronic instability patterns of the glenohumeral joint. Compared with DCAT, arthroscopy was reported to

be more accurate in the diagnosis of intra-articular lesions associated with a painful shoulder.[13] An additional benefit is that arthroscopy can be used for both diagnosis and treatment of shoulder problems of the glenohumeral joint and the subacromial region. Debridement of rotator cuff tears in elderly patients, resection of the subacromial bursa, debridement of labrum tears, and removal of loose bodies have become standard arthroscopic procedures in the shoulder. The use of the arthroscope for repairing torn rotator cuffs and for stabilization of a dislocating shoulder is still in the investigative phase.[32]

Magnetic Resonance Imaging

MRI has been used to diagnose partial-thickness and full-thickness rotator cuff tears, impingement of the rotator cuff, synovitis, articular cartilage damage, and labrum pathology associated with glenohumeral instability.[33–35] In rheumatoid arthritis, MRI is reported to be more sensitive than plain radiographs in determining soft tissue abnormalities and osseous abnormalities of the glenoid and humeral head.[36]

The best use of MRI is in the diagnosis of rotator cuff pathology. Morrison and Offstein[37] studied 100 patients with chronic subacromial impingement syndrome using arthrography and MRI. MRI was 100 percent sensitive but only 88 percent specific in confirming arthrography-proved rotator cuff tears. Nelson et al.[38] studied 21 patients with shoulder pain and found MRI to be more accurate than arthro-CT or US in identifying partial-thickness cuff tears. These authors also reported MRI to be as accurate as arthro-CT in the diagnosis of abnormalities of the glenoid labrum.[38]

The characteristic MRI findings in rotator cuff tears include a hypointense gap within the supraspinatus muscle tendon complex on T_1-weighted films, absence of a demonstrable supraspinatus tendon with narrowing of the subacromial space, and an increased signal in the supraspinatus tendon on T_2-weighted images.[39] Seeger et al.,[40] reporting on 170 MRI scans, found T_1-weighted images to be highly sensitive for identifying abnormalities in the supraspinatus tendon but that T_2-weighted images were required to differentiate tendinitis from a small supraspinatus tendon tear. Large full-thickness tears, however, could be identified on both T_1 and T_2 images. Figures 26–10 and 26–11 depict common shoulder pathology as seen by MRI. MRI is nearly as sensitive and certainly more specific than scintigraphy in the diagnosis of osteonecrosis and neoplastic lesions about the shoulder.

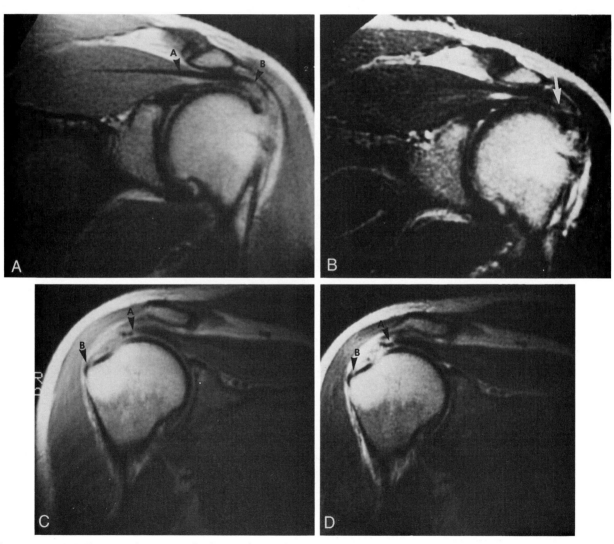

Figure 26–10. *A,* MRI proton density–weighted coronal view showing (A) supraspinatus tendon as a black band that has an increased signal (B) as it nears insertion on the greater tuberosity. *B,* Similar view in T_2-weighted image showing increased signal as gray *(arrow),* indicating partial thickness tear or tendinitis. *C,* MRI proton density–weighted coronal view showing (A) abrupt end of supraspinatus tendon as it courses right to left. From (A) to (B) is area of increased signal followed by short portion of tendon (B) inserting at greater tuberosity. *D,* Similar view in T_2-weighted image showing increased signal as white (fluid density), indicating fluid in the gap of a complete rotator cuff tear.

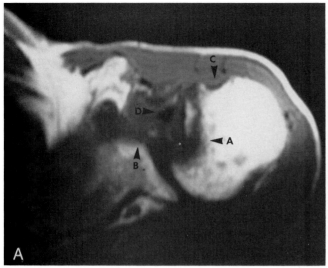
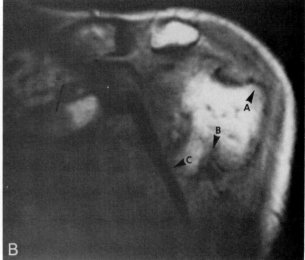

Figure 26–11. *A,* MRI T$_1$-weighted transverse view of patient with recurrent anterior and posterior dislocation and chronic dislocation of the long head of the biceps tendon, showing (A) large reverse Hill-Sachs lesion (anterior humeral defect from posterior dislocation), (B) Bankart lesion of anterior glenoid rim indicating anterior instability, (C) the bicipital groove, and (D) the biceps tendon, which is chronically dislocated from the groove. *B,* Coronal view of same patient showing (A) greater tuberosity, (B) bicipital groove, and (C) long head of biceps tendon *(broad black band)* that is dislocated from the groove.

Electromyography and Nerve Conduction Velocity Studies

EMG and nerve conduction velocity (NCV) studies can be helpful in differentiating shoulder pain from pain of neurogenic origin (see Chapter 40). They may also be beneficial in determining the localization of neurogenic pain to a particular cervical root, the brachial plexus, or a peripheral nerve.[41, 42]

Injection

Injection of local anesthetics and glucocorticoids is a useful technique for both diagnosis and treatment of shoulder pain (see Chapter 35). The physician must have a thorough knowledge of the anatomy of the shoulder girdle and a presumptive diagnosis to direct the injection properly. Injection of referred pain areas may be misleading. For example, in the patient with lateral arm pain owing to deltoid bursal involvement from calcific tendinitis of the supraspinatus tendon, injection should be in the subacromial space and not the area of referred pain in the deltoid muscle.

It is often better to use a posterior subacromial approach when injecting a rotator cuff tendinitis in a patient with anterior impingement symptoms because it is not only easier to enter the subacromial region posteriorly but also less traumatic to the contracted anterior structures.

The instillation of rapidly acting local anesthetics can be beneficial in determining the source of shoulder pain. Obliteration of pain, for instance, by injection of a local anesthetic along the bicipital groove can confirm a diagnosis of bicipital tendinitis. The use of local anesthetics is somewhat less helpful when injecting the subacromial space, owing to its extensive communications with the rest of the shoulder girdle, but relief of symptoms by such an injection can rule out pain from conditions such as cervical radiculopathy or an entrapment neuropathy.

Author's Preferred Diagnostic Tests

Table 26–2 lists the relative costs of various shoulder diagnostic tests based on 1992 estimates at a single institution. Choice of a specific test depends on its sensitivity, specificity, and cost-benefit analysis. In considering arthroscopy, it must be remembered that concomitant therapy can be delivered. For instance, in patients with symptoms of internal derangement and presumed labrum tears, arthroscopy can be used both to confirm and to treat (debride) the pathologic abnormality. History and physical examination are the most important factors in establishing diagnosis of the painful shoulder. Plain radiographs (three views) should be the first radiographic test performed. Although not as sensitive as the more sophisticated tests, plain radiographs can iden-

Table 26–2. RELATIVE COSTS OF SHOULDER DIAGNOSTIC PROCEDURES (1992)

Office visit (30 minutes): diagnostic examination	$ 75.00
Plain radiography	$ 89.00
Arthrography	$477.00
Ultrasonography	$303.00
Magnetic resonance imaging	$909.00
Computed tomography	$545.00
Tomography	$328.00

tify arthritic change, calcific tendinitis, established osteonecrosis, and most neoplasms. If interarticular pathology is suspected (labrum tear, capsular tear, loose body, chondral defect), arthro-CT is preferable to MRI. In diagnosing acute rotator cuff tears in the younger patient, US is the most cost-effective test to confirm a clinical suspicion. In cases of impingement syndrome, MRI is sensitive, but it is difficult to differentiate tendinitis, partial tears, and small complete tears. In deciding between an arthroscopic or open decompression for chronic impingement, the author prefers arthrography to MRI, as open decompression is favored if there is a repairable full-thickness tear.

PERIARTICULAR DISORDERS

Rotator Cuff Tendinitis/Impingement Syndrome

The majority of painful nontraumatic conditions about the shoulder joint are caused by tendinitis of the rotator cuff. Codman[1] published his classic text reviewing the nature of these lesions and pointed out their importance in work-related disabilities. Degenerative tendinitis has been labeled pericapsulitis, subacromial bursitis, subdeltoid bursitis, supraspinatus tendinitis, rotator cuff tear, and impingement syndrome. The variation in clinical description, method of treatment, and response to treatment perhaps is due to description of the same condition at different periods of its pathophysiology. Neer[43] has clarified this condition by pointing out the various stages of this disorder. Although stratified into three stages, the process represents a continuum of inflammation, degeneration, and attrition of the rotator cuff by impingement on the anterior edge and undersurface of the anterior third of the acromion, the coracoacromial ligament, and occasionally the AC joint.[44] The wear and attritional tears of the cuff occur in the supraspinatus tendon and may extend into the infraspinatus and long head of the biceps.[45] The mechanical impingement of the rotator cuff may be influenced by variations in the shape and slope of the acromion.[45, 46] According to Neer,[43] the three stages of impingement are as follows: *Stage I, edema and hemorrhage,* usually occurs in active individuals younger than age 25 years who engage in activities requiring excessive overhead arm usage. In stage I, treatment is conservative, and the patient generally responds to rest, nonsteroidal anti-inflammatory agents (NSAIDs), and occasional glucocorticoid injection. *Stage II, fibrosis and tendinitis,* represents the biologic response of fibrosis and thickening owing to repeated episodes of mechanical impingement. This stage is usually seen in active individuals between 25 and 40 years of age. They may respond to conservative treatment as in stage I but generally experience recurrent attacks. *Stage III, rotator cuff tears, biceps rupture, and bone changes,* rarely appears before the age of 40 years. Stage III represents the attritional

wear of the supraspinatus tendon and occasionally the infraspinatus and long head of the biceps from repeated impingement. Patients with stage III disease present with varying weakness, crepitus, and supraspinatus atrophy, depending on the extent of the tear and its chronicity.

The predominant feature of degenerative tendinitis is pain. The pain can be sudden and incapacitating or may be a dull ache. It can be focal and pinpointed as an area of tenderness along the anterior edge of the acromion (see Fig. 26–1). It also may present as a diffuse pain around the anterolateral or even posterior edge of the acromion or, at times, radiate to the subdeltoid bursa. This pain can be differentiated from other nontraumatic painful conditions about the shoulder by its position and response to treatment. For instance, the tenderness from bicipital tendinitis will follow the bicipital groove as the arm is externally rotated. Tenderness from a glenoid labrum tear is generally beneath the coracoid and over the anterior edge of the glenoid. The impingement sign as illustrated in Figure 26–12 is useful in the diagnosis of rotator cuff tendinitis. The patient with stage I and even stage II disease will frequently describe a catch as the arm is brought to an overhead position. The patient frequently raises the arm by abduction and rotation to bypass the painful "spot." This observation underscores the Codman paradox, which states that the arm can be brought fully overhead from a neutral position by either external rotation and abduction in the coronal plane or internal rotation and forward flexion in the sagittal plane.[1] In patients with focal tenderness of the supraspinatus, the tender area may disappear under the edge of the acromion as the arm is abducted (Dawbarn's sign).[3] Instillation of short-acting

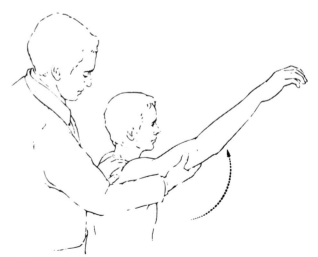

Figure 26–12. The impingement sign is elicited by forced forward elevation of the arm. Pain results as the greater tuberosity impinges on the acromion. The examiner's hand prevents scapular rotation. This maneuver may be positive in other periarticular disorders. (Reproduced with permission from Neer, C. S., II: Impingement lesions. Clin. Orthop. 173:70, 1983.)

local anesthetics into the subacromial space can frequently obliterate the symptoms and confirm the diagnosis of degenerative tendinitis with impingement. It is important to remember that trigger point injection alone can be misleading and that injection of the subacromial space is necessary to assure validity of this diagnostic test.

Radiographs in the early stages of degenerative tendinitis with impingement are normal. As the disease progresses, there may be some sclerosis, cyst formation, and eburnation of the anterior third of the acromion and the greater tuberosity. An anterior acromial traction spur may appear on the undersurface of the acromion lateral to the AC joint and represent contracture of the coracoacromial ligament. The late radiographic findings include narrowing of the acromiohumeral gap, superior subluxation of the humeral head in relationship to the glenoid, and erosive changes of the anterior acromion.[47] Arthrography, MRI, and US, as discussed earlier, may be helpful in diagnosing a full-thickness tear of the rotator cuff in association with stage III disease. In some cases of untreated stage III impingement, proximal migration of the humeral head leads to a pattern of degenerative arthritis known as cuff tear arthropathy.

The choice of treatment, and frequently its result, is a function of the stage of the impingement. In stage I disease, in which there is little mechanical impingement, most patients respond to rest. It is important not to immobilize the shoulder for any period of time because contraction of the shoulder capsule and periarticular structures can produce an adhesive capsulitis. After a period of rest, a progressive program of stretching and strengthening exercises generally restores the shoulder to normal function. Use of aspirin and other NSAIDs may shorten the symptomatic period. Modalities such as US, neuroprobe, and transcutaneous electric nerve stimulation (TENS) are generally not helpful. Patients with stage I and stage II disease may have a dramatic response to local injection of glucocorticoids and local anesthetic agents. In stage II disease, in which there is fibrosis and thickening anteriorly, it is frequently better to inject through a posterior approach. The author prefers a combination of 3 ml of 1 percent lidocaine (Xylocaine), 3 ml of 0.5 percent bupivacaine, and 20 mg of triamcinolone. This combines a short-acting anesthetic for diagnostic purposes, a longer-acting anesthetic for analgesic purposes, and a steroid preparation in a depot form.

An integrated program of occupational and physical therapy often precludes the need for surgery in patients with stage II disease. Job modification for individuals with impingement syndrome secondary to overuse may alleviate symptoms. A report of a 53-year-old woman who in 2 years stacked over 20 tons of cheese from a conveyor belt to shoulder height underscores this point. Because of poor assembly line ergonomics, this patient developed intractable impingement and was forced to take a disability pension. Management is becoming more aware of the cost savings associated with proper job ergonomics.[48, 49]

The initial rehabilitation in stage II impingement is the cessation of repetitive overhand activity. Additionally, ice, NSAIDs, and local injections may be beneficial. The initial physical therapy includes passive active assisted and active range of motion combined with stretching and mobilization exercises to prevent contracture. As pain and inflammation subside, isometric or isotonic exercises are used to strengthen the rotator cuff musculature. Isokinetic training at variable speeds and in variable positions is instituted before returning the patient to full activity. In patients with a job-related injury, it is critical to review and modify job mechanics to prevent recurrent episodes that cause further disability and may precipitate a need for surgery.[49]

Neer[43] has suggested that the patient with refractory stage II disease may respond to division of the coracoacromial ligament and bursectomy of the subacromial bursa. Division of the coracoacromial ligament alone has been performed under a local anesthetic.

Treatment of stage III disease depends on the chronicity of the symptoms and the presence or absence of a rotator cuff tear. Neer[43] recommends arthrography in those patients over 40 years of age who fail to respond to conservative treatment or experience sudden weakness of abduction and external rotation, suggesting extension of a tear. Alternatively, US or MRI may be used to clarify rotator cuff pathology.

The surgical treatment of choice is an anterior acromioplasty, although some investigators have reported adequate results with acromionectomy. Bosley[50] reported a 20-year experience using total acromionectomy for treatment of impingement. In this study of 34 shoulders at 5-year follow-up, 25 were excellent, four were good, three were fair, and one was poor. The author stressed the importance of repair of the deltoid muscle to achieve a good functional result. Most investigators prefer acromioplasty and believe that lateral acromionectomy or complete acromionectomy unnecessarily weakens the deltoid muscle and predisposes the patient to proximal migration of the humeral head.[47]

The indication for anterior acromioplasty is based on symptoms that fail to respond to at least 1 year of conservative therapy. There is controversy as to the role of open versus arthroscopic acromioplasty for stage II/III disease. Gartsman[51] reviewed 154 arthroscopic acromioplasties in patients with stage II or stage III impingement. Eighty-two of 89 stage II shoulders with an intact rotator cuff improved. In stage II disease with a partial rotator cuff tear, 33 of 40 shoulders improved. In stage III disease with a complete rotator cuff tear, only 14 of 25 patients improved. It was the author's conclusion that arthroscopic acromioplasty is effective in treatment of stage II disease, but that open acromioplasty was preferred in patients with full-thickness tears.[51]

Another prognostic indicator of the effectiveness of arthroscopic decompression is the presence of an osseous component of impingement. In a study of 80 arthroscopic subacromial decompressions, patients who underwent soft tissue rather than bone decompression had a better final outcome.[52]

Arthroscopy may be of value in elderly patients with stage III disease even with full-thickness rotator cuff tears. In these patients with stage III disease and no functional weakness, arthroscopic debridement without repair of full-thickness tears can be associated with a good functional result.[53, 54]

The results of open acromioplasty for impingement with an intact rotator cuff are gratifying.[55, 56] Hawkins et al.[55] reported an 87 percent success rate following anterior acromioplasty in 108 patients with intact rotator cuffs. In this study, the procedure was less successful in women, patients with limited motion, patients whose injury was due to direct trauma, and in workmen's compensation claims.[55] Stuart et al.[56] reported an overall 77 percent pain relief in 66 shoulders undergoing open acromioplasty. This study reported no significant difference in results with or without an associated rotator cuff tear. Bigliani et al.[57] reported 81 percent good to excellent results in 26 patients younger than 40 years of age who underwent open acromioplasty for subacromial impingement. Bjorkenheim et al.[58] reviewed 78 decompression and rotator cuff reconstructions for patients with long-standing impingement and a cuff tear. In this study, 71 percent of patients were excellent or satisfactory, and 29 percent were unsatisfactory.

A review of 67 failed anterior acromioplasties found diagnostic and operative errors to be a common cause of failure.[59] The authors point out the importance of identifying associated abnormalities such as intra-articular pathology that may be overlooked during a subacromial approach. Subsequent surgery was 75 percent successful in patients not receiving workmen's compensation but only 46 percent successful in the compensation group.

It is important to point out that not all rotator cuff tears require operative intervention.[60] The indication for surgery is intractable pain and functional impairment. In elderly individuals, symptomatic treatment and physical therapy are generally sufficient, and most cuff tears are treated conservatively.[61]

Calcific Tendinitis

Although most rotator cuff tendinitis probably represents one of the stages of mechanical impingement, there appears to be a group of patients predisposed to inflammation in this area. These patients frequently have bilateral disease and give a history of other periarticular conditions such as trochanteric bursitis of the hip or symptoms of fibrositis. One particular subset within this group is made up of those individuals with calcific tendinitis.

Calcific tendinitis is a painful condition about the rotator cuff in association with deposition of calcium salts, primarily hydroxyapatite.[62–64] It is most common in patients over 30 years of age and shows a predilection for females.[62, 65] Although it is more common in the right shoulder, there is at least a 6 percent incidence of bilaterality.[62] Patients with bilateral shoulder involvement often have the syndrome of calcific periarthritis, in which calcium hydroxyapatite crystals are found at multiple sites.[69]

Codman[1] pointed out the localization of the calcification within the tendon of the supraspinatus. He provided a detailed description of the symptoms and natural history of this condition. In describing the phases of pain, spasm, limitation of motion, and atrophy, he noted the lack of correlation between symptoms and the size of the calcific deposit. According to Codman, the natural history includes degeneration of the supraspinatus tendon, calcification, and eventual rupture into the subacromial bursa. During this latter phase, pain and decreased motion can lead to adhesive capsulitis (see Fig. 26–7).

The pathogenesis of calcific tendinitis of the supraspinatus is recognized as a degenerative process with secondary calcification within the tendon fibers.[62–64] The localization of the calcium within the supraspinatus may be due to several factors. Many of these patients have an early stage of impingement, compressing the supraspinatus tendon on the anterior portion of the acromion.[43, 44] This long-standing impingement may lead to local degeneration of the tendon fibers. In patients without impingement, the localization of the calcium within the supraspinatus may be related to the blood supply of the rotator cuff, which normally is derived from an anastomotic network of vessels from either the greater tuberosity or the bellies of the short rotator muscles.[63] The watershed of these sources is just medial to the tendinous attachment of the supraspinatus.[66] Rathburn and Macnab[67] referred to this watershed as the *critical zone* and pointed out that during abduction this area was rendered ischemic.

The stimulation for calcification in calcific tendinitis has been the focus of considerable study.[63, 64, 66] Steinbrocker[68] postulated that the process begins with necrosis and fraying of the tendon fibers, with secondary formation of a fibrinoid mass surrounded by leukocytes. This mass then serves as a template for calcification. Others have suggested that the process of degeneration of the tendon causes formation of small particles consisting primarily of calcium salts.[4] The hyperemia associated with the acute episode would cause coalescence of the calcium with formation of a liquefied calcium mass. As the increased vascularity subsides, this calcified mass would return to its "dry state."

It is also possible that the hypervascularity may, in fact, "wash out" an inhibitor substance and allow calcification to occur on the denuded fibers of the frayed tendon. It would be attractive to consider proteoglycans in this inhibitory role because they are ubiquitous in tendons and articular cartilage, both of which do not calcify in the normal state.

Uhthoff et al.[63] have proposed that the pathogenesis of this process is not associated with inflammation or scarring but suggests that the primary stimulus is hypoxia, which results in transformation of portions of the tendon into fibrocartilage. The chrondrocytes then would mediate calcification in a way similar to that occurring in the calcifying zone of the epiphyseal plate. In a subsequent study, it was pointed out that the ultrastructure of calcifying tendinitis failed to demonstrate the arrangement or cell types seen in the epiphyseal plate.[64] The calcification occurred in extracellular matrix vesicles located in areas that had undergone fibrocartilaginous transformation. The authors pointed out the similarity to extracellular vesicles noted in other normal and pathologic conditions.[64] After calcification, the foci became surrounded by mononuclear and multinucleate cells, with phagocytized material within the cytoplasm.[63] Vascular invasion occurred as part of the repair process. By restoring normal perfusion and oxygen tension to the tissue, the calcium could then be resorbed and the tendon returned to its normal state.[63] Calcific tendinitis has also been identified at the insertion of the long head of the biceps on the superior glenoid and in the long head of the biceps at the junction of the tendon and the muscle. Of 119 cases of calcific tendinitis reviewed between 1980 and 1988, 20 had calcification in the region of the biceps tendon (nine at the glenoid insertion and 11 adjacent to the humeral shaft). In the 11 cases with distal calcification, all had small homogeneous deposits, and the major differential diagnosis was with loose bodies trapped in the biceps tendon sheath.[67]

Treatment of calcific tendinitis depends on the clinical presentation and the presence of associated impingement. These patients can have an acute inflammatory reaction that may resemble gout. The acute inflammation can be treated with local glucocorticoid injection, the use of NSAIDs, or both. On occasion, US may be of some benefit. If there is associated impingement, treatment depends on the stage of presentation. The radiographic appearance of the calcification can direct and perhaps predict the response to therapy. In the resorptive phase, the deposits appear floccular, suggesting that the process is in the phase of repair and that a conservative program is indicated. Those patients with discrete calcification, and perhaps associated adhesive capsulitis (see Fig. 26–7), may be at a stable phase at which the calcium produces a mechanical block and is unlikely to be resorbed. In these patients, mechanical removal of the calcific deposits and correction of associated pathologic lesions may be necessary. Percutaneous disruption of the calcified areas may be performed using a needle directed by fluoroscopy. This technique allows lavage and injection but does not treat associated impingement. Subacromial arthroscopy allows the mechanical needle disruption of calcific deposits under direct visualization. Moreover, this technique can be combined with arthroscopic removal of the inflamed bursa and decompression of associated impingement. In many cases of refractory calcific tendinitis associated with impingement, open acromioplasty, subacromial bursectomy, and decompression are indicated.

Rotator Cuff Tear

Spontaneous tear of the rotator cuff in an otherwise normal individual is rare.[43] It can occur in patients with rheumatoid arthritis or lupus as part of the pathologic process with invasion from underlying pannus. Metabolic conditions such as renal osteodystrophy or agents such as glucocorticoids are occasionally associated with spontaneous cuff tears. Most patients report a traumatic episode such as falling on an outstretched arm or lifting a heavy object. The usual presenting symptoms are pain and weakness of abduction and external rotation. There may be associated crepitus and even a palpable defect. Long-standing tears are generally associated with atrophy of the supraspinatus and infraspinatus muscles. It may be difficult to differentiate a partial-thickness cuff tear from a painful tendinitis.

Plain radiographs are helpful only during a later stage of the process, when there may be narrowing of the acromiohumeral gap, proximal subluxation of the humeral head, and even erosion on the undersurface of the acromion.[71] US and MRI are helpful in evaluating acutely torn rotator cuffs. Arthrography, however, is more selective in differentiating full-thickness tears from partial tears.

Because of the overlap in diagnosis of complete tears and incomplete lesions, it is difficult to develop a rational form of treatment. DePalma[72] reports that 90 percent of patients with rotator cuff tears respond to conservative measures such as rest, analgesics, anti-inflammatory agents, and physiotherapy.

During the acute phase of pain, the arm may be supported in a sling, but early restoration of motion is important to prevent adhesive capsulitis. Instillation of glucocorticoids into the subacromial bursa may provide dramatic relief of symptoms.

Consideration of surgical treatment depends on the patient's symptoms, functional demand, and the cause of the tear. Most acute tears represent extension of a tear associated with chronic impingement and are reviewed previously in this chapter.[43] Patients in this group who fail to respond to conservative means should be treated by an anterior acromioplasty with rotator cuff repair.

In elderly patients whose pain and weakness do not create a functional problem, a conservative program is preferable. Wolfgang[73] pointed out that surgical results were less satisfactory with advancing patient age. Earnshaw et al.[74] reviewed 37 patients who had undergone rotator cuff repair and found an overall 65 percent with good results. Patients in the fourth and fifth decades of life generally did well, whereas only 60 percent of patients in the sixth and seventh decades had a good result. In their study, the mechanism of injury, the extent of the tear, and the timing of repair had no influence on the outcome. The authors pointed out that most shoulders showed radiographic progression of proximal subluxation despite surgical repair. In this small series, good functional results were reported in two patients with irreparable tears and in some patients with postoperative arthrograms showing leakage of contrast material. They concluded that relief of impingement and debridement of the edge of the tear were important determinants in the relief of symptoms.[74]

Acute traumatic tears of the rotator cuff in active patients may occur without long-standing impingement. These tears can occur with an acute episode and even can be associated with other pathologic changes such as dislocation or fracture. The presence of weakness to initiation of abduction and external rotation in a neutral position following injury should suggest the possibility of an acute rotator cuff tear. Acute full-thickness rotator cuff tears associated with functional weakness should be considered for immediate surgical repair. The surgical approach, technique of repair, and postoperative management are beyond the scope of this discussion and are well covered in other sources.[2, 3, 72, 74, 75]

Bicipital Tendinitis and Rupture

Bicipital tendinitis, subluxation/dislocation of the biceps tendon within the bicipital groove, and rupture of the long head of the biceps are generally associated with anterior shoulder pain. The long head of the biceps is an intracapsular and extrasynovial structure. It passes through the bicipital groove, over the head of the humerus, and inserts on the superior rim of the glenoid[76] (see Fig. 26–1A). The biceps tendon aids in flexion of the forearm, supination of the pronated forearm if the elbow is flexed, and forward elevation of the shoulder.[3] As it crosses the humeral head, the biceps tendon is fixed within the bicipital groove. Meyer[77] described a bony ridge on the lesser tuberosity and suggested this as a source of tendon wear and eventual rupture. Shallowness of this groove has been reported as a cause of subluxation and dislocation of the bicipital tendon.[78]

Peterson[79] reported a dissection study to determine the incidence of medial displacement of the biceps tendon. In 77 cadaver dissections, the biceps tendon was found to be medially displaced in five cases (6.5 percent). Displacement was always found in association with a full-thickness tear of the supraspinatus tendon. Moreover, in most cases, the tendon displaced deep to a disrupted subscapularis tendon rather than over the subscapularis tendon as commonly believed.[79]

Crenshaw and Kilgore[80] reported that the early phases of bicipital tendinitis were associated with hypervascularity, edema of the tendon, and tenosynovitis. Persistence of this process leads to adhesions between the tendon and its sheath, with impairment of the normal gliding mechanism in the groove. Stretching of these adhesions may be associated with chronic bicipital tendinitis.[78] The diagnosis of bicipital tendinitis is based on the localization of tenderness (see Fig. 26–1). It is often confused with impingement symptoms and in fact is frequently seen in association with an impingement syndrome.[23] Isolated bicipital tendinitis can be differentiated by the fact that the tender area will migrate with the bicipital groove as the arm is abducted and externally rotated. There are many eponyms associated with tests to identify bicipital tendinitis.[3] Yergason's supination sign refers to pain in the bicipital groove when the examiner resists supination of the pronated forearm with the elbow at 90 degrees. Ludington's sign refers to pain in the bicipital groove when the patient interlocks the fingers on top of the head and actively abducts the arms.

Treatment is generally conservative and consists of rest, analgesics, NSAIDs, and local injection of glucocorticoids. The use of US and neuroprobe is more beneficial in this condition than in isolated rotator cuff tendinitis. Patients with refractory bicipital tendinitis and recurrent symptoms of subluxation are treated by opening the bicipital groove and resecting the proximal portion of the tendon with either tenodesis of the distal portion into the groove or transfer to the coracoid process. The proponents of tenodesis believe that this prevents proximal migration of the humeral head, whereas those who advocate transfer to the coracoid think that the procedure maintains biceps power.

Becker and Cofield[81] reviewed the results of tenodesis of the long head of the biceps for chronic bicipital tendinitis in 54 shoulders. In this study, the authors report initial short-term relief but found that recurrent symptoms occurred in a disproportionate number of patients.

Rupture of the long head of the biceps is easily diagnosed by the appearance of the contracted belly of the biceps muscle (*Popeye sign*). The patient frequently relates a snap and acute pain in association with lifting an object. In older patients, in whom rupture is due to attrition, presentation is frequently spontaneous and is associated with minimal symptoms. Acute ruptures in young active individuals are best treated surgically with either tenodesis of the distal stump into the bicipital groove or transfer to the coracoid. Patients with long-standing symptoms of impingement and acute biceps tendon rupture are treated with anterior acromioplasty and tenodesis of the distal stump into the bicipital groove. In older patients without symptoms of impingement, a conservative program is preferable because these patients are generally asymptomatic and have sufficient strength. Mariani et al.[82] compared surgical versus nonsurgical treatment of a ruptured long head of biceps tendon. These authors found pain relief was equivalent in both groups. Residual subjective weakness at the elbow was reported in four of 27 patients in the surgical group and in 20 of 30 patients treated nonsurgically. The surgically treated patients returned to work later than the nonsurgical group, but 11 patients in the nonsurgical group were unable to return to full work capacity. On biomechanical testing, the nonsurgical group lost an average of 21 percent supination strength and 8 percent of elbow flexion strength. The surgical group lost no strength to biomechanical testing.[82]

Acromioclavicular Arthritis

The majority of painful conditions about the AC joint are caused by trauma with resultant AC joint instability, meniscal tears, and secondary degenerative change.[83] Most patients have a history of direct trauma to the shoulder girdle. The pain may be generalized, but tenderness and at times crepitus can be palpated directly over the AC joint. The pain is increased by abduction of the arm and particularly adducting the arm across the chest and compressing the joint.[2]

Plain radiographs may be normal unless there is a true dislocation or degenerative change. It is important to differentiate the traction spur at the insertion of the coracoacromial ligament from an osteophyte associated with degenerative change of the joint. MRI can frequently demonstrate impingement of an AC joint osteophyte or the tendon of the rotator cuff.

Acute traumatic instability is best studied by plain radiographs. An anteroposterior radiograph with the patient holding a weight in the ipsilateral hand may demonstrate joint instability in acute cases. Acute injuries are treated by rest, strapping, or surgical repair, depending on the degree of instability and the functional demand of the patient. Acute injuries without subluxation (grade I) or partial subluxation (grade II) are treated by conservative means. Complete dislocations (grade III) are treated by early mobilization, strapping to reduce the dislocation, or surgical repair according to the patient's functional demand and the surgeon's preference.[83–87]

Patients with degenerative change in the AC joint and symptoms that cannot be controlled by conservative means are best treated by debridement of the joint and resection of the distal clavicle.[84, 86] At no time should this joint be surgically fused.

GLENOHUMERAL DISORDERS

The various arthritides that affect the shoulder joint are discussed in detail in other chapters. They are presented here to discuss aspects that are unique to the glenohumeral joint. The usual presentation of intra-articular disorders is pain with motion and symptoms of internal derangement such as locking and clicking. The pain is generalized throughout the shoulder girdle and at times referred to the neck, back, and upper arm. The usual response to pain is to decrease glenohumeral motion and substitute with increased scapulothoracic mobility. Patients with adequate elbow and scapulothoracic motion require little glenohumeral motion for activities of daily living; in fact, patients with glenohumeral arthrodesis can achieve adequate function.[87, 88] The response to pain, therefore, is diminution of motion and secondary soft tissue contractures with muscle atrophy. With increasing weakness and involvement of adjacent joints, pain, limitation of motion, and weakness cause a substantial functional deficit.

Inflammatory Arthritis

Although the most common inflammatory arthritis involving the shoulder joint is rheumatoid arthritis, other systemic disorders such as systemic lupus erythematosus (SLE), psoriatic arthritis, ankylosing spondylitis, Reiter's syndrome, and scleroderma may cause glenohumeral degeneration. The pathogenesis of the joint involvement in these conditions is discussed in detail in other chapters. All patients with significant involvement have pain. The limitation of motion is either due to splinting of the joint with secondary soft tissue contractures or attributable to primary soft tissue involvement with scarring or rupture. Plain radiographs confirm glenohumeral involvement (Fig. 26–13A). There is narrowing of the glenohumeral joint space, with erosion and cyst formation without significant sclerosis or osteophytes. As the disease progresses, superior and posterior erosion of the glenoid with proximal subluxation of the humeral head may occur. Eventually there may be secondary degenerative changes and even osteonecrosis of the humeral head.

Treatment is initially conservative and directed toward controlling pain, inducing a systemic remission (see Chapter 56), and maintaining joint motion by physical therapy. The use of intra-articular glucocorticoids may be beneficial in controlling local synovitis. In rheumatoid arthritis, the involvement of periarticular structures with subacromial bursitis and rupture of the rotator cuff magnifies the functional deficit. When the synovial cartilage interactions produce significant symptoms and radiographic changes that cannot be controlled by conventional therapy, glenohumeral resurfacing should be considered.

When following a rheumatoid patient with shoulder involvement, the rheumatologist should carefully assess range of motion and obtain periodic radiographs. Patients with progressive loss of motion or radiographic destruction should be referred for orthopedic evaluation.

The treatment of choice is an unconstrained shoulder arthroplasty of the type reported in detail

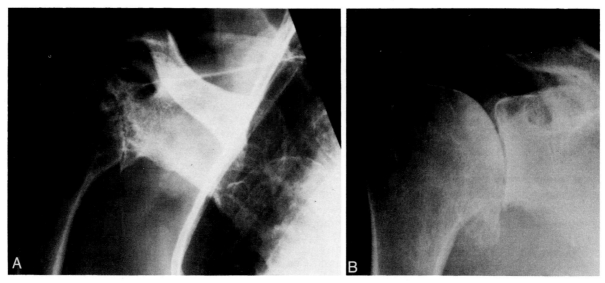

Figure 26–13. Plain radiographs. *A,* Rheumatoid arthritis with loss of joint space, cyst formation, glenohumeral erosion, and early proximal subluxation of the humerus indicating a rotator cuff tear. *B,* Osteoarthritis with narrowing of the glenohumeral joint space, sclerosis, and osteophyte formation. Note the preservation of the subacromial space, suggesting an intact rotator cuff.

in Chapter 107.[89, 90] Total shoulder arthroplasty is best performed in patients with rheumatoid arthritis before end-stage bony erosion and soft tissue contractions have occurred.[91, 92]

Acute inflammatory arthritis of the glenohumeral joint may also occur in association with gout, pseudogout, hydroxyapatite deposition of renal osteodystrophy, and recurrent hemophilic hemarthrosis.

Osteoarthritis

Osteoarthritis of the glenohumeral joint is less common than in the hip, its counterpart in the lower extremity. This is a result of both the non–weight-bearing characteristics of the shoulder joint and the distribution of forces throughout the shoulder girdle. Osteoarthritis is divided into those conditions associated with high unit loading of articular cartilage and those in which there is an intrinsic abnormality within the cartilage that causes abnormal wear at normal loads. Because the shoulder is normally a non–weight-bearing joint and is less susceptible to repeated high loading, the presence of osteoarthritis of the glenohumeral joint should alert the physician to consider other associated factors. Has the patient engaged in unusual activities such as boxing, heavy construction, or chronic use of a pneumatic hammer? Is there some disorder such as epiphyseal dysplasia that has created joint incongruity with high unit loading of the articular cartilage? Is this a neuropathic process caused by diabetes, syringomyelia, or leprosy? Is there associated hemochromatosis, hemophilia, or gout that may have altered the ability of articular cartilage to withstand normal loading? Is unrecognized chronic dislocation responsible? Osteoarthritis is generally associated with a history of trauma with residual instability and articular cartilage damage. Pain is the usual presentation, but it is generally not as acute or associated with the spasm seen in inflammatory conditions. Plain radiographs show narrowing of the glenohumeral joint, osteophyte formation, sclerosis, and some cyst formation (see Fig. 26–13B). Because the rotator cuff is generally intact, there is less bone erosion of the glenoid and proximal subluxation of the humerus. Patients with osteoarthritis of the glenohumeral joint frequently do well by functional adjustment and conservative therapy. Analgesics and NSAIDs may provide symptomatic relief. The use of glucocorticoid injections is less beneficial unless there is evidence of synovitis. Those patients with severe involvement who fail to respond are best treated by shoulder arthroplasty[89–91] (see Chapter 107).

Osteonecrosis

Osteonecrosis of the shoulder refers to necrosis of the humeral head seen in association with a variety of conditions. Symptoms are due to synovitis and joint incongruity resulting from resorption, repair, and remodeling. The pathogenesis and various causes are discussed in Chapter 97.

The most common cause of osteonecrosis of the shoulder is avascularity owing to a fracture through the anatomic neck of the humerus.[93] Fracture through this area disrupts the intramedullary and capsular blood supplies to the humeral head. Another common cause of osteonecrosis of the shoulder is steroid therapy in conjunction with organ transplantation, SLE, or asthma. The mechanism by which steroids are associated with osteonecrosis is unknown. There appears to be a host susceptibility, which may be genetically predetermined. Patients will generally develop osteonecrosis shortly after steroid use, although symptoms may not present for a considerable period. At least in renal transplant patients, the association of osteonecrosis is independent of steroid dosage. The proposed pathogenesis of steroid-induced osteonecrosis includes increased free fatty acids with obliteration of intramedullary blood supply and steroid-induced vasculitis. This may elevate the intramedullary pressures within the humeral head and cause bone ischemia and death.[94] Other conditions associated with osteonecrosis of the humeral head include SLE, hemoglobinopathies, pancreatitis, and hyperbarism.

Early diagnosis is difficult because there is frequently a considerable delay until symptoms are present. Bone scans may be helpful in early cases before radiographic changes are present. MRI is highly sensitive and more specific than scintigraphy. Plain radiographs demonstrate progressive phases of necrosis and repair as discussed in detail in Chapter 97. In the early stages, the films may be normal or show either osteopenia or bone sclerosis. A crescent sign representing subchondral fracture or demarcation of the necrotic segment appears during the reparative process. Patients who fail to remodel show collapse of the humeral head with secondary degenerative changes. There is often a considerable discrepancy between symptoms and radiographic involvement. Patients with extensive bone changes may be asymptomatic. Treatment should be directed by the patient's symptoms rather than the radiographs and is similar to that for osteoarthritis. On occasion, arthroscopy can be helpful by removing loose chondral fragments and debriding chondral incongruities.[95] Patients with severe symptoms that cannot be controlled by conservative means are best treated with an unconstrained shoulder arthroplasty or hemiarthroplasty.[89]

Cuff Tear Arthropathy

In 1873, Adams described the pathologic changes in rheumatoid arthritis of the shoulder as well as a condition that has since been referred to as *Milwaukee shoulder* or cuff tear arthropathy. The original lithographs of this report have been reproduced.[96] McCarty termed the condition Milwaukee shoulder and reported that factors predisposing to this syndrome include deposition of calcium pyrophosphate dihydrate crystals, direct trauma, chronic joint overuse, chronic renal failure, and denervation.[97] Patients with Milwaukee shoulder have been reported to have elevated levels of synovial fluid 5'-nucleotidase activity as well as elevated levels of synovial fluid inorganic pyrophosphate and nucleotide pyrophosphohydrolase activity.[98]

Neer et al.[46] have reported a similar condition in which untreated massive tears of the rotator cuff

with proximal migration of the humeral head are associated with erosion of the humeral surface. The erosion of the humeral head is different from that seen in other arthritides and is presumed to be due to a combination of mechanical and nutritional factors acting on the superior glenohumeral cartilage.

Patients with cuff tear arthropathy present a difficult therapeutic problem because the bone erosion and disruption of the cuff jeopardize the functional result from an unconstrained prosthesis.[91] In such patients, a hemiarthroplasty or even a constrained total shoulder arthroplasty may be indicated.[100, 101]

The major question in cuff tear arthropathy is to determine which patients with massive rotator cuff tears will proceed to the syndrome of cuff tear arthropathy. Patients with massive rotator cuff tears who develop localized calcium pyrophosphate disease may be predisposed to further proximal migration and further joint destruction. This situation poses a dilemma for the treating physician. Many patients with massive rotator cuff tears will remain stable and require little or no treatment. Occasionally, symptomatic patients can be treated by arthroscopic debridement of the cuff tear. It is critical to define the patient who is going to proceed to the syndrome of cuff tear arthropathy. If crystal deposition disease predisposes patients to proximal migration and joint destruction, joint aspiration with crystal analysis or scintigraphy to determine synovial reaction may be helpful diagnostic tools.

Hamada et al.[102] followed 22 patients with massive rotator cuff tears treated conservatively. The radiographic findings included narrowing of the acromiohumeral interval and degenerative changes of the humeral head, tuberosities, acromion, AC joint, and glenohumeral joint. Five of seven patients followed for more than 8 years progressed to cuff tear arthropathy. The authors concluded that progressive radiographic changes were associated with repetitive use of the arm in elevation, rupture of the long head of the biceps, impingement of the humeral head against the acromion, and weakness of external rotation.[102]

Septic Arthritis

Septic arthritis can masquerade as any of the conditions classified as periarticular or glenohumeral disorders. Sepsis must be included in any differential diagnosis of shoulder pain because early recognition and prompt treatment are necessary to achieve a good functional result. The diagnosis is confirmed by joint aspiration with synovial fluid analysis and culture. Cultures should include aerobic, anaerobic, mycobacterial, and fungal studies. Septic arthritis is extensively covered in Chapters 86 to 89.

Glenoid Labrum Tears

The growing popularity of throwing sports and racket sports in 25- to 60-year-old individuals has increased the incidence of tears of the glenoid labrum as a cause of anterior shoulder pain (see Fig. 26–1). This diagnosis is easily confused with rotator cuff tendinitis or bicipital tendinitis and can best be confirmed by arthro-CT, double-contrast arthrotomography,[11] or arthroscopy (see Fig. 26–6). Glenoid labrum tears may be seen in association with anterior or even posterior instability.

Labrum tears can be divided into those associated with symptoms of internal derangement and those associated with instability. The SLAP lesion (superior labrum anterior and posterior) is associated with internal derangement but not instability. These tears involve the biceps tendon and labrum complex. The most common mechanism of injury is a compressive force to the shoulder as a result of a fall on an outstretched arm with the shoulder positioned in abduction and forward elevation. Depending on the size of the tear, it may be treated arthroscopically by debridement or by arthroscopic stapling.[103, 104] If a glenoid labrum tear is associated with instability, care must be taken in debriding the lesion because it may increase the symptoms of instability. Swimmer's shoulder, long thought to be an impingement syndrome, is often due to anterior labrum changes that respond well to conservative arthroscopic debridement.[105]

Adhesive Capsulitis

Adhesive capsulitis, or *frozen shoulder*, is a condition characterized by limitation of motion of the shoulder joint with pain at the extremes of motion. It was first described by Putnam in 1882[106] and later by Codman.[1] The initial presentation is pain, which is generalized and referred to the upper arm, back, and neck. As the pain increases, loss of joint motion ensues. The process is generally self-limiting and in most cases resolves spontaneously within 10 months unless there is an underlying problem.

Adhesive capsulitis is slightly more common in females than in males.[107] There is usually an underlying condition producing pain and restricted motion of the glenohumeral joint. Adhesive capsulitis may be seen as an end result of rotator cuff tendinitis, calcific tendinitis (see Fig. 26–7), bicipital tendinitis, and glenohumeral arthritis.[108, 109] It is also seen in a variety of conditions, including apical lung tumors, pulmonary tuberculosis, cervical radiculopathy, and postmyocardial infarction.[108, 110, 111] In a review of frozen shoulder, three of 140 patients with this syndrome had local primary invasive neoplasms.[112] Another study reviewed three patients presenting with the syndrome of adhesive capsulitis who subsequently were found to have neoplastic lesions of the midshaft of the humerus.[113]

DePalma[109] reported that any condition that hindered scapulohumeral motion would cause muscular inactivity and predispose the patient to adhesive capsulitis. Neviaser[114] found capsular adhesions to the underlying humeral head on surgical exploration for adhesive capsulitis. Wiley[115] described the arthroscopic findings associated with the diagnosis of primary adhesive capsulitis. These included a patchy vascular reaction around the biceps tendon and the opening into the subscapularis bursa. The capacity of the joint was reduced. In no case was the infraglenoid recess obliterated, and no adhesions were observed.[115] Morris et al.[116] described erosions of the humeral head in association with the clinical syndrome of adhesive capsulitis.

It is unclear whether the contracture of the shoulder capsule is a passive process related to lack of motion or an active process associated with capsular inflammation. Bulgen et al.[117] reported an association between adhesive capsulitis and HLA-B27 antigen positivity. They also reported decreased IgA levels in patients with the condition.[118] Lundberg[119] and Neviaser[114] failed to demonstrate synovitis or capsular inflammation when surgically exploring patients with adhesive capsulitis.

Treatment of adhesive capsulitis is directed toward pain relief, restoration of function, and correction of the underlying cause. Many patients have associated depression or emotional lability either as an underlying problem or as a result of pain and functional limitation. The physician must direct a long-term therapy program and reassure the patient that this condition is usually self-limiting. Because symptoms may last for 1 to 2 years, daily visits to the physical therapist become impractical, and a home program should be outlined.

Fareed and Gallivan[120] reported good results with hydraulic distention of the glenohumeral joint using local anesthetic agents. Rizk et al.[121] performed a prospective randomized study to assess the effect of steroid or local anesthetic injection in 48 patients with frozen shoulder. In this study, there was no significant difference in outcome between those individuals who received intrabursal versus interarticular injections. Moreover, steroid with lidocaine had no advantage over lidocaine alone in restoring shoulder motion. Transient pain relief, however, occurred in two thirds of the steroid-treated patients.[121]

In patients with restriction of motion that prevents activities of daily living, a closed manipulation may be indicated. This is best achieved at the time of arthrography (to confirm the diagnosis) and entails passive manipulation after the joint is inflated with a local anesthetic. The combination of inflating the joint and passive manipulation may free some adhesions and improve joint motion. On occasion, a general anesthetic is indicated for closed manipulation. Hill and Bogumill[122] reported the results of manipulation of 17 frozen shoulders in 15 patients who did not respond to physical therapy. Seventy-eight percent of the individuals working before their shoulder problems returned to work at an average of 2.6 months following manipulation. The authors concluded that manipulation allowed patients to return to a normal lifestyle and to work sooner than the reported natural history of the condition.[122] Surgical intervention for adhesive capsulitis should be limited to treatment of an underlying problem such as calcific tendinitis or an impingement syndrome.

Glenohumeral Instability

Dislocation of the glenohumeral joint in association with trauma has characteristic clinical and radiographic findings that are beyond the scope of this chapter and have been reviewed in detail elsewhere.[123] Anterior dislocation generally occurs with the arm in an abducted and externally rotated position, and the diagnosis is usually obvious. Posterior dislocation may be difficult to diagnose and is frequently seen in association with convulsive disorders or unusual trauma with the arm in a forward flexed and internally rotated position. There is often a significant delay in the recognition of a posterior dislocation, and this diagnosis should be suspected in patients who are unable to externally rotate from a neutral position.

Recurrent subluxation without dislocation may be difficult to diagnose and be mistakenly identified as impingement with chronic rotator cuff tendinitis. Jobe et al.[124] described the syndrome of shoulder pain in overhand or throwing athletes that presents as impingement but is due to anterior subluxation of the joint with the humeral head impinging on the anterior aspect of the coracoacromial arch. Fu et al.[125] underscored this distinction by dividing the etiology of rotator cuff tendinitis into primary impingement of the supraspinatus tendon on the coracoacromial arch and anterior subluxation with secondary impingement in young athletes performing overhead movements.

The diagnosis of glenohumeral instability with subluxation in one or multiple directions is made by a combination of a detailed history, careful physical examination, and use of adjuncts such as arthrography, CT, and arthroscopy. The syndrome of multidirectional instability has been recognized in those patients who are unstable in more than one direction.[126] This syndrome frequently occurs in young athletic patients and in particular in the dominant arm of pitchers, racket sport players, and swimmers. The most common presentation in these individuals is pain, often mistakenly considered as rotator cuff tendinitis. The patient may relate a history of a minor trauma causing acute pain and a "dead arm" syndrome lasting for minutes or hours. Other associated symptoms include a sense of instability, weakness, and even radicular symptoms suggestive of neuropathy. There may be few, if any, positive physical findings in association with chronic subluxation or multidirectional instability. The patient may have signs of generalized ligamentous laxity, and pain may be reproduced by placing the arm in an evocative position of abduction and external rotation. At times, the arm may be excessively subluxated in one direction during physical examination. One particularly helpful sign is the "sulcus" sign, which refers to a subacromial indentation occurring with subluxation of the arm inferiorly with longitudinal traction or weights. Because this syndrome frequently occurs in athletes with highly developed musculature about the shoulder girdle, these physical findings of subluxation may be difficult to reproduce.[124]

Plain radiographs are generally normal, although some inferior subluxation may be reproduced by obtaining a plain radiograph with the patient carrying a weight and relaxing the shoulder musculature. Special radiographs as discussed earlier may demonstrate Bankart's lesion (avulsion of the anterior inferior glenoid rim) or a Hill-Sachs lesion (osteochondral defect of the posterior humeral head) occurring with subluxation of the humeral head in front of the anterior glenoid rim. Arthro-CT scan may demonstrate a glenoid labrum tear, laxity of the anterior glenohumeral ligaments, or a Hill-Sachs lesion (see Fig. 26–9). Arthroscopy may be of further help to delineate these pathologic abnormalities seen in association with the syndrome of multidirectional instability.

Treatment of chronic subluxation or multidirectional instability is first directed toward rehabilitation. Strengthening exercises of the shoulder girdle under the supervision of an experienced therapist may control symptoms, stabilize the glenohumeral joint, and obviate the need for surgical intervention. If a conservative treatment program fails, surgery is directed toward tightening of the capsular structures to stabilize the glenohumeral joint.

REGIONAL DISORDERS

Because the shoulder girdle connects the thorax with the upper extremity and the major neurovascular structures pass in close proximity to the joint, shoulder pain is a hallmark of many nonarticular conditions.

Cervical Radiculopathy

Cervical neck pain, with or without radiculopathy, may be associated with shoulder pain.[127] When cervical radiculopathy presents as shoulder pain, it is frequently due to involvement of the upper cervical roots. It can be differentiated from shoulder pain on the basis of history, physical examination, EMG, cervical radiographs, and myelography when indicated. Because conditions causing cervical neck pain and those causing shoulder pain, such as calcific tendinitis and cervical radiculopathy, may coexist, it is often difficult to distinguish which lesion is responsible for the symptoms. These conditions can often be differentiated by injection of local anesthetics to block certain components of the pain. As cervical neck pain is reviewed extensively in Chapter 25, its diagnosis and treatment are not discussed.

Hawkins et al.[128] reported 13 patients who underwent both subacromial shoulder decompressions or rotator cuff repairs and anterior cervical spine fusions. Eight of the 13 patients presented with nearly equal neck and shoulder pain, whereas five patients had predominantly neck symptoms. Following anterior cervical fusion, these five patients secondarily developed shoulder pain, which required subsequent surgical intervention.[128]

Brachial Neuritis

In the 1940s, Spillane[129] and Parsonage and Turner[130, 131] described a painful condition of the shoulder associated with limitation of motion. As the pain subsided and motion improved, muscle weakness and atrophy became apparent. The deltoid, supraspinatus, infraspinatus, biceps, and triceps are the most frequently involved muscles,[132] although diaphragmatic paralysis has also been reported.[131, 133] The cause remains unclear, but the clustering of cases suggests a viral or postviral syndrome.[130, 131] Occasionally an associated influenza-like syndrome or previous vaccination has been reported.[132]

Hershman et al.[134] reported on acute brachial neuropathy in athletes. The findings that suggest an acute brachial neuropathy include an acute onset of pain without trauma, persistent severe pain that continues despite rest, and patchy neurologic signs. The diagnosis is confirmed by EMG and nerve conduction studies.[134]

The prognosis for recovery is excellent, although full recovery may take 2 to 3 years. Tsiaris et al.[135] reported 80 percent recovery within 2 years and more than 90 percent by the end of 3 years.

Nerve Entrapment Syndromes

Entrapment of peripheral nerves as either a primary or a secondary process may cause pain about the shoulder girdle. The clinical picture and neurophysiology of nerve entrapment syndromes are covered in Chapter 37 and in other detailed sources.[136–138] Two entrapment neuropathies, axillary nerve entrapment and suprascapular nerve entrapment, are frequently overlooked and bear further discussion.

The axillary nerve arises from the posterior cord of the brachial plexus and exits posteriorly through the quadrilateral space. This space is bordered superiorly by the teres major, inferiorly by the teres minor, medially by the long head of the triceps, and laterally by the humeral shaft and lateral triceps heads. After sending a sensory branch to the upper lateral cutaneous surface and a motor branch to the teres minor, the nerve courses anteriorly to innervate the deltoid.[76]

Entrapment of the axillary nerve as it exits

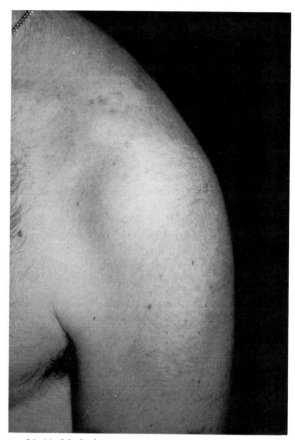

Figure 26–14. Marked anterior deltoid atrophy in the dominant arm of a professional tennis player with chronic axillary nerve entrapment.

through the quadrilateral space is an infrequent cause of pain, weakness, and atrophy about the shoulder girdle. It is most commonly seen in the dominant shoulder of young athletic individuals such as pitchers, tennis players, and swimmers who function with excessive overhead activity. Fig. 26–14 depicts severe anterior deltoid atrophy in the dominant arm of a world class tennis player with axillary nerve entrapment at the quadrilateral space. The pain may occur throughout the shoulder girdle and radiate down the arm in a nondermatomal pattern. It may be elicited by abduction and external rotation or by palpation of the quadrilateral space (see Fig. 26–1). This condition represents entrapment of the axillary nerve as it leaves the posterior cord, penetrates the quadrilateral space, and moves anteriorly to innervate the deltoid. On surgical exploration, the nerve was found to be tethered on the aponeurosis of the hypertrophied triceps muscle or by fibrous bands encroaching on the quadrilateral space.[140]

The suprascapular nerve is a branch of the upper trunk of the brachial plexus formed by the fifth and sixth cervical nerves. It passes obliquely beneath the trapezius and crosses the scapula through the suprascapular notch.[76] The suprascapular nerve has no cutaneous sensory branches but supplies motor branches to the supraspinatus and infraspinatus muscles.

The suprascapular nerve entrapment syndrome is the result of compression and tethering of the nerve as it passes through the suprascapular notch. Rengachary et al.[141] described variations in the size and shape of the fossa and the suprascapular ligament, which forms its superior border. The authors demonstrated variations in the fossa from a complete bony foramen to a smooth depression on the upper border of the scapula.[141] Patients with a true bony foramen or a deep notch should be more susceptible to the development of entrapment in this area. The entrapment may result from direct or indirect trauma, fracture of the neck of the scapula, compression by a ganglion, or from anatomic variants in the shape of the notch.[142]

The primary symptom is pain, which generally is described as a deep ache felt over the upper border and body of the scapula. The pain is well localized and does not radiate down the arm. Any activity that brings the scapula forward, such as reaching across the chest, may aggravate the pain.[142] Palpation of the suprascapular notch may elicit local tenderness (see Fig. 26–1).

Because the suprascapular nerve has no cutaneous innervation, there is no associated numbness, tingling, or paresthesias. With time, patients develop atrophy and weakness of the supraspinatus and infraspinatus muscles.[142] This syndrome must be differentiated from rotator cuff tendinitis, which also could be associated with a similar pattern of pain and muscle atrophy.[143] It also must be differentiated from brachial neuritis and a cervical radiculopathy involving the fifth and sixth roots.[144] Selective EMG examinations of the supraspinatus and infraspinatus may reveal polyphasic potentials, which are decreased in amplitude and increased in distal latency.[142] Instillation of local anesthetics into the supraspinous notch may relieve the symptoms.[142] As with axillary nerve entrapment, this syndrome is often seen in young athletic individuals with excessive overhead activity. It has also been reported in association with trauma.[145, 146] After the diagnosis is confirmed, the surgical treatment of choice is decompression of the suprascapular notch. If the entrapment is associated with trauma, a substantial period of time should be given to rule out a neuropraxia, which is likely to resolve.

Post and Mayer[147] reviewed eight patients treated surgically for suprascapular nerve entrapment. The trapezius muscle was detached from the spine of the scapula and the suprascapular ligament released. All patients in this series were reported to have good or excellent results.

Sternoclavicular Arthritis

Occasionally, traumatic, nontraumatic, or infectious conditions can cause pain about the sternoclavicular joint (see Fig. 26–1). The most common problem is ligamentous injury and painful subluxation or dislocation. This can be diagnosed by palpable instability and crepitus over the sternoclavicular joint. Sternoclavicular views may radiographically demonstrate dislocation.[84]

Inflammatory arthritis of the sternoclavicular joint has been seen in association with rheumatoid arthritis, ankylosing spondylitis, and septic arthritis. The association of palmoplantar pustulosis and sternoclavicular arthritis has been reported.[148] Seven of 15 patients who underwent biopsies for this condition had cultures positive for *Propionibacterium acnes*, suggesting an infectious origin to this condition.[148]

Two other conditions involving the sternoclavicular joint are Tietze's syndrome, a painful nonsuppurative swelling of the joint and adjacent sternochondral junctions, and Friedrich's syndrome, a painful osteonecrosis of the sternal end of the clavicle.[3] Additionally, condensing osteitis of the clavicle is a rare benign idiopathic lesion of the medial one third of the clavicle. This condition, better described as aseptic enlarging osteosclerosis of the clavicle, is most commonly seen in middle-aged women and presents as a tender swelling over the medial one third of the clavicle.[149]

Reflex Sympathetic Dystrophy

Since its original description by Mitchell in 1864,[150] reflex sympathetic dystrophy (RSD) has remained a poorly understood and frequently overlooked condition. Its cause is unknown but may be related to sympathetic overflow or short-circuiting of impulses through the sympathetic system. Any clinician dealing with painful disorders must be familiar with the diagnosis and treatment of this condition. Bonica[151] has provided an excellent review, which covers the clinical presentation, various stages of the disease, and importance of early intervention to ensure a successful outcome.

RSD has been confusingly called causalgia, shoulder-hand syndrome, and Sudeck's atrophy. It is generally associated with minor trauma and is to be differentiated from causalgia that involves trauma to major nerve trunks.[151] RSD is divided into three phases, which are important in the determination of the stage of involvement and the mode of treatment.[152] Phase one is characterized by sympathetic overflow with diffuse swelling, pain, increased vascularity, and radiographic evidence of demineralization. If left untreated for 3 to 6 months, this may progress to phase two, which is characterized by atrophy. The extremity may now be cold and shiny, with atrophy of the skin and muscles. Phase three refers to progression of the trophic changes, with irreversible flexion contractures and a pale, cold, painful extremity. It has been speculated that phase one is related to a peripheral short-circuiting of nerve impulses, phase two represents short-circuiting through the internuncial pool in the spinal cord, and phase three is controlled by higher thalamic centers.[151, 152]

Steinbrocker[153] reported that as long as there is evidence of vasomotor activity with swelling and hyperemia, there remains a chance for recovery. Once the trophic phase two or three is established, the prognosis for recovery is poor. Prompt recognition of the syndrome is important because early intervention to control pain is mandatory. Careful supervision and reassurance are critical because many of these patients are emotionally labile as a result of either the pain or an underlying problem. The syndrome may be remarkably reversed by a sympathetic block. Patients who receive transient relief from sympathetic blockade may be helped by surgical sympathectomy.

Fibrositis

Fibrositis and other diffuse musculoskeletal syndromes are characterized by multiple trigger points about the shoulder girdle. This subject is discussed in Chapter 29.

Neoplasms

Primary and metastatic neoplasms may cause shoulder pain by direct invasion of the musculoskeletal system or by compression with referred pain.[2, 138] Primary tumors are more likely to occur in younger individuals. The more common lesions have a typical distribution, such as the predilection of a chondroblastoma for the proximal humeral epiphysis or of an osteogenic sarcoma for the metaphysis.[154] The differential diagnosis of spontaneous onset of shoulder pain in older individuals should include metastatic lesions and myeloma. Neoplasms are best identified by plain radiographs, MRI, ^{99m}Tc-MDP scintigraphy, and CT.

Pancoast's syndrome or apical lung tumor may present as shoulder pain or cervical radiculitis owing to invasion of the brachial plexus or invasion of the C-8, T-1 roots.[109, 155, 156] With invasion of the cervical sympathetic chain, the patient may also develop Horner's syndrome.

Miscellaneous Conditions

A variety of other conditions may present as shoulder pain and should be mentioned in this discussion. Acute abdominal disorders such as gallbladder disease, splenic injuries, and subphrenic abscess can refer pain to the shoulder. The pain of acute angina and myocardial infarction may be referred to the left shoulder and down the inner aspect of the left arm. Metabolic disorders such as hypothyroidism and hyperthyroidism,[156] diabetes mellitus,[157–159] and secondary hyperparathyroidism in association

with renal osteodystrophy are infrequently associated with pain about the shoulder girdle.

With the increasing numbers of patients undergoing long-term maintenance hemodialysis, a shoulder pain syndrome known as dialysis shoulder arthropathy has been described. This consists of shoulder pain, weakness, loss of motion, and functional limitation. The cause and pathogenesis of this syndrome are unclear, although rotator cuff disease, pathologic fracture, bursitis, and local amyloid deposition have been implicated as causative factors.[160] To date, there are insufficient surgical or necropsy data to confirm any specific diagnosis. These patients generally respond poorly to local measures of injection, heat, and NSAIDs but may improve with correction of underlying metabolic disorders such as osteomalacia and secondary hyperthyroidism.

References

1. Codman, E. A.: The Shoulder-Rupture of the Supraspinatus Tendon and Other Lesions in or About the Subacromial Bursa. Boston, Thomas Todd Company, 1934.
2. Bateman, E.: The Shoulder and Neck. 2nd ed. Philadelphia, W. B. Saunders Company, 1978.
3. Post, M.: The Shoulder—Surgical and Non-surgical Management. Philadelphia, Lea & Febiger, 1988.
4. Cailliet, R.: Shoulder Pain. 2nd ed. Philadelphia, F. A. Davis Company, 1981.
5. Greep, J. M., Lemmens, H. A. J., Roos, D. B., and Urschel, H. C.: Pain in Shoulder and Arm. An Integrated View. The Hague, Martinus Nijhoff, 1979.
6. Jobe, F. W., Kvitne, R. S., and Giangarra, C. E.: Shoulder pain in the overhand or throwing athlete. The relationship of anterior instability and rotator cuff impingement. Orthop. Rev 18(9):963, 1989.
7. Dalton, S. E., and Snyder, S. J.: Glenohumeral instability. Baillieres Clin. Rheumatol. 3(3):511, 1989.
8. Goldman, A. B.: Shoulder Arthrography. Boston, Little, Brown & Company, 1982.
9. Goldman, A. B., and Ghelman, B.: The double contrast shoulder arthrogram. A review of 158 studies. Radiology 127:655, 1978.
10. Mink, J., and Harris, E.: Double contrast shoulder arthrography: Its use in evaluation of rotator cuff tears. Orthop. Trans. 7:71, 1983.
11. Braunstein, E. M., and O'Connor, G.: Double-contrast arthrotomography of the shoulder. J. Bone Joint Surg. 64A:192, 1982.
12. el-Khoury, G. Y., Kathol, M. H., Chandler, J. B., and Albright, J. P.: Shoulder instability: Impact of glenohumeral arthrotomography on treatment. Radiology 160(3):669, 1986.
13. Kneisl, J. S., Sweeney, H. J., and Paige, M. L.: Correlation of pathology observed in double contrast arthrotomography. Arthroscopy 4(1):21, 1988.
14. Strizak, A. M., Danzig, L., Jackson, D. W., Greenway, D., Resnick, D., and Staple, T.: Subacromial bursography. J. Bone Joint Surg. 64A:196, 1982.
15. Lie, S.: Subacromial bursography. Radiology 144:626, 1982.
16. Fukuda, H., Mikasa, M., and Yamanaka, K.: Incomplete thickness rotator cuff tears diagnosed by subacromial bursography. Clin. Orthop. 223:51, 1987.
17. Rafii, M., Minkoff, J., Bonano, J., Firooznia, H., Jaffe, L., and Golimbu, C.: Computed tomography (CT) arthrography of shoulder instabilities in athletes. Am. J. Sports Med. 16(4):352, 1988.
18. Mack, L. A., Matsen, F. A., Kilcoyne, R. F., Davies, P. K., and Sickler, M. E.: US evaluation of the rotator cuff. Radiology 157:206, 1985.
19. Crass, J. R., Craig, E. V., Bretzke, C., and Feinberg, S. B.: Ultrasonography of the rotator cuff. Radiographics 5:941, 1985.
20. Middleton, W. D., Edelstein, G., Reinus, W. R., Melson, G. L., and Murphy, W. A.: Ultrasonography of the rotator cuff: Technique and normal anatomy. J. Ultrasound Med. 3:549, 1984.
21. Bretze, C. A., Crass, J. R., Craig, E. V., and Feinberg, S. B.: Ultrasonography of the rotator cuff. Normal and pathologic anatomy. Invest. Radiol. 20:311, 1985.
22. Crass, J. R., Craig, E. V., Thompson, R. C., and Feinberg, S. B.: Ultrasonography of the rotator cuff: Surgical correlation. J. Clin. Ultrasound 12:487, 1984.
23. Middleton, W. D., Edelstein, G., Reinus, W. R., Melson, G. L., Totty,

Table 27–1. SUMMARY OF THE CHARACTERISTICS OF LOW BACK PAIN OF VARIOUS ORIGINS

Source of Pain	Distribution	Nature	Aggravating Factors	Neurologic Changes
Spinal pain	Sclerotomal Local	Sharp Dull	Motion	None
Discogenic pain	Sclerotomal	Deep, aching	Increased intradiscal pressure, e.g., bending, sitting, Valsalva maneuver	None
Nerve root pain	Radicular	Paresthesias Numbness	Root stretching	Present
Multiple lumbar spinal stenosis pain	Radicular Sclerotomal	Paresthesias Spinal claudication pattern	Lumbar extension Walking	Present
Referred visceral pain	Dermatomal	Deep, aching	Related to affected organ	None

the referral area has the same embryonic origin as the mesodermal tissue involved.

Radicular pain relates to a spinal nerve root distribution, worsens with root stretching maneuvers such as bending, and usually improves with rest. (If pain is worsened or not relieved by rest, particularly at night, a spinal cord tumor may be suspected.) The pain has neurologic characteristics of paresthesias and numbness, and there may be associated motor weakness. The characteristic of walking giving rise to the spinal claudication symptom of spinal stenosis should be noted, as well as the effect of sitting, which will improve spinal stenosis symptoms but worsen those of disc herniation. Bladder, bowel, and sexual function should be determined, as they are involved in central midline herniations of the disc, conus tumors, and occasionally spinal stenosis. Pain from muscular spasm will have cramping, achy characteristics, usually in the sacrospinalis and gluteus maximus. A summary of the characteristics of back pain of various origins is given in Table 27–1.

A useful analysis of back pain arises out of an evaluation of further mechanical relationships of the pain. These mechanical relationships reflect the pathophysiologic origins of the pain. Low back pain and the pain of disc herniation tend to worsen with postural positions of prolonged duration. Positions that increase intradiscal pressure exacerbate pain; those that decrease pressure improve the pain, as outlined by the intradiscal pressure measurements done by Nachemson.[70] However, it is not established that intradiscal pressure causes pain, only that this relationship exists. Another pattern of pain, commonly seen in degenerative spinal stenosis, is that of neurogenic claudication, pain produced in the back or leg by walking or by assuming an erect position. This pain tends to be more diffuse than the pain caused during root entrapment by a herniated lumbar disc. In neurogenic claudication, when the spine is in flexion, room in the lumbar canal enlarges and the pain lessens. A summary of mechanical relationships is given in Table 27–2.

A past medical history of medications, other medical conditions, and a family history, especially of arthritic diseases, is necessary. It is useful at the initial encounter to ascertain work status, compen-sation, litigation, disability at work and home, and the patients' own assessments of how well they are coping with their afflictions, as these factors can markedly alter the assessment, management, and outcome of treatment.[25-28] A recent study of aircraft workers suggests that psychosocial factors are the most important determinants of work disability from low back pain.[28a]

Physical Examination. Examination is preferably done with the patient undressed. The spine and stance are inspected while the patient is standing, to note lumbar lordosis, thoracic kyphos, scoliosis, tilt from "sciatic scoliosis," flexed lower extremities to relieve root tension, muscle spasm, and skin nevi over the spine. Gait and motion are noted, including toe and heel gait, to determine muscular weakness and to observe any inconsistent or exaggerated posturing.

Forward bending is measured and can be crudely quantitated by an estimate of flexion or the distance of the fingers from the floor. Lateral bending may be asymmetric with unilateral root entrapment. Hyperextension will elicit pain from inflamed facet joints. The spine is palpated to determine local tenderness, the stepoff of spondylolisthesis, or the defect of spina bifida, and percussed to produce local pain or sciatica and in the costovertebral angle to elicit pain of renal origin. The iliac crests are palpated and may be tender, particularly over the posterior iliac spine where local injection may give symptomatic relief. The sciatic nerve is palpated in its notch and along

Table 27–2. MECHANICAL RELATIONSHIPS NOTED IN DISCOGENIC LOW BACK PAIN AND HERNIATED NUCLEUS PULPOSUS AS COMPARED WITH SPINAL STENOSIS

	Herniated Nucleus Pulposus/Discogenic Low Back Pain	Spinal Stenosis
Standing/walking	▼	▲
Sitting	▲	▼
Valsalva maneuver	▲	—
Bending	▲	—
Lifting	▲	—
Bed rest	▼	▼

Table 27–3. NERVE ROOT FINDINGS

Nerve Root	Pain and Dysesthesia	Weakness and Atrophy	Decreased Reflexes
L4	Posterolateral thigh across knee Anteromedial leg	Quadriceps	Knee jerk
L5	Posterior thigh	Tibialis anterior	None or decreased tibialis posterior
	Anterolateral leg Medial foot and hallux	Extensor hallucis longus Atrophied anterior compartment of the leg	
S1	Posterior thigh Posterior leg Posterolateral foot Lateral toes	Gastrosoleus	Ankle jerk
Sacral roots S2–S4	Buttocks and perineum Posterior thigh	Gluteus maximus Hamstrings	Ankle jerk Absent plantar toe responses
	Posterior leg Plantar foot	Gastrosoleus Foot intrinsics and long flexors Anal and bladder sphincters	

its course to determine hyperesthesia and tenderness. Calf tenderness may be found, reflecting sciatic hyperesthesia.

A thorough neurologic examination is done for objective signs of lumbar root involvement. In disc herniations, L5–S1 and L4–L5 are most commonly affected, followed by L3–L4. Disc herniations at L5–S1 usually involve the S1 root; L4–L5, the L5 root; and L3–L4, the L4 root. L4–L5 herniation may involve both the L5 and S1 roots, and there is a 10 percent incidence of two-level herniations.[29] The neurologic findings are summarized in Table 27–3. The findings according to level should be regarded as guidelines because, although these patterns are generally accurate as to level of entrapment, they can be misleading. The distribution of paresis in the lower extremity in herniated discs at the L4–L5 and L5–S1 levels was studied by Weber,[30] who noted that, although there is localization of paresis according to nerve root, 30 to 40 percent of other muscle groups in the lower extremity are also affected. Impairment of the knee jerk has been shown to be caused more often by L4–L5 herniations than by those at L3–L4.[31] Neurologic assessment must be done carefully, as often only subtle motor weakness is present and must be elicited by repetitive testing. This is particularly true for the gastrosoleus, which is so powerful that manual testing may not demonstrate weakness. Repetitive toe lifts while standing on one foot are useful in this respect, as is examining a toe-toe and heel-heel gait. Reflexes can be enhanced by an isometric maneuver with the hands or, in the case of the ankle jerk, having the patient kneel on a chair. Sensory findings are often confusing and must be mapped carefully. It is of value to perform both pin and vibration tests to ascertain that all columns of the cord are intact.

The patient can then be placed supine, and thigh and leg girths measured for atrophy. Leg lengths are measured, as leg length inequality may be associated with back pain that can be helped symptomatically with a shoe lift. Maneuvers are then done to stretch the sciatic nerve and elicit pain. Straight leg raising is done by lifting the leg by the heel with the knee extended until the patient expresses pain and the hamstrings tighten. The site of the pain is asked, as only radicular pain, not back pain, is indicative of a herniated disc. The test is of value only with distal roots and is therefore most accurate with lesions involving the L5 and S1 roots. Young patients have a marked tendency toward a positive straight leg raising test result with disc herniations. Its absence fairly accurately excludes a disc herniation up to the age of 30, when it no longer excludes the diagnosis.[32] Variations of the straight leg raising test include dorsiflexion of the foot at the end-point of straight leg arising to further stretch the sciatic nerve. Lasègue's test is done by having the hip and knee flexed and then slowly extending the knee. It can also be done with the patient seated over the side of the examining table. The crossed straight leg raising test is done by elevating the leg contralateral to the symptomatic side. Reproduction of radicular pain by this maneuver is considered the most indicative sign of disc herniation.[31]

To stretch the more proximal roots to the femoral nerve, the patient is turned prone and the Ely test for rectus femoris contracture done. The knee is flexed, and the hip is hyperextended. This motion will be limited by irritation of the L3 and L4 roots. The Patrick or fabere test, to implicate the sacroiliac rather than the hip joint, is done by *flexing, ab*ducting, *externally rotating,* and *ex*tending the hip (giving rise to the mnemonic fabere).[33] A painful response points to the sacroiliac joint as the source of the complaint.

If it is thought that the patient has too much emotional overlay, is too coached in examination by multiple previous consultations, or is guilty of outright malingering, there are some tests to help reveal this. In straight leg raising, the foot is both dorsiflexed and plantar flexed to ascertain the correct anatomic result. When the patient is sitting on the table, the knees are casually extended to note the presence of Lasègue's sign and to see if the patient sits back to relax sciatic tension. With the patient supine, he or she is asked to do an active straight leg raising maneuver while the examiner's hand is under the contralateral heel. A true effort will give a downward push on the opposite heel, while a feigned attempt will not produce it. A true list will persist while the patient is bending forward in a chair. These and other useful tests are reviewed elsewhere.[34, 35]

An assessment of peripheral circulation should be performed, as well as an abdominal, rectal, and pelvic examination, as the source of some back pain may be found in these areas. Chest expansion is measured with a tape measure as a screen for ankylosing spondylitis; it is highly significant when chest excursion is reduced to 1 inch.

Laboratory Examination. Laboratory examination provides little useful information on low back pain unless specifically utilized for the evaluation of metabolic and selective abnormalities causing back pain. There is no laboratory screening test for back pain.

Psychologic Evaluation. For better or worse, back pain involves a significant number of emotional factors, and it is necessary to recognize them early in assessing pain. When personality factors are unfavorable, management will be unsuccessful no matter how skillfully performed.[27] Fortunately, identification of emotional factors can be made more objective by psychologic testing. The Minnesota Multiphasic Personality Inventory (MMPI) has been the most accurate guideline for detecting personality traits that will predict poor results.[28, 36] The hysteria (Hy) and hypochondriasis (Hs) scales of the MMPI have been shown to be the best predictors of the symptomatic result of surgery and chemonucleolysis for disc disease. A simple pain diagram has been correlated with the MMPI.[37] This makes it possible to have a quick, simple office assessment of personality traits that may confuse pain assessment. Specific examination techniques can be incorporated in the evaluation of acute and chronic low back pain. Nonorganic physical signs include superficial tenderness, simulated axial loading, distracted straight leg raising, regional motor and sensory deficits suggesting functional disturbance, and over-reaction patterns.[55] These tests cannot be used in an absolute sense to rule in or out functional versus organic pain[38] but help in deciding whether to pursue invasive therapy, to seek psychologic or psychiatric consultation, or, in the case of chronic pain, to enter into behavior modification by operant conditioning.[39, 40] The presence of psychologic traits of chronic pain syndromes and nonorganic physical findings indicate that traditional strategies will not succeed.

Anatomically based aid is given by the thiopental (Pentothal) interview,[41] utilizing the straight leg raising test. The patient's straight leg raising end-point is established, and she or he is then given intravenous thiopental anesthesia until a noxious stimulus such as toe squeeze or heel cord pinching no longer produces a response. The anesthetic is allowed to wear off, and at intervals the noxious stimulus, given in the limb examined, is tested. On return of a response such as a grimace, deep sigh, or withdrawal, the straight leg raising is repeated. If there is organic disease and lumbar root irritation, an appropriate response to this noxious stimulus will be registered. In this manner, further information as to the severity and organic nature of the pain described is gained.

Radiologic Evaluation
Plain Radiographs and Common Anomalies of the Low Back. A lateral lumbosacral radiograph delivers a 2-rem skin dose, which is 15 times the exposure delivered by a chest radiograph.[42] It should therefore be obtained with some discretion. One study has shown that the risks and costs of obtaining a lumbar radiograph at the initial visit do not justify the small associated benefit.[43] Nonetheless, the lumbosacral spine film is a necessary part of early evaluation to exclude serious conditions such as tumor and infection. The anteroposterior, lateral, and coned-down lateral views are standard. Oblique views can offer added information.[56] Early signs of disc degeneration are decreased height of the anterior disc space and anteroposterior intervertebral shift on flexion-extension lateral views.[44] The so-called vacuum sign of intranuclear gas also reflects disc degeneration.[45] Later radiographic signs of disc degeneration are further collapse of the disc space, sclerosis, and osteophyte formation. Osteophytes also occur in Reiter's syndrome, ankylosing spondylitis, and psoriatic arthritis. The presence of disc degeneration radiographically does not imply that a disc is the cause of pain. Lawrence surveyed lumbosacral spine films in persons 35 years of age and older.[46] Sixty-five percent of the males and 52 percent of the females showed disc degeneration, but in only 13 percent were there symptoms of pain. Nerve root involvement occurred in only 10 percent of those with signs of moderate to severe degeneration. In a large series of disc herniations proved at operation, the plain radiograph predicted a correct diagnosis in only 34 percent of cases.[47] Epstein found 46 percent narrowing at L5–S1 and only 25 percent narrowing at L4–L5 in 300 proved herniations.[48] Therefore a disc can often appear radiographically normal when it is symptomatic, and when a disc is symptomatic, radiography is not an accurate predictor of the symptomatic level. Plain radiographs offer little in the assessment of low back pain, and positive findings do not provide specific information as to the cause of the pain.[57, 58]

Various structural anomalies, definable on plain radiographs and associated with back pain and disc degeneration, have been reviewed.[49] A defect in the pars interarticularis (spondylolysis) increases the likelihood of symptomatic back pain by about 25 percent. Disc herniation, however, is unusual. The incidence of disc degeneration defined by discogram is increased by bilateral pars defects, and the degeneration is thought to be more rapidly progressive. Wiltse believes that unilateral pars defects increase the rate of disc degeneration.[49] Tropism, or a rotational asymmetry of the lumbosacral facets from a sagittal to a coronal direction, produces accelerated disc degeneration. Farfan and Sullivan found a 23 percent incidence of asymmetry in asymptomatic backs.[50] In symptomatic backs they found a high incidence of asymmetry and disc herniations on the side of the more coronal facet.

Scoliosis in the thoracolumbar region does not increase the incidence of low back pain in individuals up to the age of 56 years.[4, 5, 51] There is progressive disc degeneration at the apex of the curve in progressive scoliotic curves. Lumbar lordosis does increase the incidence of back pain.[1, 5] Lumbosacral tilt from a unilateral anomalous lumbosacral facet or unilateral hypoplasia of the sacrum and pelvis is not known to produce rapid disc degeneration, although it might be expected to.[49] Leg length discrepancy producing tilt is known not to cause symptoms with up to 1 to 2 cm of discrepancy.[1, 5] With greater than 4.5 cm of discrepancy, the incidence of back pain increases.[49]

Spina bifida occulta does not produce back pain.[1, 5] Transitional vertebrae are either a sacralized lumbar vertebra or a lumbarized sacral vertebra, and neither produces increased back pain.[1, 5] Five percent of people have six lumbar vertebrae, 2.5 percent have four, and the rest have the usual five.[52] Wiltse advances a guideline that the more sacralized a vertebra, the more vestigial its disc and the less likely it is to herniate.[49] If there is disc herniation, it is usually at the level above the transitional vertebra.

Bone Scan. Bone scanning with technetium-99m diphosphonate can be of use in defining the origin of back pain in some situations. It can demonstrate bony infections or tumors and is useful in detecting early evidence of ankylosing spondylitis with increased activity in the sacroiliac, facet, and costovertebral joints. A developing pars interarticularis defect, not visible on plain radiography, can be demonstrated by bone scan. Advanced degenerative disc and facet disease produces increased uptake, and bone scan yields little useful information.[53] Gallium citrate scanning offers the possibility of early diagnosis of infections.[54] Indium-labeled leukocyte imaging provides a newer technique for the early detection of infection.[59]

Myelography. Myelography is used as a preoperative investigation, not as a diagnostic technique.[29, 41] It is recommended preoperatively for two reasons: (1) it will reveal a tumor presenting as a disc herniation, which might be missed if it is not at the level examined at surgery; and (2) it more precisely localizes the site of disc herniation and root entrapment. Lateral bony root entrapments may be present

with a normal myelogram. Diffuse anular bulges will give a waisted, hourglass appearance. Multiple disc herniations occur with a 5 to 10 percent incidence.[42] Myelographic information will thus allow the surgeon to modify the approach so that excessive exposure will be avoided, minimizing postoperative perineural scarring. As has been previously noted, neurologic examination is not completely accurate in localizing the level of involvement. In disc herniations, neurologic symptoms associated with the last two lowest spaces point to the correct level only about 60 percent of the time.[31] Neurologic signs are more accurate, reaching 75 to 80 percent.[31] Myelography is accurate 80 to 90 percent of the time,[47, 65, 66] but it is not foolproof in that lateral disc herniations are detected in only 70 to 80 percent of myelograms,[42] and 11 percent of cases of sciatica have a normal myelogram as well as a normal neurologic examination.[67] Over two thirds of disc herniations with false-negative myelography are in the L5–S1 space,[31] because the dural sac may be short or may lie away from the disc by 3 to 4 mm.

Traditional myelography was done with iodophenylundelic acid (Pantopaque), which is an oil-soluble contrast medium. The complications are numerous and include fever, headache, nausea, meningismus, backache, urinary changes, paresthesias, ileus, and acute and chronic arachnoiditis. Complications related to technique include extradural injections, epidural hematomas, contrast retention, venous intravasation, pulmonary embolism, epidermoid cyst formation, chronic dural leaks, chemical arachnoiditis secondary to the mixing of blood with Pantopaque, and others that are well reviewed.[68, 69] Complications are infrequent, but the most common are the acute, transient systemic reactions secondary to inflammation caused by the Pantopaque, the extradural or mixed injection, and retention of contrast caused by faulty technique.[68]

Water-soluble myelography has replaced oil-soluble myelography and has been used extensively in Europe. Oil-soluble contrasts are now banned in Scandinavia.[70] Meglumine[69] and more recently metrizamide[60] are the agents used. These water-soluble contrast media are found to fill the root sleeves more completely because of their solubility in cerebrospinal fluid and their low viscosity. Therefore lateral disc herniations are more readily detected. These agents are less inflammatory and they are resorbed, leaving no retained contrast. The major complications are those of meningeal irritation, increased radicular symptoms, transient hypotension, and seizures.[69] Metrizamide is the most improved of the contrast agents but is still regarded as epileptogenic. It is reported to have 95 percent accuracy in identifying disc herniations.[70] Iohexol is the newest of the water-soluble contrast agents and has a lower frequency of adverse reactions than metrizamide.[60]

The abnormalities noted on myelography vary with the size and location of the lesion. Lateral disc herniations usually cause incomplete filling of the

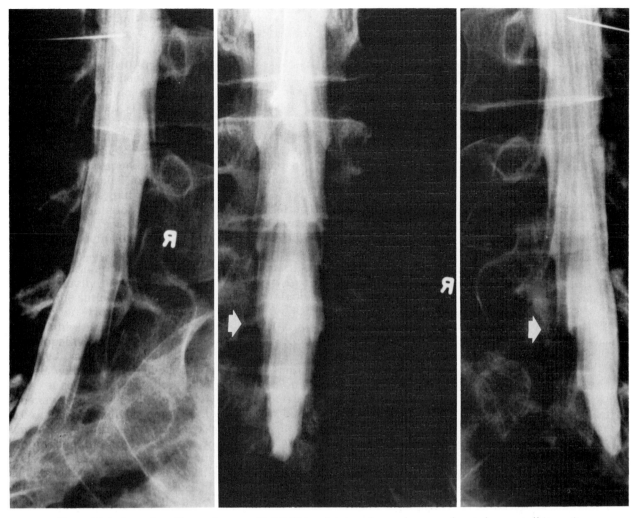

Figure 27–2. A metrizamide myelogram with L5–S1 herniated nucleus pulposus and root sleeve cutoff (*arrows*).

root sleeve, lateral dural sac indentation, and a double density of the sac (Fig. 27–2). Central midline herniations often give a complete block with ventral indentation. Sequestered free fragments may migrate and will be seen as circumscribed masses. Chronic degeneration with a diffuse annular bulge will give a waisted, hourglass appearance at the level of the disc space and osteophytes (Fig. 27–3). Artifacts encountered are from the needle, hematomas, and scarring from previous surgery.

Computed Tomography. Computed tomography (CT) has replaced many of the alternative methods of radiologic imaging. With fourth-generation scanners, the need for myelography has decreased and therefore the morbidity of investigation has decreased. CT scanning has the disadvantage of not being useful as a screening procedure, as myelography is, and it may not visualize intradural lesions unless contrast is present intrathecally. The reliability of CT scanning in detecting herniated disc appears to be well over 95 percent. Herniated disc can be easily visualized on a thin-cut CT scan, as seen in Figure 27–4. Spinal stenosis can be visualized as in

Figure 27–5, with bulging of the disc, thickening of the ligamentum flavum, osteophytic entrapment from the facets, and the obliteration of epidural fat.

These techniques should be reserved for cases in which there is clinical suspicion of an anatomic lesion.[71a] Imaging techniques should not be used to find a lesion and thereby provide a presumptive diagnosis of the cause of pain. If one uses this latter approach, false-positive results from asymptomatic degeneration will confuse the evaluation. Such degeneration in the cervical and lumbar region was found following myelography in 28 percent of patients who had no spinal symptoms but were being studied for other reasons.[72]

A study of CT scans in asymptomatic patients demonstrated abnormal findings in 35.4 percent. In patients younger than 40, 19.5 percent had a CT diagnosis of herniated disc. In patients older than 40 years, 50 percent had abnormal findings, primarily of herniated disc, spinal stenosis, and facet degeneration.[61] The studies emphasize the importance of clinical correlation.

Magnetic Resonance Imaging. Magnetic reso-

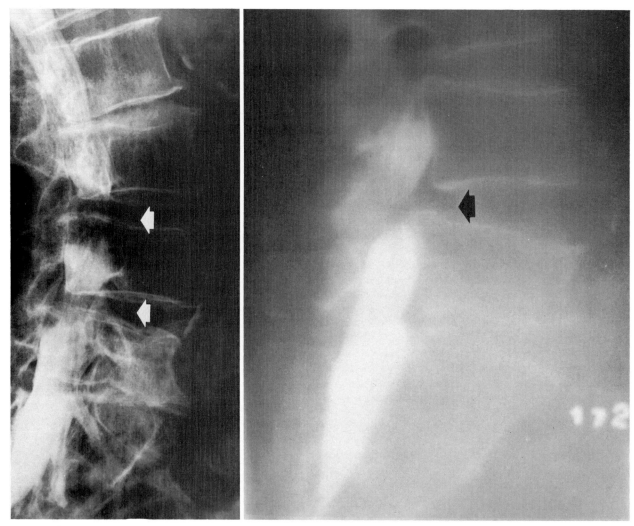

Figure 27–3. A metrizamide myelogram of a patient with degenerative spinal stenosis demonstrating central exclusion of the contrast with the hourglass configuration at the level of the discs (*arrows*). Tomography was used to enhance visualization.

nance imaging (MRI) has excellent soft tissue contrast and the ability to provide multiplanar images. The vertebrae, discs, and spinal canal over an entire anatomic region can be displayed without contrast. The normal disc has increased signal intensity on T_2-weighted images because of its water content. With degeneration, height and signal intensity are lost. Sagittal images are valuable in assessing disc herniation.[62] MRI may be sensitive and specific in the assessment of vertebral osteomyelitis[63] and has become the imaging modality of choice in the assessment of patients with persistent or recurrent symptoms following spinal surgery.[63a] Further studies are needed to compare MRI and CT evaluations of low back disorders.

Other Techniques. Lumbar epidural venography has been replaced in the era of CT scanning but was previously of significant value.[71] Epidurography is a technique of injecting epidural water-soluble contrast medium to outline the dural sac and root sleeves. It is placed via the sacral hiatus, but in one series 7.5 percent of patients could not be injected successfully.[66] Subarachnoid injections carry a risk of seizure and death.

Nerve root infiltration is of value in localizing the level of root involvement.[41] It is done under image intensification with oil-soluble contrast medium injected into the sleeve for definition and lidocaine (Xylocaine) injected to determine if clinical relief of pain occurs.

Facet blocks offer both a diagnostic and a therapeutic measure for relief of back pain.[21, 53] Under image intensification a needle is placed into the facet joint. Water-soluble contrast can be used to outline the facet, and a local anesthetic and/or a depot steroid injected for prolonged relief of symptoms. The relief of pain is the only end-point of significance.

DISEASE STATES

Spinal Stenosis and Lumbar Root Entrapment. Intervertebral disc degeneration is the central factor

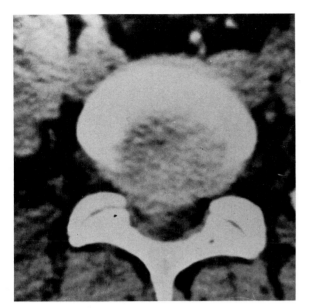

Figure 27–4. Computed tomographic scan of a herniated intervertebral disc with unilateral obliteration of the root by disc material.

Table 27–4. CLASSIFICATION OF SPINAL STENOSIS

Congenital
    Idiopathic
    Achondroplastic
Acquired stenosis
    Degenerative
        Central portion of the spinal canal
        Lateral portion of the spinal canal
        Degenerative spondylolisthesis
    Combined—any combination of congenital,
        degenerative, and disc herniations
Spondylolytic, spondylolisthetic
Iatrogenic
    Postlaminectomy
    Postfusion
    Postchemonucleolysis
Post-traumatic
Miscellaneous
    Paget's disease
    Fluorosis

in many of the conditions of age-related degenerative disease of the lumbar spine. As already noted, disc degeneration progresses with age and with progression down the lumbar spine. Mixter and Barr first emphasized the role of herniation of the nucleus pulposus in producing lumbar root entrapment.[13] Much work has focused on disc degeneration itself and lumbar root entrapment as a result of anatomic changes secondary to disc degeneration. Clinically, lumbar root entrapment is now encompassed in the broad classification of spinal stenosis,[74] which includes narrowing of the spinal canal, nerve root

canals, and intervertebral foramina. The process may be local, segmental, or generalized. It may be secondary to soft tissue or bone encroachment and may involve the canal, dural sac, or both. This definition includes classic disc herniation and a variety of entrapment syndromes described by Macnab.[75] The classification of spinal stenosis is outlined in Table 27–4.[74]

Historically, spinal stenosis was originally used to describe root entrapment caused by a congenital narrowing of the spinal canal produced by thickening of the neural arches, interpedicular narrowing, and a trefoil configuration of the canal.[76, 77] The term was subsequently extended[78, 79] to include degenerative and other changes causing root entrapment (illustrated in Figure 27–6). Prior to their inclusion in the definition of spinal stenosis, it was already known that degenerative changes caused root entrapment,[80] and it had been shown that in an already compromised canal, small changes causing further root entrapment can have marked neurologic consequences.[81] Iatrogenic spinal stenosis has been shown to produce symptomatic narrowing of the canal by thickening of the laminae after decortication—particularly after posterior fusion. Scar tissue from laminectomy may cause compression. Epidural fat involved in lipomatosis can cause spinal stenosis.[82] Degenerative stenosis is the most common kind of spinal stenosis encountered.[83]

Clinical States. Clinical complaints involving the lumbar spine can present with backache and no nerve root entrapment or with nerve root involvement with or without backache. As the disc degenerates, segmental instability is produced and abnormal degrees of motion are permitted. This produces excessive motion and subluxation in the facet joints, which undergo small degrees of trauma. As the disc loses height, further subluxation of the facets occurs, and degenerative arthritis in these joints is the sequela. Disc degeneration may remain asymptomatic, may be symptomatic because of changes in the disc itself,

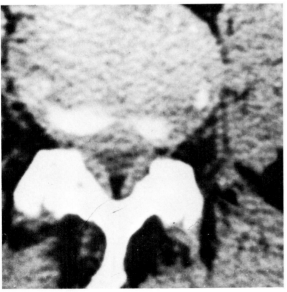

Figure 27–5. Computed tomographic scan of spinal stenosis with bulging of the annulus, osteophytic overgrowth of the facet joints, and annulus thickening of the ligamentum flavum.

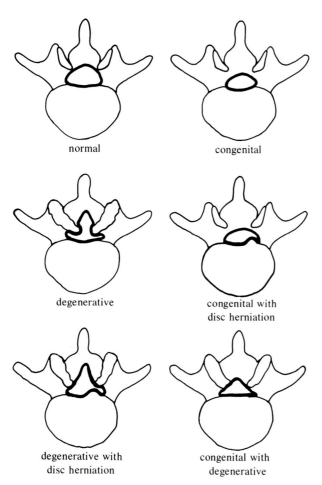

normal   congenital

degenerative   congenital with
                               disc herniation

degenerative with   congenital with
disc herniation   degenerative

Figure 27–6. Outlines of the cross section of the spinal canal in different types of spinal stenosis.

or may be symptomatic because of trauma in the facet joints and ligaments. Root entrapment occurs when roots are involved in disc herniations or entrapment by settling structures or osteophytic processes, yielding pain with discogenic or neurogenic claudication mechanics. The differences are presumably on the basis of different pathophysiologic mechanisms involving nociception to a radicular irritation or inflammatory phenomenon versus radicular ischemia.

Treatment. Backache without nerve involvement is managed conservatively. Pain can be prolonged, lasting up to 3 months in 87 percent of those affected,[8] and has a 60 percent incidence of recurrent bouts within the first year of an attack. It is managed with bedrest, analgesics, muscle relaxants, corsets, weight loss, and exercises that emphasize back stretching and abdominal strengthening. Bedrest can decrease discomfort and hasten recovery, but analgesics do not speed recovery and nonsteroid anti-inflammatory drugs (NSAIDs) are ineffective.[85] Bedrest is recommended for 2 to 7 days. Beyond this time and certainly beyond 2 weeks, bedrest is deleterious in the management of acute low back pain. Outlines of treatment programs vary with the treat-

ing physician but usually follow these measures.[34, 86] Spinal fusion may be warranted in cases of chronic backache, but thorough investigation of the patient, including a psychologic assessment,[86, 87] is required to give some preoperative estimate of the likelihood of success.

Lumbar Disc Herniation. Lumbar nerve root entrapment in disc degeneration was classically ascribed to disc herniation.[13] With annular radial fissures, the nucleus, as long as it is mobile, can herniate. The nomenclature describing disc herniations has been confusing, but certain patterns are established (Fig. 27–7). If the nucleus is confined by a few outer annular fibers so that it does not enter the epidural space, it may present as a concealed disc with a localized or diffuse annular bulge. If the annular fibers are disrupted so that the nucleus leaves the confines of the annulus and enters the epidural space, it is prolapsed. If a piece of herniated material breaks off and is free in the epidural space, it is a sequestered disc or free fragment. The mechanism of root pain is not clear. Originally it was thought to be compression, but root compression is not necessarily found at surgery. All observers agree that involved roots exhibit stages of inflammation and that these inflamed roots will reproduce sciatic symptoms when stimulated. There is biopsy substantiation of intraneural inflammation.[84] Possible mechanisms of neural damage have been reviewed by Murphy.[88]

Symptoms of disc herniation may include back-

Concealed

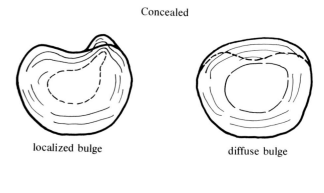

localized bulge   diffuse bulge

Prolapsed

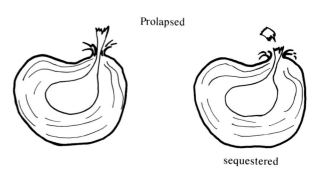

sequestered

Figure 27–7. A classification of disc herniations.

ache, backache and sciatica, sciatica, and those of cauda equina compression. The onset can be sudden and severe. Sciatic symptoms are radicular in nature and are exacerbated by activities such as Valsalva maneuvers and bending, which increase intradiscal pressure. Signs present are those reflecting root tension (see above). The phenomenon of sciatic scoliosis may suggest the relation of the herniation to the root. If the herniation is lateral to the root, the patient leans away from the symptomatic side. The patient leans toward the symptomatic side if the herniation is medial to the root. The clinical examination is directed toward establishing the diagnosis as accurately as possible. Neurologic symptoms give the correct level only 46 percent of the time,[47] whereas signs raise the accuracy to about 75 percent. Complete loss of a reflex is much more reliable as a diagnostic sign than simple depression.[31] A positive straight leg raising test is 75 to 80 percent diagnostically accurate, with pain on crossed straight leg raising almost pathognomonic for disc herniation. Electromyography raises diagnostic accuracy to 80 percent.[89] Plain radiographs are essentially nondiagnostic. Water-soluble myelography raises accuracy to 90 to 95 percent, as does CT imaging.

Conservative therapy for disc herniation centers on bedrest, analgesics, muscle relaxants, and anti-inflammatory medications. Pelvic traction may be of benefit in some patients. The degree of bedrest is dependent on the severity of symptoms. Once they abate, a program of exercises and back protection is started. For severe symptoms more enforced bedrest over a 2-week period is used. Most disc herniations respond to conservative therapy, but in those that are unresponsive further measures may be needed.[89a]

Chemonucleolysis is the injection of chymopapain into the disc space. When previously in use it had about a 75 percent rate of good results, about the same as laminectomy and discectomy.[90] More recent studies indicate good results in 89 percent of cases.[91] It is indicated in patients with a proven disc herniation who would otherwise be surgical candidates. The primary risk of chymopapain has been allergic reaction, with anaphylaxis the most threatening form. The small risk of transverse myelitis, with irreversible paraplegia, has led to the decline in the use of chemonucleolysis in the United States. Other techniques available for symptomatic relief are facet blocks[21] and radiofrequency facet denervation.[53] Intrathecal and epidural steroids have had some success in the symptomatic relief of discogenic pain,[92] although some authors find them no better than placebo.[93] Nerve root sleeve infiltrations with steroid may give relief.[86] Intradiscal steroids have been used.[94]

The one indisputable indication for surgery for removal of a disc is the cauda equina syndrome, in which a central midline herniation causes paralysis of the sacral roots, with bladder and bowel dysfunction and inability to walk (see Table 27–2). It occurs in about 2.4 percent of operative disc herniations.[95]

The loss of bladder and bowel function is disastrous and return is limited, so this entity is a true surgical emergency. There is seldom recovery from perineal anesthesia, and bladder paralysis may have a worse rate of recovery than somatic sensory deficits.[96]

Other indications for laminectomy are marked muscular weakness and progressive neurologic deficit in spite of bedrest.[86, 87] There have been studies to dispute these indications as absolute. Andersson and Carlsson found that the time since onset, duration of symptoms, and operative findings have no relationship to the return of minor activity in foot drop secondary to disc herniation.[97] Estimates of motor return after loss from disc herniation range from 50 percent[23] to 80 percent[98] and are not different in operative compared with nonoperative patients. After 1 year of follow-up the prognosis of motor return is no better after delayed surgery than with conservative therapy. Immediate surgical treatment is regarded as adequate therapy for the pain of disc herniation, but there is some doubt as to the use of paresis as an indication.[30]

Relative indications for laminectomy are intolerable pain unrelieved by bedrest, and recurrent episodes of incapacitating pain. Laminectomy for definite disc herniation remains a highly successful procedure.[2, 67, 95] Hirsch and Nachemson reported that if disc herniation is a prolapse, 96 percent of operative patients have improvement.[67] If concealed disc herniation is found with scarring and inflammation the predominant findings, 70 percent of patients have relief regardless of whether or not the disc is removed. Improvement in these patients is a matter of degree, and only 15 percent have complete and permanent relief. The remainder are improved but have recurrent symptoms. About one third will have persistent backache after discectomy.[95] The relationship between complete prolapse and a high degree of relief after surgery has been substantiated in other series.[95] Negative explorations prolong disability.[23] The overall long-term relief of sciatica has been shown to be the same in operative versus nonoperative patients, although the operative patients achieve their degree of relief more rapidly.[23] A 10-year prospectively randomized study of operative versus nonoperative treatment of disc herniation has shown no difference in the relief of symptoms after 4 years.[64] These studies imply that a relative indication for surgery offering optimal results is the emotionally stable patient with unequivocal disc herniation who for personal and socioeconomic reasons cannot sustain prolonged or repeated bouts of incapacitating pain. The most common cause for surgical failure is poor initial patient selection.[99]

Adhesive radiculitis is a condition in which the nerve root is found to be extensively involved in fibrous tissue in proximity to a disc space. It is presumably the result of chronic inflammation and clinically presents with persistent sciatic pain. Neurolysis is the only treatment, but the results are variable.

Spinal Stenosis. The remainder of the lumbar root entrapment syndromes fall into the broad definition of degenerative spinal stenosis.[99a] They are predominantly bony entrapments. As these are changes resulting from more advanced disc degeneration, they usually occur in patients over age 50.[99b] Before age 50, disc herniation is the common cause of radicular pain, but over age 50 bony entrapment predominates. The entrapment may be more lateral, giving only root symptoms, or more central, giving cauda equina symptoms. Unlike those with disc herniations, patients with these spinal stenosis syndromes have a long history of back pain and more recent history of sciatica. There is often a claudicating character to the pain, with pain in the back or in the legs while walking. The pain is not relieved by standing still but rather by flexing the back, as in sitting. Therefore these patients can walk up hills more easily than down and can bicycle, but cannot tolerate lumbar extension. These changes are usually progressive. There may be bowel and bladder symptoms, with the latter mimicking prostatic bladder outlet obstruction. These patients do not give marked root tension signs such as straight leg raising and may have multiple levels of root involvement. Radiographs reveal changes of degenerative disc disease with disc height narrowing, facet subluxation and degeneration, retrolisthesis, and pseudospondylolisthesis. The cross section of the spinal canal is difficult to visualize but can be done with transverse axial tomography,[100] and computed tomography[101] has dramatically lessened the difficulty. Myelography[83] reveals the canal diameter. In the anteroposterior dimension it is normally a minimum of 14 to 15 mm.[102, 103] Degenerative stenotic changes are noted centrally at the discs, producing hourglass waisting of the contrast column by a thickened ligamentum flavum and bulging degenerative discs (see Fig. 27–3). Peripherally the facets produce "cut-off" root sleeves by subluxation and osteophyte formation, leading to canal and foraminal encroachment. Water-soluble contrast media will give better definition of lateral entrapment by filling the root sleeve more fully. CT scan (see Fig. 27–5) easily demonstrates the entrapment via disc, bone, and ligamentum flavum.

Macnab has described a variety of root entrapment syndromes resulting from degenerative changes.[41, 75, 86] Central stenosis can occur with the bulging degenerative disc and posteriorly with a "shingling" overlap of the laminae, thickening of the ligamentum flavum, and subluxation and osteophyte formation in the facet joints. Subarticular entrapment occurs when the superior articular facet enlarges and compresses the root against a bulging disc or against the dorsum of a vertebral body. Foraminal encroachment occurs in the foramen where the superior facet lies in close relationship to the root. With subluxation and osteophytic outgrowths from the facet and the vertebral body, the root may be entrapped. Pedicular kinking occurs when there is loss of disc height, particularly asymmetrically whereby the root is kinked by the descending pedicle and commonly is entrapped between a bulging disc and a pedicle about it. Extraforaminal entrapment occurs after the root has left the foramen, where it may be involved in diffuse or discrete annular bulge and, in the case of L5, trapped by the corporotransverse ligament against the sacral ala.

For patients with mild symptoms and disability, or those who are not operative candidates for medical reasons, epidural steroid injections may be useful. One study, however, found that approximately 50 percent of patients with radicular symptoms received temporary relief with steroid injection. However, long-term relief occurred in fewer than 25 percent of patients.[103a] The treatment of all these spinal stenosis syndromes with severe symptoms is surgical, with emphasis placed on adequate decompression of the entrapped roots.[75, 104] When the symptoms are severe, they tend not to improve. If symptoms are not severe, regimens of back protection, isometric exercises, back supports, and anti-inflammatory medications are used. Operation is withheld until symptoms are no longer tolerable. Neurologic changes are not usually severe enough to warrant surgery. The symptomatic relief offered by adequate surgical decompression is considered particularly good,[104] with positive results expected in about 85 percent of patients.[104a]

Systemic Inflammatory Disease of the Low Back. Rheumatoid arthritis is known to involve the lumbar spine. An increased incidence of subluxation and disc narrowing, apophyseal destruction, and osteoporosis has been found in rheumatoid patients.[105] Rheumatoid erosions in facet joints have been demonstrated by stereoscopic radiographic examination.[106]

The inflammatory spondyloarthropathies, of which ankylosing spondylitis is the prototype, produce back pain of a diffuse and often severe nature.[107–111] They are discussed in detail in Section VIII.

Hyperostotic spondylosis, described by Forestier and Rotes-Querol,[112] is a disease of new bone formation in the thoracic and thoracolumbar spine. The spine stiffens and spurs form at multiple levels, often causing a bony ankylosis more marked on the right side of the spine. The disc spaces remain intact.[113] There may be subperiosteal new bone formation in the pelvis.[114] The cause is unknown, but there is associated glucose intolerance, diabetes, and obesity.[115]

Infections

Pyogenic Vertebral Osteomyelitis. Hematogenous osteomyelitis has a predilection for the vertebral column,[116, 117] and pyogenic vertebral osteomyelitis has a predilection for older adults.[118] This is believed to be attributable to the marked vascularity of adult vertebra[116] with seeding of the capillary beds at the end-plate, while the disc has no vascular channels in the adult.[119] An associated causative factor is that the incidence of urinary tract infections rises in adults, and these organisms may be seeded to the vertebrae by Batson's plexus, the vertebral, ascending lumbar, and sacral veins, freely communicating with the external vertebral, internal vertebral, and intraosseous vertebral veins.[120, 121] Pyogenic infection then starts in the vertebral body and frequently involves the next body by spread to the epidural space and formation of an abscess, with compression, fracture, and collapse of the involved vertebra and spinal cord vascular compromise. These complications, plus bacteremia, accounted for most of the deaths in the older literature. Mortality now is expected to be less than 10 percent.[122, 122a]

Staphylococcus aureus traditionally has been the responsible organism, but gram-negative bacilli, especially related to genitourinary manipulations, are increasingly common.[118, 123–125]

Patients present with backache of slow onset with or without radicular symptoms, low-grade fever, night sweats, and weight loss.[126] Paravertebral and hamstring spasms are present. Diabetes is frequently associated and should be sought.[117, 127] The erythrocyte sedimentation rate (ESR) is elevated, but the white blood cell count may be normal. Early radiographic signs are an eroded subchondral end-plate, followed by involvement of the adjacent vertebra and loss of disc height. There is progressive loss of disc height over 6 to 8 weeks, progressive bony destruction, and reactive bone formation. Serial radiographs help to confirm the diagnosis.[128] Bone scan is useful in early detection. Multiple blood cultures and urine cultures should be obtained to determine the responsible organism. A biopsy for culture, either by closed Craig needle biopsy or open biopsy, is strongly advised, especially if blood cultures are negative. Antibiotics are recommended for 6 weeks[118] with monitoring of blood levels of the appropriate antibiotic to achieve bactericidal levels. The ESR can be used to follow the disease course.[127, 129] Bedrest is used during the treatment period, and a plaster jacket is used for 3 months. Fusion occurs in half the patients within 1 year, and in most patients the disc space is obliterated over 2 years.

Disc Space Infections. Disc space infections can result from any procedure inoculating the disc space. The most common is disc excision, the incidence of which is estimated to be 1 to 2.8 percent.[130, 131] The hallmark of the disease is severe, excruciating pain, which may have an onset as late as 3 months postoperatively; in some cases, however, postoperative pain may not disappear but increase. There is marked muscle spasm. Laboratory evidence is not present or is obscured by the recent operation, although an elevated ESR after operation will normally fall over a period of 3 months. Aspiration biopsy of the disc space is needed to determine the specific organism and its antibiotic sensitivity. Radiographic signs include dissolution of the subchondral bone, but these signs lag behind clinical signs by 2 to 3 weeks. There is a progression of loss of disc space height and

sclerotic bony reaction.[132] Bone scan is of no diagnostic value because of operative changes. The disc space often becomes fused when infected.[133] Treatment is with antibiotics and cast immobilization.

Disc space infections in children are different from pyogenic vertebral osteomyelitis and offer a different prognosis.[134] They also differ from adult postoperative disc space infections. An irritable child will have progressive backache or a limp, or refuse to walk. Night pain is common. There is paravertebral spasm. Early radiographic findings are absent. Later, progressive loss of disc space height with irregularity of the vertebral end-plates is seen. The ESR is elevated. *Staphylococcus aureus* is the most common organism. Gallium bone scan may be useful for early detection.[54] Treatment is aimed toward 6 to 12 weeks of immobilization in a body jacket or spica cast. Antibiotics are not necessarily indicated and may not affect prognosis. They should be used when pain is not relieved by immobilization, when paravertebral spasm does not subside, or if the ESR remains elevated and the child is systematically ill. Aspiration biopsy is recommended if there are progressive and prolonged symptoms despite prolonged immobilization.

Other Infections of the Spine. Nontubercular granulomatous infections of the spine are widely reported and have been reviewed by Pritchard.[135] Blastomycosis in the vertebrae infects the disc space, adjacent bodies, and frequently the adjacent ribs. Cryptococcosis of the spine is uncommon and is thought to be hematogenous in origin. It produces little periosteal reaction and has lucent lesions. Actinomycosis may involve the anterior and posterior elements and has a tendency toward paravertebral abscesses. The vertebral body produces a "soap bubble" radiographic appearance, and the disc is spared. Coccidioidomycosis usually causes multiple vertebral lesions with relative sparing of the disc space. Brucellosis has a spondylitic form with involvement of the disc and adjacent vertebra.

Tuberculosis of the spine is now found primarily in Third World countries. The spine accounts for about half the cases of bone and joint tuberculosis. There is a predilection for L1 to be the most commonly involved vertebra, and this is thought to be due to invasion by bacteria transported from the urinary tract via Batson's plexus.[136] The vertebral body is invaded, and the disc is spared. The primary symptom is insidious backache, increasing over many months. Constitutional symptoms can usually be elicited and paravertebral spasm with an acute kyphosis is found on examination. The ESR is elevated. Radiographs initially reveal osteopenia, followed by erosion on each side of the disc. Vertebral collapse follows, producing a variety of radiographic signs described by Hodgson[136] as concertina collapse, aneurysmal syndrome, lateral deviation, bony bridging, reversal of height to width ratio of the body, and wedging of the intervertebral disc. Paraplegia is a relatively frequent complication. Management is

Table 27–5. CLASSIFICATION OF SPONDYLOLYSIS AND SPONDYLOLISTHESIS

Dysplastic—congenital abnormalities of the upper sacrum or the arch of L5 allow the olisthesis
Isthmic—a pars interarticularis lesion of one of three types:
    Lytic—fatigue fracture of the pars
    Elongated, but intact pars
    Acute fracture
Degenerative—secondary to long-standing intervertebral instability
Traumatic—secondary to bony fractures in areas other than the pars
Pathologic—secondary to generalized or local bone disease

with multiple drug therapy; there is debate about the role of surgery and immobilization.[135] Long-term results were equally good in patients treated with chemotherapy and those undergoing anterior spinal fusion in a 10-year study. Surgery does have the advantage of maintaining better vertebral height and reducing kyphosis. Anterior surgery is indicated for neurologic deficit, instability, and failed medical therapy.

Syphilitic spondylitis is rare and occurs secondary to gummatous destruction with vertebral collapse and a great deal of reactive bone. The more common manifestation is that of destructive change with excessive bony reaction from Charcot's neuropathic arthropathy, usually at the thoracolumbar junction.

Hydatid disease of bone is known but rare. The midthoracic spine is usually involved, and the vertebral body is permeated by cysts, which often progress into the spinal canal. Vertebral collapse is common because of pathologic fractures. The incidence of paraplegia is high, as is the mortality.[139]

Spondylolysis and Spondylolisthesis. Spondylolysis indicates a separation at the pars interarticularis, permitting the slippage or "olisthesis." Spondylolisthesis designates a slipping of one vertebra forward on the one below. A classification of spondylolysis and spondylolisthesis has been proposed[140] (Table 27–5). Spondylolysis and, more frequently, spondylolisthesis can be involved with back pain. As previously noted, a pars interarticularis defect increases the incidence of back pain.[49] A vertebra may slip forward on the one below as a whole, or it may separate at the isthmus and slip. The entire unit may slip with subluxated posterior facets in degenerative or pseudospondylolisthesis. The slippage is graded either as a percentage of subluxation or I to IV by quarterly increments of slipping.

In the dysplastic type there is congenital dysplasia of the upper sacrum or the neural arch of L5 and the lowest free lumbar vertebra slips forward, usually in adolescence. The pars may remain unchanged, and the slippage will not exceed 25 percent, preventing cauda equina paralysis. Usually the pars elongates or separates. Dysplastic changes of the upper sacrum with inadequate development of the L5 to S1 facets most commonly produce the instability.[141] The pars is often dysplastic, and the sacrum and L5 may have a wide spinal bifida, giving rise to a high-grade slippage. It appears to be twice as common in girls as in boys.[140]

Isthmic spondylolisthesis involves a lesion in the pars interarticularis. The lytic lesion is a separation of the pars and is a fatigue fracture.[142] It is the most common type in patients younger than 50 years and is rarely seen in those younger than 5 years. The incidence in white children is 5 percent at 7 years and increases to 5.8 percent by 18 years of age, mostly during the 11- to 15-year age period.[140] There is a hereditary component,[143] the incidence increasing to 35 percent in families in which one member has spondylolysis or spondylolisthesis. Female gymnasts have been noted to have a fourfold increase in pars defects and spondylolisthesis,[144] and football interior linemen have an even higher incidence over the normal population.[145] Of the mechanical forces involved—flexion overload, unbalanced shear forces, and forced rotation—it is not yet known[146, 147] which is primarily responsible for the slippage.

Elongation of the pars without separation is the same disease as the lytic lesion, but with repeated microfractures healing in an elongated position. The pars may taper out and then separate, in which case the defect is reclassified as lytic. Acute pars fractures are secondary to trauma and usually involve only spondylolysis without slippage.

Degenerative spondylolisthesis is secondary to degenerative disc disease, with intersegmental instability[80] producing a local spinal stenosis. It is seldom seen before the age of 50, is ten times more frequent at L4 than at L5 or L3, is six times more frequent in women, and is three times more frequent in blacks. Sacralization is four times more frequent in individuals with degenerative spondylolisthesis than in the general population. It does not occur with spina bifida or isthmic spondylolisthesis, and the slippage is never more than 30 percent. A predisposing factor is a straight, stable lumbosacral joint putting more stress on the L4–L5 facets. The disc and ligaments degenerate and allow hypermobility and facet degeneration, permitting forward slipping.[148]

Traumatic spondylolisthesis is caused by a fracture in the posterior elements other than the pars, such as a facet or pedicle.[140]

Pathologic spondylolisthesis is due to a local or generalized bone disease in the pedicle, pars, or facets, where the forward forces are inadequately opposed and forward slippage results. It is found in osteopetrosis with pars fractures giving spondylolysis, arthrogryposis in Eskimos,[149] Paget's disease with pars elongation, syphilis secondary to gummas,[150] neurogenic arthropathies, tuberculous spondylitis, giant cell tumors of the posterior elements, and metastatic tumors.[141] Spondylolysis and spondylolisthesis aquisita are known to occur at the upper end of lumbar spine fusions[151–156] and have been reported below a thoracolumbar scoliosis fusion.[157] These are complications that are not seen with lateral fusions.[140]

Management of spondylolisthesis is age and lesion dependent. Wiltse and Jackson have provided guidelines for the management of children with spondylolisthesis.[158] A child, especially if younger than 10 years, who is found to have an isthmic spondylolisthesis is examined, and radiographs obtained, every 4 months for a year, then every 6 months up to the age of 15 years, then annually until growth is completed. This is especially important in girls, who have twice the incidence of high-grade olisthesis (slippage). In cases with up to 25 percent slippage and without symptoms, the child is followed and advised to avoid a career of heavy labor. In those with up to 50 percent slippage without symptoms, avoidance of traumatic sports is recommended. Those children with symptoms, but recovery by conservative measures, are followed. In a child with greater than 50 percent slippage, fusion is recommended regardless of symptoms. A child with persistent symptoms regardless of degree of slippage is advised to undergo fusion. A child younger than 10 years with a 50 percent slippage is often fused. Slippage will usually occur before 18 years of age if it is going to occur and rarely past 25 years of age. The most rapid slippage is between 9 and 15 years of age.[159] The onset of pain may be sudden and produce a "listhetic crisis" with the sudden onset of backache. On examination, a rigid lumbar spine, spastic scoliosis, flattened sacrum, and often hamstring spasm are found. There is usually no nerve root involvement; but if such involvement is present, laminectomy and possibly decompression will be required in addition to lumbosacral fusion.[86] A prospective study of spondylolisthesis demonstrated that the incidence was 44 percent at age 6, decreasing to 6 percent by adulthood. Progression of the slippage was unusual, and pain was not a factor in the population studied. No restriction of activities was recommended.

The presence of a pars defect does not mean that it is always the cause of back pain. Macnab examined a large series of patients with backache and found a 7.6 percent incidence of pars defects, similar to the overall incidence in asymptomatic individuals.[86] Dividing these patients by age, he showed that for those older than 40 years of age the incidence is the same as in the general population. However, about 19 percent of symptomatic individuals younger than 26 years of age had a defect. Therefore if the patient is younger than 26, the defect is probably the cause of the back pain. Between ages 26 and 40 it is possibly the cause. In persons older than 40 years it is rarely the cause.

Root irritation can occur with lytic spondylolisthesis by a variety of mechanisms. The neural arch of L5 may rotate forward on the sacrum and encroach on the foramen. Small ossicles and traction spurs make foraminal encroachment worse. Bony entrapment, described by Macnab,[86] occurs with forward and downward descent. The pedicles may kink the roots. Disc degeneration with bulging may cause entrapment lateral to the foramen. The corporotransverse ligament of L5 may compress the L5 root against the sacral ala with descent of L5. Disc herniation of L4–L5 may involve the L5 root. Disc degeneration itself may be painful, and in patients older than 35 years of age lumbodorsal disc degeneration may be symptomatic.[86] Therefore clinical evaluation with myelography and root sleeve injection is necessary in the older patient with back pain and spondylolisthesis. Foraminotomy may be necessary with fusion if there is a long history of backache. In this case discography is used to determine the upper extent of the fusion. If there is L4–L5 degeneration or the slip is greater than 50 percent, an L4–S1 fusion is indicated.

In adults older than 40 years with painful spondylolisthesis, Gill's procedure of removal of the loose posterior elements has been successful.[161] In adults without evidence of root entrapment and minimal slip, Newman recommends direct repair of the defect.[162]

Degenerative spondylolisthesis is a form of local spinal stenosis and a result of disc degeneration. It produces root entrapment and cauda equina symptoms with back pain, sciatic symptoms, and occasionally spinal claudication symptoms. Ten percent of Rosenberg's series came to decompression.[148] The question of fusion is unresolved. Guidelines of management are essentially those for degenerative disc disease and spinal stenosis.

Nonspinal Sources of Back Pain. Back pain can occur from disorders of the abdominal, retroperitoneal, and pelvic viscera, but it is rarely the only symptom. Pain is referred in a dermatomal distribution from viscera and is not aggravated by activity or relieved by rest, as is most pain of spinal origin. Peptic ulcer disease; gastric, duodenal, and pancreatic tumors; retroperitoneal lymphoma; sarcoma; and colonic tumors all can give rise to back pain. Retroperitoneal bleeding in anticoagulated patients can cause back pain. In the pelvis, endometriosis and uterine, cervical, and bladder invasive carcinoma may produce back pain, and tumors invading the lumbosacral plexus give rise to radicular pain. Sacral menstrual pain occurs, and uterine malposition and prolapse can give rise to sacral pain on standing. Fibroids may cause back pain. Chronic prostatitis can result in sacral pain. Renal pain is located in the costovertebral angle and frequently radiates to the groin and testis.

Abdominal aortic aneurysm may give rise to back pain, which is particularly acute during dissection. Intermittent claudication of peripheral vascular disease may mimic sciatic pain and can be confused with spinal stenosis, but can be differentiated by the relief of vascular claudication pain on standing still.

References

1. Horal, J.: The clinical appearance of low back disorders in the city of Gothenburg, Sweden. Acta Orthop. Scand. Suppl. 118, 1969.

2. Hirsch, C.: Efficiency of surgery in low-back disorders. J. Bone Joint Surg. 47A:991, 1965.

3. Kelsey, J. L., and White, A. A.: Epidemiology and impact of low back pain. Spine 5:133, 1980.

4. Wood, P. H. N., and MacLeish, C. L.: Digest of data on the rheumatic diseases. 5. Morbidity in industry and rheumatism in general practice. Ann. Rheum. Dis. 33:93, 1974.

5. Hult, L.: The Munk Fors investigation. Acta Orthop. Scand. Suppl. 16, 1954.

6. Anderson, J. A. D.: Back pain in industry. In Jayson, M. (ed.): The Lumbar Spine and Back Pain. London, Sector Publishing, Ltd., 1976.

7. Glover, J. R.: Prevention of back pain. In Jayson, M. (ed.): The Lumbar Spine and Back Pain. London, Sector Publishing, Ltd., 1976.

8. Berquist-Ullman, M., and Larsson, U.: Acute low back pain in industry. Acta Orthop. Scand. Suppl. 170, 1977.

9. Wood, P. H. N.: Epidemiology of back pain. In Jayson, M. (ed.): The Lumbar Spine and Back Pain. London, Sector Publishing Ltd., 1976.

10. Benn, R. T., and Wood, P. H. N.: Pain in the back: An attempt to estimate the size of the problem. Rheum. Rehab. 14:121, 1975.

11. Frymoyer, J. W., Pope, M. H., Cogtanza, M. C., Rosa, J. C., Goggin, J. E., and Wilder, D. G.: Epidemiologic studies of low back pain. Spine 5:419, 1980.

12. Akeson, W. H., and Murphy, R. W.: Low back pain. Clin. Orthop. 129:2, 1977.

12a. Cats-Baril, W. L., and Frymoyer, J. W.: The economics of spinal disorders. In Frymoyer, J. W. (ed.): The Adult Spine. New York, Raven Press, 1991, p. 103.

13. Mixter, W. J., and Barr, J. S.: Rupture of the intervertebral disc with involvement of the spinal canal: N. Engl. J. Med. 211:210, 1934.

14. Hirsch, C.: Etiology and pathogenesis of low back pain. Israel J. Med. Sci. 2:362, 1966.

15. Kelsey, J. L.: An epidemiological study of acutely herniated lumbar intervertebral discs. Rheum. Rehab. 14:144, 1975.

16. Edgar, M. A., and Ghadially, J. A.: Innervation of the lumbar spine. Clin. Orthop. 115:35, 1976.

17. Luschka, H.: Die Nerven des menschlichen Wibelkanales. Verlag der H. Lappschen Buchhandelung P. V. 4850:8:1, 1850.

18. Smyth, M. J., and Wright, V. J.: Sciatica and the intervertebral disk. An experimental study. J. Bone Joint Surg. 40A:1401, 1958.

19. Kellgren, J. H.: Observations on referred pain arising from muscle. Clin. Sci. 3:175, 1938.

20. Hirsch, C., Ingelmark, B., and Miller, M.: The anatomical basis for low back pain. Acta Orthop. Scand. 33:1, 1963.

21. Mooney, V., and Robertson, J.: The facet syndrome. Clin. Orthop. 115:149, 1976.

22. Nachemson, A. L.: The natural course of low back pain. In White, A. A., and Gordon, S. L. (eds.): A.A.O.S. Symposium on Idiopathic Low Back Pain. St. Louis, C. V. Mosby Company, 1982, p. 46.

23. Hakelius, A.: Long term follow-up in sciatica. Acta Orthop. Scand. Suppl. 129, 1972.

24. Mankin, H. J., and Adams, R. D.: Pain in the back and neck. In Thorn, G. W., Adams, R. D., Braunwald, E., Isselbacher, K. J., and Petersdorf, R. G. (eds.): Harrison's Principles of Internal Medicine. 8th ed. New York, McGraw-Hill Book Company, 1977.

25. Macnab, I.: The "whiplash syndrome." Orthop. Clin. North Am. 2:389, 1971.

26. Wilfling, F. J., Klonoff, H., and Kokan, P.: Psychological, demographic and orthopaedic factors associated with prediction of outcome of spinal fusion. Clin. Orthop. 90:153, 1973.

27. White, A. W. M.: The compensation back. Applied Therap. 8:871, 1966.

28. Wiltse, L. L., and Rocchio, P. D.: Preoperative psychologic tests as predictors of success of chemonucleolysis in the treatment of low-back syndrome. J. Bone Joint Surg. 57A:478, 1975.

28a. Bigos, S. J., Battie, M. C., Spengler, D. M., Fisher, L. D., Fordyce, W. E., Hansson, T. H., Nachemson, A. L., and Wortley, M. D.: A prospective study of work perceptions and psychosocial factors affecting the report of back injury. Spine 16:1, 1991.

29. Rothman, R. H., and Simeone, F. A.: Lumbar disc disease. In Rothman, R. H., and Simeone, F. A. (eds.): The Spine. Philadelphia, W. B. Saunders Company, 1975.

30. Weber, H.: The effect of delayed disc surgery on muscular paresis. Acta Orthop. Scand. 46:631, 1975.

31. Hakelius, A., and Hindmarsh, J.: The significance of neurologic signs and myelographic findings in the diagnosis of lumbar root compression. Acta Orthop. Scand. 43:239, 1972.

32. Sprangfort, E.: Lasègue's sign in patients with lumbar disc herniation. Acta Orthop. Scand. 42:459, 1971.

33. Hoppenfeld, S.: Physical Examination of the Spine and Extremities. New York, Appleton-Century-Crofts, 1976.

34. Finneson, B. E.: Low Back Pain. Philadelphia, J. B. Lippincott Company, 1973.

35. Wiltse, L. L.: Lumbosacral strain and instability. In American Academy of Orthopedic Surgeons: Symposium on the Spine. St. Louis, C. V. Mosby Company, 1969.

36. Caldwell, A. B., and Chase, C.: Diagnosis and treatment of personality factors in low back pain. Clin. Orthop. 129:141, 1977.

37. Ransford, A. O., Cairns, D., and Mooney, V.: The pain drawing as an aid to the psychologic evaluation of patients with low back pain. Spine 1:127, 1976.

38. Sternbach, R. A.: Psychologic aspects of chronic pain. Clin. Orthop. 129:150, 1977.

39. Fordyce, W. E., Fowler, R. S., Lehman, J. F., DeLateur, B. J., Sand, P. L., and Trieschmann, R. B.: Operant conditioning in the treatment of chronic pain. Arch. Phys. Med. Rehab. 54:399, 1973.

40. Anderson, T. P., Cole, T. M., Gullickson, G., Hudgens, A., and Roberts, A. H.: Behavior modification of chronic pain: A treatment program by a multidisciplinary team. Clin. Orthop. 129:97, 1977.

41. Macnab, I.: Surgical treatment of degenerative disc disease of the lumbar spine. In McKibbin, B. (ed.): Recent Advances in Orthopaedics. Edinburgh, Churchill Livingstone, 1975.

42. Park, W.: Radiological investigation of the intervertebral disc. In Jayson, M. (ed.): The Lumbar Spine and Back Pain. London, Sector Publishing, Ltd., 1976.

43. Liang, M., and Komaroff, A. L.: Roentgenograms in primary care patients with acute low back pain. A cost-effective analysis. Arch. Intern. Med. 142:1108, 1982.

44. Harris, R. I., and Macnab, I.: Structural changes in the lumbar intervertebral discs. Their relationship to low back pain and sciatica. J. Bone Joint Surg. 36B:304, 1954.

45. Edeiken, J., and Pitt, M. J.: The radiologic diagnosis of disc disease. Orthop. Clin. North Am. 2:405, 1971.

46. Lawrence, J. S.: Disc degeneration. Its frequency and relationship to symptoms. Ann. Rheum. Dis. 28:121, 1969.

47. Hakelius, A., and Hindmarsh, J.: The comparative reliability of preoperative diagnostic methods in lumbar disc surgery. Acta Orthop. Scand. 43:234, 1972.

48. Epstein, B.: The Spine. A Radiological Text and Atlas. 3rd ed. Philadelphia, Lea & Febiger, 1969.

49. Wiltse, L. L.: The effect of common anomalies of the lumbar spine upon disc degeneration and low back pain. Orthop. Clin. North Am. 2:569, 1971.

50. Farfan, H. F., and Sullivan, J. D.: The relation of facet orientation to intervertebral disc failure. Can. J. Surg. 10:179, 1967.

51. Collis, D. K., and Ponseti, I. V.: Long term followup of patients with idiopathic scoliosis not treated surgically. J. Bone Joint Surg. 51A:425, 1969.

52. Roche, M. B., and Rowe, G. G.: The incidence of separate neural arch and coincident bone variations. Anat. Rec. 109:233, 1951.

53. Shealy, C. N.: Facet denervation in the management of back and sciatic pain. Clin. Orthop. 115:157, 1976.

54. Norris, S. H., Ehrlich, M. G., McKusick, K., and Provine, H.: The radioisotope study of an experimental model of disc space infection. J. Bone Joint Surg. 60B:281, 1978.

55. Waddell, G., McCulloch, J. A., Kummel, E., and Venner, R. M.: Nonorganic physical signs in low-back pain. Spine 5:117, 1980.

56. Gehweiler, J. A., Jr., and Daffner, R. H.: Low back pain: The controversy of radiologic evaluation. Am. J. Radiol. 140:109, 1983.

57. Frymoyer, J. W., Newberg, A., Pope, M. H., Wilder, D. G., Clements, J., and MacPherson, B.: Spine radiographs in patients with low-back pain: An epidemiological study in men. J. Bone Joint Surg. 66A:1048, 1984.

58. Witt, I., Vestergaard, A., and Rosenklint, A. A comparative analysis of x-ray findings of the lumbar spine in patients with and without lumbar pain. Spine 9:298, 1984.

59. Merkel, K. B., Brown, M. L., Dewanjee, M. K., and Fitzgerald, R. H., Jr.: Comparison of indium-labeled-leukocyte imaging with sequential technetium-gallium scanning in the diagnosis of low-grade musculoskeletal sepsis: A prospective study. J. Bone Joint Surg. 67A:465, 1985.

60. Hindmarsh, T., Ekholm, S. E., Kido, D. K., Sahler, L., and Sands, M.: Lumbar myelography with iohexol and metrizamide: A double-blind clinical trial. Acta Radiol. 25:365, 1984.

61. Wiesel, S. W., Tsourmas, N., Feffer, H. L., Citrin, C. M., and Patronas, N.: A study of computer assisted tomography, I. The incidence of positive CAT scans in an asymptomatic group of patients. Spine 9:549, 1984.

62. Modic, M. T., Pavilcek, W., Weinstein, M. A., Boumphrey, F., Ngo, F., Hardy, R., and Duchesneau, P. M.: Magnetic resonance imaging of intervertebral disk disease: Clinical and pulse sequence considerations. Radiology 152:103, 1984.

63. Modic, M. T., Feiglin, D. H., Piraino, D. W., Boumphrey, F., Weinstein, M. A., Duchesneau, P. M., and Rehm, S.: Vertebral osteomyelitis: Assessment using MR. Radiology 157:157, 1985.

63a. Djukic, S., Lang, P., Morris, J., Hoaglund, F., and Genant, H. K.: The postoperative spine. Magnetic resonance imaging. Orthop. Clin. North Am. 21:603, 1990.

64. Weber, H.: Lumbar disc herniation: A controlled, prospective study with ten years of observation. Spine 8:131, 1983.

65. Friberg, S., and Hult, L.: Comparative study of Abrodil myelogram and operative findings in low back pain and sciatica. Acta Orthop. Scand. 20:303, 1951.

66. Luyendijk, W., and Van Voorthuisen, A. E.: Contrast examination of the spinal epidural space. Acta Radiol. Scand. 5:1051, 1966.
67. Hirsch, C., and Nachemson, A.: The reliability of lumbar disc surgery. Clin. Orthop. 29:189, 1963.
68. Post, M. J. D., Brown, M. D., and Gargano, F. P.: The technique and interpretation of lumbar myelograms. Spine 2:214, 1977.
69. McNeill, T. W., Huncke, B., Kornblatt, I., Stiehl, J., and Kahn, H. A.: A new advance in water-soluble myelography. Spine 1:72, 1976.
70. Nachemson, A.: The lumbar spine. An orthopaedic challenge. Spine 1:59, 1976.
71. Macnab, I., St. Louis, E. L., Grabias, S. L., and Jacob, R.: Selective ascending lumbosacral venography in the assessment of lumbar-disc herniation. J. Bone Joint Surg. 58A:1093, 1976.
71a. Deyo, R. A., Bigos, S. J., and Maravilla, K. R.: Diagnostic imaging procedures for the lumbar spine Ann. Intern. Med. 111:865, 1989.
72. Hitselberger, W. A., and Witten, R. M.: Abnormal myelograms in asymptomatic patients. J. Neurosurg. 32:132, 1970.
73. Mathews, J. A.: Epidurography—a technique for diagnosis and research. In Jayson, M. (ed.): The Lumbar Spine and Back Pain. London, Sector Publishing, Ltd., 1976.
74. Arnoldi, C. C., Brodsky, A. E., Cauchoix, J., Crock, H. V., Dommisse, G. F., Edgar, M. A., Gargano, F. P., Jacobson, R. E., Kirkaldy-Willis, W. H., Kurihara, A., Langerskjold, A., Macnab, I., McIvor, G. W. D., Newman, P. H., Paine, K. W. E., Russin, L. A., Sheldon, J., Tile, M., Urist, M. R., Wilson, W. E., and Wiltse, L. L.: Lumbar spinal stenosis and nerve root entrapment syndrome. Definition and classification. Clin. Orthop. 115:4, 1976.
75. Macnab, I.: Negative disc exploration. An analysis of causes of nerve-root involvement in sixty-eight patients. J. Bone Joint Surg. 53A:891, 1971.
76. Verbeist, H.: A radicular syndrome from developmental narrowing of the lumbar vertebral canal. J. Bone Joint Surg. 36B:230, 1954.
77. Verbeist, H.: Further experiences on the pathological influence on the developmental narrowness of the lumbar vertebral canal. J. Bone Joint Surg. 37B:576, 1955.
78. Kirkaldy-Willis, W. H., Paine, K. W. E., Cauchoix, J., and McIvor, G. W. D.: Lumbar spinal stenosis. Clin. Orthop. 99:30, 1974.
79. Schatzker, J., and Pennal, G. F.: Spinal stenosis. A cause of cauda equina compression. J. Bone Joint Surg. 50B:606, 1968.
80. Macnab, I.: Spondylolisthesis with an intact neural arch. The so-called pseudospondylolisthesis. J. Bone Joint Surg. 32B:325, 1950.
81. Schlesinger, E. B., and Taveres, J. M.: Factors in the production of "cauda equina" syndromes in lumbar discs. Trans. Am. Neurol. Assoc. 78:263, 1953.
82. Lipson, S. J., Naheedy, M. H., Kaplan, M. M., and Bienfang, D. C.: Spinal stenosis caused by epidural lipomatosis in Cushing's syndrome. N. Engl. J. Med. 302:36, 1980.
83. McIvor, G. W. D., and Kirkaldy-Willis, W. H.: Pathologic and myelographic changes in the major types of lumbar spinal stenosis. Clin. Orthop. 115:72, 1976.
84. Lindahl, O., and Rexed, G.: Histologic changes in spinal nerve roots of operated cases of sciatica. Acta Orthop. Scand. 20:215, 1951.
85. Wiesel, J. W., Cuckler, J. M., DeLuca, F., James, F., Zeide, M. S., and Rothman, R. H.: Acute low back pain. An objective analysis of conservative therapy. Spine 5:324, 1980.
86. Macnab, I.: Backache. Baltimore, Williams & Wilkins, 1977.
87. Wiltse, L. L.: Surgery for intervertebral disk disease of the lumbar spine. Clin. Orthop. 129:22, 1977.
88. Murphy, R. W.: Nerve roots and spinal nerves in degenerative disk disease. Clin. Orthop. 129:47, 1977.
89. Knuttson, B.: Comparative value of electromyographic, myelographic and clinical neurological examination in diagnosis of lumbar root compression syndrome. Acta Orthop. Scand. Suppl. 49, 1961.
89a. Curd, J. G., and Thorne, R. P.: Diagnosis and management of lumbar disk disease. Hosp. Pract. (Off. Ed.) 24:135, 1989.
90. Nordby, E. J., and Brown, M. D.: Present status of chymopapain and chemonucleolysis. Clin. Orthop. 129:79, 1977.
91. McCulloch, J. A.: Chemonucleolysis: Experience with 2000 cases. Clin. Orthop. 146:128, 1980.
92. Brown, F. W.: Management of diskogenic pain using epidural and intrathecal steroids. Clin. Orthop. 129:72, 1977.
93. Snoek, W., Weber, H., and Jorgensen, B.: Double blind evaluation of extradural methylprednisolone for herniated lumbar discs. Acta Orthop. Scand. 48:635, 1977.
94. Feffer, H. L.: Therapeutic intradiscal hydrocortisone. A long term study. Clin. Orthop. 67:100, 1969.
95. Spangfort, E. V.: The lumbar disc herniation. A computer aided analysis of 2,504 operations. Acta Orthop. Scand. Suppl. 142, 1972.
96. Scott, R. J.: Bladder paralysis in cauda equina lesions from disc prolapse. J. Bone Joint Surg. 47:224, 1965.
97. Andersson, H., and Carlsson, C. A.: Prognosis of operatively treated lumbar disc herniation causing foot extensor paralysis. Acta Chir. Scand. 132:501, 1966.
98. Weber, H.: An evaluation of conservative and surgical treatment of lumbar disc protrusion. J. Oslo City Hosp. 20:81, 1970.

99. Spengler, D. M., Freeman, C., Westbrook, R., and Miller, J. W.: Low back pain following multiple spine procedures. Failure of initial selection? Spine 5:356, 1980.
99a. Haglund, M. M., Schumacher, J. M., and Loeser, J. D.: Spinal stenosis: an annotated bibliography. Pain 35:1, 1988.
99b. Lipson SJ: Spinal stenosis. Rheum. Dis. Clin. North Am. 14:613, 1988.
100. Sheldon, J. J., Russin, L. A., and Gargano, F. P.: Lumbar spinal stenosis. Radiographic diagnosis with special reference to transverse axial tomography. Clin. Orthop. 115:53, 1976.
101. Hammerschlag, S. B., Wolpert, S. M., and Carter, B. L.: Computed tomography of the spinal canal. Radiology 121:361, 1976.
102. Eisenstein, S.: Measurements of the lumbar spinal canal in 2 racial groups. Clin. Orthop. 115:53, 1976.
103. Paine, K. W. E., and Huang, P. W. H.: Lumbar disc syndrome. J. Neurosurg. 37:75, 1972.
103a. Rosen, C. D., Kahanovitz, N., Bernstein, R., and Viola, K.: A retrospective analysis of the efficacy of epidural steroid injections. Clin. Orthop. 228:270, 1988.
104. Wiltse, L. L., Kirkaldy-Willis, W. H., and McIvor, G. W. D.: The treatment of spinal stenosis. Clin. Orthop. 115:83, 1976.
104a. Nakai, O., Ookawa, A., and Yamaura, I.: Long-term roentgenographic and functional changes in patients who were treated with wide fenestration for central lumbar stenosis. J. Bone Joint Surg. [Am.] 73:1184, 1991.
105. Lawrence, J. S., Sharp, J., Ball, J., and Bier, F.: Rheumatoid arthritis of the lumbar spine. Ann. Rheum. Dis. 23:205, 1964.
106. Sims-Williams, H., Jayson, M. I. V., and Baddeley, H.: Rheumatoid involvement of the lumbar spine. Ann. Rheum. Dis. 36:524, 1977.
107. West, H. F.: The aetiology of ankylosing spondylitis. Ann. Rheum. Dis. 8:143, 1949.
108. Lawrence, J. S.: The prevalence of arthritis. Br. J. Clin. Pract. 17:699, 1963.
109. deBlecourt, J. J., and deBlecourt-Meindersma, T.: Hereditary factors in rheumatoid arthritis and ankylosing spondylitis. Ann. Rheum. Dis. 20:215, 1961.
110. Schlosstein, L., Terasaki, P. I., Bluestone, R., and Pearson, C. M.: High association of HL-A antigen W27 with ankylosing spondylitis. N. Engl. J. Med. 288:704, 1973.
111. Brewerton, D. A., Caffrey, M., Hart, F. D., James, D. C. O., Nicholls, A., and Sturrock, R. D.: Ankylosing spondylitis and HL-A-27. Lancet 1:904, 1973.
112. Forestier, J., and Rotes-Querol, J.: Senile ankylosing hyperostosis of the spine. Ann. Rheum. Dis. 9:321, 1950.
113. Vernon-Roberts, B., Pirie, C. J., and Trenwith, V.: Pathology of the dorsal spine in ankylosing hyperostosis. Ann. Rheum. Dis. 33:281, 1974.
114. Harris, J., Carter, A. R., Glick, R. N., and Storey, G. O.: Ankylosing hyperostosis: Clinical and radiological features. Ann. Rheum. Dis. 33:210, 1974.
115. Julkunen, H., Heinonen, O. P., and Pyorala, K.: Hyperostosis of the spine in an adult population. Its relation to hyperglycemia and obesity. Ann. Rheum. Dis. 30:605, 1971.
116. Wiley, A. M., and Trueta, J.: The vascular anatomy of the spine and its relation to pyogenic vertebral osteomyelitis. J. Bone Joint Surg 41B:796, 1959.
117. Stone, D. B., and Bonfiglio, M.: Pyogenic vertebral osteomyelitis: A diagnostic pitfall for the internist. Arch. Intern. Med. 112:491, 1963.
118. Waldvogel, F. A., Medoff, G., and Swartz, M. N.: Osteomyelitis: A review of clinical features, therapeutic considerations and unusual aspects (third of three parts). N. Engl. J. Med. 282:316, 1970.
119. Crock, H. V., Yoshzava, H., and Kame, S. K.: Observations on the venous drainage of the human vertebral body. J. Bone Joint Surg. 55B:528, 1973.
120. Batson, O. V.: The function of the vertebral veins and their role in the spread of metastasis. Ann Surg. 112:138, 1940.
121. Batson, O. V.: The vertebral vein system. Am. J. Roentgenol. 78:195, 1957.
122. Musher, D. M., Thorsteinsson, S. B., Minuth, J. N., and Luchi, R. J.: Vertebral osteomyelitis: Still a diagnostic pitfall. Arch. Intern. Med. 136:105, 1976.
122a. Wisneski, R. J.: Infectious disease of the spine. Diagnostic and treatment considerations. Orthop. Clin. North Am. 22(3):491, 1991.
123. Stauffer, R. N.: Pyogenic vertebral osteomyelitis. Orthop. Clin. North Am. 6:1015, 1975.
124. Wedge, J. H., Onyschak, A. F., Robertson, D. E., and Kirkaldy-Willis, W. H.: Atypical manifestations of spinal infections. Clin. Orthop. 123:155, 1977.
125. Ross, P. M., and Fleming, J. L.: Vertebral body osteomyelitis: Spectrum and natural history. Clin. Orthop. 118:190, 1976.
126. Bonfiglio, M., Lange, T. A., and Kim, Y. M.: Pyogenic vertebral osteomyelitis. Clin. Orthop. 96:234, 1973.
127. Garcia, A., and Grantham, S. A.: Hematogenous pyogenic vertebral osteomyelitis. J. Bone Joint Surg. 42A:429, 1960.

128. Guri, J. P.: Pyogenic osteomyelitis of the spine. Differential diagnosis through clinical and roentgenographic observations. J. Bone Joint Surg. 28A:29, 1946.

128a. Appel, B., Moens, E., and Lowenthal, A.: MRI of the spine and spinal cord: infectious and inflammatory pathology. J. Neuroradiol. 15:325, 1988.

129. Griffiths, H. E. D., and Jones, D. M.: Pyogenic infection of the spine. J. Bone Joint Surg. 53B:383, 1971.

130. Ford, L. T., and Key, J. A.: Postoperative infection of the intervertebral disc space. South. Med. J. 48:1295, 1955.

131. Pilgaard, S.: Discitis (closed space infection) following removal of lumbar intervertebral disc. J. Bone Joint Surg. 51A:713, 1969.

132. Thibodeau, A. A.: Closed space infection following removal of lumbar intervertebral disc. J. Bone Joint Surg. 50A:400, 1968.

133. Sullivan, C. R., Bickel, W. H., and Svien, H. J.: Infections of vertebral interspaces after operations on the intervertebral disks. J.A.M.A. 166:1973, 1958.

134. Boston, H. C., Bianco, A. J., and Rhodes, K. H.: Disk space infections in children. Orthop. Clin. North Am. 6:953, 1975.

135. Pritchard, D. J.: Granulomatous infections of bones and joints. Orthop. Clin. North Am. 6:1029, 1975.

136. Hodgson, A. R.: Infectious disease of the spine. In Rothman, R. H., and Simeone, F. A. (eds.): The Spine. Philadelphia, W. B. Saunders Company, 1975.

137. Medical Research Council Working Party in Tuberculosis of the Spine: A 10-year assessment of a controlled trial comparing debridement and anterior spinal fusion in the management of tuberculosis of the spine in patients on standard chemotherapy in Hong Kong. J. Bone Joint Surg. 64B:393, 1982.

138. Lifeso, R. M., Weaver, P., and Harder, E. H.: Tuberculous spondylitis in adults. J. Bone Joint Surg. 67A:1405, 1985.

139. Alldred, A. J., and Nisket, N. W.: Hydatid disease of bone in Australasia. J. Bone Joint Surg. 46B:260, 1964.

140. Wiltse, L. L., Newman, P. H., and Macnab, I.: Classification of spondylolysis and spondylolisthesis. Clin. Orthop. 117:30, 1976.

141. Taillard, W. F.: Etiology of spondylolisthesis. Clin. Orthop. 117:30, 1976.

142. Wiltse, L. L., Widell, E. H., and Jackson, D. W.: Fatigue fracture: The basic lesion in isthmic spondylolisthesis. J. Bone Joint Surg. 57A:17, 1975.

143. Wiltse, L. L.: Etiology of spondylolisthesis. Clin. Orthop. 10:45, 1957.

144. Jackson, D. W., Wiltse, L. L., and Cirincione, R. J.: Spondylolysis in the female gymnast. Clin. Orthop. 117:68, 1976.

145. Ferguson, R. J.: Low-back pain in college football linemen. J. Bone Joint Surg. 56A:1300, 1974.

146. Farfan, H. F., Osteria, V., and Lamy, C.: The mechanical etiology of spondylolysis and spondylolisthesis. Clin. Orthop. 117:40, 1976.

147. Troup, J. D. G.: Mechanical factors in spondylolisthesis and spondylolysis. Clin. Orthop. 117:59, 1976.

148. Rosenberg, N. J.: Degenerative spondylolisthesis. J. Bone Joint Surg. 57A:4, 1975.

149. Petajan, J., Momberger, G., Aase, J., and Wright, D. G.: Arthrogryposis syndrome (Kusokwim disease) in the Eskimo. J.A.M.A. 209:1481, 1969.

150. Karaharjii, E., and Hummuksela, M.: Possible syphilitic spondylitis. Acta Orthop. Scand. 44:289, 1973.

151. Anderson, C. E.: Spondyloschisis following spine fusion. J. Bone Joint Surg. 38A:1142, 1956.

152. Harris, R. I., and Wiley, J. J.: Acquired spondylolisthesis as a sequel to spine fusion. J. Bone Joint Surg. 45A:1159, 1963.

153. Unander-Scharin, L.: A case of spondylolisthesis lumbalis aquisita. Acta Orthop. Scand. 19:536, 1950.

154. DePalma, A. F., and Marme, P. J.: Spondylolysis following spine fusion. Clin. Orthop. 15:208, 1959.

155. Harrington, P. R., and Tullos, H. S.: Spondylolisthesis in children. Clin. Orthop. 79:75, 1971.

156. Strayer, L. M., Risser, J. C., and Waugh, T. R.: Results of spine fusion for scoliosis twenty-five years or more after surgery. J. Bone Joint Surg. 51A:205, 1969.

157. Tietjen, R., and Morgenstern, J. M.: Spondylolisthesis following surgical fusion for scoliosis. Clin. Orthop. 117:176, 1976.

158. Wiltse, L. L., and Jackson, D. W.: Treatment of spondylolisthesis and spondylolysis in children. Clin. Orthop. 117:92, 1976.

159. Laurent, L. E., and Einola, S.: Spondylolisthesis in children and adolescents. Acta Orthop. Scand. 82:45, 1961.

160. Frederickson, B. E., Baker, D., McHolick, W. J., Yuan, H. A., and Lubicky, J. P.: The natural history of spondylolysis and spondylolisthesis. J. Bone Joint Surg. 66A:699, 1984.

161. Osterman, K., Lindholm, T. S., and Laurent, L. E.: Late results of removal of the loose posterior element (Gill's operation) in the treatment of lytic lumbar spondylolisthesis. Clin. Orthop. 117:121, 1976.

162. Newman, P. H.: Surgical treatment for spondylolisthesis in the adult. Clin. Orthop. 117:106, 1976.

Chapter 28

Foot Pain

Jonathan T. Deland
Bruce Wood

INTRODUCTION

Ambulatory patients with foot and ankle problems can be reminded of their problem each time they take a step. They are therefore appreciative of a physician who can be helpful. Correct diagnosis and treatment require an awareness of the many foot and ankle problems that exist. Fortunately, interest in this field has increased and improvements in treatment have been accomplished. The purpose of this chapter is to convey this knowledge to the rheumatologist so that the appropriate care can be initiated. The emphasis, therefore, is on updating the clinician on how to diagnose the problem and direct treatment.

The first section of this chapter deals with biomechanics of the foot, the second with general foot problems, and the third with involvement of the foot in rheumatoid arthritis. The interested reader should also refer to Chapter 110 for a discussion of foot surgery.

BIOMECHANICS OF THE NORMAL FOOT AND ANKLE

Because the foot functions as a dynamic shock-absorbing mechanism, its ailments cannot be understood or treated without appreciating its biomechanics. Full function means that the foot has the flexibility to adapt to different terrains as well as the rigidity necessary for locomotion. The foot and ankle complex must be able not only to dorsiflex and plantarflex but also to invert and evert (motions not often appreciated). At the same time, the foot must have the ability to accommodate an impact force averaging 63 tons per mile. To understand how the foot is able to accommodate these different requirements, the various joints within the foot and ankle complex will be described along with their function.

The ankle allows dorsiflexion for heel-strike and plantar flexion for push-off. A normal range of motion is more than 10 degrees of dorsiflexion and 30 degrees of plantar flexion from the neutral position (neutral means that the foot is perpendicular to the tibia). The ankle is a joint whose axis is externally rotated in relation to the leg and can be approximated by placing the tips of the index fingers just below the malleoli.[1-3] For proper function, the ankle acts in concert with the subtalar joint complex to give greater

flexibility. The subtalar joint primarily adds the motion of inversion or eversion about the talus. When the motions of the ankle joint and the subtalar complex are combined, they become a universal or ball-and-socket type of motion, allowing some degree of tilting of the foot in each direction. The subtalar complex includes the talocalcaneal, talonavicular, and calcaneocuboid joints (Fig. 28–1). The term *subtalar joint* is most often used for just the talocalcaneal joint. However, each one of these joints within the complex is necessary for the inversion and eversion motion that is characteristic of a normal foot. If any one of these three joints is restricted, 70 per cent or more of the total inversion-eversion motion will be restricted.[4, 5]

The naviculocuneiform and tarsometatarsal joints provide a small amount of motion (10 to 15 degrees). More critical motion is provided by the metatarsophalangeal joints. At the metatarsophalangeal joint, dorsiflexion of 70 to 90 degrees allows for push-off, with the remainder of the foot locked as a rigid lever for propulsion. For push-off, the foot becomes locked in inversion, making the medial

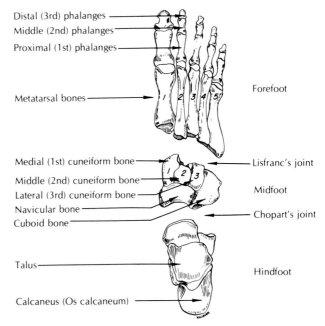

Distal (3rd) phalanges
Middle (2nd) phalanges
Proximal (1st) phalanges

Metatarsal bones

Forefoot

Medial (1st) cuneiform bone
Middle (2nd) cuneiform bone
Lateral (3rd) cuneiform bone
Navicular bone
Cuboid bone

Lisfranc's joint

Midfoot

Chopart's joint

Talus

Hindfoot

Calcaneus (Os calcaneum)

Figure 28–1. AP view of the foot. Diagram is divided into the forefoot, midfoot, and hindfoot. (From Rockwood, C. A., et al. [eds.]: Fractures: Vols. 1 and 2, Fractures in Adults. 3rd ed. Philadelphia, J. B. Lippincott, 1991, pp. 2042–2043. Used by permission.)

longitudinal arch higher and stiff. The inversion is accomplished through the subtalar joint complex by contraction of the posterior tibialis muscle and external rotation of the tibia. When the foot hits the ground again, the heel will go into eversion under the body weight, causing some collapse or pronation in the arch. This controlled collapse, along with dorsiflexion of the ankle, constitutes an important part of the shock-absorption mechanism. If stiffness occurs in these various joints, there will be increased stress on the remaining joints and the possibility of earlier degenerative change.

PHYSICAL EXAMINATION AND RADIOGRAPHS

Delineating the precise location of the patient's problem and appreciating its cause are the hallmarks of a successful foot and ankle evaluation. The physical examination brings about the accurate diagnosis more often than a long history or multiple radiographs. The examination is commenced by observing the foot and ankle under full weight bearing from a frontal view. The medial longitudinal arch is assessed by looking at the height of the medial border of the midfoot. The alignment of the forefoot in relation to the hindfoot is observed. The relationship should be viewed when the patient is standing and also when the patient is seated. When the patient is seated, the heel is grasped and held in the normal 5 degrees of valgus. Excessive tilting (more than 10 to 15 degrees) of the free-floating forefoot can then be noted. Valgus position of the hindfoot is best appreciated from the posterior view of the standing patient. A valgus deformity at the ankle joint can mislead the examiner into concluding that there is an excessive valgus in the calcaneus or subtalar joint when, in reality, the deformity is at the ankle. With the help of physical examination and standing radiographs, the examiner should be able to conclude which joint or bone is responsible for any deformity present.

Swelling should be looked for on both the frontal and posterior views. If appropriate, the patient is asked to walk, and when seated, the range of motion is checked. With the knee in 90 degrees' flexion, the ankle should be able to dorsiflex over 10 degrees. With the knee in extension, the ankle should be able to at least reach 0 degrees dorsiflexion (neutral).[6] To check the subtalar complex, the examiner should hold the heel with one hand and the forefoot with the other and then move the entire foot as a unit in an arc of motion inward and under the talus for inversion and outward for eversion (Fig. 28–2). There is normally no more than 30 degrees of inversion and 10 degrees of eversion, starting from the neutral or plantigrade (as-if-standing) position. The range of motion in the tarsometatarsal joints and naviculocuneiform joints is too small to be assessed on physical examination. The metatarsophalangeal joints, however, should be checked, especially that of the great

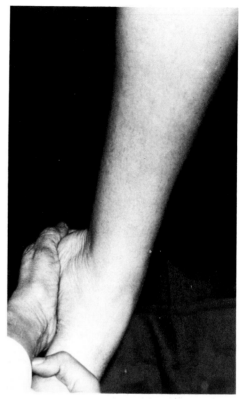

Figure 28–2. Examination for subtalar motion (eversion-inversion). Note that the hindfoot, midfoot, and forefoot are swung as a unit under the talus. (From Jahss, M. H.: Examination. *In* Jahss, M. H. [ed.]: Disorders of the Foot and Ankle. 2nd ed. Philadelphia, W. B. Saunders, 1991, p. 42.)

toe. There is normally at least 70 degrees of dorsiflexion to the metatarsal shaft.

Critical in the physical examination is the palpation of various parts of the foot to determine the point of maximum tenderness. For example, in differentiating ankle from talocalcaneal pain, ankle joint line tenderness is compared to that produced by pressing low in the sinus tarsi toward the posterior facet of the talocalcaneal joint. Even this method of palpation is not totally specific to the subtalar joint. The sinus tarsi is somewhat uncomfortable even when normal. The talonavicular joint is also located close to the ankle but on the medial side and should be differentiated from the ankle joint. Identifying the prominent bony landmarks is helpful in locating the position of these joints. On the medial side of the midfoot and ankle, besides the medial malleolus, the most prominent landmark is the medial tubercle of the navicular, just inferior and anterior to the medial malleolus. On the lateral side, besides the lateral malleolus, the most prominent structure is the base of the fifth metatarsal. In between these two structures on the lateral side is the anterior process of the calcaneus, just at the front of the sinus tarsi, and it is easily palpable. Palpation of these landmarks can be critical in getting a location of the problem, leading to the correct diagnosis.

The anteroposterior (AP) and lateral radiographic examination should be done whenever possible with the patient standing fully weight bearing on the foot.[7, 8] A full set of foot radiographs, therefore, would be a standing AP, a standing lateral, and a supine lateral oblique of the foot. A common mistake is to neglect the ankle joint and forget to evaluate it radiographically when there may be a related problem. The reverse is also true. For the ankle examination, the patient can be supine for the AP, lateral, and mortise views. However, a standing AP of the ankle is invaluable to assess the alignment of the talus within the ankle mortise in cases of varus or valgus hindfoot deformities. Evaluation of the talocalcaneal joint is difficult on routine radiograph, but can sometimes be adequately viewed on a mortise view of the ankle or even better, a Broden's view, if the technician is familiar with that view. Often a computed tomography (CT) scan with coronal cuts is necessary for the most detailed evaluation.[9]

For the assessment of cartilage injuries within the ankle joint or osteochondral lesions, a magnetic resonance imaging (MRI) scan will delineate lesions that are missed on plain films.[10, 11] An MRI scan may also reveal an identifiable cause for symptoms suggesting tarsal tunnel syndrome. Most importantly, treatment should be directed to the problem as delineated by the physical examination rather than just the radiographs.

COMMON CAUSES OF FOOT AND ANKLE PAIN

Forefoot

In the forefoot, hallux valgus is the leading cause of pain; however, tenderness may not be elicited over the metatarsal head. With the shoes off, patients often do not have tenderness at this joint because it is shoe pressure that contributes to the pain. Hallux valgus can also cause pain in the forefoot by pushing against the second and other lesser toes, causing problems more lateral than the first toe. The valgus position of the first toe also unweights the first ray, placing more pressure under the lesser metatarsal heads.

The conservative treatment of hallux valgus is footwear of adequate width and without high heels. The distance across the metatarsal heads when weight bearing should be equal or, at most, within 1/4 inch of the same distance on the sole of the shoes. Although it is difficult for some patients to accept, finding the right shoe may require an extensive search or ordering via a catalog for shoes with a proper forefoot and heel width. These methods can give enough relief to avoid surgery.[12] Patients with the deformity and without pain do not need surgery. The exception to this is the patient who presents with a progressive problem at the second toe caused by the hallux valgus.[13]

Of the lesser toes, the second is the most fre-quently a problem. This ray is often the longest and will be the first to be pushed on by tight shoes and the great toe. A hammer toe (plantar flexion of the proximal interphalangeal joint) or claw toe (plantar flexion of the proximal and distal interphalangeal joints) is often accompanied by a dorsiflexion contracture of the metatarsophalangeal joint. The flexion contractures may vary from totally flexible to totally fixed. An isolated distal interphalangeal joint flexion contracture is termed a *mallet toe* and may cause pain at the tip of the toe where it hits the ground rather than over the dorsal prominence. In all of these deformities, footwear with adequate room (a deep toe box) is the best treatment. Paring of corns and padding around the dorsal prominence (or in the case of a mallet toe, padding underneath the toe) can be quite helpful. These measures should all be tried before surgery is suggested. Painless deformities should not be referred for surgery.

Midfoot

Maladies of the midfoot (from the head of the talus to metatarsotarsal joints), usually consist of arthritic change or deformities that involve the arch. The longitudinal arch should be inspected on the lateral standing radiograph. If the line bisecting the neck of the talus is dorsiflexed in relation to the first metatarsal shaft (by 10 degrees or more), a cavus deformity is present.[14, 15] Patients with a cavus foot often suffer from deficiency of the shock-absorption mechanism. In general, they have less subtalar motion, and with the high arch, the heel and/or metatarsals become more prominent. The foot can be quite stiff with the bad combination of less weight-bearing area and less flexibility. The cause of the cavus foot should be identified and may require neurologic workup and consultation. The most common causes include Charcot-Marie-Tooth disease and spinal disorders. Appropriate padding, possibly orthotics, and ankle support may be necessary. Recurrent ankle sprains may require extensive corrective surgery.

If the line bisecting the neck of the talus is plantarflexed by 10 degrees or more, a flatfoot deformity is present. If this deformity has been progressive in the adult, it is usually caused by posterior tibial tendon insufficiency with ligament disruption, a neuropathic (Charcot) foot, or an arthritic foot from various causes.[16] The posterior tibial tendon should be palpated along its course, from proximal to the medial malleolus down to its insertion on the navicular. Resistance against inversion as a measurement of posterior tibial strength should be tested with the foot in the everted position. When standing, the combination of heel valgus and forefoot abduction, although not diagnostic, is highly suggestive of posterior tibial tendon insufficiency.[17, 18] These patients should be referred to an orthopedist. The orthopedist may elect to use a combination of rest in a cast, an orthotic with a medial heel wedge, or even an ankle foot orthosis (AFO). For severe or progressive deformities the shoe orthotic even with the medial heel wedge is not enough support. Failure of these conservative measures, continuation of pain, or progression of deformity will necessitate surgery.

A neuropathic foot, although most frequently seen in diabetics, can be from a wide variety of neurologic conditions.[19, 20] The presentation is usually a fracture or subtle disruption of the foot that does not have the usual amount of pain. Position and vibratory sense are decreased as well as deep pain. If allowed to progress, loss of the foot can result. In general, conservative treatment with prolonged non–weight-bearing casting is used. Isolated arthritis in the talonavicular or talocalcaneal joints most often results from trauma or rheumatic disease. Conservative treatment with medication is helpful, and orthotics of a more rigid type may give some relief. As in other arthritic deformities of the foot and ankle, fusions may be necessary, but only when the pain necessitates it and the conservative approaches have failed.

Care should be taken to differentiate ankle pain from pain in the talocalcaneal or talonavicular joints, because they are often confused. With inflammation in the ankle joint, careful palpation of the anteromedial and anterolateral portions of the ankle joint line should elicit greater tenderness than that in the sinus tarsi or over the navicular. Motion of the subtalar joint should be carefully checked for and will be decreased in disorders involving the subtalar joint complex. An example of such a disorder that may go unrecognized in routine radiographs is a tarsal coalition. Such a coalition, or abnormal linkage between bones, is most frequently found between the navicular and calcaneus or the talus and calcaneus.[21, 22] These somewhat stiff feet can be painful and may be a cause of frequent ankle sprains. Radiographic identification of a coalition usually requires a lateral oblique view of the foot for a calcaneonavicular coalition or a CT scan for a talocalcaneal coalition. Resection of the coalition is not uniformly successful in adults. Fusions may be necessary in patients whose symptoms warrant it.

Although seemingly benign, ankle sprains themselves can cause chronic disability. It is important that moderate and severe sprains be treated appropriately, at least with some form of initial splinting and formal physical therapy. Ankle sprains can cause osteochondral damage to the joint that may not be detected on routine radiographs. A bone or MRI scan may be necessary for the diagnosis of such a lesion. If an osteocartilaginous fragment is detected, orthopedic referral is indicated. Surgical treatment can be helpful, although complete relief of symptoms does not necessarily result. Rarely, the inferior edge of the anterior tibiofibular ligament or part of the anterior talofibular ligament can be caught in the joint and cause soft tissue impingement and necessitate debridement for pain relief. Arthroscopy has been quite

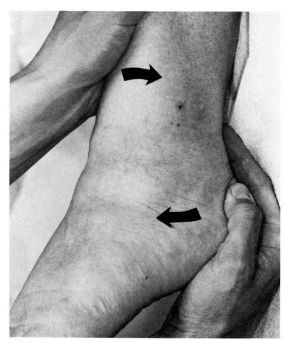

Figure 28–3. The anterior drawer test. Tibia is held by the left hand while the foot is pushed anteriorly by the right hand in a gradual, gentle manner to avoid splinting by the patient. The ankle is in slight plantarflexion.

successful in dealing with this soft tissue impingement. Chronic lateral instability of the ankle presents with pain on inversion, tenderness over the collateral ligaments and, most important a positive anterior drawer test (Fig. 28–3).[23, 24] If peroneal strengthening and protective ankle support, such as a canvas lace-up ankle brace, relieve symptoms, surgery may be avoided.

Several other disorders can cause pain on the lateral side of the ankle. One such disorder is subluxation of the peroneal tendons, which causes a snapping over the distal fibula with eversion and dorsiflexion of the ankle. Although a period of casting may be helpful, surgery may be necessary if symptoms warrant.[25, 26] A cause of chronic lateral foot and ankle pain after trauma can be an unhealed anterior process of the calcaneus fracture. This may not be visible on normal radiographs.[27] A bone scan or tomogram should be obtained if there is tenderness directly over the anterior process and plain radiographs are unrevealing. Rarely, the peroneus longus or brevis tendon may have a tear.[28, 29] This could necessitate surgery if the patient fails to improve after an "ankle sprain" and there is appropriate tenderness over the peroneal tendons.

NERVE COMPRESSION-DEGENERATION SYNDROMES

Morton's neuroma, or perineural fibrosis of a plantar interdigital nerve, is the most common nerve problem of the foot and ankle (for this and other

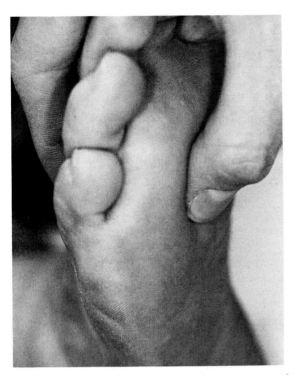

Figure 28–4. Morton's neuroma. Interdigital pressure is used to push the nerve up dorsally against the intermetatarsal ligament, causing impressive tenderness. Comparison with tenderness in the other web space and tenderness over the metatarsal head is used.

nerve compression-degeneration syndromes, also see Chapter 101). The nerves to the second or third web spaces are almost exclusively affected, and these are sensory nerves. The vast majority of cases are in women.[30] The patient complains of plantar discomfort, sometimes with tingling or burning radiating out into the appropriate toes. Advanced cases may have some sensory deficits in the plantar quadrants of the forefoot, although this is not common.

The diagnosis is best made by history and careful palpation of the web space. The thumb is used plantarly to press up between the metatarsal heads against the intermetatarsal ligament (Fig. 28–4). This should elicit fairly impressive pain because the nerve is being rubbed between the thumb and the ligament. If the tenderness is more impressive directly over the metatarsal head or the metatarsophalangeal joint itself, the diagnosis should be questioned because synovitis or metatarsophalangeal joint instability may be present. It is rare to have more than one interdigital neuroma in the same foot.[31] In some patients, the condition is well enough tolerated to be treated by wide shoes or a pad placed proximal to the neuroma to unweight it. Surgical excision may not be necessary. Cortisone injections can be performed well before any operation, but the patient should be told that such injections often do not give permanent relief.

Tarsal tunnel syndrome is an overused diagnosis. The flexor retinaculum is not as thick a structure as a transverse carpal ligament in the hand, and the incidence of this disease is low. As outlined by Mann,[32] criteria for the diagnosis should be pain in the distribution of the tibial nerve, a positive Tinel's sign, a positive electromyograph with prolonged terminal latency of the medial or lateral plantar nerve, and the exclusion of other diagnoses.[33] Other diagnoses, such as an associated posterior tibial tendon insufficiency or a neuropathy/sacral radiculopathy, should be sought for. Because surgery is unreliable, conservative measures should be given a full trial. Conservative treatment may involve the use of anti-inflammatory agents or a brace to correct a deformity. Surgical treatment is most likely to be beneficial when an exostosis, ganglion, synovitis, or lipoma is identified by special radiographic studies such as an MRI scan.

Several nerves in the foot, such as the superficial peroneal or sural nerves, are quite superficial and therefore particularly susceptible to local trauma. Tight shoes can cause compression on the dorsum, irritating the superficial peroneal nerve, especially if an exostosis is present. The sural nerve is susceptible not only to inadvertent surgical trauma but also to closed injuries. In patients with hallux valgus, the most medial branch of the medial plantar nerve can be compressed by a tight shoe causing a burning or numbness along the medial aspect of the great toe. In athletes, the medial branch of the tibial nerve can be trapped in fibrosis under the medial aspect of the navicular, causing medial arch and plantar pain. There is tenderness in this area, and conservative treatment with an orthotic should be tried before surgery is recommended.[34]

HEEL PAIN

Heel pain is a common and frustrating condition for both the patient and physician. The patient most often describes the pain on the plantar aspect of the heel, either directly plantarly or somewhat medially over the medial tubercle of the calcaneus. Plantar fasciitis with appropriate tenderness in the plantar fascia can be an accompanying finding. The examiner should not only look for the point of maximal tenderness but also determine whether there are any extrinsic causes, such as inflammatory disease (Reiter's syndrome, ankylosing spondylitis) or pain referred from the back. Spurs are more common in patients with heel pain but are not necessarily the full explanation for the problem. Many patients without spurs have the same pain and tenderness. Simple excision of the spur does not reliably alleviate the pain. Time is perhaps the most reliable treatment and should be supplemented with a trial of heel cord–stretching exercises, shoes with soft impact–absorbing heels, and possibly cushions within the shoes. Orthotics can be helpful, especially if the patient pronates excessively. An overall guide to the use of orthotics is given in Table 28–1. The patient

Table 28–1. ORTHOSES

Problem	Orthotic Treatment
Pronation (flexible); often presents with a medial tibial syndrome or fibular fracture	A longitudinal flexible arch support; can also be treated with an ⅛–¼-inch medial heel and medial sole wedge built into the midsole of the shoe
Cavovarus deformity of the foot; often presents with plantar fasciitis	An ⅛–¼-inch lateral heel wedge with a molded longitudinal arch support
Forefoot supination with a neutral heel; often presents with posterior tibial tendinitis	A longitudinal arch support with an ⅛–¼-inch lateral heel wedge and an ⅛-inch extension under the first metatarsal head (Morton's extension)
Forefoot pronation with a neutral heel; often presents with sesamoid pain	A longitudinal arch support with an ⅛–¼-inch lateral forefoot wedge
Strain of the posterior tibial tendon	A medial sole and ⅛–¼-inch heel wedge in the midsole of the shoe
Strain of the medial fibers of the Achilles tendon	A ½-inch heel lift with an ⅛-inch additional medial heel wedge in the midsole of the shoe
Strain of the lateral fibers of the Achilles tendon	A ½-inch heel lift with an ⅛-inch additional heel wedge in the midsole of the shoe
Plantar fasciitis; presents in the medial proximal plantar fascia	A longitudinal arch support with an ⅛-inch medial heel wedge; if pain is localized, a relief area can be removed from the orthosis and this area reformed with a soft rubber material
Leg length inequality; usually the short leg develops problems such as stress fractures, Achilles tendinitis, and medial knee strain	Leg length inequality should be gradually corrected at ½-inch increments; up to ½ inch can be added to the inner sole of the shoe and ½ inch can be added to the outer sole of the shoes as needed
Metatarsalgia or neuritic metatarsal pain (Morton's neuromas, etc.)	A longitudinal arch support with a ³⁄₁₆-inch metatarsal lift proximal to the second, third, and fourth metatarsal heads; also possible to use a rocker bottom placed on the outer sole of the midsole of the shoe proximal to the metatarsal heads
Black toenails	A ³⁄₁₆-inch metatarsal pad placed proximal to the metatarsal heads of the affected toes, making sure the shoe is long enough; by using a metatarsal pad, the toes do not hyperextend while running and do not slide forward in the shoe and cause the loss of toenails
Metatarsal calluses and blisters	An innersole to decrease friction, ⅛-inch metatarsal pad proximal to the affected areas; also possible to wear two pairs of socks and use a lubricant on the calluses prior to running; calluses should be debrided with a pumice stone
Sesamoiditis	A longitudinal arch support with a ³⁄₁₆-inch lateral forefoot wedge and an ⅛-inch metatarsal elevation under the second and third metatarsals and proximal to the first metatarsal head
Anterior ankle pain with impingement or synovitis	A ½-inch heel lift to the inner sole or the outer sole of the shoe
Medial tibial syndrome or a stress fracture of the fibula	A ³⁄₁₆–¼-inch medial sole and heel wedge in the midsole of the shoe

From Baxter, D. E.: Running injuries. *In* Jahss, M. H. (ed.): Disorders of the Foot. Vol. III, 2nd ed. W. B. Saunders Company, 1991, p. 2455. Used by permission.

with heel pain should be informed that it usually resolves in 3 to 12 months or sometimes longer.

Spurs on the back side of the calcaneus in the region of the Achilles tendon insertion or calcification in the tendon itself can be another cause of discomfort.[35] Again, conservative measures should be tried first and include 1/2 inch heel lift and relief of any impingement against the back of the shoe. Some of these patients eventually need surgery and attain acceptable relief.

Baxter and Thigpen[36] have described impingement of the nerve to the adductor digiti quinti as a cause of medial and plantar heel pain. They have had good results after surgical release around this nerve. This procedure is appropriate in the young athletic population with tenderness medially at the abductor hallucis as well as farther plantarly. The usefulness of this procedure in older patients with recalcitrant pain requires further study.

RHEUMATOID ARTHRITIS

The management and prevention of pain, deformity, and dysfunction in the rheumatoid arthritic foot have become increasingly important as total knee and hip joint replacement procedures provide significant and predictable improvement in lower extremity function.

It is important to differentiate between dysfunction resulting from an active inflammatory process and that resulting from structural or mechanical changes and certain pre-existing biomechanical defects. Within a large cross section of people, foot problems and minor disabilities are common, and when rheumatoid arthritis is superimposed, it is too easy to ascribe all foot pain to the arthritis. This consideration is particularly important in the patient who has a pre-existing peripheral vascular disease, neuropathy, diabetes mellitus, or structural abnormality.[37]

Patterns of Involvement

Initial symptoms of rheumatoid arthritis are reported to appear in the feet in 17 to 20 percent of patients, whereas during the course of the disease, foot involvement may reach 90 percent (for this and other patterns of involvement, also see Chapter 101). The early symptoms are most frequent in the forefoot.[38] Initial swelling is often noted with the need, particularly by women, to change to a larger shoe size but without improvement of symptoms. Because of the diffuse nature of pain in the arthritic foot, patients are often unable to identify, locate, and quantify specific areas of pain; therefore, close manual examination is needed. Pre-existing abnormalities, such as calcaneovalgus or flatfeet, should be evaluated and managed. Left untreated, such problems may further exacerbate the structural complications within the feet. Early intervention with orthotic devices may be appropriate and necessary.[39–41]

Evaluation

Early diagnostic and evaluative processes should include documenting gait function, deformity, range of motion, and relative muscle strengths. This baseline information is an essential reference point for measuring both progress and future treatment requirements. Note that the posterior tibial pulse may often be obscured by swelling and thickening in the tarsal tunnel area and that, occasionally, the posterior tibial nerve may be compressed in this same area.[42]

It is helpful to observe the walking gait both with and without shoes, but pain may limit this examination to stance only. The rheumatoid patient with forefoot involvement often fails to push off from the ball of the foot and toes but rather slides, shuffles, or lifts the foot and places it forward. With rearfoot deformity, the foot may remain pronated (flattened) throughout the gait cycle. Biomechanically, long-term weight bearing on a pronated foot may encourage the development of further forefoot deformity and pain, especially hallux valgus, splaying, and metatarsalgia. Excessive pronation may also increase the internal rotatory motion of the entire lower extremity, with resulting torsional stresses having an effect at both the knee and hip joints.[43]

Observe the standing and walking foot from both the anterior and posterior view. The rheumatoid foot, particularly with subtalar or talonavicular joint involvement, often presents a valgus attitude of the calcaneus and flattening of the medial longitudinal arch. In addition, the navicular becomes prominent medially and small skin creases may appear lateral to the heel. Typical forefoot deformities are easily recognized and consist of dorsally contracted digits

or the so-called cock-up toe deformity with dorsiflexion at the metatarsophalangeal joint and flexion of one or both of the interphalangeal joints. Occasionally, the interphalangeal joints resemble swan neck or boutonnière deformities as seen in fingers. Hallux valgus or hallux abductus, in which the great toe deviates laterally, is frequently seen, as is the prominent medial bunion whose apparent size is often accentuated by a splaying of the forefoot in the region of the metatarsal heads. The lesser toes, in addition to dorsal contraction, may also deviate laterally (fibular deviation) and often overlap one another or the great toe.

Associated with cock-up toes, the anatomic plantar fat pad that protects the ball of the foot from shearing and impact stress is displaced anteriorly to a position where it is ineffective. The plantar surface should be palpated to evaluate both the quality and quantity of the fat pad, the prominence of the metatarsal heads, and the presence of keratoses, bursae, and rheumatoid nodules. In addition, the fat pads under the heel may become atrophic. The plantar surface of the heel is a common site for the occurrence of symptomatic rheumatoid nodules. Common sites for inflammation include the Achilles tendon along its distal portion and at its insertion. Localized tenderness anterior to the tendon, just proximal to its insertion, may represent a bursitis as well as tendinitis of the Achilles and its sheath. Compression of the heel and palpation of the plantar surface of the os calcis may elicit pain, especially with Reiter's syndrome and psoriatic arthritis. Palpation medially and laterally at the talocalcaneal joint yields confusing results. Thickening of the joint synovium may cause pain, but along the medial aspect, other sources of pain could be tendinitis or nerve entrapment in the tarsal tunnel, whereas lateral pain may be secondary to bony soft tissue impingement. Compressing the metatarsal bones together elicits pain between metatarsal heads in the presence of synovitis but is a nonspecific sign. Further confirmation of metatarsophalangeal joint synovitis is made by palpating in the intermetatarsal head space. A more selective procedure to localize inflammatory pain consists of dorsiflexing the toes, if not already in a cock-up position, and applying direct digital pressure plantarly and distally at the point where the base of the toe joins the metatarsal head (Fig. 28–5). This test can be used to distinguish between synovial joint pain and metatarsal head pain secondary to mechanical problems, which is noted by applying pressure directly on the plantar weight-bearing surface of the metatarsal head. Extensor tendinitis can be appreciated by applying gentle pressure over each extensor tendon while putting the digit through a full range of motion. Pain may be elicited and, additionally, a fine crepitus may be felt. Plantar metatarsal head pain secondary to mechanical forces occurs most often under the second and third head and somewhat less frequently under the fourth head. Excessively pronated feet place considerable mechanical stress

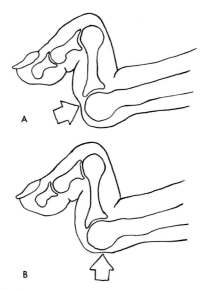

Figure 28–5. *A,* Pressure applied at the joint space and capsule may differentiate pain secondary to synovitis. *B,* Pain in response to pressure directly on the metatarsal head is more likely to be of mechanical origin.

on the second metatarsal head. Radiography of the chronically pronated foot may demonstrate a relative hypertrophy of the second metatarsal shaft.[44]

Skin Changes

The skin and its lesions are a good barometer of foot health and may indicate the extent of occlusive vascular disease, rheumatoid vasculitis, and the locations and effects of weight-bearing and shoe pressure stresses. Note the locations and severity of pressure-related skin lesions such as corns, callouses, ulcers, and hematomas. These lesions are not only painful but, with continued mechanical stress, may easily become infected. Such lesions are especially common and significant in patients on long-term steroid treatment as well as patients with diabetes mellitus, peripheral vascular disease, vasculitis, plantar nodules, and absent or atrophic plantar fat pads.[45, 46] Proper care and management of these lesions are essential to avoid infection in the patient with pending or actual joint replacements.

Rheumatoid nodules are frequently noted in the foot, appearing usually adjacent to the bony prominences in both the forefoot and heel areas. They may be a source of pain from shoe and weight-bearing pressure and may also occasionally ulcerate or become abscessed.

General Principles of Conservative Management

During stages 1 and 2, when secondary deformity is less likely to be a problem, pre-existing mechanically induced lesions and deformities, especially chronic pronation and calcaneovalgus, should

be dealt with because in the presence of rheumatoid arthritis, these deformities are likely to increase. Although inflammatory processes are active, particularly if multiple foot joints are involved, local mechanical therapy is of limited value; however, this is an appropriate time to outline changes in both foot use and footwear. A change to shoes designed for function and comfort is helpful, especially for women patients, whose shoes are often uncomfortable even for a normal foot. Appropriate exercise and activity programs should be encouraged as tolerated. Inappropriate exercise and activity would include contact sports and activities involving high foot-to-ground impact and shearing forces such as tennis and racquetball; more suitable activities include bicycling, either stationary or two or three wheeled, swimming, and certainly walking on a compliant, yet smooth surface such as a golf course or well-groomed park. Rough and uneven surfaces requiring compensatory inversion and eversion may be difficult, especially with later stages of disease. Static active, passive, and isometric exercise of all joints, but especially the ankle, subtalar, and metatarsophalangeal joints, is encouraged within reasonable limits for maintaining both muscle tone and strength and joint mobility. The use of moist heat applications may be helpful for temporary relief of pain and stiffness. Polypropylene ankle-foot orthoses may be used as a night or resting splint. When used as a night splint, these devices generally do not require custom fabrication, although stock splints may require the addition or modification of Velcro strapping for both comfort of fit and maintenance of position.

Footwear

Comfort is the essential quality for footwear in rheumatoid arthritis. A comfortable shoe should be lightweight and flexible, with room to accommodate forefoot deformity; it should have a low heel of 3/16 to 1/2 inch of height and a sole thick enough to protect the foot from mechanical surface trauma and compliant enough to cushion impact. The upper leather should be soft and pliable with a minimum of stitching and decoration and should have a laced or Velcro closure. The traditional so-called "orthopedic shoe" is of limited value except in the presence of minimal deformity and discomfort. With more severe deformity, this shoe is often uncomfortable until the supporting counter has broken down, at which point the initial supportive value of the shoe is lost. Custom-fabricated stabilizing or supportive devices can be added to the comfortable shoe when needed without compromising comfort and fit. Adding inserts or orthoses to deal with forefoot problems usually increases the difficulty of shoe fitting. The Extra-Depth Shoe (P. W. Minor & Sons, Inc., Batavia, New York) has a removable innersole that, when removed, increases the depth of the shoe by 1/4 inch, which is usually ample to accept both

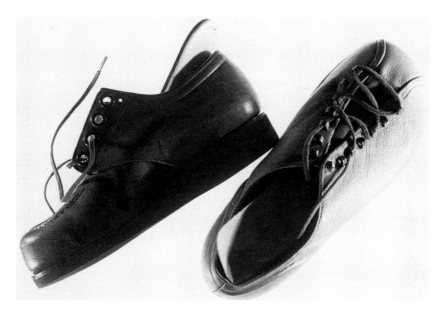

Figure 28–6. Extra-Depth Shoes showing removable inner sole and variations of style and closure (manufactured by P. W. Minor & Son, Inc., Batavia, New York 14020).

deformed toes and an effective plantar insert (Fig. 28–6). Molded or "space" shoes, although good conceptually, have definite limitations with rheumatoid feet because they are usually too stiff and noncompliant. Any increase of deformity or swelling results in an uncomfortably poor fit. Manufacturers are now using removable molded Plastazote (Alimed, Inc., Boston, Massachusetts) or Aliplast inserts, which are an improvement. This shoe is most suitable for the fixed, rigid deformity or for some osteoarthritic feet. The Plastazote sandal introduced by Paul Brand, M.D. has been successfully adapted as either a shoe or sandal for many patients other than those with the neuropathic lesions of Hansen's disease for whom it was originally designed. The experience at the Brigham and Women's Hospital has demonstrated a 25 percent reduction in surgery on the rheumatoid foot since the introduction of this material. Some manufacturers have developed a nonmolded shoe and sandal utilizing Plastazote (Fig. 28–7).

ORTHOTICS

In later stages when deformity and muscle weakness or imbalance may be present, the opportunity for effective nonsurgical care is at its greatest. If advanced beyond the point when alteration of shoes or a change in style or fit is effective, the skillful design and fabrication of orthotic devices can be of significant value. There are four principal functions of orthotics as applied to the rheumatoid patient. An appreciation of these functions, one or all of which may be required in any given application, can be helpful in attempting to prescribe appropriate orthotics. Each orthotic function is determined by the requirements of the individual patient.[47]

Function 1 is the transfer of weight-bearing forces. In the presence of a painful lesion, prominent metatarsal head, or synovitis in the region of the second metatarsal head, a device with an aperture under the head and/or with an increase in the height of the device under and behind the other metatarsal

Figure 28–7. AliMed Plastazote Shoe showing removable inner sole and Velcro closure (manufactured by AliMed, Inc., Boston, Massachusetts 02111).

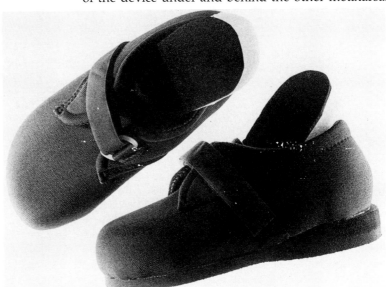

heads has the effect of reducing weight-bearing forces under the second head. Variations of the mechanical approach can be used to reduce weight bearing on one or all metatarsal heads. In general, the fewer heads involved, the more effective this will be. These devices can be used together with various metatarsal bars attached to the sole of a shoe to transfer weight away from the metatarsal heads.

Function 2, reduction of deformity, function 3, stabilization and immobilization, and function 4, prevention of deformity, may utilize similar orthotic materials and design. These last three functions require an accurately molded firm to rigid apparatus capable of forcibly maintaining an alignment position, principally in the subtalar joint complex. The stabilizing orthotic is fabricated most often from a plaster model or cast impression that has been made while the foot is maintained in the "correct" position or attitude.

It should be noted that the biomechanical principles and considerations that typically guide the orthotics laboratory apply to a limited degree in the rheumatoid patient. The goals are not to correct or create biomechanical perfection but rather to increase function and comfort and decrease pain. Correct anatomic alignment and stylish footwear are sacrificed to achieve these goals.

Orthotics attempting to improve rear and midfoot alignment are often bulky, and finding footwear to accommodate the orthotic can be difficult. However, the Extra-Depth Shoe and many athletic shoes with removable innersoles are of value. An occasional source of pain is lateral impingement occurring when a calcaneal valgus is so severe that there is soft tissue impingement between the calcaneous and the styloid of the fibula. A rigid rearfoot stabilizer may reduce the valgus deformity enough to eliminate the impingement and its associated pain.[48]

Talonavicular disease or destructive changes to any or all components of the subtalar joint complex may cause significant foot and leg pain, including peroneal muscle spasm with weight bearing and function. A rigid, stable orthotic may reduce motion and pain enough to enable continued function. Because the alternative approach to significant rear and midfoot disease is arthrodesis, a trial with the orthotic device often has merit.[49] There is considerable variety of material, technique, fabrication, and quality found in orthotic devices, and there are no reliable standards or criteria used in ordering or prescribing these devices. This lack of consistency is often frustrating to both patients and prescribing physicians. The best solution may be to develop a working relationship with a person capable of meeting the orthotic needs of your patients. The physician should recognize when orthotic devices or shoe modifications may be indicated and should describe clearly the problem being addressed as well as treatment goals and expectations.

SHOE MODIFICATION

The same principles of redistribution of weight can be applied directly to the sole of the shoe. Plantation/crepe or Vibram soles (Quabaug Corp., No. Brookfield, MA) can be added to almost any shoe to cushion impact. Metatarsal bars likewise provide a quick and simple modification to take weight off the metatarsal heads. To be effective, the front edge of the bar must be located proximal to the metatarsal heads. Many orthopedic shoe repair shops and orthotic laboratories have a shoe-stretching apparatus (e.g., a Eupedus device [Schein Orthopedic Products, New York]) that can selectively stretch a shoe to accommodate a digital deformity. The molded Plastazote shoe provides the ultimate in forefoot protection. When the need to protect the forefoot maximally is combined with rearfoot deformity requiring stabilization, a shoe using a polypropylene rearfoot stabilizer in addition to the Plastazote forefoot can be made.

Splinting and protective padding or shielding of the toes are helpful in reducing irritation of the soft tissues caused by pressure from shoes. An effective device for both splinting and protection can be molded from MPC (Siebe Norton, Inc., Pawtucket, RI) or Accumold (Premier Medical, Norristown, PA). Splints can be used to maintain these digital alignments during forefoot postoperative periods. The use of splints and wedges to correct hallux valgus deformity is of no value; because of the great forces acting on this deformity, a wedge between the great and second toes may increase the fibular displacement of the lesser toes. Hyperextension occasionally occurs at the interphalangeal joint of the great toe with or without hallux valgus or rigidis. This is a painful deformity, and the site is subject to chronic ulceration. Although surgical intervention is often required, an accommodative orthotic (MPC or Accumold) protective splint may be of value.

INJECTIONS

Polyarticular inflammatory foot pain is best managed with rest, heat, and systemic treatment; however, recalcitrant pain, particularly when located within a specific joint or joints, may be selectively treated with an injection of steroids, as can bursae and tendon sheaths. The foot, particularly its plantar and interdigital spaces, is a potentially dirty area surgically, and careful skin preparation is essential. Steroid injections into deep areas, particularly the plantar heel area, are easier when preceded by injections of anesthetic. With the exception of the ankle and subtalar joints, the foot joints should be treated as small joints in terms of quantity and strength of steroid to be injected. Tuberculin syringes provide excellent control of both insertion and introduction of fluid when dealing with small joints, superficial bursae, and tendon sheaths. The smaller joints, except in the presence of significant effusion, can be more difficult to enter for either aspiration or injections. The metatarsophalangeal and talonavicular joints are most readily entered by attempting to follow the natural joint contours rather than through a vertical approach to the joint space. Steroid injections within the Achilles tendon or its sheath are not recommended.

The subtalar joints can be entered with a 1 1/2-inch needle inserted at a point anterior to the fibula approximately 1 cm from its tip, directing the needle in a posterior, plantar, and medial direction. This provides entrance into the sinus tarsi. From this point, redirecting to a medial direction permits entrance into the extensive capsular complex, which includes the middle and anterior facets of the talocalcaneal as well as the talonavicular joints. Redirecting to a more posterior angle from the original insertion will locate the posterior talocalcaneal joint.

Other midfoot joints are difficult to locate and inject. Intermetatarsal head synovitis or bursitis does not require direct joint penetration, but a deposit along the sides of the joint may be helpful. Plantar heel injections, whether for bursitis, fasciitis, or heel spurs, are simplest when approached medially. Entrance is made just above the junction of the thick, tough plantar skin and the much more delicate skin of the upper foot and at a point medial to the attachment of the plantar fascia. Skin in this area is much more readily prepped, and the injection is far less painful. In addition, because spurs, fasciitis, or bursae are rarely limited to pencil point of bone spur seen on radiograph, medial injection allows a broader deposition of steroid in the region of pain and inflammation. When properly located, this injection site is posterior and inferior to the posterior tibial tendon nerve and vessels. Deep injections are often made easier by detaching the syringe from the well-placed needle and reloading with steroid. This procedure is likely to be less traumatic and usually more accurate.

In addition to rheumatoid arthritis, Reiter's disease and psoriasis may present painful inflammatory periosteal changes, particularly in the rearfoot area. Reiter's disease, especially, presents a frustrating problem as attempts are made to resolve or reduce heel pain. Psoriatic and Reiter's periostitis of the heel are usually not mechanical in origin and therefore do not respond well to orthotics designed to reduce traction on the plantar fascia. The use of Plastazote inserts, heel cups, and cushion-soled shoes is helpful. Rest, application of moist heat, and occasionally the timely injection of steroids may be of benefit.

JUVENILE RHEUMATOID ARTHRITIS

The patient with juvenile rheumatoid arthritis presents difficult challenges from the standpoint of both preventing and accommodating foot deformities. Early detection of structural changes and institution of appropriate shoes, orthoses, splints, and physical therapy are necessary. The physically active child should be watched for any tendency toward deformity, particularly in the rear and midfoot, where in contrast to the adult calcaneal valgus deformity, equinovarus deformity is more frequently encountered. Appropriate shoes or orthoses, or both, should be used to minimize this deformity. Night splints and foot boards may also be needed. The patient with juvenile rheumatoid arthritis is often an unreliable historian and reporter, and treatment requirements and decisions must be based largely on clinical judgment. Correction of deformities before the occurrence of fibrous ankylosis is essential if proper functional alignments are to be achieved and maintained. Active and passive range of motion and muscle strengthening exercises should be encouraged at an early stage. Once fibrous or bony ankylosis has occurred, correction is difficult at best, and surgical revision may ultimately be required.[50, 51]

SUMMARY

Early detection and treatment of deformity and pain with proper shoes, exercise, orthoses, and splints when needed may prevent, delay, or minimize disability. Soft, compliant, nonrestrictive footwear with low heels and crepe or Vibram soles, together with accommodative orthoses and shoe modifications, often increase levels of function and comfort. The management of the rheumatoid arthritic foot requires that patients be informed of the nature and course of treatment and that realistic goals and limitations be set. The criteria for lower extremity surgical intervention are such that major foot surgical procedures can be delayed at least until conservative measures have failed.

References

1. Lundberg, A.: Kinematics of the ankle and foot. Acta Orthop. Scand. Suppl. 233:60, 1989.
2. Hicks, J. H.: The mechanics of the foot. I. The joints. J. Anat. 87:345, 1953.
3. Mann, R. A.: Overview of foot and ankle biomechanics. In Jahss, M. H. (ed.): Disorders of the Foot and Ankle. 2nd ed. Philadelphia, W. B. Saunders Company, 1991, pp. 385–408.
4. Manter, J. B. T.: Movements of the subtalar and transverse tarsal joints. Anat. Rec. 80:397, 1941.
5. Huson, A.: Functional anatomy of the foot. In Jahss, M. H. (ed.): Disorders of the Foot and Ankle. 2nd ed. Philadelphia, W. B. Saunders Company, 1991, pp. 409–431.
6. Jahss, M. H.: Examination. In Jahss, M. H. (ed.): Disorders of the Foot and Ankle. 2nd ed. Philadelphia, W. B. Saunders Company, 1991, pp. 35–51.
7. Drabocky, I. Z.: Radiologic examination of the normal foot. In Mann, R. A. (ed.): Surgery of the Foot. 5th ed. St. Louis, C. V. Mosby, 1986, pp. 50–64.
8. Renton, P., and Stripp, W. J.: The radiology and radiography of the foot. In Klenerman, L. (ed.): The Foot and Its Disorders. 2nd ed. Oxford, Blackwell Scientific, 1982, pp. 305–399.
9. Martinez, S., Hergenberg, J. E., and Apple, J. S.: Computed tomography of the hindfoot. Orthop. Clin. North Am. 16:481, 1985.
10. Yao, L., and Lee, J. K.: Occult interosseous fracture: Detection with MR imaging. Radiology 167:749, 1988.
11. Yulish, B. S., Mulopulos, G. P., Goodfellow, D. B., et al.: MR imaging of osteochondral lesions of talus. J. Comput. Assist. Tomogr. 11:296, 1987.

12. Jahss, M. H.: Disorders of the hallux and the first ray. *In* Jahss, M. H. (ed.): Disorders of the Foot and Ankle. 2nd ed. Philadelphia, W. B. Saunders Company, 1991, pp. 943–1174.
13. Coughlin, M. J.: Crossover second toe deformity. Foot Ankle 8:29, 1987.
14. Giannestras, N. J.: Foot Disorders: Medical and Surgical Management. 2nd ed. Philadelphia, Lea & Febiger, 1973.
15. Shereff, M. D.: Radiographic analysis of the foot and ankle. *In* Jahss, M. H. (ed.). Disorders of the Foot and Ankle. 2nd ed. Philadelphia, W. B. Saunders Company, 1991, pp. 91–108.
16. Mann, R. A.: Acquired Flatfoot in Adults. Clin. Orthop. Rel. Res. 181:46, 1983.
17. Mann, R. A., and Thompson, F. M.: Rupture of the posterior tibial tendon causing flatfoot. J. Bone Joint Surg. 67A:556, 1985.
18. Johnson, K. A.: Surgery of the Foot and Ankle. New York, Raven Press, 1989.
19. Dyck, P. T., Stevens J. L., O'Brien, P. C. et al.: Neurogenic arthropathy and recurring fractures with subclinical inherited neuropathy. Neurology 33:357, 1983.
20. Kristiansen, B.: Ankle and foot fractures in diabetics provoking neuropathic joint changes. Acta Orthop. Scand. 51:975, 1980.
21. Deutsch, A. L., Resnick, D., and Campbell, G.: Computed tomography and bone scintigraphy in the evaluation of tarsal coalition. Radiology 144:137, 1982.
22. Herzenberg, J. E., Goldner, J. L., Martinez, S., and Silverman, P. M.: Computerized tomography of talocalcaneal tarsal coalition: A clinical and anatomic study. Foot Ankle 6:273, 1986.
23. Siligson, D., Gassman, J., and Pope, M: Ankle instability: Evaluation of the lateral ligaments. Am. J. Sports Med. 8:39, 1980.
24. Smith, R., and Reischl, S.: Treatment of ankle sprains in young athletes. Am. J. Sports Med. 14:465, 1986.
25. Zoellner, G., and Clancy, W., Jr.: Recurrent dislocations of the peroneal tendon. J. Bone Joint Surg. 61A:292, 1979.
26. Pöl, R., and Duyfjes, F.: The treatment of recurrent dislocation of the peroneal tendons. J. Bone Joint Surg. 66B:98, 1984.
27. Gellmen, M.: Fractures of the anterior process of the calcaneus. J. Bone Joint Surg. 33B:382, 1951.
28. Thompson, F. M., and Patterson, A. H.: Rupture of the peroneus longus tendon. J. Bone Joint Surg. 71A:293, 1984.
29. Sammarco, G. J., and DiRaimondo, C. V.: Chronic peroneus brevis tendon lesions following ankle trauma. Foot Ankle 9:163–170, 1989.
30. Mann, R. A., and Reynolds, J. D.: Interdigital neuroma: A critical analysis. Foot Ankle 3:238, 1983.
31. Thompson, F. M., and Deland, J. T.: Second Neuroma Same Foot. Presented at the Summer Meeting of the American Orthopedic Foot and Ankle Society, 1990.
32. Mann, R. A.: Diseases of the nerves of the foot. *In* Mann, R. A. (ed.): Surgery of the Foot. 5th ed. St. Louis, C. V. Mosby, 1984, pp. 199–208.
33. Kaplan, J.: Modern electrodiagnostic studies. *In* Jahss, M. H. (ed.): Disorders of the Foot and Ankle. 2nd ed. Philadelphia, W. B. Saunders Company, 1991, pp. 2026–2043.
34. Baxter, D. E.: Running injuries. *In* Jahss, M. H. (ed.): Disorders of the Foot and Ankle. 2nd ed. Philadelphia, W. B. Saunders Company, 1991, pp. 2446–2465.
35. Pfeffer, G. G., and Baxter, D. E.: Surgery of the adult heel. *In* Jahss, M. H. (ed.): Disorders of the Foot and Ankle. 2nd ed. Philadelphia, W. B. Saunders Company, 1991, pp. 1396–1416.
36. Baxter, D. E., and Thigpen, C. M.: Heel pain: Operative results. Foot Ankle 5:16, 1984.
37. Hall, O. C., and Brand, P. W.: The etiology of the neuropathic ulcer. J. Am. Podiatr. Assoc. 69:173, 1979.
38. Black, J. R., Cahalin, C., and Germain, B. F.: Pedal morbidity in rheumatic diseases. J. Am. Podiatr. Assoc. 72:360, 1982.
39. D'Amico, J. C.: The pathomechanics of adult rheumatoid arthritis affecting the foot. J. Am. Podiatr. Assoc. 66:227, 1976.
40. Curwen, C. H. M., Du Toit, L., Heywood, A. B., and Mills, C.: Studies of rheumatoid foot deformities. J. Bone Joint Surg. 68B:505, 1986.
41. Keenan, M. A. E., Peabody, T. D., Granley, M. A., and Perry, J.: Valgus deformities of the feet and characteristics of gait in patients who have rheumatoid arthritis. J. Bone Joint Surg. 73A:237, 1991.
42. Chater, E. H.: Tarsal tunnel syndrome in rheumatoid arthritis. Br. Med. J. 3:406, 1970.
43. Sgarlato, T. E.: A Compendium of Podiatric Biomechanics. San Francisco, College of Podiatric Medicine, 1971.
44. Root, M., Orien, W., and Weed, J.: Abnormal Function of the Foot. Los Angeles, Clinical Biomechanics, 1978.
45. Wilkinson, M., and Torrance, W. N.: Clinical background of rheumatoid vascular disease. Ann. Rheum. Dis. 26:475, 1967.
46. Soter, N. A., Austen, K. F., and Gigli, I.: Urticaria and arthralgias as manifestations of necrotizing angiitis (vasculitis). J. Invest. Dermatol. 63:485, 1974.
47. Levin, M. E., and O'Neal, L. W.: The Diabetic Foot. St. Louis, C. V. Mosby, 1983.
48. King, J., Burke, D., and Freeman, M. A.: The incidence of pain in the rheumatoid hindfoot and the significance of calcaneofibular impingement. Int. Orthop. 2:255, 1978.
49. Dalziel, R. E., Thornhill, T. S., and Thomas, W. H.: Talonavicular fusion of for hindfoot arthritis. J. Bone Joint Surg. 65B:667, 1983.
50. Schaller, J.: Chronic arthritis in children. Clin. Orthop. Rel. Res. 182:79, 1983.
51. Swann, M.: Juvenile rheumatoid arthritis. Treatment and principles. Clin. Orthop. Rel. Res. 219:38, 1987.

The Fibromyalgia Syndrome: Myofascial Pain and the Chronic Fatigue Syndrome

INTRODUCTION

Not all patients complaining of musculoskeletal pain have arthritis.[1] Bursitis, tendinitis, bone pain, fasciitis, enthesopathy, and peripheral neuropathies are well-accepted causes of nonarticular musculoskeletal pain. The muscle origin of nonarticular pain has only recently been rediscovered and gained some acceptance.[2-11] The notion that musculoskeletal pain is often of a myogenic origin is not surprising; there are approximately 696 individual muscles in the human body, and this tissue accounts for about 40 percent of body weight. Over the last decade it has become increasingly apparent that many patients presenting with elusive musculoskeletal pain have a consistency of symptoms and physical findings that are best described in terms of the fibromyalgia syndrome or a myofascial pain syndrome.[2, 3, 7, 12-17] Not all nonarticular pain can be thus characterized, but the ability to describe two distinctive rheumatic disease syndromes and their close association with the chronic fatigue syndrome has been the stimulus for an exponential growth of research into this controversial area of medicine.

CLINICAL FEATURES OF THE FIBROMYALGIA SYNDROME

Comprehensive epidemiologic studies of the fibromyalgia syndrome have not yet been reported. Its prevalence in one rheumatologic practice was 15 percent,[18] in a primary care practice 2 percent,[19] in a general medical outpatient clinic 5 percent,[20] and 3.7 to 20 percent in rheumatic disease clinics.[3, 21] Its overall prevalence in Sweden has been estimated at 1 percent.[22] The typical patient with fibromyalgia syndrome is a woman between the ages of 25 and 45; the preponderance of women to men is 8- to 20-fold. An identical syndrome may be seen in children[23-26] and in the elderly.[27, 28] One of the confusing features of many patients with the fibromyal-

gia syndrome is their reporting of multiple symptoms.[3, 12, 29-32] The full spectrum of the fibromyalgia syndrome encompasses core features that are present in every patient, typical features that are seen in most patients, and common features that are present in more than 25 percent of patients[12] (Fig. 29-1). By definition, all patients with fibromyalgia have the core features of widespread pain and multiple tender points. Most patients have the typical symptoms of fatigue, morning stiffness, nonrefreshing sleep, and postexertional muscle pain. About one third of patients have commonly associated problems such as irritable bowel syndrome, tension headaches, premenstrual syndrome, female urethral syndrome, numbness and tingling, sicca symptoms, and Raynaud's phenomenon; many other associations have been described (Table 29-1).[2, 3, 5, 20, 28, 30-59]

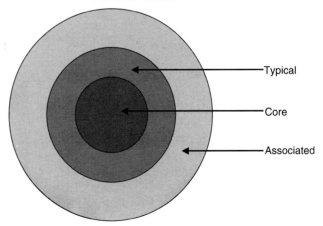

FIBROMYALGIA SYNDROME

Typical

Core

Associated

Figure 29–1. All fibromyalgia patients, by definition, have a history of widespread musculoskeletal pain and multiple tender points—the "core" features. Most patients also complain of fatigue, stiffness, and postexertional exacerbation of symptoms—the "typical" features. About 30 per cent of patients have a confusing amalgam of other symptoms, most commonly irritable bowel syndrome, Raynaud's phenomenon, paresthesia, etc.—the "associated symptoms."

Table 29–1. FIBROMYALGIA AND ASSOCIATED CONDITIONS

Feature	Reference(s)
Irritable bowel syndrome*	3, 5, 28, 30, 31, 33
Raynaud's phenomenon*	5, 31, 32, 34, 35
Chest pain	36, 37
Female urethral syndrome	38
Primary dysmenorrhea	3, 30, 39
Breathlessness	40, 41
Mitral valve prolapse	42
Vestibular dysfunction	43–45
Temporomandibular joint dysfunction	44, 46, 47
Neurologic symptoms*	3, 5, 45, 48–50
Hypothyroidism	51–53
Increased bone turnover	54
Sjögren's syndrome/sicca symptoms	32, 55
"Tension" headache*	2, 3, 5, 20, 30, 31, 39, 44
Facial pain	44, 56, 57
Leg/foot pain	44, 58
Carpal tunnel syndrome	59

*These features have been consistently reported as associated problems.

Most patients pinpoint their pain as arising from muscle. Some patients maintain their pain comes from their joints and may describe joint swelling; however, this is never observed by a clinician, and ^{99m}Tc diphosphonate joint scans are negative.[60]

Fatigue is often the predominant complaint of fibromyalgia patients. The commonest cause of chronic fatigue is a major depression.[61–63] Other causes of fatigue are viral infections, poor aerobic conditioning, chronic anxiety, overwhelming situational stresses, malignancy, eating disorders, and the diffuse connective tissue diseases. Analysis of the symptoms and fatigue in fibromyalgia patients does not implicate any one consistent interpretation. It is now apparent that many patients with the chronic fatigue syndrome also fit the criteria for fibromyalgia and vice versa (see later).

The physical examination of the typical patient with fibromyalgia is characteristically unrewarding unless attention is directed toward the presence of tender points. In 1990, the American College of Rheumatology (ACR) published criteria for the classification of fibromyalgia; the results from a multicenter study indicated that 11 or more out of 18 "specified" tender points in association with a history of widespread musculoskeletal pain provided the best diagnostic sensitivity (88.4 percent) and specificity (81.1 percent).[5] In these criteria, *widespread* pain is strictly specified as (1) pain in an axial distribution; (2) pain on the left and right sides of the body; and (3) pain above and below the waist. The specific tender points as well as the control points recommended by the ACR diagnostic criteria are shown in Figure 29–2. These points should be palpated with moderate pressure with the pulp of the thumb or forefinger; the amount of pressure recommended is 4 kg, as judged by a spring-loaded dolorimeter.[20] It is important to intersperse the examination of tender points with that of control points as the patient may

exhibit an anticipation reaction if every point is associated with pain. Although the ACR criteria specifies 18 tender points to be examined, many fibromyalgia patients have multiple tender points in other locations[3, 31, 64]; some patients with typical fibromyalgia symptoms have fewer than 11 tender points.

An important consideration in using tender points as the preeminent clinical feature of the fibromyalgia syndrome arises from the existence of a "second tender point" syndrome, most commonly referred to as *myofascial pain*.

MYOFASCIAL PAIN SYNDROME

The old term *fibrositis* may be viewed as an umbrella for two distinctive tender point syndromes, namely fibromyalgia and regional myofascial pain.[65] Much of the earlier literature on fibrositis and muscular rheumatism has probably referred mainly to regional myofascial pain problems. It is evident that these two conditions are closely related; indeed, it is not uncommon to see a patient with a regional myofascial pain syndrome evolve into the typical syndrome of widespread musculoskeletal pain, fa-

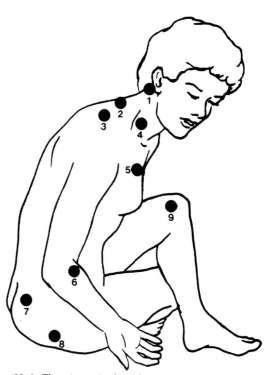

Figure 29–2. The nine paired tender points recommended by the 1990 ACR Criteria Committee for establishing a diagnosis of fibromyalgia are (1) insertion of nuchal muscles into occiput; (2) upper border of trapezius—midportion; (3) muscle attachments to upper medial border of scapula; (4) anterior aspects of the C5, C7 intertransverse spaces; (5) second rib space about 3 cm lateral to the sternal border; (6) muscle attachments to lateral epicondyle—about 2 cm below bony prominence; (7) upper outer quadrant of gluteal muscles; (8) muscle attachments just posterior to greater trochanter; and (9) medial fat pad of knee proximal to joint line. Eleven or more tender points in conjunction with a history of widespread pain are characteristic of the fibromyalgia syndrome.

Table 29–2. TRIGGER POINT CHARACTERISTICS

Always
Persistent pain (sometimes numbness and paresthesia); usually in a nondermatomal distribution*
Point tenderness of muscle to pressure
Increased pain on contraction of muscle
Increased pain on stretching of muscle; often results in a reduced range of motion

Often
Referred pain in a peripheral distribution on trigger point palpation
Indurated feel to muscle (the "palpable band" or "fibrositic nodule")
Involuntary contraction of muscle on needling a trigger point
Variable relief of pain after injection of trigger point with a local anesthetic

*Local tenderness without pain is often referred to as a *latent trigger point*.

tigue, and tender points consistent with a diagnosis of fibromyalgia.

Regional myofascial pain syndromes are probably the commonest cause of musculoskeletal pain; these problems often occur in the neck and low back but may also affect the peripheries.[44, 66] The overall prevalence of myofascial pain has been estimated to be 12 percent[67]; in a general medical population, it was found in 30 percent of patients.[68] The diagnosis of a myofascial pain syndrome is critically dependent on the demonstration of trigger point(s). A trigger point is generally considered to be an irritative focus within a muscle that is painful to palpation, often results in referred pain, induces shortening of the muscle, and causes pain on muscle contraction (Table 29–2). The precise location of a trigger point and its injection with approximately 1 to 2 ml of a local anesthetic (usually 1 per cent procaine) results in a temporary improvement, the restoration of normal range of motion, and an ability passively to stretch the muscle without causing pain.[44] Trigger points are so-called because they often refer pain in distal distribution, although this is not an invariable characteristic. Referred pain from trigger points is a common cause for so-called tension headaches and atypical arm pain.[44, 69–73] Trigger points in the gluteal muscles, particularly the gluteus medius and piriformis, commonly refer pain down the leg in a sciatic distribution; this is often the cause of diagnostic confusion and inappropriate investigations.[73–76] In many instances myofascial pain syndromes seem to be initiated by injuries or overuse. Most patients with myofascial pain syndromes have a good prognosis; however, some develop a chronic problem that is often refractory to treatment. The basic regimen for treating myofascial pain is stretching of the muscle harboring the trigger point after either a local injection or the use of a vapocoolant spray.[44, 66, 77, 78] Trigger point inactivation and stretching usually need to be repeated several times over a period of months. It is essential that the patient desist from vocational or avocational pursuits that cause strong contractions

in the involved muscle. It is not infrequent to see patients in whom recovery has been hampered by good-intentioned physical therapists who have tried to "strengthen" the involved muscles.

THE CHRONIC FATIGUE SYNDROME

Over the centuries, since the time of Hippocrates, physicians have struggled to treat patients with inexplicable fatigue. Sir Richard Manningham called the problem "Febricula" and describes the following symptoms: listlessness with great lassitude . . . low fever . . . weariness all over the body . . . little flying pains . . . [and] transient chilliness.[79] Over the years many terms have been used to describe these patients (Table 29–3).

It is important not to equate all chronic fatigue with the *chronic fatigue syndrome*.[80, 81] The basic premise underlying the concept of the chronic fatigue syndrome is that the acute onset of persistent and disabling fatigue is associated with symptoms and findings suggestive of an infectious process; these ideas were embodied in a "working case definition" by a panel of chronic fatigue syndrome experts.[82] Persistent, chronic fatigue is a common symptom; in a family practice survey from the United Kingdom, 25 percent of women and 20 percent of men always felt "tired."[83] In a U.S. study, chronic fatigue was a major problem in 24 percent of all adults attending primary care clinics.[84] In contradistinction, the *chronic fatigue syndrome* has an estimated prevalence of 37:100,000 in Australia.[85] A reduction in energy is an integral part of the *Diagnostic and Statistical Manual III Revised* (DSM IIIR) criteria for depression, and, indeed, as much as 80 percent of patients with chronic fatigue have been found to have a psychiatric diagnosis, such as depression, anxiety, or a somatization disorder.[62, 63, 84, 86–91] The concept that some patients with chronic fatigue have a preceding viral illness as a cause for their symptoms remains an active area for research; to date no one agent has been definitively implicated in the etiology of chronic fatigue syndrome.[92–100]

Many patients with chronic fatigue syndrome have chronic musculoskeletal pain and a sleep disturbance[101, 102]; it is evident that a large subset of these patients fits current criteria for fibromyalgia. Goldenberg et al.[103] reported that 94 percent of 500

Table 29–3. SYNONYMS FOR THE CHRONIC FATIGUE SYNDROME

Febricula	Hypoglycemia
Nervous exhaustion	"Total allergy" syndrome
Neurasthenia	Chronic candidiasis
Da Costa's syndrome	Chronic Epstein-Barr virus
Effort syndrome	infection
Autonomic imbalance	Chronic fatigue syndrome
syndrome	Chronic fatigue and immune
Chronic brucellosis	dysfunction syndrome

patients diagnosed as having chronic fatigue also had a history of musculoskeletal pain, and most had tender points. It is evident that whether a patient is labeled as having fibromyalgia or chronic fatigue is partly a matter of referral bias.

Moldofsy et al.[104, 105] reported that patients diagnosed as having chronic fatigue syndrome have the same alpha, delta (α, δ) sleep anomaly that they originally described in fibromyalgia.[104, 105] There is currently much interest in the notion that patients with chronic fatigue syndrome may have altered immune function; deficiencies in IgG subsets and changes in T cell subsets have been most frequently reported.[106-114] Therapeutically, the use of intravenous immunoglobulins has yielded conflicting results,[108, 109] and one trial of acyclovir was unsuccessful.[115] Hopefully, the basic research being pursued into the etiology of chronic fatigue syndrome will be applicable to fibromyalgia and vice versa.

DIFFERENTIAL DIAGNOSIS OF FIBROMYALGIA

Fibromyalgia patients often undergo an extensive workup before the correct diagnosis is considered or accepted. This is partly a reflection of inexperience in making this diagnosis; it is also a result of the multiple somatic complaints on presentation (see Table 29–1). The rationale for extensive investigation is often based on (1) the possibility that the fibromyalgia symptoms may be the prodrome of another illness; (2) the patient may have an associated condition that, if adequately treated, would lead to an improvement in the fibromyalgia symptoms[116]; and (3) the patients' insistence that they have a condition other than fibromyalgia. It is apparent that fibromyalgia can occur in association with a wide variety of conditions, and it is not uncommonly linked with rheumatoid arthritis, systemic lupus erythematosus (SLE), and primary Sjögren's syndrome. Yet, anecdotally, the effective treatment of the associated condition has seldom led to an amelioration of the fibromyalgia symptoms. Furthermore, there is no evidence to suggest that fibromyalgia represents the prodromal symptoms of an underlying connective tissue disease. Those patients who have multiple somatic symptoms as part of the wider spectrum of the fibromyalgia syndrome often present with a confusing amalgam of symptoms.[29] For instance, a patient with widespread musculoskeletal pain who perceives swollen joints, has a history of Raynaud's phenomenon, and complains of dry mouth and itchy eyes would be a prime suspect for having early SLE or primary Sjögren's syndrome. However, if the patient does not already have a well-documented connective tissue disease, and the only finding on physical examination is multiple tender points, the most likely diagnosis will be fibromyalgia. An intensive work-up (e.g., extensive serologic testing, muscle biopsy, electromyography, imaging, and

so forth) is unlikely to lead to an alternative diagnosis. A useful clue to considering this diagnosis is an apparent discrepancy between the patient's self-report of pain and disability.[117-120]

TREATMENT OF FIBROMYALGIA

In contradistinction to most rheumatic disorders, patients with the fibromyalgia syndrome are seldom helped by nonsteroidal anti-inflammatory agents and do not respond to corticosteroids.[121, 122] Longitudinal studies of individual patients treated and followed up in an academic setting have not shown a significant improvement over the course of some 5 years.[123, 124] This gloomy outlook may be related to center referral bias, because it is those patients with the severest and most long-standing disease who are most likely to be seen in academic centers. Because of the difficulty of successfully treating fibromyalgia patients with the traditional remedies of medications and physical therapy, there is a growing trend toward the use of a multidisciplinary approach.[125, 126] The principal components of such a program are discussed in the following sections.

Patient Education. Effective education is ideally based on the firm foundations of altered physiology. Given our ignorance of the underlying pathophysiologic basis for the fibromyalgia syndrome, educational efforts must be based on a compromise. It is reasonable to develop plausible hypotheses regarding the etiology of fibromyalgia based on contemporary research.[126] At the Oregon Health Sciences University, we have developed one such hypothesis that is employed in a fibromyalgia treatment program. This hypothesis is based on the concept that the pain experienced by fibromyalgia patients results from muscle microtrauma.[65, 126-129] It is envisaged that patients destined to develop fibromyalgia have a predisposition to muscle microtrauma (either acquired or genetic), which is accentuated by a persistence of the α δ sleep anomaly.[126] The resulting pain inhibits physical activity, which further enhances the predisposition to muscle microtrauma as a result of muscle deconditioning.[127] The educational value of this paradigm lies in its implicit assumption that the patient is part of a treatment team; as such, the patient's cooperation in attaining improved aerobic conditioning, in stress reduction programs, and in treatment of psychologic problems is central to effective management.

Sleep Disturbance. Virtually all patients with fibromyalgia give a history of nonrefreshing sleep. There may be an obvious cause for the sleep disturbance, and, ideally, this should be corrected before resorting to medications (Fig. 29–3). Most people find that regular exercise helps promote restorative sleep, and this has a scientific basis in that aerobic conditioning enhances non–rapid eye movement sleep.[130, 131] The α δ sleep anomaly in most fibromyalgia patients seems to be helped by use of one

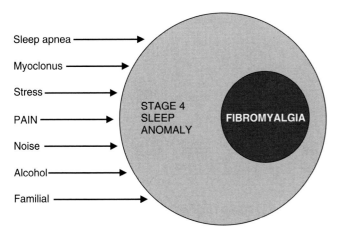

Figure 29–3. The $\alpha\delta$ sleep anomaly has been associated with fibromyalgia in patients with several provocateurs. If the sleep anomaly is central to the development of fibromyalgia, it is evident that its etiology is multifactorial.

of the tricyclic antidepressant agents. The dose required for improving restorative sleep is much less than required effectively to treat depressive disorders; however, normal sleep is seldom fully reestablished. The effectiveness of tricyclic antidepressants in improving restorative sleep depends on their ability to block the reuptake of epinephrine and serotonin[132, 133]; conversely, their side effects are dependent on their blocking acetylcholine and histamine receptors. For instance, the tendency to a morning hangover is related to antihistamine activity, whereas dry mouth, constipation, and tachycardia are associated with anticholinergic effects. The newer serotonin receptor antagonists, such as fluoxetine, lack these side effects; however, they may be poorly tolerated by fibromyalgia patients due to increased anxiety and insomnia.

Aerobic Exercise. McCain[134] has shown that fibromyalgia patients benefit from a program of aerobic conditioning. This may be related to the effect of aerobic exercise on restorative sleep[130, 131, 135–137] and a relative resistance to the musculoskeletal effects of α δ sleep.[138, 139] Patients with fibromyalgia are reluctant to exercise on account of muscle pain and fatigue. When they do exercise, they seem to suffer more postexercise pain than do normal persons and will often experience a sense of malaise for several days following a bout of unusual exertion. It is therefore critical that the prescription of an exercise program emphasizes (1) non-impact loading exercises, such as walking, swimming, and the use of an exercycle; (2) a very gentle progression of exercise intensity; and (3) adherence to a lifelong exercise regimen. One useful strategy for prescribing exercise is to use the concept of a training index. This is the product of exercise intensity (measured as a percentage of the maximum heart rate), the duration of exercise (in minutes), and the frequency of exercise each week (number of days). To maintain a reasonable aerobic fitness, the training index should be at least 42.

Because most fibromyalgia patients have become inactive, it is necessary to set a much lower goal initially and gradually achieve the desired amount of work over a period of 3 to 6 months.[140] The logic for this strategy is that the patient should have a tangible goal; this can be achieved by varying the proportion of the three products. For instance, patients who have a lot of postexercise soreness should initially work at a very low intensity and rest every other day; but this would necessitate increasing the duration of each exercise session, and so forth.

Myofascial Therapy. Heat, massage, and stretching have been a time-honored approach to treating patients with fibromyalgia.[141] These modalities are often of temporary benefit and hence are useful adjuncts to any program. The technique of myofascial spray and stretch as advocated by Travell and Simons[44] for the treatment of regional myofascial pain syndromes is anecdotally of benefit in alleviating the muscle soreness and stiffness experienced by patients with fibromyalgia. At the Oregon Health Sciences University, we initially evaluate the efficacy of spray and stretch for a particular patient and then continue therapy at home, after teaching friends or family members the basics of the technique.

The injection of tender areas with a local anesthetic (1 to 2 ml 1 percent procaine plus 0.3 ml Hydeltra-TBA) followed by stretching of the muscle harboring the tender point is another technique, which is used mainly in the treatment of regional myofascial pain; anecdotally, it also seems to be of benefit in selected muscles of some fibromyalgia patients.[142] The injection is a prelude to muscle stretching; the stretch, *not* the injection, is the critical therapeutic maneuver.

Treatment of Psychiatric Disorders. Twenty to 30 percent of fibromyalgia patients seen in an academic setting meet the criteria for a DSM IIIR diagnosis, the most common being depression, anxiety states, panic attacks, and somatization disorders.[95, 143–147] It is important to recognize these disorders and treat them appropriately in conjunction with psychiatric help when necessary.

Cognitive Restructuring. Many patients with fibromyalgia perceive themselves to be significantly disabled and have a reduced quality of life that rivals conditions such as terminal emphysema, rheumatoid arthritis, and colostomy patients.[119, 148, 149] Fibromyalgia patients seem to have difficulty coping with the stress of "daily hassles,"[150] and this, in turn, has been related to increased psychologic distress.[151] Cognitive behavioral therapy seeks to provide patients with an increased sense of control over their disease. Strategies for evaluating the effect of cognitive behavioral intervention in fibromyalgia patients have been outlined by Bradley.[152]

FIBROMYALGIA AND DISABILITY

The fibromyalgia syndrome is a common cause of disability claims.[12, 153] An analysis of claims at a major Canadian life insurance company indicated that fibromyalgia was the principal diagnosis in 9 percent of disability payments.[154] In Sweden 24 percent of one group of fibromyalgia patients were receiving a pension; in the same analysis, 44 percent were unable to manage household work.[31] In an analysis of American patients, 17 percent considered themselves disabled and 5.7 percent were receiving disability benefits; 30 percent had changed jobs on account of fibromyalgia.[155] An ergometric assessment of various work tasks indicated that fibromyalgia patients were rated at the same amount of disability as rheumatoid arthritis patients, in that both groups were able to perform only about 60 percent of the work done by normal controls.[156] Many fibromyalgia patients have difficulties sustaining a steady work pace and remaining employed[157, 158]; their reduced work capacity is usually due to limitation by pain.[156]

Physicians participating in the disability determination process are faced with a dilemma; the immediate patient-oriented goal is not to improve health but to emphasize impairment, inefficacy of treatment, and a poor prognosis. There is currently no way objectively to quantify impairment in fibromyalgia patients. Disability represents a subtle interplay between the patients' actual impairment and their perceived functional loss resulting from that impairment. Psychosocial issues inevitably become an important component in the decision to seek disability, but these are seldom appreciated by the applicant; however, the oft-quoted perception that improvement will follow a generous settlement has not be substantiated.[159] Physicians should be wary of filling out disability assessment forms that attempt to quantitate impairment of specific functions. One strategy is to send a letter documenting that the patient has fibromyalgia according to the 1990 ACR guidelines and point out that fibromyalgia patients have a diminished work capacity on account of exercise-induced pain and fatigue. A constructive dialogue between physicians, insurers, and disability assessors is urgently needed to provide unbiased guidelines for resolving this contentious issue.

PATHOPHYSIOLOGY OF FIBROMYALGIA

Although there is now widespread acceptance of fibromyalgia being a distinctive rheumatic syndrome, there is less certainty regarding its being due to distinctive pathophysiology. As a result of the lack of obvious physical findings and absence of investigational abnormalities, often coupled with the multiple somatic complaints, many patients were formerly diagnosed as having "psychogenic rheumatism." These ideas are still prevalent,[160–165] although many physicians now regard the term *psychogenic rheumatism* as being pejorative and unhelpful in physician-patient communications.[1, 2, 166, 167] If there is an important relationship between the mind and the body in the etiology of fibromyalgia symptoms,

as many investigators now believe, it is essential to understand this interplay at the level of its effect on altered physiology.

Nonrestorative Sleep

Nonrestorative sleep, or awakening unrefreshed, has been reported in 75 to 100 percent of patients with the fibromyalgia syndrome. The seminal studies of Moldofsky and colleagues[168] showed that patients with fibromyalgia had a non-REM stage 4 sleep electroencephalograph (EEG) pattern (1 to 2 cycles per second) that was disrupted by a superimposed pattern of α intrusion (10 to 12 cycles per second; Fig. 29–4). The association of this sleep disturbance with fibromyalgia has now been confirmed by others.[20, 169–171] Normal people and patients with chronic insomnia and dysthymia will often show some evidence of the α EEG sleep anomaly, but its duration is only about 25 percent of non-REM sleep. In contradistinction, patients with fibromyalgia have more than 60 percent of their non-REM sleep disrupted by the α sleep anomaly.[172, 173] Although α δ sleep is commonly associated with fibromyalgia, it is not specific; the original description was in psychologically disturbed patients.[174] It has also been described in some healthy people[175, 176]; as a familial trait[177]; as a response to emotional stress following trauma[173]; in patients with sleep apnea,[169] rheumatoid arthritis,[178] osteoarthritis,[179, 180] and nocturnal myoclonus[181, 182]; and in association with fever.[104, 105] It is of interest that the fibromyalgia syndrome has been associated with most of these diverse causes of α δ sleep. Support for its central role comes from Moldofsky and Scarisbrick's[183] observations that the production of an α δ sleep anomaly in healthy volunteers produced a syndrome of musculoskeletal pain and tender points reminiscent of the fibromyalgia syndrome.

The pathways involved in mediating non-REM sleep use gamma-aminobutyric acid and serotonin as neurotransmitters.[133, 184–186] Serotonin is formed in the brain after its precursor amino acid, tryptophan, crosses the blood-brain barrier and is acted on by oxidative and carboxylase enzymes. Parachlorophenylalanine (an inhibitor of serotonin production) can produce a syndrome of musculoskeletal pain akin to fibromyalgia.[187] Early studies suggested that the plasma concentration of unbound tryptophan was inversely related to the severity of fibromyalgia symptoms.[188] More recently, preliminary studies from two separate centers have shown that cerebrospinal fluid levels of the tryptophan metabolite, 5 hydroxyindole acetic acid, is lower in fibromyalgia patients than controls.[189, 190] If confirmed, this finding will be an important stepping stone in our understanding of the α non-REM sleep disturbance at a basic biochemical level. There is currently no unifying theory that links the occurrence of α δ sleep with the

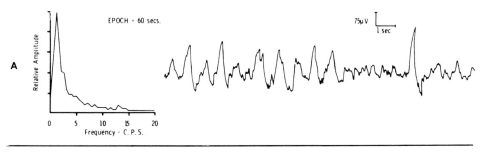

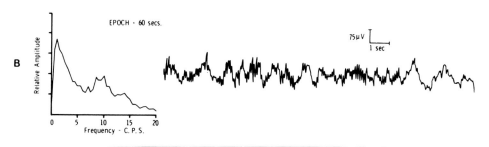

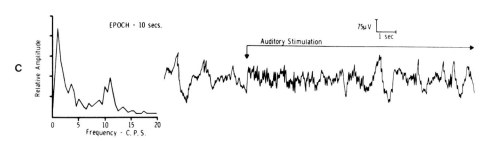

Figure 29–4. *A,* Frequency spectra and raw EEG from non-REM (stage 4) sleep in a healthy 25-year-old subject. The spectrum shows that most amplitude is concentrated at 1 cps (δ). *B,* Non-REM sleep in a 42-year-old "fibrositis" patient. The spectrum shows amplitude at both 1 cps (δ) and 8–10 cps (α). *C,* Non-REM sleep of a healthy 21-year-old subject during stage 4 sleep deprivation. In the EEG there is a clear association between external arousal (auditory stimulation) and α onset. Again, the frequency spectrum (obtained by 10-second analysis from stimulus onset) shows amplitude concentrated in the δ and α bands. (From Moldofsky, H., et al.: Musculoskeletal symptoms and non-REM sleep disturbance in patients with "fibrositis syndrome" and healthy subjects. Psychosomat. Med. 37:341, 1975. Copyright © by American Psychosomatic Society.)

widespread tender points of the fibromyalgia syndrome.

Psychological Dysfunction

The contention that many patients with fibromyalgia have a psychological disturbance such as depression, anxiety, somatization, hypochondriasis, or poor coping strategies is a common perception that is partly supported by several reports. Studies of patients seeing rheumatologists in academic setting have revealed that 30 to 100 percent have a psychiatric diagnosis.[95, 143–147, 191–196] The commonest diagnoses are depression, anxiety, somatization, and hypochondriasis. However, studies done in patients attending a general outpatient clinic or patients with mild fibromyalgia symptomatology have not revealed an increased prevalence of psychological diagnoses.[197–200] It would appear that an abnormal psyche is not a prerequisite for the development of fibromyalgia. The psychiatric diagnoses noted in some patients with fibromyalgia have much the same prevalence as those seen in patients with other medical conditions.[201]

Many fibromyalgia patients relate the onset of their illness and flares to major life stresses, and this has been confirmed by recent studies.[150, 194] Yunus et al.[202] correlated clinical features of fibromyalgia with psychological status on Minnesota Multiphasic Personality Inventory testing; the core features of fibromyalgia were unrelated to psychological status, but pain severity appeared to be influenced by psychological factors.[202] This conclusion is intuitively appealing; it suggests that the perceived severity of symptoms and the decision to seek medical help will be determined by the patient's personality, upbringing, psychological profile, and coping strategies.

Muscle Abnormalities

Contemporary studies looking at patients with a clinical picture consistent with the modern definition of the fibromyalgia syndrome have not yielded any distinctive histologic features that could be termed diagnostic.[203–205] However, one recent paper on single cell morphology reported a distinctive "banding" of several sarcomeres spaced throughout the muscle fibers of fibromyalgia patients.[206] Bengtsson et al.[207] have reported reduced levels of adenosine triphosphate in tender point areas of the trapezius but not in the tibialis anterior.[207] Similar findings have been noted in the trigger point areas with regional myofascial pain syndrome involving the head and neck.[208] If confirmed, these results would indicate

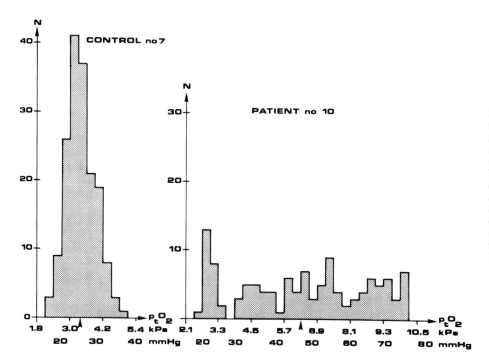

Figure 29–5. Oxygen pressure histogram obtained from the trapezius muscle of a patient with fibrositis (10) and a healthy control subject (7). The histogram distribution types are statistically different (p < 0.001). The arrow on the abscissa indicates the mean tissue oxygen pressure. (From Lund, N., et al.: Muscle tissue oxygen pressure in primary fibromyalgia. Scand. J. Rheumatol. 15:165, 1986. Used by permission.)

that tender point areas in fibromyalgia and in regional myofascial pain syndromes have the same basic underlying defect.

The concept that there might be a focal anoxia due to a disruption of capillary blood flow was supported by a study using a multipoint oxygen electrode placed over tender point areas exposed at surgery[209] (Fig. 29–5). Reduced blood flow to exercising muscle[210] but not resting muscle[211] has also been reported. The old concept that reduced blood flow is due to muscle spasm is unfounded[128]; electromyographic studies have shown fibromyalgic muscles to be electrically silent.[212]

Patients with fibromyalgia often complain of muscle weakness. Although they usually demonstrate reduced strength on formal testing,[213] this may not represent a true physiologic weakness; they are able to generate a normal force pattern on electrical stimulation.[31, 214] Similar findings have been reported in the chronic fatigue syndrome.[215] It is hypothesized that the pain experienced on exertion is the cause for this reflex inhibition. When exercised to volitional exhaustion, most patients have a poor aerobic capacity.[210]

Raynaud's Phenomenon

Many patients with fibromyalgia experience an exacerbation of pain during periods of cold, damp weather.[216] It has also been noted that fibromyalgia patients often complain of being colder than other household members and need to wear warmer clothes and turn up the thermostat. Interestingly, some patients with fibromyalgia have symptoms compatible with classic Raynaud's phenomenon.[5, 32,]

[217, 218] Bennett et al.[35] have provided objective evidence of increase in cold-induced vasospasm and correlated this with an up-regulation of α_2 adrenergic receptors.

Psycho-neuro-immuno-endocrine Axis

The fibromyalgia syndrome is commonly considered to have a psychosomatic etiology. The precise mechanism whereby the psyche could influence the soma in this condition has not been resolved. Three groups have found abnormalities in the dexamethasone suppression test in subsets of fibromyalgia patients.[219–221] Whether these changes represent a physiologic response to stress or depression has not yet been clarified. The possibility that the hypothalamic-pituitary axis may be disrupted by the stage 4 sleep anomaly is an appealing notion because growth hormone and prolactin are both secreted during stage 4 sleep.

Substance P, a major neurotransmitter in ascending pain pathways, was shown to have an almost fourfold elevation in the cerebrospinal fluid of fibromyalgia patients compared with published levels in a normal population[217]; if confirmed with appropriate controls, this observation could be seminal to understanding the increased "sensitivity" of fibromyalgia patients. The antidromic release of substance P has also been implicated in the exaggerated skin reactivity (the triple response) in patients with fibromyalgia.[222]

Miscellaneous

Several preliminary studies have suggested a possible role for autoimmunity in the fibromyalgia

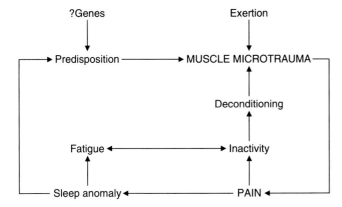

Figure 29–6. The cause of fibromyalgia is unknown; this is a paradigm that has been used to rationalize current treatment modalities. The crux of this schema is that the pain component of fibromyalgia is due to muscle microtrauma. In fibromyalgia patients it is envisioned that relatively low levels of exertion cause muscle microtrauma due to a predisposition for this type of injury. The predisposition to microtrauma is postulated to stem from (1) neurohumoral changes resulting from the stage 4 sleep anomaly; (2) deconditioning due to inactivity; and (3) a defect (?inherited/?acquired) in sarcolemmal membrane integrity. It is hypothesized that there are several "feedback loops"; if these are not interrupted, there will be a progressive worsening of symptoms.

syndrome.[31, 32, 113, 223–229] More comprehensive studies have not shown any increased prevalence of antinuclear antibodies in patients with fibromyalgia,[230] and changes in lymphocyte subsets may result from the sleep disturbance.[231–233]

The possibility that fibromyalgia patients may have a basic abnormality of collagen is suggested by the observation of low serum levels of procollagen type III aminoterminal peptide[234] and 75 percent prevalence of mitral valve prolapse in one series.[42] Elevated levels of myoglobin have been found in the serum of "fibrositis" patients after massage.[235] This result suggests that the integrity of muscle cells may be easily compromised in patients with fibromyalgia. This notion forms the basis for an hypothesis that equates fibromyalgic muscle pain with postexertional microtrauma[65, 126–129] (Fig. 29–6).

There appear to be multiple triggers to the development of fibromyalgia: posttraumatic pain and distress,[173, 236] human immunodeficiency virus infection,[237–239] Lyme disease,[192, 240–242] persistent noise,[243] Cocksackie virus infection,[244] silicone breast implants,[245] interleukin-2 adjunctive chemotherapy,[246] and the toxic oil syndrome.[247] It is possible that the interaction of certain *triggers* with a genetically susceptible host is a relevant paradigm because an inherited predisposition to fibromyalgia has been reported.[248, 249] The final common pathway, which may link these positive factors to the stage 4 sleep anomaly and muscle pain, remains elusive.

References

1. Bennett, R. M.: Nonarticular rheumatism and spondyloarthropathies: Similarities and differences. Postgrad. Med. 87:97, 102–104, 1990.
2. Goldenberg, D. L.: Fibromyalgia syndrome: An emerging but controversial condition. J.A.M.A. 257:2782, 1987.
3. Yunus, M., Masi, A. T., Calabro, J. J., Miller, K. A., and Feigenbaum, S. L.: Primary fibromyalgia (fibrositis): Clinical study of 50 patients with matched normal controls. Semin. Arthritis Rheum. 11:151, 1981.
4. Bennett, R. M.: Fibrositis: Evolution of an enigma. J. Rheumatol. 13:676, 1986.
5. Wolfe, F., Smythe, H. A., Yunus, M. B., Bennett, R. M., Bombardier, C., Goldenberg, D. L., Tugwell, P., Campbell, S. M., Abeles, M., Clark, P., Fam, A. G., Farber, S. J., Fiechtner, J. J., Franklin, C. M., Gatter, R. A., Hamaty, D., Lessard, J., Lichtbroun, A. S., Masi, A. T., McCain, G. A., Reynolds, W. J., Romano, T. J., Russell, I. J., and Sheon, R. P.: The American College of Rheumatology 1990 criteria for the classification of fibromyalgia: Report of the Multicenter Criteria Committee. Arthritis Rheum. 33:160, 1990.
6. Coulehan, J. L.: Primary fibromyalgia. Am. Family Phys. 32:170, 1985.
7. Campbell, S. M., and Bennett, R. M.: Fibrositis. Dis. Mon. 32:653, 1986.
8. Bennett, R. M.: Proceedings of The Palm Springs Fibromyalgia Syndrome Symposium, Palm Springs, CA, March 18–20, 1988. Introduction. J. Rheumatol. Suppl. 19:1, 1989.
9. Bennett, R. M.: Fibrositis (Editorial). J.A.M.A. 257:2802, 1987.
10. Bennett, R. M.: The fibrositis/fibromyalgia syndrome: Current issues and perspectives. Am. J. Med. 81:1, 1986.
11. Rogers, E. J., and Rogers, R.: Pain clinic no. 14. Fibromyalgia and myofascial pain: Either, neither, or both? Orthop. Rev. 18:1217, 1989.
12. Wolfe, F.: Fibromyalgia: The clinical syndrome. Rheum. Dis. Clin. North Am. 15:1, 1989.
13. Simons, D. G.: Fibrositis/fibromyalgia: A form of myofascial trigger points. Am. J. Med. 81:93, 1986.
14. Smythe, H. A., and Moldofsky, H.: Two contributions to understanding of the "fibrositis" syndrome. Bull. Rheum. Dis. 28:928, 1977.
15. Sheon, R. P.: Regional myofascial pain and the fibrositis syndrome (fibromyalgia). Compr. Ther. 12:42, 1986.
16. Kolar, E., Hartz, A., Roumm, A., Ryan, L., Jones, R., and Kirchdoerfer, E.: Factors associated with severity of symptoms in patients with chronic unexplained muscular aching. Ann. Rheum. Dis. 48:317, 1989.
17. Thompson, J. M.: Tension myalgia as a diagnosis at the Mayo Clinic and its relationship to fibrositis, fibromyalgia, and myofascial pain syndrome. Mayo Clin. Proc. 65:1237, 1990.
18. Wolfe, F., and Cathey, M. A.: Prevalence of primary and secondary fibrositis. J. Rheumatol. 10:965, 1983.
19. Hartz, A., and Kirchdoerfer, E.: Undetected fibrositis in primary care practice. J. Family Pract. 25:365, 1987.
20. Campbell, S. M., Clark, S., Tindall, E. A., Forehand, M. E., and Bennett, R. M.: Clinical characteristics of fibrositis: I. A "blinded," controlled study of symptoms and tender points. Arthritis Rheum. 26:817, 1983.
21. Muller, W.: The fibrositis syndrome: Diagnosis, differential diagnosis and pathogenesis. Scand. J. Rheumatol. 65(Suppl):40, 1987.
22. Jacobsson, L., Lindgärde, F., and Manthorpe, R.: The commonest rheumatic complaints of over six weeks' duration in a twelve-month period in a defined Swedish population: Prevalences and relationships. Scand. J. Rheumatol. 18:353, 1989.
23. Calabro, J. J.: Fibromyalgia (fibrositis) in children. Am. J. Med. 81:57, 1986.
24. Yunus, M. B., and Masi, A. T.: Juvenile primary fibromyalgia syndrome: A clinical study of thirty-three patients and matched normal controls. Arthritis Rheum. 28:138, 1985.
25. Calabro, J. J., and Perry, R. F.: Juvenile primary fibromyalgia syndrome (Letter). Arthritis Rheum. 29:452, 1986.
26. Cicuttini, F., and Littlejohn, G. O.: Female adolescent rheumatological presentations: The importance of chronic pain syndromes. Aust. Paediatr. J. 25:21, 1989.
27. Wolfe, F.: Fibromyalgia in the elderly: Differential diagnosis and treatment. Geriatrics 43:57, 65, 68, 1988.
28. Yunus, M. B., Holt, G. S., Masi, A. T., and Aldag, J. C.: Fibromyalgia syndrome among the elderly: Comparison with younger patients. J. Am. Geriatr. Soc. 36:987, 1988.
29. Bennett, R. M.: Confounding features of the fibromyalgia syndrome: A current perspective of differential diagnosis. J. Rheumatol. Suppl. 19:58, 1989.
30. Yunus, M. B., Masi, A. T., and Aldag, J. C.: A controlled study of primary fibromyalgia syndrome: Clinical features and association with other functional syndromes. J. Rheumatol. 19(Suppl.):62, 1989.
31. Bengtsson, A., Henriksson, K. G., Jorfeldt, L., Kågedal, B., Lennmarken, C., and Lindstrom, F.: Primary fibromyalgia: A clinical and laboratory study of 55 patients. Scand. J. Rheumatol. 15:340, 1986.
32. Dinerman, H., Goldenberg, D. L., and Felson, D. T.: A prospective evaluation of 118 patients with the fibromyalgia syndrome: Prevalence of Raynaud's phenomenon, sicca symptoms, ANA, low complement, and Ig deposition at the dermal-epidermal junction. J. Rheumatol. 13:368, 1986.
33. Romano, T. J.: Coexistence of irritable bowel syndrome and fibromyalgia. W.V. Med. J. 84:16, 1988.

34. Vaeroy, H., Qiao, Z. -G., Morkrid, L., and Forre, O.: Altered sympathetic nervous system response in patients with fibromyalgia (fibrositis syndrome). J. Rheumatol. 16:1460, 1989.
35. Bennett, R. M., Clark, S. R., Campbell, S. M., Ingram, S. B., Burckhardt, C. S., Nelson, D. L., and Porter, J. M.: Raynaud's symptomatology in patients with the fibromyalgia syndrome: A study utilizing the Nielsen test, digital photoplethysmography and measurements of platelet alpha 2 adrenergic receptors. Arthritis Rheum. 34:264, 1991.
36. Pellegrino, M. J.: Atypical chest pain as an initial presentation of primary fibromyalgia. Arch. Phys. Med. Rehabil. 71:526, 1990.
37. Fam, A. G.: Approach to musculoskeletal chest wall pain. Prim. Care 15:767, 1988.
38. Wallace, D. J.: Genitourinary manifestations of fibrositis: An increased association with the female urethral syndrome. J. Rheumatol. 17:238, 1990.
39. Yunus, M. B.: Primary fibromyalgia syndrome: Current concepts. Compr. Ther. 10:21, 1984.
40. Caidahl, K., Lurie, M., Bake, B., Johansson, G., and Wetterqvist, H.: Dyspnoea in chronic primary fibromyalgia. J. Intern. Med. 226:265, 1989.
41. Lurie, M., Caidahl, K., Johansson, G., and Bake, B.: Respiratory function in chronic primary fibromyalgia. Scand. J. Rehabil. Med. 22:151, 1990.
42. Pellegrino, M. J., Van Fossen, D., Gordon, C., Ryan, J. M., and Waylonis, G. W.: Prevalence of mitral valve prolapse in primary fibromyalgia: A pilot investigation. Arch. Phys. Med. Rehabil. 70:541, 1989.
43. Hadj-Djilani, A., and Gerster, J. C.: Meniere's disease and fibrositis syndrome (psychogenic rheumatism): Relationship in audiometric and nystagmographic results. Acta Otolaryngol. Suppl. 406:67, 1984.
44. Travell, J. G., and Simons, D. G.: Myofascial Pain and Dysfunction: The Trigger Point Manual. Baltimore, Williams & Wilkins, 1983.
45. Rosenhall, U., Johansson, G., and Orndahl, G.: Neuroaudiological findings in chronic primary fibromyalgia with dysesthesia. Scand. J. Rehabil. Med. 19:147, 1987.
46. Blasberg, B., and Chalmers, A.: Temporomandibular pain and dysfunction syndrome associated with generalized musculoskeletal pain: A retrospective study. J. Rheumatol. Suppl. 19:87, 1989.
47. Truta, M. P., and Santucci, E. T.: Head and neck fibromyalgia and temporomandibular arthralgia. Otolaryngol. Clin. North Am. 22:1159, 1989.
48. Simms, R. W., and Goldenberg, D. L.: Symptoms mimicking neurologic disorders in fibromyalgia syndrome. J. Rheumatol. 15:1271, 1988.
49. Gerster, J. C., and Hadj Djilani, A.: Hearing and vestibular abnormalities in primary fibrositis syndrome. J. Rheumatol. 11:678, 1984.
50. Rosenhall, U., Johansson, G., and Orndahl, G.: Eye motility dysfunction in chronic primary fibromyalgia with dysesthesia. Scand. J. Rehabil. Med. 19:139, 1987.
51. Wilke, W. S., Sheeler, L. R., and Makarowski, W. S.: Hypothyroidism with presenting symptoms of fibrositis. J. Rheumatol. 8:626, 1981.
52. Carette, S., Lefrancois, L.: Fibrositis and primary hypothyroidism. J. Rheumatol. 15:1418, 1988.
53. Trommer, P. R.: Hypothyroidism with presenting symptoms of fibrositis (Letter). J. Rheumatol. 9:335, 1982.
54. Appelboom, T., and Schoutens, A.: High bone turnover in fibromyalgia. Calcif. Tissue. Int. 46:314, 1990.
55. Vitali, C., Tavoni, A., Neri, R., Castrogiovanni, P., Pasero, G., and Bombardieri, S.: Fibromyalgia features in patients with primary Sjögren's syndrome: Evidence of a relationship with psychological depression. Scand. J. Rheumatol. 18:21, 1989.
56. Donlon, W. C., Kaplan, H., Javid, B., Harness, M., Shultz, P., Rome, H., Hwang, R., and Santucci, E.: Multifactorial facial pain—differential diagnosis: a case report. J. Am. Dent. Assoc. 120:315, 1990.
57. LeLiever, W. C.: Nonotologic otalgia. J.A.M.A. 264:2302, 1990.
58. Gohil, P., Young, J. R., Gohil, J. P., and Graham, J. L.: Tension fibrositis of the legs. J. Am. Podiatr. Med. Assoc. 71:136, 1981.
59. Richards, A. J.: Carpal tunnel syndrome and subsequent rheumatoid arthritis in the "fibrositis" syndrome. Ann. Rheum. Dis. 43:232, 1984.
60. Yunus, M. B., Berg, B. C., and Masi, A. T.: Multiphase skeletal scintigraphy in primary fibromyalgia syndrome: A blinded study. J. Rheumatol. 16:1466, 1989.
61. Broadhead, W. E., Blazer, D. G., George, L. K., and Tse, C. K.: Depression, disability days, and days lost from work in a prospective epidemiologic survey. J.A.M.A. 264:2524, 1990.
62. Wessely, S., and Powell, R.: Fatigue syndromes: A comparison of chronic "postviral" fatigue with neuromuscular and affective disorders. J. Neurol. Neurosurg. Psychiatry 52:940, 1989.
63. Hickie, I., Lloyd, A., Wakefield, D., and Parker, G.: The psychiatric status of patients with the chronic fatigue syndrome. Br. J. Psychiatry 156:534, 1990.
64. Simms, R. W., Goldenberg, D. L., Felson, D. T., and Mason, J. H.: Tenderness in 75 anatomic sites: Distinguishing fibromyalgia patients from controls. Arthritis Rheum. 31:182, 1988.
65. Bennett, R. M.: Myofascial pain syndromes and the fibromyalgia syndrome: A comparative analysis. J. Manual Med. 6:1, 1990.
66. Campbell, S. M.: Regional myofascial pain syndromes. Rheum. Dis. Clin. North Am. 15:31, 1989.
67. Blasberg, B., and Chalmers, A.: Temporomandibular pain and dysfunction syndrome associated with generalized musculoskeletal pain: A retrospective study. J. Rheumatol. Suppl. 19:87, 1989.
68. Skootsky, S. A., Jaeger, B., and Dye, R. K.: Prevalence of myofascial pain in general internal medicine practice. West. J. Med. 151:157, 1984.
69. Graff-Radford, S. B., Reeves, J. L., and Jaeger, B.: Management of head and neck pain: Effectiveness of altering factors precipitating myofascial pain. Headache 27:186, 1987.
70. Graff-Radford, S. B., Jaeger, B., and Reeves, J. L.: Myofascial pain may present clinically as occipital neuralgia. Neurosurgery 19:610, 1986.
71. Grosshandler, S. L., Stratas, N. E., Toomey, T. C., et al.: Chronic neck and shoulder pain: Focusing on myofascial origins. Postgrad. Med. 77:149, 1985.
72. Sola, A. E., Rodenberger, M. L., and Gettys, B. B.: Incidence of hypersensitive areas in posterior shoulder muscles. Am. J. Phys. Med. 34:585, 1955.
73. Slocumb, J. C.: Neurological factors in chronic pelvic pain: Trigger points and the abdominal pelvic pain syndrome. Am. J. Obstet. Gynecol. 149:536, 1984.
74. Simons, D. G., and Travell, J. G.: Myofascial origins of low back pain: II. Torso muscles. Postgrad. Med. 73:81, 1983.
75. Simons, D. G., and Travell, J. G.: Myofascial origins of low back pain: III. Pelvic and lower extremity muscles. Postgrad. Med. 73:99, 1983.
76. Zohn, D. A.: The quadratus lumborum: Unrecognized source of back pain. Orthopaed. Rev. 15:87, 1985.
77. Simons, D. G.: Muscle pain syndromes: II. Am. J. Phys. Med. 55:15, 1976.
78. Travell, J., and Rinzler, S. H.: The myofascial genesis of pain. Postgrad. Med. 11:425, 1952.
79. Straus, S. E.: History of chronic fatigue syndrome. Rev. Infect. Dis. 13:S2, 1991.
80. Manu, P., Lane, T. J., and Matthews, D. A.: The frequency of chronic fatigue syndrome in patients with symptoms of persistent fatigue. Ann. Intern. Med. 109:554, 1988.
81. Solberg, L. I.: Lassitude: A primary care evaluation. J.A.M.A. 251:3272, 1984.
82. Holmes, G. P., Kaplan, J. E., Gantz, N. M., Komaroff, A. L., Schonberger, L. B., Straus, S. E., Jones, J. F., Dubois, R. E., Cunningham-Rundles, C., Pahwa, S., Tosato, G., Zegans, L. S., Purtilo, D. T., Brown, N., Schooley, R. T., and Brus, I.: Chronic fatigue syndrome: A working case definition. Ann. Intern. Med. 108:387, 1988.
83. David, A., Pelosi, A., McDonald, E., Stephens, D., Ledger, D., Rathbone, R., and Mann, A.: Tired, weak, or in need of rest: Fatigue among general practice attenders. Br. Med. J. 301:1199, 1990.
84. Kroenke, K., Wood, D. R., Mangelsdorff, D., Meier, N. J., and Powell, J. B.: Chronic fatigue in primary care: Prevalence, patient characteristics, and outcome. J.A.M.A. 260:929, 1988.
85. Lloyd, A. R., Hickie, I., Boughton, C. R., Spencer, O., and Wakefield, D.: Prevalence of chronic fatigue syndrome in an Australian population. Med. J. Aust. 153:522, 1990.
86. Stricklin, A., Sewell, M., and Austad, C.: Objective measurement of personality variables in epidemic neuromyasthenia patients. South Afr. Med. J. 77:31, 1990.
87. Black, D. W., Rathe, A., and Goldstein, R. B.: Environmental illness: A controlled study of 26 subjects with "20th century disease." J.A.M.A. 264:3166, 1990.
88. Lloyd, A. R.: Muscle versus brain: Chronic fatigue syndrome. Med. J. Aust. 153:530, 1990.
89. Greenberg, D. B.: Neurasthenia in the 1980s: Chronic mononucleosis, chronic fatigue syndrome, and anxiety and depressive disorders. Psychosomatics 31:129, 1990.
90. Altay, H. T., Toner, B. B., Brooker, H., Abbey, S. E., Salit, I. E., and Garfinkel, P. E.: The neuropsychological dimensions of postinfectious neuromyasthenia (chronic fatigue syndrome): A preliminary report. Int. J. Psychiatry Med. 20:141, 1990.
91. Manu, P., Matthews, D. A., and Lane, T. J.: The mental health of patients with a chief complaint of chronic fatigue: A prospective evaluation and follow-up. Arch. Intern. Med. 148:2213, 1988.
92. Miller, N. A., Carmichael, H. A., Calder, B. D., Behan, P. O., Bell, E. J., McCartney, R. A., and Hall, F. C.: Antibody to coxsackie B virus in diagnosing postviral fatigue syndrome. Br. Med. J. 302:140, 1991.
93. Hellinger, W. C., Smith, T. F., Van Scoy, R. E., Spitzer, P. G., Forgacs, P., and Edson, R. S.: Chronic fatigue syndrome and the diagnostic utility of antibody to Epstein-Barr virus early antigen. J.A.M.A. 260:971, 1988.
94. Yousef, G. E., Bell, E. J., Mann, G. F., Murugesan, V., Smith, D. G., McCartney, R. A., and Mowbray, J. F.: Chronic enterovirus infection in patients with postviral fatigue syndrome. Lancet 1:146, 1988.
95. Payne, T. C., Leavitt, F., Garron, D. C., Katz, R. S., Golden, H. E., Glickman, P. B., and Vanderplate, C.: Fibrositis and psychologic disturbance. Arthritis Rheum. 25:213, 1982.

96. Gold, D., Bowden, R., Sixbey, J., Riggs, R., Katon, W. J., Ashley, R., Obrigewitch, R., and Corey, L.: Chronic fatigue: A prospective clinical and virologic study. J.A.M.A. 264:48, 1990.
97. Palca, J.: Does a retrovirus explain fatigue syndrome puzzle? (News). Science 249:1240, 1990.
98. Read, R., Larson, E., Harvey, J., Edwards, A., Thomson, B., Briggs, M., and Fox, J.: Clinical and laboratory findings in the Paul-Bunnell negative glandular fever-fatigue syndrome. J. Infect. 21:157, 1990.
99. Straus, S. E., Tosato, G., Armstrong, G., Lawley, T., Preble, O. T., Henle, W., Davey, R., Pearson, G., Epstein, J., Brus, I., and Blaese, M.: Persisting illness and fatigue in adults with evidence of Epstein-Barr virus infection. Ann. Intern. Med. 102:7, 1985.
100. Cunningham, L., Bowles, N. E., Lane, R. J., Dubowitz, V., and Archard, L. C.: Persistence of enteroviral RNA in chronic fatigue syndrome is associated with the abnormal production of equal amounts of positive and negative strands of enteroviral RNA. J. Gen. Virol. 71:1399, 1990.
101. Goldenberg, D. L.: Fibromyalgia and other chronic fatigue syndromes: Is there evidence for chronic viral disease? Semin. Arthritis Rheum. 18:111, 1988.
102. Goldenberg, D. L.: Fibromyalgia and its relation to chronic fatigue syndrome, viral illness and immune abnormalities. J. Rheumatol. Suppl. 19:91, 1989.
103. Goldenberg, D. L., Simms, R. W., Geiger, A., and Komaroff, A. L.: High frequency of fibromyalgia in patients with chronic fatigue seen in a primary care practice. Arthritis Rheum. 33:381, 1990.
104. Moldofsky, H.: Nonrestorative sleep and symptoms after a febrile illness in patients with fibrositis and chronic fatigue syndromes. J. Rheumatol. Suppl. 19:150, 1989.
105. Moldofsky, H., Saskin, P., Salem, L., et al.: Sleep and symptoms of post-infectious neuromyasthenia and fibrositis syndrome. Sleep Res. 16:492, 1987.
106. Gin, W., Christiansen, F. T., and Peter, J. B.: Immune function and the chronic fatigue syndrome. Med. J. Aust. 151:117, 1989.
107. Lloyd, A. R., Wakefield, D., Boughton, C. R., and Dwyer, J. M.: Immunological abnormalities in the chronic fatigue syndrome. Med. J. Aust. 151:122, 1989.
108. Peterson, P. K., Shepard, J., Macres, M., Schenck, C., Crosson, J., Rechtman, D., and Lurie, N.: A controlled trial of intravenous immunoglobulin G in chronic fatigue syndrome [see Comments]. Am. J. Med. 89:554, 1990.
109. Straus, S. E.: Intravenous immunoglobulin treatment for the chronic fatigue syndrome (Editorial; Comment). Am. J. Med. 89:551, 1990.
110. Straus, S. E., Dale, J. K., Peter, J. B., and Dinarello, C. A.: Circulating lymphokine levels in the chronic fatigue syndrome (Letter). J. Infect. Dis. 160:1085, 1989.
111. Wakefield, D., Lloyd, A., and Brockman, A.: Immunoglobulin subclass abnormalities in patients with chronic fatigue syndrome. Pediatr. Infect. Dis. J. 9:S50, 1990.
112. Klimas, N. G., Salvato, F. R., Morgan, R., and Fletcher, M. A.: Immunologic abnormalities in chronic fatigue syndrome. J. Clin. Microbiol. 28:1403, 1990.
113. Caligiuri, M., Murray, C., Buchwald, D., et al.: Phenotypic and functional deficiency of natural killer cells in patients with chronic fatigue syndrome. J. Immunol. 139:3306, 1987.
114. Prieto, J., Subira, M. L., Castilla, A., and Serrano, M.: Naloxone reversible monocyte dysfunction in patients with chronic fatigue syndrome. Scand. J. Rheumatol. 30:13, 1989.
115. Straus, S. E., Dale, J. K., Tobi, M., Lawley, T., Preble, O., Blaese, R. M., Hallahan, C., and Henle, W.: Acyclovir treatment of the chronic fatigue syndrome: Lack of efficacy in a placebo-controlled trial. N. Engl. J. Med. 319:1692, 1988.
116. Forslind, K., Fredriksson, E., and Nived, O.: Does primary fibromyalgia exist? Br. J. Rheumatol. 29:368, 1990.
117. Perry, F., Heller, P. H., and Levine, J. D.: Differing correlations between pain measures in syndromes with or without explicable organic pathology. Pain 34:185, 1988.
118. Leavitt, F., Katz, R. S., Golden, H. E., Glickman, P. B., and Layfer, L. F.: Comparison of pain properties in fibromyalgia patients and rheumatoid arthritis patients. Arthritis Rheum. 29:775, 1986.
119. Nolli, M., Ghirelli, L., and Ferraccioli, G. F.: Pain language in fibromyalgia, rheumatoid arthritis and osteoarthritis. Clin. Exp. Rheumatol. 6:27, 1988.
120. Callahan, L. F., and Pincus, T.: A clue from a self-report questionnaire to distinguish rheumatoid arthritis from noninflammatory diffuse musculoskeletal pain: The P-VAS:D-ADL ratio. Arthritis Rheum. 33:1317, 1990.
121. Yunus, M. B., Masi, A. T., and Aldag, J. C.: Short term effects of ibuprofen in primary fibromyalgia syndrome: A double blind, placebo controlled trial [Erratum appears in J. Rheumatol. 16:855, 1989]. J. Rheumatol. 16:527, 1989.
122. Clark, S., Tindall, E., and Bennett, R. M.: A double blind crossover trial of prednisone versus placebo in the treatment of fibrositis. J. Rheumatol. 12:980, 1985.

123. Felson, D. T., and Goldenberg, D. L.: The natural history of fibromyalgia. Arthritis Rheum. 29:1522, 1986.
124. Ongchi, D. R., Dill, E. R., and Katz, R. S.: How often do fibromyalgia patients improve (Abstract)? Arthritis Rheum. 33:S136, 1990.
125. Masi, A. T., and Yunus, M. B.: Fibromyalgia: Which is the best treatment? A personalized, comprehensive, ambulatory, patient-involved management programme. Baillieres Clin. Rheumatol. 4:333, 1990.
126. Bennett, R. M.: Beyond fibromyalgia: Ideas on etiology and treatment. J. Rheumatol. Suppl. 19:185, 1989.
127. Bennett, R. M.: Physical fitness and muscle metabolism in the fibromyalgia syndrome: An overview. J. Rheumatol. Suppl. 19:28, 1989.
128. Bennett, R. M.: Muscle physiology and cold reactivity in the fibromyalgia syndrome. Rheum. Dis. Clin. North Am. 15:135, 1989.
129. Bennett, R. M.: Etiology of the fibromyalgia syndrome: A contemporary hypothesis. Intern. Med. Special. 11:48, 1990.
130. Griffin, S. J., and Trinder, J.: Physical fitness, exercise and human sleep. Psychophysiology 15:447, 1978.
131. Shapiro, C. M., Bortz, R., Mitchell, D., Bartel, P., and Jooste, P.: Slow-wave sleep: A recovery period after exercise. Science 214:1253, 1981.
132. Idzikowksi, C., Mills, F. J., and Glennard, R.: 5-Hydroxytryptamine-2 antagonist increases human slow wave sleep. Brain Res. 378:164, 1986.
133. Willner, P.: Antidepressants and serotonergic neurotransmission: An integrative review. Psychopharmacology 85:387, 1985.
134. McCain, G. A.: Role of physical fitness training in the fibrositis/fibromyalgia syndrome. Am. J. Med. 81:73, 1986.
135. Herne, J. A.: Sleep and body restitution. Experientia 36:11, 1980.
136. Adam, K.: Sleep as restorative process and a theory to explain why. Prog. Brain Res. 53:289, 1980.
137. Adam, K., and Oswald, I.: Sleep is for tissue restoration. J. R. Coll. Phys. 11:376, 1977.
138. Krueger, S. M., and Karnovsky, M. L.: Sleep and the immune response. Ann. N.Y. Acad. Sci. 496:510, 1987.
139. Moldofsky, H.: Sleep and fibrositis syndrome. Rheum. Dis. Clin. North Am. 15:91, 1989.
140. Klug, G. A., McAuley, E., and Clark, S.: Factors influencing the development and maintenance of aerobic fitness: Lessons applicable to the fibrositis syndrome. J. Rheumatol. Suppl. 19:30, 1989.
141. Isomaki, H.: The sauna and rheumatic diseases. Ann. Clin. Res. 20:271, 1988.
142. Sheon, R. P., Moskowitz, R. W., and Goldberg, V. M.: Intralesional soft tissue injection technique. In Soft Tissue Rheumatic Pain: Recognition, Management, Prevention. Philadelphia, Lea & Febiger, 1987, p. 293.
143. Hudson, J. I., Hudson, M. S., Pliner, L. F., Goldenberg, D. L., and Pope, H. G., Jr.: Fibromyalgia and major affective disorder: A controlled phenomenology and family history study. Am. J. Psychiatr. 142:441, 1985.
144. Ahles, T. A., Yunus, M. B., Riley, S. D., Bradley, J. M., and Masi, A. T.: Psychological factors associated with primary fibromyalgia syndrome. Arthritis Rheum. 27:1101, 1984.
145. Wolfe, F., Cathey, M. A., Kleinheksel, S. M., Amos, S. P., Hoffman, R. G., Young, D. Y., and Hawley, D. J.: Psychological status in primary fibrositis and fibrositis associated with rheumatoid arthritis. J. Rheumatol. 11:500, 1984.
146. Burckhardt, C. S., Wiens, A. N., O'Reilly, C. A., Clark, S. R., Campbell, S. M., and Bennett, R. M.: Psychological status of women with fibromyalgia (FMS) (Abstract). Arthritis Rheum. 33:S136, 1990.
147. Goldenberg, D. L., Hudson, I. T., Keck, P. E., and Pope, H. G.: Depression, panic disorder, migraine and irritable bowel syndrome in patients with fibromyalgia syndrome (FIB) (Abstract). Arthritis Rheum. 33:S136, 1990.
148. Gaston-Johansson, F., Gustafsson, M., Felldin, R., and Sanne, H.: A comparative study of feelings, attitudes and behaviors of patients with fibromyalgia and rheumatoid arthritis. Soc. Sci. Med. 31:941, 1990.
149. Burckhardt, C. S., Clark, S. R., and Bennett, R. M.: The impact of fibromyalgia on quality of life: A comparative analysis. J. Rheumatol. 1992 (in press).
150. Dailey, P. A., Bishop, G. D., Russell, I. J., and Fletcher, E. M.: Psychological stress and the fibrositis/fibromyalgia syndrome. J. Rheumatol. 17:1380, 1990.
151. Uveges, J. M., Parker, J. C., Smarr, K. L., McGowan, J. F., Lyon, M. G., Irvin, W. S., Meyer, A. A., Buckelew, S. P., Morgan, R. K., Delmonico, R. L., Hewett, J. E., and Kay, D. R.: Psychological symptoms in primary fibromyalgia syndrome: Relationship to pain, life stress, and sleep disturbance. Arthritis Rheum. 33:1279, 1990.
152. Bradley, L. A.: Cognitive-behavioral therapy for primary fibromyalgia. J. Rheumatol. Suppl. 19:131, 1989.
153. Littlejohn, G. O.: Fibrositis/fibromyalgia syndrome in the workplace. Rheum. Dis. Clin. North Am. 15:45, 1989.
154. McCain, G. A., Cameron, R., and Kennedy, J. C.: The problem of longterm disability payments and litigation in primary fibromyalgia: The Canadian perspective. J. Rheumatol. 16 Suppl. 19:174, 1989.

155. Cathey, M. A., Wolfe, F., Kleinheksel, S. M., et al.: Functional ability and work status in patients with fibromyalgia. Arthritis Care Res. 1:85, 1988.
156. Cathey, M. A., Wolfe, F., Kleinheksel, S. M., and Hawley, D. J.: Socioeconomic impact of fibrositis: A study of 81 patients with primary fibrositis. Am. J. Med. 81:78, 1986.
157. Cathey, M. A., Wolfe, F., Roberts, F. K., Bennett, R. M., Caro, X., Goldenberg, D. L., Russell, I. J., and Yunus, M. B.: Demographic, work disability, service utilization and treatment characteristics of 620 fibromyalgia patients in rheumatologic practice (Abstract). Arthritis Rheum. 33:S10, 1990.
158. Hawley, D. J., Wolfe, F., and Cathey, M. A.: Pain, functional disability, and psychological status: A 12-month study of severity in fibromyalgia. J. Rheumatol. 15:1551, 1988.
159. Romano, T. J.: Clinical experiences with post-traumatic fibromyalgia syndrome. W.V. Med. J. 86:198, 1990.
160. Hart, F. D.: Fibrositis (fibromyalgia): A common non-entity? Drugs 35:320, 1988.
161. Beetham, W. P. J.: Diagnosis and management of fibrositis syndrome and psychogenic rheumatism. Med. Clin. North Am. 63:433, 1979.
162. Rotes-Querol, J.: The syndromes of psychogenic rheumatism. Clin. Rheum. Dis. 5:797, 1979.
163. Reynolds, M. D.: Psychogenic rheumatism and fibrositis (Letter). Arthritis Rheum. 28:1435, 1985.
164. Boland, E. W.: Psychogenic rheumatism: The musculoskeletal expression of psychoneurosis. Ann. Rheum. Dis. 6:195, 1947.
165. Colton, R. S.: Psychogenic rheumatism. Minn. Med. 64:365, 1981.
166. Merskey, H.: Physical and psychological considerations in the classification of fibromyalgia. J. Rheumatol. Suppl. 19:72, 1989.
167. Turk, D. C., and Flor, H.: Primary fibromyalgia is greater than tender points: Toward a multiaxial taxonomy. J. Rheumatol. Suppl. 19:80, 1989.
168. Moldofsky, H., Scarisbrick, P., England, R., and Smythe, H.: Musculoskeletal symptoms and non-REM sleep disturbance in patients with "fibrositis syndrome" and healthy subjects. Psychosom. Med. 37:341, 1975.
169. Molony, R. R., MacPeek, D. M., Schiffman, P. L., Frank, M., Neubauer, J. A., Schwartzberg, M., and Seibold, J. R.: Sleep, sleep apnea and the fibromyalgia syndrome. J. Rheumatol. 13:797, 1986.
170. Ware, J. C., Russel, J., and Campos, E.: Alpha intrusions into the sleep of depressed and fibromyalgia syndrome (fibrositis) patients. Sleep Res. 15:210, 1986.
171. Shackell, B. S., Horne, J. A.: The alpha sleep anomaly and related phenomena. Sleep Res. 16:432, 1987.
172. Gupta, M. A., and Moldofsky, H.: Dysthymic disorder and rheumatic pain modulation disorder (fibrositis syndrome): A comparison of symptoms and sleep physiology. Can. J. Psychiatr. 31:608, 1986.
173. Saskin, P., Moldofsky, H., and Lue, F. A.: Sleep and posttraumatic rheumatic pain modulation disorder (fibrositis syndrome). Psychosom. Med. 48:319, 1986.
174. Hauri, P., and Hawkins, D. R.: Alpha-delta sleep. Electroencephalogr. Clin. Neurophysiol. 34:233, 1973.
175. Dumermuth, G., Walz, W., and Lavizzari, G. S.: Spectral analysis of EEG activity in different sleep stages in normal adults. Eur. Neurol. 7:265, 1972.
176. Scheuler, W., Stinshoff, D., and Kubicki, S.: The alpha sleep pattern. Neuropsychobiol. 10:183, 1983.
177. Scheuler, W., Kubicki, S., and Marquardt, J.: The alpha sleep pattern-quantitative analysis and functional aspects. In Koella, W. P., Obal, F., and Schulz, H., (eds.): Sleep. Stuggart, Gustav Fischer Verlag, 1988, p. 86.
178. Moldofsky, H., Lue, F. A., and Smythe, H. A.: Sleep and morning symptoms in rheumatoid arthritis. J. Rheumatol. 10:373, 1983.
179. Moldofsky, H.: Sleep influences on regional and diffuse pain syndromes associated with osteoarthritis. Semin. Arthritis Rheum. 18:18, 1989.
180. Moldofsky, H., Lue, F. A., and Saskin, P.: Sleep and morning pain in primary osteoarthritis. J. Rheumatol. 14:124, 1987.
181. Moldofsky, H., Tullis, C., Lue, F. A., Quance, G., and Davidson, J.: Sleep-related myoclonus in rheumatic pain modulation disorder (fibrositis syndrome) and in excessive daytime somnolence. Psychosom. Med. 46:145, 1984.
182. Moldofsky, H., Tullis, C., and Lue, F. A.: Sleep related myoclonus in rheumatic pain modulation disorder (fibrositis syndrome). J. Rheumatol. 13:614, 1986.
183. Moldofsky, H., and Scarisbrick, P.: Induction of neurasthenic musculoskeletal pain syndrome by selective sleep stage deprivation. Psychosom. Med. 38:35, 1976.
184. Jones, B. E.: The sleep-wake cycle: Basic mechanisms. J. Rheumatol. 16:49, 1989.
185. Moldofsky, H.: Rheumatic pain modulation syndrome: The interrelationships between sleep, central nervous system serotonin, and pain. Adv. Neurol. 33:51, 1982.
186. Chase, T. N., and Murphy, D. I.: Serotonin and central nervous system function. Annu. Rev. Pharmacol. Toxicol. 13:181, 1983.
187. Sicuteri, F., Anselmi, B., Del Bene, E., and Galli, P.: 5-Hydroxytryptamine and pain modulation in man: A clinical pharmacological approach with tryptophan and parachlorophenylalanine. Acta Vitaminol. Enzymol. 29:66, 1975.
188. Moldofsky, H., and Warsh, J. J.: Plasma tryptophan and musculoskeletal pain in non-articular rheumatism ("fibrositis syndrome"). Pain 5:65, 1978.
189. Houvenagel, E., Forzy, G., Cortet, B., and Vincent, G.: 5-Hydroxy indol acetic acid in cerebro spinal fluid in fibromyalgia. Arthritis Rheum. 33:S55, 1990.
190. Russell, I. J., Vaeroy, H., Javors, M., and Nyberg, F.: Cerebrospinal fluid biogenic amines in fibrositis/fibromyalgia syndrome. Arthritis Rheum. 33:S55, 1990.
191. Tariot, P. N., Yocum, D., and Kalin, N. H.: Psychiatric disorders in fibromyalgia (Letter). Am. J. Psychiatry 143:812, 1986.
192. Ahles, T. A., Yunus, M. B., Gaulier, B., Riley, S. D., and Masi, A. T.: The use of contemporary MMPI norms in the study of chronic pain patients. Pain 24:159, 1986.
193. Goldenberg, D. L.: Psychological symptoms and psychiatric diagnosis in patients with fibromyalgia. J. Rheumatol. Suppl. 19:127, 1989.
194. Uveges, J. M., Parker, J. C., Smarr, K. L., McGowan, J. F., Lyon, M. G., Irvin, W. S., Meyer, A. A., Buckelew, S. P., Morgan, R. K., Delmonico, R. L., Hewett, J. E., and Kay, D. R.: Psychological symptoms in primary fibromyalgia syndrome: Relationship to pain, life stress, and sleep disturbance. Arthritis Rheum. 33:1279, 1990.
195. Robbins, J. M., Kirmayer, L. J., and Kapusta, M. A.: Illness worry and disability in fibromyalgia syndrome. Int. J. Psychiatry Med. 20:49, 1990.
196. Hudson, J. I., and Pope, H. G., Jr.: Fibromyalgia and psychopathology: Is fibromyalgia a form of "affective spectrum disorder?" J. Rheumatol. Suppl. 19:15, 1989.
197. Clark, S., Campbell, S. M., Forehand, M. E., Tindall, E. A., and Bennett, R. M.: Clinical characteristics of fibrositis: II. A "blinded," controlled study using standard psychological tests. Arthritis Rheum. 28:132, 1985.
198. Darby, P. L., and Schmidt, P. J.: Psychiatric consultations in rheumatology: A review of 100 cases. Can. J. Psychiatry 33:290, 1988.
199. Kirmayer, L. J., Robbins, J. M., Kapusta, M. A.: Somatization and depression in fibromyalgia syndrome. Am. J. Psychiatry 145:950, 1988.
200. Fishbain, D. A., Goldberg, M., Steele, R., and Rosomoff, H.: DSM-III diagnoses of patients with myofascial pain syndrome (fibrositis). Arch. Phys. Med. Rehabil. 70:433, 1989.
201. Wells, K. B., Golding, J. M., and Burnam, M. A.: Psychiatric disorder in a sample of the general population with and without chronic medical conditions. Am. J. Psychiatry 145:976, 1988.
202. Yunus, M. B., Ahles, T. A., Aldag, J. A., and Masi, A. T.: Relationship of clinical features with psychological status in primary fibromyalgia. Arthritis Rheum. 34:15, 1991.
203. Yunus, M. B., and Kalyan-Raman, U. P.: Muscle biopsy findings in primary fibromyalgia and other forms of nonarticular rheumatism. Rheum. Dis. Clin. North Am. 15:115, 1989.
204. Henriksson, K. G.: Muscle pain in neuromuscular disorders and primary fibromyalgia. Eur. J. Appl. Physiol. 57:348, 1988.
205. Kalyan Raman, U. P., Kalyan Raman, K., Yunus, M. B., and Masi, A. T.: Muscle pathology in primary fibromyalgia syndrome: A light microscopic, histochemical and ultrastructural study. J. Rheumatol. 11:808, 1984.
206. Jacobsen, S., Bartels, E. M., and Danneskiold-Samsøe, B.: Single cell morphology of muscle in patients with chronic muscle pain. Scand. J. Rheumatol. 20:336, 1991.
207. Bengtsson, A., Henriksson, K. G., and Larsson, J.: Reduced high-energy phosphate levels in the painful muscles of patients with primary fibromyalgia. Arthritis Rheum. 29:817, 1986.
208. Larsson, S. E., Bengtsson, A., Bodegard, L., Henriksson, K. G., and Larsson, J.: Muscle changes in work-related chronic myalgia. Acta Orthop. Scand. 59:74, 1988.
209. Lund, N., Bengtsson, A., and Thorborg, P.: Muscle tissue oxygen pressure in primary fibromyalgia. Scand. J. Rheumatol. 15:165, 1986.
210. Bennett, R. M., Clark, S. R., Goldberg, L., Nelson, D., Bonafede, R. P., Porter, J., and Specht, D.: Aerobic fitness in patients with fibrositis: A controlled study of respiratory gas exchange and 133xenon clearance from exercising muscle. Arthritis Rheum. 32:454, 1989.
211. Klemp, P., Nielsen, H. V., Korsgard, J., et al.: Blood flow in fibromyotic muscles. Scand. J. Rehabil. Med. 14:81, 1982.
212. Zidar, J., Bäckman, E., Bengtsson, A., and Henriksson, K. G.: Quantitative EMG and muscle tension in painful muscles in fibromyalgia. Pain 40:249, 1990.
213. Jacobsen, S., and Danneskiold Samse, B.: Isometric and isokinetic muscle strength in patients with fibrositis syndrome: New characteristics for a difficult definable category of patients. Scand. J. Rheumatol. 16:61, 1987.
214. Jacobsen, S., Wildschiodtz, G., and Danneskiold-Samsoe, B.: Isokinetic and isometric muscle strength combined with direct electrical muscle stimulation in primary fibromyalgia syndrome. J. Rheumatol. 18:1390, 1991.

215. Stokes, M. J., Cooper, R. G., and Edwards, R. H. T.: Normal muscle strength and fatiguability in patients with effort syndromes. Br. Med. J. 297:1014, 1988.
216. Guedj, D., and Weinberger, A.: Effect of weather conditions on rheumatic patients. Ann. Rheum. Dis. 49:158, 1990.
217. Vaeroy, H., Helle, R., Forre, O., Kass, E., and Terenius, L.: Elevated CSF levels of substance P and high incidence of Raynaud phenomenon in patients with fibromyalgia: New features for diagnosis. Pain 32:21, 1988.
218. Ingram, S., Nelson, D., Porter, J., Bennett, R. M., et al.: An association of cold induced vasospasm and fibrositis. Arthritis Rheum. 30:513, 1987.
219. Hudson, J. I., Pliner, L. F., Hudson, M. S., Goldenberg, D. L., and Melby, J. C.: The dexamethasone suppression test in fibrositis. Biol. Psychiatry 19:1489, 1984.
220. Ferraccioli, G., Cavalieri, F., Salaffi, F., Fontana, S., Scita, F., Nolli, M., and Maestri, D.: Neuroendocrinologic findings in primary fibromyalgia (soft tissue chronic pain syndrome) and in other chronic rheumatic conditions (rheumatoid arthritis, low back pain). J. Rheumatol. 17:869, 1990.
221. McCain, G. A., and Tilbe, K. S.: Diurnal hormone variation in fibromyalgia syndrome: A comparison with rheumatoid arthritis. J. Rheumatol. Suppl. 19:154, 1989.
222. Littlejohn, G. O., Weinstein, C., and Helme, R. D.: Increased neurogenic inflammation in fibrositis syndrome. J. Rheumatol. 14:1022, 1987.
223. Caro, X. J.: Immunofluorescent detection of IgG at the dermal-epidermal junction in patients with apparent primary fibrositis syndrome. Arthritis Rheum. 27:1174, 1984.
224. Caro, X. J.: Immunofluorescent studies of skin in primary fibrositis syndrome. Am. J. Med. 81:43, 1986.
225. Caro, X. J., Wolfe, F., Johnston, W. H., and Smith, A. L.: A controlled and blinded study of immunoreactant deposition at the dermal-epidermal junction of patients with primary fibrositis syndrome. J. Rheumatol. 13:1086, 1986.
226. Enestrom, S., Bengtson, A., Lindstrom, F., and Johan, K.: Attachment of IgG to dermal extracellular matrix in patients with fibromyalgia. Clin. Exp. Rheumatol. 8:127, 1990.
227. Russell, I. J., Vipraio, G. A., Tovar, Z., et al.: Abnormal natural killer cell activity in fibrositis syndrome is responsive in vitro IL-2. Arthritis Rheum. 31:S24, 1988.
228. Russell, I. J., Vipraio, G. A., Michalek, J., et al.: Abnormal T cell subpopulations in fibrositis syndrome. Arthritis Rheum. 31:S99, 1988.
229. Peter, J. B., and Wallace, D. J.: Abnormal immune regulation in fibromyalgia. Arthritis Rheum. 31:S24, 1988.
230. Bengtsson, A., Ernerudh, J., Vrethem, M., and Skogh, T.: Absence of autoantibodies in primary fibromyalgia. J. Rheumatol. 17:1682, 1990.
231. Moldofsky, H., Lue, F. A., Davidson, J. R., and Gorczynski, R.: Effects of sleep deprivation on human immune functions. F.A.S.E.B. J. 3:1972, 1989.
232. Moldofsky, H., Lue, F. A., and Saskin, P.: The effect of sleep deprivation on immune functions in humans: II. Interleukin-1 and 2–like activities. Sleep Res. 17:34, 1988.
233. Moldofsky, H., Lue, F. A., and Saskin, P.: The effect of sleep deprivation on immune functions in humans: I. Mitogen and natural killer activities. Sleep Res. 16:531, 1987.
234. Jacobsen, S., Jensen, L. T., Foldager, M., and Danneskiold-Samsoe, B.: Primary fibromyalgia: Clinical parameters in relation to serum procollagen type III aminoterminal peptide. Br. J. Rheumatol. 29:174, 1990.
235. Danneskiold-Samsoe, B., Christiansen, E., Lund, B., and Anderson, R. B.: Regional muscle tension and pain ("fibrositis"): Effect of massage on myoglobin in plasma. Scand. J. Rehabil. Med. 15:17, 1983.
236. Solomon, Z., Mikolincer, M., and Kotler, M.: A two year follow up of somatic complaints among Israeli combat stress reaction casualties. J. Psychosom. Res. 31:463, 1987.
237. Simms, R. W., Ferrante, N., and Craven, D. E.: High prevalence of fibromyalgia syndrome (FMS) in human immunodeficiency virus type 1 (HIV) infected patients with polyarthralgia (Abstract). Arthritis Rheum. 33:S136, 1990.
238. Rowe, I. F., Forster, S. M., Seifert, M. H., Youle, M. S., Hawkins, D. A., Lawrence, A. G., and Keat, A. C.: Rheumatological lesions in individuals with human immunodeficiency virus infection. Q. J. Med. 73:1167, 1989.
239. Buskila, D., Gladman, D. D., Langevitz, P., Urowitz, S., and Smythe, H. A.: Fibromyalgia in human immunodeficiency virus infection. J. Rheumatol. 17:1202, 1990.
240. Dinerman, H., and Steere, A. C.: Fibromyalgia following Lyme disease: Association with neurologic involvement and lack of response to antibiotic therapy (Abstract). Arthritis Rheum. 33:S136, 1990.
241. Brier, S. R.: Lyme disease. J. Manipulative Physiol. Ther. 13:337, 1990.
242. Logigian, E. L., Kaplan, R. F., and Steere, A. C.: Chronic neurologic manifestations of Lyme disease. N. Engl. J. Med. 323:1438, 1990.
243. Tarnapolsky, A., Watkin, G., and Hand, D. J.: Aircraft noise and mental health: I. Prevalence of individual symptoms. Psychol. Med. 10:683, 1980.
244. Nash, P., Chard, M., and Hazleman, B.: Chronic coxsackie B infection mimicking primary fibromyalgia. J. Rheumatol. 16:1506, 1989.
245. Weisman, M. H., Vecchione, T. R., Albert, D., Moore, L. T., and Mueller, M. R.: Connective tissue disease following breast augmentation: A preliminary test of the human adjuvant disease hypothesis. Plast. Reconstr. Surg. 82:626, 1988.
246. Wallace, D. J., Margolin, K., and Waller, P.: Fibromyalgia and interleukin-2 therapy for malignancy (Letter). Ann. Intern. Med. 108:909, 1988.
247. Alonso-Ruiz, A., de la Hoz-Martinez, A., Zea-Mendoza, A. C.: Fibromyalgia syndrome as a late complication of toxic-oil syndrome (Letter). J. Rheumatol. 12:1207, 1985.
248. Pellegrino, M. J., Waylonis, G. W., and Sommer, A.: Familial occurrence of primary fibromyalgia. Arch. Phys. Med. Rehabil. 70:61, 1989.
249. Simons, D. G.: Familial fibromyalgia and/or myofascial pain syndrome (Comment)? Arch. Phys. Med. Rehabil. 71:258, 1990.

Chapter 30

Joel M. Kremer

Nutrition and Rheumatic Diseases

INTRODUCTION

Although it has been appreciated for some time that disease processes can interfere with adequate nutrition, we are only beginning to understand how altered nutritional status may contribute to the pathogenesis of disease. As a corollary, we can now say that certain dietary manipulations may result in improvements in the inflammatory disease process. These principles represent an evolution of thinking from the relatively recent past when contributors to the field were stating that it was extremely unlikely that dietary manipulation could affect patients with inflammatory disease. Indeed, an informational bulletin of the Arthritis Foundation states, "The simple proven fact is: no food has anything to do with causing arthritis and no food is effective in treating or 'curing' it."[1] In spite of such pronouncements, appreciation of the possible role of nutritional manipulations in inflammatory disease has increased, along with the significant enhanced understanding of immunity, eicosanoid metabolism, and cellular biology.[2, 3] Epidemiologic studies have confirmed the role of diet in other disease processes such as vascular and gastrointestinal disease.[4, 5, 5a, 5b] Surprisingly, improvements in rates of mortality from cardiovascular disease in some large population studies are not linked solely to favorable changes in cholesterol, hypertension, or smoking profiles but to alteration of other biologic processes through the intake of dietary fatty acids.[6] Simultaneous with the emergence of data on the role of diet in disease states is the realization that our current dietary habits are indeed altered from the diet to which our species has adapted over almost the entire span of human history[7] (Table 30–1). Circumstantial evidence has linked an increased incidence of cancer and cardiovascular and gastrointestinal disease to high-fat, low-fiber diets.

NUTRITION IN RHEUMATOID ARTHRITIS

Interest in the possible role of nutrition in the pathogenesis of the rheumatic diseases is not new. Analysis of dietary intake in the period prior to the onset of rheumatoid arthritis[8] indicated that there were no significant differences in diet between patients who developed arthritis and a control population. When the nutritional status of patients with rheumatoid arthritis was compared with those with osteoarthritis,[9] patients with osteoarthritis were found to be 15 lb overweight on average, whereas rheumatoid patients averaged 10.3 lb underweight.

Table 30–1. COMPARISON OF THE LATE PALEOLITHIC DIET, CURRENT AMERICAN DIET, AND U.S. DIETARY RECOMMENDATIONS

	Late Paleolithic Diet	Current American Diet	U.S. Senate Select Committee Recommendations*
Total dietary energy (%)			
Protein	34	12	12
Carbohydrate	45	46	58
Fat	21	42	30
P:S ratio	1.41	0.44	1
Cholesterol (mg)	591	600	300
Fiber (g)	45.7	19.7	30–60
Sodium (mg)	690	2300–6900	1100–3300
Calcium (mg)	1580	740	800–1200
Ascorbic acid (mg)	392.3	87.7	45

*Select Committee on Nutrition and Human Needs, United States Senate: Dietary Goals for the United States. Washington, D.C., Government Printing Office, 1977.

P:S, polyunsaturated:saturated fats.

From Eaton, S. B., and Konner, M.: Paleolithic nutrition. A consideration of its nature and current implications. N. Engl. J. Med. 312:283, 1985. Reprinted with permission from *The New England Journal of Medicine*.

Deficient dietary intake of folic acid, zinc, magnesium, and pyridoxine have been described in patients with rheumatoid arthritis.[10, 11]

A nutritional assessment of 50 patients with rheumatoid arthritis was performed using anthropometric measurements, including triceps skinfold thickness and body-mass index calculated from height, weight, and upper arm muscle circumference (UAMC), as well as biochemical measurements of nutrition.[12] Thirteen patients (26 per cent) were found to be malnourished. Malnourished patients were more likely to have severe rheumatoid arthritis than those without malnutrition. Decreased weight and triceps skinfold thickness occurred twice as frequently as a significant reduction in UAMC. No differences in dietary intake were found for those who were malnourished, which suggested that the increased demand of the inflammatory state placed a greater burden on the metabolism of certain essential nutrients.

JUVENILE ARTHRITIS

Biochemical and anthropometric measurements were examined in 26 11- to 16-year-old girls with juvenile chronic arthritis and matched healthy control subjects.[13, 14] UAMC and serum creatinine were lower in the children with arthritis. Significant inverse correlations were observed between disease activity and concentrations of albumin, prealbumin, and retinol-binding protein. Using the same definition of malnutrition as in the study of adult rheumatoid patients previously discussed,[12] researchers found five girls with chronic arthritis (19 per cent) fit their definition of malnutrition. An analysis of nutrient intake by means of a 4-day dietary history in the same population failed to reveal any significant differences from controls. Children with arthritis, however, were noted to derive a greater percentage of their energy requirements from fat and a lower percentage from carbohydrates than controls.

Independent investigations have reached similar conclusions regarding the nutritional status of patients with rheumatoid and juvenile chronic arthritis: patients with active disease require increased dietary energy and protein and frequently exhibit deficiencies in micronutrients, including selenium, zinc, magnesium, and vitamins C and A. They have a high intake of fat and, in particular, saturated fatty acids that could have significant effects on immune function. These nutritional alterations may at times be associated with frank malnutrition. Considerable potential may exist for improving general well-being with a greater attention to the overall nutritional status of patients with rheumatic problems.[14a, 14b, 14c]

FREE RADICALS AND NUTRITION

A compound with unpaired free electrons is termed a *free radical*, and some of the most reactive

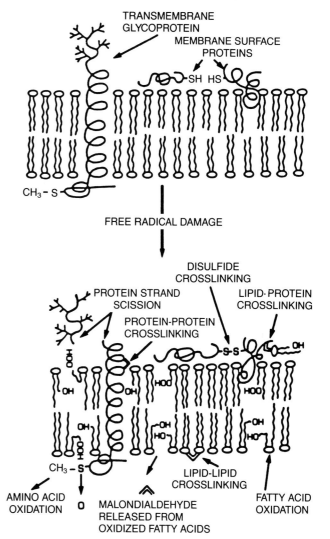

Figure 30–1. Free radical damage to lipid membranes and proteins associated with cell membranes. (From Bendich, A.: Antioxidant micronutrients and immune functions. Ann. N.Y. Acad. Sci. 587:168–180, 1990. Used by permission.)

of these compounds contain oxygen. Free radicals abstract electrons from stable compounds in an attempt to stabilize themselves and in the process create new free radicals.[15] The rapidly proliferating cells of the immune system are uniquely prone to oxidative damage from free radicals, which can also affect the activity of thromboxane (TX), prostaglandin (PG), and leukotriene species.[16]

The phospholipid bilayer of cell membranes contains polyunsaturated fatty acids that can be common sites for free radical reactions (Fig. 30–1). Membrane damage from lipid peroxidation results in the formation of unstable lipid peroxyl radicals, which can further damage the membrane in a snowball-like effect.[15] Potentially toxic products of lipid membrane peroxidation include molondialdehyde, volatile substances such as ethane and pentane, cross-linked membrane lipids, conjugated dienes, and protein-lipid adducts.[17]

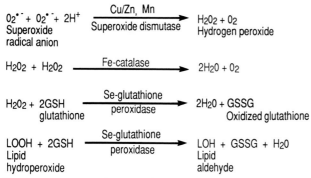

Figure 30–2. Antioxidant metalloenzyme reactions. Nutritionally essential elements are not antioxidants until they are incorporated into their metalloenzyme ligand. Cu = copper; Zn = zinc; Mn = manganese; Fe = iron; Se = selenium. (From Bendich, A.: Antioxidant micronutrients and immune functions. Ann. N.Y. Acad. Sci. 587:168–180, 1990. Used by permission.)

Free radicals are also essential to normal immune competence.[18, 19] Intracellular free radical production is part of the host response necessary for the killing of invading micro-organisms. Free radical reactions are associated with the release of arachidonic acid and the conversion of arachidonate to eicosanoids and subsequent eicosanoid metabolism.[20] These substances are, in turn, essential in the functioning of a normal immune system.[21] When considering the production and modulation of free radicals, therefore, the critical issue is the balance between potentially destructive reactions and naturally occurring free radical generation, which is essential for normal immune competence.

There are several naturally occurring enzymes that serve to inactivate reactive oxygen molecules. Antioxidant metalloenzymes interfere with the production of free radicals by inactivating precursor molecules. Superoxide dismutase exists in two forms, and either can inactivate the superoxide anion. There is a manganese-containing superoxide dismutase in mitochondria and a copper-zinc–containing superoxide dismutase in the cytoplasm (Fig. 30–2). Both of these reactions produce H_2O_2. An iron-containing catalase found in cytoplasmic peroxisomes catalyzes the decomposition of H_2O_2 to oxygen and water. Selenium is an essential component of two glutathione peroxidases that inactivate H_2O_2, lipid peroxides, and phospholipid peroxides.

The nutritionally essential mineral elements copper, zinc, iron, manganese, and selenium are not antioxidants until they are incorporated into the antioxidant enzymes.[15] Further addition of these elements to the system by dietary intake does not enhance the activity of the antioxidative enzymes once the system is saturated. Circulating levels of these enzymes are low when compared with intracellular concentrations. The balance between extracellular free radical formation and release and antioxidant enzyme protection may be important in the inflammation and tissue destruction of several immune-mediated inflammatory diseases.

ANTIOXIDANT VITAMINS

Vitamin A

Adequate amounts of dietary vitamin A are required for normal growth and development. Vitamin A is also necessary for adequate hematopoiesis. Severe infections in vitamin A–deficient animals have recently been shown to correlate with depressed helper T lymphocyte activity.[22] Vitamin A itself is a poor antioxidant compared with beta (β) carotene or vitamin E and cannot inactivate free oxygen radicals.[23]

Vitamin A is transported from the liver to tissues by retinol-binding protein, a specific transport protein whose levels reflect the amount of vitamin A available to the tissues. Retinol-binding protein is low in protein energy malnutrition. It is also low in patients with rheumatoid arthritis[12] and active ankylosing spondylitis.[24] Zinc is necessary for a normal vitamin A concentration in plasma due to its key role in the synthesis of retinol-binding protein. A study of 61 patients with rheumatoid arthritis demonstrated reduced levels of vitamin A, which correlated significantly with depressed levels of both retinol-binding protein and zinc by regression analysis.[25]

β Carotene

The carotenoids are red-yellow pigments found in all photosynthesizing plants. There are more than 500 carotenoids, but only a small number of these compounds can be synthesized to vitamin A. Cleavage of β carotene, however, results in two molecules of vitamin A, making it unique among the carotenoids. In contrast to vitamin A, β carotene is a potent antioxidant and can also function as an immunostimulant. Enhancement of activation markers of human peripheral blood mononuclear cells was observed in vitro after exposure to carotenoids.[26] In models of animal tumorigenesis, both cytotoxic T lymphocyte functions and macrophage secretion of tumor necrosis factor were increased following carotenoid administration.[27] These findings are part of a body of evidence that suggests that carotenoid ingestion is associated with important chemoprotective effects that are separate from their provitamin A activity.[23]

Vitamin E

Vitamin E (alpha [α] tocopherol) is the major lipid-soluble antioxidant found in cells. Vitamin E protects the unsaturated double bonds of the fatty acids in the phospholipid bilayer from oxidation. It accomplishes this task by donating electrons to lipid peroxide and other radicals, and in this way can interrupt the chain reaction of free radical damage to the cell membrane. The antioxidant activity of vitamin E is regenerated by electron donation from vitamin C, glutathione, and other antioxidants. Human lymphocytes are protected from lipid peroxidation when cultured with vitamin E.[28]

Vitamin E is critical to maintaining the normal function of the immune system. T cells are more susceptible to membrane peroxidative damage than B cells, and peroxidative damage has been associated with the loss of certain T cell receptor activities.[29] T cells are therefore more sensitive to vitamin E status, even though vitamin E content of both T and B lymphocytes is more than ten times that found in red blood cells.[30] The macrophage membrane expresses decreased Ia antigen in the vitamin E–deficient state. Phagocytic function is diminished in the presence of vitamin E deficiency in both animal and human studies.[31]

Vitamin C

Vitamin C (ascorbic acid) is water soluble and is important in decreasing free radical reactions in both intracellular and extracellular fluids. It is also required for the hydroxylation of proline and lysine in the production of collagen and is involved in several enzymatic reactions in the formation of neuropeptides. Neutrophils and mononuclear cells maintain concentrations of vitamin C that are approximately 150 times that found in serum.[32] Vitamin C has been shown to increase neutrophil and monocyte chemotaxis in in vitro[33] experimental models. Similar results have been observed in humans ingesting the vitamin.[34]

Plasma and platelet ascorbic acid levels have been demonstrated to be low in patients with rheumatoid arthritis taking high doses of aspirin.[35] The decrease was thought to be from either impaired tissue uptake or increased urinary excretion. Lowered ascorbate levels may be caused by superoxide associated oxidation at inflammatory sites.[36] Scorbutic guinea pigs develop lesions resembling rheumatoid arthropathy, prompting a suggestion that synovial vitamin C deficiency could contribute to rheumatoid synovitis.[35] However, a study of vitamin C supplementation in patients with rheumatoid arthritis failed to show any effect.[37]

Free radicals derived from phagocytes are autotoxic to cells in their immediate environment, causing inhibition of chemotaxis, phagocytosis, and antimicrobial activity.[38] Reactive oxygen species also inhibit proliferation of T and B lymphocytes as well as the cytotoxic activity of natural killer cells.[39] Neutrophil derived production of hydrogen peroxide and hypochlorous acid (HClO) are the most potent mediators of immunosuppression.[40] Ascorbate, at physiologically relevant concentrations, protects neutrophil metabolic activity and function from HClO, but not H_2O_2, mediated inhibition.[41] Ascorbate is the first-line plasma antioxidant in the defense against phagocyte-derived reactive oxidants, and only when it is depleted does lipid peroxidation occur.[42] By neutral-izing granulocyte-derived HClO, ascorbate maintains host defenses by sustaining the function of phagocytes and bystander lymphocytes by protecting them from oxidative damage.[41] Vitamin C may also enhance immune responses indirectly by maintaining optimal levels of vitamin E. It does this by donating an electron to the α tocopherol molecule to reestablish the latter's antioxidant activity.

Vitamin D

Dietary deficiency of vitamin D may contribute to osteopenia in patients with rheumatoid arthritis and has been linked to cortical thinning and spontaneous fractures of long bones in this condition.[43] Recent studies have indicated a possible role of vitamin D supplementation in the treatment of psoriasis.[44] 1,25 (OH)$_2$ D3 has some inhibitory effects in vitro on psoriatic fibroblast proliferation.[45] It has significant effects on the T lymphocyte proliferative response to mitogen stimulation[46] and has demonstrated effects on cytokine production.[47] 1,24 (OH)$_2$ D3 can potentiate the inhibitory effects of cyclosporin A on helper T cells from patients with rheumatoid arthritis.[48] An open, uncontrolled study using increasing dosages of 1,25 (OH)$_2$ D3 over a period of 6 months showed significant improvement in several clinical parameters of disease activity in a small number of patients with psoriatic arthritis completing the study.[49]

TRACE ELEMENTS

Before considering the effects of certain trace elements on the immune response and inflammatory disease, it is appropriate to first examine certain related areas of their metabolism and processing. Copper, zinc, and iron are bound to metallothionein, which are metal-binding proteins found within the intestinal mucosa.[50] Because these different metals compete for binding with the same proteins, there is a reciprocal relationship between high dietary levels of certain elements and a deficiency in others. It has been noted that low levels of dietary zinc result in greatly enhanced copper accumulation in tissues and copper toxicity.[51] This reciprocal relationship has not been observed by all investigators.[52] It is, however, possible that an attempt to ameliorate a deficiency of one of the elements could result in insufficient absorption of another.

Increased circulating levels of the cytokines interleukin-1, interleukin-6 and tumor necrosis factor may affect the availability of trace elements by inducing the production of increased metalloproteinases within the liver and intestine. This increased metalloproteinase production results in sequestration of these elements so that they are less readily available to peripheral tissues.[51] Thus, there may be adequate iron and zinc in the diet of patients with inflammatory disease but inadequate levels at metabolically important sites, with iron bound to increased cytokine-induced ferritin within the macrophages and liver and zinc bound to the excess metallothionein in liver and gut.[53] Teliologically, the cytokine-induced decreased concentrations of iron and zinc may have enhanced host defenses against infection or parasitism because iron is required for bacterial replication and zinc has a natural anti-inflammatory role.[53]

Zinc

Zinc has been known to be an essential element for growth for more than 100 years. It is essential for a large and diverse collection of enzymes involved in multiple areas of normal metabolic functioning. Only iron exceeds zinc in total body tissue concentrations. It is considerably less reactive and less toxic than copper. Dietary sources include protein derived from meat, fish, or dairy products, and total body storage reserves are thought to be somewhat limited. Absorption of zinc is diminished by ingestion of copper or iron. As is the case with iron and copper, increased cytokine production in inflammatory disease can result in increased binding of zinc to metallothioneins and decreased serum and leukocyte zinc concentrations.[54, 55] This may be compounded in patients who consume chronic iron supplementation because this will interfere with zinc absorption.

The unexpected incidence of autoimmune disease after treatment with D-penicillamine has been linked to its ability to chelate zinc, as well as magnesium and pyridoxine.[56] Zinc can function as a lymphocyte mitogen when added in vitro to experimental systems.[57] The process of activation is thought to be initiated through monocyte processing of a zinc-transferrin complex. Zinc has been demonstrated to enhance natural killer cell activity in vitro in the presence of interferon-α or gamma (γ).

The rationale for trials using zinc in inflammatory diseases has been summarized by Whitehouse.[58] It is derived from a collection of evidence showing (1) a tendency for decreased zinc concentrations at critical tissue stores in inflammatory disease; (2) decreased absorption associated with iron therapy; (3) the importance of zinc to normal immune functioning; (4) the tendency of certain drugs such as D-penicillamine and glucocorticoids to suppress zinc concentrations; (5) depressed oral intake of zinc in dietary surveys[11, 12] and serum measurements of patients with rheumatoid arthritis; and (6) the anti-inflammatory effect of zinc complexes in chronic models of inflammation.[59] The clinical studies of zinc supplementation, however, have yielded unconvincing mixed results.[60] A single investigation found that significant reductions in plasma zinc concentrations in women patients with rheumatoid arthritis correlated with the degree of radiographic osteoporosis.[61] Because zinc plays an important role as a cofactor in collagen synthesis, it has been proposed that zinc deficiency contributes to altered collagen metabolism and the osteoporosis seen in patients with rheumatoid arthritis. Researchers in the field retain a good deal of interest in the potential role of zinc therapy in the rheumatic diseases.

Selenium

Selenium was recognized to be an essential nutrient in 1957. It exerts a myriad of effects on the immune system and functions through several different pathways, which have been extensively reviewed.[62] Spallholz and colleagues[63] have summarized its three major functions: (1) reduction of organic and inorganic peroxides; (2) metabolism of hydroperoxides—these compounds are intermediate steps in the metabolism of PGs and leukotrienes derived from arachidonic acid; and (3) modulation of the respiratory burst through the control of superoxide and hydrogen peroxide generation.

The effect of selenium on immune function is derived from the selenium-dependent enzymes glutathione peroxidase and phospholipid-hydroperoxidase. The latter enzyme catalyzes the reduction of lipid hydroperoxides in cellular membranes.[64] Glutathione peroxidase is responsible for antioxidant activities in reactions described earlier in this chapter in the section on free radicals and nutrition (Fig. 30–2). Both enzymes participate in the reduction of PGG_2 in the arachidonic acid cascade leading to the production of $TX-A_2$, prostacyclin, and PGs.[63] They also participate in the production of leukotrienes and lipoxins through the reduction of the hydroperoxy intermediates.[63] Eicosanoid synthesis is significantly diminished in the absence of selenium.[65] It is likely that both the anti-inflammatory and immune-modulating effects of selenium are mediated via the effect of its ligand enzymes on the production of eicosanoids and the reduction of hydroperoxides. Selenium has also been shown to have anticarcinogenic and antitumor activity,[66] and dietary supplementation is associated with increased production of superoxide in an animal model.[67] It may therefore exert cytotoxic, protective, or modulatory effects in different biologic systems.

Because selenium's ligand enzyme glutathione peroxidase catalyzes the reduction of peroxides and increased levels of these reactive elements are found in serum and synovial fluid of some patients with rheumatoid arthritis, there has been some interest in the selenium status of patients with rheumatoid arthritis and other arthritic conditions. There are conflicting reports of selenium–glutathione peroxidase status in patients with rheumatoid arthritis.[68, 69] Some evidence suggests that glucocorticoid administration may result in a reduction of plasma selenium concentrations.[70] Selenium has been administered to patients with rheumatoid arthritis[71] and osteoarthritis[72] without apparent effect. An improved pain score was observed in one study of selenium supplementation in patients with rheumatoid arthritis but not osteoarthritis.[73]

Copper

Copper is an essential nutrient for biologic systems, including the immune system. Copper is present in abundance in the body as it is the third largest trace element found in human tissues after iron and zinc. Free copper ion is rapidly complexed to specific ligands through which it expresses its biologic activity. Most serum copper is bound to ceruloplasmin, which increases as part of the acute-phase response.

The mechanisms of the effects of copper on the immune system are unknown, although several hypotheses are plausible. As mentioned earlier, copper along with zinc and manganese are cofactors in the enzyme superoxide dismutase, which has an essential role in inhibiting free radical damage in tissues and the immune system (Fig. 30–2). In addition, altered glutathione levels have recently been reported in copper-deficient rats.[74] The circulating cuproenzyme ceruloplasmin also has antioxidant properties. Increased levels of ceruloplasmin produced as a result of the acute-phase response to inflammation may directly scavenge superoxide, although this is thought to be inefficient.[58] Of more importance, ceruloplasmin can oxidize Fe^{2+} to Fe^{3+}, thus inhibiting the Fe^{2+}–catalyzed reactions of lipid peroxidation and scavenging of reactive hydroxyl radicals. It also transports copper for synthesis of intracellular copper-zinc superoxide dismutase, which is critical in the reduction of highly reactive oxygen free radical species.

Immune function may be directly affected by effects on two copper-dependent enzymes present within lymphocytes: cytochrome C oxidase and sulfydryl oxidase. The former is important in intracellular energy metabolism, and the latter is located in lymphocyte plasma membranes and is important in pentamer IgM formation and B cell differentration.[75]

Iron

It is generally accepted that asymptomatic tissue iron deficiency is the most common nutritional deficiency in the world. It occurs along with the more severe iron deficiency anemia and is particularly common in infants, children, pregnancy, and menstruating women. Iron-deficient populations have been observed to have a high rate of infectious diseases, which may be paradoxically worsened with iron supplementation. This is thought to be due to the improved replication of many micro-organisms that also require iron for optimal growth.[76]

Iron has many well-documented effects on immune function. The iron-containing enzyme catalase is found in cytoplasmic peroxisomes and catalyzes the decomposition of hydrogen peroxide to water and O_2, protecting the cellular environment from free radical–induced damage (Fig. 30–2). Like zinc, serum levels of iron decrease in inflammation and infection, probably by a mechanism of cytokine-stimulated withdrawal from the circulation and enhanced synthesis of ferritin.[76] The immune effects of iron may be at least partially mediated through alterations in PG synthesis. PG endoperoxide synthase is an iron-dependent enzyme critical in the synthesis of PG species.[76] As PGE_2 can, in turn, regulate the production of interleukin 1, impaired PG production secondary to iron deficiency could affect the production of this important cytokine. The precise mechanism responsible for the effects of iron on the immune response is not currently established and may have to do with a general role in cellular growth and protein synthesis as well as more specific effects on the immune system.

FATTY ACIDS

Background

Fatty acids are designated with a number followed by a colon, another lesser number, the Greek letter omega (ω), and yet another number; for example, 18:2, ω-6. The first number designates the number of carbon atoms in the molecule. The number appearing after the colon represents the number of double bonds. The number after the ω indicates the position of the first double bond starting from the methyl, or omega (ω), end of the fatty acid chain. Linoleic acid, 18:2, ω-6, thus has 18 carbons and 2 double bonds, and the first double bond is found 6 carbon atoms from the terminal methyl group. It is therefore an ω-6 fatty acid. In discussing fatty acid dietary studies in inflammatory disease, we will consider ω-6 and ω-3 intervention separately.

Certain long-chain fatty acids are termed essential in our diet because their deficiency can result in severe growth retardation and death. Early experiments showed that rats fed a fat-free diet failed to grow or reproduce and eventually died. Linoleic acid (18:2, ω-6) was found to be the primary essential fatty acid, together with its derivative ω-6 fatty acid compounds. The ω-3 fatty acids have also been found to be essential. They represent the largest species of fatty acids in the cerebral cortex and retina and can be derived only from the diet. Animals lack two important desaturase enzymes that are present in plants and phytoplankton, which convert the monounsaturate oleic acid (18:1, ω-9) to linoleic acid and linoleic acid to α-linolenic acid (18:3, ω-3). Once animals and humans consume linoleic acid or α-linolenic acid, the basic ω-6 and ω-3 fatty acids, they can then be metabolized to the larger-chain fatty acids, including arachidonic (20:4, ω-6), eicosapentaenoic (20:5, ω-3), and docasahexaenoic acid (22:6, ω-3).

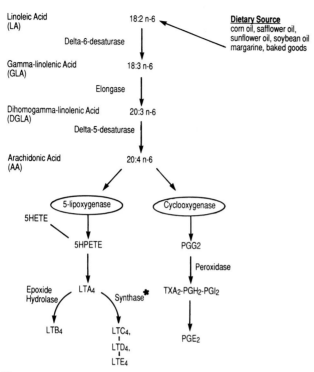

Figure 30–3. Metabolism of linoleic acid to eicosanoids. 5-HPETE = 5S-hydroperoxyeicosatetraenoic acid; 5-HETE = 5S-hydroxyeicosatetraenoic acid; LT = leukotriene; PG = prostaglandin; TXA_2 = thromboxane A_2; PGI_2 = prostacylin I_2. *Also known as glutathione S transferase.

Because of the mammalian inability to interconvert ω-3 and ω-6 fatty acids, the composition of phospholipids in cellular membranes is determined by nutritional intake.[77] The fatty acids found in the membrane bilayer are substrates for the production of PG and leukotriene species essential for many biologic activities, including modulation of the inflammatory and immune response. It is becoming widely recognized that reproducible metabolic alterations in these pathways can be engineered by consistent modifications in dietary fatty acid content. These fatty acid–induced changes have been documented in animal[78] and normal humans trials[79] and large epidemiologic studies of populations consuming relatively homogeneous diets.[80]

ω-6 Fatty Acids

By far the most common fatty acid constituents in the Western diet are the ω-6 fatty acids. They are derived predominantly from terrestrial sources and are ubiquitous in plant seeds. Linoleic acid, 18:6, ω-3, is essential to life because it is the precursor of arachidonic acid (20:4, ω-6; Fig. 30–3). Arachidonate is present in cellular membranes, where it is esterified

to phospholipids. It is released by phospholipase A_2 to then form the eicosanoid derivatives of the PG and leukotriene families through the enzymes cyclooxygenase and 5-lipoxygenase, respectively, which catalyze the insertion of molecular oxygen into arachidonic acid. γ-Linolenic acid (GLA; 18:3, ω-6) is found in seeds from the evening primrose and borage plants. It may be converted by an elongase enzyme to dihomogamma-linolenic acid (DGLA; 20:3, ω-6). DGLA is oxidized by cyclooxygenase to PGE_1 (Fig. 30–4), a monoenoic PG that has altered biologic activities from the dienoic PGE_2. For example, PGE_1 can inhibit platelet aggregation in humans and rats in vivo and in vitro, whereas PGE_2 cannot.[81] PGE_1 dietary supplementation can suppress inflammation and joint tissue injury in several animal models of inflammation[82] and can inhibit neutrophil function in vitro.[83] GLA dietary supplementation can suppress acute and chronic inflammation in several experimental animal models.

The subcutaneous air pouch model of inflammation was used to assess response to monosodium urate crystals or Freund's adjuvant in Sprague-Dawley rats consuming diets enriched with either safflower oil as a source of linoleic acid or borage seed

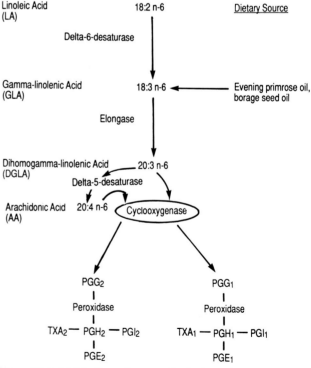

Figure 30–4. Metabolism of gamma-linolenic acid (GLA) to prostaglandin species with one double bond. Dihomogamma-linolenic acid (DGLA) cannot be converted to a leukotriene compound. Instead, it is converted by 15-lipoxygenase to 15-hydroxy DGLA (reaction not shown), which can inhibit 5-lipoxygenase activities.[131]

oil as a source of GLA.[84] Animals consuming GLA had a marked reduction of neutrophil exudate and lysosomal enzyme activity compared with those fed sunflower oil. PGE_2 and leukotriene B_4 concentrations were significantly diminished in pouch exudates in the GLA-fed rats. The fatty acid profiles in the serum and inflammatory cells from animals consuming primrose oil exhibited significant increases in GLA and DGLA.

When DGLA is added to human synovial cells grown in tissue culture, interleukin-1β–stimulated growth is suppressed fivefold compared with cells grown in medium supplemented with arachidonic acid.[85] Cells incubated with DGLA exhibited a 14-fold increase in PGE_1 and a 70 percent decrease in PGE_2 compared with cells in control medium. The increase in PGE_1 concentrations was associated with significantly enhanced levels of cyclic adenosine monophosphate, which the authors suggested was responsible for the antiproliferative effects. The inhibiting effect could be blocked by indomethacin, lending further support to PGE_1 mediation of growth suppression.

Human Studies

Studies of dietary supplementation with GLA in humans have shown somewhat mixed and disappointing results. An open study of only 20 patients with rheumatoid arthritis treated with GLA in combination with various vitamins showed no significant changes of any clinical or laboratory parameters over a period of 12 weeks.[86] An investigation comparing evening primrose oil, as a source of GLA, to olive oil in 20 patients with rheumatoid arthritis over a period of 13 weeks failed to show any significant difference between groups.[87]

A 12-month investigation compared daily dietary supplementation of 540 mg of GLA versus GLA and a very small dose of eicosapentaenoic acid (or fish oil) versus a third group taking an inert oil.[88] The GLA was derived from evening primrose oil in this randomized and double-blinded study. None of the 49 patients with active rheumatoid arthritis who participated were taking slow-acting antirheumatic medications. The stated outcome measured in this investigation was the ability of patients to reduce or discontinue their nonsteroidal anti-inflammatory drug (NSAID) therapy. After 12 months, no significant changes were seen in clinical measurements in any of the groups, although 11 of 15 evening primrose oil patients, 12 of 15 evening primrose oil/fish oil patients, and 5 of 15 placebo subjects were able to reduce their NSAID dosage. Only a few patients actually discontinued NSAID therapy. The authors commented on a "very definite" subjective improvements despite the lack of objective improvements in the patients on experimental dietary supplementation.

In a more recent investigations 1.1 g per day of GLA, derived from borage seed oil, was administered to seven patients with rheumatoid arthritis and seven normal subjects in an open 12-week uncontrolled study.[89] Patients with rheumatoid arthritis were receiving NSAIDS but not slow-acting agents. Significant clinical improvement in joint pain and morning stiffness was observed. Significant increases in total and phospholipid DGLA occurred in peripheral blood monocytes and mononuclear cells. Total PGE production (PGE_1 and PGE_2) was diminished in both normal subjects and rheumatoid arthritis patients, and leukotriene B_4 production from stimulated monocytes was moderately reduced in the normal subjects. In summary, the theoretical underpinnings of dietary therapy with GLA in inflammatory disease are well established, yet convincing clinical evidence of the effectiveness of these ω-6 fatty acids in patients with rheumatic disease has not yet emerged.

ω-3 Fatty Acids

Omega-3 fatty acids have their first double bond at the third carbon atom from the methyl end of the molecule. The primary dietary source of this class of fatty acids in our diets is fish and other marine sources that derive the ω-3 fatty acids from phytoplankton and zooplankton at the base of the food chain. Eicosapentaenoic acid (20:5, ω-3) and docosahexaenoic acid (22:6, ω-3) are the ω-3 fatty acids derived from marine sources. Omega-3 fatty acids may also occur naturally in terrestrial sources in the form of α-linolenic acid (18:3, ω-3) commonly found in chloroplasts of green leaves and in some plant oils, including flax, canola, and soybean oils. The ability to synthesize the longer-chain ω-3 fatty acids eicosapentaenoic acid and docosahexaenoic acid from α-linolenic acid is slow in humans and may diminish even further with aging or certain disease states[90] owing to a loss of the delta-6 (δ-6) and δ-5 desaturase enzyme activity (Fig. 30–5). The shorter-chain ω-3 fatty acids must also compete for these enzymes with the much larger amounts of ω-6 fatty acids found in the typical Western diet.[91] The ω-6 fatty acids can competitively inhibit the formation of eicosapentaenoic acid and docosahexaenoic acid from α-linolenic acid.[6, 91] The primary source of ω-3 fatty acids in the Western diet is therefore nonterrestrial, a reversal of the pattern of most of human prehistory in which large sources of ω-3 fatty acids were obtained in hunter-gatherer societies from wild game.[7] Fat of wild animals contains approximately 9 percent eicosapentaenoic acid and five times more polyunsaturated fat per gram than is found in domestic livestock,[92] which contains almost undetectable amounts of eicosapentaenoic acid. Throughout most of human history, hunter-gatherer societies consumed a higher percentage of polyunsaturated fat, more ω-3 fatty acids, more fiber, and less total fat than the present Western diet (see Table 30–1). Our current dietary fatty acid intake must be properly viewed as a relatively recent alteration of long-standing dietary pat-

n-3 Fatty Acid Derived Alterations in Eicosanoid Metabolism

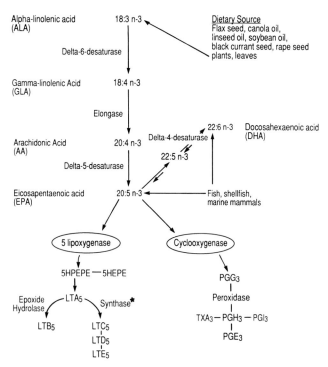

* Also known as glutathione S-Transferase

Figure 30–5. Metabolism of ω-3 fatty acids to eicosanoids. α-Linolenic acid (ALA) is derived from terrestrial sources and eicosapentaenoic acid (EPA), and docosahexaenoic acids (DHA) are derived from marine sources. Omega-3 fatty acids are converted to prostaglandin species with three double bonds and leukotriene species with five double bonds. They also compete with arachidonic acid as the substrate for cyclooxygenase and may selectively inhibit the epoxide hydrolase enzyme converting LTA_4 to LTB_4. 5-HPEPE = 5S-hydroperoxyeicosapentaenoic acid; 5-HEPE = 5S-hydroxyeicosapentaenoic acid; LT = leukotriene; PG = prostaglandin; TXA_3 = thromboxane A_3; PGI_3 = prostacyclin I_3.

terns that the human species had adapted to over tens of thousands of years. Speculation has thus arisen over the possible influence of our changing dietary patterns on the development of some major chronic diseases of industrialized society.[7]

Eicosapentaenoic acid can be metabolized through both the cyclooxygenase and 5-lipoxygenase metabolic pathways to form end-products with altered biologic activity. Eicosapentaenoic acid is acted on by cyclooxygenase to form thromboxane A_3 (TXA_3) and prostacyclin I_3 (PGI_3) (Fig. 30–5).[93] PGI_3 retains its antiaggregatory platelet activity, but TXA_3 is not nearly as potent as TXA_2 in inducing platelet aggregation. This may partially account for the diminished risk of cardiovascular morbidity and mortality that is associated with fish consumption.[4–6] Eicosapentaenoic acid will also compete with arachidonate for cyclooxygenase, with the consequent decreased production of PGE_2.[3] PGE_2 stimulates osteoclast activity, resulting in bone resorption,[94] a process of significance in rheumatoid arthritis. The dienoic PGs also increase vascular permeability in a synergistic effect

with serotonin and bradykinin.[3] PGE series PGs have important functions in blood pressure regulation, fertility, and modulation of the immune response. Omega-3 fatty acid ingestion has been documented to have significant effects in all of these areas[3, 6] as well as cardiovascular health and well-being. Moreover, the E series PGs are not localized to specific tissues as is the case with TX and prostacyclin, which are limited to platelets and vascular endothelium, respectively. Therefore, the effect of altering PGE content in any specific site will vary, depending on the tissue where the synthesis takes place.[95]

Of possibly greater importance than the altered end-products of ω-3 fatty acids ingestion is their effect on inhibiting arachidonate metabolism. They can inhibit the synthesis of arachidonic acid from its linoleic acid substrate[91] possibly through competition for the 2-position occupied by arachidonate in membrane phospholipids. Eicosapentaenoic acid will also directly compete with arachidonic acid as the substrate for cyclooxygenase and inhibit its metabolism into eicosanoids.[96] Omega-3 fatty acid ingestion thus results in the production of compounds with altered biologic activity as well as a decrease in the usual amounts of biologically active arachidonate derivatives (Fig. 30–5).

Ingestion of eicosapentaenoic acid is associated with the production of leukotrienes with five double bonds such as leukotriene B_5 (Fig. 30–5) which has greatly attenuated proinflammatory activities.[97, 98] Leukotriene B_5 is usually undetectable in humans consuming a Western diet. Simultaneous with the production of small amounts of leukotriene B_5 from stimulated neutrophils of normal subjects consuming fish oil, there are large decreases in the production of neutrophil leukotriene B_4.[99] Neutrophil chemotaxis was significantly suppressed in subjects after 6 weeks of fish oil ingestion and returned to normal after the supplements were discontinued.

Other investigators have found evidence of a selective inhibition of the epoxide hydrolase enzyme (Fig. 30–5) in neutrophils from normal subjects[98] and rheumatoid arthritis patients[100] consuming fish oil because of unaltered quantities of 5-hydroxyeicosatetraenoic acid (5-HETE) and 5-hydroxyeicosapentaenoic (5-HEPE) relative to the corresponding arachidonic acid product generated before dietary supplementation.

Chemotactic activity of neutrophils from rheumatoid arthritis patients who had ingested fish oil was found to be enhanced compared with the pretreatment state.[100] This is seemingly paradoxical in view of the suppression of neutrophil chemotaxis after fish oil ingestion in normal subjects.[99] The improved chemotaxis in rheumatoid arthritis patients represents a partial correction of a reduced chemotactic activity of peripheral blood neutrophils of subjects with this disease. Sperling et al.[100] believe that the increased neutrophil chemotaxis after fish oil ingestion in patients with rheumatoid arthritis is due to a reversal of an abnormal desensitization of neutrophils to the chemotactic factor leukotriene B_4. Platelet activating factor-acether (PAF-acether) generation of stimulated monocytes is significantly diminished[99] after fish oil ingestion, suggesting an ω-3 fatty acid–induced inhibitory effect of phospholipase A_2 activity on substrate alkyl phospholipids that would affect PAF generation. This is of considerable interest in the context of inflammation in that PAF can stimulate tumor necrosis factor as well as other cytokines in endothelial tissue[101] and is 1000 times more potent than histamine in inducing vascular permeability.[102] Evidence suggests that PAF can also modulate T cell and monocyte function.[101]

Omega-3 fatty acid ingestion is associated with significant changes in the fatty acid profiles of cellular lipids.[2] Neutrophil arachidonic acid content is reduced by 33 percent, and eicosapentaenoic acid content is enhanced 20-fold compared with presupplement values obtained in rheumatoid arthritis patients ingesting fish oil.[100] Omega-3 fatty acid ingestion is thus associated with reproducible changes in the biochemical composition of cell membranes of neutrophils and monocytes and striking alterations in the production of the metabolic end-products of a myriad of inflammatory and immunologically active compounds that may influence the course of rheumatic disease.

The lipid bilayer of cellular membranes is composed primarily of phospholipids and cholesterol (Fig. 30–6). Because cellular receptors, enzymes, and transport proteins are embedded in the phospholipid bilayer, a change in its structure could have significant implications for cellular function that extend beyond the alterations in eicosanoid and PAF-acether biosynthesis[2] described herein. A recent investigation demonstrated a significant reduction of interleukin-1 from monocytes of normal volunteers ingesting fish oil for 6 weeks.[103] The precise mechanism of this effect is speculative but could be associated with membrane changes in phospholipid fatty acid content leading to diminished amounts of eicosanoid products such as leukotriene B_4.[99]

Animal Studies

Dietary modifications containing ω-3 fatty acids reduce the severity of diffuse proliferative glomerulonephritis in several autoimmune strains of mice including the NZBxNZWF1, BxSB/Mpj, and MRL/lpr strains.[78, 104] Dietary ω-3 fatty acids reduce the severity of glomerulonephritis even when they are withheld until after the renal disease has begun to evolve.[104] Not all observed effects of fish oil have been beneficial in the laboratory; an increased incidence of arthritis was observed in rats immunized with type II collagen who consumed a fish oil–enriched diet compared with animals ingesting beef tallow, although the severity of the arthritis was the same in each group.[105] An increased incidence of necrotizing vasculitis was noted in renal arteries of MRL/lpr mice with systemic lupus erythematosus–like disease, even while their glomerulonephritis was alleviated

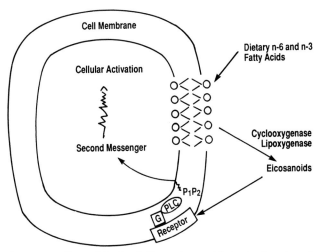

Figure 30–6. Potential role of dietary fatty acids in the function of the membrane phospholipid bilayer of cells. Dietary fatty acids will be incorporated into the phospholipid bilayer of cells, where they can be metabolized to eicosanoids. Biologically modified eicosanoids derived from feeding ω-3 or ω-6 fatty acids may have a role in modulating receptor-ligand activity and cellular activation to various stimuli. Fatty acid changes in the lipid bilayer may also result in changes in membrane fluidity that could have potential effects on the function of other receptor-related membrane activities. The stimulated receptor transmits a signal via a G-protein to phospholipase C (PLC), which splits phosphatidylinositol-4,5-biphosphate (PIP_2) to products that eventually lead to second-messenger generation and cellular activation (biochemical steps not shown). (Modified from Weber, P. C.: Membrane phospholipid modification by dietary ω-3 fatty acids: Effects on eicosanoid formation and cell function. *In* Karnovsky, M. L. [ed.]: Biological Membranes: Aberrations in Membrane Structure and Function. New York, Alan R. Liss, 1988, pp. 263–274. Copyright © 1988 Wiley-Liss. Reprinted by permission of Wiley-Liss, A Division of John Wiley & Sons, Inc.)

on a fish oil diet.[104] Conversely, the severity of type II collagen–induced arthritis in mice is reduced significantly by menhaden oil as a source of ω-3, but the reduction is only seen in female mice.[106] The effects of ω-3 fatty acids are thus species specific in laboratory animals, and it cannot be said that they have generalized beneficial effects. In addition, some of the salutory effects are dose dependent as they were lost when the concentration of menhaden oil in the diet was reduced from 25 per cent to 5.5 per cent.[107] Studies indicate that a mixture of ω-3 fatty acids containing both eicosapentaenoic acid and docosahexaenoic acid may be more effective than either of these ω-3 fatty acids by themselves.[108]

Human Studies

In a pilot study published in 1985, 17 patients with rheumatoid arthritis consumed an experimental diet high in polyunsaturated fat and low in saturated fat, with a daily supplement of 1.8 g of eicosapentaenoic acid and 0.9 g of docosahexaenoic acid.[109] A control group consumed a diet with a ratio of polyunsaturated to saturated fat of 1:4, as in a typical Western diet, and indigestible paraffin wax. The results showed a significant improvement in the number of tender joints after 12 weeks in the group consuming fish oil, with a subjective significant worsening in this group after discontinuing these supplements.

In a subsequent investigation, rheumatoid arthritis patients received 2.8 g of eicosapentaenoic acid and 1.8 g of docosahexaenoic acid in a blinded cross-over format in which subjects received fish oil–derived ω-3 fatty acids or olive oil for a period of 14 weeks before crossing over to receive the opposite dietary supplement.[110] Patients were observed to have a highly statistically significant decrease in their number of tender joints on fish oil compared with when they consumed olive oil. Fatigue, which was quantitated as the time interval from awakening to the first feeling of tiredness, also improved significantly in patients consuming fish oil. All of 12 clinical parameters measured favored fish oil, although only two achieved statistical significance. Leukotriene B$_4$ from stimulated neutrophils decreased by 57.8 percent in patients while receiving the fish oil ω-3 supplement compared with when they consumed olive oil. A significant correlation was observed between the decrease in the number of tender joints and the decrease in neutrophil leukotriene B$_4$ production in individual patients.

A recent investigation demonstrated that leukotriene B$_4$ production from stimulated neutrophils was significantly reduced at week 4 in patients on fish oil even though significant clinical improvement did not occur until week 12.[111] There is thus an asynchrony between ω-3–induced decreases in neutrophil leukotriene B$_4$ production that occur after only 4 to 6 weeks[99, 100, 111] and the clinical benefits that are delayed until at least week 12.[109–111] It is possible that this could be due, in part, to the delayed suppressive effects of fish oil ingestion on the production of interleukin-1.[103]

A recent investigation examined the effects of different doses of fish oil versus olive oil in a 6-month randomized, double-blinded, parallel study of 49 patients with active rheumatoid arthritis.[112] Fish oil supplements were supplied according to body weight, not as a uniform dose as in previous studies. A "low-dose" group consumed 27 mg per kg per day of eicosapentaenoic acid and 18 mg per kg per day of docosahexaenoic acid and a "high dose" group ingested exactly twice that amount. Patients maintained their background medications and diets without change as in the previously described studies in patients with rheumatoid arthritis. Multiple clinical parameters improved from baseline in the groups consuming fish oil, with statistically significant improvements in joint swelling and tenderness scores, morning stiffness, and physician evaluation of global disease activity occurring with significantly greater frequency in the high-dose group. Significant decreases were also observed in stimulated neutrophil production of leukotriene B$_4$ and monocyte interleukin-1, with the greatest decreases in interleukin-1 observed in the patients consuming the higher dose

of fish oil. It thus appears that the beneficial effects of ω-3 fatty acid ingestion in humans with inflammatory disease are dose dependent as in the autoimmune animal model[108] and studies of the antihypertensive effects of fish oil ingestion in humans.[113] Significant clinical benefits were observed more commonly after 18 and 24 weeks of fish oil ingestion.

VASCULAR DISEASES

The role of ω-3 fatty acids in cardiovascular disease is well established and has been recently reviewed.[6] Effects of ω-3 fatty acids that may improve the status of patients with impaired circulation include (1) improved rheologic status secondary to increased erythrocyte deformability; (2) decreased plasma viscosity; (3) a more favorable vascular response to ischemia; (4) a reduced vasospastic response to catecholamines and angiotensin; (5) increased levels of tissue plasminogen activator; and (6) increased endothelial-dependent relaxation of arteries in response to bradykinin, serotonin, adenine diphosphate, and thrombin. Fish oil dietary intervention thus differs from present interventions for vascular disease because of the potential for beneficial benefits at multiple physiologic loci.

In a recent investigation of the effect of fish oil ingestion in patients with Raynaud's phenomenon, 32 patients with primary or secondary disease consumed daily dietary supplements of 3.96 g of eicosapentaenoic acid and 2.64 g of docosahexaenoic acid or olive oil for 12 weeks.[114] Digital systolic blood pressure and blood flow were evaluated by a strain-gauge plethysmograph in room air and in water baths of 40°C, 25°C, 15°C, and 10°C. Results showed significant improvements in the time interval to the onset of Raynaud's phenomenon and digital systolic pressure in the cold water baths in patients with primary, but not secondary, Raynaud's phenomenon. The mechanism of these benefits was not studied.

ALLERGIC ARTHRITIS

The idea that rheumatologic disease could be etiologically linked to ingestion of food is not a new one.[115, 116] The idea has gained some support from sporadic but convincing case reports of the reproducible onset of joint symptoms shortly after the ingestion of certain foodstuffs. Patients with Behçet's syndrome were observed to have striking exacerbations of disease within 48 hours of ingestion of English walnuts.[117] Lymphocytes from these patients also exhibited significantly decreased reactivity to a walnut extract ex vivo within 2 days of ingestion of English walnuts, whereas leukocyte incorporation of tritiated thymidine after mitogen stimulation was increased.[117] A hypersensitivity to certain foods has been speculated to be the cause of at least some cases of palindromic rheumatism[116] and was documented to occur in a case report of a person with hypersensitivity to sodium nitrate in food preservatives.[118] L-Canavanine, a nonprotein amino acid found in alfalfa, has been linked to exacerbations of systemic lupus erythematosus in both monkeys[119] and humans.[120]

For a response to food to be linked plausibly to a hypersensitivity reaction resulting in articular symptoms, it is necessary to implicate an altered intestinal permeability that would allow passage of intact food antigens into the circulation. Studies documenting this possible effect are tantalizing, although not numerous. Circumstantial evidence exists to link arthritis to damaged intestinal function in ulcerative colitis,[121] Crohn's disease,[122] and the polyarthritis that occurs after jejunal bypass surgery for obesity.[123] Moreover, immune complexes containing intact food antigens complexed to IgE or IgG have been documented in normal and atopic subjects[124] and have been observed to cause bronchospasm and pruritis in allergic patients. A study of intestinal absorption using oral ^{51}Cr-EDTA (edetic acid) showed that only rheumatoid arthritis patients taking NSAIDs exhibited increased absorption from the gut.[125] Patients not taking NSAIDs did not exhibit increased absorption. Indium 111–labeled leukocyte scans showed ileocecal inflammation in six of nine patients on NSAIDs.

A food antigen can be convincingly linked to arthritis if a flare of clinical symptoms occurs within 48 hours of a blinded challenge with the putative offending antigen. An elimination diet in which a patient totally discontinues ingestion of the food in question with total clearing of articular symptoms would also provide implicative evidence, albeit weaker than a flare-up after a blinded challenge. Two patients have been reported who had significant flares in articular symptoms after ingestion of milk or dairy products.[126, 127] The challenges were open[126] and blinded,[127] and symptoms peaked within 24 to 48 hours. IgE antibodies to milk were demonstrated using the radioallergosorbent test in one patient,[126] whereas large amounts of IgG4 anti-milk antibodies directed to α-lactalbumin were detected in the other.[127] A flare-up in articular disease manifestations has also been documented after blinded challenges with shrimp and nitrates.[128]

Interest in the possible role of food intolerance in the etiology of arthritic symptoms has been renewed[129, 130] as a result of these case reports. It is difficult to assess the incidence of this syndrome in that patients may not necessarily be aware of possible sensitivities to commonly ingested foods in their diet. Because of the small number of documented cases of food intolerance in the literature, however, the syndrome is probably rare.

References

1. Arthritis: The Basic Facts. Atlanta, Arthritis Foundation, 1981.
2. Weber, P. C.: Membrane phospholipid modification by dietary ω-3 fatty acids: Effects on eicosanoid formation and cell function. In Karnovsky, M. L. (ed.): Biological Membranes: Aberrations in Membrane Structure and Function. New York, Alan R. Liss, 1988, pp. 263–274.
3. Robinson, D. R., Tateno, S., Balkrishna, P., and Hirai, A.: Lipid mediators of inflammatory and immune reactions. JPEN 12:375, 1988.
4. Hirai, A., Terano, T., Saito, H., et al.: Eicosapentaenoic acid and platelet function in Japanese. In Lovenburg, W., Yamori, Y., (eds.): Nutritional Prevention of Cardiovascular Disease. New York, Academic Press, 1984, pp. 231–239.
5. Kromhout, D., Bosschieter, E. B., and de Lezenne Coulander, C.: The inverse relation between fish consumption and 20-year mortality from coronary heart disease. N. Engl. J. Med. 312:1205, 1985.
5a. Stenson, W. F., Cort, D., Rodgers, J., et al.: Dietary supplementation with fish oil in ulcerative colitis. Ann. Intern. Med. 116:609, 1992.
5b. Donadio, J. U.: Omega-3 polyunsaturated fatty acids: A potential new treatment of immune renal disease. Mayo Clin. Proc. 66:1018, 1991.
6. Leaf, A., and Weber, P. C.: Cardiovascular effects of ω-3 fatty acids. N. Engl. J. Med. 318:549, 1988.
7. Eaton, S. B., and Konner, M.: Paleolithic nutrition: A consideration of its nature and current implications. N. Engl. J. Med. 312:283, 1985.
8. Bayles, T. B., Richardson, H., and Hall, F. C.: The nutritional background of patients with rheumatoid arthritis. N. Engl. J. Med. 229:319, 1943.
9. Eising, L.: Dietary intake in patients with arthritis and other chronic diseases. J. Bone Joint Surg. 45A:69, 1963.
10. Kowsari, B., Finnie, S. K., Carter, R. L., et al.: Assessment of the diet of patients with rheumatoid arthritis and osteoarthritis. J. Am. Diet. Assoc. 82:657, 1983.
11. Bigaouette, J., Timchalk, M. A., and Kremer, J.: Nutritional adequacy of diet and supplements in patients with rheumatoid arthritis who take medications. J. Am. Diet. Assoc. 87:1687, 1987.
12. Helliwell, M., Coombes, E. J., Moody, B. J., et al.: Nutritional status in patients with rheumatoid arthritis. Ann. Rheum. Dis. 43:386, 1984.
13. Johansson, U., Portinsson, S., Akesson, A., et al.: Nutritional status in girls with juvenile chronic arthritis. Hum. Nutr. 40C:57, 1986.
14. Portinsson, S., Akesson, A., Svantesson, H., et al.: Dietary assessment in children with juvenile chronic arthritis. J. Hum. Nutr. Diet. 1:133, 1988.
14a. Kjeldseu-Kragh, J., Hangen, M., and Borchgreviak, C. F.: Controlled trial of fasting and one-year vegetarian diet in rheumatoid arthritis. Lancet 338:899, 1991.
14b. Van de Laar, M. A., Nieuweuhuis, J. M., Former-Boon, M., et al.: Nutritional habits of patients suffering from seropositive rheumatoid arthritis: a screening of 93 Dutch patients. Clin. Rheumatol. 9:483, 1990.
14c. Buchanan, H. M., Preston, S. T., Brooks, P. M., and Buchanan, W. W.: Is diet important in rheumatoid arthritis? Br. J. Rheumatol. 30:125, 1991.
15. Bendich, A.: Antioxidant nutrients and immune functions. Adv. Exp. Med. Biol. 262:1, 1990.
16. Tengerdy, R. P., Mathias, M. M., and Nockels, C. F.: Effect of vitamin E on immunity and disease resistance. In Prasad, K. N. (ed.): Vitamins, Nutrition and Cancer. Basel, Karger, 1984, pp. 118–122.
17. Halliwell, B., and Gutteridge, J. M. C.: Lipid peroxidation: A radical chain reaction. In Halliwell, B., and Gutteridge, J. M. C. (eds.): Free Radicals in Biology and Medicine. Oxford, Clarendon Press, 1985, pp. 139–189.
18. Fidelius, R. K.: The generation of oxygen radicals: A positive signal for lymphocyte activation. Cell. Immunol. 113:175, 1988.
19. Dornand, J., and Gerber, M.: Inhibition of murine T-cell responses by antioxidants: The targets of lipoxygenase pathway inhibitors. Immunology 68:384, 1989.
20. Austen, K. F., and Soberman, R. J.: Perspectives on additional areas for research in leukotrienes. Ann. N.Y. Acad. Sci. 524:xi, 1988.
21. Goodwin, J. S., and Behrens, T.: Role of lipoxygenase metabolites of arachidonic acid in T cell activation. Ann. N.Y. Acad. Sci. 524:201, 1988.
22. Carmen, J. A., Smith, S. M., and Hayes, C. E.: Characterization of a helper T lymphocyte defect in vitamin A-deficient mice. J. Immunol. 142:388, 1989.
23. Bendich, A., and Olson, J. A.: Biological actions of carotenoids. FASEB J. 3:1927, 1989.
24. Mezes, M., Bartosiewicz, G., and Nemeth, J.: Comparative investigations on vitamin A level in some rheumatic diseases. Clin. Rheum. 5:221, 1986.
25. Honkanen, V., Konttinen, Y. T., and Mussalo-Rauhamaa, H.: Vitamins A and E, retinol-binding protein and zinc in rheumatoid arthritis. Clin. Exp. Rheum. 7:465, 1989.
26. Bendich, A.: A role for carotenoids in immune function. Clin. Nutr. 7:113, 1988.
27. Boxer, L. A.: The role of leukocyte antioxidants in modulating neutrophil functional responses. Adv. Exp. Med. Biol. 262:19, 1990.

28. Topinka, J., Binkova, B., Sram, R. J., et al.: The influence of alpha-tocopherol and pyritinol on oxidative DNA damage and lipid peroxidation in human lymphocytes. Mutat. Res. 225:131, 1989.

29. Grever, M. R., Thompson, V. N., Balcerzak, S. P., et al.: The effect of oxidant stress on human lymphocyte cytotoxicity. Blood 56:284, 1980.

30. Hatam, C. J., and Cayden, H. J.: A high-performance lipid chromatographic method for the determination of tocopherol in plasma and cellular elements of the blood. J. Lipid Res. 20:639, 1979.

31. Boxer, L. S., Oliver, J. M., Spielberg, S. P., et al.: Protection of granulocytes by vitamin E in glutathione synthetase deficiency. N. Engl. J. Med. 301:901, 1979.

32. Moser, J., and Weber, F.: Uptake of ascorbic acid by human granulocytes. Int. J. Vit. Nutr. Res. 54:47, 1983.

33. Goetzl, E. J., Wasserman, S. I., Gigli, I., and Austen, K. F.: Enhancement of random migration and chemotactic response of human leukocytes by ascorbic acid. J. Clin. Invest. 53:813, 1974.

34. Weening, R. S., Schorrel, E. P., Roos, D., et al.: Effect of ascorbate on abnormal neutrophil, platelet, and lymphocyte function in a patient with the Chediak-Higashi syndrome. Blood 57:856, 1981.

35. Sahud, M. A., and Cohen, R.: Effect of aspirin ingestion on ascorbic acid levels in rheumatoid arthritis. Lancet 1:937, 1971.

36. Rowley, D. A., and Halliwell, B.: Formation of hydroxyl radicals from hydrogen peroxide and iron salts by superoxide- and ascorbate-dependent mechanisms: Relevance to the pathology of rheumatoid disease. Clin. Sci. 64:649, 1983.

37. Hall, M. G., Darling, R. C., and Taylor, F. H.: The vitamin C requirement in rheumatoid arthritis. Ann. Intern. Med. 13:415, 1939.

38. Baehner, R. L., Boxer, A., Allen, J. M., et al.: Autooxidation as a basis for altered function by polymorphonuclear leukocytes. Blood 50:327, 1977.

39. El-Hag, A., Lipsky, P. E., Bennett, M., et al.: Immunomodulation by neutrophil myeloperoxidase and hydrogen peroxide: Differential susceptibility of human lymphocyte functions. J. Immunol. 136:3420, 1986.

40. El-Hag, A., and Clark, R. A.: Immunosuppression by activated human neutrophils: Dependence on the myeloperoxidase system. J. Immunol. 139:2406, 1987.

41. Anderson, R., Smit, M., Joone, G. K., and VanStaden, A. M.: Vitamin C and cellular immune functions. Ann. N.Y. Acad. Sci. 587:34–48, 1990.

42. Frei, B. R., Stocker, R., and Ames, B. N.: Antioxidant defenses and lipid peroxidation in human blood plasma. Proc. Natl. Acad. Sci. U.S.A. 85:9748, 1988.

43. Maddison, P. J., and Bacon, P. A.: Vitamin D deficiency, spontaneous fractures and osteopenia in rheumatoid arthritis. Br. Med. J. 4:433, 1974.

44. Smith, E. L., Pincus, S. H., Donovan, L., et al.: A novel approach for the evaluation and treatment of psoriasis. J. Am. Acad. Dermatol. 19:516, 1988.

45. MacLaughlin, J. A., Gange, W., Taylor, D., et al.: Cultured psoriatic fibroblasts from involved and uninvolved sites have a partial but not absolute resistance to the proliferation-inhibition activity of 1,25-dihydroxyvitamin D_3. Proc. Natl. Acad. Sci. U.S.A. 82:5409, 1985.

46. Rigby, W. F. C., Stacy, T., and Ganger, M. W.: Inhibition of T lymphocyte mitogenesis by 1,25-dihydroxyvitamin D_3 (calcitriol). J. Clin. Invest. 74:1451, 1984.

47. Ghalla, A. K., Amento, E. P., and Krane, S. M.: Differential effects of 1,25-dihydroxyvitamin D_3 on human lymphocytes and monocyte/macrophages: Inhibition of interleukin-2 and augmentation of interleukin-1 production. Cell. Immunol. 98:311, 1986.

48. Gepner, P., Amor, B., and Fournier, C.: 1,25-dihydroxyvitamin D_3 potentiates the in vitro inhibitory effects of cyclosporin A on T cells from rheumatoid arthritis patients. Arthritis Rheum. 32:31, 1989.

49. Huckins, D., Felson, D. T., and Holick, M.: Treatment of psoriatic arthritis with oral 1,25-dihydroxyvitamin D_3: A pilot study. Arthritis Rheum. 33:1732, 1990.

50. Fukushima, T., Iijima, Y., and Kosaka, F.: Endotoxin-induced zinc accumulation by liver cells is mediated by metallothionein synthesis. Biochem. Biophys. Res. Comm. 152:874, 1988.

51. Cousins, R. J.: Absorption, transport and hepatic metabolism of copper and zinc: Special reference to metallothionein and ceruloplasmin. Physiol. Rev. 65:238, 1985.

52. Mussalo-Rauhamaa, H., Konttinen, Y. T., Lehto, J., et al.: Predictive clinical and laboratory parameters for serum zinc and copper in rheumatoid arthritis. Ann. Rheum. Dis. 47:816, 1988.

53. Kluger, M. J., and Rothenburg, B. A.: Fever and reduced iron: Their interaction as a host defense response to bacterial infection. Science 203:374, 1979.

54. Svenson, K. L. G., Hallgren, R., and Johansson, E.: Reduced zinc in peripheral blood cells from patients with inflammatory connective tissue diseases. Inflammation 9:189, 1985.

55. Hallgren, R., Fettelins, N., and Lindh, H.: Redistribution of minerals and trace elements in chronic inflammation: A study on isolated blood cells from patients with ankylosing spondylitis. J. Rheumatol. 14:548, 1987.

56. Seelig, M. S.: Auto-immune complications of D-penicillamine: A possible result of zinc and magnesium depletion and of pyridoxine inactivation. J. Am. Coll. Nutr. 1:207, 1982.

57. Ruhl, J., and Kirshner, H.: Monocyte-dependent stimulation of human T cells by zinc. Clin. Exp. Immunol. 32:484, 1978.

58. Whitehouse, M. W.: Trace element supplements for inflammatory disease. In Dixon, J., Furst, D. (eds.): Second Line Agents in the Rheumatic Diseases. New York, Marcel Dekker, 1992, pp. 549–578.

59. Whitehouse, M. W., Rainsford, K. D., Taylor, R. M., and Vernon-Roberts, B.: Zinc monoglycerolate: A slow-release source of zinc with anti-arthritic activity in rats. Agents Actions 31:47, 1990.

60. Cimmino, M. A., Mazzucotelli, A., Rovetta, G., and Cutolo, M.: The controversy over zinc sulphate efficacy in rheumatoid and psoriatic arthritis. Scand. J. Rheumatol. 13:191, 1984.

61. Kennedy, A. C., Fell, G. S., Rooney, P., et al.: Zinc: Its relationship to osteoporosis in rheumatoid arthritis. Scand. J. Rheum. 4:243, 1975.

62. Spallholz, J. E.: Anti-inflammatory immunologic and carcinostatic attributes of selenium in experimental animals. Adv. Exp. Med. Biol. 135:43, 1981.

63. Spallholz, J. E., Boyland, L. M., and Larsen, H. S.: Advances in understanding selenium's role in the immune system. Ann. N.Y. Acad. Sci. 587:123, 1990.

64. Ursini, F., Maiorino, M., and Gregolin, C.: The selenoenzyme phospholipid hydroperoxide glutathione peroxidase. Biochem. Biophys. Acta 839:62, 1985.

65. Bryant, R. W., Bailey, J. M., King, J. C., and Levander, O. A.: Altered platelet glutathione peroxidase activity and arachidonic acid metabolism during selenium repletion in a controlled human study. In Spallholz, J. E., Martin, J. L., and Ganther, H. E. (eds.): Selenium in Biology and Medicine. Westport, CT, AVI Publishing, 1981, pp 395–399.

66. Medina, D.: Mechanisms of selenium inhibition of tumorigenesis. J. Am. Coll. Toxicol. 5:21, 1986.

67. Spallholz, J. E., and Boylan, L. M.: Effect of dietary selenium on peritoneal macrophage chemiluminescence. Fed. J. 3:A778, 1989.

68. Sonne, M., Helleberg, L., and Jenson, P. T.: Selenium status in patients with rheumatoid arthritis. Scand. J. Rheumatol. 14:318, 1985.

69. Borgland, M., Akesson, A., and Adesson, B.: Distribution of selenium and glutathione peroxidase in plasma compared in healthy subjects and rheumatoid arthritis patients. Scand. J. Clin. Lab. Invest. 48:27, 1988.

70. Peretz, A., Neve, J., Vertangen, F., Famaey, J. P., and Molle, L.: Selenium status in relation to clinical variables and corticosteroid treatment in rheumatoid arthritis. J. Rheumatol. 14:1104, 1987.

71. Tarp, U., Overvad, K., Thorling, E. B., Grandal, H., and Hansen, J. C.: Selenium treatment in rheumatoid arthritis. Acta Pharmacol. Toxicol. 59 Suppl. 7:382, 1986.

72. Hill, J., and Bird, H. A.: Failure of selenium-ACE to improve osteoarthritis. Br. J. Rheumatol. 29:211, 1990.

73. Wagner, E., and Gruber, F. O.: The trace element selenium in rheumatic diseases. Abstract P-682, XVII ILAR Congress of Rheumatology, Rio, 1989.

74. Allen, K. G. D., Arthur, J. R., Morrice, P. C., et al.: Copper deficiency and tissue glutathione concentration in the rat. Proc. Soc. Exp. Biol. Med. 187:38, 1988.

75. Roth, R. A., and Koshland, M. E.: Identification of a lymphocyte enzyme that catalyzes pentamer immunoglobulin M assembly. J. Biol. Chem. 256:4633, 1981.

76. Sherman, A. R.: Influence of iron on immunity and disease resistance. Ann. N.Y. Acad. Sci. 587:140–146, 1990.

77. Weber, P. C.: Membrane phospholipid modification by dietary ω-3 fatty acids: Effects on eicosanoid formation and cell function. In Karnovsky, M. L. (ed.): Biological Membranes: Aberrations in Membrane Structure and Function. New York, Alan R. Liss, 1988, pp. 263–274.

78. Prickett, J. D., Robinson, D. R., and Steinberg, A. D.: Dietary enrichment with the polyunsaturated fatty acid eicosapentaenoic acid prevents proteinuria and prolongs survival in NZBxNZW F1 mice. J. Clin. Invest. 68:556, 1981.

79. Lee, T. H., Hoover, R. L., Williams, J. D., et al.: Effect of dietary enrichment with eicosapentaenoic and docosahexaenoic acids on in vitro neutrophil and monocyte leukotriene generation and neutrophil function. N. Engl. J. Med. 312:1217, 1985.

80. Shekelle, R. B., Missell, L. V., Paul, O., et al.: Fish consumption and mortality from coronary heart disease. N. Engl. J. Med. 313:820, 1985.

81. Willis, A. L., Comai, K., Kuhn, D. C., et al.: Dihomogammalinolenate suppresses platelet aggregation when administered in vitro or in vivo. Prostaglandins 7:509, 1974.

82. Zurier, R. B.: Prostaglandins, immune responses, and murine lupus. Arthritis Rheum. 25:804, 1982.

83. Smolen, J. E., Korchak, H. M., and Weissmann, G.: Increased levels of cyclic adenosine-3', 5'-monophosphate in human polymorphonuclear leukocytes after surface stimulation. J. Clin. Invest. 65:1077, 1980.

84. Tate, G. A., Mandell, B. F., Karmali, R. A., et al.: Suppression of

monosodium urate crystal–induced acute inflammation by diets enriched with gammalinolenic acid and eicosapentaenoic acid. Arthritis Rheum. 31:1543, 1988.

85. Baker, D. G., Krakauer, K. A., Tate, G., et al.: Suppression of human synovial cell proliferation by dihomogammalinolenic acid. Arthritis Rheum. 32:1273, 1989.

86. Hansen, T. M., Lerche, A., Kassis, V., et al.: Treatment of rheumatoid arthritis with prostaglandin E$_1$ precursors cis-linoleic acid and gamma-linolenic acid. Scand. J. Rheum. 12:85, 1983.

87. Jantti, J., Nikkari, T., Solakivi, T., et al.: Evening primrose oil in rheumatoid arthritis: Changes in serum lipids and fatty acids. Ann. Rheum. Dis. 48:124, 1989.

88. Belch, J. J., Ansell, D., Madhok, R., et al.: Effects of altering essential fatty acids on requirements for non-steroidal anti-inflammatory drugs in patients with rheumatoid arthritis: A double-blind placebo-controlled study. Ann. Rheum. Dis. 47:96, 1988.

89. Pullman-Mooars, S., Laposata, M., Lem, D., et al.: Alteration of the cellular fatty acid profile and the production of eicosanoids in human monocytes by gammalinolenic acid. Arthritis Rheum. 33:1526, 1990.

90. Lands, W. E. M.: Fish and Human Health. Orlando, Academic Press, 1986, p. 103.

91. Holman, R. T.: Nutritional and metabolic interrelationships between fatty acids. Fed. Proc. 23:1062, 1964.

92. Crawford, M. A.: Fatty-acid ratios in free-living and domestic animals. Lancet 1:1329, 1968.

93. Fischer, S., and Weber, P. C.: Prostaglandin I$_3$ is formed in vivo in man after dietary eicosapentaenoic acid. Nature 307:165, 1984.

94. Robinson, D. R., Tashjian, A. H., Jr., and Levine, L.: Prostaglandin-stimulated bone resorption by rheumatoid synovia. J. Exp. Med. 150:338, 1979.

95. Ferretti, A., and Flanagan, V. P.: Modification of prostaglandin metabolism in vivo by longchain omega-3 polyunsaturates. Biochem. Biophysic. Acta 1045:299, 1990.

96. Simopoulos, A. P., Kifer, R. R., and Martin, R. E. (eds.): Health Effects of Polyunsaturated Fatty Acids in Seafoods. New York, Academic Press, 1986.

97. Strasser, T., Fischer, S., and Weber, P. C.: Leukotriene B$_5$ is formed in human neutrophils after dietary supplementation with eicosapentaenoic acid. Proc. Natl. Acad. Sci. U.S.A. 82:1540, 1984.

98. Lee, T. H., Mencia-Huerta, J. M., Shih, C., et al.: Characterization and biologic properties of 5, 12-dihydroxy derivatives of eicosapentaenoic acid, including leukotriene B$_5$ and the double lipoxygenase product. J. Biol. Chem. 259:2383, 1984.

99. Lee, T. H., Hoover, R. L., Williams, J. D., et al.: Effect of dietary enrichment with eicosapentaenoic and docosahexaenoic acids on in vitro neutrophil function. N. Engl. J. Med. 312:1217, 1985.

100. Sperling, R. I., Weinblatt, M., Robin, J. L., et al.: Effects of dietary supplementation with marine fish oil on leukocyte lipid mediator generation and function in rheumatoid arthritis. Arthritis Rheum. 30:988, 1987.

101. Dulioust, A., Salem, P., Vivier, E., et al.: Immunoregulatory functions of PAF-Acether (platelet-activating factor). In Karnovsky, M. L. (ed.): Biological Membranes: Aberrations in Membrane Structure and Function. New York, Alan R. Liss, 1988, pp. 87–96.

102. Humphrey, D. M., McManase, L., Satouchi, K., et al.: Vasoactive properties of acetyl glyceryl ether phosphorylcholine and analogs. Lab. Invest. 46:422, 1982.

103. Endres, S., Chorbani, R., Kelley, V. E., et al.: The effects of dietary supplementation with ω-3 polyunsaturated fatty acids on the synthesis of interleukin-1 and tumor necrosis factor by mononuclear cells. N. Engl. J. Med. 320:265, 1989.

104. Robinson, D. R., Prickett, J. D., Makoul, G. T., Steinberg, A. D., and Colvin, R. B.: Dietary fish oil reduces progression of established renal disease in (NZBxNZW) F1 mice and delays renal disease in BXSB and MRL/1 strains. Arthritis Rheum. 29:539, 1986.

105. Prickett, J. D., Trentham, D. E., and Robinson, D. R.: Dietary fish oil augments the induction of arthritis in rats immunized with type II collagen. J. Immunol. 132:725, 1984.

106. Leslie, C. A., Gonnerman, W. A., Ullman, M. D., et al.: Dietary fish oil modulates macrophage fatty acids and decreases arthritis susceptibility in mice. J. Exp. Med. 162:1336, 1985.

107. Robinson, D. R., Prickett, J. D., Polisson, R., et al.: The protective effect of dietary fish oil on murine lupus. Prostaglandins 30:51, 1985.

108. Robinson, D. R., Tateno, S., Knoell, C., et al.: Dietary marine lipids suppress murine autoimmune disease. J. Int. Med. 225(Suppl. 1):211, 1989.

109. Kremer, J. M., Bigauoette, J., Michalek, A. U., et al.: Effects of manipulating dietary fatty acids on clinical manifestations of rheumatoid arthritis. Lancet 1:184, 1985.

110. Kremer, J. M., Jubiz, W., Michalek, A., et al.: Fish-oil fatty acid supplementation in active rheumatoid arthritis: A double-blinded, controlled crossover study. Ann. Intern. Med. 106:498, 1987.

111. Cleland, L. G., French, J. K., Betts, W. H., et al.: Clinical and biochemical effects of dietary fish-oil supplements in rheumatoid arthritis. J. Rheumatol. 15:1471, 1988.

112. Kremer, J. M., Lawrence, D. A., Jubiz, W., et al.: Dietary fish oil and olive oil supplementation in patients with rheumatoid arthritis: Clinical and immunologic effects. Arthritis Rheum. 33:810, 1990.

113. Knapp, H. R., and FitzGerald, G. A.: The antihypertensive effects of fish oil: A controlled study of polyunsaturated fatty acid supplements in essential hypertension. N. Engl. J. Med. 320:1037, 1989.

114. DiGiacomo, R. A., Kremer, J. M., and Shah, D. M.: Fish oil supplementation in patients with Raynaud's phenomenon: A double-blind controlled prospective study. Am. J. Med. 86:158, 1989.

115. Lewis, P., and Taub, S. J.: Allergic synovitis due to ingestion of English walnuts. J.A.M.A. 106:21444, 1936.

116. Zeller, M.: Rheumatoid arthritis food allergy as a factor. Ann. Allergy 7:200, 1947.

117. Marquardt, J. C., Snyderman, R., and Oppenheim, J. J.: Depression of lymphocyte transformation and exacerbation of Behçet's syndrome by ingestion of English walnuts. Cell. Immunol. 9:263, 1973.

118. Epstein, S.: Hypersensitivity to sodium nitrate: A major causative factor in case of palindromic rheumatism. Ann. Allergy 27:343, 1969.

119. Malinow, M. R., Bardana, E. J., Pirofsky, B., et al.: Systemic lupus erythematosus-like syndrome in monkeys fed alfalfa sprouts: Role of a nonprotein amino acid. Science 216:415, 1982.

120. Roberts, J. L., and Hayashi, J. A.: Exacerbation of SLE associated with alfalfa ingestion (Letter). N. Engl. J. Med. 308:1361, 1983.

121. Wright, V., and Watkinson, G.: The arthritis of ulcerative colitis. Br. Med. J. 2:670, 1965.

122. von Potter, W. N.: Regional enteritis. Gastroenterology, 26:347, 1954.

123. Wands, J. R., LaMont, J. T., Mann, E., and Isselbacher, K.: Arthritis associated with intestinal by-pass procedure for morbid obesity: Complement activation and character of circulating cryoproteins. N. Engl. J. Med. 294:121, 1976.

124. Paganelli, R., Levinsky, R. J., Brostoff, J., et al.: Immune complexes containing food proteins in normal and atopic subjects after oral challenge and effect of sodium cromoglycate on antigen absorption. Lancet 1:1270, 1979.

125. Bjarnason, I., So, A., Levi, A. J., et al.: Intestinal permeability and inflammation in rheumatoid arthritis: Effects of non-steroidal anti-inflammatory drugs. Lancet 2:1171, 1984.

126. Parke, E. L., and Hughes, G. R. V.: Rheumatoid arthritis and food: A case study. Br. Med. J. 282:2027, 1981.

127. Panush, R. S., Stroud, R. M., and Webster, E. M.: Food-induced (allergic) arthritis. Arthritis Rheum. 29:220, 1986.

128. Panush, R. S.: Food induced ("allergic") arthritis: Clinical and serologic studies. J. Rheumatol. 17:291, 1990.

129. Darlington, L. G.: Does food intolerance have any role in the aetiology and management of rheumatoid disease? Ann. Rheum. Dis. 44:801, 1985.

130. Panush, R. S.: Possible role of food sensitivity in arthritis. Ann. Allergy, 19(Suppl.):31, 1988.

131. Ziboh, V. A., and Chapkin, R. S.: Biologic significance of polyunsaturated fatty acids in the skin. Arch. Dermatol. 123:1686, 1987.

Hyperuricemia

Evaluation of the patient with hyperuricemia is directed toward answering the following questions: (1) Does the patient really have hyperuricemia? (2) Has damage to tissues or organs occurred as a result? (3) Are associated findings present? (4) What is the cause? (5) What, if anything, should be done? From a practical standpoint, these inquiries are pursued simultaneously, because decisions about the significance of hyperuricemia and about therapy depend on the answers to all of them.

WHAT IS HYPERURICEMIA, AND DOES THE PATIENT HAVE IT?

The serum urate value is elevated in an absolute sense when it exceeds the limit of solubility of monosodium urate in serum. At 37°C the saturation value of urate in plasma is about 7 mg per dl; a value above this concentration represents supersaturation in a physicochemical sense. The serum urate concentration is elevated in a relative sense when it exceeds the upper limit of an arbitrary normal range, which is usually defined as the mean serum urate value plus two standard deviations in a sex- and age-matched healthy population. In most epidemiologic studies, the upper limit has been rounded off at 7 mg per dl in men and 6 mg per dl in women. Finally, a serum urate value in excess of 7 mg per dl begins to carry an increased risk of gouty arthritis or renal stones.

Many factors, including sex and age, have an important influence on the serum urate concentration. The serum urate concentration before puberty in both boys and girls averages approximately 3.6 mg per dl. After the onset of puberty, the levels rise in males more than in females. Values in males reach a plateau in the early 20s and are essentially stable thereafter. Values in females are constant at a lower level than those found in males from age 20 through 40. With menopause, the values in women rise and approach or equal those in men. Differences in the serum urate levels with sex and age are thought to be related to differences in the renal clearance of urate, perhaps determined, in turn, by the endogenous levels of estrogens and androgens. In addition, there may be substantial variation over time in any single person, an observation attributable to many causes, including some of the variables described earlier, dietary alterations, medication usage, and seasonal changes. Accordingly, a single serum urate value is of considerably less value than several determinations over time.

Hyperuricemia by one or more of the aforementioned definitions has been described in 2.3 to 17.6 percent of the populations studied. In one hospitalized population in the United States, 13.2 percent of all adult men exhibited a serum urate concentration in excess of 7 mg per dl.[1]

HAS TISSUE OR ORGAN DAMAGE OCCURRED AS A RESULT OF THE HYPERURICEMIA?

Assessment of tissue damage that might be attributed to hyperuricemia is of major importance in the patient with arthritis, subcutaneous nodules, erosions or other changes on radiographs, nephrolithiasis, or renal insufficiency. Any other clinical signs and symptoms that might result from sustained hyperuricemia would be rare in the absence of at least one of these conditions.

Arthritis. Hyperuricemia can result in both acute and chronic forms of arthritis. In the hyperuricemic patient with acute joint disease, the most useful diagnostic test is direct examination of the synovial fluid, provided it is done properly.[2, 3] According to current dogma, the demonstration of intracellular monosodium urate crystals establishes the diagnosis of gout; it does not, of course, exclude other diseases that may occur simultaneously, e.g., septic arthritis, pseudogout, calcific tendinitis or periarthritis, osteoarthritis, fractures, or torn ligaments or tendons, and these possibilities may have to be excluded.[4, 5] Intracellular monosodium urate crystals can be demonstrated in virtually all patients with gout if synovial fluid from the appropriate joint is carefully examined using compensated polarized light microscopy within the first 24 to 48 hours after onset of the attack. Thus, failure to demonstrate intracellular urate crystals in synovial fluid obtained from an acutely inflamed joint makes the diagnosis of gout highly unlikely as the cause of an acute episode of synovitis. However, when patients are examined several days after the onset of acute synovitis, the likelihood of finding urate crystals declines and the urate crystals observed may not be located in polymorphonuclear leukocytes. Extracellular urate crystals can be found in synovial fluid of 70 percent of gouty patients even

498

during the intercritical period when they are asymptomatic.[6] The finding of extracellular urate crystals in synovial fluid does not carry the same degree of specificity for diagnosing gout as does the demonstration of intracellular urate crystals. This conclusion is based on the following observations. Although the patient with uncomplicated, asymptomatic hyperuricemia rarely (5 percent) exhibits extracellular urate crystals in synovial fluid, as many as 20 percent of patients with hyperuricemia secondary to renal failure may have extracellular urate crystals in the absence of any history of arthritis.[6]

When synovial fluid cannot be obtained or active joint disease is not present at the time of examination, the relationship of hyperuricemia to the clinical symptoms may be more difficult to evaluate. If there is a history of classic podagra or of an acute monoarticular arthritis strongly suggestive of gouty arthritis and dramatically responsive to colchicine, a working assumption that the patient has gout is justified. The diagnosis should be documented with demonstration of urate crystals at the first opportunity.

Sustained hyperuricemia can lead to a chronic, persistent arthritis with symptoms identical to those of osteoarthritis. This complication of hyperuricemia is extremely rare in the absence of andecedent attacks of acute inflammatory arthritis. Typically, chronic gouty arthritis is accompanied by a history of intermittent acute inflammatory attacks and visible tophi; however, this is not always the case. In some instances, the frequent use of a nonsteroidal anti-inflammatory agent or low-dose colchicine may attenuate symptoms. Furthermore, tophi develop in bone and cartilage before they are apparent as subcutaneous nodules and, therefore, may not be identified on physical examination.[7] Thus, the role of hyperuricemia in patients with chronic arthritis may be difficult to determine. Although the presence of hyperuricemia in a patient with chronic arthritis should alert one to the possibility of gout, antihyperuricemic therapy should not be initiated unless there is convincing evidence of the diagnosis.

Nodules. The finding of subcutaneous nodules in the hyperuricemic subject raises the possibility that these are tophaceous deposits. The history is important in this connection, because tophi rarely occur without preceding gouty arthritis. However, if a question exists as to the nature of the nodule or deposit, material should be obtained for microscopic examination. This may be done most easily by closed aspiration of the nodule under aseptic conditions, using a sterile 22-gauge needle. Injection of a small amount of sterile saline may enhance the recovery of urate crystals if no material is obtained with aspiration alone. Suspected tophi in the helix of the ear can be confirmed by gentle abrasion of the skin and blotting the denuded surface with a sterile slide. If urate crystals are demonstrated, the nodule represents a tophus. If crystals are not demonstrated with this procedure, open surgical biopsy of the lesion may be performed. The tissue obtained at that time

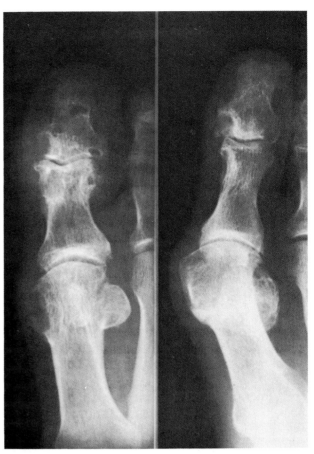

Figure 31–1. These panels show changes typical for bony tophi, including soft tissue distortion, erosions with sclerotic margins, and overhanging edges. Joint space narrowing is minimal despite the large erosions. (From Nakayama, D. A., et al.: Tophaceous gout: A clinical and radiographic assessment. Arthritis Rheum. 27:469, 1984. Used by permission.)

should be fixed in absolute alcohol to avoid dissolution of crystals, if present.

Serologic tests for rheumatoid factor are minimally helpful in evaluating the patient with subcutaneous nodules. If the lesion is a rheumatoid nodule, more than 90 percent of patients will have a positive screening test for rheumatoid factor and the test will usually remain positive at serum dilutions of 1:80 or greater. On the other hand, 30 percent of patients with gout exhibit positive screening tests for rheumatoid factor, and these are usually of low titer.

Radiographic Findings. Bony erosions seen on roentgenograms in a patient with hyperuricemia can present a difficult diagnostic problem. The radiographic appearance of the erosions may be of some help in determining the cause of the lesion. In fact, the bony erosions in gout may be pathognomonic.[8] The classic gouty erosion has a sclerotic border that produces a "punched out" appearance, has an elevated margin or "overhanging lip" that extends outward in the soft tissue apparently carrying the tophaceous nodule, and is proximate to a well-preserved joint space (Fig. 31–1). One should ordinarily assume that the erosions are not due to deposition of monosodium urate crystals unless the history is consistent with gout and the radiologic features are typical. Biopsy may be indicated, particularly if a neoplastic lesion or infection is possible.

Tophi in the subcutaneous tissues are usually radiolucent, but they can become radiopaque if calcium is deposited in these lesions. In the latter circumstances, radiographic examination may reveal the presence of tophaceous deposits, but physical examination will usually detect tophi localized in subcutaneous tissues before they are evident on roentgenograms.

Nephrolithiasis. A history or laboratory finding indicative of a renal calculus provides information important to the future management of the patient. In contrast to the situation observed with tophi, renal calculi may antedate the onset of gouty arthritis. The typical uric acid stone is radiolucent and, therefore, is not visible on routine radiologic examination of the abdomen. It will appear as a filling defect with the use of radiopaque contrast material. As such it may be confused with other radiolucent stones, such as those composed of xanthine or adenine, as well as with tumors or blood clots. If a stone is passed or retrieved at surgery, it is important that it be subjected to chemical analysis.

The importance of hyperuricemia in patients with radiopaque stones deserves emphasis. First, radiopaque stones occur more commonly in patients with gout than in a nongouty population. In addition, reduction of uric acid production (and hence concentration in the urine) with allopurinol is associated with a striking decrease in the frequency of radiopaque stones containing calcium oxalate in both hyperuricemic and hyperuricaciduric subjects (see Chapter 76). It is possible that the initial nidus for opaque stones in this setting is crystals of urate or uric acid. Whether or not this hypothesis accounts for the observation, the therapeutic implications are clear. Hyperuricemic subjects with calcium oxalate stones but not other radiopaque stones, such as magnesium ammonium phosphate or cystine, may benefit from a trial with allopurinol. In normouricemic subjects with hyperuricosuria (800 and 750 mg of uric acid excreted per 24 hours for men and women, respectively) who repetitively form calcium-containing stones, a trial of allopurinol may be indicated.[9]

Renal Insufficiency. One of the most difficult problems facing the clinician lies in the attempt to determine the relationship of hyperuricemia and renal insufficiency in the patient presenting with both abnormalities. In assessing the relationship between hyperuricemia and renal insufficiency, it is important to consider the mechanisms by which urate or uric acid, or both, may injure the kidney. Urate can precipitate in the interstitium of the kidney, leading to slowly progressive renal insufficiency referred to as *urate nephropathy;* uric acid can precipitate in the collecting tubules, leading to acute renal failure,

which is referred to as *uric acid nephropathy;* or uric acid crystals can grow into calculi, which leads to obstruction or infection, or both, of the kidney.

The relationship among hyperuricemia, gout, and renal insufficiency is complex. Autosomal dominant polycystic kidney disease is one cause of renal failure clearly associated with gout.[10] This association cannot be attributed to a special defect of renal urate clearance and, therefore, is probably related to renal insufficiency alone.[11] Interestingly, gout is less common in other types of renal disease, despite the fact that these diseases also progress to renal insufficiency. If the patient has a history of gout preceding renal insufficiency and there is no evidence to suggest another cause such as hypertension or lead exposure, one may assume that urate nephropathy is the cause of the renal failure. Attempts to reduce uric acid production are justified in that setting to prevent further progression of the putative urate nephropathy. The patient with hyperuricemia and renal disease without a previous history of gout presents a more difficult problem. Because an understanding of the relationship of asymptomatic hyperuricemia to chronic renal disease is an important element in the management of the former, this issue is discussed extensively later in this chapter.

In the patient with acute renal failure, uric acid nephropathy should be considered. This entity is more likely to be encountered in patients with malignancies who are undergoing chemotherapy or radiation treatment than in gouty patients, with the exception of those persons with inherited enzyme abnormalities leading to marked purine overproduction.[12] The uric acid to creatinine ratio in a random urine sample from such a patient may help in the evaluation. The finding of a ratio in excess of 1.0 in a patient with acute renal insufficiency is indicative of a substantial increase in uric acid production and raises the possibility that uric acid deposition in the nephron or collecting system may be contributing to the renal insufficiency.[13] In this situation, vigorous therapy is indicated. The more common finding in acute renal failure is a ratio of less than 1.0. In this situation the hyperuricemia may be due entirely to the renal disease and associated factors such as acidosis and dehydration. A history of renal calculi, especially if the stone is demonstrated to contain uric acid or calcium, or both, may be another indication for antihyperuricemic therapy in the patient with renal insufficiency.

A general approach to the hyperuricemic patient is summarized in Figure 31–2. Most hyperuricemic patients will have no evidence of end-organ damage and thus have asymptomatic hyperuricemia. Management of asymptomatic hyperuricemia depends on the associated findings and the cause of the hyperuricemia, as discussed in the following sections.

ARE ASSOCIATED FINDINGS PRESENT?

Hyperuricemia and gout are associated with obesity, ethanol consumption, and hypertension in a

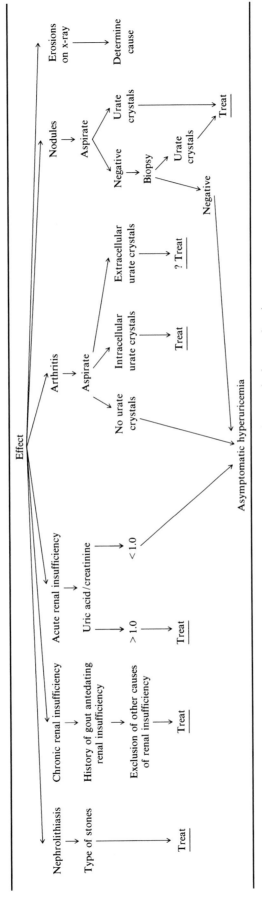

Figure 31–2. Treatment decision diagram for hyperuricemia.

significant percentage of patients.[14] As a consequence, it is not uncommon also to find glucose intolerance, hypertriglyceridemia, atherosclerosis, and renal, hepatic, and ischemic heart disease in hyperuricemic patients. In evaluating hyperuricemic subjects, it is important to keep these associated problems in mind. It may be justified to include a complete blood count, urinalysis, 2-hour postprandial blood sugar, fasting triglycerides, creatinine, liver panel, electrocardiogram, and chest radiograph in the evaluation of the hyperuricemic patient who is overweight or hypertensive or who consumes significant amounts of ethanol. In the normotensive hyperuricemic patient who is not overweight and does not drink, a search for these associated findings probably would not be cost effective.

WHAT IS THE CAUSE OF HYPERURICEMIA?

Hyperuricemia may be defined as primary, first in order of time or development, or secondary, second in order of time or development (see Chapter 76).[15] In the latter setting, the hyperuricemia develops in the course of another disease or as a consequence of its therapy. Hyperuricemia, whether primary or secondary, may be due to overproduction of purines, reduced renal clearance of uric acid, or a combination of the two processes.

In 70 percent of hyperuricemic patients, an underlying cause of hyperuricemia can be readily defined by history and physical examination. Hyperuricia may be the initial clue to the presence of a previously unsuspected disorder. In addition, the nature of the underlying cause may be useful in predicting the potential consequence, if any, of the chemical abnormality. Thus, the possibility of an underlying cause should be explored in every hyperuricemic patient.

A schema for investigating the cause of hyperuricemia, including the secondary causes, is summarized in Figure 31–3. It would seem most reasonable that one be guided by the initial history and physical examination.[1] If an acquired cause commonly associated with normal uric acid excretion is present in the patient with asymptomatic hyperuricemia, further evaluation is probably unnecessary. If the patient has an underlying disorder usually associated with an overproduction of uric acid, determination of 24-hour urinary uric acid may be useful. The higher the urinary uric acid in this group of patients, the higher the incidence of renal calculi[16] and acute uric acid nephropathy,[17] and thus the more likely that treatment will be indicated. If no findings suggestive of a secondary cause are forthcoming, then 24-hour urinary uric acid should be measured in those patients with a serum urate in excess of 11 mg per dl. Further rationale underlying this approach is described later in this chapter under "Management of Hyperuricemia."

THE GENERAL WORK-UP

At this point the general work-up of the patient with hyperuricemia may be reviewed.

History. In beginning to sort out clues that will help direct the physician toward a correct understanding of the problem, it is useful to formulate questions that will decide the following:

1. Is the hyperuricemia primary or secondary? (a) Is the patient obese? If so, for how long? (b) Does the patient consume alcohol regularly and liberally? (c) Has the patient consumed unbonded alcohol? (d) Is the patient taking thiazide diuretics, salicylates, or other drugs? (e) Is there evidence of volume depletion? (f) Is there a history suggestive of renal disease? (g) Is there a history suggestive of a myeloproliferative syndrome, chronic hemolytic anemia, or solid tumor malignancy? (h) Is there a history of lead exposure?
2. Is there a history of acute arthritic attacks? If so, what was their character? Was there a response to colchicine? Has the patient noted any tophi?
3. Is there a history of kidney stones?
4. Has there been hypertension or any history of cardiovascular disease?
5. Is there a family history of hyperuricemia, gout, kidney stones, or renal disease?

Physical Examination. Special attention should be directed toward the following:

1. Habitus should be noted, and height and weight recorded.
2. Is there plethora or pallor? Is there lymphadenopathy, splenomegaly, or hepatomegaly?
3. What is the status of the vascular system? Is there evidence of present or previous hypertension?
4. Are there tophi present in the ears, tendons, joints, or fingertips? Is joint disease present?

Laboratory Data. The need for laboratory studies depends on the severity of the hyperuricemia and the findings elicited from history and physical examination. In general, the laboratory studies will be those that would be indicated because of the basic disease process, whether or not the patient had hyperuricemia or gout. Some of these have been reviewed earlier in the chapter. Several special tests, however, are worthy of emphasis.

1. The most useful of special tests in determining whether the hyperuricemic patient has gout are those that may disclose urate crystals: (a) Synovial fluid analysis—note should be made of gross appearance, viscosity, total and differential cell count, as well as bacteria or crystals, if present[18]—the fluid should be examined with standard light as well as with polarized light microscopy (see Chapter 36). (b) Needle aspiration or biopsy of suspected superficial or bony tophus with search for urate crystals. (c) Radiographs of chronically symptomatic joints may show erosive changes characteristic of gout but are

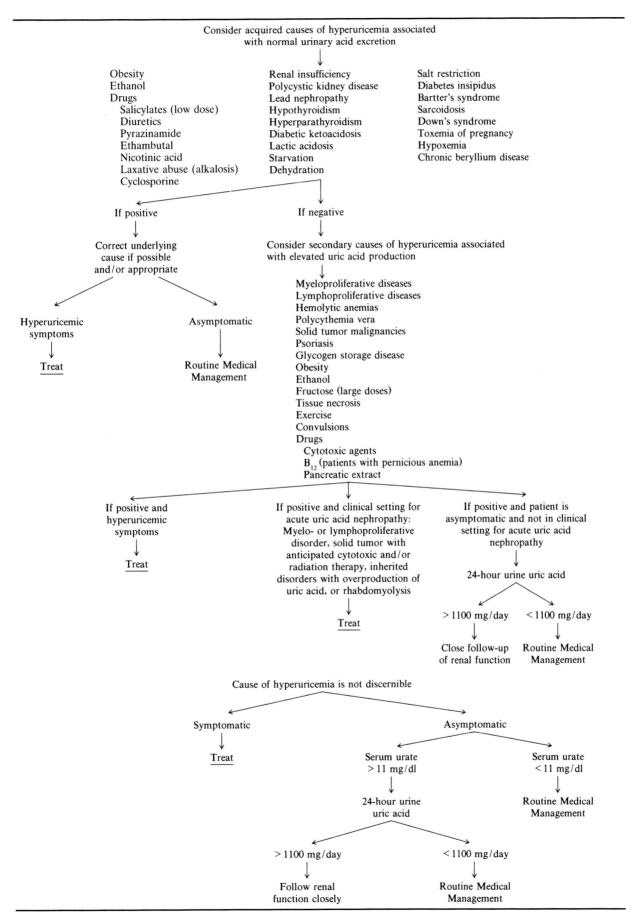

Figure 31–3. Evaluation of the patient with hyperuricemia.

not recommended as part of the routine evaluation of hyperuricemic patients.

2. If a renal stone is recovered, it should be analyzed for uric acid and other constituents by the most definitive methods available. If there is a history of renal colic, an intravenous pyelogram or ultrasound examination may be required to identify calculi.

3. If there is a suspicion of lead-induced hyperuricemia or gout, one should perform a calcium EDTA infusion test with measurement of urinary lead, or analyze erythrocyte–aminolevulinic acid dehydratase activity.

MANAGEMENT OF HYPERURICEMIA

The management of patients with symptoms related to hyperuricemia is discussed in detail in Chapter 76. In general, such patients should be treated with antihyperuricemic agents. The decision of whether to treat hyperuricemia uncomplicated by articular gout, urolithiasis, or nephropathy is an exercise in clinical judgment on which there is less than universal agreement among physicians. The lack of unanimity reflects the paucity of firm data on hyperuricemia as an independent risk factor for hypertension, atherosclerosis, and renal disease. The weight of evidence favors the view that hyperuricemia is directly important only as it may predispose to articular tophi, gout, urate nephropathy, uric acid stones, and acute uric acid nephropathy. Accordingly, the risks engendered by asymptomatic hyperuricemia can be reduced to the statistical risks of development of these manifestations and their consequences.

The magnitude of the risk of articular gout or tophi is related to the degree and duration of hyperuricemia and the sex and age of the patient. Gouty arthritis and tophi are treatable and reversible whenever they occur and by themselves are not life threatening. It would be reasonable to withhold antihyperuricemic therapy in patients with hyperuricemia if the only goal of such therapy was to prevent the development of gout. Clearly, such therapy could be instituted when these manifestations occur.

Urate nephropathy is an entity that may not be reversible. This manifestation is difficult to document, is probably a very late event, and is rarely reported to occur in the absence of previous episodes of gouty arthritis. Several studies have failed to show a relationship between hyperuricemia and urate nephropathy. For example, in one study renal function was monitored prospectively with serum creatinine determinations for 8 years in 113 asymptomatic hyperuricemic subjects and 193 normouricemic patients.[19] During this extended follow-up, the development of azotemia, as reflected by an increase in serum creatinine concentration, was not different in the hyperuricemic and control subjects. To the extent that an increase in serum creatinine concentration

can be used to detect urate nephropathy, we conclude from this study that this particular abnormality is not a major contributor to renal dysfunction in hyperuricemic subjects who do not have articular manifestations of gout.

Urate nephropathy may not be a common cause of renal dysfunction even in the patient with gout. In one study of 524 gouty patients followed for up to 12 years, hyperuricemia alone appeared to have no deleterious effect on renal function.[20] Renal functional deterioration was mainly associated with aging, renal vascular disease, renal calculi, and pyelonephritis, and the correlation with hypertension and resultant nephrosclerosis was much stronger than with hyperuricemia. In another study of 168 gouty patients followed for 10 years, the development of azotemia was uncommon, mild when it occurred, and appeared unrelated to the control of the hyperuricemia.[19] Thus, although an association appears to exist between gout and renal disease, a causal role of the hyperuricemia, per se, in the production of urate nephropathy has yet to be established.

The lack of proof of a direct causal role of hyperuricemia in the genesis of urate nephropathy serves to emphasize the importance of a study designed to determine if control of hyperuricemia has an effect on renal function. One such short-term study exists: a study of 116 patients followed for a mean of 2.5 years compared the effects of allopurinol and placebo therapy in nongouty patients matched for serum urate concentration, mean creatinine clearance, blood pressure, and body weight.[21] No statistically significant differences were consistently found between the placebo- and allopurinol-treated groups, and it was concluded that normalization of the plasma urate concentration did not significantly alter renal function.

Currently available data, which are admittedly incomplete, suggest that (1) renal function is not necessarily affected in an adverse manner by an elevated serum urate concentration; (2) the renal disease that accompanies hyperuricemia may often be related to inadequately controlled hypertension; and (3) correction of hyperuricemia has no apparent effect on renal function. When these observations are coupled with the expense and side effects of the antihyperuricemic drugs, our current recommendation is that asymptomatic hyperuricemia, per se, is not an indication for antihyperuricemic agents if the goal is to prevent urate nephropathy.

Uric acid nephrolithiasis and calcium oxalate nephrolithiasis occur more commonly in patients with hyperuricemia or hyperuricaciduria. Fessel[19] found an incidence of one stone per 114 patients per year in gouty patients, one stone per 295 patients per year in subjects with asymptomatic hyperuricemia, and one stone per 852 patients per year in normouricemic control subjects. In a careful long-term follow-up of gouty patients by Yu and Gutman,[22] the risk of uric acid nephrolithiasis was related to the height of the serum urate level and, to a greater degree, to the magnitude of urinary uric acid excretion. For example, risk of stone formation was less than 20 percent if the serum urate level was 7.1 to 9 mg per dl and reached 50 percent if it was over 13 mg per dl. In similar patients the risk of nephrolithiasis was less than 21 percent if urinary uric acid excretion was less that 700 mg per day and increased substantially with uric acid excretion over 700 mg per day, reaching 50 percent if the excretion was over 1100 mg per day.

The most common type of stone in patients with gout is a uric acid calculus, but gouty subjects also have an increased prevalence of calcium-containing stones. From 1 to 3 percent of the gouty population have a history of calcium stone formation as compared with an overall prevalence of calcium stones in the population of about 0.1 percent. In addition, patients selected because of calcium oxalate or calcium phosphate stones have a high prevalence of hyperuricemia. In one series the mean serum urate in 67 patients with calcium oxalate stones was 7.2 mg per dl compared with the mean serum urate in 10 patients with uric acid stones of 7.8 mg per dl.[23] Perhaps more importantly, Coe and Kavalach[24] noted that 46 of 105 male patients and 9 of 41 female patients with idiopathic recurrent calcium stone disease had a urinary uric acid value over 750 (females) or 800 (males) mg per day while on an unrestricted diet. Hyperuricemia occurred in only 26 of the 55 hyperuricosuric patients. These studies have clearly identified a relationship between hyperuricemia, hyperuricaciduria, and idiopathic calcium oxalate nephrolithiasis. The incidence of calcium oxalate stone disease in a group of patients with asymptomatic hyperuricemia, however, has not been determined.

Although both uric acid and calcium nephrolithiasis are often responsive to appropriate therapeutic regimens, including allopurinol, several observations militate against routine antihyperuricemic prophylaxis in asymptomatic patients at putative risk for developing renal stone disease: (1) the actual prevalence of stone disease in the asymptomatic patient with hyperuricemia is only twice as high as it is in the normouricemic population; and (2) when a stone is formed, it rarely produces a life-threatening or irreversible series of events. In fact, stone disease related to hyperuricemia or hyperuricaciduria, or both, is often reversible with appropriate therapy. At this point, antihyperuricemic therapy should not be instituted as prophylaxis against the development of stone disease but should be started promptly with discovery of a stone in the hyperuricemic or hyperuricaciduric patient. Identification of the patient with a substantial risk of developing a stone in the future may be valuable to the physician in counseling the patient and in recommending frequency of follow-up visits (see later).

Uric acid nephropathy is a severe form of acute renal failure that may occur in hyperuricemic subjects as a result of the precipitation of uric acid crystals in collecting ducts and ureters. This condition occurs most commonly (1) in patients with profound overproduction of uric acid, particularly those with leukemia or lymphoma subjected to aggressive chemotherapy; (2) in patients with gout and marked hyperuricaciduria; and possibly (3) in patients after severe exercise or convulsions. Postmortem studies in patients with acute uric acid nephropathy reveal intraluminal precipitates of uric acid with dilatation of proximal tubules. Therapy designed to decrease the formation of uric acid and to increase the fraction of uric acid present as the more soluble ionized form, monosodium urate, is highly effective in the prevention or reversal of this process. Indeed, it is in this small group of patients that prophylactic antihyperuricemic therapy may be useful.

An approach to the hyperuricemic patient, based on the considerations discussed earlier, is summarized in Figure 31–3. Determine, if possible, whether the patient has one of the conditions listed that might account for the hyperuricemia. If the underlying cause cannot be corrected, a decision regarding therapy and future management is required. When a condition such as articular gout, tophi, bone lesions, or renal calculi is documented, antihyperuricemic therapy is justified. In the absence of these conditions, the following guidelines are helpful:

1. If the hyperuricemia is associated with one of the conditions that leads to a decrease in renal clearance of urate, the patient can be observed, without instituting urate-lowering therapy, at intervals dictated by his or her other medical problems.

2. If the hyperuricemia is related to one of the conditions associated with increased uric acid production, these patients may be at greater risk of developing renal calculi or acute uric acid nephropathy. In clinical settings in which acute uric acid nephropathy is likely, prophylactic treatment is probably justified. In other situations, although immediate antihyperuricemic therapy may not be indicated, quantification of 24-hour urine uric acid excretion may be helpful in directing future management of the hyperuricemic subject. Based on studies of gouty patients and subjects with malignancies, we have selected 1100 mg of uric acid excreted per day as a cutoff for potentially identifying those patients at higher risk for developing renal calculi and acute uric acid nephropathy. In our opinion, those patients who excrete more than 1100 mg of uric acid per day warrant close follow-up of their renal function and immediate therapy at the first onset of symptoms or evidence of renal dysfunction.

3. If the probable cause of hyperuricemia cannot be determined, one should endeavor to identify those patients with increased uric acid production and excretion. The serum urate concentration may be indicative of the amount of uric acid excreted in the urine. Studies in nongouty subjects with normal renal function have demonstrated that there is an abrupt increase in the rate of excretion of urinary uric acid when the serum urate concentration is increased to more than 11 mg per dl, and the amount

of uric acid excreted at these rates exceeds 1000 mg per day.[25] In our opinion, those patients with serum urate concentrations of more than 11 mg per dl in whom a secondary cause of hyperuricemia cannot be determined deserve further evaluation with quantitation of 24-hour urine uric acid excretion. This level of serum urate concentration should not lead to the unnecessary evaluation of large numbers of asymptomatic hyperuricemic subjects but should identify those patients who need further evaluation and close follow-up of their renal function.

References

1. Paulas, H. E., Coutts, A., Calabro, J. J., et al.: Clinical significance of hyperuriciemia in routinely screened hospitalized men. J.A.M.A. 211:277, 1970.
2. Gordon, G., Swan, A, and Dieppe, P.: Detection of crystals in synovial fluids by light microscopy: Sensitivity and reliability. Ann. Rheum. Dis. 48:737, 1989.
3. Schumacher, H. R., Sieck, M., and Clayburne, G.: Development and evaluation of a method for preservation of synovial fluid wet preparations for quality control testing of crystal identification. J. Rheumatol. 17:1369, 1990.
4. Bomalaski, J. S., and Schumacher, H. R.: Podagra is more than gout. Bull. Rheum. Dis. 34:1, 1984.
5. McCarty, D. J.: Podagra due to calcific periarthritis in a young woman. Ann. Intern. Med. 12:70, 1991.
6. Rouault, T., Caldwell, D. S., and Holmes, E. W.: Aspiration of the asymptomatic metatarsal joint in gouty patients and hyperuricemic controls. Arthritis Rheum. 25:209, 1982.
7. Nakayama, D. A., Barthelemy, C., Carrera, G., Lightfoot, R. W., and Wortmann, R. L.: Tophaceous gout: A clinical and radiographic assessment. Arthritis Rheum. 27:468, 1984.
8. Martel, W.: The overhanging margin of bone: A roentgenologic manifestation of gout. Radiology 91:755, 1968.
9. Coe, F. L.: Hyperuricosuric calcium oxalate nephrolithiasis. Contemp. Issues Nephrol. 5:116, 1980.
10. Mejias, E., Navas, J., Lluberes, R., and Martinez-Maldonado, M.: Hyperuricemia, gout, and autosomal dominant polycystic kidney disease. Am. J. Med. Sci. 297:145, 1989.
11. Kaehny, W. D., Tangel, D. J., Johnson, A. M., Kimberling, W. J., Schrier, R. W., and Gabow, R. A.: Uric acid handling in autosomal dominant polycystic kidney disease with normal filtration rates. Am. J. Med. 89:49, 1990.
12. Conger, J. D.: Acute uric acid nephropathy. Med. Clin. North Am. 74:859, 1990.
13. Kelton, J., Kelley, W. N., and Holmes, E. W.: A rapid method for the diagnosis of acute uric acid nephropathy. Arch. Intern. Med. 138:612, 1978.
14. Roubenoff, R.: Gout and hyperuricemia. Rheum. Dis. Clin. North Am. 16:539, 1990.
15. Wyngaarden, J. B., and Kelley, W. N.: Gout and Hyperuricemia. New York, Grune & Stratton, 1976.
16. Boyce, W. H., Garvey, F. K., and Strawcutter, H. E.: Incidence of urinary calculi among patients in general hospitals, 1948 to 1952. J.A.M.A. 161:1437, 1956.
17. Rieselbach, R. E., Bentzel, C. J., Cotlove, E., et al.: Uric acid excretion and renal function in the acute hyperuricemia of leukemia: Pathogenesis and therapy of uric acid nephropathy. Am. J. Med. 37:872, 1964.
18. Shmerling, R. H., Delbanco, T. L., Tosteson, A. N., and Trentham, D. E.: Synovial fluid tests: What should be ordered? J.A.M.A. 264:1009, 1990.
19. Fessel, W. J.: Renal outcomes of gout and hyperuricemia. Am. J. Med. 67:74, 1979.
20. Berger, L., and Yu, T.-F.: Renal function in gout: IV. An analysis of 524 gouty subjects including long-term follow-up studies. Am. J. Med. 59:605, 1975.
21. Rosenfeld, J. B.: Effect of long-term allopurinol administration on serial GFR in normotensive and hypertensive hyperuricemic subjects. In Sperling, O., de Vries, A., and Wyngaarden, J. B. (eds.): Purine Metabolism in Man. New York, Plenum Press, 1974, p. 581.
22. Yu, T.-F., and Gutman, A. B.: Uric acid nephrolithiasis in gout: Predisposing factors. Ann. Intern. Med. 67:1133, 1967.
23. Smith, M. J. V., Hunt, L. D., King, J. S., Jr., et al.: Uricemia and urolithiasis. J. Urol. 101:637, 1969.
24. Coe, F. L., and Kavalach, A. G.: Hypercalcemia and hyperuricosuria in patients with calcium nephrolithiasis. N. Engl. J. Med. 291:1344, 1974.
25. Wyngaarden, J. B.: Gout. Advances Metab. Dis. 2:1, 1965.

Chapter 32

Andrew P. Ferry

The Eye and Rheumatic Diseases

INTRODUCTION

Not many of the detailed clinical studies of rheumatic diseases reported in the literature include a detailed ocular examination by an ophthalmologist as an integral part of the study. Although most rheumatologists are aware of eye involvement in rheumatic disease, they are not necessarily well informed about how often the eyes are affected in patients with rheumatic diseases, which ocular abnormalities are most likely to be present in each of these conditions, and what the management should entail. Many of the associated ocular lesions are potentially blinding. In some instances (e.g., rheumatoid scleritis), the presence of an ocular abnormality may be obvious on casual examination; in other cases, however, ocular abnormality may be overlooked on careful rheumatologic examination. For example, it is well known that the uveitis that leads to cataract formation in juvenile rheumatoid arthritis is usually asymptomatic. This situation *demands* ocular examination as part of the management protocol for children with this disease. Furthermore, even when ocular symptoms are present, the patient may not report them to the rheumatologist. Patients seldom relate their ocular symptoms to their nonocular disorders.

Detailed ophthalmic examination should be included in the protocol for future prospective studies of the rheumatic diseases. This benefits the individual patients involved and helps fill some of the many gaps that remain in our understanding of the various types of ocular lesions that develop in patients afflicted with rheumatic disease.

In some of the diseases within the purview of the rheumatologist (e.g., the mucopolysaccharidoses, ochronosis, and Marfan's syndrome), ocular involvement is an integral part of the disorder. These ocular abnormalities are described in the chapters of this book devoted to these particular rheumatic diseases. Ocular involvement may also occur in certain other diseases (e.g., hemochromatosis) that are not included in this chapter because of their rarity.

The entities discussed here are rheumatoid arthritis, juvenile rheumatoid arthritis, ankylosing spondylitis, Reiter's syndrome, systemic lupus erythematosus, connective tissue diseases other than rheumatoid arthritis and lupus erythematosus (scleroderma, periarteritis nodosa, and polymyositis), Wegener's granulomatosis, relapsing polychondritis, enteropathic arthropathy, sarcoidosis, and Lyme disease. Ocular manifestations of rheumatic fever, giant cell arteritis and polymyalgia rheumatica, amyloidosis, and gout are discussed in the previous edition of this book.[1]

RHEUMATOID ARTHRITIS

Keratoconjunctivitis sicca is the most common ocular complication of rheumatoid arthritis in adults.[2] But the most dramatic complications occur in the sclera, episclera, and corneal periphery. Anterior uveitis, band keratopathy, secondary cataract, palpebral edema, orbital myositis, and transitory palsies of the oculomotor nerves are all uncommon complications (although anterior uveitis and band keratopathy do occur with increased frequency in juvenile rheumatoid arthritis).

Keratoconjunctivitis Sicca

Immunocytochemical studies of lacrimal gland biopsies in patients who have Sjögren's syndrome show a predominantly lymphoid infiltrate consisting chiefly of B cells and Leu-3+ helper T cells.[3] It is hypothesized that destruction of the lacrimal gland tissue is secondary to this lymphoproliferation. The resultant atrophic and cirrhotic changes in the lacrimal glands cause a decreased elaboration of tears and a corresponding reduction of the normal precorneal tear film, the latter becoming attenuated and more viscous. Patients with keratoconjunctivitis sicca have tear lysozyme levels that are below normal.

Dryness of the mouth and oropharynx consequent to salivary gland atrophy is a frequent associated finding. This combination of xerostomia and keratoconjunctivitis sicca is commonly referred to as the *sicca syndrome*.[4, 5] When associated with rheumatoid arthritis or another connective tissue disorder, the resultant triad is known as *Sjögren's syndrome*.

Supported in part by a grant from Research to Prevent Blindness, Inc.

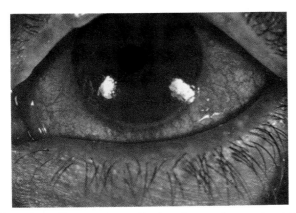

Figure 32–1. Keratoconjunctivitis sicca. Intense hyperemia of the conjunctival vessels accounts for the prominent redness. Dryness of the corneal epithelium causes the reflection from the photographic flash to be dull and irregular rather than normally sharp and highly polished.

Keratoconjunctivitis sicca is usually of insidious onset and is bilateral, occurs far more commonly in women than in men (about 90 percent of cases occur in women), and is extremely uncommon in those below age 40 years. Affected patients usually complain of itching or burning of the eyes. Photophobia is another common symptom. When first seen by the ophthalmologist, only a minority of these patients complain of ocular dryness. Because itching and burning of the eyes are such common symptoms among the general population, the presence of keratoconjunctivitis sicca often goes unsuspected by the ophthalmologist for months or years. Treatment of the supposed infection or allergy with various types of ointment only worsens the condition.

The eyes often appear slightly to moderately red and irritated (Fig. 32–1; see color section at front of this volume). On slit-lamp biomicroscopic examination, tiny, punctate, gray opacities are seen that stain prominently with fluorescein solution. This epithelial keratopathy is usually most prominent in the portion of the cornea located in the interpalpebral fissure. Because this area is not covered by the lids during most of the waking hours, it is particularly subject to drying.

In keratoconjunctivitis sicca, the conjunctival goblet cells are stimulated to secrete an overabundance of mucus. A common finding is the presence of ropelike strands of mucus, often 1 cm or longer, arrayed over the eye or resting in the inferior fornix. Less often a so-called filamentary keratitis may develop. Plaques of diseased epithelium desquamate but remain attached to the adjacent epithelium at one end, forming epithelial filaments that may reach several millimeters in length and that simulate strands of mucus on clinical examination. A relatively rare complication of keratoconjunctivitis sicca is severe corneal opacification resulting from an infectious ulcer developing in the dry cornea.

When keratoconjunctivitis sicca is suspected, the Schirmer test of tear secretion often helps establish the diagnosis. This procedure can be carried out by the internist as well as by the ophthalmologist. Although there are many variables, such as the patient's age, wetting of 5 mm or less in 5 minutes is regarded as strongly indicative of abnormally low tear secretion.

Treatment of keratoconjunctivitis sicca is unsatisfactory. Chronic replacement of tears by artificial substances is required. A variety of such agents are available. Some of the most popular ones are Adsorbotear (Burton, Parsons), Tears Naturale (Alcon), and Liquifilm Tears (Allergan). These are helpful in mild to moderate cases and typically must be instilled at least four times daily. In severe cases, the ophthalmologist must resort to other forms of therapy.

Scleritis and Episcleritis

Anatomy of Sclera and Episclera

The sclera is composed of three layers (from without inward)—the episcleral tissue, the sclera proper, and the lamina fusca. The episclera is a loose structure of delicate fibrous and elastic tissue that is continuous superficially with the loose trabeculae of Tenon's space. (Tenon's capsule is covered, in turn, by the bulbar conjunctiva.) The loose structure of the episclera gradually gives way to a denser arrangement as the episclera merges with the sclera proper. The peculiar feature of the episclera is the large number of small vessels that it possesses in contrast to the sclera proper, which is almost avascular. The episcleral vessels are not seen easily in the uninflamed eye. But as soon as the eye becomes congested, three separate vascular plexuses become readily visible.[6]

The sclera proper is made up of a dense mass of fibrous tissue arranged in compact bundles. Each bundle consists of parallel collagenous fibers, interspersed among which are numerous elastic fibers. Between the bundles are the fixed cells of the scleral tissue. They are fibroblasts with small nuclei and long, branching processes.

Incidence of Scleritis and Episcleritis in Rheumatoid Arthritis

It has been known for many years that the incidence of scleritis and episcleritis is higher in patients with rheumatoid arthritis than it is in the general population. In an attempt to determine the incidence of these inflammatory lesions in patients with rheumatoid arthritis and to differentiate rheumatoid scleritis and episcleritis from nonrheumatoid scleritis and episcleritis, a cooperative study was undertaken by the Center for Rheumatic Diseases in Glasgow, Scotland, and the Tennent Institute of Ophthalmology in that city.[7]

Between 1965 and 1973, 4210 patients with rheumatoid arthritis were examined at the Center for

Rheumatic Diseases. Twenty-eight (0.67 percent) had scleritis, and seven (0.17 percent) had episcleritis.[7] (One can assume that some patients in this cohort with rheumatoid arthritis who did not have episcleritis or scleritis at the time of initial examination will develop one of these lesions in the future, thereby increasing the overall incidence of scleritis and episcleritis in the group of 4210 patients.)

Correspondingly, in 1971 and 1972, a total of 27 patients with scleritis and 35 patients with episcleritis were seen at the Tennent Institute of Ophthalmology. Of the 27 patients with scleritis, nine (33 percent) had clinical and radiologic evidence of rheumatoid arthritis. Of the 35 patients with episcleritis, two (6 percent) had rheumatoid arthritis.[7] Of the 159 patients with episcleritis reported from London by Watson and Hayreh,[6] seven (4 percent) had rheumatoid arthritis, as did 21 (10 percent) of their 207 patients with scleritis.

Combining their patients, investigators at the two cooperating institutions in Glasgow found that all nine of their patients with rheumatoid episcleritis, and 25 of their 37 patients with rheumatoid scleritis, were women. Among nonrheumatoid patients with episcleritis, men and women were affected equally. But among nonrheumatoid patients with scleritis, women were affected about five times as often as were men.

The mean age of all patients with rheumatoid scleritis, rheumatoid episcleritis, and nonrheumatoid scleritis was in the sixth decade. Patients with nonrheumatoid episcleritis were younger, with a mean age of 45 years. With regard to bilaterality, among patients with rheumatoid scleritis, both eyes were involved in 25 of 37 cases (68 percent). Among patients with rheumatoid episcleritis, both eyes were affected in about half the cases.[7]

Rheumatoid scleritis and rheumatoid episcleritis generally occur in patients whose arthritis is of longer duration than that of rheumatoid control patients. Moreover, patients with rheumatoid scleritis and episcleritis usually have more widespread systemic disease—particularly of the cardiovascular and respiratory systems—and have radiologic evidence of more advanced joint disease than do rheumatoid control patients. Subcutaneous granulomatous nodules and atrophy of the skin are much more common in patients with rheumatoid scleritis and episcleritis than in rheumatoid control patients.[7]

The erythrocyte sedimentation rate is significantly higher in patients with rheumatoid scleritis and episcleritis than in rheumatoid control patients. Autoantibody studies in patients with rheumatoid scleritis and episcleritis show little variation from results expected in patients with rheumatoid arthritis.[7]

Signs and Symptoms of Scleritis and Episcleritis

Inflammatory lesions of the sclera and episclera have been subjected to a variety of classifications.[8]

Table 32–1. CLASSIFICATION OF EPISCLERITIS AND SCLERITIS

Episcleritis			217 eyes
Simple episcleritis	170		
Nodular episcleritis	47		
Scleritis			301 eyes
Anterior scleritis	295		
Diffuse scleritis		119	
Nodular scleritis		134	
Necrotizing scleritis		42	
With inflammation		29	
Without inflammation		13	
(scleromalacia perforans)			
Posterior scleritis	6		

From Watson, P. G., and Hayreh, S.S.: Scleritis and episcleritis. Br. J. Ophthalmol. 60:163, 1976. Used by permission.

Scleritis and episcleritis are clinically distinct, with different symptoms, signs, and prognoses. They require different forms of management. From a series involving many years of experience in treating patients with scleral inflammatory disease, Watson and Hayreh[6] have put forth a simplified classification that is useful clinically and that has gained wide acceptance (Table 32–1).

Episcleritis rarely or never causes *loss of vision*. Scleritis may cause loss of vision by leading to one or more of a variety of complications such as uveitis, keratitis, or secondary cataract formation. In the series of Watson and Hayreh,[6] 14 percent of patients with scleritis lost a significant amount of vision after the disease had been present for 1 year.

Scleritis is one of the few diseases that cause severe ocular *pain*. Some 60 percent of patients with scleritis have severe ocular pain. Although about half the patients with episcleritis complain of ocular discomfort, severe pain is not a clinical feature of episcleritis.

In simple episcleritis, the onset of *redness* is often extremely rapid, the eye becoming flushed within several minutes of the beginning of symptoms. In nodular episcleritis and scleritis, the onset is much more gradual. In episcleritis, the color is salmon pink to bright red (Fig. 32–2; see color section at the front of this volume); in scleritis, the redness has a deeper, purple hue (Fig. 32–3; see color section at the front of this volume). In scleromalacia perforans, there often is little or no redness of the eye at all.

Conjunctival discharge is not a feature of either scleritis or episcleritis. Indeed, if there is a discharge, and if it is anything but watery, the patient probably has neither of these disorders.

Scleral defects, as opposed to scleral thinning or increased scleral translucency, occur only in the severest forms of necrotizing disease. In *necrotizing scleritis with adjacent inflammation* (see Table 32–1), the disease begins as a localized area of scleritis associated with severe congestion. About one fourth of these patients also exhibit avascularity of a patch of episcleral tissue overlying or adjacent to the area of

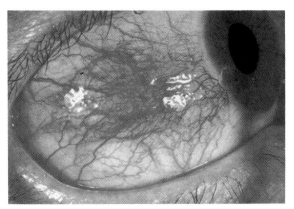

Figure 32–2. Severe episcleritis involving the temporal aspect of the right eye in the region of the interpalpebral fissure. Congestion of the episcleral vessels accounts for the bright red appearance.

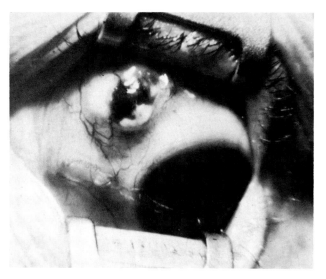

Figure 32–4. Scleromalacia perforans (necrotizing scleritis without adjacent inflammation) in a 54-year-old woman with severe rheumatoid arthritis. The left upper and lower eyelids are separated by a speculum, and the eye is directed inferotemporally. The sclera has perforated superonasally, and the underlying uveal tissue bulges through the scleral defect. (Courtesy of Milton Boniuk, M. D.)

scleral edema. The inflammation may remain localized or may spread in both directions around the globe. In areas where necrosis has occurred, there is scleral thinning or even absence of the sclera, with exposure of the underlying uvea (see Fig. 32–3).

In *necrotizing scleritis without adjacent inflammation* (*scleromalacia perforans;* see Table 32–1), many patients initially have no ocular symptoms. Either the patient or an acquaintance may notice a grayish or yellow scleral patch that already may have progressed to a complete loss of scleral tissue in a localized area. Any clinical evidence of inflammatory change is minimal. After a variable period, the yellowish gray area, together with the overlying episclera, separates as a sequestrum. The resulting defect is covered by a thin layer of conjunctiva. Although unsupported by sclera, the underlying uvea tends not to bulge through the defect unless the intraocular pressure becomes elevated (Fig. 32–4).

About half the patients with scleromalacia perforans have rheumatoid arthritis, usually of long standing. Virtually all of these patients are women.

In episcleritis, severe *uveitis* is rare. In scleritis,

about one third of the patients have anterior uveitis (iridocyclitis) and a smaller number have posterior uveitis (choroiditis). The uveitis is believed to be caused by inflamed sclera overlying the uveal tract. In adult rheumatoid arthritis, when scleritis is not present, the incidence of uveitis is thought to be no greater than it is in the nonrheumatoid population.

Marginal corneal ulcer ("ring ulcer" or "limbal guttering") is the most important type of *keratitis* that occurs in patients who have scleritis.[6] Marginal corneal ulcers (see Fig. 32–8) are potentially devastating because of the risk of perforation. They occur in about 5 percent of all patients with scleritis. Marginal corneal ulcers are more common in patients whose scleritis is associated with rheumatoid arthritis and other connective tissue diseases than they are in nonrheumatoid patients with scleritis. Immune-associated antigen–positive (Ia+) macrophages have been found in conjunctiva adjacent to corneal ring ulcers of patients with rheumatoid arthritis. This observation is regarded as evidence for involvement of the immune system in the pathogenesis of corneal stromal loss in rheumatoid arthritis.

Pathology of Scleritis and Episcleritis

The characteristic histologic picture in rheumatoid scleritis is a zonal type of granulomatous inflammatory reaction (Fig. 32–5). A central area of necrotic scleral collagen is surrounded by a palisade of epithelioid cells and giant cells. These epithelioid and giant cells are in turn surrounded by a mantle of chronic inflammatory cells, chiefly plasma cells and lymphocytes, which often involve the overlying episclera and the underlying uvea. In eyes with scleromalacia perforans, the nongranulomatous com-

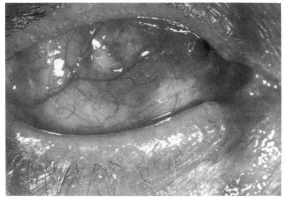

Figure 32–3. Necrotizing scleritis. The eye is adducted and slightly elevated. Destruction of sclera has rendered visible the underlying ciliary body, which has a bluish gray color.

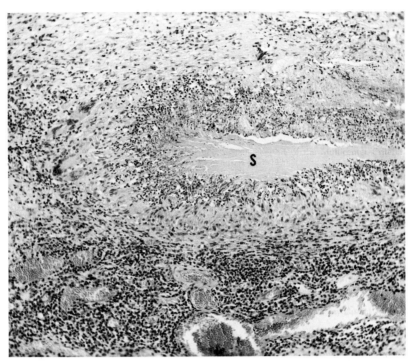

Figure 32–5. Granulomatous scleritis. In this field only a small island of necrotic sclera (*S*) remains. It is being attacked and surmounted by polymorphonuclear neutrophils and a mantle of epithelioid cells. Several well-developed giant cells are present at the left side of the field, directly opposite the scleral fragment. The granulomatous inflammatory reaction is surrounded, in turn, by an outpouring of inflammatory cells consisting chiefly of plasma cells and lymphocytes. These are seen best in the lower portion of the field. Hematoxylin and eosin stain (115 ×); Armed Forces Institute of Pathology Negative Number 57–1163. (Courtesy of Lorenz E. Zimmerman, M. D.)

ponent of the inflammatory reaction is often inconspicuous.

In simple episcleritis and in most cases of nodular episcleritis, the usual histologic changes consist of hyperemia, edema, and infiltration by lymphocytes and plasma cells. However, some rheumatoid episcleral nodules have exhibited all the features of subcutaneous rheumatoid nodules on pathologic examination.[9]

Treatment

Episcleritis is a benign, self-limiting disorder for which no therapy is necessary in most patients. There is a tendency for recurrence in many cases. Should it seem desirable to treat a particular patient, topical glucocorticoids may be used briefly.

Scleritis is a much more serious condition and requires skilled management. Topical glucocorticoids alone are seldom effective in arresting the disease. Topical therapy with glucocorticoids (e.g., prednisolone or dexamethasone) must be supplemented in most cases with systemic anti-inflammatory agents such as indomethacin or prednisone. Complications of the scleritis (e.g., uveitis and secondary glaucoma) require appropriate treatment by the ophthalmologist.

In extreme cases, more heroic forms of medical and surgical treatment have been used. A variety of antimetabolites and alkylating compounds—including methotrexate, 5-fluorouracil, azathioprine, chlorambucil, nitrogen mustard, duazomycin, and cyclophosphamide—have been used with favorable results. Among these drugs, the one now believed to be most effective is cyclophosphamide (Cytoxan).

Scleral grafting has been done to bridge gaps that have developed at the site of necrotizing scleritis. Donor sclera, fascia lata, and periosteum are some of the substances that have been used for this purpose.

JUVENILE RHEUMATOID ARTHRITIS

Juvenile rheumatoid arthritis differs from adult rheumatoid arthritis in many ways well known to the rheumatologist. These two disorders also differ in the nature of associated ocular involvement. In juvenile rheumatoid arthritis, the classic triad of ocular lesions consists of anterior uveitis, band keratopathy, and secondary cataract. In adults with rheumatoid arthritis, uveitis (except as a complication of scleritis) probably occurs no more often than it does in the general population. Except for individuals who have scleritis or who have drug-induced lenticular opacities, cataract is no more common in these adults than in normal persons. Nor is band keratopathy a feature of adult rheumatoid arthritis. Conversely, scleritis and keratitis, both of which are major problems in adult rheumatoid arthritis, are seldom seen in patients with juvenile rheumatoid arthritis. Keratitis sicca, which is so common in adults who have rheumatoid arthritis, occurs only rarely in afflicted children.

The known risk factors for developing *uveitis* are young age, female sex, antinuclear antibody positivity, rheumatoid factor seronegativity, and pauciarticular onset. In virtually all cases, the uveitis involves predominantly the anterior portion of the uveal tract and is therefore an iridocyclitis. Iridocyclitis occurred in 36 of 210 patients (17 percent) with juvenile rheumatoid arthritis reported by Chylack and co-workers in Boston.[10] In a report from England of 160 patients who had anterior uveitis and seronegative juvenile arthritis, chronic uveitis was present in 131.[11] In the remaining 29 patients, 27 of whom were boys, the anterior uveitis was of an *acute* form.

Fifty-one patients who had juvenile rheumatoid arthritis and uveitis were studied in long-term follow-up at the University of Michigan to determine prognostic factors.[12] The average duration of follow-up was 12.7 years. Eighty-nine eyes had uveitis. In all cases, the iridocyclitis was of chronic type. It was bilateral in 75 percent. The initial ocular examination had been completely normal in 41 of the 89 eyes that had uveitis. Of the 89 eyes with uveitis, 22 percent had visual loss to 20/200 or worse, 46 percent had cataracts, 30 percent had band keratopathy, and 27 percent were glaucomatous. The eventual severity of visual loss and ocular complications correlated with the degree of inflammation that had been present on initial ocular examination.[12]

Band keratopathy is not pathognomonic of juvenile rheumatoid arthritis. It occurs in a variety of other disorders and results from deposition of calcium in Bowman's layer (Fig. 32–6). Typically, the first areas of the cornea to be involved are located just inside the limbus nasally and temporally. Calcification of Bowman's layer then progresses across the cornea, eventually connecting the two original sites of involvement. The result is a bandlike opacity located in the interpalpebral fissure. Although a slit-lamp biomicroscope is required to detect the incipient stage of the lesion, the opacity soon becomes visible to the naked eye. In the three series reported above, the incidence of band keratopathy ranged from 13 to 41 percent of eyes that had chronic anterior uveitis.[10–12]

Cataract is caused both by the chronic uveitis and by the glucocorticoids that many children receive for treatment of the uveitis. The incidence of cataract in eyes afflicted with chronic iridocyclitis in the three series mentioned here ranged from 22 to 46 percent.[10–12]

Treatment of eyes affected with the *acute* form of anterior uveitis is usually relatively simple, the inflammation responding well to topical medications. In Kanski's study of 29 patients with the acute type of anterior uveitis,[11] the mean age at onset of arthritis was 11.5 years. Thus, these patients tend to be older at the onset of ocular inflammation than are those afflicted with iridocyclitis of chronic type. They are more likely to complain of ocular pain and discomfort. Their symptoms, together with the redness that is characteristic of the acute form of iridoycyclitis, usually makes it obvious to the parents and to the rheumatologist that an ocular abnormality is present and there seldom is any delay in beginning treatment. Serious ocular complications (e.g., cataract and band keratopathy) seldom occur.[11] Follow-up examination of Kanski's 29 patients with the acute type of

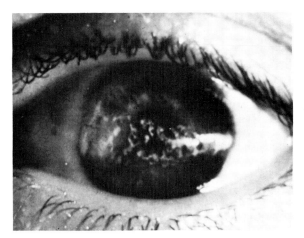

Figure 32–6. Band keratopathy in a 12-year-old girl with severe juvenile rheumatoid arthritis.

anterior uveitis disclosed that 21 of them had developed typical ankylosing spondylitis, and five had sacroiliitis.

Treatment of the *chronic* form of uveitis is often difficult. The degree of ocular disease that is present on initial examination is the critical factor in long-term prognosis.[12] Topical glucocorticoids and atropine are the mainstays of therapy. Systemic glucocorticoids may be required to treat eyes that fail to respond to topical medications. Immunosuppressive drugs other than glucocorticoids have seldom been used in treating iridocyclitis that occurs in patients with juvenile rheumatoid arthritis.[11, 12]

Chelation of the calcium in Bowman's layer with topically applied sodium versenate solution results in clearing of band keratopathy and improvement of vision in many cases. In children who eventually require ocular surgery (e.g., for a cataract dense enough to cause major visual loss or for glaucoma consequent to synechia formation), the results are often discouraging.

Many observers have commented on the lack of symptoms reported by children with the chronic form of uveitis when the ocular inflammation begins. Only a minority report symptoms of iridocyclitis or exhibit evidence of ocular inflammation that is apparent to their parents or to the rheumatologist. In view of this often asymptomatic onset of ocular inflammation, and because treatment of the uveitis at an early stage often forestalls development of complications such as band keratopathy and cataract, it is of great importance that children with rheumatoid arthritis be subjected to periodic examination by an ophthalmologist in a search for anterior uveitis. A 6-month interval between ophthalmic examinations is appropriate in most cases. The children who are at greatest risk are young girls with the pauciarticular form of the disease and antinuclear antibodies. They should be seen, at least initially, at even more frequent intervals.

ANKYLOSING SPONDYLITIS

In various series, 4 to 50 percent of patients with ankylosing spondylitis have anterior uveitis, 25 percent being perhaps the most commonly accepted figure. Studies indicate that among patients with ankylosing spondylitis, uveitis occurs far more commonly in those who have positive histocompatibility antigen HLA-B27 determinations than it does in those who are HLA-B27 negative.[13] Although uveitis may be the presenting sign of the disease, the ocular inflammation characteristically develops in a patient already known to have spondylitis. Typically, the inflammation is an acute, nongranulomatous anterior uveitis. The signs and symptoms include photophobia, some decrease in visual acuity, a variable degree of ocular pain, congestion of the episcleral vessels, fine cellular precipitates on the corneal endothelium, cells and flare in the anterior chamber, and miosis. A severe plastic iritis, with formation of dense synechiae, is decidedly uncommon.

Treatment of the iridocyclitis consists of the usual topical glucocorticoids, cycloplegics (e.g., atropine), and mydriatics. The iritis generally runs a favorable course and tends to clear in 3 to 6 weeks, with few sequelae. Relapses are typical of the disease and may occur repeatedly over the course of many years.

REITER'S SYNDROME

Reiter's syndrome is discussed in detail in Chapter 57. Self-limited conjunctivitis, either papillary or mucopurulent in nature, is the most common ophthalmic manifestation. In a series of 113 patients with Reiter's syndrome, conjunctivitis occurred in 66 (58 percent), iridocyclitis in 13 (12 percent), and keratitis in four (4 percent).[14]

SYSTEMIC LUPUS ERYTHEMATOSUS

In the realm of the ophthalmologist, the most common manifestation of this disease is the *butterfly eruption*,[15] which occurs in about 40 percent of cases and which is discussed in Chapter 72. Signs and symptoms of *central nervous system* involvement occur in some 30 percent of patients with systemic lupus erythematosus, and some of these individuals are seen by the ophthalmologist because of ptosis, diplopia, or nystagmus.[16]

With regard to the *eye* itself, cotton wool patches in the retina often have been cited as being the most common lesion, followed in frequency by corneal and conjunctival involvement, with only an occasional patient exhibiting uveitis or scleritis. But one encounters difficulty in attempting to determine the incidence of ocular involvement in systemic lupus erythematosus. For example, many observers have remarked that the retinal lesions occur much more

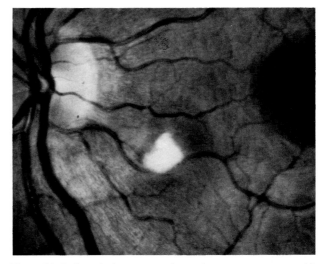

Figure 32–7. A typical cotton wool spot in a young woman with systemic lupus erythematosus. The lesion is situated along the upper border of a retinal arteriole, about midway between the optic nerve head and the macula.

often in acutely ill patients than they do in those who are in remission or who have only a relatively mild form of the disease. Another consideration in determining the incidence of ocular involvement in systemic lupus erythematosus is the greater clinical awareness and better laboratory diagnostic aids that have led to the detection of many mild cases of lupus. These patients are the ones who are least likely to exhibit ocular complications.

Retinopathy

Cotton wool spots occur in lupus and in a variety of other disorders, most notably the connective tissue diseases, vascular hypertension, central retinal vein occlusion, diabetic retinopathy, papilledema, the dysproteinemias, leukemia, and severe anemia.[17] On ophthalmoscopic examination, one or more (but usually fewer than ten) cotton wool spots are seen. They occur preferentially in the posterior part of the retina, rendering them detectable by casual examination. The optic nerve head is often involved. Each cotton wool spot appears as a grayish white, soft, fluffy exudate, usually situated more closely to the arterioles than to the veins, lying in the inner layers of the retina and bulging slightly toward the vitreous body (Fig. 32–7). They are small, averaging about one third of a disc diameter in width. (The diameter of the normal optic nerve head is 1.5 to 2.0 mm.) Cotton wool spots usually clear within 1 to 3 months of their appearance.

Pathologic examination of cotton wool spots discloses disciform thickening of the retinal nerve fiber layer. In this region, some of the nerve fibers have been interrupted, leading to formation of *cytoid bodies*. The latter are globular structures, 10 to 20 μm in diameter. Each bears a superficial resemblance to a cell because of a centrally located structure simulating a nucleus. (Thus, *cotton wool spot* is an ophthalmo-scopic term, and cytoid body is a histologic feature of a cotton wool spot.[17])

Hemorrhages in the inner retinal layers are another feature of the retinopathy that occurs in systemic lupus erythematosus. As is true of cotton wool spots, they are not necessarily mere reflections of a concomitant vascular hypertension. They can result from an independent effect of the disease on the retinal tissues, and they are found in the absence of hypertension.

Corneal and Conjunctival Lesions

A variety of these have been described.[18] The most common are *conjunctivitis* (3 to 20 percent of cases) and mild *epithelial degeneration*, rendering the affected cells stainable with topical fluorescein. *Sjögren's syndrome* has been documented in association with various connective tissue diseases, including systemic lupus erythematosus, and any of these may replace rheumatoid arthritis in the classic triad of Sjögren's syndrome.[5]

CONNECTIVE TISSUE DISEASES OTHER THAN RHEUMATOID ARTHRITIS AND LUPUS ERYTHEMATOSUS

Scleroderma (systemic sclerosis) is a rare disease. Some three to five new cases per million people appear each year in the United States. In this disorder, the ocular adnexa and the outer coats of the eye are affected relatively often, but involvement of the inner eye, particularly the retina, is unusual.[19] The most common finding is tightness of the eyelids. Keratoconjunctivitis sicca and Sjögren's syndrome occur less often.

Ocular involvement is uncommon in *periarteritis nodosa* (polyarteritis nodosa). Reported abnormalities of the outer coats of the eye include chemosis (conjunctival edema), subconjunctival hemorrhages, conjunctivitis, keratitis, scleritis, marginal corneal ulceration, and Sjögren's syndrome. Choroidal angiitis has been found in many eyes examined after death, but clinical signs of choroidal involvement are seldom seen. Retinal lesions are rarer than choroidal involvement, and most of these result from the effects of vascular hypertension on the retinal vessels.[20]

Involvement of the eye is rare in *polymyositis* and in *dermatomyositis*. Conjunctivitis, episcleritis, iritis, and retinal cotton wool spots have been reported. The eyelids are involved more often. A peculiar bluish to violaceous (heliotrope) erythematous suffusion develops in the eyelids in many cases and is often associated with closely set telangiectasias of the palpebral skin and with marked palpebral edema. The orbicularis oculi muscles and the extraocular muscles may participate in the widespread myositis, leading to pain, tenderness, oculomotor palsies, and nystagmus.[21]

WEGENER'S GRANULOMATOSIS

The classic triad of Wegener's granulomatosis consists of granulomas of the upper or lower respiratory tract, focal necrotizing glomerulonephritis, and arteritis. But, as Wegener has emphasized, the condition should not be considered primarily an angiitis.[22] Angiitis is a prominent feature in the lungs in some patients, but it is not responsible for the extravascular granulomatous lesions. In some cases, it is difficult or impossible to demonstrate angiitis.

Ocular involvement is common in Wegener's granulomatosis and may be the first sign of the disease. Haynes and colleagues[23] reported the ocular findings in 29 patients with Wegener's granulomatosis seen at the National Institutes of Health during a 15-year span and reviewed ocular involvement in cases reported in the English language literature since 1957. Of the overall total of 342 patients, 39 percent had ocular disease. In 286 of the 342 patients (83 percent), the nature of the ocular involvement had been recorded. The most common abnormalities among these 286 patients were proptosis (18 percent); conjunctivitis, scleritis, episcleritis, or corneoscleral ulcer (16 percent); vasculitis of retina or optic nerve (8 percent); dacryocystitis (inflammation of the tear sac; 3 percent); and uveitis (2 percent). Among 140 patients with Wegener's granulomatosis seen from 1966 to 1982 at the Mayo Clinic, ocular or orbital involvement or both occurred in 40 (29 percent).[24] Orbital inflammatory disease was most common, followed in descending order by scleritis, keratitis, nasolacrimal duct obstruction, and various other lesions.

In some patients, ring ulcers of the corneal periphery are the initial sign of Wegener's granulomatosis. The woman whose eye is shown in Figure 32–8 (see color section at the front of this volume) had been treated initially for conjunctivitis. When first examined, 3 weeks after the onset of her ocular symptoms, she had a deep ring ulcer in the superotemporal periphery of her cornea. She also gave a history of recent weight loss and had several areas of cutaneous ulceration over her lower legs. Urinalysis disclosed the presence of albuminuria and erythrocyte casts. Pulmonary cavities were demonstrated on roentgenography. The corneal lesion progressed, and she soon developed a necrotizing scleritis of the type seen in rheumatoid arthritis. Death occurred from a cerebral hemorrhage 14 months after the onset of her symptoms. On pathologic examination of the affected eye, a granulomatous reaction to collagen fibers was found in the corneal ring ulcer and in the broad area of necrotizing scleritis. There was no evidence of vasculitis in serial sections of the entire eye.

Although topical and systemic glucocorticoids often are helpful in controlling some of the ocular lesions that occur in Wegener's granulomatosis, cyclophosphamide is regarded as the drug of choice in treating this disorder.[23, 24]

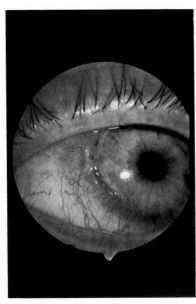

Figure 32–8. Wegener's granulomatosis. Deep ring ulcer in corneal periphery superotemporally in patient with previously undiagnosed Wegener's granulomatosis. Note also the episcleritis adjacent to the corneal lesion. Necrotizing scleritis developed in this area within several weeks after the photograph was made.

RELAPSING POLYCHONDRITIS

Relapsing polychondritis is a rare disorder characterized by inflammation and destruction of cartilage. The condition has some features of rheumatoid arthritis, Wegener's granulomatosis, and midline lethal granuloma. The cause and pathogenesis are unknown.

The human eye and eyelid do not contain cartilage, nor does the orbit, except for the minuscule amount that constitutes the trochlea. This absence of cartilage notwithstanding, involvement of the eye and its adnexa is common in relapsing polychondritis. In a series of 112 patients with this disorder, 21 had ocular or ocular adnexal symptoms or both at the outset, and 57 others developed ocular or ocular adnexal symptoms later in the course of their disease.[25] Scleritis and episcleritis are the most common ocular manifestations. Proptosis and chemosis simulating orbital pseudotumor, and inflammation of the eyelids, are the most common forms of ocular adnexal involvement.[25]

Hyaline cartilage, such as articular cartilage, contains exclusively type II collagen. Type II collagen is found in sclera,[26] retina, and vitreous body, but of these three tissues only the sclera is an ocular site of predilection for involvement in relapsing polychondritis.

ENTEROPATHIC ARTHROPATHY

The disorders of main interest in this group are ulcerative colitis, Crohn's disease, and Whipple's disease.

The reported incidence of arthritis complicating *ulcerative colitis* and *Crohn's disease* is generally in the range of 10 percent, although Greenstein and associates[27] reported involvement in 53 (26 percent) of 202 patients with ulcerative colitis and in 111 (22 percent) of 498 patients with Crohn's disease. The most common rheumatic pattern is an asymmetric polyarthritis involving a few joints. The reported incidence of spondylitis, which is indistinguishable from ankylosing spondylitis, in patients with ulcerative colitis and Crohn's disease varies from 2 to 6 percent. In contrast to Crohn's disease, the extraintestinal manifestations of ulcerative colitis (involvement of joints, eyes, and skin) seldom precede the intestinal symptoms.

There is an increased incidence of uveitis, particularly iritis, in patients with ulcerative colitis. Episcleritis and (rarely) marginal ring ulceration of the cornea are other types of ocular abnormalities that occur in these individuals. Patients with ulcerative colitis and spondylitis are much more likely to have iritis than are those without such joint involvement.

Ocular involvement was found in 41 of 820 patients (5 percent) with Crohn's disease.[27, 28] (But because not all of the 820 individuals had undergone ophthalmologic examination, the prevalence of ocular involvement was undoubtedly higher than the reported 5 percent.) The most common ocular disorders were conjunctivitis, episcleritis, uveitis (especially iridocyclitis), and peripheral corneal ulceration.[27, 28] Ocular lesions were much more common in those patients whose disease affected the colon than in those whose disease was in the small intestine.[27] (Similarly, joint involvement was also much more prevalent in patients whose Crohn's disease occurred in the colon than in those whose disease was limited to the small bowel.[27]) There was a striking association of ocular involvement with joint involvement: Patients with Crohn's disease who had joint lesions were far more likely to also have ocular lesions than were patients with Crohn's disease whose joints were unaffected.[28]

In patients with *Whipple's disease*, there is heavy infiltration of the intestinal wall and lymphatics by macrophages filled with glycoprotein. Steatorrhea and diarrhea are frequent signs. Nondeforming migratory arthritis is common and is often the initial complaint. Fever occurs in about one third of patients with Whipple's disease. Many of these individuals have been regarded erroneously as having rheumatoid arthritis.

Opacities in the vitreous body are the most common ocular abnormality in patients with Whipple's disease. They consist of macrophages that have migrated from the inner layers of the retina into the vitreous body. Thus, the basic abnormality is a retinitis. The strong periodic acid–Schiff positivity of the macrophages' cytoplasm is attributed to the high content of polysaccharides present in bacterial wall remnants that are located within the cytoplasmic granules.[29] Electron microscopic examination of these macrophages in the retina and vitreous body has displayed intracytoplasmic, degenerating, rod-shaped bacteria and membranous structures identical with those seen in the intestine, brain, heart, and other tissues of patients with Whipple's disease.[29]

SARCOIDOSIS

The eyes and ocular adnexa are involved in many patients with sarcoidosis. The precise incidence varies widely in different studies and depends on several factors. Involvement of the eyes in 25 percent of patients with sarcoidosis is a widely accepted approximation. Considerable suffering and visual loss often occur.

Uveitis is the most common type of ocular involvement.[30] It is granulomatous in nature, is usually bilateral, and characteristically affects the anterior uvea (iris and ciliary body) more often and more severely than it does the posterior uvea (choroid). The severe inflammation leads to cataract formation and—by adhesion of the iris to the corneal periphery (anterior synechia formation) or by adhesion of the iris to the lens (posterior synechia formation)—may result in chronic secondary glaucoma (Fig. 32–9). Much less often inflammation of the posterior portion of the uveal tract (choroid) predominates. A relatively common event is the development of *retinal perivasculitis*. The inflammatory cells aggregated about the retinal vessels account for the ophthalmoscopic picture known as "candle wax drippings." *Optic neuritis* and central nervous system sarcoidosis occur more

often in patients with retinal perivasculitis than in those who do not have retinal lesions. Topical and systemic glucocorticoids and topical atropine are the mainstays in treating sarcoid uveitis.

Involvement of the *outer coats* of the eye occurs much less often than do uveitis and retinitis. Major scleral lesions are great rarities. Particularly in patients with erythema nodosum, however, small granulomatous lesions may develop in the episclera or in the outer scleral layers. Band keratopathy caused by calcium deposition in Bowman's layer may occur in patients with hypercalcemia.

Involvement of the *ocular adnexa* is common. The eyelids often are affected. The lacrimal glands and fornical conjunctiva also are involved frequently. Although sarcoidosis of the main and accessory lacrimal glands may lead to diminished tear formation and thereby to keratoconjunctivitis sicca in a small minority of patients, in most cases, involvement of the lacrimal gland and conjunctiva is asymptomatic. However, simple clinical inspection of the conjunctiva, especially the conjunctiva in the inferior fornix, and the lacrimal gland often reveals abnormalities in the form of conjunctival nodules and lacrimal gland enlargement (Fig. 32–10).

The lacrimal gland and conjunctiva are located superficially and are readily available for *biopsy*. At the Medical College of Virginia, lacrimal gland biopsies were performed on 60 patients who had uveitis of the type seen in sarcoidosis. Thirty-three percent of the biopsies contained noncaseating epithelioid cell tubercles, affording a tissue diagnosis of sarcoidosis. In the same study, 11 of 50 other patients (22 percent) who did not have uveitis but who had been referred for lacrimal gland biopsy by internists because of systemic or roentgenographic findings suggestive of sarcoidosis had abnormal biopsy findings.

Biopsy of the conjunctiva or lacrimal gland has many advantages over such invasive procedures as biopsy of a scalene lymph node, mediastinoscopy, or transbronchial biopsy of the lung. These procedures require hospitalization and, in the case of mediastinoscopy, subjection of the patient to general anesthesia. The yield of positive abnormal biopsy findings is higher with the invasive procedures, in which abnormal results are obtained in 70 to 90 percent of cases, than it is in biopsies of the conjunctiva or lacrimal gland. The yield of abnormal results in patients with proven sarcoidosis whose conjunctiva and lacrimal glands appear normal on clinical examination ranges from 25 to 55 percent.[31] The yield is even higher in patients with obvious conjunctival nodules or with frank lacrimal gland enlargement. Biopsy of the conjunctiva or lacrimal gland is accomplished in a matter of a few minutes on an outpatient basis, using a local anesthetic. Conjunctival biopsy is well known to be a safe procedure, and none of the 160 patients who have undergone lacrimal gland biopsy on my service has developed any complication. Therefore, when at-

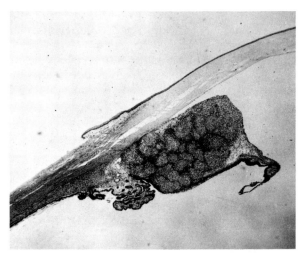

Figure 32–9. Iridocyclitis in sarcoidosis. The peripheral and mid zones of the iris are massively infiltrated by discrete, noncaseating epithelioid cell tubercles. The pupillary zone of the iris is uninvolved and, in this plane of section, only the most anterior aspect of the ciliary body participates in the inflammatory reaction. Peripheral anterior synechia formation (adhesion of the iris to the anterior chamber angle structures and to the corneal periphery) has caused obstruction of the major outflow channels of the aqueous humor, resulting in intractable secondary glaucoma. Hematoxylin and eosin stain (20 ×). (Courtesy of Lorenz E. Zimmerman, M. D.)

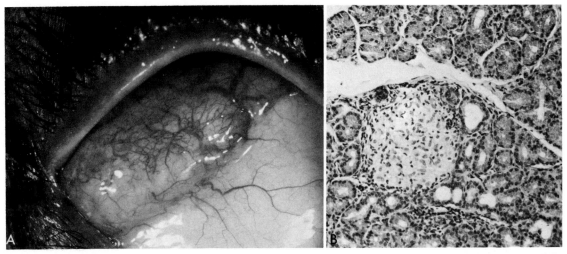

Figure 32–10. Sarcoidosis of the lacrimal gland. *A*, The right upper lid is partially everted for photographic purposes, and the patient is directing her gaze inferonasally. The palpebral lobe of the lacrimal gland is moderately to markedly enlarged. *B*, Biopsy of the lacrimal gland revealed many discrete, noncaseating epithelioid cell tubercles of the type seen near the center of the field. Hematoxylin and eosin stain (150 ×).

tempting to establish histologic confirmation in a patient suspected of having sarcoidosis, it seems prudent to perform biopsy of the lacrimal gland or conjunctiva. Should results of these simple procedures prove normal (the results will be available within a day or two), the patient can then be subjected to the more formidable invasive procedures involving thoracic surgery. Thus, instead of merely referring the patient with suspected sarcoidosis to the ophthalmologist for ocular examination, the internist should suggest that biopsy of the lacrimal gland or conjunctiva, or both, be done if a histologic diagnosis has not been established already.

LYME DISEASE

Lyme disease is a tick-borne illness caused by the spirochete *Borrelia burgdorferi* and manifested by cutaneous rash and neurologic and arthritic findings. Most publications in the ophthalmic literature pertaining to this disorder have been clinical case reports. Ocular manifestations of Lyme disease include blepharitis, photophobia, conjunctivitis, keratitis, episcleritis, iritis, choroiditis, orbital myositis, retinal edema, papilledema, and the pseudotumor cerebri syndrome.[32] Other neuro-ophthalmologic manifestations that have been reported include meningitis, optic neuritis, neuroretinitis, and cranial nerve palsies.[33]

Antibiotic therapy is the mainstay in treating ocular involvement in Lyme disease,[34] but addition of glucocorticoids or other anti-inflammatory agents has been advocated for some patients.[35]

References

1. Kelley, W. N., Harris, E. D., Ruddy, S., and Sledge, C. B. (eds.): Textbook of Rheumatology. 3rd ed. Philadelphia, W. B. Saunders Company, 1989, p. 579.

2. Duke-Elder, S., and Soley, R. E.: Arthritis. In Duke-Elder, S. (ed.): System of Ophthalmology. Vol. 15. Summary of Systemic Ophthalmology. St. Louis, C. V. Mosby Company, 1976, p. 15.

3. Pepose, J. S., Akata, R. F., Pflugfelder, S. C., and Voigt, W.: Mononuclear cell phenotypes and immunoglobulin gene rearrangements in lacrimal gland biopsies from patients with Sjögren's syndrome. Ophthalmology 97:1599, 1990.

4. Farris, R. L.: Sjögren's syndrome. In Gold, D. H., and Weingeist, T. A. (eds.): The Eye in Systemic Disease. Philadelphia, J. B. Lippincott Company, 1990, pp. 70–71.

5. Duke-Elder, S., and MacFaul, P. A.: Atrophies of the lacrimal gland. In Duke-Elder, S. (ed.): System of Ophthalmology. Vol. 13. The Ocular Adnexa. St. Louis, C. V. Mosby Company, 1974, pp. 625–635.

6. Watson, P. G., and Hayreh, S. S.: Scleritis and episcleritis. Br. J. Ophthalmol. 60:163, 1976.

7. McGavin, D. D., Williamson, J., Forrester, J. V., Foulds, W. S., Buchanan, W. W., Dick, W. C., Lee, P., Macsween, R. N., and Whaley, K.: Episcleritis and scleritis: A study of their clinical manifestations and association with rheumatoid arthritis. Br. J. Ophthalmol. 60:192, 1976.

8. Duke-Elder, S., and Leigh, A. G.: Inflammation of the sclera. In Duke-Elder, S. (ed.): System of Ophthalmology. Vol. 8. Diseases of the Outer Eye. St. Louis, C. V. Mosby Company, 1965, pp. 1003–1050.

9. Ferry, A. P.: The histopathology of rheumatoid episcleral nodules: An extraarticular manifestation of rheumatoid arthritis. Arch. Ophthalmol. 82:77, 1969.

10. Chylack, L. T., Bienfang, D. C., Bellows, A. R., and Stillman, J. S.: Ocular manifestations of juvenile rheumatoid arthritis. Am. J. Ophthalmol. 79:1026, 1975.

11. Kanski, J. J.: Anterior uveitis in juvenile rheumatoid arthritis. Arch. Ophthalmol. 95:1794, 1977.

12. Wolf, M. D., Lichter, P. R., and Ragsdale, C. G.: Prognostic factors in the uveitis of juvenile rheumatoid arthritis. Ophthalmology 94:1242, 1987.

13. Perkins, E. S.: Ankylosing spondylitis. In Gold, D. H., and Weingeist, T. A. (eds.): The Eye and Systemic Disease. Philadelphia, J. B. Lippincott, 1990, pp. 43–45.

14. Lee, D. A., Barker, S. M., Su, W. P., Allen, G. L., Liesegang, T. J., and Ilstrup, D. M.: The clinical diagnosis of Reiter's syndrome: Ophthalmic and non-ophthalmic aspects. Ophthalmology 93:350, 1986.

15. Duke-Elder, S., and MacFaul, P. A.: Connective tissue diseases. In Duke-Elder, S. (ed.): System of Ophthalmology. Vol. 13. The Ocular Adnexa. St. Louis, C. V. Mosby Company, 1974, pp. 321–327.

16. Lessell, S.: The neuro-ophthalmology of systemic lupus erythematosus. Doc. Ophthalmol. 47:13, 1979.

17. Ferry, A. P.: Retinal cotton wool spots and cytoid bodies. Mt. Sinai J. Med. 39:604, 1972.

18. Duke-Elder, S., and Leigh, A. G.: In Duke-Elder, S. (ed.): System of Ophthalmology. Vol. 8. Diseases of the Outer Eye. St. Louis, C. V. Mosby Company, 1965, pp. 1098–1100.

19. Duke-Elder, S., and Soley, R. E.: In Duke-Elder, S. (ed.): System of Ophthalmology. Vol. 15. Summary of Systemic Ophthalmology. St. Louis, C. V. Mosby Company, 1976, p. 145.

20. Duke-Elder, S., and Soley, R. E.: In Duke-Elder, S. (ed): System of Ophthalmology. Vol. 15. Summary of Systemic Ophthalmology. St. Louis, C. V. Mosby Company, 1976, p. 129.

21. Duke-Elder, S., and Soley, R. E.: *In* Duke-Elder, S. (ed.): System of Ophthalmology. Vol. 15. Summary of Systemic Ophthalmology. St. Louis, C. V. Mosby Company, 1976, p. 43.

22. Wegener, F.: About the so-called Wegener's granulomatosis, with special reference to the generalized vascular lesions. Morgagni 1:5, 1968.

23. Haynes, B. F., Fishman, M. L., Fauci, A. S., and Wolff, S. M.: The ocular manifestations of Wegener's granulomatosis: Fifteen years experience and review of the literature. Am. J. Med. 63:131, 1977.

24. Bullen, C. L., Liesegang, T. J., McDonald, T. J., and DeRemee, R. A.: Ocular complications of Wegener's granulomatosis. Ophthalmology 90:279, 1983.

25. Isaak, B. L., Liesegang, T. J., and Michet, C. J.: Ocular and systemic findings in relapsing polychondritis. Ophthalmology 93:681, 1986.

26. Hoang-Xuan, T., Foster, C. S., and Rice, B. A.: Scleritis in relapsing polychondritis: Response to therapy. Ophthalmology 97:892, 1990.

27. Greenstein, A. J., Janowitz, H. D., and Sachar, D. B.: The extraintestinal complications of Crohn's disease and ulcerative colitis: A study of 700 patients. Medicine 55:401, 1976.

28. Hopkins, D. J., Horan, E., Burton, I. L., Clamp, S. E., de Dombal, F. T., and Goligher, J. C.: Ocular disorders in a series of 332 patients with Crohn's disease. Br. J. Ophthalmol. 58:732, 1974.

29. Font, R. L, Rao, N. A., Issarescu, S., and McEntee, W. J.: Ocular involvement in Whipple's disease: Light and electron microscopic observations. Arch. Ophthalmol. 96:1431, 1978.

30. Green, W. R.: Sarcoidosis. *In* Spencer, W. H. (ed.): Ophthalmic Pathology: An Atlas and Textbook. 3rd ed. Philadelphia, W. B. Saunders Company, 1986, pp. 1966–1990.

31. Nichols, C. W., Eagle, R. C., Yanoff, M., and Menocal, N. G.: Conjunctival biopsy as an aid in the evaluation of the patient with suspected sarcoidosis. Ophthalmology 87:287, 1980.

32. Flach, A. J., and Lavoie, P. E.: Episcleritis, conjunctivitis, and keratitis as ocular manifestations of Lyme disease. Ophthalmology 97:973, 1990.

33. Lesser, R. L., Kornmehl, E. W., Pachner, A. R., Kattah, J., Hedges, T. R., Newman, N. M., Ecker, P. A., and Glassman, M. I.: Neuro-ophthalmologic manifestations of Lyme disease. Ophthalmology 97:699, 1990.

34. Aaberg, T. M.: The expanding ophthalmologic spectrum of Lyme disease. Am. J. Ophthalmol. 107:77, 1989.

35. Baum, J., and Barza, M.: The expanding ophthalmologic spectrum of Lyme disease (letter). Am. J. Ophthalmol. 107:684, 1989.

Chapter 33

Nicholas A. Soter
Andrew G. Franks, Jr.

The Skin and Rheumatic Diseases

INTRODUCTION

Dermatologic lesions may indicate associated disorders of organ systems other than the skin. The presence of skin lesions is especially noteworthy in patients with rheumatic diseases. Thus, the integument should be assessed with the same precision that is devoted to an examination of the joints and musculoskeletal system.

INTERPRETATION OF ALTERATIONS IN THE SKIN

Examination of the Skin

Skin lesions may be the presenting complaint of the patient, may occur in association with other symptoms and signs such as fever or arthralgia, or may be incidental findings observed during the routine physical examination. Eruptions may be localized or generalized. When the eruption occurs in a bilateral or symmetric distribution, the pathologic stimulus is usually endogenous or is hematogenously disseminated.

Certain signs are recognized more easily by magnification of the skin lesions. Nail-fold capillary changes may be better visualized with an ophthalmoscope. The technique known as diascopy is performed by firmly pressing a piece of glass, such as a microscope slide, over a skin lesion; in the examination of erythematous lesions, blanching reflects capillary dilation and lack of blanching reflects extravasated blood. Diascopy thus permits the differentiation of purpura from the erythema of vasodilation. Diascopy performed on dermal papules may have a yellow-brown appearance that is characteristic of granulomas, which occur in disorders such as sarcoid. A Wood's lamp, which emits long-wave ultraviolet light (360 nm), is useful in the assessment of variations in skin pigmentation.

All lesions that consist of crusts and purulent exudates should be examined with Gram's stain and bacterial cultures.

The application of 10 percent potassium hydroxide to a portion of scale, which is then gently heated

and examined with a light microscope, is used to search for fungi.

Microscopic examination of skin lesions is particularly useful, since biopsy specimens are easily obtained for diagnosis by the use of a skin trephine or punch. Specimens from nodular lesions, such as panniculitis, are best obtained by incision with a scalpel.

Classification of Skin Lesions

A *macule* is a circumscribed area of altered skin color without elevation or depression of its surface relative to the surrounding skin. Macules may be of any size and are the result of pigmentary or vascular abnormalities of the skin.

A *papule* is a solid lesion, most of which is elevated above, rather than deep within, the plane of the surrounding skin. The elevation may be caused by a localized increase of cellular elements in the dermis or epidermis, by metabolic deposits in the dermis, or by dermal edema.

A *nodule* is a solid, round, or ellipsoidal lesion usually located in the dermis or subcutaneous tissue, but it may occur in the epidermis. The depth of involvement rather than the diameter primarily differentiates a nodule from a papule. Nodules result from infiltrates, neoplasms, or metabolic deposits in the dermis or subcutaneous tissue and often indicate systemic disease.

A *plaque* is an elevation above the skin surface that occupies a relatively large surface area in comparison with its height above the skin. Frequently, it is formed by the confluence of papules.

A *wheal* is an edematous, flat-topped, erythematous elevation of the skin that is evanescent. Wheals reflect edema in the superficial layer of the dermis; when the edema occurs in the deep dermis or subcutaneous tissue, the term *angioedema* is used.

Vesicles and *bullae* are circumscribed, elevated lesions that contain fluid. They arise either from separation within the epidermis (intraepidermal vesiculation) or from separation at the dermoepidermal junction (subepidermal vesiculation).

A *pustule* is a circumscribed elevation of the skin that contains an infiltrate of cells, usually neutrophils

519

that may be white, yellow, or greenish yellow. These lesions may be sterile, as in psoriasis, or may reflect a purulent exudate. All pustules should be examined with Gram's stain and culture.

Erosions are superficial lesions in which there is destruction of the epidermis; when there is extension into the dermis, the lesion becomes an *ulcer*.

CUTANEOUS MANIFESTATIONS OF CERTAIN RHEUMATIC DISORDERS

Rheumatoid Arthritis

A variety of skin alterations occur in patients with rheumatoid arthritis; the most frequently recognized lesion is the rheumatoid nodule (Fig. 33–1).[1, 2] These lesions occur over areas subjected to trauma or pressure, especially the ulnar aspect of the forearm and the lumbosacral area. They are up to several centimeters in diameter, are firm in consistency, may be movable or fixed to underlying structures, and may ulcerate after trauma. These subcutaneous nodules occur in approximately 20 percent of patients with rheumatoid arthritis, especially in those individuals with severe forms of the disease and rheumatoid factor.

The skin is often pale, translucent, and atrophic, especially over the hands, fingers, and toes. The presence of swelling of the proximal interphalangeal joints in addition to the atrophic skin may mimic the appearance of sclerodactyly. Palmar erythema is a frequent feature; however, its presence does not imply underlying liver disease. Some patients manifest abnormal telangiectases of the nail folds. Ray-

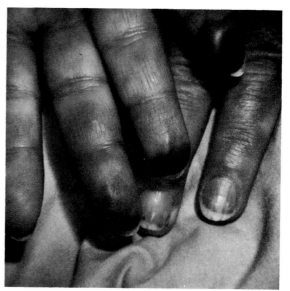

Figure 33–2. Necrotizing arteritis. Necrosis of the fingers in a patient with rheumatoid arthritis. Note bulla at top right.

naud's phenomenon may occur, as well as a blue coloration over the distal portions of the toes, sometimes associated with pitting edema of the legs. Occasionally, erythematous papules and plaques are present on the extremities and histologically contain neutrophilic infiltrates.[3] Pyoderma gangrenosum occasionally may occur in individuals with severe rheumatoid arthritis.[4]

Vasculitis in patients with rheumatoid arthritis appears as a variety of syndromes; the clinical and pathologic features reflect involvement of vessels of different sizes.[5] Rheumatoid vasculitis is frequently described as an arteritis that involves the small arteries, such as the vasa nervorum and the digital arteries (Fig. 33–2). The clinical features of vasculitis in patients with severe rheumatoid arthritis include a peripheral neuropathy, digital gangrene, nail-fold infarcts, cutaneous ulcers, and, in some instances, pericarditis as well as coronary or mesenteric arteritis.[6, 7] Patients with nodular and erosive disease and high titers of rheumatoid factor are particularly prone to develop arteritis.[8]

Occasional patients experience involvement of medium rather than small arteries. The segmental pathologic lesions in these instances resemble those of polyarteritis nodosa.[9] These individuals manifest a form of arteritis with clinical features similar to that of patients with vasculitis of small arteries.

A common form of necrotizing vasculitis in patients with rheumatoid arthritis involves the venules, especially of the skin. *Cutaneous necrotizing venulitis* is recognized as erythematous papules (palpable purpura), in which the erythema does not blanch when pressed (Fig. 33–3). The venular lesions are not related to the duration of the arthritis but rather are associated with severe articular disease, which is generally but not invariably seropositive. The duration and evolution of the venulitis do not seem to

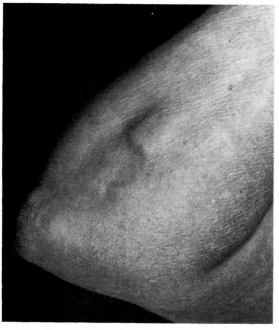

Figure 33–1. Rheumatoid nodule. Subcutaneous nodule over the ulnar aspect of the forearm in a patient with rheumatoid arthritis.

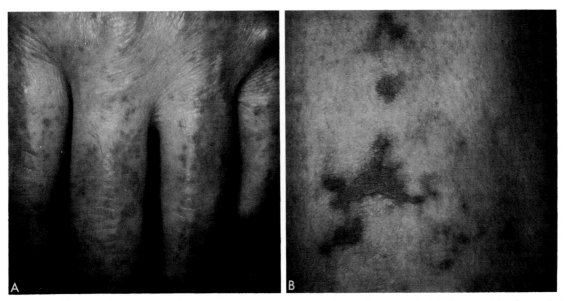

Figure 33–3. Necrotizing venulitis. *A,* Palpable purpura over the dorsa of the fingers in a patient with rheumatoid arthritis. *B,* Necrosis in a reticulate array over the thigh in a patient with systemic lupus erythematosus.

correlate with the levels of the rheumatoid factor and involvement of the complement system.[10] Arteritic, arteriolar, and venular lesions may coexist in the same patient.

Sjögren's Syndrome

The dermatologic manifestations in patients with Sjögren's syndrome reflect glandular dysfunction with desiccation of the skin and mucous membranes and frequently are a manifestation of involvement of blood vessels. Approximately 50 percent of individuals manifest dry skin (xerosis), but the ability to sweat is normal.[11] The mucous membranes of the eyes, oral cavity, and vagina usually are involved in the sicca complex. A burning sensation of the eyes may occur with erythema, pruritus, a decreased ability to form tears, and the accumulation of inspissated ropelike material most prominent at the inner canthus. The lack of tears is suggested by decreased wetting of a measured distance of filter paper strips placed under the eyelids (Schirmer's test); however, this test should be used only for screening patients inasmuch as false positive results may be obtained in elderly persons. The oral cavity and tongue may be red and dry with oral erosions and decreased amounts of saliva. Scaling of the lips and fissures at the angles of the mouth may be noted; the teeth readily decay. Desiccation of the vagina results in burning, pruritus, and dyspareunia. Enlargement of parotid and accessory salivary glands is frequently seen; minor salivary gland biopsy often confirms the diagnosis. Raynaud's phenomenon may occur.

Cutaneous necrotizing venulitis[10] occurs in patients with Sjögren's syndrome[12] and appears as episodes of either palpable purpura or urticaria.[13]

The venular lesions are present predominantly over the lower extremities, appear after exercise, and are associated with hyperpigmentation and cutaneous ulcers. Anti-Ro (SS-A) antibodies are noted in most patients with primary Sjögren's syndrome, especially when associated with systemic or cutaneous necrotizing vasculitis with hematologic and serologic abnormalities.[13, 14] Sjögren's syndrome occurs in association with other disorders such as hypergammaglobulinemic purpura, systemic lupus erythematosus, scleroderma, biliary cirrhosis, and lymphoproliferative disorders[15]; certain dermatologic features may thus reflect the coexistent disorder.

Reiter's Syndrome

Reiter's syndrome[16] is recognized as a clinical symptom complex that consists of conjunctivitis, urethritis, arthritis, and skin lesions and that usually occurs in men. An association between infection with human immunodeficiency virus and Reiter's syndrome has been noted,[17–19] especially in individuals with the histocompatability antigen HLA-B27.[20] Postdysenteric forms of Reiter's syndrome have been reported and often are not diagnosed because of the lack of the classical tetrad of features.[21, 22] The conjunctivitis and urethritis tend to be transient in contrast to the arthritis and skin manifestations. Some 50 to 80 percent of patients experience mucocutaneous alterations[23] with involvement of the acral regions, especially the soles, toes, and fingers. The most characteristic skin lesions, which are rare, begin as vesicles on erythematous bases, become sterile pustules, evolve to manifest keratotic scale, and are known as *keratoderma blennorrhagicum* (Fig. 33–4). In addition, keratotic papules and plaques occur on the

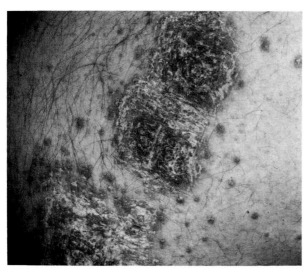

Figure 33–4. Keratoderma blennorrhagicum. Keratotic plaques and nodules in a patient with Reiter's syndrome.

scalp and elsewhere on the skin. These plaques are reminiscent of psoriasis. Indeed, patients have been reported on with both Reiter's syndrome and psoriasis, yet the skin lesions in these two disorders are often difficult or impossible to distinguish clinically and histologically.[24] This relation between Reiter's syndrome and psoriasis takes on even greater importance because of the association of the histocompatibility antigen HLA-B27 with each disorder.[25, 26] Sterile pustules develop beneath the nail plate; onychodystrophy frequently is noted.

Conjunctivitis, which occurs in 50 percent of patients,[27, 28] is usually bilateral; a sterile purulent exudate frequently is noted. Balanitis occurs in 25 percent of individuals; it appears as papules and plaques with scale over the glans. Mouth erosions have been noted.

Psoriatic Arthritis

Psoriasis occurs in a variety of patterns and may be associated with several forms of arthritis. Classical psoriasis appears as papules and plaques with layers of scales; the individual lesion (Fig. 33–5) is erythematous, covered with layers of silver-white scale, and rather sharply demarcated from adjacent uninvolved skin. Removing the scale results in punctate bleeding that reflects rupture of the superficial blood vessels in the tips of the dermal papillae (Auspitz's sign). Individual lesions may heal with transient hyperpigmentation or hypopigmentation.

Psoriasis occurs in two distinct forms: one is hereditary with an onset in the second and third decades, and the other is sporadic with an onset in the sixth decade.[29] Psoriasis may occur over any portion of the integument, especially the elbows, knees, lumbosacral area, scalp, gluteal cleft, and genitalia. The glans penis is frequently affected; the

oral mucosa is infrequently involved; and the tongue is rarely affected.[30] The extent of involvement varies from minimal lesions of the elbows and knees to extensive numbers of lesions scattered over the skin. At times, there are considerable numbers of small, droplike plaques designated as *guttate psoriasis,* which may occur after infections.[31, 32] Rarely, fissures and scale of the distal portions of the fingers may be a predominant manifestation.[33] The skin lesions often appear at sites of trauma (Koebner's reaction or isomorphic phenomenon).[34, 35] Although the stimulus is usually mechanical, excessive exposure to sunlight and the administration of drugs have been implicated.

The nails are frequently affected[36]; the extent of involvement varies in severity and may include one or several nails. The nail plate manifests a translucent quality with a yellow or brown coloration. There may be subungual accumulations of keratotic material, which frequently contains *Candida* or *Pseudomonas* species; however, dermatophyte infections are rare.[37] The most widely recognized alteration of the nail plate is the presence of discrete pits (Fig. 33–6).

Generalized erythroderma or exfoliative dermatitis may develop spontaneously or occur after systemic illness, the administration of medications, or prolonged exposure to the sun.[38–41] Associated abnormalities include abnormal thermoregulation, increased transepidermal water loss, enhanced absorption of topically applied medicaments, loss of protein and iron,[42] and the possibility of high-output cardiac failure in persons with heart disorders.[43]

Pustular types of psoriasis are uncommon and occur in two forms: one is generalized,[44, 45] and the other is localized to the palms and soles.[46] Patients with generalized pustular psoriasis manifest an extensive sterile pustular eruption that may involve the mucous membranes. The onset is sudden, with py-

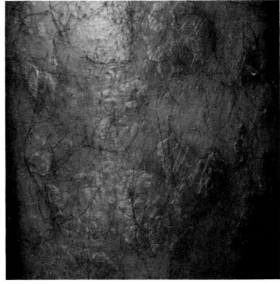

Figure 33–5. Psoriasis. Erythematous plaques with layers of scales.

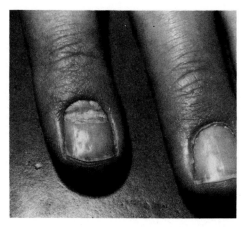

Figure 33–6. Psoriasis. Onychodystrophy of the proximal portion of the nail plate with pits.

rexia and other signs of systemic toxicity, such as myalgia and arthralgia. The skin lesions consist of superficial pustules that may evolve into large purulent areas; existing psoriatic plaques may also contain sterile pustules. The episodes of pustules may continue over intervals of days to weeks. It has been suggested that patients with psoriatic arthritis are more likely to develop generalized pustular psoriasis than are patients without arthritis.[47, 48]

Localized pustular psoriasis of the palms and soles is bilateral and recalcitrant without systemic manifestations. Onychodystrophy is common, and the plaques of ordinary psoriasis may be found elsewhere.

There are increased numbers of *Staphylococcus aureus* on lesional skin of patients with psoriasis.[49] Shedding of scale has been suggested as a source of hospital infection.[50] Surgical intervention through psoriatic plaques, such as in prosthetic joint replacement, also has been associated with increased risk of local infection.[51]

Psoriasis may occur in association with various forms of inflammatory arthritis[52, 53] (see Chapter 58), which include asymmetric oligoarthritis, symmetric arthritis, spondyloarthritis, and arthritis mutilans. The presence of psoriasis in patients with rheumatoid arthritis is considered to be the coincidental association of two common disorders. Onychodystrophy including pits in patients with symmetric psoriatic arthritis may help to differentiate them from patients with rheumatoid arthritis.

Especially severe forms of psoriasis have been reported in individuals with acquired immunodeficiency syndrome.[17, 54, 55]

Lupus Erythematosus

Lupus erythematosus may occur as a systemic disease or as a disorder in which the lesions are restricted to the skin. The term *discoid lupus erythematosus*[56, 57] has been used to refer to disease restricted to the skin as well as to the gross appearance of the atrophic skin lesions irrespective of whether there is systemic disease. The term *subacute cutaneous lupus erythematosus* defines a mild systemic form with symmetric, nonscarring skin lesions.[58] When lupus erythematosus initially is restricted to the skin, particularly involving only the head and neck, data suggest that these individuals are low at risk of developing systemic disease. However, widespread cutaneous involvement, in contrast to local disease, is more likely to be associated with extracutaneous manifestations.

The skin is involved at some time during the course of disease in approximately 80 percent of patients with lupus erythematosus.[59] The most widely recognized manifestation is an erythematous eruption (butterfly rash) over the malar areas of the face (Fig. 33–7), which occurs in patients with acute exacerbations of systemic lupus erythematosus. Rarely, bullous skin lesions occur that contain infiltrates of neutrophilis in the superficial dermis.[60]

The discoid skin lesion in patients with lupus erythematosus is a circumscribed, slightly indurated, red-purple plaque that manifests scaling, follicular plugs, telangiectases, atrophy, and hyperpigmentation or hypopigmentation (Fig. 33–8). The pigmentary alterations are especially prominent in black patients, in whom the cosmetic alteration may be disfiguring. The cutaneous lesions may be single but

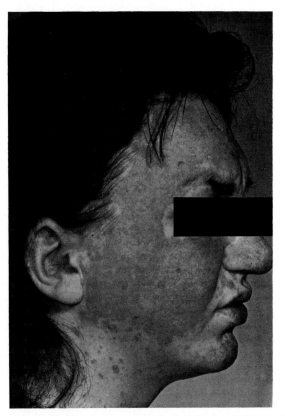

Figure 33–7. Systemic lupus erythematosus. Erythema with slight scale over the malar areas and forehead. Note that the distribution is determined by exposure to sunlight.

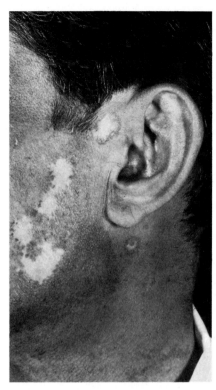

Figure 33–8. Cutaneous lupus erythematosus. Circumscribed atrophic patches with hypopigmentation and hyperpigmentation on the face.

are usually multiple and occur over any portion of the body, including the scalp, the nasolabial folds usually being spared. There is a predilection for sun-exposed areas in some individuals. The skin lesions are usually asymptomatic.

Skin lesions in *subacute cutaneous lupus erythematosus* are symmetric and predominantly affect the neck, the extensor surfaces of the arms, and the upper portions of the trunk. The early lesions are edematous and erythematous papules and plaques that evolve into lesions with scales, producing a psoriasiform picture, or into annular polycyclic or figurate configurations.[58, 61] These individuals have a mild systemic illness with fever, arthralgia, and malaise without central nervous system and progressive renal disease. There is an association with HLA-B8 and DR3 as well as anti-Ro and anti-La antibodies.[62, 63]

A variant of cutaneous lupus erythematosus called *tumid lupus erythematosus* is present as erythematosus, indurated papules, plaques, and nodules without surface changes. Histologically, mucin deposition and inflammatory-cell infiltrates are present in the dermis without alterations of the basement membrane zone or epidermis.[64, 65]

Alopecia is common in patients with lupus erythematosus; it occurs in both scarring and nonscarring forms. Atrophic patches are present as solitary or multiple areas with the characteristic features of erythema, scale, follicular plugs, and pigmentary

alterations. Recession of the frontal hairline progressing to diffuse hair loss without scarring may occur, especially in individuals with subacute cutaneous lupus erythematosus or with systemic lupus erythematosus.

Although many patients with subacute or systemic lupus erythematosus develop telangiectases over the nail folds, this sign also occurs in patients with rheumatoid arthritis, dermatomyositis, and scleroderma.[66] Whereas in systemic lupus erythematosus and rheumatoid arthritis, these telangiectases usually are linear, in dermatomyositis and scleroderma, wide polygonal mats with areas of vascular dropout develop.

A variety of other skin lesions occur in patients with lupus erythematosus. Raynaud's phenomenon is reported to occur in 10 to 30 percent, and episodes of urticaria or angioedema may be a manifestation[67] in some instances of underlying necrotizing venulitis.[68] Another manifestation of cutaneous necrotizing venulitis is palpable purpura, which occurs during exacerbations of the systemic disease.[10] Involvement of larger arterial blood vessels may be present as peripheral gangrene.[69] In addition, flat purpura and petechiae may occur as manifestations of thrombocytopenia or as a result of the administration of glucocorticoid preparations. Livedo reticularis may be present as a reticulate, erythematous mottling of the skin and may signal necrotizing vasculitis or anticardiolipid antibodies.

Photosensitivity[70, 71] occurs in at least one third of patients with systemic lupus erythematosus and may be associated with flares of both the cutaneous and the systemic manifestations of the disease. Skin lesions in patients with discoid lupus erythematosus, subacute cutaneous lupus erythematosus, and systemic lupus erythematosus have been experimentally induced by exposure to ultraviolet B (290 to 320 nm) and ultraviolet A (320 to 400 nm) from artificial light sources.[72, 73]

The oral and lingual lesions are more common in patients with systemic lupus erythematosus and consist of erythematous patches, dilated blood vessels, and erosions, which are frequently painful. Ulcers of the nasal septum and palate may occur.

A rare skin manifestation is panniculitis (*lupus profundus*),[74] which appears as firm, deep nodules that have a predilection for the face, buttocks, and upper arms. The overlying skin may be normal, erythematous, atrophic, or ulcerated. Healing results in a depressed scar.

Alterations in the integument are prominent features in classifying patients with systemic lupus erythematosus. Noteworthy features include the presence of an erythematous macular eruption, atrophic plaques with follicular plugs, photosensitivity, and oral or nasopharyngeal ulcers. Alopecia and Raynaud's phenomenon are excluded as a result of their lack of specificity and sensitivity as discriminating factors.[75, 76]

Direct immunofluorescence techniques have

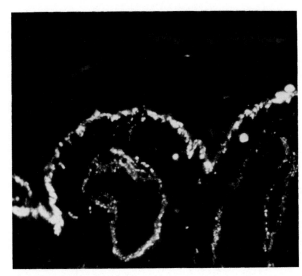

Figure 33–9. Positive lupus band test. Note bright intensity of granular deposits of IgM along basement membrane zone. Vascular staining is likewise present (× 25). (Courtesy of Terrence J. Harrist, M.D.)

been applied to the study of the skin of patients with lupus erythematosus as an aid in diagnosis and prognosis.[77–81] This procedure is known as the *lupus band test* (Fig. 33–9). In the skin lesions of both systemic and cutaneous lupus erythematosus, immunoglobulins and complement proteins are deposited in a granular pattern along the dermoepidermal junction in 90 to 95 percent of patients, whereas these immunoreactants are detected in uninvolved non–sun-exposed skin of approximately 50 percent of patients with systemic but not cutaneous lupus erythematosus—an important distinguishing feature. When uninvolved sun-exposed skin is examined, the lupus band test is usually negative in cutaneous lupus erythematosus and is positive in about 80 percent of individuals with systemic lupus erythematosus.[82]

The types of immunoglobulins detected in the deposited materials include mainly IgG and IgM. Complement proteins from both the classical activating and the amplification pathways are deposited at the same site,[83–85] notably C1q, C4, C3, properdin, and B as well as those of the terminal membrane attack complex, C5b, C6–C9.[86]

It has been suggested that the deposition of immunoreactants in uninvolved non–sun-exposed skin of patients with systemic lupus erythematosus can be correlated with renal disease.[87–89] Moreover, the suggestion has been offered that direct immunofluorescence techniques may have value as an indicator of the efficacy of therapy, especially with immunosuppressive agents in experimental animals.[90] In a longitudinal analysis of 10 years' duration to assess the relation between the deposition of cutaneous immunoreactants and renal disease in systemic lupus erythematosus, an initial positive lupus band test identified patients with renal disease

and a decreased survival.[91] Also, it appears that the specificity and predictive value of the lupus band test depend, at least in part, on the nature and number of the immunoreactants detected at the dermoepidermal junction.[92]

Mixed Connective Tissue Disease

Mixed connective tissue disease has clinical features of systemic lupus erythematosus, scleroderma, or polymyositis in association with circulating antibody to a soluble ribonuclear protein (nRNP).[93] The dermatologic manifestations include a diffuse non-scarring alopecia, areas of hyperpigmentation and hypopigmentation, sclerodactyly, sclerosis reminiscent of the alterations observed in patients with scleroderma, and a variety of skin changes similar to those observed in patients with lupus erythematosus.[94] Raynaud's phenomenon is frequently present. These patients are considered to have a good prognosis with a low incidence of renal disease.[95]

Necrotizing Vasculitides

Necrotizing angiitis or *vasculitis* is a term applied to disorders in which there is segmental inflammation with fibrinoid necrosis of the blood vessels. Clinical syndromes are based on criteria that include the gross and histologic appearance of the vascular lesions, the caliber of the affected blood vessels,[96–100] the frequency of involvement of specific organs, and the presence of hematologic, serologic, and immunologic abnormalities. Although all sizes of blood vessels may be affected, necrotizing vasculitis of the skin in most instances involves venules.[101–103] Cutaneous necrotizing venulitis may occur in association with coexistent chronic diseases, may be precipitated by infections or drugs, or may develop for unknown reasons.[104]

Although the manifestations of cutaneous necrotizing venulitis are polymorphous, the most characteristic lesion is an erythematous papule, in which the erythema does not blanch when the skin is pressed (*palpable purpura*) (see Fig. 33–3; Fig. 33–10*A*, see color section at the front of this volume).[10, 105] Transient areas of urticaria or angioedema are less frequent manifestations.[106–110] Nodules, pustules,[111] vesicles, ulcers, necrosis, and a netlike mottling of the skin (livedo reticularis) may occur. Occasionally, there is subcutaneous edema in the area of the vascular lesions.

The vascular eruption most often appears on the lower extremities and frequently over dependent portions of the body or areas under local pressure. The lesions may occur anywhere on the skin but are uncommon on the face, palms, soles, and mucous membranes. The skin lesions occur in episodes that may recur for various periods ranging from weeks to years. Palpable purpuric lesions persist for 1 to 4

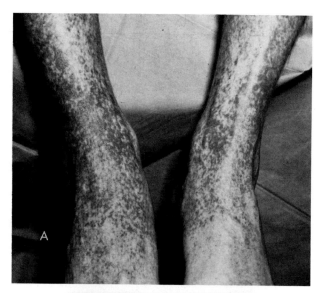

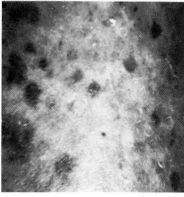

Figure 33–10. *A,* Necrotizing venulitis. Palpable purpura distributed over the lower extremities. *B,* Close-up view of the lesions.

weeks and then resolve, leaving hyperpigmentation or atrophic scars. An episode of cutaneous vascular lesions may be attended by pyrexia, malaise, arthralgias, or myalgias. When present, associated systemic involvement of the small blood vessels most commonly occurs in the joints, muscles, peripheral nerves, gastrointestinal tract, and kidneys.

Involvement of large blood vessels occurs in periarteritis nodosa, which is recognized in the skin as nodular lesions over an artery,[112–114] and giant cell (temporal) arteritis, which is present as erythema overlying the affected vessel.[115] Both Wegener's granulomatosis[116] and allergic angiitis and granulomatosis (Churg-Strauss syndrome)[117, 118] affect large and small vessels; the skin lesions in both disorders are present as erythematous nodules with or without necrosis and a variety of less specific erythematous, edematous, purpuric, papular, and pustular lesions. Patients with systemic necrotizing vasculitis and involvement of blood vessels of various sizes in whom the skin is involved are referred to as having systemic polyangiitis.[119]

Cutaneous necrotizing venulitis has been associated with collagen vascular diseases, notably rheu-

matoid arthritis, Sjögren's syndrome, and systemic lupus erythematosus, as previously mentioned.

Hypergammaglobulinemic purpura,[120] occurs predominantly in older women and may be associated with Sjögren's syndrome, systemic lupus erythematosus, and chronic lymphocytic lymphoma.[121] The recurrent purpuric skin lesions are a manifestation of necrotizing venulitis.

Cutaneous necrotizing venulitis also has been reported in association with lymphoproliferative disorders, especially Hodgkin's disease, lymphosarcoma, myelofibrosis, and acute and chronic myelogenous leukemia.[122, 123]

Cryoglobulins may occur in patients with cutaneous necrotizing venulitis with and without concomitant collagen vascular and lymphoproliferative disorders,[10, 124] in patients with hepatitis B virus,[125, 126] and idiopathically.[127]

Infections and drugs are known to precipitate cutaneous necrotizing venulitis. The most commonly recognized infectious agents are hepatitis B virus,[125, 126, 128] group A streptococci,[129] *S. aureus,*[129] and *Mycobacterium leprae.*[129–132] In hepatitis B virus disease, transient urticaria may be present early in the course and represents immune complex–induced vasculitis.[126] Episodes of palpable purpura may occur in patients with chronic active hepatitis.[133]

The most commonly incriminated medications are sulfonamides, thiazides, penicillin, and serum. Inasmuch as this is an infrequent form of drug-induced reaction, the literature consists of case reports rather than prospective or retrospective studies.

Genetic C2 deficiency has been noted in patients with cutaneous necrotizing venulitis[134, 135] that was labeled anaphylactoid purpura.

In perhaps half of instances, the cause of cutaneous necrotizing venulitis remains unknown. The Henoch-Schönlein syndrome or anaphylactoid purpura is the most widely recognized subgroup. A history of upper respiratory tract symptoms and signs is occasionally obtained. The syndrome, which occurs predominantly in children[136] and less frequently in adults,[137] includes involvement of the skin, joints, gastrointestinal tract, and kidneys. IgA is deposited around blood vessels in the skin, synovium, kidneys, and gastrointestinal tract in the Henoch-Schönlein syndrome and has been detected in circulating immune complexes.[138–140]

The urticarial form of cutaneous necrotizing venulitis (Fig. 33–11; see color section at the front of this volume)[106–110] affects mainly women and is associated with episodic arthralgias that are related in time to the appearance of the skin lesions. General features may include fever, malaise, myalgia, and enlargement of the lymph nodes, liver, and spleen. Other features may include renal involvement in the form of glomerulitis or glomerulonephritis; gastrointestinal tract manifestations in the form of nausea, vomiting, diarrhea, and pain; respiratory tract involvement as laryngeal edema and chronic obstructive pulmonary disease; eye involvement as conjunctivitis, episcleri-

Figure 33–11. Necrotizing venulitis. Circumscribed area of edema (urticaria).

tis, and uveitis; and central nervous system involvement as headaches and benign intracranial hypertension (pseudotumor cerebri).[110, 141–146] Additional skin manifestations include macular erythema, angioedema, and foci of purpura. This array of cutaneous lesions has led to the description of similar patients with hypocomplementemia and C1q precipitins under the terms *unusual systemic lupus erythematosus-like syndrome, hypocomplementemic urticarial vasculitis,* and *atypical erythema multiforme.*[147–151]

Erythema elevatum diutinum[152, 153] consists of erythematous papules, plaques, and nodules predominantly disposed over the buttocks and extensor surfaces and is often accompanied by arthralgias of the associated joint. Other systemic manifestations are lacking.

Nodular vasculitis occurs as painful red nodules over the lower extremities, especially the calves.[154] Recurrent episodes are common, and ulcers may occur at times. Erythema induratum, which once was associated with tuberculosis, probably represents a form of nodular vasculitis.[155]

Livedoid vasculitis[156–158] occurs in women as recurrent, painful ulcers of the lower legs associated with a persistent livedo reticularis that often is deep purple. Healing results in sclerotic pale areas surrounded by telangiectases that have been called *atrophie blanche.*[159] Livedoid vasculitis may occur in patients with systemic lupus erythematosus who develop central nervous system involvement[160]; it is associated with anticardiolipin antibodies.[161] Moreover, a similar clinical syndrome of livedo reticularis and transient cerebral ischemia with circulating anticardiolipin antibodies has been reported.[162, 163]

Dermatomyositis–Polymyositis

A variety of cutaneous lesions, which develop insidiously or abruptly, occur in patients with dermatomyositis–polymyositis. Inasmuch as the clinical features and histopathologic alterations in involved muscles are similar in the absence or presence of skin lesions, dermatomyositis and polymyositis are considered as manifestations of a single disease. Dermatomyositis occurs in approximately 25 percent of patients with polymyositis. The most characteristic skin changes are periorbital edema and a purple-red color of the eyelids, which is frequently described as heliotrope.[164] Erythematous macules with scale occur on the face, scalp, neck, upper back, and shoulders (shawl sign). In contradistinction to lupus erythematosus, the malar eruption frequently involves the nasolabial folds. Especially characteristic are purple-red papules that evolve into atrophic plaques with telangiectases and pigmentary alterations (Fig. 33–12); these lesions, known as Gottron's sign, occur over the dorsal aspects of the interphalangeal joints. Bright erythema arising in a linear pattern on extensor surfaces and fissures and scale of the hands also may occur. Ulcers of the oral mucous membranes may occur[165]; less frequently, the conjunctivae and genitalia are affected. Various degrees of alopecia may be present; dilated and tortuous telangiectases are noted frequently over the nail folds.

Calcification has been noted in both muscle and subcutaneous tissues; this change is more frequent when the disease begins in childhood.[166] Calcification occurs especially over the shoulders, elbows, and buttocks, and is rare over the fingers in contrast to scleroderma.[167] Cutaneous ulcers and sinuses may develop after the extrusion of deposited calcium.

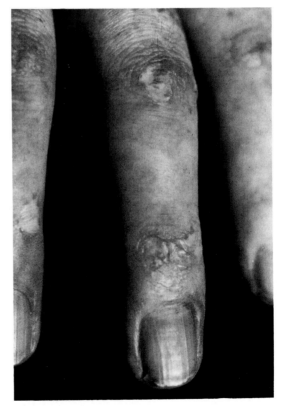

Figure 33–12. Dermatomyositis. Atrophic plaques with telangiectases and pigmentary alterations over the interphalangeal joints of the fingers. Note telangiectases of the nail folds.

Raynaud's phenomenon may be present in adults but is rare in children. Children often manifest facial erythema[168] and vasculitis involving the gastrointestinal tract leading to intestinal perforation.

The skin manifestations in patients with dermatomyositis are at times reminiscent of those occurring in individuals with systemic lupus erythematosus and scleroderma.[169] Occasionally, a reticulated erythema known as *poikiloderma* is noted, with telangiectases, atrophy, and pigmentary alterations.

Although the emergence of dermatomyositis in persons past middle age has been associated with the presence of internal malignant disorders, the reported frequency is undoubtedly too high.

Scleroderma

Scleroderma may occur as a systemic disorder or as various localized forms that primarily affect the skin. The most common type is *morphea*, in which the skin lesions are present as circumscribed areas of atrophy with an ivory color in the center and a violet hue at the periphery. The lesions of morphea commonly persist for years; they may disappear spontaneously, however, healing with or without residual pigmentary alterations.

Linear scleroderma appears in a bandlike distribution. The lower extremities are most frequently affected.[170] In addition to the skin, underlying muscles and bones may be involved with deformities. Linear scleroderma begins most frequently during the first two decades of life. It has been associated with abnormalities of the axial skeleton, especially occult spina bifida.[171] Other variants of scleroderma include frontal or frontoparietal involvement of the head known as *en coup de sabre,* which is characterized by an atrophic furrow that extends below the plane of the skin, and progressive facial hemiatrophy (Parry-Romberg syndrome).

Although proximal involvement is characteristic in systemic scleroderma[172] or systemic sclerosis, cutaneous alterations of the face and hands may be especially prominent. Features include a masklike expressionless face with a fixed stare, inability to wrinkle the forehead, tightening of the skin over the nose with a beaklike appearance, and restriction of the mouth with radial folds and loss of tissue such that the teeth are prominent. An early sign is indolent nonpitting edema over the dorsa of the fingers, hands, and forearms. Sclerodactyly is noted with tapered fingers over which the skin is atrophic; flexion contractures may be present, especially about the fingers, elbows, and knees. When calcification occurs in association with Raynaud's phenomenon (Fig. 33–13), esophageal abnormalities, sclerodactyly, and telangiectases, the clinical symptom complex is known as the CREST syndrome. Although this form of scleroderma was alleged to pursue a more benign course,[173] pulmonary hypertension[174] and biliary cirrhosis[175] have been reported.

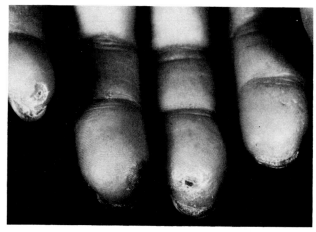

Figure 33–13. Scleroderma. Ulcers and scars of the tips of the digits in an individual with Raynaud's phenomenon.

Telangiectases occur commonly on the nail folds; telangiectatic macules, which are square, may involve the face, lips, tongue, and hands (Fig. 33–14). Other features may include generalized hyperpigmentation and alopecia.

Disorders with cutaneous sclerosis that should be considered in the differential diagnosis of scleroderma include eosinophilic fasciitis,[176, 177] porphyria cutanea tarda, papular muninosis (scleromyxedema),[178] lichen sclerosus et atrophicus, melorheostosis,[179, 180] the chronic form of graft-versus-host disease,[181] and eosinophilia–myalgia syndrome related to L-tryptophan ingestion (see Chapter 68).[182–185]

Juvenile Rheumatoid Arthritis

The cutaneous eruptions that occur in association with juvenile rheumatoid arthritis are not adequately characterized. The most frequently recog-

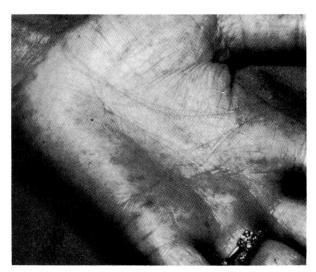

Figure 33–14. Scleroderma. Telangiectases and telangiectatic macules over the palms.

nized form is an evanescent, erythematous eruption that accompanies the late afternoon temperature rise in 25 to 40 percent of patients.[186, 187] The skin lesions appear as small erythematous or salmon-colored macules and papules distributed over the face, trunk, and extremities. They are usually not pruritic and once formed do not move or enlarge. They occur when the disease is active, subside with remission, and heal without residua. Subcutaneous nodules may be noted and must be differentiated from the subcutaneous form of granuloma annulare.[188]

Rheumatic Fever

A variety of erythematous eruptions have been noted in patients with rheumatic fever.[189] The most specific eruption is *erythema marginatum*.[190, 191] It appears as erythematous rings, usually with raised margins, that rapidly spread peripherally to form a polycyclic or geographic outline, leaving a pale or pigmented center. The essential feature is the rapid spread, which may be 2 to 10 mm in 12 hours.[192] The lesions occur on the trunk and extremities; they are rarely pruritic. The flat or macular form is known as *erythema circinatum*. Both erythema marginatum and erythema circinatum are usually associated with carditis and are unaffected by treatment of the underlying disease. Small, multiple subcutaneous nodules may be noted, especially in patients with carditis.[193–195]

A rare manifestation is *erythema papulatum*, which appears as indolent, asymptomatic papules, especially over the elbows and knees.[196]

Lyme Disease

Lyme disease is an immune complex–mediated multisystem disorder caused by the spirochete *Borrelia burgdorferi* and transmitted by the tick *Ixodes dammini* (see Chapter 88). The cutaneous hallmark is the expanding erythematous skin lesion *erythema chronicum migrans*, which may be followed weeks to months later by joint, neurologic, or cardiac manifestations.[197–199] Erythema chronicum migrans is an expanding ring of erythema with partial central clearing. The average diameter is 15 cm. Approximately 50 percent of patients have one or more annular lesions, urticaria, and morbilliform eruptions. The skin manifestations may clear without treatment.

Amyloid

Amyloid may be present as a primary cutaneous disease, may occur with multiple myeloma or genetic disorders, or may be associated in a secondary fashion with chronic inflammatory conditions.[200, 201] Skin lesions occur in primary amyloid; secondary amyloid rarely has skin lesions. However, clinically unin-volved skin may contain amyloid deposits in both primary and secondary types, suggesting that a skin biopsy of such uninvolved skin can have a high diagnostic yield.[202] Moreover, cutaneous but not systemic forms of amyloid contain SH groups and can be differentiated by staining techniques.[203]

The skin lesions appear as firm papules that are translucent and occur on the face (especially about the eyes), neck, intertriginous areas, and extremities. They vary in color from rose to yellow to brown; pruritus is absent. A conspicuous feature is hemorrhage; in fact, the tendency to develop purpura is the basis for a diagnostic maneuver, in which purpura develops after a blunt instrument is used to traumatize the lesions.[204] Ecchymoses may occur in the absence of papules. Macroglossia is present in 25 to 40 percent of patients and appears with papules of the tongue; it is occasionally accompanied by ulcers and purpura.

Other clinical disorders associated with amyloid include familial Mediterranean fever, in which erythema and lesions resembling those of erysipelas occur; the syndrome of amyloid, urticaria, and deafness,[205, 206] in which papules are present over the trunk; the Portuguese form, in which hyperkeratosis and ulcers of the feet occur[207]; and the carpal tunnel syndrome.

Sarcoid

A variety of cutaneous manifestations have been noted in patients with sarcoid.[208] Skin lesions occur in 25 percent of patients, and erythema nodosum occurs in 30 percent.[209–211] The most characteristic lesions observed in the United States are yellow-brown to violaceous papules and plaques with a predilection for the face, especially the alae nasi and the periocular areas (Fig. 33–15). Similar lesions may be widely distributed over the trunk and extremities. The papules may arise in a scar,[210] a valuable diagnostic sign. Especially in Europe, livid purple plaques have been described on the nose (nasal rim lesions), cheeks, and lobes of the ear; these lesions are known as *lupus pernio*,[208] which is associated with involvement of the respiratory tract[212] and kidneys.[213] Other skin manifestations include an ichthyosiform dermatosis over the lower legs, subcutaneous calcification,[214] and areas of hypopigmentation.[215] Black patients with sarcoid and patients with skin manifestations other than erythema nodosum should be observed closely, since white patients with erythema nodosum have less progressive disease.[216]

Panniculitis

Panniculitis is the term used to describe disorders in which inflammation occurs in the subcutaneous tissue. Panniculitis of all types is recognized as erythematous or violaceous nodules, which may

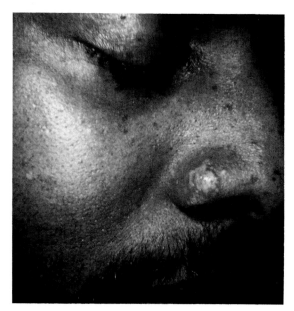

Figure 33–15. Sarcoid. Firm papules and plaques of the face.

or may not ulcerate. *Erythema nodosum* is the most widely recognized form of panniculitis. The age and sex distribution for erythema nodosum varies throughout the world, depending on the eliciting etiologic agents, which include a variety of infections and systemic diseases.

The relation between infections with beta (β)-hemolytic streptococci and erythema nodosum has been well established.[217, 218] Other associations include tuberculosis and *Yersinia* infections.[219, 220] In endemic areas, blastomycosis, coccidioidomycosis, and histoplasmosis are associated with erythema nodosum. Infectious mononucleosis, lymphogranuloma venereum, cat-scratch disease, leptospirosis, paravaccinia, psittacosis, and tularemia also have been implicated.

Drugs implicated in causing erythema nodosum include sulfonamides and oral contraceptives.[221] Erythema nodosum can occur in association with enteropathies, notably ulcerative colitis and, less frequently, regional enteritis.[222] Sarcoidosis is a well-recognized cause of erythema nodosum.[210] On rare occasions, erythema nodosum has been reported in association with Behçet's syndrome and malignant disorders such as leukemia and Hodgkin's disease.[223] Erythema nodosum has also been observed to develop after radiation therapy of malignant conditions.

The clinical eruption usually appears as tender, erythematous nodules over the extensor aspects of the lower extremities. The onset of lesions may be accompanied by fever, chills, malaise, and leukocytosis. The erythema often becomes violet blue during the second week of the eruption. Individual nodules usually resolve spontaneously in 3 to 6 weeks without ulcers or scars. Patients with erythema nodosum often have arthralgias, which may persist after the cutaneous lesions have resolved. Episcleral lesions also may develop with the cutaneous nodules.

Erythema nodosum migrans and subacute nodular migratory panniculitis[224–226] are imprecise terms used to designate clinical variants of erythema nodosum.

Weber-Christian disease is the term applied to a relapsing form of idiopathic panniculitis associated with systemic manifestations.[227, 228] The cutaneous lesions occur as recurrent episodes of erythematous, sometimes tender, subcutaneous nodules that appear at intervals of weeks to months. The lesions are symmetric in distribution, and the thighs and lower legs usually are affected. Occasionally, necrosis of the overlying skin occurs, and an oily yellow-brown liquid is discharged. Individual nodules involute over the course of a few weeks, resulting in a hyperpigmented and atrophic scar.

The episodes of cutaneous lesions usually are accompanied by malaise, fever, and arthralgias.[229] Nausea, vomiting, abdominal pain, weight loss, and hepatomegaly may occur. In severe instances, the inflammation can involve the lungs, heart, gastrointestinal tract, spleen, kidneys, and adrenal glands.[230–233]

The prognosis in patients with Weber-Christian disease displays a spectrum ranging from self-limited or intermittent disease to persistent disease with a fatal outcome. A clinical course characterized by frequent remissions and exacerbations of cutaneous lesions, with eventual permanent remission after several years, is common. Prominent visceral involvement may eventuate in death; the major causes of death are sepsis, hepatic failure, hemorrhage, and thrombosis.[234]

Physical trauma of a thermal, mechanical, or chemical nature can result in panniculitis. The most common physical factors are exposure to cold or direct physical or chemical trauma; sometimes these traumatic factors are factitious and consequent to self-induced diseases.

Lobular panniculitis may be associated with pancreatic carcinoma or pancreatitis.[235] Elevated lipase and amylase levels have been detected in fluid aspirated from the skin lesions as well as in pleural, pericardial, and ascitic fluid. Painful erythematous nodules may appear in any location, but there is a predilection for the legs. The nodules occasionally drain an oily substance. Arthritis occurs in about 60 percent of the cases, and a polyserositis can be manifested as pleuritis, pericarditis, or synovitis.[236]

Panniculitis may be a sign of underlying systemic diseases, such as lupus erythematosus, lymphomas and leukemia, sarcoidosis, granuloma annulare, and fungal and bacterial infections. Panniculitis secondary to jejunoileal bypass surgery has been reported.[237]

References

1. Collins, D. H.: The subcutaneous nodule of rheumatoid arthritis. J. Pathol. Bacteriol. 45:97, 1937.
2. Bennett, G. A., Zeller, J. W., and Bauer, W.: Subcutaneous nodules

of rheumatoid arthritis and rheumatic fever: A pathologic study. Arch. Pathol. 30:70, 1940.

3. Sanchez, J. L., and Cruz, A.: Rheumatoid neutrophilic dermatitis. J. Am. Acad. Dermatol. 22:922, 1990.

4. Stolman, L. P., Rosenthal, D., Yaworsky, R., and Horan, F.: Pyoderma gangrenosum and rheumatoid arthritis. Arch. Dermatol. 111:1020, 1975.

5. Glass, D. N., Soter, N. A., and Schur, P. H.: Rheumatoid vasculitis. Arthritis Rheum. 19:950, 1976.

6. Sokoloff, L., Wilens, S. L., and Bunim, J. J.: Arteritis of striated muscle in rheumatoid arthritis. Am. J. Pathol. 27:157, 1951.

7. Schmid, F. R., Cooper, N. S., Ziff, M., and McEwen, C.: Arteritis in rheumatoid arthritis. Am. J. Med. 30:56, 1961.

8. Mongan, E. S., Cass, R. M., Jacox, R. F., and Vaughan, J. H.: A study of the relation of seronegative and seropositive rheumatoid arthritis to each other and to necrotizing vasculitis. Am. J. Med. 47:23, 1969.

9. Sokoloff, L., and Bunim, J. J.: Vascular lesions in rheumatoid arthritis. J. Chronic Dis. 5:668, 1957.

10. Soter, N. A., Austen, K. F., and Gigli, I.: The complement system in necrotizing angiitis of the skin: Analysis of complement component activities in serum of patients with concomitant collagen-vascular diseases. J. Invest. Dermatol. 63:219, 1974.

11. Bloch, K. J., Buchanan, W. W., Wohl, M. J., and Bunim, J. J.: Sjögren's syndrome: A clinical, pathological, and serological study of sixty-two cases. Medicine 44:187, 1965.

12. Shearn, M. A.: Sjögren's syndrome. Semin. Arthritis Rheum. 2:165, 1972.

13. Alexander, E. L., and Provost, T. T.: Cutaneous manifestations of primary Sjögren's syndrome: A reflection of vasculitis and association with anti-Ro (SS-A) antibodies. J. Invest. Dermatol. 80:386, 1983.

14. Alexander, E. L., Arnett, F. C., Provost, T. T., and Stevens, M. B.: Sjögren's syndrome: Association of anti-Ro (SS-A) antibodies with vasculitis, hematologic abnormalities, and serologic hyperreactivity. Ann. Intern. Med. 98:155, 1983.

15. Bloch, K. J., and Bunim, J. J.: Sjögren's syndrome and its relation to connective tissue diseases. J. Chronic Dis. 16:915, 1963.

16. Weinberger, H. W., Ropes, M. W., Kulka, J. P., and Bauer, W.: Reiter's syndrome, clinical and pathologic observations: A long-term study of 16 cases. Medicine 41:35, 1962.

17. Duvic, M., Johnson, T. M., Rapini, R. P., Freese T., Brewton G., and Rios A.: Acquired immunodeficiency syndrome–associated psoriasis and Reiter's syndrome. Arch. Dermatol. 123:1622, 1987.

18. Winchester, R., Bernstein, D. H., Fischer, H. D., Enlow R., and Solomon G.: The co-occurrence of Reiter's syndrome and acquired immunodeficiency. Ann. Intern. Med. 106:19, 1987.

19. Lin, R. Y.: Reiter's syndrome and the human immunodeficiency virus. Dermatologica 176:39, 1988.

20. Winchester, R., Brancato, L., Itescu, S., et al.: Implications from the occurrence of Reiter's syndrome and related disorders in association with advanced HIV infection. Scand. J. Rheumatol. 74:89, 1988.

21. Inman, R. D., Johnston, M. E., Hodge, M., Falk, J., and Helewa, A.: Postdysenteric reactive arthritis. Arthritis Rheum. 31:1377, 1988.

22. Stieglitz, H., Fosmire, S., and Lipsky, P. E.: Bacterial epitopes involved in the induction of reactive arthritis. Am. J. Med. 85:56, 1988.

23. Montgomery, M. M., Poske, R. M., Barton, E. M., Foxworthy, D. T., and Baker, L. A.: The mucocutaneous lesions of Reiter's syndrome. Ann. Intern. Med. 51:99, 1959.

24. Wright, V., and Reed, W. B.: The link between Reiter's syndrome and psoriatic arthritis. Ann. Rheum. Dis. 23:12, 1964.

25. Brewerton, D. A., Caffrey, M., Nicholls, A., Walters, D., and James, D. C. O.: Acute anterior uveitis and HLA-27. Lancet 2:994, 1973.

26. Lambert, J. R., Wright, V., Farjah, S. M., and Moll, J. M. H.: Histocompatibility antigens in psoriatic arthritis. Ann. Rheum. Dis. 35:526, 1976.

27. Csonka, G. W.: The course of Reiter's syndrome. Br. Med. J. 1:1088, 1958.

28. Hancock, J.: Surface manifestations of Reiter's disease in the male. Br. J. Vener. Dis. 36:36, 1960.

29. Henseler, T., and Christophers, E.: Psoriasis of early and late onset: Characterization of two types of psoriasis vulgaris. J. Am. Acad. Dermatol. 13:450, 1985.

30. Schuppner, H. J.: Das klinische Bild der Schleimhautbeteiligung bei Psoriasis pustulosa. Arch. Klin. Exp. Dermatol. 209:600, 1960.

31. Whyte, H. J., and Baughman, R. D.: Acute guttate psoriasis and streptococcal infection. Arch. Dermatol. 89:350, 1964.

32. Honig, P. J.: Guttate psoriasis associated with perianal streptococcal disease. J. Pediatr. 113:1037, 1988.

33. Baer, R. L., and Witten, V. H.: Psoriasis: A discussion of selected aspects. In Baer, R. L., and Witten, V. H. (eds.): Yearbook of Dermatology, 1961–1962 Series. Chicago, Year Book Medical Publishers, 1962, p. 9.

34. Farber, E. M., Roth, R. J., Aschheim, E., Eddy, D. D., and Epinette, W. W.: Role of trauma in isomorphic response in psoriasis. Arch. Dermatol. 91:246, 1965.

35. Reinertson, R. P.: Vascular trauma and pathogenesis of the Koebner reaction in psoriasis. J. Invest. Dermatol. 30:283, 1958.

36. Zaias, N.: Psoriasis of the nail: A clinical-pathologic study. Arch. Dermatol. 99:567, 1969.

37. White, C. J., and Laipply, T. C.: Histopathology of nail diseases. J. Invest. Dermatol. 19:121, 1952.

38. Montgomery, H.: Exfoliative dermatitis and malignant erythroderma: The value and limitations of histopathologic studies. Arch. Dermatol. Syphilol. 27:253, 1933.

39. Wilson, H. T. H.: Exfoliative dermatitis: Its etiology and prognosis. Arch. Dermatol. Syphilol. 69:577, 1954.

40. Gentele, H., Lodin, A., and Skog, E.: Dermatitis exfoliativa. Acta Derm. Venereol. (Stockh.) 38:296, 1958.

41. Abrahams, I., McCarthy, J. T., and Sanders, S. L.: 101 cases of exfoliative dermatitis. Arch. Dermatol. 87:96, 1963.

42. Marks, J., and Shuster, S.: Iron metabolism in skin disease. Arch. Dermatol. 98:469, 1968.

43. Fox, R. H., Shuster, S., Williams, R., Marks, J., Goldsmith, R., and Condon, R. E.: Cardiovascular, metabolic, and thermoregulatory disturbances with patients with erythrodermic skin diseases. Br. Med. J. 1:619, 1965.

44. von Zumbusch, L. R.: Psoriasis und pustuloses exanthem. Arch. Dermatol. Syphilis 99:335, 1909–1910.

45. Tolman, M. M., and Moschella, S. L.: Pustular psoriasis (von Zumbusch). Arch. Dermatol. 81:400, 1960.

46. Barber, H. W.: Acrodermatitis continua vel perstans (dermatitis repens) and psoriasis pustulosa. Br. J. Dermatol. Syphilol. 42:500, 1930.

47. Ingram, J. T.: Pustular psoriasis. Arch. Dermatol. 77:314, 1958.

48. Champion, R. H.: Generalized pustular psoriasis. Br. J. Dermatol. 71:384, 1959.

49. Marples, R. R., Heaton, C. L., and Kligman, A. M.: Staphylococcus aureus in psoriasis. Arch. Dermatol. 107:568, 1973.

50. Payne, R. W.: Severe outbreak of surgical sepsis due to Staphylococcus aureus of unusual type and origin. Br. Med. J. 4:17, 1967.

51. Stern, S. H., Insall, J. N., Windsor, R. E., Inglis, A. E., and Dines, D. M.: Total knee arthroplasty in patients with psoriasis. Clin. Orthop. 248:108, 1989.

52. Moll, J. M. H., and Wright, V.: Psoriatic arthritis. Semin. Arthritis Rheum. 3:55, 1963.

53. Kammer, G. M., Soter, N. A., Gibson, D. J., and Schur, P. H.: Psoriatic arthritis: A clinical, immunologic and HLA study of 100 patients. Semin. Arthritis Rheum. 9:75, 1979.

54. Johnson, T. M., Duvic, M., Rapini, R. P., and Rios, A.: AIDS exacerbates psoriasis. N. Engl. J. Med. 313:1415, 1985.

55. Lazar, A. P., and Roenigk, H. H.: Acquired immunodeficiency syndrome (AIDS) can exacerbate psoriasis. J. Am. Acad. Dermatol. 18:144, 1988.

56. Rothfield, N. F., March, C. H., Miescher, P., and McEwen, C.: Chronic discoid lupus erythematosus: Study of 65 patients and 65 controls. N. Engl. J. Med. 269:1155, 1963.

57. Beck, J. S., and Rowell, N. R.: Discoid lupus erythematosus: A study of clinical features and biochemical and serological abnormalities in 120 patients with observation on relationship of this disease to systemic lupus erythematosus. Q. J. Med. 35:119, 1966.

58. Sontheimer, R. D., Thomas, J. R., and Gilliam, J. N.: Subacute cutaneous lupus erythematosus: A cutaneous marker for a distinct LE subset. Arch. Dermatol. 115:1409, 1979.

59. Tuffanelli, D. L., and Dubois, E. L.: Cutaneous manifestations of systemic lupus erythematosus. Arch. Dermatol. 90:377, 1964.

60. Hall, R. P., Lawley, T. J., Smith, H. R., and Katz, S. I.: Bullous eruption of systemic lupus erythematosus: Dramatic response to dapsone therapy. Ann. Intern. Med. 97:165, 1982.

61. Gilliam, J. N., and Sontheimer, R. D.: Distinctive cutaneous subsets in the spectrum of lupus erythematosus. J. Am. Acad. Dermatol. 4:471, 1981.

62. Sontheimer, R. D., Stastny, P., and Gilliam, J. N.: HLA associations in subacute cutaneous lupus erythematosus. J. Clin. Invest. 67:312, 1981.

63. Sontheimer, R. D., Stastny, P., Maddison, P., Reichlin, M., and Gilliam, J. N.: Anti-Ro and La antibodies and further HLA associations in subacute cutaneous lupus erythematosus (SCLE). Arthritis Rheum. 23:750, 1980.

64. Ackerman, A. B.: Superficial and deep perivascular dermatitis. In Ackerman, A. B. (ed.): Histologic Diagnosis of Inflammatory Skin Disease: A Method by Pattern Analysis. Philadelphia, Lea & Febiger, 1978, p. 315.

65. Franks, A. G., Jr.: Identifying dermatologic manifestations of lupus erythematosus. J. Musculoskel. Med. 5:59, 1988.

66. Ross, J. P.: Nail fold capillaroscopy: A useful aid in the diagnosis of collagen vascular diseases. J. Invest. Dermatol. 47:282, 1966.

67. Harvey, A. M., Shulman, L. E., Tumulty, P. A., Conley, C. L., and Schoenrich, E. H.: Systemic lupus erythematosus: Review of the literature and clinical analysis of 138 cases. Medicine 33:291, 1954.

68. O'Loughlin, S., Schroeter, A. L., and Jordan, R. E.: Chronic urticaria-

like lesions in systemic lupus erythematosus: A review of 12 cases. Arch. Dermatol. 114:879, 1978.

69. Dubois, E. L., and Arterberry, J. D.: Gangrene as a manifestation of systemic lupus erythematosus. JAMA 181:366, 1962.

70. Epstein, J. H., Tuffanelli, D. L., and Dubois, E. L.: Light sensitivity and lupus erythematosus. Arch. Dermatol. 91:483, 1965.

71. Baer, R. L., and Harber, L. C.: Photobiology of lupus erythematosus. Arch. Dermatol. 92:124, 1965.

72. Freeman, R. G., Knox, J. M., and Owens, D. W.: Cutaneous lesions of lupus erythematosus induced by monochromatic light. Arch. Dermatol. 100:677, 1969.

73. Lehmann, P., Hölzle, E., Kind, P., Goerz, G., and Plewig, G.: Experimental reproduction of skin lesions in lupus erythematosus by UVA and UVB radiation. J. Am. Acad. Dermatol. 22:181, 1990.

74. Tuffanelli, D. L.: Lupus erythematosus panniculitis (profundus): Clinical and immunologic studies. Arch. Dermatol. 103:231, 1971.

75. Tan, E. M., Cohen, A. S., Fries, J. F., Masi, A. T., McShane, D. J., Rothfield, N. F., Schaller, J. G., Talal, N., and Winchester, R. J.: The 1982 revised criteria for the classification of systemic lupus erythematosus. Arthritis Rheum. 25:1271, 1982.

76. Levin, R. E., Weinstein, A., Peterson, M., Testa, M. A., and Rothfield, N. F.: A comparison of the sensitivity of the 1971 and 1982 American Rheumatism Association criteria for the classification of systemic lupus erythematosus. Arthritis Rheum. 27:530, 1984.

77. Burnham, T. K., Neblett, T. R., and Fine, G.: The application of the fluorescent antibody technique to the investigation of lupus erythematosus and various dermatoses. J. Invest. Dermatol. 41:451, 1963.

78. Cormane, R. H.: "Bound" globulin in the skin of patients with chronic discoid lupus erythematosus and systemic lupus erythematosus. Lancet 1:534, 1964.

79. Tan, E. M., and Kunkel, H. G.: An immunofluorescent study of the skin lesions in systemic lupus erythematosus. Arthritis Rheum. 9:37, 1966.

80. Tuffanelli, D. L., Kay, D., and Fukuyama, K.: Dermal-epidermal junction in lupus erythematosus. Arch. Dermatol. 99:652, 1969.

81. Harrist, T. J., and Mihm, M. C., Jr.: The specificity and clinical usefulness of the lupus band test. Arthritis Rheum. 23:479, 1980.

82. Provost, T. T., Andres, G., Maddison, P. J., and Reichlin, M.: Lupus band test in untreated SLE patients: Correlation of immunoglobulin deposition in the skin of the extensor forearm with clinical renal diseases and serological abnormalities. J. Invest. Dermatol. 74:407, 1980.

83. Jordon, R. E., Schroeter, A. L., and Winkelmann, R. K.: Dermoepidermal deposition of complement components and properdin in systemic lupus erythematosus. Br. J. Dermatol. 92:263, 1975.

84. Schrager, M. A., and Rothfield, N. F.: Clinical significance of serum properdin levels and properdin deposition in the dermo-epidermal junction in systemic lupus erythematosus. J. Clin. Invest. 57:212, 1976.

85. Provost, T. T., and Tomasi, T. B.: Evidence for complement activation via the alternate pathway in skin diseases. I. Herpes gestationis, systemic lupus erythematosus, and bullous pemphigoid. J. Clin. Invest. 52:1779, 1973.

86. Biesecker, G., Lavin, L., Ziskind, M., and Koffler, D.: Cutaneous localization of the membrane attack complex in discoid and systemic lupus erythematosus. N. Engl. J. Med. 306:264, 1982.

87. Pohle, E. L., and Tuffanelli, D. L.: Study of cutaneous lupus by immunohistochemical methods. Arch. Dermatol. 97:520, 1968.

88. Gilliam, J. N., Cheatum, D. E., Hurd, E. R., Stastny, P., and Ziff, M.: Immunoglobulin in clinically uninvolved skin in systemic lupus erythematosus: Association with renal disease. J. Clin. Invest. 53:1434, 1974.

89. Dantzig, P. I., Mauro, J., Rayhanzadeh, S., and Rudofsky, U. H.: The significance of a positive cutaneous immunofluorescence test in systemic lupus erythematosus. Br. J. Dermatol. 93:531, 1975.

90. Gilliam, J. N.: The significance of cutaneous immunoglobulin deposits in lupus erythematosus and NZB/NZW F_1 hybrid mice. J. Invest. Dermatol. 65:154, 1975.

91. Davis, B. M., and Gilliam, J. N.: Prognostic significance of subepidermal immune deposits in uninvolved skin of patients with systemic lupus erythematosus: A 10-year longitudinal study. J. Invest. Dermatol. 83:242, 1984.

92. Smith, C. D., Marino, C., and Rothfield, N. F.: The clinical utility of the lupus band test. Arthritis Rheum. 27:382, 1984.

93. Sharp, G. C., Irvin, W. S., LaRoque, R. L., Velez, C., Daly, V., Kaiser, A. D., and Holman, H. R.: Association of antibodies to different nuclear antigens with clinical patterns of rheumatic disease and responsiveness to therapy. J. Clin. Invest. 50:350, 1971.

94. Gilliam, J. N., and Prystowsky, S. D.: Mixed connective tissue disease syndrome: Cutaneous manifestations of patients with epidermal nuclear staining and high titer serum antibody to ribonuclease-sensitive extractable nuclear antigen. Arch. Dermatol. 113:583, 1977.

95. Nimelstein, S. H., Brody, S., McShane, D., and Holman, H. R.: Mixed connective tissue disease: Subsequent evaluation of the original 25 patients. Medicine 59:239, 1980.

96. Zeek, P. M.: Periarteritis nodosa: A critical review. Am. J. Clin. Pathol. 22:777, 1952.

97. Zeek, P. M.: Periarteritis nodosa and other forms of necrotizing angiitis. N. Engl. J. Med. 248:764, 1953.

98. Fauci, A. S., Haynes, B. F., and Katz, P.: The spectrum of vasculitis: Clinical, pathologic, immunologic, and therapeutic considerations. Ann. Intern. Med. 89:660, 1978.

99. af Ekenstam, E., and Callen, J. P.: Cutaneous leukocytoclastic vasculitis: Clinical and laboratory features of 82 patients seen in private practice. Arch. Dermatol. 120:484, 1984.

100. Sanchez, N. P., VanHale, H. M., and Su, W. P.: Clinical and histopathologic spectrum of necrotizing vasculitis: Report of findings in 101 cases. Arch. Dermatol. 121:220, 1985.

101. Copeman, P. W. M., and Ryan, T. J.: The problem of classification of cutaneous angiitis with reference to histopathology and pathogenesis. Br. J. Dermatol. 82(Suppl 5):2, 1970.

102. Soter, N. A., Mihm, M. C., Jr., Gigli, I., Dvorak, H. F., and Austen, K. F.: Two distinct cellular patterns in cutaneous necrotizing angiitis. J. Invest. Dermatol. 66:344, 1976.

103. Braverman, I. M., and Yen, A.: Demonstration of immune complexes in spontaneous and histamine-induced lesions and in normal skin of patients with leukocytoclastic angiitis. J. Invest. Dermatol. 64:105, 1975.

104. Soter, N. A., and Austen, K. F.: Cutaneous necrotizing venulitis. In Samter, M., et al. (eds.): Immunological Diseases, 4th ed. Boston, Little, Brown & Company, 1988, pp. 1267–1280.

105. Braverman, I. M.: The angiitides. In Skin Signs of Systemic Disease. Philadelphia, W. B. Saunders Company, 1970, p. 199.

106. McDuffie, F. D., Sams, W. M., Jr., Maldonado, J. E., Andreini, P. H., Conn, D. L., and Samayoa, E. A.: Hypocomplementemia with cutaneous vasculitis and arthritis: Possible immune complex syndrome. Mayo Clin. Proc. 48:340, 1973.

107. Soter, N. A., Austen, K. F., and Gigli, I.: Urticaria and arthralgias as manifestations of necrotizing angiitis (vasculitis). J. Invest. Dermatol. 63:485, 1974.

108. Soter, N. A.: Chronic urticaria as a manifestation of necrotizing venulitis. N. Engl. J. Med. 296:1440, 1977.

109. Monroe, E. W.: Urticarial vasculitis: An updated review. J. Am. Acad. Dermatol. 5:88, 1981.

110. Sanchez, N. P., Winkelmann, R. K., Schroeter, A. L., and Dicken, C. H.: The clinical and histopathologic spectrums of urticarial vasculitis: Study of 40 cases. J. Am. Acad. Dermatol. 7:599, 1982.

111. Diaz, L. A., Provost, T. T., and Tomasi, T. B., Jr.: Pustular necrotizing angiitis. Arch. Dermatol. 108:114, 1973.

112. Borrie, P.: Cutaneous polyarteritis nodosa. Br. J. Dermatol. 87:87, 1972.

113. Diaz-Perez, J. L., and Winkelmann, R. K.: Cutaneous periarteritis nodosa. Arch. Dermatol. 110:407, 1974.

114. Kussmaul, A., and Maier, R.: Uber eine bisher nicht beschriebene eigenthumliche Arterienerkrankung (Periarteritis nodosa), die mit Morbus brightii und rapid fortschreitender allgemeiner Muskellahmung einhergeht. Dtsch. Arch. Klin. Med. 1:484, 1866.

115. Hamilton, C. R., Jr., Shelley, W. M., and Tumulty, P. A.: Giant cell arteritis: Including temporal arteritis and polymyalgia rheumatica. Medicine 50:1, 1971.

116. Fauci, A. S., and Wolff, S. M.: Wegener's granulomatosis: Studies in eighteen patients and a review of the literature. Medicine 52:535, 1973.

117. Churg, J., and Strauss, L.: Allergic granulomatosis, allergic angiitis and periarteritis nodosa. Am. J. Pathol. 27:277, 1951.

118. Chumbley, L. C., Harrison, E. G., and DeRemee, R. A.: Allergic granulomatosis and angiitis (Churg-Strauss syndrome): Report and analysis of 30 cases. Mayo Clin. Proc. 52:447, 1977.

119. Leavitt, R. Y., and Fauci, A. S.: Polyangiitis overlap syndrome: Classification and prospective experience. Am. J. Med. 81:79, 1986.

120. Capra, J. D., Winchester, R. J., and Kunkel, H. G.: Hypergammaglobulinemic purpura: Studies on the unusual anti-γ-globulins characteristic of the sera of these patients. Medicine 50:125, 1971.

121. Kyle, R. A., Gleich, G. J., Bayrd, E. D., and Vaughan, J. H.: Benign hypergammaglobulinemic purpura of Waldenström. Medicine 50:113, 1971.

122. Sams, W. M., Jr., Harville, D. D., and Winkelmann, R. K.: Necrotising vasculitis associated with lethal reticuloendothelial diseases. Br. J. Dermatol. 80:555, 1968.

123. Longley, S., Caldwell, J. R., and Panush, R. S.: Paraneoplastic vasculitis: Unique syndrome of cutaneous angiitis and arthritis associated with myeloproliferative disorders. Am. J. Med. 80:1027, 1986.

124. Brouet, J.-C., Claurel, J.-P., Danon, F., Klein, M., and Seligmann, M.: Biologic and clinical significance of cryoglobulins: A report of 86 cases. Am. J. Med. 57:775, 1974.

125. Levo, Y., Gorevic, P. D., Kassab, H., Zucker-Franklin, D., Gigli, I., and Franklin, E. C.: Mixed cryoglobulinemia: An immune complex disease often associated with hepatitis B virus infection. Trans. Assoc. Am. Physicians 90:167, 1977.

126. Dienstag, J. L., Rhodes, A. R., Bhan, A. K., Dvorak, A. M., Mihm, M. C., Jr., and Wands, J. R.: Urticaria associated with acute viral hepatitis type B. Ann. Intern. Med. 89:34, 1978.

127. Meltzer, M., and Franklin, E. C.: Cryoglobulinemia: A study of twenty-nine patients. I. IgG and IgM cryoglobulins and factors affecting cryoprecipitability. Am. J. Med. 40:828, 1966.

128. Gower, R. G., Sausker, W. F., Kohler, P. F., Thorne, G. E., and McIntosh, R. M.: Small vessel vasculitis caused by hepatitis B virus immune complexes: Small vessel vasculitis and HBsAg. J. Allergy Clin. Immunol. 62:222, 1978.

129. Parish, W. E.: Cutaneous vasculitis: The occurrence of complexes of bacterial antigens with antibody, and of abnormalities associated with chronic inflammation. In Beutner, E. H., Chorzelski, T. P., Bean, S. F., and Jordon, R. E. (eds.): Immunopathology of the Skin: Labelled Antibody Studies. Chicago, Year Book Medical Publishers, 1974, p. 153.

130. Moschella, S. L.: The lepra reaction with necrotizing skin lesions: A report of six cases. Arch. Dermatol. 95:565, 1967.

131. Quismorio, F. P., Jr., Rea, T., Chandor, S., Levan, N., and Frious, G. J.: Lucio's phenomenon: An immune complex deposition syndrome in lepromatous leprosy. Clin. Immunol. Immunopathol. 9:184, 1978.

132. Murphy, G. F., Sanchez, N. P., Flynn, T. C., Sanchez, J. L., Mihm, M. C., Jr., and Soter, N. A.: Erythema nodosum leprosum: Nature and extent of the cutaneous microvascular alterations. J. Am. Acad. Dermatol. 14:59, 1986.

133. Duffy, J., Lidsky, M. D., Sharp, J. T., Davis, J. S., Person, D. A., Hollinger, F. B., and Min, K.-W.: Polyarthritis, polyarteritis, and hepatitis B. Medicine 55:19, 1976.

134. Sussman, M., Jones, J. H., Almeida, J. D., and Lachmann, P. J.: Deficiency of the second component of complement associated with anaphylactoid purpura and presence of Mycoplasma in the serum. Clin. Exp. Immunol. 14:531, 1973.

135. Gelfand, E. W., Clarkson, J. E., and Minta, J. O.: Selective deficiency of the second component of complement in a patient with anaphylactoid purpura. Clin. Immunol. Immunopathol. 4:269, 1975.

136. Gairdner, D.: The Schönlein-Henoch syndrome (anaphylactoid purpura). Q. J. Med. 66:95, 1948.

137. Cream, J. J., Gumpel, J. H., and Peachey, R. D. G.: Schönlein-Henoch purpura in the adult: A study of 77 adults with anaphylactoid or Schönlein-Henoch purpura. Q. J. Med. 34:461, 1970.

138. Baart de la Faille-Kuyper, E. H., Kater, L., Kooiker, C. J., and Dorhout Mees E. J.: IgA deposits in cutaneous blood-vessel walls and mesangium in Henoch-Schönlein syndrome. Lancet 1:892, 1973.

139. Giangiacomo, J., and Tsai, C. C.: Dermatologic and glomerular deposition of IgA in anaphylactoid purpura. Am. J. Dis. Child. 131:981, 1977.

140. Maggiore, G., Martini, A., Grifeo, S., De Giacomo C., and Scotta M. S.: Hepatitis B virus infection and Schönlein-Henoch purpura. Am. J. Dis. Child. 138:681, 1984.

141. Sissons, J. G. P., Williams, D. G., Peters, D. K., Boulton-Jones, J. M., and Goldsmith, H. J.: Skin lesions, angio-oedema, and hypocomplementaemia. Lancet 2:1350, 1974.

142. Feig, P. U., Soter, N. A., Yager, H. M., Caplan, L., and Rosen, S.: Vasculitis with urticaria, hypocomplementemia, and multiple system involvement. JAMA 236:2065, 1976.

143. Schultz, D. R., Perez, G. O., Volanakis, J. E., Pardo V., and Moss S. H.: Glomerular disease in two patients with urticaria: Cutaneous vasculitis and hypocomplementemia. Am. J. Kidney Dis. 1:157, 1981.

144. Schwartz, H. R., McDuffie, F. C., Black, L. F., Schroeter A. L., and Conn D. L.: Hypo-complementemic urticarial vasculitis: Association with chronic obstructive pulmonary disease. Mayo Clin. Proc. 57:231, 1982.

145. Ludivico, C. L., Myers, A. R., and Maurer, K.: Hypocomplementemic urticarial vasculitis with glomerulonephritis and pseudotumor cerebri. Arthritis Rheum. 22:1024, 1972.

146. Ramirez, G., Saba, S. R., and Espinoza, L.: Hypocomplementemic vasculitis and renal involvement. Nephron 45:147, 1987.

147. Agnello, V., Winchester, R. J., and Kunkel, H. G.: Precipitin reactions of the C1q component of complement with aggregated γ-globulin and immune complexes in gel diffusion. Immunology 19:909, 1970.

148. Agnello, V., Koffler, D., Eisenberg, J. W., Winchester, R. J., and Kunkel, H. G.: C1q precipitins in the sera of patients with systemic lupus erythematosus and other hypocomplementemic states: Characterization of high and low molecular weight types. J. Exp. Med. 134:228s, 1971.

149. Agnello, V., Ruddy, S., Winchester, R. J., Christian, C. L., and Kunkel, H. G.: Hereditary C2 deficiency in systemic lupus erythematosus and acquired complement abnormalities in an unusual SLE-related syndrome. Birth Defects 11:312, 1975.

150. Agnello, V.: Association of systemic lupus erythematosus and SLE-like syndromes with hereditary and acquired complement deficiency states. Arthritis Rheum. 21(Suppl. 5):S146, 1978.

151. Marder, F. J., Burch, F. X., Schmid, F. R., Zeiss, C. R., and Gewurz, H.: Low molecular weight C1q-precipitins in hypocomplementemic vasculitis–urticaria syndrome: Partial purification and characterization as immunoglobulin. J. Immunol. 121:613, 1978.

152. Mraz, J. P., and Newcomer, V. D.: Erythema elevatum diutinum: Presentation of a case and evaluation of laboratory and immunological status. Arch. Dermatol. 96:235, 1967.

153. Katz, S. I., Gallin, J. I., Hertz, K. C., Fauci, A. S., and Lawley, T. J.: Erythema elevatum diutinum: Skin and systemic manifestations, immunologic studies, and successful treatment with dapsone. Medicine 56:443, 1977.

154. Montgomery, H., O'Leary, P. A., and Barker, N. W.: Nodular vascular diseases of the legs: Erythema induratum and allied conditions. JAMA 128:335, 1945.

155. Andersen, S. C.: Erythema induratum (Bazin) treated with isoniazid. Acta Derm. Venereol. (Stockh.) 50:65, 1970.

156. Bard, J. W., and Winkelmann, R. K.: Livedo vasculitis: Segmental hyalinizing vasculitis of the dermis. Arch. Dermatol. 96:489, 1967.

157. Su, W. P., and Winkelmann, R. K.: Livedoid vasculitis. In Wolff, K., and Winkelmann, R. K. (eds.): London, Lloyd-Luke Medical Books, 1980, p. 297.

158. Stiefler, R. E., and Bergfeld, W. F.: Atrophie blanche. Int. J. Dermatol. 21:1, 1982.

159. Milian, M. G.: Les atrophies cutanées syphilitiques. Bull. Soc. Fr. Dermatol. Syphiligr. 36:865, 1929.

160. Yasue, T.: Livedoid vasculitis and central nervous system involvement in systemic lupus erythematosus. Arch. Dermatol. 122:66, 1986.

161. Sammartino, L. R., Gharavi, A. E., and Lockshin, M. D.: Antiphospholipid antibody syndrome: Immunologic and clinical aspects. Semin. Arthritis Rheum. 20:81, 1990.

162. Sneddon, I. B.: Cerebro-vascular lesions and livedo reticularis. Br. J. Dermatol. 77:180, 1965.

163. Grattan, C. E. H., Burton, J. L., and Boon, A. P.: Sneddon's syndrome (livedo reticularis and cerebral thrombosis) with livedo vasculitis and anticardiolipin antibodies. Br. J. Dermatol. 120:441, 1989.

164. Keil, H.: The manifestations in the skin and mucous membranes in dermatomyositis, with special reference to the differential diagnosis from systemic lupus erythematosus. Ann. Intern. Med. 16:828, 1942.

165. O'Leary, P. A., and Waisman, M.: Dermatomyositis: A study of 40 cases. Arch. Dermatol. Syphilol. 41:1001, 1940.

166. Muller, S. A., Winkelmann, R. K., and Brunsting, L. A.: Calcinosis in dermatomyositis: Observations on course of diseases in children and adults. Arch. Dermatol. 79:660, 1959.

167. Everett, M. A., and Curtis, A. D.: Dermatomyositis: A review of nineteen cases in adolescents and children. Arch. Intern. Med. 100:70, 1957.

168. Banker, B. Q., and Victor, M.: Dermatomyositis (systemic angiopathy) of childhood. Medicine 45:261, 1966.

169. Christianson, H. B., Brunsting, L. A., and Perry, H. O.: Dermatomyositis: Unusual features, complications, and treatment. Arch. Dermatol. 74:581, 1956.

170. Christianson, H. B., Dorsey, C. S., O'Leary, P. A., and Kierland, R. R.: Localized scleroderma: A clinical study of two hundred thirty-five cases. Arch. Dermatol. 74:629, 1956.

171. Rubin, L.: Linear scleroderma: Association with abnormalities of spine and nervous system. Arch. Dermatol. Syphilol. 58:1, 1948.

172. Tuffanelli, D. L., and Winkelmann, R. K.: Systemic scleroderma: Clinical study of 727 cases. Arch. Dermatol. 84:359, 1961.

173. Carr, R. D., Heisel, E. B., and Stevenson, T. D.: CRST syndrome: Benign variant of scleroderma. Arch. Dermatol. 92:519, 1965.

174. Salerni, R., Rodnan, G. P., Leon, D. F., and Shaver, J. A.: Pulmonary hypertension in the CREST syndrome variant of progressive systemic sclerosis (scleroderma). Ann. Intern. Med. 86:394, 1977.

175. McHugh, N. J., James, I. E., Fairburn, K., and Maddison, P. J.: Autoantibodies to mitochondrial and centromere antigens in primary biliary cirrhosis and systemic sclerosis. Clin. Exp. Immunol. 81:244, 1990.

176. Schulman, L. E.: Diffuse fasciitis with eosinophilia: A new syndrome? Trans. Assoc. Am. Physicians 88:70, 1975.

177. Schumacher, H. R.: A scleroderma-like syndrome with fasciitis, myositis, and eosinophilia. Ann. Intern. Med. 84:49, 1976.

178. Rudner, E. J., Mehregan, A., and Pinkus, H.: Scleromyxedema: A variant of lichen myxedematosus. Arch. Dermatol. 93:3, 1966.

179. Morris, J. M., Samilson, R. L., and Corley, C. L.: Melorheostosis: Review of the literature and report of an interesting case with a nineteen-year follow-up. J. Bone Joint Surg. [Am.] 45:1191, 1963.

180. Wagers, L. T., Young, A. W., Jr., and Ryan, S. F.: Linear melorheostotic scleroderma. Br. J. Dermatol. 86:297, 1972.

181. Hood, A. F., Soter, N. A., Rappeport, J., and Gigli, I.: Graft-versus-host reaction: Cutaneous manifestations following bone marrow transplantation. Arch. Dermatol. 113:1087, 1977.

182. Sternberg, E. M., Van Woert, M. H., Young, S. N., Magnussen, I., Baker, H., Gauthier, S., and Osterland, C. K.: Development of a scleroderma-like illness during therapy with L-5-hydroxytryptophan and carbidopa. N. Engl. J. Med. 303:782, 1980.

183. Centers for Disease Control: Eosinophilia myalgia syndrome: New Mexico. M.M.W.R. 38:765, 1989.

184. Hertzman, P. A., Blevins, W. L., Mayer, J., Greenfield B., Ting M., and Gleich G. J.: Association of the eosinophilia–myalgia syndrome with the ingestion of tryptophan. N. Engl. J. Med. 322:869, 1990.

185. Silver, R. M., Heyes, M. P., Maize, J. C., Quearry, B., Vionnet-Fuasset, M., and Sternberg, E. M.: Scleroderma, fasciitis, and eosinophilia associated with the ingestion of tryptophan. N. Engl. J. Med. 322:874, 1990.

186. Isdale, I. C., and Bywaters, E. G. L.: The rash of rheumatoid arthritis and Still's disease. Q. J. Med. 25:377, 1956.

187. Calabro, J. J., and Marchesano, J. M.: Rash associated with juvenile rheumatoid arthritis. J. Pediatr. 72:611, 1968.

188. Taranta, A.: Occurrence of rheumatic-like subcutaneous nodules without evidence of joint or heart disease: Report of a case. N. Engl. J. Med. 266:13, 1962.

189. Canizares, O.: Cutaneous lesions of rheumatic fever: A clinical study in young adults. Arch. Dermatol. 76:702, 1957.

190. Perry, C. B.: Erythema marginatum (rheumaticum). Arch. Dis. Child. 12:233, 1937.

191. Kiel, H.: The rheumatic erythemas: A critical survey. Ann. Intern. Med. 11:2223, 1938.

192. Bywaters, E. G. L.: Skin manifestations of rheumatic diseases. In Fitzpatrick, T. B., et al. (eds.): Dermatology in General Medicine. New York, McGraw-Hill, 1971, p. 1534.

193. Bywaters, E. G. L., and Thomas, G. T.: Bed rest, salicylates and steroid in rheumatic fever. Br. Med. J. 1:1628, 1961.

194. Laitinen, O., Leirisalo, M., and Allander, E.: Rheumatic fever and Yersinia arthritis: Criteria and diagnostic problems in a changing disease pattern. Scand. J. Rheumatol. 4:145, 1975.

195. Barnert, A. L., Terry, E. E., and Persellin, R. H.: Acute rheumatic fever in adults. JAMA 232:925, 1975.

196. Bass, M. H.: The cutaneous manifestations of acute rheumatic fever in childhood. Med. Clin. North Am. 2:201, 1918.

197. Berger, B. W.: Erythema chronicum migrans of Lyme disease. Arch. Dermatol. 120:1017, 1984.

198. Berger, B. W., Kaplan, M. H., Rothenberg, I. R., and Barbour A. G.: Isolation and characterization of the Lyme disease spirochete from the skin of patients with erythema chronicum migrans. J. Am. Acad. Dermatol. 13:444, 1985.

199. Steere, A. C.: Lyme disease. N. Engl. J. Med. 321:586, 1989.

200. Goltz, R. W.: Systematized amyloidosis: A review of the skin and mucous membrane lesions and a report of two cases. Medicine 31:381, 1952.

201. Rukavina, J. G., Block, W. D., Jackson, C. E., Falls, H. F., Carey, J. H., and Curtis, A. C.: Primary systemic amyloidosis: A review and an experimental, genetic, and clinical study of 29 cases with particular emphasis on the familial form. Medicine 35:239, 1956.

202. Rubinow, A., and Cohen, A. S.: Skin involvement in generalized amyloidosis: A study of clinically involved and uninvolved skin in 50 patients with primary and secondary amyloidosis. Ann. Intern. Med. 88:781, 1978.

203. Mukai, H., Kanzaki, T., and Nishiyama, S.: Sulfhydryl and disulfide staining in amyloids of skin-limited and systemic amyloidoses. J. Invest. Dermatol. 82:4, 1984.

204. Hurley, H. J., and Weinberg, R.: Induced intralesional hemorrhage in primary systemic amyloidosis. Arch. Dermatol. 89:678, 1964.

205. Muckle, T. J., and Wells, M.: Urticaria, deafness and amyloidosis: A new heredo-familial syndrome. Q. J. Med. 31:235, 1962.

206. Black, J. T.: Amyloidosis, deafness, urticaria, and limb pains: A hereditary syndrome. Ann. Intern. Med. 70:989, 1969.

207. Andrade, C.: A peculiar form of peripheral neuropathy: Familial atypical generalized amyloidosis with special involvement of peripheral nerves. Brain 75:408, 1952.

208. James, D. G.: Dermatological aspects of sarcoidosis. Q. J. Med 28:109, 1959.

209. James, D. G., Thomson, A. D., and Willcox, A.: Erythema nodosum as a manifestation of sarcoidosis. Lancet 2:218, 1956.

210. Löfgren, S.: Erythema nodosum: Studies on etiology and pathogenesis in 185 adult cases. Acta Med. Scand. (Suppl.) 174:1, 1946.

211. Wood, B. T., Behlen, C. H., and Weary, P. E.: The association of sarcoidosis, erythema nodosum, and arthritis. Arch. Dermatol. 94:406, 1966.

212. Jorizzo, J. L., Koufman, J. A., Thompson, J. N., White, W. L., Shar, G. G., and Schreiner, D. J.: Sarcoidosis of the upper respiratory tract in patients with nasal rim lesions: A pilot study. J. Am. Acad. Dermatol. 22:439, 1990.

213. Spiteri, M. A., Matthey, F., Gordon, T., Carstairs, L. S., and James, D. G.: Lupus pernio: A clinico-radiological study of thirty-five cases. Br. J. Dermatol. 112:315, 1985.

214. Kroll, J. J., Shapiro, L., Koplon, B. S., and Feldman, F.: Subcutaneous sarcoidosis with calcification. Arch. Dermatol. 106:894, 1972.

215. Cornelius, C. E., Stein, K. M., Hanshaw, W. J., and Spolt, D. A.: Hypopigmentation and sarcoidosis. Arch. Dermatol. 108:249, 1973.

216. Olive, K. E., and Kataria, Y. P.: Cutaneous manifestations of sarcoidosis: Relationship to other organ system involvement, abnormal laboratory measurements, and disease course. Arch. Intern. Med. 145:1811, 1985.

217. MacPherson, P.: A survey of erythema nodosum in a rural community between 1954 and 1968. Tubercle 51:324, 1970.

218. Favour, C. B., and Sosman, M. C.: Erythema nodosum. Arch. Intern. Med. 80:435, 1947.

219. Debois, J., Vandepitte, J., and Degreef, H.: Yersinia entercolitica as a cause of erythema nodosum. Dermatologica 156:65, 1978.

220. Hannuksela, M.: Human yersiniosis: A common cause of erythematous skin eruptions. Int. J. Dermatol. 16:665, 1977.

221. Salvatore, M. A., and Lynch, P. J.: Erythema nodosum, estrogens and pregnancy. Arch. Dermatol. 116:557, 1980.

222. Jacobs, W. H.: Erythema nodosum in inflammatory diseases of the bowel. Gastroenterology 37:286, 1959.

223. Sumaya, C. V., Babu, S., and Reed, R. J.: Erythema nodosum–like lesions of leukemia. Arch. Dermatol. 110:415, 1974.

224. Bafverstedt, B.: Erythema nodosum migrans. Acta Derm. Venereol. (Stockh.) 34:181, 1954.

225. Vilanova, X., and Pinol-Aguade, J.: Subacute nodular migratory panniculitis. Br. J. Dermatol. 71:45, 1959.

226. Perry, H. O., and Winkelmann, R. K.: Subacute nodular migratory panniculitis. Arch. Dermatol. 89:170, 1964.

227. Weber, E. P.: A case of relapsing non-suppurative nodular panniculitis, showing phagocytosis of subcutaneous fat-cells by macrophages. Br. J. Dermatol. Syphilol. 37:301, 1925.

228. Christian, H. A.: Relapsing febrile nodular nonsuppurative panniculitis. Arch. Intern. Med. 42:338, 1928.

229. Milner, R. D. G., and Mitchinson, M. J.: Systemic Weber-Christian diseases. J. Clin. Pathol. 18:150, 1965.

230. DeLor, C. J., and Martz, R. W.: Weber-Christian disease with bone marrow involvement. Ann. Intern. Med. 43:591, 1955.

231. Pinals, R. S.: Nodular panniculitis associated with an inflammatory bone lesion. Arch. Dermatol. 101:359, 1970.

232. Oram, S., and Cochrane, G. M.: Weber-Christian disease with visceral involvement: An example with hepatic enlargement. Br. Med. J. 2:281, 1958.

233. Wilkinson, P. J., Harman, R. R. M., and Tribe, C. R.: Systemic nodular panniculitis with cardiac involvement. J. Clin. Pathol. 27:808, 1974.

234. Aronson, I. K., West, D. P., Variakojis, D., Malkinson, F. D., Wilson, H. D., and Zeitz, H. J.: Fatal panniculitis. J. Am. Acad. Dermatol. 12:535, 1985.

235. Potts, D. E., Mass, M. F., and Iseman, M. D.: Syndrome of pancreatic disease, subcutaneous fat necrosis and polyserositis: Case report and review of literature. Am. J. Med. 58:417, 1975.

236. Schrier, R. W., Melman, K. L., and Fenster, L. F.: Subcutaneous nodular fat necrosis in pancreatitis. Arch. Intern. Med. 116:832, 1965.

237. Williams, H. J., Samuelson, C. O., Jr., and Zone, J. J.: Nodular nonsuppurative panniculitis associated with jejunoileal bypass surgery. Arch. Dermatol. 115:1091, 1979.

Psychosocial Management of Rheumatic Diseases

The humane and effective care of patients with chronic rheumatic illnesses requires that the physician plan the medical management and also attend to the psychological needs of the patient to facilitate their coping with the disease and to optimize their functioning.[1] For most rheumatic disorders, patients and their physicians are involved in a life-long relationship in which the vagaries of the disease and normal life interact in a complex manner. Many of these psychological problems can be managed without consultation. When major psychiatric illness occurs, it is usually a manifestation of premorbid problems or is coincidental.[2, 3]

This chapter outlines a conceptual framework for understanding the psychosocial and functional impact of rheumatic disorders and clinical approaches to its management.

THE EXPERIENCE OF RHEUMATIC ILLNESS

In chronic disease, the most mundane activities of daily life cannot be taken for granted.[4-8] The simplest tasks may become so overwhelming that one's time and resources may be totally absorbed in attempts to accomplish them. It is difficult to capture the suffering, frustration, and poverty of an existence characterized by pain and loss of physical capacity with numbers and statistics alone.

The patients' expressions about how a rheumatic disorder affects the fabric of their lives and what helps them evoke common themes.

I have found that much changes in the 25-year course of chronic illness. Since my [joint replacement] surgery, I have returned to college and earned a BFA, started a demanding full-time job, and settled down with a human being I thought I could create only in my imagination. But I still have active JRA [juvenile rheumatoid arthritis]. Presently, with a friend whose daughter is in Saudi, a grown man who sits in his wheelchair and actually asks *me* how I deal with disability and feelings of inadequacy, and others close to me with AIDS and cancer struggling for their lives, it is honestly very difficult for me to find words that explain (justifiably in my own mind) how arthritis has an impact on my life.

What follows is a page from a journal I started when I was working on a screenplay. I feel this, as a writer, best describes what life is like for me now:

'. . . I'm through the second draft, despite my stiff and swollen hands that keep cramping up when I need them to type another paragraph. I didn't brush my long snarled hair this morning—I *wouldn't* tolerate the pain. So it's a little messy but curlier.

'Yesterday I met a woman recently diagnosed with RA. She told me her goal was to get out and visit more, like she used to, because now she stays home. She doesn't like her friends and family to see her wince in pain, or have such difficulty putting on a coat. And she's afraid of driving because even though she has power steering she has trouble making corners. Two weeks or so ago she was unable to press the toasting lever down on her toaster. This week she can do it—this small thing, toasting a slice of bread, makes her happy today. I know how she feels. I could hold a mug of tea made for me this morning, almost with one hand.

'I had trouble getting my lace shirt pulled down over my head and wondered why I'd chosen it. Sometimes I forget—I can't think of every potential problem, so when they come, they come; then they go, often leaving me with new ideas: I won't buy clothes like that anymore, nothing tight that needs to be pulled; no tiny buttons that come close to my neck, where my hands can't reach because my elbows won't bend enough, like on the blouse I gave away last month.

'Besides, I have other things to wear. . . .

'I have friends who can get up at 5 a.m. to write. How I envy them. Morning stiffness (that lasts sometimes till noon) challenges the day as I work at my job (even if I've taken all my meds), just enough to wear me out, making me quiet when I get home as I try to hide my grumpiness and frustration in knowing I should rest when I'd rather get more things done. I would like to be able to find no excuses not to write. But this arthritis seems to dangle my ideas just beyond my range of motion so I can't get a good hold of them—today. But on good days I am able to stretch a little farther and get back on schedule—*my* schedule—which is the most constant reminder of the necessity I have to make adjustments.'

> An editorial assistant, age 31,
> with JRA since age 6

Beyond the obvious day-to-day discomfort, the most significant effect on my life from the spondylitis is that which it has on my self-image. This image is directly related to how I feel at any given moment. When I feel good, and am essentially unaware of symptoms, I am who I always have been—young, energetic, capable. But when my symptoms are present, my self-image changes—I am aging, tentative, dependent, tinged with self-pity and regret. I am more willing to accept, rather than strive. In short, my confidence in my life and myself is reduced by how I feel physically.

535

Despite this, a part of me rebels against this lowered self-esteem. It effectively refuses to accept the disease, to admit to not being able to do things I once did with ease or even skill. These two conflicting personae—the hesitant, reflective sick person, and the unaccepting person who does what he wants despite how he feels—arise from each other in a constant, uninterrupted shifting pattern. The self-pity, which is the last stage of my "sick person," awakens my "healthy person." When he is eventually confronted with a task, however mundane, which symptoms prevent him from doing, the "sick person" re-emerges and the cycle begins anew. Maintaining equilibrium about my condition—emotional balance—is essential, and the best way to maintain it is to understand the disease, as it affects you, in a realistic manner, including realistic expectations of the future. It is thus most important that the treating physician be open and honest with the patient regarding treatment, diagnosis, prognosis, and symptoms.

A lawyer, age 45, with spondylitis
since age 20

Health professionals usually deal with the negative impact of diseases, but they must realize that most patients persevere and stay active,[9] and some inspire the healthy with their accomplishments. Well-known examples of people with arthritis who have achieved much include Pierre Auguste Renoir, E. Power Biggs, Dr. Christiaan Barnard, Gail Riggs, Sara Lynn Allaire, Byron Janus (with psoriatic arthritis), and Flannery O'Connor (with systemic lupus erythematosus), but less well-known heroes and heroines abound.

PSYCHOLOGICAL FRAMEWORK

In rheumatic disease, as in other chronic illnesses, the vagaries of the disease interact with the patients' stage in life; their life experience, personality, and home and work environment; and their social and cultural systems. The interaction of these factors defines the meaning of the disease to the patient (the "illness experience").

Persons with chronic rheumatic diseases experience a series of adaptations. The responses seen in acute life-threatening illnesses (shock, anger, denial, resignation, and acceptance) are mirrored in the course of having a chronic disease. Reaction to the initial diagnosis is influenced by the degree of incapacity and the immediate threat to the patient's lifestyle. Patients with insidious-onset rheumatoid arthritis or systemic lupus erythematosus may be relieved to have a diagnosis after frustrating efforts to be diagnosed or lack of sympathy for their symptoms. Patients commonly ask themselves, "Why did this happen to me?" and attempt their own explanation as a way of rationalizing their illness or relieving uncertainty. The disease may be attributed to emotional or physical trauma or punishment for some misdeed. The patient may seek confirmation of the diagnosis by consulting others or reading medical sources. At this stage, the most helpful

approach is to provide support, reassurance, a plan, and a discussion of what to expect. Denial is another common reaction that may help the patient adapt to the disease and to be as functional as possible.

During periods of stable or quiescent disease activity, resignation and acceptance are more prominent adaptive mechanisms. During exacerbations, anger, denial, anxiety, and depression may recur. Anger, frequently toward the bearer of bad news, may manifest itself in demanding behavior or nonadherence.

Adjustments in chronic arthritis occur against the background of the patients' stage in life. For the physician, sensitivity to the psychological meaning of the illness starts with an awareness of the usual concerns and growth and development issues in that stage.

A common age for arthritis to occur during childhood is between 2 and 4 years, which is a period of great physical and psychological change. The critical developmental milestone during this period is that the child must bond to the mother, and the resultant physical satisfaction and warmth lay the foundation for developing trust in others. Other critical developmental tasks are to gain new motor and mental skills and a basic control of self and environment, which promote a sense of confidence and mastery. Between ages 3 and 6, a child begins to explore a wider environment and to develop a conscience. In the years between 6 and 12, the normal child is exploring the world beyond the home at school and must begin to master intellectual and social skills and to increase in physical strength.

One fourth of children with rheumatic disorders experience psychosocial problems in addition to the impaired function and delayed physical growth that may occur with inflammatory arthritis. Systemic illness and polyarthritis interfere with the ability of the parents to provide warmth and comfort. They also limit the child's involvement in school, the most important social experience in youth, which may lead to social isolation and psychosocial growth retardation. A study by Stoff et al.[10] suggests that school achievement in children with rheumatic diseases is related more to inattention and distractibility than impaired mobility or fatigue. Children typically do not complain of pain and may not limit their activities in accordance with their symptoms.[11]

Normal family dynamics are challenged.[12-15] The affected child's normal siblings may feel abandoned because of the interest shown in the child with illness, which increases sibling rivalry and conflict. Fathers are often uninvolved with the day-to-day health care of their child and may feel estranged and bewildered by the experience. Parents and teachers may overprotect and deprive the child of the chance to be strong and to feel independent. Children with less obvious physical impairment, such as monoarticular or pauciarticular disease, may have more psychosocial problems than children who have more extensive disease.[16] The latter group may have a legitimized disability and have allowances made for them by adults; children with minimal disease may not be perceived as sick or disabled, and this discrepancy may cause conflict in roles and interpersonal relationships. Less functional incapacity, higher family income, and higher educational level of the mother are factors that lessen the impact of a child's illness on the family.[13]

Public Law 94–142 (The Education for All Handicapped Children Act) emphasizes mainstreaming and mandates that support services be available in schools for all children. Because childhood arthritis disorders are relatively rare, the school system, the teachers, or the school nurse will not likely have any experience in accommodating or helping such patients. Ensuring smooth integration into the school may require follow-up by the health care team to educate school personnel in the nuances of the disease.

Polyarthritis affects the critical issues of adolescence, which are separation from parents and home, career training, career choice, achievement of economic independence, peer relationships, and selection of a mate. Adolescence is normally a tumultuous time for the person and their family, and with the additional stress of a chronic illness, many problems become manifest. Adolescents with arthritis refuse to take their pills or to do prescribed exercises.[17–20] This "push-pull" of adolescence can create many problems for the parents and health care providers and requires a coordinated, consistent approach to management. The adolescent must be treated as an adult whenever possible. The physical examination should be done without the parent in the room. Giving some young patients choices from a menu of equivalent therapy or control over when they are administered is another way of making them feel like adults. Adolescents do not want to appear different from their peers, and the use of devices, aids, or splints might be encouraged at home or at night as a trade-off between what is necessary and what is responsive to their feelings.[17, 18]

Spondylitis disability seen in patients with ankylosing spondylitis, spondylitis associated with Reiter's disease, psoriasis, inflammatory bowel disease, or juvenile arthritis are characterized by stiffness and restrictive movement of the spine with occasional involvement of the shoulder, hip, or knee; difficulties sitting or standing for extended periods; stiffness and fatigue on awakening; its male predominance; onset in young and middle-aged adults; and the episodic nature of the peripheral arthritis. Spondylitis disability is usually compatible with good function except when it involves peripheral joints. Iritis, aortic insufficiency, or apical fibrosis of the lungs, or associated systemic diseases, such as inflammatory bowel disease, may be even more limiting in some patients. Spondylitis in young adults affects self-esteem, body image, leisure and athletic activities, and peer and sexual relationships.

Patients with spondylitis are frequently lost to follow-up, perhaps because the disease is insidious and generally compatible with good function. Physical therapy programs to maintain or improve spinal mobility are poorly complied with unless they are perceived as being useful, and most importantly, unless they are incorporated into normal activities. In Reiter's disease, the connection with venereal infection and urethritis may raise anxiety or guilt about sexual intercourse in the patient or their partners.

In late mid-life, rheumatic disorders may intensify the perception of aging and accelerate physical dependence. After mid-life, the dominant issue is maintaining one's independence. Old age is a time when people look forward to activities previously deferred because of work or family commitments, and a chronic illness may make this deferral permanent.

The most common rheumatic condition of the late middle age, the elderly, and the oldest old is osteoarthritis with its involvement of the small joints of the hand, the hips, knees, or back, its lack of systemic symptoms, and its monoarticular or pauciarticular involvement.

Osteoarthritis disability unfolds slowly, paralleling the aging process, and its impact is not as apparent as rheumatoid disability. Indeed, many patients (and physicians) assume that musculoskeletal symptoms from osteoarthritis are an inevitable part of aging. In old-old age, osteoarthritis is the most common form of chronic arthritis and is the major reason for dependence and being homebound. Its impact is particularly devastating in this group because this is also the time of many losses: general health, friends, family, and resources.

COMMON PSYCHOLOGICAL PROBLEMS

In patients with rheumatoid arthritis, seronegative polyarthritis, and psoriatic arthritis, the disease is usually characterized by polyarticular involvement, chronicity, variability, and constitutional symptoms. Common psychological problems include the fear of becoming disabled and dependent, uncertainty about the disease process, altered body image, devaluation of self, and frustration and depression.

The fear of becoming disabled or helpless may be harder to endure than the event itself. Seeing other patients or knowing someone with handicapping arthritis can be frightening to a newly diagnosed person. The best antidotes are being frank, giving information to demystify the illness, and discussing the range of treatments available. The way in which patients resolve the dilemma of independence versus dependence depends on disease activity, the quality of their interactions with others, their financial resources, and their capacity to receive and ask for help. Having the ability to modify a work schedule or hire additional help, or not to work, aids adjustment. In time, most patients discover that they can gain more independence by both acknowledging and accepting help from others.

A patient's reaction may center around specific losses, such as physical limitations, and abstract losses, such as expectations for the future, self-image, and self-esteem. Grief over such losses may lead to depression that is generally limited to a few days or weeks. Prolonged grief or depression may require antidepressant medication and referral for psychotherapy. Indications for a referral include impaired function; vegetative symptoms; sleep disturbance; loss of appetite; and ruminating, intractable hopelessness, or preoccupation with suicide.

The physician's understanding of what is significant to the patient is aided by knowing the most meaningful aspects of the patient's life. For example, for a person whose primary identity and social interactions are through work, loss of a job will be more devastating than for a person with other outlets. Grief over the losses can be compensated for by substitution of something else valued.

Sexuality may be altered by pain, discomfort, and constitutional symptoms such as fatigue or poor self-image from deformities or from medications such as steroids.[21] The unaffected partner may fear causing discomfort to the partner with arthritis, who may view unwillingness to engage in sexual activity as a loss of attraction. Systemic symptoms impair libido. A physician can legitimize the subject by raising the issue or by appropriate referral if sexuality is a concern.

Patients with rheumatoid vasculitis or with rheumatoid arthritis and extra-articular manifestations, systemic lupus erythematosus, and other systemic vasculitides are troubled by the uncertainty and the potential life-threatening nature of the disease. Symptoms and functional capacity in rheumatoid arthritis may change from day to day and even from morning to afternoon. Joint symptoms and even sleep apnea may cause disturbed sleep and contribute to the fatigue.[22] The phenomena of morning stiffness and fatigue need to be explained to the family and other contacts because the patient may not have any visible signs to validate the symptoms to others. The patient may be able to work but have less energy for other activities. This difficulty can be mitigated to a degree if the patient can explain the problem without feeling guilty about being unable to fulfill commitments.

In systemic lupus erythematosus, a number of neuropsychiatric manifestations are described,[6, 23-25] such as psychoaffective disorders, psychosis, cognitive disorders, and organic brain syndrome. In the individual patient, whether the manifestation is due to systemic lupus erythematosus itself, a side effect of treatment, a reaction to having a serious illness, or a concomitant psychiatric disorder, is always a challenge to differential diagnosis. When a specific cause can be found, it is treated, but for many serious psychiatric symptoms, psychotherapy or pharmacotherapy is necessary. Measures of psychological characteristics such as the Minnesota Multiphasic Personality Inventory do not show any differences among patients with lupus, rheumatoid arthritis, or other chronic disorders.[6]

Some patients with chronic rheumatic disorders attempt to conceal their disability for fear their arthritis will make them less attractive to others or cost them a job. Denial and acting no differently from others are the most healthy behaviors in many situations. Patients who maintain their own identity as distinct from that of an "arthritis patient" seem to adapt better, function better, and to be in a better psychological state. On the other hand, concealment of symptoms may not allow others to help or to understand what the patient is going through. The physician should try to make the patient not feel pitied and help friends and family to understand that talking about the disorder will not upset the patient.

Distracting pain leads to lower tolerance, irritability, self-preoccupation, and loss of concentration. Nevertheless, considering the chronic pain experienced by persons with various forms of chronic arthritis, few become patients who use narcotic analgesics and have lifestyles dominated by pain behavior. Behavioral techniques for pain secondary to structural damage may be helpful in increasing the pain threshold.

Finally, undergoing surgery is a major event in a patient's life and an opportunity for the physician to relieve anxiety. A discussion about what to expect before and after surgery can maximize a successful outcome. A meta-analysis of 49 studies showed that psychological and educational preparation for surgery can consistently reduce pain and discomfort, use of medications, and length of stay after surgery by an average of 1.25 days.[26] Despite this finding, and published standards for developing and managing such programs, there is little evidence that many physicians have developed formal programs for their own patients.

Dealing with chronic disorders affects caregivers as well, but there is little understanding of how the disappointments and the inability to help some patients with incurable illnesses might affect them and their effectiveness. Those who provide care for the chronically ill face their limitations daily, and it takes a unique temperament to maintain equanimity and commitment. One must be able to derive satisfaction from helping patients make small adjustments, having modest goals and being satisfied with them, and being available through the vicissitudes of flares.

Medical care occupies a major role in the lives of the chronically ill, and patients with rheumatic diseases cite the central importance of being able to communicate with their physician. Despite their awareness of the limitations of medicine, they continue to look to the medical system for ways of minimizing pain and providing support. The physician's knowledge provides a framework for dealing with the experience. Even if people who are impaired have a diminished status in society, they do have a role within the context of medical care and a physician's continued concern in their condition *and* their personal lives gives meaning and value to the patient.

SOCIAL POLICY AND PSYCHOSOCIAL DISABILITY

Descriptions of the impact of rheumatic disease indicate that disability is strongly influenced by social and environmental circumstances and presents an opportunity to buffer the consequences of these disorders for people so affected on a societal level.[27]

Society's challenge is to provide services to meet these needs and to do it in a manner that does not create dependency and devalued status. It is likely that these solutions will not take place in medical institutions. Many appropriate services are available for arthritis patients, but they are inaccessible or fragmented, and there is need for specially trained clinicians, frequently the physician, to coordinate the appropriate mix of services for patients.[28]

People with rheumatic disabilities are bound to be disadvantaged and less economically well off in a competitive society with its values on physical attractiveness, independence, and productivity. Although social policy may redress some of the disadvantages arising from chronic rheumatic disease, some types of deprivation are much less amenable to change. Attitudes and settings that alienate the person with rheumatic disabilities and contribute to their sense of social isolation are important examples. But even in this instance, it is possible to identify ways of helping families to contain or manage conflict, to adapt to new roles and responsibilities, and to change the attitudes of the nondisabled toward the disabled.

When people no longer have the strength or dexterity to perform everyday tasks or are immobilized by pain, the resources they command affect their lives and their self-perception profoundly. Available social supports and financial resources determine whether a valued activity can be maintained. Buying help is preferable to help provided by community programs because the buyer retains control and can choose the kind and timing of the help, which reinforces their independence at a time when it is undermined. Health care benefits, in kind, create dependency and limit choice; cash benefits might have problems also, but they allow patients with rheumatic disease to maintain their self-determination and dignity.

The meaning of a rheumatic disease is not the same even to those with identical impairments. The problems that arise from a disease may be more or less managable according to available resources. Knowledge, money, social supports, aids and appliances, and adapted environments are powerful determinants of patients' ability to function in their home or at work and their access to society's opportunities. These resources are variably distributed in the society, and people from some social strata are less able to manage the effects of disability than others. The relationship, however, is not simple, because neither hardship nor happiness is exclusively the fate of lower socioeconomic groups. Opportunities for remaining in work following the onset of disability are not markedly different for those employed in manual and nonmanual occupations, and the availability of social support is not limited to one social class. Location of activities that offer alternatives to work seems to be influenced most by previous occupation.

Other social policy gambits include removing inequality in the quality of treatment; targeting psychoeducational programs to improve self-management, coping, adherence, and social supports; developing programs to provide more than subsistence income to disabled people; improving physical access to the community; and providing meaningful work and independence in living. These priorities overlap, and accomplishing one helps to fulfill the others.

PSYCHOLOGICAL RESEARCH

Psychological research in rheumatic diseases has focused on the following areas: the impact of rheumatic diseases on psychological development and health; the relationship of psychological factors to the onset of illness; psychological factors as modifiers of outcome; adherence to medical regimens; the evaluation of behavioral techniques (behavior modification, autogenic training, relaxation response, etc.) in the management of rheumatic symptoms; and the evaluation of psychological techniques in treating psychological distress. Much of the literature prior to the 1970s did not clearly distinguish the type of arthritis; used cross-sectional, uncontrolled studies with highly selected samples; applied nonstandard psychosocial measures of unknown validity and inappropriate analytic techniques; or dwelt on the negative aspects of psychological health.

Psychological Factors in Disease Pathogenesis

Earlier work focused on a unique rheumatoid personality and on the psychological factors that were thought to induce rheumatoid arthritis or juvenile rheumatoid arthritis, but a critical review of the evidence casts doubt on this hypothesis.[5, 8, 29] Fibrositis has been considered a psychosomatic illness or as having a psychological cause, but the evidence is similarly wanting.[30] However, it is possible that stress modifies the expression of the disease or lowers the patient's pain threshold. A body of tantalizing studies links psychological phenomena with immune functions.[31]

Psychosocial Impact

There are few diseases in which patients suffer as much pain and discomfort over a prolonged period as they do with arthritis. Patients with rheumatoid arthritis consistently report that pain relief is their primary objective in seeking medical care. Pain is a major determinant of the health perceptions of both patients and physicians and is strongly related to future disability in patients with chronic rheumatic diseases.

Although patients with chronic rheumatic disorders have a greater burden imposed on them than healthy people, longitudinal studies suggest that psychological and physical adaptation among patients with arthritis and other chronic illnesses is remarkably effective[9, 22] and that most people prevail. This is in contrast to much of the literature that emphasizes the negative aspects of personality and psychoaffective disturbances. Although there are setbacks and stress, given guidance, support, and time, many, perhaps more than is generally appreciated, do well despite physical impairment. For health care providers, this is a reminder that medicalizing problems, overmanaging, and making patient's more dependent may undermine their learning to cope and the innate resourcefulness of patients and their families.

Patients with rheumatoid arthritis appear to have more depression as measured by psychological testing than normal people and disease controls. However, these findings reflect arthritis symptoms such as fatigue, which may be also seen in depression and probably represent a reaction to the experience of the illness rather than an integral part of the disease.[32] Indeed, no differences have been found between rheumatoid arthritis patients' self-reports of depression and those of patients with other chronic diseases.[6]

COMPLIANCE

Reviews of adherence to treatment in arthritis management adds to a large literature from other chronic illnesses.[33–37] Estimates of self-reported nonadherence to medications range from 22 percent to 67 percent and to physical therapy range from 33 percent to 66 percent. Long-term compliance with medications, physical therapy, and physical modalities is about 50 percent for each, which is also the rate seen in other chronic illness. In contrast to the vast descriptive literature, little attention has been paid to evaluating strategies to enhance adherence.[38] Because prescribed arthritis regimens are rarely curative and their side effects are neither predictable nor trivial, nonadherence may be the best solution for the patient.[39] Not surprisingly, nonadherence is increased when patients doubt a regimen's effectiveness or have erroneous beliefs about the medication[40] or when the medication requires multiple doses. The

literature on compliance in other illness is relevant to arthritis management. Adherence is generally improved when the patient and physician agree on the problem, the disease model, and treatment goals; when the patient perceives a threat and an effective treatment exists; when there is a simple technique for self-monitoring; when there is social reinforcement; when the regimen is not disruptive to normal patterns of activities; and when the disease is of more recent onset. Writing down the prescribed regimen is a simple and effective way to enhance compliance.

PSYCHOEDUCATIONAL TECHNIQUES

A number of psychoeducational approaches for arthritis pain and disability have been tested.[41–44] These include educational approaches, group psychotherapy, structured group support, electromyography or alpha biofeedback training, and relaxation training. These techniques teach patients to recognize and alter the association between environmental stimuli and pain and place therapy under the control of the patient. Cognitive-behavioral interventions are considered as a general class within self-control programs; they emphasize the patients' role in reduction of pain and disability and involve them in their own appraisal of efficacy. Biofeedback training has been used in patients with chronic arthritis pain and in Raynaud's phenomenon and disease. Critical review of the literature shows that a wide variety of psychoeducational interventions reduce pain and improve function and psychological well-being.[41–44] A behavioral component added to an educational program increases the effectiveness of the program, and even "experienced" patients, that is, patients followed by specialists and who have had the disease for years, appear to benefit in increased knowledge about their disease and its treatment with organized patient education programs.[43] With few exceptions, studies usually do not examine the cost effectiveness or durability of the results.

Although it is believed that perceived or actual social support is a strong mitigating factor against psychological distress, prospective clinical trials show that increasing social support alone produces mixed results,[45–47] perhaps because of small sample size, insensitive instruments, or weak educational programs. Patients' knowledge about arthritis may improve after educational and social support programs, but that increased knowledge does not always lead to improved coping and occasionally produces a negative effect.

Exceptions to these studies are those evaluating the arthritis self-management program for patients with a variety of rheumatic conditions.[48] This program consists of six 2-hour sessions led by lay volunteers and is based on concepts derived from research in learned helplessness. The program provides information and home practice instructions on topics such as range of motion, isometric exercise, relaxation techniques, joint protection, and nutrition. When the effects of the program in patients waiting to receive it were compared with the effects in those who received the intervention, it was found that there was significant reduction in pain, greater practice of arthritis-related exercise and relaxation, and diminished dependence on the health care system but no improvement in self-reported function. The effects appear to persist up to 4 years after the program.

A study using lay instructors and health professionals for a program modeled after Lorig et al.'s self-management program[48] showed that both patient educational programs improved participants' knowledge of arthritis and therapeutic exercise compared to a nonintervention control group. The groups led by professional instructors had the same outcome as those led by lay instructors. However, neither intervention was any more effective than nonintervention in lessening pain, improving function, enhancing social support, and lessening depression.[50]

The link between a health behavior that is changed by any intervention and a beneficial outcome is not straightforward any more than the relationship between increased knowledge and improved outcome. Controlled studies of health education have demonstrated that although experimental groups adopt more of the desired behaviors and exhibit greater improvements in health outcome, there is not a clear path between the performance of behaviors with their health outcomes.[49] Participants in such programs are taught a variety of skills and may use only those that are applicable or effective for them. Also, training in behavioral skills may give patients a sense of control and mastery, which can produce benefits.

A randomized clinical trial evaluated three interventions in patients with rheumatoid arthritis: a biofeedback-assisted cognitive-behavioral psychological intervention; a structured group social support therapy group; and a control group. It was shown that the psychological intervention produced statistically significant reductions in pain behavior and the Rheumatoid Activity Index at 3 months. Relaxation training was believed to be the most important component of the intervention. Anxiety was reduced at the 6-month follow-up.[51]

In another randomized clinical trial in a Veteran's Administration hospital population with rheumatoid arthritis, a 12-month cognitive-behavioral pain management group, an attention-placebo group, and a control group were evaluated.[52] The group that received the psychological intervention showed significantly greater use of coping strategies and more confidence in their ability to manage pain. However, the impact of the program on disease activity and functional or psychological status was minimal and occurred only in the most adherent group.

Goeppinger et al.[53] also evaluated two models of arthritis self-care in a rural Southern population with a variety of arthritis disorders and showed a beneficial and statistically significant effect on arthritis knowledge, self-care behavior, perceived helplessness, and pain.

Structured group support for patients with rheumatic disease and their families provides a milieu to verbalize and share concerns, to learn about the disease, to realize that others have similar experiences and emotional reactions, and to strengthen coping strategies through problem solving. Therapeutic groups for arthritis patients were first described by Henkle.[54] Since then, evaluations of many groups offering psychological support and education have been reported. Groups with different emphasis, organization, and leadership exist. All have educational goals and emphasize communication skills, coping, and mutual support, but some focus more on one aspect than another. Groups emphasizing psychological support are usually led by psychiatrists, psychologists, social workers, and other health professionals with special group training. One study reported improvement in joint tenderness in groups receiving stress management and mutual support.[55]

Schwartz et al.[56] described a group that sought to improve the education of physicians concerning the emotional impact of chronic disease. Observed improvement occurred in compliance with treatment, communication with families and physicians, and modifications in lifestyle.

Groups are probably not effective for the people with the most resourcefulness and who already have the appropriate values and attitudes, and for others the change may be short lived and dependent on participation. Evidence from programs designed to enhance compliance with hypertensive medications suggests that participation in group programs may actually have the worst compliance in the long term.

The effectiveness of psychotherapy group assertion and relaxation training was compared with no treatment in rheumatoid arthritis.[57] Fifty-seven rheumatoid arthritis patients were randomized to each of the three groups. The dependent variables were standardized items taken from self-reported measures of satisfaction and physical, psychological, and social function and a physician global evaluation of disease activity. Measurement occurred at baseline, immediately after the intervention, and 12 months after baseline. There were a few outcome measures for which either treatment resulted in significantly higher scores than seen in the control group, although there were more improvements noted in patients who received conventional group psychotherapy.

Rheumatoid arthritis patients randomized to educational sessions and to 12 weekly group counseling plus education showed that the group receiving the counseling improved their scores on two areas of self-concept and in factual knowledge but not in amount of depression.[58]

In a controlled study of an educational support group for patients with ankylosing spondylitis,[59] patients in the experimental group had significant increased knowledge and observed compliance with exercise programs. Verbal feedback concerning improved coping abilities was given in most instances. Control patients showed no substantial changes in knowledge or compliance.

SUMMARY

Psychological and social problems are an integral feature of chronic rheumatic diseases and a key to understanding how these diseases affect the individual patient and family. In the absence of true cures for many disorders, patients and their advocates must find ways of dealing with the psychosocial consequences. These include a commitment to dealing with these consequences, a caring attitude, and an understanding of how the life cycle interacts with a chronic illness, how social and environmental factors modify the resultant handicap, and how specific interventions might be employed to ameliorate these effects. Psychoeducational interventions can often improve pain management and coping skills above and beyond what the individual clinician can offer.

References

1. Rogers, M. P., Liang, M. H., and Partridge, A. J.: Psychological care of adults with RA. Ann. Intern. Med. 96:344, 1982.
2. Rogers, M. P., Reich, P., Kelly, J. H., and Liang, M. H.: Psychiatric consultation among hospitalized arthritis patients. Gen. Hosp. Psychiatry 2:89, 1980.
3. Murphy, S., Creed, F., and Jayson, M. I. V.: Psychiatric disorder and illness behavior in rheumatoid arthritis. Br. J. Rheum. 27:357, 1988.
4. Meenan, R., Yelin, E., Nevitt, M., and Epstein, W.: The impact of chronic disease: A sociomedical profile of rheumatoid arthritis. Arthritis Rheum. 24:544, 1981.
5. Bradley, L. A.: Psychological aspects of arthritis. Bull. R. U. Dis. 35:1, 1985.
6. Liang, M. H., Rogers, M., Larson, M., Eaton, H. M., Murawski, B. J., Taylor, J. E., Swafford, J., and Schur, P. H.: The psychosocial impact of systemic lupus erythematosus and rheumatoid arthritis. Arthritis Rheum. 27:13, 1984.
7. Ehrlich, G. E.: Social, economic, psychologic, and sexual outcomes in rheumatoid arthritis. Am. J. Med. 75:27, 1983.
8. Baum, J.: A review of the psychological aspects of rheumatic diseases. Semin. Arthritis Rheum. 11:352, 1982.
9. Cassileth, B. R., Lusk, E. J., Strouse, T. B., Miller, D. S., Brown, L. L., Gross, P. A., and Tenaglia, A. N.: Psychosocial status in chronic illness: A comparative analysis of six diagnostic groups. N. Engl. J. Med. 311:506, 1984.
10. Stoff, E., Bacon, M. L., and White, P. H.: The effects of fatigue, distractibility, and absenteeism on school achievement in children with rheumatoid diseases. Arthritis Care Res. 2:49, 1990.
11. Beales, J. C., Keen, J. H., and Holt, P. J.: The child's perception of the disease and the experience of pain in juvenile chronic arthritis. J. Rheumatol. 10:16, 1983.
12. Henoch, M., Batson, J., and Baum, J.: Psychosocial factors in JRA. Arthritis Rheum. 21:229, 1978.
13. McCormick, M. C., Stemmoer, M. M., and Athreya, B. H.: The impact of childhood rheumatic diseases on the family. Arthritis Rheum. 29:872, 1986.
14. Quirk, M. E., and Young, M. H.: The impact of JRA on children, adolescents, and their families: Current research and implications for future studies. Arthritis Care Res. 3:36, 1990.
15. Miller, J. J., Spitz, P. W., Simpson, U., and Williams, G. F.: The social function of young adults who had arthritis in childhood. J. Pediatr. 100:378, 1982.
16. McAnarney, E. R., Pless, I. B., Satterwhite, B., and Friedman, S. B.: Psychological problems in children with chronic juvenile arthritis. Pediatrics 53:523, 1974.
17. Litt, I. F., Cuskey, W. R., and Rosenberg, A.: Role of self-esteem and

18. Rapoff, M. A., Lindsley, C. B., and Christophersen, E. R.: Parents' perceptions of problems experienced by their children in complying with treatments for JRA. Arch. Phys. Med Rehabil. 66:427, 1985.
19. Rapoff, M. A.: Compliance with treatment regimens for pediatric rheumatoid diseases. Arthritis Care Res. 2:S40, 1989.
20. Hayford, J. R., and Ross, C. K.: Medical compliance in juvenile rheumatoid arthritis: Problems and perspectives. Arthritis Care Res. 1:190, 1989.
21. Yoshino, S., and Uchida, S.: Sexual problems of women with a rheumatoid arthritis. Arch. Phys. Med. Rehabil. 62:122, 1981.
22. Mahowald, M. W., Mahowald, M. L., Burdlie, S. R., and Ytterberg, S. R.: Sleep fragmentation in rheumatoid arthritis. Arthritis Rheum. 32:974, 1989.
22a. Tack, B. B.: Fatigue in rheumatoid arthritis. Arthritis Care Res. 3:2, 1990.
23. Ganz, V. H., Gurland, B. J., Deming, W. E., and Fisher, B.: The study of the psychiatric symptoms of SLE: A biometric study. Psychosom. Med. 34:207, 1972.
24. Kremer, J. M., Rynes, R. I., Bartholomew, L. E., Rodichok, L. D., Pelton, E. W., Block, E. A., Tassnari, R. B., and Silver, R. J.: Non-organic non-psychotic psychopathology in patients with SLE. Semin. Arthritis Rheum. 11:182, 1981.
25. Ginsburg, K. S., Wright, E. A., Larson, M. G., Fossel, A. H., Albert, M., Schur, P. H., and Liang, M. H.: A controlled study of the prevalence of cognitive dysfunction in randomly selected patients with systemic lupus erythematosus. Arthritis Rheum. Vol. 32, 1992 (in press).
26. Devine, E. C., and Cook, T. D.: A meta-analytic analysis of effects of psycho-educational interventions on length of post-surgical hospital stay. Nurs. Res. 32:267, 1983.
27. Liang, M. H., and Daltroy, L. H.: The impact of inflammatory arthritis on society and the individual. In Hadler, N. M., and Gillings, D. B. (eds.): Options for Public Health Programs in Arthritis and Society. London, Butterworths, 1985, pp. 1–16.
28. Liang, M. H., Phillips, E. E., Scamman, M. D., Lurye, C. S., Keith, A., Cohen, L., and Taylor, G.: Evaluation of a pilot program for rheumatic disability in an urban community. Arthritis Rheum. 24:937, 1981.
29. Wallace, D. J.: The role of stress and trauma in rheumatoid arthritis and systemic lupus erythematosus. Semin. Arthritis 16:153, 1987.
30. Bradley, L. A., Anderson, H. O., Young, L. D., and McDaniel, L. K.: Is psychological disturbance highly associated with primary fibrositis? Evidence that primary fibrosis is not a form of "psychogenic rheumatism." Behav. Med. Abstr. 6:145, 1985.
31. Ader, R., and Cohen, N.: CNS–immune system interactions: Conditioning phenomena. Behav. Brain Sci. 8:379, 1985.
32. Pincus, T., Callahan, L. F., Bradley, L. A., Vaughn, W. K., and Wolfe, F.: Elevated MMPI scores for hypochondriasis, depression, and hysteria in patients with RA reflect disease rather than psychological status. Arthritis Rheum. 29:1456, 1986.
33. Ferguson, K., and Bole, G. G.: Family support, health belief, and therapeutic compliance in patients with rheumatoid arthritis. Patient Counsel. Health Ed. 2:101, 1979.
34. Jette, A. M.: Improving patient cooperation with arthritis treatement regimens. Arthritis Rheum. 25:447, 1982.
35. Katz, W. A.: Compliance. Semin. Arthritis Rheum. 12:132, 1982.
36. Belcon, M. C., Haynes, R. B., and Tugwell, P.: A critical review of compliance studies in rheumatoid arthritis. Arthritis Rheum. 27:1227, 1984.
37. Bradley, L. A.: Adherence with treatment regimens among rheumatoid arthritis patients: Current status and future directions. Arthritis Care Res. 2:S33, 1989.
38. Waggoner, C. D., and LeLieuvre, R. B.: A method to increase compliance to exercise regimens in rheumatoid arthritis patients. J. Behav. Med. 4:191, 1981.
39. Liang, M. H.: Compliance and quality of life: Confessions of a difficult patient. Arthritis Care Res. 2:S71, 1989.
40. Lorish, C. D., Richards, B., and Brown, S. Jr.: Perspective of the patient with rheumatoid arthritis on issues related to missed medication. Arthritis Care Res. 3:78, 1990.
41. Winfield, J. B., and ACR/AHPA/AF/NAAB Task Force on Arthritis Patient Education: Arthritis patient education: Efficacy, implementation, and financing. Arthritis Rheum. 32:1330, 1989.
42. Mullen, P. D., Laville, E. A., Biddle, A. K., and Lorig, K.: Efficacy of psycho-educational interventions on pain, depression, and disability with arthritic adults: A meta-analysis. J. Rheumatol. 15:33, 1987.
43. Mazzuca, S. A.: Does patient education in chronic disease have therapeutic value? J. Chronic Dis. 35:521, 1982.
44. Lorig, K., Konkol, L., and Gonzalez, V.: Arthritis patient education: A review of the literature. Patient Educ. Counsel. 10:207, 1987.
45. Potts, M., and Brandt, K. D.: Analysis of education-support groups for patients with rheumatoid arthritis. Patient Counsel. Health Educ. 4:161, 1983.
46. Parker, J. C., Singsen, B. H., Hewett, J. E., Walker, S. E., Hazelwood,

S. E., Hall, P. J., Holstein, D. J., and Rodon, C. M.: Educating patients with rheumatoid arthritis: A prospective analysis. Arch. Phys. Med. Rehabil. 65:771, 1984.

47. Kaye, R. L., and Hammond, A. H.: Understanding rheumatoid arthritis: Evaluation of a patient education program. J.A.M.A. 239:2466, 1978.

48. Lorig, K., Lubeck, D., Kraines, R. G., Seleznick, M., and Holman, H. R.: Outcomes of self-help education for patients with arthritis. Arthritis Rheum. 28:680, 1985.

49. Lorig, K., Seleznick, M., Lubeck, D., Ung, E., Chastain, R. L., and Holman, H. R.: The beneficial outcomes of the arthritis self-management course are not adequately explained by behavior change. Arthritis Rheum. 32:91, 1989.

50. Cohen, J. L., Sauter, S., DeVellis, R. F., and DeVellis, B. M.: Evaluation of arthritis self-management courses led by lay persons and by professionals. Arthritis Rheum. 29:388, 1986.

51. Bradley, L. A., Young, L. D., Anderson, K. O., McDaniel, L. K., Pisko, E. J., Samble, E. L., and Morgan, T. M.: Effects of psychological therapy on pain behavior of rheumatoid arthritis patients: Treatment outcomes and six-month follow-up. Arthritis Rheum. 30:1105, 1987.

52. Parker, J. C., Frank, R. G., Beck, N. C., Smarr, K. L., Buescher, K. L., Phillips, L. R., Smith, E. I., Anderson, S. K., and Walker, S. E.: Pain management in rheumatoid arthritis patients: A cognitive-behavioral approach. Arthritis Rheum. 31:593, 1988.

53. Goeppinger, J., Arthur, M. W., Baglioni, A. J., Jr., Brunk, S. E., and Brunner, C. M.: A reexamination of the effectiveness of self-care education for persons with arthritis. Arthritis Rheum. 32:706, 1989.

54. Henkle, C.: Social groupwork as a treatment modality for hospitalized people with rheumatoid arthritis. Rehabil. Liter. 36:334, 1975.

55. Shearn, M. A., and Fireman, B. H.: Stress management and mutual support group in rheumatoid arthritis. Am. J. Med. 78:771, 1985.

56. Schwartz, J. H., Marcus, R., and Gordon, R.: Multidisciplinary group therapy for rheumatoid arthritis. Psychosomatics 19:289, 1978.

57. Strauss, G. D., Spiegel, J. S., Daniels, M., Spiegel, T., Landsverk, J., Roy-Byrne, P., Edelstein, C., Ehlhardt, J., Falke, R., Hinden, L., and Zackler, L.: Group therapies for rheumatoid arthritis: A controlled study of two approaches. Arthritis Rheum. 29:1203, 1986.

58. Kaplan, S., and Kozin, F.: A controlled study of group counselling in rheumatoid arthritis. J. Rheumatol. 8:91, 1981.

59. Gross, M., and Brandt, K. D.: Educational support groups for patients with ankylosing spondylitis: A preliminary report. Patient Counsel. Health Educ. 3:6, 1981.

Diagnostic Tests and Procedures in Rheumatic Diseases

Chapter 35

Duncan S. Owen, Jr.

Aspiration and Injection of Joints and Soft Tissues

INTRODUCTION

Synovial fluid analysis is an important diagnostic procedure and is thoroughly covered in Chapter 36. The purpose of this chapter is to discuss the soft tissue and intra-articular injections of glucocorticoids and their benefits and contraindications. The techniques of injections are extensively covered, and illustrations of many joints are presented. For rapid review, if needed, the illustration legends include brief descriptions of techniques.

An interesting survey was conducted by the Mayo Clinic in 1990. It was directed to former medical residents in their internal medicine program. The study revealed that 65 percent of general internists trained at Mayo Clinic after 1970 perform arthrocenteses; however, 64 percent responded that they needed more training in these procedures.[1] Therefore, it is hoped this chapter will be helpful not only to rheumatologists and orthopedists but to all physicians who perform or are interested in learning diagnostic and therapeutic injections of the musculoskeletal system.

Shortly after systemic cortisone and hydrocortisone were first used in the management of rheumatoid arthritis, Thorn injected 10 mg of hydrocortisone into the knee joint of a patient with rheumatoid arthritis.[2] The knee improved locally, but the patient also improved generally; it was concluded that the improvement resulted from systemic absorption of the intra-articularly injected material. No further studies of intra-articular glucocorticoid injections were done until the early 1950s.[3, 4] Ten years later, a series of more than 100,000 injections of joints, bursae, or tendon sheaths in 4000 patients was reported

by Hollander et al.[5] They called attention to the usefulness of intra-articular glucocorticoids as temporary, palliative, repeatable, local adjunctive treatments for a variety of rheumatic conditions[6] and to the more prolonged benefits afforded by preparations less rapidly hydrolyzed than hydrocortisone.

MECHANISM(S) OF ACTION OF INTRA-ARTICULAR GLUCOCORTICOIDS

The anti-inflammatory mechanisms of systemically administered glucocorticoids are still not fully understood. There is less known about the mechanisms of intra-articular glucocorticoids. Also, the mechanisms of action of systemic glucocorticoids (discussed in Chapter 48) may not be analogous to those administered intra-articularly. Early studies after intra-articular glucocorticoid administration demonstrated a decrease in erythema, swelling, heat, and tenderness of the inflamed joints.[4] An increase in viscosity and hyaluronate concentration of the synovial fluid was observed.[7]

One study of intra-articular glucocorticoids demonstrated a transient decrease in synovial fluid complement.[8] In another study, 12 patients received intra-articular methylprednisolone. Six patients showed no alteration of synovial fluid total hemolytic complement, C4 protein level, or rheumatoid factor titer. The other six showed a 50 percent or greater change in only one of the synovial fluid values. Most had reductions in total leukocyte counts, polymorphonuclear leukocyte counts, and acid phosphatase levels.[9]

Dick et al. in 1970[10] reported the results of studies

using intra-articular radioactive xenon (^{133}Xe). They demonstrated a fall in the rate of disappearance of ^{133}Xe after an intra-articular injection of hydrocortisone hemisuccinate. They believed that glucocorticoids diminish synovial permeability. In 1979, a study from this same laboratory of patients with rheumatoid arthritis,[11] using intra-articular ^{133}Xe and triamcinolone hexacetonide in one group and ^{133}Xe and lidocaine in a second group, revealed no difference in the rate of clearance of ^{133}Xe after 40 minutes in the triamcinolone-treated group. Therefore, these investigators believed that triamcinolone had no immediate effect on synovial blood vessels. However, the lidocaine-treated group showed a decrease in the rate of ^{133}Xe clearance.

Eymontt et al. in 1982[12] reported the effects of intra-articular triamcinolone hexacetonide, prednisolone tebutate, and a saline administration on both synovial permeability and synovial fluid leukocyte counts in patients with symptomatic osteoarthritis. In their study they employed a radioactive blood-pool tracer, ^{99m}Tc human serum albumin. Their results indicated that glucocorticoids decrease synovial permeability but produce an increase in synovial fluid leukocytes.

POTENTIAL SEQUELAE

This section discusses the potential sequelae of intra-articular and soft tissue glucocorticoid injections, which are summarized in Table 35–1.

In the late 1950s, a few reports of Charcot-like arthropathy attributed to intra-articular glucocorticoid therapy first appeared.[13, 14] One study by Mankin and Conger in 1966[15] reported that intra-articularly administered hydrocortisone acetate reduced the incorporation of glycine-^{3}H into rabbit articular cartilage to approximately one third of control values within 6 hours. They interpreted the decrease in utilization to a decrease in matrix protein synthesis caused by hydrocortisone.

In 1969, Bentley and Goodfellow[16] advised strongly against recurrent intra-articular injections because of potential severe arthropathy. In 1970,

Table 35–1. POTENTIAL SEQUELAE FROM INTRA-ARTICULAR AND SOFT TISSUE GLUCOCORTICOID INJECTIONS

Radiologic deterioration of joints: "steroid arthropathy"; Charcot-like arthropathy; osteonecrosis—low incidence
Iatrogenic infection—very low incidence
Tendon rupture
Tissue atrophy, fat necrosis, calcification
Nerve damage, e.g., inadvertent injection of median nerve in carpal tunnel syndrome
"Postinjection flare"
Uterine bleeding
Pancreatitis—rare
Erythema, warmth, diaphoresis of face and torso
Posterior subcapsular cataracts

Moskowitz et al.[17] showed that intra-articular triamcinolone acetonide produced nuclear degeneration of chondrocytes and prominent cyst formation. In 1972, Mankin et al.[18] reported that intramuscular cortisone reduced the incorporation of glycine-^{3}H and ^{35}SO$_4$ and was associated with a progressive decline in the concentration of hexosamine. In 1975, Behrens et al.[19] found an increased number of fissures in rabbit cartilage after intra-articular injections of hydrocortisone. Hexosamine incorporation decreased, as did synthesis of proteoglycans; collagen production was reduced to one fifth. They hypothesized that the antianabolic effects of the glucocorticoids cause a massive decrease in the synthesis of all major matrix components. The loss of proteoglycan content led to a decrease in cartilage stiffness such that the impact of cyclic loading with weight-bearing caused death of cells, cystic degeneration of matrix, and fissuring in the midzonal areas of weight-bearing surfaces.

Completely different data were reported in 1976 by Gibson et al.[20] They repeatedly injected the knee joints of ten *Macaca irus* monkeys with either methylprednisolone or a control solution. Minor degenerative changes of femoral condyles were shown by India ink staining and by a system of histochemical grading, but changes in the joints injected with glucocorticoids were *not* significantly different from those seen in control joints. Additionally, in 1985, Williams and Brandt[21] reported that triamcinolone hexacetonide protects against fibrillation and osteophyte formation following chemically induced articular cartilage damage. Protective effects were reported in 1989 on cartilage lesions and osteophyte formation in the Pond-Nuki dog model of osteoarthritis by Pelletier and Martel-Pelletier.[22]

In 1981, Tenenbaum et al.[23] reported on continuing study of the long-term effects of intra-articular dexamethasone TBA on rabbit knee cartilage. There was an acceleration of the calcific degenerative arthropathy that occurs in mature New Zealand rabbits. Under these experimental conditions, the cartilage injury seemed limited and did not progress with repeated injections.

The concept of "glucocorticoid arthropathy" is based largely on subprimate animal studies and anecdotal case reports. Studies of primate models have shown no long-term adverse effect on cartilage.[24] Gray et al.[25] reported a case of a 51-year-old woman who received 100 glucocorticoid injections into each knee over a span of 10 years, with no deleterious effects being noted on knee radiographs taken before and after these treatments.

In 1969, Sweetnam[26] cautioned against steroid injection of inflamed tendons in athletes because of the possibility of tendon rupture. In 1954, Wrenn et al.[27] demonstrated a 40 percent reduction in tensile strength of a tendon after the use of glucocorticoids. (We have rarely observed a rupture of the long head of the biceps tendon or Achilles tendon following the injection of the tendon sheath for tendinitis.) Other complications include soft tissue atrophy, especially noted when the small joints, such as finger proximal interphalangeal joints, are injected. Periarticular calcifications and ecchymoses around the atrophied areas have been reported.[26, 28] The locations of the calcification seemed to be related to the site of needle perforation.[29]

The intra-articular injection of corticosteroids occasionally produces what has been called a *postinjection flare*.[30] This increase in local inflammation may develop a few hours after injection and last up to 48 hours. The difficulty of distinguishing this reaction from an iatrogenic infection may be worrisome. The flare is noted more frequently with the needle-shaped glucocorticoid crystals and may be a form of crystal-induced arthritis produced by synovial fluid leukocytes phagocytosing the crystals and subsequently releasing lysosomal enzymes and other mediators of inflammation. These flares, however, may be caused by preservatives in the suspension.

Systemic absorption of intra-articular glucocorticoids or absorption from other soft tissue injections occurs in almost all patients. Usually, this is clinically manifested, e.g., in a patient with rheumatoid arthritis, by subjective and objective improvement of inflamed joints other than the one(s) injected. There may be other effects, such as eosinopenia, lymphopenia, and, depending on the glucocorticoid injected, changes in serum and urine cortisol levels. There may be suppression of the hypothalamic-pituitary-adrenal axis.[31, 32] Patients with diabetes mellitus may note a short-lived severalfold rise in their blood glucose levels.

Prominent erythema, warmth, and diaphoresis of the face and torso may occur within minutes to hours after an intra-articular glucocorticoid injection.[33] It is noted mainly with triamcinolone acetonide. Some believe that it is an uncommon reaction, but we note it in greater than 10 percent of patients injected with this medication. Some of these patients note headache. In this regard, it resembles the nitritoid reaction occasionally observed with the injection of gold salts, especially gold sodium thiomalate. These glucocorticoid reactions may last a few minutes to a few days. However, some patients are so frightened by these reactions that they refuse further injections. Local skin eruptions have been reported.[34]

Abnormal uterine bleeding may occur from injection of glucocorticoids, especially triamcinolone acetonide. The exact mechanisms are unknown, but ovulation may be inhibited.[35, 36] Also, glucocorticoids may produce uterine bleeding in a postmenopausal patient. This alarms both patient and physician.

Pancreatitis, apparently induced by injectable glucocorticoids, is rarely noted.

Cushing's syndrome is rare, but Gray et al.[25] have observed posterior subcapsular cataracts in a number of middle-aged patients receiving frequent intra-articular glucocorticoid injections. We concur with these observations.

An interesting side effect of intra-articular glucocorticoids is the transient fall in serum salicylate levels in patients with rheumatoid arthritis. This probably is related to an increase in glomerular filtration rate.[37]

PRECAUTIONS

Strict adherence to aseptic procedures is required when performing arthrocenteses or soft tissue injections. The physician should use the same precautions as for a lumbar spinal puncture. Iatrogenic infections may be disastrous but are rare if these precautions are taken. At the Medical College of Virginia we have observed one, or possibly two, infections in more than 65,000 injections.

In theory, arthrocentesis may provide a focus for septic arthritis in a patient with bacteremia, such as staphylococcal endocarditis.[38] It is well known that a patient with damaged joints from, for example, rheumatoid arthritis is more susceptible to developing spontaneous septic arthritis from blood-borne bacteria. Arthrocentesis in such instances has enabled rapid diagnosis and prevented the patient's joint from being destroyed. "Routine" therapeutic arthrocenteses should be avoided, however, if the patient is being treated for a condition associated with bacteremia.

Because of tissue atrophy with glucocorticoids, one should use extreme caution when injecting near peripheral nerves. For example, carpal tunnel syndrome, either idiopathic or rheumatoid arthritis induced, may be benefited by glucocorticoid injection in the carpal tunnel. An injection directly into the median nerve could result in nerve necrosis or atrophy.

Gottlieb[39] reported two cases of hypodermic needle separations during arthrocentesis. He recommended that the needles be inspected after arthrocentesis to ascertain that they are intact, and he advised keeping a hemostat within easy access to enable the operator to remove a separated needle from the soft tissues.

EFFICACY OF INJECTIONS

Intra-articular Injections

Despite the fact that thousands of intra-articular glucocorticoid preparations have been injected in thousands of patients, there are few good studies of their efficacy.[40] The length of symptomatic improvement appears to be related to the particular preparation used. Most patients with rheumatoid arthritis will benefit from an injection, but the effect may last for only days. Hydrocortisone acetate may give improvement for a few days to a week or more and prednisolone tebutate for 2 weeks or more. Triamcinolone hexacetonide, which is poorly water soluble and one of the longest-acting agents, has been shown to provide reversal of inflammation in some patients for longer periods.[28] As with oral nonsteroidal anti-inflammatory drugs, responses among patients are extremely varied. If one or two injections prove ineffective or give only short-lived benefit, there is no logic in persistently injecting the same joint.

Results of injections in osteoarthritic joints conflict. The data range from outstanding benefit to no benefit.[2, 41-47] The differences may relate, in part, to the joint injected. For example, degenerative arthritis of the first carpometacarpal joint is a fairly common and painful condition in which there is little synovial thickening or increase in synovial fluid. The injection of glucocorticoid is often painful, probably because of the moderate or marked decrease in joint space, but dramatic symptomatic improvement usually occurs within 12 hours and may last many months. This contrasts with injection for osteoarthritis of the hip, in which it is difficult to know if the hip joint space has been entered even with use of the fluoroscope as a guide. Improvement of hip symptoms within 12 to 24 hours after injection probably indicates that the glucocorticoid was injected intra-articularly, but benefit often lasts only 2 days to a week. The mechanical problem of bone rubbing against bone in a weight-bearing joint may be the reason for the short-lived benefit, and repeated injections may be expected to have little efficacy.

Osteoarthritis of the knee may be extremely painful and associated with large volumes of synovial fluid. Even though it is the usual practice to remove as much synovial fluid as possible, the efficacy of this procedure in osteoarthritis is questionable. The glucocorticoid injection usually is associated with dramatic symptomatic relief that lasts days to weeks or more. If the injections give short-lived benefit, repeated injections are probably contraindicated because the primary problem is in the cartilage, and repeated injections could hasten cartilage deterioration for reasons previously outlined.

A weight-bearing joint probably should be rested as much as possible for 48 to 72 hours after injection. Neustadt[48] recommends the use of crutches or a cane for another 3 weeks. Others advise resting all glucocorticoid-injected joints for a longer period.[49] There is no consensus, however.

Nonarticular Injections

In contrast to the situation with intra-articular injections, which are used adjunctively, certain soft tissue inflammatory conditions may be more or less permanently eradicated by judicious injections of glucocorticoids with or without local anesthetics.[50-53] The conditions having the longest benefit from injections are those precipitated by trauma, especially when the activity causing the inflammation is avoided. For example, a patient troubled by recurrent lateral epicondylitis who derives short-lived benefit from a glucocorticoid injection into the inflamed area may improve more permanently by discontinuing the precipitating physical activity, e.g., tennis or racquetball.

Many cases of apparent tendinitis and bursitis may be secondary manifestations of rheumatoid arthritis, in which injections may give outstanding initial benefit that, unfortunately, is temporary. In such patients, appropriate treatment of the underlying disease should be instituted, and the injections must be considered as adjunctive management.

The poorly understood but apparently quite common fibromyalgia syndrome[54, 55] is associated with various "tender points" and is discussed in detail in Chapter 29. These exaggerated tender areas may respond dramatically to the injection of a local anesthetic directly into the most tender area, but the addition of a glucocorticoid in the same syringe may give more lasting relief.

TYPES OF PREPARATIONS

The original intra-articular glucocorticoid, hydrocortisone acetate, is still available, widely used, and inexpensive. Other preparations of various potency and solubility are now available (Table 35-2). Few comparative studies of the efficacy or duration of action of the various agents have been reported. As previously mentioned, McCarty[28] has noted long-term benefits with triamcinolone hexacetonide and thinks this is the least soluble and produces the most prolonged effect of the agents commercially available. Such "longer-acting and more potent" suspensions are much more expensive than hydrocortisone. Some investigators have the opinion that the more potent preparations are also more efficacious,[40] but the evidence for this is only moderate.

Many clinicians, over months or years of practice, have settled on a preparation that seems to have, in their opinion, good benefit and few side effects. Some prefer, for example, a preparation of a "short-acting" solution and a "long-acting" suspension of betamethasone (Celestone Soluspan). They believe the solution works rapidly and prevents the

Table 35–2. GLUCOCORTICOIDS AND PREDNISONE EQUIVALENTS*

Intra-articular Preparations†	Prednisone Equivalents
Betamethasone sodium phosphate and acetate suspension 6 mg/ml (Celestone Soluspan)	10
Dexamethasone sodium phosphate 4 mg/ml (Decadron and Hexadrol)	8
Dexamethasone acetate 8 mg/ml (Decadron-LA)	16
Hydrocortisone acetate 25 mg/ml (Hydrocortone)	1
Methylprednisolone acetate 20, 40, and 80 mg/ml (Depo-Medrol)	5, 10, and 20
Prednisolone tebutate 20 mg/ml (Hydeltra-TBA)	4
Triamcinolone acetonide 10 and 40 mg/ml (Kenalog-10 and Kenalog-40)	2.5 and 10
Triamcinolone hexacetonide 20 mg/ml (Aristospan)	5

*One equivalent = 5 mg prednisone.
†Generic drug name is followed by trade name in parentheses.

possibility of a postinjection flare. For the same reason, others prefer to inject a "short-acting" solution, such as dexamethasone sodium phosphate, together with a more "long-acting" suspension.

Mixing the glucocorticoid suspension with a local anesthetic, particularly procaine or lidocaine, may be helpful when injecting small joints and tendon sheaths; this avoids the injection of a very concentrated suspension in a single area, which could produce soft tissue atrophy. (Some clinicians prefer to inject the glucocorticoid first. Then, with the needle in the joint, they remove the syringe and inject the local anesthetic. This technique may prevent pericapsular calcifications in small joints.) However, one must be concerned over the compatibility of the two preparations. In the Lederle section of the 1990 *Physicians' Desk Reference*, the following is written: "Aristospan suspension may be mixed with 1 percent or 2 percent lidocaine hydrochloride, using the formulations which do not contain parabens. Similar local anesthetics may also be used. Diluents containing methylparaben, propylparaben, phenol, etc., should be avoided since these compounds may cause flocculation of the steroid."[55a] A review of package inserts of intra-articular glucocorticoids from the larger pharmaceutical companies revealed that most do not recommend the use of a mixture of glucocorticoids and local anesthetics containing preservatives. Some manufacturers are less specific. In addition, we have observed flocculation with certain generic brands but not with the trade name product.

Local anesthetics usually contain preservatives. Ones without them are usually more expensive and are usually not available on the average arthrocentesis tray. Lidocaine for intravenous use does not contain preservatives. A brief survey of several rheumatologists and orthopedic surgeons throughout the country revealed that approximately one half used a glucocorticoid–local anesthetic mixture, and only one was aware of the potential problem of flocculation. A few orthopedists, however, reported finding "steroid chalk" in joints, especially wrists, that had been injected with the "older steroids." There is no way of knowing if these joints had been injected with glucocorticoid–local anesthetic combinations. Also, we wonder if the chalk might represent formations of hydroxyapatite, apparently from injections of only glucocorticoids.

There is no consensus concerning the amount of material that should be injected into the various sizes of joints. Some clinicians tend to inject a smaller amount in volume of the "more potent" glucocorticoids, but many, probably the majority, tend to inject 1 ml in the large joints and a lesser amount in the medium and small joints. Table 35–3 is a rough guide to the amount to be injected.

INDICATIONS

Intra-articular or soft tissue glucocorticoid injections, or both, are considered adjunctive therapy.

Table 35–3. AMOUNT OF INTRA-ARTICULAR GLUCOCORTICOID TO BE INJECTED

Size of Joint	Examples	Range of Dosage (ml)
Large	Knees	1–2
	Ankles	
	Shoulders	
Medium	Elbows	0.5–1
	Wrists	
Small	Interphalangeal	0.1–0.5
	Metacarpophalangeal	

Rarely are they considered primary therapy. Exceptions, as previously noted, include bursitis, tendinitis, or documented gout in a single joint. Table 35–4 lists the indications for intra-articular glucocorticoid injections. This therapeutic list is not in any particular order of preference or likelihood of response. The intra-articular injections of experimental drugs, including radioisotopes, are not discussed in this chapter.

Articular

Rheumatoid Arthritis, Adult and Juvenile. Rheumatoid arthritis (with the possible exception of tendinitis and bursitis) is probably the illness for which the most injections are given by rheumatologists. The efficacy of such injections is controversial, for reasons previously discussed. If systemic regimens were uniformly efficacious in patients with rheumatoid arthritis, there would be no need to inject glucocorticoids in the joints. Because this is not the case, the judicious use of intra-articular glucocorticoids may enable the patients to lead a more productive life and one of better quality. Most rheumatologists are quite enthusiastic about the injections.[56, 57] Injections may be indicated especially when the patient has failed to respond or when there are contraindications to nonsteroidal anti-inflammatory drugs, hydroxychloroquine, gold salts, or other systemic agents. The injections usually will enable the patient to participate more fully in physical ther-

Table 35–4. INDICATIONS FOR INTRA-ARTICULAR GLUCOCORTICOID INJECTIONS

Rheumatoid arthritis (adult and juvenile)
Crystal deposition disease (gout and pseudogout)
Systemic lupus erythematosus and mixed connective tissue disease
Acute traumatic "arthritis"
Osteoarthritis
Synovitis of ipsilateral knee following total hip arthroplasty
Miscellaneous conditions with joint manifestations: inflammatory bowel disease, ankylosing spondylitis, psoriatic arthritis, Reiter's disease (injections probably should be avoided in cases of Reiter's disease associated with HIV infections)
Shoulder periarthritis (adhesive capsulitis, frozen shoulder)
Tietze's syndrome

apeutic procedures. The number of injections on a single day should be limited to two, but other joints may be injected on other days. There are no data as to how often the same joint may be safely reinjected. Not more than three times a year seems prudent.

In children with rheumatoid arthritis, the number of systemic drugs that can be administered is limited. The judicious use of intra-articular glucocorticoids may prove quite helpful. This is especially true when only a few joints are involved, e.g., in the pauci (oligo)-articular type.[57a]

Crystal Deposition Diseases (Gout and Pseudogout). Acute gouty arthritis (monosodium urate monohydrate crystal deposition disease) occasionally is refractory to so-called conventional regimens, i.e., colchicine and nonsteroidal anti-inflammatory drugs. If this is the case, and if phagocytosed sodium urate crystals continue to be present in the synovial fluid, complete aspiration of the inflamed joint followed by glucocorticoid injection may be helpful. One has to be certain that an infectious process is not the reason for the persistent inflammation.

The diagnosis of pseudogout (calcium pyrophosphate dihydrate crystal deposition disease) requires the identification of calcium pyrophosphate crystals in synovial fluid. Aspirating as much fluid as possible may alleviate not only pain but also inflammation. That is, aspiration may remove a sufficient number of crystals to reduce the inflammatory process. On occasion, however, the inflammation does not respond to this or the usual nonsteroidal anti-inflammatory drugs, and intra-articular glucocorticoids prove efficacious. In older patients, especially those with even mild renal insufficiency, serious sequelae from colchicine and nonsteroidal anti-inflammatory drugs may occur. For example, nonsteroidal anti-inflammatory drugs may produce worsening renal failure, hypertension, and congestive heart failure.[58] Colchicine is an especially dangerous drug in these circumstances and may produce bone marrow abnormalities, septicemia, and death.[59] The use of intra-articular glucocorticoids seems to be a much safer regimen.

Systemic Lupus Erythematosus and Mixed Connective Tissue Disease. These diseases may be associated with polyarticular or pauciarticular synovitis that persists despite good control of the systemic disorder. Intra-articular glucocorticoids may be quite helpful.

Acute Traumatic "Arthritis." Acute trauma to joints is usually treated with a conservative regimen of cold packs, rest, and, after an appropriate time, an increase in activity. Many believe that injuries to the soft tissue of the shoulder and ankle will cause serious sequelae if range of motion exercise is not instituted after a short period of rest. Intra-articular glucocorticoids may help in these situations by allowing early movement.

Osteoarthritis. Osteoarthritic joints, as previously discussed, can be extremely painful. The efficacy of intra-articular glucocorticoids is debated; on occasion, however, injections give outstanding and prolonged benefit. This is especially true if inflammation is present and there is little cartilage loss. If one or two injections do not give benefit, there is no good reason to keep injecting the joint.

Synovitis of Knee After Hip Arthroplasty. Synovitis of the ipsilateral knee after total hip arthroplasty is noted occasionally and may resolve spontaneously after a few days. It may persist, however, and injection of the knee with a glucocorticoid usually is quite beneficial.

Miscellaneous. Inflammatory gastrointestinal diseases may be associated with peripheral or axial arthritis, or both. Sometimes, depending on the type of intestinal disorder, an exacerbation of the intestinal problem is associated with an exacerbation of the joint symptoms. In certain situations, control of the intestinal disease also controls the joint disease. If the arthropathy is not helped, however, injections of intra-articular glucocorticoids may give rapid and prolonged relief.

Peripheral joint manifestations of other inflammatory arthritides, such as ankylosing spondylitis, psoriatic arthritis, and Reiter's disease, may also be benefited by intra-articular glucocorticoids. If the patient with Reiter's disease has a human immunodeficiency virus (HIV) infection, intra-articular glucocorticoid injections are probably contraindicated.

Shoulder Periarthritis (Adhesive Capsulitis, Frozen Shoulder). This condition may improve, sometimes dramatically, with intra-articular and tendinous sheath glucocorticoid injections.[60-64] Many clinicians, however, combine the treatment with nonsteroidal anti-inflammatory drugs and physical therapy.

Tietze's Syndrome. Tietze's syndrome, an "illness" associated with pain and tenderness of the parasternal joints, may be helped by injections of a combination of glucocorticoid and local anesthetic.[65]

Nonarticular

Nonarticular inflammatory conditions may be greatly benefited by the injection of a glucocorticoid with or without a local anesthetic. Table 35–5 lists various soft tissue conditions that may benefit from injections.

Shoulder. The main shoulder problems are bicipital tendinitis, subacromial bursitis, and supraspinatus tendinitis. As previously mentioned, these problems can be primary or part of a systemic problem, e.g., rheumatoid arthritis. Injection of the specifically inflamed tendon sheath or bursa usually gives relief within a few hours. However, when glucocorticoids are mixed with a local anesthetic, relief is usually immediate if the physician injected the correct area.

The possible sequelae of intratendinous injections have previously been mentioned. If the inflammatory problems involve the bicipital tendon or sub-

Table 35–5. INDICATIONS FOR NONARTICULAR GLUCOCORTICOID INJECTIONS

Shoulder
  Bicipital tendinitis
  Subacromial bursitis
  Supraspinatus tendinitis
  Periarthritis (adhesive capsulitis, frozen shoulder)
Elbow
  Lateral epicondylitis ("tennis elbow")
  Medial epicondylitis ("golfer's elbow")
  Olecranon bursitis
  Cubital tunnel syndrome
Wrist and Hand
  Ganglion
  DeQuervain's disease (stenosing tenosynovitis of extensor
    pollicis brevis and abductor pollicis longus)
  Trigger (snapping) fingers
  Carpal tunnel syndrome
Hip
  Trochanteric bursitis
Knee
  Anserine bursitis
  Prepatellar bursitis
Pelvis
  Ischial bursitis
  Iliopectineal bursitis
Back
  "Fibromyalgia" trigger points
  Herniated presacral fat pads (Stockman's nodules)
Foot
  Achilles tendinitis
  Achilles bursitis
  Calcaneal bursitis
  Morton's neuroma
  Tarsal tunnel syndrome

acromial bursa, some physicians prefer to inject the shoulder joint directly. This seems especially true in patients with rheumatoid arthritis because arthrographic studies in these patients have frequently shown a communication between the subacromial bursa, the bicipital tendon sheath, and the shoulder joint. Thus, the drug can have a local effect in all these areas. Shoulder periarthritis is discussed earlier.

Elbow. Inflammation of the elbow epicondylar areas is frequently noted in patients who are active in sports, especially tennis and golf. Lateral epicondylitis is frequently a sequela of these activities and can be quite painful. Injecting the inflamed region can give good to excellent results. Some clinicians prefer a more conservative approach.[66] Mixing the glucocorticoid with local anesthetic can give immediate benefit; however, when the effect of the anesthetic subsides, there is frequently a marked exacerbation of pain lasting 6 to 24 hours, which apparently is a crystal-induced postinjection flare. Medial epicondylitis also can be extremely painful and usually responds well to an injection. However, one should be careful not to inject the nearby ulnar nerve.

Olecranon bursitis may be a primary condition, probably from trauma, but may be secondary to conditions such as gout, infection, and rheumatoid arthritis. Because septic olecranon bursitis is common, aspiration of the fluid and synovial fluid analysis are essential before glucocorticoids are injected. Cubital tunnel syndrome, an entrapment of the ulnar nerve at the elbow, may be caused by tenosynovitis. The symptoms are usually more motor related than sensory. Injections can be administered by experienced operators; however, surgical decompression is usually necessary.[67]

Wrist and Hand. A ganglion on the dorsal aspect of the wrist can be treated by aspiration and injection. Again, there may be considerable discomfort several hours after injection. Between two thirds and three fourths of patients have their ganglia "cured" by this conservative approach.[30, 68]

Stenosing tenosynovitis of the extensor pollicis brevis and abductor pollicis longus (de Quervain's disease) may cause considerable discomfort over the distal aspect of the radius. Conservative management with glucocorticoid and local anesthetic injection may be quite helpful.[53, 69, 69a] If immediate benefit is noted, this usually indicates that the injection was in the proper area. Recurrence is common, according to some operators, but Harvey et al.[70] report complete and lasting relief in 40 percent of cases.

Trigger and snapping fingers may be caused by a primary nonspecific hand flexor tenosynovitis or tenosynovitis with rheumatoid arthritis. The tendinous sheath injection of glucocorticoid and local anesthetic has been shown to be efficacious in more than 90 percent of the cases, and the median length of relief has been 2 years.[51, 71–73] Carpal tunnel syndrome has multiple etiologies, but the rheumatoid and idiopathic types may be helped by glucocorticoid injections. Extreme care is necessary to prevent median nerve damage.[69, 74, 75, 75a] Personal instruction in the technique is recommended.

Hip. Trochanteric bursitis can give considerable discomfort and may be relieved by injections. There are one or more bursae about the femoral trochanter at the gluteal insertion. The tender region is easily palpated unless there is obesity.

Knee. The anserine bursa is present on the medial aspect of the knee, where the tendons of the sartorius, semitendinosus, and gracilis muscles insert on the tibia.[76] When inflamed, there is pain, tenderness, and usually swelling over the medial anterior aspect of the tibia just below the knee. There may be associated degenerative arthritis of the knee, obesity, or a history of physical activity such as jogging, frequent knee bending, or frequent going up and down stairs. Some authors do not consider the condition a true bursitis and classify it as Dercum's disease (painful adiposity) or place it in the "fibrositis syndrome" category.[54] I disagree with this opinion and consider it a commonly misdiagnosed condition. In addition, there are other bursae close by that may become inflamed. Most cases are greatly benefited by injection of glucocorticoid and local anesthetic. If the material is injected in the proper place, immediate relief is usually experienced.

Prepatellar bursitis may be secondary to trauma,

e.g., "housemaid's knee," or could be secondary to systemic illness such as rheumatoid arthritis or gout. It may be asymptomatic or quite painful. Some patients request treatment for cosmetic reasons. If clinically indicated, the bursal fluid can be examined in a similar manner to synovial fluid. Injections are usually effective.[74]

Pelvis. Ischial or ischiogluteal bursitis may be more common than is generally thought and may be misdiagnosed as herniated nucleus pulposus, lumbosacral strain, or thrombophlebitis.[77] The ischiogluteal bursa overlies the sciatic nerve and the posterior femoral cutaneous nerve. Therefore, the pain may radiate and the wrong diagnosis be made. Palpation over the ischial tuberosity should cause significant pain. Injections are helpful but are not recommended for the inexperienced operator.

Iliopectineal (iliopsoas) bursitis is an inflammation of the bursa that is located between the iliopsoas muscle and the iliopectineal eminence. It may communicate with the hip joint. There is tenderness over the anterior aspect of the hip in the region of the middle portion of the inguinal ligament. Hyperextension, adduction, or internal rotation of the hip elicits pain. Differential diagnoses include femoral hernia, psoas abscess, and septic arthritis of the hip. When these other diagnoses have been excluded, and if more conservative regimens have failed or are not practical, an injection of glucocorticoid with or without local anesthetic can be tried.[78]

Back. Painful subjective and objective areas of the back that may be difficult to explain anatomically may be noted. Areas tender to moderately deep palpation, the so-called tender points, may be noted, especially around the upper medial border of the trapezius, various periscapular areas, inferior posterior cervical area, and presacral regions. The latter may represent herniated presacral fat pads (Stockman's nodules). Some of these painful areas may be part of the fibrositis syndrome.[54] An injection of glucocorticoid, local anesthetic, or a combination of the two, into the tender points frequently gives relief.

Foot. Achilles tendinitis may be secondary to trauma or to systemic illness such as rheumatoid arthritis or gout. The former may be associated with rheumatoid nodules in the tendon and the latter with tophi. Rest, analgesics, and anti-inflammatory medications are preferable to injections. If little benefit is obtained from these conservative measures, a small amount of a mixture of glucocorticoid and local anesthetic in the tendon sheath may be injected.

Achilles bursitis may represent inflammation of the retrocalcaneal bursa between the calcaneus and Achilles tendon or a subcutaneous bursitis between the skin and tendon. One should not forget the possibility of gout being the cause, and if the bursae are punctured, an attempt at aspiration is a good idea. The contents should then be examined. Reiter's syndrome should be suspected when inflammatory fluid is aspirated from the retrocalcaneal bursa, examination for crystals is negative, and there is no other obvious diagnosis.[79] Conservative management of nonspecific bursitis is similar to that of Achilles tendinitis, but if this is ineffective, an injection may prove beneficial.

Calcaneal bursitis is an inflammation of the bursa at the attachment of the plantar fascia to the os calcis. Pain is present in the center of the plantar aspect of the heel. Conservative management, such as a rubber doughnut, may help. If not, an intrabursal injection of glucocorticoid mixed with local anesthetic usually gives good relief, although the injection frequently causes considerable pain.

Tarsal tunnel syndrome is an entrapment neuropathy of all or part of the posterior tibial nerve as it passes under the flexor retinaculum of the ankle. Burning pain and paresthesias in the affected foot are the symptoms. It may be associated with the hypermobile joint syndrome.[80] Injections by an experienced operator may help, but relief is usually temporary.[81]

An excellent review on the syndromes of bursitis was written by Larsson and Baum.[82] They believe that glucocorticoids with local anesthetic injection are the most successful treatment.

The metatarsalgia from Morton's neuroma may be greatly relieved by the direct injection of a combination of glucocorticoid–local anesthetic mixture.[83]

CONTRAINDICATIONS TO INTRA-ARTICULAR GLUCOCORTICOID INJECTIONS

The main contraindications to intra-articular glucocorticoid injections are listed in Table 35–6. As previously stated, even though they are rare, iatrogenic infections occur. Therefore, it is essential to adhere to strict aseptic procedures, and certainly the physician must avoid inserting a needle through any areas of cellulitis and active psoriasis.

The previously mentioned bacteremia, as would be noted in certain cases of pneumonia, endocarditis, and pyelonephritis, is considered a contraindication by some. Therefore, if a patient hospitalized for a condition that may be associated with bacteremia concomitantly has active rheumatoid arthritis, it is probably wise not to institute therapeutic arthrocenteses and glucocorticoid injections because of the

Table 35–6. CONTRAINDICATIONS TO INTRA-ARTICULAR GLUCOCORTICOID INJECTIONS

Periarticular sepsis
Bacteremia
Unstable joints
Most spinal joints
Intra-articular fracture
Septic joint—do *not* forget possibility of tuberculosis
Difficult access to nondiarthrodial joints, e.g., symphysis pubis (sternomanubrial injections may prove helpful)
Marked juxta-articular osteoporosis
Failure to respond to prior injections
Blood clotting disorders

possibility of an iatrogenic infection. (If one is concerned that bacteremia may have produced septic arthritis, arthrocentesis and special studies on the synovial fluid are mandatory.)

Instability of joints possibly may be part of a Charcot-like arthropathy from multiple intra-articular glucocorticoid injections. Theoretically, further injections could make the instability worse. In general, joints such as spinal are considered inaccessible, and injections are contraindicated because of potential sequelae. However, facet joint arthropathy is believed to be a common cause of low back and cervical spine pain. The injection of these joints by an experienced operator may give long-lasting benefit.[84, 85]

One should keep in mind that articular pain following trauma could represent an intra-articular fracture. Glucocorticoid injection is contraindicated because the healing of a fracture could be retarded.

Injection of a septic joint with a glucocorticoid could greatly increase the morbidity of the infection. Purulent appearance of synovial fluid should alert the physician to this possibility, but tuberculous synovitis, for example, may produce synovial fluid with minimal inflammatory findings, and the physician may thus be misled. The possibility of infection should always be kept in mind, and further studies of synovial fluid and even percutaneous synovial biopsy or arthroscopy with biopsy should be considered.

Nondiarthrodial joints, such as the symphysis pubis, are involved with certain arthritides, but these joints are difficult to inject. If they are accessible, injections occasionally are helpful, but several punctures may be necessary.

Juxta-articular osteoporosis of a marked degree may be worsened by intra-articular glucocorticoid. This type of osteoporosis is more commonly seen in the patient with rheumatoid arthritis, and the arthritis itself plus lack of motion in the joint may be the main cause of the osteoporosis. Therefore, theoretically, one or two glucocorticoid injections may improve the problem. If one or two glucocorticoid injections in the same joint provide no benefit, there is no sound reason to continue, because one could be producing more harm than good.

Blood clotting disorders, such as factor VIII deficiency, may produce a destructive type of arthritis. Arthrocentesis could produce both intra-articular and external hemorrhage. This problem should definitely be considered when undiagnosed synovitis is noted in a child. Arthrocenteses can be performed with caution on patients receiving anticoagulants if the joint is immobilized for 24 to 48 hours after the injection. Applying ice and wrapping the joint with an elastic bandage may be helpful.

Patients with rheumatoid arthritis who have had total joint arthroplasties, especially of the knees, may subsequently have an exacerbation of synovitis in these joints. In the past, because there is an increased incidence of infections in such joints, we have been very reluctant to inject glucocorticoids. However, at the Medical College of Virginia, more than 400 joints with replacements that developed recurrent rheumatoid synovitis have been injected with glucocorticoids with benefit and without sequelae. In these cases, we recommend that synovial fluid analysis, including culture, be performed prior to the injection of glucocorticoids.

ANESTHESIA

As previously discussed, some physicians prefer mixing the glucocorticoid with a local anesthetic, usually procaine or lidocaine, for two reasons. First, when injecting a bursa, tendon sheath, or periarticular region, this combination usually gives immediate relief if the materials are injected in the proper space. This immediate benefit, of course, would be from the local anesthetic, not the glucocorticoid; patients should be told that they may experience further pain in an hour or two but should improve a few hours later, when the anti-inflammatory actions of the glucocorticoids begin. Second, a mixture may be preferable because the glucocorticoid is diluted, and there should be less soft tissue atrophy at the sites of injection.

A physician experienced in arthrocentesis may elect not to use any anesthesia when injecting large joints. If the patient is cooperative and relaxed, and if disposable needles are used, there should be little pain associated with the arthrocenteses. If the physician is inexperienced or the patient anxious and tense, a short burst of ethyl chloride spray on the skin over the joint to be injected is helpful.

The injection of a local anesthetic is the other option. First, a skin wheal should be made followed by infiltration of the subcutaneous tissue and joint capsule. After a few minutes, arthrocentesis can be done and should be painless.

TECHNIQUES

To perform an arthrocentesis, the specific area of the joint to be aspirated is palpated and is then marked with firm pressure by a ballpoint pen that has the inked portion retracted. This will leave an impression that will last 5 to 15 minutes. (The ballpoint pen technique can also be used with soft tissue injection.) Strict asepsis is important and deserves re-emphasis. The area to be aspirated or injected, or both, should be carefully cleansed with a good antiseptic, such as one of the iodinated compounds. Then the needle can be inserted through the ballpoint pen impression. This method does not require the use of rubber gloves. For self-protection, I strongly recommend the operator be immunized against hepatitis B. If there is concern that the patient may have HIV infection, the use of gloves is probably a good idea.

A tray for arthrocentesis can be prepared and

kept available for use. This includes the following items: alcohol sponges; iodinated solution and surgical soap; gauze dressings (2 × 2); sterile disposable 3-, 10-, and 20-ml syringes; 18- and 20-gauge, 1 ½-inch needles; 20-gauge spinal needles; 25-gauge, ⅝-inch needles; plain test tubes; heparinized tubes; clean microscope slides and coverslips; heparin to add to heparinized tubes if a large amount of inflammatory fluid is to be placed in the tube; fingernail polish to seal wet preparation/slide cover slip; chocolate agar plates or Thayer-Martin medium; tryptic soy broth for most bacteria; anaerobic transport medium (replace periodically to keep culture media from becoming outdated); tubes with fluoride for glucose; plastic adhesive bandages; ethyl chloride; hemostat; tourniquet for drawing of simultaneous blood samples; and 1 percent lidocaine.

Articular

Knee. The knee is the easiest joint to inject. If fluid is to be aspirated, the patient should be in a supine position with the knee fully extended. The puncture mark is made just posterior to the medial portion of the patella, and an 18- to 20-gauge, 1 ½-inch needle directed slightly posteriorly and slightly inferiorly. The joint space should be entered readily and synovial fluid easily aspirated. On occasion, thickened synovium or villous projections may occlude the opening of the needle, and it may be necessary to rotate the needle to facilitate aspiration of the knee when using the medial approach. An infrapatellar plica, a vestigial structure that is also called the *ligamentum mucosum,* may prevent adequate aspiration of the knee when the medial approach is used.[86] However, the plica should not adversely affect aspiration from the lateral aspect. If glucocorticoid is administered, one should not have any feeling of obstruction as it is being injected. Parenthetically, a medial synovial shelf plica may become thickened and inflamed. Rovere[87] believes that this diagnosis can be made by physical examination and the plica itself injected, with relief of symptoms. Others disagree. A review of the subject is presented by Schonholtz and Magee.[88]

The supine technique is illustrated in Figure 35–1. The patient should be relaxed if this technique is used. An anxious patient may tighten the patella to the point of making arthrocentesis extremely difficult. If this is the case or if fusion or osteophytes make the medial or lateral approach to the knee joint difficult, an easy technique that usually avoids these problems is to inject the knee while the patient sits with the knee flexed. The mark is made at the medial aspect of the distal border of the patella, and the needle is directed slightly superiorly toward the joint cavity. It is usually difficult to obtain fluid with this technique.

The suprapatellar "bursa" may be distended if a large amount of synovial fluid is present. In this

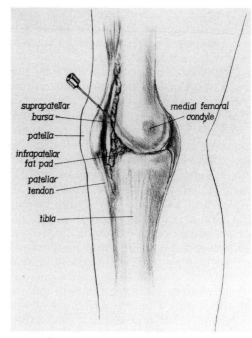

Figure 35–1. Knee arthrocentesis. The needle is inserted just posterior to the medial portion of the patella and is directed slightly posteriorly and slightly inferiorly.

instance, the bursa may be aspirated in an easy and essentially asymptomatic fashion.

Shoulder. The shoulder arthrocentesis is most easily accomplished with the patient sitting and the shoulder externally rotated. A mark is made just medial to the head of the humerus and slightly inferiorly and laterally to the coracoid process. A 20- to 22-gauge, 1 ½-inch needle is directed posteriorly and slightly superiorly and laterally. One should be able to feel the needle enter the joint space. If bone is hit, the operator should pull back and redirect the needle at a slightly different angle. This technique is illustrated in Figure 35–2.

The acromioclavicular joint may be palpated as a groove at the lateral end of the clavicle just medial to the shoulder. A mark is made, and a 22- to 25-gauge, ⅝- to 1-inch needle is carefully directed inferiorly. Rarely is synovial fluid obtained.

The sternoclavicular joint is most easily entered from a point directly anterior to the joint. Caution is necessary to avoid a pneumothorax. The space is fibrocartilaginous, and rarely can fluid be aspirated.

Ankle Joint. The patient should be supine and the leg-foot angle at 90 degrees. A mark is made just medial to the tibialis anterior tendon and lateral to the medial malleolus. A 20- to 22-gauge, 1 ½-inch needle is directed posteriorly and should enter the joint space easily without striking bone. Figure 35–3 illustrates injection of the ankle joint.

Subtalar Ankle Joint. Again the patient is supine and the leg-foot angle at 90 degrees. A mark is made just inferior to the tip of the lateral malleolus. A 20- to 22-gauge, 1 ½-inch needle is directed perpendic-

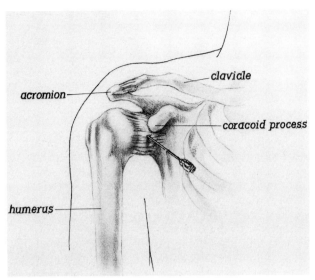

Figure 35–2. Shoulder arthrocentesis. With the shoulder externally rotated, the needle is inserted at a point just medial to the head of the humerus and slightly inferior and lateral to the coracoid process. The needle is then directed posteriorly and slightly superiorly and laterally.

ular to the mark. With this joint the needle may not enter the first time, and another attempt or two may be necessary. Because of this and the associated pain, local anesthesia may be helpful. Figure 35–4 illustrates injection of this joint.

Wrist. This is a complex joint, but fortunately most of the intercarpal spaces communicate. A mark is made just distal to the radius and just ulnar to the so-called anatomic snuff box. Usually a 24- to 26-gauge, ⅝- to 1-inch needle is adequate, and the

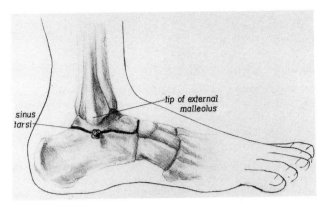

Figure 35–4. Ankle subtalar arthrocentesis. With the leg-foot angle at 90 degrees, the needle is inserted at a point just inferior to the tip of the lateral (external) malleolus, and is directed perpendicularly.

injection is made perpendicular to the mark. If bone is hit, the needle should be pulled back and slightly redirected toward the thumb. This type of injection is illustrated in Figure 35–5.

First Carpometacarpal Joint. Degenerative arthritis often involves this joint. The joint space is often quite narrowed, and arthrocenteses may be difficult and painful. A few simple maneuvers may make the injection fairly easy, however. The thumb is flexed across the palm toward the tip of the fifth finger. A mark is made at the base of the first metacarpal bone away from the border of the snuff box. A 22- to 26-gauge, ⅝- to 1-inch needle is inserted at the mark and directed toward the proximal end of the fourth metacarpal. This approach avoids hitting the radial artery. Figure 35–6 illustrates injection of this joint.

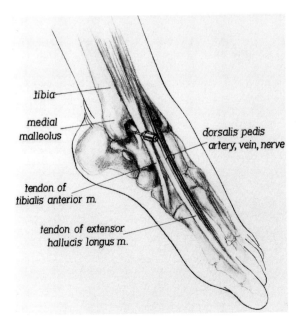

Figure 35–3. Ankle arthrocentesis. With the leg-foot angle at 90 degrees, the needle is inserted at a point just medial to the tibialis anterior tendon and just lateral to the medial malleolus. The needle is then directed posteriorly.

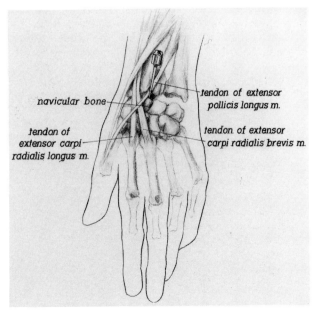

Figure 35–5. Wrist arthrocentesis. The needle is inserted at a point just distal to the radius and just ulnar to the anatomic snuff box. It is then directed perpendicularly. If bone is hit, the needle should be pulled back and slightly redirected toward the thumb.

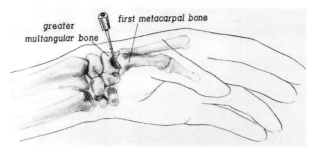

Figure 35–6. First carpometacarpal arthrocentesis. The thumb is flexed across the palm toward the tip of the fifth finger. The needle is inserted at the base of the metacarpal bone away from the border of the snuff box. It is then directed toward the proximal end of the fourth metacarpal.

Metacarpophalangeal Joints and Finger Interphalangeal Joints. Synovitis in these joints usually causes the synovium to bulge dorsally, and a 24- to 26-gauge, ½- to ⅝-inch needle can be inserted on either side just under the extensor tendon mechanism. It is not necessary for the needle to be interposed between the articular surfaces. Some clinicians prefer having the fingers slightly flexed when injecting the metacarpophalangeal joints. It is unusual to obtain synovial fluid. When injecting glucocorticoids, consider mixing them with a small amount of local anesthetic using the precautions previously discussed. This will distend the joint on all sides and possibly help prevent soft tissue atrophy. These injections are illustrated in Figure 35–7.

Metatarsophalangeal Joints and Toe Interphalangeal Joints. The techniques are quite similar to those of the metacarpophalangeal and finger interphalangeal joints, but many prefer to inject more dorsally and laterally to the extensor tendons. Marking the area(s) to be injected is helpful as is gentle traction on the toe of each joint that is injected.

Elbow. A technique preferred by many clinicians is to have the elbow flexed at 90 degrees. The joint capsule will bulge if there is inflammation. A mark is made just below the lateral epicondyle of the humerus. A 22-gauge, 1- to 1 ½-inch needle is inserted at the mark and directed parallel to the shaft

of the radius or directed perpendicular to the skin. Figure 35–8 illustrates these two approaches.

Hip. The hip is an extremely difficult joint to inject even when using a fluoroscope as a guide. Rarely is the physician quite sure that the joint has been entered; synovial fluid is rarely obtained. Two approaches can be used: anterior or lateral. A 20-gauge, 3 ½-inch spinal needle should be used for both approaches.

For the anterior approach, the patient is supine and the extremity fully extended and externally rotated. A mark should be made about 2 to 3 cm below the anterior superior iliac spine and 2 to 3 cm lateral to the femoral pulse. The needle is inserted at a 60 degree angle to the skin and directed posteriorly and medially until bone is hit. The needle is withdrawn slightly, and possibly a drop or two of synovial fluid can be obtained, indicating entry into the joint space.

Many clinicians prefer the lateral approach because the needle can "follow" the femoral neck into the joint. The patient is supine, and the hips should be internally rotated—the knees apart and toes touching. A mark is made just anterior to the greater trochanter, and the needle is inserted and directed medially and sightly cephalad toward a point slightly below the middle of the inguinal ligament. One may feel the tip of the needle slide into the joint. Figure 35–9 illustrates the lateral approach to the hip joint.

Temporomandibular Joint. The temporomandibular joint is palpated as a depression just below the zygomatic arch and 1 to 2 cm anterior to the tragus. The depression is more easily palpated by having the patient open and close the mouth. A mark is made and, with the patient's mouth open, a 22-gauge, ½- to 1-inch needle is inserted perpendicular to the skin and directed slightly posteriorly and superiorly. Figure 35–10 illustrates injection of the temporomandibular joint.

Nonarticular

Shoulder. Bicipital tendinitis can be treated by injecting the shoulder joint or by injecting the tendon

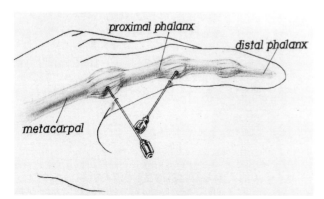

Figure 35–7. Metacarpophalangeal and finger interphalangeal arthrocenteses. With the digit straight or slightly flexed, a small and short needle is inserted on either side just under the extensor tendon mechanism. It is not necessary for the needle to be interposed between the articular surfaces.

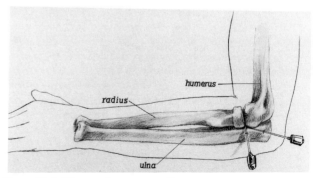

Figure 35–8. Elbow arthrocenteses illustrating parallel and perpendicular techniques. With the elbow flexed at 90 degrees, the needle is inserted just below the lateral epicondyle of the humerus and is directed parallel to the shaft of the radius; it may also be directed perpendicular to the skin.

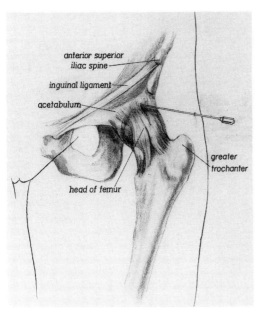

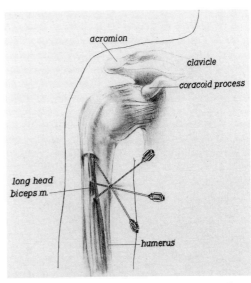

Figure 35–9. Hip arthrocentesis illustrating lateral technique. In this technique, the patient is supine with the hips internally rotated—knees apart and toes touching. The needle is inserted just anterior to the greater trochanter and is directed medially and slightly cephalad toward a point slightly below the middle of the inguinal ligament. One may feel the needle slip into the joint. For the *anterior approach,* the patient is supine and the extremity fully extended and externally rotated. A mark is made 2 to 3 cm below the anterior superior iliac spine and 2 to 3 cm lateral to the femoral pulse. The needle is inserted at a 60-degree angle to the mark and directed posteriorly and medially until bone is hit.

Figure 35–11. Bicipital tendon sheath injections. At the point of maximal tenderness, the needle is inserted just under the sheath and glucocorticoid, with or without local anesthetic, is injected. The needle is directed superiorly and then inferiorly, with further injections at each site.

sheath. The tendon is tender, is easily palpated in the bicipital groove of the humerus, and can be rolled from side to side. If it is elected to inject the sheath, the point of maximal tenderness is marked. A 22-gauge, 1½-inch needle is inserted in the sheath at

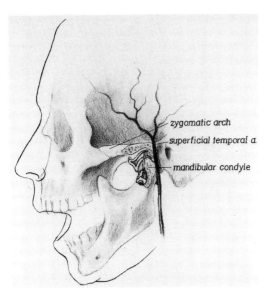

Figure 35–10. Temporomandibular arthrocentesis. With the patient's mouth open, the joint space is palpated as a depression just below the zygomatic arch and 1 to 2 cm anterior to the tragus. The needle is inserted just perpendicular to the skin and directed slightly posteriorly and superiorly.

the mark, and a portion of 0.5 ml of glucocorticoid, with or without local anesthetic, is injected at this site. Then the needle is directed superiorly along the tendon, in the sheath, for about 2 to 3 cm, and more material is injected. The needle is then partially withdrawn and redirected inferiorly along the tendon for about 2 to 3 cm, and the remainder of the material is injected. Figure 35–11 illustrates the bicipital tendon sheath injection.

Subacromial bursitis can be treated by injecting the shoulder joint or the bursa. The bursitis is frequently secondary to supraspinatus tendinitis. If only the subacromial bursa is to be injected, the most tender area is marked; using a 20- to 22-gauge, 1- to 1½-inch needle, 0.5 ml of glucocorticoid, with or without local anesthetic, is injected. Calcification of the supraspinatus tendon may be present, and there may be an acute and severe pain. In this circumstance, one should consider aspirating and irrigating the bursa using a 16- to 18-gauge, 1½-inch needle. Then 0.5 to 1 ml of glucocorticoid, with or without local anesthetic, can be injected. Figure 35–12 illustrates the injection of the subacromial bursa.

The supraspinatus tendon can be directly injected by palpating the groove between the acromium and the humerus on the lateral aspect of the shoulder and marking this spot. Then a 20- to 22-gauge, 1- to 1½-inch needle is directed medially on a horizontal plane for about 2.5 cm, and 0.5 ml of glucocorticoid and 2.5 to 4 ml of local anesthetic is injected. The technique of injecting the supraspinatus tendon is illustrated in Figure 35–12.

Elbow. Lateral epicondylitis, or "tennis elbow," can be quite painful, disabling, and chronic. With the elbow flexed and pronated, there is usually marked tenderness to palpation of a small area on the anterolateral surface of the external condyle of

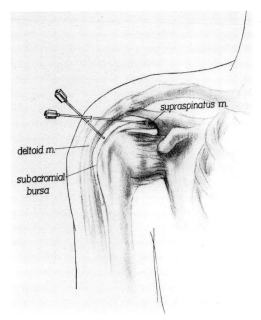

Figure 35–12. Subacromial bursa and supraspinatus tendon injections. For the subacromial bursa, the most tender area is palpated, and the needle is inserted directly into this area. To inject the supraspinatus tendon, the groove between the acromium and the humerus on the lateral aspect of the shoulder is palpated. The needle is inserted at this point and directed medially on a horizontal plane for 2.5 cm; the materials are injected at this point.

the humerus. This spot should be marked. A 20- to 22-gauge, 1- to 1½-inch needle is inserted about 2 cm distal to the mark; 0.5 ml of glucocorticoid mixed with 4 to 4.5 ml of local anesthetic is administered in several small doses by injecting, withdrawing, redirecting the needle, and reinjecting the mixture. The injection of the tennis elbow is illustrated in Figure 35–13.

"Nodule." A nodule, e.g., in the olecranon region or on the proximal aspect of the extensor

surface of the ulna, may be a diagnostic dilemma: is it a tophus or a rheumatoid nodule? A simple punch needle biopsy should answer the question. Figure 35–14 illustrates the technique. Prepare the nodule with an antiseptic solution. Then insert an 18- to 20-gauge, 1- to 1½-inch needle at a 90-degree angle, and rotate it. The needle is then retracted almost completely and is inserted at a 45-degree angle and again rotated (Fig. 35–14A). Repeat this in three other quadrants of the nodule. Remove the needle from the nodule and slightly loosen it. Pull back on the syringe plunger to the 2- to 3-ml level, tighten the needle, and expel the contents onto a microscopic slide. In addition, use a 25-gauge needle to pick out collected material from the biopsy needle (Fig. 35–14B). Examine the specimen under the microscope for sodium urate crystals, preferably using polarizing filters. With a little experience, you can virtually exclude the possibility of a tophus if no crystals are observed.

Wrists and Hands. Aspiration of a ganglion on the dorsal aspect of the wrist is done by using an 18-gauge, 1½-inch needle. After as much material as possible is aspirated, 0.5 to 1 ml of an intra-articular glucocorticoid is injected.

De Quervain's disease (stenosing tenosynovitis of the extensor pollicis brevis and abductor pollicis longus) may be helped by injection. The most tender area in the region of the radial styloid is located by performing a modified Finkelstein's test: clasping the fingers over the thumb and gradually flexing the

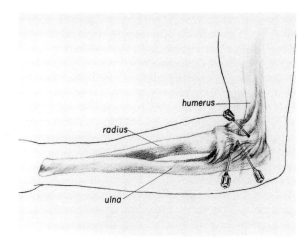

Figure 35–13. "Tennis elbow" injection(s). With the elbow flexed and pronated, the needle is inserted at the most tender area on the anterolateral aspect of the external condyle of the humerus. A combination of glucocorticoid and local anesthetic is injected in several areas.

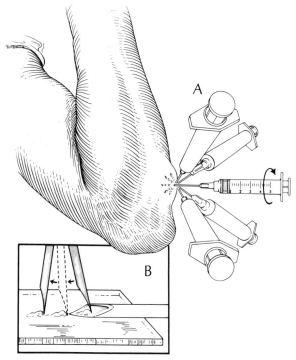

Figure 35–14. Punch needle biopsy of forearm nodule. The needle is inserted at a 90-degree angle and is rotated. The needle is then retracted almost completely and is inserted at a 45-degree angle. This is repeated in three other quadrants (A). The contents of the needle are placed on a microscopic slide (B) and examined.

wrist in ulnar deviation. The most tender point is marked. Then a 22-gauge, 1½-inch needle is inserted about 1 cm proximal to the most tender spot and directed almost parallel to the skin toward the styloid process. As the needle is being advanced, in the tendon sheath, 0.5 ml of glucocorticoid and 2.5 ml of local anesthetic can be injected.

Trigger fingers are usually associated with chronic stenosing tenosynovitis of the finger flexor tendons. The main pathology usually lies over the head of the metacarpal bones in the palm, and a localized swelling may be palpated in this area. A mark is made over the palmar aspect of the metacarpal head; a 22-gauge, 1½-inch needle is inserted at a 45-degree angle and then directed proximally, almost parallel to the skin; and a mixture of 0.5 ml of both glucocorticoid and local anesthetic is injected. Lack of resistance during injection should indicate proper needle placement.

Carpal tunnel syndrome injections should not be done by an inexperienced operator. Theoretically, an injection of a long-acting glucocorticoid directly into the median nerve will damage it. If one elects to perform the procedure, a mark is made over the carpal tunnel just on the ulnar side of the long palmar tendon. A 25-gauge, ⅝-inch needle is directed perpendicular to the mark and inserted its full length. If the needle meets obstruction, or if the patient experiences paresthesias, the needle should be withdrawn and redirected in a more ulnar fashion. An injection of 0.5 ml glucocorticoid may give benefit. The carpal tunnel may be injected again, but if relief is short-lived, surgery should be considered.

Hip. With trochanteric bursitis, there is an area that is tender to palpation in the region of the greater trochanter of the femur. After marking this area, a 20- to 22-gauge, 1½- to 3½-inch needle is inserted perpendicular to the skin directly into the tender area(s). Because several bursae may be inflamed, it is usually more effective to inject several areas superior and inferior to the mark with a mixture of 0.5 to 1 ml glucocorticoid and 4 to 4.5 ml local anesthetic.

Knee. Anserine bursitis produces pain on the medial aspect of the tibia. In this same region may be noted pain from a fat pad, from another bursa, or from medial collateral ligament strain. All may benefit from injection. The point of maximal tenderness is marked. A 20- to 22-gauge, 1½-inch needle is inserted perpendicular to the skin and continued until bone is hit. It is then withdrawn slightly, and 0.25 to 0.5 ml glucocorticoid and 2.5 to 4.5 ml local anesthetic is injected.

The prepatellar bursa is easily aspirated. An 18-gauge, 1½-inch needle is recommended because sometimes the fluid is quite gelatinous and difficult to obtain through a small-bore needle. After aspirating as much fluid as possible, 0.5 to 1 ml glucocorticoid is injected. On occasion, little fluid is obtained during the initial aspiration, but reaspiration 24 hours after glucocorticoid injection may yield a large amount of fluid.

Pelvis. When inflamed, the ischial (ischiogluteal) bursa is usually easily palpated as a tender area when the patient is lying on his or her side with the knees flexed. This position theoretically will make the ischium more exposed as gluteal muscles and sciatic nerve are pulled away. The point of maximal tenderness is marked, and 0.5 to 1 ml of glucocorticoid and 2.5 to 4 ml of local anesthetic are mixed in a syringe with a 20-gauge, 3½-inch needle attached. It is helpful to "fix" the skin over the mark. Then the needle is inserted into the mark until bone is hit. The needle is withdrawn slightly and all the mixture injected; alternatively, the needle is redirected in one or two other directions and portions of the mixture injected.

Iliopectineal (iliopsoas) bursitis, as previously mentioned, must be differentiated from psoas abscess, femoral hernia, and septic arthritis of the hip. If one elects to inject the bursa, a 20- to 22-gauge, 3½-inch spinal needle is used. Many use the technique of hip arthrocentesis. A dose of 0.5 to 1 ml of glucocorticoid is injected, with or without 4 to 4.5 ml of local anesthetic.

Back. The fibrositis syndrome and the tender points of the back have been discussed briefly. These tender points can be marked and each injected with 0.25 ml of glucocorticoid or 1 ml or more of local anesthetic or, as many physicians prefer, a combination of the two. The shorter-acting glucocorticosteroids, in contrast to the repository forms, have been recommended.[55] The physician must be careful to avoid injury to the underlying structures.

Foot. Achilles tendinitis may respond to injection. If this is done, a 22-gauge, 1½-inch needle is inserted just under the tendon sheath and a mixture of 0.25 ml of glucocorticoid and 2.5 ml of local anesthetic injected. Direct injection of the tendon should be avoided.

An inflammation of the subcutaneous Achilles bursa between the skin and tendon is usually readily palpable, can be marked, and should be easily aspirated with a 20-gauge, 1-inch needle. The retrocalcaneal bursa is located between the Achilles tendon and the posterior facet of the calcaneus. A lateral or medial approach is probably best. Careful injection of either location with 0.25 to 0.5 ml of glucocorticoid, with or without local anesthetic, is usually beneficial.

Calcaneal bursitis can be treated by inserting a 20-gauge, 1½-inch needle perpendicular to the plantar surface of the midcalcaneal region, pushing the needle in until bone is hit, withdrawing slightly, and injecting 0.5 ml of glucocorticoid and 3.5 ml of local anesthetic.

References

1. Nelson, R. L., McCaffrey, L. A., Nobrega, F. T., et al.: Altering residency curriculum in response to a changing practice environment: Use of the Mayo internal medicine residency alumni survey. Mayo Clin. Proc. 65:809, 1990.
2. Hollander, J. L.: Arthrocentesis and intrasynovial therapy. In McCarty, D. J. (ed.): Arthritis and Allied Conditions. 9th ed. Philadelphia, Lea & Febiger, 1979.
3. Hollander, J. L.: The local effects of compound F (hydrocortisone) injected into joints. Bull. Rheum. Dis. 2:3, 1951.

4. Young, H. H., Ward, L. E., and Henderson, E. D.: The use of hydrocortisone acetate (compound F acetate) in the treatment of some common orthopedic conditions. J. Bone Joint Surg. 36A:602, 1954.

5. Hollander, J. L., Jessar, R. A., and Brown, E. M., Jr.: Intrasynovial corticosteroid therapy: A decade of use. Bull. Rheum. Dis. 11:239, 1961.

6. Hollander, J. L.: Intrasynovial corticosteroid therapy in arthritis. Md. State Med. J. 19:62, 1970.

7. Jessar, R. A., Ganzell, M. A., and Ragan, C.: The action of hydrocortisone in synovial inflammation. J. Clin. Invest. 32:480, 1954.

8. Hunder, G. G., and McDuffie, F. C.: Effect of intra-articular hydrocortisone on complement in synovial fluid. J. Lab. Clin. Med. 79:62, 1972.

9. Goetzl, E. J., Bianco, N. E., Alpert, J. S., et al.: Effects of intra-articular corticosteroids *in vivo* on synovial fluid variables in rheumatoid synovitis. Ann. Rheum. Dis. 33:62, 1974.

10. Dick, W. C., Whaley, K., St. Onge, R. A., et al.: Clinical studies on inflammation in human knee joints: Xenon (Xe[133]) clearances correlated with clinical assessment in various arthritides and studies on the effect of intra-articular administered hydrocortisone in rheumatoid arthritis. Clin. Sci. 38:123, 1970.

11. DeCeulaer, K., Balint, G., El-Ghobarey, A., et al.: Effects of corticosteroids and local anaesthetics applied directly to the synovial vascular bed. Ann. Rheum. Dis. 38:440, 1979.

12. Eymontt, M. J., Gordon, G. V., Schumacher, H. R., et al.: The effects on synovial permeability and synovial fluid leukocyte counts in symptomatic osteoarthritis after intra-articular corticosteroid administration. J. Rheumatol. 9:198, 1982.

13. Chandler, G. N., and Wright, V.: Deleterious effect of intra-articular hydrocortisone. Lancet 2:661, 1958.

14. Chandler, G. N., Wright, V., and Hartfall, S. J.: Intra-articular therapy in rheumatoid arthritis: Comparison of hydrocortisone tertiary butyl-acetate and hydrocortisone acetate. Lancet 2:659, 1958.

15. Mankin, H. J., and Conger, K. A.: The acute effects of intra-articular hydrocortisone on articular cartilage in rabbits. J. Bone Joint Surg. 48A:1383, 1966.

16. Bentley, G., and Goodfellow, J. W.: Disorganization of the knees following intra-articular hydrocortisone injections. J. Bone Joint Surg. 51B:498, 1969.

17. Moskowitz, R. W., Davis, W., Sammarco, J., et al.: Experimentally induced corticosteroid arthropathy. Arthritis Rheum. 13:236, 1970.

18. Mankin, H. J., Zarins, A., and Jaffe, W. L.: The effect of systemic corticosteroids on rabbit articular cartilage. Arthritis Rheum. 15:593, 1972.

19. Behrens, F., Shepard, N., and Mitchell, N.: Alteration of rabbit articular cartilage by intra-articular injections of glucocorticosteroids. J. Bone Joint Surg. 57A:70, 1975.

20. Gibson, T., Barry, H. C., Poswillo, D., et al.: Effect of intra-articular corticosteroid injections on primate cartilage. Ann. Rheum. Dis. 36:74, 1976.

21. Williams, J. M., and Brandt, K. D.: Triamcinolone hexacetonide protects against fibrillation and osteophyte formation following chemically induced articular cartilage damage. Arthritis Rheum. 28:1267, 1985.

22. Pelletier, J.-P., and Martel-Pelletier, J.: Protective effects of corticosteroids on cartilage lesions and osteophyte formation in the Pond-Nuki dog model of osteoarthritis. Arthritis Rheum. 32:181, 1989.

23. Tenenbaum, J., Pritzker, K. P. H., Gross, A. E., et al.: The effects of intra-articular corticosteroids on articular cartilage. Semin. Arthritis Rheum. 11 (Suppl. 1):140, 1981.

24. Gray, R. G., and Gottlieb, N. L.: Intra-articular corticosteroids: An updated assessment. Clin. Orthop. Rel. Res. 177:235, 1983.

25. Gray, R. G., Tenenbaum, J., and Gottlieb, N. L.: Local corticosteroid injection treatment in rheumatic disorders. Semin. Arthritis Rheum. 10:231, 1981.

26. Sweetnam, R.: Corticosteroid arthropathy and tendon rupture (Editorial). J. Bone Joint Surg. 51B:397, 1969.

27. Wrenn, R. N., Goldner, J. L., and Markee, J. L.: An experimental study of the effect of cortisone on the healing process and tensile strength of tendons. J. Bone Joint Surg. 36A:588, 1954.

28. McCarty, D. J.: Treatment of rheumatoid joint inflammation with triamcinolone hexacetonide. Arthritis Rheum. 15:157, 1972.

29. Gilsanz, V., and Bernstein, B. H.: Joint calcification following intra-articular corticosteroid therapy. Radiology 151:647, 1984.

30. McCarty, D. J., Jr., and Hogan, J. M.: Inflammatory reaction after intrasynovial injection of microcrystalline adrenocorticosteroid esters. Arthritis Rheum. 7:359, 1964.

31. Koehler, B. F., Urowitz, M. B., and Killinger, D. W.: The systemic effects of intra-articular corticosteroid. J. Rheumatol. 1:117, 1974.

32. Armstrong, R. D., English, J., Gibson, T., et al.: Serum methylprednisolone levels following intra-articular injection of methylprednisolone acetate. Ann. Rheum. Dis. 40:571, 1981.

33. Gottlieb, N. L., and Riskin, W. G.: Complications of local corticosteroid injections. J.A.M.A. 243:1547, 1980.

34. Konttinen, Y. T., Friman, C., Tolvanen, E., et al.: Local skin rash after intra-articular methylprednisolone acetate injection in a patient with rheumatoid arthritis. Arthritis Rheum. 26:231, 1983.

35. Carson, T. E., Daane, T. A., Lee, P. A., et al.: Effect of intramuscular triamcinolone acetonide on the human ovulatory cycle. Cutis 19:633, 1977.

36. Cunningham, G. R., Goldzieher, J. W., de la Pena, A., et al.: The mechanism of ovulation inhibition by triamcinolone acetonide. J. Clin. Endocrinol. Metab. 46:8, 1978.

37. Baer, P. A., Shore, A., and Ikeman, R.: Transient fall in serum salicylate levels following intra-articular injection of steroid in patients with rheumatoid arthritis. Arthritis Rheum. 30:345, 1987.

38. McCarty, D. J., Jr.: A basic guide to arthrocentesis. Hosp. Med. 4:77, 1968.

39. Gottlieb, N. L.: Hypodermic needle separation during arthrocentesis. Arthritis Rheum. 24:1593, 1981.

40. Fitzgerald, R. F., Jr.: Intrasynovial injection of steroids. Mayo Clin. Proc. 51:655, 1976.

41. Miller, J. H., White, J., and Norton, T. H.: The value of intra-articular injections in osteoarthritis of the knee. J. Bone Joint Surg. 40B:636, 1958.

42. Friedman, D. M., and Moore, M. F.: The efficacy of intra-articular corticosteroid for osteoarthritis of the knee. Arthritis Rheum. 21:556, 1978.

43. Utsinger, P. D., Resnick, D., Shapiro, R. F., et al.: Roentgenologic, immunologic, and therapeutic study of erosive (inflammatory) osteoarthritis. Arch. Intern. Med. 138:693, 1978.

44. Huskisson, E. C.: The drug treatment of osteoarthritis. Scand. J. Rheumatol. 43(Suppl.):57, 1982.

45. Friedman, D. M., and Moore, M. E.: The efficacy of intra-articular steroids in osteoarthritis: A double-blind study. J. Rheumatol. 7:850, 1980.

46. Neustadt, D. H.: Intra-articular steroid therapy. In Moskowitz, R. W., Howell, D. S., Goldberg, V. M., and Mankin, H. J. (eds.): Osteoarthritis: Diagnosis and Management. 1st ed. Philadelphia, W. B. Saunders Company, 1984.

47. Dieppe, P. A., Sathapatayavongs, B., Jones, H. E., et al.: Intra-articular steroids in osteoarthritis. Rheumatol. Rehabil. 19:212, 1980.

48. Neustadt, D. H.: Intra-articular therapy for rheumatoid synovitis of the knee: Effects of the postinjection rest regimen. Clin. Rheumatol. Pract. 3:65, 1985.

49. McCarty, D. J.: Intrasynovial therapy with adrenocorticosteroid esters. Wis. Med. J. 77:S75, 1978.

50. Henderson, E. D., and Henderon, C. C.: The use of hydrocortisone acetate (compound F acetate) in the treatment of post-traumatic bursitis of the knee and elbow. Minn. Med. 36:142, 1953.

51. Gray, R. G., Kiem, I. M., and Gottlieb, N. L.: Intratendon sheath corticosteroid treatment of rheumatoid arthritis-associated and idiopathic hand flexor tenosynovitis. Arthritis Rheum. 21:92, 1978.

52. Steinbrocker, O.: Management of some non-articular rheumatic disorders. Mod. Treatment 1:1254, 1964.

53. Steinbrocker, O., and Neustadt, D. H.: Aspiration and injection therapy in arthritis and musculoskeletal disorders. Hagerstown, Harper & Row, 1972.

54. Smythe, H. A., and Moldofsky, H.: Two contributions to understanding of the "fibrositis" syndrome. Bull. Rheum. Dis. 28:928, 1977.

55. Brown, B. B., Jr.: Diagnosis and therapy of common myofascial syndromes. J.A.M.A. 239:646, 1978.

55a. Physicians' Desk Reference (Lederle Laboratories). Oradell, NJ, Medical Economics Company, Inc., 1990.

56. Geborek, P., Mansson, B., Wollheim, F. A., et al.: Intra-articular corticosteroid injection into rheumatoid arthritis knees improves extensor muscle strength. Rheumatol. Int. 9:265, 1990.

57. Owen, D. S., Jr., Weiss, J. J., and Wilke, W. S.: When to aspirate and inject joints. Patient Care 24:128, 1990.

57a. Hertzberger-ten, C. R., de Vries van der Vlugt, B. C. M., and Van Suijlekom-Smit, L. W. A.: Intra-articular steroids in pauciarticular juvenile chronic arthritis, type 1. Eur. J. Pediatr. 150:170, 1991.

58. Gurwitz, J. H., Avorn, J., Ross-Degnan, D., et al.: Nonsteroidal anti-inflammatory drug-associated azotemia in the very old. J.A.M.A. 264:471, 1990.

59. Roberts, W. N., Liang, M. H., and Stern, S. H.: Colchicine in acute gout: Reassessment of risks and benefits. J.A.M.A. 257:1920, 1987.

60. Steinbrocker, O., and Argyros, T. G.: Frozen shoulder treatment by local injection of depot corticosteroids. Arch. Phys. Med. 55:209, 1974.

61. Roy, S., and Oldham, R.: Management of painful shoulder. Lancet 1:1322, 1976.

62. Weiss, J. J., and Ting, Y. M.: Arthrography-assisted intra-articular injection of steroids in treatment of adhesive capsulitis. Arch. Phys. Med. 59:285, 1978.

63. Kozin, F.: Painful shoulder and the reflex sympathetic dystrophy syndrome. In McCarty, D. J. (ed.): Arthritis and Allied Conditions. 10th ed. Philadelphia, Lea & Febiger, 1985.

64. Lee, P. N., Lee, M., Hag, A. M., et al.: Periarthritis of the shoulder: Trial of treatments investigated by multivariate analysis. Ann. Rheum. Dis. 33:116, 1974.

65. Jelenko, C.: Tietze's syndrome at the xiphisternal joint. South. Med. J. 67:818, 1974.

66. Kamien, M.: A rational management of tennis elbow. Sports Med. 9:173, 1990.
67. Clark, C. B.: Cubital tunnel syndrome. J.A.M.A. 241:801, 1979.
68. Lapidus, P. W., and Guidotti, F. P.: Report on the treatment of one hundred and two ganglions. Bull. Hosp. Joint Dis. 28:50, 1967.
69. Phalen, G. S.: Soft tissue affection of the hand and wrist. Hosp. Med. 7:47, 1971.
69a. Anderson, B. C., Manthey, R., and Brouns, M. C.: Treatment of de Quervain's tenosynovitis with corticosteroids. Arthritis Rheum. 34:793, 1991.
70. Harvey, F. J., Harvey, P. M., and Horsley, M. W.: De Quervain's disease: Surgical or nonsurgical treatment. J. Hand Surg. (Am.) 15:83, 1990.
71. Marks, M. R., and Gunther, S. F.: Efficacy of cortisone injection in treatment of trigger fingers and thumbs. J. Hand Surg. (Am.) 14:722, 1989.
72. Canoso, J. J.: Bursitis, tenosynovitis, ganglions, and painful lesions of the wrist, elbow, and hand. Curr. Opin. Rheum. 2:276, 1990.
73. Fauno, P., Anderson, H. J., and Simonsen, O.: A long-term follow-up of the effect of repeated corticosteroid injections for stenosing tenosynovitis. J. Hand Surg. (Br.) 14:242, 1989.
74. Blau, S. P.: All those joint pains may not be arthritis. Drug Ther. (Nov):144, 1976.
75. Schuchmann, J. A., Melvin, J. L., Duran, R. J., et al.: Evaluation of local steroid injection for carpal tunnel syndrome. Arch. Phys. Med. Rehabil. 51:253, 1971.
75a. Dehaan, M. R., and Wilson, R. L.: Diagnosis and management of carpal tunnel syndrome. J. Musculoskeletal Med. 6:47, 1989.
76. Larsson, L.-G., and Baum, J.: The syndrome of anserina bursitis: An overlooked diagnosis. Arthritis Rheum. 28:1062, 1985.
77. Swartout, R., and Compere, E. L.: Ischiogluteal bursitis. J.A.M.A. 227:551, 1974.
78. Hucherson, D. C., and Freeman, G. E., Jr.: Iliopectineal bursitis—a cause of hip pain frequently unrecognized. Am. J. Orthop. 4:220, 1962.
79. Canoso, J. J., Wohlgethan, J. R., Newberg, A. H., et al.: Aspiration of the retrocalcaneal bursa. Ann. Rheum. Dis. 43:308, 1984.
80. Francis, H., March, L., Terenty, T., et al.: Benign joint hypermobility with neuropathy: Documentation and mechanism of tarsal tunnel syndrome. J. Rheumatol. 14:577, 1987.
81. Kaplan, P. E., and Kernahan, W. T.: Tarsal tunnel syndrome. J. Bone Joint Surg. 63A:96, 1981.
82. Larsson, L.-G., and Baum, J.: The syndromes of bursitis. Bull. Rheum. Dis. 36:1, 1986.
83. Strong, G., and Thomas, P. S.: Conservative treatment of Morton's neuroma. Orthop. Rev. 16:97, 1987.
84. Roy, D. R., Fleury, J., Fontaine, S. B., et al.: Clinical evaluation of cervical facet joint infiltration. Can. Assoc. Radiol. J. 39:118, 1988.
85. Warfield, C. A.: Facet syndrome and the relief of low back pain. Hosp. Prac. 23:41, 1988.
86. Hardaker, W. T., Whipple, T. L., and Bassett, F. H.: Diagnosis and treatment of the plica syndrome of the knee. J. Bone Joint Surg. 62A:221, 1980.
87. Rovere, G. D.: Medial synovial shelf plica syndrome. Am. J. Sports Med. 13:382, 1984.
88. Schonholtz, G. J., and Magee, C. M.: The synovial plicae of the knee joint. Contemp. Orthop. 12:31, 1986.

Chapter 36

H. Ralph Schumacher, Jr.

Synovial Fluid Analysis and Synovial Biopsy

The actual disease process in a given joint can be defined only by direct study of that joint. Evaluation of every patient with arthritis should include some morphologic investigation of the joint. Abnormal results of blood tests such as those for rheumatoid factor, antinuclear antibodies, and elevated uric acid can be misleading and do not establish the nature of disease in the joint. Because crystal-induced arthritis can closely mimic rheumatoid disease, at least one joint fluid specimen should be examined for crystals. Nearly 100 other diseases can also involve joints; in many, the study of fluid or tissue is the only way to establish the diagnosis. In addition, not all joints in each patient need have the same findings. Some joints in patients with rheumatoid arthritis (RA) may be totally spared or affected only by coincidental osteoarthritis, whereas others may have a superimposed infectious arthritis.

Full information from aspiration or biopsy or both may suggest major changes in management. Unexpected findings can suggest a variety of less common but often specifically treatable causes of arthritis. Expertise in joint fluid analysis and interpretation of synovial tissue study is not widely available, and these skills should be developed by anyone specializing in the care of joint disease.

SYNOVIAL FLUID ANALYSIS

Joint fluid examination[1, 2] is even more important in the evaluation of joint disease than urinalysis is in renal disease. Analysis of joint fluid should be per-formed as part of the diagnostic evaluation in any patient with joint disease. Examination of joint fluid is especially important in monoarticular arthritis in which septic arthritis must be distinguished from a wide variety of different possible causes (see Table 22–3). Even small amounts of joint fluid can be aspirated and systematically examined. A few drops or more of synovial fluid can often be obtained from normal joints and virtually any joint that is even equivocally swollen.[3]

Some common diseases such as gout, pseudogout, septic arthritis, and systemic lupus erythematosus (SLE) as well as other less common diseases, can be quickly and almost definitively diagnosed by examination of joint fluid. In one study, joint fluid examination changed clinically suspected diagnoses (and often planned treatments) in about 20 percent of individuals seen for initial evaluation.[4] Even if joint fluid examination is not diagnostic in other patients, it can be one of the most useful of a battery of clinical and laboratory tests used in differential diagnosis. Gross examination and leukocyte count allow narrowing of diagnostic possibilities to the diseases causing "noninflammatory" effusions, "inflammatory" fluids including septic effusions, and hemarthroses (Tables 36–1 to 36–4).

Even in patients in whom the diagnosis has been established, synovial fluid analysis can show clues to new developments such as low-grade infection in a joint of a patient with lupus erythematosus or rheumatoid disease, superimposition of calcium pyrophosphate or apatite crystal deposition in osteoarthritis, or crystals of intra-articularly injected gluco-

Table 36–1. CLASSIFICATION OF SYNOVIAL EFFUSIONS*

Gross Examination	Normal	"Noninflammatory"	Inflammatory	Septic
Volume (knee)	< 1 ml	Often > 1 ml	Often > 1 ml	Often > 1 ml
Viscosity	High	High	Low	Variable
Color	Colorless to straw	Straw to yellow	Yellow	Variable
Clarity	Transparent	Transparent	Translucent	Opaque
WBCs/mm³†	< 200	200–2000	2000–75000	Often > 100,000 +
PMN†	< 25%	< 25%	Often > 50%	> 85%
Culture	Negative	Negative	Negative	Often positive
Mucin clot	Firm	Firm	Friable	Friable
Glucose (A.M. fasting)	Nearly equal to blood	Nearly equal to blood	< 50 mg/dl lower than blood	> 50 mg/dl lower than blood

*See Tables 36–2 and 36–3 for diseases in the "noninflammatory" and inflammatory groups.
†WBC count and PMN percentage are less if organism is less virulent or partially treated.

Table 36–2. RELATIVELY NONINFLAMMATORY JOINT EFFUSIONS (LEUKOCYTE COUNT FEWER THAN 2000 PER MM³)

Osteoarthritis
Traumatic arthritis
Acromegaly
Gaucher's disease
Hemochromatosis
Hyperparathyroidism
Ochronosis
Paget's disease
Mechanical derangement
Erythema nodosum
Villonodular synovitis, tumors
Aseptic necrosis
Ehlers-Danlos syndrome
Sickle cell disease
Amyloidosis
Hypertrophic pulmonary osteoarthropathy
Pancreatitis
Osteochondritis dissecans
Charcot's joints
Wilson's disease
Epiphyseal dysplasias
Glucocorticoid withdrawal

Table 36–3. INFLAMMATORY JOINT EFFUSIONS (LEUKOCYTE COUNT MORE THAN 2000 PER MM³)

Rheumatoid arthritis
Psoriatic arthritis
Reiter's syndrome
Ulcerative colitis
Regional enteritis
Post–ileal bypass arthritis
Ankylosing spondylitis
Juvenile rheumatoid arthritis
Rheumatic fever
Collagen-vascular disease
  Systemic lupus erythematosus
  Scleroderma
  Polymyositis
  Polychondritis
  Polyarteritis
Polymyalgia rheumatica
Giant cell arteritis
Sjogren's syndrome
Wegener's granulomatosis
Goodpasture's syndrome
Henoch-Schönlein purpura
Familial Mediterranean fever
Whipple's disease
Behçet's sydrome
Erythema nodosum
Sarcoidosis
Multicentric reticulohistiocytosis
Erythema multiforme (Stevens-Johnson)
Post-*Salmonella*, post-*Shigella*, post-*Yersinia* arthritis
Infectious arthritis
  Parasitic
  Viral (hepatitis, mumps, rubella, human immunodeficiency virus, others)
  Fungal
  Mycoplasmal
  Bacterial (staphylococcal or gonococcal infection, tuberculosis, others)
  Spirochetal (Lyme disease, syphilis)
Carcinoid
Subacute bacterial endocarditis
Crystal-induced arthritis
  Gout
  Pseudogout
  Post–intra-articular steroid injection
  Apatite arthritis
  Oxalosis
Hyperlipoproteinemias
Serum sickness
Hypogammaglobulinemia
Leukemia
Hypersensitivity angiitis
Palindromic rheumatism

corticoids that cause a transient crystal-induced synovitis.

Discrepancies between laboratories examining the same fluids are common.[5] It is best to examine fluids personally and to be certain of quality-control mechanisms established in your own laboratory.[6]

Normal joint fluid is described in detail in Chapter 1. Briefly, normal synovial fluid is an ultrafiltrate of plasma—with only small amounts of higher-molecular-weight proteins such as fibrinogen, complement, globulin, and other immunoglobulins—to which has been added hyaluronate protein produced in the synovial membrane. Normal fluid is compared with that seen in various diseases in Table 36–1.

Technique for Arthrocentesis

The techniques used, appropriate precautions, and routes for arthrocentesis are described in Chapter 35. If no fluid is identified in the syringe after attempted aspiration, try to express a drop of blood or tissue fluid from the needle. One can use such a single drop for examination for crystals, Gram's stain, or culture. If no fluid is obtained and infection is suspected, irrigate the joint with a small amount of normal saline and culture this irrigating fluid.

Consider the studies most likely to be helpful in each case before arthrocentesis, and prepare a list of priorities for the fluid obtained. By no means must all tests be performed on each specimen. Because leukocyte counts can fall and artefactual crystals may develop over several hours, the importance of prompt examination of fluid is emphasized.[7]

Gross Examination

Gross examination can be done at bedside to help plan which of the other studies are most pertinent.

Table 36–4. HEMARTHROSES

Trauma with or without fractures
Pigmented villonodular synovitis
Tumors
Hemangioma
Charcot's joint or other severe joint destruction
Hemophilia or other bleeding disorders
Von Willebrand's disease
Anticoagulant therapy
Myeloproliferative disease with thrombocytosis
Thrombocytopenia
Scurvy
Ruptured aneurysm
Arteriovenous fistula
Idiopathic
Intense inflammatory disease

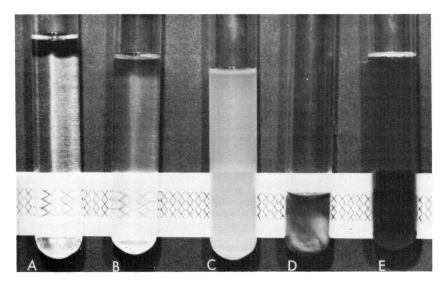

Figure 36–1. Synovial effusions. *A*, Normal or edema fluid is clear, pale yellow, or colorless. Print is easily read through the tube. *B*, Fluid from noninflammatory joint disease is yellow and clear. *C*, An inflammatory effusion is cloudy and yellow. Print may be blurred or completely obliterated, depending on the number of leukocytes. The effusion is translucent. *D*, A purulent effusion from septic arthritis contains a dense clump that does not even allow light through the many leukocytes. *E*, Hemorrhagic fluid is red. The supernatant may be darker yellow-brown (xanthochromic). A traumatic tap is less uniform and often has blood streaks.

Volume. The amount of effusion can help serve as one measure of the severity of arthritis and can be used for comparison with previous arthrocentesis results. Low volume does not mean absence of an important intra-articular process. Effusions may be difficult to aspirate because of thick fibrin, rice bodies, and other debris. Fluid may be loculated and not accessible by the route chosen.

Viscosity. Although estimation of viscosity is now known to be less reliable than previously thought in classification of effusions,[8] it can be estimated by watching the synovial fluid as it is slowly expressed from the syringe or by manipulating several drops of fluid between the gloved thumb and finger. Fluid of normal viscosity holds together and stretches to a string of 1 to 2 inches before separating. Low-viscosity fluid drips from a syringe like water. Very viscous fluid is seen in hypothyroid effusions and in ganglia or osteoarthritic mucous cysts. Viscosity is generally decreased in inflammation (see Table 36–1) but also is low in edema fluid. Viscosity tends to parallel the concentration of hyaluronate. In purulent effusions, the massive numbers of leukocytes may make the fluid seem more viscous. Hyaluronidase or dilution with saline can be used to decrease synovial fluid viscosity before performing other tests, provided the normal values using this enzyme have been standardized in the laboratory[9] and that the dilution factor is considered.

Color and Clarity (Fig. 36–1). If print cannot be read easily through the fluid, the effusion is cloudy, and this finding should suggest an inflammatory process. The plastic of some syringes makes fluids appear falsely cloudy, so fluids should be examined in glass. Generally, the more cloudy fluids have more cells, but not all cloudy or opaque fluids are inflammatory. Microscopic examination is needed to be certain that the opacity is not due to massive numbers of crystals, lipids, fibrin, or amyloid. Sometimes chronically inflamed joints have effusions that contain rice bodies, which might also be confused grossly with pus. Rice bodies are end-results of synovial proliferation and degeneration; they contain collagen, cell debris, and fibrin (Fig. 36–2; see color section at the front of this volume).

Ochronotic fluid may be speckled with dark particles (ground pepper sign).[10] Black or gray debris from metal or plastic fragments after prosthetic arthroplasty can also discolor the fluid.[11]

Fluid in pigmented villonodular synovitis can be grossly bloody or may have an orange-brown color. Urate- or apatite-laden fluids can be white or yellow and pasty. Cholesterol-containing fluids may be golden. Streaks of blood are the result of injury to a small vessel during the procedure. Causes of diffusely bloody fluids are listed in Table 36–4. Lipid floating on the top of the erythrocytes is often a result of fracture to the joint. Partially treated or low-

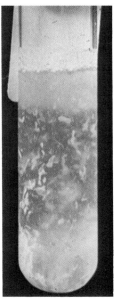

Figure 36–2. Synovial fluid rice bodies containing fibrin and debris from degenerated villi are especially common in rheumatoid arthritis but can also be seen in other conditions such as tuberculous arthritis.

grade infection can make the synovial fluid like any other moderately inflammatory but not purulent fluid. Slightly inflammatory or clear fluids are common in SLE, rheumatic fever, polymyositis, and scleroderma, and can be seen in the interim between attacks of gout and pseudogout.

Leukocyte Count

Quantitation of the synovial fluid leukocyte count is an important part of synovial fluid analysis, especially because it is the major basis for classification of an effusion as septic, inflammatory, or noninflammatory (see Table 36–1). Synovial fluid leukocyte counts, along with volumes, can be used as a rough measure of the intensity of inflammation in sequential samples.

The standard leukocyte-counting chamber and techniques are used, except that ordinary counting fluid should be replaced with normal or 0.3 percent saline, which will lyse erythrocytes. The acid of ordinary leukocyte-counting fluid clots synovial fluid and gives inaccurate counts. A small amount of fluid should be placed in a heparinized tube and shaken to mix it thoroughly. The count must be done promptly, as there may be some spontaneous clotting and clumping of leukocytes. Methylene blue can be added for easier identification of leukocytes. RA fluid usually has leukocyte counts from 2000 to 75,000. Counts over 60,000 should raise a suspicion of infection. However, partially treated infections or low-grade infections with gonococci, mycobacteria, and fungi often have lower leukocyte counts. Patients with rheumatoid disease, psoriatic arthritis, Reiter's syndrome, and crystal-induced arthritis may have leukocyte counts over 100,000 cells per mm³. Small joints, such as finger joints, may have unusually high counts, because less volume dilutes the cell in such joints.

Leukocyte counts of 200 to 2000 per mm³ have generally been termed *noninflammatory*. Actually, truly normal joint fluid usually has only up to 50 to 100 leukocytes per mm³, so that counts over 200 clearly represent at least a low-grade inflammatory response, which is seen, for example, in some patients with osteoarthritis. Patients who have predominantly degenerative arthritis, as in hemochromatosis, can have inflammatory effusions with high leukocyte counts if associated chondrocalcinosis leads to crystal-induced arthritis.

Microscopic Studies

Wet Preparation. Probably the single most important step in synovial fluid analysis is prompt microscopic examination of a fresh drop of synovial fluid as a wet preparation. Even if only a single drop of fluid is obtained with aspiration, it can be examined for crystals and other constituents as a wet preparation and then the same fluid allowed to dry

for staining with Gram's stain if required. Express 1 to 2 drops of unadulterated synovial fluid from the syringe or transfer the fluid with a pipette or loop onto an ultraclean glass slide. The author usually examines uncentrifuged fluids, but examination of a pellet after centrifugation can help concentrate rare crystals or cells in clear-appearing fluid. Dirty slides can be washed in acetone and air dried. Lens paper used to clean slides can introduce birefringent paper fibrils.

Cover the drop of synovial fluid with a glass coverslip. If any delay is expected before examination, the coverslip margins may be sealed with nail polish. This allows several hours of delay, but slides may still dry out and produce birefringent-drying artifacts if left overnight. Remember that the nail polish at the margins is birefringent with polarized light.

Regular Light Microscopy. First, examine each joint fluid with regular light microscopy. Erythrocytes and leukocytes can be seen and their numbers estimated. Fragments of cartilage or synovium may contain crystals and, if numerous enough, can be concentrated by centrifugation and fixed for staining as a biopsy. Some leukocytes contain cytoplasmic inclusions (Fig. 36–3) that are thought to represent distended phagosomes or lipid droplets. Such cytoplasmic inclusion-containing cells,[12] or ragocytes, were first detected in RA but are also seen in other inflammatory arthropathies. Erythrocytes may be seen to be sickled in patients with sickle cell disease or trait, but this does not establish that the current effusion is due to the sickle cell disease.

A variety of fibrillar materials can be seen in joint fluids. Some of these fibrils are fibrin, whereas others can be shown to be collagen from synovium or cartilage fragments.[13, 14] Such fibrils (and crystals) often can be seen better by lowering the condenser or closing the diaphragm to produce a partial phase effect. Both collagen and fibrin are faintly birefringent. Dark, irregularly shaped metal fragments can be seen in effusions of patients with implant arthroplasties.[11] Polymer fragments might also be seen. The rare shards of ochronotic cartilage are yellow or ochre fragments with regular transmitted light microscopy[15] (Fig. 36–4; see color section at the front of this volume).

Large numbers of lipid droplets may be seen in

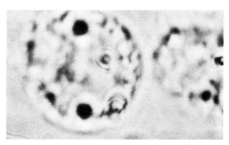

Figure 36–3. Synovial fluid leukocytes with cytoplasmic inclusions, "ragocytes," which have been felt to represent phagocytic vacuoles. Inclusions can appear pale or dark, depending on focus.

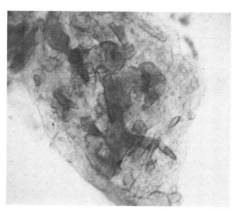

Figure 36–4. Shards of golden or ochre cartilage fragments embedded in detached synovium found floating in synovial fluid in a patient with ochronotic arthropathy.

traumatic arthritis,[16] in inflammatory effusions of various types, including some otherwise unexplained effusions, and in pancreatic fat necrosis,[17] or a few droplets can simply result from the arthrocentesis. In trauma, some lipid presumably comes from marrow and synovium. Bone spicules may be found if fracture into the joint has occurred. Such spicules tend to adhere to glass and must be sought carefully.[18]

Amorphous globular and irregular material, usually without birefringence, can be seen and can be due to amyloid masses[19] in patients with primary amyloid, multiple myeloma, and Waldenström's macroglobulinemia or in patients with chronic renal failure who are treated with dialysis regimens. Congo red stains this material pink or red on the wet preparation. Apple-green birefringence is seen with polarized light. Other shiny globular or coin-like clumps can be seen from apatite aggregates in joint and bursa fluids.[20] Clumps of apatites and other calcium-containing crystals can be stained red with alizarin red S as an additional screening aid.[21]

Crystals can be seen with regular light microscopy. Urate crystals are usually 2- to 20-μm long rods or needles. Calcium pyrophosphate crystals can be thin or thick rods or rhomboids, are rarely as long as urates, and may occasionally be best seen with regular light as they are often faintly birefringent. Oxalate crystals as a complication of renal failure can be pleomorphic but usually include some bipyramidal forms.[22] These and other crystals can be further differentiated with compensated polarized light.

Compensated Polarized Light Microscopy (Table 36–5).[23, 24] In a polarized light microscope, ordinary incandescent light is oriented in a single plane by a polarizer over the light source. When a second polarizer is added and rotated 90 degrees to the first, all light is blocked and the microscope field viewed through the ocular appears totally dark. If crystalline (birefringent) material is placed in the light path between the polarizers, light is deflected and split into fast and slow rays that vibrate at different angles from the incident light. The vibration planes of these two new rays are mutually perpendicular, but neither is parallel to the original ray of plane polarized light. Some of these rays now pass through the second polarizer (also termed the *analyzer*) and are brightly visible on the dark field. This brightness is common to all birefringent material.

In clinical use, different birefringent materials such as crystals can be distinguished in part by the altered behavior of light that passes through another birefringent structure (the *compensator*) placed between the first polarizer and the specimen. The compensator generally used is a first-order red plate, which eliminates green from the background and produces a rose-colored, instead of black, background field. The first-order red compensator quality and thickness can be expressed numerically as 540 nm. If the slow ray of a birefringent crystal is parallel to the slow ray from the compensator, the additive effect of a urate or pyrophosphate crystal creates a value of about 700 nm and a blue color. If the same crystal is now rotated 90 degrees so that its fast ray is parallel to the compensator's slow ray, a color subtraction of the same number of nanometers gives a yellow color.

Table 36–5. MORPHOLOGIC FEATURES OF SOME SYNOVIAL FLUID CRYSTALS ASSOCIATED WITH JOINT DISEASE

Crystals	Size (μm)	Morphology	Birefringence	Diseases
MSU	2–10	Needles, rods	Intensely negative	Acute and chronic gout
CPPD	2–10	Rhomboids, rods	Weakly positive	CPPD crystal deposition disease, osteoarthritis
Apatite-like clumps	5–20	Round, irregular clumps	None	Periarthritis, acute or chronic arthritis, osteoarthritis
Calcium oxalate	2–10	Polymorphic, dipyramidal shapes	Intensely or weakly positive	Renal failure
Cholesterol	10–80	Rectangles, often with missing corners, needles	Negative or positive	Chronic rheumatoid or osteoarthritic effusions
Depot glucocorticoids	4–15	Irregular rods, rhomboids	Intensely positive or negative	Iatrogenic postinjection flare
Lipid liquid crystals	2–8	Maltese crosses	Intensely positive	Acute arthritis, bursitis
Charcot-Leyden	17–25	Spindles	Positive and negative	Eosinophilic synovitis
Immunoglobulins	3–60	Polymorphic, rods	Positive and negative	Multiple myeloma, cryoglobulinemia

MSU = monosodium urate; CPPD = calcium pyrophosphate dihydiate.

Monosodium urate crystals can be differentiated from calcium pyrophosphate dihydrate (CPPD) crystals because with urate crystals the fast ray is in the long axis of the crystal, giving a yellow color when the crystal axis is parallel to the slow ray of the compensator. This is termed a *negative optical sign* or *negative elongation*. CPPD crystals have their slow ray in the long axis of the crystal; thus, when parallel to the axis of slow vibration of the compensator, they appear blue (positive elongation).

Monosodium urate crystals of gout tend to be brightly negatively birefringent (Fig. 36–5; see color section at the front of this volume). Crystals are generally identifiable within cells during active gouty arthritis. Crystals obtained from puncturing a tophus in a joint or elsewhere are often longer needles that are predominantly extracellular. Microtophi may occasionally be seen in tissue fragments found floating in the fluid. CPPD crystals have a weaker birefringence and positive elongation (Fig. 36–6; see color section at the front of this volume).

A variety of other birefringent materials are seen on polarized light examinations of joint fluids. Depot corticosteroid preparations are crystalline[25] and can contaminate fluids during injections or occasionally remain in joints or adjacent connective tissue for variable periods after local injections. These crystals can be phagocytized and occasionally induce a transient inflammation several hours after intra-articular injections (Fig. 36–7; see color section at the front of this volume). Corticosteroid crystals can appear as positively or negatively birefringent rods similar in size to urates or CPPD crystals, as granules, or as irregular debris.

Cholesterol crystals can be seen in chronic joint effusions, especially in RA.[26] Crystals are usually platelike with a notch in one corner (Fig. 36–8; see color section at the front of this volume) and larger than a cell, but crystals in cholesterol-laden effusions can occasionally also be needles with negative elongation. Some lipid droplets appear as positively birefringent Maltese crosses,[27] and these may be phlogistic in some cases.

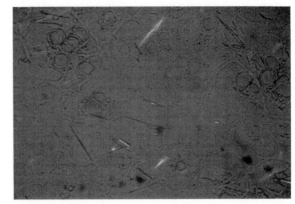

Figure 36–5. Monosodium urate crystals from a gouty synovial fluid as viewed with compensated polarized light. The crystals are yellow parallel to the axis of slow vibration marked on the compensator (negative birefringence).

Calcium hydrogen phosphate dihydrate crystals are brightly positively birefringent and have been identified in joint fluids and tissues.[28] These crystals might be confused with CPPD and can best be definitely differentiated by x-ray diffraction. Apatite crystal clumps occasionally have some birefringence. Spindle-shaped Charcot-Leyden crystals can be seen in fluids with eosinophils. Rarely, cryoglobulin (or other immunoglobulins), hemoglobin, and hematoidin derived from RBCs can be a cause of joint fluid crystals.

Most other irregular birefringent material is artifact, such as dust from the slide or glass fragments from the coverslip. Powder from rubber gloves is birefringent and generally shows a Maltese cross appearance. Artifactual needle-shaped or irregular crystals can develop in time, so prompt examination of fluid is important. Erroneous use of an ethylenediaminetetraacetic acid, oxalate,[29] or lithium heparin[30] anticoagulant can introduce anticoagulant-derived crystals. Such crystals can be phagocytized by WBCs in vitro and can thus be seen intracellulary.

Commercial polarizing microscopes are readily available and should generally be used.[20] One can

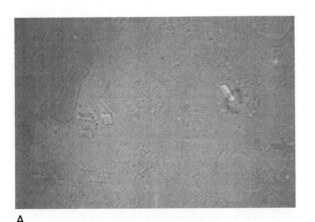

A

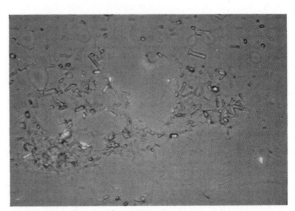

B

Figure 36–6. CPPD crystals can be needle, rod, or rhomboid shaped but usually have blunt ends (*A*). They often have fainter birefringence than is seen with urates (*B*). CPPD are blue when aligned longitudinally with the axis of slow vibration of the compensator (positive birefringence).

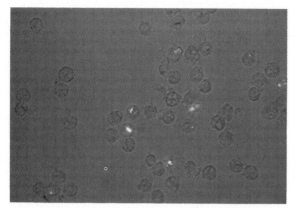

Figure 36–7. Triamcinolone acetonide (Aristospan) crystals phagocytized by synovial fluid cells after intra-articular injection.

also obtain polarizing filters to be inserted in a regular light microscope. One filter is placed between the light source and condenser; another is placed above the objective or in the eyepiece. Filters are rotated until a black field is obtained. This produces the white birefringence that shows crystals more easily than ordinary light but cannot separate positive and negative birefringence. An effect similar to that obtained with a commercial compensated polarizing microscope can be achieved by applying two layers of cellophane tape to the top of a clean glass slide and placing this over the polarizing filter above the light source.[31] The long axis of the slide then is substituted for the axis of slow vibration of the first-order red compensator. Tapes that appear semi-opaque before use do not appear to work. Before using such a setup, findings should be clinically compared on several crystals with findings obtained with a commercial compensator.

Absolutely definitive diagnosis of crystals can be made by x-ray diffraction, but sufficient numbers of crystals are needed for this. Uricase digestion may be helpful in that urates but not other crystals are digested with uricase.[32] Fortunately, this is rarely required. Occasionally crystals of urate or CPPD are so few or so small that they are detected only by electron microscopy.[33] Urate crystals are dissolved out in usual electron microscopic preparations, leaving only typical clefts, but CPPD crystals are not. Individual apatite crystals can only be seen by electron microscopy. Electron diffraction or electron probe elemental analysis can be done on apatites and other basic calcium phosphates.[1] Atomic force microscopy is being tested to identify crystals by their surface molecular structure. Infrared spectroscopy using Fourier's transformation or electron microscopy can identify small amounts of crystals mixed with other predominant crystals.

Dried Smears for Staining. Synovial smears are made using one or two drops of heparinized fluid on slides in the same manner as with peripheral blood smears. If the WBC count is greater than approximately 2500 per mm[3], a good smear can generally be made from the whole fluid. Fluids with lower counts often produce better smears if the fluid is cytocentrifuged or centrifuged and the button is resuspended in a few drops of the supernatant before smearing. Smears should be allowed to air dry and can be stained the same day or the next. Some fluids with very few cells can be best examined for cellular features in a wet preparation with a supravital stain.[34]

Wright's stain is the single most useful stain.[35, 36] Smears should be examined briefly under low magnifications to look for such findings as lupus erythematosus cells. Lupus erythematosus cells have so far been reported frequently in SLE and only rarely in RA, but they need not be present in typical SLE. Cartilage and synovial fragments may be seen and should be examined for any characteristic changes such as tophi. Iron-laden chondrocytes have been seen in cartilage fragments in hemochromatosis. Brown-pigmented debris or cytoplasmic granules can be seen in ochronosis. Bone marrow spicules with fat cells or other marrow elements may also be seen.

The smear is next examined carefully under oil immersion. Cells can be fairly easily separated into polymorphonuclear leukocytes (PMNs), macrophages, small lymphocytes, and large mononuclear cells. The latter probably include some transformed lymphocytes, monocytes, natural killer cells, and synovial lining cells. Although classification of individual large mononuclear cells may be difficult, it may be worth attempting, since transformed lymphocytes tend to be seen in RA and not in acute gout or pseudogout.[35] Most other diseases have received insufficient study. Atypical lymphocytes with nuclear indentations have been seen in HTLV-1–associated arthritis.[37] Synthetic-type synovial lining cells (Fig. 36–9; see color section at the front of this volume) typically are 20 to 40 μm in diameter, with an eccentric nucleus that occupies less than half of the cytoplasm. Some large monocyte-derived cells are similar in size, although they often have larger nuclei. Other large cells (15 to 25 μm in diameter) that have nuclei filling most of the cytoplasm are the transformed lymphocytes or lymphoblasts (Fig. 36–10; see color section at the front of this volume). Both the lining cells and lymphoblasts often have prominent

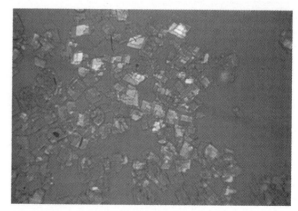

Figure 36–8. Cholesterol crystals from a chronic rheumatoid olecranon bursal effusion. These are most often flat plates with notched corners.

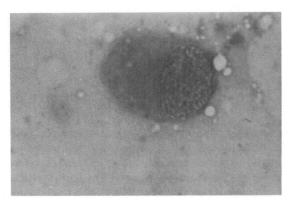

Figure 36–9. Synovial lining cell. The prominent homogeneous blue cytoplasm is typical of type B or synthetic cells. Other large cells with a nucleus:cytoplasm ratio of less than 50 percent have vacuolated cytoplasm and are either phagocytic lining cells or large monocytes (macrophages).

nucleoli. Mononuclear cells in joint fluid can now also be classified by monoclonal antibodies, and there are preliminary suggestions that this may be helpful in diagnosis.[38] The percentage of PMNs is helpful in distinguishing some diseases (see Table 36–1). Even among noninflammatory fluids, higher percentages of PMNs should raise consideration that one is seeing crystal-associated disease between acute attacks or another low-grade inflammatory disease.[34] Among the inflammatory effusions, lower PMN counts have been seen in some early RA, SLE, rheumatic fever, scleroderma, and fungal and other chronic infections. Recent studies suggest that drugs may account for some variation in joint fluid differentials, with use of nonsteroidal anti-inflammatory drugs alone being associated with the presence of more lymphocytes in the fluid.[39] Lining cells or large monocytes can be seen to have phagocytized PMNs in a variety of diseases in which there is both exudation of neutrophils and lining cell proliferation. Such cells are common in Reiter's syndrome but are by no means diagnostic (Fig. 36–11). Typical plasma cells with or without Russell's body cytoplasmic inclusions are uncommon but have been suggested to be more

common in reactive or psoriatic arthritis,[40] as have cells in mitosis. Mast cells can be seen in RA and probably other diseases but require toluidine blue or other special staining. Multinucleated cells can be seen in pigmented villonodular synovitis and multicentric reticulohistiocytosis but also occasionally in RA, osteoarthritis, and other states. Dark purple inclusions in phagocytic cells can be from cell debris but also can be clumps of apatite crystals. Bacteria can occasionally be seen in cells, even with Wright's stain. Urate or CPPD crystals can often be seen in Wright-stained specimens, although the urates are dissolved out of some smears.

Eosinophils are uncommon in differential counts but have been reported after arthrography with just air or contrast medium, in angioedema, in parasitic diseases, in tumors, after radiation, in RA, and in hypereosinophilic syndrome but also occasionally in a variety of other effusions, including infections such as Lyme disease[41] and in rheumatic fever. Malignant cells can occasionally be identified in synovial fluid with Wright's or Papanicolaou's stain or immunocytochemistry.[36, 42]

Smears for Gram's stain are made as for Wright's stain. Bacteria can be quickly classified into broad groups, but mucin and cell debris artifacts can be confusing. The absence of bacteria on Gram's stain is much too common in infection and does not exclude the possibility of a septic joint. Kinyoun carbofulchsin stain may be helpful in evaluation of possible tuberculosis, but culture and synovial biopsy are often needed. A periodic acid–Schiff (PAS) stain may show deposits in synovial macrophages in Whipple's disease. A Prussian blue stain can identify iron in synovial lining cells in pigmented villonodular synovitis or in hemochromatosis.

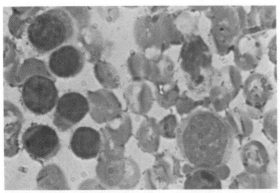

Figure 36–10. Synovial fluid small lymphocytes with one activated lymphocyte, the larger cell with nucleus filling most of the cytoplasm.

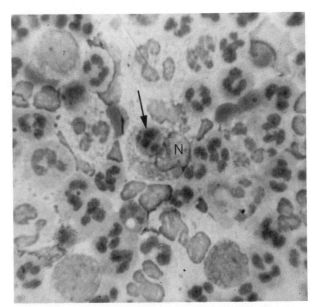

Figure 36–11. "Reiter's cell." This is a phagocytic mononuclear cell with its nucleus marked (*N*) that has phagocytized a polymorphonuclear leukocyte (*arrow*) with a pyknotic nucleus.

Special Tests

Mucin Clot Test. The mucin clot test[43] is largely of historical interest. Several drops of synovial fluid are added to about 20 ml of 5 percent acetic acid in a small beaker. Normal or osteoarthritis fluid forms a firm mass that does not fragment on shaking. A poor clot, such as those that result from many inflammatory effusions, fragments easily. A poor clot generally indicates both dilution and destruction of hyaluronate protein (see Table 36–1).

Proteoglycans. Actual measurements of hyaluronate or of sulfated glycosaminoglycans presumably derived from cartilage can be made but do not yet convincingly correlate with any clinical findings.[44]

Glucose. Synovial fluid glucose if measured should be done simultaneously on fasting serum and synovial fluid for comparison.[43] Synovial fluid glucose concentration is normally slightly less than that of blood. Equilibration between blood and synovial fluid after a meal is slow and unpredictable so that fasting levels are most reliable. Effusions for glucose should be placed in a fluoride tube to stop glucose metabolism in vitro by the synovial fluid leukocytes. A very low level of glucose in the synovial fluid suggests joint infection. Most effusions in RA have a synovial fluid glucose level of less than half that of the blood, and some are as low as in infections.

Complement. Synovial fluid complement is predominantly of value when compared with serum levels and with serum and synovial fluid protein determinations.[45] Fluid must be centrifuged promptly and the supernatant stored at $-70°C$ if total hemolytic complement is to be measured. In RA, the serum complement level is usually normal, but the synovial fluid level is often less than 30 percent of this. In SLE and hepatitis, both serum and synovial fluid levels may be low. Synovial fluid complement levels in infectious arthritis, gout, and Reiter's syndrome may be high, but this is largely the result of elevated serum levels. Complement components C3 or C4 can also be measured by immunodiffusion in addition to or instead of hemolytic complement. Measurement of activation fragments such as C5a may be of more interest.[46] Synovial fluid complement level may be low in normal or noninflammatory fluids in which there is little escape of complement or other proteins into the joint space from the circulation.

Cultures. Prompt and careful culture of synovial fluid is important if there is any suspicion of infection. Most laboratories prefer that fluid is delivered immediately in the syringe rather than handled outside the microbiology laboratory. Try to obtain laboratory help in planning cultures needed for fastidious organisms.

Other Tests. Antinuclear antibodies, rheumatoid factor immunoglobulins, and other substances involved in immune reactions can be measured in synovial fluid, but these assays have so far added little to the studies described here. Antinuclear antibodies, and latex fixation tests for rheumatoid factor are occasionally positive in effusions when negative in the serum. However, the significance of such positive synovial fluids is not established. Several causes for false positive results for rheumatoid factor in synovial fluid have been described.[47] Immune complexes can be measured with a variety of techniques, but the implications are not clear.

Cytokines, their inhibitors, and other mediators can be measured in joint fluid but have not generally been clinically helpful. Some potential is suggested by studies such as those showing that soluble interkeukin-2 receptor levels parallel disease activity in RA.[48]

The pH of normal fluid is 7.4, and this is slightly lower in inflammation.[49] Joint fluid PO_2 also falls in many inflammatory conditions. This tends to correlate with severity of leukocytosis and also with synovial fluid volume, which may lower PO_2 by affecting blood flow to the joint.[50] Relative ischemia may also be a factor in RA. Total protein normally averages only 1.7 g per dl, but this rises with inflammation. Protein levels, however, have not been shown to be of any diagnostic value. Uric acid, electrolytes, and urea nitrogen tend to reflect the serum values. Fibrinogen and its products are normally absent, so that normal fluid does not clot on standing. Bence Jones kappa light chains have been demonstrated in amyloid arthropathy secondary to multiple myeloma.

Gas chromatography on synovial fluid has been suggested as an aid in identifying bacterial products in culture-negative infections.[51] Elevated synovial fluid lactic acid measurements have been found in untreated nongonococcal septic arthritis. Succinic acid levels are also elevated in septic arthritis and tend to persist even after treatment. Neither lactic nor succinic acid is specific for infection but may complement other tests for early diagnosis of infectious arthritis. Bacterial antigens can also be sought in synovial fluid by counterimmunoelectrophoresis, and recently developed molecular probes can detect DNA or RNA sequences of a growing list of organisms.[52, 53]

SYNOVIAL BIOPSY AND PATHOLOGY

Biopsy of the synovial membrane should be considered in patients in whom the diagnosis is not clear after clinical evaluation. Synovial fluid analysis should generally be performed before consideration of a biopsy if a synovial effusion can be aspirated. Examination of synovial tissue may be the only way to make a definite diagnosis in some infectious, infiltrative, and deposition diseases of joints such as granulomatous infections, sarcoidosis, osteochondromatosis, the rare synovial leukemia or other malignancy, multicentric reticulohistiocytosis, pigmented villonodular synovitis, hemochromatosis, Whipple's disease, ochronosis, and amyloidosis. Although the diagnosis of gout or pseudogout is best made by joint fluid analysis, occasionally these or other crystals are first found in synovial membrane when joint fluid is absent or not noted to contain crystals.[54]

Synovial membrane findings of villous proliferation, superficial fibrin, marked lining cell increase, focal necrosis, plasma cells, and lymphoid follicles may strongly suggest RA but are not specific. In RA, as with several other systemic rheumatic diseases, diagnosis is often made by accumulation of criteria. A synovial biopsy showing a definite inflammatory process may help, as, for example, in the previous American Rheumatism Association (ARA) diagnostic criteria.[55] Even if not giving a definite diagnosis, by illustrating the presence or absence of inflammation, synovial biopsy may help guide symptomatic treatment. Synovial fluid findings can help in the same way, but both inflammatory and infiltrative synovial membrane lesions are not infrequently found with noninflammatory effusions.[56] About 35 percent of needle biopsies performed in diagnostic problems are of clinical assistance.[56]

Methods for Obtaining Synovium

Needle Biopsy. Probably the most popular technique for diagnostic synovial biopsy is use of the 14-gauge Parker-Pearson needle[56] (Fig. 36–12) for closed synovial biopsy. Needle synovial biopsy can be performed in the hospital or in the clinic or office. The knee is by far the most frequent joint to undergo biopsy, but synovial tissue can also be obtained successfully from shoulders, elbows, wrists, ankles, olecranon bursae, and occasionally even smaller joints if they are sufficiently swollen. The route of entry is generally that described for arthrocentesis. The procedure can be performed by a single operator with one assistant. Meperidine is occasionally used for anxious patients; young children may even need general anesthesia. The biopsy area is widely prepared with soap and then iodine and is washed with alcohol. The operator then dons gloves and drapes a transparent plastic drape with a 2-inch hole over the biopsy site. The skin and subcutaneous tissue are infiltrated to the capsule with 1 percent lidocaine, using a 25-gauge needle. Caution is exercised to avoid instilling anesthetic into the joint space, which would distort the findings of the synovial fluid analysis. Next, a 20-gauge needle is passed through the anesthetized area into the joint space. Fluid is aspirated for analysis. Two to 4 ml of 1 percent lidocaine can be instilled into the joint space, but biopsy can also be done without this if it is believed important to avoid any possible artifact that might be introduced by the local anesthetic. As the needle is withdrawn, lidocaine can be infiltrated into the needle track. The trochar is inserted and the biopsy needle is inserted through it. The side with the hooked notch is approximated against the synovium, and suction is applied with a 20-ml Luer-Lok syringe. The needle is always directed away from the site of initial lidocaine infiltration, to avoid possible artifacts in this area. Five to eight specimens (to minimize sampling error) from the various parts of the joint are taken by angling the needle without reinserting

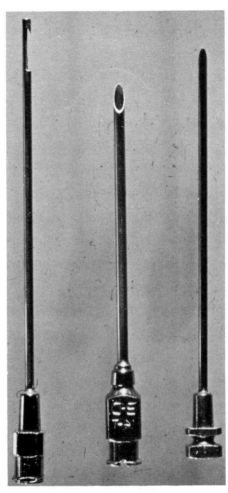

Figure 36–12. Parker-Pearson synovial biopsy needle. The hooked biopsy needle on the left is inserted through the center 14-gauge needle, and tissue is drawn into the notch proximal to the hook by suction.

the outer needle. Suction is maintained with one hand on the syringe while the other retracts the inner needle through the outer with a slight twist. One must become familiar with the appearance of the specimens, so as not to mistake fibrin or necrotic material (yellow-white) for synovial tissue (pink). Specimens may be transferred carefully from the needle to the fixative on a small piece of sterile paper by a 25-gauge needle. Patients are instructed to rest the joints until the following day, when they are permitted to resume usual activity, provided no increased pain or swelling has been noted. Hemarthrosis and infection are rare complications. To avoid needle tips' breaking off in the joint,[57] care must be taken before biopsy to check that the needle fits easily through the trochar and that the tip is not bent or weakened. Other needles that have been used for synovial biopsy are those of Cope, Williamson and Holt,[58] and Franklin and Silverman.[59]

Other Methods of Synovial Biopsy

Arthroscopy. Arthroscopy has the advantage of identifying discrete localized lesions, which can then undergo biopsy with a needle technique under direct visualization. The procedure is generally limited to larger joints, although thinner arthroscopes can even be used in digits (see Chapter 38).

Open Surgical Biopsy. If one is concerned about the possibility of focal granulomas or tumors, deeper lesions such as a vasculitis in larger capsular vessels, or other lesions that might have been missed on needle biopsy, open surgical biopsy can be considered. Surgical biopsy is also useful at small joints not suitable for needle biopsy. A small incision over a metacarpophalangeal joint is effective and offers virtually no morbidity. Open biopsy even of a knee can be done with a small incision. If one wants the advantage of the full joint exploration, however, a large surgical incision and some postoperative immobilization are obviously needed.

Found Fragments of Synovial Membrane. Synovial membrane fragments can occasionally be found floating in joint fluid after arthrocentesis. These can be examined in a wet smear for crystals and can also be collected by centrifugation and fixed for processing as with any biopsy specimen.

Specimens from Previous Procedures. Tissue from a previous carpal tunnel release, meniscectomy, or other exploration may be reviewed and found to contain helpful information. Even clinically uninvolved joints may have significant inflammatory changes in RA.[60]

Methods of Handling Tissue

The multiple small pieces of synovium from needle biopsy or the large specimens obtained at operation should be distributed among several methods of handling, depending on the questions being asked. Specimens for routine light microscopy are placed into neutral buffered formalin. Some slides should be stained with hematoxylin and eosin and other tissue saved for consideration of special stains. If gout is a possibility, a portion of the biopsy should be placed in absolute alcohol, since urates are water-soluble. Specimens then should be processed without water and stained with the DeGolantha stain for urate; unstained sections can be examined with compensated polarized light. Frozen sections of unfixed specimens can also be used for polarized light examination for urates.

Immunofluorescent or other immunocytochemical study of synovium has not been of any convincing clinical value but is of research interest. Studies have suggested that demonstration of prominent extravasated immunoglobulins may favor the diagnosis of RA.[61] Detailed characterization of mononuclear cell subsets is still under study. Specimens for such study should be placed in saline until transferred to OCT compound (Miles Inc., Elkhart, IN) on a cryostat chuck, which is then quick-frozen by immersion in liquid nitrogen.

Electron microscopy of synovium is also largely of research interest. For example, it can show still

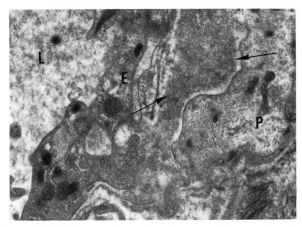

Figure 36–13. Electron-dense deposit (*arrows*) in vessel wall of synovium of patient with rheumatoid arthritis of recent onset. E = vascular endothelium, L = lumen, P = pericyte. Electron micrograph (16,000 ×).

unexplained electron-dense deposits in vessel walls in early RA[62] and in palindromic rheumatism[63] and also in the syndrome of hypertrophic pulmonary osteoarthropathy[64] (Fig. 36–13). Of more immediate value, electron microscopy may be a major diagnostic aid in identifying apatite crystals (Fig. 36–14), viruses including human immunodeficiency virus,[65] small amounts of amyloid, bacilliform bodies of Whipple's disease, chlamydial elementary bodies in Reiter's syndrome,[66] Lyme spirochetes,[67] and Gaucher's cell tubules. Any specimen for electron microscopy should be placed immediately in a fixative such as 3

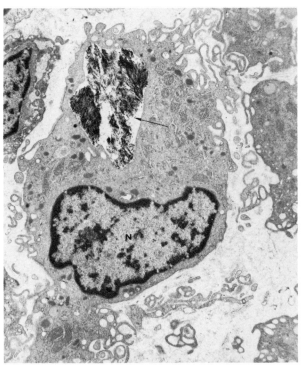

Figure 36–14. Apatite crystals (*arrows*) in vacuole of a synovial lining cell in a patient with osteonecrosis of the knee. N = nucleus of cell. Electron micrograph (17,000 ×).

percent glutaraldehyde or half-strength paraformaldehyde glutaraldehyde. Specimens should be minced into 0.5 × 0.5–mm pieces, ideally fixed for up to 4 hours, and then switched into a buffer before processing. Specimens for research involving immunocytochemical electron or light microscopic studies are best handled by gentle fixation in 1 percent glutaraldehyde for only 1 hour or by quick-freezing, respectively. Tissue for molecular probes or polymerase chain reaction is also quick-frozen.

Culture of synovial membrane can sometimes be more useful than that of synovial fluid, especially with mycobacteria, fungi, and gonococci. Synovial membrane can also be grown in tissue culture for investigative purposes. Biopsy specimens so designated are placed promptly in tissue culture medium and taken to the laboratory.

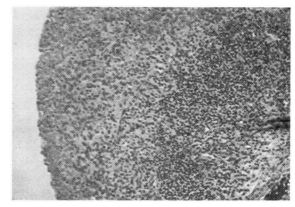

Figure 36–16. Rheumatoid arthritis synovium showing many layers of synovial lining cells on the left and infiltration of lymphocytes and plasma cells on the right. × 100. Hematoxylin and eosin stain.

Findings on Light Microscopic Examination of Synovial Biopsy Specimens

Normal. Normal synovial membrane (Fig. 36–15; see color section at the front of this volume) consists of one or two layers of synovial lining cells overlying a richly vascular areolar or fibrous connective tissue. A biopsy specimen that contains several pieces of normal synovium does not absolutely exclude intra-articular disease but should direct the search toward focal disease or extrasynovial processes. Failure to identify a characteristic lesion does not exclude diagnosable diseases. For example, gouty, tuberculous, or ochronotic synovium can show only mild proliferation or changes indistinguishable from those of RA in tissue adjacent to a tophus, granuloma, or typical pigmented shard.

Rheumatoid Arthritis and Spondylarthropathies. In RA, the combination of villous hypertrophy, lining cell proliferation, infiltration by lymphocytes and plasma cells (Fig. 36–16; see color section at the front of this volume) with a tendency to form lymphoid nodules, fibrin deposition, and focal necrosis

is typical. This is not diagnostic, similar changes being sometimes seen in SLE and other diseases. Especially in RA of recent onset, all the aforementioned findings may not be present, and vascular occlusion or mild vasculitis may be especially prominent.[62] Rheumatoid nodules are seen only rarely in synovium. There may be multinucleated giant cells beneath the lining cells. Effects of drugs on findings are just beginning to be studied but must be taken into consideration.[68]

Psoriatic arthritis and ankylosing spondylitis can show synovial changes indistinguishable from those in RA; large numbers of plasma cells are actually more common in spondylitis than in RA.[69] Early Reiter's syndrome has a typical superficial congestion and PMN infiltration, which can, however, also be seen in some patients with early RA, familial Mediterranean fever, Behçet's disease, and enteritis, as well as other conditions. Synovium from patients with chronic Reiter's syndrome is indistinguishable from that of patients with RA.

Collagen–Vascular Diseases. The synovial membrane in SLE typically shows less intense lining cell hyperplasia and less leukocyte infiltration than in RA,[70] although, as noted, inflammation may occasionally mimic RA. In polyarteritis, synovial inflammation is usually mild, and inflammatory cell infiltration of medium-sized vessel walls is only a rare finding.[71] Early scleroderma[72] shows sparse lining cells, superficial fibrin, and chronic inflammatory cell infiltration (Fig. 36–17; see color section at the front of this volume). Similar findings with paucity of lining cells can be seen also in some SLE, polymyositis, rheumatic fever, and some infections. In later scleroderma, synovial fibrin and fibrosis predominate.

Infectious Arthritis and Sarcoidosis. Infection is one of the types of joint disease that can be definitively diagnosed by synovial biopsy.[73] In acute bacterial arthritis, clusters or sheets of neutrophils can be seen (Fig. 36–18). Bacteria can sometimes be demonstrated in synovium with a tissue Gram's stain. Cultures may be positive on synovial biopsy

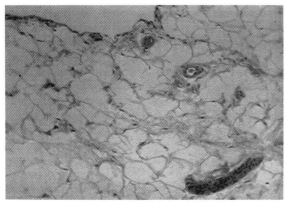

Figure 36–15. Normal synovial membrane of the knee. There is a single layer of flattened synovial cells overlying areolar connective tissue. Note the small synovial vessels immediately under the lining layer and the larger vessel in the lower right corner. × 100. Hematoxylin and eosin stain.

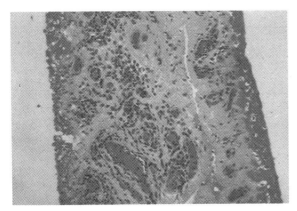

Figure 36–17. Synovial membrane in early scleroderma shows massive superficial fibrin, loss of lining cells, and infiltration with lymphocytes and plasma cells. × 100. Hematoxylin and eosin stain.

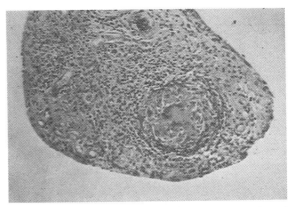

Figure 36–19. Granuloma in superficial synovium in tuberculous arthritis. Some superficial granulomas such as this one do not show caseation. There is also scattered chronic inflammatory cell infiltration. × 100. Hematoxylin and eosin stain.

specimens when they have been negative on blood and synovial fluid.[74] In chronic or resolving infections, there are often large numbers of lymphocytes and plasma cells.

Chronic infections such as tuberculosis and fungus disease can produce focal lesions that may be missed on limited biopsies. Mycobacterial granulomas in the superficial synovium do not always show caseation (Fig. 36–19; see color section at the front of

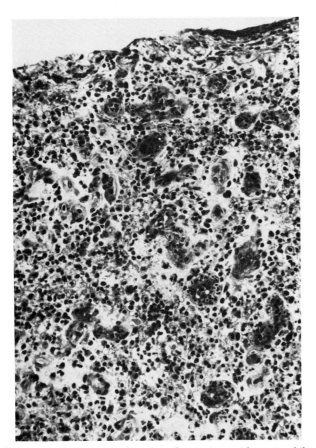

Figure 36–18. Massive infiltration of synovium with neutrophils and some lymphocytes in untreated septic arthritis of 10 days' duration. Hematoxylin and eosin stain (100 ×).

this volume). Kinyoun stains can show acid-fast organisms. Staining for fungi should be attempted with Grocott-Gomori and Gridley's stains. Spirochetes can be sought in Lyme disease and secondary syphilis with fluorescent and silver stains or with electron microscopy. Monoclonal antibodies and molecular probes can also identify many organisms.[75] Sarcoidosis can involve the synovium with typical granulomas[76]; other patients, however, especially those with erythema nodosum, more often have predominantly periarthritis or only scattered lymphocytes in the synovium.

Infiltrative and Deposition Diseases. Infiltrative and deposition diseases have specific findings that are amenable to diagnosis by synovial biopsy.

Crystal-Induced Arthritis. Both gout and pseudogout often have tophus-like deposits in synovial membrane (Fig. 36–20; see color section at the front of this volume). Precautions for tissue handling to demonstrated urate tophi were described earlier. CPPD crystals are not as water-soluble but can be dissolved by decalcification in specimens submitted along with bone. Thus, pseudogout synovium occasionally can have lucent areas where crystals were

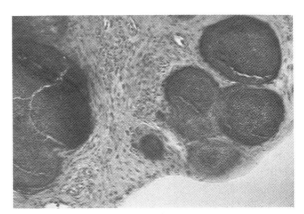

Figure 36–20. Tophus-like deposits in synovium containing positively birefringent crystals in pseudogout. × 100. Hematoxylin and eosin stain.

lost, as in gout. Usually only a fibrous capsule, a few histiocytes, and giant cells surround the tophi. In acute crystal-induced arthritis, there are areas of neutrophil infiltration; in chronic disease, however, large numbers of lymphocytes and plasma cells can be seen. Clumps of apatite crystals in synovium can appear as hematoxyphilic areas.[77] The tiny crystals that form these clumps are identifiable by electron microscopy. Oxalate crystals have also been found as pleomorphic birefringent bodies in the synovia of patients receiving hemodialysis for chronic renal failure.[78]

Amyloidosis. In patients with primary amyloidosis, multiple myeloma, and Waldenstrom's disease, amyloid may be deposited in the synovium. It appears pink on hematoxylin and eosin stain, and red with Congo red. The Congo red–stained material has an apple-green birefringence when viewed with plain polarized light.[79] Most amyloid has been on the synovial surface (Fig. 36–21; see color section at the front of this volume) and in the interstitium, but rarely in vessel walls. Synovial amyloid deposits can also complicate hemodialysis.[80]

Ochronosis. The synovial membrane in ochronosis is embedded with brownish shards from the friable cartilage[81] (Fig 36–22; see color section at the front of this volume). Macrophages adjacent to the cartilage fragments often contain pigment granules. Clusters of lymphocytes can be seen and can also be found in areas of synovium in other patients with cartilage degeneration, such as in primary or secondary osteoarthritis. Cartilage and bone fragments without the ochronotic pigment can also be seen embedded in synovium in osteoarthritis, RA, and other destructive arthropathies.[82]

Hemochromatosis. Golden brown hemosiderin pigment deposition in synovial lining cells and, to a lesser degree, in deeper phagocytes is characteristic of hemochromatosis[83] and other diseases with systemic iron overload. Iron in synovium from bleeding into the joint space or extravasation or erythrocytes into tissue produces hemosiderin mainly in deep macrophages. Iron stains blue with Prussian blue for

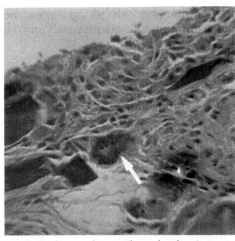

Figure 36–22. Dark, angular cartilage shards pigmented brown with homogentisic acid polymer are embedded in ochronotic synovium. Note also a giant cell *(arrow)* and mild proliferation of synovial lining cells. × 400. Hematoxylin and eosin stain.

confirmation (Fig. 36–23; see color section at the front of this volume). CPPD crystals can be seen in these synovia as well as in several other metabolic joint diseases.

Tumors. A variety of benign and malignant tumors or tumor-like conditions can involve the synovial membrane. Metastatic malignancies are occasionally identified in synovium.[84] Blast forms or overt lymphomatous cells have been found infiltrating synovium in a few, but by no means all, patients with leukemia or lymphoma and arthritis.[85] Monoclonal populations can be established by T cell–receptor gene rearrangement analysis.[86] Malignant synovioma is an extra-articular tumor that is rarely seen in joint synovium. Osteochondromas developing in synovium can be seen as foci of metaplasia to bone and chondrometaplasia in the synovial connective tissue. Pigmented villonodular synovitis, generally involving a single joint or tendon sheath, is characterized by giant cells, foamy cells, and hemosiderin deposits predominantly in the deep synovium (Fig. 36–24; see color section at the front of this volume). There is

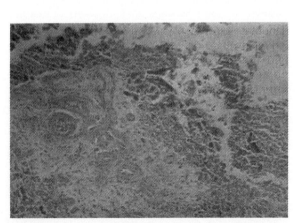

Figure 36–21. Amyloid arthritis as seen here in a patient with multiple myeloma is characterized by Congo red staining on the surface and sparing the synovial vessels (V). × 100. Congo red stain.

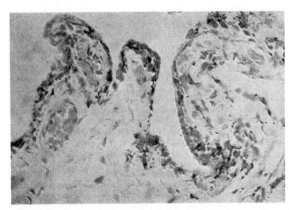

Figure 36–23. Iron stain of synovial membrane in idiopathic hemochromatosis shows blue (dark) staining predominantly in the lining cells. × 100. Prussian blue stain.

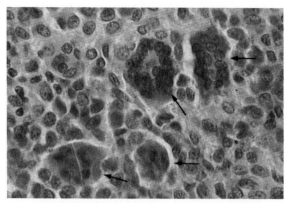

Figure 36–24. Pigmented villonodular synovitis is characterized by golden brown hemosiderin in deep macrophages, giant cells (marked by arrows), monotonous proliferation of deep cells with pale nuclei, and, not illustrated here, foam cells, lining cell hyperplasia (dark), and villous proliferation. × 400. Hematoxylin and eosin stain. (Courtesy of Schumacher, H. R.: Semin. Arthritis Rheum. 12:32, 1982.)

villous or nodular proliferation with areas also showing some lymphocytes and plasma cells.

Other Diseases. *Multicentric reticulohistiocytosis*[87] shows extensive infiltration of synovium with large foamy cells or multinucleated cells with eosinophilic ground-glass cytoplasm. *Whipple's disease* synovial membrane often shows just mild lining cell hyperplasia and scattered lymphocytes and neutrophils, but PAS-positive macrophages can be seen in some cases to suggest the diagnosis.[88] Electron microscopy can show suggestions of bacilliform bodies.[89] Despite large painful effusions, early *hypertrophic osteoarthropathy* tends to have virtually no inflammatory cell infiltration in synovium but marked vascular congestion.[64] In chronic hypertrophic osteoarthropathy, infiltration is reported. *Scurvy* of the synovium shows edema, estravasation of erythrocytes, and large fibrocytes that have been unable to release their collagen precursors because of the lack of vitamin C.[90] A *familial arthropathy* with synovial coating with fibrin-like material and giant cells has been described in children.[91] Synovium in *sickle cell disease* can show obliterated vessels and occasionally some lymphocyte and plasma cell infiltration.[92]

Exogenous particles such as thorns or animal spines can occasionally penetrate into joints and be visible in biopsy specimens; they can also produce a chronic synovitis.[93] Lead particles from bullets have been identified in joints. Metallic or silicone prosthetic particles or polymethacrylate cement in patients with joint arthroplasties or prosthetic ligaments can also commonly be found embedded in synovium.[94, 95]

Synovial fat necrosis and lipid-laden macrophages can be associated with *pancreatic disease*.[96] Rare, unexpected new findings occasionally are encountered if biopsy is done in undiagnosed cases. For example, an eosinophilic infiltration with fibrin deposition was found in a patient later determined to have the *hypereosinophilic syndrome*.[97]

Conclusions. Synovial biopsy specimens obtainable by a variety of mechanisms can give specific diagnoses in some diseases or can provide additional criteria to support diagnoses in other situations. Future studies of synovium should continue to provide important ideas about pathogenesis and therapy. Careful consideration of the questions to be asked before performing a diagnostic biopsy allows optimal handling of the tissue.[98]

References

Synovial Fluid Analysis

1. Schumacher, H. R., and Reginato, A. J.: Atlas of Synovial Fluid Analysis and Crystal Identification. Philadelphia, Lea & Febiger, 1991.
2. Gatter, R. A., and Schumacher H. R.: A Practical Handbook of Joint Fluid Analysis. 2nd ed. Philadelphia, Lea & Febiger, 1991.
3. Bomalaski, J. S., Lluberas, G., and Schumacher, H. R.: Monosodium urate crystals in the knee joints of patients with asymptomatic nontophaceous gout. Arthritis Rheum. 29:1480, 1986.
4. Eisenberg, J. M., Schumacher, H. R., Davidson, P. K., and Kaufmann, L.: Usefulness of synovial fluid analysis in the evaluation of joint effusions. Arch. Intern. Med. 144:715, 1984.
5. Schumacher, H. R., Sieck, M. S., Rothfuss, S., Clayburne, G. M., Baumgarten, D. F., Mochan, B. S., and Kant, J. A.: Reproducibility of synovial fluid analysis: A study among 4 laboratories. Arthritis Rheum. 29:770, 1986.
6. Schumacher, H. R., Sieck, M. S., and Clayburne, G.: Development and evaluation of a method for presentation of synovial fluid wet preparations for quality control testing of crystal identification. J. Rheumatol. 17:1369, 1990.
7. Kerolus, G., Clayburne, G., and Schumacher, H. R.: Is it mandatory to examine synovial fluids promptly after arthrocentesis? Arthritis Rheum. 32:271, 1989.
8. Hasselbacher, P.: Measuring synovial fluid viscosity with a white blood cell diluting pipette. Arthritis Rhuem. 19:1358, 1978.
9. Palmer, D. G.: Total leukocyte enumeration in pathologic synovial fluids. Am. J. Clin. Pathol. 49:812, 1968.
10. Hunter, T., Gordon, D. A., and Ogryzlo, M. A.: The ground pepper sign of synovial fluid: A new diagnostic feature of ochronosis. J. Rheumatol. 1:45, 1974.
11. Kitridou, R., Schumacher, H. R., Sbarbaro, J. L., and Hollander, J. L.: Recurrent hemarthrosis after prosthetic knee arthoplasty: Identification of metal particles in the synovial fluid. Arthritis Rheum. 12:520, 1969.
12. Hollander, J. L., McCarthy, D. J., and Rawson, A. J.: The "RA cell," "ragocyte," or "inclusion body cell." Bull. Rheum. Dis. 16:382, 1965.
13. Kitridou, R., McCarthy, D. J., Prokop, D. J., and Hummeler, K.: Identification of collagen in synovial fluid. Arthritis Rheum. 12:580, 1969.
14. Cheung, H. S., Ryan, L. M., Kozin, F., and McCarthy, D. J.: Identification of collagen subtypes in synovial fluid sediments from arthritic patients. Am. J. Med. 68:73, 1980.
15. Schumacher, H. R., and Holdsworth, D. E.: Ochronotic arthropathy. I. Clinicopathologic studies. Semin. Arthritis Rheum. 6:207, 1977.
16. Weinberg, A., and Schumacher, H. R.: Experimental joint trauma: Synovial response to blunt trauma and inflammatory response to intraarticular injection of fat. J. Rheumatol. 8:380, 1981.
17. Gibson, T., Schumacher, H. R., Pascual, E., and Brighton, C.: Arthropathy, skin and bone lesions in pancreatic disease. J. Rheumatol. 2:7, 1975.
18. Lawrence, C., and Seife, B.: Bone marrow in joint fluid: A clue to fracture. Ann. Intern. Med. 74:740, 1971.
19. Gordon, O. A., Pruzanski, W., and Orgyzlo, M. A.: Synovial fluid examination from the diagnosis of amyloidosis. Ann. Rheum. Dis. 32:428, 1973.
20. Schumacher, H. R., Somlyo, A. P., Tse, R. L., and Maurer, K.: Apatite crystal–associated arthritis. Ann. Intern. Med. 87:411, 1977.
21. Paul, H., Reginato, A. J., and Schumacher, H. R.: Alizarin red S staining as a screening test to detect calcium compounds in synovial fluid. Arthritis Rheum 26:191, 1983.
22. Reginato, A. J., and Kurnik, B. R. C.: Calcium oxalate and other crystals associated with kidney diseases and arthritis. Semin. Arthritis Rheum. 18:198, 1989.
23. Phelps, P, Steele, A. D., and McCarthy, D. J.: Compensated polarized light microscopy. J. A. M. A. 203:508, 1968.
24. Gatter, R. A.: Use of the compensated polarized microscope. Clin. Rheum. Dis. 3:91, 1977.
25. Kahn, C. B., Hollander, J. L., and Schumacher, H. R.: Corticosteroid crystals in synovial fluid. J. A. M. A. 211:807, 1970.

26. Zuckner, J., Uddin, J., Gantner, G., and Dorner, R. W.: Cholesterol crystals in synovial fluid. Ann. Intern. Med. 60:436, 1964.
27. Trostle, D. C., Schumacher, H. R., Medsger, T. A., and Kapoor, W. N.: Lipid microspherule-associated acute monoarticular arthritis. Arthritis Rheum. 29:1166, 1986.
28. Gaucher, A., Faure, G., Netter, P., Pourel, J., and Ducheille, J.: Identification des cristaux observes dans les arthropathies destructrices de la chondrocalcinose. Rev. Rheumatol. 44:407, 1977.
29. Schumacher, H. R.: Intracellular crystals in synovial fluid anticoagulated with oxalate. N. Engl. J. Med. 274:1372, 1966.
30. Tanphaichitr, K., Spielberg, I., and Hahn, B.: Lithium heparin crystals simulating calcium pyrophosphate dihydrate crystals in synovial fluid (Letter). Arthritis Rheum. 19:966, 1976.
31. Fagan, T. J., and Lidsky, M. D.: Compensated polarized light microscopy using cellophane adhesive tape. Arthritis Rheum. 17:256, 1974.
32. McCarthy, D. J., and Hollander, J. L.: Identification of urate crystals in gouty synovial fluid. Ann. Rheumatol. 54:452, 1961.
33. Honig, S., Gorevic, P., Hoffstein, S., and Weissman, G.: Crystal deposition disease: Diagnosis by electron microscopy. Am. J. Med. 63:161, 1977.
34. Louthrenoo, W., Sieck, M., Clayburne, G., et al.: Supravital staining of cells in non-inflammatory synovial fluids. J. Rheumatol. 18:409, 1991.
35. Traycoff, R. B., Pascual, E., and Schumacher, H. R.: Mononuclear cells in human synovial fluid: Identification of lymphoblasts in rheumatoid arthritis. Arthritis Rheum. 19:743, 1976.
36. Villanueva, T. G., and Schumacher, H. R.: Cytologic examination of synovial fluid. Diagn. Cytopathol. 3:141, 1987.
37. Ijich, S., Matsuda, T., Maruyama, I., et al.: Arthritis in a human T lymphotrophic virus type I (HTLV-I) carrier. Ann. Rheum. Dis. 49:718, 1990.
38. Poulter, L. W., Ai-Shakarchi, H. A. A., Campbell, F. D. R., Goldstein, A. J., and Richardson, A. T.: Immunocytology of synovial fluid cells may be of diagnostic and prognostic value in arthritis. Ann. Rheum. Dis. 45:584, 1986.
39. Bahremand, M., and Schumacher, H. R.: Effect of medication on synovial fluid leukocyte differentials in patients with rheumatoid arthritis. Arthritis Rheum. 34:1173, 1991.
40. Freemont, A. J., Denton, J., Chuck, A., et al.: Diagnostic value of synovial microscopy: A reassessment and rationalization. Ann. Rheum. Dis. 50:101, 1991.
41. Kay, J., Eichenfield, A., Arthreya, B., et al: Synovial fluid eosinophilia in Lyme disease. Arthritis Rheum. 31:1384, 1988.
42. Fam, A. G., Voornevelt, C., Robinson, J. B., et al.: Synovial fluid immunocytology in the diagnosis of leukemic synovitis. J. Rheumatol. 18:293, 1991.
43. Ropes, M. M., and Bauer, W.: Synovial Fluid Changes in Joint Disease. Cambridge, MA, Harvard University Press, 1953.
44. Silverman, B., Cawston, T. E., Page Thomas, D. P., et al.: The sulfated glycosaminoglycan levels in synovial fluid aspirates in patients with acute and chronic joint disease. Br. J. Rheumatol. 29:340, 1990.
45. Bunch, T. W., Hunder, G. G., McDiffie, F. C., O'Brien, P. C., and Markowtiz, H.: Synovial fluid complement determination as a diagnostic aid in inflammatory joint disease. Mayo Clin. Proc. 49:715, 1974.
46. Jose, P. J., Moss, I. K., Maini, R. N., and Williams, T. J.: Measurement of the chemotactic complement fragment C5a in rheumatoid synovial fluids by radioimmunoassay: Role of C5a in the acute inflammatory phase. Ann. Rheum. Dis. 49:747, 1990.
47. Seward, C. W., and Osterland, C. K.: The pattern of anti-immunoglobulin activities in serum, pleural and synovial fluids. J. Lab. Clin. Med. 81:230, 1973.
48. Moisse, C. P., Elhamiani, M., and Edmonds-Alt, X.: Functional studies of soluble low-affinity interleukin-2 receptors in rheumatoid synovial fluid. Arthritis Rheum. 33:1688, 1990.
49. Ward, T. T.: Acidosis of synovial fluid correlates with synovial fluid leukocytosis. Am. J. Med. 64:933, 1978.
50. Richman, A. L., Su, E. Y., and Ho, G.: Reciprocal relationship of synovial fluid volume and oxygen tension. Arthritis Rheum. 24:701, 1981.
51. Borenstein, D. G., Gibbs, C. A., and Jacobs, R. B.: Gas–liquid chromatographic analysis of synovial fluid. Arthritis Rheum. 25:947, 1982.
52. Rahman, M. U., Cheema, M. A., Schumacher, H. R., and Hudson, A. P.: Molecular evidence for the presence of Chlamydia in the synovium of patients with Reiter's syndrome. Arthritis Rheum. 35:521, 1992.
53. Vitanen, A. M., Arstila, T. P., Lahesmaa, R., et al.: Application of the polymerase chain reaction and immunofluorescence techniques to the detection of bacteria in yersinia-triggered reactive arthritis. Arthritis Rheum. 34:89, 1991.

Synovial Biopsy and Pathology

54. Agudelo, C., and Schumacher, H. R.: The synovitis of acute gouty arthritis. Hum. Pathol. 4:265, 1973.
55. Ropes, M. W., Bennett, G. A., Cobbs, S., et al.: 1958 revision of diagnostic criteria for rheumatoid arthritis. Arthritis Rheum. 2:16, 1959.
56. Schumacher, H. R., and Kulka, J. P.: Needle biopsy of the synovial membrane: Experience with the Parker-Pearson technique. N. Engl. J. Med. 286:416, 1972.
57. Bocanerga, T. S., McClelland, J. J., Germain, B. F., et al.: Intraarticular fragmentation of a new Parker-Pearson synovial biopsy needle. J. Rheumatol. 7:248, 1980.
58. Williamson, N., and Holt, L. P. T.: A synovial biopsy needle. Lancet 1:799, 1966.
59. Moon, M. S., and Kim, J. M.: Synovial biopsy by Franklin-Silverman needle. Clin. Orthop. 150:224, 1980.
60. Soden, M., Rooney, M., Cullen, A., et al.: Immunohistologic features in the synovium obtained from clinically uninvolved knee joints of patients with rheumatoid arthritis. Br. J. Rheumatol. 28:287, 1989.
61. Fritz, P., Laschner, W., Saal, J. G., et al.: Histological classification of synovitis. Zentralblatt Algemeine Pathol. Anat. 135:729 1989.
62. Schumacher, H. R.: Synovial membrane and fluid morphologic alterations in early rheumatoid arthritis: Microvascular injury and virus-like particles. Ann. N. Y. Acad. Sci. 256:39, 1975.
63. Schumacher, H. R.: Palindromic onset of rheumatoid arthritis: Clinical synovial fluid and biopsy studies. Arthritis Rheum. 25:361, 1982.
64. Schumacher, H. R.: The articular manifestations of hypertrophic pulmonary osteoarthropathy in bronchogenic carcinoma. Arthritis Rhuem. 19:629, 1876.
65. Bentin, J., Feremans, W., Pasteels, J. L., et al.: Chronic acquired immunodeficiency syndrome–associated arthritis: A synovial ultrastructural study. Arthritis Rheum. 33:268, 1990.
66. Schumacher, H. R., Magge, S., Cherian, P. V., et al.: Light and electron microscopic studies on the synovial membrane in Reiters' syndrome. Arthritis Rheum. 31:937, 1988.
67. Valesova, M., Tranvsky., K., Hulinska, D., et al.: Detection of Borrelia in the synovial tissue from a patient with Lyme borreliosis by electron microscopy. J. Rheumatol. 16:1502, 1989.
68. Haraoui, B., Pelletier, J. P., Clouther, J. M., et al.: Synovial membrane histology and immunopathology in rheumatoid arthritis and osteoarthritis: In vivo effects of antirheumatic drugs. Arthritis Rheum. 34:153, 1991.
69. Chang, C.-P., and Schumacher, H. R.: The synovium and synovial fluid in ankylosing spondylitis. Semin Arthritis Rheum. (in press).
70. Labowitz, R. and Schumacher, H. R.: Articular manifestations of SLE. Ann. Intern. Med. 74:911, 1974.
71. Smuckler, N. M., and Schumacher, H. R.: Chronic non-destructive arthritis associated with cutaneous polyarteritis. Arthritis Rheum. 20:1114, 1977.
72. Schumacher, H. R.: Joint involvement in progressive systemic sclerosis (scleroderma). Am. J. Clin. Pathol. 60:593, 1973.
73. Schumacher, H. R.: Joint pathology in infectious arthritis. Clin. Rheum. Dis. 4:33, 1978.
74. Wofsy, D.: Culture-negative septic arthritis and bacterial endocarditis: Diagnosis by synovial biopsy. Arthritis Rheum. 23:605, 1980.
75. Espinoza, L. R., Aguilar, J. L., Espinoza, C. G., et al: HIV-associated arthropathy: HIV demonstration in the synovial membrane. J. Rheumatol. 17:1195, 1990.
76. Sokoloff, L., and Bunim, J. J.: Clinical and pathological studies of joint involvement in sarcoidosis. N. Engl. J. Med. 260:841, 1959.
77. Reginato, A. J., and Schumacher, H. R.: Synovial calcification in a patient with collagen–vascular disease: Light and electron microscopic studies. J. Rheumatol. 4:261, 1977.
78. Hoffman, G. S., Schumacher, H. R., Paul, H., et al.: Calcium oxalate microcrystalline–associated arthritis in end-stage renal disease. Ann. Intern. Med. 97:36, 1982.
79. Canoso, J. J., and Cohen, A. S.: Rheumatological aspects of amyloid disease. Clin. Rheum. Dis. 1:149, 1975.
80. Bardin, T., Kuntz, D., Zingraff, J., et al.: Synovial amyloidosis in patients undergoing long-term hemodialysis. Arthritis Rheum. 28:1052, 1985.
81. Schumacher, H. R., and Holdsworth, D. E.: Ochronotic arthropathy. Semin. Arthritis Rheum. 6:207, 1977.
82. Resnick, D., Weisman, M., Goergan, T. G., and Feldman, P. S.: Osteolysis with detritic synovitis. Arch. Intern. Med. 138:1003, 1978.
83. Schumacher, H. R.: Ultrastructural characteristics of the synovial membrane in idiopathic hemochromatosis. Ann. Rheum. Dis. 31:465, 1972.
84. Goldenberg, D. L., Kelley, W., and Gibbons, R. B.: Metastatic adenocarcinoma of synovium presenting as an acute arthritis. Arthritis Rheum. 18:107, 1975.
85. Spilberg, I., and Myer, G. J.: The arthritis of leukemia. Arthritis Rheum. 15:630, 1972.
86. Yancey, W. B., Dolson, L. H., Oblon, D., et al.: HTLV-1 associated T-cell leukemia/lymphoma presenting with nodular synovial masses. Am. J. Med. 89:676, 1990.
87. Krey, P. R., Comerford, F. R., and Cohen, A. S.: Multicentric reticulohistocytosis. Arthritis Rheum. 17:615, 1974.
88. Delcambre, B., Luez, J., Leonardelli, J., et al.: Les manifestations articulaires de la maladie de Whipple. Semin. Hop. Paris 50:847, 1974.
89. Rubinow, A., Canoso, J. J., Goldenberg, D. L., and Cohen, A. S.: Synovial fluid and synovial membrane pathology in Whipple's disease. Arthritis Rheum. 19:820, 1976.

90. Bevilaqua, F. A., Hasselbacher, P., and Schumacher, H. R.: Scurvy and hemarthrosis. J. A. M. A. 235:1874, 1976.
91. Athreya, B., and Schumacher, H. R.: Pathologic features of a recently recognized form of familial arthropathy. Arthritis Rheum. 21:429, 1978.
92. Schumacher, H. R.: Rheumatological manifestations of sickle cell disease and other hereditary hemoglobinopathies. Clin. Rheum. Dis. 1:37, 1975.
93. Reginato, A. J., Ferreiro, J. L., O'Connor, O. R., et al.: Clinical and pathologic studies of 26 patients with penetrating foreign body injury to the joints, bursae and tendon sheaths. Arthritis Rheum. 33:1753, 1990.
94. Kitridou, R. C., Schumacher, H. R., Sbarbaro, J. L., and Hollander, J. L.: Recurrent hemarthrosis after knee arthroplasty. Arthritis Rheum. 12:520, 1969.
95. Christie, A. J., Pierre, G., and Levitan, J.: Silicon synovitis. Semin. Arthritis Rheum. 19:166, 1989.
96. Smuckler, N. M., Schumacher, H. R., Pascual, E., et al.: Synovial fat necrosis associated with ischemic pancreatic disease. Arthritis Rheum. 22:547, 1979.
97. Brogadir, S. P., Goldwein, M. I., and Schumacher, H. R.: A hypereosinophilic syndrome mimicking rheumatoid arthritis. Am. J. Med. 69:799, 1980.
98. Schumacher, H. R.: Exploring the synovium in 1990. Br. J. Rheumatol. 29:3, 1990.

Chapter 37
Imaging

Donald Resnick
Marie-Josée Berthiaume
David Sartoris

INTRODUCTION

The routine radiographic examination is a keystone in the diagnosis and management of the patient with articular disease. In some patients, the diagnosis may initially be suggested by standard radiographic films, whereas in other patients with a known clinical diagnosis, the extent and the severity of the disease process may be documented by such techniques. Furthermore, serial radiographic examinations provide evidence of the therapeutic response of the disease process. In this chapter, we discuss routine radiographic techniques and additional imaging methods, cardinal roentgen signs of articular disease, and the radiographic findings at specific "target" areas of the major articular disorders. As the major advances in imaging of musculoskeletal disorders in the last 5 years have involved computed tomography, (CT) and magnetic resonance (MR) techniques, these two methods are emphasized in this chapter.

IMAGING TECHNIQUES AND METHODS

Plain Film Examination. Appropriately selected plain films form the initial step in the radiographic evaluation of the articular disease. The choice of radiographic projections for each anatomic area is a decision that deserves careful consideration. The need for a comprehensive examination to document the extent and configuration of the disease process must be balanced with the consideration of expense, comfort, and radiation exposure to the patient, who may be expected to have numerous radiation examinations over many years.

In most instances, multiple radiographic projections of a number of joints are indicated. Table 37–1 lists the suggested radiographic projections for the optimal evaluation of specific anatomic areas. In the patient with monoarticular or pauciarticular disease, such a protocol may be followed closely. In the patient with polyarticular disease, however, obtaining the numerous radiographic views listed in Table 37–1 would be considered excessive in almost all instances. In these patients, the initial radiographic examination should be individually tailored to as great an extent as possible.

A "tailored" arthritis series is useful in those patients with polyarthritis who have either a known or a highly likely clinical diagnosis. In this setting, plain films are selected that most optimally show the major target areas of the disease as well as additional areas of clinical significance. For example, the patient with rheumatoid arthritis requires careful radiographic evaluation of the hands, wrists, feet, knees, shoulders, and cervical spine, whereas the patient with calcium pyrophosphate dihydrate (CPPD) crystal deposition disease usually requires analysis of only the hands, wrists, knees, and symphysis pubis.

The situation often arises in which a patient has polyarthritis without a specific clinical diagnosis. In this instance, a so-called standard arthritis series is useful; projections are selected to provide adequate visualization of a large number of major target areas with a minimum of radiation exposure. A suggested standard arthritis series, consisting of 15 radiographs, is listed in Table 37–2.

The follow-up radiographic examination obtained during the course of treatment need not be as extensive as the initial survey. In many instances it can be limited to a few symptomatic areas or areas where unsuspected progression of disease may lead to catastrophic consequences, such as the cervical spine in patients with rheumatoid arthritis.

Use of intensifying screen in a radiographic film cassette combined with double-emulsion radiographic film allows formation of a radiographic image with considerably less radiation exposure to the pa-

Table 37–1. RADIOGRAPHIC PROJECTIONS

Hand	Posteroanterior, oblique
Wrist	Posteroanterior, oblique, lateral
Elbow	Anteroposterior, lateral
Shoulder	Anteroposterior with internal rotation of the humerus; anteroposterior with external rotation of the humerus
Foot	Anteroposterior, oblique, lateral (including calcaneus)
Ankle	Anteroposterior, lateral
Knee	Anteroposterior, lateral, "tunnel" (anteroposterior in semiflexion), axial patellar ("sunrise")
Hip	Anteroposterior of pelvis, anteroposterior of hip with internal rotation of leg, anteroposterior of hip with external rotation of leg ("frog leg")
Sacroiliac joint	Anteroposterior, anteroposterior with 30 degrees cephalic angulation of central ray
Lumbar spine	Anteroposterior, obliques, lateral, lateral coned down to L5–S1
Thoracic spine	Anteroposterior, lateral
Cervical spine	Anteroposterior, obliques, lateral with neck in flexion, lateral with neck in extension, "open-mouth" odontoid view

Table 37–2. ARTHRITIS SURVEY

Area	Projection
Hand and wrist	Posteroanterior, obliques
Foot	Anteroposterior, obliques, lateral
Knee	Anteroposterior, lateral
Pelvis and hips	Anteroposterior
Thorax and shoulders	Anteroposterior
Cervical spine	Lateral with neck in flexion

tient. A small decrease in radiographic resolution, however, is the price paid for this considerable diminution in radiation exposure. Occasionally, in evaluating diseases such as rheumatoid arthritis, osteomyelitis, septic arthritis, or hyperparathyroidism, greater resolution may be important in establishing a diagnosis at an early stage.[1-3] In these instances, increased radiation exposure to a relatively radioresistant area of the body, such as the hand, the wrist, or the foot, may be acceptable for the important diagnostic information that is obtained. With virtually any radiographic unit, use of single-emulsion film and a nonscreen vacuum-packed cassette, refered to as the *mammographic technique,* allows high-resolution images to be obtained. Furthermore, optical or radiographic magnification can be extremely helpful. With the magnification technique, images may be obtained using microfocal spot radiographic tubes, such as are present on many angiographic units, or specially designed magnification units. It should be emphasized that these are specialized techniques and should be used only in selected clinical situations.

Radiographs of an articulation obtained during weight bearing or the application of stress or traction may provide valuable supplemental information to the plain film radiographic examination. Weight-bearing views of the knees are especially valuable in the evaluation of patients with osteoarthritis[4] and may allow a more exact delineation of cartilaginous loss as well as abnormal varus or valgus angulation of the joint. Stress radiographs may be used to assess soft tissue and bony stability following injury to the knee, ankle, acromioclavicular joint, or first metacarpophalangeal joint.[5] Upright lateral radiographs of the lumbar spine obtained after prolonged standing may accentuate bony neural arch defects (spondylolysis) or intervertebral slippage (spondylolisthesis). Radiographs of the pelvis obtained with the patient standing on one leg at a time may demonstrate instability of the sacroiliac joint or symphysis pubis.[6]

Radiographs obtained during application of traction across a joint also may prove useful in selected circumstances. Demonstration of subtle transchondral fractures in osteonecrosis of the femoral head may be improved with this technique.[7] Such traction may also stimulate the release of gas, primarily nitrogen, into the joint cavity, an occurrence that usually will rule out the presence of a joint effusion and allows visualization of a portion of the cartilaginous surface. This method is mostly used in children to rule out a septic arthritis.

Conventional Tomography. Conventional tomography can aid both in the identification of subtle abnormalities and in the more precise delineation of previously identified lesions. In some anatomic areas such as the temporomandibular joint (TMJ) and sternoclavicular and costovertebral articulations, plain radiographs are rarely adequate and conventional tomography is often indicated.

Arthrography and Bursography. Injection of radiopaque contrast material, air, or both, into a joint or bursa may be essential in evaluating a number of articular disorders.[8] Contrast arthrography is most often used in the knee and shoulder to identify surgically repairable soft tissue injuries such as meniscal or rotator cuff tears. Aspiration arthrography allows confirmation of suspected joint sepsis; fluoroscopically guided intra-articular needle placement is particularly useful in recovering fluid from deep articulations such as the glenohumeral joint or the hip. Subsequent instillation of a small amount of radiographic contrast agent allows verification that the joint space was indeed entered and may also yield important information concerning the extent of periarticular soft tissue destruction. An important indication for aspiration arthrography is evaluation of the patient with a painful total hip or knee prosthesis to differentiate conclusively between chronic infection and aseptic loosening of the prosthesis.[9] Air arthrography, usually combined with conventional tomography, often is of great value in the identification of transchondral fractures and intra-articular osteocartilaginous bodies. Arthrography also may provide a firm diagnosis in cases of pigmented villonodular synovitis[10] or idiopathic synovial osteochondromatosis.[11] Finally, arthrography can serve as a method of treatment with the "brisement" procedure, or distension arthrography in cases of adhesive capsulitis, in which the articular capsule is progressively distended with a mixture of lidocaine or bupivacaine hydrochloride and steroids until the capsule ruptures or relief of symptoms is obtained.

Bursography has its greatest value in evaluating lesions of the subacromial bursa in the shoulder.[12, 13] In this location, bursitis, intrabursal osteocartilaginous bodies, partial rotator cuff tears, and causes of shoulder impingement may be identified. At the same time, instillation of local anesthetic agents or anti-inflammatory medications directly into the bursa can serve both diagnostic and therapeutic purposes.

Computed Tomography

Introduction and Technical Considerations. In an age in which MR imaging is increasingly being employed, CT remains an excellent investigative tool for musculoskeletal disorders used either solely or in combination with MR. CT permits cross-sectional images to be displayed with excellent structural definition of both soft tissues and bones. In most circumstances, CT scans provide more than sufficient information and obviate any other imaging examination. Nevertheless, significant drawbacks limit its performance. For instance, artefacts caused by the presence of metallic objects greatly diminish image quality. Also, direct images obtainable during CT are generally in the transaxial plane. Although most CT units have software capable of reconstructing original image data in any plane or in three dimensions,[14] sometimes this requires increased patient radiation exposure or an increase of examination time, and often a significant loss of definition in the reconstructed images.

CT frequently serves as a supplement to conventional imaging techniques. Because different factors often reduce its availability, it is of the utmost importance that clinical and imaging records be reviewed prior to CT to select the most appropriate examination protocol for any given condition.

Each examination begins with a scout film covering the area of interest. It is important to note that although CT generally is limited with regard to initial imaging plane, the patient's body or specific regions of the body can, to some extent, be positioned in such a way that different planes other than transaxial can be produced. As a rule, the more distal the body part to be studied, the greater the number of possible planes that can be obtained. For example, transaxial views are required for the lumbar spine, whereas virtually all planes are obtainable for a hand, elbow, or foot. Positioning of the subject also may be limited by the patient's comfort, physical state, and cooperation. The next important step relates to the choice of slice thickness and interval. Although slice thickness and interval are included as part of many standard protocols, it is important to tailor these specific aspects of the procedure whenever necessary. The choice depends primarily on the type, size, and location of the lesion, the need for further reformation of the images, the duration of the examination, and the resulting radiation exposure.

CT images are digitalized and depict various structures in terms of different densities on a standard gray scale. The distribution within the range of the gray scale can be modified to enhance soft tissue relationships or bony structures but not both of these at the same time on one image. Generally, two sets of images are obtained at different "window" levels to show optimally bone and soft tissue structures. The relative densities of all structures are expressed in Hounsfield units (HU). Arbitrarily, gas has the lowest density at −1000 HU and bone or metal the highest at +1000 HU. Water is considered being neutral with a value of 0 HU. CT depicts the shape, structure, content and, above all, the extent of a lesion with a precision that is far beyond that of any conventional imaging technique. It is possible to rely on the Hounsfield values to predict the nature of a given lesion, including cysts (Fig. 37–1), fat, and calcification; however, density alone should not be regarded as a precise histologic indicator. One must rely on the results of a combination of clinical, laboratory, conventional, and other imaging techniques.

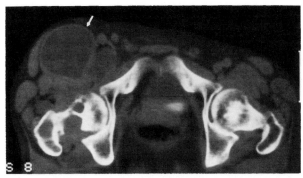

Figure 37–1. Synovial cyst of the hip in a patient with rheumatoid arthritis. Observe the erosion of the femoral head and femoral neck and a large cystic mass located anterior to the hip *(arrow)*.

In some specific clinical settings, the simultaneous use of positive or negative contrast material enhances the value of CT. In the musculoskeletal system, this has been most true for spine studies in which intrathecal positive contrast material is used. Because of the invasiveness and the risks related to the injection of intrathecal iodinated material and the more extensive use of MR, this type of procedure has been used less frequently in the past few years. Nevertheless, injection of positive contrast material into the intrathecal space in combination with CT remains extremely useful in acute or emergency settings when patients cannot undergo an MR examination because of clinical status or because of medical equipment attached to them. Intravenous contrast material is mainly used to characterize soft tissue masses or the vascular status of a given lesion, and positive or negative contrast material (air), or both, is used frequently in articular studies in which it is particularly useful to evaluate the articular surface; to detect intra-articular bodies, such as in primary synovial osteochondromatosis; and to study other articular components. The software for three-dimensional reconstruction of image data is not yet generally available. Nevertheless, it holds great promise and is especially useful in the study of areas of complex anatomy, such as the facial bones, pelvis, spine, and hindfoot. Moreover, it has important applications in trauma, reconstructive surgery, and prosthetic design.[15, 16]

Clinical Indications. CT is efficient and practical in studying axial structures such as the spine, pelvis, sacrum and sacroiliac joints, sternum and sternoclavicular joints, hip (Fig. 37–2), shoulder, hindfoot, and midfoot. The wrist (Fig. 37–3) and TMJ are now better studied by MR imaging. Some specific indications and applications of CT scanning are discussed briefly here.

Trauma. CT has its greatest advantage in the evaluation of the acutely traumatized patient, especially when the injury involves axial structures. It allows the identification of fractures and dislocations. It is extremely useful in the investigation of acute spinal trauma[17, 18] and, in that regard, is superior to plain films. Standard CT slices at the suspected level

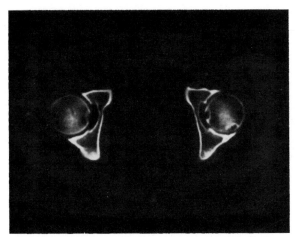

Figure 37–2. Pigmented villonodular synovitis. Multiple erosions of the right femoral head, well demonstrated with CT, are consistent with the diagnosis of pigmented villonodular synovitis.

of injury with multiplanar reformated images will accurately determine the extent of vertebral fractures and provide information on their stability, simultaneous dislocation, cord compression by bone fragments in the spinal canal, and the integrity of posterior elements below and above the injured level.[19–22] In most instances, this information can be obtained rapidly, without significant risk to the patient.

The value of CT also is evident in the analysis of injuries to the pelvis and hip.[23] Pelvic and sacral fractures often are difficult to assess on plain films, whereas CT depicts them and their extent with great precision. Particularly in the evaluation of the acetabulum, for femoral head dislocation, loose bodies, and

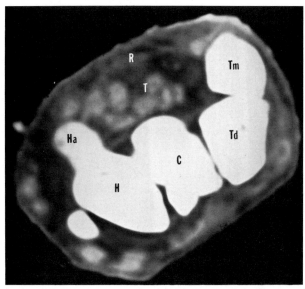

Figure 37–3. Normal wrist. The individual musculotendinous and neurovascular units are well delineated on both the volar and the dorsal aspects. Of particular clinical importance is the optimal depiction of the relationships between structures beneath the flexor retinaculum (R) within the carpal tunnel (T) and the adjacent bones. (H = hamate; Ha = hamulus; C = capitate; Td = trapezoid; Tm = trapezium.)

acetabular fragment displacement, CT again is superior to plain films or even conventional tomograms.[24, 25] Furthermore, the pelvis is frequently the site of complex fractures that can be well delineated only by CT, often with multiplanar or three-dimensional images.[26]

Other traumatized articulations also benefit from CT evaluation. The sternum and sternoclavicular joints often are poorly demonstrated by conventional imaging techniques, but CT reveals their anatomy with great precision. Furthermore, it has the advantage of providing information about the mediastinum at the same time.[27, 28] The injured glenohumeral joint is much better studied with CT than with plain films. Humeral head dislocation[29] is a frequent diagnosis. Although the diagnosis can be made on plain films, the associated bone injury and cartilaginous injuries are better assessed with CT. The Bankart deformity, a cartilaginous or bone lesion of the inferior glenoid rim cavity, and the Hill-Sachs deformity, an impaction fracture of the posterior aspect of the humeral head at the level of the coracoid process, usually indicate previous anterior glenohumeral dislocation and frequently are not detected when plain films alone are used.[30]

CT is of more limited use in the evaluation of trauma to the foot, hand, or elbow,[31] although this imaging method is widely used for the assessment of calcaneal,[32] talar (Fig. 37–4), and wrist fractures and the presence of loose bodies in the elbow. MR studies have replaced CT for evaluation of traumatic damage to ligaments, articular cartilage, and menisci of the knee.

Infections. CT plays a significant role in the diagnosis of osteomyelitis. Although such a diagnosis still relies on the combination of clinical, scintigraphic, and plain film findings, CT features characteristic of infection include single or multiple sequestra, delineation of sinus tracts, and rarely intraosseous (pneumatocysts)[33] or soft tissue gas. Although the presence of gas always is suggestive of infection, gas density in the intervertebral disc and vertebral bodies in disc degeneration and vertebral body osteonecrosis (Kummell's disease), respectively, are well known. CT also allows the physician to choose the most appropriate site for an eventual biopsy or aspiration (Fig. 37–5).

Bone and Soft Tissue Neoplasms. MR imaging is the preferred technique in the evaluation of tumors; CT, however, remains useful in this setting.[34] CT is able to determine (1) whether the neoplasm is fatty, produces bone or cartilage, or has a nidus surrounded by bone sclerosis (osteoid osteoma) or a fluid level (cyst, giant cell tumor, etc.); or (2) the thickness of the cartilaginous cap of an osteochondroma (the thicker the cap, the more likely the presence of a chondrosarcoma).[35–37] Soft tissue neoplasms are much better studied by MR. MR is quite sensitive but not specific for these neoplasms, whereas CT is neither sensitive nor specific. On the other hand, if the presence of calcified matrix in a soft tissue neoplasm must be evaluated, the use of

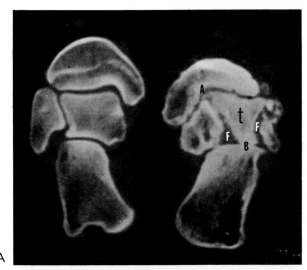

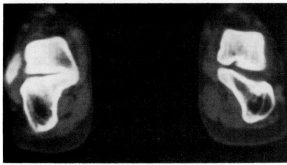

Figure 37–4. Ankle and hindfoot disease. *A,* Degenerative alterations following talar fracture. Articular irregularity and narrowing of the tibiotalar (A) and posterior subtalar (B) joints are evident in the right foot. Multiple persistent fracture lines (F) can be identified within the talus (t), indicative of nonunion. *B,* Talocalcaneal tarsal coalition. A bony bridge extending between the sustentaculum tali of the calcaneus and the middle facet of the talus is indicative of a bony coalition. Compare the appearance with that of the opposite normal side.

CT is still recommended. Finally, CT allows accurate diagnostic biopsy if necessary.

Articular Diseases. Generally, CT is not required for the diagnosis of articular disorders but, in some instances, it may be employed to define the extent of bone involvement in these disorders. This is particularly true in joints that are difficult to assess by conventional imaging techniques, such as apophyseal, costovertebral, sternoclavicular, and temporomandibular joints.

Temporomandibular Joint (TMJ). Exquisite TMJ anatomic detail can be obtained with CT using high-resolution techniques and multiplanar reconstructed images[38] (Fig. 37–6). Previous studies have shown that CT findings correlate well with arthrographic and surgical abnormalities. CT can demonstrate indirect signs of internal derangement of the TMJ, such as post-traumatic alterations and meniscus dislocation.[39] MR imaging, however, is actually the preferred imaging technique for this articulation. Nevertheless, if MR is not available, CT is definitely the best alternative. The examination protocol should include open- and closed-mouth 1.5-mm transaxial

contiguous slices, the use of bone and soft tissue window images, and coronal and sagittal reformatted images, although direct sagittal images[40–42] can be obtained with some specialized software. Direct sagittal CT has 92 percent sensitivity and 87 percent accuracy, for a predictive value of 93 percent in the diagnosis of meniscal displacement. Direct sagittal CT allows assessment of the range of motion, osseous abnormalities of the temporal eminentia and the mandibular condyle, joint space narrowing, meniscal configuration, and positional abnormalities without the technical problems and limitations of reconstructing sagittal images from transaxial slices.

Sternoclavicular Joint. The sternoclavicular joint can be affected by a wide variety of pathologic processes ranging from trauma to inflammatory or neoplastic diseases (Fig. 37–7). CT, when compared with conventional imaging techniques, is much less time consuming, is less uncomfortable for the patient, and provides detailed information about the articulation and the surrounding soft tissues. CT remains the preferred examination for sternoclavicular joint disorders.[27]

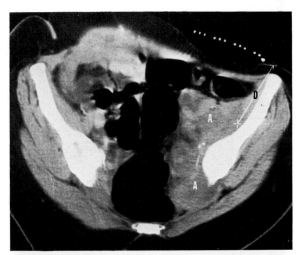

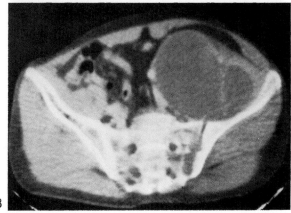

Figure 37–5. *A,* CT-guided needle aspiration of an abscess (A) involving the left iliacus muscle and pararectal fossa secondary to septic sacroiliitis in an intravenous drug abuser. Depth (D) of process can be accurately determined using computer software. *B,* Tuberculosis of the sacroiliac joints. Observe the destruction of the left sacroiliac joint and a large cystic mass anterior to the articulation, representing soft tissue extension of the infection.

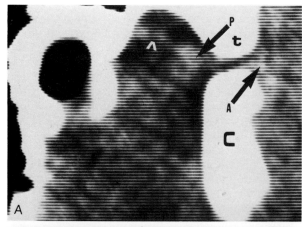

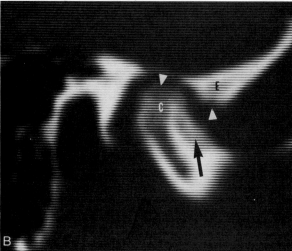

Figure 37–6. Temporomandibular joint imaging. *A,* Direct sagittal image of a normal articulation in the open-mouth position reveals the anterior (A, *arrow*) and posterior (P, *arrow*) bands of the meniscus superior to the mandibular condyle (C). The bilaminar zone of posterior attachment *(arrowhead)* is also visualized (t = temporal eminentia). *B,* Direct sagittal image in the closed-mouth position from a patient with postoperative septic arthritis demonstrates poorly defined erosions *(arrowheads)* involving the articular surface of the mandibular condyle (C) and the temporal eminentia (E). Prominent periostitis *(arrow)* is also noted along the anterior aspect of the condylar neck.

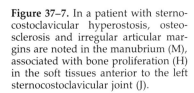

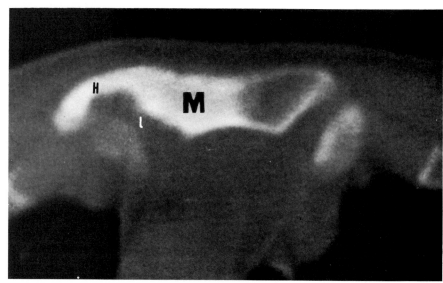

Figure 37–7. In a patient with sterno-costoclavicular hyperostosis, osteo-sclerosis and irregular articular margins are noted in the manubrium (M), associated with bone proliferation (H) in the soft tissues anterior to the left sternocostoclavicular joint (J).

Lumbar Facet Joint. Facet, or zygapophyseal, joints are diarthrodial synovial articulations that can be affected by a wide variety of diseases, including inflammatory and degenerative disorders,[43, 44] trauma, and neoplasms. CT constitutes one of the best imaging modalities to investigate apophyseal joint disorders. Because these joints have varying anatomic orientations at different levels, CT is particularly well suited for their study. Furthermore, if necessary, reformatted sagittal, coronal, or oblique views can be obtained. Standard protocols include nontilted transaxial contiguous 3- to 5-mm slices. Intraspinal synovial cysts,[45, 46] which result from a herniation of the capsule of the apophyseal joint within the spinal canal, are clearly demonstrated by CT. They are seen as homogeneous, low-density posterolateral masses in the spinal canal with or without cord compression. These synovial cysts can contain a certain amount of gas. Synovial cysts have been seen in association with degenerative spondylolisthesis and osteoarthritis involving apophyseal joints with or without radiculopathy. It is important to note that the clinical manifestations of synovial cysts can mimic those of a disc herniation. CT evaluation is important because it discloses the correct diagnosis and thus prevents unnecessary exploratory laminectomy. Furthermore, CT-guided intra-articular injection of glucocorticoids may lead to relief of symptoms and cause the cyst to decrease in size. In patients with ankylosing spondylitis[47] and the cauda equina syndrome, careful CT examination of the lumbar posterior elements may reveal multiple scalloped erosions involving the laminae. These result from thecal diverticula (Fig. 37–8).

Sacroiliac Joint. The contribution of CT in the investigation of sacroiliac joint disorders,[48, 49] especially sacroiliitis,[50] has been evaluated in numerous studies. Certain normal CT variants have been established by studying asymptomatic subjects prospec-

tively. These studies showed asymmetry in the sacroiliac joints in 77 percent of asymptomatic subjects over the age of 30 years and in 87 percent of those over 40 years of age. Poor indicators of sacroiliitis consist of nonuniform iliac sclerosis, focal joint space loss, ill-defined areas of subchondral sclerosis (mostly on the iliac side), and vacuum phenomena (indicative of lack of joint effusion). Good indicators of sacroiliitis include increased subchondral sclerosis in patients under 40 years of age, unilateral or bilateral diffuse joint space loss (<2 mm), and erosions and intra-articular ankylosis. The superiority of CT over plain films and tomograms in the study of sacroiliitis is controversial. In most patients with clinical signs of sacroiliitis, high-quality radiographs of the sacroiliac joints will be diagnostic. When CT is used, however, it often will reveal that the disease is more advanced than had been suspected. CT also allows aspiration and arthrography of the sacroiliac joint in instances of suspected infection.[51]

Hip. CT plays little diagnostic role in the evaluation of disorders of the hip.[52] Nevertheless, CT still is useful in demonstrating the extent of synovial osteochondromatosis prior to therapy. Although CT had been widely used to investigate the possibility of osteonecrosis of the femoral head, the emergence of MR imaging, which is a far more sensitive and specific diagnostic method for ischemic necrosis, has led to a decline in the use of CT for this indication.

Glenohumeral Joint. CT, alone or combined with arthrography, is an excellent diagnostic tool for shoulder trauma and specifically for instability of the glenohumeral joint[53, 54] (Fig. 37–9). For the investigation of soft tissue structures such as the rotator cuff, MR is the preferred imaging method.

Knee. MR imaging is better suited than CT[55] to the evaluation of soft tissue structures, and because the most common pathologic processes affecting the knee involve the menisci and ligaments, MR imaging is now the best imaging method for evaluation of a great variety of internal derangements of the knee. CT, however, represents an efficient technique for examination of the femoropatellar articulation, especially when malalignment is suspected. Different CT protocols have been described for the investigation of this problem. Dynamic investigation of this compartment can be accomplished by imaging the knee sequentially at different degrees of knee flexion (e.g., from 0 to 30 degrees of flexion). By reformatting these images, it is then possible to obtain a "cinematic" view of patellofemoral motion and thereby assess the possibility of malalignment during this motion. Some investigators have tried to evaluate the degree of lateral or medial displacement of the patella in relation to the anterior tibial tuberosity. This is done by obtaining contiguous 5-mm slices of the knee with the patient lying supine in a neutral position, with a lead marker placed on the anterior tibial tuberosity. Two images then are selected for each knee, one that shows the marker and one that includes both the patella and the femoral condyles. These selected images are then superimposed by a

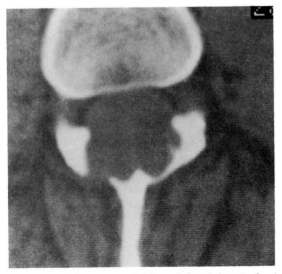

Figure 37–8. Ankylosing spondylitis and thecal diverticula. A CT image of a lumbar vertebra demonstrates scalloped erosions of the posterior elements, diagnostic of thecal diverticula.

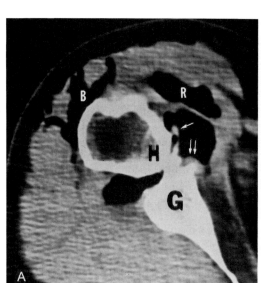
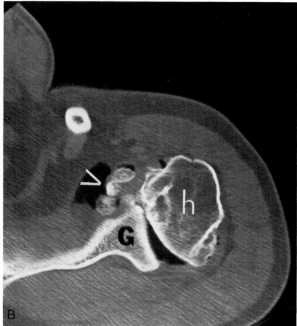

Figure 37–9. Computed air arthrotomography of the shoulder joint. *A,* Following introduction of air into the glenohumeral articulation, communication with the subacromion-subdeltoid bursa (B) is indicative of a full-thickness rotator cuff tear. The anterior portion of the cartilaginous labrum is blunted *(double arrow),* and the anterior capsular recesses (R) appear prominent owing to prior anterior dislocation. An intra-articular osteochondral body *(single arrow)* is also evident. (G = glenoid; H = humerus.) *B,* In another patient, multiple intra-articular osteochondral bodies *(arrowhead)* are demonstrated, along with post-traumatic and degenerative deformity of the humeral head (h). (G = glenoid.)

computer to ensure a common relation to the reference frame. It is then possible to measure the actual projection of the femoral groove and the patella in relation to the anterior tibial tuberosity. These measurements are corrected for any imaging magnification. Angles between the patella and the femoral groove also are measured. A more detailed description of this procedure and the normal reference values are available elsewhere.[56, 57]

Miscellaneous Regions and Disorders

Spine. Retrospective review of cervical myelograms and CT scans of patients with cervical radiculopathy secondary to disc herniation or spondylosis has indicated that CT, with or without the use of intrathecal metrizamide, is more accurate in the identification of causative lesions. In certain patients, CT can obviate cervical myelography.[58] Metrizamide CT myelography provides significant information, including improved characterization of the abnormality and lateralization, when the conventional myelogram is indeterminate. In patients with cervical myelopathy, a cross-sectional diameter of the cord equaling less than 50 percent of the subarachnoid space is predictive of poor patient response to surgical intervention.[59]

Unilateral flattening of the cord by a spondylitic mass or bulging disc in a normally wide spinal canal on CT myelography is considered nonspecific, because nerve root signs are contralateral nearly as often as they are ipsilateral to the radiologic findings. Concentric compression of the cord in a narrow canal produces long tract signs only after the cross-sec-

tional area of the cord had been reduced by about 30 percent (to a value of 60 mm^2 or less). Strong correlation exists between the side of disc herniation with occlusion of the corresponding neural foramen and the side of nerve root symptoms. If stenosis of the spinal canal and disc herniation are considered reliable CT myelographic signs of nerve root symptoms, a specific diagnosis can be made in about 40 percent of cases.[60] Posterior displacement of the epidural veins and epidural enhancement following high-dose intravenous contrast administration provide excellent delineation of disc extrusion and may allow demarcation of free fragments. Although noninfusion scans are usually adequate, the improved anatomic information available from infusion CT may increase diagnostic certainty and, in selected cases, makes myelography unnecessary in patients with focal cervical radiculopathy.[61]

Criteria have been established for distinguishing between a herniated nucleus pulposus and a bulging annulus fibrosus by CT. In anatomically or surgically verified cases of bulging annulus, CT reveals generalized extension of the disc border beyond the vertebral body margin. A herniated nucleus pulposus, conversely, exhibits a focal, usually posterolateral, protrusion of the disc margin, which may be calcified[62] (Fig. 37–10). The demonstration of intradiscal gas by CT is virtually diagnostic of degenerative disease (Fig. 37–11), because rarely is gas observed in the setting of infection.[63]

Retrospectively, poor correlation has been found between CT and myelography in the diagnosis of a

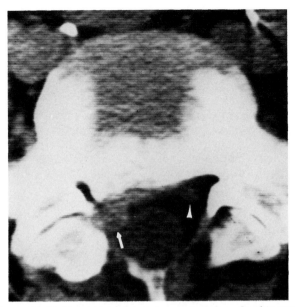

Figure 37–10. Herniation of an intervertebral disc. On this cross-sectional image at the level of the intervertebral disc, observe a soft tissue density protruding into the spinal canal *(arrow)*, obliterating the adjacent nerve root. The root on the opposite site *(arrowhead)* is visible.

slightly bulging lumbar disc. A major discrepancy rate of less than 1 percent among patients without prior surgery has been reported, and the two methods agree on definite abnormalities in 70 percent of cases.[64] CT has been shown to demonstrate normal and herniated intervertebral discs as effectively as myelography in a prospective comparative study.[65]

Transaxial CT scans are most sensitive and specific, whereas sagittal reformations are helpful in evaluating the size of a disc bulge into the spinal canal (especially at the L5–S1 level) and spondylolisthesis. Coronal reformations are least informative. Myelography and sagittal reformations are equally useful in the detection of a herniated disc, but transaxial CT scans are superior to either.[66]

CT of the lumbar spine has exhibited 93 percent agreement with surgical findings in revealing the presence or absence of a herniated nucleus pulposus, including posterior disc protrusion and extruded disc fragments. Discrepancy is most likely in the setting of previous surgery, spondylolisthesis, or spinal stenosis.[67] In patients with low back pain or sciatica, CT findings also correlate well with clinical response to intra-articular facet block. CT can thus effectively differentiate between lumbar facet arthropathy and a herniated disc.[68]

CT has been shown to be useful in diagnosing posterolateral as well as central lumbar disc herniations. Because it can image the disc margin and free disc fragments irrespective of dural sac or root sheath deformity, CT is more effective than myelography for demonstrating the presence and extent of lateral disc herniation. The CT features of a lateral herniated disc include (1) focal protrusion of the disc margin; (2) displacement of epidural fat within the intervertebral foramen; (3) absence of dural sac deformity; and (4) soft tissue mass within or lateral to the intervertebral foramen.[69]

An extruded or free disc fragment commonly appears on CT scans as an epidural mass, and a

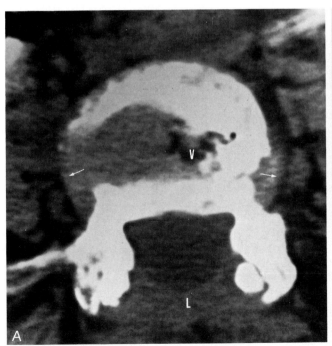
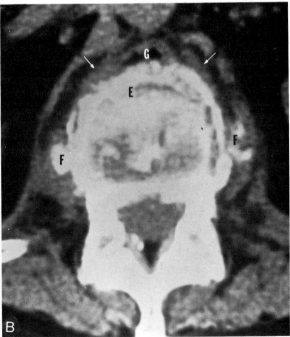

Figure 37–11. CT Identification of gas as a diagnostic aid in the spine. *A,* Intradiscal gas or vacuum phenomenon (V) in association with diffuse annular bulge *(arrows)* is a classic finding of degenerative intervertebral disc disease. The site of a previous laminectomy (L) can also be appreciated. Demonstration of gas within a collapsed vertebral body by CT should suggest ischemic necrosis as the underlying etiology. *B,* Pyogenic infection of the lumbar spine. Low-density areas (G) in the soft tissues anterior to the spine are typical of gas-forming organisms. Vertebral end-plate destruction (E) with osseous fragmentation (F) is characteristic. Prevertebral soft tissue swelling *(arrows)* is also evident.

normal posterior disc margin does not exclude herniation when the nuclear fragment is extruded. Free disc fragments can be differentiated from root sheath anomalies and tumors in most instances by measuring tissue densities and analyzing adjacent bone.[70] The CT appearance of conjoined nerve roots has been described, including the resemblance between this condition and herniated nucleus pulposus as well as differentiation between the two using the "blink mode."[71] CT features of conjoined lumbar nerve roots include asymmetry of the bony spinal canal, manifested as slight dilatation of the ipsilateral lateral recess. This alteration is not typically associated with extruded free intervertebral disc fragments and thus serves as a distinguishing feature between these two entities.[72]

Patients with unequivocal regression or disappearance of a herniated lumbar disc on follow-up CT study have recently been reported. More frequent use of sequential CT scans has thus been advocated to determine whether regression of herniated disc is a frequent occurrence among patients who recover with conservative therapy.[73]

CT has also been shown to be an effective noninvasive means of imaging the lumbar spine in patients with suspected recurrent disc disease. Intravenous contrast material significantly increases the diagnostic accuracy and level of confidence in differentiating between recurrent herniated disc and hypertrophic extradural scar by CT.[74] Enhancement occurs with scar but not with recurrent disc herniation. The method is advocated by some investigators for more accurate evaluation of failed back surgery and can assist in the recognition of discitis.[75]

Patient selection for chymopapain chemonucleolysis is based partially on the CT demonstration of morphologic criteria for a herniated nucleus pulposus, which favors a successful therapeutic outcome. CT findings have been found to correlate closely with objective clinical parameters used to assess therapeutic response.[76] In a prospective evaluation, changes in the size, location, shape, homogeneity, and density of the disc herniation after chemonucleolysis were uncommon on 6-week follow-up CT studies.[77] The most common findings at this time were vacuum phenomena, increased disc attenuation, and a slight decrease (1 to 3 mm) in the size of the disc herniations.[77] At 3 months, the compression produced by the herniated disc was eliminated or reduced, with development of diffuse annular bulging in most patients. No evidence for osseous alterations or epidural fibrosis has been detected by CT.[78] A successful response on 6-month follow-up CT scans has been characterized by decreased disc height, vacuum phenomena, and a more impressive decrease in the size of the disc herniations.[77]

Articular Sepsis. The diagnostic role of CT in septic arthritis is based primarily on its ability to guide proper access to joints that are difficult to image otherwise, e.g., intervertebral discs, sacroiliac joints (see Fig. 37–5). CT also allows evaluation of soft tissues around these anatomically complex areas

and thereby excludes the presence of a periarticular abscess. CT makes diagnostic aspiration possible in difficult cases. Extension of an infectious process through an intervertebral disc to adjacent vertebral bodies with or without surrounding soft tissue abscess formation is well depicted by CT, although MR imaging often can give equal or superior information.

Congenital Diseases. CT plays an important role in the diagnosis and evaluation of many congenital diseases involving the musculoskeletal system. Examples include leg length discrepancy, femoral neck anteversion, tibial torsion, scoliosis with rotation, coalitions, and congenital hip dysplasia.[79, 80] In congenital hip dysplasia, CT can outline the interposition of the iliopsoas tendon between the femoral head and the acetabulum, which could prevent reduction of the dislocation or cause instability. CT with three-dimensional reconstructed images also is of great importance in surgical decision making and postoperative follow-up evaluation. Spinal dysraphism likewise can be evaluated by CT. Although spondylolysis and spondylolisthesis can be detected on plain radiographs, CT allows an accurate evaluation of the posterior elements of the involved vertebra and the adjacent apophyseal joints.

MAGNETIC RESONANCE IMAGING

The indications for MR have increased dramatically in the last several years. Multiplanar MR imaging is extremely rewarding in the study of many musculoskeletal disorders. Newly designed surface coils are more specifically adapted to each part of the body, thereby enhancing image quality. MR imaging's advantages are its ability to depict physical differences among tissues and fluids, expressing these differences in terms of image contrast; the apparent lack of significant biologic hazard; the capacity to select any direct imaging plane closely adapted to the anatomic or pathologic structure under study; the close correlation of the images with actual normal anatomy; and outstanding sensitivity. Its main drawback, however, is that it often lacks specificity. For many reasons, MR imaging is employed as the sole imaging method only infrequently; in most instances, it is used as an adjunct to conventional imaging techniques or even CT. It is beyond the scope of this chapter to discuss in great detail the physics and examination protocols of MR. However, it should be mentioned that primary pulse sequences include T_1- and T_2-weighted spin-echo and gradient-echo methods and 5-mm thick multiplanar images.[81–83]

Spine. Anatomic areas of interest in the spine that are frequently studied with MR imaging include intervertebral discs, spinal canal, neural foramina, and apophyseal joints. In addition, a variety of axial conditions or disorders can be studied with MR, including degenerative disc disease, disc herniation, spinal stenosis, the postoperative spine, discitis, vertebral osteomyelitis, and spinal dysraphism.

Degenerative Disc Disease. The basic chemical constitution of vertebral discs is a combination of proteoglycans and collagen. The nucleus pulposus has a greater proportion of proteoglycans, whereas the surrounding annulus fibrosus has more collagen. This is reflected by a different signal intensity of these structures on MR images. The disc is attached superiorly and inferiorly to the fused physeal ring of the adjacent vertebral body surfaces by strong annular fibers, and anteriorly and posteriorly, it is loosely attached to the corresponding longitudinal ligaments. The normal intervertebral disc has a concave contour on a sagittal view and a symmetric appearance on a transaxial view. The annulus fibrosus shows low signal intensity (dark) with all pulse sequences, whereas the nucleus pulposus shows a moderate signal intensity (gray) on T_1-weighted images and a high signal intensity (bright) on both T_2-weighted and gradient-echo images. With aging, the intervertebral disc is subject to biochemical and structural changes, resulting in an imbalance in which the proteoglycans lose their close association with collagen fibers and the disc loses 15 to 20 percent of its water content. At the same time, the adjacent end-plates of the vertebral bodies become thinner.[84] When this process is more advanced, the distinction between the nucleus pulposus and the annulus fibrosus disappears as dense, disorganized, fibrous tissue replaces the normal fibrocartilaginous structure of the nucleus pulposus. Fissures then develop within the cartilaginous end-plates and granulation tissue appears in this area. A correlative study of cadavers and MR images by Yu et al.[85] demonstrated three types of tears in the annulus fibrosus: radial, concentric, and transverse.

These biochemical and structural changes in the intervertebral disc are reflected on MR images by a change in signal intensity, mainly a decreased signal in gradient-echo and T_2-weighted images. A *bulging* disc refers to a symmetric circumferential enlargement of the disc without major disruption of the annulus fibrosus. *Protrusion* refers to an eccentric bulging of the disc, indicating a focal weakening of the annulus fibers with consequent thinning of the involved area (Fig. 37–12). This may potentially predispose to disc herniation. Disc *herniation* refers to a rupture of the annulus fibrosus with consequent extrusion of the disc through the annular defect while the extruded part remains in contact with the parent disc. A disc *prolapse* describes a herniated disc still covered with a few remaining annular fibers.[86] Finally, *sequestration* refers to a disc fragment that is no longer in contact with the parent disc; such a fragment can be located either above or below the involved disc level. To study discal abnormality, transaxial and sagittal MR images are usually obtained. In neither plane does a normal disc project beyond the posterior margin of the vertebral bodies. Sagittal views are better suited to the analysis of disc herniation. The herniated disc has an hourglass appearance

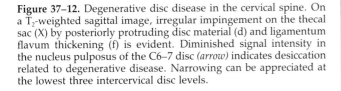

Figure 37–12. Degenerative disc disease in the cervical spine. On a T_2-weighted sagittal image, irregular impingement on the thecal sac (X) by posteriorly protruding disc material (d) and ligamentum flavum thickening (f) is evident. Diminished signal intensity in the nucleus pulposus of the C6–7 disc (arrow) indicates desiccation related to degenerative disease. Narrowing can be appreciated at the lowest three intercervical disc levels.

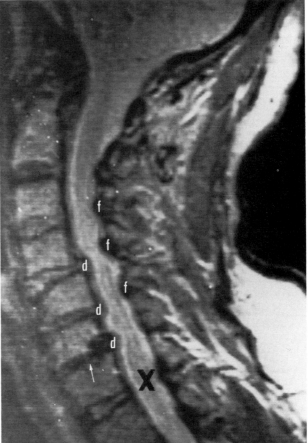

along the posterior disc margin. On transaxial views, the posterior disc margin will show some asymmetry and often a soft tissue mass displacing the adjacent nerve root or thecal sac to a varying extent.[87] Anatomic contact with the parent disc is still apparent. Sequestrated discs do not have such contact, although other findings are similar to those of a simple disc herniation. Disc fragments are more often located on the anterolateral aspect of the spinal canal because the lateral portion of the posterior longitudinal ligament is somewhat weaker than its central part.

Spinal Stenosis. Spinal stenosis is either congenital or acquired. The congenital form is related to developmental aberrations such as short pedicles, whereas the acquired form results from a reduction in diameter of the spinal canal caused by any combination of disc bulging, ligamentum flavum hypertrophy, postoperative modifications, and facet hypertrophy. The most common form of spinal stenosis that is studied by MR imaging is the acquired form.[88, 89] It is best displayed by MR using sagittal gradient-echo–pulsed images. In this sequence, the thecal sac, which displays a high-intensity signal, appears compressed or even obliterated by bulging discs, osteophytes, and a hypertrophied ligamentum flavum. The resulting appearance of the thecal sac is an hourglass deformity. Multilevel disc degeneration illustrated by an abnormally low signal intensity for these discs and disc space narrowing also may be present. On transaxial images, the stenotic spinal canal has a triangular shape owing to an encroachment by hypertrophied facets.

Postoperative Spine. One of the most common and often difficult tasks in diagnostic radiology is the evaluation of patients with a failed back surgery syndrome. These are patients who have residual or recurrent back pain after back surgery.[90, 91] MR imaging now is recognized as the imaging method of choice for analysis of the postoperative spine.[92–94] Furthermore, recent experience with Gadolinium DTPA (Gd-DTPA)–enhanced MR imaging in combination with noncontrast MR imaging has revealed unprecedented sensitivity and accuracy in the investigation of such patients.[95, 96] The main causes of failed back surgery syndrome are lateral spinal stenosis, recurrent or residual disc herniation, fibrosis, scar formation, arachnoiditis, infection, surgical nerve injury, pseudomeningocele formation, and incorrect choice of level of surgery. MR studies obtained in the early postoperative period are exceedingly difficult to interpret. The presence of various types of materials at the site of surgery, such as gas, Gelfoam, blood, and fat graft, lead to complex imaging alterations. The topographic features and signal intensity of recurrent disc herniation and epidural scar are very similar. After a 1-month delay, however, it is easier to distinguish a scar from recurrent or residual disc herniation. Recurrent or residual disc herniation is associated with a mass that is still in contact with the parent disc. The signal intensity is the same for both herniated disc material and the parent disc on both T_1- and T_2-weighted images unless the herniated material has been separated, surgically or not, from the parent disc, thus becoming sequestered. Also, a discontinuity in the fibers of the annulus fibrosus can reflect the presence of disc disease, or it can be secondary to the surgical incision. Finally, herniated discs are usually well delineated and are sometimes circumscribed by a rim of low-signal intensity. The margins of an epidural scar are usually poorly defined. The MR signal of a scar is either isointense or hypointense to the disc signal in T_1-weighted images and hyperintense on T_2-weighted images.[92] The latter tends to be attenuated months or years after surgery. Scar also causes retraction of soft tissues with displacement of the thecal sac on the same side as the surgery. With Gd-DTPA–enhanced MR imaging, epidural scar shows greater enhancement than adjacent disc or nerve root structures. Gd-DTPA is incorporated into inflammatory material, therefore allowing clearer depiction of the scar and enabling it to be distinguished from adjacent disc and nerve roots, even if the latter are incorporated within the scar.

Postsurgical Infection. Infections after back surgery are uncommon but may have severe consequences. They usually consist of vertebral osteomyelitis with or without adjacent discitis or epidural abcess. MR imaging is an excellent diagnostic method in this clinical setting. Changes that are encountered in cases of infection include confluent areas of low-signal intensity in vertebral bone marrow and adjacent disc on T_1-weighted images, increased signal intensity of the bone marrow and adjacent disc on T_2-weighted images, the loss of the normal demarcation between vertebral body and intervertebral disc, and abnormal disc shape. Epidural abscesses (Fig. 37–13) form a mass of variable size that is usually easy to separate from the thecal sac; abscesses appear isointense to the thecal sac on T_1-weighted images and hyperintense on T_2-weighted images. The use of Gd-DTPA–enhanced MR imaging greatly improves the sensitivity for the diagnosis of such abcesses. Viable inflammatory tissue enhances on T_1-weighted images after administration of contrast material.

Bone Marrow. Bone marrow historically has been poorly evaluated with conventional imaging techniques. Although CT represented a strong improvement in the investigation of the bone marrow, MR now is regarded as the state-of-the-art imaging method for this purpose.[97] A number of pathologic processes involve the bone marrow and can be broadly classified into five groups: (1) reconversion; (2) infiltration by neoplasia, infection, or other processes; (3) myeloid depletion; (4) edema; and (5) ischemia (Fig. 37–14A and B). Normal bone marrow provides a continuous supply of red and white blood cells, platelets, and other cells to meet the body's demand for oxygenation, immunity, and coagulation. It also plays a role in bone biomechanics in terms of mechanical support and mineral deposit. Nerves, fat cells, and blood and lymphatic vessels

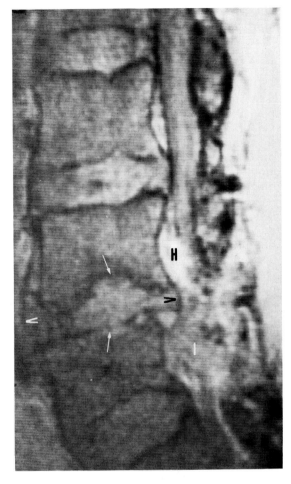

Figure 37–13. Intervertebral disc space infection. On a T$_2$-weighted sagittal image of the lumbar spine, narrowing and bulging *(arrowheads)* of the L4–5 interspace is apparent, in association with irregular destruction of the adjacent end-plates *(arrows)*. Posterior extension of the process has resulted in an epidural abscess, characterized by mixed areas of intermediate (I) and high (H) signal intensity.

are also part of the bone marrow. At birth, red marrow is present almost throughout the bones of the body, but it will progressively be converted to yellow marrow. In the adult, the largest red marrow reservoirs reside in the axial skeleton (spine, pelvis, and ribs), skull, and proximal portions of the humeri and femora. Other bones have yellow marrow. Normal yellow marrow has a signal that is isointense to subcutaneous fat on T$_1$-weighted and T$_2$-weighted images. Normal red marrow has a low-signal intensity on T$_1$-weighted images as compared to subcutaneous fat, although it has a higher-signal intensity than that of muscle. On T$_2$-weighted images, red marrow remains of relatively low-signal intensity.

Reconversion is a response to the depletion of the body's red marrow related to a number of different causes, such as anemia and myelofibrosis. The reconversion process will involve successively the spine, the flat bones, and, finally, the long bones. With MR imaging, marrow appears focally or diffusely hypointense on T$_1$-weighted images, depending on the extent of the disease process. On T$_2$-weighted images, the appearance varies depending on the water content of the process; it may appear hypointense, isointense, or hyperintense in comparison to yellow marrow.[98, 99] Bone marrow infiltration or replacement by infection, leukemia, lymphoma, metastasis, or primary bone tumors may occur throughout the body according to the relative prev-

alence of red and yellow marrow. Certain infiltrating conditions of bone marrow have a low-signal intensity on T$_1$-weighted images, but signal intensity varies greatly on T$_2$-weighted images (i.e., high-signal intensity for most primary tumors and infection, low-signal intensity for leukemia, lymphoma, myelofibrosis, and Gaucher's disease).[100] Thus, MR imaging is extremely sensitive in the diagnosis of bone marrow involvement, but it is not specific.[101] Once a histologic diagnosis is made, MR imaging is useful in determining the extent and the response to treatment for many pathologic processes that involve the bone marrow.

Disorders resulting in myeloid depletion (e.g., irradiation) involve red marrow in such a way that the signal pattern of the diseased areas is transformed to that of yellow marrow on both T$_1$- and T$_2$-weighted images.[102]

Several conditions, such as trauma (Fig. 37–15) and the reflex sympathetic dystrophy syndrome, can induce bone marrow edema. This edema is thought to be secondary to hypervascularity causing a regional increase in the concentration of extracellular fluid. This increase in water content appears as a lower signal intensity on T$_1$-weighted images and an increase in signal intensity on T$_2$-weighted images.[103, 104]

The sensitivity of MR imaging for bone marrow ischemia is extremely high. In this condition the

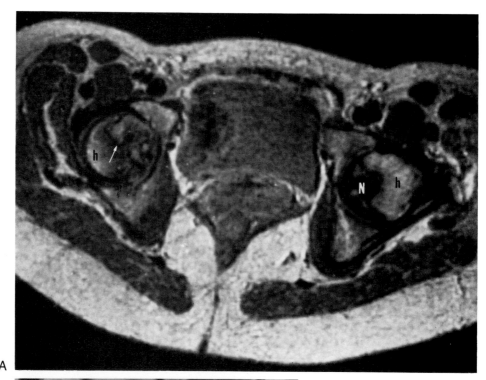

A

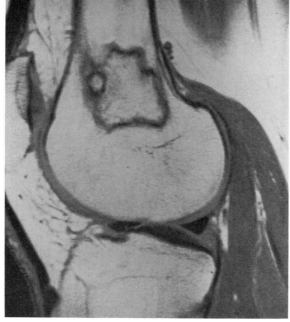

B

Figure 37–14. *A,* Steroid-induced ischemic necrosis affecting the hip joints in a patient with systemic lupus erythematosus. On a T_1-weighted transaxial image, an inhomogeneous pattern is noted in the weight-bearing aspects of both femoral heads (h). On the right, a curvilinear geographic pattern is evident *(arrow),* whereas the left femoral head exhibits more widespread loss of the normally intense marrow signal intensity in the necrotic zone (N). *B,* Bone infarct. MR imaging of the distal femur: T_1-weighted sagittal image revealing a serpentine-shaped metaphyseal lesion with marginal area of decreased signal intensity.

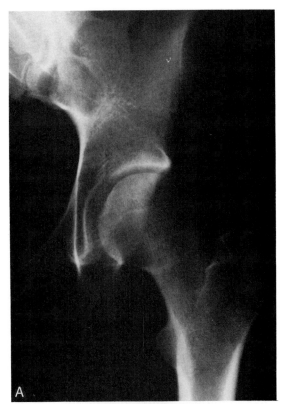

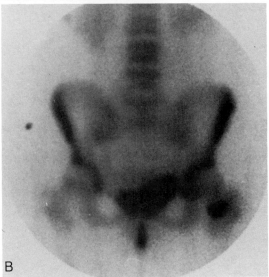

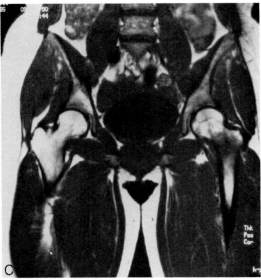

Figure 37–15. Stress fracture. *A,* Anteroposterior radiograph of the left hip showing a horizontal band of sclerosis at the medial aspect of the left femoral neck. *B,* Bone scan: abnormal radionuclide uptake at the same area. *C,* MR imaging: T_1-weighted coronal image, with a band of low signal intensity along the femoral neck suggesting bone marrow edema.

marrow reveals a low-signal intensity on T_1-weighted images and variable signal intensity on T_2-weighted images, probably depending on the stage of the disease[105] (see Fig. 37–14A and B).

Temporomandibular Joint. The MR examination of TMJ usually includes sagittal closed- and open-mouth T_1-weighted images. Because of the relatively high frequency (26 percent) of lateral or medial displacement of the meniscus, many authors also advocate coronal MR images.[106] The normal TMJ meniscus is a biconcave structure of low signal intensity with a thinner central portion. With the mouth closed, the posterior band is in contact with the mandibular condyle, and with the mouth open, the intermediate zone of the meniscus is in contact with the condyle. During motion, a complex movement of anterior translation and rotation occurs. MR abnormalities include abnormal position of the mandibular condyle or the meniscus, or both, in relation to the temporal eminence.[107]

Currently, MR is considered the best imaging method for analysis of the TMJ. It depicts, with great precision, the meniscus and the rest of the articulation, and it allows the visualization of the surrounding muscular apparatus, notably the mastication muscles (Fig. 37–16). Multiplanar views and the use of surface coils allow detection of anterior, medial, or lateral displacement of the meniscus, detection of which is not possible by simple arthrography. MR imaging also allows assessment of the underlying bone, joint effusion, and postoperative complications. Because of the functional similarity of this joint and the femoropatellar joint, real-time assessment of joint mechanics with MR imaging can be useful and is accomplished by scanning during incremental opening and closing of the mouth.[108]

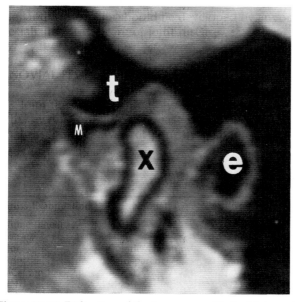

Figure 37–16. Dislocation of the temporomandibular joint meniscus. On a T_1-weighted sagittal image, the fibrocartilaginous disc (M) of low signal intensity is displaced anterior to the mandibular condyle (X), limiting its range of forward excursion. (t = temporal eminentia; e = external auditory canal.)

Shoulder. MR imaging has had a great impact in the evaluation of the shoulder owing to the possibility of studying soft tissue and osseous anatomy (muscles, tendons, cartilage, and bones) with a multiplanar approach.[109] With its contrast sensitivity, MR can be used to assess a whole spectrum of disorders commonly leading to shoulder pain: rotator cuff pathology, impingement syndrome, bicipital tendon abnormalities, bone marrow disease, and intra-articular osteochondral bodies. CT in combination with arthrography, however, has proved to be as accurate as MR imaging in the evaluation of shoulder instability.

The impingement syndrome is a well-recognized clinical entity that is defined as the entrapment of soft tissues in the subacromial space between the humeral head and the coracoacromial arch; these soft tissues include the rotator cuff (particularly the supraspinatus muscle), the tendon of the long head of the biceps, and the subacromial bursa. According to Neer,[110] most rotator cuff problems are secondary to chronic impingement of tendons by a prominent coracoacromial ligament, abnormal slope or shape of the acromion, the presence of enthesophytes at the tip of the acromion, or degenerative changes of the acromioclavicular joint. A grading system for severity of impingement has been instituted: edema and hemorrage (grade I); inflammation and fibrosis (grade II); and rotator cuff tear (grade III). This syndrome is strongly associated with participation in sports that involve overhead motion. The MR findings of the early stages of impingement include thickening of the subacromial bursa and decreased thickness of the supraspinatus tendon with an increased signal intensity within the tendon indicative of tendinopathy.[111] Further damage to the tendon is manifested by a partial tear involving only the articular or bursal surface. Partial tears are often mistaken for full-thickness tears or tendinopathy with MR imaging. MR findings of full-thickness tear include the presence of fluid in the subacromial or subdeltoid bursa, or both, (bright signal on T_2-weighted images), increased signal intensity within the supraspinatus tendon on T_2-weighted images, loss of the normal fat plane surrounding the subdeltoid-subacromial bursa, musculotendinous retraction, joint effusion, and a high-riding humeral head.[112, 113]

MR arthrography, with Gd-DTPA as the intra-articular contrast medium, has recently been introduced as an additional tool for the evaluation of partial tears, with encouraging results.[114] This technique is particularly helpful in the evaluation of partial tears of the undersurface of the cuff and also in the evaluation of the glenoid labrum and the search for intra-articular bodies. The rationale for using an intra-articular contrast medium in cases of shoulder instability relates to the fact that labral morphology is hard to depict when the glenohumeral joint is free of fluid. Recent studies have emphasized the "many faces" of the normal labrum. Indeed, the normal labrum can be triangular in shape, rounded, or bifid. The best MR images are those in the transaxial plane, in which the labrum is depicted as a structure devoid of signal because of its fibrocartilaginous nature. Labral tears may appear as regions of increased signal intensity extending to the labral surface. The region of increased signal intensity can be diffuse in nature, and the labrum may appear blunted or frayed.

Wrist. MR has established itself as a new imaging tool for a limited range of bony and soft tissue wrist abnormalities.[115] In the carpal tunnel syndrome, the median nerve can be damaged by compression or entrapment as it passes through the carpal tunnel, which is delineated dorsally by the carpal bones, volarly by the flexor retinaculum, ulnarly by the hook of the hamate and the pisiform, and radially by the scaphoid and the trapezium. A variety of causes of the carpal tunnel syndrome can be depicted by MR imaging, including fluid collections (synovitis), fibrosis, and space-occupying lesions (e.g., neuroma and ganglion). Compression of the median nerve induces nerve edema that will be reflected by an increase in the size of the nerve on T_1-weighted images and a bright signal intensity within the nerve on T_2-weighted images. Other findings include distortion of the normal ovoid shape of the nerve, swelling of the flexor tendon sheaths, and palmar convexity of the flexor retinaculum.[116] Failure of surgery to relieve the carpal tunnel syndrome also can be studied with MR imaging.

Other causes of wrist pain that can be demonstrated by MR include joint effusions, synovial inflammatory processes,[117, 118] and bone marrow abnormalities, such as ischemic necrosis of the proximal pole of the scaphoid and Kienbock's disease.[119] Although T_1-weighted MR images reveal great anatomic detail, this technique has not yet supplanted the use of wrist arthrography in the assessment of intracarpal ligamentous pathology. The triangular fibrocartilage, however, is usually well demonstrated with coronal T_1-weighted images, and both the normal and the pathologic appearance of the triangular fibrocartilage with MR imaging have been well documented.[120]

Foot and Ankle. Direct multiplanar images of the foot and ankle are obtainable with both CT and MR. MR is an efficient imaging technique for the evaluation of muscles and tendons; it depicts their anatomy with great precision and documents the presence of tenosynovial fluid or intratendinous fluid collections.[121] Normal tendons appear as smooth, well-defined, hypointense structures on T_1- and T_2-weighted images.[122] In addition, a recent partial tear of a tendon is typically diagnosed with MR imaging by the presence of fluid within the tendon and tendon sheath, creating a bright signal on T_2-weighted images. A complete tear manifests itself by tendon discontinuity secondary to its retraction.[123] Chronic tendon tears or chronic tendinitis appear as a diffusely thickened tendon that has low-signal intensity on both T_1 and T_2-weighted images. Associated tenosynovial fluid collections are seen as areas of intermediate signal intensity on T_1-weighted images and of high-signal intensity on T_2-weighted images.

Posterior tibial tendon rupture[124] and Achilles tendinitis[125] are two entities that can be specifically studied with MR. The posterior tibial tendon is one of the main stabilizers of the hindfoot. Chronic inflammation involving this tendon may lead to a complete tear. Plain film signs of tenosynovitis or rupture of the posterior tibial tendon are subtle and include periostitis of the medial aspect of the distal tibia. The normal posterior tibial tendon appears on MR images as a dark, homogeneous, ovoid to round structure passing posterior to the medial malleolus. It is twice as large as the adjacent flexor digitorum longus or flexor hallucis longus tendon. Classification of posterior tibial tendon tears using MR imaging correlates well with surgical findings. In type I tears, the tendon appears enlarged in comparison to the normal contralateral side (both ankles are usually studied at the same time for comparison). Type I tears may also reveal foci of high signal intensity on proton density weighted images and of somewhat lesser signal intensity on T_2-weighted images. In type II tears, the tendon appears atrophic and its size approaches that of the adjacent flexor digitorum longus tendon. Also, hypertrophy of the tendon segments above and below the ruptured area may be evident. Type III tears are manifested by a gap in the tendon itself and retraction of the proximal muscle-tendon complex.

Causes of Achilles tendinitis are multiple: strenuous athletic training, gout, rheumatoid arthritis, systemic or local use of glucocorticoids, and chronic renal failure. All of these conditions eventually can lead to rupture of this tendon. MR imaging provides important information about this tendon and the surrounding structures. The actual site of rupture generally is located 3 to 5 cm proximal to its distal insertion on the posterior aspect of the calcaneus. It is at this point that the anterior and posterior fibers cross, in a region of relative hypovascularity. Achilles tendon rupture is clinically misdiagnosed in approximately 25 percent of cases. MR imaging, therefore, plays an important role as a diagnostic tool. The optimal images are those in the transaxial plane. The normal tendon has a crescentic shape, with the concave aspect projected anteriorly; it reveals a signal void on all MR imaging sequences. A complete tear is seen as an area of increased signal intensity on T_2-weighted images, discontinuity of the tendon, and retraction of the muscle-tendon junction. Tendinitis appears as a small focus of increased signal intensity within an enlarged tendon without any tendon discontinuity. Surrounding edema is seen as a brightening of the loose connective tissue anterior to the tendon. Partial tears are difficult to differentiate from tendinitis with MR imaging.

Arthrography allows accurate assessment of ligamentous integrity about the ankle. Indeed, specific patterns of contrast extravasation permit differentiation among injuries of the anterior inferior tibiofibular, anterior and posterior talofibular, calcaneofibular, and deltoid ligaments. Experience with MR imaging in the evaluation of these ligaments is limited, but findings strongly suggestive of disruption of the anterior inferior tibiofibular ligament have been described, consisting of disorganization of the soft tissues between the tibia and fibula, fluid above the expected syndesmosis, and slight subluxation of the fibula.

Lesions responsible for chronic ankle pain and disability include osseous, osteocartilaginous and cartilaginous abnormalities such as osteonecrosis, osteochondritis dissecans, and osteochondral fractures. *Osteochondritis dissecans* refers to fragmentation and partial to complete separation of a portion of the articular surface of a joint. Trauma is the proposed cause in most instances. Indeed, the term *transchondral fracture* is frequently used as a synonym for this condition. The fracture is parallel to the articular surface and may involve either cartilage alone or cartilage and subchondral bone. Osteochondritis dissecans may involve the medial or lateral portion of the talus. The fragment may remain in place and heal in situ or it may undergo resorption. Furthermore, it may become detached. The fragment may enlarge by means of bone proliferation on its surface or it may be resorbed. The fragment also may become loose within the joint cavity, perhaps becoming embedded elsewhere on the synovial surface. MR imaging is useful in the detection of radiographically occult lesions, in the assessment of the integrity of the overlying cartilage, in the detection of intraarticular bodies, in the definition of the exact location and extension of the process, and in the prediction of the stability of the osteochondral fragment.

As is the case with all synovial articulations, inflammatory diseases and other synovial disorders that may involve the ankle, such as rheumatoid arthritis, juvenile rheumatoid arthritis,[126] hemophilic arthropathy,[127] or pigmented villonodular synovitis, can be studied with MR imaging.

Knee. MR imaging has been used increasingly in the investigation of many disorders involving the knee. A standard MR examination of the knee requires about 30 to 45 minutes and includes coronal and sagittal T_1- and T_2-weighted images.[128] The protocol permits an extensive evaluation of the ligaments, menisci, articular surfaces, and bone marrow.[129] Transaxial views also are frequently obtained.

The normal signal intensity for ligaments, tendons, and menisci is low on all pulse sequences. Menisci normally have a triangular shape on sagittal and coronal planes and a C shape in the transaxial plane. The posterior horn of the medial meniscus is larger than the anterior horn. Also, the height of the meniscus is greater at the periphery than at its central part.[130] Abnormalities in the menisci are depicted as foci of increased signal intensity. Various attempts to classify abnormal signals within the meniscus have been recorded in recent literature.[131, 132] Grades I and II changes represent foci of bright signal in the meniscus that represent sites of degenerative myxoid

changes without tear. Grade III changes represent abnormally increased signal that extends to the articular surface, indicative of meniscal tear. Meniscal tears can be classified according to their morphology. Chronic degenerative tears are frequently horizontal in configuration, whereas acute tears tend to be vertical or oblique. Acute tears, however, also may be radial, transverse, or complex in appearance.[128] The bucket-handle tear represents a vertical tear in which the inner portion of the damaged meniscus is displaced into the intercondylar notch,[133] thus causing locking of the knee. The accuracy and specificity of MR in the analysis of internal derangement of the knee are highly dependent on the experience of the interpreter. The reported values for these with regard to meniscal tears have ranged from 75 to 100 percent.[134, 135] MR imaging can obviate exploratory arthroscopy.[136] If performed preoperatively, MR imaging can facilitate the detection or treatment, or both, of some lesions. In patients with residual or recurrent symptoms after a previous meniscectomy, MR also is useful in detecting incompletely excised meniscal tears or fragments and in disclosing a new tear in the residual meniscus.

With MR imaging, ligaments are depicted as structures of low signal intensity on all imaging sequences. Anterior and posterior cruciate and collateral ligaments are well studied with MR imaging. Findings suggestive of tears are an abnormal signal within these structures or nonvisualization. The anterior cruciate ligament extends from the medial aspect of the lateral femoral condyle to the anterior tibial spine. Because of this oblique course, sagittal images spaced each 3 mm through the intercondylar notch with 10 degrees of external rotation of the knee are often necessary for better visualization of this structure.[130] An acute complete tear often appears as an area of discontinuity in the normal course of the anterior cruciate ligament, and the ligament appears globular with an intermediate to high signal intensity on T_2-weighted images.[129, 130, 135] Edema and hemorrhage within and about the ligament are responsible for the foci of increased signal intensity. Secondary signs of anterior cruciate ligament tear are related to knee instability and include anterior bowing of the posterior cruciate ligament.[137, 138] Ninety percent of the tears typically occur in the midportion of the ligament or near its proximal femoral insertion. Avulsion of the ligament is less commonly seen (7 percent from its femoral attachment and 3 percent from its tibial attachment). MR imaging has a 95 percent accuracy in the diagnosis of anterior cruciate ligament tears and a negative predictive value of up to 100 percent.[129–135] Tears of the posterior cruciate ligament often lead to significant clinical instability of the knee. MR findings of posterior cruciate ligament tear most commonly consist of foci of increased signal intensity on T_2-weighted images, similar to the appearance of anterior cruciate ligament tears. Because the posterior cruciate ligament is thicker than its anterior counterpart, this ligament may appear widened in the area of the tear but is less likely to have a mass-like appearance. Posterior cruciate ligament tears are associated with other serious intra-articular injuries, including detachment of the posterior horn of the medial meniscus, disruption of the medial and lateral capsular ligaments, tears of the medial and lateral collateral ligaments, and avulsion of the tibial insertion site.[129]

Tears of lateral and medial collateral ligaments of the knee are well studied by MR imaging. They appear as disruptions of the normal low signal intensity of the ligament on T_1-weighted images with infiltration of the surrounding area by edema and blood, resulting in a high signal intensity on T_2-weighted images. Ligamentous sprain results in surrounding edema without ligamentous discontinuity. The Segond fracture represents traumatic detachment of the lateral capsule.[139] The resulting fragment of bone is usually small and minimally displaced.

MR imaging is well established as a sensitive means of evaluation of the bone marrow of the knee. It can detect abnormalities before they can be visualized on plain films and even before they can be detected by scintigraphy. MR is particularly sensitive in the detection of osteonecrosis, osteochondritis dissecans (Fig. 37–17), occult bone fractures, or bone contusion.[140] Osteochondritis dissecans usually involves the lateral aspect of the non–weight-bearing articular surface of the medial femoral condyle and is usually unilateral in distribution. Many hypotheses have been proposed to explain its pathogenesis, including acute or chronic trauma. Some authors report a familial incidence of osteochondritis dissecans of the knee.

MR evaluation of the articular cartilage has not yet been perfected. The transaxial plane is the preferred one to study the patellar cartilage, which is often poorly visualized in the sagittal plane. Fat suppression images (e.g., short tau inversion recovery, or STIR) are helpful if an effusion is present because with this technique, hyaline cartilage appears gray and fluid appears white, allowing distinction between the two. Patellofemoral joint malalignment also can be detected by obtaining multiple sequential transaxial images while the knee is positioned at various increments of flexion from 0 to 30 degrees, the range of flexion during which subluxation or dislocation of the patella most commonly appears. These images can be displayed in a cine-loop fashion to obtain a dynamic evaluation of the femoropatellar joint.[141]

MR imaging can aid in the investigation of patients with arthritis. Although early bone erosions can be depicted with MR imaging, the main application of this technique lies in the demonstration of the inflammatory pannus, which is depicted as a thickened, irregular synovium of intermediate signal intensity on T_1-weighted images. Acutely inflamed synovium has an increased signal intensity on T_2-weighted images, rendering it difficult to distinguish from an adjacent joint effusion. In chronically inflamed synovium, the pannus may appear as an area of low or intermediate signal intensity on T_2-weighted images, whereas the adjacent effusion appears brighter on the same imaging sequence.[142] Recent literature suggests that the intravenous injection of Gd-DTPA in patients with rheumatoid arthritis enhances the inflamed synovium, thereby helping in the detection of acute synovitis and its distinction

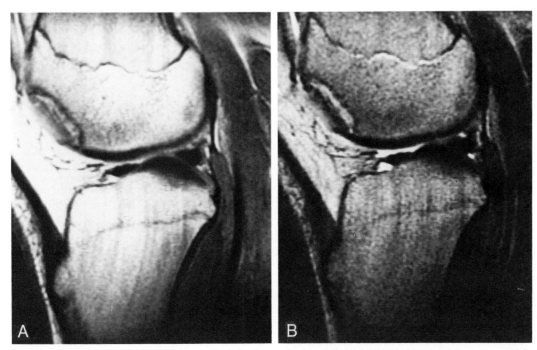

Figure 37–17. Osteochondritis dissecans. MR imaging of the knee: *A,* T_1-weighted sagittal image revealing an ovoid lesion, whose marginal zone has decreased signal intensity. B, T_2-weighted sagittal image with increase in signal intensity compatible with fluid or granulation tissue.

from accompanying effusion.[143] This procedure also can allow monitoring of the inflammatory process, as well as of the response to therapy.

MR imaging allows the detection of cysts about the knee. Three types of cysts are commonly found: popliteal, meniscal, and ganglionic cysts. Popliteal cysts (Fig. 37–18) are synovial cysts arising in the medial aspect of the popliteal fossa. They are caused by a communication between the posterior portion of the joint capsule and the normal gastrocnemiosem-imembranous bursa. Any condition associated with increased intra-articular pressure (such as knee effusion) can result in a popliteal cyst. These conditions include rheumatoid arthritis, degenerative joint disease, gout, pigmented villonodular synovitis (Fig. 37–19), and idiopathic synovial chondromatosis. Meniscal cysts are common (Fig. 37–20). They are associated with an underlying meniscal abnormality. The proposed pathogenesis relates to the intrusion of synovial fluid through a horizontal tear of the meniscus.[144] Lateral meniscal cysts occur more frequently than medial cysts. Ganglionic cysts usually contain a gelatinous material that has a high protein content. They may appear isointense to muscle on T_1-weighted images but bright on T_2-weighted images.[144] They most commonly appear as masses close to a joint, with which they may have a fibrous connection. They are not associated with meniscal tears.

RHEUMATOID ARTHRITIS

General Radiographic Features

Symmetry. The symmetry of rheumatoid arthritis constitutes an important diagnostic criterion for this disease. Asymmetric involvement may be noted in male patients and in men and women with early disease or neurologic deficit.[145]

Osteoporosis. Osteoporosis is a characteristic feature of rheumatoid arthritis. Early in the course of the disease, it tends to be localized to the juxta-articular region of the small peripheral joints. Later, generalized osteoporosis may be present in the axial and appendicular skeleton, often exacerbated by medications (i.e., salicylates, glucocorticoids) and disuse or immobilization. In a few patients with rheumatoid arthritis, osteomalacia may be observed.[146]

Soft Tissue Changes. Radiographic changes in the soft tissues can be of diagnostic importance in the patient with rheumatoid arthritis. Diffuse (fusiform) periarticular soft tissue swelling (Fig. 37–21) is an early finding about the small joints of the hands and feet. Intra-articular effusions are common radiographic findings in the knees, elbows, and ankles, producing characteristic displacements of adjacent fat planes. Occasionally, similar effusions in the small joints of the hand may lead to mild joint space widening. Bursal involvement can be identified as

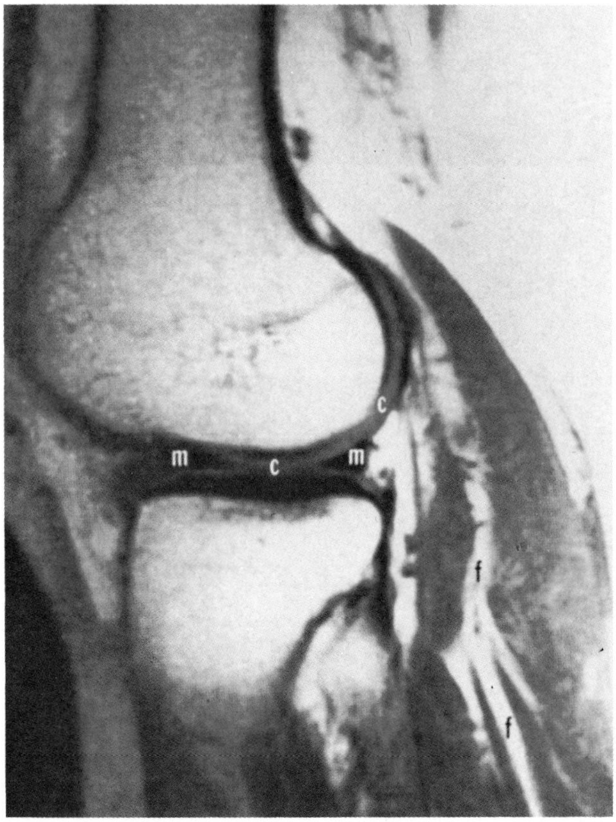

Figure 37–18. Ruptured popliteal cyst. On a T_2-weighted sagittal image of the knee following contrast arthrography, linear fluid collections (f) are noted within the calf musculature. The femoral and tibial hyaline articular cartilage (c) as well as the fibrocartilaginous lateral meniscus (m) is well visualized.

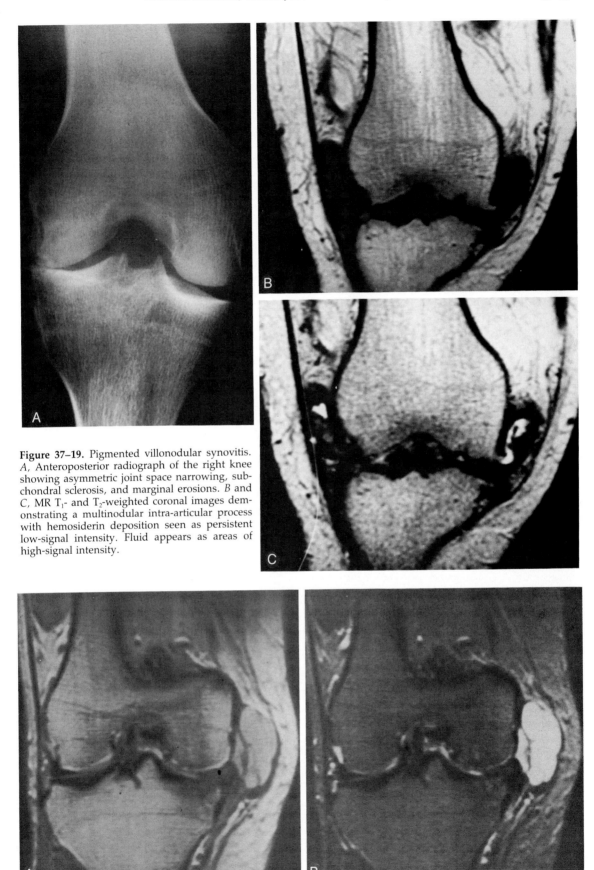

Figure 37–19. Pigmented villonodular synovitis. *A,* Anteroposterior radiograph of the right knee showing asymmetric joint space narrowing, subchondral sclerosis, and marginal erosions. *B* and *C,* MR T_1- and T_2-weighted coronal images demonstrating a multinodular intra-articular process with hemosiderin deposition seen as persistent low-signal intensity. Fluid appears as areas of high-signal intensity.

Figure 37–20. Meniscal cyst. MR imaging of the right knee. *A,* T_1-weighted coronal image with a low signal intensity mass adjacent to the medial femorotibial compartment associated with abnormal medial meniscus morphology. *B,* T_2-weighted coronal image with homogenous brightening suggesting a cystic mass.

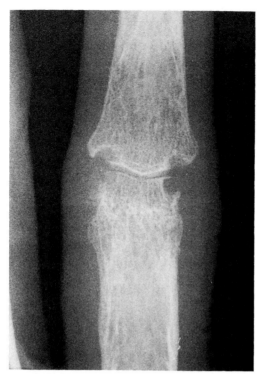

Figure 37–21. Rheumatoid arthritis. Marginal erosions are present on both sides of the interphalangeal joint. Joint space narrowing and fusiform soft tissue swelling are also evident.

asymmetric soft tissue prominence, particularly in the knee (prepatellar bursa), elbow (olecranon bursa), heel (retrocalcaneal bursa), and shoulder (subacromial bursa). Tendinitis and tenosynovitis are most frequently identified in the wrist when involvement of the extensor carpi ulnaris tendon and its synovial sheath causes prominent soft tissue swelling adjacent to the ulnar styloid process. Rheumatoid nodules may occasionally be observed on radiographs as noncalcified, eccentric, lobular soft tissue masses, which may cause pressure erosion of adjacent bones.

Joint Space Narrowing. Progressive joint space narrowing due to destruction of articular cartilage by pannus is another hallmark of rheumatoid arthritis, which may allow its differentiation from gout, a disease in which preservation of joint width is typical. In rheumatoid arthritis, the diffuse cartilaginous loss and the tendency toward pancompartmental involvement of complex joints, such as the knee and the wrist, limit additional diagnostic possibilities. Bony ankylosis is common only in the wrist and in the midfoot; it is distinctly unusual at other sites.

Bony Erosions. Three types of bony erosions may be identified in rheumatoid arthritis. *Marginal erosions* occur at intra-articular sites that are not protected by overlying cartilage. Typically these "bare" areas are the initial points of attack by the proliferating synovial tissue (see Fig. 37–21). *Compressive erosions* occur when collapse of osteoporotic subchondral bone leads to invagination of one bone into another. These changes occur at articulations exposed to strong muscular actions or significant

weight-bearing forces. The most characteristic site of compressive erosion is the hip, where protrusio acetabuli may be identified (Fig. 37–22). Other important sites are at the metacarpophalangeal joints, where collapse of the base of a proximal phalanx by a metacarpal head produces a ball-in-socket type articulation, and the radiocarpal joint of the wrist, where the scaphoid may appear to be "countersunk" into the distal radius. The third type of erosion seen in rheumatoid arthritis is *surface resorption*, usually related to inflammation of an adjacent tendon sheath (Fig. 37–23). This is an important finding in the wrist, where a characteristic erosion of the outer margin of the ulnar styloid process, due to extensor carpi ulnaris tenosynovitis, provides an early radiographic sign of rheumatoid arthritis.

Bony Cysts. Subchondral cystic lesions are frequent in rheumatoid arthritis and have been described as cysts, pseudocysts, geodes, and granulomas. Most commonly, multiple small, ill-defined subchondral radiolucencies are identified at any articulation involved in rheumatoid arthritis. The identification of larger cystic areas, especially in the hands and wrists of physically active men, has been termed *rheumatoid arthritis of the robust reaction pattern.*[147] Occasionally, very large cystic lesions may be encountered in the elbow (olecranon process of ulna, distal humerus), femoral neck, or knee (distal femur, proximal tibia, patella) and have been described as pseudocystic rheumatoid arthritis (Fig. 37–24).[148] These large lesions may subsequently fracture.

Deformities and Instabilities. Many types of articular deformity and instability are observed in rheumatoid arthritis (Fig. 37–25). Most of these relate to tendinous or ligamentous laxity or disruption, with alteration of the normal muscle pull across one or

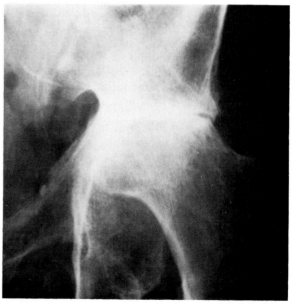

Figure 37–22. Rheumatoid arthritis. Symmetric destruction of the cartilaginous surface has resulted in axial migration of the femoral head. The femoral head has become small and flattened. Sclerosis is apparent.

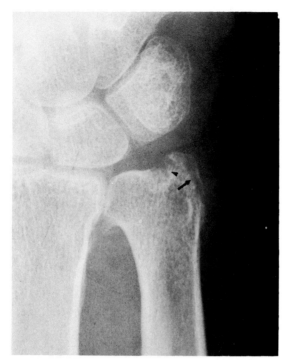

Figure 37–23. Rheumatoid arthritis. An osseous erosion is present in the outer margin of the ulnar styloid (surface erosion) *(arrow)* owing to synovitis of the extensor carpi ulnaris tendon sheath. A second erosion is present at the point of insertion of the triangular fibrocartilage on the ulnar head *(arrowhead).* (From Resnick, D., and Niwayama, G: Diagnosis of Bone and Joint Disorders. Philadelphia, W. B. Saunders Co., 1988.)

more articulations (e.g., boutonniére or swan-neck deformity of the fingers, ulnar deviation at the metacarpophalangeal joints, fibular deviation at the metatarsophalangeal joints, or atlantoaxial subluxation). In some cases, however, the abnormality may relate directly to bone or cartilage destruction (e.g., protrusion acetabuli). These characteristic deformities and instabilities are summarized in Table 37–3.

Abnormalities at Specific Sites

Hand. The target areas of rheumatoid arthritis in the hands are the metacarpophalangeal and proximal interphalangeal joints. The earliest changes consist of fusiform soft tissue swelling, juxta-articular osteoporosis, diffuse joint space loss, and marginal bony erosions (see Fig. 37–21). A particularly characteristic finding is indistinctness and focal loss of continuity of the dorsoradial subchondral bone plate (dot-dash pattern) of the metacarpal head.[149] In general, these radiographic findings appear initially at the second and third metacarpophalangeal joints and third proximal interphalangeal joint. The marginal osseous erosions tend to be more prominent on the proximal bone of the articulation, which tends to have a larger bare area. With progression of the disease, large erosions, complete joint space obliteration, and finger deformities appear. The end stage is usually fibrous ankylosis of the articular cavity; bony ankylosis is rare in the hand but, when present, almost exclusively involves the proximal interphalangeal joints.[145]

Wrist. The wrist is a complex articulation that should properly be viewed as a series of distinct synovial compartments: (1) radiocarpal, (2) inferior radioulnar, (3) midcarpal, (4) pisotriquetral, (5) common carpometacarpal, and (6) first carpometacarpal. Rheumatoid arthritis demonstrates distinctive pancompartmental involvement of the wrist, which helps to differentiate it from other arthropathies.[150] The least commonly involved area is the first carpometacarpal compartment, which may be spared even in the presence of advanced disease elsewhere in the wrist.

The distal ulna, being bounded by three impor-

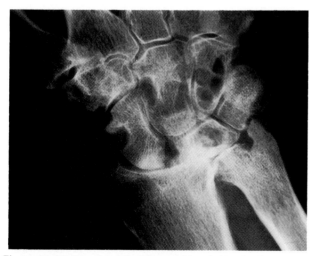

Figure 37–24. Pseudocystic rheumatoid arthritis. In this patient, large cystic erosions are present, giving the appearance of "hollow" carpal bones. Also note the narrowing of the radiocarpal joint with ulnar translocation of the carpus. (From Resnick, D., and Niwayama, G.: Diagnosis of Bone and Joint Disorders. Philadelphia, W. B. Saunders Co., 1988.)

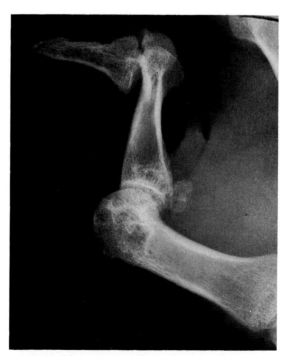

Figure 37–25. Rheumatoid arthritis. In this patient, note the prominent thumb deformity with flexion at the metacarpophalangeal joint and extension of the interphalangeal joint. This constitutes the boutonnière deformity.

Table 37–3. INSTABILITIES AND DEFORMITIES IN RHEUMATOID ARTHRITIS

Site	Name	Abnormality
Hand		
DIP joint	Mallet finger	Flexion DIP
PIP and DIP joints	Boutonnière deformity	Flexion PIP, extension DIP
	Swan-neck deformity	Extension PIP, flexion DIP
MCP joint		Ulnar deviation
		Volar subluxation
Wrist		
Distal radioulnar joint	Caput ulna	Subluxation/dislocation distal radioulnar joint
Radiocarpal joint		Radial deviation
		Ulnar translocation
Intercarpal joints	Scapholunate dissociation	Scapholunate space >2 mm
	Dorsal intercalary segment instability	Dorsiflexion lunate, volar flexion scaphoid
	Volar intercalary segment instability	Volar flexion lunate, dorsiflexion scaphoid
		Subluxation extensor carpi ulnaris tendon
Hip	Protrusio acetabuli	Acetabular wall medial to ilioischial line
		>3 mm in male
		>6 mm in female
Knee	Genu varus	Inward deviation of tibia
	Genu valgus	Outward deviation of tibia
Foot		
First MTP joint	Hallux valgus (bunion)	Lateral deviation first MTP joint
MTP (all)		Lateral deviation MTP joints (I–IV)
		Plantar subluxation MTP joints
	Cock-up toe	Hyperextension and dorsal subluxation MTP
PIP and DIP	Hammer toe	Hyperflexion PIP or DIP
Cervical spine		
Atlantoaxial joint	Atlantoaxial subluxation	Atlanto-odontoid space >3 mm
	Vertical atlantoaxial subluxation	Superior displacement odontoid
All levels	Stair-step deformity	Subluxation apophyseal joints

DIP, distal intephalangeal; PIP, proximal interphalangeal; MCP, metacarpophalangeal; MTP, metatarsophalangeal.

tant sites of synovial proliferation, occupies a prominent role as a target area in rheumatoid arthritis[151] (see Fig. 37–23). Erosions along the outer margin of the ulnar styloid are related to tenosynovitis of the extensor carpi ulnaris tendon; erosions of the styloid tip are related to involvement of the prestyloid recess of the radiocarpal compartment; and erosions of the base and juxta-articular area of the distal ulna indicate inferior radioulnar compartment involvement.

Early erosions may involve any bone in the wrist; in addition to the distal ulna, some of the more characteristic sites[152, 153] include the radial styloid, lateral scaphoid waist, triquetrum, and pisiform. These changes may be manifested as distinct erosions or as cystic lesions that give the radiographic appearance of hollow carpal bones. With time, the characteristic pancompartmental involvement becomes evident with loss of articular spaces. Bony ankylosis of the carpus is a relatively common end result of advanced rheumatoid arthritis. In some cases diffuse carpal destruction may occur, culminating in complete disintegration of the wrist.

Numerous deformities related to soft tissue destruction and muscular imbalances may be seen. The most characteristic wrist deformities consist of ulnar translocation of the proximal carpal row, related to destruction of the triangular fibrocartilage-meniscus homologue complex, and radial deviation at the radiocarpal joint (Fig. 37–26).[154]

Elbow. The elbow is a frequent site of abnormality, particularly in patients with advanced disease. In this area a common radiographic finding

consists of a positive "fat pad" sign, representing displacement of the fat pads anterior and posterior to the distal humerus owing to intra-articular effusion or synovial hypertrophy.[155, 156] Soft tissue swelling

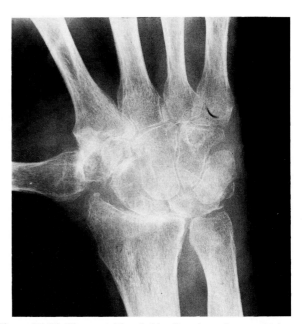

Figure 37–26. Rheumatoid arthritis. Prominent juxta-articular osteoporosis is present with radial deviation of the radiocarpal joint and ulnar translocation of the carpus. Extensive erosive changes of the radial and ulnar styloid processes and multiple carpal bones are also present. (From Resnick, D., and Niwayama, G.: Diagnosis of Bone and Joint Disorders. Philadelphia, W. B. Saunders Co., 1988.)

over the ulnar olecranon, related to olecranon bursitis, and about the proximal ulna, related to rheumatoid nodules, is another frequent finding. Eventually, extensive osteolysis of the humerus, radius, and ulna may resemble the findings in neuroarthropathy. Large medullary cystic lesions of the distal humerus and ulnar olecranon may be the sites of pathologic fracture.[157]

Shoulder. Two main anatomic sites are frequently involved in rheumatoid arthritis of the shoulder: the glenohumeral and acromioclavicular joints. In the former location, changes of rheumatoid arthritis are prominent joint space narrowing, bony sclerosis, and cyst formation.[152] Osseous erosions are most prominent along the superolateral margin of the humerus, adjacent to the greater tuberosity, and may resemble the Hill-Sachs fracture associated with anterior shoulder dislocation. Erosions may be present at other sites on the proximal humerus and glenoid region of the scapula. Subacromial bursitis, bicipital tendinitis, and rotator cuff tears are frequent complications.

At the acromioclavicular joint, soft tissue swelling and erosions, which tend to be more prominent on the clavicular side of the joint, are early findings.[146] Later, destruction of a large portion of the distal clavicle may be seen.

Foot. Sites of foot involvement in rheumatoid arthritis may be divided into the forefoot, the midfoot, and the heel. The forefoot is very commonly affected (80 to 90 percent) in rheumatoid arthritis, especially the metatarsophalangeal joints.[158–160] The earliest changes involve the metatarsal heads at the first and fifth metatarsophalangeal articulations (Fig. 37–27).[145] At the fifth metatarsophalangeal joint, an early and characteristic erosion occurs on the dorsolateral aspect of the metatarsal head and may be

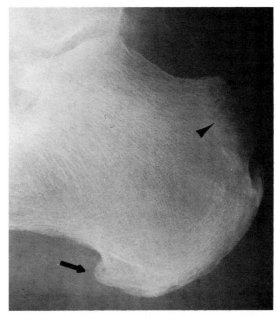

Figure 37–28. Rheumatoid arthritis. Erosions are present on the posterior *(arrowhead)* calcaneal surface. A plantar calcaneal spur is evident *(arrow).*

visualized only on oblique radiographs. At the first metatarsophalangeal joint, the earliest involvement is along the medial aspect of the metatarsal head, with later erosions involving the adjacent sesamoid bones. With progression, diffuse joint space loss and larger erosions may be seen. Forefoot deformities in rheumatoid arthritis include hallux valgus, hammer toes, and "cock-up" toes, as well as fibular deviation of the digits and plantar subluxation of the metatarsal heads.

In the midfoot, rheumatoid arthritis is characterized by diffuse joint space loss, bony sclerosis, and osteophytosis, with osseous erosions being uncommon.[145] Osseous fusion in long-standing disease is relatively common. Differentiation of this disease from degenerative, post-traumatic, or neuropathic disorders may be difficult in this region.

In the heel, abnormalities of rheumatoid arthritis are related to involvement of the retrocalcaneal bursa, Achilles tendon, and plantar fascia. With the utilization of soft tissue–enhancing radiographic techniques, swelling of the Achilles tendon (>1 cm in diameter at the level of the posterosuperior margin of the calcaneus) or soft tissue masses adjacent to the posterosuperior margin of the calcaneus as the result of an engorged retrocalcaneal bursa may be early findings.[145, 161, 162] Osseous erosions at the posterosuperior margin of the calcaneus (Fig. 37–28) are subsequently noted. Well-defined plantar calcaneal enthesophytes, which are identical to those seen in "normal" persons, can be distinguished from the fluffy, proliferative calcaneal excrescences seen in the seronegative spondyloarthropathies.

Ankle. Although the ankle may be the site of radiographically identifiable joint effusions in the patient with rheumatoid arthritis, bony changes at

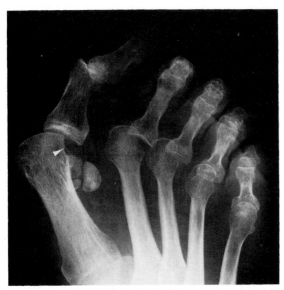

Figure 37–27. Rheumatoid arthritis. The classic forefoot deformities are well illustrated in this patient. Note the subluxation and fibular deviation at the MTP joints and the prominent marginal erosions of the first metatarsal head *(arrowhead).* (From Resnick, D., and Niwayama, G.: Diagnosis of Bone and Joint Disorders. Philadelphia, W. B. Saunders Co., 1988.)

this site are relatively uncommon. In some cases diffuse osteoporosis and joint space narrowing as well as marginal and central bony erosions may be seen.[163] Rarely, with severe disease, loss of integrity of the ankle mortise may occur.

Knee. The knee is commonly affected in rheumatoid arthritis. Engorgement of the suprapatellar space of the knee joint by effusion or synovial hypertrophy is noted on the lateral radiographic projection. Small erosions along the medial and lateral margins of the tibia and femur are the earliest bony changes and are followed by joint space loss involving the medial femorotibial, lateral femorotibial, and patellofemoral compartments.[145] Subchondral cysts may be seen in the femoral condyles or proximal tibia, and subchondral sclerosis due to bony collapse may be prominent.[164] Varsus or valgus deformity of the knee joint or patellar instability may be present. Rupture of the quadriceps or patellar tendon may occur with corresponding abnormalities of the soft tissue shadows about the knee. The knee is also a common site of large synovial cysts, especially in the popliteal region.[165] These synovial cysts may extend along fascial planes for a considerable distance in a proximal or distal direction.

Hip. Hip involvement in rheumatoid arthritis is less common than knee involvement. A characteristic radiographic abnormality is diffuse concentric loss of articular space, with migration of the femoral head along the plane of the axis of the femoral neck.[166] Radiolucent zones at the bone cartilage junction of the femoral head are related to circumferential marginal erosions.[145] Central erosions of the femoral head and, less commonly, of the acetabulum may be seen. Occasionally large pseudocystic lesions of the femoral neck occur and are liable to pathologic fracture. Acetabular protrusion is present if the inner margin of the acetabulum is medial to the ilioischial line by 3 mm or more in men or 6 mm or more in women. Mild sclerosis and small osteophytes may be noted, related to secondary degenerative disease (osteoarthritis). Osteonecrosis of the femoral heads may be encountered in rheumatoid arthritis, usually in association with glucocorticoid therapy.[167]

Sacroiliac Joints. Asymptomatic sacroiliac joint changes are common in rheumatoid arthritis of long duration.[168] In general the findings consist of bilateral but asymmetric bony erosions that primarily involve the iliac side of the synovial articulation.

Spine. The cervical spine is one of the more common and important areas of involvement in rheumatoid arthritis. The apophyseal joints of the cervical spine are diffusely affected with bony erosion, joint space narrowing and, eventually, subluxation that leads to a "stair-step" type of deformity (Fig. 37–29), with contiguous vertebral bodies being offset like the steps of a staircase.[169] Erosions and destruction involving the uncovertebral joints (Luschka) as well as the discovertebral junctions are also common. Between the spinous processes, the formation of adventitious bursae and their subsequent inflammation lead to characteristic erosions and a "sharpened"

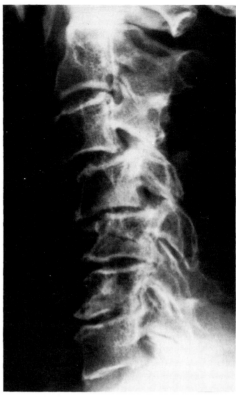

Figure 37–29. Rheumatoid arthritis. The "stair-step" deformity of the cervical spine is present with subluxation at multiple contiguous levels. Diffuse loss of intervertebral disc height and erosion of articular surfaces of the apophyseal joints are also present. (From Resnick, D., and Niwayama, G.: Diagnosis of Bone and Joint Disorders. Philadelphia, W. B. Saunders Co., 1988.)

appearance of these processes on lateral radiographs of the cervical spine.

The most important site of cervical spine abnormality is the craniocervical junction. Erosions involving the anterior or posterior margins of the odontoid process as well as joint space narrowing and marginal osseous erosions involving the lateral occipito-atlantoaxial articulations are early findings.[169] Subsequently, laxity or destruction of the transverse atlantoaxial ligament can lead to horizontal (in the sagittal plane) atlantoaxial subluxation with encroachment of the odontoid process on the vertebral canal during flexion of the neck.[170, 171] The diagnosis of this complication is based on the identification of an abnormally wide space (>3 mm in the adult) between the posterior margin of the anterior arch of the atlas and the anterior surface of the odontoid process on lateral radiographs of the cervical spine exposed during flexion of the patient's neck. Large odontoid erosions may predispose to pathologic fracture. A second, less common but potentially fatal, pattern of cevical instability in rheumatoid arthritis is vertical atlantoaxial subluxation in which compression of the lateral masses of the atlas in association with disease of the lateral atlantoaxial and atlanto-occipital joints allows the odontoid process to be elevated vertically, becoming intimate with the brainstem.[171, 172] Furthermore, occipito-atlantoaxial instability in the coronal plane can lead to lateral tilting of the head.

In contrast to the frequency of cervical spine involvement, changes in the thoracic and lumbar spine are uncommon in rheumatoid arthritis. However, erosive and destructive abnormalities about the lumbar apophyseal joints are well documented, as are irregularity, erosion, and loss of definition of the bony vertebral end-plates.[145] Synovial cysts arising from the apophyseal joints are rare causes of neurologic symptoms and signs.[173]

Other Locations. Other synovial joints that may be involved in rheumatoid arthritis include the TM and sternoclavicular joints. Not infrequently, cartilaginous articulations, such as the sternomanubrial joint and symphysis pubis, may show erosive change and narrowing.

JUVENILE CHRONIC ARTHRITIS

General Radiographic Features. *Juvenile chronic arthritis* (JCA) is a generic term used to describe a group of childhood articular disorders that share, to a variable degree, certain clinical, laboratory, and radiologic features. Each specific subgroup of JCA has its own distinctive radiographic appearance. However, many of the changes are nonspecific and related to effects of the disorder on growth and development of the immature skeleton. It is useful to first consider these general features of childhood arthritis prior to considering abnormalities in specific subgroups of disease.

Growth Disturbances.[174-176] Epiphyseal enlargement is a common feature of JCA and is related to growth stimulation associated with epiphyseal hyperemia. The changes occur diffusely but often are most marked at the femoral condyles, humeral condyles, and radial head. Epiphyseal overgrowth is combined with subnormal growth of the diaphyseal portion of the bone, resulting in a constricted appearance to the diaphysis with "ballooning" of the epiphysis (Fig. 37–30). The time of appearance and the size of individual bones in the wrist and midfoot may be increased. In some cases, overall bone length may be diminished owing to premature closure of the physis or, in other cases, increased owing to hyperemia.

Periostitis.[176] Periostitis is a common and nonspecific component of virtually all forms of JCA. This is in contrast to the specificity of periostitis in the differential diagnosis of adult arthropathies. In childhood the periosteum is relatively loosely attached to the underlying bone, a situation that allows it to be easily lifted and stimulated to produce new bone in response to inflammation. Periostitis is most common in the phalanges, metacarpals, and metatarsals but may occasionally be seen in the metaphyses and diaphyses of long tubular bones. In the small bones of the hands and feet, exuberant periosteal new bone formation may result in a "squared" appearance.

Epiphyseal Compression Fractures.[176] Flattening

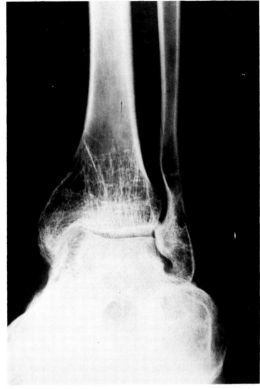

Figure 37–30. Juvenile chronic arthritis. Note the prominent juxta-articular osteoporosis with "ballooning" of the distal tibial and fibular epiphyses and a constricted appearance to the bone shafts.

and deformity of the epiphyseal centers in weight-bearing articulations are common in JCA. Cupping of the epiphyseal centers of the proximal phalanges is also frequent. These changes are related to the abnormal stresses associated with joint contracture and subluxation acting on the osteoporotic epiphyses.

Osteopenia. Osteopenia, representing increased skeletal radiolucency, is generally most striking in the metaphyseal region of a bone, resulting in the formation of horizontally oriented radiolucent metaphyseal bands.[176] These lucent bands are commonly noted in the femur, tibia, fibula, and radius and are identical to those seen in childhood leukemia, metastatic neuroblastoma, and congenital infections. With time, diffuse osteoporosis can develop. Growth recovery lines (Fig. 37–31) are thin, horizontally oriented radiodense bands visualized in the diametaphyseal region of tubular bones in children with chronic illness. Presumably they are manifestations of accelerated bone growth in the intervals following exacerbations of disease. Occasionally, widespread metaphyseal sclerosis is seen (see Fig. 37–31).

Juvenile-Onset Adult-Type (Seropositive) Rheumatoid Arthritis. Soft tissue swelling, juxta-articular osteoporosis, and marginal erosions are present, as in the typical adult case.[174] However, two features help differentiate this disorder from adult-onset rheumatoid arthritis: the presence of periostitis, especially of the small bones of the hands and feet, and the frequent occurrence of prominent

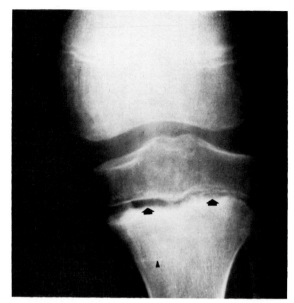

Figure 37–31. Juvenile chronic arthritis. There is overgrowth of the epiphyses about the knee. Juxta-articular osteoporosis is evident, with several horizontally oriented growth recovery lines *(arrowhead)*. Metaphyseal sclerosis *(arrows)* can be visualized in the proximal tibia.

marginal erosions without associated joint space narrowing.[177, 178]

Seronegative Chronic Arthritis (Still's Disease).[179] Classic systemic Still's disease is an acute systemic illness that rarely manifests radiographic articular changes.

Polyarticular disease may occur in the presence or absence of classic Still's disease. Symmetric involvement of the hands, wrists, knees, ankles, feet, and cervical spine is common. In the hands and feet, osteoporosis is associated with joint space narrowing, and the small bones assume a "squared" shape as a result of new bone formation. Osseous erosions are unusual in this disorder and, when present, are usually of small size. Intra-articular bony ankylosis (Fig. 37–32) is a common late complication in the small joints, in contrast to its rarity in adult-onset rheumatoid arthritis. In the larger articulations such as the knee and the hip, osteoporosis and epiphyseal overgrowth are the most typical manifestations, often occurring without joint space narrowing or bony erosions. The cervical spine is frequently the only spinal level involved in this disorder (Fig. 37–33); abnormalities predominate in the upper cervical region. The growth disturbance results in a constriction of vertebral body width and depth with relatively normal height, resulting in a slender, gracile appearance. Apophyseal joint space narrowing, bony ankylosis, and osseous erosions occur with hypoplasia of the intervertebral discs and bony ankylosis of vertebral bodies. As in adults, atlantoaxial subluxation is a frequent complication in children.

Pauciarticular and monoarticular forms of seronegative chronic arthritis are occasionally seen.[178, 180] Changes are generally confined to the larger articulations such as the knee, hip, ankle, elbow, and

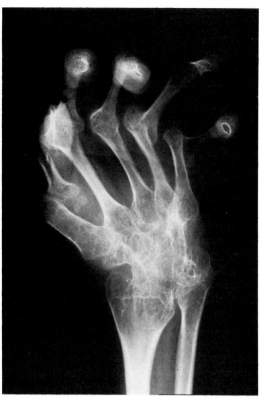

Figure 37–32. Juvenile chronic arthritis. There are prominent finger deformities, osteoporosis, and bony ankylosis, especially in the carpus. Note the elongated, slender appearance of the tubular bones, which is related to growth disturbance.

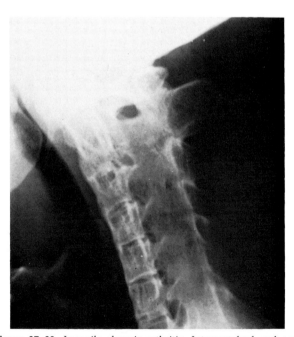

Figure 37–33. Juvenile chronic arthritis. Intervertebral and apophyseal joint bony ankylosis is present at multiple levels. The overall appearance of the cervical spine is gracile, owing to the relatively normal height of the vertebral bodies and the diminished anteroposterior vertebral diameter. (From Resnick, D., and Niwayama, G.: Diagnosis of Bone and Joint Disorders. Philadelphia, W. B. Saunders Co., 1981.)

wrist; the small joints of the hands and feet are spared. Radiographic abnormalities are the same as those in the polyarticular pattern of disease.

Juvenile-Onset Ankylosing Spondylitis. Juvenile-onset ankylosing spondylitis is generally first manifest in the articulations of the lower extremity, particularly the hips, knees, ankles, and small joints of the feet.[174] The joints of the upper extremities are relatively spared. Sacroiliitis and spondylitis occur but are usually identified later in the course of the disease, in contrast to adult-onset ankylosing spondylitis. In the spine, thoracic and lumbar involvement is common, with involvement of the cervical spine being distinctly unusual.

Radiographic changes in the peripheral skeleton consist of joint space narrowing, bony erosions and proliferation, and intra-articular osseous fusion.[181] Osteoporosis is frequently not prominent. In the sacroiliac articulations and the thoracolumbar spine, the radiographic changes are identical to those of adult-onset ankylosing spondylitis.[182] Useful features in differentiating this disorder from other types of JCA include the absence of diffuse osteoporosis, relative sparing of the articulations of the upper extremity and cervical spine, and sacroiliitis and spondylitis.

Juvenile-Onset Psoriatic Arthritis. Juvenile-onset psoriatic arthritis is occasionally encountered. Radiographic changes simulate those in adults. Hand involvement is characterized by resorption of the terminal tufts of the distal phalanges and interphalangeal joint destruction.[179] Although sacroiliitis is common in this disorder, the normal indistinct appearance of the sacroiliac articulations in children and adolescents makes accurate radiographic diagnosis of sacroiliitis difficult.

Adult-Onset Still's Disease. Rarely, an adult patient may be encountered with a febrile illness identical to classic Still's disease.[183] When present, radiographic changes involve the wrists, knees, and fingers. Bony erosions are unusual. A peculiar tendency toward narrowing or ankylosis of the common carpometacarpal joint, especially that portion at the level of the second and third metacarpal bases, and the intercarpal joint in a pericapitate distribution has been reported.[184]

Others. Enteropathic arthropathy may be identified in childhood accompanying regional enteritis, ulcerative colitis, or bowel infections (*Salmonella, Shigella*). Its appearance is identical to that of juvenile-onset ankylosing spondylitis. Other rare causes of childhood arthropathy include systemic lupus erythematosus and familial Mediterranean fever.

SERONEGATIVE SPONDYLOARTHROPATHIES

Ankylosing Spondylitis. Synovial and cartilaginous joints as well as sites of tendon and ligament insertion (entheses) may be involved in ankylosing spondylitis and the other seronegative spondyloarthropathies.[185, 186] Axial skeletal involvement is characteristic, with a predilection for the sacroiliac, apophyseal, discovertebral, and costovertebral articulations. The initial sites of involvement are the sacroiliac joints and lumbosacral and thoracolumbar vertebral junctions. Subsequently, ascending and descending spinal disease may be encountered.[187, 188] Peripheral joint involvement, although frequent (50 percent), is usually mild.[182] The hips and glenohumeral joints are the most common extraspinal locations of disease.

Sacroiliac Joints. Involvement of the sacroiliac joint is the hallmark of ankylosing spondylitis. It is difficult to verify the diagnosis of this disease in the absence of such involvement. Rarely, spinal disease occurs in the absence of significant sacroiliac joint abnormality. Sacroiliitis occurs early in the course of ankylosing spondylitis and is characteristically bilateral and symmetric in its distribution.[187-190] On rare occasions, initial unilateral or asymmetric sacroiliac joint changes are observed. Changes occur both in the synovial and in the ligamentous portions of the joint, with the abnormalities being more prominent on the iliac side of the articulation.[186] Osteoporosis, subchondral bony resorption with loss of definition of the articular margins, and superficial osseous erosions are interspersed with focal areas of bony sclerosis. Radiographically, in this stage, the articulation may appear widened. With progression of the disease, a wide, ill-defined band of sclerosis is seen on the iliac side of the joint with larger subchondral erosions (Fig. 37–34). In the late proliferative stage, bony bridges traverse the joint space, initially isolating islands of intact cartilage. Such segmental ankylosis may be followed by complete intra-articular bony fusion (Fig. 37–35) and disappearance of the periarticular sclerosis. The ligamentous (syndesmotic) portions of the sacroiliac joint may also be affected, leading to bony erosions and proliferation. In general, involvement of the ligamentous portion of the articulation is less prominent in ankylosing spondylitis than in psoriatic arthritis and Reiter's syndrome.

Spine. The initial sites of spinal involvement, especially in men, are the lumbosacral and thoracolumbar junctions. In women, the cervical spine may be affected at an early stage of disease. "Osteitis" is an initial finding, related to inflammation of the anterior portion of the discovertebral junction.[186] A focal erosive lesion at the anterosuperior and anteroinferior vertebral margins leads to loss of the normal concavity of the anterior aspect of the vertebral body, resulting in a "squared" configuration of the vertebral body in the lateral radiographic projection. This appearance is more easily identified in the lumbar spine, as the thoracic vertebral bodies may normally have a squared appearance. In ankylosing spondylitis, bony sclerosis adjacent to the sites of erosion produces a "shiny corner" sign on radiographs.

Syndesmophytes are vertically oriented bony excrescences, which represent ossification of the outer fibers of the annulus fibrosus of the intervertebral disc.[191] They predominate on the anterior and

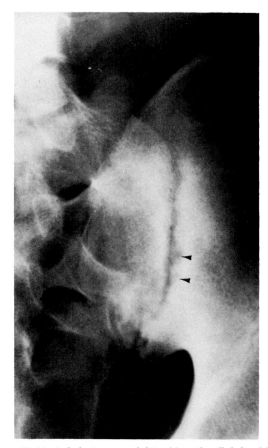

Figure 37–34. Ankylosing spondylitis. Note the ill-defined band of sclerosis and prominent erosions of the subchondral bone plate *(arrowheads)*, which are most conspicuous on the iliac side of the articulation.

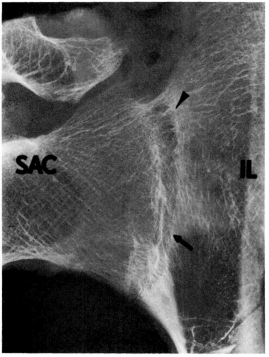

Figure 37–35. Ankylosing spondylitis. A specimen radiograph from a cadaver with the disease demonstrates complete intra-articular ankylosis of the ligamentous *(arrowhead)* and synovial *(arrow)* portions of the joint. (SAC = sacrum; IL = ilium.)

lateral aspects of the spine and eventually bridge the intervertebral disc (Fig. 37–36A). In the late stages of the disease, extensive syndesmophytic formation produces a smooth, undulating spinal contour, the "bamboo" spine.

It is of critical importance that the syndesmophytes that characterize ankylosing spondylitis (and enteropathic spondyloarthritis) be differentiated from other spinal and paraspinal bony excrescences (Fig. 37–36; also see Figs. 37–43, 37–58, and 37–59). Vertebral excrescences in spondylosis deformans arise several millimeters from the discovertebral junction, are triangular in shape, and demonstrate a horizontally oriented segment of variable length at their point of origin. In diffuse idiopathic skeletal hyperostosis (DISH), bone formation in the anterior longitudinal ligament results in a flowing pattern of ossification, thicker than that seen in ankylosing spondylitis. Such ossification is best demonstrated on lateral spine radiographs. Furthermore, in DISH, there is absence of erosion or widespread bony ankylosis in the sacroiliac joints. The paravertebral ossifications that characterize psoriatic arthritis and Reiter's syndrome arise in an asymmetric fashion in the soft tissues adjacent to the outer layer of the annulus fibrosus. They are initially unattached to the vertebral body but, with time, they fuse with the margins of the vertebral body at a point several millimeters from the discovertebral junction.

Erosions at one or more discovertebral junctions can be prominent radiographic findings in ankylosing spondylitis. These may be classified as focal or diffuse.[192] Focal lesions may relate to intraosseous displacement of disc material (cartilaginous or Schmorl's node) or enthesitis. Diffuse destruction of the discovertebral junction may be related to a pseudarthrosis following fracture. Discal calcification is common and usually seen in association with apophyseal joint ankylosis at the same spinal level.

Early alterations in the apophyseal joints in the lumbar, thoracic, and cervical segments consist of ill-defined erosions accompanied by reactive sclerosis. Capsular ossification or intra-articular bony ankylosis may subsequently occur. On frontal radiographs of the spine, such ossification produces vertically oriented, parallel, radiodense bands, which, when combined with a central radiodense band related to ossification of the interspinous and supraspinous ligaments, lead to the "trolley-track" sign (Fig. 37–36B).[186]

Erosions of the odontoid process and atlantoaxial subluxation may be observed in ankylosing spondylitis, although with less frequency than in rheumatoid arthritis.[171, 187] Ankylosis of the atlantoaxial articulation, either in its normal position or in a position of subluxation, may occasionally be noted. At other levels in the cervical spine, the changes, when present, are identical to those in the thoracolumbar spine.

Extraspinal Locations. The hip is the most commonly involved peripheral articulation in ankylosing spondylitis, with the changes most frequently being

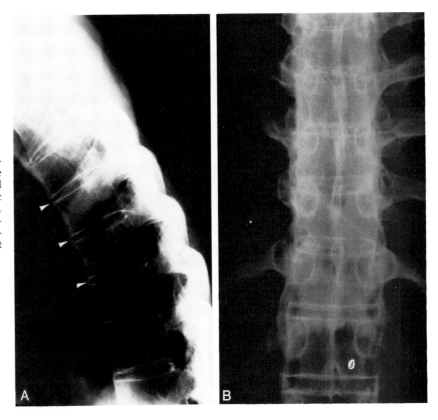

Figure 37–36. Ankylosing spondylitis. Lateral *(A)* and frontal *(B)* radiographs of the spine demonstrate complete intervertebral ankylosis, which produces the characteristic "bamboo spine" appearance. Note the thin, vertically oriented syndesmophytes *(arrowheads)* arising from the discovertebral junction, owing to ossification in the outermost layer of the annulus fibrosus.

bilateral and symmetric in distribution.[193] Concentric joint space narrowing with axial migration of the femoral head and marginal osteophyte formation characterizes the hip disease of ankylosing spondylitis (Fig. 37–37). Osteophytes are first observed at the lateral margin of the femoral head-neck junction and, with progression, proliferate circumferentially to produce a characteristic "ring osteophyte."[193, 194] Subchondral cysts and erosions as well as intra-

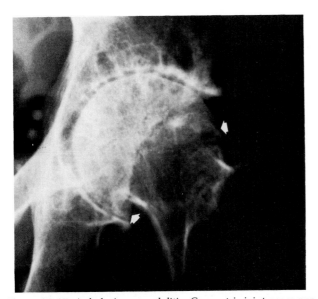

Figure 37–37. Ankylosing spondylitis. Concentric joint space narrowing with axial migration of the femoral head is present. Osteophytes *(arrows)* are present at the medial and lateral margins of the femoral head.

articular bony ankylosis may be seen in some cases. Such hip disease can lead to significant clinical manifestations requiring surgical intervention. However, patients with ankylosing spondylitis who undergo hip surgery, including total joint replacement, are prone to develop exuberant deposits of juxta-articular heterotopic bone, which may severely restrict postoperative hip motion.[195]

The shoulder is the second most common peripheral site of involvement in ankylosing spondylitis.[182] Bilateral involvement is common; changes are osteoporosis, joint space narrowing, bony erosions, and rotator cuff disruption. A characteristic large destructive abnormality involving the superolateral aspect of the humeral head in this disease has been termed the "hatchet" sign (Fig. 37–38).[196]

Changes in other peripheral joints occur with variable frequency. In general, these changes, which are similar to but less extensive than those in the other seronegative spondyloarthropathies, include soft tissue swelling, mild osteoporosis, joint space narrowing, bony erosions, and osseous proliferation.[186] The erosions tend to be less prominent than in rheumatoid arthritis. The presence of bone proliferation (whiskering) and periostitis in ankylosing spondylitis (and the other seronegative spondyloarthropathies) is another helpful diagnostic feature.

Inflammation with bony proliferation at sites of tendon and ligament insertion (enthesopathy), especially those of the pelvis, patella, and calcaneus, is prominent in ankylosing spondylitis (as well as in the other seronegative spondyloarthropathies). Plantar and posterior calcaneal spurs are common and

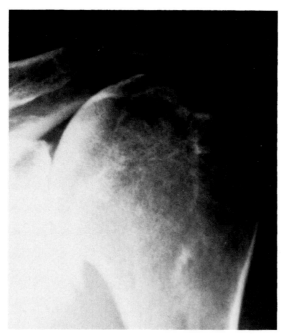

Figure 37–38. Ankylosing spondylitis. There is disruption of the musculotendinous rotator cuff with superior migration of the humeral head. The large erosion *(arrow)* of the superolateral aspect of the humeral head ("hatchet deformity") is a characteristic radiographic sign of the disease.

may be either well defined or indistinct with feathery margins, representing the combination of erosive and proliferative change. Erosions of the posterior calcaneal margin due to inflammation in the retrocalcaneal bursa and thickening of the Achilles tendon may be present (Fig. 37–39).[161] The inflammatory enthesopathy of the seronegative spondyloarthropathies[186, 197] differs from the degenerative enthesopathy seen in DISH (see Fig. 37–61). In the latter disease, bony outgrowths (enthesophytes) are sharply marginated and well defined.

Other sites of involvement in ankylosing spondylitis[186] include the symphysis pubis and manubriosternal, TM, and sternoclavicular joints.

Psoriatic Arthritis. In general, psoriatic arthritis is asymmetric or unilateral with involvement of synovial and cartilaginous joints as well as entheses.[198] The most common sites of involvement are the interphalangeal joints of the hands and feet, metatarsophalangeal joints, metacarpophalangeal joints, sacroiliac joints, and spine. Changes in the knees, ankles, elbows, and wrists and manubriosternal, acromioclavicular, and sternoclavicular joints, as well as pelvic entheses, are not uncommon. Hip or glenohumeral joint involvement is rare.

The arthritis of psoriasis is associated with periarticular soft tissue swelling, which in some cases may be manifested by diffuse, sausage-like enlargement of an entire digit.[199] The absence of osteoporosis is remarkable in many cases of psoriatic arthritis and is an important consideration in the differential diagnosis. However, osteoporosis may occasionally be evident; thus, its presence does not exclude the

diagnosis of psoriatic arthritis. Joint space narrowing or widening may be encountered, the latter being more common in the small joints of the hands and feet. Erosions progress from marginal areas in a central direction, often resulting in a "whittled" or "pencil-in-cup" deformity of the involved articulation.[200] In cases in which this severe destructive change is predominant, in combination with marked joint deformity, the term *arthritis mutilans* is frequently used. Bony proliferation is a striking feature of psoriatic arthritis and the other seronegative spondyloarthropathies (Fig. 37–40).[201] Proliferation around erosions produces a "whiskered" appearance. Diaphyseal and metaphyseal periostitis is also common.[202] In fact, osseous proliferation involving the distal phalanges may produce diffuse increased radiodensity, termed the *ivory phalanx*.[203] Intra-articular bony fusion, especially involving the proximal and distal interphalangeal joints of the hands and feet, is a common finding. An inflammatory enthesopathy consisting of fine, feathery, bony proliferation at sites of tendon and ligament insertion is also prominent in many cases.

Hands. In the hands, involvement of the distal interphalangeal joints is frequent and may be unilateral or bilateral, symmetric or asymmetric in distribution (Fig. 37–40). Erosions occur at the joint margins and progress centrally, with irregular destructive changes. Protrusion of one joint surface into its articular counterpart produces the pencil-in-cup deformity. Resorption of the terminal tufts of the distal phalanges may be seen. Psoriatic arthritis can lead

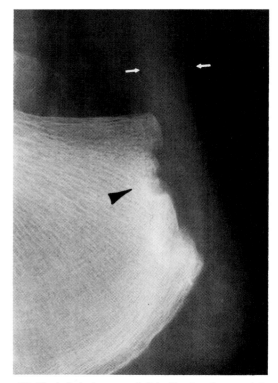

Figure 37–39. Ankylosing spondylitis. Erosive change of the posterior calcaneal margin is present *(arrowhead)* as well as thickening of the Achilles tendon *(between arrows)*.

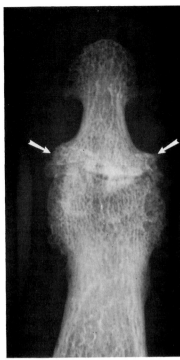

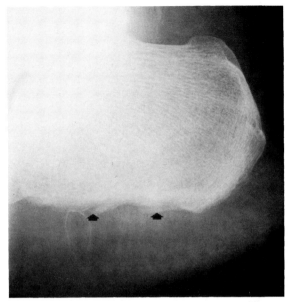

Figure 37–41. Psoriatic arthritis. The inferior surface of the calcaneus reveals the characteristic combination of erosive and proliferative changes *(arrows)* that are the hallmark of the seronegative spondyloarthropathies.

Figure 37–40. Psoriatic arthritis. The distal interphalangeal joint is narrowed, with proliferative bony erosions *(arrows)*. Also note the prominent soft tissue swelling and the abnormality of the fingernail.

to intra-articular bony ankylosis, a finding that is rare in rheumatoid arthritis.

Feet. Psoriatic arthritis involves two major areas in the foot: the forefoot and the calcaneus.[198] In the forefoot, changes are usually bilateral and asymmetric, predominating at the interphalangeal and metatarsophalangeal articulations. Marginal erosion, joint space narrowing (or widening), and bony proliferation are present, characteristically without significant osteoporosis. Severe destruction of the interphalangeal articulation of the great toe can be seen in psoriatic arthritis (and in Reiter's syndrome). Sesamoid involvement is also common in the foot as well as in the hand.

As in the other seronegative spondyloarthropathies, the combination of proliferative and erosive changes in the posterior and inferior surfaces of the calcaneus is an important radiographic finding of psoriatic arthritis. Erosions of the posterior surface of the calcaneus with surrounding proliferation adjacent to the retrocalcaneal bursa are common. Irregular and poorly defined spurs are typically present at the insertion of the plantar aponeurosis (Fig. 37–41), although in time, such spurs may become relatively well defined.

Sacroiliac Joints. A bilateral and symmetric distribution constitutes the most common radiographic pattern of sacroiliac joint abnormalities in psoriatic arthritis, although asymmetric involvement is not rare (Fig. 37–42).[197, 204] Initially subchondral bony erosions and ill-defined sclerosis with apparent joint space widening are noted, abnormalities identical to

those in ankylosing spondylitis. However, the frequency of intra-articular bony ankylosis in psoriatic arthritis is less than that in ankylosing spondylitis or the spondyloarthritis associated with inflammatory bowel diseases. Furthermore, in psoriatic arthritis (as in Reiter's syndrome), blurring and eburnation of apposing sacral and iliac surfaces within the ligamentous portion of the sacroiliac joint are more common than in ankylosing spondylitis.

Spine. The characteristic spinal lesion of psoriatic arthritis (as well as Reiter's syndrome) is paravertebral ossification.[205] These ossifications initially appear as either thick and irregular or thin and curvilinear densities, asymmetrically distributed parallel to the

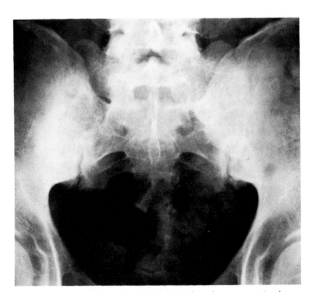

Figure 37–42. Psoriatic arthritis. Bilateral and asymmetric changes of the sacroiliac joints are present with erosions and sclerosis of the subchondral bone plate.

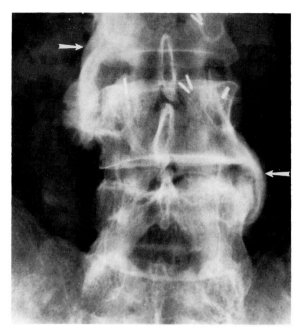

Figure 37–43. Psoriatic arthritis. Note the thick asymmetric paravertebral ossifications *(arrows)* arising from the vertebral margins in this patient with psoriatic spondylitis. These lesions, which are best visualized in the anteroposterior projection of the spine, are characteristic of psoriatic arthritis and Reiter's syndrome.

lateral surface of the intervertebral disc and vertebral body (Fig. 37–43). At this stage, the outgrowths are not attached to the vertebral body, although in later stages, the ossific densities merge with the lateral margins of the vertebral body several millimeters distal to the discovertebral junction. Occasionally, syndesmophytes identical to those in ankylosing spondylitis do occur in psoriatic arthritis[198] and Reiter's syndrome; however, in the great majority of cases, they are interspersed with the more characteristic paravertebral ossifications. "Corner osteitis," vertebral body "squaring," and apophyseal joint ankylosis are less common than in ankylosing spondylitis.

Cervical spine changes in psoriatic arthritis may be dramatic, even in patients with minimal thoracolumbar spinal involvement.[204, 206] Discovertebral joint irregularity with extensive bony proliferation about the anterior aspect of the vertebra and extensive apophyseal joint erosion and narrowing may be seen. Atlantoaxial subluxation is common.[204]

Other Locations. In long-standing or severe disease, virtually any articulation may be involved. In most sites, the characteristic combination of erosive and proliferative change is present.

Reiter's Syndrome. Radiographic alterations occur in approximately 60 to 80 percent of patients with Reiter's syndrome.[207] These radiographic changes demonstrate morphologic characteristics that are virtually indistinguishable from those in the other seronegative spondyloarthropathies, especially psoriatic arthritis; differentiation is usually possible only by means of the distribution of abnormalities and the clinical history. Synovial joints, cartilaginous joints,

and entheses may be affected. Characteristically, these changes are bilateral and asymmetric, with a predilection for involvement of the lower extremity.[207]

The most common sites of involvement are the small joints of the foot and the posterior and inferior calcaneal surfaces, followed, in order of frequency, by the ankle and the knee. Involvement of the hip and upper extremity is considerably less common. In the axial skeleton the sacroiliac joints, spine, symphysis pubis, and manubriosternal joints are the most common sites of alteration.

The general radiographic features of Reiter's syndrome are soft tissue swelling, joint space narrowing, and bony erosion and proliferation. Osteoporosis is variable in frequency and extent but may be present during acute exacerbations of arthritis. Osseous proliferation at insertions of tendons and ligaments is a frequent finding, especially in the pelvis and the calcaneus.

Feet and Ankles. Asymmetric abnormalities of the metatarsophalangeal and interphalangeal joints of the forefoot are the most common manifestations of Reiter's syndrome (Fig. 37–44).[208] Frequently, effusions in the retrocalcaneal bursa may be identified as radiodense shadows obliterating the normal fat plane between the posterosuperior aspect of the calcaneus and the Achilles tendon.[162] Thickening of this tendon may also be evident. Ill-defined plantar calcaneal enthesophytes are characteristic but, as in

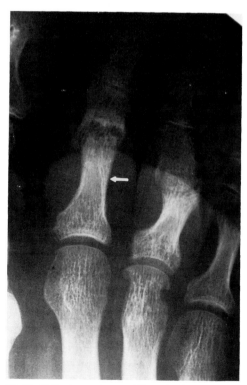

Figure 37–44. Reiter's syndrome. There is destructive change in the second and third proximal interphalangeal joints with subperiosteal proliferative reaction along the phalangeal shafts *(arrow)*. Marginal erosions of the metatarsal heads and proximal phalanges are also evident.

the other seronegative spondyloarthropathies, the outgrowths may be relatively well defined in the later stages of the disease. Marginal erosions are somewhat uncommon about the ankle, but joint space narrowing, with adjacent soft tissue swelling, and fluffy periostitis of the distal tibia and fibula are seen.[207]

Knee. The most common abnormality in the knee in Reiter's syndrome is the presence of a joint effusion, which in some instances becomes massive. Osteoporosis, joint space narrowing, and periostitis of the patella and distal femoral shaft also occur. Bony erosions in the femur or tibia are rare.

Sacroiliac Joints. Sacroiliac joint abnormalities are common and may be bilateral and asymmetric or unilateral in distribution. These abnormalities are identical to those of psoriatic arthritis.

Spine. Spinal involvement is less frequent in Reiter's syndrome than in ankylosing spondylitis and psoriatic arthritis. Although in some instances the changes may be identical to those of ankylosing spondylitis, a more characteristic finding consists of asymmetrically distributed paravertebral ossifications involving the thoracolumbar spine.[209] Cervical spine involvement is unusual, and atlantoaxial subluxation is rare.

Other Locations. In the cartilaginous manubriosternal and pubic symphyseal articulations, the changes of Reiter's syndrome consist of erosions of the articular surfaces with adjacent bony proliferation and sclerosis.[206]

Severe and diffuse involvement of joints of the upper extremity is rare in Reiter's syndrome,[207] although scattered lesions, particularly in the proximal interphalangeal joints of the hands, may occasionally be seen. Distal interphalangeal or metacarpophalangeal joint alterations are less frequent. Fusiform or "sausage-like" soft tissue swelling, joint space narrowing, periarticular osteoporosis, and bony erosion and proliferation are observed.

Enteropathic Arthropathies and Related Conditions. The frequency of peripheral joint involvement in enteropathic arthritis is variable. Several types of involvement are seen[210–214]: a mild, inflammatory, self-limited peripheral arthritis in which the radiographic changes consist principally of soft tissue swelling and juxta-articular osteoporosis; a progressive, destructive peripheral arthropathy characterized by soft tissue swelling, variable osteoporosis, joint space narrowing, osseous erosions, bony proliferation; and sacroiliitis or spondylitis. In patients with spondyloarthritis, the changes are identical to those in ankylosing spondylitis, although the male predominance of ankylosing spondylitis is less marked in this group of disorders and isolated sacroiliitis without spinal involvement is more common.

In primary biliary cirrhosis, a severe destructive arthropathy of the hands has been described,[215] characterized by the asymmetric distribution of well-defined marginal erosions primarily involving the proximal and distal interphalangeal joints with relative sparing of the metacarpophalangeal joints.

Chondrocalcinosis may be present in some patients, and occasionally, severe involvement of the hips and shoulders resembling osteonecrosis has been noted.[216]

A number of pancreatic diseases, including carcinoma, inflammation, and pancreatic duct calculi, may be associated with a syndrome characterized by subcutaneous nodules, polyarthritis, and medullary fat necrosis.[217, 218] The polyarthritis is radiographically nonspecific, with osteoporosis and soft tissue swelling being most commonly encountered. The radiographic appearance of medullary fat necrosis consists of diffuse osteolytic lesions with a "moth-eaten" appearance and periostitis. These changes closely resemble those of osteomyelitis and osteonecrosis.

OTHER CONNECTIVE TISSUE DISEASES

A number of other connective tissue disorders, including systemic lupus erythematosus, progressive systemic sclerosis, dermatomyositis, polymyositis, periarteritis nodosa, and mixed connective tissue disease, may be associated with musculoskeletal radiographic abnormalities.

Systemic Lupus Erythematosus. The roentgenographic changes of systemic lupus erythematosus (SLE) include symmetric polyarthritis, deforming nonerosive arthropathy, spontaneous tendon rupture, osteonecrosis, soft tissue calcification, infection, acrosclerosis, and tuftal resorption.[219–228] With the polyarthritis the radiographic changes are nonspecific and consist of soft tissue swelling and periarticular osteoporosis.[219, 220]

Joint space narrowing and bony erosions are unusual. Deforming nonerosive arthropathy is seen in 5 to 40 percent of patients with SLE.[220] Symmetric involvement of the hands is typical. The specific type of deformity is variable.[219–221] Swan-neck or boutonnière deformity can be evident. Other deformities include hyperextension of the interphalangeal joint of the thumb, ulnar drift at the metacarpophalangeal joints, and subluxation of the first carpometacarpal joint (Fig. 37–45). It is the prominent thumb deformity that is especially characteristic of lupus arthropathy. Although bony and cartilaginous abnormalities are generally not present, joint space narrowing, "hooklike" erosions of the radial and volar aspects of the metacarpal heads, and subchondral cyst formation are occasionally encountered (Fig. 37–46).[223] The radiographic findings of osteonecrosis in patients with SLE include transchondral fractures, subchondral sclerosis with cyst formation, and osseous collapse. Secondary osteoarthritis may eventually be prominent.

Linear or nodular calcific deposits in the subcutaneous tissues, particularly in the lower extremities, may occasionally be seen in SLE.[225] Sclerosis (acrosclerosis) or resorption of the tufts of the terminal phalanges also is occasionally evident in SLE.[228]

Progressive Systemic Sclerosis (Scleroderma). Soft tissue or bony involvement in progressive sys-

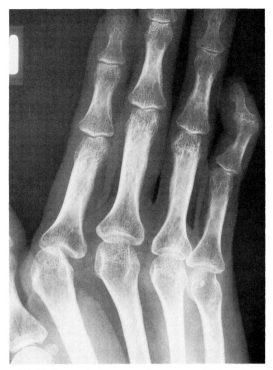

Figure 37–45. Systemic lupus erythematosus. This patient demonstrates juxta-articular osteoporosis with ulnar deviation at the metacarpophalangeal joints. No erosions are present.

temic sclerosis (PSS) is common. The radiographic abnormalities can be divided into four main categories[228]: (1) soft tissue resorption, (2) soft tissue calcification, (3) osteolysis, and (4) erosive articular disease.

Soft tissue resorption is most commonly noted in the fingertips in association with Raynaud's phenomenon (Fig. 37–47). Early changes can be identified by noting a reduction in the normal distance between the phalangeal tips and the skin (normal ≥20 percent of the transverse diameter of the base of the same distal phalanx).[229] In time, the fingertip assumes a conical shape and soft tissue calcification is often present.

Soft tissue calcification is most common in the hand but may occur at virtually any site.[230, 231] Calcification may be present in subcutaneous tissue, joint capsule, tendons, or ligaments (Fig. 37–48). The calcification typically is composed of hydroxyapatite crystals and has a soft, cloudlike radiographic appearance. Occasionally large tumoral collections may be present adjacent to a joint. Intra-articular or intraosseous calcification may also be noted (Fig. 37–49).

Extra-articular osteolysis is a frequent manifestation of PSS. The most common site is the tuft of the distal phalanx of the hand or occasionally the foot, usually in association with Raynaud's phenom-

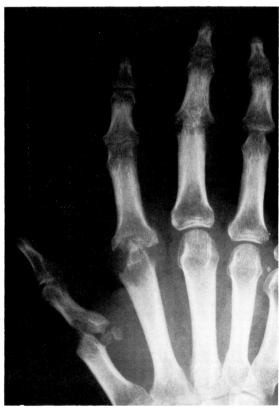

Figure 37–46. Systemic lupus erythematosus. An unusual pattern of involvement is seen. Severe erosive changes are present in the first and second metacarpophalangeal joints and third PIP joint. Juxta-articular osteoporosis is prominent.

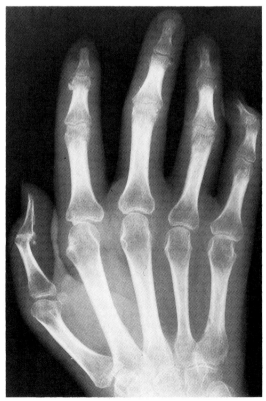

Figure 37–47. Scleroderma. Juxta-articular osteoporosis, soft tissue calcification, and resorption of the terminal tufts of the distal phalanges are present. Also note the tapered appearance of the soft tissues of the second finger and a hooklike erosion in the radial aspect of the third metacarpal head.

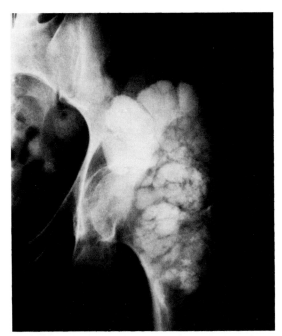

Figure 37–48. Scleroderma. A large tumoral calcific collection is present adjacent to the hip.

enon and soft tissue calcification. The earliest change is in the volar aspect of the tuft with continuing resorption leading to a "sharpened" appearance of the phalanx (Fig. 37–50).[228] Elsewhere, thickening of

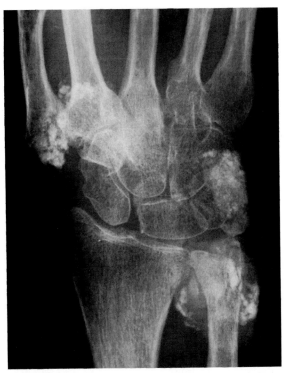

Figure 37–49. Scleroderma. Prominent soft tissue calcification and intra-articular calcification are present as well as severe erosive change of the first carpometacarpal joint. This is a characteristic "target" area of scleroderma. (From Resnick, D., and Niwayama, G.: Diagnosis of Bone and Joint Disorders. Philadelphia, W. B. Saunders Co., 1981.)

the periodontal membrane about the roots of the teeth[232] or localized mandibular osteolysis may be seen, the latter predisposing to pathologic fracture.[233] Localized osteolysis involving the ribs, acromion, clavicle, radius, ulna, and cervical spine has also been reported.[233–236]

A severe articular disease consisting of joint space narrowing, marginal and central osseous erosions, and deformity may occur.[237] There is a distinctive tendency toward involvement of the first carpometacarpal joint (see Fig. 37–49).[238] Indeed, bilateral destructive changes of the first carpometacarpal articulation with joint subluxation should arouse suspicion of PSS. Other relatively common sites of joint involvement in PSS include the distal interphalangeal, proximal interphalangeal, inferior radioulnar, and metatarsophalangeal joints.[239]

Dermatomyositis and Polymyositis. Articular abnormalities in dermatomyositis and polymyositis are usually without radiographic manifestations, although periarticular soft tissue swelling and osteoporosis may occasionally be noted.[240] More dramatic roentgenographic changes occur in the skeletal musculature, especially the large proximal muscle groups of the thorax, arm, forearm, thigh, and calf. Initial inflammation produces increased bulk and radiodensity of muscles with loss of the normal intermuscular fat planes.[241] In later stages, muscle atrophy or contractures may be prominent. The most characteristic soft tissue abnormality is calcification[242] in subcutaneous tissue, intermuscular fascia, tendons, or fat (Fig. 37–51). Subcutaneous calcific deposits simulate those of progressive systemic sclerosis, but the presence of marked linear calcific collections favors the diagnosis of polymyositis or dermatomyositis.

Periarteritis Nodosa. Plain film radiographic findings are unusual in this disorder, although joint effusions or periostitis of the tubular bones identical to that of hypertrophic osteoarthropathy may occasionally be seen.[243] Angiography is an important

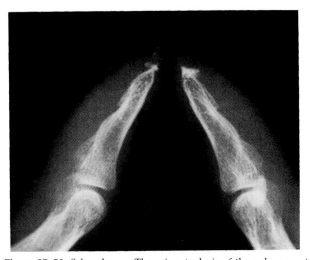

Figure 37–50. Scleroderma. There is osteolysis of the volar aspect of the distal phalanges of the thumbs with adjacent soft tissue calcification. Also note the tapered appearance of the adjacent soft tissues.

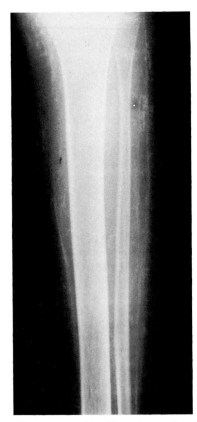

Figure 37–51. Dermatomyositis. There is prominent calcification of the subcutaneous tissue and the muscle in the leg.

diagnostic modality in evaluating the extent of vascular damage in this disease.

Mixed Connective Tissue Disease and "Overlap" Syndromes. A broad spectrum of radiographic abnormalities may be present in mixed connective tissue disease (MCTD),[244, 245] including soft tissue swelling and calcification, osteoporosis, joint space narrowing, bony erosions, and joint deformity. Useful radiographic clues include (1) a radiographic pattern suggestive of more than one collagen vascular disease, (2) an erosive arthropathy with an asymmetric distribution or with prominent involvement of the distal interphalangeal joints, and (3) sausage-like soft tissue swelling of a digit. However, none of these changes is specific for MCTD.

There is a group of patients with clinical and radiographic features of more than one collagen vascular disease in whom serologic testing fails to document the presence of MCTD. Such patients are considered to have an "overlap" syndrome. Roentgenographic alterations generally indicate findings of rheumatoid arthritis, SLE, PSS, and dermatomyositis in various combinations.

DEGENERATIVE JOINT DISEASE

The most characteristic sites of osteoarthritis (OA) include the proximal and distal interphalangeal joints of the hand, first carpometacarpal and trape-

zioscaphoid joints of the wrist, acromioclavicular and sacroiliac joints, hip, knee, and first metatarsophalangeal joint of the foot. Degenerative joint disease may also affect cartilaginous joints (such as the manubriosternal joint and symphysis pubis) and tendinous and ligamentous attachments to bone or entheses (such as in the pelvis, patella, and calcaneus). Degenerative disease of the spine is a separate subject and will be discussed later.

Osteoarthritis. In spite of a diversity of etiologies of OA, certain common radiographic characteristics allow a confident diagnosis in most instances. Joint space narrowing is a key diagnostic feature of the disease (Fig. 37–52).[246] In contrast to the inflammatory arthropathies, in which diffuse joint space narrowing of an involved articulation is expected, the joint space loss in OA tends to involve the portion of the joint exposed to the greatest stress (i.e., the lateral aspect of the hip, the medial compartment of the knee). Subchondral bone abnormalities are also characteristic of OA and include sclerosis (eburnation) and cyst formation, both of which predominate in the stressed area of the articulation. Subchondral eburnation results from cartilage denudation with subsequent bone-to-bone contact. The origin of subchondral cysts remains in debate.[247, 248]

Osteophytes are the single most characteristic radiographic and pathologic abnormality in OA.[246] They tend to arise from endochondral ossification in areas of low stress where islands of cartilage are preserved, most commonly at joint margins. In some cases osteophytes may arise from the synovium or joint capsule.

Hand and Wrist. The interphalangeal joints of the hand are frequent target areas of OA (Fig. 37–52). The appearance of articular space narrowing with closely apposed interdigitating bony surfaces

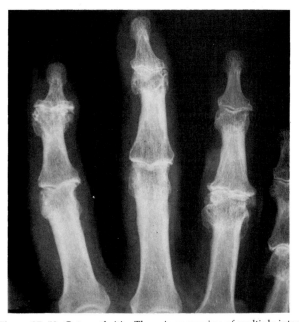

Figure 37–52. Osteoarthritis. There is narrowing of multiple interphalangeal joints with interdigitating osteophytes.

and marginal osteophytes is characteristic. Metacarpophalangeal joint involvement may also occur but not as an isolated event; rather, such involvement is associated with alterations at interphalangeal articulations. At the metacarpophalangeal joints, it is interosseous space narrowing that is the predominant abnormality. Osseous erosions are not apparent. The first carpometacarpal (trapeziometacarpal) joint is the characteristic site of degenerative abnormalities in the wrist (Fig. 37–53). Joint space narrowing with bony eburnation, subchondral cysts, and osteophyte formation is typical. Radial subluxation of the first metacarpal base is common. The trapezioscaphoid space is the only other common site of OA in the wrist; involvement at this site is generally combined with that at the first carpometacarpal joint. Trapezioscaphoid joint disease in the absence of first carpometacarpal joint involvement should suggest another diagnosis, especially CPPD crystal deposition disease. Similarly, a degenerative disease–like arthropathy elsewhere in the wrist, especially at the radiocarpal joint, in the absence of significant occupational or accidental trauma, is generally related to a disease other than OA.

Sacroiliac Joint. OA of the sacroiliac joint is extremely common in the older age group. Joint space narrowing with a thin, well-defined band of subchondral sclerosis, especially in the ilium, is typically present. Osteophyte formation is most common at the superior and inferior margins of the synovium-lined portion of the joint. At the former location, these osteophytes may appear as localized radiodensities projected over the joint in the anteroposterior radiographic projection. Bony erosion and intra-articular osseous fusion are not features of OA of the sacroiliac joint.

Hip. OA of the hip is exceedingly frequent and may lead to significant patient disability. In the typical case, cartilage loss is focal, involves the superolateral aspect of the joint, and leads to upward migration of the femoral head[249] (Fig. 37–54). Osteophyte formation is most prominent at the lateral acetabular and medial femoral margins, often in combination with thickening (buttressing) of the cortex in the medial aspect of the femoral neck. Subchondral sclerosis and cyst formation on both sides of the joint space may be marked. Focal loss of cartilage on the medial aspect of the articulation occurs in approximately 20 percent of patients with OA. Diffuse loss of cartilage with axial migration of the femoral head (along the axis of the femoral neck) is rare in OA. This latter feature is important in the differentiation of OA from inflammatory arthropathies such as rheumatoid arthritis.

Knee. The knee is a common site of OA. The most characteristic pattern of disease consists of involvement of the medial femorotibial compartment with joint space narrowing, osseous eburnation, subchondral cysts, and marginal osteophytes.[250] Sharpening of the tibial spines or the presence of osteophytes arising from the intercondylar notch of the femur may also be observed. A true assessment of cartilage destruction may not be possible on standard anteroposterior radiographs (obtained with the patient supine) but is better provided by radiographs obtained either in the "tunnel" projection (Fig. 37–55) or with the patient in a weight-bearing position.[251] Varus angulation of the knee is the most common deformity in OA, reflecting the more severe involvement of the medial femorotibial compartment compared with the lateral one. Symmetric medial and lateral femorotibial compartment disease is unusual. Osteoarthritic changes in the patellofemoral compartment are also common, either in isolation or accompanying medial femorotibial compartment disease.

Osseous or cartilaginous debris may be present as intra-articular bodies ("joint mice") either free within the joint cavity or embedded in the synovial membrane. Degeneration of the fibrocartilaginous menisci is a typical feature of advanced OA.

Foot. OA in the foot typically affects the first metatarsophalangeal joint. Articular space narrowing, bony eburnation, osteophyte formation, and subchondral cysts are common. Hallux rigidus is a specific pattern of OA, which may be seen in adolescents or young adults; there is painful restriction of dorsiflexion at the first metatarsophalangeal joint.[252] Hallux valgus is another common pattern of OA about this joint, with lateral angulation of the first toe and prominent sclerosis, cyst formation, and osteophytosis on the medial aspect of the first metatarsal head.

Other Locations. Typical osteoarthritic changes in the elbows, acromioclavicular and glenohumeral joints, and ankles may be encountered, usually in

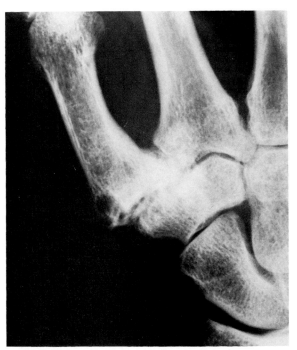

Figure 37–53. Osteoarthritis. Narrowing of the articular space and subchondral sclerosis about the first carpometacarpal joint are apparent.

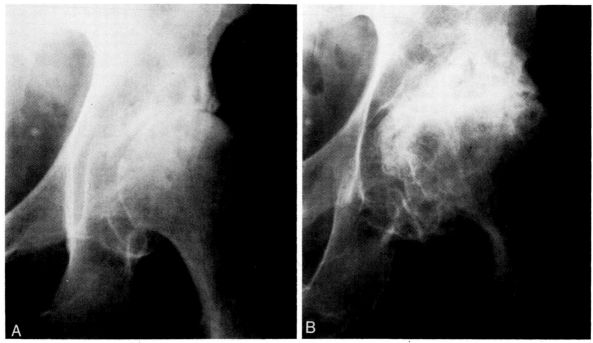

Figure 37–54. Osteoarthritis. Moderately advanced osteoarthritic changes are present in *A,* with asymmetric joint space narrowing and superior migration of the femoral head. Eburnation and cystic changes are seen in the subchondral region. In *B,* advanced changes have occurred, with collapse of the superior articular surface and the formation of large marginal osteophytes.

patients with a history of trauma or pre-existing disease. In general, without such a history, a radiographic pattern consistent with OA[246] at an unusual site should suggest another disease process, including acromegaly, CPPD crystal deposition disease, ochronosis, and epiphyseal dysplasia.

Inflammatory Osteoarthritis. Inflammatory osteoarthritis is a disease most common in middle-aged women. It is characterized by acute episodic inflammation of the interphalangeal joints of the hand.[253] On roentgenograms, typical marginal osteophytes with or without bony erosions are seen. The erosions

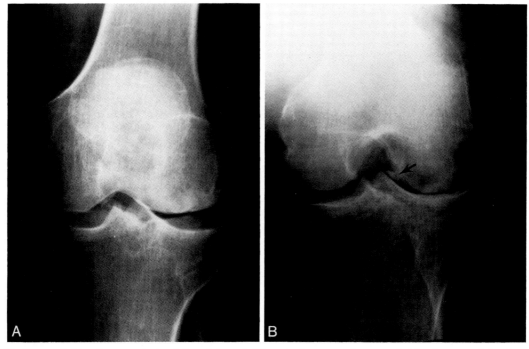

Figure 37–55. Osteoarthritis. Anteroposterior *(A)* and tunnel *(B)* projections reveal osteoarthritic changes of the knee. Note the asymmetric involvement with subchondral eburnation of the lateral articular surfaces. In this case the actual degree of joint space narrowing is much more apparent in the tunnel projection. An osteophyte arising from the intercondylar notch is identified *(arrow).*

are first evident in the central portion of the subchondral bone, appearing as sharply marginated defects (Fig. 37–56).[246] Intra-articular ankylosis may subsequently result.[254] It must be emphasized that the clinical syndrome of inflammatory osteoarthritis can occur in the absence of radiographically demonstrable bony erosions; therefore, the term *erosive osteoarthritis* is not an ideal one for this disorder.

Degenerative Enthesopathy. Coarse, bony proliferation at sites of ligamentous and tendinous attachment is a manifestation of a degenerative enthesopathy. This is most commonly observed in the pelvis, patella, ulnar olecranon, and calcaneus. The resulting bony excrescences are identical to those encountered in diffuse idiopathic skeletal hyperostosis. They are usually coarser and better defined than the outgrowths accompanying the inflammatory enthesopathy of the seronegative spondyloarthropathies.

Degenerative Disease of the Spine. The vertebral column is composed of a complex series of synovial, cartilaginous, and fibrous articulations. Degenerative diseases of the spine can involve any of these articulations as well as ligamentous insertions (entheses).[255, 256] Many distinct degenerative processes can be identified.

Intervertebral (Osteo)chondrosis. Primary degenerative disease of the nucleus pulposus of the intervertebral disc, termed *intervertebral (osteo)chon-*

drosis, is a common disorder, especially in the elderly, which may occur at any spinal level but is more commonly identified in the lumbar and cervical regions.[1]

The earliest radiographic change consists of linear or circular collections of gas ("vacuum phenomena") within the disc substance (Fig. 37–57).[257] These gas collections are more prominent on radiographs obtained with the spine in extension and may disappear in flexion. The presence of a vacuum phenomenon is a useful observation, because it virtually excludes the possibility of infection.[258] Progressive narrowing of the intervertebral disc and sclerosis beneath the subchondral bone plate are additional manifestations of intervertebral (osteo)chondrosis. Herniation of portions of the intervertebral disc into the adjacent vertebral body (Schmorl's node, cartilaginous node) is a further radiographic sign. Small triangular osteophytes at the discovertebral junction are also seen (Fig. 37–57).

Spondylosis Deformans. Spondylosis deformans[255] refers to the formation of multiple large osteophytes predominantly along the anterior and lateral aspects of the vertebral bodies (Fig. 37–58).[259] These osteophytes may occur at any level; in the thoracic spine, they predominate on the right side, presumably because their formation is inhibited on the left side by the constant pulsation of the descending thoracic aorta.[260] Narrowing of the intervertebral disc space, vacuum phenomena, and end-plate bony sclerosis are not features of spondylosis deformans. The differentiation of the osteophytes of spondylosis deformans from the vertebral lesions of the seronegative spondyloarthropathies has been discussed previously.

Apophyseal Joint Osteoarthritis. The synovium-lined apophyseal joint is a frequent site of degenerative disease.[256] Changes are most common in the mid- and lower cervical spine, the midthoracic spine, and the lower lumbar spine. The radiographic changes are identical to those of OA in peripheral articulations,[261] with joint space narrowing, osseous eburnation, and marginal osteophyte formation. Capsular laxity may result in apophyseal joint malalignment. In this setting or with large osteophytes arising from the joint margins, impingement of a spinal nerve root within the neural foramen may occur.

Uncovertebral Arthrosis. Degenerative changes in the cervical uncovertebral articulations (Luschka) are often identified on the frontal radiograph of the cervical spine. The nature of this process is debated, because these articulations have been shown to represent intervertebral disc extensions in early life and to contain synovium-like tissue in later life. Radiographic changes consist of osseous sclerosis, joint space loss, and osteophyte formation.

Costovertebral Osteoarthritis. Osteoarthritic changes of the synovium-lined costovertebral joints are extremely common, especially at the level of the 11th and 12th ribs.[256] Radiographic demonstration of these abnormalities (joint space narrowing, bony

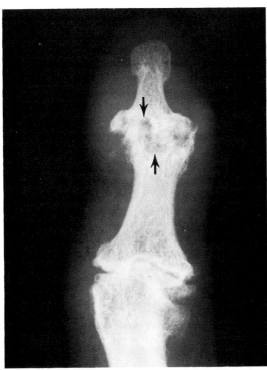

Figure 37–56. Inflammatory osteoarthritis. The combination of interphalangeal joint involvement, prominent marginal osteophytes, and central erosions of the articular surfaces *(arrows)* is characteristic of this disease. (From Resnick, D., and Niwayama, G.: Diagnosis of Bone and Joint Disorders. Philadelphia, W. B. Saunders Co., 1981.)

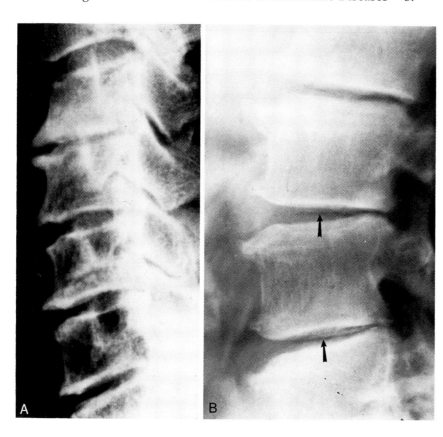

Figure 37–57. Intervertebral osteochondrosis. Lateral projections of the cervical spine *(A)* and lumbar spine *(B)* reveal typical abnormalities of intervertebral (osteo)chondrosis. Intervertebral disc space narrowing with sclerosis of the vertebral end-plates and the formation of small triangular osteophytes from the anterior vertebral margins are evident. Prominent vacuum phenomena *(arrows)* are present in the lumbar spine. (From Resnick, D., and Niwayama, G.: Diagnosis of Bone and Joint Disorders. Philadelphia, W. B. Saunders Co., 1981.)

sclerosis, osteophytes) is frequently difficult, owing to the superimposition of ribs and vertebral bodies over the articulations on conventional radiographic studies. Hypertrophy of adjacent ribs may accompany this disease.

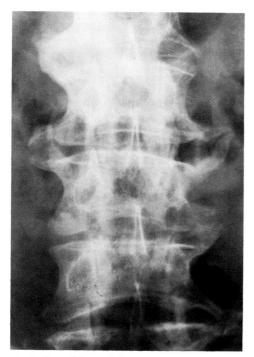

Figure 37–58. Spondylosis deformans. The frontal projection of the spine reveals multiple, large interdigitating osteophytes arising from the lateral margins of the vertebral bodies. Note that the initial portion of the osteophytes has a horizontal orientation.

Diffuse Idiopathic Skeletal Hyperostosis. DISH is a common degenerative enthesopathy and has been described under a variety of terms,[262–264] including *Forestier's disease, spondylitis ossificans ligamentosa, spondylosis hyperostotica,* and *ankylosing hyperostosis of the spine.* Although radiographic changes are evident in both the axial and the appendicular skeleton, the diagnosis of DISH is based on the presence of characteristic spinal alterations. In fact, the radiographic change in the vertebral column must fulfill three criteria before a diagnosis of DISH can be made: (1) the presence of flowing calcification or ossification along the anterolateral aspects of at least four contiguous vertebral levels; (2) relative preservation of intervertebral disc height in the involved vertebral segments without extensive changes of primary degenerative disc disease; and (3) the absence of apophyseal joint ankylosis or sacroiliac joint erosions, sclerosis, or intra-articular bony ankylosis.

The most characteristic radiographic abnormality of DISH is calcification and ossification of the anterior longitudinal ligament of the spine.[265] This is most commonly identified in the midthoracic spine but is also evident in the cervical and lumbar levels. Early in the disease, an undulating radiodense band forms along the anterolateral aspect of the spine separated from the anterior aspect of the vertebral body by a thin radiolucent line (Fig. 37–59); with progression of the disease, the lucency may disappear. These changes, which are best demonstrated in the lateral radiographic projection of the thoracic spine, may resemble the "bamboo spine" of ankylosing spondylitis, but several important diagnostic features exist. Syndesmophytes arise from the anterosuperior

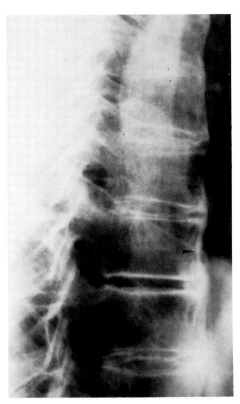

Figure 37–59. Diffuse idiopathic skeletal hyperostosis (DISH). The lateral view of the thoracic spine in this patient with DISH demonstrates ossification of the anterior longitudinal ligament (ALL). Note the characteristic lucencies between the ossified ALL and the anterior vertebral margin *(arrowheads).*

soft tissues between the anterior ribs, medial clavicle, and sternum is evident.

In the lumbar spine, changes of DISH resemble those in the cervical region; osteophytes are present.

Extraspinal manifestations of DISH[269] are especially common in the pelvis. Bony proliferation at sites of ligamentous and tendinous attachment (enthesopathy) results in the formation of coarse, well-marginated bony excrescences, in contrast to the fine, spiculated, ill-defined bony proliferative changes of the seronegative spondyloarthropathies (Fig. 37–61). Calcification of the iliolumbar and sacrotuberous ligaments is an additional characteristic feature (Fig. 37–62). Para-articular osteophytes are commonly noted about the hip and along the inferior aspect of the sacroiliac joints.

Other extraspinal sites of prominent bony proliferation include the patellar poles, calcaneus, and olecranon process of the ulna. The "spurs" that form at these sites may be identical in appearance to localized degenerative changes in otherwise normal persons, but they demonstrate a tendency toward increased size and multiplicity. In the hand, hyperostotic changes of the metacarpal and phalangeal heads, with proliferation in the terminal tufts, may be noted. Irregular excrescences may also be seen at the femoral trochanters, deltoid tuberosity of the humerus and anterior tibial tuberosity, and about the interosseous membranes of the forearm and leg.

NEUROARTHROPATHY

Neuroarthropathy (Charcot joint) refers to destructive and productive articular abnormalities occurring

and anteroinferior margins of the vertebral body, whereas the ossification in DISH attaches to the vertebral body several millimeters from these margins. In addition, syndesmophytes may be best seen in the frontal radiographic projection, in contrast to DISH, in which changes are most prominent on the lateral radiographic projection. The presence of sacroiliac joint erosions and extensive intra-articular bony ankylosis of the sacroiliac or apophyseal joints in ankylosing spondylitis constitutes another important differential diagnostic point.

In the cervical spine, bony outgrowths characteristically appear at the anteroinferior margin of the vertebral body and extend inferiorly around the disc space. With progression, a thick, armor-like mass of bone bridges the intervertebral disc, leading to markedly diminished cervical motion and, in some cases, dysphagia (Fig. 37–60).[266] Linear or Y-shaped radiolucencies in the bony mass may be noted at the level of the intervertebral disc space owing to displacement of disc material into the ossific mass. Ossification adjacent to the inferior margin of the anterior arch of the atlas is common and may be confused with traumatic changes. Ossification of the posterior longitudinal ligament may be seen as a distinct entity but occurs with increased frequency in patients with DISH (Fig. 37–60).[267] DISH may also be associated with a rare syndrome, sternocostoclavicular hyperostosis,[267, 268] in which extensive ossification of the

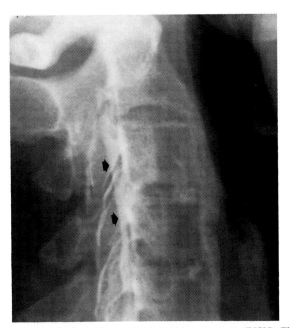

Figure 37–60. Diffuse idiopathic skeletal hyperostosis (DISH). The lateral view of the cervical spine in this patient demonstrates thick, flowing ossification along the anterior margins of the vertebral bodies. Ossification of the posterior longitudinal ligament (OPLL) is also present *(arrows).*

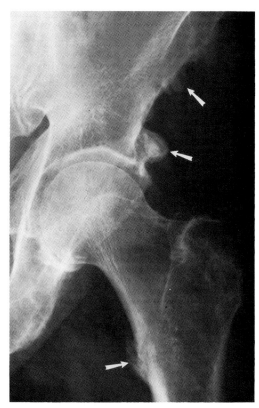

Figure 37–61. Diffuse idiopathic skeletal hyperostosis (DISH). The degenerative enthesopathy of DISH is well demonstrated with coarse bony excrescences arising from sites of ligament and tendon insertion along the lateral aspect of the ilium, superior acetabular margin, and lesser trochanter *(arrows)*. This appearance differs from that of the finely spiculated inflammatory enthesopathy of the seronegative spondyloarthropathies.

in association with loss of pain or proprioceptive sensation, or both. Although debate exists as to the precise pathogenesis of neuroarthropathy, it is believed that the cumulative effect of trauma and joint laxity due to relaxation of periarticular supporting structures is contributory.

One of the early radiographic changes of neuroarthropathy is the presence of a joint effusion, which may become large. Mild joint subluxation may

then appear.[270] Subsequently, fragmentation of the articular surface occurs with eburnation of bony surfaces, leading, in time, to complete joint disorganization. These radiographic abnormalities have been subdivided into hypertrophic and atrophic types. The hypertrophic reaction is more common in central lesions, as in tabes dorsalis and syringomyelia. There is prominent periosteal new bone formation as well as metaplasia of the synovium with the formation of bone and cartilage within its deeper layers. Large osteocartilaginous bodies of synovial origin, in combination with fragments originating from the articular surfaces, result in a fragmented, disorganized articulation with a great deal of osseous debris (Fig. 37–63). The atrophic reaction occurs more commonly with diseases, such as diabetes mellitus, in which the abnormality involves the peripheral nerve (Fig. 37–64). Fragmentation occurs, but the osteocartilaginous debris is resorbed, resulting in disappearance of the articular surfaces. It should be emphasized that hypertrophic and atrophic patterns are not completely reliable in identifying the level of neurologic abnormality, because exceptions to these rules are common.

A great number of disorders lead to neuropathic changes. In general the morphologic aberrations produced by these disorders are similar; however, there are differences in articular distribution among these disorders, which provide clues to the specific diagnosis.

Tabes Dorsalis.[270–272] Five to 10 percent of patients with tabes dorsalis demonstrate neuroarthropathy. The articulations of the lower extremity are most commonly affected, with the knee and the hip being the most frequent target sites (see Fig. 37–63). Other sites include the ankle and the articulations in both the upper extremity and the spinal column. In peripheral joints, typical radiographic features are large effusions, bony eburnation, and fragmentation. Bilateral and symmetric changes are not uncommon. In the axial skeleton, intervertebral disc space narrowing, vertebral body sclerosis, and formation of large osteophytes may resemble the changes of unusually severe degenerative disease.

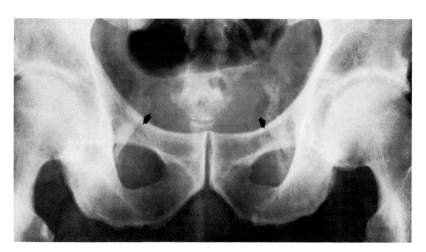

Figure 37–62. Diffuse idiopathic skeletal hyperostosis (DISH). Calcification of the sacrotuberous ligaments *(arrows)* has occurred.

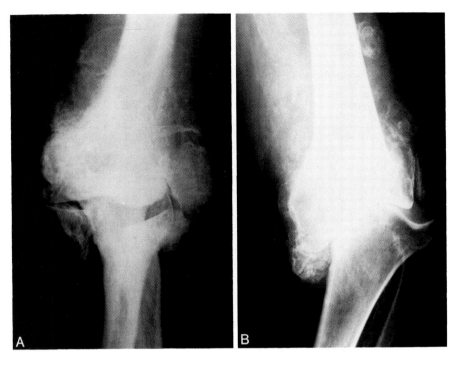

Figure 37–63. Tabes dorsalis with neuroarthropathy. Radiographs of the elbow (A) and knee (B) in patients with tabes dorsalis demonstrate changes of neuroarthropathy. Bony sclerosis, fragmentation, and instability of the joints are present with dramatic soft tissue swelling.

Syringomyelia.[273] Approximately 20 to 50 percent of patients with syringomyelia develop neuroarthropathy. There is a distinct predilection for upper extremity involvement, especially the glenohumeral joint, elbow, and wrist. Lower extremity or spinal alterations may occur in some cases. Bilateral and symmetric involvement is less frequent in syringomyelia than in tabes dorsalis.

Diabetes Mellitus.[274–276] Diabetes mellitus is probably the most common cause of neuroarthropathy, although less than 1 percent of patients with this disease develop such changes. The articulations of the foot are affected in the majority of cases, although the ankle, knee, spine, and joints of the upper extremity may occasionally be affected. Abnormalities predominate in the tarsal and tarsometatarsal articulations, consisting of bony eburnation and fragmentation. Spontaneous fractures are common, and a Lisfranc fracture-dislocation pattern may be seen (see Fig. 37–64). In the forefoot, a resorptive pattern is most typical, with tapering or "sharpening" of metatarsal and phalangeal shafts. Concurrent or superimposed infection is a common problem in the diabetic patient. There is great difficulty in differentiating the radiographic changes of neuroarthropathy from those of infection; however, the indistinctness of bony margins in infection compared with the sharp margins in neuroarthropathy aids in correct diagnosis.

Other Disorders. Although peripheral neuropathy is common in the alcoholic patient, neuroarthropathy is rare. It resembles that in diabetes mellitus with characteristic involvement of the articulations of the foot.[277] In amyloidosis, knee and ankle involvement is most typical.[278] Neuropathic changes in childhood should suggest the possibility of congenital indifference to pain or meningomyelocele.[269] In both of these disorders, involvement of the ankle and tarsal articulations is seen, and changes may appear at the physis, or growth plate, with osseous irregularity, sclerosis, epiphyseal separation, and periostitis. An idiopathic form of neuroarthropathy of the elbow has been described, and neuroarthropathic

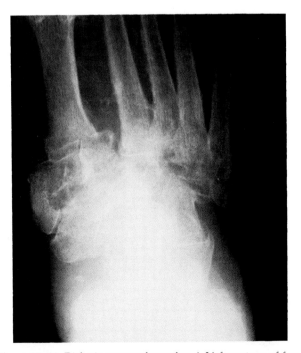

Figure 37–64. Diabetic neuroarthropathy. A Lisfranc type of fracture-dislocation has occurred as a complication of neuroarthropathy in this diabetic patient. Note the lateral displacement of the second through fifth metatarsal bases with sclerosis and fragmentation of the adjacent tarsal bones.

changes have been observed following intra-articular administration of steroids.

CRYSTAL-RELATED ARTHROPATHIES

Several types of articular disease are related to abnormal deposition or accumulation of crystalline material in and about articulations. These include gout, CPPD crystal deposition disease, hemochromatosis, and hydroxyapatite crystal deposition disease (HADD).[279] Two other entities that may be included in this group are Wilson's disease and ochronosis (alkaptonuria).

Gout. The earliest radiographic change in gout consists of reversible soft tissue swelling about the involved articulation during an acute gouty attack. With chronicity of disease, tophi lead to nodular, lobulated soft tissue densities, especially in the feet, ankles, knees, elbows, and hands. Calcification within a tophus may be evident, particularly in patients with gouty nephritis, whereas ossification of a tophus is rare.[279, 280] Bony erosions are common in long-standing gout and may be intra-articular or extra-articular in location. Intra-articular erosions most commonly involve the joint margins and proceed centrally (Fig. 37–65). Extra-articular erosions involve the cortex of the bone, frequently in association with a soft tissue mass (tophus) (Fig. 37–66). These erosions are usually round or oval, often with a sclerotic border and a "punched-out" appearance.[281] The presence of an "overhanging lip" of

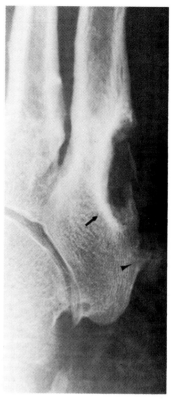

Figure 37–66. Gout. A large extra-articular erosion of the lateral aspect of the fifth metatarsal shaft is bordered by reactive bony sclerosis *(arrow)*. A smaller erosion is present more proximally *(arrowhead)* with an adjacent calcified soft tissue tophus. (From Resnick, D., and Niwayama, G.: Diagnosis of Bone and Joint Disorders. Philadelphia, W. B. Saunders Co., 1981.)

bone at the margin of an erosion is a characteristic feature of gout. Occasionally, a more extensive proliferative bony reaction, presumably due to a reparative process, may be noted, typically at the first metatarsophalangeal joint, intertarsal joints, and knee.[282, 283] The joint space is usually preserved in gouty arthritis until the late stages of the disease. In fact, the presence of prominent intra-articular osseous erosions with relative preservation of the joint space suggests the diagnosis of gout. Intra-articular bony ankylosis is occasionally seen, especially involving the interphalangeal joints of the hands and feet as well as the carpal region.[282] Although transient localized osteoporosis may be present during an acute gouty attack, extensive osteoporosis is not a feature of this disease.

The general radiographic features of gout are similar at all sites; however, involvement at several specific areas may be of diagnostic importance.[279] The first metatarsophalangeal joint is the most characteristic site of involvement (see Fig. 37–65). Erosions are most frequent on the dorsal and medial aspects of the metatarsal head, usually in association with a hallux valgus deformity. They are best demonstrated in the oblique radiographic projection. In the hand, proximal and distal interphalangeal joint involvement is more common than metacarpophalangeal joint involvement. Wrist abnormality is frequently

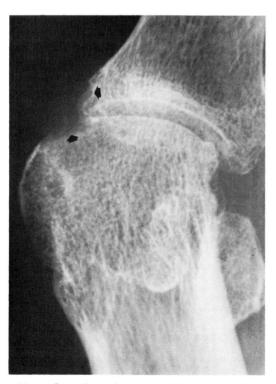

Figure 37–65. Gout. Typical erosions of the metatarsal head and proximal phalangeal base *(arrows)* are present in this patient with gouty arthritis of the first metatarsophalangeal joint.

pancompartmental, but extensive involvement of the common carpometacarpal articulation is important, because this area is relatively spared in most other arthropathies. Erosions of the olecranon process of the elbow and the dorsal surface of the patella strongly suggest gouty bursitis.

Chondrocalcinosis is occasionally seen in patients with gout. It is usually localized to a few articulations and predominates in fibrocartilage.

Secondary gout is associated with a wide variety of situations, including glycogen storage disease (type I),[284] Lesch-Nyhan syndrome,[285] myeloproliferative disorders,[286] endocrine diseases,[287] and the administration of certain drugs.[288] In general, secondary gout resembles primary gout radiographically, although unusual sites may be affected.[284-288]

Calcium Pyrophosphate Dihydrate Crystal Deposition Disease. CPPD crystal deposition disease is characterized by the deposition of CPPD crystals in hyaline cartilage and fibrocartilage as well as in synovium, capsule, tendons, and ligaments.[279] *CPPD crystal deposition disease* is a general term indicating the presence of CPPD crystal in or around joints. *Chondrocalcinosis* refers to calcification of hyaline cartilage or fibrocartilage, regardless of its etiology. *Pyrophosphate arthropathy* refers to a pattern of structural joint damage with or without radiographically demonstrable chondrocalcinosis. There are two main types of radiographic abnormalities in CPPD crystal deposition disease: (1) abnormal calcification and (2) destructive arthropathy. These changes may be present in combination or in isolation.

Abnormal calcification related to CPPD crystal deposition disease may be identified in articular or periarticular structures. The most common intra-articular site of calcification is within cartilage, either hyaline cartilage or fibrocartilage (Fig. 37–67). Hyaline cartilage calcification may occur in any joint but is most common in the wrist, knee, elbow, and hip. It appears as thin curvilinear radiodensities parallel to, but distinct from, the subchondral bone plate.[279] Fibrocartilage calcification most commonly involves

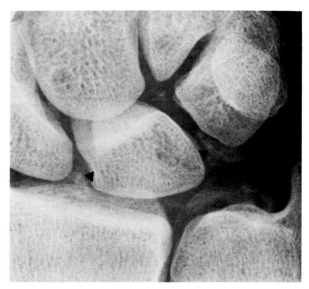

Figure 37–68. Calcium pyrophosphate crystal deposition disease. A frontal radiograph of the wrist demonstrates calcification of the triangular fibrocartilage *(open arrow)* and several intercarpal ligaments *(arrowheads)*. (From Resnick, D., and Niwayama, G.: Diagnosis of Bone and Joint Disorders. Philadelphia, W. B. Saunders Co., 1981.)

the menisci of the knee, triangular fibrocartilage of the wrist, symphysis pubis, annulus fibrosus of the intervertebral disc, or labra of the glenoid and acetabulum (Fig. 37–68). It appears as thick, irregular radiodensities within the involved structure. Cloud-like or speckled radiodensities, representing calcific deposits within synovium, may be seen at many locations, including bursal cavities, but are most common about the wrist. Additional sites of calcification include joint capsule, tendons, bursae, and ligaments.[289] Calcification at these sites is less frequent than within cartilage.

Pyrophosphate arthropathy exhibits a degenerative disease-type pattern of structural joint damage. Its general radiographic features include a bilateral symmetric or asymmetric distribution and changes characterized by joint space narrowing, bony sclerosis, and prominent subchondral cysts.[289] The last, representing an important diagnostic feature of the arthropathy, are frequently numerous and large and may simulate neoplasm. These cysts may progress rapidly in size, undermining the articular surface and resulting in collapse and deformity of the joint. At times, this progression may be so rapid as to resemble infection or neuroarthropathy (Fig. 37–69). In some patients, large osteophytes may be present about involved articulations.

Pyrophosphate arthropathy is most commonly seen in the knee, wrist, and metacarpophalangeal joints, although any joint may be involved. The relatively common involvement of the wrist, elbow, and shoulder contrast with the situation in degenerative joint disease, in which these areas are usually spared. In the hand there is a tendency toward selective involvement of the second and third metacarpophalangeal joints. In the wrist, the radioscaph-

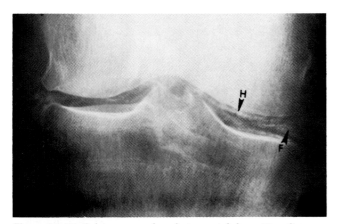

Figure 37–67. Calcium pyrophosphate crystal deposition disease. A frontal radiograph of the knee reveals calcification of hyaline articular cartilage (H) as well as fibrocartilaginous menisci (F). (From Resnick, D., Niwayama, G., Goergen, T. G., et al.: Radiology 122:1, 1977.)

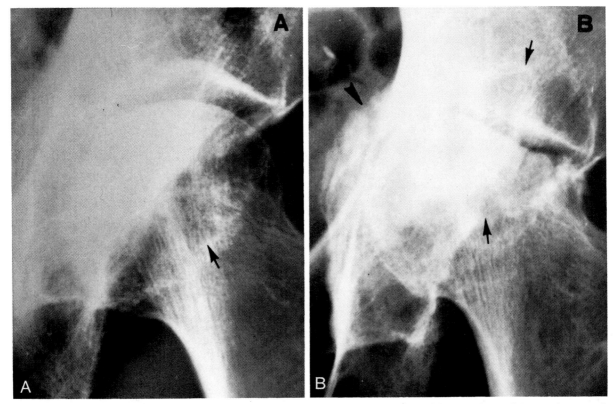

Figure 37–69. Calcium pyrophosphate crystal deposition disease. *A* and *B* are radiographs of the hip obtained 16 months apart. In *A*, there is preservation of the joint space with subtle cystic change within the femoral head *(arrow)*. In *B*, there is collapse of the femoral head with large cystic lesions *(arrows)* and fragmentation of the acetabulum *(arrowhead)*. This rapidly progressive arthropathy is characteristic of pyrophosphate arthropathy. (From Resnick, D., Niwayama, G., Goergen, T. G., et al.: Clinical, radiographic, and pathologic abnormalities in calcium pyrophosphate dihydrate deposition disease (CPPD): pseudogout. Radiology 122:1, 1977.)

oid space is frequently involved, with collapse of the proximal pole of the scaphoid into the distal radial articular surface (Fig. 37–70). Narrowing of the capitolunate space is also frequent, as is involvement of the trapezioscaphoid articulation with or without involvement of the first carpometacarpal joint. Associated calcification of the triangular fibrocartilage, intercarpal ligaments, or articular cartilage may be encountered. In the knee, the distribution of abnormalities may mimic that of osteoarthritis with involvement of the medial femorotibial and patellofemoral compartments. At times, there is isolated involvement of the patellofemoral space. In the hip, superior joint space narrowing, mimicking osteoarthritis, or axial migration of the femoral head, simulating rheumatoid arthritis, can be seen.

Calcium Hydroxyapatite Crystal Deposition Disease. HADD may be a primary idiopathic disorder or secondary to other diseases and is characterized by the deposition of calcium hydroxyapatite crystals in periarticular or, rarely, intra-articular structures. In idiopathic disease, calcification is most commonly seen about the shoulder, although involvement of the hand, wrist, hip, foot, and paraspinal tissues may be seen. Hydroxyapatite deposits appear on radiographs as soft, cloudlike densities within tendons, ligaments, joint capsules, bursae, and periar-

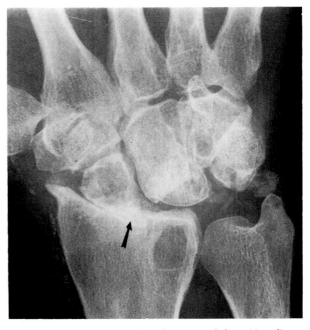

Figure 37–70. Calcium pyrophosphate crystal deposition disease. In this patient, the changes of pyrophosphate arthropathy include narrowing of the radiocarpal joint with collapse of the scaphoid into the radial articular surface *(arrow)* as well as the presence of numerous subchondral cystic lesions. Calcification of the triangular fibrocartilage can also be noted.

ticular soft tissues. These deposits may vary in size from small collections, 1 to 2 mm in diameter, to large lobulated masses, many centimeters in diameter. On serial radiographs, deposits may enlarge, remain unchanged, or diminish in size. They can even disappear completely.

In the shoulder, HADD is most commonly identified in the supraspinatus tendon of the fibromuscular rotator cuff. Here, it is frequently referred to as calcific tendinitis, peritendinitis calcarea, or hydroxyapatite rheumatism (Fig. 37–71).[279] Other sites of calcification in the shoulder include the infraspinatus, teres minor, subscapularis, and bicipital tendons.[290] It should be emphasized that in most instances these deposits are not symptomatic; most patients with shoulder discomfort and periarticular calcific deposits will have another cause of pain, frequently subacromial bursitis or rotator cuff tendinitis.

Intra-articular HADD may be seen as an isolated event or in association with osteoarthritis or collagen vascular disease. Radiographically, cloudlike calcific collections within the joint are apparent. Rarely, severe articular destruction, especially in the glenohumeral joint, may be an associated feature.

Periarticular calcification, representing hydroxyapatite crystal deposition, is seen in a variety of disorders,[279] including hyperparathyroidism, renal osteodystrophy, collagen vascular diseases, hypoparathyroidism, milk-alkali syndrome, hypervitaminosis D, and sardoidosis.

Hemochromatosis. Radiographically, the manifestations of hemochromatosis may be divided into three major categories: (1) osteoporosis, (2) articular calcification, and (3) structural joint damage.

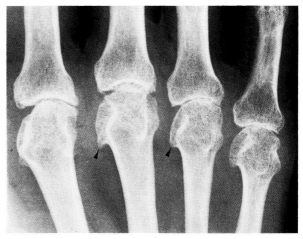

Figure 37–72. Hemochromatosis. There is joint space narrowing with erosive change about the second through fifth metacarpophalangeal joints. "Hook" osteophytes (arrowheads) occur at the radial margins of the metacarpal heads. (From Resnick, D., and Niwayama, G.: Diagnosis of Bone and Joint Disorders. Philadelphia, W. B. Saunders Co., 1981.)

Diffuse osteoporosis is an important feature of hemochromatosis,[291] in contrast to idiopathic CPPD crystal deposition disease,[292] and may involve the axial and appendicular skeleton. In the spine, collapse of the vertebral end-plates leads to biconcave deformities of the vertebral body ("fish" vertebra). Osteoporosis in the appendicular skeleton tends to be diffuse without a tendency toward a periarticular distribution.[293]

Articular calcification, related to CPPD crystal deposition (chondrocalcinosis), occurs in approximately 30 percent of patients with hemochromatosis.[279] In general this calcification is identical to that of idiopathic CPPD crystal deposition disease, but several characteristics may help to distinguish between these two disorders. In hemochromatosis, hyaline cartilage calcification tends to be more prominent and the fibrocartilage of the symphysis pubis is more commonly involved than in idiopathic CPPD crystal deposition disease.[279]

Structural articular alterations in hemochromatosis occur in slightly less than half of the cases.[294, 295] In general, the arthropathy of hemochromatosis is similar to that of idiopathic CPPD crystal deposition disease, with joint space narrowing and subchondral cyst formation being prominent features. Although the two disorders cannot be absolutely separated on a radiographic basis, several features may be useful in differential diagnosis.[279] "Hook" osteophytes are distinctive bony excrescences, most commonly identified at the radial margins of the metacarpal heads, in patients with hemochromatosis. These osteophytes tend to be small, triangular, and sharply defined (Fig. 37–72). They are not prominent in osteoarthritis or idiopathic CPPD crystal deposition disease. The distribution of abnormalities may also be a useful diagnostic feature. In both CPPD crystal deposition disease and hemochromatosis, the second and third metacarpophalangeal joints are the most

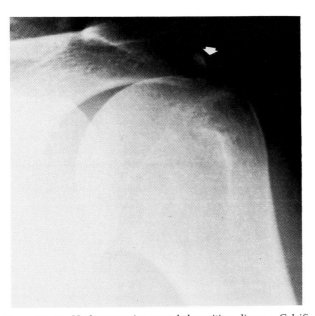

Figure 37–71. Hydroxyapatite crystal deposition disease. Calcification (arrow) of the supraspinatus tendon of the musculotendinous rotator cuff is present. This constitutes the single most common manifestation of this disorder. (From Resnick, D., and Niwayama, G.: Diagnosis of Bone and Joint Disease. Philadelphia, W. B. Saunders Co., 1981.)

commonly involved sites in the hands, but additional alterations of the fourth and fifth metacarpophalangeal joints are more frequent in hemochromatosis. In addition, the radiocarpal joint may be spared in hemochromatosis, whereas it is almost always involved in idiopathic CPPD crystal deposition disease. The arthropathy of hemochromatosis is usually slowly progressive, in contrast to idiopathic pyrophosphate arthropathy, in which a rapidly progressive arthropathy may be seen.

Wilson's Disease. Wilson's disease is a rare inherited disorder characterized by abnormal accumulation of copper in body tissues. The age of onset is typically the first through fourth decades of life. The general radiographic features consist of osteopenia and arthropathy.[279, 296] Chondrocalcinosis has been considered an important feature of this disorder, but it appears to be very rare. Osteopenia, present in approximately 50 percent of patients, is most prominent in the hands, feet, and spine. It may relate to osteoporosis or osteomalacia, or both. Changes of rickets, with Looser's zones or "pseudofractures," are prominent in some cases.[297]

The arthropathy of Wilson's disease is most commonly identified in the wrist, hand, foot, hip, shoulder, elbow, and knee. Irregularity and indistinctness of the subchondral bone plate ("paintbrush" appearance) in combination with focal radiodense excrescences at the central and peripheral joint margins are characteristic. Subchondral cysts and focal areas of fragmentation of the articular surface may also be observed. An additional manifestation is the occurrence of small, distinctly corticated ossicles about affected joints, especially prominent in the wrist. These structures resemble the accessory ossicles frequently seen in normal persons but are more numerous and appear in unusual locations. Joint effusions are not prominent, but spiculated bony proliferative changes are frequently noted at entheses, resembling the inflammatory enthesopathy seen in the seronegative spondyloarthropathies.

Ochronosis (Alkaptonuria). The major radiographic features of ochronosis consist of osteoporosis, abnormal calcification and ossification, and arthropathy.[279] Osteoporosis, although generally diffuse in nature, is most evident in the spine, where it may be associated with vertebral body collapse.[298]

Abnormal calcification and ossification are most prominent in the intervertebral discs, especially those in the lumbar spine. Additional sites of calcification and ossification include the symphysis pubis, costal cartilage, helix of the ear, and peripheral tendons and ligaments.[299] The crystals are composed of calcium hydroxyapatite and demonstrate a typical "cloudlike" appearance.

In the spine, osteoporosis with wafer-like calcification of the intervertebral disc is an early radiographic finding. Intervertebral disc narrowing with the formation of radiolucent discal collections (vacuum phenomena) is also common, often obscuring the calcification.[300] Progressive discal ossification and the formation of peripheral bony bridges in the

outermost layer of the annulus fibrosus may lead to the appearance of a "bamboo spine," similar to that in ankylosing spondylitis. At some levels, osteophytes may also be prominent.

In the peripheral skeleton, the knees, hips, and shoulders are most commonly involved, with relative sparing of the small joints of the hands and feet.[300] In these locations, changes resemble those of degenerative joint disease; however, osteophytes and subchondral cysts are not prominent in ochronosis. In addition, the location of abnormalities, such as the lateral femorotibial compartment of the knee, may help in differentiating ochronosis from OA. Occasionally, a rapidly progressing destructive peripheral arthropathy characterized by fragmentation of articular surfaces may be observed.

SEPTIC ARTHRITIS

Mechanisms. In general, the radiographic features of joint sepsis consist of periarticular soft tissue swelling, intra-articular effusions, cartilage destruction with joint space narrowing, and irregular erosions of the subchondral bone plate.[301–303] In the initial stage of disease, the joint may appear widened, owing to the presence of a large effusion, but rapid cartilage destruction results in articular space narrowing with confluent irregular erosions of the subchondral bone plate (Fig. 37–73). In children, epiphyseal centers may completely disappear as a result of the hyperemia associated with the infected joint. Diabetic patients are prone to develop indolent, slowly progressive joint infections, usually adjacent to soft

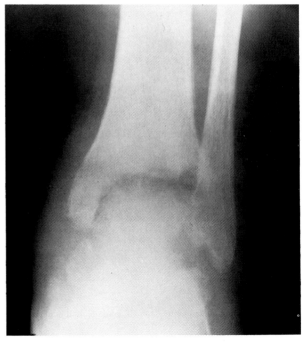

Figure 37–73. Septic arthritis. In this patient with a pyogenic arthritis of the ankle, note the soft tissue swelling, joint space loss, and large confluent subchondral erosions.

tissue ulcerations. In this setting the loss of distinctiveness of articular margins may be the only radiographic manifestation of infection (Fig. 37–74).

In contrast to bacterial infection, granulomatous infection (tuberculosis and fungal) may demonstrate a more slowly progressive pattern of joint destruction (Fig. 37–75). Osseous erosions first appear at the joint margins ("bare" areas), where synovial inflammatory tissue is in direct contact with bone. In fact, prominent juxta-articular osteoporosis and marginal bone erosions, in the absence of significant joint space loss, are characteristics of granulomatous infection. The late complications of joint sepsis include intra-articular fibrous or bony ankylosis as well as joint instability. In the spine the latter complication may result in spinal cord or nerve root compromise.

The role of various imaging modalities in the diagnosis of joint sepsis should be emphasized. Early detection is important to avoid irreversible joint destruction, or in the child, significant growth disturbance. Radionuclide studies are useful in this regard, both in detecting infection early in the course of the disease and in documenting the extent of involvement. However, adjacent soft tissue or bone infections, recent surgery, or post-traumatic changes may render this important tool useless in some cases. Recognition of articular effusions and periarticular soft tissue swelling on roentgenograms is of critical importance in the early diagnosis of joint infection. Magnification radiography may provide additional diagnostic information, especially in the diabetic patient with a foot infection. Fluoroscopically guided aspiration may play an important role in the evalu-

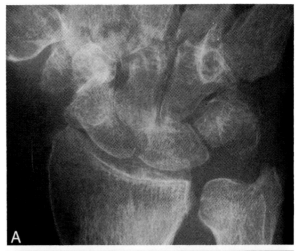

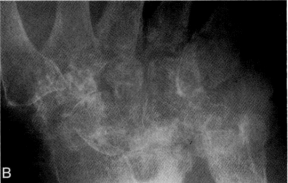

Figure 37–75. Tuberculosis. Note the gradual progression of destructive changes in radiographs obtained 18 months apart. In *A*, there is prominent soft tissue swelling and osteoporosis with marginal osseous erosions at multiple sites. In *B*, the process has progressed to virtually complete destruction of the carpus. A large erosion of the distal radius is also present.

ation of joint sepsis, especially in deep joints such as the hip or the shoulder or in sites such as the spine, where surgical exploration may be required. Although the principal aim of this procedure is to procure a specimen for laboratory analysis, instillation of a small amount of radiopaque contrast agent may be helpful in ascertaining the extent of articular destruction and in detecting extra-articular spread of contaminated material.

MISCELLANEOUS ARTHROPATHIES

Osteonecrosis. Early in the course of epiphyseal osteonecrosis, radiographic changes are not evident. Subsequently, a characteristic progression of radiographic changes will be seen. The earliest findings are a subtle, arclike radiolucent subchondral band (crescent sign) and the formation of patchy subchondral lucent and sclerotic foci (Fig. 37–76). Fragmentation and collapse of the articular surface follow. The joint space is usually preserved until late in the course of the disease, when secondary osteoarthritis may supervene.

A peculiar form of spontaneous osteonecrosis is

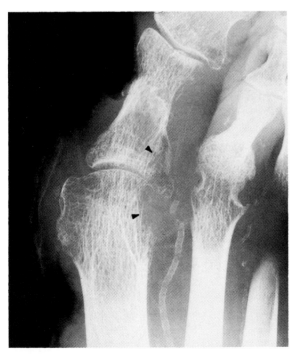

Figure 37–74. Septic arthritis. In this specimen radiograph of an infected foot in a diabetic patient, note the erosions of the lateral margins of the articular surfaces of the first metatarsal head and proximal phalanx *(arrowheads)*.

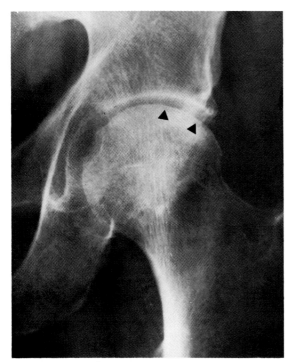

Figure 37–76. Osteonecrosis. An early radiographic change of osteonecrosis is an arclike radiolucent band *(arrowheads)* parallel to the articular surface.

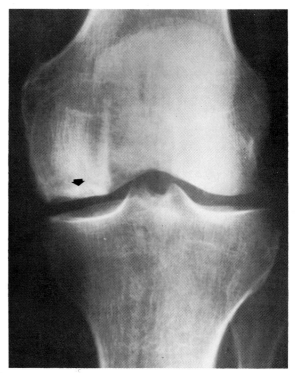

Figure 37–77. Spontaneous osteonecrosis. In this adult with the sudden onset of knee pain, the frontal radiograph demonstrates a defect in the articular surface of the medial femoral condyle *(arrow)*. This is the characteristic location of this lesion. (From Resnick, D., and Niwayama, G.: Diagnosis of Bone and Joint Disorders. Philadelphia, W. B. Saunders Co., 1988.)

seen in the knee, most commonly involving the medial femoral condyle. It is manifested by the sudden appearance of pain and the radiographic changes of sclerosis, flattening, and irregularity of the femoral surface (Fig. 37–77).

Paget's Disease. Articular disease is a recognized complication of Paget's disease. Gout,[304] CPPD crystal deposition disease,[305] and rheumatoid arthritis[304] have each been observed in patients with Paget's disease. More importantly, patients with this disease demonstrate an increased incidence of OA in association with juxta-articular pagetic bony involvement.[249] This is most common in the hip and knee. Although radiographic features resemble those in idiopathic osteoarthritis (Fig. 37–78), more specific changes, such as acetabular protrusion, may be seen.

Acromegaly. Acromegalic arthropathy most closely resembles degenerative joint disease. Some features that aid in its recognition are (1) increased soft tissue thickness (e.g., heel pad > 21 mm) (Fig. 37–79), (2) prominent phalangeal tufts and bases ("arrowhead" phalanges) (Fig. 37–80), (3) "hooklike" osteophytes in the metacarpal heads, (4) joint space widening, (5) exuberant spinal osteophytosis with widened intervertebral discs (Fig. 37–81), and (6) prominent thoracic kyphosis.[306, 307] In the later stages of the disease, loss of joint space becomes apparent. Acromegaly should be considered if a degenerative process occurs in an unusual articulation, such as the glenohumeral joint.

Hemoglobinopathies. Hemoglobinopathies may affect articular structures. The major changes in sickle

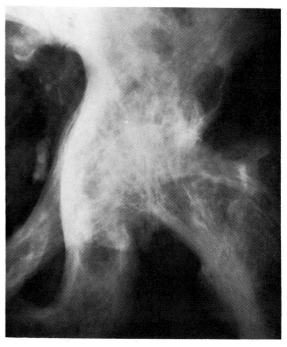

Figure 37–78. Paget's disease. Observe the prominent osteoarthritis-like changes of the hip with asymmetric joint space loss and large marginal osteophytes. The juxta-articular bone is coarsened and enlarged.

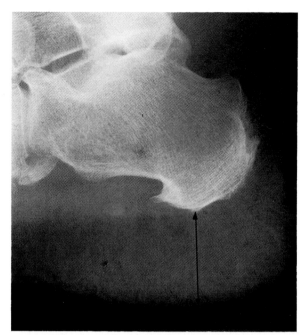

Figure 37–79. Acromegaly. Note the soft tissue prominence of the heel pad with the formation of multiple enthesophytes from the plantar and posterior surfaces of the calcaneus. (From Resnick, D., and Niwayama, G.: Diagnosis of Bone and Joint Disorders. Philadelphia, W. B. Saunders Co., 1988.)

cell anemia relate to vascular occlusion with osteonecrosis, which may involve epiphysis, metaphysis, or diaphysis of a tubular bone as well as flat bones. In sickle cell dactylitis (hand-foot syndrome), the changes of bone infarction are accompanied by prom-

inent soft tissue swelling and exuberant periosteal reaction.[308] Osteomyelitis and, less commonly, septic arthritis can be seen in sickle cell anemia. *Salmonella* is frequently implicated.

Amyloidosis. Radiographically, the diagnosis of amyloidosis is suggested by the occurrence of a bilateral, symmetric erosive arthropathy similar to rheumatoid arthritis but without joint space narrowing.[309, 310] Large soft tissue masses and osteolytic defects in the diaphyses of tubular bones are other prominent findings in this disorder (Fig. 37–82).

Hemophilia. The arthropathy of hemophilia is related to destructive changes associated with repeated episodes of intra-articular hemorrhage (hemarthrosis).[311] Any joint may be involved, but changes in the knee, ankle, and elbow are most frequently identified. The earliest finding consists of juxta-articular soft tissue swelling with large intra-articular effusions. This is followed by prominent osteoporosis and, in the immature skeleton, by epiphyseal overgrowth (Fig. 37–83). Subchondral cysts and bony erosions appear, initially with preservation of the cartilaginous coat, and subsequently with cartilage destruction and joint space narrowing. Late abnormalities include complete joint disorganization with obliteration of the articular space, large bony erosions, and joint instability. In the knee, radiographic features of hemophilia include widening of

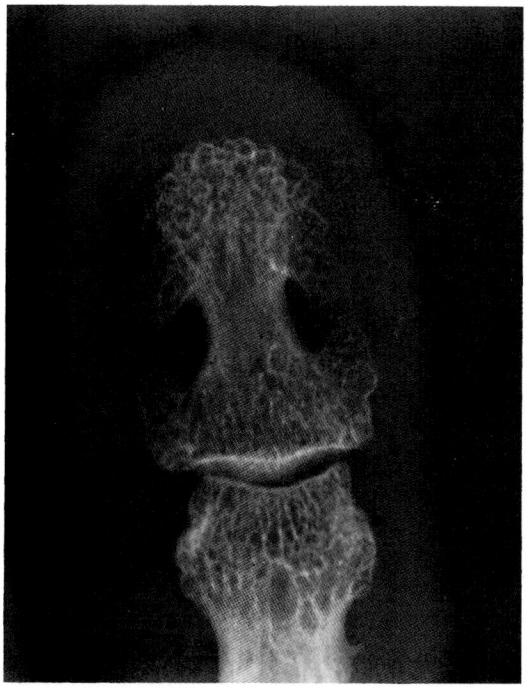

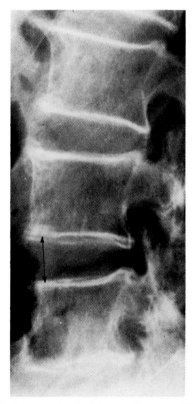

Figure 37–81. Acromegaly. In this case, the most striking finding is the abnormally increased height of the intervertebral disc spaces *(between arrowheads).* Note posterior concavity of the vertebral bodies and degenerative changes.

Figure 37–80. Acromegaly. There is proliferation of the margins of the base and terminal tuft of the distal phalanx, resulting in the classic "arrowhead" appearance.

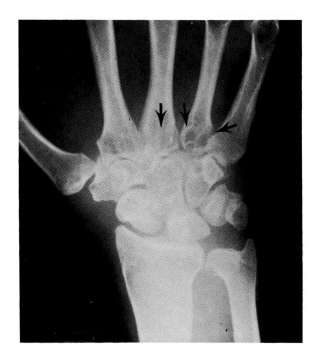

Figure 37–82. Amyloidosis. Observe the diffuse soft tissue swelling and the presence of destructive lesions in the third and fourth metacarpal bases *(arrows)*, radius, and ulna.

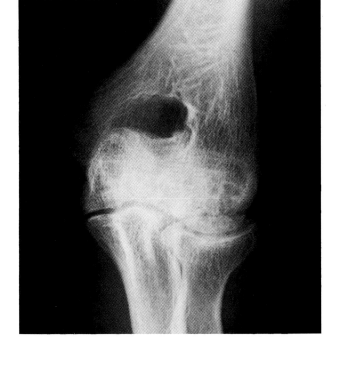

Figure 37–83. Hemophilia. There is overgrowth of the epiphyses, especially the radial head. Joint space narrowing and subchondral cysts are seen.

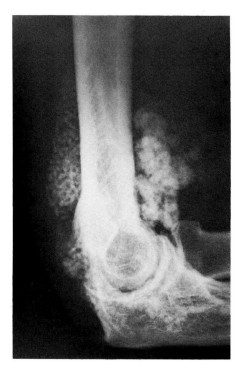

Figure 37–84. Idiopathic synovial (osteo)chondromatosis. A radiograph of the elbow reveals multiple calcified bodies of varying sizes within the confines of an enlarged joint capsule.

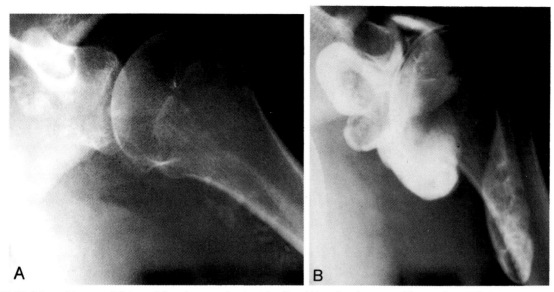

Figure 37–85. Idiopathic synovial (osteo)chondromatosis. A plain film *(A)* and arthrogram *(B)* reveal typical changes. In *A,* observe intra-articular calcified bodies along the synovial sheath of the bicipital tendons. The arthrogram defines multiple radiolucent filling defects.

the intercondylar notch of the distal femur and squaring of the inferior patellar pole. The radiographic features of hemophilia may be difficult to differentiate from those of juvenile chronic arthritis.

Synovial (Osteo)chondromatosis and Pigmented Villonodular Synovitis. The typical radiographic picture of synovial (osteo)chondromatosis is that of numerous calcific densities confined to the articular cavity (Fig. 37–84). Pressure erosions of adjacent bony surfaces may be seen. Osteoporosis and joint space narrowing are generally not prominent. In cases in which the bodies are not calcified, arthrography may confirm the diagnosis (Fig. 37–85).

Multiple erosions and cysts on both sides of the joint are seen in pigmented villonodular synovitis. Osteoporosis and joint space narrowing are usually not prominent.[312–314] During arthrography, nodular soft tissue masses may be demonstrated, and aspiration of joint fluid will yield a characteristic "rusty" fluid. MR imaging will reveal signal characteristics diagnostic of hemosiderin deposition.

Synovial Sarcoma. The typical roentgenographic finding of a synovial sarcoma is a soft tissue mass, which contains calcification in approximately 30 percent of cases. Erosion of neighboring bone is seen in 25 to 35 percent of lesions.

References

1. Mall, J. C., Genant, H. K., Silcox, D. C., and McCarty, D. J.: The efficacy of fine-detail radiography in the evaluation of patients with rheumatoid arthritis. Radiology 112:37, 1974.
2. Genant, H. K.: Magnification radiography. *In* Resnick D., and Niwayama, G. (eds.): Diagnosis of Bone and Joint Disorders. Philadelphia, W. B. Saunders Company, 1981, p. 335.
3. Genant, H. K., Valdez Horst, J., Lanzl, L. H., Mall, J. C., and Doi, K.: Skeletal demineralization in primary hyperparathyroidism. *In* Mazeski, R. B. (ed.): Proceedings of the International Conference on Bone Mineral Measurement. Washington, D.C., National Institute of Arthritis, Metabolism and Digestive Diseases, 1973, p. 177.
4. Leach, R. E., Grett, T., and Ferris, J. S.: Weight-bearing radiography in osteoarthritis of the knee. Radiology 97:265, 1970.
5. Resnick, D., and Danzig, L.: Arthrographic evaluation of injuries at the first metacarpophalangeal joint: Gamekeeper's thumb. Am. J. Roentgenol. 126:1046, 1976.
6. Chamberlain, W. E.: The symphysis pubis in the roentgen evaluation of the sacroiliac joint. Am. J. Roentgenol. 24:621, 1930.
7. Martel, W., and Poznanski, A. K.: The value of traction during roentgenography of the hip. Radiology 94:497, 1970.
8. Resnick, D.: Arthrography, tenography, and bursography. *In* Resnick, D., and Niwayama, G. (eds.): Diagnosis of Bone and Joint Disorders. Philadelphia, W. B. Saunders Company, 1981, p. 510.
9. Gelman, M., Coleman, R. E., Stevens, P. M., and Davey, B. W.: Radiography, radionucleide imaging, and arthrography in evaluation of painful total hip and knee replacements. Radiology 128:677, 1978.
10. Wolfe, R. D., and Giuliano, V. J.: Double-contrast arthrography in the diagnosis of pigmented villonodular synovitis of the knee. Am. J. Roengenol. 110:793, 1970.
11. Prager, R. J., and Mall, J. C.: Arthrographic diagnosis of synovial chondromatosis. Am. J. Roentgenol. 127:344, 1976.
12. Strizak, A. M., Danzig, L. A., Jackson, D. W., Greenway, G., Resnick, D., and Staple, T.: Subacromial bursography: An anatomic and clinical study. J. Bone Joint Surg. 64A:196, 1982.
13. Cone, R., Danzig, L., and Resnick, D.: The shoulder impingement syndrome. Radiology 150:29, 1984.
14. Totty, W. G., and Vannier, M. W.: Complex musculoskeletal anatomy using 3-D surface reconstruction. Radiology 150:173, 1985.
15. Sartoris, D. J., Pate, D., Andre, M., and Resnick, D.: 3-D display of CT data. New aid to pre-op surgical planning. Diagn. Imag. 8:74, 1986.
16. Fishman, E. K., Drebin, B., Magid, D., Scoot, W. N., Jr., Ney, D. R., Brooker, A. F., Jr., Riley, L. H., et al.: Volumetric rendering techniques: Applications for 3-D imaging of the hip. Radiology 163:737, 1987.
17. Cacayorin, E. D., and Kieffer, S. A.: Applications and limitations of CT of the spine. Radiol. Clin. North Am. 20:185, 1982.
18. Harris, J. H., and Edeiken-Monroe, B.: The Radiology of Acute Cervical Spine Trauma. 2nd ed. Baltimore, Williams & Wilkins, 1982.
19. Guerra, J., Jr., Garfin, S. R., and Resnick, D.: Vertebral burst fractures: CT analysis of the retropulsed fragment. Radiology 153:769, 1984.
20. Daffner, R. H.: Thoracic and lumbar vertebral trauma. Orthop. Clin. North Am. 21:463, 1990.
21. Kaye, J. J., and Nance, E. P.: Cervical spine trauma. Orthop. Clin. North Am. 21:449, 1990.
22. Perch, P., Kilgore, D. P., Pojima, K. W., and Haughton, V. M.: Cervical spine fractures: CT detection. Radiology 157:117, 1985.
23. Pitt, M. J., Lund, P. J., and Speer, D. P.: Imaging of the pelvis and hip. Orthop. Clin. North Am. 21:545, 1990.
24. Harley, J. D., Mack, L. A., and Winquist, R. A.: CT of acetabular fractures: A comparison with conventional radiography. A.J.R. 138:413, 1982.
25. Harley, J. D., Mack, L. A., and Winquist, R. A.: CT of acetabular fractures: Analysis of fracture patterns. A.J.R. 138:407, 1982.

26. Burk, D. L., Jr., Mears, D. C., Kennedy, W. H., Cooperstein, L. H., and Herbert, D. L.: 3-D CT of acetabular fractures. Radiology 155:183, 1985.

27. Destonet, J. M., Gibula, L. A., Murphy, W. A., and Sagel, S. S.: CT of sternoclavicular joint and sternum. Radiology 138:123, 1981.

28. Vukich, D. J., and Markovichick, V. J.: Pulmonary and chest wall injuries. In Rosen, P., Baker, F. J., II, Barkin, R. M., et al. (eds.): Emergency Medicine: Concepts and Clinical Practice. 2nd ed. St. Louis, C. V. Mosby, 1988, pp. 473–486.

29. Singson, R. D., Feldman, F., and Bibliani, L.: CT arthrographic patterns in recurrent glenohumeral instability. A.J.R. 149:749, 1987.

30. Beltran, J.: The shoulder: New approaches. Radiology 5:7, 1990.

31. Singson, R. D., Feldman, F., and Rosenberg, Z. S.: Elbow joint: Assessment with double contrast CT arthrography. Radiology 160:167, 1986.

32. Gilmer, P. W., Herzenberg, J., Frank, L., Silverman, P., et al.: CT analysis of acute calcaneal fractures. Foot Ankle 6:184, 1986.

33. Ramirez, H. Jr., Blatt, E. S., Cable, H. F., McComb, B. L., Zornoza, J., and Hibri, N. S.: Intraosseous pneumatocysts of the ilium. Radiology 150:503, 1984.

34. Soye, I., Levine, E., Desmet, A. A., and Weff, J. R.: CT of preoperative evaluation of masses arising in or near the joints of the extremities. Radiology 143:727, 1982.

35. Heiken, J. P., Lee, J. K. T., Smothers, R. L., Totty, W. G., and Murphy, W. A.: CT of benign soft tissue masses of extremities. A.J.R. 142:575, 1984.

36. Aisen, A. M., Martel, W., Braunstein, E. M., et al.: MRI and CT evaluation of primary bone and soft tissue tumors. A.J.R. 146:749, 1986.

37. Zimmer, W. D., Berquist, T. H., Mcload, R. A., Sim, F. H., Pritchard, D. J., Shives, T. C., Wold, L. E., and May, G. R.: Bone tumors: MRI vs CT. Radiology 155:709, 1985.

38. Thompson, J. R., Christiansen, E., Hasso, A. N., and Hinshaw, D. B., Jr.: TMJ: High resolution CT evaluation. Radiology 150:105, 1984.

39. Thompson, J. R., Christiansen, E., Hasso, A. N., and Hinshaw, D. B., Jr.: Dislocation of the TMJ meniscus: Contrast arthrography vs CT. A.J.R. 144:171, 1985.

40. Sartoris, D. J., Neumann, C. H., and Riley, R. N.: The TMJ: True sagittal with meniscus visualization. Radiology 150:250, 1984.

41. Simon, D. C., Hess, M. R., Similak, M. S., and Beltran, J.: Direct sagittal CT of the TMJ. Radiology 157:545, 1985.

42. Manco, L. G., Messing, S. G., Busine, L. J., Faculo, C. P., and Sordill, W. C.: Internal derangements of TMJ evaluated by direct sagittal CT: A prospective study. Radiology 157:407, 1985.

43. Dussault, R. G., and Lander, P. H.: Imaging of facet joints. Radiol. Clin. North Am. 28:1033, 1990.

44. Carrera, G. F., Haughton, V. M., Syvertsen, A., et al.: CT of lumbar facet joints. Radiology 134:134, 1981.

45. Bjorkengren, A. G., Kurz, L. T., Resnick, D., et al.: Symptomatic intraspinal synovial cysts: Opacification and treatment by percutaneous injection. A.J.R. 149:105, 1987.

46. Hemminghytt, S., Daniels, D. L., Williams, A. L., and Haughton, V. M.: Intraspinal synovial cysts: Natural history and diagnosis by CT. Radiology 145:395, 1982.

47. Russel, A. S., and Jackson, F.: CT of apophyseal changes in patients with ankylosing spondylitis. J. Rheumatol. 13:581, 1986.

48. Forrester, D. M.: Imaging of sacroiliac joints. Radiol. Clin. North Am. 28:1055, 1990.

49. Durback, M. A., Edelstein, G., and Shumacher, H. R.: Abnormalities of the sacroiliac joints in DISH: Demonstration by CT. J. Rheumatol. 15:1506, 1988.

50. Vantiggelen, R., et al.: Sacroiliitis: Difficulties in the radiographic diagnosis: Advantage of CT? Preliminary report. J. Belge Radiol. 70:1, 1987.

51. Guyst, D. R., Mandi, A., and Kling, G. A.: Pyogenic sacroiliitis in drug abusers. A.J.R. 149:1209, 1987.

52. Sartoris, D. J., Resnick, D., Gershumi, D., Bielecki, D., and Meyers, M.: CT with multiplanar reformation and 3-D image analysis in the preoperative evaluation of ischemic necrosis of the femoral head. J. Rheumatol. 13:153, 1986.

53. Deutsch, A. L., Resnick, D., Mink, J. H., Berman, J. L., Cone, R. O., III, Resnik, C. S., Danzig, L., and Guerra, J., Jr.: CT and conventional arthrotomography of the glenohumeral joint: Normal anatomy and clinical experience. Radiology 153:603, 1984.

54. Beltran, J., Gray, L. A., Bools, J. C., et al.: Rotator cuff lesions of the shoulder: Evaluation by direct sagittal CT arthrography. Radiology 160:161, 1986.

55. Gundry, C. R., Schils, J. P., Resnick, D., and Sartoris, D. J.: Arthrography in post-traumatic knee, shoulder, and wrist: Current status and future trends. Radiol. Clin. North Am. 27:957, 1989.

56. Reikeiras, O., and Hoiseth, A.: Patellofemoral relationship in normal subjects determined by computed tomography. Skeletal Radiol. 19:591, 1990.

57. Inoue, M., Shino K., et al.: Subluxation of the patella: CT of patellofemoral congruence. J. Bone Joint Surg. 70:1331, 1988.

58. Daniels, D. L., Grogan, J. P., Johansen, J. G., Meyer, G. A., Williams, A. L., and Haughton, V. M.: Cervical radiculopathy: Computed tomography and myelography compared. Radiology 151:109, 1984.

59. Badami, J. P., Norman, D., Barbaro, N. M., Cann, C. E., Weinstein, P. R., and Sobel, D. F.: Metrizamide CT myelography in cervical myelopathy and radiculopathy: Correlation with conventional myelography and surgical findings. A.J.R. 144:675, 1985.

60. Penning, L., Wilmink, J. T., van Woerden, H. H., and Knol, E.: CT myelographic findings in degenerative disorders of the cervical spine: Clinical significance. A.J.R. 146:793, 1986.

61. Russell, E. J., D'Angelo, C. M., Zimmermann, R. D., Czervionke, L. F., and Huckman, M. S.: Cervical disk herniation CT demonstration after contrast enhancement. Radiology 152:703, 1984.

62. Williams, A. L., Haughton, V. M., Meyer, G. A., and Ho, K. C.: Computed tomographic appearance of the bulging annulus. Radiology 142:403, 1982.

63. Bielecki, D. K., Sartoris, D., Van Lom, K., Resnick, D., Fierer, J., and Haghighi, P.: Intraosseous and intradiscal gas in association with spinal infection: Report of three cases. A.J.R. 147:83, 1986.

64. Raskin, S. P., and Keating, J. W.: Recognition of lumbar disk disease: Comparison of myelography and computed tomography. A.J.R. 139:49, 1982.

65. Haughton, V. M., Eldevik, O. P., Magnaes, B., and Amundsen, P.: A prospective comparison of computed tomography and myelography in the diagnosis of herniated lumbar disks. Radiology 142:103, 1982.

66. Rosenthal, D. I., Stauffer, A. E., Davis, K. R., Ganott, M., and Taveras, J. M.: Evaluation of multiplanar reconstruction in CT recognition of lumbar disk disease. A.J.R. 143:169, 1984.

67. Firooznia, H., Benjamin, V., Kricheff, I. I., Rafii, M., and Golimbu, C.: CT of lumbar disk herniation: Correlation with surgical findings. A.J.R. 142:587, 1984.

68. Carrera, G. F., Williams, A. L., and Haughton, V. M.: Computed tomography in sciatica. Radiology 137:433, 1980.

69. Williams, A. L., Haughton, V. M., Daniels, D. L., and Thornton, R. S.: CT recognition of lateral lumbar disk herniation. A.J.R. 139:345, 1982.

70. Williams, A. L., Haughton, V. M., Daniels, D. L., and Grogan, J. P.: Differential CT diagnosis of extruded nucleus pulposus. Radiology 154:119, 1985.

71. Helms, C. A., Dorwart, R. H., and Gray, M.: The CT appearance of conjoined nerve roots and differentiation from a herniated nucleus pulposus. Radiology 148:141, 1983.

72. Hoddick, W. K., and Helms, C. A.: Bony spinal changes that differentiate conjoined nerve roots from herniated nucleus pulposus. Radiology 154:119, 1985.

73. Teplick, J. G., and Haskin, M. E.: Spontaneous regression of herniated nucleus pulposus. A.J.R. 145:371, 1985.

74. Braun, I. F., Hoffman, J. C., Jr., Davis, P. C., Landman, J. A., and Tindall, G. T.: Contrast enhancement in CT differentiation between recurrent disk herniation and postoperative scar: Prospective study. A.J.R. 145:371, 1985.

75. Teplick, J. G., and Haskin, M. E.: Intravenous contrast-enhanced CT of the postoperative lumbar spine: Improved identification of recurrent disk herniation, scar, arachnoiditis, and discitis. A.J.R. 143:845, 1984.

76. Brown, B. M., Stark, E. H., Dion, G., and Ono, H.: Computed tomography and chymopapain chemonucleolysis: Preliminary findings. A.J.R. 144:667, 1985.

77. Gentry, L. R., Turski, P. A., Strother, C. M., Javid, M. J., and Sackett, J. F.: Chymopapain chemonucleolysis: CT changes after treatment. A.J.R. 145:361, 1985.

78. Konings, J. G., Williams, F. J. B., and Deutman, R.: The effects of chemonucleolysis as demonstrated by CT. J. Bone Joint Surg. 3:417, 1984.

79. Hernandez, R. J., Taehdjian, M. O., and Dias, L. S.: Hip CT in congenital dislocation: Appearance of tight iliopsoas tendon and pulvinar hypertrophy. A.J.R. 139:335, 1982.

80. Lafferty, C. M., Sartoris, D. J., Tyson, R., Resnick, D., Kursunoglu, D., Pate, D., and Sutherland, D.: Acetabular alterations in untreated congenital hip dysplasia: CT with multiplanar reformation and 3-D analysis. J. Comput. Assist. Tomogr. 4:493, 1980.

81. Berquist, T. H., and Ehman, R. L.: MRI evaluates diseases of musculoskeletal system. Diagn. Imag. 10:88, 1985.

82. Burk, D. L., Jr., Dalinka, M. K., Schiebler, M. L., et al.: Strategies for musculoskeletal magnetic resonance imaging. Radiol. Clin. North Am. 26:653, 1988.

83. Bradley, W. G. Jr., and Tsuruda, J. S.: MR sequences parameter optimization: An algorithmic approach. A.J.R. 149:815, 1987.

84. Modic, M. T., Masaryk, T. J., Ross, J. S., and Carter, J. R.: Imaging of degenerative disk disease. Radiology 168:177, 1988.

85. Yu, S., Haughton, V. M., Sether, L. A., and Wagner, M.: Annulus fibrosus in bulging intervertebral disks. Radiology 169:761, 1988.

86. Masaryk, T. J., Ross, J. S., Modic, M. T., et al.: High-resolution MR imaging of sequestered lumbar intervertebral disks. A.J.N.R. 9:351, 1988.

87. Lee, S. H., Coleman, P. E., and Hahn, F. J.: Magnetic resonance imaging of degenerative disk disease of the spine. Radiol. Clin. North Am. 26:949, 1988.

88. Grenier, N., Kressel, H. Y., Schiebler, M. L., et al.: Normal and degenerative posterior spinal structures: MR imaging. Radiology 165:517, 1987.

89. Heithoff, K. B., Ray, C. D., Schellhas, K. P., and Fritts, H. M.: CT and MRI of lateral entrapment syndromes. In Genant, H. K. (ed.): Spine Update 1987. San Francisco, Radiology Research and Education Foundation, 1987, pp. 203–234.

90. Burton, C. V.: Avoiding the failed back surgery syndrome. In Cauthen, J. C. (ed.): Lumbar Spine Surgery. Baltimore, Williams & Wilkins, 1988, pp 331–341.

91. White, A. H., and Hsu, K.: Failed Posterior Spine Surgery. St. Louis, C. V. Mosby, 1987.

92. Bundschuh, C. V., Modic, M. T., Ross, J. S., et al.: Epidural fibrosis and recurrent disk herniation in the lumbar spine: Assessment with magnetic resonance. A.J.N.R. 5:169, 1988.

93. Sotiropoulos, S., Chafetz, N., Winkler, M., et al.: Differentiation between postoperative scar and recurrent disk herniation: Prospective comparison of MR, CT and contrast-enhanced CT. A.J.N.R. 10:639, 1989.

94. Djukic, S., Genant, H. K., Helms, C. A., and Holt, R. G.: Magnetic resonance imaging of the postoperative lumbar spine. Radiol. Clin. North Am. 28:341, 1990.

95. Hueftle, M. G., Modic, M. T., Ross, J. S., et al.: Lumbar spine: Postoperative MR imaging with Gd-DTPA. Radiology 167:817, 1988.

96. Ross, J. S., et al.: Gadolinium-DTPA–enhanced MR imaging of the postoperative lumbar spine: Time course and mechanism of enhancement. A.J.R. 152:825, 1989.

97. Vogler, J. B., III, and Murphy, W. A.: State of the art: Bone marrow imaging. Radiology 168:679, 1988.

98. Kricun, M. E.: Red-yellow marrow conversion: Its effects on the location of some solitary bone lesions. Skeletal Radiol. 14:10, 1985.

99. Rao, V. M., Fishman, M., Mitchell, D. G., et al.: Painful sickle cell crisis: Bone marrow patterns observed with MR imaging. Radiology 161:211, 1986.

100. Moore, S. G., Gooding, C. A., Brasch, R. C., et al.: Bone marrow in children with acute lymphocytic leukemia: MR relaxation times. Radiology 160:237, 1986.

101. Sugimura, K., Yamasaki, K., Kitagaki, H., Tanaka, Y., Kono, M.: Bone marrow diseases of the spine: Differentiation with T_1 and T_2 relaxation times in MRI. Radiology 165:541, 1987.

102. McKinstry, C. S., Steiner, R. E., Young, A. T., Jones, L., Swirsky, D., and Aber, V.: Bone marrow in leukemia and aplastic anemia: MR imaging before, during and after treatment. Radiology 162:701, 1987.

103. Yao, L., and Lee, J. K.: Occult intraosseous fracture: Detection with MRI. Radiology 167:749, 1988.

104. Bloem, J. L.: Transient osteoporosis of the hip: MRI. Radiology 167:753, 1988.

105. Beltran, J., Herman, L. J., Burk, J. M., et al.: Femoral head avascular necrosis: MRI with clinical-pathologic correlation. Radiology 166:215, 1988.

106. Katzberg, R. W., Westesson, P. L., Tallents, R. L. H., et al.: Temporomandibular joint: MR assessment of rotational and sideways disk displacements. Radiology 169:741, 1988.

107. Katzberg, R. W.: Temporomandibular joint imaging. Radiology 170:297, 1989.

108. Conway, W. F., Hayes, C. W., and Campbell, R. L.: Dynamic MRI of the temporomandibular joint using FLASH sequences. J. Oral Maxillofac. Surg. 46:930, 1988.

109. Huber, D. J., Sauter, R., Mueller, E., et al.: MR imaging of the normal shoulder. Radiology 158:405, 1986.

110. Neer, C. S. II: Impingement lesions. Clin. Orthop. Rel. Res. 173:70, 1983.

111. Seeger, L. L., Gold, R. H., Bassett, L. W., et al.: Shoulder impingement syndrome: MR findings in 53 shoulders. A.J.R. 150:343, 1988.

112. Zlatkin, M. B., Iannotti, J. P., Roberts, M. C., et al.: Rotator cuff tears: Diagnostic performance of MR imaging. Radiology 172:223, 1989.

113. Kursunoglu-Brahme, S., and Resnick, D.: MR imaging of the shoulder. Radiol. Clin. North Am. 28:941, 1990.

114. Flannigan, B., Kursunoglu-Brahme, S., Snyder, S., Karzel, R., et al.: MR arthrography of the shoulder: Comparison with conventional MR imaging. A.J.R. 155:829, 1990.

115. Weiss, K. L., Beltran, J., Shaman, O. M., Stilla, R. F., and Levey, I. M.: High-field MR surface-coil imaging of the hand and wrist: I. Normal anatomy. Radiology 160:143, 1986.

116. Middleton, W. D., Kneeland, J. B., Kellman, G. M., Cates, J. D., Sanger, J. R., Jesmanowic, A., et al.: MRI of carpal tunnel: Normal anatomy and preliminary findings in the carpal tunnel syndrome. A.J.R. 148:307, 1987.

117. Stoller, D. W.: MRI in Orthopedics and Rheumatology. Philadelphia, J.B. Lippincott Company, 1989.

118. Gilkeson, G., Polisson, R., Sinclair, H., Vogler, J., et al.: Early detection of carpal erosions in patients with rheumatoid arthritis: A pilot study of MRI. J. Rheumatol. 15:1361, 1988.

119. Reinus, W. R., Conway, W. F., Totty, W. G., Gilula, L. A., et al.: Carpal avascular necrosis: MRI. Radiology 160:689, 1986.

120. Baker, L. L., Hajek, P. C., Bjorkengren, A., et al.: High resolution MRI of the wrist. Skeletal Radiol. 16:128, 1987.

121. Beltran, J., Noto, A. M., Herman, L. J., et al.: Tendons: High field-strength surface coil MRI. Radiology 162:735, 1987.

122. Kneeland, B., Macrander, S., Middleton, W. D., et al.: MR imaging of the normal ankle: Correlation with anatomic sections. A.J.R. 151:117, 1988.

123. Daffner, R. H., Reimer, B. L., Lupetin, A. R., et al.: MRI in acute tendon ruptures. Skeletal Radiol. 15:619, 1986.

124. Alexander, I. J., Johnson, K. A., and Berquist, T. H.: MRI in the diagnosis of disruption of the posterior tibial tendon. Foot Ankle 8:144, 1987.

125. Mink, J. H., and Deutsch, A. (eds.): MRI of the Musculoskeletal System: A teaching file. New York, Raven Press, 1990.

126. Yulish, B. S., Lieberman, J. M., Neuman, A. J., et al.: JRA: Assessment with MRI. Radiology 165:149, 1987.

127. Yulish, B. S., Lieberman, J. M., Strandjord, S. E., et al.: Hemophilic arthropathy: Assessment with MRI. Radiology 164:759, 1987.

128. Burk, D. L., Dalinka, M. K., Kanal, E., et al.: High resolution MR imaging of the knee. In Kressel, H. Y. (ed.): Magnetic Resonance Annual. New York, Raven Press, 1988, pp. 1–36.

129. Langer, J. E., Meyer, S. J., and Dalinka, M. K.: Imaging of the knee. Radiol. Clin. North Am. 28:977, 1990.

130. Mink, J. H., Reicher, M. A., and Crues, J. V.: MRI of the knee. New York, Raven Press, 1987.

131. Stoller, D. W., Martin, C., Crues, J. V., et al.: Meniscal tears: Pathologic correlation with MRI. Radiology 163:731, 1987.

132. Mink, J. H., Levy, T., and Crues, J. V.: Tears of anterior cruciate ligament and menisci of the knee: MR imaging evaluation. Radiology 167:769, 1988.

133. Deutsch, A. L., and Mink, J. H.: Articular disorders of the knee. Top. Magn. Reson. Imag. 1:43, 1989.

134. Crues, J. V., Mink, J., Levy, T., et al.: Meniscal tears of the knee: Accuracy of MRI 164:445, 1987.

135. Kursunoglu-Brahme, S., and Resnick, D.: Magnetic resonance imaging of the knee. Orthop. Clin. North Am. 21:564, 1990.

136. Reicher, M. A., Hartzman, S., Basset, L. W., et al.: MR imaging of the knee: Traumatic disorders. Radiology 162:547, 1987.

137. Jackson, D. W., Jennings, L. D., Maywood, R. M., et al.: Magnetic resonance imaging of the knee. Am. J. Sports Med. 16:29, 1988.

138. Mink, J. H., and Deutsch, A. L.: MRI of Musculo-skeletal System: A Teaching File. New York, Raven Press, 1990.

139. Dietz, G. W., Wilcox, D. M., and Montgomery, J. B.: Second tibial condyle fracture: Lateral capsular ligament avulsion. Radiology 159:467, 1986.

140. Mink, J. H., and Deutsch, A. D.: Occult osseous and cartilagenous injuries at the knee: MR detection, classification and assessment. Radiology 170:823, 1989.

141. Shellock, F. G., Mink, J. H., and Fox, J. M.: Patellofemoral joint: Kinematic MR imaging to assess tracking abnormalities. Radiology 168:551, 1988.

142. Senac, M. O., Deutsch, D., Bernstein, B. H., et al.: MRI in juvenile rheumatoid arthritis. A.J.R. 150:843, 1988.

143. Bjorkengren, A. G., Geborek, P. L., Rydholm, U., Holtas, S., et al.: MR imaging of the knee in acute rheumatoid arthritis: Synovial uptake of Gadolinium-DTPA. A.J.R. 155:329, 1990.

144. Burk, D. L., Dalinka, M. K., Kanal, E., et al.: Meniscal and ganglion cysts of the knee: MR evaluation. A.J.R. 150:331, 1988.

145. Resnick, D., and Niwayama, G.: Rheumatoid arthritis. In Resnick, D., and Niwayama, G. (eds.): Diagnosis of Bone and Joint Disorders. Philadelphia, W. B. Saunders Company, 1981, p. 906.

146. O'Driscoll, S., and O'Driscoll, M.: Osteomalacia in rheumatoid arthritis. Ann. Rheum. Dis. 39:1, 1980.

147. DeHaas, W. H. D., DeBoer, W., Griffin, F., and Oosten-Elst, P.: Rheumatoid arthritis of the robust reaction type. Ann. Rheum. Dis. 33:81, 1974.

148. Renneic, C., Mainzer, F., Multz, C. V., and Genant, H. K.: Subchondral pseudocysts in rheumatoid arthritis. Am. J. Roentgenol. 129:1069, 1977.

149. Norgaard, F.: Tidligste rontgenoligiske forandringer ved polyarthritis. Ugeskr. Laeger 125:1312, 1963.

150. Resnick, D.: Rheumatoid arthritis of the wrist: The compartmental approach. Med. Radiog. Photog. 52:50, 1976.

151. Resnick, D.: Rheumatoid arthritis of the wrist: Why the ulnar styloid? Radiology 112:29, 1974.

152. Berens, D. L., and Lin, R. K.: Roentgen Diagnosis of Rheumatoid Arthritis. Springfield, Ill., Charles C Thomas, 1969.

153. Resnick, D.: Early abnormalities of the pisiform and triquetrum in rheumatoid arthritis. Ann. Rheum. Dis. 35:46, 1976.
154. Linscheid, R. L.: The mechanical factors affecting deformity at the wrist in rheumatoid arthritis. In Proceedings of the Twenty-Fourth Annual Meeting of the American Society for Surgery of the Hand. New York, Jan. 17–18, 1969. J. Bone Joint Surg. 51A:790, 1969.
155. Jackman, R. J., and Pugh, D. G.: The positive elbow fat pad sign in rheumatoid arthritis. Am. J. Roentgenol. 108:812, 1970.
156. Weston, W. J.: The synovial changes at the elbow in rheumatoid arthritis. Aust. Radiogr. 15:170, 1971.
157. Rappaport, A. S., Sosman, J. L., and Weissman, B. N.: Spontaneous fractures of the olecranon process in rheumatoid arthritis. Radiology 119:83, 1976.
158. Short, C. L., Bauer, W., and Reynolds, W. E.: Rheumatoid Arthritis. Cambridge, Massachusetts, Harvard University Press, 1957.
159. Thould, A. K., and Simon, G.: Assessment of the radiological changes in the hands and feet in rheumatoid arthritis. Ann. Rheum. Dis. 25:220, 1966.
160. Calabro, J. J.: The feet as an aid in the differential diagnosis of arthritis (Abstract). Arthritis Rheum. 3:435, 1960.
161. Bywaters, E. G. L.: Heel lesions in rheumatoid arthritis. Ann. Rheum. Dis. 13:42, 1954.
162. Resnick, D., Feingold, M. L., Curd, J., Niwayama, G., and Goergen, T. G.: Calcaneal abnormalities in articular disorders: Rheumatoid arthritis, ankylosing spondylitis, psoriatic arthritis, and Reiter's Syndrome. Radiology 125:355, 1977.
163. Kirkup, J. R.: Ankle and tarsal joints in rheumatoid arthritis. Scand. J. Rheumatol. 3:50, 1974.
164. Magayar, E., Talerman, A., Feher, M., and Wouters, H. W.: Giant bone cysts in rheumatoid arthritis. J. Bone Joint Surg. 56B:121, 1974.
165. Genovese, G. R., Jayson, M. I. J., and Dixon, A. S.: Protective value of synovial cysts in rheumatoid knees. Ann. Rheum. Dis. 31:179, 1972.
166. Resnick, D.: Patterns of migration of the femoral head in osteoarthritis of the hip: Roentgenographic-pathologic correlation and comparison with rheumatoid arthritis. Am. J. Roentgenol. 124:62, 1975.
167. Armbuster, T., Guerra, J., Resnick, D., Georgen, J. G., Feingold, M. L., Niwayama, G., and Danzig, L.: The adult hip: An anatomic study: I. The bony landmarks. Radiology 128:1, 1978.
168. Sievers, K., and Caine, V.: The sacroiliac joint in rheumatoid arthritis in adult females. Acta Rheum. Scand. 9:222, 1963.
169. Martel, W.: The occipito-atlanto-axial joints in rheumatoid arthritis. In Carter, M. E. (ed.): Radiological Aspects of Rheumatoid Disease. Proceedings of an international symposium. Amsterdam, 1963. Amsterdam, Excerpta Medica, 1964, p. 189.
170. Mathews, J. A.: Atlanto-axial subluxation in rheumatoid arthritis: A 5-year follow-up study. Ann. Rheum. Dis. 33:526, 1974.
171. Martel, W.: The occipito-atlanto-axial joints in rheumatoid arthritis and ankylosing spondylitis. Am. J. Roentgenol. 86:223, 1961.
172. Rana, N. A., Hancock, D. O., Taylor, A. R., and Hill, A. G. S.: Upward translocation of the dens in rheumatoid arthritis. J. Bone Joint Surg. 55B:471, 1973.
173. Linquist, P. R., and McDonnell, D. E.: Rheumatoid cyst causing extradural compression. J. Bone Joint Surg. 52A:1235, 1970.
174. Ansell, B. M., and Kent, P. A.: Radiological changes in juvenile chronic polyarthritis. Skeletal Radiol. 1:129, 1977.
175. Ansell, B. M., and Bywaters, E. G .L.: Growth in Still's disease. Ann. Rheum. Dis. 15:295, 1956.
176. Martel, W., Holt, J. F., and Cassidy, J. T.: Roentgenologic manifestations of juvenile rheumatoid arthritis. Am. J. Roentgenol. 88:400, 1962.
177. Resnick, D., and Niwayama, G.: Juvenile chronic arthritis. In Resnick, D., and Niwayama, G. (eds.): Diagnosis of Bone and Joint Disease. Philadelphia, W. B. Saunders Company, 1981, p. 1008.
178. Ansell, B. M.: Chronic arthritis in childhood. Ann. Rheum. Dis. 37:107, 1978.
179. Schaller, J., and Wedgewood, R. J.: Juvenile rheumatoid arthritis: A review. Pediatrics 50:940, 1972.
180. Cassidy, J. T., Brody, G. L., and Martel, W.: Monoarticular juvenile rheumatoid arthritis. J. Pediatr. 70:867, 1967.
181. Kleinman, P., Rivelas, M., Schneider, R., and Kaye, J. J.: Juvenile ankylosing spondylitis. Radiology 125:775, 1977.
182. Resnick, D.: Patterns of peripheral joint disease in ankylosing spondylitis. Radiology 110:523, 1977.
183. Bywaters, E. G. L.: Still's disease in the adult. Ann. Rheum. Dis. 30:121, 1971.
184. Medsger, T. A., Jr., and Christy, W. C.: Carpal arthritis with ankylosis in late onset Still's disease. Arthritis Rheum. 19:232, 1976.
185. Bluestone, R.: Histocompatibility antigens and rheumatic disease. In Current Concepts. Kalamazoo, Michigan, Upjohn Company, 1978, p. 17.
186. Resnick, D., and Niwayama, G.: Ankylosing spondylitis. In Resnick, D., and Niwayama, G. (eds.): Diagnosis of Bone and Joint Disorders. Philadelphia, W. B. Saunders Company, 1981, p. 1040.
187. Wilkinson, M., and Bywaters, E. G. L.: Clinical features and course of ankylosing spondylitis as seen in a follow-up of 222 hospital referred cases. Ann. Rheum. Dis. 17:209, 1958.
188. Rosen, P. S., and Graham, D. C.: Ankylosing (Strumpell-Marie) spondylitis (A clinical review of 128 cases). A.J.R. 5:158, 1962.
189. Berens, D. L.: Roentgen features of ankylosing spondylitis. Clin. Orthop. Rel. Res. 74:20, 1971.
190. Resnick, D., Niwayama, G., and Goergen, T. G.: Comparison of radiographic abnormalities of the sacro-iliac joint in degenerative joint disease and ankylosing spondylitis. Am. J. Roentgenol. 128:189, 1977.
191. Forestier, J., Jacqueline, F., and Rotes-Querol, J.: Ankylosing Spondylitis. Springfield, Ill., Charles C Thomas, 1956.
192. Cawley, M. I. D., Chalmers, T. M., Kellgren, J. H., and Ball, J.: Destructive lesions of vertebral bodies in ankylosing spondylitis. Ann. Rheum. Dis. 31:345, 1972.
193. Dwosh, I. L., Resnick, D., and Becker, M. P.: Hip involvement in ankylosing spondylitis. Arthritis Rheum. 19:683, 1976.
194. Glick, E. N.: A radiological comparison of the hip joint in rheumatoid arthritis and ankylosing spondylitis. Proc. R. Soc. Med. 59:1229, 1976.
195. Resnick, D., Dwosh, I. L., Goergen, T. G., Shapiro, R. F., and D'Ambrosia, R.: Clinical and radiographic "reankylosis" following hip surgery in ankylosing spondylitis. Am. J. Roentgenol. 216:1181, 1976.
196. Rosen, P. S.: A unique shoulder lesion in ankylosing spondylitis: Clinical Comment. J. Rheumatol. 7:109, 1980.
197. Ball, J.: Enthesopathy of rheumatoid and ankylosing spondylitis. Ann. Rheum. Dis. 30:213, 1971.
198. Resnick, D., and Niwayama, G.: Psoriatic arthritis. In Resnick, D., and Niwayama, G. (eds.): Diagnosis of Bone and Joint Disorders. Philadelphia, W. B. Saunders Company, 1981, p. 1103.
199. Wright, V.: Psoriatic arthritis. In Scott, J. T. (ed.): Copeman's Textbook of the Rheumatic Diseases. 5th ed. Edinburgh, Churchill Livingstone, 1978, p. 537.
200. Zaias, N.: Psoriasis of the nail: A clinico-pathological study. Arch. Dermatol. 99:567, 1967.
201. Resnick, D., and Niwayama, G.: On the nature and significance of bony proliferation in "rheumatoid variant" disorders. Am. J. Roentgenol. 129:275, 1977.
202. Forrester, D. M., and Kirkpatrick, R. W.: Periostitis and pseudoperiostitis. Radiology 118:597, 1976.
203. Resnick, D., and Broderick, R. W.: Bony proliferation of terminal phalanges in psoriasis: The "ivory" phalanx. J. Can. Assoc. Radiol. 28:187, 1977.
204. Killebrew, K., Gold, R. H., and Sholkoff, S. D.: Psoriatic spondylitis. Radiology 108:9, 1973.
205. Sundaram, M., and Patton, J. T.: Paravertebral ossification in psoriasis and Reiter's disease. Br. J. Radiol. 48:628, 1975.
206. Kaplan, D., Plotz, C. M., Nathanson, L., and Frank, L.: Cervical spine in psoriasis and psoriatic arthritis. Ann. Rheum. Dis. 23:50, 1964.
207. Resnick, D., and Niwayama, G.: Reiter's syndrome. In Resnick, D., and Niwayama, G. (eds.): Diagnosis of Bone and Joint Disorders, Philadelphia, W. B. Saunders Company, 1981, p. 1130.
208. Sholkoff, S. D., Glickman, M. G., and Steinback, H. L.: Roentgenology of Reiter's syndrome. Radiology 97:497, 1970.
209. Cliff, J. M.: Spinal bony bridging and carditis in Reiter's disease. Ann. Rheum. Dis. 30:171, 1971.
210. Resnick, D., and Niwayama, G.: Enteropathic arthropathies. In Resnick, D., and Niwayama, G. (eds.): Diagnosis of Bone and Joint Disorders. Philadelphia, W. B. Saunders Company, 1981, p. 1149.
211. Jayson, M. I. V., Salmon, P. R., and Harrison, W. J.: Inflammatory bowel disease in ankylosing spondylitis. Gut 11:506, 1970.
212. McEwen, C., Ditata, D., Lingg, C., Porini, A., Good, A., and Rankin, T.: Ankylosing spondylitis and spondylitis accompanying ulcerative colitis, regional enteritis, psoriasis, and Reiter's disease. Arthritis Rheum. 14:291, 1971.
213. Haslock, I.: Enteropathic arthritis. In Scott, J. T. (ed.): Copeman's Textbook of the Rheumatic Diseases. 5th ed. Edinburgh, Churchill Livingstone, 1978, p. 567.
214. Ferguson, R. H.: Enteropathic arthritis. In Hollander, J. L., and McCarty, D. J. (eds.): Arthritis and Allied Conditions. 8th ed. Philadelphia, Lea & Febiger, 1972, p. 846.
215. O'Connell, D. J., and Marx, W. J.: Hand changes in primary biliary cirrhosis. Radiology 129:31, 1978.
216. Clarke, A. K., Galbraith, R. M., Hamilton, E. B. D., and Williams, R.: Rheumatic disorders in primary biliary cirrhosis. Ann. Rheum. Dis. 37:42, 1978.
217. Lucas, P. F., and Owen, T. K.: Subcutaneous fat necrosis, "polyarthritis", and pancreatic disease. Gut 3:146, 1962.
218. Gibson, T. J., Schumacher, H. R., Pascual, E., Brighton, E., and Brighton, C.: Arthropathy, skin and bone lesions in pancreatic disease. J. Rheumatol. 2:7, 1975.
219. Labowitz, R., and Schumacher, H. R., Jr.: Articular manifestations of systemic lupus erythematosus. Ann. Intern. Med. 74:911, 1971.
220. Weissman, B. N., Rappoport, A. S., Sosman, J. L., and Schur, P. H.: Radiographic findings in the hands in patients with systemic lupus erythematosus. Radiology 126:313, 1978.
221. Bleifield, C. J., and Inglis, A. E.: The hand in systemic lupus erythematosus. J. Bone Joint Surg. 56A:1207, 1974.

222. Bywaters, E. G. L.: Jaccoud's syndrome: A sequel to the joint involvement in systemic lupus erythematosus. Clin. Rheum. Dis. 1:125, 1975.
223. Twinning, R. H., Marcus, W. Y., and Garey, J. L.: Tendon rupture in systemic lupus erythematosus. J.A.M.A. 189:377, 1964.
224. Klippel, J. H., Gerber, L. H., Pollack, L., and Decker, J. L.: Avascular necroses in systemic lupus erythematosus: Silent symmetric osteonecrosis. Am. J. Med. 67:83, 1979.
225. Budin, J. A., and Feldman, F.: Soft tissue calcifications in systemic lupus erythematosus. Am. J. Roentgenol. 124:358, 1975.
226. Staples, P. J., Gerding, D. N., Decker, J. L., and Gordon, R. S., Jr.: Incidence of infection in systemic lupus erythematosus. Arthritis Rheum. 17:1, 1971.
227. Goodman, N.: The significance of terminal phalangeal osteosclerosis. Radiology 89:709, 1967.
228. Resnick, D.: Scleroderma (progressive systemic sclerosis). In Resnick, D., and Niwayama, G. (eds.): Diagnosis of Bone and Joint Disorders. Philadelphia, W. B. Saunders Company, 1981, p. 1204.
229. Poznanski, A. K.: The Hand in Radiologic Diagnosis. Philadelphia, W. B. Saunders Company, 1974, p. 531.
230. Thibierge, G., and Weissenbach, R. J.: Concretions calcare souscutanees et sclerodermie. Ann. Dermatol. Syphiligr. 2:129, 1911.
231. Muller, S. A., Brunsting, L. A., and Winkelmann, R. K.: Calcinosis cutis: Its relationship to scleroderma. Arch. Dermatol. 80:15, 1959.
232. Rowell, N. R., and Hopper, F. E.: The periodontal membrane in systemic lupus erythematosus. Br. J. Dermatol. 93(Suppl.):23, 1975.
233. Seifert, M. H., Steigerwald, J. C., and Cliff, M. M.: Bone resorption of the mandible in progressive systemic sclerosis. Arthritis Rheum. 18:507, 1977.
234. Keats, T. E.: Rib erosions in scleroderma. Am. J. Roentgenol. 100:530, 1967.
235. Mezarsos, W. T.: The regional manifestations of scleroderma. Radiology 70:313, 1958.
236. Kemp Harper, R. A., and Jackson, D. C.: Progressive systemic sclerosis. Br. J. Radiol. 38:825, 1965.
237. Haverbush, T. J., Wilde, A. H., Hawk, W. A., Jr., and Scherbel, A. L.: Osteolysis of the ribs and cervical spine in progressive systemic sclerosis (scleroderma): A case report. J. Bone Joint Surg. 56A:637, 1974.
238. Lovell, C. R., and Jayson, M. I. V.: Joint involvement in systemic sclerosis. Scand. J. Rheumatol. 8:154, 1979.
239. Resnick, D.: Dermatomyositis and polymyositis. In Resnick, D., and Niwayama, G. (eds.): Diagnosis of Bone and Joint Disorders. Philadelphia, W. B. Saunders Company, 1981, p. 1230.
240. Schumacher, H. R., Schimmer, B., Gordon, G. V., Bookspan, M. A., Brogadir, S., and Dorwart, B. B.: Articular manifestations of polymyositis and dermatomyositis. Arthritis Rheum. 23:491, 1980.
241. Ozonoff, M. B., and Flynn, F. J., Jr.: Roentgenologic features of dermatomyositis of childhood. Am. J. Roentgenol. 118:206, 1973.
242. Sewell, J. R., Liyanage, B., and Ansell, B. M.: Calcinosis in juvenile dermatomyositis. Skeletal Radiol. 3:137, 1978.
243. Resnick, D.: Polyarteritis nodosa and other vasculitides. In Resnick, D., and Niwayama, G. (eds.): Diagnosis of Bone and Joint Disorders. Philadelphia, W. B. Saunders Company, 1981, p. 1242.
244. Bennet, R. M., and O'Connell, D. J.: The arthritis of mixed connective tissue disease. Ann. Rheum. Dis. 37:397, 1978.
245. Ramos-Niembro, F., Alarcon-Segovia, D., and Hernandez-Ortiz, J.: Articular manifestations of mixed connective tissue disease. Arthritis Rheum. 22:43, 1979.
246. Resnick, D., and Niwayama, G.: Degenerative disease of extraspinal locations. In Resnick, D., and Niwayama, G. (eds.): Diagnosis of Bone and Joint Disorders. Philadelphia, W. B. Saunders Company, 1981, p. 1270.
247. Landells, J. W.: The bone cysts of osteoarthritis. J. Bone Joint Surg. 35B:643, 1953.
248. Ferguson, A. B.: The pathologic changes in degenerative arthritis of the hip and treatment by rotational osteotomy. J. Bone Joint Surg. 46A:1337, 1964.
249. Resnick, D.: Patterns of migration of the femoral head in osteoarthritis of the hip: Roentgenographic-pathologic correlation and comparison with rheumatoid arthritis. Am. J. Roentgenol. 124:62, 1975.
250. Thomas, R. H., Resnick, D., Alazraki, N. P., Daniel, D., and Greenfield, R.: Compartmental evaluation of osteoarthritis of the knee: A comparative study of available diagnostic modalities. Radiology 116:585, 1975.
251. Leach, R. E., Gregg, T., and Siber, F. J.: Weight-bearing radiography in osteoarthritis of the knee. Radiology 97:265, 1970.
252. Mann, R. A., Coughlin, M. J., and DuVries, H. L.: Hallux rigidus: A review of the literature and a method of treatment. Clin. Orthop. Rel. Res. 142:57, 1979.
253. Crain, D. C.: Interphalangeal osteoarthritis characterized by painful inflammatory episodes resulting in deformity of the proximal and distal articulations. J.A.M.A. 175:1049, 1961.
254. McEwen, C.: Osteoarthritis of the fingers with ankylosis. Arthritis Rheum. 11:734, 1968.
255. Resnick, D., and Niwayama, G.: Degenerative disease of the spine. In Resnick, D., and Niwayama, G. (eds.): Diagnosis of Bone and Joint Disorders. Philadelphia, W. B. Saunders Company, 1981, p. 1368.
256. Schmorl, G., and Junghanns, H.: The Human Spine in Health and Disease. 2nd ed. Translated by E. F. Besemann. New York, Grune & Stratton, 1971, p. 138.
257. Knutsson, F.: The vacuum phenomenon in the intervertebral discs. Acta Radiol. 23:173, 1942.
258. Kroker, P.: Sichtbare Rissbildungen in den Bandscheiben der Wirbelsaule. Fortschr. Geb. Roentgenstr. Nuklearmed. 72:1, 1949.
259. Bick, E. M.: Vertebral osteophytosis: Pathologic basis of its roentgenology. Am. J. Roentgenol. 73:979, 1955.
260. Goldberg, R. P., and Carter, B. L.: Absence of thoracic osteophytosis in the area adjacent to the aorta: Computed tomography demonstration. J. Comput. Assist. Tomogr. 2:173, 1978.
261. Hadley, L. A.: Anatomico-roentgenographic studies of the posterior spinal articulations. Am. J. Roentgenol. 86:270, 1961.
262. Resnick, D., and Niwayama, G.: Diffuse idiopathic skeletal hyperostosis (DISH): Ankylosing hyperostosis of Forestier and Rotes-Querol. In Resnick, D., and Niwayama, G. (eds.): Diagnosis of Bone and Joint Disorders. Philadelphia, W. B. Saunders Company, 1981, p. 1416.
263. Forestier, J., and Rotes-Querol, J.: Senile ankylosing hyperostosis of the spine. Ann. Rheum. Dis. 9:321, 1950.
264. Oppenheimer, A.: Calcification and ossification of vertebral ligaments (spondylosis ossificans ligamentosa): Roentgen study of pathogenesis and clinical significance. Radiology 38:160, 1940.
265. Resnick, D., and Niwayama, G.: Radiographic and pathologic features of spinal involvement in diffuse idiopathic skeletal hyperostosis (DISH). Radiology 119:559, 1976.
266. Bauer, F.: Dysphagia due to cervical spondylosis. J. Laryngol. Otol. 67:615, 1953.
267. Resnick, D., Guerra, J., Jr., Robinson, C. A., and Vint, V. C.: Association of diffuse idiopathic skeletal hyperostosis (DISH) and calcification and ossification of the posterior longitudinal ligament. Am. J. Roentgenol. 131:1049, 1978.
268. Kohler, H., Uehlinger, E., Kutzner, J., and West, T. B.: Sternocostoclavicular hyperostosis: Painful swelling of the sternum, clavicles, and upper ribs. Ann. Intern. Med. 87:192, 1977.
269. Resnick, D., Shaul, S. R., and Robins, J. M.: Diffuse idiopathic skeletal hyperostosis (DISH): Forestier's disease with extraspinal manifestations. Radiology 115:513, 1975.
270. Resnick, D.: Neuroarthropathy. In Resnick, D., and Niwayama, G. (eds.): Diagnosis of Bone and Joint Disorders. Philadelphia, W. B. Saunders Company, 1981, p. 2422.
271. Key, J. A.: Clinical observations on tabetic arthropathies (Charcot joints). Am. J. Syph. 14:429, 1932.
272. Pomeranz, M. M., and Rothberg, A. S.: A review of 58 cases of tabetic arthropathy. Am. J. Syph. 25:103, 1941.
273. Jaffe, H. L.: Metabolic, Degenerative and Inflammatory Diseases of Bones and Joints. Philadelphia, Lea & Febiger, 1972, p. 847.
274. Clouse, M. E., Gramm, H. F., Legg, M., and Flood, T.: Diabetic osteoarthropathy: Clinical and roentgenographic observations in 90 cases. Am. J. Roentgenol. 121:22, 1974.
275. Gray, R. G., and Gottlieb, N. L.: Rheumatic disorders associated with diabetes mellitus: Literature review. Semin. Arthritis Rheum. 6:19, 1976.
276. Giesecke, S. B., Dalinka, M. K., and Kyle, G. C.: Lisfranc's fracture-dislocation: A manifestation of peripheral neuropathy. Am. J. Roentgenol. 131:139, 1978.
277. Thornhill, H. L., Richter, R. W., Shelton, M. L., and Johnson, C. A.: Neuropathic arthropathy (Charcot forefeet) in alcoholics. Orthop. Clin. North Am. 4:7, 1973.
278. Peitzman, S. J., Miller, J. L., Ortega, L., Schumacher, H. R., and Fernandez, P. C.: Charcot arthropathy secondary to amyloid neuropathy. J.A.M.A. 235:1345, 1976.
279. Resnick, D., and Niwayama, G.: Crystal-induced and related diseases. In Resnick, D., and Niwayama, G. (eds.): Diagnosis of Bone and Joint Disorders. Philadelphia, W. B. Saunders Company, 1981, p. 1463.
280. Talbott, J. H.: Gout. 3rd ed. New York, Grune & Stratton, 1967.
281. Vyhanek, L., Lavicka, J., and Blahos, J.: Roentgenological findings in gout. Radiol. Clin. North Am. 28:256, 1960.
282. Good, A. E., and Rapp, R.: Bony ankylosis: A rare manifestation of gout. J. Rheumatol. 5:335, 1978.
283. Kawenoki-Minc, E., Eyman, E., Leo, W., and Werynska-Przybylska, J.: Zwyrodnienie stawow i kregoslupa u chorych na dne. Analiza 262 przypadkowdny. Reumatoligia 12:267, 1974.
284. von Hoyningen-Huene, C. B. J.: Gout and glycogen storage disease in preadolescent brothers. Arch. Intern. Med. 118:471, 1966.
285. Riley, J. D.: Gout and cerebral palsy in a three-year-old boy. Arch. Dis. Child. 35:293, 1960.
286. Gutman, A. B.: Primary and secondary gout. Ann. Intern. Med. 39:1062, 1953.
287. Grahme, R., Sutor, D. J., and Mitchener, M. B.: Crystal deposition in hyperparathyroidism. Ann. Rheum. Dis. 30:597, 1971.
288. Dmartini, F. E.: Hyperuricemia induced by drugs. Arthritis Rheum. 8:823, 1965.

289. Resnick, D., Niwayama, G., Goergen, T. G., Utsinger, P. D., Shapiro, R. F., Hasselwood, D. H., and Wiesner, K. B.: Clinical, radiographic and pathologic abnormalities in calcium pyrophosphate dihydrate deposition disease (CPPD): Pseudogout. Radiology 122:1, 1977.

290. Vigario, D. G., and Keats, T. E.: Localization of calcific deposits in the shoulder. Am. J. Roentgenol. 108:806, 1970.

291. Schumacher, H. R., Jr.: Hemochromatosis and arthritis. Arthritis Rheum. 7:41, 1964.

292. Hamilton, E., Williams, R., Barlow, K. A., and Smith, P. M.: The arthropathy of hemochromatosis. Q. J. Med. 37:171, 1968.

293. Atkins, C. J., McIvor, J., Smith, P. M., Hamilton, E., and Williams, R.: Chondrocalcinosis and arthropathy: Studies in haemochromatosis and in idiopathic chondrocalcinosis. Q. J. Med. 39:71, 1970.

294. Seze, S. de, Solnica, J., Mitrovic, D., Miravet, L., and Dorfmann, H.: Joint and bone disorders and hypoparathyroidism in hemochromatosis. Semin. Arthritis Rheum. 2:71, 1972.

295. Hirsch, J. H., Killien, C., and Troupin, R. H.: The arthropathy of hemochromatosis. Radiology 118:591, 1976.

296. Feller, E. R., and Schumacher, H. R.: Osteoarticular changes in Wilson's disease. Arthritis Rheum. 15:259, 1972.

297. Finby, N., and Bearn, A. G.: Roentgenographic abnormalities of the skeletal system in Wilson's disease (hepatolenticular degeneration). Am. J. Roentgenol. 79:603, 1958.

298. Cervenansky, J., Sitaj, S., and Urbanek, T.: Alkaptonuria and ochronosis. J. Bone Joint Surg. 41A:1169, 1959.

299. Mueller, M. N., Sorenson, L. B., Strandjord, N., and Kappas, A.: Alkaptonuria and ochronotic arthropathy. Med. Clin. North Am. 49:101, 1965.

300. Martin, W. J., Underahl, L. O., Mathieson, D. R., and Pugh, D. G.: Alkaptonuria: Report of 12 cases. Ann. Intern. Med. 42:1052, 1955.

301. Resnick, D., and Niwayama, G.: Osteomyelitis, septic arthritis, and soft tissue infection: the mechanisms and situations. In Resnick, D., and Niwayama, G. (eds.): Diagnosis of Bone and Joint Disorders. Philadelphia, W. B. Saunders Company, 1981, p. 2042.

302. Chuinard, R. G., and D'Ambrosia, R.: Human bite infections of the hand. J. Bone Joint Surg. 59A:416, 1977.

303. Patterson, F. P., and Brown, C. S.: Complications of total hip replacement arthroplasty. Orthop. Clin. North Am. 4:503, 1973.

304. Franck, W. A., Bress, N. M., Singer, F. R., and Krane, S. M.: Rheumatic manifestation of Paget's disease of bone. Am. J. Med. 56:592, 1974.

305. McCarty, D. J., Jr.: Pseudogout: articular chondrocalcinsis. In Hollander, J. L., and McCarty, D. J., Jr. (eds.): Arthritis and Related Disorders. 8th ed. Philadelphia, Lea & Febiger, 1972, p. 410.

306. Steinbach, H. L., and Russell, W.: Measurements of the heel pad as an aid to diagnosis of acromegaly. Radiology 82:418, 1964.

307. Lang, E. K., and Bessler, W. T.: The roentgenologic features of acromegaly. Am. J. Roentgenol. 86:321, 1961.

308. Watson, R. J., Burko, H., Megas, H., and Robinson, M.: Hand-foot syndrome in sickle cell disease in young children. Pediatrics 31:975, 1963.

309. Grossman, R. E., and Hensley, G. T.: Bone lesions in primary amyloidosis. Am. J. Roentgenol. 101:872, 1967.

310. Weinfield, A., Stern, M. H., and Marx, L. H.: Amyloid lesions of bone. Am. J. Roentgenol. 108:799, 1970.

311. Pettersson, H., Ahlberg, A., and Nilsson, I. M.: A radiologic classification of hemophilic arthropathy. Clin. Orthop. Rel. Res. 149:153, 1980.

312. Resnick, D.: Tumors and tumor-like lesions in or about joints. In Resnick, D., and Niwayama, G. (eds.): Diagnosis of Bone and Joint Disorders. Philadelphia, W. B. Saunders Company, 1981, p. 2638.

313. Prager, R. J., and Mall, J. C.: Arthrographic diagnosis of synovial chondromatosis. Am. J. Roentgenol. 127:344, 1976.

314. Breimer, C. W., and Freiberger, R. H.: Bone lesions associated with villonodular synovitis. Am. J. Roentgenol. 79:618, 1958.

Chapter 38

Robert W. Metcalf*

Arthroscopy

INTRODUCTION

Arthroscopy is an accurate, reliable method for atraumatically examining the interior structures of joints. It can be performed with the patient under either general or local anesthesia, usually in an out-patient operating room environment, utilizing a rigid telescope (about the size and diameter of an ordinary pencil) that has remarkable optic capabilities and fiberoptic illumination. The arthroscope is attached to a small solid-state television camera that transmits a magnified image to a monitor in the operating room, where the arthroscopist and assistants can view the procedure together. A videotape record of the operation allows patient instruction, clinical follow-up studies, and physician education.

CHANGE FROM DIAGNOSTIC TO SURGICAL EMPHASIS

From 1918, when Takagi[1] performed the first diagnostic knee-joint exploration using a rudimentary cystoscope, to the mid-1970s, arthroscopy was, with few exceptions, considered to be primarily a diagnostic technique. In fact, over that 60-year period, arthroscopy received scant attention from those interested in joint problems (i.e., rheumatologists and orthopedic surgeons) because of the common view that helpful information was seldom gained. Also, the technique had inherent problems, such as breakage inside a joint of the tungsten bulb used for illumination. Nonetheless, Watanabe's color atlas of arthroscopy, first published in 1957,[2] is still a classic demonstration of the accuracy and clarity of examination obtainable in virtually every joint in the body.

From 1974 to the present, there has been a dramatic reversal of interest in the arthroscope[3] and its capabilities stimulated by

1. Development of surgical techniques in which operations have been converted from "open" arthrotomy to "closed" percutaneous methods.[4–7]
2. Technologic improvements, such as fiberoptic illumination, improved optics, and a myriad of instruments specifically designed for surgical intervention in specific joints.[8]
3. Patient demand for these less invasive procedures, concurrent with the growth of "oscopies" in other specialties.
4. Potential cost savings, including outpatient surgery, reduced rehabilitation expense, and less time lost from work and sports.[9]

Arthroscopy has thus taken a prominent place among the operative skills practiced by a majority of orthopedic surgeons, even to the point of fostering organizations devoted to the technique, such as the Arthroscopy Association of North America (AANA) and the International Arthroscopy Association (IAA). A quarterly journal, *Arthroscopy*, is sponsored by these organizations, as well as numerous postgraduate courses, motor-skills labs, and instructional videotape series.

LEARNING ARTHROSCOPY

In common with endoscopy in other parts of the body, the examination of joints with an arthroscope can be difficult to learn. The process requires patience and persistence and is largely self-taught.[10] There are postgraduate seminars, including hands-on motor skills courses, that can provide high-quality instruction in both basic and advanced techniques, but the best method of teaching is still one-to-one tutelage with an experienced arthroscopist through residency and fellowship programs.

Orthopedic surgeons regard arthroscopy as a surgical skill entirely different from traditional open surgery. It is a form of microsurgery where tiny instruments are manipulated within the narrow confines of a joint under fiberoptic illumination with magnification that can create significant problems of interpretation. However, there is a systematic order in the development of arthroscopic competence. Such a graduated step-by-step progression in this education process helps the trainee build toward a reliable method for examining a particular joint. In fact, attempts to learn these new endoscopic procedures without recognizing the importance of a patient, step-by-step approach can produce so much frustration that some eventually abandon the technique.

The following skills are enumerated in a progressive order to give a brief overview of what is involved in learning basic arthroscopy.

Use of Basic Portals. For each joint, there are now established standard percutaneous portals of entry for the arthroscope through which the majority

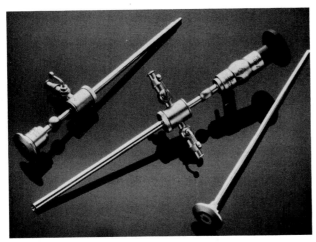

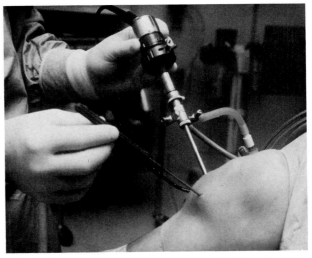

Figure 38–1. Standard 4.5-mm diameter arthroscope inserted into irrigation cannula (center) with blunt obturator (left) and sharp trochar (right) used initially in various percutaneous entries into the knee, shoulder, ankle, and hip joints. Smaller diameter (1.9 mm) arthroscopes are used for elbow, wrist, and subtalar and temporomandibular joints.

Figure 38–2. Solid-state television camera attached to arthroscope. Camera is sterilized and transmits magnified image of interior of joint to monitor at head of operating table.

of the joint interior can be visualized. Obviously, the first step is to know the anatomy of the particular joint and the relationship of these entry incisions to its interior. After years of experience, arthroscopists have learned that even slight variance from the ideal sites of joint entry can produce problems of poor visualization and restricted maneuverability.

Managing Joint Distention and Irrigation. Arthroscopy requires a constant flow of irrigation solution, such as Ringer's lactate, to distend and constantly clear the joint. The solution flows by gravity through the sleeve of the arthroscope and exits from a separate cannula in another part of the joint. (Some arthroscopists prefer the opposite set-up, with flow going through a cannula and exiting around the arthroscope.) Infusion pumps are also used and are especially helpful in the shoulder. Learning to manage this basic part of arthroscopy examination is critical to seeing clearly.

Use of a Television System. Today, nearly all arthroscopy is done using a rigid arthroscope, 4 to 5 mm in diameter, that has a small, sterilizable solid-state television camera that is either attached or incorporated into the optics of the scope itself (Figs. 38–1 and 38–2). The arthroscopist manipulates the scope-camera at the joint while looking at the image of the interior of the joint magnified on a television monitor at the head or side of the operating table. This requires a unique type of hand-eye coordination that can be developed only with experience. Once learned, the use of video arthroscopy is actually easier than looking with eye to arthroscope in a hunched-over position that was once required of the arthroscopist. Now the surgeon and assistants all can stand or sit comfortably while viewing the procedure together on the television monitor, which has made arthroscopic surgery much more like traditional open surgery with respect to operating team participation (Fig. 38–3).

Ability to Utilize Multiple Portals. In order to see all parts of a joint and also to insert probes and surgical instruments, multiple entry portals are needed. Once the basic entry portals are mastered, the trainee is next introduced to the principle of triangulation, in which he or she learns to position the viewing arthroscope on one side of the joint and bring in another instrument from an opposite site. This type of stereoscopic skill is at the core of proficient arthroscopic technique and eventually becomes so automatic that an instrument is brought to a desired location within the joint without the struggle often encountered at first.

Use of a Probe. During diagnostic examination, a rigid probe with a 4-mm, right-angled blunt tip is used to manipulate normal and pathologic anatomy,

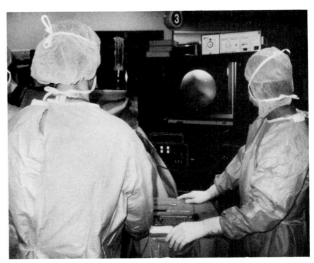

Figure 38–3. Surgeon and assistants viewing arthroscopic image on television monitor. Most arthroscopists now use this method of visualization rather than looking directly through the eyepiece of the arthroscope.

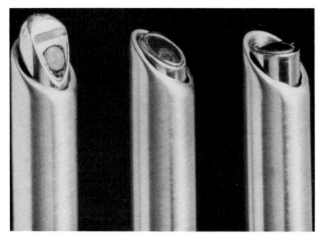

Figure 38–4. Series of 4.5-mm diameter arthroscopes showing varying tip angles (left, 70 degrees; middle, 30 degrees; right, 5 degrees) useful in looking either straight ahead or around condyles in a joint. Each arthroscope is inside a slightly larger diameter protective cannula where irrigation fluid flows to continually clear the lens.

thus providing an essential additional element to the evaluation. Diagnostic accuracy is enhanced by appreciating the texture, tension, mobility, or compressibility of a particular tissue. Because the arthroscopic view is monocular, depth-perception is difficult, and the ability to palpate within the joint enhances the examiner's sense of dimension and size relationships. Probing is also a precursor to using surgical tools. The blunt tip does not scratch the articular surfaces and is therefore safe in practicing triangulation and positioning of an instrument within the joint. Every routine diagnostic arthroscopy should include the use of a probe even though an additional portal is needed.

Use of a Variety of Arthroscopes. The standard viewing arthroscope, which is 4 or 5 mm in diameter and has a viewing angle of 30 degrees, is used in perhaps 80 per cent of arthroscopic work (see Fig. 38–1). It is large enough to give a wide field of vision (110 degrees), and the slight inclination of view is just enough to see "around corners" when the scope is rotated but not so much as to create confusion for the viewer. However, there are other types of arthroscopes that are useful for special situations, and proficiency with these variations is the next important skill (Fig. 38–4). For example, an arthroscope with a tip angle of 70 degrees is useful where joint recesses are harder to reach, such as in the posterior compartments of the knee joint. In addition, there are times when an arthroscope that is 4 mm in diameter is too large, and a smaller diameter is needed, even down to 1.8 mm. Obviously, proper use of these specialized scopes requires additional experience. The 70-degree (or even, rarely, a 120-degree) angulation of view can be disorienting. The small-diameter scopes have a very limited angle of view and reduced illumination.

Use of Hand-Operated Instruments. There is now available a wide variety of hand-operated (as opposed to motorized) equipment used primarily for surgical techniques. Proper utilization of these scissors, knives, and forceps involves an additional level of dexterity and experience. Care must be taken to avoid scuffing the articular surfaces of the joint or cutting into normal adjacent structures, such as ligaments and neurovascular bundles. Eventually the arthroscopist uses many specialized tools, such as rasps, osteotomes, grasping forceps, suturing devices, punches, and the like.

Use of Motorized Equipment. These instruments can morselize either soft or hard tissues within a joint and suction the pieces away. Their use requires another type of dexterity, because they are even more capable of damaging normal structures. Some beginning arthroscopists believe that these motorized instruments can do most of the operative work in a joint, thereby providing a simple short cut to developing arthroscopic skills (Fig. 38–5). Such a notion is incorrect. The development of the finely controlled motions used in manipulating manual instruments is far more important, because such manipulation gives more tactile feedback. While motorized devices are an important adjunct to manual instruments, they will never replace the need for the type of delicate manual dexterity required for most arthroscopic procedures.

DIAGNOSTIC ARTHROSCOPY

Indications. Although there are specific indications for diagnostic arthroscopy in each joint,[11, 12] these can also be categorized generally. Before listing these indications, it should be emphasized that arthroscopy should not be used indiscriminately. Unfortunately, as is the case with most new techniques, there has been a tendency on the part of a few

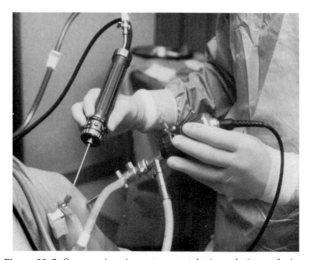

Figure 38–5. Surgeon is using a two-portal triangulation technique in the anterior compartments of the knee, guiding a motorized cutter with one hand while positioning the small television camera and arthroscope with the other.

practitioners to overuse arthroscopy and disregard reasonable indications. Such practice is to be condemned. The fact that arthroscopy is a minimally invasive procedure and is relatively painless and easy for the patient should never be an indication alone for its use. Such abuse of indications only detracts from the cost savings and many other advantages that arthroscopy affords.

The goal of diagnostic arthroscopy is both to establish an accurate diagnosis and to prevent unnecessary surgery. McGinty and Freedman[13] demonstrated that one third of planned knee arthrotomies were canceled on the basis of arthroscopic findings.

There are five basic general indications for diagnostic arthroscopy:

1. When a thorough history, physical examination, and suitable noninvasive and radiographic studies[14, 15] have failed to establish a diagnosis needed for appropriate treatment.
2. When treatment of a specific joint problem has failed and there is a need for additional information that radiographic or other studies cannot provide.
3. When specific additional diagnostic information can be obtained in a less traumatic way (i.e., biopsy).
4. To investigate the reasons for the failure (or success) of a previous surgical procedure where it is desirous to avoid trauma to the joint.[16]
5. Immediately prior to any arthroscopic surgical procedure, as a means of confirming the suspected pathologic condition and indications for surgery (or lack thereof).

With present videotaping capabilities, the presence or absence of joint pathology can be recorded and documented in a dynamic way during diagnostic arthroscopy and saved for future reference. Such video recordings are especially helpful in medicolegal and workers' compensation cases, often resolving controversies.[17]

Direct vision of a joint through an arthroscope is not entirely free of error, being dependent on the interpretive skill and thoroughness of the examiner, but its accuracy is greater than that of any other diagnostic technique, including magnetic resonance imaging.[18, 19]

Contraindications. Any potentially infected skin lesion in the areas where the arthroscope will be introduced requires that the procedure be delayed until the lesion has been treated. Examples include abrasions, small furuncles or pustules, acne vulgaris, and rashes; these are usually temporary. Joint sepsis was once thought to preclude arthroscopy, but it is now an indication, allowing biopsy for tissue culture, joint lavage, and instillation of closed suction irrigation of antibiotics. Ankylosis was also previously considered a contraindication, but it is now possible to use the arthroscope for lysis of adhesions. Bleeding disorders can be controlled during the arthroscopy,

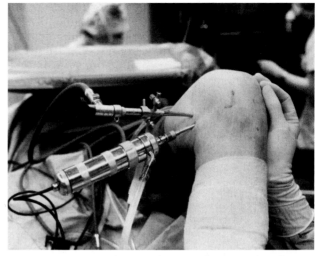

Figure 38–6. Motorized synovial resector being used in the posteromedial compartment of the left knee during arthroscopic synovectomy. Double puncture technique allows arthroscope to view the synovium in an area difficult to reach with an arthrotomy.

and hemophiliac synovitis may now be excised with arthroscopy rather than arthrotomy.

Advantages. Diagnostic and operative arthroscopy would not have flourished so dramatically over the past 10 years were there not significant advantages to both physicians and patients. These benefits include minimal disruption of the normal tissues surrounding joints, more accurate diagnosis, the unique ability to observe joint mechanics, and improved planning of operative approaches whether by endoscopy or by arthrotomy. Fewer postoperative problems occur. Joint and muscle strength are regained more quickly; and complications,[20] such as thrombophlebitis and fibrous ankylosis, can be reduced.

Arthroscopy also enables the surgeon to perform certain operations that previously were difficult even with an arthrotomy. Examples include repair of meniscal tears at the posterior roots of the menisci, lysis of adhesions in the temporomandibular joint and distal radioulnar carpal complex, and synovectomy in relatively inaccessible regions, such as the submeniscal and posterior compartments of the knee (Fig. 38–6).

Disadvantages. As already mentioned, arthroscopy requires time, patience, and much experience to learn and can be difficult to perform. Arthroscopic tools are expensive and fragile. Equipping an arthroscopy unit costs upwards of $60,000, including television systems, motorized equipment, arthroscopes, and cutting forceps, knives, scissors, and probes. Upkeep and replacement costs can also be high. It is estimated that the average cost of arthroscopy equipment is about $150 per case. For the patient, these overall costs are more than offset by the decreases in hospitalization, physical therapy, and time lost from employment. Yet, the cost of equipment and postgraduate education is significant to the individual physician contemplating arthroscopic practice.

Anesthesia. Local, regional, and general anesthesia all have been utilized for arthroscopy. General anesthesia is most commonly used because muscles relax, and joints can be stressed open for better viewing. Shoulder arthroscopy almost always requires a general anesthetic because of the difficulty in obtaining an effective regional block or infiltration of local anesthetics into a joint that is more deeply surrounded by muscle and fascial layers.

Spinal anesthesia is sometimes used in knee arthroscopy but is not favored by most patients. It is otherwise a satisfactory method, providing good muscle relaxation without tourniquet discomfort.

Local anesthetics[21] can be used by infiltrating skin portals with one per cent lidocaine (Xylocaine) with epinephrine and by injecting 10 ml of 0.5 per cent bupivacaine (Marcaine) without epinephrine intra-articularly. This technique is adequate for simpler procedures, such as diagnostic arthroscopy, synovial biopsy, resection of a synovial plica or adhesion, partial meniscectomy, and limited débridement. The main disadvantage of local anesthesia is the lack of muscle relaxation, which may preclude adequate joint opening and visibility. In addition, patients may experience discomfort and become restless, especially if a tourniquet has to be used, such as in knee, ankle, and elbow arthroscopy.

TECHNIQUE OF DIAGNOSTIC KNEE ARTHROSCOPY

Arthroscopy is done in the operating room of an out-patient surgery center under strict sterile technique. With the patient supine on the operating table, an anesthetic is administered, and a tourniquet is placed around the upper thigh for inflation as needed. A thigh-holding device is used to give a fulcrum for stressing open the knee joint in either the varus or the valgus direction. The end of the table is flexed to 90 degrees, allowing the knee to flex. The skin from midthigh distally is prepared and draped as for any limb procedure. Two assistants are ideal, one to handle instruments and the other to help hold and maneuver the limb.

The arthroscope is never forced about the joint or used to pry against any tissue. Instruments used in the joint are always kept in view. Blind cutting can cause articular damage or even laceration of adjacent nerves or vessels. Also, failure to follow a systematic plan of examination is often the reason for a missed diagnosis.

The 4.5 mm–diameter arthroscope is inserted anterolaterally through a small skin incision, using a trocar first to pierce the fascial layers and then an obturator to enter the synovial cavity and avoid scoring the articular cartilage. This anterolateral portal is just lateral to the patellar tendon at a level 1.5 cm above the anterior edge of the tibia. Ringer's lactate is used as a continuous irrigation fluid, entering the joint through the sleeve of the arthroscope and exiting through a cannula that has been inserted into the suprapatellar pouch. When searching for a loose body, the direction of flow is reversed. The joint is examined systematically, beginning first with the suprapatellar pouch. The synovium is scanned with the knee in extension. Normal synovium is usually thin, flat, and somewhat transparent, with little vascularity. Delicate villi may be seen superiorly or adjacent to patellar borders. A few transverse folds may appear as ridges over the femur. Occasionally, there is a more prominent crescent-shaped fold extending transversely from the superior roof (the suprapatellar plica).

The patella is examined next. Its articular surfaces should be smooth, glistening, and firm to palpation with a probe. As the knee is flexed, tracking in the femoral groove can be observed for proper central alignment; to give a better perspective of this gliding action, the arthroscope is often moved to a lateral suprapatellar portal. A small fringe of synovium rings the patella, sometimes with a fold.

The 30-degree arthroscope scans medially, then laterally to view the paracondylar gutters. Loose bodies may lie at the base of these gutters, especially laterally where joint debris often collects in a series of small transverse folds. A medial plica, running longitudinally along the medial synovial wall to insert into the infrapatellar fat pad, is seen in about 50 per cent of knees.[22] This fold is normally less than 5 mm wide; however, in pathologic states, it can be up to 2 cm wide, projecting into the patellofemoral interface or bowstringing across the femoral condyle during flexion.

With the knee extended, the femoral condyles and patellofemoral groove are scanned for any articular disruption. Normal articular cartilage is white, glistening, compressible yet resilient, and remarkably smooth. Any irregularities can be readily observed with the tangential magnified view provided by the arthroscope. In older patients, the hyaline cartilage looks somewhat granular and takes on a yellowish, less shiny character. It often loses its ability to rebound quickly from pressure deformation.

Next, the arthroscope is rotated inferiorly along the lateral wall of the femur to view the edge of the posterior horn of the lateral meniscus. The popliteal tendon can be seen as it obliquely passes through a synovium-lined hiatus. Here the meniscus lacks an attachment to the capsule, and this cleft permits a mobility of the posterior horn that is sometimes confused with a tear. Loose bodies may be hidden in this synovial sheath.

With the knee slightly flexed and a varus internal rotational stress applied to the tibia, the lateral compartment of the joint can be examined. The articular cartilage of the tibial plateau is usually the first site of fibrillation or fissuring as individuals age. As the knee is flexed and extended, the convexity of the femoral condyle is studied, and the meniscal rim is probed for tears. There is a small recess palpable underneath the posterior horn, which is formed by the slightly offset attachment of the meniscotibial ligament. This normal cleft can be confused with a tear and sometimes requires a direct posteromedial approach for clarification.

The knee is flexed to about 60 degrees for the arthroscope's entry into the intercondylar notch. The ligamentum mucosa and infrapatellar fat pad must often be pulled aside with a probe to view the anterior cruciate ligament, whose synovial covering is rich with a plexus of vessels. The bands of the ligament traverse at an angle from anteromedial to posterolateral with a slight spiral configuration, often in two bundles. Ligament tension can be palpated while performing an anterior drawer test—a forward pull on the tibia with the knee at 90 degrees of flexion. Sometimes the anterior cruciate ligament can be pulled aside to permit a clear view of the posterior cruciate ligament, but the latter is better viewed from a direct posteromedial portal.

The knee is brought to a position of 20 degrees of flexion, and a valgus external rotation stress is applied to the tibia by outward rotation of the foot. Care must be taken to avoid excessive stress lest the medial collateral ligament tear. Except for the posterior capsular corner, the entire medial meniscus can usually be seen from the anterior approaches. A torn mobile flap may have rolled posteriorly, where it is easily missed. However, a 70-degree arthroscope is often angled across the intercondylar notch into the posterior compartments for direct vision. This eliminates blind spots and aids in finding tears of the meniscus or loose fragments. (The posterior compartments are especially difficult to see with an arthrotomy.)

The arthroscopic examination is completed by scanning the medial femoral condyle for any articular defects. Occasionally, a direct posteromedial puncture is made to evaluate the meniscocapsular junction or the posterior cruciate ligament. Other approaches include a transpatellar tendon central approach and suprapatellar and lateral patellar entry. In fact, any point around the anterior joint line may be used as an entry portal if necessary. Postoperative morbidity is not increased by this multiple puncture method.

At the conclusion of the diagnostic inspection, any required surgery is completed. The joint is thoroughly irrigated and vacuumed with a motorized suction-cutting instrument. Then the tiny incisions are closed with either a single stitch or an adhesive strip. An elastic bandage is applied for mild compression. If the tourniquet has been inflated, it is released prior to the final irrigation and skin closure.

DIAGNOSTIC EXAMINATIONS IN OTHER JOINTS

Shoulder. For diagnostic arthroscopy, the patient is turned to the side opposite the involved shoulder.[23] The limb is placed in a special traction-abduction support that gently distracts the glenohu-

meral joint. Anterior,[24] superior, and posterior approaches all may be used, but commonly the first insertion is posterior, just inferior to the acromion process.[25] In order, the examination focuses on biceps tendon, humeral head and glenoid, glenoid labrum, glenohumeral ligaments, subscapular tendon and recess, rotator cuff attachments, and superior recess.[26, 27] The subacromial bursa can also be entered through a separate portal to view the bursa, rotator cuff, coracoacromial ligament, and undersurface of the acromion process.

In addition to diagnostic examination, operative procedures include removal of loose bodies, débridement of labral tears or a ruptured long head of the biceps, acromioplasty for impingement syndromes, and stapling or suturing of lax capsular ligaments in instability problems. Little can be done for degenerative arthritis, but synovectomy may be of benefit in the rheumatoid shoulder. Lavage and débridement give temporary relief. Shoulder arthroscopy is now a major procedure, and its use has expanded dramatically.

Elbow. This small joint is less commonly examined, but there are a few diagnostic and surgical problems that can be solved. The removal of loose bodies is the most common operative procedure. However, fibrous adhesion lysis, resection of osteophytes, synovectomy, and reattachment of osteochondritis dissecans fragments have been reported. The joint can be entered medially, laterally, and at the tip of the olecranon. The elbow is usually in a flexed position, suspended by the hand at the side of the supine anesthetized patient. A tourniquet is routinely used for hemostasis. Poehling and associates[28] have reported a new method of elbow arthroscopy in which the patient lies prone, and the elbow is flexed over the end of an arm board at the side of the operating table. They claim that this position allows easier access to the joint, especially posteriorly.

Wrist. Regional anesthesia is preferred inasmuch as infiltration of a local anesthetic can obscure the small spaces of the wrist. This joint is entered through dorsal portals using a small-diameter (1.9-mm) arthroscope.[29] Diagnosis of a torn triradiate cartilage, resection of loose bodies, débridement of torn capsular ligaments, partial synovectomy, and carpal tunnel release[30] are currently performed arthroscopically. These techniques are being used with increasing frequency, especially by hand surgeons.

Hip. The hip is difficult to examine because it is surrounded by large muscles, tendon insertions, and a thick, tough capsule and has a deep acetabular socket, all of which combine to create problems in distracting the femur sufficiently to allow space for visualization. The procedure is done with the patient under general anesthesia on a fracture table so that controlled traction can be applied to the lower limb. Glick and colleagues[31] have recently developed a special frame and distraction device to make the procedure easier. Baseline observations have been

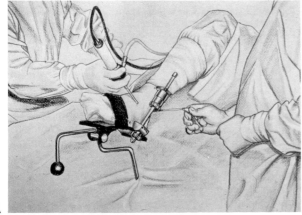

A

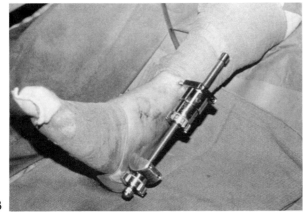

B

Figure 38–7. *A* and *B*, Arthroscopic examination of the ankle is facilitated by the use of a mechanical distracting device to create a space between the talus and the tibial plafond. (Courtesy of James F. Guhl, M.D.)

made of pathologic changes in degenerative and rheumatoid arthritis, aseptic necrosis, and osteochondromatosis, especially in children. Arthroscopic removal of loose bodies can be done, and other procedures are being developed by a few surgeons, but for now, hip arthroscopy is not commonly done.

Ankle. With distraction, most of this joint can be clearly visualized (Fig. 38–7). However, viewing the extreme posterior portion of the joint remains difficult. Guhl[32] has developed a mechanical distraction device utilizing a pin in the tibia and another in the calcaneus; it gives better distraction to the joint but also introduces the potential for pin track infections to an otherwise uncomplicated procedure. Osteochondritis dissecans of the talus, loose bodies, synovitis,[33] and chondral fractures have been managed with arthroscopic technique.

Postoperative Care. After diagnostic arthroscopy, isometric exercises and gentle active range of motion are begun immediately. Because the percutaneous portals do not disrupt normal muscle function, the extremity can be returned to full function rapidly. Normal activities, including sports, are permitted when the joint shows no effusion, pain is absent, and there is full range of motion and strength. Occasionally, the help of a physical thera-

pist is needed to reach these goals. Postoperative regimens will vary if operative arthroscopy is performed; in general, rehabilitation after any arthroscopic procedure is much faster and easier than after arthrotomy.[34]

Complications. Although uncommon, complications can occur. Small[35] has reported an overall complication rate of 1.60 percent in more than 10,000 arthroscopic surgical procedures studied prospectively among experienced arthroscopists. As low as this rate is, it is still very important to inform the patient of possible complications, such as thrombophlebitis, infections, neurovascular damage, loss of knee motion, broken instruments within the joint, tourniquet damage to thigh muscles, excessive bleeding requiring further operative procedures, and anesthetic complications including death. Arthroscopy is an invasive procedure, and as in any operation, such risks are inherent and must be acknowledged by both the patient and the physician. Nevertheless, when done with reasonable care, arthroscopy is safe and effective.

Pathologic Findings in Arthritis. Rheumatoid synovial villi are larger than normal, club shaped, pale, edematous, and numerous; in the knee they proliferate in the suprapatellar roof, along the edges of the femoral condyles, beneath the menisci, and in the intercondylar notch (Fig. 38–8). Early, the creeping pannus can be pulled from articular edges with a probe, demonstrating the erosion of underlying hyaline cartilage. Later stages may show extensive fibrillation, ulcers, or craters, often in an irregular pattern over the femoral condyles and patellofemoral groove. The joint often contains thick, yellowish synovial fluid with numerous, small, opaque white fragments, so-called rice bodies.

Osteoarthritic synovium is less fibrillated and not nearly as proliferative as that seen in rheumatoid

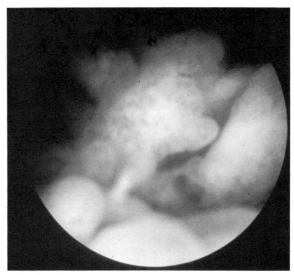

Figure 38–8. Typical arthroscopic appearance of rheumatoid synovium in the suprapatellar pouch of the knee. The villi are hypertrophied and club shaped.

arthritis. Fronds may be hyperemic or yellowish. Free-floating debris is also seen but is finer and more irregular in size.[36] Articular changes include fibrillation, fissuring, and loss of normal thickness. The patella, central femoral condyles, and tibial plateaus are common sites of wear. There may be craters revealing bare bone, and the articular edges of the joint may show osteophytic spurring, especially in the knee, shoulder, and ankle. The glenoid labrum or knee menisci are often softened and shaggy, with frank tears and mobile fragments protruding and catching in the joint and producing erosion of articular cartilage.

Pigmented villonodular synovitis is extremely prolific and dense, having a reddish-brown or even orangish color. Its nodular character is unique.[37] Articular erosion and meniscal pathology are less common but do occur. Hemophiliac arthropathy can show extensive articular destruction and a florid, hemosiderin-stained synovium that proliferates into every recess of the joint. The synovium is friable on probing and easily peels away from subsynovial layers. In later stages, one sees osteophytic spurring, joint flattening, and subchondral cysts that visibly open into the joint. Gouty arthritis can erode the articular edges in much the same way as does rheumatoid arthritis. Crystalline deposits in synovium are seen in both gout and pseudogout, but those in the latter more often coat otherwise normal-appearing articular cartilage. Calcium pyrophosphate dehydrate deposits can completely cover the menisci or fill the intercondylar notch extensively.

Synovial chondromatosis[38] is characterized by multiple cartilaginous bodies that are free within the joint. These may be small and resemble the rice bodies of rheumatoid arthritis, but usually there is an extraordinary arthroscopic picture of large, irregular loose bodies so numerous that they nearly fill the suprapatellar pouch. There may be an associated villous synovitis that resembles that seen in osteoarthritis.

Mild forms of synovial inflammation cannot be differentiated arthroscopically. The early stages of rheumatoid arthritis may mimic post-traumatic synovitis. Hypertrophy and hyperemia, in moderate degree, are common in most acute and chronic trauma; thus, biopsies are routinely taken for accurate synovial diagnosis by microscopic sections.

OPERATIVE ARTHROSCOPY

Table 38–1 summarizes arthroscopic procedures possible for arthritic joints. Avoidance of long incisions through skin, fascia, and muscle makes arthroscopic technique attractive in arthritis management.[39] The early results of these procedures are encouraging, and some evidence suggests that the long-term results of arthroscopic surgery will equal or exceed those of open surgery. (Arthroscopic synovectomy is discussed in Chapter 39.)

Table 38–1. TYPES OF ARTHROSCOPIC SURGERY USED IN ARTHRITIC JOINTS

Synovial Cavity
  Lavage
  Biopsy
  Removal of loose bodies
  Lysis of adhesions
  Synovectomy, partial or total
Bursae
  Bursectomy (e.g., prepatellar, olecranon, subdeltoid)
Articular Cartilage
  Shaving, débridement (partial thickness)
  Drilling, burring (full thickness)
  Pinning, stabilization (chondral fractures)
Fibrocartilage (e.g., menisci, glenoid labrum, distal radial-ulnar triradiate)
  Partial resection, débridement
  Repair
  Total excision
Ligament and Tendon
  Trimming of fragmented or ruptured ends (anterior cruciate, long head of biceps)
  Division, release (coracoacromial ligament, lateral patellar retinaculum)
Bone
  Acromioplasty for shoulder impingement
  Osteophyte resection, burring
  Stabilization, pinning of osteochondritis dissecans and osteochondral fractures

FUTURE DEVELOPMENTS

During the 1980s there was dramatic growth in the use of arthroscopy, leading to its present status of being one of the most common operative procedures done by orthopedic surgeons. There is certainly no evidence that arthroscopic usage is leveling. Rather, this trend shows signs of becoming stronger over the next decade, primarily because of new and innovative operative procedures that are being done either entirely through the arthroscope or with arthroscopic control of a portion of the operation. Operations thought impossible to perform endoscopically are becoming routine, such as suturing of torn menisci,[40] fixation of the unstable shoulder,[41] acromioplasty,[42] and reduction of intra-articular fractures.[43] These types of surgical advances are not unique to arthroscopists but are part of a general trend among all the endoscopic surgical subspecialties to adopt ever-expanding, ingenious methods of converting open procedures to these less invasive techniques.

Also, improvements in instrument technology seem to set the pace of these developments. Better metallurgy allows sharper, more durable, and smaller cutting forceps. Inventive tools can now place sutures inside joints through an arthroscopic cannula. Motorized resectors, such as those used in synovectomy and meniscal resection, cut more rapidly and efficiently (Fig. 38–9). Perhaps the greatest impetus to increased arthroscopic usage has come from patients themselves. The public is much more demanding and knowledgeable, insisting on treatment methods

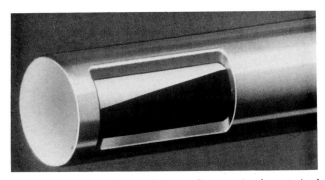

Figure 38–9. Magnified view of 6.5-mm diameter tip of a motorized suction-cutter used for synovectomy. The synovium is pulled into the window in the outer sheath by suction, then cut by the rotation of the sharp inner blade. The resected fragment is then drawn up through the center of the device and exits through tubing to a suction bottle.

that are less costly and that allow them to return to work and sports sooner.

One notable exception in this technologic advancement is the use of lasers in arthroscopy. At first glance, this high-energy modality seems ideally suited for transmission through a lens-oriented, fiberoptic system, such as an arthroscope. However, the use of lasers in arthroscopy has remained limited for nearly a decade, even though there has been considerable research and development by many companies and individuals. Lasers still present more problems than solutions to the arthroscopist,[44] such as their high cost, being more time consuming and less efficient as compared with motorized cutters, and their production of carbonaceous debris that is difficult to remove and can cause synovitis and the possibility of rapid ablation of normal articular cartilage from errant aim within the joint. Perhaps further research with new types of lasers, such as the contact neodinium:yttrium-aluminum-garnet (YAG)[45, 46] will solve these problems, but for now the use of lasers in arthroscopy is regarded as experimental by most arthroscopists.

ARTHROSCOPY AND THE RHEUMATOLOGIST

While there are a few rheumatologists who now use the technique of arthroscopy, in most communities a referral is made to an orthopedic surgeon who specializes in this technique. This may be more a result of economic factors than anything else. For example, arthroscopy is usually performed in an operating room with the patient under general anesthesia where the practitioner is required to have malpractice insurance at a cost-risk level several times that required for standard rheumatology practice. Also the cost of buying and maintaining arthroscopy equipment can be prohibitive if the technique is used only occasionally.

There is also the dilemma of what to do if a lesion is discovered at diagnostic arthroscopy that is treatable by surgical arthroscopy during the same period of anesthesia. Should only the diagnostic portion be completed, and the patient then referred to an arthroscopic surgeon? Obviously this is not practical, and so the person performing diagnostic arthroscopy increasingly finds himself or herself needing to learn further surgical techniques. This may be comfortable for some rheumatologists but not for others.

The decision to learn arthroscopy, therefore, is an individual one based on practice preferences, hospital requirements, and cost-insurance issues as well as, most importantly, an interest in the technique itself. The Arthroscopy Association of North America (AANA) has issued guidelines[47] for the practice of arthroscopic surgery that could apply to either a rheumatologist or an orthopedic surgeon. Also, membership in AANA is open to rheumatologists. The first executive board formed by AANA in 1982 included a rheumatologist who made many outstanding contributions to the growth of this association.

Office arthroscopy is being developed using smaller-diameter and flexible arthroscopes that can be used with the patient receiving local anesthesia. The patient can comfortably watch the examination on a television monitor, and the findings can be discussed immediately. Although there are many problems yet to be solved with this idea, it seems entirely possible that all diagnostic arthroscopy will one day be done in an office setting, which may overcome most of the current objections that rheumatologists have to doing the procedure.

References

1. Takagi, K.: Practical experiences using Takagi's arthroscope. J. Jpn. Orthop. Assoc. 8:132, 1933.
2. Watanabe, M., Takeda, S., and Ideuchi, H.: Atlas of Arthroscopy. New York, Springer-Verlag, 1957.
3. Alm, A., Gillquist, J., and Liljedahl, S. C.: The diagnostic value of arthroscopy of the knee joint. Injury 5:319, 1974.
4. O'Connor, R. L.: Arthroscopy. Philadelphia, J. B. Lippincott Company, 1977.
5. Ikeuchi, H.: Surgery under arthroscopic control. Rheumatologie 33:57, 1976.
6. Metcalf, R. W.: Operative arthroscopy of the knee. Instructional Course Lectures. Vol. 30. Chicago, American Academy of Orthopedic Surgeons, 1981.
7. Dandy, D. J.: The impact of arthroscopic surgery on the management of disorders of the knee. Arthroscopy 6:96, 1990.
8. Roth, J. H., Poehling, G. G., and Whipple, T. L.: Hand instrumentation for small joint arthroscopy. Arthroscopy 4:126, 1988.
9. Rosenberg, T. D., and Wong, H. C.: Arthroscopic knee surgery in a free-standing outpatient surgery center. Orthop. Clin. North Am. 13:277, 1982.
10. Metcalf, R. W.: Education in arthroscopy. In McGinty, J. B. (ed.): Operative Arthroscopy. New York, Raven Press, 1990.
11. Dandy, D. J.: Arthroscopic Management of the Knee. 2nd ed. New York, Churchill Livingstone, 1987.
12. Buss, D. D., Warren, R. F., and Galinat, B. J.: Indications for shoulder arthroscopy. In McGinty, J. B. (ed.): Operative Arthroscopy. New York, Raven Press, 1990.
13. McGinty, J. B., and Freedman, P. A.: Arthroscopy of the knee. Clin. Orthop. 121:171, 1976.
14. Selernich, F. H., Noble, H. B., Bachman, D. C., and Steinberg, F. L.: Internal derangement of the knee: Diagnosis by arthrography, arthroscopy, and arthrotomy. Clin. Orthop. 198:26, 1985.
15. Barronian, A. D., Zoltan, J. D., and Bucon, K. A.: Magnetic resonance

imaging of the knee: Correlation with arthroscopy. Arthroscopy 5:187, 1989.

16. Wasilewski, S. A., and Frankl, U.: Arthroscopy of the painful dysfunctional total knee replacement. Arthroscopy 5:294, 1989.

17. Jackson, D. W., and Ovadia, D. N.: Video arthroscopy: Present and future developments. Arthroscopy 1:116, 1985.

18. Fischer, S. P., Fox, J. M., Del Pizzo, W., Friedman, M. J., Snyder, S. J., and Ferkel, R. D.: Accuracy of diagnoses from magnetic resonance imaging of the knee. J. Bone Joint Surg. 73-A:2, 1991.

19. Raunest, J., Oberle, K., Loehnert, J., and Hoetzinger, H.: The clinical value of magnetic resonance imaging in the evaluation of meniscal disorders. J. Bone Joint Surg. 73-A:11, 1991.

20. Sprague, N. F.: Complications in arthroscopy. New York, Raven Press, 1989.

21. Yacobucci, G. N., Bruce, R., Conahan, T. J., Kitz, D. S., and Torg, J. S.: Arthroscopic surgery of the knee under local anesthesia. Arthroscopy 6:3, 1990.

22. Jackson, R. W., Marshall, D. J., and Fujisawa, Y.: The pathologic medial shelf. Orthop. Clin. North Am. 13:2, 1982.

23. Andrews, J. R., and Heckman, M. M.: Basic Techniques for Shoulder Arthroscopy. In McGinty, J. B. (ed.): Operative Arthroscopy. New York, Raven Press, 1991.

24. Wolf, E. M.: Anterior portals in shoulder arthroscopy. Arthroscopy 5:210, 1989.

25. Johnson, L. L.: Shoulder arthroscopy. In Arthroscopic Surgery: Principles and Practice. 3rd ed. St. Louis, C. V. Mosby, 1986.

26. Matthews, L. S., Terry, G., and Vetter, W. L.: Shoulder anatomy for the arthroscopist. Arthroscopy 1:83, 1985.

27. Johnson, L. L.: The shoulder joint: An arthroscopist's perspective of anatomy and pathology. Clin. Orthop. 223:113, 1987.

28. Poehling, G. G., Whipple, T. L., Sisco, L. S., and Goldman, B.: Elbow arthroscopy: A new technique. Arthroscopy 5:222, 1989.

29. Whipple, T. L., Poehling, G. G., and Roth, J. H.: Surgical technique for wrist arthroscopy. In McGinty, J. B. (ed.): Operative Arthroscopy. New York, Raven Press, 1991.

30. Chow, J. C. Y.: Endoscopic release of the carpal ligament: A new technique for carpal tunnel syndrome. Arthroscopy 5:11, 1989.

31. Glick, J. M., Sampson, T. G., Gordon, R. B., Behr, J. T., and Schmidt, E.: Hip arthroscopy by the lateral approach. Arthroscopy 3:4, 1987.

32. Guhl, J. F.: Portals and techniques: Mechanical distraction. In Guhl, J. F. (ed.): Ankle Arthroscopy: Pathology and Surgical Technique. Thorofare, NJ, Slack, 1987.

33. Martin, D. F., Curl, W. W., and Baker, C. L.: Arthroscopic treatment of chronic synovitis of the ankle. Arthroscopy 5:101, 1989.

34. Paulos, L. E., Rosenberg, T. D., and Beck, C. L.: Postsurgical care for arthroscopic surgery of the knee and shoulder. Orthop. Clin. North Am. 19:715, 1988.

35. Small, N. C.: Complications in arthroscopy: The knee and other joints. Arthroscopy 2:253, 1986.

36. Jackson, R. W., Marans, H. J., and Silver, R. W.: The arthroscopic treatment of degenerative arthritis of the knee. J. Bone Joint Surg. 70B:332, 1988.

37. Beguin, J., Locker, B., Vielpeau, M. D., and Souquieres, G.: Pigmented villonodular synovitis of the knee: Results from 13 cases. Arthroscopy 5:62, 1989.

38. Dorfmann, H., De Bie, B., Bonvarlet, J. P., and Boyer, T.: Arthroscopic treatment of synovial chondromatosis of the knee. Arthroscopy 5:48, 1989.

39. Altman, R. D., and Gray, R.: Diagnostic and therapeutic uses of the arthroscope in rheumatoid arthritis and osteoarthritis. Am. J. Med. 75:4B, 1983.

40. Hanks, G. A., Gause, T. M., Sebastianelli, W. J., O'Donnell, C. S., and Kalenak, A.: Repair of peripheral meniscal tears: Open versus arthroscopic technique. Arthroscopy 7:72, 1991.

41. Morgan, C. D., and Bodenstab, A. B.: Arthroscopic Bankart suture repair. Arthroscopy 3:111, 1987.

42. Altchek, D. W., Warren, R. F., Wickiewicz, T. L., Skyhar, M. J., Ortiz, G., and Schwartz, E.: Arthroscopic acromioplasty. J. Bone Joint Surg. 72A:1198, 1990.

43. Jennings, J. E.: Arthroscopic management of tibial plateau fractures. Arthroscopy 1:160, 1985.

44. Metcalf, R.: Orthopedic application of lasers. In Dixon, J. (ed.): Laser Surgery. Surgical Applications of Lasers. Chicago, Yearbook Medical Publishers, 1987, pp. 275–286.

45. Bickerstaff, D. R., Wyman, A., Laing, R. W., and Smith, T. W. D.: Partial meniscectomy using the neodymium:YAG laser. An in vitro study. Arthroscopy 7:63, 1991.

46. Miller, D. V., O'Brien, S. J., Arnoczky, S. S., Kelly, A., Fealy, S. V., and Warren, R. F.: The use of the contact Nd:YAG laser in arthroscopic surgery: Effects on articular cartilage and meniscal tissue. Arthroscopy 5:245, 1989.

47. Lidge, R. E.: Suggested guidelines for the practice of arthroscopy. Arthroscopy 1:74, 1985.

Chapter 39

Alan P. Newman

Synovectomy

INTRODUCTION

Synovial disorders are a frequent cause of pain, swelling, and functional impairment. Although these conditions often are responsive to a wide range of physical and pharmacologic modalities, their management sometimes may require operative intervention. Over the past 20 years, the development of arthroscopic instrumentation and techniques has been responsible for renewed interest in the surgical, *yet conservative*, approach to these problems. Owing to the decreased morbidity and increased precision of the closed, arthroscopic approach, the risk-benefit ratio of débridement and synovectomy has improved dramatically (Figs. 39–1 and 39–2, see color section at the front of this volume; see Table 39–2).

PATHOPHYSIOLOGY

For more than 100 years, removal of an inflamed synovial membrane *(synovectomy)* has been a cornerstone of management for joint inflammation refractory to medical management. Arthroscopy has dramatically changed the role of this modality in recent years. A careful understanding of the theory and principles of synovectomy, as well as its applications in a variety of disorders and joints, is crucial to its proper utilization. The remainder of this chapter is devoted to this topic.

SYNOVECTOMY IN RHEUMATOID ARTHRITIS

History

Volkmann[1] is generally credited with the original concept of the removal of inflamed periarticular soft tissues, which he performed in 1877 for a tuberculous knee joint. Subsequently, many other physicians in Europe and North America have utilized synovectomy and synoviorthesis for a multitude of diagnostic entities and joints, and with a variety of techniques (Table 39–1). Interest in this procedure markedly increased during the 1950s (and has remained high), primarily because it was seen as a means of preventing the recurrent and progressive damage frequently observed in rheumatoid arthritis (RA). The development of open, arthroscopic, chemical, and radioisotope methods for the removal of synovial tissue has been a logical consequence of our understanding of synovial disorders. As the various technologies have evolved, there has been a general trend toward more effective procedures, with less associated morbidity.

Theory

Swett[2] and Gschwend[3] have based the theoretical rationale of synovectomy on two principles: the improvement of the *mechanical function* of inflamed joints and the removal of the *pathologic tissue* from the joints. Even if the surgical procedure is not curative, synovectomy allows the return (at least temporarily) of more normal joint function by the elimination of boggy, swollen tissues, chronic effusions, fibrinous exudates and adhesions, and other mechanical obstacles. This direct benefit is probably responsible for the short-term improvement noted in patients soon after synovectomy.

Whether the synovium is primarily involved in the disease process (as in RA) or secondarily (as in hemophilia), it plays an important role in the pathophysiology of joint destruction. In RA, synovium is the "immunocompetent tissue,"[3] being infiltrated with large numbers of lymphocytes and plasma cells. These cells produce many of the products (immunoglobulins and complement) responsible for tissue inflammation and damage. The synovial tissue of a hemophiliac is intrinsically normal, but secondary to the phagocytosis of large amounts of iron products, it hypertrophies and becomes a major factor in progressive articular destruction. In both these situations, synovial ablation should therefore stall, if not completely halt, further deterioration. Goldie[4] has demonstrated that the level of inflammation (as evaluated by changes in temperature and pH) decreased significantly after synovectomy in patients with RA. The principle of removal of diseased tissue suggests that long-term improvement can be maintained in this fashion.

In the case of RA, there is another potential advantage of synovectomy. In the early stages of synoviocyte proliferation and metaplasia into fibroblastic cells, the comparative avascularity of this tissue should make it relatively refractory to traditional medical management with anti-inflammatory medications. Surgical removal of these cells is theoretically the most effective method of dealing with this phase of the rheumatoid process.[5, 6]

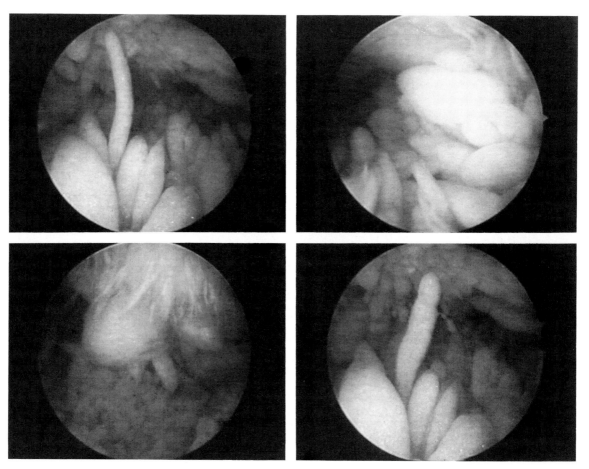

Figure 39–1. Arthroscopic view of rheumatoid synovium.

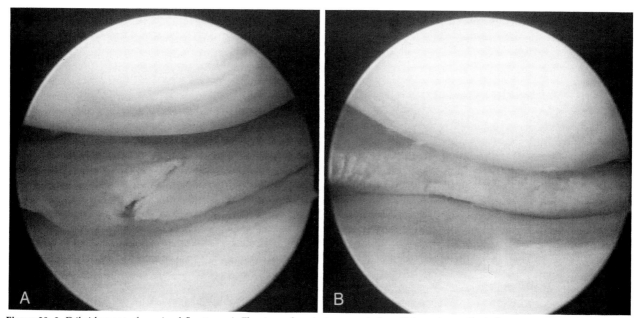

Figure 39–2. Débridement of meniscal flap tear. *A*, Flap tear of posterior aspect of medial meniscus. *B*, Arthroscopic view after resection of the tear, removing all unstable tissue and leaving behind as much normal meniscus as possible, in order to preserve the mechanical function of the joint.

Table 39–1. HISTORY OF SYNOVECTOMY

Investigator	Year	Technique	Comments
Volkmann	1877	Open	Tuberculous knee
Schuller	1887	Open	Chronic rheumatic inflammation
Muller	1894	Open	Rheumatoid arthritis
Mignon	1900	Open	Rheumatoid arthritis, tuberculous knee
Goldwaith	1900	Open	Nontuberculous arthritis
Murphy	1916	Open	Hypertrophic villous synovitis
Swett	1923	Open	Chronic "infectious" arthritis
Von Reis and Swensson	1951	Chemical	Osmic acid
Fellinger and Schmid	1952	Radioisotope	Radioactive gold
Flatt	1962	Chemical	Thiotepa
Mori	1963	Open	Modified anterior synovectomy
Ansell et al.	1963	Radioisotope	Radioactive gold
Matsui	1969	Arthroscopic	Manual punch forceps
Aritomi	1972	Arthroscopic	Electric resectoscope
Gumpel	1975	Radioisotope	Radioactive yttrium
Highgenboten	1977	Arthroscopic	Motorized suction cutters
Sledge et al.	1983	Radioisotope	Radioactive dysprosium

Finally, there are some reasons why synovectomy should *not* provide lasting improvement, particularly in the case of rheumatoid processes. A number of investigators have demonstrated the regrowth of synovial tissue within 1 to 3 years following synovectomy.[7-11] Paus and Pahle[12] have shown, by follow-up arthroscopy, complete synovial regeneration within 6 months of surgery, with some areas involved with recurrent synovitis. Patzakis and colleagues[13] observed that following open synovectomy in patients with RA, the synovial membrane that regenerated was histologically abnormal as early as 1 month postoperatively. The regrown tissue may remain quiescent for some time, but reactivation is always a possibility. Although the regenerated tissue is presumably normal in nonrheumatoid disorders, it can later become secondarily affected by the underlying disease process, as it did originally. Aschan and Moberg,[14] furthermore, have shown that synovial tissue that has invaded bone (e.g., in even minor bone erosions), which is often not removed at the time of a synovectomy, can be responsible for the recurrence of a generalized synovitis.

Open Techniques

Although the theoretical goal of any synovectomy is the complete removal of all synovial tissue, proponents of open techniques have realized that this is unachievable in practice. A more realistic goal of open synovectomy is the radical removal of as much synovium as possible, at least 80 to 90 per cent of that present.[15-17] The most critical locations occur at the chondrosynovial junctions,[3, 18, 19] where the pathologic synovial membrane does its worst damage, participating in the formation of pannus and marginal erosions.

Although a superficially located joint, the knee possesses certain anatomic features that make complete open synovectomy a difficult challenge. Mori and Ogawa[20] recognized that the extensor mechanism was compromised by long incisions into the quadriceps muscle bellies and advocated a modified anterior synovectomy utilizing two shorter medial and lateral parapatellar incisions. The parameniscal synovium often is markedly involved and is difficult to eradicate with the menisci in place. Some authors advocated total meniscectomy[12, 18, 19, 21-24] as a means of exposing this tissue, but more recent reports have suggested meniscectomy only if the menisci are torn or severely damaged.[7, 15, 16] Removal of posterior compartment synovium has also proved to be demanding. Gschwend[3] recommends incisions at the posterior corners of the joint, approached with the knee flexed through a long, extensile anterior skin incision. In an effort to minimize adhesions in the suprapatellar pouch, with subsequent stiffness, Marmor[19, 21] advised retaining the pouch. However, that certainly compromises the primary goal of removing as much synovial tissue as possible and, with current methods of aggressive postoperative management (see later), should not be necessary.[17]

One of the most significant disadvantages to open techniques is the morbidity of the procedure. For certain joints located deep beneath musculature (e.g., the hip and shoulder), the exposure itself creates significant bleeding and, postoperatively, the chance for substantial pain, scarring, and loss of motion. Once the joint is exposed, the dissection required to perform a radical synovectomy necessitates further surgical trauma to important capsular and ligamentous structures. These points are responsible for the frequent need for prolonged hospitalization and intensive physical therapy as well as occasional manipulations.[17, 25] Graham and Checketts[26] reported a loss of motion following open synovectomy in 31 per cent of their patients, while in a study by Paradies,[18] 64 per cent of patients lost motion. Ranawat and Desai[23] reported on a series of 32 open knee synovectomies in 26 patients with RA in which 50 per cent required manipulations.

Despite these problems with intraoperative completeness and postoperative morbidity, the experience with open methods of synovectomy has been quite good (see Table 39–2 and the section on results that follows). Certain features common to the practices of different authors and different joints have evolved over time. Prophylactic antibiotics are commonly employed, as these procedures are associated with large soft tissue dissections (and resultant dead spaces) and occasional hematomas and are often performed on immunocompromised patients. The use of a tourniquet (except in the hip and shoulder) is routine, in order to promote atraumatic and thorough resection. To prevent a postoperative hemarthrosis or hematoma, the tourniquet should be deflated prior to wound closure for hemostasis.

The actual removal of the synovium is facilitated by carefully dissecting the synovial layer and separating it from the underlying areolar tissue.[21] This allows "en bloc" removal of large segments of the membrane rather than a piecemeal excision. Sharp dissection is usually employed, but over some surfaces (e.g., cruciate ligaments, chondral edges) curettes and rongeurs are helpful.

Postoperatively, compressive dressings are utilized, along with suction drains for the first 24 to 48 hours. Early postoperative physical therapy to restore motion and strength are imperative in order to minimize morbidity.[7, 16, 19, 21, 23, 24] The surgeon may opt for either a splint to support the limb while it is not involved in physical therapy, or a continuous passive motion device, but the need for prompt and frequent exercise is essential.

Arthroscopy

With the growing interest in the arthroscope in the 1970s, attention quickly turned to its application to synovial disorders. Use of arthroscopy for diagnostic visualization (Table 39–2) and biopsy soon led to early attempts at synovectomy. Matsui and associates[27] reported on an arthroscopic technique that they began to use in 1969, removing synovium with manual punch forceps. Aritomi[28] utilized an electric resectoscope (a modified urologic instrument) in 1972. In the 1980s, two technical developments occurred that tremendously facilitated synovial resection. Motorized suction cutting instruments made the removal of the synovial membrane fast and thorough, and the introduction of video technology to arthroscopy improved the ability of the surgeon to carefully proceed through a long and sometimes tedious operation as well as improved the sterile technique of arthroscopic synovectomy.

The arthroscope is well suited to addressing the specific problems surgeons encounter with open synovectomy: the *completeness* of synovial resection and the *morbidity* of the procedure. With the use of multiple accessory portals and arthroscopes with lenses of varying obliquity, it is possible to guide cutting instruments, under direct visualization, to cover virtually the entire interior of the knee, shoulder, elbow, and ankle. For example, in the knee the synovial membrane in the parameniscal regions and posterior compartments proved difficult to approach with open techniques (without meniscectomy and multiple capsular incisions). These areas are easily within the reach of arthroscopic synovial resectors (Fig. 39–3A and B; see color section at the front of this volume), making total synovectomy at least a theoretical possibility.

The morbidity of open synovectomy has been one major factor against its utilization early in a disease process. With arthroscopy, the surgical trauma is greatly minimized, with attendant decreases in pain, medications, and length of hospitalization. Many surgeons now perform arthroscopic synovectomies as outpatient procedures.[25] Since postoperative pain is diminished, the risk of loss of motion and the need for intensive physical therapy are reduced,[7] and manipulations to regain motion are rarely needed.[25]

Table 39–2. ARTHROSCOPIC APPEARANCE OF ARTHRITIC DISORDERS

Disorder	Synovium	Articular Cartilage	Menisci
Rheumatoid arthritis	Boggy, hyperemic, with large, edematous club-shaped villi	Softened, friable, shallow, but few ulcerations until late. Pannus formation is classic	Frayed central edge
Osteoarthritis	Slightly hyperemic, slender villi with entrapped cartilage debris	Rough, irregular, fibrillated; exposed bone in advanced cases. Osteophytes present	Horizontal cleavage tears, cyst formation, second-degree complex tears
Hemophilia	Resembles RA, but with marked hemosiderin staining	Fibrillations and erosions late in the process	
PVNS	Similar to hemophilia, villi may cluster into nodular formations	Fibrillation and erosions late in the process	
Gout/pseudogout		Flecks of crystalline deposits on articular surface	Flecks of crystalline deposits on surface of menisci
Osteochondromatosis	Numerous, tightly packed villi in bulbous shapes (multiple osteocartilaginous loose bodies)		

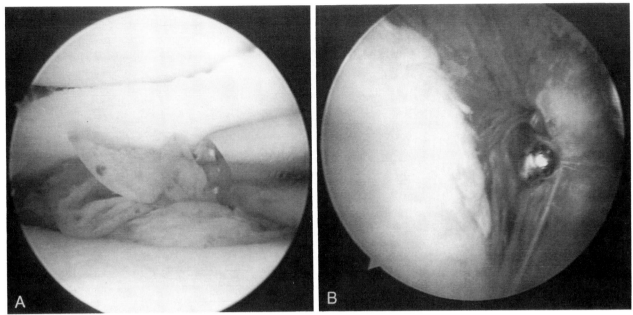

Figure 39–3. *A,* Arthroscopic view of motorized synovial resector tip approaching the perimeniscal synovium beneath the lateral meniscus (in a case of PVNS). *B,* Visualization of the posteromedial compartment of a knee with hemophilic arthropathy, with the synovial resector inserted through a separate posteromedial portal.

The primary disadvantage of closed synovectomy is that it is one of the more technically demanding arthroscopic procedures and should not be attempted by the inexperienced arthroscopist.[25, 29] Familiarity with multiple portals, basic triangulation skills, and motorized instrumentation are essential to a successful synovectomy. Furthermore, closed synovectomy requires patience and persistence on the part of the surgeon, as a total arthroscopic synovectomy may take 90 minutes or longer, and deviation from a methodical approach will result in a subtotal synovectomy.

Prophylactic antibiotics generally are not used, as there is no soft tissue dissection, and rarely a significant hematoma. As with open methods, removal of the synovial membrane is facilitated by dissecting the interval between the intimal and subintimal layers.[30] This can be done bluntly with the tip of a motorized cutter used as a probe. Tourniquets are usually employed, but hemostasis is typically achieved solely by the use of a compression dressing postoperatively. Physical therapy is managed on an outpatient basis, and most authors[25, 28, 31] report that patients regain their preoperative range of motion and are off crutches by 7 to 10 days after an arthroscopic knee synovectomy.

Chemical Agents and Radioisotopes

Interest has developed in nonoperative methods of synovectomy as ways of avoiding the hospitalization, cost, and potential complications that both closed and open techniques share. Over the last 30 years, both chemical and radioactive agents have been utilized to ablate synovial tissue. The earliest experience with synoviorthesis began with chemicals such as osmic acid[32, 33] (a protein denaturant) and thiotepa[34, 35] (an alkylating agent). Despite promising early results, they did not achieve widespread usage because of concerns over potential damage to articular cartilage.

The first reported use of radioactive material to remove inflamed synovium was by Fellinger and Schmid[36] in 1952. Since then many different isotopes ([198]gold, [90]yttrium, [186]rhenium, [169]erbium, [32]phosphorus, [224]radium, and [165]dysprosium) in various preparations have been employed.[3] Radionuclides have been selected on the basis of their predominance of beta (β)-particle emission, along with an absence of alpha (α)-particle and a relative lack of gamma (γ)-particle emission[3, 37–39] (β-particle emissions are preferred because their depth of tissue penetration is usually quite small). Those isotopes with particularly deeply penetrating β-particles, such as [90]yttrium, are suitable for larger joints well covered by soft tissue (knee, hip, and shoulder) but would not be appropriate for the smaller joints of the fingers.[40]

A major issue with the use of these materials has been the potential for leakage from the joint after injection,[41] with resultant damage to other parts of the body. In order to minimize this concern, these materials are generally injected in a colloidal or particulate form.[38, 39, 41, 42] Although radionuclides with long half-lives have maximum therapeutic benefit, their risk to the patient is also greater. Thus, radioisotopes with shorter half-lives are generally favored, in the event that significant leakage does occur. It is for these reasons that Sledge and associates[37, 41] have employed [165]dysprosium ferric hydroxide macroaggregates (FHMAs). [165]Dysprosium has a half-life of 2.3 hours and is almost a pure β-particle emitter, with maximum soft tissue penetration of 5.7 mm. Since the FHMAs are very large, their rate of joint leakage is very low. In animal studies,[43] of the original injected dose, 0.1 per cent had leaked to the liver, and 0.001 per cent leaked to the regional lymph nodes. On the other hand, the extremely short half-life of [165]dysprosium mandates the proximity of a nuclear reactor capable of producing this material.[41]

Onetti and colleagues[38] observed the effect of [32]phosphorus on the synovial membrane and found that phagocytic activity of type A cells was generally increased, while the synthetic properties of type B cells was decreased. They also suggested that immunologic activity was suppressed at the synovial level. Because these agents require dispersal throughout the joint cavity to exert their effect, they are not applicable to multiloculated joints, either on a physiologic (e.g., the wrist) or pathologic (e.g., any inflamed joint with a thick exudate or a hypertrophic villous synovitis) basis.[3]

The primary benefit of synoviorthesis compared with operative synovectomy is the relative simplicity of the procedure.[3, 44] Hospitalization is reduced, and anesthetic and surgical complications are avoided. Although most investigators have reported frequent flare-ups of synovitis[45] after injection, pain is much less than that with either closed or open techniques, and there is no need for narcotics. Postinjection mobilization is accomplished easily, without the need for physical therapy. The cost of synoviorthesis, therefore, reflects all these differences and is significantly less.[44, 46]

A particular disadvantage of this method is that none of these agents are selective for synovium[3, 47]; one can expect ultrastructural changes in articular cartilage, menisci, and subchondral bone as well as in synovium. Besides possible intraarticular side effects, other local problems have been identified, such as skin eruptions, needle track burns, radionecrosis, and scar formation.[48] A more serious potential problem is that of leakage outside the target joint, with the risk of chromosome damage to regional lymph nodes and circulating lymphocytes.[3, 39, 42] Although chromosome damage has been reported,[49–51] its clinical significance is unknown, as there has not been a single malignancy linked to radioisotope synoviorthesis in almost 30 years of clinical use.[41, 42] However, because of the potential for mutagenesis, it has been suggested that this technique is suitable only for those patients older than 45 years of age.[3, 37, 42, 44, 45, 47, 51, 52] This is because the theoretical risk of cancer induction is quite small compared with the risk of naturally occurring neoplasia at that age, and also the risk of inducing and transmitting germinal chromosomal damage beyond the ordinary child-bearing years is negligible.[51]

Meticulous attention needs to be directed to the proper handling of radioactive materials. Goggles are recommended for transfer and injection of the material.[47] Since many patients experience an increase in pain and swelling after injection, most advocate simultaneous injection of a glucocorticoid along with a local anesthetic.[3, 47] A period of immobilization after injection is recommended (the length of which is dependent on the half-life) to minimize leakage from the joint.[3, 37, 39, 40, 42, 44, 45–47, 49, 50]

Results

Synovectomy has been a popular treatment for RA as well as other inflammatory joint conditions for the last 40 years. Designed to treat the symptomatic joint, it has also enjoyed some enthusiasm as a prophylactic measure to prevent the progressive articular damage that so often occurs in these conditions.[15, 16] In spite of this, significant controversies remain concerning the efficacy of this procedure. These questions persist partly because of the lack of controlled studies and partly because of the nature of RA. Owing to the frequent asymmetry of involvement and the variable natural history of the disease (punctuated by intermittent flare-ups and remission), it is difficult unequivocally to ascribe good results to the synovectomy itself. McEwen[53, 54] illustrated this in the multicenter, controlled study that he directed. He reported that most patients had less pain at 1, 3, and 5 years after knee synovectomies, but this trend was also observed in the control subjects.

Most studies (Table 39–3) document a favorable response in regard to pain, swelling, and function, with 75 to 80 per cent good results commonly reported after 2 postoperative years.[17] These initially positive outcomes tend to deteriorate somewhat to about 60 to 70 per cent good results after 5 years.[15, 17] Despite these reasonable functional results, radiographic progression of disease (particularly degenerative changes) is common after synovectomy.[3, 16, 24, 26, 53, 55]

There is virtually complete agreement that results are improved if synovectomy is performed early, prior to the development of severe articular damage.[3, 15, 16, 19, 21, 22, 24, 56] Synovectomy should not be performed in cases with stage IV (American Rheumatism Association [ARA] classification) involvement. Geens and associates[55] have emphasized that in advanced cases, instability implies a particularly bad prognosis. Laurin and colleagues[15] observed that the presence of flexion deformities tended to adversely affect results. However, these deformities usually occur in more advanced cases, so it is difficult to separate the effects of those two factors. Doets and associates[56] concluded that early synovectomy provided symptomatic relief but questioned whether there was any prophylactic effect (due to progressive deterioration during their 7-year follow-up). They also stated that late synovectomy had an unacceptably high failure rate.

Two recent controlled, multicenter studies do

Table 39–3. RESULTS OF OPEN KNEE SYNOVECTOMY IN RA

Author(s)	Patients	Cases	Follow-Up	Results
Geens et al.[55] (1969)	20	28	23 months avg.; range: 7–49 months	Subjective: 22 improved (79%) Objective: 18 improved (64%)
Ranawat et al.[24] (1972)	46	60	2.8 years avg.; range: 1–8 years	Subjective: 46 improved (77%) Objective: 44 improved (73%)
Conaty[144] (1973)	32	39	4 years avg.; 1 year minimum	30 successful (77%) 9 failures (23%)
Marmor[19] (1973)	142	175	4 years avg.; range: 12–108 months	93 successful (53%)
Laurin et al.[15] (1974)	49	66	7.5 years avg.; range: 5–17 years	26 good/18 satisfactory (67%) 13 unsatisf./9 poor (33%)
Ranawat and Desai[23] (1975)	26	32	3 years avg.; range: 1–6 years	Subjective: 25 improved (78%) Objective: 23 improved (72%)
Kohler et al.[145] (1985)	32	41	10.6 years avg.; range: 9–16 years	30 satisfactory (73%) 24 no pain/26 no effusion
Brattstrom et al.[146] (1985)	—	508	10 year minimum	329 good (65%)
Ishikawa et al.[16] (1986)	55	78	14.1 years avg.; range: 10–23 years	17 excellent/31 satisfactory (61.5%) 18 unsatisf./12 poor (38.5%)
Doets et al.[56] (1989)	65	83	7 years avg.; range: 3–11 years	34/67 satisfactory (50.8%) 2/16 satisfactory (12.5%)

shed some doubt on the otherwise generally favorable reports in the rest of the literature. A British study,[57] by the Arthritis and Rheumatism Council and the British Orthopaedic Association, and an American study,[53, 54] by the Arthritis Foundation, both compared the results of open knee and metacarpophalangeal (MCP) synovectomy to conservative management of a matched set of control patients. The U.K. trial[57] demonstrated, at 3-year follow-up, no clinical benefit of the MCP synovectomies, but the patients with knee synovectomies had less pain, swelling, and less frequent bony erosions. The U.S. study[53, 54] showed similar findings at 1 year. However, by 3 years the postoperative knees were better only with regard to the amount of swelling, and by 5 years there was no statistically significant difference between the synovectomy and control patients. Interestingly, in both these studies the patients who underwent synovectomy overwhelmingly were satisfied subjectively with their results.

It is difficult at this time to analyze the results of arthroscopic synovectomy as critically as those of open methods. The follow-up period is shorter, and the series, to date, have often presented groups of patients with multiple diagnoses, making conclusions and comparisons complicated. Furthermore, there has been a steady evolution and improvement of motorized instrumentation over the last 10 years, so the series with the longest periods of follow-up also were done with the least effective equipment. Table 39–4 lists some of the arthroscopic series published to date, and in general the results are comparable to those from the open synovectomy literature. There have been few complications, and the anticipated decrease in morbidity has been gratifying. None of the arthroscopy studies reported any loss of motion, and Cleland and associates[58] actually observed increased motion postoperatively in 5 of their 6 patients. Ogilvie-Harris and Basinski[30] found a statistically significant decrease in pain and synovitis at 4-year follow-up of 96 patients. In the study of Klein and Jensen,[59] patients who had one knee syn-

Table 39–4. RESULTS OF ARTHROSCOPIC KNEE SYNOVECTOMY IN RA

Author(s)	Patients	Cases	Follow-Up	Results
Aritomi[28] (1984)	31	38	42 months avg.; range: 5 months–6 years	12 excellent/15 good (71%) 8 fair/3 poor (29%)
Wilkes[147] (1985)	30	30	57 months avg.	Good/satisfactory (56.7%) Unsatisfactory/poor (43.3%)
Cohen and Jones[7] (1987)	8	9	24 months	4 of 5 satisfactory (80%) 0 of 4 satisfactory (0%)
Matsui et al.[27] (1989)	27	41	12 years avg.; range: 2–17 years	Good—after 3 years (82.9%) Good—after 8 years (45.9%)
Smiley and Wasilewski[149] (1990)	19	25	55 months avg.; range: 6 months–6 years	24 of 25 good—after 6 months (96%) 19 of 21 good—at 2–4 years (90%) 8 of 14 good—after 4 years (57%)

Table 39–5. RESULTS OF CHEMICAL/RADIOISOTOPE KNEE SYNOVIORTHESIS IN RA

Author(s)	Patients	Cases	Agent	Follow-up	Results
Sheppeard et al.[47] (1981)	67	91	Osmic acid	3 years	69 satisfactory—after 1 year (76%) 62 satisfactory—after 2 years (68%) 57 satisfactory—after 3 years (63%)
Sheppeard et al.[47] (1981)	59	84	^{90}Yttrium	3 years	58 satisfactory—after 1 year (69%) 48 satisfactory—after 2 years (57%) 40 satisfactory—after 3 years (48%)
Onetti et al.[38] (1982)		112	^{32}Phosphorus	1 year	90 improved—after 1 year (80%)
Sledge et al.[37] (1984)	44	53	^{165}Dysprosium	1 year	Improvement–after 1 year (80%)
Aeckerle and Heisel[148] (1985)	68	72	^{90}Yttrium	Up to 4 years	Good (77.6%)
Boerbooms et al.[45] (1985)		49	^{198}Gold	1 year	Excellent/good—after 1 year (55%) Excellent/good—after 5 years (40%)
Boerbooms et al.[45] (1985)		15	^{90}Yttrium	1 year	Excellent/good—after 1 year (60%)
Sledge et al.[41] (1986)	63	74	^{165}Dysprosium	1 year	Good (61%) Fair (23%)

ovectomy performed arthroscopically while the contralateral knee was done closed uniformly favored the arthroscopic method. Continued investigations (particularly controlled trials) will be helpful in answering the remaining questions about this procedure.

The results from a number of studies of synoviorthesis are listed in Table 39–5. In general, the results are again comparable to those seen after open synovectomy, with up to 80 per cent improved at 1 year and a gradual deterioration to about 40 to 50 per cent improved in later years. Again, these studies suffer from lack of adequate controls. As with operative synovectomy, the results are usually better in the early stages of disease when there is little articular damage. Similar to the findings after arthroscopic synovectomy, there are virtually no problems regaining motion, and patient satisfaction with the procedure is extremely high.[46]

Indications and Contraindications

Synovectomy is indicated (in inflammatory conditions) for a chronic synovitis that has been refractory to aggressive medical management for 6 months or longer.[3, 7, 12, 15–18, 21, 30, 37, 45, 56, 60] Because of the potential (unproven, see earlier) for preventing progression of articular changes, some authors[21] suggest earlier synovectomy when dealing with a young patient who already has some radiographic changes present. Gschwend[3] has written of a "biomechanical" indication for surgical synovectomy, as opposed to

chemical or radioisotope synoviorthesis, when there are loculations or fibrinous exudates present. These represent intra-articular obstacles that block the free dispersal of the pharmacologic agents throughout the joint, limiting their effectiveness.

Although most surgeons agree that synovectomy should be deferred if the patient is "toxic" from floridly active RA,[17, 21] it is not necessary to wait for the disease to become quiescent (e.g., as confirmed by erythrocyte sedimentation rate [ESR]).[3, 16, 21] It is important, however, to ensure that the skin around the operative site is healthy and intact, and any rashes or skin infections should be treated until clear prior to surgery.[3] Rheumatoid nodules should be avoided in any operative approach, particularly with open techniques.

General policies of preoperative evaluation should be followed, and any medical problem that substantially increases perioperative risk should be treated. The patient with RA on maintenance steroid management should be given a preoperative steroid "booster".[21] Other contraindications specific to the disease or the procedure itself should be carefully considered. Patients with advanced articular damage (stage IV destruction)[3, 16, 21, 53, 56] are not candidates for synovectomy, nor are patients with significant fixed deformities.[21] Synovectomy should be avoided in the patient who is judged to be poorly motivated,[3, 15, 19, 21] as a good result is dependent on some measure of compliance with postoperative physical therapy. Although this factor may not be as critical with arthroscopic synovectomy as with the open technique, it is still important to consider.

The indications for radioisotope synoviorthesis are, in general, the same as those for operative methods: early cases without evidence of advanced articular damage.[3, 37, 40, 41, 44, 45] In addition, synoviorthesis does not work well in multiloculated joints and cases with hypertrophic villous synovitis and is not applicable to tenosynovitis. One important contraindication is the patient who is of child-bearing age,[3, 37, 39, 43, 45, 47, 52] which in practice often makes it difficult to utilize this method before significant joint destruction has occurred.

SYNOVECTOMY IN CONDITIONS OTHER THAN RA

Hemophilia

Hemophilia (see also Chapter 90) comprises a group of bleeding diatheses characterized by deficiencies of specific clotting factors.[61] The two most common disorders associated with spontaneous hemarthroses are classic hemophilia (hemophilia A, caused by factor VIII deficiency) and Christmas disease (hemophilia B, caused by factor IX deficiency). The likelihood of spontaneous joint bleeding is related to the functional plasma level of the deficient clotting factor; patients with moderately severe (plasma levels between 1 and 5 percent of normal) and severe (plasma levels below 1 percent) hemophilia have bleeding episodes frequent enough to generate the typical picture of hemophilic arthropathy.[61] The most commonly afflicted joints include the knee, elbow, and ankle, with the hip and shoulder less commonly involved.[62, 63]

Intra-articular bleeding of a recurrent nature leads to synovial hypertrophy, along with deposition of hemosiderin within the synovial membrane (Fig. 39–4; see color section at the front of this volume). This causes a number of changes in the subintimal layer, among them an inflammatory response, vascular hyperplasia, and, ultimately, synovial fibrosis.[63, 64] The synovium can become markedly infolded and engorged, creating a more friable membrane that is more easily traumatized and results in an ever-increasing frequency of hemarthroses. At some point in this process, pannus formation and lysosomal enzyme release lead to articular cartilage breakdown.[65] This chronic arthropathy can produce rapid joint destruction, all too frequently leading to severe deformities, contractures, and even ankylosis before the third decade.[61, 65]

Although the advent of various factor concentrates has dramatically improved the medical management of these patients, many still are faced with progressive joint deterioration. Hemophilia is an excellent example of a disease process that secondarily affects the synovium (as opposed to those disorders, such as RA, in which the synovium is primarily

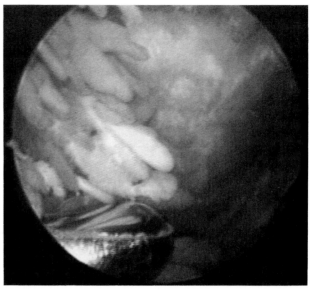

Figure 39–4. Arthroscopic view of synovial membrane in hemophilia. Note the orange pigmentation and the marked synovial hypertrophy.

involved). It is therefore tempting to speculate that removal of the hypertrophic synovium not only may produce short-term benefit but also may actually have a protective effect on the articular surface by interrupting the vicious pathophysiologic cycle.[63]

Since 1969, surgeons have utilized synovectomy in the cases that have been refractory to the most aggressive medical management. The experience with open synovectomy (Table 39–6), as reported by many authors,[63, 64, 66–73] has been very gratifying in regard to decreasing the frequency and severity of bleeding episodes and also in terms of functional improvement. However, as in the case of synovectomies performed for RA, there have been problems with maintaining motion postoperatively.[67–69, 73–75] Indeed, the problem has been more profound following synovectomy in hemophiliacs, for a number of reasons. The age of the patient undergoing the procedure is perhaps the most important factor; many of these patients are young teenagers, who may not comply with the requisite postoperative rehabilitation. The potential for perioperative complications in these patients also makes their recovery more difficult, as postoperative hemarthroses, adhesions, and infections all may compromise the final range of motion.[67–69, 72]

The early 1980s saw orthopedic surgeons turn to arthroscopy in an effort to decrease the morbidity of this procedure and, thereby, widen its application. Although the experience, to date, has been somewhat limited (Table 39–7), it mirrors that observed for arthroscopic synovectomy for RA.[76–78] The desired therapeutic effect (in this case, decreasing the frequency and severity of joint bleeding) is achieved, with an attendant decrease in morbidity. The arthroscopic experience suggests that motion is not com-

Table 39–6. RESULTS OF OPEN KNEE SYNOVECTOMY IN HEMOPHILIA

Author(s)	Patients	Cases	Follow-up	Recurrent Hemarthroses	Postoperative Motion
Pietrogrande et al.[73] (1972)	14	15	16 months avg.	Marked reduction	3 of 15 increased ROM (avg. 33°) 1 of 15 had no change in ROM 11 of 15 decreased ROM (avg. 31°)
Dyszy-Laube et al.[64] (1974)	14	14	Range: several weeks–2 years	None	All improved
Storti and Ascari[63] (1975)		51	36.5 months avg.	Marked reduction	Increased ROM in 55% No change in ROM in 33% Decreased ROM in 12%
Kay et al.[68] (1981)	8	11	52 months avg.; range: 29–76 months	Marked reduction	9 of 11 lost avg. of 42° ROM
Montane et al.[69] (1986)	13	13	7.3 years avg.; minimum: 2 years	Marked reduction	10 of 13 lost avg. of 41° ROM
Post et al.[70] (1986)		12	Range: 10–120 months	Marked reduction	8 of 12 increased ROM (avg. 25°) 1 of 12 had no change in ROM 3 of 12 decreased ROM (max. 10°)
Nicol and Menelaus[72] (1986)	10	10	Range: 4 months–11 years	Marked reduction	8 of 10 lost avg. of 51° ROM
Canale et al.[71] (1988)	14	16	30.6 months avg.; range: 6–93 months	Marked reduction	5 of 16 increased ROM 6 of 16 had no change in ROM

promised to the extent that it is following open synovectomy in this population,[79] but it is striking to note that some patients still have had motion difficulties after arthroscopic synovectomy. This underscores the serious problems and complications one may encounter when operating on a patient with hemophilia, any of which can create substantial hurdles for regaining motion.

Despite the medical and surgical challenges that these cases represent, it is unanimously agreed that arthroscopic synovectomy is a valuable adjunct to therapy for these conditions. The major indication is a joint that has experienced recurrent hemarthroses despite the most aggressive medical management.[80] A major dilemma is when to intervene surgically. All authors acknowledge that it is best to operate early, prior to irreversible articular damage.[61, 63, 71, 76, 77, 81–83] However, problems with regaining motion postoperatively increase as the age of the patient decreases.[69] The best results are seen in cooperative, well-motivated patients who will follow through with a structured and demanding rehabilitation program.[76]

Table 39–7. RESULTS OF ARTHROSCOPIC KNEE SYNOVECTOMY IN HEMOPHILIA

Author(s)	Patients	Cases	Follow-up	Recurrent Hemarthroses	Postoperative Motion
Wiedel[77] (1985)	5	5	??	Marked reduction	5 of 5 regained preop ROM
Limbird and Dennis[78] (1987)	5	5	24–38 months	Marked reduction	2 of 5 increased ROM 1 of 5 had no change in ROM 2 of 5 decreased ROM
Klein et al.[83] (1987)	7	7	50 months avg.; range: 20–72 months	Marked reduction	3 of 7 increased ROM (avg. 20°) 1 of 7 had no change in ROM 3 of 7 decreased ROM (avg. 9°)
Poggini et al.[86] (1989)	7	7	7–24 months	Marked reduction	7 of 7 increased ROM (avg. 36°)

The decision as to when to treat hemophilic arthropathy surgically must be individualized according to a judgment of the patient's maturity, compliance, articular disease, and overall medical condition.

The prevalence of seropositivity for the human immunodeficiency virus in this population must be taken into account. One estimate has placed the incidence as high as 90 percent.[81] This not only influences life expectancy but also may increase the risk of postoperative infection. Greene and colleagues[84] have demonstrated a correlation between the CD4 lymphocyte count and the risk of nosocomial infection in the postoperative patient. If the CD4 lymphocyte count is more than 400×10^9 cells per liter, the risk is only slightly increased. With a cell count between 200 and 400×10^9 cells per liter, the risk of infection is substantially increased, and if the CD4 lymphocyte count is fewer than 200×10^9 cells per liter, surgery should be avoided, if possible.

The surgical technique[76-78] for arthroscopic synovectomy is identical to that utilized in other conditions. Preoperatively, the patient must be tested for the presence of a circulating inhibitor to the deficient clotting factor.[71] A high titer of inhibitor is an absolute contraindication to elective surgery.[81] Immediately prior to an operation, adequate concentrate is infused to achieve a plasma level of 75 to 100 percent of normal, which is continued for the first 5 postoperative days. The level may be decreased at that time, but it is usually kept between 25 and 50 per cent until the end of the second week. Subsequently, the concentrate is administered as a bolus shortly before daily physical therapy (usually for the third and fourth postoperative weeks).[81]

A suction drain is used,[71, 77, 83, 85] and its removal is timed to coincide with a bolus of concentrate, usually on the second postoperative day. Most surgeons[71, 72, 77, 81, 86] advocate the use of a continuous passive-motion device while the patient is in the hospital, and they generally report superior results in final range of motion with this approach.

Pigmented Villonodular Synovitis

Pigmented villonodular synovitis (PVNS) is a locally invasive, proliferative lesion involving the synovial membrane of joints, bursae, and tendon sheaths.[87-89] Although there is some controversy about its actual cause—whether it represents a reactive phenomenon or a true neoplasm—it has never been observed to metastasize. Macroscopic involvement of the synovium is described as either localized (nodular) or diffuse,[87, 89] and Jaffe and associates[89] believe that these two categories represent the same disorder in different states of maturity. The pathologic picture[88, 90] is marked by proliferation of synovial cells and histiocytes, commonly associated with the appearance of multinucleated giant cells. Foam cells and hemosiderin granules are usually present. Because of the pigmentation and synovial hypertrophy, this process is virtually indistinguishable from hemophilic arthropathy (see Fig. 39–3A).

Patients typically present with a long (approximately 5 years, average) history of painful monarticular swelling, with no episode of prior trauma. Articular involvement is typically in the lower extremities, with the knee the most common site. The diffuse form usually affects the knee (although nodular lesions can also occur there), while the most common location for the nodular form is the fingers.[90] The process usually starts between the second and fifth decades.[90, 91] Radiographs may show nonspecific juxta-articular osteoporosis, degenerative changes, and, more important, intracapsular cystic changes indicating bony invasion of the proliferative process. Magnetic resonance imaging (MRI) can be useful in establishing the margins of the diseased synovium[92] and, thus, can be helpful in classifying the process as nodular or diffuse (although it cannot histologically distinguish PVNS from other synovial proliferative lesions, such as synovial sarcoma, synovial chondromatosis, hemophilia, and rheumatoid synovitis).

The treatment of PVNS has always been the ablation of involved tissue. There are no well-controlled studies in the literature with any technique other than surgical excision. In general, marginal excision of the pathologic nodules has been advocated for the localized form of the disease,[93] and complete synovectomy is the treatment of choice for the diffuse form.[94, 94a] To date, there is no large-scale experience with arthroscopic synovectomy in PVNS, but the same concepts and issues that have been discussed earlier in this chapter make this an attractive modality when the physician is faced with the need for surgical intervention in a joint that is amenable to the arthroscopic technique.

Since PVNS is not a malignant process, the main issue with regard to treatment is local recurrence. Most reports in the literature document a recurrence rate between 14 per cent[91] and 44 per cent.[95] In a carefully designed retrospective study employing very rigid criteria for recurrent disease, Schwartz and associates[88] reported a 15 per cent recurrence rate at 5 years, and a plateau at 35 per cent at 25 years. The only joint in which they observed recurrence was the knee, and the mean interval to recurrence was 4.9 years. In this study, factors that were associated with higher recurrence rates were a shorter duration of preceding symptoms (3.9 years in the recurrence group, compared with 5 years in the overall study) and the history of a previous surgical procedure that did not completely remove the diseased synovium. Other factors did not seem to influence the rate of recurrence, among them the gross pathologic architecture (nodular versus diffuse) and the presence of bony involvement. Byers and colleagues[90] believed that recurrences and unsatisfactory results were much more common with the diffuse form than with the nodular form.

Synovial Chondromatosis

Synovial chondromatosis is a disorder of the synovial membrane of joints, bursae, and tendon sheaths in which foci of cartilage develop as a result of metaplasia within the subintimal zone.[96, 97] It is intra-articular in approximately 80 per cent of cases.[98] Milgram[99] suggested that cartilage metaplasia was an indication of active intrasynovial disease, whereas cartilage loose bodies may be present when the synovium is quiescent. On this basis, he classified synovial chondromatosis into three phases: early (active intrasynovial disease with no loose bodies), transitional (active disease with loose bodies), and late (loose bodies with no intrasynovial disease).

Clinically, the patient typically presents with a history (of variable duration) of local pain and swelling. Mechanical symptoms of locking, clicking, or both are present in about one third of patients.[98] Although the diagnosis is confirmed by histology, it can often be made preoperatively by plain radiographs,[96, 100] in which multiple radiodense shadows with the typical stipled calcification of cartilaginous lesions are seen. Double-contrast arthrography has been utilized, which can demonstrate the presence of both intra-articular loose bodies and a nodular synovium.[98, 101]

The treatment of this condition has focused on the surgical removal of loose bodies and of involved synovium, but there is controversy about the role synovectomy plays in preventing recurrences. Some authors contend that since this is a proliferative synovial disorder, complete synovectomy is required to permanently eradicate the process.[97, 102] Others feel that for localized intra-articular disease, excision of abnormal or active synovium alone is all that is required,[98] while still others propose that removal of loose bodies without synovectomy gives results equal to those obtained with synovectomy.[103, 104] Milgram[99] has based his treatment algorithm on the stage of activity of the synovium: in early and transitional cases he suggests loose body removal in conjunction with a synovectomy, but for late cases (with inactive synovium), he favors loose body removal alone. However, Dorfmann and colleagues[104] concluded that there was no statistically significant difference in the results between patients with active synovium and those with inactive synovium, even when the treatment consisted of loose body removal alone. Maurice and associates[98] rely more on the presenting symptoms to guide treatment: if the patient primarily has mechanical symptoms, loose body removal alone should be sufficient, while the patient who complains of pain and swelling is best served by both loose body removal and synovectomy.

Since arthroscopic synovectomy does not carry the morbidity and potential loss in mobility that sometimes follows open synovectomy, it is logical to consider the removal of all involved or active synovium at the time of surgery.[98, 99] Maurice and colleagues[98] reported a recurrence rate of 12 per cent, with recurrences limited to those patients who had generalized intra-articular disease and an active synovium at the time of surgery. However, one should be aware that results are most strongly influenced by a thorough removal of all loose intra-articular osteocartilaginous bodies. In addition, Dorfmann and associates[104] have shown a significant correlation between the state of the tibiofemoral articular surfaces at the time of surgery and the long-term results.

Septic Arthritis

Septic arthritis (see Chapter 86) can be a devastating process, leading to virtually complete destruction of a joint in a very short period of time. Whether the process begins hematogenously, postoperatively, or through penetrating trauma, the same pathophysiologic steps take place. The synovium hypertrophies and generates a serofibrinous exudate. Vascular permeability of the synovial membrane increases, with increasing intra-articular levels of plasma proteins, coagulative elements, and fibrin. Adhesions and loculations quickly form, which makes drainage more difficult and can be responsible for loss of motion. Lysosomal enzymes are released, the source of much of the ensuing cartilage damage. During the first 3 to 5 days much of this process is reversible, but beyond that period complete recovery of the articular surfaces and joint function becomes increasingly improbable.

The clinical signs are pain, swelling, and a marked decrease in motion. There is usually an elevated temperature, along with increases in the sedimentation rate and peripheral white blood cell count. Joint aspiration typically yields turbid fluid, with the white cell count often more than 100,000 and demonstrating a marked left shift (rarely, an inflammatory process, such as gout or RA, can also yield as high a cell count). The fluid should also be sent for Gram stain and culture, although treatment must be instituted prior to the return of culture reports. Since radiographic changes appear quite late, they are of no help in making the diagnosis acutely. Radionuclide scanning with gallium can be helpful in securing the diagnosis in questionable cases.

In the past, the standard treatment for septic arthritis has been immobilization, antibiotics, and drainage. In recent years, both the concept of immobilization and the optimal form of drainage have come under scrutiny and discussion. There has been a definite trend away from immobilization and toward more "functional" forms of treatment, preferably earlier mobilization, weightbearing, and so forth. In regard to the most effective method of drainage, many internists have favored repeated needle aspirations (in joints amenable to this technique), and most orthopedists prefer open débridement. The argument in support of serial aspirations is that it avoids the morbidity of an arthrotomy and delayed wound closure, whereas advocates of open drainage point to the limited decompression that results from serial aspirations. It is precisely for these reasons that arthroscopic débridement of infected joints is so attractive a concept, since it can accomplish a complete and thorough débridement with minimal morbidity.

In 1970, Kelly and colleagues[105] reported on a series of 25 patients treated with open drainage. Only five patients obtained 90 degrees or more of flexion, while six joints spontaneously ankylosed and 13 joints required surgical fusion. The series of Ballard and associates[106] utilized functional treatment after open drainage of 34 infected cases, and had 16 good, 12 moderate, and 6 bad results. Tscherne and colleagues[107] stressed the importance of early motion after arthrotomy, and in their series 24 of 25 patients obtained 90 degrees or more of flexion.

In 1985, Jackson[108] reported on the arthroscopic treatment of septic knees, in which he advocated the use of a distention-irrigation system. In this method, the arthroscopic sheath (with blunt obturator) is maneuvered around the interior of the joint to bluntly break up any adhesions. Arthroscopic irrigation is then carried out, with motorized instrumentation aiding in the removal of residual debris, although a formal synovectomy is not carried out. Two sets of tubes are placed in the joint postoperatively, and the joint is alternately maximally distended with an antibiotic solution for 3 hours, and then suctioned for 1 hour. This distention-irrigation system is continued for about 1 week. Jackson[108] believed that this would avoid the loculations that can occur and would help to adequately débride the joint. He obtained 100 per cent good and excellent results in 14 cases after a minimum follow-up of 2 years.

Ivey and Clark[109] and Smith[110] both reported excellent results with a similar arthroscopic approach, although they did not utilize the distention-irrigation method. Smith[110] placed a suction drain for 48 hours postoperatively and stressed the importance of employing motorized instrumentation to adequately remove all debris and foreign particles (in the case of penetrating trauma). As was the case with Jackson,[108] they did not perform a synovectomy in acute cases, although removal of the synovial membrane is probably necessary in chronic cases. Ivey and Clark[109] reported excellent results in 11 of 11 cases. Smith[110] achieved excellent results (with full motion) in 28 of 30 patients, and good results in the other two patients. As further proof of the advantage of the arthroscopic approach in this problem, the children in Smith's series had an average hospital stay of 3.5 days, whereas the adults' average length of hospitalization was 9.5 days. This is in contrast with most series of open drainage, which are associated with much more lengthy hospital stays.

The arthroscopic management of infected joints is based on a thorough débridement and copious irrigation of the entire interior of the joint. This includes, in the knee, the posterior compartments, which necessitates supplementary posterior portals.

All fibrinous debris and loculations must be removed, and the decision as to whether to perform a synovectomy is based on the chronicity of the process and the assessment of synovial involvement. A suction drain should be placed postoperatively. If there is question as to the adequacy of the original débridement, or a more difficult organism is encountered, a repeat arthroscopic lavage can be carried out in another 2 or 3 days. Postoperatively, the use of continuous passive motion is extremely helpful, in order to achieve better motion, to facilitate fluid evacuation through the suction system, and to enhance cartilage nutrition. Parenteral antibiotics are administered between 3 and 7 days, and oral antibiotics are continued for an additional 3 to 5 weeks (provided that serum levels prove adequate).

Other Conditions

Arthroscopy may be helpful in a variety of other articular conditions, such as crystal-induced synovitis and osteoarthritis. Lavage and débridement can provide dramatic, although temporary, relief in selected patients who have failed aggressive medical management. However, synovectomy has not been studied adequately in these conditions to suggest its routine use.

TECHNIQUE OF ARTHROSCOPIC SYNOVECTOMY

General Considerations

Arthroscopic synovectomy is a procedure that should be done only by the experienced arthroscopist.[25, 29, 60] It is a deceptively difficult operation, with many potential pitfalls and complications. Although it may appear to be a technically easy surgical exercise, requiring little more than familiarity with basic triangulation skills and facility with multiple portals, in reality it is quite demanding. A complete synovectomy can be a lengthy, tedious undertaking, sometimes taking between 90 and 120 minutes. This requires an abundance of patience and persistence on the part of the surgeon. Rigid adherence to a systematic approach is mandatory in order to avoid leaving behind islands of pathologic synovium. Motorized cutting instruments greatly facilitate synovial removal, but care must be taken to monitor the depth of resection, to prevent damage to muscles, tendons, and neurovascular structures. Finally, knowledge of the specific disease processes (e.g., rheumatoid disease, hemophilia) is fundamental to eliminating potentially disastrous sequelae of surgical procedures in these patients.

Local anesthesia is not suitable for arthroscopic synovectomy, because of the multiple portals, length of the procedure, and the need for a tourniquet.[60] Although regional anesthesia provides the requisite muscular relaxation to allow sufficient exposure of the medial and lateral compartments, many surgeons prefer (in the absence of any medical contraindications) general anesthesia.[111, 112] This is because of the complete lack of tourniquet pain and patient discomfort (regardless of the length of the operation) with general anesthesia as well as the rapidity with which the patient is able to be discharged from an ambulatory surgery setting.

A tourniquet is essential (except in the shoulder) for efficient synovial excision.[112] During the early stages of removal of an inflamed synovial membrane, there may be considerable bleeding without tourniquet control. Tourniquet pressure can be set at 100 mm Hg above systolic pressure,[113–115] although the pressure may need to be somewhat higher (to prevent venous bleeding) in a patient with a large thigh. If the procedure lasts more than 90 minutes, the tourniquet should be deflated for 15 minutes to allow for reperfusion.[113] Reinflation for another 30 minutes is then permissible.

A high-flow irrigation system is mandatory because of the use of motorized suction instruments during virtually the entire procedure, the need to clear large amounts of debris and blood, and the need for continuous capsular distention.[112] Although high flow is possible with a gravity system and large-bore inflow cannulae, an infusion pump with independent controls over pressure and flow rate simplifies the procedure. Care must be taken to avoid excessive joint distention, with subsequent capsular rupture and soft tissue extravasation.

A combination of manual and motorized instrumentation is essential. Probes are utilized during the diagnostic phase to palpate and investigate the status of menisci, ligaments, and articular cartilage. Pituitary rongeurs are useful for obtaining tissue for biopsy. Synovial membrane removal is accomplished by a motorized suction device with a series of cutting heads (Fig. 39–5A and B). The development of this particular tool has made arthroscopic synovectomy feasible. Ranging in size from 2.7 mm to 5.5 mm (outer diameter), the cutting tips consist of an outer hollow sleeve with a window near the tip and an inner, motor-driven cutting head that rotates. Suction pulls the tissue to be cut into the window, and the inner cutting head resects the tissue, which is then cleared down the hollow assembly into a suction reservoir. Working at speeds between 200 and 900 rpm, these devices are fast and efficient.

It is helpful to have a number of arthroscopes available. The primary arthroscope has an objective lens angled 25 degrees or 30 degrees away from the long axis of the scope. Rotation of the arthroscope then increases the conical field of vision (Fig. 39–6). It is important to have at least one additional scope with a higher angle of inclination (usually 70 degrees) to facilitate looking around corners and into recesses.

Familiarity with multiple portals is critical to a complete synovial excision, regardless of the joint being addressed. The need to visualize the entire

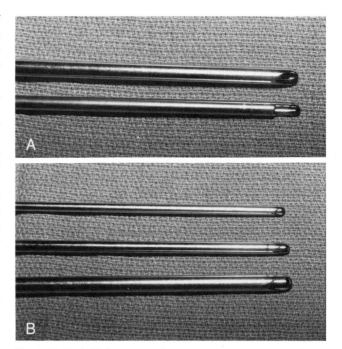

Figure 39–5. *A,* Each motorized cutting piece is composed of two elements: an outer sleeve and an inner hollow cutting head that rotates. *B,* Assembled synovial resectors, in 3.5-mm, 4.2-mm, and 5.5-mm sizes.

interior of the joint, along with the ability to cover the complete extent of the synovial surface area with the cutting instrument dictates the use of all standard, and many accessory portals. Inability to deliver the arthroscope and cutting instrument into every region of a joint limits the procedure to a partial synovectomy.

Knee

The patient is placed supine on the operating table, and general or regional anesthesia is induced (Fig. 39–7). A pneumatic tourniquet is placed around the proximal thigh, and the thigh is placed in an

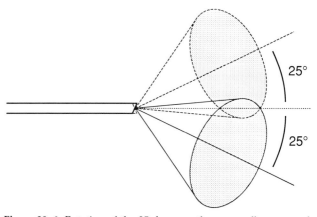

Figure 39–6. Rotation of the 25-degree arthroscope allows a much greater conical field of vision.

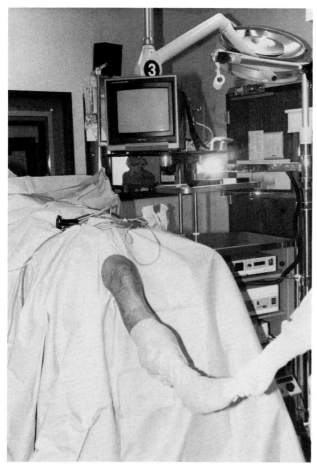

Figure 39–7. Operative set-up for arthroscopic synovectomy of the knee.

Since a systematic approach is critical to avoiding incomplete synovial removal, it is helpful to conceptualize the synovectomy as a procedure with six distinct steps.[60, 111]

Step 1. The first step is to carry out a thorough diagnostic arthroscopy to catalogue the extent of pathology present within the joint. Any articular or meniscal lesions should be noted, and plans should be made at some point during the procedure to débride these accordingly (see Fig. 39–2). The quantity and quality of abnormal synovial tissue is observed, as well as its distribution. Tissue is biopsied with a pituitary rongeur, sampling in the region of most florid involvement (usually the floor of the suprapatellar pouch, or in the medial or lateral recesses).

Step 2. The synovectomy begins in the anterior compartment. The suprapatellar pouch and medial and lateral gutters contain the largest volume of synovial membrane to be excised, and it is best to approach these areas first, to preserve tourniquet time and before fatigue is a factor. With the 25-degree arthroscope in the anterolateral portal and the motorized cutter in the anteromedial portal, resection of the membrane is carried out in a sequential fashion. Care is taken to stay in one area until the membrane is completely removed, rather than skipping around (Fig. 39–8; see color section at the front of this volume). When no more synovial membrane can be reached with the instruments in one set of portals, others are then used. All four of the anterior portals (anteromedial, anterolateral, medial, and lat-

arthroscopic leg-holding device.[111] It is important to position the tourniquet and leg holder more proximally on the thigh to achieve more clearance space for use of the arthroscope and the motorized cutting heads alternately in each of the suprapatellar portals. The contralateral limb is placed on a well leg support to prevent hyperextension of the hip[111] (and possible femoral neuropraxia) and is padded adequately to guard against excess pressure.

The tourniquet is inflated after exsanguination of the extremity (although this can be deferred until after the initial diagnostic arthroscopy is carried out, in order to minimize the total tourniquet time). The 25-degree arthroscope is inserted through the anterolateral portal, just lateral to the patellar tendon and just above the lateral meniscus. The joint is then insufflated with irrigating fluid, and the outflow cannula–pressure-monitoring device is placed in the medial suprapatellar portal. The anteromedial portal is usually positioned 1 cm medial to the patellar tendon and immediately above the medial meniscus. Correct location of this portal is best checked by trial placement of an 18-gauge spinal needle, to verify that the posterior horn of the medial meniscus can be reached by an instrument inserted through the portal.[116]

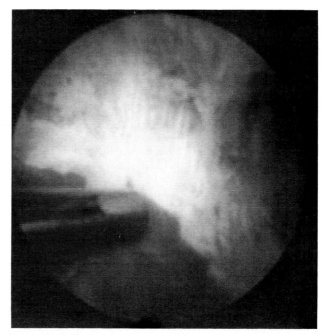

Figure 39–8. Synovial resector working on the anteromedial synovial membrane. Note the boundary between the remaining abnormal synovium and the exposed subsynovial layer. It is important to make every effort to keep working at this boundary in one location rather than skip around to different areas.

eral suprapatellar) are utilized, with the arthroscope and cutting device alternating between them until no more pathologic synovium is visible. Excision of the membrane in the distal gutters is facilitated by inserting the arthroscope into the suprapatellar portals, and the cutters in the anteromedial and anterolateral portals.

Step 3. The third step removes the synovium from the intercondylar notch and the back of the fat pad. This is actually started during step 2 but is continued by triangulation with the scope and cutter alternately in the anteromedial and anterolateral portals. The synovium over the cruciate ligaments and on the inner faces of the condyles is often involved, and a small cutting tip can delicately strip the membrane away without damaging the underlying ligaments. The synovium over the fat pad must be thoroughly excised, and this excision is continued laterally and medially to connect with the resection in the gutters performed in step 2. It is helpful to use a 70-degree arthroscope in this position to help view the midline. Extreme care must be taken not to carry the resection too deeply. There is a report of resection of the patellar tendon during an arthroscopic synovectomy.[117]

Step 4. Excision of the perimeniscal synovium takes place in step 4. Again, the instruments are alternately placed in the two anterior portals. By opening the medial and lateral compartments, the small-diameter cutter can remove the synovium both above and below the meniscus.

Steps 5 and 6. Steps 5 and 6 remove the synovium from the posterolateral and posteromedial compartments, respectively. This is technically the most challenging part of the procedure, but also the most important, as the posterior compartments are the most common site of incomplete removal of the synovial membrane. The arthroscope cannula with blunt obturator is placed in the anteromedial compartment and is directed through the intercondylar notch, between the lateral femoral condyle and the anterior cruciate ligament. The blunt obturator is then withdrawn, and the 70-degree arthroscope inserted. While viewing the posterolateral corner of the joint from the inside, correct placement of the posterolateral portal is verified with an 18-gauge needle. In a thin person, the general vicinity of the portal can be chosen by observing the area of arthroscopic transillumination through the skin. An alternative method is to palpate with a finger on the outside, and observe with the arthroscope on the inside the area of palpation. An absolute rule is that the portal must be anterior to the biceps femoris tendon with the knee flexed, in order to avoid the peroneal nerve. Once the correct site has been selected, the portal is made with a no. 11 scalpel, and the motorized cutter is passed into the joint (see Fig. 39–3B). The synovium is removed from the entire posterolateral compartment. Rotation of the scope allows visualization of the extreme corner of the joint, as well as the midline, but can leave a blind spot in between these two

regions (Fig. 39–9A). This can be remedied by leaving the arthroscopic cannula in the posterolateral compartment and exchanging the 70-degree scope with the 25-degree scope (see Fig. 39–9B).

The posteromedial compartment synovectomy is carried out in an analogous fashion. The blunt obturator and sheath are placed in the anterolateral portal, and then through the intercondylar notch between the medial femoral condyle and the posterior cruciate ligament. The 70-degree scope is inserted, and the posteromedial portal created, first with an 18-gauge needle, followed by a no. 11 scalpel. Use of the 25-degree scope is often helpful here, also.

Pitfalls. Some common mistakes can occur during arthroscopic synovectomy. One mistake is failure to budget operative time appropriately, which, because of the lack of tourniquet time, forces the surgeon to rush through the final stages and end up with an incomplete excision. It is very important to work quickly and systematically and always to keep in mind the stage of the operation in relation to the amount of tourniquet time remaining. Another error is to skip around to areas that are most affected by hypertrophic synovium rather than to concentrate on one area at a time. The best approach is to define a leading edge of the resection and stay with it until no further resection can be carried out with the instruments in those portals. The instruments are then switched, and the resection is resumed at the same location at which it was halted.

High inflow and outflow rates are mandatory. The volume of hypertrophic synovium may be so large that even the 5.5-mm cutting heads may become clogged or dull. Frequent cleaning and occasional replacement with fresh cutting heads are necessary to keep the rate of resection sufficiently high. Finally, one must always see the tip of the cutting head when it is in operation.[30] Although rare, reports of damage to important tendon and neurovascular structures by motorized instrumentation emphasize the importance of not cutting what you cannot see.

Postoperatively, most surgeons decline the use of a suction drain, except in cases of hemophilic arthropathy. A compression dressing is applied, and mild analgesics are used for the first 48 to 72 hours. Some surgeons have their patients use continuous passive-motion devices at home, some advocate supervised physical therapy, and some do not utilize either one. The choice of how to regain postoperative motion should be individualized, based on the specific diagnosis as well as the age, compliance, and overall status of the patient.

Shoulder

Most orthopedists prefer the lateral decubitus position for shoulder arthroscopy. After general anesthesia is induced, the patient is rolled onto his or her side, supported on a vacuum bean bag and

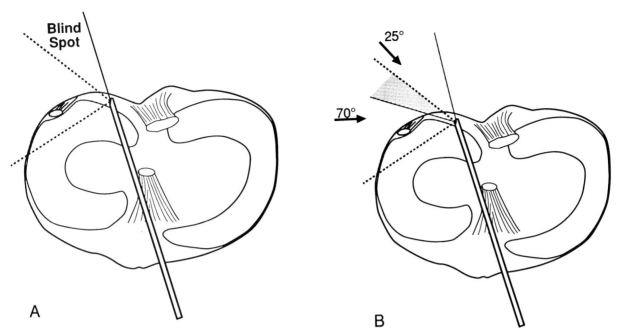

Figure 39–9. Use of both the 25-degree and the 70-degree arthroscopes to completely visualize the posterior compartments. *A,* The 70-degree arthroscope provides excellent visualization of the extreme corners of the joint but leaves a "blind spot," even after rotation of the scope, between the corner and the midline. *B,* Substitution of the 25-degree arthroscope for the 70-degree system. This helps eliminate the blind spot caused by the 70-degree inclined lens.

supplemented with kidney rests.[118] Rolling the patient backwards about 15 degrees allows easier access to the anterior shoulder during the procedure.[119] An axillary pad is placed beneath the unaffected arm, and all bony prominences (including the lower extremities) are adequately padded. The entire shoulder region is then sterilely prepared, and the upper extremity is draped free. A sterile wrist gauntlet or stockinette is utilized to apply skin traction to the wrist and forearm. The shoulder is abducted to approximately 70 degrees and 10 to 15 pounds of traction is applied.[118, 120] There is the possibility of causing a neuropraxia with higher weights.[121]

Some surgeons advocate the use of the seated, beach-chair position.[122, 123] In this technique, the table is flexed so that the patient's torso is elevated to 70 degrees to the horizontal. A pad is placed behind the medial border of the scapula, and the patient is moved to the side of the table so that the shoulder is free. The advantages of this approach include better airway management and the ability to use scalene block anesthesia in certain instances. Other benefits are the ability to perform an anterior open procedure without the need to reprepare and drape the surgical area, easier manipulation of the upper extremity by an assistant, and a more anatomic appearance of intra-articular anatomy.

A complete glenohumeral synovectomy can be accomplished with the use of three portals: posterior, anterior, and superior.[124] Portal placement is facilitated by drawing the superficial bony landmarks on the skin before starting, including the acromion,

clavicle, acromioclavicular joint, and the coracoid process.[125] The typical site of the posterior portal is 3 cm inferior and 1 to 2 cm medial to the posterolateral tip of the acromion.[122, 125] An 18-gauge spinal needle is placed at this location and is then advanced into the glenohumeral space, by aiming for the coracoid process. The joint is then distended with 30 to 60 ml of irrigating solution. A 5-mm skin incision is made, and the arthroscopic cannula with sharp trocar is placed along the same path down to the level of the capsule. A blunt obturator is replaced in the cannula, and the capsule is penetrated. The superior portal is used for inflow or outflow, and its location is determined by palpating the soft spot bordered by the posterior edge of the clavicle, the medial margin of the acromion, and the scapular spine.[122, 126] Again, an 18-gauge spinal needle is useful in verifying the position, and after arthroscopic confirmation, the inflow-outflow cannula is placed.

Care in making an anterior portal is necessary because of the danger of damaging important neurovascular structures. There are two methods of making this portal, one starting on the inside of the joint and the other starting on the outside. The most popular technique is to visualize the anterior capsule with the arthroscope in the posterior portal.[126, 127] There is a triangular space formed by the long head of the biceps tendon, the subscapularis tendon, and the anterosuperior border of the glenoid rim. The arthroscope is advanced into this triangle, and the scope is removed and replaced by a Wissinger rod (a long, straight, conical tipped pin). The rod is advanced through the anterior capsule and subcutaneous tissue and tents the skin. Making sure that the portal passes *lateral* to the coracoid process and conjoined tendon, make the portal and pass another cannula in retrograde fashion over the Wissinger rod and back into the joint. Alternatively, this portal can be established from the outside, selecting a location lateral to the coracoid process and midway between the coracoid and the anterior acromion.[125] An 18-gauge spinal needle is then placed through the anterior soft tissues into the joint, with arthroscopic confirmation that it enters the joint in the triangular space previously described.

The procedure begins with the arthroscope in the posterior portal and the motorized cutter in the anterior portal. Synovial resection in the entire anterior half of the joint (including the superior and inferior aspects) is possible with this arrangement. To resect the synovium in the posterior joint, the instruments are reversed. This is expedited by use of a switching stick (a long rod with blunt tips).[127] Since there is considerable soft tissue between the skin and the glenohumeral capsule, it is best not to remove the arthroscopic cannulae once they are in place. The motorized cutting device is removed from the anterior portal, and a switching stick is placed in the cannula. With the switching stick in the joint, the cannula is removed and replaced over the switching stick by an arthroscopic cannula, followed by placement of the arthroscope itself through the newly inserted cannula in the anterior portal. In a similar fashion, the cannula for the motorized cutter is replaced over a switching stick for the arthroscopic cannula in the posterior portal.

In some cases the subacromial bursa may be affected by the same process as the glenohumeral joint. Subacromial bursoscopy can evaluate the involvement in this area, and a synovectomy can be carried out if necessary.[122] The same posterior skin incision can be utilized, with the arthroscopic cannula (and blunt obturator) redirected immediately underneath the acromion. A lateral portal is helpful and is made 1 to 2 cm below the midlateral acromion.[122] A second anterior portal is occasionally useful, located at the anterior tip of the acromion. Attention must be given to the location of the axillary nerve. It ramifies on the undersurface of the deltoid muscle, approximately 5 cm distal to the acromion. An aggressive resection of the bursa can jeopardize this structure.

Excessive bleeding is sometimes encountered in the glenohumeral and subacromial spaces. This can be controlled in most instances with adequate distention by an infusion pump or by gravity inflow.[122] Caution is recommended, as too high an irrigating pressure can result in large amounts of fluid extravasation into the soft tissues. Electrocautery is also of some benefit. Although most orthopedists advocate use of a nonconducting fluid (e.g., glycine or sterile water), others have safely utilized electrocautery with electrolyte solutions. If bleeding is still excessive, dilute solutions of epinephrine can be employed, if there are no medical or anesthetic contraindications to its use.

A compression dressing and sling are utilized postoperatively. Range-of-motion exercises are instituted on the first postoperative day. Since many of these patients have had restricted motion preoperatively, it is generally helpful to enlist the aid of a physical therapist.

Elbow

Arthroscopy of the elbow shares many of the same advantages as that of other joints, with increased visualization compared with open methods as well as decreased postoperative recovery times.[128, 130] However, the neurovascular anatomy about the elbow makes arthroscopy of this joint somewhat more hazardous than that in other locations.[128–130] Lynch and colleagues[129] carried out a cadaver study and demonstrated the danger of neurovascular injury with incorrect portal placement, direction of entry of instruments, or elbow position, and inadequate joint distention. In addition, there are a number of clinical reports[129, 131–133] of nerve damage following arthroscopy of the elbow.

Elbow arthroscopy is most commonly performed with the patient supine and under general anesthesia.[128] A tourniquet is used, and the elbow is flexed to 90 degrees.[128, 129] The forearm and wrist are attached to an overhead suspension device via a prefabricated wrist gauntlet or stockinette, and traction is applied. This allows access to both the medial and the lateral sides of the elbow, and the forearm can be pronated and supinated.

The bony landmarks should be traced out on the skin prior to incision. The three main portals utilized are the anteromedial, posterolateral, and anterolateral. Accessory portals include straight lateral, straight posterior, and proximal medial. The posteromedial approach is *never* employed, because of the risk to the ulnar nerve. To facilitate insertion of instruments, the joint is first distended with irrigating solution, via an 18-gauge spinal needle inserted in the soft spot of the elbow laterally.[128, 129] The anterolateral portal is made with the elbow flexed 90 degrees and is located 3 cm distal and 1 to 2 cm anterior to the lateral humeral epicondyle.[128, 134] A no. 11 scalpel is used to incise the skin, and the arthroscopic cannula is inserted with the aid of the blunt obturator, being directed to the center of the joint. If the portal is too anterior, the radial nerve is at jeopardy, and if the angle of insertion of the cannula is too anterior, the median nerve and brachial artery can be damaged.[129]

The anteromedial portal is made after the arthroscope has been inserted anterolaterally. The insertion point is 2 cm distal and 2 cm anterior to the medial humeral epicondyle, while the elbow is still flexed 90 degrees.[128, 134] An 18-gauge spinal needle is inserted at this point and is observed with the scope to pass easily into the joint space. The medial antebrachial cutaneous nerve is in close proximity to this portal.[129]

The posterolateral portal is positioned 3 cm proximal to the tip of the olecranon, and just lateral to the triceps muscle.[128] The arthroscopic cannula and blunt obturator are used for insertion, and the elbow should be between 20 degrees and 30 degrees of flexion when this portal is made. There are no major neurovascular structures in association with this portal.[129]

Most of the synovium can be excised using these three portals.[130] Caution must be exercised when removing the synovectomy within this joint. Too aggressive a resection in the midline anteriorly could cause penetration through the capsule, with possible damage to the median nerve and brachial artery. Similarly, the ulnar nerve is at risk when the shaver is in the posterior portal and working toward the medial side of the joint.

Elbow synovectomy can be done on an outpatient basis, and a compressive dressing and sling are utilized for the first few postoperative days for comfort. Postoperative paresthesias and dysesthesias are common and can be due to the use of a tourniquet, extravasation of fluid or local anesthetic through the capsular portals, or traction on a nerve.[128] As soon as the patient is comfortable, an active range-of-motion exercise program is instituted.

Ankle

With current techniques, most synovial lesions of the ankle can be addressed arthroscopically. In addition to routine inflammatory conditions, a syndrome of anterior soft tissue impingement of the ankle has been described. It is believed to be secondary to trauma, usually a severe lateral ligament sprain. Martin and colleagues[135] reported on a series of 16 patients who underwent anterior synovectomy for this condition, with good or excellent results in 75 per cent of patients after a minimum follow-up of 2 years.

As with the elbow and shoulder, thorough familiarity with the soft tissue anatomy about the ankle joint aids greatly in safe, efficient arthroscopic procedures. General or regional anesthesia is employed. There are a number of different methods of positioning the patient.[136] Andrews[137] described a set-up much like that employed in knee arthroscopy, with the knee flexed to 90 degrees over the end of the operating table, and the thigh placed in a knee holder. Parisien[138] has utilized a lateral decubitus position, with the ankle elevated on a padded box. Guhl[139] places the flexed hip and knee of the supine patient over a padded support, while the foot is held in a specially designed ankle holder. One of the easiest and most versatile methods was described by Sweeney.[140] He breaks the end of the operating table

to about 45 degrees, and the arthroscopic knee holder is placed distally, to support the calf. It is well padded, and the tourniquet is still placed around the thigh. In this way, the leg is parallel to the floor, and the surgeon can comfortably operate from a standing position, is free to manipulate the ankle, and has easy access to all sides of the ankle.

Most ankle arthroscopic surgery is performed with the use of three portals. The anterolateral portal is made 5 mm distal to the joint line, and just lateral to the extensor tendons.[141] Through this portal, one can see the entire anterior compartment. The joint is usually distended with 15 to 30 ml of irrigating solution, and the blunt obturator with cannula is inserted into the portal. The anteromedial portal is next created; it is helpful for initial placement of an outflow cannula, and to begin anterior débridement with motorized instrumentation. It is located 5 mm distal to the joint line and just medial to the tibialis anterior tendon.[141] The portal must be lateral to the saphenous vein and nerve; transillumination of this region with the arthroscope in the anterolateral portal is sometimes helpful in identifying these structures. An anterocentral portal has been described but is rarely used, as it is too close to the course of the dorsalis pedis artery and the deep peroneal and medial branch of the superficial peroneal nerves.[141]

The posterolateral portal is often beneficial when instrumentation in the posterior compartment is necessary. It is positioned in the space between the Achilles and peroneal tendons. In order to avoid the sural nerve, it is best to stay close to the lateral border of the Achilles tendon. This portal is usually located about 1 cm distal to the anterolateral portal, since posteriorly the joint line is more distal.

Maneuvering within the ankle joint is sometimes challenging, in part because of the talar dome. The use of an external skeletal distraction apparatus greatly assists working in the posterior compartment. The apparatus is most commonly based laterally,[136, 139] but it can be utilized medially[142] in certain special circumstances. A threaded 3/16-inch pin is placed into the anterior tibia and the calcaneus[136] (or in the talus if the distraction is medially based). The distractor is then attached to the pins, and force is slowly applied until the joint is separated 7 to 8 mm. This allows passage of both the arthroscope and the motorized instrument from anterior to posterior, or the arthroscope can visualize the cutter working through the posterolateral portal.

The synovectomy is begun in the anterior compartment, with the arthroscope and the synovial resector alternating between the anteromedial portal and the anterolateral portal to accomplish a thorough resection anteriorly. Attention needs to be directed inferiorly into the paramalleolar gutters to remove the synovium in these locations. The posterior compartment is then addressed, with the arthroscope visualizing from anterior, and the resector is placed through the three portals as required. The 70-degree arthroscope is occasionally needed to see the extremes of the posterior corners, and into the para-malleolar gutters.

Postoperatively a compression dressing is applied, and the ankle is splinted at neutral for 48 hours. The splint is then removed, and active and passive range-of-motion exercises are started. Partial weightbearing is allowed within the first 48 hours, and progression to full weightbearing is usually possible by 4 to 7 days.

Other Locations

Open synovectomy has been performed in other joints (hip, wrist, small joints of the hand and foot) and in tendon sheaths, with well-documented results.[3] The general indications and contraindications for these regions are the same as those previously discussed. The arthroscopic technique has not been applied to these areas as commonly as in the knee, ankle, shoulder, and elbow, but experience is accumulating.[143]

References

1. Volkmann, R. von: Cited by Hoffmann, R.: Die Synovektomie unter besonderer Berucksichtigung der an der Erlanger Chirurgischen Universitatsklinik erzielten Erfolge. Dissertation, Erlangen, 1952.
2. Swett, P. P.: Synovectomy in chronic infectious arthritis. J. Bone Joint Surg. 5:110, 1923.
3. Gschwend, N.: Synovectomy. In Kelley, W. N., Harris, E. D., Ruddy, S., and Sledge, C. B. (eds.): Textbook of Rheumatology. 3rd ed. Philadelphia, W. B. Saunders Company, 1989.
4. Goldie, I.: A synopsis of surgery for rheumatoid arthritis (excluding the hand). Clin. Orthop. 191:185, 1984.
5. Fassbender, H. G.: Pathologie Rheumatischer Erkrankungen. Berlin, Springer, 1975.
6. Harris, E. D., Jr.: Recent insights into the pathogenesis of the proliferative lesions in rheumatoid arthritis. Arthritis Rheum. 19:68, 1976.
7. Cohen, S., and Jones, R.: An evaluation of the efficacy of arthroscopic synovectomy of the knee in rheumatoid arthritis: 12–24 months results. J. Rheumatol. 14:452, 1987.
8. Barnes, C. G., and Mason, R. M.: Synovectomy of the knee joint in rheumatoid arthritis. Ann. Phys. Med. 9:83, 1957.
9. Goldie, I.: Pathomorphologic features in original and regenerated synovial tissues after synovectomy in rheumatoid arthritis. Clin. Orthop. 77:295, 1971.
10. Ranawat, C. S., Straub, L. R., Freyburg, R., Granda, J. L., and Rivelis, M.: A study of regenerated synovium after synovectomy of the knee in rheumatoid arthritis. Arthritis Rheum. 14:117, 1971.
11. Mitchell, N. S., and Shepard, N.: The effect of synovectomy on synovium and cartilage in early rheumatoid arthritis. Orthop. Clin. North Am. 4:1057, 1973.
12. Paus, A. C., and Pahle, J. A.: Arthroscopic evaluation of the synovial lining before and after open synovectomy of the knee joint in patients with chronic inflammatory joint disease. Scand. J. Rheumatol. 19:193, 1990.
13. Patzakis, M., Mills, D., Bartholomew, B., Clayton, M. L., and Smyth, C. J.: A visual, histological, and enzymatic study of regenerating rheumatoid synovium in the synovectomized knee. J. Bone Joint Surg. 55A:287, 1973.
14. Aschan, W., and Moberg, E.: A long-term study of the effect of early synovectomy in rheumatoid arthritis. Bull. Hosp. Jt. Dis. Orthop. Inst. 44:106, 1984.
15. Laurin, C. A., Desmarchais, J., Daziano, L., Gariepy, R., and Derome, A.: Long-term results of synovectomy of the knee in rheumatoid patients. J. Bone Joint Surg. 56A:521, 1974.
16. Ishikawa, H., Osamu, O., and Hirohata, K.: Long-term results of synovectomy in rheumatoid patients. J. Bone Joint Surg. 68A:198, 1986.
17. Sim, F. H.: Synovial proliferative disorders: Role of synovectomy. Arthroscopy 1:198, 1985.
18. Paradies, L. H.: Synovectomy for rheumatoid arthritis of the knee. J. Bone Joint Surg. 57A:95, 1975.
19. Marmor, L.: Surgery of the rheumatoid knee: Synovectomy and débridement. J. Bone Joint Surg. 55A:535, 1973.
20. Mori, M., and Ogawa, R.: Anterior capsulectomy in the treatment of rheumatoid arthritis of the knee joint. Arthritis Rheum. 6:130, 1963.
21. Marmor, L.: Synovectomy of the knee joint. Orthop. Clinic North Am. 10:211, 1979.
22. Bryan, R. S., and Peterson, L. F.: Synovectomy of the knee. Orthop. Clin. North Am. 2:705, 1971.
23. Ranawat, C. S., and Desai, K.: Role of early synovectomy of the knee joint in rheumatoid arthritis. Arthritis Rheum. 18:117, 1975.
24. Ranawat, C. S., Ecker, M. L., and Straub, L. R.: Synovectomy and débridement of the knee in rheumatoid arthritis (a study of 60 knees). Arthritis Rheum. 15:571, 1972.
25. Highgenboten, C. L.: Arthroscopic synovectomy. Orthop. Clinic North Am. 13:399, 1982.
26. Graham, J., and Checketts, R. G.: Synovectomy of the knee joint in rheumatoid arthritis. J. Bone Joint Surg. 55B:786, 1973.
27. Matsui, N., Taneda, Y., Ohta, H., Itoh, T., and Tsuboguchi, S.: Arthroscopic versus open synovectomy in the rheumatoid knee. Int. Orthop. 13:17, 1989.
28. Aritomi, H.: Arthroscopic synovectomy of the knee joint with the electric resectoscope. Scand. J. Haematol. (Suppl.) 40:249, 1984.
29. Meyers, J. F.: Surgical technique for arthroscopic synovectomy. Contemp. Orthop. 10:41, 1985.
30. Ogilvie-Harris, D. J., and Basinski, A.: Arthroscopic synovectomy of the knee for rheumatoid arthritis. Arthroscopy 7:91, 1991.
31. Highgenboten, C. L.: Arthroscopic synovectomy. Arthroscopy 1:190, 1985.
32. Von Reis, G., and Swensson, A.: Intra-articular injections of osmic acid in painful joint affections. Acta Med. Scand. 140(Suppl. 259):27, 1951.
33. Nissila, M., Anttila, P., Hamalainen, M., and Jalava, S.: Comparison of chemical, radiation, and surgical synovectomy for knee joint synovitis. Scand. J. Rheumatol. 7:225, 1978.
34. Fearnley, M. E.: Intra-articular thiotepa in rheumatoid arthritis. Ann. Phys. Med. 7:294, 1963.
35. Flatt, A. E.: Intra-articular thiotepa in rheumatoid disease of the hands. Rheumatism 18:70, 1962.
36. Fellinger, K., and Schmid, J.: Die Lokale Behandlund der rheumatischen erkraankungen. Wein Z. Inn. Med. 33:351, 1952.
37. Sledge, C. B., Atcher, R. W., Shortkroff, S., Anderson, R. J., Bloomer, W. D., and Hurson, B. J.: Intra-articular radiation synovectomy. Clin. Orthop. 182:37, 1984.
38. Onetti, C., Guitierrez, E., Hilba, E., and Aguirre, C. R.: Synoviorthesis with ^{32}P colloidal chromic phosphate in rheumatoid arthritis: Clinical, histopathologic, and arthrographic changes. J. Rheumatol. 9:229, 1982.
39. Gumpel, J. M., Beer, T. C., Crawley, J. C. W., and Farran, H. E. A.: Yttrium 90 in persistent synovitis of the knee—a single centre comparison. The retention and extra-articular spread of four ^{90}Y radiocolloids. Br. J. Radiol. 48:377, 1975.
40. Beatson, T. R.: Radiation synovectomy (synoviorthesis) for rheumatoid arthritis in the Isle of Man. Gerontology 28:258, 1982.
41. Sledge, C. B., Zuckerman, J. D., Zalutsky, M. R., Atcher, R. W., Shortkroff, S., Lionberger, D. R., Rose, H. A., Hurson, B. J., Lankenner, P. A., Jr., Anderson, R. J., and Bloomer, W. A.: Treatment of rheumatoid synovitis of the knee with intra-articular injection of dysprosium 165–ferric hydroxide macroaggregates. Arthritis Rheum. 29:153, 1986.
42. Gumpel, J. M., and Stevenson, A. C.: Chromosomal damage after intra-articular injection of different colloids of ^{90}yttrium. Rheumatol. Rehab. 14:7, 1975.
43. Sledge, C. B., Noble, J., Hnatowich, D. J., Kramer, R., and Shortkroff, S.: Experimental radiation synovectomy by ^{165}Dy ferric hydroxide macroaggregate. Arthritis Rheum. 20:1334, 1977.
44. Spooren, P. F., Rasker, J. J., and Arens, R. P.: Synovectomy of the knee with ^{90}Y. Eur. J. Nucl. Med. 10:441, 1985.
45. Boerbooms, A. M. Th., Buijs, W. C. A. M., Danen, M., van de Putte, L. B. A., and Vandenbroucke, J. P.: Radio-synovectomy in chronic synovitis of the knee joint in patients with rheumatoid arthritis. Eur. J. Nucl. Med. 10:446, 1985.
46. Gumpel, J. M., and Roles, N. C.: A controlled trial of intra-articular radiocolloids versus surgical synovectomy in persistent synovitis. Lancet 1:488, 1975.
47. Sheppeard, H., Aldin, A., and Ward, D. J.: Osmic acid versus yttrium-90 in rheumatoid synovitis of the knee. Scand. J. Rheumat. 10:234, 1981.
48. Menkes, C. J., et al.: Le traitement des rhumatismes par les synoviotheses. Rhumatologie 1(Suppl.):61, 1972.
49. de la Chapelle, A., Oka, M., Rekonen, A., and Ruotsi, A.: Chromosome damage after intra-articular injection of radioactive yttrium. Effect of immobilisation on the biological dose. Ann. Rheum. Dis. 31:508, 1972.

50. Stevenson, A. C.: Chromosomal damage in human lymphocytes from radio-isotope therapy. Ann. Rheum. Dis. 32(Suppl.):19, 1973.

51. Doyle, D. V., Glass, J. S., Gow, P. J., Daker, M., and Grahame, R.: A clinical and prospective chromosomal study of 90yttrium synovectomy. Rheumatol. Rehab. 16:217, 1977.

52. Gumpel, J. M.: Review of published and personal results. Ann. Rheum. Dis. 32:29, 1973.

53. McEwen, C.: Multicenter evaluation of synovectomy in the treatment of rheumatoid arthritis. Report of results at the end of five years. J. Rheumatol. 15:764, 1988.

54. Arthritis Foundation Committee on Evaluation of Synovectomy: Multicenter evaluation of synovectomy in the treatment of rheumatoid arthritis. Arthritis Rheum. 20:765, 1977.

55. Geens, S., Clayton, M. L., Leidholt, J. D., Smyth, C. J., and Bartholomew, B. A.: Synovectomy and débridement of the knee in rheumatoid arthritis: Part II. Clinical and roentgenographic study of thirty-one cases. J. Bone Joint Surg. 51A:626, 1969.

56. Doets, H., Bierman, B., and Soesbergen, R.: Synovectomy of the rheumatoid knee does not prevent deterioration. Acta Orthop. Scand. 60:523, 1989.

57. Arthritis and Rheumatism Council and British Orthopaedic Association: Controlled trial of synovectomy of knee and metacarpophalangeal joints in rheumatoid arthritis. Ann. Rheum. Dis. 35:437, 1976.

58. Cleland, L. G., Treganza, R., and Dobson, P.: Arthroscopic synovectomy: A prospective study. J. Rheumatol. 13:907, 1986.

59. Klein, W., and Jensen, K.-U.: Arthroscopic synovectomy of the knee joint: Indications, technique, and follow-up results. Arthroscopy 4:63, 1988.

60. Rosenberg, T. D., Tearse, D. S., and Kolowich, P. A.: Synovectomy of the knee. In McGinty, J. B. (ed.): Operative arthroscopy. New York, Raven Press, 1991.

61. Arnold, W. D., and Hilgartner, M. W.: Hemophilic arthropathy: Current concepts of pathogenesis and management. J. Bone Joint Surg. 59A:287, 1977.

62. DePalma, A. F.: Hemophilic arthropathy. Clin. Orthop. 52:145, 1967.

63. Storti, E., and Ascari, E.: Surgical and chemical synovectomy. Ann. N.Y. Acad. Sci. 240:316, 1975.

64. Dyszy-Laube, B., Kaminski, W., Gizycka, I., Kaminska, D., Sekowska-Zmuda, J., and Luder, E.: Synovectomy in the treatment of hemophilic arthropathy. J. Pediatr. Surg. 9:123, 1974.

65. Stein, H., and Duthie, R. B.: The pathogenesis of chronic haemophilic arthropathy. J. Bone Joint Surg. 63B:601, 1981.

66. Storti, E., Traldi, A., Tosatti, E., and Davoli, P. G.: Synovectomy, a new approach to hemophilic arthropathy. Acta Haematol. 41:193, 1969.

67. McCollough, N. C., Enis, J. E., Lovitt, J., Lian, E. C.-Y., Niemann, K. N. W., and Loughlin, E. C.: Synovectomy or total replacement of the knee in hemophilia. J. Bone Joint Surg. 61A:69, 1979.

68. Kay, L., Stainsby, D., Buzzard, B., Fearns, M., Hamilton, P. J., Owen, P., and Jones, P.: The role of synovectomy in the management of recurrent haemarthroses in haemophilia. Br. J. Haematol. 49:53, 1981.

69. Montane, I., McCollough, N. C., and Lian, E. C.-Y.: Synovectomy of the knee for hemophilic arthropathy. J. Bone Joint Surg. 68A:210, 1986.

70. Post, M., Watts, G., and Telfer, M.: Synovectomy in hemophilic arthropathy: A retrospective review of 17 cases. Clin. Orthop. 202:139, 1986.

71. Canale, S. T., Dugdale, M., and Howard, B. C.: Synovectomy of the knee in young patients with hemophilia. South. Med. J. 81:1480, 1988.

72. Nicol, R. O., and Menelaus, M. B.: Synovectomy of the knee in hemophilia. J. Pediatr. Orthop. 6:330, 1986.

73. Pietrogrande, V., Dioguardi, N., and Mannucci, P. M.: Short-term evaluation of synovectomy in haemophilia. Br. Med. J. 2:378, 1972.

74. Bussi, L., Silvello, L., Baudo, F., and DeCataldo, F.: Results of synovectomy of the knee in haemophilia. Haematologica (Pavia)59:81, 1974.

75. Clark, M. W.: Knee synovectomy in hemophilia. Orthopedics 1:285, 1978.

76. Wiedel, J. D.: Arthroscopic synovectomy in hemophilic arthropathy of the knee. Scand. J. Haematol. (Suppl.)40:263, 1984.

77. Wiedel, J. D.: Arthroscopic synovectomy for chronic hemophilic synovitis of the knee. Arthroscopy 1:205, 1985.

78. Limbird, T. J., and Dennis, S. C.: Synovectomy and continuous passive motion in hemophilic patients. Arthroscopy 3:74, 1987.

79. Luck, J. V., and Kasper, C. K.: Surgical management of advanced hemophilic arthropathy: An overview of 20 years' experience. Clin. Orthop. 242:60, 1989.

80. Green, W. B., and McMillan, C. W.: Nonsurgical management of hemophilic arthropathy. In Barr, J. S. (ed.): Instructional Course Lectures, Vol. XXXVIII. Park Ridge, IL, American Academy of Orthopaedic Surgeons, 1989.

81. DeGnore, L. T., and Wilson, F. C.: Surgical management of hemophilic arthropathy. In Barr, J. S. (ed.): Instructional Course Lectures, Vol. XXXVIII. Park Ridge, IL, American Academy of Orthopaedic Surgeons, 1989.

82. Casscells, C. D.: Commentary: The argument for early arthroscopic synovectomy in patients with severe hemophilia. Arthroscopy 3:78, 1987.

83. Klein, K. S., Aland, C. M., Kim, H. C., Eisele, J., and Saidi, P.: Long term follow-up of arthroscopic synovectomy for chronic hemophilic synovitis. Arthroscopy 3:231, 1987.

84. Greene, W. B., DeGnore, L. T., and White, G. C.: Orthopaedic procedures and prognosis in hemophilic patients who are seropositive for human immunodeficiency virus. J. Bone Joint Surg. 72A:2, 1990.

85. Kim, H. C., Klein, K., Hirsch, S., Seibold, J. R., Eisele, J., and Saidi, P.: Arthroscopic synovectomy in the treatment of hemophilic synovitis. Scand. J. Haematol. (Suppl.)40:271, 1984.

86. Poggini, L., Chistolini, A., Mariani, G., and Mariani, P. P.: Arthroscopic synovectomy in the treatment of haemophilic arthropathy: Preliminary results in eight patients. Ital. J. Orthop. Traumatol. 15:457, 1989.

87. Flandry, F., and Norwood, L. A.: Pigmented villonodular synovitis of the shoulder. Orthopedics 12:715, 1989.

88. Schwartz, H. S., Unni, K. K., and Pritchard, D. J.: Pigmented villonodular synovitis: A retrospective review of affected larger joints. Clin. Orthop. 247:243, 1989.

89. Jaffe, H. L., Lichenstein, L., and Sutro, C. J.: Pigmented villonodular synovitis, bursitis, and tenosynovitis. Arch. Pathol. 31:731, 1941.

90. Byers, P. D., Cotton, R. E., Deacon, O. W., Lowy, M., Newman, P. H., Sissons, H. A., and Thomson, A. D.: The diagnosis and treatment of pigmented villonodular synovitis. J. Bone Joint Surg. 50B:290, 1968.

91. Myers, B. W., Masi, A. T., and Feigenbaum, S. L.: Pigmented villonodular synovitis and tenosynovitis: A clinical epidemiologic study of 166 cases and literature review. Medicine 59:223, 1980.

92. Poletti, S. C., Gates, H. S., Martinez, S. M., and Richardson, W. J.: The use of magnetic resonance imaging in the diagnosis of pigmented villonodular synovitis. Orthopedics 13:185, 1990.

93. Johansson, J. E., Ajjoub, S., Coughlin, L. P., et al.: Pigmented villonodular synovitis of joints. Clin. Orthop. 163:159, 1982.

94. Jones, F. E., Soule, E. H., and Coventry, M. B.: Fibrous xanthoma of synovium (giant cell tumor of tendon sheath pigmented nodular synovitis). J. Bone Joint Surg. 51A:76, 1969.

94a. Ogilvie-Harris, D. J., McLean, J., and Zarnett, M. E.: Pigmented villonodular synovitis of the knee. J. Bone Joint Surg. 74A:119, 1992.

95. Wright, C. J. E.: Benign giant cell synovioma: An investigation of 85 cases. Br. J. Surg. 38:257, 1951.

96. Sim, F. H., Dahlin, D. C., and Ivins, J. C.: Extra-articular synovial chondromatosis. J. Bone Joint Surg. 59A:492, 1977.

97. Jaffe, H. L.: Tumors and Tumorous Conditions of the Bones and Joints. Philadelphia, Lea & Febiger, 1958.

98. Maurice, H., Crone, M., and Watt, I.: Synovial chondromatosis. J. Bone Joint Surg. 70B:807, 1988.

99. Milgram, J. W.: Synovial osteochondromatosis: A histopathological study of thirty cases. J. Bone Joint Surg. 59A:792, 1977.

100. Zimmerman, C., and Sayegh, V.: Roentgen manifestations of synovial osteochondromatosis. A. J. R. 83:680, 1960.

101. Prager, R. J., and Mall, J. C.: Arthrographic diagnosis of synovial chondromatosis. A.J.R. 127:344, 1976.

102. Murphy, F. P., Dahlin, D. C., and Sullivan, C. R.: Articular synovial chondromatosis. J. Bone Joint Surg. 44A:77, 1962.

103. Jeffreys, T. E.: Synovial chondromatosis. J. Bone Joint Surg. 49B:530, 1967.

104. Dorfmann, H., DeBie, B., Bonvarlet, J. P., and Boyer, T.: Arthroscopic treatment of synovial chondromatosis of the knee. Arthroscopy 5:48, 1989.

105. Kelly, P. J., Martin, W. J., and Coventry, M. B.: Bacterial (suppurative) arthritis in the adult. J. Bone Joint Surg. 1:1595, 1970.

106. Ballard, A., Burkhalter, W. E., Mayfield, G. W., Dehne, E., and Brown, P.: The functional treatment of pyogenic arthritis of the adult knee. J. Bone Joint Surg. 57A:1119, 1975.

107. Tscherne, H., Giebel, G., Muhr, G., and Howell, C.: Synovectomy as treatment for purulent joint infection. Arch. Orthop. Trauma Surg. 103:162, 1984.

108. Jackson, R. W.: The septic knee—arthroscopic treatment. Arthroscopy 1:194, 1985.

109. Ivey, M., and Clark, R.: Arthroscopic débridement of the knee for septic arthritis. Clin. Orthop. 199:201, 1985.

110. Smith, M. J.: Arthroscopic treatment of the septic knee. Arthroscopy 2:30, 1986.

111. Rosenberg, T. D., Paulos, L. E., Parker, R. D., and Abbott, P. J.: Arthroscopic surgery of the knee. In Chapman, M. W. (ed.): Operative Orthopaedics. Philadelphia, J. B. Lippincott Company, 1988.

112. Dandy, D. J.: Basic technique: The standard approach. In McGinty, J. B. (ed.): Operative Arthroscopy. New York, Raven Press, 1991.

113. Milford, L.: Surgical technique and aftercare. In Crenshaw, A. H. (ed.): Campbell's Operative Orthopaedics. 7th ed. St. Louis, C. V. Mosby, 1987.

114. Crenshaw, A. H.: Surgical techniques. In Crenshaw, A. H. (ed.): Campbell's Operative Orthopaedics. 7th ed. St. Louis, C. V. Mosby, 1987.

115. Estersohn, H. S., and Sourifman, H. A.: The minimum effective midthigh tourniquet pressure. J. Foot Surg. 21:281, 1982.
116. Carson, W. G.: Arthroscopic techniques to improve access to posterior meniscal lesions. Clin. Sports Med. 9:619, 1990.
117. Bachner, E. J., Parker, R. D., and Zaas, R. D.: Resection of the patellar ligament: A complication of arthroscopic synovectomy. Arthroscopy 5:76, 1989.
118. Andrews, J. R., and Heckman, M. M.: Shoulder arthroscopy operating room set-up. In McGinty, J. B. (ed.): Operative Arthroscopy. New York, Raven Press, 1991.
119. Andrews, J. R., Carson, W. G., and Ortega, K.: Arthroscopy of the shoulder: Technique and normal anatomy. Am. J. Sports Med. 12:1, 1984.
120. Caspari, R. B.: Shoulder arthroscopy: A review of the present state of the art. Contemp. Orthop. 4:523, 1982.
121. Klein, A. H., France, J. C., Mutschler, T. A., and Fu, F. H.: Measurement of brachial plexus strain in arthroscopy of the shoulder. Arthroscopy 3:45, 1987.
122. Altchek, D. W., Warren, R. F., and Skyhar, M. J.: Shoulder arthroscopy. In Rockwood, C. A., and Matsen, F. A. (eds.): The Shoulder. Philadelphia, W. B. Saunders Company, 1990.
123. Skyhar, M. J., Altchek, D. W., Warren, R. F., Wickiewicz, T. L., and O'Brien, S. J.: Shoulder arthroscopy with the patient in the beach-chair position. Arthroscopy 4:256, 1988.
124. Matthews, L. S., Wolock, B. S., and Martin, D. F.: Arthroscopic management of inflammatory arthritis and synovitis of the shoulder. In McGinty, J. B. (ed.): Operative Arthroscopy. New York, Raven Press, 1991.
125. Andrews, J. R., and Heckman, M. M.: Basic techniques for shoulder arthroscopy. In McGinty, J. B. (ed.): Operative Arthroscopy. New York, Raven Press, 1991.
126. Caspari, R. B.: Anatomy and portals for arthroscopic surgery of the shoulder. In McGinty, J. B. (ed.): Arthroscopic Surgery Update: Techniques in Orthopaedics. Rockville, MD, Aspen Systems Corporation, 1985.
127. Johnson, L. L.: Shoulder arthroscopy. In Arthroscopic Surgery: Principles and Practice. St. Louis, C. V. Mosby Company, 1986.
128. Carson, W. G., and Meyers, J. F.: Diagnostic arthroscopy of the elbow: Surgical technique and arthroscopic and portal anatomy. In McGinty, J. B. (ed.): Operative Arthroscopy. New York, Raven Press, 1991.
129. Lynch, G. J., Meyers, J. F., Whipple, T. L., and Caspari, R. B.: Neurovascular anatomy and elbow arthroscopy: Inherent risks. Arthroscopy 2:191, 1986.
130. Andrews, J. R., and McKenzie, P. J.: Arthroscopic surgical treatment of elbow pathology. In McGinty, J. B. (ed.): Operative Arthroscopy. New York, Raven Press, 1991.
131. Cascells, S. W.: Neurovascular anatomy and elbow arthroscopy: Inherent risks (editor's comments). Arthroscopy 2:190, 1986.
132. Thomas, M. A., Fast, A., and Shapiro, D.: Radial nerve damage as complication of elbow arthroscopy. Clin. Orthop. 215:130, 1987.
133. Guhl, J. F.: Arthroscopy and arthroscopic surgery of the elbow. Orthopaedics 8:290, 1985.
134. Andrews, J. R., and Carson, W. G.: Arthroscopy of the elbow. Arthroscopy 1:97, 1985.
135. Martin, D. F., Curl, W. W., and Baker, C. L.: Arthroscopic treatment of chronic synovitis of the ankle. Arthroscopy 5:110, 1989.
136. Guhl, J. F.: Ankle arthroscopy: Special equipment, operating room set-up, and technique: In McGinty, J. B. (ed.): Operative Arthroscopy. New York, Raven Press, 1991.
137. Andrews, J. R.: Seminar given at The American Foot and Ankle Society. San Francisco, CA, January, 1987.
138. Parisien, J. S.: Instrumentation in arthroscopic surgery of the ankle. In Guhl, J. F. (ed.): Ankle Arthroscopy: Pathology and Surgical Indications. Thorofare, NJ, Slack, Inc., 1988.
139. Guhl, J. F.: Portals and techniques. In Guhl, J. F. (ed.): Ankle Arthroscopy: Pathology and Surgical Indications. Thorofare, NJ, Slack, Inc., 1988.
140. Sweeney, H.: Ankle Arthroscopy. Presented at "Arthroscopic Surgery—1986." Salt Lake City, UT, January, 16–18, 1986.
141. Morgan, C. D.: Gross and arthroscopic anatomy of the ankle. In McGinty, J. B. (ed.): Operative Arthroscopy. New York, Raven Press, 1991.
142. Morgan, C. D.: Arthroscopic tibiotalar arthrodesis. In McGinty, J. B. (ed.): Operative Arthroscopy. New York, Raven Press, 1991.
143. McGinty, J. B. (ed.): Operative Arthroscopy. New York, Raven Press, 1991.
144. Conaty, J.: Surgery of the hip and knee in patients with rheumatoid arthritis. J. Bone Joint Surg. 55A:301, 1973.
145. Kohler, G., Coldewey, J., and Richter, R.: Zur Fruhsynovektomie des Kniegelenkes (Stadium I nach Steinbrocker) bei chronischer Polyarthritis. Akt. Rheumatol. 10:129, 1985.
146. Brattstrom, et al., Czurda, et al., Gschwend, et al., Hagena, et al., Kinell, et al., Kohler, G., Mori, et al., Pavlov, et al., and Thabe, et al.: Long-term results of knee synovectomy in early cases of rheumatoid arthritis. Clin. Rheumatol. 4:19, 1985.
147. Wilkes, L. L.: Arthroscopic synovectomy in the rheumatoid knee. J. Med. Assoc. Ga. 74:582, 1985.
148. Aeckerle, J., and Heisel, J.: Die Behandlung chronisch arthrotischer Reizergusse des Kniegelenkes durch die radiologische Synoviorthese mit Yttrium-90. Orthop. Praxis 8:619, 1985.
149. Smiley, P., and Wasilewski, S. A.: Arthroscopic synovectomy. Arthroscopy 6:18, 1990.

Chapter 40

Stanley P. Ballou
Irving Kushner

Laboratory Evaluation of Inflammation

INTRODUCTION

The inflammatory process occupies a central pathophysiologic role in many rheumatic diseases. Although examination of histopathology can provide information concerning the presence and extent of inflammatory changes, from a clinical viewpoint the laboratory evaluation of inflammation ordinarily involves assessment of elements of the *acute phase response*, the array of systemic and metabolic changes that occur following tissue injury or infection.[1] The acute phase response has been noted following a large variety of inflammatory or injurious stimuli, including surgery, trauma, tissue ischemia, bacterial (and, less frequently, viral) infections, rheumatic and other systemic inflammatory diseases, advanced malignancies, childbirth, and even extremely vigorous physical exercise.[2] The major changes noted are in the concentrations of a heterogeneous group of plasma proteins: the *acute phase proteins*. If the inflammatory stimulus is self-limited or is treated, acute phase protein levels return to normal within days or weeks, whereas tissue alterations that continue may lead to persistent "acute phase" changes.

The proteins that participate in this response display variable acute phase behavior. The concentrations of some proteins, such as ceruloplasmin and several complement components, rise to levels 50 percent greater than normal, while others, such as haptoglobin, α_1-protease inhibitor (α_1-antitrypsin), and fibrinogen, may increase several fold. The major acute phase reactants in humans are C-reactive protein (CRP) and serum amyloid A (SAA). In both cases, concentrations several hundredfold above those found in normal individuals occur commonly, and concentrations one-thousandfold or more above normal may be seen in severe inflammatory states, usually infections. In contrast, the concentrations of several plasma proteins fall. Of these "negative" acute phase proteins, the most prominent is albumin. These acute phase changes are of great interest, both because their measurement can be of clinical value and because of the questions they raise concerning the mechanisms that regulate their synthesis and the functions served by these proteins.

Mechanisms, Teleology, and Clinical Usefulness

The changes in concentration of acute phase proteins following inflammatory stimuli have been shown to result primarily from alterations in synthesis by hepatocytes.[3] In vitro studies have shown that cytokines, the polypeptide regulatory mediators secreted by activated monocytes, macrophages, fibroblasts, endothelial cells, and certain other cells, play a central role in the regulation of acute phase protein synthesis.[4, 5] Among these cytokines are interleukin-6, interleukin-1, tumor necrosis factor-α, and γ-interferon. The mechanisms of acute phase protein induction at the molecular level have been the subject of great interest and may involve both transcriptional and post-transcriptional events.[6, 7] Acute phase reactant levels do not always rise coordinately, suggesting heterogeneous and independently regulated inducing mechanisms. Recent data indicate that various acute phase proteins respond differently to different combinations of cytokines and that the potential exists for highly specific regulation of synthesis of individual plasma proteins by cytokine interactions.[4, 8]

Teleologic considerations suggest that the changes in concentration of these proteins permit improved functional capacity to cope with the consequences of tissue injury or infection. Thus, CRP has been identified at local sites of inflammation,[9, 10] and administration of this acute phase protein is protective against experimentally induced pneumonia in mice.[11, 12] As is the case with many defense mechanisms, the acute phase response may, in some cases, be injurious; for example, the deposition of amyloid A in parenchymal tissue consequent to prolonged elevation of SAA.[13] The precise role played by the individual acute phase proteins in the response to tissue injury may be inferred from the known functional capabilities of these proteins but is difficult to establish with certainty, since in vitro effects may not always be relevant to in vivo phenomena.

The most widely employed indicators of the acute phase response in clinical medicine are measurement of the erythrocyte sedimentation rate (ESR) and serum CRP concentration. These tests have been employed clinically to gauge the presence and degree of inflammation, and to monitor the course of disease in individual patients, as guides to management. The bulk of this chapter deals with these two tests and their clinical significance.

ERYTHROCYTE SEDIMENTATION RATE

In this test, anticoagulated blood is placed in a vertical cylindrical tube, and the ESR is measured. It has been known since the time of the ancient Greeks that the sedimentation rate may be altered in disease states, and this test has been widely employed in clinical medicine for nearly 70 years. The ESR should be viewed as an indirect way of screening for increased concentrations of fibrinogen and, to a lesser extent, of other acute phase proteins; such changes cause increased aggregation of erythrocytes suspended in plasma (rouleaux formation), causing them to fall more rapidly.

Two types of changes in plasma proteins may lead to an elevation in ESR: either a moderate increase in concentration of extremely asymmetric proteins (e.g., fibrinogen) or a major increase in concentration of only moderately asymmetric molecules (e.g., the immunoglobulins). The first of these is characteristic of the acute phase response. Fibrinogen is the most asymmetric of the acute phase proteins in plasma and has the greatest effect on the ESR. Other acute phase proteins show lesser degrees of asymmetry and have less effect on erythrocyte aggregation. The second type of plasma protein abnormality leading to elevation of the ESR is the massive increase in concentration of a single molecular species of immunoglobulin that occurs in multiple myeloma or Waldenström's macroglobulinemia.

Method of ESR Determination. It is now well established that Westergren's method is the preferred method of ESR determination. The International Committee for Standardization in Hematology has recommended that this technique be designated as the standardized selected method.[14] Correction for anemia has been abandoned, since it is only approximate, misleading, and an artificial ultrarefinement. The widely accepted upper limits of normal in young adults are 15 mm per hour for males and 20 mm per hour for females. With aging, higher values seem to be the norm, although specific standards are uncertain. A simple formula to calculate the maximum normal ESR at any age has been proposed.[15] Values up to 40 mm per hour are not uncommon in healthy elderly people.[16]

Current Status of the ESR. The use of the ESR has been attacked as unsuitable, imprecise, and outmoded for a variety of reasons: (1) Alterations in the shape and size of red blood cells influence the ability of these cells to sediment. Anisocytosis, poikilocytosis (such as that seen in sickle cell anemia), microcytosis, spherocytosis, and acanthocytosis all physically interfere with rouleaux formation and thus may

result in the finding of a paradoxically normal ESR when major acute phase plasma protein abnormalities are, in fact, present. In addition, alterations in the concentration of erythrocytes, such as with anemia or polycythemia, may affect the ESR, leading to a more rapid rate of fall of red cells or a spuriously slow ESR, respectively. Unfortunately, it is impossible to correct accurately for alterations in size, shape, or concentration of erythrocytes. (2) The ESR is abnormal in the presence of monoclonal immunoglobulins irrespective of acute phase proteins; an elevation does not necessarily reflect inflammation or tissue injury. (3) The administration of certain drugs to patients or to blood from patients may alter the ESR. For example, the ESR is spuriously elevated when determined on heparinized specimens of blood or on blood from patients who have received heparin.[17] (4) The ESR is merely an indirect reflection of acute phase protein concentration. Direct measurement of a number of acute phase proteins themselves is now readily available and provides more accurate assessment than the indirect information provided by the ESR. (5) There is uncertainty about the effect of age and sex on the ESR; no one is quite sure what the range of normal is, particularly in the elderly. (6) Serum CRP levels rise and fall faster than ESR and therefore reflect the current status of a patient more accurately. (7) The range of abnormal CRP levels is much greater than the ESR and is clinically useful, since marked CRP elevation has greater diagnostic specificity.

Nonetheless, the ESR still manages to retain an important place in medical practice. The continued widespread use of the ESR stems from its relative simplicity, its familiarity, and the wealth of information about its clinical significance that has accumulated over many years. In the current era of sophisticated and automated laboratory testing, the fact that a practitioner can easily perform this familiar test himself in the simplest of laboratory settings probably ensures a place for the ESR for some time to come. Some relative advantages and disadvantages of ESR and CRP determinations are enumerated in Table 40-1.

C-REACTIVE PROTEIN

History, Structure, and Function. C-reactive protein (CRP) was originally detected in human serum because of its ability to precipitate with the somatic C-polysaccharide of the pneumococcus.[18] The most characteristic feature of CRP—its dramatic acute phase behavior in humans—was recognized at the time of discovery. CRP is an aggregate of five identical, noncovalently linked subunits arranged in cyclic pentameric symmetry.[19] It is encoded on human chromosome 1,[20] and based on cDNA studies a molecular weight of about 117,500 daltons can be computed.[21, 22]

The likelihood that CRP plays an important

Table 40–1. ADVANTAGES AND DISADVANTAGES OF CLINICAL TESTS USED TO ASSESS INFLAMMATION

Advantages	Disadvantages
Erythrocyte Sedimentation Rate (ESR)	
Easy	Value affected by age
Inexpensive	Value affected by RBC morphology
Reproducible	Value affected by RBC number
Familiar	Value affected by serum proteins, not involved in inflammation
	Slow response to acute inflammatory stimulus and recovery
	An indirect measure of APP levels
	Fresh sample required
C-reactive Protein (CRP)	
Value unaffected by age	Limited clinical experience reported
Reflects quantity of single APP	Quantitation more technically complex
Wide range of clinically important values detectable	Requires antisera
Rapid response to acute inflammatory stimulus and recovery	
Can be precisely quantitated	
Can be measured on stored sera	

RBC, red blood cell; APP, acute phase protein.

biologic role is supported by the conservation of this protein over hundreds of millions of years of evolution; proteins displaying structural and functional characteristics of CRP have been found in most mammals, as well as chickens and fish,[23] and in the ancient organism *Limulus polyphemus*, the horseshoe crab.[24] It is of interest, however, that CRP does not demonstrate acute phase behavior in all these species.

The magnitude and rapidity of the CRP response in humans suggest that an important physiologic role is played by this protein. While the precise functions of CRP during the acute phase are not known, this protein has been shown to exhibit important *recognition* and *activation* capacities that have the potential for influencing inflammation and other defense mechanisms.[25] Among the major biologic ligands recognized by CRP are phosphocholine, a ubiquitous component of some bacterial cell walls and eukaryotic cell membranes[26]; constituents of cell nuclei, including chromatin, histones, and small nuclear ribonucleoprotein[27, 28]; connective tissue matrix proteins, such as fibronectin[29]; and certain biologic polycations.[30]

Two types of activation functions are of particular interest. The interaction of CRP with the ligands described previously leads to activation of the complement system,[31] with generation of a group of inflammatory mediators. The other important activation capacity of CRP is related to its influence on phagocytic cell function. Binding of CRP to polymorphonuclear cells[32, 33] and to monocytes[34, 35] has been demonstrated. Both CRP and peptide fragments of CRP with structural similarity to the immunomodulatory tetrapeptide tuftsin have been reported to modulate neutrophil and monocyte functions, including chemotaxis, phagocytosis, and superoxide production.[36] The ability of CRP to induce monocyte production of cytokines[37, 38] and to enhance mono-

cyte-macrophage cytotoxicity[39, 40] has also been reported.

The potential effects of CRP on lymphocytes and platelets have been less well documented, although CRP has been reported to augment lymphocyte-mediated cytotoxicity,[41] inhibit the activity of platelet-activating factor,[42] and play a role in platelet-mediated cytotoxicity.[43]

This plethora of observations makes it unlikely that CRP serves only a single function and strongly implies that CRP plays a broad range of physiologic roles in response to tissue injury and infection. Although a precise delineation of its function in vivo is not yet possible, a synthesis of these observations suggests that the role of CRP may be to recognize and combine with foreign configurations (both endogenous and exogenous), with consequent activation of the complement system, and adherence to and activation of phagocytic cells.

Magnitude and Time Course of the CRP Response. The true range of normal serum CRP levels is difficult to define, since even minor degrees of injury in normal persons during the course of everyday life probably cause slight degrees of CRP elevation. Although most apparently healthy adults have CRP levels of less than 0.2 mg per dl,[44] concentrations as high as 1 mg per dl are found often enough in normal persons to justify regarding concentrations lower than this value as clinically insignificant.

Following acute inflammatory stimuli, a dramatic increase in serum concentration of CRP occurs, usually beginning within a few hours (Fig. 40–1) and resulting from a progressive increase in the number of hepatocytes producing CRP. The magnitude of the CRP rise reflects the extent of tissue injury; more extensive lesions cause longer periods of rising CRP levels and higher concentrations. As a useful approximation, concentrations of less than 1 mg per dl are regarded as normal or *insignificant elevations*; con-

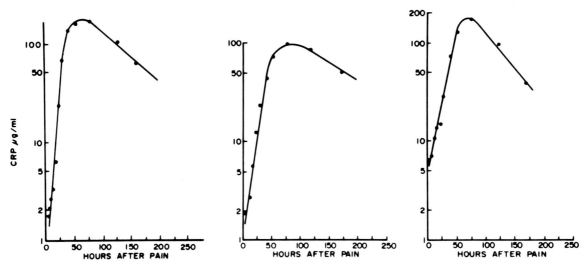

Figure 40–1. Serum concentrations of CRP following onset of chest pain in three patients with acute myocardial infarction. (From Kushner, I., et al.: Control of the acute phase response. Serum C-reactive protein kinetics after acute myocardial infarction. J. Clin. Invest. 61:235, 1978. Reproduced from the *Journal of Clinical Investigation* by copyright permission of the American Society of Clinical Investigation.)

centrations between 1 and 10 mg per dl, as *moderate increases*; and concentrations over 10 mg per dl, as *marked increases*. The majority of patients with very high levels have bacterial infection.[45, 46] Patients with severe acute inflammatory states, usually infections, may display serum CRP levels greater than 30 mg per dl; such levels are over 1000 times the concentrations found in most normal individuals. No other acute phase protein, with the exception of SAA, is known to increase in concentration this markedly. Examples of clinical conditions associated with CRP elevations of varying degrees are shown in Table 40–2.

Serum CRP levels generally reach a peak in 2 or 3 days following acute stimuli and then fall relatively rapidly. Recent studies (M. Pepys, personal communication) indicate that the half-life of CRP is about 18 hours in humans. However, persistently elevated serum CRP concentrations are often seen in chronic inflammatory states, such as active rheumatoid arthritis (RA) or pulmonary tuberculosis, or in the presence of extensive malignant disease.

Methods of CRP Detection. Serum levels of CRP can be accurately and reproducibly measured by a variety of methods, including radioimmunoassay, radial immunodiffusion, enzyme immunoassay, and laser nephelometry.[47] These methods can detect levels as low as 0.2 mg per dl. The semiquantitative latex agglutination used in the past is not particularly helpful. Recently, a rapid, semiquantitative solid-phase immunoassay for use in the physician's office has been introduced in Europe.

OTHER ACUTE PHASE REACTANTS

Although changes in concentration of the other acute phase proteins do tend to reflect inflammatory states, they are rarely employed clinically for this purpose. None of them offers an advantage over CRP determination; except for SAA, their concentrations rise more slowly, and the magnitude of the rise is nowhere near as great. Levels of SAA may be even more sensitive to minor degrees of tissue injury than are CRP levels, and several recent reports have focused on the clinical value of SAA determination in a number of disorders, including RA,[48] acute gout,[49] inflammatory bowel disease,[50] and myocardial infarction.[51] Such testing, however, is not widely available for clinical purposes.

A novel approach to assessment of the acute phase response in clinical circumstances involves

Table 40–2. EXAMPLES OF CONDITIONS ASSOCIATED WITH ELEVATED CRP LEVELS

Normal or Insignificant Elevation (<1 mg/dl)	Moderate Elevation (1–10 mg/dl)	Marked Elevation (>10 mg/dl)
Vigorous exercise	Myocardial infarction	Acute bacterial infection (80–85%)
Common cold	Malignancies	Major trauma
Pregnancy	Pancreatitis	Systemic vasculitis
Gingivitis	Mucosal infection (bronchitis, cystitis)	
Cerebrovascular accident	Most connective tissue diseases	
Seizures		
Angina		

measurement of the pattern of glycosylation of some of the acute phase proteins. It has been observed that the microheterogeneous glycosylation patterns of some acute phase proteins, such as α_1-acid glycoprotein (orosomucoid) and α_1-protease inhibitor, may vary during the acute phase response, independently of the actual concentration of these proteins.[52] Thus, the microheterogeneity of α_1-acid glycoprotein has been reported to be helpful in the detection of intercurrent infection in patients with active systemic lupus erythematosus (SLE)[53] and in differentiating acute inflammatory states from chronic ones.[54]

CLINICAL VALUE OF ASSESSMENT OF ACUTE PHASE REACTANTS

Elevation of the ESR or CRP has no diagnostic specificity but tends to reflect the presence of tissue injury and inflammation. In general, mild elevations reflect mild tissue alterations, whereas marked elevations reflect major tissue injury. In a number of protracted or chronic illnesses, the course of the disease process is reflected by the rise and fall of the acute phase reactants.

Measurements of ESR and CRP are of little use for diagnostic screening purposes in asymptomatic individuals or patients with trivial complaints. There are certain clinical circumstances, however, in which measurement of acute phase reactants has some diagnostic value. For example, the finding of a normal ESR or CRP argues against the diagnosis of active polymyalgia rheumatica–giant cell arteritis (although such cases have been reported[55]), deep vein thrombosis,[56] or acute appendicitis.[57] Similarly, extreme elevation of these reactants may provide useful diagnostic information in some circumstances. Specifically, marked elevations of CRP (levels greater than 10 mg per dl) have been associated with acute bacterial infection in 80 to 85 percent of cases.[45, 46]

Acute phase reactant determinations are felt to be of greatest diagnostic value in differentiating between diseases in which substantial amounts of inflammation or tissue injury occur and those in which inflammation is absent or minimal. This is most true for CRP, for which the broad range of possible values permits a relatively greater degree of confidence in differentiating between states with mild and severe tissue injury.[57a] Thus, CRP has been reported to be of value in distinguishing acute myocardial infarction from atypical angina,[58] pyelonephritis from cystitis,[59] bacterial pneumonia from bronchitis,[45] bacterial meningitis from viral meningitis,[60] and pulmonary tuberculosis from active pulmonary sarcoidosis.[61] In addition, CRP determinations may be of value in suggesting the diagnosis of occult bacterial infection in neonates[62] or patients with certain chronic disease states.[63, 64] In the assessment of such clinical situations, CRP levels should be expressed quantitatively, since differing degrees of CRP elevation have different implications. For example, while serum CRP levels may be elevated in both Behçet's disease and Still's disease, CRP elevation in Behçet's disease is usually modest, with levels rarely exceeding 2 mg per dl.[65] However, CRP levels as high as 20 mg per dl may occur in Still's disease. Still lacking are systematic studies in which the specificity, sensitivity, predictive value, and cost-effectiveness of these tests are addressed for a variety of clinical enigmas. Only a few such studies have been reported,[53, 66–68] and one of these suggested that both the ESR and CRP may have limited clinical utility for the diagnosis of infection or inflammation in elderly individuals.[69]

In clinical practice, physicians who treat chronic illnesses have found that quantitation of acute phase reactants is most valuable for monitoring the course of disease activity over time. The greatest experience has been obtained with the ESR, which is recognized to be an excellent indicator of disease activity in polymyalgia rheumatica–giant cell arteritis, very good in RA, and less reliable but occasionally helpful in other inflammatory diseases, such as SLE. Since the ESR is only an indirect measure of the acute phase response and is influenced by a host of confounding variables, its reliability has been limited in many disorders.[47] An increasing number of clinical studies have therefore focused on the potential value of serial determinations of CRP levels in both acute and chronic inflammatory diseases.[70] Such reports have emphasized the benefits of CRP detection and follow-up in such diverse disorders as acute gout,[49] RA,[71–76] spondyloarthropathies,[77] SLE,[78–83] systemic vasculitis,[84] polymyalgia rheumatica–giant cell arteritis,[85] juvenile arthritis,[86, 87] bacterial endocarditis,[88] inflammatory bowel disease,[50, 89] and pancreatitis[90] and in patients following renal transplantation[91, 92] or surgical operations.[93] The ability quickly and precisely to quantitate CRP levels will undoubtedly lead to much needed clinical studies in which the role of serial determinations of CRP in the evaluation of chronic inflammatory diseases will be more clearly defined. A tabulation of reports describing the clinical value of CRP determinations in a number of disorders is shown in Table 40–3.

Rheumatoid Arthritis. A time-honored method of distinguishing RA from other varieties of arthritis, particularly osteoarthritis, is the detection of an elevated ESR. Today, this practice must be regarded as of limited value for a variety of reasons. Not all patients with RA have an elevated ESR. Many of the diseases from which RA must frequently be differentiated are themselves often accompanied by an elevated ESR. Most patients with osteoarthritis are in an age group in which an elevated ESR is frequently found as a result of associated diseases, and aging itself is not infrequently associated with elevated ESR. Most important, careful history and physical examination usually permit the diagnosis of RA to be made without the need for determination of the ESR or CRP. It has been found that an abnormal ESR increases the probability of RA (and decreases the probability of osteoarthritis), but not by much![67]

Table 40–3. DISORDERS IN WHICH MEASUREMENT OF CRP HAS BEEN REPORTED TO BE OF CLINICAL VALUE

For Differential Diagnosis*	Reference
Pyelonephritis *versus* cystitis	45, 59
Pneumonia *versus* bronchitis	45
Rheumatoid arthritis *versus* osteoarthritis	48
Myocardial infarction *versus* angina	58
Bacterial *versus* aseptic meningitis	45, 60
Acute appendicitis	57
Deep vein thrombosis	56
Pulmonary tuberculosis *versus* sarcoidosis	61
Presence of occult infection	
In neonates	62
In postoperative patients	93
Superimposed on chronic disease	53, 54, 63, 64
For Follow-Up of Disease Activity	
Rheumatic Diseases	
Gout	49
Reumatoid arthritis	71–76
Polymyalgia rheumatica–giant cell arteritis	85
Systemic lupus erythematosus	79–83
Ankylosing spondylitis	77
Reiter's syndrome	77
Juvenile arthritis	86, 87
Systemic vasculitis	84
Other Diseases	
Inflammatory bowel disease	50, 89
Pancreatitis	90
After renal transplantation	91, 92

*The precise sensitivity and specificity of elevated CRP levels for diagnosis in these disorders are uncertain.

While assessment of the acute phase proteins is only occasionally of value in diagnosis, it is more often helpful in the management of RA by aiding in the monitoring of disease activity. Studies employing both the ESR and CRP have generally suggested that CRP levels correlate better with degree of activity than does the ESR,[73, 74, 94–97] although a recent consensus analysis suggested that the ESR, which is influenced by multiple factors such as anemia of chronic disease, may be the single most useful test clinically.[98] CRP levels average about 3 to 4 mg per dl in adult RA patients with moderate disease activity, but there is considerable variation: about 7 percent of such patients have values in the normal range, while a few patients with severe disease activity show levels of 14 mg per dl or more.

The clinical usefulness of acute phase protein determination as a prognostic indicator and as an aid to selection of therapeutic agents is a subject of great current interest. In general, high levels of acute phase reactants at the onset of disease are correlated with a relatively poor prognosis and progressive erosive disease.[73, 99–101] Serum CRP and ESR levels frequently fall in patients manifesting clinical improvement while receiving treatment with slow-acting antirheumatic agents (e.g., gold and methotrexate) and glucocorticoids,[74, 102–104] while these levels may fall in only a proportion of those receiving nonsteroidal anti-inflammatory drugs.[76, 105] It has been suggested that erosive disease will be prevented if ESR or CRP

are controlled.[100, 106, 107] One recent, nonrandomized study does suggest that progressive radiologic deterioration is less likely to occur in patients in whom the ESR and CRP are consistently lowered.[72] However, such a correlation could simply represent nothing more than an association between two different reflectors of disease activity that one might expect. There is insufficient evidence, at present, to conclude with confidence that treatment that lowers acute phase reactants to normal levels will affect the array of chronic inflammatory and biochemical mechanisms that lead to destruction of bone and cartilage. Even so, a number of rheumatologists regard the finding of moderate to marked CRP elevation as a signal to use "second-line" drugs rather than nonsteroidal anti-inflammatory drugs alone.

The determination of acute phase reactants such as the ESR and CRP in the evaluation of new drugs for RA is also of value. A decrease in CRP levels during the treatment of RA has the advantage of being an objective indication that anti-inflammatory effects have been achieved, in contrast with the relatively subjective changes in signs and symptoms that we more commonly employ to measure effectiveness. This is particularly important when as many as 40 percent of patients with RA claim to experience improvement while receiving placebo therapy. Thus, the ESR is the most important laboratory criterion in the American Rheumatism Association criteria for determining remission.[108] In addition, a fall in acute phase reactants probably reflects greater degrees of improvement in elements of the local inflammatory process than does clinical improvement without an accompanying fall in acute phase reactants.

Polymyalgia Rheumatica and Giant Cell Arteritis. The diagnoses of polymyalgia rheumatica and giant cell arteritis are supported by the finding of an elevated ESR, often over 100 mm per hour. Such elevations are no longer regarded as a sine qua non of these disorders, since a number of reports have described patients with polymyalgia rheumatica and giant cell arteritis who have a normal ESR.[55] Extreme elevation of the ESR in the absence of symptoms of polymyalgia rheumatica or giant cell arteritis is not likely to be due to these conditions; the majority of such patients have underlying infection, malignancy, or renal disease.[68]

In patients with polymyalgia rheumatica or giant cell arteritis, the return of the ESR to normal levels following initial treatment usually indicates that inflammation has been brought under control. Disease activity may be monitored by following the ESR; elevation in the ESR would suggest recurrence of activity and call for more aggressive therapy. Determinations of the CRP and ESR appear to be of approximately equal value in assessing disease activity.[85] Of course, clinical manifestations of disease, even in the presence of a normal ESR, should not be ignored.

Systemic Lupus Erythematosus. While CRP levels are elevated above the normal range in most patients with active SLE and tend to fall and rise as the disease improves or becomes more active, a number of patients with active SLE do not show even mild CRP elevation, and median CRP levels in series of patients with SLE are lower than in patients with RA who are thought to have comparable degrees of disease severity.[79] However, markedly elevated CRP levels occur in some patients with SLE, particularly those with acute serositis or chronic synovitis.[80–83, 109–111] The use of serum CRP levels as a diagnostic criterion to distinguish SLE from RA does not seem to be a practical suggestion, in view of the considerable overlap in CRP concentrations observed in patients with these disorders.

The suggestion that CRP elevation in the course of SLE is more likely to be due to superimposed bacterial infection than to activation of lupus can be addressed directly if CRP levels are expressed in quantitative terms. It has now become clear that markedly elevated serum CRP levels in the hospitalized population are seen most frequently, but not exclusively, with bacterial infection. Occurrence of CRP levels in excess of 6 to 8 mg per dl in the course of SLE should serve as a stimulus to rule out the possibility of infection, just as it should in other diseases.[78] However, such values should not be regarded as proof of infection; as indicated previously, marked CRP elevation due to active SLE is frequently seen.[110]

References

1. Kushner, I.: The phenomenon of the acute phase response. Ann. N. Y. Acad. Sci. 389:39, 1982.
2. Taylor, C., Rogers, G., Goodman, C., et al.: Hematologic, iron-related, and acute-phase protein responses to sustained strenuous exercise. J. Appl. Phys. 62:464, 1987.
3. Kushner, I., and Feldman, G.: Control of the acute phase response. Demonstration of C-reactive protein synthesis and secretion by hepatocytes during acute inflammation in the rabbit. J. Exp. Med. 148:466, 1978.
4. Ganapathi, M. K., Rzewnicki, D., Samols, D., et al.: Effect of combinations of cytokines and hormones on synthesis of serum amyloid A and C-reactive protein in Hep 3B cells. J. Immunol. 147:1261, 1991.
5. Castell J. V., Gomez-Lechon, M. J., David, M., et al.: Recombinant human interleukin-6 (IL-6/BSF-2/HSF) regulates the synthesis of acute phase proteins in human hepatocytes. FEBS Lett. 232:347, 1988.
6. Kushner, I., and Mackiewicz, A.: Acute phase proteins as disease markers. Dis. Markers 5:1, 1987.
7. Rogers, J. T., Bridges, K. R., Durmowicz, G. P., et al.: Translational control during the acute phase response. Ferritin synthesis in response to interleukin-1. J. Biol. Chem. 265:14572, 1990.
8. Mackiewicz, A. J., Speroff, T., Ganapathi, M. K., et al.: Effects of cytokine combinations on acute phase protein production in two human hepatoma cell lines. J. Immunol. 146:3032, 1991.
9. Gitlin, J. D., Gitlin, J. I., and Gitlin, D.: Localization of C-reactive protein in synovium of patients with rheumatoid arthritis. Arthritis Rheum. 20:1491, 1977.
10. Duclos, T. W., Mold, C., Paterson, P. Y., et al.: Localization of C-reactive protein in inflammatory lesions of experimental allergic encephalomyelitis. Clin. Exp. Immunol. 43:565, 1981.
11. Mold, C., Nakayama, S., Holzer, T. J., et al.: C-reactive protein is protective against fatal Streptococcus pneumoniae infection in mice. J. Exp. Med. 154:1703, 1981.
12. Horowitz, J., Volanakis, J. E., and Briles, D. E.: Blood clearance of Streptococcus pneumoniae by C-reactive protein. J. Immunol. 138:2598, 1987.
13. McAdam, K. P. W. J., and Sipe, J. D.: Murine model for human secondary amyloidosis: genetic variability of the acute-phase serum protein SAA response to endotoxins and casein. J. Exp. Med. 144:1121, 1976.
14. International Committee for Standardization in Hematology: Recommendation for measurement of erythrocyte sedimentation rate of human blood. Am. J. Clin. Pathol. 68:505, 1977.
15. Miller, A., Green, M., and Robertson, D.: Simple rule for calculating normal erythrocyte sedimentation rate. Br. Med. J. 286:266, 1983.
16. Shearn, M. A., and Kang, I. Y.: Effect of age and sex on the erythrocyte sedimentation rate. J. Rheum. 13:297, 1986.
17. Penchas, S., Stern, Z., Bar-Or, D.: Heparin and the ESR. Arch. Intern. Med. 138:1864, 1978.
18. McCarty, M.: Historical perspective on C-reactive protein. Ann. N. Y. Acad. Sci. 389:1, 1982.
19. Osmand, A. P., Friedenson, B., Gewurz, H., et al.: Characterization of C-reactive protein and the complement subcomponent C1t as homologous proteins displaying cyclic pentameric symmetry (pentraxins). Proc. Natl. Acad. Sci. U. S. A. 74:739, 1977.
20. Whitehead, A. S., Bruns, G. A. P., Markham, A. F., et al.: Isolation of human C-reactive protein complementary DNA and localization of the gene to chromosome 1. Science 221:69, 1983.
21. Lei, K. J., Liu T., Zon, G., et al.: Genomic DNA sequence for human C-reactive protein. J. Biol. Chem. 260:1377, 1985.
22. Woo, P., Korenberg, J. R., and Whitehead, A. S.: Characterization of genomic and complementary DNA sequences of human C-reactive protein, and comparison with complementary DNA sequence of serum amyloid P component. J. Biol. Chem. 260:13384, 1985.
23. Baltz, M. L., de Beer, F. C., Feinstein, A., et al.: Phylogenetic aspects of C-reactive protein and related proteins. Ann. N. Y. Acad. Sci. 389:49, 1982.
24. Robey, F., and Liu, T.-Y.: Limulin: A C-reactive protein from Limulus polyphemus. J. Biol. Chem. 256:969, 1981.
25. Volanakis, J. E., Xu, Y., and Macon, K. J.: Human C-reactive protein and host defense. In Marchalonis, J. J., and Reinisch, C. L. (eds.): Defense Molecules. New York, Wiley-Liss, Inc., 1990.
26. Volanakis, J. E., and Kaplan, M. H.: Specificity of C-reactive protein for choline phosphate residues of pneumococcal c-polysaccharide. Proc. Soc. Exp. Biol. Med. 163:612, 1971.
27. Robey, F. A., Jones, K. D., Tanaka, T., et al.: Binding of C-reactive protein to chromatin and nucleosome core particles. J. Biol. Chem. 259:7311, 1984.
28. DuClos, T. W.: C-reactive protein reacts with the U_1 small nuclear ribonucleoprotein. J. Immunol. 143:2553, 1989.
29. Tseng, J., and Mortensen, R. F.: The effect of human C-reactive protein on the cell-attachment activity of fibronectin and laminin. Exp. Cell Res. 180:303, 1989.
30. DiCamelli, R., Potempa, L. A., and Siegel, J.: Binding reactivity of C-reactive protein for polycations. J. Immunol. 125:1933, 1980.
31. Kaplan, M. H., and Volanakis, J. E.: Interaction of C-reactive protein complexes with the complement system. I. Consumption of human complement associated with the reaction of C-reactive protein with pneumococcal C-polysaccharide and with choline phosphatides, lecithin, and sphingomyelin. J. Immunol. 112:2135, 1974.
32. Müller, H., and Fehr, J.: Binding of C-reactive protein to human polymorphonuclear leukocytes: evidence for association of binding sites with Fc receptors. J. Immunol. 136:2202, 1986.
33. Buchta, R., Pontet, M., and Fridkin, M.: Binding of C-reactive protein to human neutrophils. FEBS Lett. 211:165, 1987.
34. Ballou, S. P., Buniel, J., and Macintyre, S. S.: Specific binding of human C-reactive protein to human monocytes in vitro. J. Immunol. 142:2708, 1989.
35. Ballou, S. P., and Cleveland, R. P.: Binding of human C-reactive protein to monocytes: analysis by flow cytometry. Clin. Exp. Immunol. 84:329, 1991.
36. Ballou, S. P., and Kushner, I.: C-reactive protein and the acute phase response. Adv. Intern. Med. 37:313, 1992.
37. Barna, B. P., Thomassen, M. J., Clements, M., et al.: Cytokine induction associated with human C-reactive protein. FASEB J. 3:A824, 1989.
38. Ballou, S. P., and Lozanski, G.: C-reactive protein (CRP) induces cytokine production by monocytes. FASEB J. 5:A634, 1991.
39. Zahedi, K., and Mortensen, R. F.: Macrophage tumoricidal activity induced by human C-reactive protein. Cancer Res. 46:5077, 1986.
40. Gautam, S., James, K., and Deodhar, S. D.: Macrophage-mediated tumoricidal activity generated by human C-reactive protein (CRP) encapsulated in liposomes is complement-dependent. Clev. Clin. Q. 53:235, 1986.
41. Vetter, M. L., Gewurz, H., and Baum, L. L.: The effects of C-reactive protein on human cell-mediated cytotoxicity. J. Leukoc. Biol. 157:301, 1986.
42. Kilpatrick, J. M., and Virella, G.: Inhibition of platelet-activating factor by rabbit C-reactive protein. Clin. Immunol. Immunopathol. 37:276, 1985.
43. Bout, D., Joseph, M., Pontet, M., et al.: Rat resistance to schistosomiasis: platelet-mediated cytotoxicity induced by C-reactive protein. Science 231:153, 1986.
44. Claus, D. R., Osmand, A. P., and Gewurz, H.: Radioimmunoassay of

human C-reactive proteins and levels in normal sera. J. Lab. Clin. Med. 87:120, 1976.

45. Morley, J. J., and Kushner, I.: Serum C-reactive protein levels in disease. Ann. N. Y. Acad. Sci. 389:406, 1982.

46. Cox, M. L., Rudd, A. G., Gallimore, R., et al.: Real-time measurement of serum C-reactive protein in the management of infection in the elderly. Age Ageing 15:257, 1986.

47. Bull, B. S., Chien, S., Dormandy, J. A., et al.: Guidelines on selection of laboratory tests for monitoring the acute phase response. J. Clin. Pathol. 41:1203, 1988.

48. Sukenik, S., Henkin, J., Zimlichman, S., et al.: Serum and synovial fluid levels of serum amyloid A protein and C-reactive protein in inflammatory and noninflammatory arthritis. J. Rheumatol. 15:942, 1988.

49. Roseff, R., Wohigethan, J. R., Sipe, J. D., et al.: The acute phase response in gout. J. Rheumatol. 14:974, 1987.

50. Chambers, R. E., Stross, P., Barry, R. E., et al.: Serum amyloid A protein compared with C-reactive protein, alpha₁-antichymotrypsin and alpha₁-acid glycoprotein as a monitor of inflammatory bowel disease. Eur. J. Clin. Invest. 17:460, 1987.

51. Marhaug, G., Harklau, L., and Olsen, B.: Serum amyloid A protein in acute myocardial infarction. Acta Med. Scand. 220:303, 1986.

52. Mackiewicz, A., Ganapathi, M. K., Schultz, D., et al.: Monokines regulate glycosylation of acute phase proteins. J. Exp. Med. 166:253, 1987.

53. Mackiewicz, A., Marcinkowska-Pieta, R., Mackiewicz, S., et al.: Microheterogeneity of alpha₁-acid glycoprotein in the detection of intercurrent infection in systemic lupus erythematosus. Arthritis Rheum. 30:513, 1987.

54. Pawlowski, T., Mackiewicz, S. H., and Mackiewicz, A.: Microheterogeneity of alpha₁-acid glycoprotein in the detection of intercurrent infection in patients with rheumatoid arthritis. Arthritis Rheum. 32:347, 1989.

55. Wong, R. L., and Korn, J. H.: Temporal arteritis without an elevated erythrocyte sedimentation rate. Case report and review of the literature. Am. J. Med. 80:959, 1986.

56. Thomas, E. A., Cobby, M. J., Rhys Davies, E., et al.: Liquid crystal thermography and C-reactive protein in the detection of deep venous thrombosis. Br. Med. J. 229:951, 1989.

57. Dueholm, S., Bagi, P., and Bud, M.: Laboratory aid in the diagnosis of acute appendicitis. A blinded, prospective trial concerning diagnostic value of leukocyte count, neutrophil differential count, and C-reactive protein. Dis. Colon Rectum 32:855, 1989.

57a. Deodhar, S. D.: C-reactive protein: the best laboratory indicator available for monitoring disease activity. Cleve. Clin. J. Med. 56:126, 1989.

58. Kushner, I., Broder, M. L., and Karp, D.: Control of the acute phase response. Serum C-reactive protein kinetics after acute myocardial infarction. J. Clin. Invest. 61:235, 1978.

59. Hellerstein, S., Duggan, E., Welchert, E., et al.: Serum C-reactive protein and the site of urinary tract infections. J. Pediatr. 100:21, 1982.

60. Valmari, P.: White blood cell count, erythrocyte sedimentation rate, and serum C-reactive protein in meningitis: magnitude of the response related to bacterial species. Infection 12:328, 1984.

61. Hind, C. R. K., Flint, K. C., Hudspith, B. N., et al.: Serum C-reactive protein concentrations in patients with pulmonary sarcoidosis. Thorax 42:332, 1987.

62. Forest, J. C., Lariviere, F., Dolce, P., et al.: C-reactive protein as biochemical indicator of bacterial infection in neonates. Clin. Biochem. 19:192, 1986.

63. Hind, C. R. K., Thomson, S. P., Winearls, C. G., et al.: Serum C-reactive protein concentration in the management of infection in patients treated by continuous ambulatory peritoneal dialysis. J. Clin. Pathol. 38:459, 1985.

64. Venditti, M., Brandimarte, C., Trobiani, P., et al.: Serial study of C-reactive protein for the diagnosis of bacterial and fungal infections in neutropenic patients with hematologic malignancies. Haematologica 73:285, 1988.

65. Adinolfi, M., and Lehner, T.: Acute phase proteins and C9 in patients with Behçet's syndrome and aphthous ulcers. Clin. Exp. Immunol. 25:36, 1976.

66. Bedell, S. E., and Bush, B. T.: Erythrocyte sedimentation rate. From folklore to facts. Am. J. Med. 78:1001, 1982.

67. Sox, H. C., and Liang, M. H.: The erythrocyte sedimentation rate. Guidlines for rational use. Ann. Intern. Med. 140:515, 1986.

68. Fincher, R. M., and Page, M. I.: Clinical significance of extreme elevation of the erythrocyte sedimentation rate. Arch. Intern. Med. 146:1581, 1986.

69. Katz, P. R., Gutman, S. I., Richman, G., et al.: Erythrocyte sedimentation rate and C-reactive protein compared in the elderly. Clin. Chem. 35:466, 1989.

70. Okamura, J. M., Miyagi, J. M., Terada, K., and Hokama, Y.: Potential clinical applications of C-reactive protein. J. Clin. Lab. Anal. 4:231, 1990.

71. Dixon, J. S., Pickup, M. E., Lowe, J. R., et al.: Discriminatory indices of response of patients with rheumatoid arthritis treated with D-penicillamine. Ann. Rheum. Dis. 39:301, 1980.

72. Dawes, P. T., Fowler, P. D., Clarke, S., et al.: Rheumatoid arthritis: treatment which controls the C-reactive protein and erythrocyte sedimentation rate reduces radiological progression. Br. J. Rheumatol. 25:44, 1986.

73. Larsen, A.: The relation of radiographic changes to serum acute-phase proteins and rheumatoid factor in 200 patients with rheumatoid arthritis. Scand. J. Rheumatol. 17:123, 1988.

74. Segal, R., Caspi, D., Tishler, M., et al.: Short-term effects of low-dose methotrexate on the acute phase reaction in patients with rheumatoid arthritis. J. Rheumatol. 16:914, 1989.

75. Walters, M. T., Stevenson, F. K., and Goswami, R., et al.: Comparison of serum and synovial fluid concentrations of β₂-microglobulin and C-reactive protein in relation to clinical disease activity and synovial inflammation in rheumatoid arthritis. Ann. Rheum. Dis. 48:905, 1989.

76. Cush, J. J., Lipsky, P. E., Postlethwaite, A. E., et al.: Correlation of serologic indicators of inflammation with effectiveness of nonsteroidal antiinflammatory drug therapy in rheumatoid arthritis. Arthritis Rheum. 33:19, 1990.

77. Nashel, D. J., Petrone, D. L., Ulmer, C. C., et al.: C-reactive protein: a marker for disease activity in ankylosing spondylitis and Reiter's syndrome. J. Rheumatol. 13:364, 1986.

78. Becker, G. J., Waldenburger, M., Hughes, G. R. V., et al.: Value of serum C-reactive protein measurement in the investigation of fever in systemic lupus erythematosus. Ann. Rheum. Dis. 39:50, 1980.

79. Pereira Da Silva, J. A., Elkon, K. B., Hughes, G. R. V., et al.: C-reactive protein levels in systemic lupus erythematosus: a classification criterion? Arthritis Rheum. 23:770, 1980.

80. Morrow, W. J. W., Isenberg, D. A., Parry, H. F., et al.: C-reactive protein in sera from patients with systemic lupus erythematosus. J. Rheumatol. 8:599, 1981.

81. Moutsopoulos, H. M., Mavridis, A. K., Acritidis, N. C., et al.: High C-reactive protein response in lupus polyarthritis. Clin. Exp. Rheumatol. 1:53, 1983.

82. Bertouch, J. V., Roberts-Thompson, P. J., Feng, P. H., et al.: C-reactive protein and serological indices of disease activity in systemic lupus erythematosus. Ann. Rheum. Dis. 42:655, 1983.

83. Sturfelt, G., and Sjoholm, A. G.: Complement components, complement activation, and acute phase response in systemic lupus erythematosus. Int. Arch. Allergy Appl. Immunol. 75:75, 1984.

84. Hind, C. R. K., Savage, C. O., Winearls, C. G., et al.: Objective monitoring of disease activity in polyarteritis by measurement of serum C-reactive protein concentration. Br. Med. J. 288:1027, 1984.

85. Kyle, V., Cawston, T. E., and Hazleman, B. L.: Erythrocyte sedimentation rate and C-reactive protein in the assessment of polymyalgia rheumatica/giant cell arteritis on presentation and during follow-up. Ann. Rheum. Dis. 48:667, 1989.

86. Gwyther, M., Schwartz, H., Howard, A., et al.: C-reactive protein in juvenile chronic arthritis: an indicator of disease activity and possibly amyloidosis. Ann. Rheum. Dis. 41:259, 1982.

87. Kunnamo, I., Kallio, P., Pelkonen, P., et al.: Clinical signs and laboratory tests in the differential diagnosis of arthritis in children. Am. J. Dis. Child. 141:34, 1987.

88. McCartney, A. C., Orange, G. V., Pringle, S. D., et al.: Serum C reactive protein in infective endocarditis. J. Clin. Pathol. 41:44, 1988.

89. Prantera, C., Davoli, M., Lorenzetti, R., et al.: Clinical and laboratory indicators of extent of ulcerative colitis. Serum C-reactive protein helps the most. J. Clin. Gastroenterol. 10:41, 1988.

90. Wilson, C., Heads, A., Shenkin, A., et al.: C-reactive protein, antiproteases and complement factors as objective markers of severity in acute pancreatitis. Br. J. Surg. 76:177, 1989.

91. Cohen, D. J., Benvenisty, A. I., Meyer, E., and Hardy, M. A.: Serum C-reactive protein concentrations in cyclosporine-treated renal allograft recipients. Transplantation 45:919, 1988.

92. Lalla, M. L. T., Eklund, B., and Ahonen, J.: The clinical significance of serum C-reactive protein after renal transplantation. Transplantation Proc. 20:402, 1988.

93. Fischer, C. L., Gill, C., Forrester, M. G., et al.: Quantitation of "acute phase proteins" postoperatively. Value in detection and monitoring of complications. Am. J. Clin. Pathol. 66:840, 1976.

94. Walsh, L., Davies, P., and McConkey, B.: Relationship between erythrocyte sedimentation rates and serum C-reactive protein in rheumatoid arthritis. Ann. Rheum. Dis. 38:362, 1979.

95. Mallya, R. D., DeBeer, F. C., Berry, H., et al.: Correlation of clinical parameters of disease activity in rheumatoid arthritis with serum concentration of C-reactive protein and erythrocyte sedimentation rate. J. Rheumatol. 9:224, 1982.

96. Dixon, J. S., Bird, H. A., Sitton, N. G., et al.: C-reactive protein in the serial assessment of disease activity in rheumatoid arthritis. Scand. J. Rheumatol. 13:39, 1984.

97. Wright, V., Dixon, J. S., and Bird, H. A.: Therapeutic significance of laboratory results in rheumatic disease. Semin. Arthritis Rheum. 15:8, 1985.

98. Bull, B. S., Westengard, J. C., Farr, M., et al.: Efficacy of tests used to monitor rheumatoid arthritis. Lancet 2:965, 1989.

99. Fleming, A., Crown, J. M., and Dorbett, M.: Prognostic value of early features in rheumatoid disease. Br. Med. J. 1:1243, 1976.

100. Amos, R. S., Constable, T. J., Crockson, R. A., et al.: Rheumatoid arthritis: relation of serum C-reactive protein and erythrocyte sedimentation rates to radiographic changes. Br. Med. J. 1:195, 1977.

101. Nusinow, S., and Arnold, W. J.: Prognostic value of C-reactive protein (CRP) levels in rheumatoid arthritis. Clin. Res. 30:474A, 1982.

102. Huskisson, E. C.: The problems of studying disease-remittive agents in RA. J. Rheumatol. 9(Supp. 18):201, 1982.

103. Forster, P. J. G., and McConkey, B.: The effect of antirheumatic drugs on circulating immune complexes in rheumatoid arthritis. Q. J. Med. 58:29, 1986.

104. Situnayake, R. D., and McConkey, B.: Clinical and laboratory effects of prolonged therapy with sulfasalazine, gold, or penicillamine: the effects of disease duration on treatment response. J. Rheumatol. 17:1268, 1990.

105. McConkey, B., Crockson, R. A., Crockson, A. P., et al.: The effects of some anti-inflammatory drugs on the acute-phase proteins in rheumatoid arthritis. Q. J. Med. 42:785, 1973.

106. Editorial: Inducing remission in rheumatoid arthritis. Lancet 1:193, 1981.

107. Amos, R. S., Crockson, R. A., Crockson, A. P., et al.: Rheumatoid arthritis: C-reactive protein and erythrocyte sedimentation rate during initial treatment. Br. Med. J. 1:1396, 1978.

108. Roth, S. H.: Remission: the goal of rheumatic disease therapy. J. Rheumatol. 9(Suppl. 8):120, 1982.

109. terBorg, E. J., Horst, G., Limburg, P. C., et al.: C-reactive protein levels during disease exacerbations and infections in systemic lupus erythematosus: a prospective longitudinal study. J. Rheumatol. 17:1642, 1990.

110. Kushner, I.: C-reactive protein in rheumatology. Arthritis Rheum. 34:1065, 1991.

111. Spronk, P. E., ter Borg, E. J., and Kallenberg, C. G. M.: Patients with systemic lupus erythematosus and Jaccoud's arthropathy: a clinical subset with an increased C-reactive protein response? Ann. Rheum. Dis. 51:358, 1992.

Chapter 41   Richard O. Day

Aspirin and Salicylates

Aspirin and its active metabolite, salicylate, were the first nonsteroidal anti-inflammatory drugs (NSAIDs), having been introduced into widespread use at the beginning of this century. They are beneficial in the rheumatic diseases because of anti-inflammatory and analgesic properties but are also antipyretic, and aspirin has important platelet inhibitory actions. In this chapter, the term *salicylate(s)* refers to the drugs that *liberate* the salicylate anion in vivo (Fig. 41–1). This definition includes aspirin but excludes diflunisal.

The ancient Greeks knew that the bitter extracts from the bark of various trees could alleviate the symptoms of rheumatism; in 1763, the Reverend Edmund Stone rediscovered the efficacy of an extract of willow bark. The active component was identified as salicin, which is metabolized to salicylate. Salicylic acid was synthesized in 1860 by Kolbe and Lautemann but caused dyspepsia and tasted bitter when administered orally. This was the stimulus for Kolbe and chemists from the Bayer Company in Germany to prepare sodium salicylate, which was shown to be effective as an analgesic and antipyretic in rheumatic fever in 1875.[1, 2] Acetylsalicylic acid was synthesized by Felix Hoffman and named "Aspirin" in 1899 by Heinrich Dresser. The *a* of aspirin refers to the acetyl grouping, while "spirin" recalls the botanical genus *Spiraea*, from which salicylates commonly can be extracted.

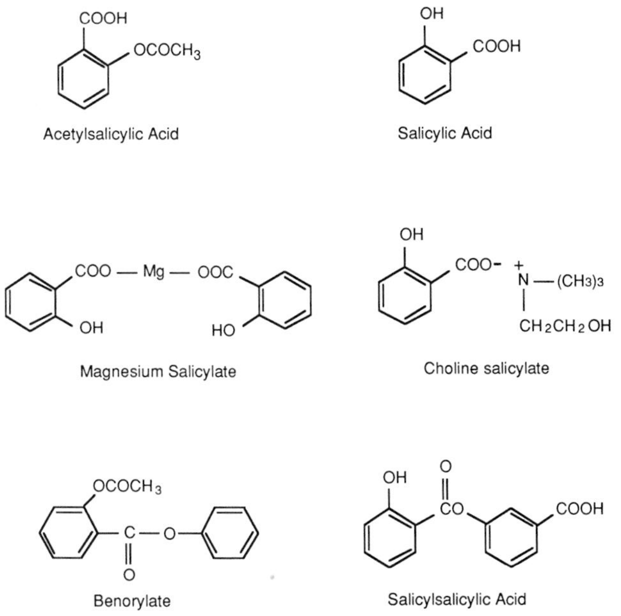

CLINICAL PHARMACOLOGY

Chemistry

Salicylic acid has a pKa of 3.0 and exists largely in the ionized form in vivo. The salicylate anion is commonly formulated as soluble salts, with sodium, magnesium, choline, or choline magnesium as cation (see Fig. 41–1). Aspirin is also acidic, with a pKa of 3.5, and is administered orally either as the free acid or as soluble salts with sodium or calcium as cation.

Salicylsalicylic acid (a dimer of salicylate), choline magnesium trisalicylate (CMT), aloxiprin (an insoluble complex salt of aluminium and aspirin), and benorylate (an ester of aspirin with acetaminophen) all are preferentially dissolved and absorbed in the neutral environment of the small intestine. These formulations are notable for their reduced gastric mucosal irritability as compared with plain aspirin.

Figure 41–1. Structures of some of the salicylates.

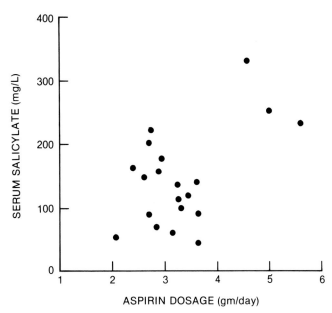

Figure 41–2. The relationship between dosage of aspirin and steady-state serum salicylate concentrations in 20 individuals with RA after 5 days dosing with buffered aspirin, approximately 50 mg/kg/day. (Adapted with permission from Gupta, N., Sarkissian, E., and Paulus, H. E.: Correlation of plateau serum salicylate level with rate of salicylate metabolism. Clin. Pharmacol. Ther. 18:350, 1975.)

Pharmacokinetics

Particular note should be taken of the major contributions of Levy, at University of California, San Francisco and State University of New York, Buffalo, to the elucidation of the pharmacokinetics of salicylates. This topic is important for two reasons: first, plasma concentrations of salicylates do relate to therapeutic and toxic effects, and, second, there is considerable intersubject variation in salicylate pharmacokinetics (Fig. 41–2).

Plasma Concentration-Response Relationships. It is widely accepted, although not proven, that the appropriate plasma concentration range for anti-inflammatory effect is 150 to 300 μg per ml (1.1 to 2.2 mmol per liter). Salicylate assays are readily available and inexpensive and a useful adjunct to clinical assessment, particularly in the evaluation of inadequate disease control or possible salicylate toxicity. For maximal utility, blood samples should be drawn at the "trough" point in the dosing interval, that is, just before a dose of salicylate.

Bioavailability. Aspirin and salicylates, once in solution, are rapidly and completely absorbed across the gastrointestinal mucosa by passive diffusion.[3, 4] The wide variety of formulations of aspirin and salicylates alter the rate of dissolution of drug and thereby determine the rate of absorption.[5, 5a] Thus, factors that hasten dissolution, such as micronizing aspirin, addition of antacids to formulations, and the use of water-soluble salts of sodium and calcium aspirin, increase absorption rates.[6] Rapidly absorbed formulations are preferred when aspirin is being used

as a simple analgesic because onset of action is faster and analgesia may be more effective and prolonged.[7] Although the acidic environment of the stomach promotes the presence of the lipid-soluble, un-ionized acid species of salicylate, which is much better absorbed than the ionized form, the bulk of absorption occurs in the upper small intestine, as a consequence of the larger surface area and abundant blood supply.

Factors that either speed up (e.g., metoclopramide) or slow down (e.g., food, anticholinergic drugs) gastric emptying will *pari pasu* perturb the rate of absorption of aspirin but generally will not reduce the amount of absorption. These effects are particularly notable with pH-sensitive, enteric-coated tablets, which are designed to reduce gastrointestinal side effects by liberating their contents in the small intestine and not in the stomach. Consequently, the onset of absorption can be quite variable, but this is not of great consequence in patients taking high doses chronically because of the stabilizing effect on plasma salicylate levels of the long half-life of salicylate at high doses (see later). Modern enteric-coated salicylate formulations are generally reliable with respect to the extent of absorption, although this may occasionally be erratic in certain individuals.[8, 9]

First-pass metabolism is considerable for the esters of salicylate, namely aspirin and salicylsalicylate. They are subject to the action of esterases in the gut wall, portal blood, and liver, resulting in liberation of salicylate. Thus, between 30 and 50 percent of aspirin is hydrolyzed during first-pass metabolism,[4] this proportion potentially increasing substantially if aspirin is administered as a slow-release formulation or after meals. As the salicylate anion is active as an anti-inflammatory drug in its own right, the high first-pass metabolism of aspirin is of little consequence for anti-inflammatory effect.

Distribution and Protein Binding. Typical of weakly acidic drugs, salicylate has a small volume of distribution (approximately 0.17 liter per kg) owing to low tissue binding but avid binding to plasma albumin. Salicylates accumulate in relatively acidic environments, such as the inflamed joint, gastric mucosa, and renal medulla, because of the phenomenon of "ion trapping" (Fig. 41–3).[10]

The "free-fraction" of salicylate refers to the ratio of free, or unbound, concentration to total plasma concentration, and it increases with increasing dose of salicylate.[11] Thus, about 10 percent is unbound at total plasma salicylate levels of 100 μg per ml, rising to 25 percent at 300 μg per ml. This increase with dose is due to two effects, namely, saturation of binding sites on albumin and also saturation of the capacity of the clearance mechanisms for unbound salicylate.[12, 12a] The latter mechanism is most significant, as this determines the unbound salicylate concentration. The unbound concentration of salicylate is most relevant because it is available to bind to its receptors. Salicylate plasma binding is reduced in hypoalbuminemic and uremic states and as a result

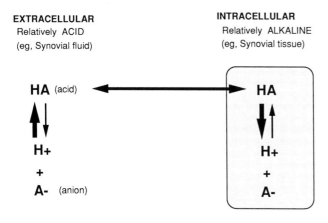

EXTRACELLULAR
Relatively ACID
(eg, Synovial fluid)

INTRACELLULAR
Relatively ALKALINE
(eg, Synovial tissue)

Relatively more acid   Relatively more anions

Figure 41–3. Weak acids such as salicylate accumulate in relatively acidic areas such as inflamed joints. (Source: Day, R. O.: Mode of action of nonsteroidal anti-inflammatory drugs. Med. J. Aust. 1988; 148:195. Copyright © *The Medical Journal of Australia* 1988. Adapted with permission.)

of competitive protein-binding interactions.[13] Reduced binding in the elderly is due to decreased albumin levels.[14]

Synovial Fluid Distribution. Aspirin and salicylate are detected in significant concentrations in synovial fluid, but peak levels are less than in plasma, and synovial fluid concentrations are sustained for longer than plasma levels, indicating slow transport of drug into and out of the synovial compartment.[15, 16] At the high dosages typically employed in rheumatic diseases, plasma and synovial fluid salicylate concentrations achieve a constant ratio because the long plasma half-life of elimination of the drug exceeds the half-lives for transport of salicylate into and out of the synovial space. Importantly, it has been shown that unbound concentrations of salicylate in plasma and synovial fluid are equal during chronic, high-dose therapy[17] (Fig. 41–4).

Metabolism and Half-Life. The half-life of aspirin in plasma is about 15 minutes, and accumulation during chronic therapy cannot occur.[18] Salicylate, liberated from aspirin by hydrolysis, is subject to renal excretion and conjugative metabolic processes in the liver, with a minor proportion being oxidized (Fig. 41–5). The total oral dose is recovered in the urine as salicylate and its metabolites. The formation of salicylurate and salicylphenolic glucuronide are "capacity limited" or "saturable" in the usual dosage ranges. This means that proportionally less salicylurate and salicylphenolic glucuronide is recovered in urine with increasing daily dose of salicylate.[19] Consequently, the overall clearance of salicylate falls as dose increases, and its plasma elimination half-life increases from about 2 hours after 250 mg of aspirin to 12 to 16 hours after 3 to 4 g of aspirin daily.

The time it takes for salicylate to reach plateau or steady-state concentrations increases with increasing daily dosages and is of the order of 3 to 5 days at the higher doses employed to treat rheumatoid arthritis. During high-dose therapy with salicylate, dosage intervals of 8 or 12 hours yield acceptable swings between peak and trough salicylate concentrations, as would be expected given the long half-life of salicylate at these doses. Saturation of metabolism leads to more than proportional increases in total plasma salicylate concentrations versus daily dosage, and this is most notable at concentrations at the lower end of the therapeutic concentration range, namely, 100 μg per ml.[12] At higher plasma concentrations, this effect is counteracted by the increasing saturation of binding to plasma albumin such that total plasma concentrations of salicylate are approximately proportional to the daily dosage of salicylate throughout most of the therapeutic range for salicylate. However, it is important to note that unbound concentrations will rise more than proportionally with increasing dose, as a result of decreasing clearance of unbound salicylate.

Steady-state levels of salicylate can fall significantly in the first few weeks of dosing, as a result of autoinduction of the formation rate of salicylurate and salicylphenolic glucuronide.[20, 21] Men may have a higher metabolic clearance of salicylate because of enhanced formation of salicylurate,[22, 23] but this has not been observed by others.[24]

Urinary Excretion. Unmetabolized salicylate is both filtered through the glomerulus and secreted by the weak acid secretory system of the proximal convoluted tubule. The lipid-soluble, un-ionized form is subject to reabsorption from the tubular lumen. Reabsorption is increased in acidic urine and decreased in alkaline urine owing to changes in the relative abundance of the lipophilic, un-ionized species. A 20-fold increase in renal clearance of salicylate results from increasing urinary pH from 5 to 8 (Fig.

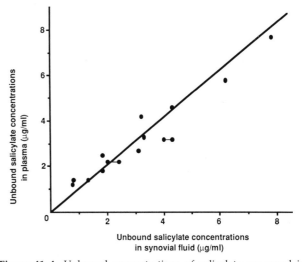

Figure 41–4. Unbound concentrations of salicylate are equal in plasma and synovial fluid during chronic dosing. The diagonal represents the line of identity and the joined points are from pairs of knees. (Reproduced with permission from Rosenthal, R. K., Boyles, T. B., and Fremont-Smith, K.: Simultaneous salicylate concentrations in synovial fluid and plasma in rheumatoid arthritis. Arthritis Rheum. 7:103, 1964.)

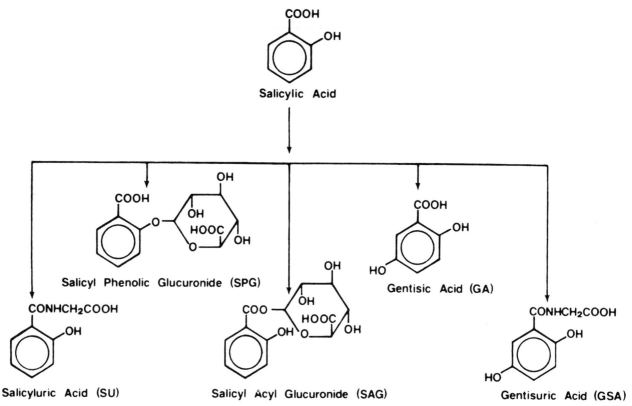

Figure 41–5. The metabolic pathways of salicylate. The major metabolite is salicylurate, a glycine conjugate which accounts for about 60% of the dose when salicylate 3-4 g/day is given. Salicyl phenolic glucuronide accounts for 20% of the dose, salicyl acyl glucuronide 10%, the oxidative product gentisate 4%, and gentisuric acid a minute percentage.

41–6).[5] These effects can be important clinically especially during high-dose therapy, in which a greater proportion of salicylate is eliminated unchanged. Even small changes in urinary pH, as occur with introduction or cessation of regular dosing with standard liquid antacids, can lead to wide swings in plasma salicylate concentrations.[25, 26]

MECHANISMS OF ANTI-INFLAMMATORY ACTION

Inhibition of the synthesis of prostaglandins is widely accepted as the major mechanism of action of aspirin as an anti-inflammatory, analgesic, antipyretic, and antiplatelet agent.[27, 28] These actions, especially the analgesic effects, are mediated peripherally, that is, at the site of the inflammatory or painful stimulus.[29] Aspirin is unique among NSAIDs in that it irreversibly acetylates the enzyme cyclooxygenase, leading to prolonged inhibition; thus, the effect on platelet function lasts the lifetime of the platelet.[30]

Aspirin is increasingly used as an antithrombotic because of its ability to inhibit thromboxane A_2 synthesis in platelets. Prostacyclin and prostaglandin E_2 synthesis by vascular endothelium is also inhibited but recovers more quickly than thomboxane A_2 synthesis.[31] It is possible, with appropriate aspirin dosing

schedules, to continuously inhibit thromboxane A_2 synthesis while prostacyclin synthesis is only briefly and intermittently inhibited. This is beneficial, as thromboxane A_2 is a potent stimulus for platelet aggregation, whereas prostacyclin is a potent vasodilator and inhibits platelet aggregation.

There are some difficulties with the hypothesis that aspirin exerts its effects solely by inhibition of prostaglandin synthesis.[32] In marked contrast with aspirin, salicylate is a weak, reversible inhibitor of cyclooxygenase; yet, when it is administered directly it is as effective as aspirin as an anti-inflammatory drug, although less potent as an antipyretic, analgesic, and antiplatelet agent.[33, 34] Thus, it has been suggested that there may be pharmacologic effects of salicylate in addition to inhibition of the synthesis of prostanoids. Vane and colleagues[35] have evidence that salicylate in high doses leads to reduction in prostaglandin synthesis, whereas other investigators find no evidence that sodium salicylate reduces prostaglandin secretion in vivo.[36] Numerous mechanisms have been canvassed as possible contributors to the anti-inflammatory actions of salicylates, including inhibition of polymorphonuclear leukocyte and monocyte functions such as chemotaxis, aggregation, and phagocytosis; inhibition of the release of lysosomal enzymes; impairment of the synthesis of various leukotrienes; scavenging of oxygen-centered free radicals; and inhibition of lymphocyte transforma-

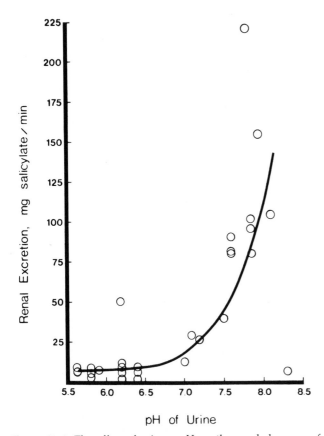

Figure 41–6. The effect of urinary pH on the renal clearance of salicylate. (Reproduced with permission from Levy, G., and Leonards, J. R.: Absorption, metabolism, and excretion of salicylates. *In* Smith, M. J. H., and Smith, P. K. [eds.]: Salicylate: A Critical Bibliographic Review. New York, Interscience Publishers, 1966.)

tion.[32, 37, 38] Recent work suggests that aspirin and the salicylate anion may act independently of prostaglandin synthesis by disrupting signal transduction across inflammatory cell membranes to a range of stimuli, such as leukotriene B_4, platelet-activating factor, and $C5_a$, particularly by interfering with the functions of various membrane G proteins.[39] None of these purported "non-prostaglandin inhibitory mechanisms" have yet been demonstrated to contribute to the anti-inflammatory effect of salicylates in vivo.

USE IN RHEUMATIC DISEASES

In the treatment of chronic rheumatic disease, salicylate formulations that are absorbed largely in the small intestine, such as slow-release or enteric-coated formulations, are optimal because they are better tolerated by the upper gastrointestinal tract. Perhaps, even better tolerated are nonacetylated salicylate formulations.

Rheumatoid Arthritis. Numerous controlled studies indicate that high-dose (3.9 g per day or more) salicylates are able to suppress the inflammation of rheumatoid arthritis rapidly and reversibly

and that the major anti-inflammatory principle is the salicylate ion.[13, 40, 41] Unlike the disease-modifying antirheumatic drugs, such as gold salts, the salicylates do not appear to appreciably slow disease progression or joint damage. At the high doses indicated for active inflammation, the long half-life of salicylate allows 8 or even 12 hourly dosing of standard salicylate preparations and also slow-release and enteric-coated formulations. Despite the availability of many newer NSAIDs, none has been shown to be notably more efficacious than salicylates in rheumatoid arthritis. Optimal results will be achieved by maintaining trough plasma salicylate concentrations between 150 and 300 µg per ml.

Spondylarthropathies. Aspirin, 4 g per day, is less effective than indomethacin, 100 g per day, or phenylbutazone, 300 mg per day, for ankylosing spondylitis.[42]

Juvenile Rheumatoid Arthritis. Aspirin is as effective as other NSAIDs, such as tolmetin, in the treatment of juvenile rheumatoid arthritis and is used in doses ranging up to 70 to 120 mg per kg per day (2.5 g per m^2 per day) in order to maintain concentrations in the high therapeutic range, namely, 200 to 300 µg per ml.[43]

Osteoarthritis. Aspirin is used extensively in osteoarthritis and is useful in the control of pain and stiffness in the short term. Considerable debate surrounds the use of salicylates or NSAIDs on a long-term basis because of possible deleterious effects on cartilage metabolism (see later). The intermittent use of salicylates during periods of increased symptomatology and, particularly, inflammation may be optimal.

Gout. Aspirin is not generally used to treat acute gout, although high-dose aspirin with plasma salicylate concentrations greater than 150 µg per ml is effective as an anti-inflammatory agent and also enhances urinary excretion of urate. On the other hand, low-dose salicylate can lead to urate retention by inhibiting renal tubular secretion of urate, thereby increasing the risk of acute gout.[44] Indomethacin is generally the drug of choice for acute gout.

Rheumatic Fever. High-dose salicylates reduce the inflammatory arthritis, fever, and erythrocyte sedimentation rate as effectively as glucocorticoids in patients with rheumatic fever.[45]

ADVERSE EFFECTS

It has been said that aspirin would not be registered if it was submitted to the U.S. Food and Drug Administration today because of its impressive list of adverse effects. There is little doubt that plain aspirin taken chronically in high dosage is much less well tolerated than newer NSAIDs, but modern aspirin and salicylate formulations are tolerated as well as, and possibly better than, other NSAIDs and are at least as effective. Overall, it appears that the acetyl group of aspirin adds little to anti-inflammatory efficacy but is associated with more adverse effects than its metabolite salicylate.[46a]

Gastrointestinal Adverse Effects

Aspirin-Induced Acute Mucosal Injury. Acute injury to the gastric mucosa by aspirin is due to aspirin-induced breaches in the gastric mucosal barrier that allow back-diffusion of hydrogen ions across the mucosa, resulting in inflammation and bleeding.[46] This effect is enhanced by alcohol, nicotine, and bile reflux. Aspirin inhibits the synthesis of mucosal prostaglandin E_2 and prostacyclin, which are important in maintaining the mucosal barrier and blood flow and inhibiting acid secretion.[47] Administration of prostaglandin analogues orally significantly reduces aspirin-induced acute mucosal injury, as will preadministration of histamine$_2$ receptor blockers such as cimetidine.

Dyspepsia. Dyspepsia is the most common adverse effect of aspirin and is expected in as many as one third of subjects taking the drug chronically. There is no good relationship between dyspepsia and observable upper gastrointestinal pathology. Thus, a considerable proportion of patients with endoscopically proven ulcers are symptom free. Indeed, it is known that the elderly who sustain a serious gastrointestinal bleed while taking NSAIDs are quite likely not to have noted dyspepsia or pain prior to the event.[48]

Administration of aspirin after meals, with water, liquid antacids, or sucralfate, may improve tolerance. Buffered preparations of aspirin are widely used; although they can reduce dyspepsia, there is little or no effect on mucosal damage.[49] Enteric-coated and slow-release preparations do decrease luminal contact of aspirin with the gastric mucosa and are associated with less dyspepsia, mucosal bleeding, and endoscopic evidence of damage than is plain aspirin[50] and have a rate of upper gastrointestinal adverse effects similar to that of other NSAIDs. Nonacetylated salicylates, such as salicylsalicylic acid and CMT, are associated with substantially less dyspepsia and gastrointestinal damage than is plain aspirin and perform similarly or better than do other NSAIDs in this respect.[51]

Occult blood loss due to aspirin and other NSAIDs is well known and is most probable with plain aspirin taken chronically in high dosage. Substantial decreases in hemoglobin are, however, uncommon.[52]

Peptic Ulceration, Major Bleeding, and Perforation. In recent years, the serious upper gastrointestinal adverse effects of aspirin and NSAIDs have been studied intensely. In the consideration of the risks of these effects, aspirin used chronically in the management of rheumatic diseases has not been differentiated from other NSAIDs used similarly. It may be that the risks associated with nonacetylated salicylate preparations are less than with other NSAIDs, but this remains to be established.

Endoscopic studies of patients taking NSAIDs indicate a very high proportion with mucosal damage, notably 10 to 20 percent with gastric, particularly antral and pre-pyloric, ulcers,[53] but, as noted, correlation with dyspeptic symptoms is poor. Aspirin, 1 g per day for 3 years, was associated with a relative risk of 10.7 times (95 percent confidence interval 2.5 to 45.5 times) for duodenal ulcer and 9.7 (1.2 to 71.4) for gastric ulcer–related hospitalizations in males.[54] Of most importance is the risk of major bleeding or perforation as a consequence of exposure to aspirin or NSAIDs. The estimates of absolute risk of serious gastrointestinal complications for NSAIDs have varied widely, from 2 to 4 percent per year,[55] to 1 percent per year risk of hospitalization due to NSAID-induced upper gastrointestinal adverse effects in patients with RA[56] and downward. A figure of the order of 3 to 6 cases per 1000 patient years of therapy is reasonable at present.[53, 57] An individual's risk of complications of peptic ulcer is low but increases two- to fivefold as a consequence of chronic NSAID intake.[53] Risk increases with age greater than 65 years and a previous peptic ulcer, particularly a recent, large, or complicated ulcer. Recent studies indicate that higher doses of NSAIDs increase the risk, which may be greatest after 3 to 4 months of therapy.[58]

Misoprostol, 100 to 200 μg four times daily, is effective in significantly reducing the appearance of NSAID-induced adverse effects, including aspirin-induced gastric ulcers, and this effect appears to be apparent for at least 3 to 12 months.[59, 60] Ranitidine, cimetidine, and sucralfate are not as effective. Histamine 2 antagonists and misoprostol are effective against the much less common NSAID-induced duodenal ulcer, and the proton-pump inhibitor omeprazole is probably highly effective against all NSAID-induced peptic ulcers.[53]

Renal Effects

Aspirin and NSAIDs are associated with a range of adverse renal effects.[61]

Acute Effects. A temporary but variable reduction in glomerular filtration rate and renal blood flow can occur during aspirin treatment, and this is more probable in subjects who are salt- and volume-depleted or who have pre-existing abnormal renal function as a result of lupus erythematosus, glomerulonephritis, cirrhosis, and heart failure. The latter patients are reliant on renal prostaglandin synthesis to counteract the vasoconstrictive effects of the renin-angiotensin and adrenergic systems. Such patients require regular monitoring of body weight, blood pressure, and urine for protein and plasma creatinine. These effects may be less with nonacetylated salicylates, although deterioration of chronic renal impairment has been observed with salicylic acid.[77] Inhibition of renal prostaglandin synthesis can also result in salt and water retention and peripheral edema.[61, 62]

Hyperkalemia. Hyperkalemia can occur with aspirin and is more probable in patients with renal insufficiency. This effect is attributed to inhibition of renin secretion and the resulting reduction in angiotensin II and aldosterone levels.[61]

Papillary Necrosis. Papillary necrosis is characteristic of "analgesic nephropathy," leading to cortical atrophy and renal failure. This lesion has been clearly related to abuse of analgesics, notably combinations of aspirin with phenacetin or possibly paracetamol.[63] More recently, the latter two agents, but not aspirin, have been implicated.[64] There has been much debate whether patients taking aspirin alone for the treatment of rheumatic diseases can develop analgesic nephropathy, and absolute and relative risks are not yet known. It seems that aspirin alone may rarely cause this problem.[65] Hematuria and azotemia are indicators of this lesion.

The effects on renal function and airways (see later) in aspirin-sensitive individuals are less with nonacetylated salicylates; however, deterioration of renal function in some high-risk patients has been observed with these salicylate formulations.[77]

Hepatotoxicity

Elevation of Hepatic Enzymes. Transient elevation of hepatic transaminase concentrations in plasma despite continued therapy is not unusual with chronic aspirin therapy, particularly in patients with juvenile rheumatoid arthritis or systemic lupus erythematosus, or patients who are elderly or have impaired renal function. This effect is enhanced by methotrexate, whereas hydroxychloroquine substantially reduces the frequency of raised enzymes.[66] In a comparison with ibuprofen in arthritic patients, aspirin was significantly more hepatotoxic.[67] The hepatic lesions are characterized by scattered necrosis, mononuclear cell infiltration of portal tracts, and, sometimes, biliary stasis. If hepatic enzyme concentrations exceed three times the upper limit of normal or if there is other evidence of hepatic damage, such as prolongation of the prothrombin time, then aspirin should be stopped.[68] Jaundice and symptomatic hepatitis due to aspirin are quite rare.

Reye's Syndrome. This is a rare and often fatal condition in children, characterized by encephalopathy and fatty degeneration of the liver and kidneys that is linked with aspirin therapy and concurrent viral illness. Children with juvenile rheumatoid arthritis probably are at greater risk for this adverse effect simply because of their greater exposure to aspirin. There has been a substantial decrease in the incidence of this syndrome in the United States and the United Kingdom since public warnings about the association between aspirin and Reye's syndrome.[69]

Bleeding

Aspirin inhibits collagen, epinephrine, and adenosine diphosphate (ADP)-induced platelet aggregation for the 5- to 7-day lifetime of the platelet[70] as a result of the irreversible inhibition of platelet cyclooxygenase. Salicylate does not inhibit platelet function, as it is a very weak, reversible cyclooxygenase inhibitor.[71] Thus, salicylsalicylic acid and CMT have no significant effect on platelets,[72] and CMT has been used successfully in treating the symptoms of hemophiliac arthropathy without bleeding occurring.[73] Aspirin prolongs the bleeding time by about 2 minutes, the effect lasting for around 24 to 48 hours. This limited effect is surprising, given the potency of aspirin-induced inhibition of platelet function in vitro, but aspirin is less effective in inhibiting thrombin-induced platelet aggregation, thrombin being important in this role in vivo.[31] About 14 percent of individuals may be "hyper-responders" to aspirin with respect to bleeding time.[74] Also, bleeding time prolongation by aspirin is likely to be very significant in subjects who are anticoagulated, have coagulation disorders, or have taken alcohol recently. Aspirin and salicylates can also lengthen the prothrombin time, but only if plasma salicylate concentrations are maintained above 300 μg per ml.

Surprisingly, there are few published data that aspirin is associated with significant hemorrhagic complications in surgical patients.[75] Many surgeons believe that aspirin increases perioperative bleeding and therefore recommend that aspirin not be taken for some days before surgery. Acetaminophen, a short-acting NSAID, or a nonacetylated salicylate could be employed before surgery. Aspirin taken within 5 days before giving birth increases the risk of bleeding complications in mothers and babies.

Anaphylactoid Reactions, Intolerance, and Skin Reactions

Aspirin Intolerance. Classically, aspirin intolerance is manifested by asthma and rhinitis associated with nasal polyposis and often accompanied by erythema and conjunctival inflammation. A wide range of reactions occurs, and the reported incidence varies, depending on the study methods employed.[76] Acute asthma, and/or angioedema or urticaria occurs minutes to hours following ingestion of aspirin and can culminate in shock and death. Aspirin intolerance is of the order of 5 to 25 percent in asthmatics, but this includes those whose asthma is simply exacerbated by aspirin.[31] Aspirin intolerance correlates with prostaglandin synthesis inhibition, and other NSAIDs are equally dangerous in susceptible individuals, whereas sodium salicylate, which is a weak prostaglandin synthesis inhibitor, often is tolerated. It is unknown whether this syndrome is due to decreased levels of prostaglandins, increased synthesis of leukotrienes, or some combination of these

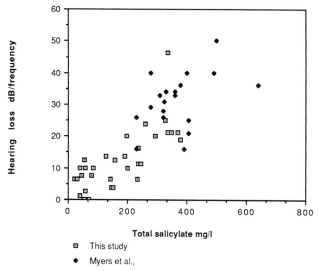

Total salicylate mg/l

□ This study

◆ Myers et al.,

Figure 41–7. Relationship between hearing loss in decibels and total plasma salicylate concentrations during chronic dosing. (From Myers, E. N., Bernstein, J. M., and Fostiropolous, G.: Salicylate ototoxicity: A clinical study. N. Engl. J. Med. 273:587, 1965. Reprinted with permission from *The New England Journal of Medicine*.)

effects in susceptible individuals.[78] Nonacetylated salicylates may be used with great caution in aspirin-sensitive subjects, as there have been reports of serious reactions even with these drugs.[79] Alternatives include acetaminophen and narcotic analgesics.

Skin Reactions. Acute or chronic urticaria may be caused by aspirin in as many as 5 to 10 percent of cases. Some patients with aspirin-sensitive chronic urticaria also react to other NSAIDs, tartrazine, and preservatives such as sodium benzoate.

Tinnitus and Deafness

Tinnitus and a reversible, sensorineural hearing deficit up to 30 to 40 decibels across all audible frequencies are common in people prescribed high doses of salicylate, and there is a linear relationship between unbound and total plasma concentrations of salicylate and these symptoms (Fig. 41–7).[80] These symptoms are part of the syndrome of *salicylism*, which includes vague neurologic symptoms, hyperventilation, and sweating, and this effect may be more difficult to diagnose in the young and elderly.

Articular Cartilage

It is known that salicylates and some other NSAIDs can suppress cartilage metabolism and the synthesis of proteoglycans by chondrocytes in vitro and ex vivo from animals, and that these effects are more marked in osteoarthritic than normal cartilage.[81, 82] Recent clinical data suggest that

NSAIDs that are potent inhibitors of prostaglandin synthesis may be more damaging to cartilage than are weak inhibitors.[83] These findings may have implications for the use of aspirin, nonacetylated salicylates, and NSAIDs chronically used in humans, but further work focusing on global clinical outcomes in addition to process measures, such as cartilage thickness, is needed to clarify the situation.[84]

Salicylate Overdose

Salicylate poisoning is common, especially in children, and can be fatal, death being probably due to toxic brain concentrations of salicylate.[85] Hyperventilation, sweating, fever, and dehydration are common signs of salicylate toxicity. Respiratory alkalosis due to hyperventilation followed by metabolic acidosis results from central and metabolic effects of salicylate. Acidosis is a poor prognostic sign and leads to sequestration of salicylate into the relatively alkaline brain cells. Alkalinization enhances renal elimination of salicylate and reduces brain salicylate levels.[85] Activated charcoal is useful to reduce the absorption of aspirin from the gastrointestinal tract, and hemodialysis may be needed in severe cases.

Pregnancy and Lactation

Pregnancy and labor can be prolonged by aspirin, as is the case with other NSAIDs that inhibit the synthesis of prostaglandins. Whether there is a risk of congenital malformations if aspirin is taken early during pregnancy is contentious, with large prospective, controlled studies generally not detecting any effect.[86] It is estimated that about 0.1 to 0.2 percent of the maternal daily dose of salicylate is available to the baby over a 24-hour period via breast milk, but no studies have examined systematically breast milk salicylate in mothers on chronic high-dose therapy. Occasional cases of infants with very high plasma salicylate concentrations acquired by this route have been reported.[87]

DRUG INTERACTIONS

Salicylate is involved in pharmacokinetic and pharmacodynamic drug interactions, in which salicylate may be either the precipitant or the object drug in these interactions.[88]

Effects of Other Drugs on Salicylates

Antacids. Antacids and sucralfate are commonly administered with salicylates either in combination products (soluble and buffered tablets) or separately to reduce gastrointestinal adverse effects. Generally, antacids may increase the rate of absorption of salicylate (e.g., soluble tablets) but not significantly affect the total absorption of salicylate.

Steroids. Concurrent low-dose glucocorticoids can lead to substantially lower steady-state concentrations of salicylate, the mechanism being uncertain but most likely due to enhanced metabolic clearance of salicylate.[22, 88, 89] This effect has also been seen after intra-articular administration of glucocorticoids.[90] Coadministration of the oral contraceptive steroids also increases metabolic clearance of salicylates, formation of both salicylurate and salicylic acid glucuronides being enhanced.[88]

Probenecid. Probenecid inhibits the renal secretion of salicylate.[91] Because little salicylate is generally excreted unchanged, this interaction is usually not clinically significant unless the urine is alkaline, when excretion of unchanged salicylate becomes substantial. Salicylate at concentrations above 50 μg per ml inhibits the uricosuric action of probenecid.

Effects of Salicylates on Other Drugs

Interactions Due To Inhibition of Renal and Vascular Prostaglandin Synthesis. A number of drug interactions relate to prostaglandin synthesis inhibition. These include reduction in natriuretic or hypotensive actions of several *diuretics* and *antihypertensive agents*. This occurs as a result of inhibition of the prostaglandin-dependent renal and vascular hemodynamic effects of these drugs and minor direct sodium-retaining actions of aspirin.[62, 92] Thus, the diuretic, natriuretic, and hypotensive effects of furosemide, thiazides (hypotensive but not natriuretic effects inhibited), spironolactone, triamterene (especially hazardous with aspirin), beta (β)-blockers, and angiotensin-converting enzyme (ACE) inhibitors (e.g., captopril) are inhibited to variable degrees by aspirin. The latter interactions are most apparent when there is underlying renal disease or reduced renal perfusion associated with hyponatremia, volume depletion, cirrhosis, and heart failure. Salicylate-induced reduction in glomerular filtration rate can lead to toxicity of *lithium, digoxin,* and *aminoglycoside,* again more likely in those with pre-existing renal impairment or volume depletion.

Concurrent use of acetazolamide and salicylates should be avoided, as unbound acetazolamide concentrations increase substantially owing to competition for secretion across the renal tubule as well as binding to plasma albumin.[88]

Anticoagulants. Aspirin has the potential to increase bleeding in patients anticoagulated with warfarin or heparin and is therefore relatively contraindicated. The propensity of aspirin to cause acute upper gastrointestinal mucosal injury and to inhibit platelet function is reason to avoid salicylates in anticoagulated individuals. Although warfarin is displaced from plasma albumin by salicylates, a long-lasting effect on prothrombin time is not expected; however, there may be a transient increase in this index after commencement of salicylates, particularly in patients with significant impairment of hepatic or renal function. Again, nonacetylated salicylates, which will not inhibit platelet function and which cause less gastrointestinal damage than does aspirin, are less likely to adversely interact with anticoagulants.

Methotrexate. A dangerous interaction can occur between methotrexate and salicylates, leading to retention of methotrexate and the potential for marrow and other toxicities. Salicylate inhibits the renal clearance of methotrexate, and, additionally, there is a competitive protein-binding reaction between these two drugs.[93] Although this interaction is much more likely with high-dosage compared with "rheumatic" regimens of methotrexate, serious interactions have occurred at "rheumatic doses" of methotrexate, particularly in the elderly and renally impaired.

Anticonvulsants. Salicylate displaces phenytoin from albumin, but unbound concentrations of phenytoin are unlikely to be substantially affected because of compensatory increases in total clearance of phenytoin. However, the total concentrations of phenytoin are lower, but dose increases are not indicated because efficacy and toxicity relate directly to unbound concentrations of phenytoin, and no substantive change in therapeutic performance is predicted.[88] Valproic acid toxicity has been reported following the introduction of aspirin therapy, which results in increases in unbound plasma concentrations of valproate owing possibly to a combination of protein-binding competition and inhibition of β-oxidation of valproate.[88]

Other NSAIDs. Aspirin has been widely used with other NSAIDs, but there seems to be little merit in this approach, particularly as anti-inflammatory doses of both drugs increase adverse effects.[94] The plasma concentrations of NSAIDs drop as a result of concurrent high-dose salicylate, owing to a competitive protein-binding interaction, but unbound NSAID concentrations probably are little altered.[88]

Oral Hypoglycemics. Moderate doses of salicylates may potentiate the actions of oral hypoglycemic drugs, perhaps related to inherent hypoglycemic effects of salicylates.[95]

CONCLUSION

The salicylates are effective and safe NSAIDs. Tolerability is significantly enhanced by slow-release and enteric-coated formulations of aspirin and by the nonacetylated salicylates. The place of salicylates in rheumatic therapy is being reassessed, as it is increasingly appreciated that the nonacetylated formulations may be advantageous in comparison not only with aspirin but also with other NSAIDs with respect to gastrointestinal and renal toxicities.

References

1. Gross, M., and Greenberg, L.: The Salicylates. New Haven, Hillhouse Press, 1948.

2. Weissmann, G.: Aspirin. Sci. Am. January:58, 1991.
3. Levy, G.: Salicylates. *In* Dixon, A. St. J., Martin, B. K., Smith, M. J. H., and Wood, P. H. N. (eds.): An International Symposium. Boston, Little Brown, 1963.
4. Rowland, M., Reigelman, S., and Harris, P., et al.: Absorption kinetics of aspirin in man following oral administration of an aqueous solution. J. Pharm. Sci. 61:379, 1972.
5. Levy, G., and Leonards, J. R.: Absorption, metabolism and excretion of salicylates. *In* Smith, M. J. H., and Smith, P. K. (eds.): Salicylate: A Critical Bibliographic Review. New York, Interscience Publishers, 1966.
5a. Bochner, F., Somogyi, A. A., and Wilson, K. M.: Bioinequivalence of our 100 mg oral aspirin formulations in healthy volunteers. Clin. Pharmacokinet. 21:394, 1991.
6. Levy, G.: Comparison of dissolution and absorption rates of different commercial aspirin tablets. J. Pharm. Sci. 50:388, 1961.
7. Levy, G.: Clinical pharmacokinetics of salicylates. A reassessment. Br. J. Clin. Pharmacol. 10:285, 1980.
8. Paull, P., Day, R., and Graham, G., et al.: Single dose evaluation of a new enteric-coated aspirin preparation. Med. J. Aust. 1:617, 1976.
9. Halla, J., Fallahi, S., and Hardin, J.: Acute and chronic salicylate intoxication in a patient with gastric outlet obstruction. Arthritis Rheum. 24:1205, 1981.
10. Brune, K., and Graf, P.: Non-steroid anti-inflammatory drugs: influence of extra-cellular pH on biodistribution and pharmacological effects. Biochem. Pharmacol. 27:525, 1978.
11. Ekstrand, R., Alvan, G., and Borga, O.: Concentration-dependent plasma protein binding of salicylate in rheumatoid patients. Clin. Pharmacokinet. 4:137, 1979.
12. Furst, D., Tozer, T., and Melmon, K.: Salicylate clearance, the resultant of protein binding and metabolism. Clin. Pharmacol. Ther. 26:380, 1979.
12a. Shen, J., Wanwimolruk, S., and Purves, R. D., et al.: Model representation of salicylate pharmacokinetics using unbound plasma salicylate concentrations and metabolite urinary excretion rates following a single oral dose. J. Pharmacokinet. Biopharm. 19:575, 1991.
13. Day, R. O., Furst, D. E., and Graham, G. G., et al.: The clinical pharmacology of aspirin and the salicylates. *In* Paulus, H. E., Furst, D. E., and Dromgoole, S. H. (eds.): Drugs for Rheumatic Disease. New York, Churchill Livingstone, 1987.
14. Roberts, M., Rumble, R., and Wanwimolruk, S., et al.: Pharmacokinetics of aspirin and salicylate in elderly subjects and in patients with alcoholic liver disease. Eur. J. Clin. Pharmacol. 25:253, 1983.
15. Sholkoff, S., Eyring, E., and Rowland, M., et al.: Plasma and synovial fluid concentrations of acetylsalicylic acid in patients with rheumatoid arthritis. Arthritis Rheum. 10:348, 1967.
16. Soren, A.: Kinetics of salicylates in blood and joint fluid. Eur. J. Clin. Pharmacol. 16:279, 1979.
17. Rosenthal, R. K., Bayles, T. B., and Fremont-Smith, K.: Simultaneous salicylate concentrations in synovial fluid and plasma in rheumatoid arthritis. Arthritis Rheum. 7:103, 1964.
18. Rowland, M., and Riegelman, S.: Pharmacokinetics of acetylsalicylic acid and salicylic acid after intravenous administration in man. J. Pharm. Sci. 57:1313, 1968.
19. Levy, G., and Tsuchiya, T.: Salicylate accumulation kinetics in man. N. Engl. J. Med. 9:430, 1972.
20. Furst, D., Gupta, N., and Paulus, H.: Salicylate metabolism in twins: evidence suggesting a genetic influence and induction of salicylurate formation. J. Clin. Invest. 60:32, 1977.
21. Day, R. O., Furst, D. E., and Dromgoole, S. H., et al.: Changes in salicylate serum concentration and metabolism during chronic dosing in normal volunteers. Biopharm. Drug Dispos. 9:273, 1988.
22. Graham, G., Champion, G., and Day, R., et al.: Patterns of plasma levels and urinary excretion of salicylates in subjects with rheumatoid arthritis. Clin. Pharmacol. Ther. 22:410, 1977.
23. Miners, J., Grgurinovich, N., and Whitehead, A., et al.: Influence of gender and oral contraceptive steroids on the metabolism of salicylic acid and acetylsalicylic acid. Br. J. Clin. Pharmacol. 22:135, 1986.
24. Montgomery, P., Berger, L., and Mitenko, P., et al.: Salicylate metabolism: effects of age and sex in adults. Clin. Pharmacol. Ther. 39:571, 1986.
25. Levy, G., Lampman, T., and Kamath, B., et al.: Decreased serum salicylate concentrations in children with rheumatic fever treated with antacid. N. Engl. J. Med. 293:323, 1975.
26. Hansten, P. D., and Hayton, W. L.: Effect of antacid and ascorbic acid on serum salicylate concentration. J. Clin. Pharmacol. 20:326, 1980.
27. Vane, J.: Inhibition of prostaglandin synthesis as a mechanism of action for aspirin-like drugs. Nature (New Biol.) 231:232, 1971.
28. Flower, R., Gryglewski, R., and Hervasczynska-Cedro, K., et al.: Effects of anti-inflammatory drugs on prostaglandin biosynthesis. Nature (New Biol.) 238:104, 1972.
29. Lim, R. K. S.: Analgesia. *In* Smith, M. J. H., and Smith, P. K. (eds.): The Salicylates. New York, John Wiley & Sons, 1966, pp. 155–202.
30. Smith, M., and Willis, A.: Aspirin selectively inhibits prostaglandin production in human platelets. Nature 231:235, 1971.
31. Oates, J. A., Fitzgerald, G. A., and Branch, R. A., et al.: Clinical implications of prostaglandin and thromboxane A_2 formation (first of two parts). N. Engl. J. Med. 319:689, 1988.
32. Atkinson, D., and Collier, H.: Salicylates: molecular mechanism of therapeutic action. Adv. Pharmacol. Chemother. 17:233, 1981.
33. Preston, S. J., Arnold, M. H., and Beller, E. M., et al.: Comparative analgesic and anti-inflammatory properties of sodium salicylate and acetylsalicylic acid (aspirin) in rheumatoid arthritis. Br. J. Clin. Pharmacol. 27:607, 1989.
34. April, P., Abeles, M., and Baraf, H., et al.: Does the acetyl group of aspirin contribute to the antiinflammatory efficacy of salicylic acid in the treatment of rheumatoid arthritis? Semin. Arthritis Rheum. 19(Suppl. 2):20, 1990.
35. Henderson, B., Higgs, G. A., and Salmon, J. J., et al.: Is aspirin a pro-drug for salicylate? Br. J. Pharmacol. Suppl. 88:400P, 1986.
36. Ritter, J. M., Cockcroft, H. S., and Doktor, J., et al.: Differential effect of aspirin on thromboxane and prostaglandin biosynthesis in man. Br. J. Clin. Pharmacol. 28:573, 1989.
37. Hichens, M.: Molecular and cellular pharmacology of the anti-inflammatory drugs: some in vitro properties related to their possible modes of action. *In* Scherrer, R. A., and Whitehouse, M. W. (eds.): Anti-inflammatory Agents: Chemistry and Pharmacology. Vol. 2. New York, Academic Press, 1974.
38. Forrest, M., and Brooks, P. M.: Mechanism of action of non-steroidal anti-rheumatic drugs. Bailliere's Clin. Rheumatol. 2(2):275, 1988.
39. Abramson, S., and Weissmann, G.: The mechanisms of action of non-steroidal anti-inflammatory drugs. Arthritis Rheum. 32:1, 1989.
40. Fremont-Smith, K., and Bayles, T.: Salicylate therapy in rheumatoid arthritis. J.A.M.A. 192:1133, 1965.
41. Boardman, P., and Hart, F.: Clinical measurement of the anti-inflammatory effect of salicylates in rheumatoid arthritis. Br. Med. J. 4:264, 1967.
42. Godfrey, R., Calabro, J., and Mills, D., et al.: A double-blind crossover trial of aspirin, indomethacin, and phenylbutazone in ankylosing spondylitis. Arthritis Rheum. 15:110, 1972.
43. Baum, J.: Aspirin in the treatment of rheumatoid arthritis. Am. J. Med. 75:10, 1983.
44. Yu, T. F., and Gutman, A. B.: Study of the paradoxical effects of salicylate in low, intermediate, and high dosage on the renal mechanisms for excretion of urate in man. J. Clin. Invest. 38:1298, 1959.
45. Bywaters, E., and Thomas, G.: Bedrest, salicylates, and steroid in rheumatic fever. Br. Med. J. 5240:1628, 1961.
46. Davenport, H. W.: Salicylate damage to the gastric mucosal barrier. N. Engl. J. Med. 276:1307, 1967.
46a. Paulus, H. E.: Aspirin versus nonacetylated salicylate. J. Rheumatol. 16:264, 1989.
47. Kauffman, G., and Grossman, M.: Prostaglandin and cimetidine inhibit the formation of ulcers produced by parenteral salicylates. Gastroenterology 75:1099, 1978.
48. Skander, M. P., and Ryan, F. P.: Non-steroidal anti-inflammatory drugs and pain-free peptic ulceration in the elderly. Br. Med. J. 297:833, 1988.
49. Silvoso, G., Ivey, K., and Butt, J., et al.: Incidence of gastric lesions in patients with rheumatic disease on chronic aspirin therapy. Ann. Intern. Med. 91:517, 1979.
50. Lanza, F., Royer, G., and Nelson, R.: Endoscopic evaluation of the effects of aspirin, buffered aspirin, and enteric-coated aspirin on gastric and duodenal mucosa. N. Engl. J. Med. 303:136, 1980.
51. Lanza, F., Rack, M. F., and Doucette, M., et al.: An endoscopic comparison of the gastroduodenal injury seen with salsalate and naproxen. J. Rheumatol. 16:1570, 1989.
52. Barager, F., and Duthie, J. J.: Importance of aspirin as a cause of anemia and peptic ulcer in rheumatoid arthritis. Br. Med. J. 1:1106, 1960.
53. Hawkey, C. J.: Non-steroidal anti-inflammatory drugs and peptic ulcers. Br. Med. J. 300:278, 1990.
54. Kurata, J. H., and Abbey, D. E.: The effect of chronic aspirin use on duodenal and gastric ulcer hospitalizations. J. Clin. Gastroenterol. 12:260, 1990.
55. Paulus, H. E.: Serious gastrointestinal toxicity of nonsteroidal antiinflammatory drugs; drug-containing renal and biliary stones; diclofenac and carprofen approved. Arthritis Rheum. 31:1450, 1988.
56. Fries, J. F., Miller, S. R., and Spitz, P. W., et al.: Towards an epidemiology of gastropathy associated with nonsteroidal antiinflammatory drug use. Gastroenterology 96(Suppl.):647, 1989.
57. Henry, D.: Side-effects of non-steroidal anti-inflammatory drugs. Bailliere's Clin. Rheumatol. 2:425, 1988.
58. Carson, J. L., Strom, B. L., and Soper, K. A., et al.: The association of non-steroidal anti-inflammatory drugs with upper gastrointestinal tract bleeding. Arch. Intern. Med. 147:85, 1987.
59. Graham, D. Y., Agrawal, N., and Roth, S. H.: Prevention of NSAID-induced gastric ulcer with misoprostol: multicentre, double-blind placebo-controlled trial. Lancet 2:1277, 1988.
60. Hopkinson, N., and Doherty, M.: NSAID-associated gastropathy—a role for misoprostol? Br. J. Rheumatol. 29:133, 1990.
61. Clive, D., and Stoff, J. S.: Renal syndromes associated with non-steroidal anti-inflammatory drugs. N. Engl. J. Med. 310:563, 1984.

62. Davis, A., Day, R. O., and Begg, E. J.: Interactions between nonsteroidal anti-inflammatory drugs and antihypertensives and diuretics. Aust. N.Z. J. Med. 16:537, 1986.
63. Prescott, L. F.: Renal damage in man from ingestion of anti-inflammatory and analgesic drugs. Adv. Inflamm Res. 6:109, 1984.
64. Sandler, D. P., Smith, J. C., and Weinberg, C. R., et al.: Analgesic use and chronic renal disease. N. Engl. J. Med. 320:1238, 1989.
65. Fries, J. F., Singh, G., and Lenert, L., et al.: Aspirin, hydroxychloroquine, and hepatic enzyme abnormalities with methotrexate in rheumatoid arthritis. Arthritis Rheum. 33:1611, 1990.
66. New Zealand Rheumatism Association Study: Aspirin and the kidney. Br. Med. J. 1:593, 1974.
67. Freeland, G. R., Northington, R. S., and Hedrich, D. A., et al.: Hepatic safety of two analgesics used over the counter: ibuprofen and aspirin. Clin. Pharmacol. Ther. 43:473, 1988.
68. Paulus, H. E.: FDA Advisory Committee Meeting. Arthritis Rheum. 26:206, 1983.
69. Glen-Bott, M. A.: Aspirin and Reye's syndrome: A reappraisal. Med. Toxicol. 2:161, 1987.
70. O'Brien, J. R.: Effects of salicylates on human platelets. Lancet 1:779, 1968.
71. Weiss, J. H., Aledort, L. M., and Kochwa, S.: The effect of salicylates on the hemostatic properties of platelets in man. J. Clin. Invest. 47:2169, 1968.
72. Morris, H., Sherman, N. A., and McQuain, C., et al.: Effects of salsalate (nonacetylated salicylate) and aspirin on serum prostaglandins in humans. Ther. Drug Monit. 7:435, 1985.
73. Steven, M. M., Small, M., and Pinkerton, L., et al.: Non-steroidal anti-inflammatory drugs in haemophilic arthritis. Haemostasis 15:204, 1985.
74. Fiore, L. D., Brophy, M. T., and Lopez, A., et al.: The bleeding time response to aspirin. Identifying the hyperresponder. Am. J. Clin. Pathol. 94:292, 1990.
75. Amrein, P. C., Ellman, L., and Harris, W. H.: Aspirin-induced prolongation of bleeding time and perioperative blood loss. J.A.M.A. 245:1825, 1981.
76. Kwoh Kent, C., and Feinstein, A. R.: Rates of sensitivity reactions to aspirin: Problems in interpreting the data. Clin. Pharmacol. Ther. 40:494, 1986.
77. Abraham, P. A., and Stillman, M. T.: Salsalate exacerbation of chronic renal insufficiency. Relation to inhibition of prostaglandin synthesis. Arch. Intern. Med. 147:1674, 1987.
78. Stevenson, D. D., and Lewis, R. A.: Proposed mechanisms of aspirin sensitivity reactions. J. Allergy Clin. Immunol. 80:788, 1987.
79. Szczeklik, A., Nizankowska, E., and Dworski, R.: Choline magnesium trisalicylate in patients with aspirin-induced asthma. Eur. Respir. J. 3:535, 1990.
80. Day, R. O., Graham, G. G., and Bieri, D., et al.: Concentration-response relationships for salicylate-induced ototoxicity in normal volunteers. Br. J. Clin. Pharmacol. 28:695, 1989.
81. Brandt, K. D.: Effects of nonsteroidal anti-inflammatory drugs on chondrocyte metabolism in vitro and in vivo. Am. J. Med. 83:29, 1987.
82. Slowman-Kovacs, S., Albrecht, M. E., and Brandt, K. D.: Effects of salicylate on chondrocytes from osteoarthritic and contralateral knees of dogs with unilateral anterior cruciate ligament transection. Arthritis Rheum. 32:486, 1989.
83. Rashad, S., Revell, P., Hemingway, A., Rainsford, K., et al.: Effect of non-steroidal anti-inflammatory drugs on the course of osteoarthritis. Lancet 2:519, 1989.
84. Doherty, M.: "Chondroprotection" by non-steroidal anti-inflammatory drugs. Ann. Rheum. Dis. 48:619, 1989.
85. Hill, J. B.: Salicylate intoxication. N. Engl. J. Med. 288:1110, 1973.
86. Needs, C., and Brooks, P.: Antirheumatic medication in pregancy. Br. J. Rheumatol. 24:282, 1985.
87. Needs, C., and Brooks, P.: Antirheumatic medication during lactation. Br. J. Rheumatol. 24:291, 1985.
88. Miners, J.: Drug interactions involving aspirin (acetylsalicylic acid) and salicylic acid. Clin. Pharmacokinet. 17:327, 1989.
89. Day, R. O., Harris, G., and Brown, M., et al.: Interaction of salicylate and corticosteroids in man. Br. J. Clin. Pharmacol. 26:334, 1988.
90. Baer, P. A., Shore, A., and Ikeman, R. L.: Transient fall in serum salicylate levels following intraarticular injection of steroids in patients with rheumatoid arthritis. Arthritis Rheum. 30:345, 1987.
91. Gutman, A. B., Yu, T. F., and Sirota, J. H.: A study by simultaneous clearance techniques, of salicylate excretion in man. Effect of alkalinization of the urine by bicarbonate administration; effect of probenecid. J. Clin. Invest. 34:711, 1955.
92. Brater, C.: Drug-drug and drug-disease interactions with nonsteroidal anti-inflammatory drugs. Am. J. Med. 80:62, 1986.
93. Furst, D. E., Herman, R. A., and Koehnke, R., et al.: Effect of aspirin and sulindac on methotrexate clearance. J. Pharm. Sci. 79:782, 1990.
94. Furst, D., Blocka, K., and Cassell, S., et al.: A controlled study of concurrent therapy with a nonacetylated salicylate and naproxen in rheumatoid arthritis. Arthritis Rheum. 30:146, 1987.
95. Richardson, T., Foster, J., and Mawer, G.: Enhancement by sodium salicylate of the blood glucose–lowering effect of chlorpropamide—drug interaction or summation of similar effects. Br. J. Clin. Pharmacol. 22:43, 1986.
96. Gupta, N., Sarkissian, E., and Paulus, H. E.: Correlation of plateau serum salicylate level with rate of salicylate metabolism. Clin. Pharmacol. Ther. 18:350, 1975.
97. Day, R. O.: Mode of action of non-steroidal anti-inflammatory drugs. Med. J. Aust. 148:195, 1988.
98. Myers, E. N., Bernstein, J. M., and Fostiropolous, G.: Salicylate ototoxicity: A clinical study. N. Engl. J. Med. 273:587, 1965.

Sulfasalazine

HISTORY

Professor Nanna Svartz of Stockholm believed that infection was the main cause of rheumatoid disease and in 1938–1939 commenced synthesizing potential antirheumatic compounds that incorporated salicylic acid and antibacterial sulfonamides. Collaboration with the Swedish Pharmaceutical Company, Pharmacia, led to salicylazosulfapyridine (now known as sulfasalazine [Salazopyrin]), consisting of salicylic acid and sulfapyridine joined by an azo bond (Fig. 42–1). Svartz observed that about 60 percent of her chronic polyarthritic patients improved and that good responses also occurred in patients with ankylosing spondylitis. Suspension of therapy in her polyarthritic patients usually led to relapse.[1] Svartz concluded that a useful antirheumatic drug had been discovered; however, in an influential but flawed study in patients with rheumatoid arthritis, Sinclair and Duthie[2] found sulfasalazine to be no more effective than general supportive treatment and less effective than intramuscular gold. Interest in the antirheumatic properties of sulfasalazine waned, whereas the efficacy of the drug in ulcerative colitis was established. Innovative studies by McConkey et al.[3, 4] refocused attention on sulfasalazine as a potential antirheumatic drug. Substantial and unequivocal evidence now exists for the effectiveness and relative safety of sulfasalazine as an antirheumatic drug in rheumatoid arthritis. Uniquely, the drug shows efficacy against ankylosing spondylitis and human leukocyte antigen (HLA)-B27–related arthropathies. Evidence is also accumulating for the efficacy of sulfasalazine in juvenile rheumatoid arthritis and psoriatic arthritis.

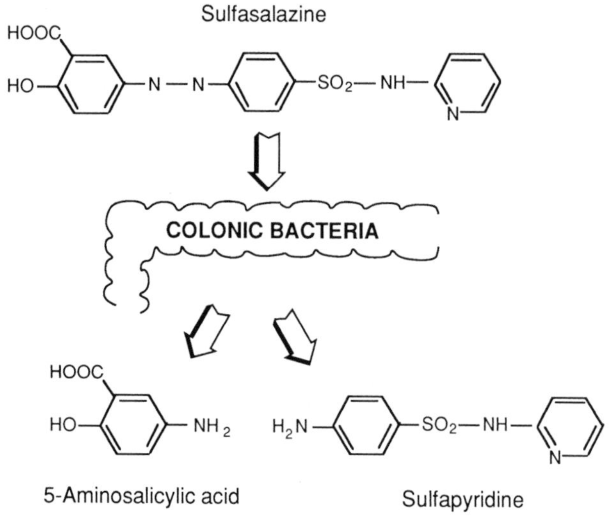

CLINICAL PHARMACOLOGY

Sulfasalazine has a molecular weight of 398.39 and consists of minute brown-yellow crystals that are practically insoluble in water. An enteric-coated formulation of the drug is used in the treatment of rheumatic diseases and is associated with a lower incidence of upper gastrointestinal adverse effects than uncoated formulations.

Absorption

Very little absorption of sulfasalazine occurs in the stomach or small bowel because of the insolubility of the drug. Most reaches the colon, where the azo bond is reduced by colonic bacteria, and sulfapyridine and 5-aminosalicylic acid are liberated (see Fig. 42–1).[5] Virtually no sulfasalazine appears in the stools unless the large bowel is removed or patients are taking antibiotics.[6] Only 10 to 20 percent of ingested sulfasalazine is absorbed intact. Sulfasalazine is highly protein bound (more than 95 percent), is excreted largely in urine and bile, and undergoes enterohepatic recirculation.[6, 7] Peak plasma concentrations occur 3 to 5 hours following a dose. The apparent plasma elimination half-life following an oral dose is variable (6 to 17 hours) and probably reflects the half-life of absorption of the drug (Fig. 42–2).[6]

Metabolism

About 30 percent of the liberated 5-aminosalicylic acid is excreted in the urine as its N-acetylation product, acetyl-5-aminosalicylic acid, whereas at least 50 percent of 5-aminosalicylic acid is recovered unchanged in feces.

Sulfapyridine appears in plasma 4 to 6 hours following a dose of sulfasalazine, reflecting the time taken for the latter to reach the colon before liberation

Figure 42–1. Sulfasalazine and its major metabolites.

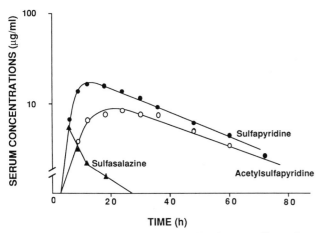

Figure 42–2. Serum concentrations of sulfasalazine, sulfapyridine, and acetylsulfapyridine after 2 g orally in a 40-year-old woman. (From Taggart, A., McDermott, B., Delargy, M., et al.: The pharmacokinetics of sulphasalazine in young and elderly patients with rheumatoid arthritis. Scand. J. Rheumatol. 64:29, 1987.)

of sulfapyridine. Sulfapyridine is extensively metabolized in the liver by N4-acetylation and ring hydroxylation with subsequent glucuronidations, and these metabolites plus unchanged sulfapyridine are recovered in urine.[8] Wide intersubject variation in metabolic rates of sulfapyridine is observed, and this is due in part to genetically determined variation in *acetylation* and *oxidative* capacities.[8] The very small proportion of patients who are classified as slow oxidizers of sulfapyridine and also slow acetylators may be expected to have significantly higher steady-state plasma sulfapyridine concentrations.[8] Age appears not to have a significant effect on the pharmacokinetics of sulfasalazine and sulfapyridine.[9]

Clinical studies suggest that sulfapyridine may be responsible for the antirheumatic actions of sulfasalazine, but sulfapyridine administered orally was more toxic than sulfasalazine.[10] On the other hand, 5-aminosalicylic acid is the active species in inflammatory bowel disease. These studies do not rule out the possibility that sulfasalazine itself is active alone or along with sulfapyridine, either in the gut or systemically.

No relationship between plasma concentrations of sulfapyridine and efficacy has been revealed from limited studies to date.[11–13] Sulfasalazine and sulfapyridine have been quantitated in synovial fluid of patients with rheumatic diseases taking sulfasalazine chronically, concentrations being similar to plasma concentrations.[14]

POSSIBLE MODES OF ACTION

As with all specific antirheumatic drugs, the detailed mechanism of the antirheumatic action of sulfasalazine is unknown. Sulfapyridine may act indirectly by suppressing inflammatory and immunologic processes in the gut, perhaps, in part, a conse-

quence of the antibacterial properties of sulfapyridine. Much work suggests that the gut may be important in the immunopathogenesis of spondyloarthropathies and rheumatoid arthritis, particularly as a site of entry and processing of antigens instrumental in the etiologies of these disorders.

Sulfasalazine and its metabolites have activity in a number of experimental systems pertinent to the immunopathogenesis of inflammatory arthritides, but proof of the relevance of these properties to the drug's antirheumatic actions in humans remains to be established. For example, sulfasalazine and to a greater extent 5-aminosalicylic acid have been shown to be scavengers of reactive oxygen species and their products, such as the hypochlorite ion, which are released from activated polymorphs and contribute to the inflammatory process.[15, 16] Early increases in thiol concentrations and decreases in superoxide dismutase levels in red cells of patients with rheumatoid arthritis treated with sulfasalazine, but also seen with other specific antirheumatic drugs, seem to suggest further that response may be related to free radical scavenging activity.[17] Sulfasalazine can inhibit the production and destruction of important prostanoid products of arachidonic acid.[18] Thus, formation of the products of the 5-lipoxygenase pathway of human leukocytes, such as leukotriene B_4 and 5 hydroxyeicosatetraenoic acid (HETE), is inhibited, as is the synthesis by platelets of thromboxane A_2.[19–21]

Evidence for immunomodulatory activity of sulfasalazine in rheumatoid arthritis is suggested by the reduction of circulating activated lymphocytes after 12 weeks of therapy and the restoration of normal responses of lymphocytes to concanavalin A (ConA) ex vivo.[22] No alterations in lymphocyte subsets were noted, but there were significant falls in gamma M immunoglobulin (IgM) and rheumatoid factor titers, further indicating that sulfasalazine perturbs lymphocyte function. The same investigators demonstrated that responses of peripheral blood mononuclear cells to various mitogens were suppressed by sulfasalazine and some of its metabolites in vitro, whereas Comer and Jasin[23] have found that sulfasalazine, but not its metabolites, inhibits activation of B lymphocytes. Similarly, Sheldon et al.[24] found that high concentrations of parent drug alone inhibited mitogen-induced transformation of mouse spleen cells in vitro and suggested that sulfasalazine may act on gut-associated lymphoid tissue.

EFFICACY

Rheumatoid Arthritis

Sulfasalazine displays specific antirheumatic properties and is approximately as effective as more traditional antirheumatic drugs such as gold and penicillamine.[25, 26] Sulfasalazine, however, acts faster and is less problematic with respect to adverse effects than gold or penicillamine, although the likelihood of patients continuing this drug over sustained periods is probably similar to other specific antirheumatic drugs. Similar to other antirheumatic drugs, patient variables usefully predictive of response to sulfasalazine have not been identified.

Sulfasalazine affected clinical and laboratory measures of rheumatoid disease activity in a pattern consistent with a specific antirheumatic drug, and significant improvements were detected as early as 4 weeks with rapid recrudescence of disease on cessation of drug.[3, 4, 27] Two short-term, randomized, double-blind, placebo-controlled studies established the efficacy of sulfasalazine, 3 g per day, but both showed relatively high rates of patient withdrawal largely owing to upper gastrointestinal adverse effects as a consequence of the high dose of sulfasalazine employed.[28, 29] Clear improvements from baseline in articular index; grip strength, an index of disease activity; erythrocyte sedimentation rate (ESR); and platelet count were demonstrated with sulfasalazine and gold sodium thiomalate (50 mg intramuscular injection weekly; unblinded) in contrast to placebo in the study of Pullar et al.[28] Nine out of 30 sulfasalazine patients withdrew owing to adverse effects, mainly nausea and vomiting. Pinals et al.[29] showed significant improvements in joint tenderness and swelling, grip strength, morning stiffness, and pain score in a 15-week study, but withdrawals from the sulfasalazine group reached 28 percent.

Comparisons with Other Specific Antirheumatic Drugs

Sulfasalazine, 2 g per day, produced equivalent effects to penicillamine, 500 mg per day, over a 16-week, double-blind, randomized study and, in contrast to penicillamine, at 4 weeks showed significant improvement in articular index, duration of morning stiffness, ESR, and C-reactive protein.[30] Longer comparisons of sulfasalazine with penicillamine over 1 year revealed comparable efficacy and numbers of patients entering remission as defined by American Rheumatology Association criteria but generally less toxicity.[31, 32] Other studies have also recognized the ability of sulfasalazine to induce remissions.[13, 33] A comparison of penicillamine and sulfasalazine in 200 general practice patients over 2 years revealed similar outcomes with respect to efficacy and continuation of therapy.[34]

A 37-week, randomized, double-blind, placebo-controlled comparison among sulfasalazine, 2 g per day; gold sodium thiomalate, 50 mg per week; and placebo in 186 patients revealed the expected and substantial improvements in disease activity parameters with gold and similar, sometimes greater, changes with sulfasalazine. The effect of sulfasalazine was measurable at 4 weeks, confirming the slightly faster onset of action of this drug. Significantly more patients were withdrawn from the gold thiomalate group (41 percent) because of adverse effects compared with the sulfasalazine (16 percent) and placebo (10 percent) groups.[35] Unexpectedly, placebo responses were much greater than predicted from the previous extensive experience of this research group and were generally indistinguishable from gold and sulfasalazine. In fact, only ESR and grip strength in the right hand were more significantly improved by the active agents compared with placebo. The authors concluded that sulfasalazine showed similar efficacy to gold, with better tolerance and less toxicity. Subsequently, an important and innovative reanalysis of the data using a composite index of response applied to individual patients did indicate a clear difference between the active drugs and placebo.[36]

An important, double-blind, 48-week study compared sulfasalazine (2 g per day) with hydroxychloroquine (400 mg per day for 24 weeks, then 200 mg per day) in 60 patients with early rheumatoid arthritis with little radiologic damage and previously untreated with specific antirheumatic drugs. Again, sulfasalazine had a faster onset of action with significant improvements in duration of morning stiffness, pain score, and grip strength observed at 4 weeks. Both drugs were associated with equally significant improvement in a wide range of disease activity variables at 48 weeks.[37] Analysis of radiologic progression, as measured by appearance of joint erosions and a composite score, revealed a significant advantage for sulfasalazine versus hydroxychloroquine at 24 and 48 weeks,[38] and this advantage was maintained at about 3 years.[39] This partially confirms other studies that have suggested that sulfasalazine retards the radiologic progression of rheumatoid disease in patients with more advanced illness.[40] The reduction of rheumatoid nodules by sulfasalazine is also suggestive of an ability to retard disease progression.[41]

Combinations with Other Specific Antirheumatic Drugs

Frustration with the apparent lack of success of single specific antirheumatic drugs to alter substantially the long-term outlook of patients with progressive rheumatoid arthritis, despite often impressive short-term improvements, has led to widespread use of combinations of specific antirheumatic drugs. Reviews of this practice emphasize the absence of rationale based on detailed understanding of the pathophysiology of rheumatoid arthritis as well as mechanisms of drug action.[42] Uncontrolled studies of combinations of sulfasalazine with penicillamine and gold[43, 44] and methotrexate[45] have been reported and suggest increased efficacy but, at least with gold and penicillamine, increased rates of withdrawal owing to toxicity. Again, in a controlled but open study, the combination of sulfasalazine with penicillamine was associated with somewhat greater efficacy but also greater toxicity.

Juvenile Rheumatoid Arthritis

Sulfasalazine has been accepted as an effective specific antirheumatic drug in juvenile rheumatoid arthritis,[46, 47] although no controlled trials have been published. The drug has been used extensively in childhood inflammatory bowel disease.

Ankylosing Spondylitis and HLA-B27–Associated Rheumatic Diseases

Because gastrointestinal infections and inflammation have been implicated in the HLA-B27–associated rheumatic diseases, investigation of the activity of sulfasalazine has been undertaken. The drug is significantly superior to placebo against clinical and laboratory abnormalities in a number of controlled, double-blind studies in ankylosing spondylitis, the duration of studies ranging from 12 to 52 weeks,[48–51] a conclusion confirmed by a meta-analysis of the five controlled studies available.[52] The rate of onset of effect was 2 to 3 months in these studies. Sulfasalazine was found to be highly effective in an open, uncontrolled study of patients with HLA-B27–associated asymmetric, pauciarticular arthritis.[53, 54]

Psoriatic Arthritis

Sulfasalazine showed promise in an open, uncontrolled study of 1 year duration in 30 patients with psoriatic arthritis, both symmetric joint disease and arthritis in association with spondyloarthritis responding, and no exacerbation of psoriatic skin disease was observed.[55] These results were confirmed in a double-blind study versus placebo.[56]

ADVERSE EFFECTS

Sulfasalazine has been used extensively since the 1950s in the treatment of inflammatory bowel disease, often at higher dosage rates than employed in rheumatic therapy. Thus, there is substantial knowledge of the adverse effects profile of sulfasalazine, although there may be some contrasts in experience between the two disease groups. In the 40 years since its introduction, a number of deaths have been associated with the use of sulfasalazine, largely in association with the use of the drug in ulcerative colitis (Table 42–1). A study of 774 rheumatoid arthritis patients followed for 1 to 11 years, however, recorded no deaths or long-term adverse effects.[57]

As Fries et al.[58] have noted, summary measures of drug toxicity taking into account frequency and severity of all adverse effects experienced by large numbers of patients as a basis for rational comparison and selection of antirheumatic agents are sorely needed. Currently, discontinuations of specific anti-

Table 42–1. SERIOUS ADVERSE EFFECTS OF SULFASALAZINE ASSOCIATED WITH DEATH

Aplastic anemia
Agranulocytosis
Fibrosing alveolitis
Hypersensitivity reactions
Irreversible neuromuscular and CNS effects
Renal damage
Hepatic damage

CNS, Central nervous system.

rheumatic drugs, owing more usually to drug toxicity than lack of efficacy, are our only crude measure of comparative utility. Studies to date suggest a discontinuation rate for sulfasalazine similar to gold and penicillamine. One year after commencing sulfasalazine, 75 percent of 200 subjects were still taking the drug, 20 percent having stopped because of an adverse reaction and 5 percent for other reasons including inefficacy. By the end of the second year, 66 percent remained on the drug, with 21 percent discontinuing owing to adverse effects and 12 percent for other reasons.[59] Capell et al.[34] found 51 percent of patients managed in conjunction with general practitioners remained on sulfasalazine after 2 years. These data contrast somewhat with the experience of others, who report continuation rates at 1 year of only approximately 50 percent, a higher proportion of discontinuations owing to inefficacy, with smaller proportions remaining on sulfasalazine after 2 years of treatment.[13, 33, 60, 61] Five years after commencing specific antirheumatic drugs, in one study fewer than 20 percent of patients were still taking gold, penicillamine, or sulfasalazine,[61] whereas Jones et al.[62] found that 22 percent of 86 patients were still taking sulfasalazine after 5 years.

Side effects with sulfasalazine are relatively few and trivial[33, 57, 59] in comparison to parenteral gold or penicillamine, and one analysis ranked sulfasalazine with antimalarials and auranofin as the best-tolerated specific antirheumatic drugs.[63] Adverse effects are most common in the first 2 to 3 months of therapy, and the nonidiosyncratic, less serious adverse reactions appear to increase with increasing dose and possibly sulfapyridine plasma concentrations.[64] Sulfapyridine concentrations are highest in patients with low oxidative and acetylation capacity for sulfapyridine. Adverse effects, particularly nausea and abdominal discomfort, have been found to be greater in slow acetylators in some studies, the combination of slow acetylator and oxidizer not having been systematically studied in this respect,[64, 65] but there appears to be no clear practical benefit in knowing a patient's acetylator status before commencing sulfasalazine in rheumatic patients.[65–67] The most common side effects involve the gastrointestinal tract and hematologic, skin, and central nervous systems (Table 42–2), and because they are often dose-dependent, simple dose reduction can be effective in reducing the adverse effect.

Table 42–2. MOST FREQUENT ADVERSE EFFECTS OF SULFASALAZINE

	Common Adverse Effects
GI	Nausea, vomiting, anorexia, malaise
	Abdominal pain, indigestion, dyspepsia
CNS	Headache
	Fever
	Lightheadedness, dizziness
	Less Common Adverse Effects
Skin	Rash (exanthemlike),
Hepatic	Marginal enzyme elevations
Hematologic	Leukopenia
	Hemolysis, mean corpuscular volume increased
	Methemoglobinemia

GI, Gastrointestinal; CNS, central nervous system.

Gastroenterologic Effects

Nausea and upper abdominal discomfort, often in association with headache and dizziness, are the most common adverse effects, and their incidence is reduced by increasing dosage gradually. If patients can persist with the drug in the first 2 to 3 months, often continued usage is less problematic.

Hematologic Effects

The incidence of leukopenia and neutropenia may be greater in rheumatoid arthritis than ulcerative colitis patients. The reported incidence varies from 1 to 5 percent, lower percentages being more common, and the drug has to be stopped in about one third to half of these patients. Although seen most often in the first 24 weeks of therapy, leukopenia and neutropenia can occur at any time, necessitating continued surveillance (Fig. 42–3).[57, 68, 69] Timely recognition is usually associated with recovery,[68, 70, 71] although a number of individual cases of agranulocytosis have been described.[72] No HLA associations have been suggested for this adverse effect of sulfa-

salazine in contrast to gold and penicillamine.[73] Thrombocytopenia is much less common than leukopenia.

There are conflicting data concerning the effect of sulfasalazine on serum or red cell folate concentrations, some studies showing lowered folate levels, whereas Grindulis and McConkey[74] found no effect in a prospective 6-month study of patients with rheumatoid arthritis. Although some degree of macrocytosis and hemolysis has been common in patients taking higher doses of sulfasalazine for ulcerative colitis, frank hemolytic anemia is unusual.[75] The latter is typically associated with methemoglobinemia, Heinz bodies, and reticulocytosis.

Skin

Skin rashes occur in 1 to 5 percent of patients. Pruritic, maculopapular, and generalized rashes are most common, but occasional patients have urticarial reactions. *Desensitization* to sulfasalazine has been successfully accomplished by employing escalating doses of drug.[76] Some cases of alopecia have been noted. Classic serum sickness with fever, generalized maculopapular rash, mouth ulcers, enlarged and tender cervical lymph nodes, marked leukocytosis, polyclonal hypergammaglobulinemia with marked elevations of gamma immunoglobulin E (IgE) and IgM, and low C3 and C4 levels in a 43-year-old woman taking sulfasalazine, 0.5 to 2 g per day for 3 weeks, has been described.[77] Rarely, toxic epidermal necrolysis (Lyell's syndrome) and Stevens-Johnson syndrome have been reported in association with sulfasalazine treatment.

Liver

Abnormal liver function tests occur, and five cases were recorded in 200 subjects with inflammatory arthritis followed for 1 year.[59] Acute hepatitic reactions sometimes accompanied by fever, rash, and lymphadenopathy are well-known adverse effects of sulfasalazine.

Pulmonary Effects

The appearance of dyspnea in a patient taking sulfasalazine raises the possibility of pulmonary adverse effects of this drug. A number of cases manifesting reversible pulmonary infiltrates accompanied by eosinophilia, fever, and weight loss have been described.[78] Fibrosing alveolitis in a 53-year-old woman 5 months after commencing sulfasalazine, 1.5 g per day, slowly resolved with prednisone therapy and cessation of sulfasalazine.[79]

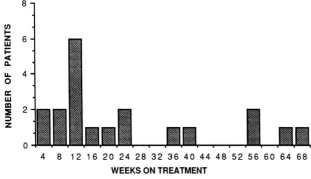

Figure 42–3. Patients developing leukopenia during sulfasalazine treatment indicating that most cases occur in the first few months of therapy. (From Marabani, M., Madhok, R., Capell, H., et al.: Leucopenia during sulphasalazine treatment for rheumatoid arthritis. Ann. Rheum. Dis. 48:505, 1989.)

Reproduction

No higher incidence of fetal abnormalities or perinatal morbidity or mortality has been observed in the offspring of males or females taking sulfasalazine at the time of conception or during pregnancy.[80, 81] Avoidance of specific antirheumatic drugs around the time of conception and during pregnancy, however, is always preferable, and the natural improvement in rheumatoid arthritis during pregnancy is of some assistance in this circumstance. In addition, because sulfasalazine is highly protein-bound and a sulfonamide, the possibility of kernicterus in fetuses or babies resulting from use of the drug in women near term or while breast feeding suggests against the use of sulfasalazine in these circumstances. In fact, little sulfasalazine enters milk, whereas sulfapyridine concentrations are 40 percent of plasma concentrations, but this metabolite does not readily displace bilirubin from albumin. Rapidly reversible male infertility has been observed in association with sulfasalazine and is related to reduction in sperm count and motility and also morphologic abnormalities of the sperm, these effects being quite common in patients taking sulfasalazine.[82] In general, however, this effect has not been considered a contraindication to therapy in young males, but the drug should be withdrawn in men wishing to sire children.

Other Adverse Effects

Changes in mood including irritability and depression are not unusual in the early months of therapy.[57] Lower extremity weakness and wide-based gait, which resolved on cessation of sulfasalazine, 3 g per day in a 73-year-old man, have been reported.[83] Hypoimmunoglobulinemia has been described.[13, 84] Drug-induced lupus and DNA antibodies have been described owing to sulfasalazine in patients with inflammatory bowel disease and in some rheumatic subjects.[13]

DRUG INTERACTIONS

Broad-spectrum antibiotics that alter gut flora may reduce the bioavailability of sulfapyridine and 5-aminosalicylic acid as the azo link between these two metabolites of sulfasalazine is cleaved by bacterial metabolism. Concomitant cholestyramine is likely to reduce the availability of sulfapyridine as it binds sulfasalazine, rendering it unavailable for bacterial digestion. Sulfasalazine absorption is reduced if coadministered with oral iron preparations, but sulfapyridine concentrations are unaffected.

DOSAGE AND MONITORING

The most common adult dosage for rheumatic disease is 2 g (range 1.5 to 3 g) daily, taken as 1 g twice a day with meals. To minimize the risk of intolerance to the drug, starting doses of 500 mg to 1 g per day are usually employed with dosage increments of 500 mg per day at intervals of a week or longer. Increases from a daily dose of 2 to 3 g per day do not seem to improve response in many patients.

Opinions vary regarding appropriate monitoring for patients taking sulfasalazine. Neutropenia if it occurs usually does so suddenly so monitoring to avoid this serious adverse effect is difficult. At a minimum, patients should be aware of the possibility of serious hematologic adverse effects, so they can immediately stop the drug and consult their physician should sore throat, mouth ulcers, fever, and significant malaise become apparent. This information can be provided in written form as well as reinforced at follow-up visits. Many groups recommend frequent blood counts, for example, every 2 to 4 weeks during the first 3 months of therapy and reducing the frequency thereafter, whereas others perform the first blood count 6 weeks after commencing therapy and then every 3 months.

SUMMARY

Sulfasalazine is approximately as effective a specific antirheumatic agent as gold or penicillamine in short-term studies, and its onset of effect is somewhat faster than either. Sulfasalazine is also efficacious in the spondyloarthropathies. The drug is associated with a lower incidence of adverse effects than gold or penicillamine, and with careful attention to individualizing dosage, the most common problem of gastrointestinal side effects can be reduced. These properties suggest a useful role for sulfasalazine, particularly early in the course of rheumatoid arthritis[26] and as part of combination regimens.

As with other specific agents, a critical question concerning sulfasalazine is the outcome of prolonged therapy in rheumatoid arthritis. We and our patients need to know the impact of this drug on quality of life and in particular longevity and ability to continue working.[85] The sobering reports of Wolfe[86] and Pincus,[85] concerning the outcome of sequential specific antirheumatic drug therapy for patients with rheumatoid arthritis followed in rheumatology clinics and practices for periods of 20 years, which indicate distressingly high morbidity, increased mortality, and low continuation rates with antirheumatic drugs, have suggested the necessity of different strategies of therapy. Wilske and Healey[87] have emphasized that prevention of joint damage correlates best with suppression of inflammation and that much damage occurs in the first 2 years of disease. Innovative experiments with combinations and cycles of specific antirheumatic drugs are needed to attempt to improve the long-term outcome of this disease while reducing the risks of drug-induced toxicity. A second critical question under intense investigation is where does sulfasalazine best fit in combinations and cycles of specific antirheumatic drugs?

References

1. Svartz, N.: Salazopyrin, a new sulfanilamide preparation. Acta Med. Scand. 110:577, 1942.
2. Sinclair, R., and Duthie, J.: Salazopyrin in the treatment of rheumatoid arthritis. Ann. Rheum. Dis. 8:226, 1948.
3. McConkey, B., Amos, R., and Butler, E.: Salazopyrin in rheumatoid arthritis. Agents Actions 8:438, 1978.
4. McConkey, B., Amos, R., Durham, S. et al.: Sulphasalazine in rheumatoid arthritis. Br. Med. J. 280:442, 1980.
5. Peppercorn, M., and Goldman, P.: The role of intestinal bacteria in the metabolism of salicylazosulfapyridine. J. Pharm. Exp. Ther. 181:555, 1972.
6. Azad Khan, A., Truelove, S., and Aronson, J.: The disposition and metabolism of sulphasalazine (salicylazosulphapyridine) in man. Br. J. Clin. Pharm. 13:523, 1982.
7. Das, K., and Dubin, R.: Clinical pharmacokinetics of sulphasalazine. Clin. Pharmacokinet. 1:406, 1976.
8. Schroder, H., and Campbell, D.: Absorption, metabolism and excretion of salicylazo-sulfapyridine in man. Clin. Pharmacol. Ther. 13:539, 1972.
9. Taggart, A., McDermott, B., Delargy, M., et al.: The pharmacokinetics of sulphasalazine in young and elderly patients with rheumatoid arthritis. Scand. J. Rheumatol. 64:29, 1987.
10. Pullar, T., Hunter, J., and Capell, H.: Which component of sulphasalazine is active in rheumatoid arthritis? Br. Med. J. 290:1535, 1985.
11. Pullar, T., Hunter, J., and Capell, H.: Sulphasalazine in the treatment of rheumatoid arthritis: Relationship of dose and serum levels to efficacy. Br. J. Rheumatol. 24:269, 1985.
12. Martin, L., Sitar, D., Chalmers, I., et al.: Sulfasalazine in severe rheumatoid arthritis: A study to assess potential correlates of efficacy and toxicity. J. Rheumatol. 12:270, 1985.
13. Chalmers, I., Sitar, D., and Hunter, T.: A one-year, open, prospective study of sulfasalazine in the treatment of rheumatoid arthritis: Adverse reactions and clinical response in relation to laboratory variables, drug and metabolite serum levels and acetylator status. J. Rheumatol. 17:764, 1990.
14. Farr, M., Brodrick, A., and Bacon, P.: Plasma and synovial fluid concentrations of sulphasalazine and two of its metabolites in rheumatoid arthritis. Rheumatol. Int. 5:247, 1985.
15. Aruoma, O., Wasil, M., Halliwell, B., et al.: The scavenging of oxidants by sulphasalazine and its metabolites: A possible contribution to their anti-inflammatory effects? Biochem. Pharmacol. 36:3739, 1987.
16. Williams, J., and Hallett, M.: Effect of sulphasalazine and its active metabolite, 5-amino-salicylic acid, on toxic oxygen metabolite production by neutrophils. Gut 30:1581, 1989.
17. Pullar, T., Zoma, A., Capell, A., et al.: Alteration of thiol and superoxide dismutase status in rheumatoid arthritis treated with sulphasalazine. Br. Med. J. 26:202, 1987.
18. Hoult, J.: Pharmacological and biochemical actions of sulphasalazine. Drugs 32:18, 1986.
19. Stenson, W., and Lobos, E.: Sulfasalazine inhibits the synthesis of chemotactic lipids by neutrophils. J. Clin. Invest. 69:494, 1982.
20. Stenson, W., and Lobos, E.: Inhibition of platelet thromboxane synthetase by sulfasalazine. Biochem. Pharmacol. 32:2205, 1983.
21. Bach, M., Brashler, J., and Johnson, M.: Inhibition by sulfasalazine of LTC synthetase and of rat liver glutathione s-transferases. Biochem. Pharmacol. 34:2695, 1985.
22. Symmons, D., Salmon, M., and Farr, M., et al.: Sulfasalazine treatment and lymphocyte function in patients with rheumatoid arthritis. J. Rheumatol. 15:575, 1988.
23. Comer, S., and Jasin, H.: In vitro immunomodulatory effects of sulfasalazine and its metabolites. J. Rheumatol. 15:580, 1988.
24. Sheldon, P., Webb, C., and Grindulis, K.: Effect of sulphasalazine and its metabolites on mitogen induced transformation of lymphocytes—clues to its clinical action? Br. J. Rheumatol. 27:344, 1988.
25. Felson, D., Anderson, J., and Meenan, F.: The comparative efficacy and toxicity of second-line drugs in rheumatoid arthritis. Results of two metaanalyses. Arthritis Rheum. 33:1449, 1990.
26. Situnayake, R., and McConkey, B.: Clinical and laboratory effects of prolonged therapy with sulfasalazine, gold or penicillamine: The effects of disease duration on treatment response. J. Rheumatol. 17:1268, 1990.
27. Bird, H., Dixon, J., and Pickup, M.: A biochemical assessment of sulphasalazine in rheumatoid arthritis. J. Rheumatol. 9:36, 1982.
28. Pullar, T., Hunter, J., and Capell, H.: Sulphasalazine in rheumatoid arthritis: A double blind comparison of sulphasalazine with placebo and sodium aurothiomalate. Br. Med. J. 287:1102, 1983.
29. Pinals, R., Kaplan, S., Lawson, J., et al.: Sulphasalazine in rheumatoid

arthritis: A double-blind placebo controlled trial. Arthritis Rheum. 29:1427, 1986.
30. Neumann, V., Grindulis, K., Hubball, S., et al.: Comparison between penicillamine and sulphasalazine in rheumatoid arthritis: Leeds-Birmingham trial. Br. Med. J. 287:1089, 1983.
31. Farr, M., Tunn, E., Crockson, A., et al.: The long term effects of sulphasalazine in the treatment of rheumatoid arthritis and a comparative study with penicillamine. Clin. Rheumatol. 3:473, 1984.
32. Carroll, G., Will, R., Breidahl, P., et al.: Sulphasalazine versus penicillamine in the treatment of rheumatoid arthritis. Rheumatol. Int. 8:251, 1989.
33. Bax, D., and Amos, R.: Sulphasalazine: A safe, effective agent for prolonged control of rheumatoid arthritis. A comparison with sodium aurothiomalate. Ann. Rheum. Dis. 44:194, 1985.
34. Capell, H., Hunter, J., and Madhok, R., et al.: What effect can be expected from sulphasalazine (SASP) and penicillamine (PEN) therapy over two years in routine setting? Br. J. Rheumatol. Suppl. 1:27, 1989.
35. Williams, H., Ward, J., Dahl, S., et al.: A controlled trial comparing sulfasalazine, gold sodium thiomalate, and placebo in rheumatoid arthritis. Arthritis Rheum. 31:702, 1988.
36. Paulus, H., Egger, M., Ward, J., et al.: Analysis of improvement in individual rheumatoid arthritis patients treated with disease-modifying antirheumatic drugs, based on the findings in patients treated with placebo. Arthritis Rheum. 33:477, 1990.
37. Nuver-Zwart, I., van Riel, P., van de Putte, L., et al.: A double blind comparative study of sulphasalazine and hydroxychloroquine in rheumatoid arthritis: Evidence of an earlier effect of sulphasalazine. Ann. Rheum. Dis. 48:389, 1989.
38. Van der Heijde, D., van Riel, P., Nuver-Zwart, E., et al.: Effects of hydroxychloroquine and sulphasalazine on progression of joint damage in rheumatoid arthritis. Lancet 1:1036, 1989.
39. Van der Heijde, D., van Riel, P., Nuver-Zwart, E., et al.: Sulphasalazine versus hydroxychloroquine in rheumatoid arthritis: 3-year follow-up. Lancet 335:539, 1990.
40. Pullar, T., Hunter, J., and Capell, H.: Effect of sulphasalazine on the radiological progression of rheumatoid arthritis. Ann. Rheum. Dis. 46:398, 1987.
41. Englett, H., Hughes, G., and Walport, M.: Sulphasalazine and regression of rheumatoid nodules. Ann. Rheum. Dis. 46:244, 1987.
42. Paulus, H.: The use of combinations of disease-modifying antirheumatic agents in rheumatoid arthritis. Arthritis Rheum. 33:113, 1990.
43. Taggart, A., Hill, J., Astbury, C., et al.: Sulphasalazine alone or in combination with d-penicillamine in rheumatoid arthritis. Br. J. Rheumatol. 26:32, 1987.
44. Farr, M., Kitas, G., and Bacon, P.: Sulphasalazine in rheumatoid arthritis: Combination therapy with D-penicillamine or sodium aurothiomalate. Clin. Rheumatol. 7:242, 1988.
45. Shiroky, J., Watts, C., and Neville, C.: Combination methotrexate and sulfasalazine in the management of rheumatoid arthritis: Case observations. Arthritis Rheum. 32:1160, 1989.
46. Grondin, C., Malleson, P., and Petty, R.: Slow-acting antirheumatic drugs in chronic arthritis of childhood. Semin. Arthritis Rheum. 18:38, 1988.
47. Ozdogan, H., Turunc, M., and Dermingol, B., et al.: Sulphasalazine in the treatment of juvenile rheumatoid arthritis: A preliminary open trial. J. Rheumatol. 13:124, 1986.
48. Nissila, M., Lehtinen, K., Leirisalo-Repo, M., et al.: Sulphasalazine in the treatment of ankylosing spondylitis. A twenty-six-week, placebo-controlled clinical trial. Arthritis Rheum. 31:1111, 1988.
49. Feltelius, N., and Hallgren, R.: Sulphasalazine in ankylosing spondylitis. Ann. Rheum. Dis. 45:396, 1986.
50. Dougados, M., Boumier, P., and Amor, B.: Sulphasalazine in ankylosing spondylitis: A double-blind controlled study in 60 patients. Br. Med. J. 293:911, 1986.
51. Taylor, H., Beswick, E., Davis, M., et al.: Sulphasalazine in ankylosing spondylitis—effective in early disease? Br. J. Rheumatol. 28:6, 1989.
52. Ferraz, M., Tugwell, P., Goldsmith, C., et al.: Meta-analysis of sulfasalazine in ankylosing spondylitis. J. Rheumatol. 17:1482, 1990.
53. Mielants, H., and Veys, E.: HLA-B27 Related arthritis and bowel inflammation. Part 1. Sulfasalazine (Salazopyrin) in HLA-B27 related reactive arthritis. J. Rheumatol. 12:287, 1985.
54. Mielants, H., Veys, E., and Joos, R.: Sulphasalazine (salazopyrin) in the treatment of enterogenic reactive arthritis and ankylosing spondylitis with peripheral arthritis. Clin. Rheumatol. 5:80, 1986.
55. Farr, M., Kitas, G., Waterhouse, L., et al.: Treatment of psoriatic arthritis with sulphasalazine: A one-year open study. Clin. Rheumatol. 7:372, 1988.
56. Farr, M., Kitas, G., Waterhouse, L., et al.: Sulphasalazine in psoriatic arthritis: A double-blind placebo-controlled study. Br. J. Rheumatol. 29:46, 1990.
57. Amos, R., Pullar, T., and Capell, H.: Sulphasalazine for rheumatoid arthritis: Toxicity in 774 patients monitored for one to 11 years. Br. Med. J. 293:420, 1986.
58. Fries, J., Spitz, P., Williams, C., et al.: A toxicity index for comparison of side effects among different drugs. Arthritis Rheum. 33:121, 1990.

59. Farr, M., Scott, D., and Bacon, P.: Side effect profile of 200 patients with inflammatory arthritis treated with sulphasalazine. Drugs 32:49, 1986.

60. Grindulis, K., and McConkey, B.: Outcome of attempts to treat rheumatoid arthritis with gold, penicillamine, sulphasalazine, or dapsone. Ann. Rheum. Dis. 43:398, 1984.

61. Situnayake, R., Grindulis, K., and McConkey, B.: Long term treatment of rheumatoid arthritis with sulphasalazine, gold or penicillamine: A comparison using life-table methods. Ann. Rheum. Dis. 46:177, 1987.

62. Jones, E., Verrier Jones, J., and Woodbury, J.: Response to sulfasalazine in rheumatoid arthritis: Life table analysis of a 5-year follow-up. J. Rheumatol. 18:195, 1991.

63. Furst, D.: Rational use of disease-modifying antirheumatic drugs. Drugs 39:19, 1990.

64. Das, K., Eastwood, M., McManus, J., et al.: Adverse reactions during salicylazosulphapyridine therapy and the relation with drug metabolism and acetylator phenotype. N. Engl. J. Med. 289:491, 1973.

65. Pullar, T., Hunter, J., and Capell, H.: Effect of acetylator phenotype on efficacy and toxicity of sulphasalazine in rheumatoid arthritis. Ann. Rheum. Dis. 44:831, 1985.

66. Bax, D., Greaves, M., and Amos, R.: Sulphasalazine for rheumatoid arthritis: Relationship between dose and acetylator phenotype and response to treatment. Br. J. Rheumatol. 25:282, 1986.

67. Kitas, G., Farr, M., Waterhouse, L., et al.: Influence of acetylator status on the efficacy and toxicity in rheumatoid arthritis. Br. J. Rheumatol. Suppl. 1:53, 1989.

68. Marabani, M., Madhok, R., Capell H et al.: Leucopenia during sulphasalazine treatment for rheumatoid arthritis. Ann. Rheum. Dis. 48:505, 1989.

69. Marouf, E., and Morris, I.: Neutropenia in patients with rheumatoid arthritis treated with sulphasalazine. Br. J. Rheumatol. 29:407, 1990.

70. Farr, M., Tunn, E., Symmons, D., et al.: Sulphasalazine in rheumatoid arthritis: Haematological problems and changes in haematological indices associated with therapy. Br. J. Rheumatol. 28:134, 1989.

71. Amos, R., and Bax, D.: Leucopenia in rheumatoid arthritis: Relationship to gold or sulphasalazine therapy. Br. J. Rheumatol. 27:465, 1988.

72. Guilleman, F., Aussedat, R., Guerci, A., et al.: Fatal agranulocytosis in sulfasalazine-treated rheumatoid arthritis. J. Rheumatol. 16:1166, 1989.

73. Bliddal, H., Eiberg, B., Helin, P., et al.: HLA types in patients with rheumatoid arthritis developing leucopenia after both gold and sulphasalazine treatment. Ann. Rheum. Dis. 48:539, 1989.

74. Grindulis, K., and McConkey, B.: Does sulphasalazine cause folate deficiency in rheumatoid arthritis? Scand. J. Rheumatol. 14:265, 1985.

75. Hopkinson, N., Saiz, G., and Gumpel, J.: Haematological side-effects of sulphasalazine in inflammatory arthritis. Br. J. Rheumatol. 28:414, 1989.

76. Farr, M., Scott, D., and Bacon, P.: Sulphasalazine desensitisation in rheumatoid arthritis. Br. Med. J. 284:118, 1982.

77. Pettersson, T., Gripenberg, M., and Molander, G., et al.: Severe immunological reaction induced by sulphasalazine. Br. J. Rheumatol. 29:239, 1990.

78. Tydd, T., and Dyer, N.: Sulphasalazine lung. Med. J. Aust. 1:570, 1976.

79. Boyd, B., Gibbs, A., and Smith, A.: Fibrosing alveolitis due to sulphasalazine in a patient with rheumatoid arthritis. Br. J. Rheumatol. 29:222, 1990.

80. Willoughby, V., and Truelove, S.: Ulcerative colitis and pregnancy. Gut 21:469, 1980.

81. Mogadam, M., Dobbins, W., Korelitz, B., et al.: Pregnancy in inflammatory bowel disease: Effect of sulphasalazine and corticosteroids on fetal outcome. Gastroenterology 80:72, 1981.

82. Toovey, S., Hudson, E., Hendry, W., et al.: Sulphasalazine and male infertility: Reversibility and possible mechanism. Gut 22:445, 1981.

83. Bhalotra, R., Loring, L., and Massarelli, J.: A case of possible sulfasalazine neurotoxicity. Dig. Dis. Sci. 35:665, 1990.

84. Farr, M., Tunn, E., and Bacon, P.: Immunodeficiency associated with sulphasalazine therapy in rheumatoid arthritis (Abstract). Br. J. Rheumatol. Suppl. 25:47, 1986.

85. Pincus, T.: Rheumatoid arthritis: Disappointing long-term outcomes despite successful short-term clinical trials. J. Clin. Epidemiol. 41:1037, 1988.

86. Wolfe, F.: 50 Years of antirheumatic therapy: The progress of rheumatoid arthritis. J. Rheumatol. 17:24, 1990.

87. Wilske, K. R., and Healey, L. A.: Remodeling the pyramid—a concept whose time has come. J. Rheumatol. 16:565, 1989.

Chapter 43

Philip J. Clements
Harold E. Paulus

Nonsteroidal Anti-Inflammatory Drugs (NSAIDs)

Nonsteroidal antirheumatic drugs reduce the signs and symptoms of established inflammation but do not in themselves eliminate the underlying causes of the inflammation. Their effects on pain, swelling, heat, erythema, and loss of function begin promptly after their absorption into the blood and become fully evident within a few weeks. Drug withdrawal is quickly followed by exacerbation of signs and symptoms of inflammation. They have no effect on the course of the basic disease process and do not protect against tissue or joint injury; thus, damage to joints continues to occur during the administration of such a drug to patients with chronic inflammatory arthritis.

Although these drugs have been sought and developed because of their effects on arthritis, their substantial analgesic, antipyretic, and antiprostaglandin effects have led to their widespread application in the symptomatic management of aches and pains of all types, fever, uterine cramps, closure of patent ductus arteriosus in infants, and other applications that derive from their suppression of prostaglandin synthesis. Drugs with these characteristics are generally referred to as nonsteroidal anti-inflammatory drugs (NSAIDs); examples include aspirin and the nonacetylated salicylates (discussed in Chapter 41), phenylbutazone, indomethacin, ibuprofen, fenoprofen, ketoprofen, flurbiprofen, naproxen, tolmetin, sulindac, meclofenamate, diclofenac, ketorolac, etodolac, diflunisal, and piroxicam.

Colchicine is discussed also in this chapter; it has some of the characteristics of the NSAIDs, although it differs in its mechanism of action and its adverse effects profile. The slowly acting antirheumatic drugs, such as gold and the immunoregulatory agents, differ in their pharmacologic characteristics and clinical applications and are discussed in subsequent chapters. To some extent, the glucocorticoids resemble NSAIDs, in that they moderate established inflammation and do not prevent the progression of joint damage; however, they have many characteristics that clearly differentiate them from the nonsteroidal antirheumatic drugs; they are discussed in Chapter 48. This chapter emphasizes similarities and class characteristics of the NSAIDs. The discussions of individual drugs are limited to unique characteristics such as their pharmacokinetics and areas in which they differ from the general characteristics of the class. Finally, a basis for clinical differentiation among the nonsteroidal antirheumatic drugs is discussed, to provide some guidance in the selection of a particular drug for an individual patient.

HISTORY

Willow and poplar barks that contain salicin have been used since antiquity to treat pain, gout, and fever. Extracts of the autumn crocus, containing colchicine, were used for treatment of acute gout as early as the 6th century A.D. Colchicine was isolated in 1820, and by 1900 salicylic acid and aspirin had been synthesized.[1] The term *nonsteroidal anti-inflammatory drug* was first applied to phenylbutazone, which was introduced into clinical practice in 1949, 3 years after the dramatic demonstration of the anti-inflammatory properties of the glucocorticoids.[2] A pharmacologic breakthrough occurred when indomethacin was selected by deliberately screening numerous chemicals for activity against inflammation induced in the rat paw by injection of carrageenan. Since it was marketed in 1965, a great many other compounds have been found to suppress the acute development of rat paw edema, following the injection of carrageenan or other irritating substances. Essentially all of the currently marketed NSAIDs were initially identified by their in vivo effects on this model of acute inflammation, and its ability to identify additional similar compounds seems limitless. Thus, the lead provided by aspirin and indomethacin has been fully exploited; however, the lead provided by colchicine has been largely ignored.

POSSIBLE MECHANISMS OF ACTION

Inflammation is essentially a local event. Normally, the chemical mediators considered central to the inflammatory process function to preserve homeostasis in the microenvironment. These mediators

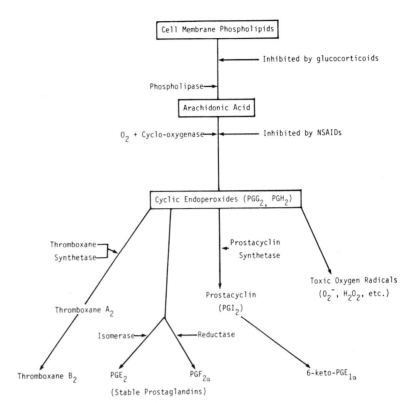

Figure 43–1. Cyclooxygenase pathway for arachidonic acid metabolism.

include products of activated leukocytes and platelets, prostaglandins, leukotrienes, complement-derived products, and products of activated mast cells. If conditions within the microenvironment exceed the normal homeostatic capacity of the chemical mediators, a full inflammatory response occurs, which may result in systemic manifestations if sufficiently severe.[3] The NSAIDs appear to act predominantly in this microenvironment.

Since the currently useful NSAIDs have been selected because of their effect on induced acute inflammation in a whole-animal model, it is apparent that these drugs successfully moderate the general process of acute inflammation in vivo. As our knowledge of the mechanisms and pathways of inflammatory processes has become increasingly sophisticated, various hypotheses have been advanced to explain the actions of NSAIDs. Under appropriate conditions, NSAIDs have been demonstrated to uncouple oxidative phosphorylation,[4] displace an endogenous anti-inflammatory peptide from plasma proteins,[5] inhibit lysomal enzyme release,[6] inhibit complement activation,[7] and antagonize the generation or activity of kinins.[8] Currently favored mechanisms of the action of NSAIDs include inhibition of cyclo-oxygenase, inhibition of lipoxygenase, and inhibition of free radicals. None of these, however, completely explains the actions of NSAIDs, and other hypotheses are emerging. For example, Weissmann[9] has estimated that in rheumatoid arthritis arachidonic acid–derived products mediate only between 25 and 30 percent of the inflammatory response; if this were true, even complete suppression of arachidonic acid metabolism would have only modest benefit in this disease.

Inhibition of Arachidonic Acid Metabolites

Prostaglandin activity was discovered in seminal fluid in 1933 by Goldblatt[10] and confirmed by von Euler,[11] but the structural identification of arachidonic acid, its metabolites, and the pertinent metabolic enzymes beginning in 1964 provided the chemical tools with which to study inter-relationships of these substances with inflammation and to characterize the effects of NSAIDs on this metabolic process.[12] This subject is discussed in detail in Chapter 11 but is summarized briefly here because of the important effects of NSAIDs on arachidonic acid metabolism and the potential for manipulation of this process in the development of new anti-inflammatory drugs.[13]

Essentially all cells in the body have the capacity to synthesize prostaglandins (Fig. 43–1). In response to inflammatory stimuli, arachidonic acid is cleaved from membrane phospholipids by specific phospholipases. Arachidonic acid is oxidized and cyclized by the enzyme *cyclooxygenase* to form a cyclic endoperoxide prostaglandin G_2 (PGG_2). PGG_2 is converted to PGH_2 by peroxidation with concomitant production of unstable toxic oxygen radicals. The cyclic endoperoxides have a half-life of about 5 minutes and demonstrate marked effects on guinea pig and rabbit aorta and promote the aggregation of platelets. PGH_2 is then converted to the stable prostaglandins E_2 and $F_{2\alpha}$, thromboxane, or prostacyclin by the appropriate

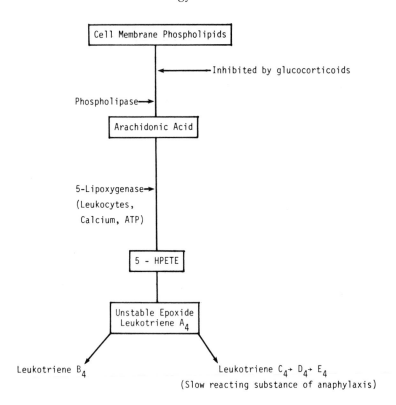

Figure 43–2. Lipoxygenase pathway for arachidonic acid metabolism.

enzymes as indicated in Figure 43–1. Thromboxane A_2 is synthesized by platelets and promotes their aggregation but has a half-life of only about 30 seconds before it is rapidly hydrolyzed to inactive thromboxane B_2. Prostacyclin (PGI_2) is synthesized within arterial walls, opposes the effects of thromboxane A_2 by inhibiting aggregation of platelets, and is a potent vasodilator.[12, 13]

Some of the biologic actions of the cyclic endoperoxides and their metabolites reproduce many of the signs of acute inflammation. Erythema is associated with the vasodilating activities of PGE_1, PGE_2, PGD_2, and PGI_2. Edema formation is promoted by increased vascular permeability induced by prostaglandins of the E series and their potentiation of bradykinin and histamine. Injection of PGE has also been demonstrated to cause pain and fever and to promote local bone resorption and cartilage destruction, depending on the sites of injection or application. Elevated levels of prostaglandins have been demonstrated in synovial effusions from untreated patients with inflammatory arthritis.[13]

Another pathway of arachidonic acid metabolism is catalyzed by *5-lipoxygenase* (Fig. 43–2). In contrast with cyclooxygenase, which is present in all tissues, 5-lipoxygenase appears to be limited to neutrophils, eosinophils, monocytes/macrophages, basophils, and certain mast cell populations.[3, 14] These cells, when activated and in the presence of calcium, adenosine triphosphate (ATP), and 5-lipoxygenase, enzymatically convert arachidonic acid to 5-hydroperoxyeicosatetraenoic acid (5-HPETE); this is further transformed enzymatically to form the unstable epoxide leukotriene A_4. In neutrophils, leukotriene A_4 is converted to leukotriene B_4, which attracts other neutrophils to the site. Leukotriene B_4, in addition to thromboxane A_2, changes the adherence properties of endothelial cells, no doubt an important factor in the chemotaxis of neutrophils to the site of injury. Eosinophils do not produce leukotriene B_4 but synthesize leukotriene C_4, which with its metabolites D_4 and E_4 forms the slowly reacting substance of anaphylaxis (SRSA), and profoundly increase the contractile activity of vascular and nonvascular smooth muscle; thus, the relationship with anaphylaxis. Leukotriene C_4 profoundly compromises guinea pig lung function, and its intradermal injection produces a wheal and flare reaction. Monocytes can produce both leukotriene B_4 and C_4. Receptor sites for leukotriene B_4 have been found on neutrophils and monocytes, and receptors for leukotriene D_4 are present in pulmonary tissue.[3] Neutrophils can inactivate leukotriene B_4, and both eosinophils and neutrophils can inactivate leukotriene C_4, D_4, and E_4.

Arachidonic acid may also be converted by 12-lipoxygenase and 15-lipoxygenase to form 15-HPETE, which when incubated with neutrophils results in the formation of *lipoxin A* and *lipoxin B*. The lipoxins are reported to inhibit the cytotoxic reaction of natural killer T cells and to cause degranulation of leukocytes and contraction of bronchial smooth muscle.[12]

Lipocortins are a family of related proteins that inhibit phospholipase A_2 in vitro and have been postulated to mimic the effect of glucocorticoids on the arachidonic acid cascade.[15] Synthetic peptides derived from human lipocortin also inhibit phospholipase A_2, show potent anti-inflammatory activity in vivo on the carrageenan-induced rat foot paw edema model of acute inflammation, and inhibit neutrophil aggregation and chemotaxis induced by complement component C5a.[16]

Paradoxically, some of the stable prostaglandins can, under appropriate circumstances, exert anti-inflammatory or regulatory functions; pharmacologic doses of PGE_1 and PGE_2 have been shown to suppress acute and chronic inflammation in several experimental models.[17] Indeed, arachidonic acid metabolites often have opposing effects on various mechanisms involved in inflammation. Thus, vessel tone is increased by $PGF_{2\alpha}$ and thromboxane A_2 and decreased by PGE_2 and PGI_2, whereas vessel permeability is increased by PGE_2, PGI_2, and LTB_4 and decreased by PGF_2. Chemotaxis is stimulated by PGE_2 and LTB_4 and is inhibited by PGI_2. It has been suggested that the generation of free radicals during arachidonic acid metabolism by cyclo-oxygenase may potentiate the inflammatory process.[18] The concentration of free radical oxidation products is higher in inflammatory synovial effusions, and the free radical scavenger, MK-477, exerts an anti-inflammatory effect in an experimental edema model without inhibiting the production of stable prostaglandins.[13] Thus, it is evident that the effects of arachidonic acid metabolism are exceedingly local, determined by the type of cell that is activated and by the tissue in which the activation takes place and probably by other less well-defined circumstances in the microenvironment.

In 1971, Vane[19] reported that aspirinlike drugs inhibit prostaglandin synthesis. Subsequent work from many studies has established that there is a good correlation between the order of potency of various NSAIDs in the suppression of prostaglandin synthesis and in the suppression of inflammation. Low concentrations of aspirin irreversibly inhibit this process by acetylating the enzyme cyclo-oxygenase; the other NSAIDs reversibly inhibit cyclo-oxygenase in a concentration-related manner by competitive inhibition. Nonacetylated salicylate is much less potent than aspirin as an inhibitor of cyclo-oxygenase, but anti-inflammatory doses (3 g) of salicylate have been reported to reduce the urinary output of prostaglandin metabolites in humans by 85 to 95 percent[20] perhaps because of the high concentrations of salicylate attained.

Thus, NSAIDs reduce the synthesis of prostaglandins, prostacyclin, and thromboxane but appear not to affect leukotriene production. In vitro studies have demonstrated marked inhibition of lipoxygenase by benoxaprofen and moderate inhibition by diclofenac and ketoprofen but no inhibition by indomethacin, flurbiprofen, piroxicam, or naproxen.[21] BW755C, a drug that will remain experimental because it causes hemolysis, inhibits both cyclo-oxygenase and 5-lipoxygenase; it suppressed leukocyte migration more effectively than indomethacin and as effectively as dexamethasone, suggesting that dual inhibition of arachidonic acid metabolism may be desirable.[20] Anti-inflammatory glucocorticoids decrease arachidonic acid production from membrane phospholipids by facilitating the release of the protein, lipocortin, that inhibits phospholipase A_2. Lipocortin itself has been isolated and is reported to be a potent anti-inflammatory agent.[20] Further studies with diclofenac demonstrate that it indirectly decreases leukotriene production by reducing arachidonic acid availability. In formyl-methionyleucylphenylaline (f-MLP)–stimulated purified rat peritoneal neutrophils, diclofenac enhanced the incorporation of free arachidonic acid into triglycerides, thus decreasing the amount of arachidonic acid available for metabolism by 5-lipoxygenase or cyclooxygenase.[22] Sulfasalazine also appears to decrease both cyclo-oxygenase and 5-lipoxygenase pathway metabolites of arachidonic acid produced by colonic mucosa obtained from inflammatory bowel disease patients.[23] A specific inhibitor of 5-lipoxygenase (Abbott 64077) has been reported to demonstrate some benefit in a preliminary trial in rheumatoid arthritis.[24] A combined lipoxygenase/cyclo-oxygenase inhibitor (Tenidap) is also undergoing clinical trials in rheumatoid arthritis, with reported favorable effects.[25]

Another indirect approach to regulation of leukotriene production involves the administration of dietary fish oil that contains docosahexanoic acid and eicosapentaenoic acid (EPA), which inhibit the conversion of arachidonic acid by cyclo-oxygenase. In addition, 5-lipoxygenase converts EPA to a pentaene rather than a tetraene series of products (LTA_5, LTB_5, LTC_5). Leukotriene B_5 is markedly less active than leukotriene B_4 in its ability to attract human neutrophils in a chemotactic assay and to cause human leukocytes to adhere to an endothelial cell monolayer, but leukotriene C_5 is no less active than leukotriene C_4. Thus, induced anaphylaxis was more severe in guinea pigs fed fish oil–enriched diets than in those on regular diets. The biochemical effects in the neutrophils of 12 patients with rheumatoid arthritis treated with fish oil capsules for 6 weeks were selective for suppression of LTB_4 generation only. Modest clinical benefit was noted after 6 weeks but was no longer present 4 weeks after fish oil supplementation was discontinued.[26]

Other Possible Mechanisms

Other proposals for the mechanism of action of NSAIDs include their effects on pro-inflammatory cell functions. Under carefully controlled in vitro conditions, various investigators have demonstrated that NSAIDs inhibit phosphodiesterase; this leads to potentiation of PGE_1-mediated increased intracellular cyclic adenosine monophosphate (AMP) levels and subsequent inhibition of pro-inflammatory cellular functions, inhibition of peripheral blood lymphocyte responses to mitogen stimulation, inhibition of neutrophil and monocyte migration, and inhibition of various neutrophil functions.[13] Weissmann and various associates have demonstrated that NSAIDs inhibit the aggregation of human neutrophils in vitro and in vivo.[27] They also have demonstrated this effect of NSAIDs in cells of the marine sponge, which do not contain cyclo-oxygenase and are unresponsive to stable prostaglandins. They suggest that NSAIDs may act by interfering with a receptor site that triggers immobilization of intracellular calcium and activation of the cell.[27]

A number of hypotheses have been proposed to explain the anti-inflammatory properties of NSAIDs, and each appears to explain some of the mechanisms of NSAID action. The exact mode of action of this class of drugs, however, is not yet completely understood, and clinical application of these drugs continues to be empirical.

Mechanism of Action of Colchicine

Colchicine appears to interfere with several steps of the inflammatory response in which neutrophils play a central role. Intracellular interference with the organization of labile fibrillar microtubular systems concerned with cell structure and movement may lead to microtubular disaggregation and to decreased neutrophil motility, chemotaxis, release of chemotactic factors, formation of digestive vacuoles, and lysosomal degranulation. The net effect seems to decrease the migration of neutrophils into an area of inflammation and to diminish the metabolic and phagocytic activity of those neutrophils that are already there, interrupting part of the inflammatory process of gout.[28] Colchicine binds to tubulin and prevents the polymerization of tubulin into functional microtubules.[29] Lumicolchicines, photoisomers of colchicine, do not bind to microtubule proteins and have no anti-inflammatory effects.[30] Most of the in vitro effects of colchicine on neutrophils have been demonstrated at concentrations of drug that far exceeded the blood levels produced in patients treated with colchicine. Chemotaxis of neutrophils, however, toward bacteria, immune complex–activated serum, or endotoxin-activated serum is suppressed by colchicine in concentrations of $10^{-8}M$, which are attained in neutrophils of patients treated with standard clinical doses of the drug.[28] Ehrenfeld et al.[31] noted that patients on colchicine have significantly fewer neutrophils at Rebuck skin window sites 24 hours after the skin was abraded, suggesting that neutrophil migration is also altered by colchicine in vivo. Neutrophils release a chemotaxic substance during phagocytosis of urate crystals; colchicine $10^{-6}M$ inhibits the release of this substance, and $10^{-8}M$ partially suppresses its release.[32] Colchicine has also been reported to suppress the release of chemotactic leukotriene B_4 by neutrophils[33] and to have corrected T suppressor cell deficiencies in five patients with familial Mediterranean fever who were

treated with 0.5 mg of colchicine twice daily.[34] The capacity for and rate of phagocytosis of yeast were significantly suppressed in neutrophils obtained from patients with acute gout after several days of treatment with oral colchicine, 1.8 mg daily, compared with baseline phagocytosis before starting colchicine.[35] Thus, investigations focused on colchicine effects on neutrophils have succeeded in demonstrating drug-induced changes in the functions of these cells, both in humans treated with clinically tolerated doses of colchicine, and in vitro with concentrations of colchicine readily attained in patients treated with the drug.

CHARACTERISTICS OF NSAIDs

The NSAIDs can be classified on the basis of their chemical structure (Table 43–1). Most of the NSAIDs are organic acids with relatively low pK_a. This property may allow higher concentrations of active drug in inflamed tissue, where the pH is lower.[36] Generally, the lower the Pk_a, the shorter the half-life of an NSAID.[37] It is not essential, however, that NSAIDs be acidic; the nonacid compounds proquazone and nabumetone have well-documented anti-inflammatory effects.[38, 39]

Almost all NSAIDs are more than 90 percent bound to plasma proteins. If total drug concentrations are increased beyond the point where the binding sites on albumin are saturated, biologically active free drug concentrations increase dispropor-

---

Table 43–1. CLASSIFICATION OF SOME NSAIDs

Acidic Agents
Arylcarboxylic acids
  Salicylic acids: aspirin in its various forms,* diflunisal* (Dolobid), choline magnesium trisalicylate* (Trilisate), salsalate* (Disalcid), benorylate, sodium salicylate*
  Anthranilic acids (fenamates): flufenamic acid, mefenamic acid* (Ponstel), meclofenamic acid* (Meclomen), niflumic acid
Arylalkanoic acids
  Arylacetic acids: diclofenac (Voltaren),* fenclofenac, alclofenac, fentiazac
  Arylpropionic acids: ibuprofen* (Motrin, Rufen, Advil, Nuprin), flurbiprofen (ANSAID),* ketoprofen* (Orudis), naproxen* (Naprosyn), fenoprofen* (Nalfon), fenbufen, suprofen, indoprofen, tiaprofenic acid, benoxaprofen, pirprofen
  Heteroarylacetic acids: tolmetin* (Tolectin), zomepirac, clopirac, ketorolac trimethamine* (Toradol)
  Indole and indene acetic acids: indomethacin* (Indocin), sulindac* (Clinoril), etodolac* (Lodine)
Enolic acids
  Pyrazolidinediones: phenylbutazone* (Butazolidine), oxyphenbutazone,* azapropazone, feprazone
  Oxicams: piroxicam* (Feldene), isoxicam, sudoxicam
Nonacidic Agents
Proquazone, fluproquazone, tiaramide, bufexamac, flunizole, epirazole, tinoridine, nabumetone* (Relifen)

---

*Available in the United States.
Modified from Dudley-Hart, F., and Huskisson, E. C.: Nonsteroidal antiinflammatory drugs: Current status and rational therapeutic use. Drugs 27:232, 1984.

tionately to the increasing total drug concentration. This effect is more pronounced for the less potent NSAIDs such as salicylate or ibuprofen, for which daily doses are measured in grams, rather than for the more potent drugs, such as piroxicam with daily doses measured in milligrams, and may help to account for apparently disproportionate increases in anti-inflammatory activity with higher doses of some NSAIDs.

The pharmacologic activities of the available NSAIDs are largely similar, although for commercial reasons, their manufacturers have chosen to emphasize certain applications for particular drugs. For example, naproxen sodium, zomepirac, suprofen, and ketorolac were marketed as analgesics, whereas diflunisal and etodolac were initially marketed for osteoarthritis.

Anti-inflammatory Effects

Historically, plants containing salicylate and colchicine were used to treat inflammatory conditions, and the dose-response relationship of aspirin in rheumatic fever was well documented. It was not until the early 1960s that aspirin was shown to have anti-inflammatory effects both in experimental models of inflammation and in clinical studies of patients with rheumatoid arthritis.[40, 41] Fremont-Smith and Bayles[41] demonstrated decreased ring size, increased range of motion, and increased grip strength in rheumatoid arthritis patients treated with aspirin. This observation was confirmed by the American Rheumatism Association Cooperating Clinics Committee in 1965,[42] and since then innumerable clinical trials of NSAIDs in rheumatoid arthritis and other rheumatic diseases have confirmed the anti-inflammatory effects of these drugs. NSAIDs have been compared with placebo, with aspirin, and with each other in double-blind randomized studies using well-defined criteria for evaluation of joint inflammation. Efficacy superior to that of placebo is easily demonstrated within 1 or 2 weeks in patients with active rheumatoid arthritis who are not receiving glucocorticoids or other anti-inflammatory medications. Comparisons of adequate doses of one NSAID with another or with aspirin almost always show comparable efficacy, but the newer NSAIDs are somewhat less toxic than aspirin at full dosage.[43] In addition to rheumatoid arthritis, the anti-inflammatory effects of NSAIDs have also been demonstrated in juvenile rheumatoid arthritis, ankylosing spondylitis, gout, and osteoarthritis. Although not as rigorously proved, their efficacy is also widely accepted in the treatment of Reiter's syndrome, psoriatic arthritis, acute and chronic bursitis, and tendinitis.

The anti-inflammatory benefit of colchicine in acute gouty arthritis is legendary. Colchicine is also used in small maintenance doses to decrease the frequency and severity of recurrent attacks of gouty arthritis.[44] Its benefit has also been demonstrated in patients with acute episodes of pseudogout[45] and in the suppression of recurrent or chronic joint inflammation owing to calcium crystal disease.[46] It is the drug of choice for prevention of attacks of familial Mediterranean fever[47] and has been used in other rheumatologic disorders such as Behçet's disease, sarcoidosis, calcific tendinitis, amyloidosis, cutaneous necrotizing vasculitis, and Sweet's syndrome.[28]

Analgesic Effects

Colchicine has no effect on pain perception, but virtually all of the NSAIDs relieve pain when used in doses substantially smaller than those required to demonstrate suppression of inflammation. Cross-circulation experiments in 1964 by Lim et al.[48] that induced pain by peripheral injection of bradykinin demonstrated that perfusion of the brain with aspirin does not decrease bradykinin-induced painful responses, whereas perfusion of the peripheral site with aspirin is analgesic, even when the aspirin does not circulate to the brain. Because prostaglandins enhance the painful response to injections of bradykinin and other peripheral chemical or mechanical stimuli, it has been suggested that NSAID suppression of the synthesis and release of prostaglandins averts their sensitization of pain receptors to chemical mediators.[49]

Antipyretic Effects

NSAIDs, but not colchicine, effectively suppress fever in humans and experimental animals. Injection of PGE into the lateral ventricles of cats, rabbits, and rats has been shown to produce fever, and increased PGE concentrations have been reported in the cerebrospinal fluid of rabbits with fever induced by endogenous pyrogen or endotoxin, leading to the hypothesis that the antipyretic effects of NSAIDs are due to their ability to suppress prostaglandin synthesis.[50]

Other Effects of NSAIDs

Both aspirin and NSAIDs inhibit platelet cyclooxygenase and thus markedly decrease platelet aggregation in response to various stimuli. Aspirin is commonly used as a platelet anticoagulant, but the NSAIDs have not been used in this way because their effects on platelets are only temporary. Cyclooxygenase suppression by NSAIDs has been useful in the prevention of menstrual cramping and assisting in the closure of patent ductus arteriosus in infants. Other applications are developing in the treatment of ocular inflammation, shock, periodontal disease, and sports injuries and as an adjunct to cancer chemotherapy.[51] Sulindac has been reported to suppress colorectal polyps completely in three patients with familial polyposis (Gardner's syndrome).[52]

ADVERSE EFFECTS OF NSAIDs

Given the widespread use of NSAIDs and their substantial pharmacologic activity, the occurrence of adverse reactions is inevitable. In general, the NSAIDs share a common spectrum of clinical toxicities, although the frequency of particular side effects varies with the compound. Both adverse effects and beneficial effects tend to be dose-related, necessitating careful evaluation of benefit-to-risk ratios. Important toxicities occur in the gastrointestinal tract, central nervous system, hematopoietic system, kidney, skin, and liver. A great deal of regulatory attention has been focused on the adverse effects of NSAIDs, and the package inserts (also found in the *Physician's Desk Reference*) now contain reliable information about the frequencies of specific adverse effects known to occur with each of the NSAIDs that is marketed in the United States. None are completely safe; aspirin is the most difficult to use effectively, has more frequent side effects, and is more dangerous if overdoses are taken. Of interest, chronopharmacologic studies suggest that in many patients, the adverse effects of NSAIDs can be minimized and their efficacy optimized by adjusting the time of day when drug doses are administered.[53]

Gastrointestinal Adverse Effects

Probably because of their suppression of prostaglandin synthesis, NSAIDs as a group tend to cause gastric irritation and exacerbate peptic ulcers. Prostaglandins have been demonstrated in laboratory animals to suppress gastric acid secretion and to help maintain the gastric mucosal barrier, thus providing gastrointestinal cytoprotection.[54] The administration of an exogenous PGE_2 analogue, misoprostil, has been shown to reduce the incidence of aspirin-induced endoscopic damage to the gastric and duodenal mucosa in humans.[55] NSAID-related symptoms include dyspepsia, epigastric pain, indigestion, heartburn, nausea, and vomiting. NSAIDs have been shown to cause mucosal lesions that may range from hyperemia to diffuse gastritis, superficial erosions, or penetrating ulcer craters. Occult blood loss may occur, especially with aspirin, or massive gastrointestinal bleeding may occur.[56] Indomethacin, sulindac, and meclofenamate sodium have an extensive enterohepatic recirculation, which increases gastrointestinal exposure to these drugs and enhances their gastrointestinal toxicity. A metered-release tablet of indomethacin was withdrawn from the market in Great Britain because of its association with intestinal perforations, apparently caused by direct local irritation by the indomethacin. Caruso and Bianchi-

Porro[57] gastroscopically evaluated the effects of 12 NSAIDs administered singly or in combinations to 164 patients with rheumatoid arthritis and to 85 patients with osteoarthritis. During 1 year of treatment with NSAIDs, 31 percent of the patients had endoscopically confirmed gastric lesions. Lesions were present in 51 percent of patients receiving multiple NSAID treatment. All of the NSAIDs caused gastric damage, the greatest offender being aspirin and the least being sulindac and diflunisal.[57] Similar findings have been reported by Lanza,[58] who found the least mucosal injury with sulindac, enteric-coated aspirin, and low-dose ibuprofen (1200 mg daily). Poor correlation has been found between subjective symptoms of dyspepsia, fecal blood loss, and endoscopic findings.[59, 60] In contrast to aspirin, the nonacetylated salicylates have not been associated with an increase in occult gastrointestinal blood loss[61] or severe gastroscopically detected mucosal injury.[62, 63]

Gastrointestinal bleeding induced by aspirin or NSAIDs tends to be more severe because these agents decrease platelet aggregation by suppressing cyclo-oxygenase. Thus, platelet anticoagulation is more prolonged with aspirin, which irreversibly acetylates platelet cyclo-oxygenase, but is also present in a concentration-related manner with the other NSAIDs, persisting as long as the platelet is exposed to adequate concentrations of the drug.

By life-table analysis of prospectively collected data from multiple NSAID submissions, the Food and Drug Administration estimates that gastrointestinal ulcers, bleeding, and perforation occur in approximately 1 to 2 percent of patients using NSAIDs for 3 months and approximately 2 to 5 percent of those using them for 1 year. Based on ARAMIS data, Fries[64] estimates that NSAID-induced gastropathy is responsible for 76,000 hospitalizations and 7600 deaths each year in the United States. The cumulative risk of these serious events appears to increase with the duration of therapy and to be greater in patients with previous peptic ulcer disease. Fatal outcomes are more likely in elderly or debilitated patients. Higher dosages of NSAIDs probably entail greater risk than lower dosages. The patient's disease, age, and degree of inflammation need to be considered in determining the optimal dosage for an individual patient, and every attempt should be made to use the lowest dose that adequately controls the patient's symptoms.[65] Other strategies to minimize NSAID gastropathy include the substitution of a nonacetylated salicylate[59, 62, 63] and supplemental gastroprotective agents such as misoprostil, carafete, H_2 receptor antagonists, or omeprazole.[66, 66a] Other reported gastrointestinal adverse effects of NSAIDs include stomatitis and diarrhea as well as rare cases of sialoadenitis, esophageal ulceration, perforation of colonic diverticula, and pancreatitis.[67]

Hepatic Effects

During prospective clinical trials reported to the Food and Drug Administration, 5.4 percent of rheumatoid arthritis patients treated with aspirin developed persistent elevations of more than one liver function test, as did 2.9 percent of patients treated with other NSAIDs.[68] Hepatic toxicity has been reported with all NSAIDs; there appears to be a higher risk with acetaminophen, diclofenac, sulindac, and phenylbutazone and a lower risk with ibuprofen and ketoprofen.[69] Patients are usually asymptomatic, and discontinuation or dose reduction generally results in normalization of the transaminase values, although rare fatal outcomes have been reported with almost all NSAIDs.[69] Advanced age, decreased renal function, multiple drug use, higher drug doses, increased duration of therapy, juvenile rheumatoid arthritis, and systemic lupus erythematosus are considered likely to increase the risk of liver toxicity from NSAIDs.[68] Prolongation of the prothrombin time or hyperbilirubinemia are poor prognostic signs and may presage progressive liver disease and possible fatal hepatic necrosis.[70] Benoxaprofen was withdrawn because of a number of fatalities related to hepatic toxicity, mostly in elderly patients receiving high doses of the drug. Phenylbutazone-induced liver injury also has resulted in a number of fatalities; hepatocellular injury, cholestasis, and granulomatous hepatitis may occur and are more common in patients more than 60 years old.[71] Therefore, the treatment of elderly patients with phenylbutazone is not recommended. After starting or changing an NSAID, it is probably prudent to monitor liver enzyme tests during the first 4 to 6 weeks.[69]

Renal Adverse Effects

The vasodilatory prostaglandins E_2 and I_2 increase or support renal blood flow and water excretion, increase sodium chloride excretion, and stimulate renin secretion. The vasoconstrictor autocoids $PGF_{2\alpha}$ and thromboxane A_2 may decrease renal function in glomerulonephritis and transplant rejection. PGE_2 and PGI_2 produced in the glomerulus have predominant effects on glomerular blood flow and filtration rate; PGI_1 produced in renal arterioles can also regulate renal blood flow. PGE_2 is synthesized by medullary interstitial cells, helping to regulate renal blood flow to the medulla; it is also synthesized in the collecting duct, where it alters the permeability of the duct to water and its responsiveness to antidiuretic hormone.[72] Experiments in dogs demonstrate that reductions of renal blood flow by infusion of angiotensin II or by constriction of the main renal artery are accompanied by increased synthesis of PGE_2 followed by a compensatory increase in blood flow. Simultaneous administration of an NSAID, however, markedly augments the reduction in renal blood flow associated with angiotensin II infusion, presumably by preventing the synthesis of vasodilatory PGE_2. In the healthy, well-hydrated individual with normal kidneys, PGE_2 and PGI_2 play little or no role in controlling renal function,[73, 74] but under certain conditions of local circulatory stress often associated with elevated levels of angiotensin II and catecholamines, locally produced vasodilatory prostaglandins become essential to the maintenance of adequate renal function.[75, 76] Experimental induction of immune glomerulonephritis in rats as well as ureteral obstruction and renal vein occlusion is associated with increased production of the vasoconstrictor, thromboxane A_2, which contributes to chronic renal vasoconstriction in these situations.[72, 74]

With this understanding of the role of products of the cyclo-oxygenase pathway of arachidonic acid metabolism and renal hemodynamics, the renal effects of NSAIDs are somewhat logical. The renal effects of these agents are directly related to their potency in inhibiting renal prostaglandin production, as reflected by inhibition of urinary prostaglandin excretion. In predisposed subjects, suppression of compensatory prostaglandin production may result in acute reduction in renal blood flow and glomerular filtration, associated with fluid retention, edema, and elevation of serum creatinine. Patients most at risk include those with congestive heart failure, systemic lupus erythematosus, chronic glomerulonephritis, liver failure with ascites, premature infants, and those receiving diuretics. Marked reductions in medullary blood flow may result in papillary necrosis. Cyclooxygenase inhibition may result in hyperkalemia, most commonly occurring in patients with diabetes mellitus, mild to moderate renal insufficiency, and patients receiving beta (β)-blockers, angiotensin-converting enzyme inhibitors, or potassium-sparing diuretics. Cyclooxygenase inhibition has also been associated with blunting of antihypertensive drug effects and blunting of diuretic drug effects.[77] Considering the huge market for aspirin and NSAIDs, there are relatively few published reports of acute nephrotoxicity associated with these drugs. The ischemic type of NSAID-induced renal insufficiency tends to occur in hospitalized patients rather than in outpatients, and NSAID-induced hyperkalemia is probably more frequent than the induction of acute renal insufficiency.[77]

Several studies have suggested that sulindac, whose active sulindac sulfide metabolite is oxidized by the kidney to the inactive sulfone metabolite or to the relatively inactive prodrug, sulindac, spares the kidney and is less likely to induce renal insufficiency.[78, 79] Others, however, have demonstrated sulindac-induced impairment in renal function or renal prostaglandin synthesis, particularly in more severely hemodynamically compromised patients and with higher doses of sulindac.[80-82] Therefore, great caution should be taken when treating high-risk patients with any NSAID, although sulindac or a nonacetylated salicylate (which is a very weak cyclo-oxygenase inhibitor) probably is preferable to the more potent cyclo-oxygenase inhibitors such as indomethacin.

A second type of renal adverse effect to NSAIDs involves an idiosyncratic reaction accompanied by massive proteinuria and acute interstitial nephritis. Hypersensitivity phenomena such as fever, skin rash, and eosinophilia are occasionally present. Renal biopsy demonstrates focal or diffuse interstitial nephritis with predominance of lymphocytic infiltration, although eosinophils may be present in the biopsy of some patients.[72, 73, 75] This syndrome has been observed with practically all NSAIDs, but the largest number of cases have been reported with fenoprofen.[83] Following discontinuation of the NSAID, complete recovery of renal function eventually occurs in almost all patients; occasionally, however, dialysis or high-dose glucocorticoid therapy has been necessary before recovering renal function.

A third possible mechanism of NSAID-induced renal toxicity may be intratubular precipitation, of uric acid in the case of suprofen or of drug metabolite in the case of benoxaprofen. The abrupt onset of severe bilateral flank pain within 2 or 3 hours after the first or second dose of suprofen, lasting 2 or 3 days and usually associated with a rise in serum creatinine, microscopic hematuria, mild proteinuria, and polyuria, was reported to the Food and Drug Administration in approximately 300 cases during 1986. Young men were most commonly affected, and in all patients the pain resolved and renal function returned to baseline within a few days to a few weeks. This syndrome has also been observed in a few patients treated with other NSAIDs. Careful study demonstrated that suprofen is a potent uricosuric, although its half-life is so short that this effect lasts for only a few hours. It has been hypothesized, however, that persons with hyperuricemia, an acid urine, and low urine flow rates may precipitate uric acid crystals and produce temporary tubular obstruction. This syndrome could be avoided by ensuring that patients are well hydrated before taking the first dose of NSAID, but the manufacturer has withdrawn suprofen from the market because of this adverse effect.[65] It has also been speculated that renal failure associated with benoxaprofen therapy may have been contributed to by similar intratubular accumulation of a metabolite of benoxaprofen that was observed to be present in the urine as microscopic globular bodies.

It is generally considered to be exceedingly unusual for end-stage renal failure to develop as a complication of NSAID therapy.[77, 84] Patients starting an NSAID should be well hydrated. Patients with predisposing diseases or patients taking predisposing drugs should be treated with the lowest effective dose of a less potent renal cyclo-oxygenase inhibitor and should be followed closely. Baseline serum creatinine and electrolyte levels with repeat measurements after 5 to 7 days have been recommended.[85] Particular care should be taken with hospitalized patients, who seem to be at much greater risk.[77]

Cutaneous Adverse Effects

A wide spectrum of cutaneous reactions has been associated with NSAIDs. The spontaneous adverse reaction reporting system of the American Academy of Dermatology in 1984 reported that adverse cutaneous reactions were most frequently reported with piroxicam, zomepirac, sulindac, meclofenamate sodium, and benoxaprofen.[86] Benign morbilliform eruptions, fixed drug reactions, photosensitivity reactions, vesiculobullous eruptions, serum sickness, and exfoliative erythroderma have been reported. Almost all the NSAIDs have been associated with erythema multiforme, Stevens-Johnson syndrome, or toxic epidermal necrolysis. Phenylbutazone and oxyphenbutazone have more reports of serious or fatal dermal reactions.[67] NSAIDs may also cause urticaria, especially in aspirin-sensitive patients. Pseudoporphyria, a photoinduced bullous dermatitis with characteristic clinical and histopathologic features, has been reported with naproxen use.[87]

Hypersensitive Reactions

In some patients with bronchial asthma, especially those with the triad of vasomotor rhinitis, nasal polyposis, and asthma, aspirin, or NSAID ingestion may precipitate an acute asthmatic attack, probably owing to drug-related inhibition of bronchodilating prostaglandins. It is also possible that inhibition of the cyclo-oxygenase metabolic pathway diverts arachidonic acid metabolism toward lipoxygenase products such as the slow-reacting substance of anaphylaxis (leukotrienes C_4 and D_4), which may precipitate bronchospasm.[88] Patients exhibiting this reaction generally are sensitive to all NSAIDs and should avoid them. Anaphylactoid reactions have been reported with many of the NSAIDs, especially with tolmetin and zomepirac, and zomepirac has been withdrawn from the market because of this adverse effect.[67] The risk of anaphylaxis appears to be accentuated for those who use NSAIDs intermittently for relief of pain.[89]

Hematologic Effects

Aplastic anemia, agranulocytosis, and thrombocytopenia rarely are associated with NSAIDs but are prominent among the causes of deaths attributed to these drugs. Based on Inman's estimate of 22 deaths from blood dyscrasia per million patients[90] and Food and Drug Administration estimates of 16 deaths per million,[91] phenylbutazone is not recommended for initial use for any condition. The risk is approximately sixfold greater in women over the age of 60.[91] Scattered reports of blood dyscrasias associated with other NSAIDs have been published, but a large case control study has shown an association only for indomethacin and for phenylbutazone, with excess risk rates of 10.1 per million and 6.6 per million.[92] In view of the rarity of these problems and their unpredictable nature, monitoring for their occurrence with frequent routine blood cell counts is not mandatory, although it should be strongly considered if phenylbutazone or oxyphenbutazone is used in women older than 60 years of age.

NSAIDs reversibly impair platelet aggregation by inhibiting platelet cyclo-oxygenase, thereby blocking synthesis of thromboxane A_2. This effect persists for only as long as the drug is present but can increase the severity of gastrointestinal bleeding in patients taking NSAIDs. Preoperatively NSAIDs should be discontinued for a long enough time before surgery to permit complete excretion of the drug, i.e., about four or five times the half-life for excretion of the drug (see Table 43–4). Thus, drugs with a short half-life such as tolmetin or ibuprofen can be discontinued 18 to 24 hours preoperatively, whereas drugs with a long half-life such as piroxicam should be discontinued about 8 days before surgery.

Central Nervous System Effects

Headaches and giddiness occur in patients taking indomethacin, and dizziness, confusion, depression, drowsiness, hallucinations, depersonalization reactions, seizures, and syncopy also have been reported. Elderly patients taking naproxen or ibuprofen have been reported to experience cognitive dysfunction, memory loss, inability to concentrate, confusion, personality change, forgetfulness, depression, sleeplessness, irritability, lightheadedness, and paranoid ideation. An acute aseptic meningitis, perhaps an unusual type of hypersensitivity reaction, has been reported in patients with systemic lupus erythematosus or mixed connective tissue disease treated with ibuprofen, sulindac, tolmetin, or naproxen.[93, 94]

Other Adverse Effects

Pulmonary edema has been reported with phenylbutazone and pulmonary infiltrates with naproxen. Gynecomastia has been associated with sulindac, alopecia with ibuprofen, and goiter with oxyphenbutazone.

Overdoses of NSAIDs

Acute overdoses of NSAIDs are much less toxic than are overdoses of aspirin or salicylate. This subject has been most carefully evaluated for ibuprofen, prompted by its approval for over-the-counter sale to the general public. A total of 201 cases of ibuprofen overdose have been reported by two poisoning control centers.[95, 96] The majority of patients did not develop symptoms; those who did developed them within 4 hours after drug ingestion. One child and one elderly woman died. Symptoms, with overdoses ranging up to 40 g, include central nervous system depression, seizures, apnea, nystagmus, blurred vision, diplopia, headache, tinnitus, bradycardia, hypotension, abdominal pain, nausea, vomiting, hematuria, abnormal renal function, coma, and cardiac arrest. Treatment includes evacuating the stomach contents, observation, and administration of fluids. Additional information about poisoning owing to specific NSAIDs is available in an encyclopedic review by Vale and Meridith.[97]

Adverse Effects of Colchicine

Colchicine does not share those adverse effects of NSAIDs that depend on the ability to suppress cyclo-oxygenase. About 80 percent of patients who take a full therapeutic dose of colchicine orally experience cramping abdominal pain, diarrhea, nausea, or vomiting, and these symptoms usually limit the dosage that can be given for acute gout. With long-term maintenance therapy, bone marrow depression, peripheral neuritis, hair loss, amenorrhea, dysmenorrhea, oligospermia, and azoospermia have been reported.[28] Colchicine should not be used in patients with inflammatory bowel disease or in pregnant or nursing patients. It should be avoided or used with great caution and in reduced dosages in patients with hepatic or renal dysfunction because it is excreted by the liver and the kidney.

Colchicine overdoses are associated with more severe and more diffuse toxic manifestations. Gastrointestinal effects include hemorrhage, dehydration, hypokalemia, metabolic acidosis, and renal shutdown. Shock may occur owing to profound dehydration or to gram-negative septicemia associated with the gastrointestinal irritation. Hepatocellular failure, seizures, myopathy, hypocalcemia, stomatitis, and coma may occur. Deaths have been seen with as little as 8 mg but are invariable after the ingestion of more than 40 mg. Treatment includes aspiration of the stomach, intensive support measures, and hemodialysis, although there is no evidence that colchicine can be removed by dialysis. Patients for whom colchicine is prescribed should be strongly advised to keep the medication in childproof containers and to store it in areas that are not accessible to irresponsible individuals.[28]

EFFECTS OF CONCOMITANT DRUGS, DISEASES, AGING, AND PATIENT CHARACTERISTICS

In view of the extensive use of NSAIDs under both prescription and nonprescription conditions for a wide variety of complaints and the substantial pharmacologic activity of these compounds, there are opportunities for the occurrence of almost any conceivable interactions of these drugs with other factors within the patients. Drug–drug and drug–disease interactions with NSAIDs have been reviewed in detail by Brater.[98]

Drug–Drug Interactions

Table 43–2 provides a partial list of potential interactions involving NSAIDs. The degree to which individual patients exhibit these interactions varies considerably, but they should be considered when prescribing potentially interacting drug combinations. With the exception of nabumetone and proquazone, the NSAIDs as a group are well absorbed when administered orally. With few exceptions, concomitant food or antacid may delay the absorption of NSAIDs but does not alter the area under the curve or overall bioavailability to any significant extent. Concomitant administration of food does, however, improve the rate of absorption but not the area under the curve of nabumetone, whereas concomitant administration of aluminum-containing antacids decreases the total absorption of diflunisal.

As most NSAIDs bind firmly to plasma proteins, they may displace other drugs from binding sites or may themselves be displaced by other agents. Aspirin and other NSAIDs may thus increase the activity or toxicity of sulfonylurea hypoglycemic agents, oral anticoagulants, phenytoin, sulfonamides, and methotrexate by displacing these drugs from their protein-binding site and increasing the free fraction of the drug in plasma.[99] Of the available NSAIDs, the ones least likely to interact with warfarin to accentuate anticoagulation include diclofenac, flurbiprofen, ibuprofen, ketorolac, tolmetin, and naproxen (Tables 43–3 through 43–5). The NSAIDs least likely to interact with oral hypoglycemic agents to accentuate hypoglycemia are diclofenac, etodolac, fenoprofen, flurbiprofen, ibuprofen, indomethacin, ketoprofen, ketorolac, meclofenamate, tolmetin, diflunisal, naproxen, and sulindac. Caution or avoidance should be exercised if considering the use of other NSAIDs with warfarin or hypoglycemics. Similarly, salicylate may compete with other NSAIDs for protein-binding sites, thus decreasing their serum level when used concomitantly.[100] In most cases, however, the increase in the unbound concentration of the displaced drug is transient because increased excretion or distribution to other tissue sites results in a new steady state in which the concentration of unbound drug is the same as it was before the displacement occurred.[98]

Drug interactions also may occur if one drug interferes with the metabolism or excretion of another drug. By this mechanism, probenecid impairs the excretion of many NSAIDs, and steady-state lithium levels may increase when it is given concomitantly with NSAIDs.[99] Induction of the hepatic microsomal enzyme system by phenylbutazone may induce the metabolism of digitoxin, dicoumarol, and hexobarbitol. Phenylbutazone also may inhibit the metabolism of carbamazepine, phenobarbital, phenytoin, tolbutamide, and warfarin.[98] As organic acids, NSAIDs may inhibit the secretion of other organic acids by the secretory pump of the proximal nephron and thus decrease their renal clearance. This may be important with methotrexate, whose excretion is inhibited by salicylate and probenecid and is potentially inhibitable by fenoprofen, naproxen, phenylbutazone, and tolmetin.[98]

As discussed earlier, suppression of renal prostaglandins by NSAIDs during administration of a loop diuretic may result in a decrease in natriuresis by preventing prostaglandin-induced increases in renal blood flow in response to the loop diuretic. NSAIDs apparently do not affect the diuretic response to thiazides.[98] Reversible acute renal failure or hyperkalemia, however, may occur when indomethacin and triamterene are combined.[101]

For unclear reasons, NSAIDs may blunt the antihypertensive effects of β-blockers, captopril, and thiazides.[98] Ethanol potentiates the gastrointestinal toxicity of NSAIDs. Enhanced bleeding also may occur in patients receiving both NSAIDs and anticoagulants. The combination of NSAID-induced gastrointestinal irritation and impaired hemostasis makes gastrointestinal bleeding more serious.

Only a tiny fraction of the possible combinations of NSAIDs with other drugs have been examined carefully. Therefore one should exercise caution when initiating multiple drug therapy and carefully observe the patient for unexpected interactions.

Drug–Disease Interactions

Conditions that decrease serum albumin concentrations or decrease NSAID binding to proteins or that impair drug metabolism or excretion by the liver or kidneys may alter the expected response of the patient to a given dose of NSAID (see Table 43–3). Most studies have shown no significant effect of rheumatoid arthritis on the clearance of NSAIDs. Cirrhosis, however, may both decrease serum albumin concentrations and impair hepatic metabolism of drugs. With sulindac, the predominant effect of cirrhosis was a fourfold increase in the area under the curve of sulindac sulfide owing to impairment of biliary excretion of this active metabolite; therefore, sulindac dosage in cirrhotics should be only one fourth of the normal dose. With naproxen, clearance of unbound drug is impaired, although clearance of total drug is unchanged by cirrhosis, and patients should receive half the normal dose of naproxen.[98] Patients with cirrhosis also may have increased susceptibility to the nephrotoxic effects of NSAIDs because maintenance of renal blood flow is more likely to depend on renal synthesis of prostaglandins in patients with portal hypertension or ascites. Thus, the changes in the pharmacokinetics of some NSAIDs in cirrhosis and the possibility of severe adverse consequences owing to inhibition of prostaglandin synthesis in these patients mandate extreme caution in their use in cirrhosis.

Renal insufficiency is associated with a decrease in serum albumin concentrations and displacement of NSAIDs from protein-binding sites by accumu-

Table 43–2. SOME DRUG–DRUG INTERACTIONS INVOLVING NSAIDs

Perturbed Drug	Perturbing Drug	Effect	Suggested Action
Salicylate	Antacids	Increased urine pH results in increased excretion with decreased salicylate levels	Review need for antacid Use low, moderate antacid doses Select another NSAID
Warfarin and other anticoagulants	Phenylbutazone Oxyphenbutazone	Significant prolongation of prothrombin time owing to inhibition of warfarin catabolism	Beware all NSAIDs and aspirin Avoid phenylbutazone, oxyphenbutazone, and aspirin Ibuprofen, naproxen, and tolmetin relatively safer
	All NSAIDs	Increased risk of bleeding owing to anticoagulant inhibition of platelet function and gastric mucosal damage	
Sulfonylurea	Phenylbutazone	Risk of hypoglycemia owing to inhibition of sulfonylurea metabolism	Choose alternative NSAID
	High-dose salicylate	Potentiates hypoglycemia by different mechanism	Choose alternative NSAID
β-Blocker	All prostaglandin-inhibiting NSAIDs	Blunting of hypotensive but not of negative chronotropic or inotropic effect	Avoid phenylbutazone, indomethacin, and aspirin Review need for and use minimum dose of NSAID (especially the elderly or renal impaired)
Peripheral vasodilators: hydralazine proazosin	All prostaglandin-inhibiting NSAIDs	Loss of hypotensive effect	Adjust dose of hypotensive for desired effect Thiazide may be preferred diuretic Sulindac may enhance hypotensive effects of thiazide New NSAIDs interact less
ACE-inhibitor	All prostaglandin-inhibiting NSAIDs	Loss of hypotensive effect	
Diuretics	All prostaglandin-inhibiting NSAIDs	Loss of natriuretic, diuretic, hypotensive effects of furosemide Loss of natriuretic effect of spironolactone Loss of hypotensive but not natriuretic or diuretic effects of thiazide	
Salicylate	Glucocorticoids	Increased salicylate metabolism lowers plasma salicylate level	Use minimum doses of glucocorticoids Adjust salicylate dose or choose alternative NSAID Check salicylate levels after changes in glucocorticoid dose
Lithium	Many NSAIDs	Increased plasma lithium levels	Elderly and renal disease patients more susceptible Review need for NSAID Use minimum dose of NSAID Reduce lithium dose; monitor plasma lithium levels
Methotrexate (MTX)	Salicylates Phenylbutazone Other NSAIDs, probenecid	Increased MTX levels owing to decreased renal clearance of MTX	Reduce MTX dose substantially Use another NSAID Monitor plasma MTX with high-dose MTX
Phenytoin	Phenylbutazone Oxyphenbutazone Salicylate	Increased phenytoin toxicity by decreased metabolism of phenytoin Displaces active phenytoin	Use alternative NSAID Monitor phenytoin plasma levels
Carbonic anhydrase inhibitor	Salicylate	Metabolic acidosis	Use alternative NSAID
NSAIDs	Probenecid	Impairs/prolongs NSAID excretion Increased potential for toxicity	Adjust dose of NSAID
Probenecid, sulfinpyrazone	Salicylate (low dose)	Inhibits uricosuria	Choose alternative NSAID
NSAIDs	Aspirin	Blood levels of many NSAIDs are reduced	Avoid concomitant use of aspirin with any other NSAIDs
Digoxin	Aspirin, ibuprofen	May increase digoxin levels	Monitor digoxin Use minimum dose of NSAID
NSAIDs	Omeprazol H$_2$ blockers Misoprostil	Decreases gastric acid secretion Replaces PGE in stomach	Use cytoprotective drugs in PUD, elderly, dyspepsia
Piroxicam	Cimetidine	Increased plasma concentrations and half-life of piroxicam	Decrease piroxicam dose [131]

ACE, Angiotensin-converting enzyme; PGE, prostaglandin E; PUD, peptic ulcer disease.
Adapted from Day, R. O., Graham, G. G., et al.: Anti-rheumatic drug interactions. Clin. Rheum. Dis. 10(2):251–275, 1984.
References:
1. Conner, C. R. and Rumack, B. H. (eds.): Drug-dex Information System. Denver, Micromedix Inc., 1992.
2. McEvoy, G. K. (ed.): AHFS Drug Information 92. Bethesda, MD, American Society of Hospital Pharmacists, 1992.

Table 43–3. SOME DRUG–DISEASE INTERACTIONS INVOLVING NSAIDs

Therapy	Interaction of NSAID with Disease States and Therapy						Dosage Adjustment of NSAID Needed for Concomitant				
	HTN	Anti-HTN* Therapy	Renal ADR*	PUD*	Plate Inhib*	ASA Hyper*	Warfarin	Hypo-glycemics	Renal Failure	Hepatic Failure	Elder (>70 years old)
Minimal PG Inhibition											
Nonacetylated salicylate	0	0	0	±	0	0	caut	caut	caut	caut	none
Minimal Renal PG Inhibition											
Sulindac	0	0	±	+	+	+	caut	none	decr	decr	decr
PG Inhibition, Short Half-life											
Aspirin	±	±	±	+ +	+ +	+ +	caut	caut	caut	caut	none
Diclofenac	+	+	+	+	+	+	none	none	none	avoid	none
Etodalac	+	+	+	+	+	+	ID	none	none	ID	none
Fenoprofen	+	+	+ +	+	+	+	caut	none	none	ID	none
Flurbiprofen	+	+	+	+	+	+	none	none	ID	ID	none
Ibuprofen	+	+	+	+	+	+	none	none	none	none	none
Indomethacin	+	+	+ +	+	+	+	caut	none	none	ID	none
Ketoprofen	+	+	+	+	+	+	caut	none	decr	decr	decr
Ketorolac	+	+	+	+	+	+	none	none	decr	ID	decr
Meclofenamate	+	+	+	+	+	+	caut	none	none	ID	none
Tolmetin	+	+	+	+	+	+	none	none	none	ID	ID
PG Inhibition, Long Half-life											
Azapropazone	+	+	+	+	+	+	avoid	avoid	decr	decr	decr
Diflunisal	+	+	+	+	+	+	caut	none	decr	ID	none
Fenbufen	+	+	+	+	+	+	caut	ID	none	ID	none
Nabumetone	+	+	+	+	+	+	ID	ID	decr	avoid	decr
Naproxen	min	+	±	+	+	+	none	none	decr	decr	decr
Phenylbutazone	+	+	+	+	+	+	avoid	avoid	decr	avoid	ID
Piroxicam	+	+	+	+	+	+	caut	none	none	decr	decr
Carprofen	+	+	+	+	+	+	none	none	none	caut	none
Proquazone	+	+	+	+	+	+	ID	ID	ID	ID	ID

*Involves prostaglandin inhibition.

HTN, Hypertension; ADR, adverse drug reaction; PUD, peptic ulcer disease; Plate inhib, inhibition platelet function; ASA hyper, aspirin hypersensitivity; PG, prostaglandin; caut, cautious use; decr, decreased dose; ID, insufficient data.

References:
1. Gelman, C. R., and Rumack, B. H. (eds.): DRUGDEX® Information System. Denver: Micromedex Inc., 1990.
2. McEvoy, G. K. (ed.): AHFS Drug Information 92. Bethesda, MD, American Society of Hospital Pharmacists, 1992.

lated endogenous organic acids. In addition, drugs such as azapropazone and nabumetone that to a considerable extent are excreted unchanged in urine may have decreased drug clearance associated with decreases in creatinine clearance. Studies in patients with renal insufficiency indicate that no change in dose is necessary for diclofenac, fenoprofen, ibuprofen, indomethacin, meclofenamate, tolmetin, piroxicam, fenbufen, or etodolac. Unbound drug concentrations of naproxen and oxaprozin, however, are doubled in patients with moderate to severe renal insufficiency, and for these drugs, doses should be half the normal dose.[98]

NSAID Use in the Elderly

Various physiologic, pharmacokinetic, and pharmacodynamic changes may occur with increased age. Drug absorption is not altered, but drug distribution may be significantly changed owing to a decrease in total body water and lean mass and an increase in body fat. In the elderly, age-related reductions in hepatic mass, blood flow, and enzymatic activity as well as in renal plasma flow, glomerular filtration rate, and tubular function may contribute to decreased drug clearance.[93] In addition, the elderly appear to be more susceptible to the development of

Table 43–4. NSAIDs WITH LONG HALF-LIVES

| Drug | Available Formulations (mg) | Maximum Daily Dose (mg) | Active Metabolite | % Bound | Time of Maximum Concentration (Hr) | Half-life (Hr) | Time to Steady State (days) | Renal Excretion Unchanged Drug (% dose) | Changes in Dose for | | | Influence on NSAID Efficacy by | | Influence of NSAID on Toxicity of | |
									Renal Failure	Hepatic Disease	Elderly	Food	Antacid	Warfarin	Hypoglycemic Agents
Diflunisal	Tabs: 250, 500	1000	—	99	2–3	7–15	3–9	<3	↓ by 50% with GFR <10 ml/min	ID	none	none	Aluminum decreases absorption	caution	none
Nabumetone	Tabs: 500	2000	6-methoxy 2-naphthyl acetic acid	99	3–6	24	3–7	<1	Probably decrease	Avoid in severe disease	Limit to 1 g every day	↑ rate of absorption	none	ID	ID
Naproxene	Tabs: 250, 375, 500	1500	—	99	2–4	12–15	2–3	<5	↓ dose with GFR <20 ml/min	↓ dose by 50% with chronic liver disease	Probably decrease	none	none	none	none
Phenylbutazone	Tabs, Caps: 100	400	Oxyphenbutazone	>90	2–8	29–140	7–15	5	Avoid with GFR <20 ml/min	avoid	none	ID	ID	avoid	avoid
Piroxicam	Caps: 10, 20	20	—	99	2–5	14–158	7–21	<10	none	↓ dose	Limit to 20 mg every day	none	none	caution	ID
Sulindac	Tabs: 150, 200	400	Sulfide	98	2–4	16–18 (sulfide) 7 (sulindac)	3	<7	↓ by 50% with GFR <10 ml/min	↓ dose	Probably decrease	none	ID	caution	none
Azapazone	Not available	900–1800	—	99	3–6	12–15	3	51–73	↓ dose	↓ dose by 50+%	↓ dose by 50+%	ID	none	avoid	avoid
Carprofen	Not available	200–600	—	99	0.5–2.0	6–16	2–3	3–12	none	none	none	none	none	none	ID
Fenbufen	Not available	1000	Hydroxy-biphenyl-butanoic acid Biphenyl acetic acid	99	1–2 (parent) 1–8 (metabolite)	10–12 (parent) 10 (metabolite)	7	4	none	ID	none	none	none	caution	ID
Proquazone	Not available	1200	m-hydroxy proquazone	98	1–2	0.6–1.3 (parent) 13.4 (metabolite)	3	<1	ID	ID	ID	↑ rate of absorption	none	ID	ID

Tabs, Tablets; Caps, capsules; GFR, glomerular filtration rate; ID, insufficient data.

References:

1. Gelman, C. R., and Rumach, B. H. (eds.): DRUGDEX® Information System. Denver, Micromedex, Inc., 1990.
2. McEvoy, G. K. (ed.): AHFS Drug Information 92. Bethesda, MD, American Society of Hospital Pharmacists, 1992.

Table 43–5. NSAIDs WITH SHORT HALF-LIVES

Drug	Available Formulations (mg)	Maximum Daily Dose (mg)	Active Metabolite	% Bound	Time of Maximum Concentrations (Hr)	Half-life (Hr)	Renal Excretion Unchanged Drug (% dose)
Diclofenac	Tabs: 25, 50, 75	200	—	99	1–3	1.2–2.0	<1
Etodolac	Caps: 200, 300	600	—	99	1	7.3	1
Fenoprofen	Caps, Tabs: 200, 300, 600	3200	—	99	1–2	2–3	2–5
Flurbiprofen	Tabs: 50, 100	300	—	99	1.5–3.0	3–4	<15
Ibuprofen	Tabs: 200, 300, 400, 600, 800	3600	—	99	1–2	2.0–2.5	<10
Indomethacin	Caps: 10, 25, 50 Sustained-release Caps: 75 Oral suspension: 25 mg/5 ml Suppositories: 50	200	—	>98	1–4	2–13	<15
Ketoprofen	Caps: 25, 50, 75	300	—	99	0.5–2.0	1–4	<10
Ketorolac	Parenteral: 15 mg/ml, 30 mg/ml Tabs: 10 mg	150 first day, 120 thereafter 40	—	99	0.3–1.0	4–9	60
Meclofenamate	Caps: 50, 100	400	Hydroxy-methyl deriva-tive	99	0.5–2.0	2–3	<4
Tolmetin	Tabs, Caps: 200, 400, 600	2000	—	99	0.5–1.0	2–7	15

adverse drug reactions. They have more illnesses and take more medications than younger patients and use more over-the-counter medications; thus, they are at greater risk for drug–drug interactions. They are more likely to self-medicate and may be more likely to make mistakes in the timing or quantity of drug doses. The effects of age on the pharmacokinetics of some NSAIDs has been studied. Brater[98] suggests that doses of naproxen, ketoprofen, and oxaprozin should be halved in the elderly but that ibuprofen and etodolac require no dosage adjustment. Conclusions regarding the effect of aging on piroxicam disposition are conflicting,[98, 102] but discretion suggests some decrease in its dosage in the elderly.

Increased attention to the aging process has emphasized the heterogeneity of older persons and the need to individualize one's approach to them. Healthy, well-nourished, elderly individuals are vastly different from sick, malnourished persons for whom death is rapidly approaching. In general, greater care must be taken when treating elderly patients with NSAIDs because increased toxicity may occur owing to unanticipated, clinically important changes in responses to drugs, related to concomitant diseases, other medications, or subclinical changes in organ function.

Individual Variability in Responses to Nonsteroidal Antirheumatic Drugs

One of the most striking findings in all careful evaluations of these drugs is the wide range of responses among the subjects studied, regardless of what variable is being measured. This is immediately apparent to the investigator who is dealing with the raw data but tends to be obscured in the statistical analysis and by the generalizations needed to produce a concise report. Fourfold to fivefold differences between subjects are frequently observed in plasma half-life and other pharmacokinetic measurements in individuals who have been given the same weight-adjusted dose of the drug. In evaluating the efficacy of established NSAIDs, responses invariably range from marked improvement to no response or even clinical deterioration. Similarly, only rarely are we able to predict which individuals will develop adverse effects to a particular drug; even when a subgroup at greater risk for an adverse effect can be identified, the adverse effect will actually occur in only a proportion of the higher risk patients. Given the genetic, dietary, and environmental diversity of humans, this wide range of individual responses is not unexpected. Genetic influences have been demonstrated in the metabolism of salicylate and of phenylbutazone[103, 104] and no doubt are factors with other drugs as well. The character and degree of inflammation being treated vary from patient to patient even when they have the same diagnosis. Concomitant drugs and environmental factors may have variable or contradictory influences on drug pharmacokinetics or pharmacodynamics. Because it is impossible to control for or even to know all of the factors impinging on the responses of a particular patient to a drug, one must be cautious in initiating treatment and increasing dosage and must maintain

Table 43–5. NSAIDs WITH SHORT HALF-LIVES *Continued*

Drug	Changes in Dose for			Influence on NSAID Efficacy by		Influence of NSAID on Toxicity of	
	Renal Failure	*Hepatic Disease*	*Elderly*	*Food*	*Antacid*	*Warfarin*	*Hypoglycemic Agents*
Diclofenac	none	avoid	none	none	none	none	none
Etodolac	none	ID	none	none	ID	caution	none
Fenoprofen	none	ID	none	none	none	caution	ID
Flurbiprofen	ID	ID	none	none	none	none	ID
Ibuprofen	none	none	none	none	none	none	none
Indomethacin	none	ID	none	none	ID	caution	ID
Ketoprofen	↓ by ½–⅓ with CrCl <10 ml/min	↓ dose	probably decrease	none	none	caution	none
Ketorolac	↓ dose by 50%	ID	↓ dose by 50%	none	none	none	ID
Meclofenamate	none	ID	none	none	none	caution (prolongs protime)	ID
Tolmetin	none	ID	ID	none	ID	none	none

Tabs, Tablets; Caps, capsules; ID, insufficient data; CrCl, creatinine clearance.
References:
1. Gelman, C. R., and Rumack, B. H. (eds.): DRUGDEX® Information System. Denver, Micromedex, Inc., 1990.
2. McEvoy, G. K. (ed.): AHFS Drug Information 92. Bethesda, American Society of Hospital Pharmacists, 1992.

close communication with and careful observation of each patient.

DISTINCTIVE CHARACTERISTICS OF INDIVIDUAL DRUGS

The following discussion highlights important individual characteristics of selected nonsteroidal antirheumatic drugs. Characteristics that conform to the general properties of this class of drugs as previously described are not repeated in the individual descriptions. As a first source for additional information about individual drugs, the reader is directed to the current package insert for that drug or its reproduction in the *Physician's Desk Reference*. No longer a throw-away item, the package insert development process for the NSAIDs has been refined to the point where it represents the most current and reliable conservative summary of the information known about the drug. It reflects not only published information, but also all of the unpublished information in the manufacturer's files and additional information about adverse effects in the Food and Drug Administration's files. Especially useful are the quantitative estimates of the frequency of adverse effects associated with the drug and the advice regarding dosage for approved conditions. Unfortunately, there is no information about use of the drug for indications that have not yet been approved by

the Food and Drug Administration, even though these may be well established in clinical practice. The language of the package insert is arrived at by negotiation between representatives of the manufacturer and the Food and Drug Administration. Determination of this language is taken seriously because drug company representatives are not allowed to deviate from this language in promoting the drug. Negotiations over its precise wording are to a considerable extent responsible for delays in the marketing of new drugs, as the manufacturer attempts to increase the flexibility of the language and the Food and Drug Administration attempts to preserve its accuracy.

It is useful to group the nonsteroidal antirheumatic drugs according to their half-life. Those with a long half-life can be given once or twice a day, whereas those with a short half-life should be given every 4 to 6 hours if one wishes to obtain maximal anti-inflammatory effects.

NONSTEROIDAL ANTIRHEUMATIC DRUGS WITH A LONG HALF-LIFE

Drugs with a half-life of 12 hours or more can be given once or twice daily (see Table 43–4). Because five half-lives are required to approach steady state, plasma concentrations of these drugs continue to rise for 3 days to several weeks depending on the half-life but thereafter tend to be fairly stable between doses. The long half-life allows ample time for equilibration of drug between plasma and synovial fluid, and synovial fluid concentrations of unbound drug usually are equal to those in plasma, whereas the sum of the bound and unbound drug concentrations is lower in synovial fluid, reflecting the lower quantity of albumin in the synovial fluid. Individual variations in drug disposition or excretion are more likely to result in excessive accumulation of drug and potentially serious side effects if the half-life is long than if it is short, although the long half-life itself does not increase the inherent toxicity of the compound. Although one would anticipate that monitoring plasma concentrations of these drugs would be helpful in avoiding problems, and drug concentrations are easily determined, this technique has not been applied to routine clinical practice as yet.

Phenylbutazone

Phenylbutazone is an exceptionally effective NSAID (Fig. 43–3) and still has a loyal following among patients who did not respond to other therapies; however, it is no longer recommended as initial therapy for any indication (and oxyphenbutazone has been withdrawn from the market by its major manufacturer) because of its well-documented serious and sometimes fatal adverse reactions and the increasing availability of alternative NSAIDs.[91, 92, 105]

Naproxen

Naproxen is the active D(+) isomer of 6-methoxy-α-methyl-2 naphthaleneacetic acid (Fig. 43–4). The inactive L(−) isomer is not contained in naproxen. Naproxen is rapidly and completely absorbed after oral administration, and with twice-daily administration steady-state concentrations are achieved after 2 or 3 days. It is readily absorbed rectally, but suppository preparations are not marketed in the United States. As with most NSAIDs, food and antacids do not alter the completeness of absorption but may change the rate of absorption to some extent.[106]

Protein binding of naproxen decreases with single doses larger than 500 mg; the resulting disproportionate increases in concentrations of unbound drug are associated with increases in excretion rates.

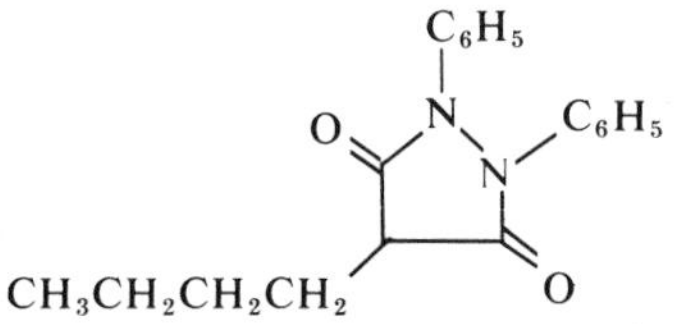

Figure 43–3. Chemical structure of phenylbutazone.

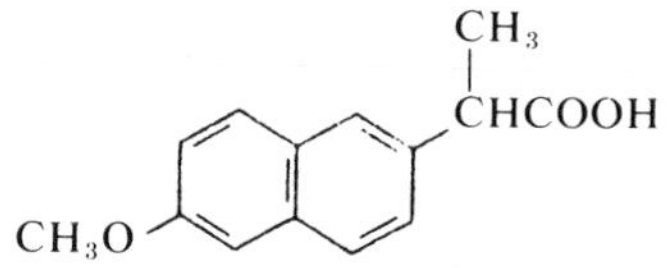

Figure 43–4. Chemical structure of naproxen.

Thus, single doses larger than 500 mg are not associated with proportionate increases in bioavailable naproxen. Naproxen does not accumulate in tissues; it has a low volume of distribution, and most of it remains in the plasma compartment bound to plasma proteins. Naproxen is cleared from plasma predominantly by metabolism to glucuronide and other conjugates of naproxen and by 6-desmethylation with subsequent conjugation of this metabolite. Almost all of the ingested drug is excreted in the urine, predominantly as inactive metabolites and conjugates.[106] Moderate renal failure has little effect on naproxen kinetics, but severe renal failure decreases naproxen protein binding, doubling unbound drug concentrations and increasing the volume of distribution. Although intrinsic clearance of the drug by hepatic metabolism increases, naproxen doses should be halved if the glomerular filtration rate is less than 20 mg per minute.[107] Patients with severe hepatic disease eliminate naproxen less rapidly because they do not metabolize it as well.[106] In one study, patients with alcoholic cirrhosis had a 60 percent decrease in clearance of unbound naproxen. Therefore, it has been suggested that naproxen doses should be decreased by 50 percent in these patients.[108] Naproxen synovial fluid levels are lower than those in simultaneous specimens of plasma.[109]

Efficacy of naproxen has been demonstrated in rheumatoid arthritis, osteoarthritis, ankylosing spondylitis, tendinitis, bursitis, and acute gout. It is also effective in juvenile rheumatoid arthritis and primary dysmenorrhea, and its sodium salt (Anaprox) has been marketed as an analgesic and for the treatment of dysmenorrhea.[110] The usual starting dose of naproxen is 250 mg to 500 mg every 12 hours with meals, but doses as high as 1500 mg daily have been used in rheumatoid arthritis without apparent increase in toxicity. Clinical efficacy has been demonstrated to correlate with plasma naproxen concentrations in one study.[111] Of patients, 76 percent responded when serum naproxen concentrations were greater than 50 µg/ml, whereas no patients responded to concentrations less than 18 µg/ml, when specimens were taken just before the next dose.

The adverse effects of naproxen are typical of those already described for NSAIDs. They occur less frequently than with aspirin or indomethacin, but essentially all of the class-related adverse effects have been observed with this drug. Gastric irritation is more likely to occur with higher doses.[106]

Aspirin decreases naproxen serum concentrations, probably as a result of its displacement from

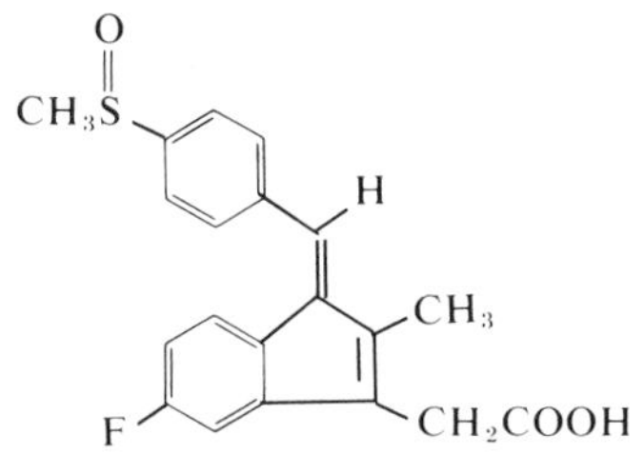

Figure 43–5. Chemical structure of sulindac.

protein-binding sites by aspirin.[106] Probenecid, 500 mg four times a day, increased the plasma half-life of a single 500-mg naproxen dose from 14 hours to 37 hours and increased steady-state naproxen concentrations by 50 percent. It decreased naproxen plasma clearance both by inhibiting naproxen glucuronide formation and by decreasing renal clearance of naproxen.[112]

Concurrent administration of naproxen, 500 mg daily, plus aspirin, 3.25 g daily, was more effective than aspirin alone in rheumatoid arthritis in one study,[113] but in another study, the efficacy of naproxen, 1500 mg daily, was not increased by adding nonacetylated salicylate in a dose sufficient to produce average plasma salicylate concentrations of 23.5 mg/dl.[114] Indeed, naproxen, 1500 mg daily, was marginally more effective and was less toxic than this high dose of salicylate.

Sulindac

Sulindac is an indene-acetic acid derivative chemically related to indomethacin and is a prodrug (Fig. 43–5).[115] The minimally active parent drug sulindac, a sulfoxide, is reversibly metabolized to sulindac sulfide, a potent cyclo-oxygenase inhibitor with a half-life of 16 to 18 hours. Sulindac is also irreversibly metabolized to the inactive sulfone metabolite. Sulindac and its metabolites undergo extensive enterohepatic recirculation.[116, 117] Twenty-five to 30 percent of the dose is excreted in the stool, primarily as the sulfone and sulfide metabolites. About 50 percent of the administered dose is excreted in the urine, almost entirely as the sulfone, sulfoxide, and sulindac glucuronide.[116] Less than 1 percent is excreted in the urine as the active sulindac sulfide. The long half-life for the biologic activity of this drug is attributed to its enterohepatic recirculation and the reversible interconversion between the active sulfide and the parent sulfoxide. However, substantial interindividual differences have been noted in drug disposition, plasma concentrations, and areas under the plasma concentration-time curves in subjects given sulindac.[118]

The adverse effects profile of sulindac is also thought to be influenced by the interrelationship of the inactive prodrug and its active metabolite. Compared with other NSAIDs, sulindac demonstrates a relatively low incidence of gastric abnormalities in gastroscopic studies, presumably because of the lack of local cyclo-oxygenase suppression by the prodrug in the stomach.[57] Animal studies demonstrate that gastrointestinal toxicity is proportional to the amount of sulindac sulfide in the gastrointestinal tract.[119] If none of the active metabolites were present in the gut, gastrointestinal toxicity should be low. Unfortunately, as already indicated, significant amounts of sulfide are present in the stool, and in clinical use sulindac has exhibited the usual range of gastrointestinal toxicities including ulcers, bleeding, and diarrhea.

Similarly, absence of the active metabolite in the urine owing to its conversion to sulfoxide by the kidney has been proposed as a mechanism to prevent acute renal toxicity mediated by cyclo-oxygenase inhibition. This is fully discussed in the earlier section on renal side effects of NSAIDs, but one cannot be sanguine in using sulindac in predisposed patients because acute renal toxicity has been observed in some patients taking sulindac, despite its theoretical advantages.[81]

Dimethyl sulfoxide (DMSO) decreases plasma levels of sulindac sulfide and in addition has been reported to cause peripheral neuropathy and should not be used with sulindac. Salicylate and diflunisal decrease plasma levels of sulindac sulfide, and their concurrent use is not advised.[117] Clinically significant interactions do not seem to occur between sulindac and tolbutamide, warfarin, probenecid, propoxyphene, or acetaminophen.

Sulindac's clinical efficacy profile is similar to that of other NSAIDs. The maximum recommended dose is 200 mg twice daily.

Diflunisal

Difluorophenyl salicylic acid, diflunisal, differs from most other salicylic acid derivatives in that it is not metabolized to salicylate (Fig. 43–6). It lacks an acetyl group, but it is more potent than aspirin in small animal studies of its analgesic, anti-inflammatory, and antipyretic activities.[120] Diflunisal resembles aspirin more than salicylate in the potency of its inhibition of cyclo-oxygenase, but lacking the acetyl group, this inhibition is reversible with diflunisal. Nevertheless, pretreatment with diflunisal can prevent the acetylation of cyclo-oxygenase by aspirin. Although aspirin irreversibly acetylates cyclooxygenase and salicylate does not inhibit this enzyme at all in moderate concentrations, diflunisal reversibly

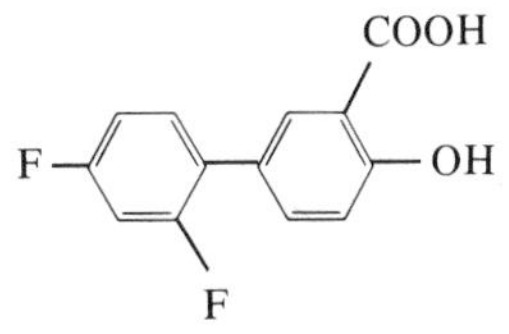

Figure 43–6. Chemical structure of diflunisal.

inhibits it, as do indomethacin and most other NSAIDs. It is 99 percent bound to albumin at moderate concentrations of drug but is displaced during renal failure when the unbound fraction may increase by as much as 370 percent.[121]

Similar to other salicylic acid derivatives, the pharmacokinetics of diflunisal are concentration-dependent. Thus, the plasma half-life following 125 mg of diflunisal twice daily is 7 or 8 hours, but it increases to 15 hours after 500 mg twice daily. Steady-state plasma levels are achieved after 3 to 9 days and increase disproportionately as the dose is increased. Ninety-five percent of ingested drug is excreted in the urine as glucuronide metabolites.[121]

Diflunisal may prolong the prothrombin time in patients taking oral anticoagulants but does not interact with tolbutamide. Pharmacokinetic interactions occur with hydrochlorothiazide, acetaminophen, aspirin, sulindac, naproxen, and indomethacin, but the clinical significance of these interactions is uncertain.[121] Coadministration of diflunisal and indomethacin has been associated with fatal gastrointestinal hemorrhage, and this combination should be avoided.[122] In patients with severe renal failure, total body clearance and protein binding of diflunisal were decreased, and its plasma half-life was markedly increased.[123]

Diflunisal is useful for the full range of NSAID indications. Similarly, the full range of NSAID adverse effects has been observed with it. Because of the dose-related disproportionate increases in plasma concentrations and plasma half-lives and the decrease in clearance associated with renal insufficiency, particular care must be taken in increasing the dose beyond the recommended maximum of 1000 mg daily, and doses should be decreased in patients with renal insufficiency.

Piroxicam

Piroxicam is a member of the oxicam family of enolic acids (Fig. 43–7). It is marketed worldwide and was first introduced in the United States in 1982. It is a potent inhibitor of cyclo-oxygenase but has no effect on lipoxygenase.[124] Its pharmacologic activity is similar to that of other cyclo-oxygenase inhibitors, but it may be a more effective inhibitor of superoxide generation in vitro by stimulated neutrophils.[125]

Piroxicam is slowly cleared from plasma by metabolism, with an average plasma half-life of about 38 hours and a wide range of 14 to 158 hours.[126] Steady-state plasma levels occur after 1 to 3 weeks of once daily dosage, depending on the half-life within the individual patient, and are two to four times higher than the peak levels after the first dose. Piroxicam is metabolized to at least seven inactive metabolites that are excreted in both urine and stool. It appears in breast milk at 1 to 3 percent of the maternal plasma concentration.[127] In rheumatoid arthritis, synovial fluid concentrations are lower than those in plasma, but the elimination half-life is the same.[128] Piroxicam levels are not elevated in patients with renal insufficiency, probably because it is cleared primarily by hepatic metabolism. Indeed, one study reported that the elimination half-life of piroxicam was decreased in patients with renal insufficiency.[129] The effect of cirrhosis on piroxicam metabolism has not been reported, but it might be expected to increase its half-life. The coadministration of aspirin has been reported to reduce piroxicam plasma levels by about 20 percent, whereas cimetidine increases plasma piroxicam levels and half-life.[130, 131] In view of the serious toxicity encountered in some elderly patients with benoxaprofen, there has been concern about possible piroxicam accumulation in elderly patients. One single-dose study of healthy subjects projected that steady-state plasma levels and half-lives of piroxicam would be greater in elderly women as compared with young women, but that there would be no difference in these measures between young and elderly men,[102] but other studies failed to demonstrate these projected differences.[93, 132]

The toxicity of piroxicam is similar to that of other NSAIDs, as confirmed by an intensive review of the entire worldwide experience with the drug in over 75,000 patients[133] and further review by the United States Food and Drug Administration. Peptic ulceration, however, is considerably more common with daily doses in excess of 20 mg, and this dose generally should not be exceeded.

Piroxicam has been approved for use in rheumatoid arthritis and osteoarthritis. Published studies also suggest that it is effective in gout, ankylosing spondylitis, acute musculoskeletal disorders, and sports injuries.[130]

Nabumetone

Nabumetone is a 2,6-disubstituted naphthylalkanone that is not acidic and is a poor inhibitor of prostaglandin synthesis. After absorption, it is rapidly metabolized in the liver to an acidic metabolite that is a potent inhibitor of prostaglandin synthesis. The active metabolite has a plasma half-life of about 21 hours, increasing to 29 hours in the elderly and to 39 hours in patients with creatinine clearance less than 30 ml per minute. It is eliminated both by direct urinary excretion and by metabolism to inactive metabolites. In animal studies, nabumetone induced less gastric damage than aspirin or comparison NSAIDs, and human studies of quantitative gastroin-

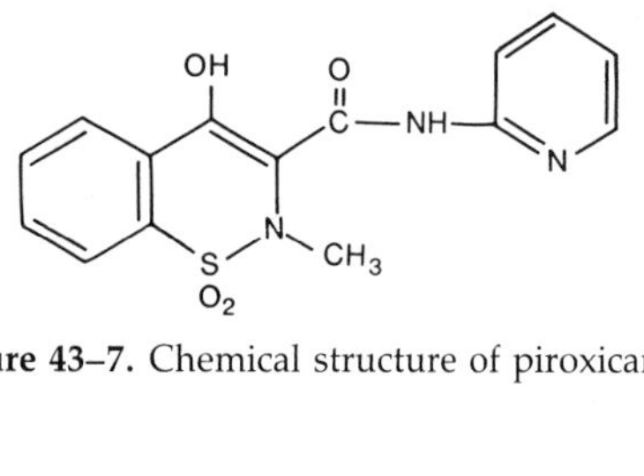

Figure 43–7. Chemical structure of piroxicam.

testinal blood loss as well as endoscopic studies suggest that it is less gastrotoxic than naproxen or aspirin. Nevertheless, peptic ulcers and gastrointestinal bleeding have been noted during long-term clinical trials, although perhaps less frequently than might have been anticipated with aspirin or some other NSAIDs. With doses of 1000 mg once daily at bedtime, anti-inflammatory efficacy has been demonstrated in patients with rheumatoid arthritis and osteoarthritis.[139]

Other NSAIDs with a Long Half-Life

Several NSAIDs with plasma half-lives long enough to justify once or twice daily dosage have not yet been approved for use or are not being marketed in the United States.

Azapropazone

Azapropazone is a pyrazolidine derivative similar to phenylbutazone but may not share its bone marrow toxicity. It is very highly bound to albumin, but this binding decreases in renal failure and severe liver disease (Fig. 43–8).[134] It is principally excreted in the urine, and elderly patients with a mean creatinine clearance of 36 ml per minute had a prolonged plasma half-life of 31 hours, mandating the use of lower doses in these patients.[135] Azapropazone appears to impair the plasma clearance of tolbutamide, warfarin, and phenytoin.[38] It has been used in doses of 900 to 1800 mg daily in the treatment of rheumatoid arthritis, osteoarthritis, psoriatic arthritis, Reiter's disease, ankylosing spondylitis, and gout.[38] It has been reported to decrease serum uric acid as effectively as allopurinol, but there were more frequent clinical and laboratory adverse effects with azapropazone, particularly upper gastrointestinal symptoms, decreases in renal function, and skin rashes.[136]

Fenbufen

Fenbufen is a phenylalkanoic acid derivative that is inactive as a prostaglandin synthetase inhibitor. Its active metabolite 4-biphenylacetic acid inhibits prostaglandin synthetase and has a much longer half-life, permitting twice-daily administration. Peak concentrations of the active metabolite are delayed until 6 to 8 hours after ingestion. The drug is excreted in both urine and stool, primarily as conjugates.[137] A second metabolite, a hydroxybiphenylbutanoic acid, is also reported to be active in animal models of inflammation, although it does not inhibit prostaglandin synthesis.[137] There are only minimal serum protein displacement interactions between fenbufen and warfarin or digoxin.[137] Fenbufen, 300 mg twice daily, is more effective than 600 mg once daily in rheumatoid arthritis. Doses of 600 mg to 1000 mg daily are reported to be effective in rheumatoid arthritis, osteoarthritis, and gout.[137] The adverse effects profile is similar to that with other NSAIDs.

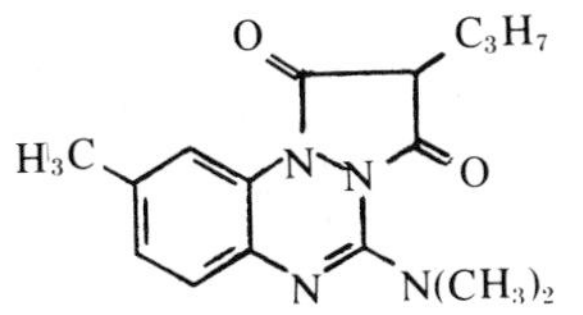

Carprofen

Carprofen is a carbazole acetic acid derivative with a terminal half-life of 12 hours (range, 6 to 27 hours).[138] It has been approved by the Food and Drug Administration but has not been marketed as yet. A reversible inhibitor of cyclo-oxygenase in vitro, it is active in standard animal models of induced inflammation. Between 50 and 80 percent is excreted in the urine, primarily as a glucuronide ester, but 15 to 25 percent is excreted in the feces, mostly as unmetabolized carprofen. Thus, enterohepatic recirculation appears to occur in humans. Carprofen concentrations in synovial fluid range from 36 to 103 percent of those in serum. The serum half-life of carprofen in the elderly was reduced to 9.4 hours as compared with 15.7 hours in younger individuals.[138] In doses of 150 mg twice daily or 100 mg two or three times daily, carprofen has been effective in rheumatoid arthritis and osteoarthritis. For gout, initial doses as high as 600 mg daily have been used.[138]

Proquazone

Proquazone is a quinazolinone but differs from other NSAIDs in that it is not acidic. Its elimination half-life is about 14 hours, and it has three pharmacologically active metabolites. Its absorption is enhanced and its bioavailability is doubled when given with food. Even though it is not an acid, it increases occult blood loss in the stool as much as aspirin does, and gastrointestinal toxicity was fairly prominent in clinical studies.[38]

Colchicine

Colchicine is absorbed fairly readily from the gastrointestinal tract, reaching an average peak plasma level of 0.32 μg per 100 ml ½ hour to 2 hours after a single 1-mg dose by mouth.[140] After intravenous administration, colchicine leaves the blood rapidly with a half-life of less than 20 minutes, owing to rapid distribution from the plasma into cells. Peripheral blood leukocytes are known to accumulate colchicine but may not be the only tissue in which the drug is concentrated. Mean white blood cell concentration reached a peak of 43 μg per 100 ml, 10 minutes after intravenous administration of 3 mg of colchicine to healthy volunteers; a plateau between

Figure 43–8. Chemical structure of azapropazone.

18 and 23 μg per 100 ml was maintained during the interval from 1/2 hour to 24 hours after administration. Seventy-two hours after the infusion of drug, the mean white blood cell concentration was 11 μg per 100 ml, and measurable concentrations were still present in leukocytes 10 days later.[141] Thus, the elimination half-life from peripheral blood leukocytes, a probable site of drug effect, is prolonged, easily permitting once-daily administration of maintenance doses of colchicine. In a study of four patients with familial Mediterranean fever given 1 mg intravenously, the mean elimination half-life from serum was 157 minutes, compared with 65 minutes in six normal subjects. Eight patients receiving 1 mg of colchicine daily orally had serum concentrations of 0.3 to 2.4 ng per ml. One patient with a poor clinical response, however, had undetectable serum levels after 2 mg daily, suggesting that lack of response may result from inadequate absorption or altered disposition of colchicine.[142] In another study of 13 patients with polyserositis receiving long-term colchicine therapy, plasma concentrations ranged from 0.8 to 7.8 ng per ml.[143]

Colchicine is excreted in the bile, feces, and urine. There is no evidence that colchicine is metabolized to any significant extent. The use of colchicine is well established in gout, pseudogout, and familial Mediterranean fever, but it also has been evaluated in Behçet's disease, amyloidosis, cutaneous necrotizing vasculitis, acute febrile neutrophilic dermatosis (Sweet's syndrome), and skin manifestations of scleroderma.[28] Its toxicity has been discussed earlier in this chapter.

NSAIDs with a Short Half-Life

This group of NSAIDs generally have a half-life of 6 hours or less in patients and are given three or four times daily (Table 43–5). Steady state is reached within 24 to 36 hours after starting the drug but is characterized by marked fluctuations in plasma levels between peak postabsorption levels and trough levels at the time of the next dosage. Peak synovial fluid concentrations are substantially lower than peak plasma concentrations, and the half-life for disappearance from synovial fluid is usually longer than the initial half-life for disappearance from plasma, suggesting that the half-life for biologic effects may be substantially longer than the short plasma half-life. Both synovial fluid and plasma concentrations are quite low during this late phase of delayed resorption of drug from synovial fluid and tissue stores into plasma, from which it is then excreted (see Fig. 43–10). Some of these short half-life drugs have been marketed in delayed-release formulations to make them more convenient for patients to use.

Indomethacin

Indomethacin is the prototype of the short half-life NSAIDs that are potent inhibitors of cyclo-oxy-

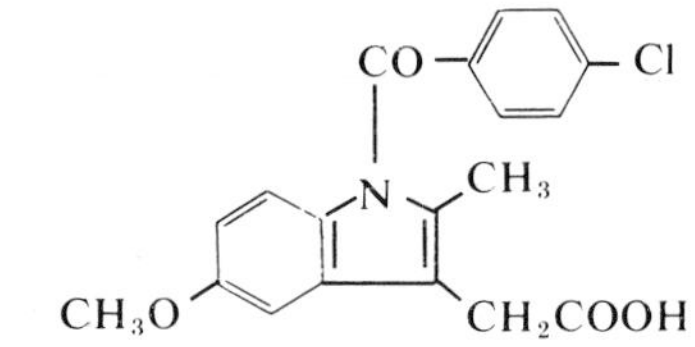

Figure 43–9. Chemical structure of indomethacin.

genase (Fig. 43–9). It is an indoleacetic acid, chemically related to sulindac. Indomethacin was identified by its effectiveness in suppressing the induction of edema when carrageenan was injected into rat paws.[144] It was marketed in the United States in 1965 and was noted by Vane to be an extremely potent inhibitor of prostaglandin synthesis when he made the original observations that the inhibition of prostaglandin synthesis was an important mechanism of action of NSAIDs.[19]

Both the standard and the sustained-release formulations of indomethacin are well absorbed.[145] Food or antacid somewhat delays absorption but does not decrease overall bioavailability. Indomethacin crosses the placenta, with equilibrium between mother and fetus reached within 5 hours.[146] Its plasma half-life is biexponential; the initial half-life includes distribution into tissue compartments and is 1 to 2 hours in duration, whereas the terminal half-life is about 13 hours.[147] Synovial fluid indomethacin concentrations show a delayed rise and lower peak compared with plasma levels, but they then remain equal to or higher than serum levels for at least 9 hours after a dose (Fig. 43–10).[148] Indomethacin is highly metabolized to compounds that lack anti-inflammatory activity. Most of an oral indomethacin dose is excreted as metabolites.[149] Indomethacin has an extensive enterohepatic recirculation; it is estimated that more than 43 percent of a dose is excreted in the bile.[150] The plasma half-life is prolonged in infants; in one study, the half-life in mothers was 2.2 hours, whereas it was 14.7 hours in their newborn infants.[151] The half-life in elderly men, however, was no different than that in younger men.[152]

Aspirin decreases indomethacin absorption, decreases its renal clearance, and increases its biliary clearance; the net effect is a slight decrease in indomethacin bioavailability when it is administered during long-term aspirin therapy.[153] In rheumatoid arthritis, however, the efficacy of indomethacin alone is not detectably different from the efficacy of the same dose of indomethacin combined with therapeutic doses of aspirin.[154] Indomethacin may prevent the acetylation of platelet cyclo-oxygenase by aspirin.[155] Probenecid appears to decrease indomethacin biliary clearance and increases bioavailability by 63 percent;[156] when given with indomethacin, clinical improvement was also noted.[157]

As a lead compound, indomethacin has been used for all of the rheumatologic and nonrheumatologic indications for NSAIDs. In those patients who

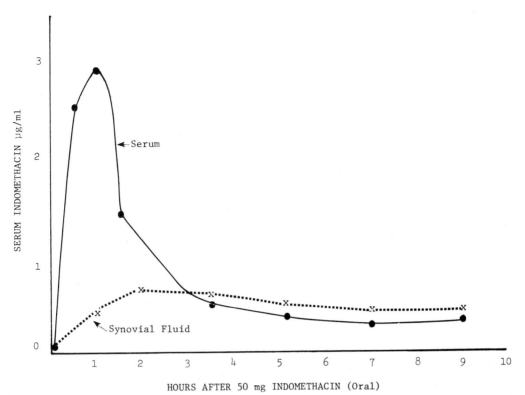

Figure 43–10. Serum and synovial fluid indomethacin concentrations in a patient, following a single 50-mg oral dose. Following equilibration, synovial fluid concentrations slightly exceed those in serum, a typical finding with short half-life NSAIDs.

tolerate it, it is generally quite effective, but upper gastrointestinal symptoms and headaches prompt discontinuation of therapy in a substantial number of patients. The 75-mg, sustained-release indomethacin capsule is designed to deliver 25 mg of drug immediately and the remaining 50 mg over the next 8 to 12 hours. Rectal suppositories, oral suspension, and intravenous preparations of indomethacin are also available.

Ibuprofen

Ibuprofen is an arylpropionic acid that is present predominantly in the ionized form at physiologic pH (Fig. 43–11). Ibuprofen as well as fenoprofen and ketoprofen has an asymmetric carbon and exists as R(−) and S(+) optical isomers. The marketed preparations of these drugs are racemic mixtures consisting of equal parts of both isomers. The S(+) isomer of ibuprofen is much more active than the R(−) isomer as an inhibitor of cyclo-oxygenase in vitro. In vivo, however, the less potent R(−) isomer is converted to the S(+) isomer; consequently it is difficult to detect differences in the pharmacologic activity of

the two isomers in whole animal studies.[158] It is more than 98 percent bound to plasma proteins, but protein-binding capacity may be exceeded with higher doses; this was noted in one study when doses exceeded 850 mg.[159] Thus, there may be disproportionate increases in biologically active unbound ibuprofen as doses increase in size. Concentrations of unbound ibuprofen are approximately equal in serum and synovial fluid; synovial fluid concentrations fluctuate less than those in plasma, and the drug is detectable for long periods of time in the synovial fluid.[160] The half-life of the active S(+) isomer is longer than the R(−) isomer, and thus a longer duration of action is possible than would be predicted by measurement of total plasma concentrations only.[161]

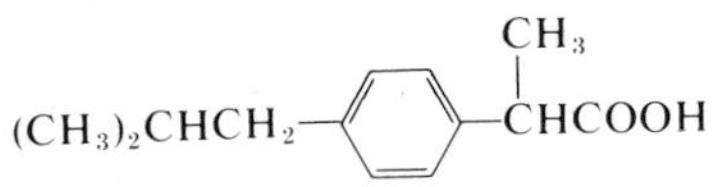

Ibuprofen is extensively metabolized to inactive metabolites. Enterohepatic recirculation is probably not significant in humans. Ibuprofen kinetics are not significantly different in elderly as compared with younger individuals,[162] and even severe hepatic disease with cirrhosis and ascites did not alter ibuprofen kinetics.[159]

Doses of 3600 to 4800 mg per day of ibuprofen increased the fraction of unbound warfarin by 10 to 30 percent, although lower doses do not alter warfarin-induced hypoprothrombinemia.[163] Probenecid does not increase plasma concentrations of ibuprofen, which is largely metabolized by oxidation, and ibuprofen does not interfere with the uricosuria induced by probenecid.[164] Ibuprofen appears to protect

$$(CH_3)_2CHCH_2-\overset{\displaystyle CH_3}{\underset{\displaystyle CHCOOH}{\bigcirc}}$$

Figure 43–11. Chemical structure of ibuprofen.

platelet cyclo-oxygenase from the irreversible effects of aspirin, presumably by a mechanism similar to that seen with indomethacin.[165]

Ibuprofen has been associated with all of the generic adverse effects reported with NSAIDs. It predominates in the small number of reports of NSAID-associated aseptic meningitis.[166]

Ibuprofen has been used for all of the indications for NSAIDs. Doses of 400 to 1200 mg daily are primarily analgesic; doses for rheumatoid arthritis generally are from 2400 to 3600 mg daily, and doses as high as 4800 mg daily have been used for the initial treatment of acute gout.[166]

Because of its greater margin of safety as compared with aspirin and acetaminophen, ibuprofen was approved for nonprescription sale to the general public. It is recommended for use as an analgesic and for symptomatic treatment of menstrual cramps, in 200-mg doses, with a maximum recommended daily dose of 1200 mg. As discussed earlier in this chapter, a number of cases of overdose of ibuprofen have been reported, but there have been very few deaths. Prospective follow-up of 43 women who were exposed to ibuprofen during pregnancy did not reveal any fetal abnormalities at the time of delivery, but retrospective reports include one case each of anencephaly, convulsions, cerebral palsy, and microphthalmia.[167]

Fenoprofen

Fenoprofen is also a substituted arylpropionic acid whose $S(+)$ enantiomer is much more active than the $R(-)$ optical isomer as an in vitro inhibitor of cyclo-oxygenase from human platelets (Fig. 43–12). In vivo, the $R(-)$ enantiomer is stereoselectively converted to the $S(+)$ isomer.[168] The marketed drug is a racemic mixture of the two isomers. Although its absorption has been reported to be reduced 30 percent by food, its total absorption is changed.[169] Both fenoprofen and its inactive metabolite hydroxy-fenoprofen are excreted in the urine as glucuronides. Its kinetics are not significantly different in elderly as compared with younger patients.[170] Fenoprofen slightly decreases warfarin protein binding.[171]

Fenoprofen is recommended in rheumatoid arthritis and osteoarthritis in doses of 300 to 600 mg three or four times a day. Aspirin and fenoprofen (900 to 1800 mg per m[2] per day) were equally effective in a 3-month study of children with juvenile rheumatoid arthritis.[172] It also has been used in ankylosing spondylitis and gout and as an analgesic.[166] Its adverse effects are spondylitis and gout and as an analgesic.[166] Its adverse effects are typical of drugs in

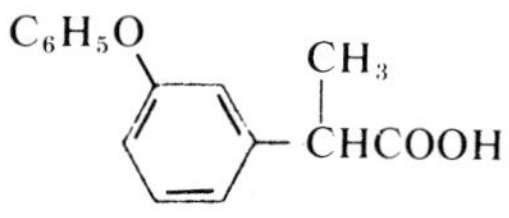

Figure 43–12. Chemical structure of fenoprofen.

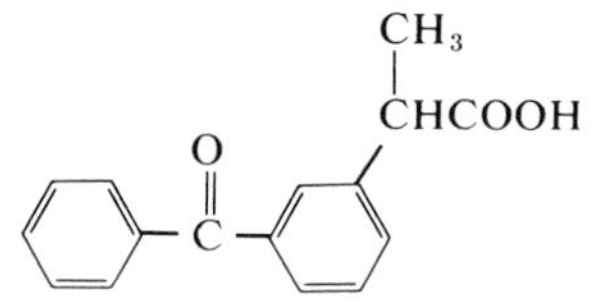

Figure 43–13. Chemical structure of ketoprofen.

its class except that idiosyncratic nephropathy has been seen more frequently with fenoprofen than with any of the other NSAIDs.[173] Days to months following the initiation of fenoprofen therapy, patients may present with renal insufficiency, edema, and either nephrotic-range proteinuria or oliguria. Both the renal failure and the proteinuria resolve following discontinuation of the NSAID, but steroid therapy may be necessary.[166] Renal biopsies have shown T lymphocyte infiltration in the renal interstitium and foot process fusion.[174] Eosinophilia is sometimes seen as part of this syndrome, and patients who have had allergic reactions to nonsteroidal drugs should be given fenoprofen only under very close observation.

Ketoprofen

Ketoprofen is another arylpropionic acid that was developed about the same time as ibuprofen and fenoprofen (Fig. 43–13). It has been used extensively in Europe since 1973 and was marketed in the United States in 1986. Although its plasma half-life is ½ to 2 hours, during long-term therapy, ketoprofen-induced inhibition of platelet aggregation does not return to normal until 36 hours after the last dose, suggesting that the elimination half-life of ketoprofen from platelets (and perhaps other tissue sites of action) may be more on the order of 6 or 7 hours.[175] Consistent with this observation, the plasma disappearance curve of ketoprofen is multiexponential, with a slower terminal phase of elimination;[176] also, ketoprofen readily enters the synovial fluid, and synovial fluid PGE_2 concentrations remain decreased for at least 24 hours after a 100-mg dose of drug.[177] Thus, administration every 6 or 8 hours appears to be reasonable on a pharmacodynamic basis.

Both ketoprofen and its hydroxylated metabolite are extensively conjugated and excreted in the urine. Although ketoprofen is excreted in the bile, essentially all is reabsorbed, and very little drug is present in the feces.[177] Initial doses of ketoprofen should be decreased in the elderly and in patients with renal failure because of decreased clearance in both situations.[178, 179] Staffanger et al.[179] found a direct correlation between creatinine clearance and ketoprofen clearance.

A number of potential drug interactions with ketoprofen have been evaluated. Two grams of probenecid daily decreased ketoprofen protein binding by 28 percent, total ketoprofen clearance by 67 percent, renal clearance of ketoprofen conjugates by 93 percent, and clearance of unbound ketoprofen by 74 percent, resulting in increased concentrations of both free and protein-bound ketoprofen in plasma.[180] Ketoprofen plasma concentrations decrease when aspirin is added to the treatment regimen; the protein binding of ketoprofen decreases, and plasma clearance increases.[181] Ketoprofen may increase plasma methotrexate concentrations with high doses of methotrexate,[182] but similar observations have not been noted with low doses of methotrexate. No interactions were noted in studies with digoxin, oral hypoglycemics, gold salts, antimalarials, or glucocorticoids.[177] Ketoprofen decreases hydrochlorothiazide-induced excretion of potassium and chloride but did not alter the diuretic or antihypertensive effects of this drug.[177]

Ketoprofen is usually used in doses of 100 to 300 mg daily and is effective in the treatment of rheumatoid arthritis, osteoarthritis, ankylosing spondylitis, and acute gout; it has also been used in juvenile arthritis.[166] The most prominent adverse effects are upper gastrointestinal toxicity, but these and other adverse effects are similar to those of other NSAIDs.

Tolmetin

Tolmetin is a pyrrole acetic acid derivative with the pharmacologic characteristics of the NSAID inhibitors of prostaglandin biosynthesis (Fig. 43–14). It has a biphasic elimination half-life from plasma; the half-life of the initial phase is about 2 hours, and the half-life of the terminal phase has been estimated to range from 2 hours to 6.8 hours.[183] Tolmetin enters the synovial fluid and is associated with depressed concentrations of PGE_2 for at least 24 hours after a dose.[184] A small amount of unchanged tolmetin is excreted in the urine, but the majority of the drug is excreted as the dicarboxylic acid metabolite or as glucuronide conjugates of tolmetin and its metabolite; the metabolites are inactive.[185] There does not appear to be any enterohepatic recirculation of tolmetin. No clinically significant interactions have been reported with warfarin, phenprocoumon, oral hypoglycemic agents, or aspirin.[186] There is no accumulation of tolmetin during long-term administration on a four times a day schedule.[183] Doses of 600 to 2000 mg daily, in three or four divided doses, are effective in rheumatoid arthritis, osteoarthritis, and ankylosing spondylitis.[186] Tolmetin has been approved by the Food and Drug Administration for use in juvenile rheumatoid arthritis; the recommended starting dose for children age 2 years and older is 20 mg per kg per day; doses larger than 30 mg per kg per day are not recommended.[186]

Gastrointestinal side effects are the most com-

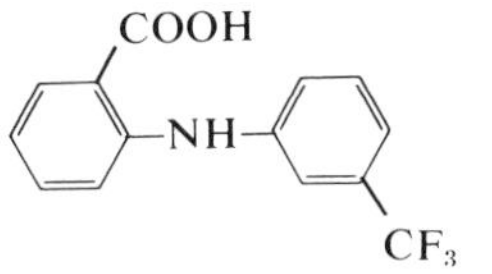

Figure 43–15. Chemical structure of flufenamic acid.

mon adverse reaction and are slightly more common in elderly patients.[187] Anaphylaxis similar to that seen with zomepirac has been reported with tolmetin, and care should be exercised when the drug is reinstituted after a hiatus in treatment.[188] Of interest, *pseudoproteinuria* is seen if sulfasalicylic acid or other acid is used as a test for urine protein. A cloudy precipitate of tolmetin and its metabolites in the acid solution causes the appearance of marked proteinuria, but tests that do not rely on acid precipitation remain negative.

Tolmetin is particularly useful in the presurgical management of patients who require an NSAID because it is almost completely excreted within 24 hours after a dose. Therefore, discontinuation of tolmetin 36 hours before surgery will avoid increased bleeding owing to inhibition of platelet cyclo-oxygenase.

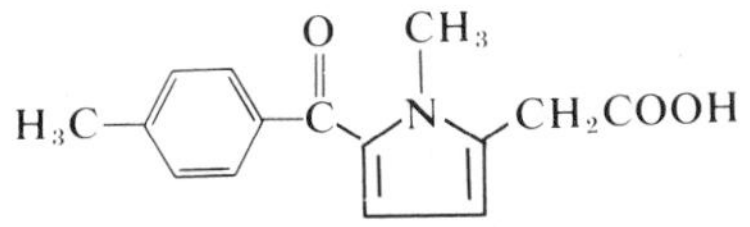

Meclofenamate Sodium and Other Fenamates

The fenamates are substituted n-phenyl anthranilic acids that were found to have anti-inflammatory activity in animal studies in the late 1950s and early 1960s.[189] Flufenamic acid (Fig. 43–15) and mefenamic acid (Fig. 43–16) have been marketed since then but have been used primarily as analgesics and for treatment of dysmenorrhea. They have not been popular for long-term therapy owing to their associations with dose-related intestinal cramping and diarrhea in up to 25 percent of patients and with rashes in up to 16 percent. Ten to 20 percent of mefenamic acid and 36 percent of flufenamic acid are excreted in feces. Overdoses of mefenamic acid may be associated with grand mal seizures. Flufenamic acid, 300 to 600 mg daily, is given in three divided doses for rheumatoid arthritis, osteoarthritis, or ankylosing spondylitis. For primary dysmenorrhea, 500 mg initially of mefenamic acid is followed by 250 mg every 6 hours.[189]

The sodium salt of meclofenamic acid has been marketed in the United States since 1982. Of interest, meclofenamate is an in vitro inhibitor of both 5-lipoxygenase and cyclo-oxygenase pathways of arachidonic acid metabolism in human neutrophils,[190]

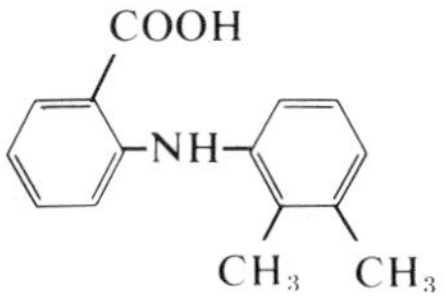

Figure 43–14. Chemical structure of tolmetin.

Figure 43–16. Chemical structure of mefenamic acid.

but the clinical significance of this observation is uncertain. In addition, the major metabolite in humans has anti-inflammatory activity, although it is less active than the parent compound. After multiple dosing, the mean half-life of unchanged drug in plasma is about 3 hours, but the half-life of the metabolites is about 24 hours.[191] About 25 percent of radioactivity associated with the drug was recovered from stool in a balance study in humans.[191] The remainder was excreted in the urine, primarily as glucuronides of the five major metabolites. Meclofenamic acid increases the prothrombin time in patients receiving warfarin.[192] Addition of aspirin increases gastrointestinal blood loss to nearly three times that seen with either drug alone.[192] No interactions were noted with propoxyphene or sulfinpyrazone.[192]

Meclofenamate sodium is used for treatment of rheumatoid arthritis, osteoarthritis, gout, and ankylosing spondylitis. Fifty-milligram and 100-mg capsules are available and are usually given in three or four divided doses, totaling 200 to 400 mg daily. Similar to the other fenamates, meclofenamate sodium causes diarrhea. This is thought to be due to the inherent laxative properties of the drug, which is a secretagogue.[189] In long-term studies, diarrhea occurred in about 15 percent of patients but required drug discontinuation in only 7 percent.[193] The occurrence of rashes with meclofenamate sodium was not as frequent as with other fenamates.[193] Other adverse effects are those expected with NSAIDs.

Diclofenac. Diclofenac is another member of the fenamate family of phenylacetic acid derivatives (Fig. 43–17). It is a potent inhibitor of platelet aggregation induced by collagen in vitro, but in doses of 75 to 100 mg daily in humans, there is no effect on platelet count, platelet adhesiveness, platelet aggregation, or activated prothrombin time.[194] It suppresses prostaglandin synthesis in vitro and in vivo and also decreases the production of leukotrienes by stimulating the uptake of arachidonic acid into triglycerides, thus inhibiting the release of intracellular arachidonic acid, although it appears to have no effect on lipoxygenase itself.[22] Diclofenac is marketed as an enteric-coated tablet, which somewhat delays its absorption. It is metabolized to an inactive metabolite that is excreted in both urine and bile.[194] Renal dysfunction does not influence the plasma levels of diclofenac significantly because it is cleared from plasma primarily by metabolism. It does not accumulate during long-term use and does not displace oral anticoagulants or hypoglycemic agents.[195] Suppression of PGE_2 in synovial fluid persists for 8 to 12 hours after a dose.[195] There is no significant

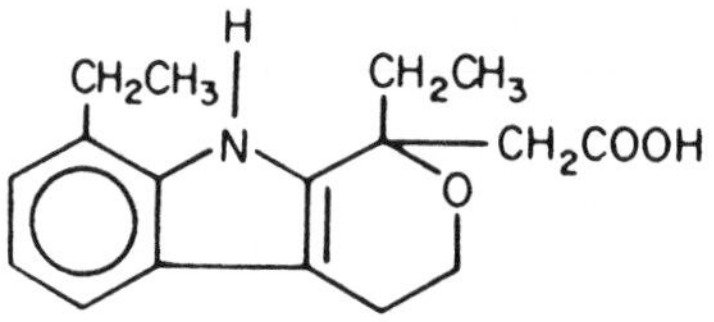

Figure 43–18. Chemical structure of etodolac.

difference in maximum plasma concentrations or overall urinary excretion in elderly as compared with younger subjects.[194]

Diclofenac in doses of 75 to 200 mg daily, divided into two to four doses, has been reported to be effective in rheumatoid arthritis, osteoarthritis, ankylosing spondylitis, gout, nonarticular rheumatism, and pain.[194] Its toxicity is generally similar to that of other NSAIDs, although monitoring of liver enzymes is recommended for several months after initiating treatment.

Etodolac. Etodolac, an indoleacetic acid, is one of a series of pyrano-carboxylic acids (Fig. 43–18). It inhibits cyclo-oxygenase but does not inhibit lipoxygenase.[196] It is extensively metabolized and excreted in both urine and bile. The kinetics of etodolac are unchanged in the elderly and apparently not significantly changed in renal impairment.[197] It has been approved by the Food and Drug Administration for treatment of osteoarthritis and pain.[197] Of interest, joint damage in rats with adjuvant arthritis has reversed after 28 days of etodolac administration, and the progression of radiographic changes in the hands and wrists of rheumatoid arthritis patients treated with etodolac for 1 year was significantly less than in patients treated with aspirin in a controlled multicenter trial.[198] This observation prompted a large, well-controlled, double-blind prospective study of radiographic changes during 3 years of treatment with etodolac or a comparison NSAID that is still awaiting analysis. At this point, the safety profile of etodolac is not readily distinguishable from that of other NSAIDs. The recommended dosage is 200 to 400 mg every 6 to 8 hours, not to exceed a total daily dose of 1200 mg.

Flurbiprofen. Flurbiprofen, a biphenylpropionic acid derivative, inhibits cyclo-oxygenase but not lipoxygenase and inhibits platelet aggregation in humans (Fig. 43–19). Flurbiprofen does not appear to interact with oral anticoagulants, sulfonamides, or phenytoin.[199] It is extensively metabolized, and more than 95 percent is excreted in urine as conjugates of the parent drug and its metabolites. About 5 percent of urinary excretion consists of unmetabolized flur-

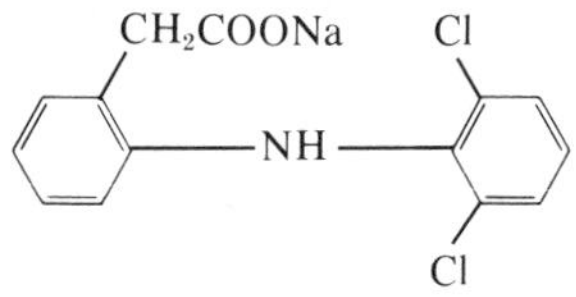

Figure 43–17. Chemical structure of diclofenac.

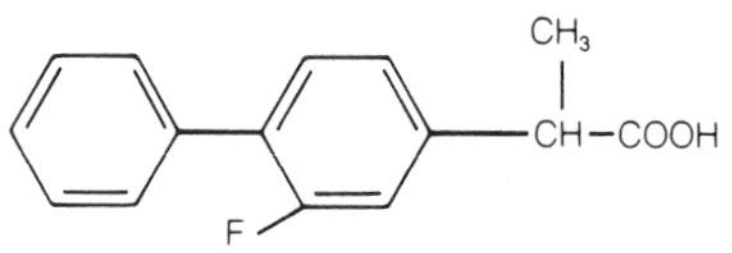

Figure 43–19. Chemical structure of flurbiprofen.

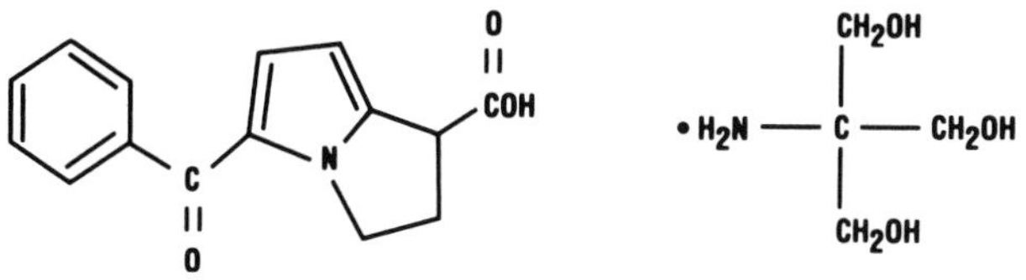

Figure 43–20. Chemical structure of ketorolac trimethamine.

biprofen. One of the metabolites has minimal anti-inflammatory activity.[200] Aspirin decreases plasma concentrations and decreases the half-life of flurbiprofen.[201]

Flurbiprofen has been found to be effective in the treatment of rheumatoid arthritis, osteoarthritis, ankylosing spondylitis, bursitis, and acute gout. The usual doses are 100 to 300 mg daily, divided into two to four doses. Acute gout is treated with 400 mg on the first day, followed by 200 mg daily. Symptoms of gastrointestinal irritation have been observed in 20 to 36 percent of patients in controlled clinical trials. Other adverse effects are those expected with this class of drugs.[199]

Ketorolac. Ketorolac trimethamine is a pyrrolo-pyrrole, an acidic NSAID that has been developed for the short-term management of pain (Fig. 43–20).[202] It inhibits cyclo-oxygenase–mediated prostaglandin production and exhibits anti-inflammatory, analgesic, and antipyretic activity in preclinical models. Pharmacodynamic and kinetic data are similar for oral and intramuscular administration with 100 percent bioavailability of the oral formulation. Peak plasma levels occur about 1 hour after intramuscular injection, and peak analgesic effect occurs 45 to 90 minutes later. It is more than 99 percent bound to plasma proteins at therapeutic concentrations and has a small volume of distribution. The terminal plasma half-life is 2 to 9 hours in young adults and 4 to 9 hours in elderly subjects. Ketorolac is 90 percent excreted in urine as unchanged drug and metabolite; thus, the plasma half-life in patients with renal impairment was approximately twice as long as in normals.[202]

In patients with postoperative pain following orthopedic, gynecologic, abdominal, or oral surgery, ketorolac, 10 mg intramuscularly, produced peak pain relief comparable to 50 mg of meperidine or 6 mg of morphine; 30 or 90 mg was comparable to 100 mg of meperidine or 12 mg of morphine, and the duration of effect was longer for ketorolac than for the narcotics.[203, 204] The maximum recommended intramuscular daily dose is 120 mg, divided into 6-hourly injections.[204] Pain management may begin with oral ketorolac, but it is usually begun with intramuscular, followed by oral. The maximum oral daily dose is 40 mg in four divided doses. Intramuscular therapy should be limited to no more than 5 days, oral for "limited duration." Other NSAID therapy should be withheld during ketorolac therapy. Ketorolac is not a narcotic and does not depress respiration or cause constipation. Adverse effects are

less frequent with short-term intramuscular ketorolac than with long-term oral administration of aspirin or other NSAIDs, but with long-term use for persistent painful conditions, the usual adverse reactions associated with NSAIDs may occur. Ketorolac causes reversible inhibition of platelet function.[202] Its use to treat acute episodes of inflammatory arthritis, such as gout, has not been evaluated.

BASIS FOR CLINICAL DIFFERENTIATION AMONG NONSTEROIDAL ANTIRHEUMATIC DRUGS

There is little evidence to suggest that one NSAID is clearly more efficacious than another. Although there is marked variation in the responses of individuals to different NSAIDs, at present there is no way to predict which NSAID will be most effective for an individual patient.[205] Combinations of NSAIDs probably are not more beneficial than single-drug therapy. Indeed, several studies have suggested either no change or a decrease in anti-inflammatory activity when a second NSAID was added,[114, 154, 206] toxicity may well be additive,[57] and costs are certain to be increased by the second drug. Because substantial individual variability is present with respect to the pharmacology and pharmacokinetics of these drugs, it is essential to adjust the dosage to the patient's response. This is especially important in the elderly, in whom age-related physiologic changes may further increase individual variability.[93]

One would anticipate that plasma drug concentrations would reflect efficacy and toxicity more accurately than dosage. This appears to be true in one study of naproxen[109] and was suggested in studies of carprofen in patients with rheumatoid arthritis[207] and indomethacin in juvenile rheumatoid arthritis[208] but has not been demonstrated with most NSAIDs.[209] Synovial fluid concentrations of NSAIDs fluctuate less than concurrent plasma concentrations[210] but have not been correlated with clinical efficacy or toxicity. Thus, at the present time, clinicians receive little help from either plasma or synovial fluid drug concentration measurements in determining the optimal dose of a NSAID to use in an individual patient.

When prescribing a nonsteroidal antirheumatic drug, consideration must be given to complicating illnesses and concurrent drug therapy. For example, if a patient has a history of peptic ulcer disease, one should use the lowest effective dose of NSAID and should give consideration to using a nonacetylated salicylate (which as a class has minimal prostaglandin-inhibiting activity) instead of a more potent cyclo-oxygenase inhibitor. Supplemental H_2 receptor antagonist, carafate, or misoprostil may be needed in some situations. In patients with persistent symptoms or ulcers, omeprazole may be used for up to 8 weeks. In addition, a drug with a short half-life is preferable to one that inhibits platelet aggregation for a prolonged time. If a patient is receiving warfarin or an oral hypoglycemic agent, the addition of an NSAID may require adjustment in its dose. In a patient with congestive heart failure, intrinsic renal disease, hepatic insufficiency, or dehydration, the potential for NSAID-induced fluid retention, electrolyte abnormalities, and renal insufficiency must be considered. Because it is impossible to know or to predict accurately the effects of every possible interaction, patients should be followed closely during the introduction of an NSAID, when doses are increased, or when the patient's condition changes. With appropriate care, the benefits of NSAIDs can be achieved even in the elderly, while avoiding irreversible serious toxicity, but inattentiveness can quickly lead to trouble.

Although there have been a number of studies published in which two or more NSAIDs have been compared, there still is no generally accepted rank order of the desirability of individual NSAIDs for particular patients. Most studies fail to show significant differences between drugs, and patient preferences vary from patient to patient and indeed often vary within the same patient from time to time. Nevertheless, available evidence and clinical experience have led to some therapeutic preferences.[211]

For rheumatoid arthritis patients who tolerate enteric-coated aspirin or a nonacetylated salicylate, plasma level–guided dosage is generally effective and relatively inexpensive. Many patients, however, are unable or unwilling to tolerate prolonged therapy with maximum salicylate dosage. When they reduce the dose to more tolerable levels, the anti-inflammatory effects decrease markedly, and better results can generally be achieved with full doses of a NSAID. In addition to having somewhat less toxicity than aspirin, patient compliance can be improved by using a once-daily or twice-daily dosage regimen with a longer half-life NSAID. If the initial dose is not sufficiently effective, it is usually better to increase the dose to the maximum permissible before trying the next drug. For specific situations, such as preoperatively, a short half-life NSAID may be preferred. Aspirin is generally effective in juvenile rheumatoid arthritis, but serum salicylate monitoring is advisable. Tolmetin, ibuprofen, and naproxen are also approved for juvenile rheumatoid arthritis, and other NSAIDs have been used by pediatric rheumatologists, although they have not been approved for this indication.

Because elderly osteoarthritis patients are more likely to experience serious adverse effects from aspirin and NSAIDs, the therapeutic approach differs from that used in rheumatoid arthritis. Generally, the lowest effective dose of a short half-life NSAID is used. If ineffective, it may be advisable to try a different NSAID before increasing to maximal doses of the first. Because osteoarthritis symptoms may fluctuate, it is advisable to try to stop the drug periodically to ascertain if the patient can get along without it. Sometimes treatment is needed only in the evening, to reduce aches and pains enough to permit a good night's sleep. When osteoarthritis is associated with acute episodes of joint inflammation, pseudogout should be considered. Even if intraarticular calcium crystals have not been documented, a trial of prophylactic colchicine, 0.6 mg twice daily, may be effective in suppressing and preventing recurrent episodes of polyarticular subacute pseudogout, and these low doses are unlikely to produce serious side effects.

Ankylosing spondylitis, Reiter's syndrome, and psoriatic arthritis are less likely to respond to salicylate than to indomethacin or to other NSAIDs. Phenylbutazone is no longer used for initial therapy of any condition but may be effective for spondyloarthropathies when all other NSAIDs have failed. High doses of a NSAID are usually preferred for the treatment of acute gout or pseudogout, although intravenous colchicine is also effective and well tolerated. High-dose oral colchicine is seldom used because it almost always causes diarrhea. After the acute attack subsides, maintenance prophylactic colchicine, 0.6 mg twice daily, is probably preferable to long-term maintenance with chronic NSAID therapy.

Most NSAIDs and salicylates are taken by healthy individuals for acute, usually self-limited musculoskeletal pain. Self-treatment with intermittent doses of aspirin or ibuprofen is used to alleviate discomfort while the condition resolves spontaneously. Similar self-treatment is fairly effective for menstrual cramps and is relatively safe in the low doses used.

Increasing understanding of the complex biochemical and cellular interactions involved in immunity and inflammation is providing many leads for the development of drugs to alter specifically certain portions of the process. These leads have not as yet been translated into useful new classes of antirheumatic therapeutic agents but may well lead to safer and more effective treatments for certain specifically defined inflammatory conditions in the not too distant future. If such drugs with drastically different mechanisms of action become available, it may then be logical to add one of these agents to one of the current cyclo-oxygenase inhibitors, just as gold or methotrexate is appropriately added at the present time.

I wish to thank my secretary, Marlene Rosensweig, for the excellent work she did on this chapter and her unflagging good humor, which she sustained even under great pressure.

References

1. Rodnan, G. P., and Benedek, T. G.: The early history of antirheumatic drugs. Arthritis Rheum. 13:145, 1970.
2. Dudley-Hart, F., and Huskisson, E. C.: Nonsteroidal antiinflammatory drugs: Current status and rational therapeutic use. Drugs 27:232, 1984.
3. Austen, K. F.: The role of arachidonic acid metabolites in local and systemic inflammatory processes. Drugs 33(Suppl. 1):10, 1987.
4. Adams, S. S., and Cobb, R.: A possible basis for the antiinflammatory

activity of salicylates and other nonhormonal antirheumatic drugs. Nature (London) 181:773, 1958.

5. Smith, M. J. H., Dawkins, P. D., and McArthur, J. N.: The relation between clinical inflammatory activity and the displacement of L-tryptophan and a dipeptide from human serum in vitro. J. Pharm. Pharmacol. 23:451, 1971.

6. Ignarro, L. J., and Colombo, C.: Enzyme release from guinea pig polymorphonuclear leukocyte lysosomes inhibited in vitro by antiinflammatory drugs. Nature (New Biol.) 239:155, 1972.

7. Harrity, T. W., and Goldlust, M. B.: Anticomplement effects of two antiinflammatory agents. Biochem. Pharmacol. 23:3107, 1974.

8. Collier, H. O. J.: New light on how aspirin works. Nature (London) 223:35, 1969.

9. Weissmann, G.: Discussion. In Dunn, M., and Weissmann, G. (eds.): Arachidonic Acid Metabolism and Inflammation: Therapeutic Implications. Drugs 33(Suppl. 1):8, 1987.

10. Goldblatt, M. W.: A depressor substance in seminal fluid. J. Soc. Chem. Ind. London 52:1056, 1933.

11. von Euler, U. S.: Zur kenntnis der pharmacologischen wirkungen von nativsekreten und extrakten mannlicher accessorischer Geblechtsdrusen. Naunyn-Schmiedebergs Archiv. Exp. Pathol. Pharmacol. 175:78, 1934.

12. Samuelsson, B.: An elucidation of the arachidonic acid cascade. Discovery of prostaglandins, thromboxane and leukotrienes. Drugs 33(Suppl. 1):2, 1987.

13. Schlegel, S. I.: General characteristics of nonsteroidal antiinflammatory drugs. In Paulus, H. E., Furst, D. E., and Dromgoole, S. (eds.): Drugs for Rheumatic Disease. New York, Churchill Livingstone, 1987, p. 203.

14. Lewis, R. A., Austin, K. F., and Soberman, R. J.: Leukotrienes and other products of the 5-lipoxygenase pathway. N. Engl. J. Med. 323:645, 1990.

15. Miele, L., Cordella-Miele, E., Facchiano, A., and Meekherjee, A. B.: Novel antiinflammatory peptides from the region of highest similarity between uteroglobin and lipocortin I. Nature 335:726, 1988.

16. Camussi, G., Tetta, C., Bussolino, F., and Baglioni, C.: Antiinflammatory peptides (antiflammins) inhibit synthesis of platelet-activating factor, neutrophil aggregation and chemotaxis, and intradermal inflammatory reactions. J. Exp. Med. 171:913, 1990.

17. Goodwin, J. S.: Are prostaglandins proinflammatory, antiinflammatory, both or neither? J. Rheumatol. 18(Suppl. 28):26, 1991.

18. Kuehl, F. A., Jr., Humes, J. L., Ham, E. A., Egan, R. W., and Dougherty, H. W.: Inflammation: The role of peroxidase-derived products. In Samuelsson, B., Ramwell, B., and Paletti, R. (eds.): Advances in Prostaglandin and Thromboxane Research. Vol. 6. New York, Raven Press, 1980, p. 77.

19. Vane, J. R.: Inhibition of prostaglandin synthesis as a mechanism of action for aspirin-like drugs. Nature (New Biol.) 231:232, 1971.

20. Vane, J.: The evolution of non-steroidal anti-inflammatory drugs and their mechanisms of action. Drugs 33(Suppl. 1):18, 1987.

21. Dawson, W., Boot, J. R., Harvey, J., and Walker, J. R.: The pharmacology of benoxaprofen with particular reference to effects on lipoxygenase product formation. Eur. J. Rheumatol. Inflamm. 5:61, 1982.

22. Ku, E. C., Lee, W., Kothari, H. V., Kimble, E. F., Liauw, L., and Tjan, J.: The effect of diclofenac sodium on arachidonic acid metabolism. Semin. Arthritis Rheum. 15:36, 1985.

23. Isselbacher, K. J.: The role of arachidonic acid metabolites in gastrointestinal homeostasis. Biochemical, histological and clinical gastrointestinal effects. Drugs 33(Suppl. 1):38, 1987.

24. Weinblatt, M., Kremer, J., Helfgott, S., Coblyn, J., Maier, A., Sperling, R., Petrillo, G., Kesterson, J., Dube, L., Henson, B., Teoh, N., and Rubin, P.: A 5-lipoxygenase inhibitor in rheumatoid arthritis (Abstract). Arthritis Rheum. 33(Suppl. 9):S152, 1990.

25. Smith, D. M., Johnson, J. A., Loeser, R., and Turner, R. A.: Evaluation of tenidap (CP-66, 248) on human neutrophil arachidonic acid metabolism, chemotactic potential and clinical efficacy in the treatment of rheumatoid arthritis. Agents Actions 31:102, 1990.

26. Sperling, R. I., Weinblatt, M., Robin, J.-L., Coblyn J., Fraser, P., Lewis, R. A., and Austen, K. F.: Effects of dietary fish oil on in vitro leukocyte function, leukotriene generation and activity of disease in rheumatoid arthritis (Abstract). Arthritis Rheum. 29(Suppl. 4):S-18, 1986.

27. Abramson, S. B., and Weissmann, G.: The mechanisms of action of nonsteroidal antiinflammatory drugs. Arthritis Rheum. 32:1, 1989.

28. Chang, Y.-H., Silverman, S. L., and Paulus, H. E.: Colchicine. In Paulus, H. E., Furst, D. E., and Dromgoole, S. (eds.): Drugs for Rheumatic Disease. New York, Churchill-Livingstone, 1987, p. 431.

29. Keates, R. A. B., and Mason, G. B.: Inhibition of microtubule polymerization by tubulin-colchicine complex: Inhibition of spontaneous assembly. Can. J. Biochem. 59:361, 1981.

30. Malawista, S. E., Chang, Y.-H., and Wilson, L.: Lumicolchicine, lack of antiinflammatory effect. Arthritis Rheum. 15:641, 1972.

31. Ehrenfeld, M., Levy, M., Bar Eli, M., Galliby, R., and Eliakim, M.: Effect of colchicine on polymorphonuclear leukocyte chemotaxis in human volunteers. Br. J. Clin. Pharmacol. 10:297, 1980.

32. Spilberg, I., Mandell, B., Mehta, J., Simchowitz, L., and Rosenberg, D.: Mechanism of action of colchicine in acute urate-induced arthritis. J. Clin. Invest. 64:775, 1979.

33. Serhan, C. N., Lundberg, U., Weissmann, G., and Samuelsson, B.: Formation of leukotrienes and hydroxy acids by human neutrophils and platelets exposed to monosodium urate. Prostaglandins 27:563, 1984.

34. Schlesinger, M., Ilfeld, D., Handzel, Z. T., Altman, Y., Kuperman, O., Levin, S., Netzer, L., and Trainin, N.: Effect of colchicine on immunoregulatory abnormalities in familial Mediterranean fever. Clin. Exp. Immunol. 54:73, 1983.

35. Dellaverde, E., Fan, P. T., and Chang, Y.-H.: Mechanisms of action of colchicine. V. Neutrophil adherence and phagocytosis in patients with acute gout treated with colchicine. J. Pharmacol. Exp. Ther. 223:197, 1982.

36. Brune, K., Glatt, M., and Graf, P.: Mechanisms of action of antiinflammatory drugs. Gen. Pharmacol. 7:27, 1976.

37. Nuki, G.: Nonsteroidal analgesic and antiinflammatory agents. Br. Med. J. 287:39, 1983.

38. Furst, D. E., and Dromgoole, S.: Other nonsteroidal antiinflammatory drugs. In Paulus, H., E., Furst, D. E., and Dromgoole, S. (eds.): Drugs for Rheumatic Disease. New York, Churchill Livingstone, 1987, p. 409.

39. Mangan, F. R.: Nabumetone. In Lewis, A. J., and Furst, D. E. (eds.): Nonsteroidal Anti-inflammatory Drugs: Mechanisms and Clinical Use. New York, Marcel Dekker, 1987, p. 439.

40. Spector, W. G., and Willoughby, D. A.: Antiinflammatory effects of salicylate in the rat. In Dixon, A. St. J., Smith M. J. H., Martin, B. K., and Wood, P. H. N. (eds.): Salicylates: An International Symposium. Boston, Little, Brown, 1963, p. 141.

41. Freemont-Smith, K., and Bayles, B.: Salicylate therapy in rheumatoid arthritis. J.A.M.A. 192:103, 1964.

42. American Rheumatism Association Cooperating Clinics Committee: Aspirin in rheumatoid arthritis, a seven-day double-blind trial—preliminary report. Bull. Rheum. Dis. 16:388, 1965.

43. Paulus, H. E.: Pharmacological considerations. In Roth, S. H. (ed.): Handbook of Drug Therapy in Rheumatology. Littleton, MA, PSG Publishing, 1985, p. 39.

44. Paulus, H. E., Schlosstein, L. H., Godfrey, R. G., Klinenberg, J. R., and Bluestone, R.: Prophylactic colchicine therapy of intercritical gout: A placebo-controlled study of probenecid-treated patients. Arthritis Rheum. 17:609, 1974.

45. Meed, S. D., and Spilberg, I.: Successful use of colchicine in acute polyarticular pseudogout. J. Rheumatol. 8:689, 1981.

46. Bowles, C., Harrington, T., Zinsmeister, S., Ellman, M., Reginato, A., McCarty, D., Ryan, L., Espinosa, L., Spilberg, I., and O'Duffy, D.: Colchicine prevents recurrent pseudogout: Multicenter trial. Arthritis Rheum. 29:S-38, 1986.

47. Ainarello, C. A., Wolff, S. M., and Goldfinger, S. E.: Colchicine therapy for familial Mediterranean fever. A double-blind study. N. Engl. J. Med. 291:934, 1976.

48. Lim, R. K. S., Guzman, F., Rodger, D. W., Goto, K., Brawn, C., Dickerson, G. D., and Engle, R. J.: Site of action of narcotic and non-narcotic analgesics determined by blocking bradykinin-evoked visceral pain. Arch. Int. Pharmacodyn. Ther. 152:25, 1964.

49. Brune, K.: Prostaglandins and the mode of action of antipyretic analgesic drugs. Am. J. Med. 75:19, 1983.

50. Feldberg, W., and Melton, A. S.: Prostaglandins and body temperature. In Vane, J. R., and Ferreira, S. H. (eds.): Inflammation. New York, Springer-Verlag, 1978, p. 617.

51. Lewis, A. J., and Furst, D. E. (eds.): Nonsteroidal Antiinflammatory Drugs: Mechanisms and Clinical Use. New York, Marcel Dekker, 1987.

52. Friend, W. G.: Sulindac suppression of colorectal polyps in Gardner's syndrome. Am. Family Physician 41:891, 1990.

53. Reinberg, A., and Levi, F.: Clinical chronopharmacology with special reference to NSAIDs. Scand. J. Rheumatol. (Suppl. 65):118, 1987.

54. Miller, T. A., and Jacobson, E. D.: Gastrointestinal cytoprotection by prostaglandins. Gut 20:75, 1979.

55. Roth, S., Agrawal, M., Nahowald, M., Swabb, E., et al.: Misoprostil heals gastroduodenal injury in patients with rheumatoid arthritis receiving aspirin. Arch. Intern. Med. 149:775, 1989.

56. O'Brien, W. M.: Pharmacology of nonsteroidal antiinflammatory drugs: Practical review for clinicians. Am. J. Med. 75(Suppl.):32, 1983.

57. Caruso, I., and Bianchi-Porro, G.: Gastroscopic evaluation of antiinflammatory agents. Br. Med. J. 280:75, 1980.

58. Lanza, F. L.: Endoscopic studies of gastric and duodenal injury after the use of ibuprofen, aspirin, and other nonsteroidal antiinflammatory agents. Am. J. Med. 77(1A):19, 1984.

59. Bianchi Porro, G., Petrillo, M., and Ardizzone, S.: Salsalate in the treatment of rheumatoid arthritis: A double-blind clinical and gastroscopic trial versus piroxicam. II. Endoscopic evaluation. J. Int. Med. Res. 17:320, 1989.

60. Hedenbro, J. L., Wetterberg, P., Vallgren, S., and Bergqvist, L.: Lack of correlation between fecal blood loss and drug-induced gastric mucosal lesions. Gastrointest. Endoscopy 34:247, 1988.

61. Cohen, A.: Fecal blood loss and plasma salicylate study of salicylsalicylic acid and aspirin. J. Clin. Pharmacol. 19:242, 1979.
62. Lanza, F. L., Rack, M. F., Doucette, M., Ekholm, B., Goldlust, B., and Wilson, R.: An endoscopic comparison of the gastroduodenal injury seen with salsalate and naproxen. J. Rheumatol. 16:1570, 1989.
63. Roth, S., Bennett, R., Calderon, P., Hartman, R., Mitchell, C., Doucette, M., Ekholm, B., Goldlust, B., Lee, E., and Wilson, R.: Reduced risk of NSAID gastropathy (GI mucosal toxicity) with nonacetylated salicylate (salsalate): an endoscopic study. Semin. Arthritis Rheum. 19:11, 1990.
64. Fries, J. F.: NSAID gastropathy: the second most deadly rheumatic disease? Epidemiology and risk appraisal. J. Rheumatol. 18(Suppl. 28):6, 1991.
65. Paulus, H. E.: Government affairs. FDA Arthritis Advisory Committee Meeting: Risks of agranulocytosis/aplastic anemia, flank pain, and adverse gastrointestinal effects with the use of nonsteroidal antiinflammatory drugs. Arthritis Rheum. 30:593, 1987.
66. Roth, S. H.: Prevention of NSAID-induced gastric mucosal damage and gastric ulcer: A review of clinical studies. J. Drug Devel. 1:255, 1989.
66a. Walan, A., Bader, J. P., Classen, M., Lamers, C. B., Piper, D. W., Rutgersson, K., and Eriksson, S.: Effect of omeprazole and ranitidine on ulcer healing and relapse rates in patients with benign gastric ulcer. N. Engl. J. Med. 320:69, 1989.
67. O'Brien, W. M., and Bagby, G. F.: Rare adverse reactions to nonsteroidal antiinflammatory drugs. J. Rheumatol. 12:13, 1985.
68. Paulus, H. E.: Government affairs: FDA Arthritis Advisory Committee Meeting. Arthritis Rheum. 25:1124, 1982.
69. Katz, L. M., and Love, P. Y.: Hepatic dysfunction in association with NSAIDs. In Famaey, J. P., and Paulus, H. E. (eds.): Nonsteroidal Antiinflammatory Drugs: Subpopulation Therapy and Drug Delivery Systems. New York, Marcel Dekker, 1991.
70. Benson, G. D.: Hepatotoxity following the therapeutic use of antipyretic analgesics. Am. J. Med. 75 (Suppl.):85, 1983.
71. Benjamin, S. B., Ishak, K. G., Zimmerman, H. J., and Grushka, A.: Phenylbutazone liver injury: A clinical-pathologic survey of 23 cases and review of the literature. Hepatology 1:255, 1981.
72. Dunn, M.: The role of arachidonic acid metabolites in renal homeostasis. Nonsteroidal antiinflammatory drugs and renal function: biochemical, histological and clinical effects and drug interactions. Drugs 33(Suppl. 1):56, 1987.
73. Blackshear, J. L., Napier, J. S., Davidman, M., and Stillman, M. T.: Renal complications of nonsteroidal antiinflammatory drugs: Identification and monitoring of those at risk. Semin. Arthritis Rheum. 14:163, 1985.
74. DiBona, G. F.: Prostaglandins and nonsteroidal antiinflammatory drugs. Effects on renal hemodynamics. Am. J. Med. 80(Suppl. 1A):12, 1986.
75. Clive, D. M., and Stoff, J. S.: Renal syndromes associated with nonsteroidal antiinflammatory drugs. N. Engl. J. Med. 310:563, 1984.
76. Stillman, M. T., Napier, J. S., and Blackshear, J. L.: Adverse effects of nonsteroidal antiinflammatory drugs on the kidney. Med. Clin. North Am. 68:371, 1984.
77. Zipser, R. D., and Henrich, W. L.: Implications of nonsteroidal antiinflammatory drug therapy. Am. J. Med. 80(Suppl. 1A):78, 1986.
78. Eriksson, L. O., Sturfelt, G., Thysell, H., and Wollheim, F. A.: Effects of sulindac and naproxen on prostaglandin excretion in patients with impaired renal function and rheumatoid arthritis. Am. J. Med. 89:313, 1990.
79. Ciabattoni, G., Cinotte, G. A., Pierucci, A., Simonetti, B. M., Manzi, M., Pugliese, F., Barsotti, P., Pecci, G., Taggi, F., and Patrono, C.: Effects of sulindac and ibuprofen in patients with chronic glomerular disease. N. Engl. J. Med. 310:279, 1984.
80. Roberts, D. G., Gerber, J. G., and Nies, A. S.: Comparative effects of sulindac and indomethacin in humans. Clin. Pharmacol. Ther. 35:269, 1984.
81. Brater, D. C., Anderson, S., Baird, B., and Campbell, W. B.: Sulindac does not spare the kidney. Clin. Pharmacol. Ther. 35:229, 1984.
82. Svendsen, G., Gerstoft, J., Hansen, T. M., Christensen, P., and Lorenzen, I. B.: The renal excretion of prostaglandins and changes in plasma renin during treatment with either sulindac or naproxen in patients with rheumatoid arthritis and thiazide-treated heart failure. J. Rheumatol. 11:779, 1984.
83. Abraham, P. A., and Keane, W. F.: Glomerular and interstitial diseases induced by nonsteroidal antiinflammatory drugs. Am. J. Nephrol. 4:1, 1984.
84. Bennett W. M., and DeBroe, M. E.: Analgesic nephropathy—a preventable renal disease. N. Engl. J. Med. 320:1269, 1989.
85. Whelton, A., Stout, R. L., Spilman, P. S., and Klossen, D. K.: Renal effects of ibuprofen, piroxicam and sulindac in patients with asymptomatic renal failure. Ann. Intern. Med. 112:568, 1990.
86. Stern, R. S., and Bigby, M.: An expanded profile of cutaneous reactions to nonsteroidal antiinflammatory drugs. J.A.M.A. 52:1433, 1984.
87. Suarez, S. M., Cohen, P. R., and De Leo, V. A.: Bullous photosensitivity to naproxen: "Pseudoporphyria." Arthritis Rheum. 33:903, 1990.
88. Szczeklik, A.: Antipyretic analgesics and the allergic patient. Am. J. Med. 75:82, 1983.
89. Strom, B. L., Carson, J. L., Morse, M. L., West, S. L., and Soper, K. A.: The effect of indication on hypersensitivity reactions associated with zomepirac sodium and other nonsteroidal antiinflammatory drugs. Arthritis Rheum. 30:1142, 1987.
90. Inman, W. H.: Study of fatal bone marrow depression with special reference to phenylbutazone and oxyphenbutazone. Br. Med. J. 1:1500, 1977.
91. Paulus, H. E.: Government affairs: FDA Arthritis Advisory Committee Meeting. Arthritis Rheum. 28:450, 1985.
92. The International Agranulocytosis and Aplastic Anemia Study: Risks of agranulocytosis and aplastic anemia. A first report of their relation to drug use with special reference to analgesics. J.A.M.A. 256:1749, 1986.
93. Schlegel, S. I., and Paulus, H. E.: Nonsteroidal and analgesic therapy in the elderly. Clin. Rheum. Dis. 12:245, 1986.
94. Sylvia, L. M., Forlenza, S. W., and Brocavick, J. M.: Aseptic meningitis associated with naproxen. Drug Intell. Clin. Pharm. 22:339, 1988.
95. Court, H., Streete, P., and Volans, G.: Acute poisoning with ibuprofen. Hum. Toxicology 2:381, 1983.
96. Hall, A. H., Smolinske, S. C., Conrad, F. L., Wruk, K. M., Kulig, K. W., Dwelle, T. L., and Rumack, B. H.: Ibuprofen overdose: 126 cases. Ann. Emerg. Med. 15:1308, 1986.
97. Vale, J. A., and Meridith, T.: Poisoning due to non-steroidal antiinflammatory drugs. In Famaey, J. P., and Paulus, H. E. (eds.): Therapeutic Applications of Nonsteroidal Antiinflammatory Drugs: Subpopulations and New Formulations. New York, Marcel Dekker, 1992, p. 67.
98. Brater, D. C.: Drug-drug and drug-disease interactions with nonsteroidal antiinflammatory drugs. Am. J. Med. 80(Suppl. 1A):62, 1986.
99. Klotz, U.: Interactions of analgesics with other drugs. Am. J. Med. 75:133, 1983.
100. Grennan, D. M., and Aarons, L.: Salicylate-NSAID interactions. Ann. Rheum. Dis. 43:351, 1984.
101. Favre, L., Glasson, P., and Vallotten, M. B.: Reversible acute renal failure from combined triamterene and indomethacin. Ann. Intern. Med. 96:317, 1984.
102. Richardson, C. J., Blocka, K. L. N., Ross, S. G., and Verbeeck, R. K.: Effects of age and sex on piroxicam disposition. Clin. Pharmacol. Ther. 37:13, 1985.
103. Furst, D. E., Gupta, N., and Paulus, H. E.: Salicylate metabolism in twins. J. Clin. Invest. 60:32, 1977.
104. Vassell, E. S., and Page, J. G.: Genetic control of drug levels in man: phenylbutazone. Science 154:1479, 1968.
105. Fowler, P. D., and Faragher, E. B.: Drug and non-drug factors influencing adverse reactions to pyrazoles. J. Int. Med. Res. 5(Suppl. 2):108, 1977.
106. Dromgoole, S. H., and Furst, D. E.: Naproxen. In Paulus, H. E., Furst, D. E., and Dromgoole, S. H. (eds.): Drugs for Rheumatic Disease. New York, Churchill Livingstone, 1987, p. 347.
107. Antilla, M., Haataja, M., and Kasanen, A.: Pharmacokinetics of naproxen in subjects with normal and impaired renal function. Eur. J. Clin. Pharmacol. 18:263, 1980.
108. Williams, R. L., Upton, R. A., Cello, J. P., Jones, R. M., Blitstein, M., Kelly, J., and Nierenburg, D.: Naproxen disposition in patients with alcoholic cirrhosis. Eur. J. Clin. Pharmacol. 27:291, 1984.
109. Jalava, S., Saarimaa, H., Antilla, M., and Sundquist, H.: Naproxen concentrations in serum, synovial fluid, and synovium. Scand. J. Rheumatol. 6:155, 1977.
110. Todd, P. A., and Clissold, S. P.: Naproxen. A reappraisal of its pharmacology and therapeutic use in rheumatic diseases and pain states. Drugs 40:91, 1990.
111. Day, R. O., Furst, D. E., Dromgoole, S. H., Kamm, B., Roe, R., and Paulus, H. E.: Relationship of serum naproxen concentration to efficacy in rheumatoid arthritis. Clin. Pharmacol. Ther. 31:733, 1982.
112. Runkel, R., Mroszczak, E., Chaplin, M., Sevelius, H., and Segre, E.: Naproxen-probenecid interaction. Clin. Pharmacol. Ther. 24:706, 1978.
113. Willkens, R. F., and Segre, E. J.: Combination therapy with naproxen and aspirin in rheumatoid arthritis. Arthritis Rheum. 19:677, 1975.
114. Furst, D. E., Blocka, K., Cassell, S., Harris, E. R., Hirschberg, J. M., Josephson, M., Lachenbruch, P. A., Paulus, H. E., and Trimble, R. B.: A controlled study of concurrent therapy with a nonacetylated salicylate and naproxen in rheumatoid arthritis. Arthritis Rheum. 38:146, 1987.
115. Duggan, D. E.: Sulindac: Therapeutic implications of the prodrug/pharmacophore equilibrium. Drug Metab. Rev. 12:325, 1981.
116. Kwan, K. C., Duggan, D. E., and Hucker, H. B.: Metabolism and pharmacokinetics of sulindac. Postgraduate Medicine Communications. McGraw-Hill Publications, 13, 1979.
117. Furst, D. E., and Dromgoole, S. H.: Indomethacin and sulindac. In Paulus, H. E., Furst, D. E., and Dromgoole, S. H. (eds.): Drugs for Rheumatic Disease. New York, Churchill Livingstone, 1987, p. 285.
118. Swanson, B. N., Boppano, V. K., Vlasses, P. H., Holmes, C. I.,

Monsell, K. C., and Ferguson, R. K.: Sulindac disposition when given once or twice daily. Clin. Pharmacol. Ther. 32:397, 1982.

119. Duggan, D. E., Hooke, K. F., Noll, R. M., Hucker, H. B., and Van Arman, C. G.: Comparative disposition of sulindac and metabolites in five species. Biochem. Pharmacol. 27:2311, 1978.

120. Steelman, S. L., Tempero, K. F., and Cirillo, V. J.: The chemistry, pharmacology, toxicology and clinical pharmacology of diflunisal. Clin. Ther. 1(Suppl. A):1, 1978.

121. Dromgoole, S. H., and Furst, D. E.: Diflunisal. In Paulus, H. E., Furst, D. E., and Dromgoole, S. H. (eds.): Drugs for Rheumatic Disease. New York, Churchill Livingstone, 1987, p. 399.

122. Davies, R. O.: Review of the animal in clinical pharmacology of diflunisal. Pharmacotherapy 3(Suppl. 1):9S, 1983.

123. Verbeeck, R., Tjandramage, T. B., Mullie, A., Verbesselt, R., Verberck-moses, R., and DeSchepper, P. J.: Biotransformation of diflunisal and renal excretion of its glucuronides in renal insufficiency. Br. J. Clin. Pharmacol. 9:273, 1979.

124. Myers, R. F., and Siegel, M. I.: Differential effects of antiinflammatory drugs on lipoxygenase and cyclo-oxygenase activities of neutrophils from a reverse passive Arthus reaction. Biochem. Biophys. Res. Commun. 112:586, 1983.

125. Kaplan, H. B., Edelson, H. S., Korchak, H. M., Given, W. P., Abramson, S., and Weissmann, G.: Effects of nonsteroidal antiinflammatory agents on human neutrophil functions in vitro and in vivo. Biochem. Pharmacol. 33:371, 1984.

126. Hobbs, D. C., and Twomey, T. M.: Piroxicam pharmacokinetics in man. Aspirin and antacid interaction studies. J. Clin. Pharmacol. 19:270, 1979.

127. Ostensen, M., Matheson, I., Loufen, H.: Piroxicam in breast milk after long-term treatment. Europ. J. Clin. Pharmacol. 35:567, 1988.

128. Kurowski, M., and Dunky, A.: Transsynovial kinetics of piroxicam in patients with rheumatoid arthritis. Eur. J. Clin. Pharmacol. 34:401, 1988.

129. Dupont, D., Dayer, P., Balant, L., Gorgia, A., and Fabre, J.: Variations intraindividuelles du comportement du piroxicam. Pharmacocinetique chez l'homme en bonne santé et chez le malade en insuffisance renale. Pharma. Acta Helv. 57:20, 1982.

130. Chang, Y.-H., and Dromgoole, S. H.: Oxicams. In Paulus, H. E., Furst, D. E., and Dromgoole, S. H. (eds.): Drugs for Rheumatic Disease. New York, Churchill Livingstone, 1987, p. 389.

131. Said, S. A., and Fodar, A. M.: Influence of cimetidine on the pharmacokinetics of piroxicam in rat and man. Arzneim. Forsch. 39:790, 1989.

132. Darrugh, A., Gordon, A. J., Byrne, H. O., Hobbs, D., and Casey, E.: Single-dose and steady-state pharmacokinetics of piroxicam in elderly vs. young adults. Eur. J. Clin. Pharmacol. 28:305, 1985.

133. Piroxicam Symposium: Piroxicam: A clinical perspective. Am. J. Med. 82(Suppl. 5B):1, 1986.

134. Jahnchen, E., Blanck, K. J., Breuing, K. H., Gilfrich, H. J., Minertz, T., and Trenk, D.: Plasma protein binding of azapropazone in patients with kidney and liver disease. Br. J. Clin. Pharmacol. 11:361, 1981.

135. Ritch, A. E. S., Perera, W. N. R., and Jones, C. J.: Pharmacokinetics of azapropazone in the elderly. Br. J. Pharmacol. 14:116, 1982.

136. Templeton, J. S.: Azapropazone or allopurinol in the treatment of chronic gout and/or hyperuricemia: A preliminary report. Br. J. Clin. Pract. 36:353, 1982.

137. Brogden, R. N., Heel, R. C., Speight, T. M., and Avery, G. S.: Fenbufen: A review of its pharmacological properties and therapeutic use in rheumatic disease and acute pain. Drugs 21:1, 1981.

138. Enthoven, D., Coffey, J. W., and Wyler-Plaut, R. S.: Carprofen. In Lewis, A. J., and Furst, D. E. (eds.): Nonsteroidal Antiinflammatory Drugs: Mechanisms and Clinical Use. New York, Marcel Dekker, 1987, p. 313.

139. Turner, R. A. (ed.): Proceedings of a symposium. Nabumetone, a new nonsteroidal antiinflammatory drug. Am. J. Med. 83(Suppl. 4B):1, 1987.

140. Wallace, S. L., and Ertel, N. H.: Plasma levels of colchicine after oral administration of a single dose. Metabolism 22:749, 1973.

141. Ertel, N. H., and Wallace, S. L.: Measurement of colchicine in urine and peripheral leukocytes. Clin. Res. 19:348, 1971.

142. Halkin, H., Dany, S., Greenwald, M., Schnaps, Y., and Tirosh, M.: Colchicine kinetics in patients with familial Mediterranean fever. Clin. Pharmacol. Ther. 28:82, 1980.

143. Levy, M., Eldor, A., Zylber-Katz, E., and Eliakim, M.: The effect of long-term colchicine therapy in patients with recurrent polyserositis on the capacity of blood platelets to synthesize thromboxane A_2. Br. J. Clin. Pharmacol. 16:191, 1983.

144. Winter, C. A., Risley, E. R., and Seller, R. H.: Anti-inflammatory activity of indomethacin and plasma corticosterone in rats. J. Pharmacol. Exp. Ther. 162:196, 1968.

145. Yeh, K. C., Berger, E. T., Breault, G. O., and Lei, B. W.: Effect of sustained release on the pharmacokinetic profile of indomethacin in man. Biopharm. Drug Dispos. 3:219, 1982.

146. Parks, B. R., Jordan, R. L., Rawson, J. E., and Douglas, B. H.: Indomethacin: Studies of absorption and placental transfer. Am. J. Obstet. Gynecol. 129:464, 1977.

147. Astier, A., and Renat, B.: Sensitive high performance liquid chromatographic determination of indomethacin in human plasma. Pharmacokinetic studies after a single oral dose. J. Chromatogr. 233:279, 1982.

148. Emori, H. W., Champion, G. D., Bluestone, R., and Paulus, H. E.: Simultaneous pharmacokinetics of indomethacin in serum and synovial fluid. Ann. Rheum. Dis. 32:433, 1973.

149. Duggan, D. E., Hogan, A. F., Kwan, K. C., and McMahon, D. G.: The metabolism of indomethacin in man. J. Pharmacol. Exp. Ther. 181:563, 1972.

150. Duggan, D. E., and Kwan, K. C.: Enterohepatic recirculation of drugs as a determinant of therapeutic ratio. Drug Metab. Rev. 9:21, 1979.

151. Traeger, A., Noschel, H., and Zaumseil, J.: Pharmacokinetics of indomethacin in pregnant and parturient women and in their newborn infants. Zentralbl. Gynakol. 95:635, 1973.

152. Traeger, A., Kunze, M., Stein, G., and Ankermann, M.: Pharmacokinetics of indomethacin in the aged. Z. Alternsforsch 27:151, 1973.

153. Kwan, K. C., Breault, G. O., Davis, R. L., Lei, B. W., Czerwinski, A. W., Besselaar, G. H., and Duggan, D. E.: Effects of concomitant aspirin administration on the pharmacokinetics of indomethacin in man. J. Pharmacokinet. Biopharm. 6:451, 1978.

154. Brooks, P. M., Walker, J. J., Bell, M. A., Buchanan, W. W., and Rhymer, A. R.: Indomethacin-aspirin interaction: A clinical appraisal. Br. Med. J. 11:69, 1975.

155. Livio, M., Del Maschio, A., Cesletti, C., and deGaetano, G.: Indomethacin prevents the long-lasting inhibitory effect of aspirin on human platelet cyclo-oxygenase activity. Prostaglandins 23:787, 1982.

156. Helleberg, L.: Clinical pharmacokinetics of indomethacin. Clin. Pharmacokinet. 6:245, 1981.

157. Brooks, P. M., Bell, M. A., Sturrock, R. D., Famaey, J. P., and Dick, W. C.: The clinical significance of indomethacin-probenecid interaction. Br. J. Clin. Pharmacol. 1:287, 1974.

158. Adams, S. S., Bresloff, P., and Mason, C. G.: Pharmacological differences between the optical isomers of ibuprofen: Evidence for metabolic inversion of the (−) isomer. J. Pharm. Pharmacol. 28:256, 1976.

159. Albert, K. S., and Gernaat, C. M.: Pharmacokinetics of ibuprofen. Am. J. Med. 77:40, 1984.

160. Whitlam, J. B., Brown, K. F., Crooks, M. J., and Room, J. F. W.: Transsynovial distribution of ibuprofen in arthritic patients. Clin. Pharmacol. Ther. 29:487, 1981.

161. Kaiser, D. G., Vangiessen, G. J., Reischer, R. J., and Wechter, W. J.: Isomeric inversion of ibuprofen R(−) enantiomers in humans. J. Pharm. Sci. 65:269, 1976.

162. Albert, K. S., Gillespie, W. R., Wagner, J. G., Pau, A., and Lockwood, G. F.: Effects of age on the clinical pharmacokinetics of ibuprofen. Am. J. Med. 77:47, 1984.

163. Slattery, J. T., and Levy, G.: Effects of ibuprofen on protein-binding of warfarin in human serum. J. Pharm. Sci. 66:1060, 1977.

164. Brooks, C. D., and Ulrich, J. E.: Effect of ibuprofen or aspirin on probenecid induced uricosuria. J. Int. Med. Res. 8:283, 1980.

165. Rao, G. H. R., Johnson, G. G., Reddy, K. R., and White, J. G.: Ibuprofen protects platelet cyclo-oxygenase from irreversible inhibition by aspirin. Atherosclerosis 3:383, 1983.

166. Day, R., and Furst, D. E.: Ibuprofen, fenoprofen, ketoprofen. In Paulus, H. E., Furst, D. E., and Dromgoole, S. H. (eds.): Drugs for Rheumatic Disease. New York, Churchill Livingstone, 1987, p. 315.

167. Barry, W. S., Meinzinger, M. M., and Howse, C. R.: Ibuprofen overdose and exposure in utero: Results from a post marketing voluntary reporting system. Am. J. Med. 77(Suppl. 1A):35, 1984.

168. Rubin, A., Knadler, M. P., Ho, P. P., Bechtol, L. D., and Wolen, R. L.: Stereoselective inversion of (R)-fenoprofen to (S)+fenoprofen in humans. J. Pharm. Sci. 74:82, 1985.

169. Chernish, S. M., Rubin, A., Rodda, B. E., Ridolfo, A. S., and Gruber, C. M., Jr.: The physiological disposition of fenoprofen in man. IV. The effects of position of subject, food ingestion and antacid ingestion on the plasma levels of orally administered fenoprofen. J. Med. (Basel) 83:249, 1972.

170. Kamal, A., and Koch, I. M.: Plasma profiles of two differing doses of fenoprofen in geriatric patients. Pharmatherapeutica 2:552, 1981.

171. Brogden, R. N., Pinder, R. M., Speight, T. M., and Avery, G. S.: Fenoprofen: A review of its pharmacological properties and therapeutic efficacy in rheumatic diseases. Drugs 13:241, 1977.

172. Brewer, E. J., Giannini, E. H., Baum, J., Bernstein, B., Fink, C. W., Emery, H. M., and Schaller, J. G.: Aspirin and fenoprofen (Nalfon) in the treatment of juvenile rheumatoid arthritis. Results of a double-blind trial. J. Rheumatol. 9:123, 1982.

173. Garella, S., and Matarese, R. A.: Renal effects of prostaglandins and clinical adverse effects of non-steroidal antiinflammatory agent. Medicine 63:165, 1984.

174. Stachura, I., Jayakumar, S., and Bourke, E.: T and B lymphocyte subsets in fenoprofen nephropathy. Am. J. Med. 75:9, 1983.

175. Gandini, R., Cunietti, E., Pappalepore, V., Ferrari, M., Deleo, B., Locatelli, E., and Fasoli, A.: Effects of intravenous high-doses of

ketoprofen on blood clotting, bleeding time and platelet aggregation in man. J. Int. Med. Res. 11:243, 1983.

176. Upton, R. A., Williams, R. L., Guentert, T. W., Buskin, J. N., and Reigelman, S.: Ketoprofen pharmacokinetics and bioavailability based on an improved and specific assay. Eur. J. Clin. Pharmacol. 20:127, 1981.

177. Vavra, I.: Ketoprofen. In Lewis, A. J., and Furst, D. E. (eds.): Nonsteroidal Antiinflammatory Drugs: Mechanisms and Clinical Use. New York, Marcel Dekker, 1987, p. 419.

178. Advenier, C., Roux, A., Gobert, C., Massais, P., Variquax, O., and Flouvat, B.: Pharmacokinetics of ketoprofen in the elderly. Br. J. Clin. Pharmacol. 16:65, 1983.

179. Staffanger, G., Larsen, H. W., Hansen, H., and Sorensen, K.: Pharmacokinetics of ketoprofen in patients with chronic renal failure. Scand. J. Rheumatol. 10:189, 1981.

180. Upton, R. A., Williams, R. L., Buskin, J. N., and Matthew-Jones, R.: Effects of probenecid on ketoprofen kinetics. Clin. Pharmacol. Ther. 31:705, 1982.

181. Williams, R. L., Upton, R. A., Buskin, J. N., and Jones, R. M.: Ketoprofen-aspirin interactions. Clin. Pharmacol. Ther. 30:226, 1981.

182. Thyss, S., Milano, G., Kubar, J., Namer, M., and Schneider, M.: Clinical and pharmacokinetic evidence of a life-threatening interaction between methotrexate and ketoprofen. Lancet 1:256, 1986.

183. Furst, D. E., Dromgoole, S. H., Fow, S., and Landaw, E. M.: Comparison of tolmetin kinetics in rheumatoid arthritis and matched healthy controls. J. Clin. Pharmacol. 23:557, 1983.

184. Dromgoole, S. H., Furst, D. E., Desiraju, R. K., Nayak, R. K., Kirschenbaum, M. A., and Paulus, H. E.: Tolmetin kinetics and synovial fluid prostaglandin E levels in rheumatoid arthritis. Clin. Pharmacol. Ther. 32:371, 1982.

185. Selley, M. L., Glass, J., Triggs, E. J., and Thomas, J.: Pharmacokinetic studies of tolmetin in man. Clin. Pharmacol. Ther. 17:599, 1975.

186. Dromgoole, S. H., and Furst, D. E.: Tolmetin. In Paulus, H. E., Furst, D. E., and Dromgoole, S. H. (eds.): Drugs for Rheumatic Disease. New York, Churchill Livingstone, 1987, p. 365.

187. O'Brien, W. M.: Long-term efficacy and safety of tolmetin sodium in treatment of geriatric patients with rheumatoid arthritis and osteoarthritis: a retrospective study. J. Clin. Pharmacol. 23:309, 1983.

188. Restivo, C., and Paulus, H. E.: Anaphylaxis from tolmetin. J.A.M.A. 240:246, 1978.

189. Dromgoole, S. H., and Furst, D. E.: Fenamates. In Paulus, H. E., Furst, D. E., and Dromgoole, S. H. (eds.): Drugs for Rheumatic Disease. New York, Churchill Livingstone, 1987, p. 379.

190. Boctor, A. M., Eickholt, M., and Pugsley, T. A.: Meclofenamate sodium is an inhibitor of both the 5-lipoxygenase and cyclo-oxygenase pathways of the arachidonic acid cascade in vitro. Prostaglandins Leukotr. Med. 23:229, 1986.

191. Glazko, A. J.: Pharmacology of the fenamates. III. Metabolism and disposition. In Kendall, P. H. (ed.): Fenamates in Medicine: A Symposium. Ann. Phys. Med. (Suppl. 8):23, 1966.

192. Baragar, F. D., and Smith, T. C.: Drug interaction studies with meclofenamate (meclomen). Curr. Ther. Res. 23(Suppl.):S51, 1978.

193. Eberl, R.: Long-term experience with meclofenamate sodium. Arzneim. Forschung 33:667, 1983.

194. Brogden, R. N., Heel, R. C., Pakes, G. E., Speight, T. M., and Avery, G. S.: Diclofenac sodium: A review of its pharmacological properties and therapeutic use in rheumatic diseases and pain of varying origin. Drugs 20:24, 1980.

195. Liauw, H. L., Moscaritola, J. D., and Burcher, J.: Diclofenac sodium (Voltaren). In Lewis, A. J., and Furst, D. E. (eds.): Nonsteroidal Antiinflammatory Drugs: Mechanisms and Clinical Use. New York, Marcel Dekker, 1987, p. 329.

196. Cayen, M. N., Kraml, M., Fernandi, E. S., Gaeselin, E., and Dvornik, D.: The metabolic disposition of etodolac in rats, dogs and man. Drug Metab. Dispos. 12:339, 1981.

197. Sanda, M., Jacob, G. B., Fliedner, L. Jr., Kennedy, J., and Gotz, M.: Etodolac. In Lewis, A. J., and Furst, D. E. (eds.): Nonsteroidal Antiinflammatory Drugs: Mechanisms and Clinical Use. New York, Marcel Dekker, 1987, p. 349.

198. Jacob, G., Sanda, M., Mullane, J., Kennedy, J., Barbette, M., and Suleski, P.: A 52-week double-blind trial of etodolac versus aspirin in the treatment of rheumatoid arthritis. Adv. Ther. 2:82, 1985.

199. Smith, R. J., Lomen, P. L., and Kaiser, D. G.: Flurbiprofen. In Lewis, A. J., and Furst, D. E. (eds.): Nonsteroidal Antiinflammatory Drugs: Mechanisms and Clinical Use. New York, Marcel Dekker, 1987, p. 393.

200. Kaiser, D. G., Brooks, C. D., Lomen, P. L.: Pharmacokinetics of flurbiprofen. Am. J. Med. 80(Suppl. 3A):10, 1986.

201. Brooks, P. M., and Khong, T. K.: Flurbiprofen-aspirin interaction: A double-blind cross-over study. Curr. Med. Res. Opin. 5:53, 1977.

202. Ketorolac Trimethamine. The Medical Letter 32:79, 1990.

203. O'Hara, D. A., Fragen, R. F., Kinzer, M., and Pemberton, D.: Ketorolac trimethamine as compared with morphine sulfate for treatment of postoperative pain. Clin. Pharmacol. Ther. 41:556, 1987.

204. Physician's Desk Reference. 45th Edition. Oradell, N. J., Medical Economics Company, 1991, pp. 2207–2209.

205. Ward, J. R.: Nonsteroidal (nonsalicylate) antiinflammatory drugs. In Roth, S. H. (ed.): Rheumatic Therapeutics. New York, McGraw-Hill, 1985, p. 363.

206. Miller, D. R.: Combination use of nonsteroidal antiinflammatory drugs. Drug Intell. Clin. Pharm. 15:3, 1981.

207. Furst, D. E., Caldwell, J. R., Klugman, M. P., and Sarkissian, E.: Dose-response relationship for carprofen in patients with rheumatoid arthritis (RA). Arthritis Rheum. 30(Suppl. 4):S95, 1987.

208. Goldsmith, D. P., Eichenfield, A. H., Drott, H. R., and Athreya, B. H.: Plasma indomethacin levels in juvenile rheumatoid arthritis. Arthritis Rheum. 30(Suppl. 4):S-35, 1987.

209. Brooks, P. M., and Day, R. O.: Plasma concentrations and therapeutic effects of antiinflammatory and antirheumatic drugs. In Lewis, A. J., and Furst, D. E. (eds.): Nonsteroidal Antiinflammatory Drugs: Mechanisms and Clinical Use. New York, Marcel Dekker, 1987, p. 189.

210. Famaey, J. P.: Synovial antiinflammatory and antirheumatic drug levels: Importance in therapeutic efficacy. In Lewis, A. J., and Furst, D. E. (eds.): Nonsteroidal Antiinflammatory Drugs: Mechanisms and Clinical Use. New York, Marcel Dekker, 1987, p. 201.

211. Schlegel, S. I., and Paulus, H. E.: NSAIDs, use in rheumatic disease, side effects and interactions. Bull. Rheum. Dis. 6(36):1, 1986.

Antimalarial Drugs

HISTORICAL PERSPECTIVE

The antimalarial medications, which are also antirheumatic drugs, are derived from the bark of the Peruvian cinchona tree. The active agents, quinine and cinchonine, were isolated by Pelletier and Caventau in 1820.[1] In 1894, J. P. Payne, physician to St. Thomas' Hospital in London, delivered a postgraduate lecture on lupus erythematosus in which he first described the successful use of quinine for a rheumatic disease.[2]

During the first half of the twentieth century, extensive efforts were undertaken to synthesize antimalarial compounds with improved therapeutic/toxicity ratios. These compounds were also successfully used to treat lupus erythematosus and have been reviewed previously.[3]

Page's seminal publication in 1951[4] provided much of the impetus for the widespread use of antimalarials to treat connective tissue diseases. He used quinacrine for patients with lupus erythematosus and noted that skin lesions improved in 17 of 18 patients. Associated "rheumatoid arthritis" also remitted in two of these patients, and systemic symptoms, including arthritis, cleared in a third. The response of Page's patients with lupus and rheumatoid arthritis influenced several groups to treat rheumatoid arthritis (RA) with antimalarials,[3, 5-8] with good results.

Chloroquine and hydroxychloroquine were used in an effort to minimize antimalarial toxicity. However, in 1959, Hobbes and associates[9] recognized that long-term treatment with antimalarials might result in serious drug-induced retinal toxicity, and this led to a marked diminution in antimalarial use (reviewed in reference 3). More recent studies have shown that retinal toxicity is related to high daily dose and not to long-term treatment.[10, 11]

In the past several years, the spectrum of connective tissue diseases reported to respond to antimalarials has increased with the addition of childhood dermatomyositis,[12, 13] palindromic rheumatism,[14-17] and eosinophilic fasciitis.[18-20] Antimalarials have also been successfully employed for other immunologically mediated diseases, such as asthma.[21]

DEFINITION AND STRUCTURE

At present, only three antimalarial compounds are used to treat rheumatic diseases (Fig. 44–1). Of these, two 4-aminoquinoline derivatives, chloroquine and hydroxychloroquine, are virtually the only drugs prescribed. The 4-aminoquinoline compounds differ only by the substitution of a hydroxyethyl group for an ethyl group on the tertiary aminonitrogen of the side chain of chloroquine. At least one survey shows that hydroxychloroquine is more commonly prescribed than chloroquine in Canada and Australia,[22] and this is also true in the United States.

Quinacrine, although not a 4-aminoquinoline, does include the chloroquine structure (see Fig. 44–1). It is occasionally used in patients with discoid lupus, but its use is limited because it may cause yellowish skin discoloration. Other antimalarials no longer utilized because of unacceptable toxicity have been described in earlier textbook editions.[3]

PHARMACOKINETICS

Chloroquine and hydroxychloroquine are rapidly absorbed after oral administration[1, 8] and are quickly cleared from plasma. Most of the absorbed medication is excreted in urine unchanged, but about one third is metabolized[23, 24] to a desethyl derivative formed by alkyl degradation of a terminal aminoethyl group in the side chain. The urinary excretory rate is increased when the urine is acidified. About 8 percent can be found in feces, some of which is a result of excretion.[23]

The half-life of chloroquine has been reported to vary from 3.5 to 12 days,[25, 26] with plateau plasma levels achieved in 2 to 5 weeks.[25, 27, 28] Some of these differences may be explained by study design or by methodology of measurement,[25, 29] but a fivefold variation in plasma levels has been noted in one series of patients treated for 2 months with 250 mg of chloroquine per day.[26] Plasma levels in patients receiving daily dosages of 250 mg of chloroquine generally range from 200 to 400 µg per liter,[27] and the plateau level of urinary excretion is 75 mg per day.[30] Hydroxychloroquine plasma plateau levels of 400[31] to 700 µg per liter are found at dosages of 400 mg per day, with a corresponding urinary excretion of 55 mg per day.[27, 30] Daily doses of 200 mg result in a proportional decrease in plasma levels of about 50 percent.[32] By the seventy-seventh day after chloroquine administration has been discontinued, urinary daily output falls to about 1 mg.[25] At this time, about 55 percent of the total ingested dose may be ac-

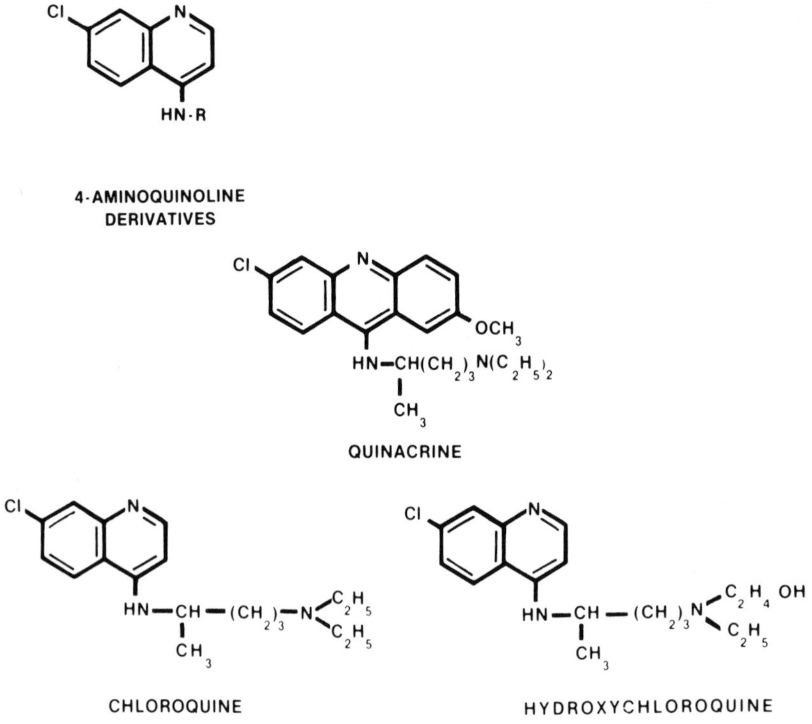

Figure 44–1. Structural formulas of antimalarials currently used to treat rheumatic disease and the basic structure of 4-aminoquinolines in which R represents the side chain.

counted for by urinary excretion.[25] However, small amounts of chloroquine may be found in plasma, red blood cells, and urine for as long as 5 years after the last dose.[33]

Tissue concentrations of chloroquine and hydroxychloroquine are much greater than plasma levels both in animal studies[34] and in the rare examples of human measurements.[35, 36] Among circulating blood cells, mononuclear cells demonstrate higher hydroxychloroquine concentration than do neutrophils in patients with RA, and monocytes have greater uptake than do lymphocytes in in vitro studies.[37] Localization of the 4-aminoquinolines in the eye assumes great importance because of retinal toxicity. In albino rats, drug concentration in the eye ranks between that in muscle and heart, but concentration in the eye of pigmented rats is 10 to 20 times greater than that in any other tissue,[34, 38] related to deposition in the iris and choroid.[39]

MECHANISM OF ACTION

Various drug actions that may affect rheumatic diseases are listed in Table 44–1 under the headings *primary actions, anti-inflammatory activity, effects on immune function, effects on infectious agents,* and *miscellaneous actions.*[3]

The most likely primary antimalarial actions are inhibition of enzyme activity and interference of cellular function in compartments in which there is an acid microenvironment, such as lysosomes, endosomes, and the Golgi complex. These basic drug actions may subsequently affect pathways of inflammation and the immune cascade. Chloroquine reduces the activity of many enzymes,[40] including phospholipase A$_2$.[41, 42] Total prostaglandin production decreases,[43] and in an experimental test system leukotriene release from lung was diminished.[44] In addition to causing direct enzyme inhibition, these

Table 44–1. ANTIMALARIAL ACTIONS

"Primary" Actions
Inhibition of enzyme activity, including phospholipase
Interference with intracellular function dependent on an acidic microenvironment

Anti-inflammatory Activity
Stabilizes lysosomal membranes
Inhibits polymorphonuclear cell chemotaxis
Inhibits polymorphonuclear cell phagocytosis
Affects superoxide generation
Inhibits connective tissue encapsulation
Decreases fibronectin production
Decreases histamine production
Decreases intravascular erythrocyte aggregation
Decreases platelet aggregation
Photoprotective
Inhibits interleukin-1–induced cartilage degradation

Effects on Immune Function
Inhibits monokine formation
Inhibits proliferative response of stimulated lymphocytes
Inhibits natural killer cell activity
Inhibits immune complex formation

Effects on Infectious Agents
Inhibits bacteria replication
Protects tissue culture from virus infection
Prevents virus replication
Induces expression of Epstein-Barr virus early antigen

Miscellaneous Actions
Complexes with deoxyribonucleic acid (DNA)
May interfere with sulfhydryl-disulfide interchange reactions

drugs stabilize lysosomal membranes, thereby inhibiting the release of lysosomal enzymes.[45]

Perhaps even more important than enzyme inhibition is the lysosomotropic action of antimalarials. Aminoquinolines, such as chloroquine and hydroxychloroquine, are weak bases. These weak bases enter the lysosome, are protonated, raise the pH,[46, 47] and interfere with enzyme activity that depends on an acid milieu. Electron micrographs of both polymorphonuclear cells and lymphocytes[48] from patients treated with chloroquine reveal abnormal lysosomal structures presumably caused by this lysosomotropic action.

Lysosomal interference can have far-reaching effects. Some cell surface receptors and ligands are internalized and transported by endosomes to lysosomes, where receptors are separated from ligands and returned to the cell surface. Antimalarials interfere with this receptor recycling.[49, 50]

Antimalarials also affect the Golgi complex. Chloroquine may inhibit protein secretion and the intracellular processing of proteins by blocking the proteolytic conversion of secretary protein precursors, such as the complement precursor component pro-C3.[51] These biochemical changes are associated with morphologic changes in the Golgi complex.[51]

Among the anti-inflammatory effects, a photoprotective effect[52–55] may explain the improvement of lupus skin lesions. Various investigators attribute this to ultraviolet radiation absorption[52] or to a modification of an abnormal tissue response[54, 55] to such radiation.

Antimalarials have been shown to affect multiple aspects of the immunologic cascade but not to exert a uniform influence. Animal studies[56, 57] suggest that they do not inhibit antibody production. Chloroquine does inhibit antigen-antibody interaction and immune complex formation,[58, 59] and immune complex levels are reduced in treated patients with RA.[60]

Interference with macrophage and lymphocyte function may be even more pertinent. Chloroquine inhibits the proliferative response of stimulated cultured human lymphocytes,[61] and decreased responsiveness to phytohemagglutinin has been demonstrated by lymphocytes of treated patients.[62] Natural killer (NK) cell action is inhibited both in vitro[63] and in vivo.[64]

Suppression of the immune system may be mediated by inhibition of interleukin-1 production by monocytes. Salmeron and Lipsky[65] observed suppression of lymphocyte proliferation by chloroquine in concentrations as low as 1 μg per ml. Proliferation was restored by adding a monokine, presumed to be interleukin-1. Using somewhat different experimental conditions but also employing a chloroquine concentration that may be present in vivo, Baker's group showed inhibition of lectin binding.[66] This may be related to the inhibition of receptor recycling already described, thus associating lysosomotropic action with immunologic effects. They further postulated that inhibition of lectin binding

may be a mechanism that causes diminished monokine production.[66] Antimalarials may also interfere with the action of interleukin-1, and hydroxychloroquine has been shown to inhibit interleukin-1–induced cartilage degradation.[67]

Among miscellaneous actions, antimalarials form complexes with DNA by binding of the quinoline ring to the phosphate groups and nucleotide bases[68] and thereby interfere with nuclear events.[69–71] Reactions between DNA and anti-DNA antibodies[72] may be blocked. This may explain the inhibition of the lupus erythematosus cell phenomenon observed by Dubois.[73]

THERAPEUTIC EFFECTIVENESS

Lupus Erythematosus

The variability of the natural course of lupus erythematosus and of the response of different manifestations of disease to various medications makes treatment evaluation difficult, but antimalarials are beneficial.

Discoid Lupus Erythematosus

Antimalarials are effective against discoid lesions. Compared with the spontaneous remissions in 15 percent, remissions or major improvements have been noted in 60 to 90 percent of treated patients.[74] However, daily dosages were often much larger than those currently acceptable.[74–77] Quinacrine is occasionally helpful when discoid lesions fail to respond adequately to hydroxychloroquine or chloroquine.[74, 78]

Chloroquine and hydroxychloroquine were used to treat discoid lupus because they did not impart the yellowish skin staining induced by quinacrine.[79] Sixty to 70 percent of patients had substantial improvement while receiving these medications.[74–76, 80] In a double-blind crossover placebo-hydroxychloroquine trial in which daily doses as high as 1200 mg were employed, the antimalarial was significantly more effective.[77]

The effectiveness of antimalarials in the treatment of skin lesions is often apparent within the first week, when erythematous changes start to regress. Follicular plugging may then disappear, and after several months thickening and induration diminish or clear. Most patients responding to antimalarial medication experience relapse after the drug is discontinued. Winkelman and associates[78] found that only 7 of 67 patients who took quinacrine or chloroquine for 10 weeks to 4 years maintained remission for 3 years after stopping their medication. Most of the 50 who had relapses responded to additional courses of treatment.

Systemic Lupus Erythematosus

The strongest evidence supporting the efficacy of antimalarials in treating systemic lupus erythematosus comes from studies in which medication was discontinued in successfully treated patients.[81, 82] However, many studies favoring antimalarial use are anecdotal. Patients with improvement of "subacute" lupus are included in larger series of patients with only discoid skin lesions.[75, 78, 79]

Dubois[83] treated 20 patients with systemic lupus erythematosus using rather high doses of quinacrine. Seven of nine patients with arthralgias and fever had remission on treatment, whereas only 3 of 11 patients with more severe acute systemic lupus erythematosus benefited. In general, the less active the disease, the more rapid and better was the improvement.

Reviewing information on 43 patients who had been treated with antimalarials for at least 2 years and then had medication discontinued because of toxicity, Rudnicki and colleagues[81] found that significantly fewer flare-ups occurred while patients were receiving treatment when the most recent years during which patients were on drug were compared with the years after the medication was discontinued. Although no significant glucocorticoid-sparing effect was found in this study, others suggest that antimalarial treatment may have a corticosteroid-sparing effect.[84]

A 6-month, double-blind, placebo-controlled drug discontinuation study provides substantial evidence that hydroxychloroquine prevents lupus flare-ups.[82] Forty-seven patients, all of whom were being treated with hydroxychloroquine, were studied. Sixteen of the 22 patients in whom placebo was substituted for hydroxychloroquine experienced flare-ups, whereas only 9 of 25 continuing hydroxychloroquine suffered a disease exacerbation (p = 0.02). Most manifestations were minor. Only one severe exacerbation occurred in the treatment group, compared with five in the placebo group (p = 0.06). Three of the placebo-treated patients required hospitalization. Overall the risk of disease flare-up was increased by a factor of 2.5 for the placebo group.

Antimalarials alone are not appropriate treatment for the more severe manifestations of systemic lupus erythematosus.[74] Although one study reported substantial benefit in patients with active diffuse proliferative glomerulonephritis treated with a combination of indomethacin (3 mg per kg per day) and hydroxychloroquine (800 mg per day),[85] these results have not been confirmed.

Rheumatoid Arthritis

The antimalarials belong to the class termed slow-acting antirheumatic drugs (SAARDs). Little or no improvement may be apparent for weeks or months after antimalarials are started. Benefits ensue gradually but may not be maximal for 6 months or

even longer.[6, 8] Analogously, when antimalarial treatment is discontinued, the disease will not flare up immediately but will gradually worsen over weeks or months.

In open studies, substantial benefit has been noted in approximately 60 to 70 percent of patients.[6, 8, 86] Adams and coworkers[86] used 400 mg per day of hydroxychloroquine and noted that 13 of 100 patients had complete remission and another 15 had more than 75 percent improvement.

Scherbel and associates[8] compared efficacy and toxicity of chloroquine and hydroxychloroquine and concluded that for the same dosage of each medication hydroxychloroquine was one half to two thirds as effective as chloroquine and one half as toxic. On the other hand, meta-analysis of placebo-controlled studies of drug effectiveness suggests that chloroquine, 250 mg per day, is superior to hydroxychloroquine, 400 mg per day.[87] It is not certain that the groups from various studies included in analysis were truly comparable.

Daily dosage may affect results, and 800 mg of hydroxychloroquine was more effective than 400 mg.[7] A year-long, double-blinded, controlled study showed no statistically significant differences between 400 mg and 200 mg per day, although improvement favored patients receiving the higher dose.

At least eight controlled studies have confirmed antimalarial benefit. Chloroquine was studied in five,[88–92] and hydroxychloroquine in three.[93–95] The dosage of active drug varied. In several studies, it did not exceed the currently recommended daily dosage,[90, 91, 95] whereas in others it was twice as much.[89, 92, 94] The length of studies ranged from 16 weeks[90] to 1 year.[89, 92, 95] One study was crossover in design.[93] In general, these controlled studies did not show as impressive results as those of open studies, but in each, definite drug benefit was observed.

The Cooperating Clinics of the American Rheumatism Association conducted a 6-month, placebo-controlled study in which 53 patients received 800 mg per day of hydroxychloroquine, twice the current recommended daily dosage, and 60 received placebo.[94] Changes in individual parameters favored the drug-treated group, but none reached statistical significance. More impressive were the changes in the overall assessments.

A year-long, placebo-controlled study of 104 patients with mild disease showed that daily doses of 400 mg of hydroxychloroquine are also effective.[95] All four clinical parameters assessed and erythrocyte sedimentation rate were significantly improved in the treated group compared with baseline values, but only morning stiffness was better in the control group. Furthermore, withdrawals for lack of efficacy were significantly higher in the placebo group, 18 against 8 (p < 0.05). Interestingly, two patients receiving placebo dropped out because of toxicity, compared with one drug-treated patient.

Favorable results with chloroquine treatment

Table 44–2. COMPARISON OF EFFICACY OF ANTIMALARIALS WITH OTHER SLOW-ACTING ANTIRHEUMATIC DRUGS (SAARDs)

Antimalarial	Other SAARD	Length of Study (mo)	Type of Study	Clinical Outcome	Comment
HCQ[98]*	Intramuscular gold	—	Retrospective life table analysis	Gold superior	See text for discussion
HCQ[99]	Intramuscular gold	—	Retrospective life table analysis	Equal	See text for discussion
C[100]	Intramuscular gold (gold thiomalate)	6	Random assignment of patients	Equal	See text for discussion
HCQ[100a]	Oral gold (auranofin)	11	Random assignment of patients	Equal	More parameters improved on HCQ
C[101]	D-Penicillamine	12	Random assignment of patients	Equal	Laboratory test results favored D-penicillamine
HCQ[99]	D-Penicillamine	—	Retrospective life table analysis	Equal	
HCQ[96]	D-Penicillamine	24	Double blinded	D-Penicillamine superior at 6 and 12 mo, equal at 24 mo	Low daily doses of each medication Marked improvement at 24 mo: 25% for HCQ and 11% for D-penicillamine
HCQ[97]	Sulfasalazine	11	Double blinded	Equal	Sulfasalazine more rapid improvement, greater number of parameters improved, less withdrawal for lack of effect
C[101a]	Dapsone	6	Random assignment of patients	C superior	
C[100]	Azathioprine	6	Random assignment of patients	Equal	
HCQ[99]	Levamisole	—	Retrospective life table analysis	HCQ superior	

HCQ = hydroxychloroquine; C = chloroquine.
*Superscripts refer to references.

were obtained in two 1-year studies in which the daily dose was twice that currently recommended.[89, 92] Freedman and Steinberg[92] noted definite general improvement in 80 percent of 107 patients who completed 1 year of chloroquine treatment, compared with 30 percent of the placebo group. Deterioration was seen in only 5 percent of chloroquine-treated patients but in 25 percent of control subjects.

Radiographic evaluation shows a difference in erosion score between treated and placebo patients in one study[92] but equal progression in two others.[89, 95]

Laboratory evaluation revealed that rheumatoid factor titers often decreased in patients on active drug for at least 6 months,[89, 92, 94] and erythrocyte sedimentation rates decreased in those treated for 1 year.[89, 92, 95]

Comparisons With Other SAARDs

Studies comparing the effectiveness of antimalarials with other SAARDs are summarized in Table 44–2. Only a few were double-blinded.[96, 97]

Two studies from one institution illustrate the difficulty of some comparisons.[98, 99] Treatment terminations were assessed using life table analysis. In

the first, gold was superior to hydroxychloroquine,[98] whereas the second showed an equal frequency of treatment termination for lack of effect.[99] Commenting on the differences between studies, the authors suggested that they may have discontinued hydroxychloroquine before full benefit or may have demanded a more complete remission in the first study.

Although equal effectiveness was found in a study comparing chloroquine, gold, and azathioprine, the authors concluded that "gold is still the drug of choice in active RA" and that chloroquine is a "moderately effective anti-rheumatic drug and should be considered early in the management of RA."[100]

Comparison of radiographic changes showed less deterioration with D-penicillamine than with chloroquine,[101] but not with hydroxychloroquine,[96] and less changes with sulfasalazine than with hydroxychloroquine.[102] Other drugs could be substituted for sulfasalazine or hydroxychloroquine after 1 year. At 3 years, radiographic changes still favored the group started on sulfasalazine, but all differences were completely accounted for by changes in the first year.[103]

Felson and colleagues[87] combined 117 treatment groups from 66 trials in a meta-analysis. Antimalarials were significantly less effective in composite treatment effect than was penicillamine (p = 0.04) but not other SAARDs or methotrexate. However, patients who had failed to respond while receiving hydroxychloroquine almost universally responded to methotrexate.[104]

Combination Therapy

Combination therapy using two or more SAARDs, cytotoxics, or immunosuppressive medications has been recently propounded as an option in the treatment of RA.[105] In the first study of the use of combination slow-acting antirheumatic drug treatment, Sievers and Hurri found that antimalarials could be given with intramuscular gold, to therapeutic advantage, compared with antimalarials alone.[106] Side effects appeared additive and, in general, could be attributed to only one medication.[107]

A 1-year, randomized, controlled study of 101 patients compared standard doses of intramuscular gold (aurothiomalate) plus either placebo or hydroxychloroquine.[108] Twenty to 25 percent greater improvement was noted in the combination therapy group, which was statistically significant for a validated overall disease activity index, articular index, duration of morning stiffness, and C-reactive protein levels. Only two patients receiving combination therapy withdrew because of lack of effect, compared with five receiving gold. Adverse reactions were greater in patients receiving combination treatment, with 18 withdrawing, compared with five. Ten of 18 withdrawals were because of skin rashes.

Although intramuscular gold and antimalarials may be more effective than either alone, combination oral gold (auranofin) and hydroxychloroquine is not.[109] Nor does combination of either hydroxychloroquine[96] or chloroquine[101] with D-penicillamine confer any advantage over D-penicillamine alone.

Low-dose combined hydroxychloroquine, cyclophosphamide, and azathioprine therapy has been reported to be beneficial, but this trial was uncontrolled.[110] The toxicity that appeared to be associated primarily with cyclophosphamide limited this program. At least one study of combination methotrexate and hydroxychloroquine is currently under way (V. Stecher, personal communication).

A recent report from the American Rheumatism Association Medical Information System (ARAMIS) data bank found that combination of hydroxychloroquine with either aspirin or methotrexate was less frequently associated with elevated serum levels of liver enzymes compared with aspirin or methotrexate taken without hydroxychloroquine.[111] Unfortunately, this study, suggesting that combination with hydroxychloroquine prevents methotrexate liver toxicity, was uncontrolled and will need to be confirmed. Hydroxychloroquine may decrease corticosteroid toxicity by lessening the hyperlipidemic effect of the steroids.[112]

Other Connective Tissue Diseases

Seronegative Arthropathies

The reports of response of psoriatic arthritis and of the peripheral arthritis of ankylosing spondylitis to antimalarials are anecdotal. Several investigators have noted responses similar to those of rheumatoid arthritis.[6, 8] Kammer and coworkers[113] reported 68 percent benefit in 50 courses of hydroxychloroquine treatment of patients with psoriatic arthritis. Exacerbation of psoriatic skin lesions may occur with antimalarial treatment.[114]

Juvenile Rheumatoid Arthritis

Several groups have found antimalarials to be efficacious in treating juvenile rheumatoid arthritis.[115, 116] In an open, parallel study, hydroxychloroquine was equal in efficacy and was better tolerated than gold sodium thiomalate or D-penicillamine.[116] However, no placebo-treated control group was included. A collaborative placebo-controlled study found neither hydroxychloroquine nor D-penicillamine more effective than placebo.[117]

Palindromic Rheumatism

Chloroquine and hydroxychloroquine each have been reported to be beneficial in treating palindromic rheumatism in uncontrolled studies.[14-17] The largest series[17] reviewed 71 patients with an average follow-up of 3.6 years. Forty-seven were treated with chloroquine, and four with hydroxychloroquine. Forty-one patients responded with a 77 percent reduction in frequency and 63 percent reduction in duration of attacks.

Eosinophilic Fasciitis

Eosinophilic fasciitis has been successfully treated with antimalarials in uncontrolled studies.[18-20] In one series of 52 patients with this disease,[20] two of eight patients failing to respond to prednisone and two of eight who had not received prednisone had complete resolution with hydroxychloroquine treatment, whereas six had a partial response, one had no response, and 5 of the 16 patients treated with hydroxychloroquine were lost to follow-up. Responses occurred in 3 to 6 months on a daily dose of 200 or 400 mg.

Childhood Dermatomyositis

Hydroxychloroquine has been effective against childhood dermatomyositis[12, 13] in patients who had been unresponsive or partially responsive to corticosteroids. All seven patients in one report[12] had improvement of skin rash, with complete clearing in three. Myositis did not appear to improve, but corticosteroid dosage was tapered in two patients. A retrospective review of nine patients showed significant improvement in skin rash and in abdominal and proximal muscle strength.[13] After 6 months of treatment with hydroxychloroquine, prednisone dosage had been significantly reduced.

Sjögren's Syndrome

Laboratory abnormalities, including protein levels and serologic abnormalities, improved in two series of patients with Sjögren's syndrome treated with hydroxychloroquine,[118, 119] one of which had a control group.[118] Sedimentation rate fell and hemolgobin rose in treated patients.[118] Clinical findings were not assessed in one study,[118] and improvement in the other could not definitely be attributed to hydroxychloroquine.[119]

SIDE EFFECTS AND TOXICITY

After it was established that antimalarials could cause loss of vision, safety became the paramount issue and the major factor limiting antimalarial use.[3] Recent studies have shown an excellent safety profile, with few discontinuations due to side effects. Comparisons with other SAARDs have consistently shown greater safety for hydroxychloroquine. In analyses of drug withdrawal for toxicity, hydroxychloroquine was better tolerated than intramuscular gold,[98, 99] D-penicillamine, or levamisole.[99] Others also found antimalarials to have fewer side effects than did D-penicillamine[96, 101] or sulfasalazine.[97] Patients treated with oral gold withdrew more frequently for side effects than did those receiving hydroxychloroquine, because of gold-induced diarrhea.[113]

Meta-analysis of 71 drug placebo-controlled trials lasting at least 2 months that contained 128 treatment arms also suggests that antimalarials have less toxicity resulting in drug withdrawal than do other SAARDs or methotrexate.[87] The drop-out rate for antimalarials was 8.5 percent, which was lower than that for any other treatment. The difference was statistically significant compared with intramuscular gold, sulfasalazine, or penicillamine but not with oral gold or methotrexate.

Although hydroxychloroquine and chloroquine are relatively safe, the list of reported side effects is extensive (Table 44–3).

The incidence of untoward effects may vary widely, depending on daily dosage. Side effects were three times greater in patients receiving a daily dose of hydroxychloroquine of 400 mg compared with those receiving 200 mg.[32] Hydroxychloroquine has been found to be half as toxic as chloroquine on a weight basis.[8] Scherbel and colleagues[8] noted reactions in 440 (55 percent) of 805 patients treated with daily doses of 250 to 500 mg of chloroquine or 400 to 600 mg of hydroxychloroquine. Sixty-seven percent were transient reactions and disappeared spontaneously. Another 26 percent responded to reductions in dosage. Only 7 percent of reactions precluded further treatment. Bagnall[6] reported similar findings. Analysis of toxicity reported in double-blind studies suggests that open studies overestimate the incidence of side effects.[92, 94, 95]

Gastrointestinal side effects of antimalarial drugs may mimic those of nonsteroidal anti-inflammatory drugs and include epigastric burning, nausea, and vomiting, but antimalarials do not cause gastrointestinal bleeding. Nausea and anorexia may begin shortly after medication is started. Abdominal cramps, bloating, and diarrhea are more unique to antimalarials.[8, 79] Significantly fewer gastrointestinal reactions occur with hydroxychloroquine than with chloroquine.[8]

Rashes are the most common side effect leading to cessation of treatment. They occur with equal frequency in patients receiving chloroquine or hydroxychloroquine.[8] The lesions may be lichenoid, urticarial, morbilliform, or maculopapular. Patients with psoriatic arthritis may experience an exacerbation of psoriatic skin lesions,[114, 120, 121] although this was not observed in one series of 50 patients.[113] Occasionally, exfoliative dermatitis has been noted.[114, 120]

Pigmentary changes of skin or hair include either grayish hypopigmentation or blue-black hyperpigmentation.[8, 74] Alopecia may develop[8, 26] and must be differentiated from the alopecia that is a disease manifestation of lupus erythematosus.

The more frequently noted neurologic manifestations are often of little significance because of their mildness and reversibility when the daily dosages are lowered.[6] These include headaches, giddiness, insomnia, and nervousness.[6, 122, 123] A reversible myasthenic syndrome has been noted.[74] More important, but also uncommon, is a neuromuscular syndrome[124–126] that includes proximal lower extremity muscle weakness (which may start months after treatment is begun), normal CPK levels,[126] a neurogenic component,[125] and abnormal muscle and nerve biopsies.[124, 126] Biopsy changes may not be specific for drug toxicity[127] and also were present in two patients with antimalarial-induced cardiomyopathy.[128] Neuromyopathy may be confused with glucocorticoid-induced muscle weakness or may be attributed to the disease being treated.

Chloroquine and hydroxychloroquine may cause three types of ocular toxicity. Defects in accommodation or convergence may cause blurred vision or difficulty in quickly changing focus[122, 123] and are probably due to a central neural effect, but diplopia may result from extraocular muscle palsy.[129] A second problem, corneal deposits, may be associated with halos around lights.[130] Similar symptoms caused by corticosteroid-induced glaucoma must be differentiated. These problems are benign and reversible. They may even improve with continued drug use. The third ocular problem, retinal toxicity, is potentially serious because it may cause permanent loss of vision.

Table 44–3. TOXIC EFFECTS OF CHLOROQUINE AND HYDROXYCHLOROQUINE

Gastrointestinal
  Anorexia*[8]
  Abdominal bloating[8]
  Abdominal cramps[8]
  Diarrhea[8]
  Heartburn[8]
  Nausea[8]
  Vomiting[8]
  Weight loss
Skin and Hair[8, 26]
  Alopecia[8, 26]
  Bleaching of hair[8, 74]
  Dryness of skin[8]
  Exacerbation of psoriasis[114, 120]
  Increased pigmentation of skin and hair[74]
  Pruritus[8]
  Rashes[8, 114, 123]
    Exfoliative
    Lichenoid
    Maculopapular
    Morbilliform
    Urticarial
Neuromuscular
  Convulsive seizures[144]
  Difficulty in visual accommodation[129]
  Headache[8]
  Insomnia[8]
  Involuntary movements[145]
  Lassitude[8]
  Myasthenic reaction[74]
  Mental confusion[8]
  Nervousness or irritability[8]
  Neuromyopathy[124–126]
  Ototoxicity
    Nerve deafness[8, 146, 147]
    Tinnitus[8, 146]
  Polyneuropathy[26]
  Toxic psychosis[148, 149]
  Vestibular dysfunction[8, 140]
  Weakness[122]

Ocular
  Corneal deposits[7, 130]
    Halos around lights
  Diplopia‡
  Defects in accommodation and convergence‡[129]
    Various mild visual difficulties[74, 123]
  Loss of corneal reflex[150, 151]
  Retinopathy[9, 10, 104, 131–136, 139]
    Loss of vision
    Pigment abnormalities
    Scotomata
    Visual field abnormalities
Miscellaneous
  Birth defects†[152]
  Blood dyscrasias
    Leukopenia[6, 78]
    Agranulocytosis[153, 154]
    Aplastic anemia[155]
    Leukemia[156]
  Death from overdosage[35, 140]
    Peripheral circulatory collapse
  Heart
    Electrocardiographic changes[123]
    Cardiomyopathy[35, 128, 157]
    Precipitation of porphyria[158]

*References for toxic effects are selected, some side effects are not discussed in text.
†Effect not conclusively related to medication.
‡May be neuromuscular toxic effect.

Retinopathy has been extensively reviewed in other textbook editions.[3] Hydroxychloroquine has caused fewer cases of retinopathy than has chloroquine. Bernstein[131] has found only 18 cases of true visual loss with hydroxychloroquine, and patients often received daily doses greater than those currently recommended.

Recent studies show that low daily dose and regular ophthalmologic examinations using the protocol outlined in Table 44–4 will prevent visual loss even with long-term treatment.[10, 11, 132]

Characteristic changes of antimalarial retinopathy include pigmentary stippling, mottling, or clumping and, occasionally, the classic bull's-eye lesion. Visual acuity may be decreased in association with central scotomata, peripheral field constriction, and, later, more dense field loss.

Retinal lesions can be divided into two groups. Those that have been termed premaculopathy[104] show mild pigmentary stippling or loss of visual field to a red test object and are generally reversible when the medication is discontinued.[10, 133, 134] True retinopathy is much more serious. Pigment changes are more prominent, often revealing a bull's-eye lesion. Loss of vision is almost always present, rarely improves, and may even progress after treatment is discontinued.[134–136] Although it is believed that premaculopathy may presage more severe changes if medication is continued, there are no cases in which premaculopathy has progressed to true retinopathy.[131]

Histologic examination shows loss of rods and cones and migration of clumps of pigment.[137] Speculation about the etiology of retinopathy centers on the binding of 4-aminoquinolines to melanin of the retinal pigment epithelium (RPE) or on lysosomal dysfunction, with subsequent diminution of RPE protective function[137] and eventual visual loss.

Newer methods to evaluate retinal toxicity appear promising. Studies are under way to assess whether patient self-testing with Amsler grids[138] or automated visual fields will be more sensitive with-

Table 44–4. OPHTHALMOLOGIC SAFETY GUIDELINES FOR ANTIMALARIAL DRUGS

Daily Dose	
Hydroxychloroquine	400 mg or 6.5 mg/kg
Chloroquine	250 mg or 4 mg/kg
Ophthalmologic Monitoring	
Frequency	Baseline, then every 6 months
Protocol for evaluation	Question patient about visual disturbance
	Determine best-corrected visual acuity
	Examine fundus for pigmentary abnormalities
	Assess visual fields with a 5-mm red test object; use 3-mm white test object at baseline and if red test object fields are abnormal
Adjunct methods of evaluation	Amsler grid (self-testing)
	Automated visual fields

out loss of specificity (V. Stecher, personal communication).

GUIDELINES FOR USE OF ANTIMALARIALS

Antimalarials may be used as the initial SAARD in patients with RA who respond insufficiently to nonsteroidal anti-inflammatory medications. Any difference in effectiveness is offset by the superior safety record of antimalarials, with decreased side effects and fewer treatment terminations for toxicity.[87, 96–99, 108–110] Another advantage is the lower cost of monitoring for toxicity. Although an ophthalmologic examination should be performed every 6 months, routine hematologic and urinary monitoring are not necessary. After the drug has been found to be well tolerated, the patient need not visit the physician more frequently than indicated by disease severity. A treatment course should not be considered to have failed until it has been tried for at least 6 months. Plasma levels do not appear to predict clinical response.[139]

Antimalarials have an important role in the treatment of skin lesions, articular disease, fever, and malaise in patients with lupus erythematosus. They have been shown to prevent flare-ups of systemic disease.[81, 82] Hydroxychloroquine may be started when the diagnosis is established and may be continued indefinitely to prevent disease flare-ups.[82] Alternatively, antimalarials may be used only in patients with those manifestations shown to be drug responsive and may be taken intermittently when the disease is active. This is especially attractive for discoid lupus erythematosus. Quinacrine in dosages of 100 mg per day may be helpful in treating resistant discoid lesions.[74, 78]

Antimalarials may be used with benefit in patients with other inflammatory arthritides and rheumatic diseases, such as eosinophilic fasciitis,[18–20] palindromic rheumatism,[14–26] childhood dermatomyositis,[12, 13] and, perhaps, Sjögren's syndrome.[118, 119]

Patients with psoriatic arthritis should be warned that their skin lesions may flare up, and they should be monitored carefully during the initial 3 months of treatment.[121] However, the potential exacerbation of skin lesions should not be considered an absolute contraindication in such patients.[113]

Effectiveness in juvenile chronic arthritis is under question.[115, 117] If antimalarials are used to treat juvenile chronic arthritis, modification of dosage, depending on the patient's weight, is mandatory.[140] It is important to remember that children are quite sensitive to antimalarial overdose. Death has resulted from ingestion of as little as 1 g (4 tablets) of chloroquine.[141]

Even with the currently recommended daily doses, retinal toxicity may occur[131, 139] and ophthalmologic examinations should be conducted regularly to detect mild changes that are reversible (see Table 44–4). If funduscopic examination shows pigmentary changes or if visual field examination demonstrates a 5-degree constriction compared with baseline or a paracentral scotoma, the medication should be discontinued. Even though this conservative ophthalmologic protocol may occasionally deny antimalarial treatment to some patients who have changes unrelated to medication,[131] strict adherence has prevented loss of vision in all patients so monitored.[10, 132]

Antimalarials are not recommended for use during pregnancy because there have been rare reports of birth defects involving loss of hearing.[142] However, it is unlikely that antimalarials present great risk to the fetus. Parke[143] has reported a number of successful births of healthy children by women treated with antimalarials.

References

1. Webster, L. T.: Drugs used in the chemotherapy of protozoal infections, malaria. In Gilman, A. J., Goodman, L. S., Rall, T. W., and Murad, E. (eds.): The Pharmacological Basis of Therapeutics. 7th ed. New York, Macmillan Publishing Co., 1985, pp. 1029–1048.
2. Payne, J. P.: A post-graduate lecture on lupus erythematosus. Clin. J. 4:223, 1894.
3. Rynes, R. I.: Antimalarials. In Kelley, W. N., et al. (eds.): Textbook of Rheumatology. 2nd ed. Philadelphia, W. B. Saunders Company, 1985.
4. Page, F.: Treatment of lupus erythematosus with mepacrine. Lancet 2:755, 1951.
5. Freedman, A., and Bach, F.: Mepacrine and rheumatoid arthritis. Lancet 2:231, 1952.
6. Bagnall, A. W.: The value of chloroquine in rheumatoid disease—a four-year study of continuous therapy. Can. Med. Assoc. J. 77:182, 1957.
7. Kersley, G. D., and Palin, A. G.: Amodiaquine and hydroxychloroquine in rheumatoid arthritis. Lancet 2:886, 1959.
8. Scherbel, A. L., Harrison, J. W., and Atdjian, M.: Further observations on the use of 4-aminoquinoline compounds in patients with rheumatoid arthritis or related diseases. Cleve. Clin. Q. 25:95, 1958.
9. Hobbs, H. E., Sorsby, A., and Freedman, A.: Retinopathy following chloroquine therapy. Lancet 2:478, 1959.
10. Tobin, D. R., Krohel, G. B., and Rynes, R. I.: Hydroxychloroquine. A seven-year experience. Arch. Ophthalmol. 100:81, 1982.
11. Mackenzie, A. H.: Dose refinements in long-term therapy of rheumatoid arthritis with antimalarials. Am. J. Med. 75:40(Suppl July 18), 1983.
12. Woo, T. Y., Callen, J. P., Voorhees, J. J., Bickers, D. R., Hanno, R.,

and Hawkins, C.: Cutaneous lesions of dermatomyositis are improved by hydroxychloroquine. J. Am. Acad. Dermatol. 10(4):592, 1984.

13. Olson, N. Y., and Lindlsey, C. B.: Adjunctive use of hydroxychloroquine in childhood dermatomyositis. J. Rheumatol. 16:12, 1989.

14. Mattingly, S., Jones, D. W., Robinson, W. M., et al.: Palindromic rheumatism. J. R. Coll. Phys. 15:119, 1981.

15. Golding, D. N.: D-Penicillamine in palindromic rheumatism. Br. Med. J. 2:1382, 1976.

16. Hannonen, P., Mottonen, T., and Oka, M.: Treatment of palindromic rheumatism with chloroquine. Br. Med. J. 294:1289, 1987.

17. Youssef, W., Yan, A., and Russell, A.: Palindromic rheumatism: a response to chloroquine. J Rheumatol. 18:1, 1991.

18. Michet, C. J., Jr., Doyle, J. A., and Ginsburg, W. W.: Eosinophilic fasciitis: Report of 15 cases. Mayo Clin. Proc. 56:27, 1981.

19. Bidula, L. P., and Myers, A. R.: Eosinophilic fasciitis associated with hematologic disorders: Case reports and a review of the literature. Clin. Rheumatol. Pract. 3:117, 1985.

20. Lakhanpal, S., Ginsburg, W. W., Michet, C. J., Doyle, J. A., and Breanndan Moore, S.: Eosinophilic fasciitis: Clinical spectrum and therapeutic response in 52 cases. Semin. Arthritis Rheum. 17:221, 1988.

21. Charous, B. L.: Open study of hydroxychloroquine in the treatment of severe symptomatic or corticosteroid-dependent asthma. Ann. Allergy 65:58, 1990.

22. Bellamy, N., and Brooks, P. M.: Current practice in antimalarial drug prescribing in rheumatoid arthritis. J. Rheumatol. 13:551, 1986.

23. McChesney, E. W., Conway, W. D., Banks, W. F., Jr., Rogers, J. E., and Shekosky, J. M.: Studies on the metabolism of some compounds of the 4-amino-7-chloroquinoline series. J. Pharmacol. Exp. Ther. 151:482, 1966.

24. Rubin, M.: The antimalarials and tranquilizers. Dis. Nerv. Syst. (Suppl.) 29:67, 1968.

25. McChesney, E. W., Fasco, M. J., and Banks, W. F., Jr.: The metabolism of chloroquine in man during and after repeated oral dosage. J. Pharmacol. Exp. Ther. 158:323, 1967.

26. Frisk-Holmberg, M., Bergkvist, Y., Domeigj-Nyberg, B., Hellstrom, L., and Jansson, F.: Chloroquine serum concentration and side effects: Evidence of dose-dependent kinetics. Clin. Pharmacol. Ther. 25:345, 1979.

27. McChesney, E. W., Banks, W. F., Jr., and McAuliff, J. P.: Laboratory studies of the 4-aminoquinoline antimalarials. II. Plasma levels of chloroquine and hydroxychloroquine after various oral dosage regimens. Antibiot. Chemother. 12:583, 1962.

28. Zvaifler, N. J., and Rubin, M.: The metabolism of chloroquine (abstract). Arthritis Rheum. 5:330, 1962.

29. Frisk-Holmberg, M.: Variation in chloroquine pharmacokinetics due to assay sensitivity and duration of sampling. Eur. J. Clin. Pharmacol. 31:743, 1987.

30. McChesney, E. W., and Rothfield, N. F.: Comparative metabolic studies of chloroquine and hydroxychloroquine (abstract). Arthritis Rheum. 7:328, 1964.

31. Tett, S. E., Cutler, D. J., and Day, R. O.: Hydroxychloroquine concentrations and clinical effects in rheumatoid arthritis patients. Eur. J. Pharmacol. 183:1035, 1990.

32. Pavelka, K., Jr., Pavelka Sen, K., Peliskova, Z., Vacha, J., and Trnavsky, K.: Hydroxychloroquine sulphate in the treatment of rheumatoid arthritis: a double-blind comparison of two dose regimens. Ann. Rheum. Dis. 48:542, 1989.

33. Rubin, M., Bernstein, H. N., and Zvaifler, N. J.: Studies on the pharmacology of chloroquine. Arch. Ophthalmol. 70:474, 1962.

34. McChesney, E. W., Banks, W. F., Jr., Fabian, R. J.: Tissue distribution of chloroquine, hydroxychloroquine and desethylchloroquine in the rat. Toxicol. Appl. Pharmacol. 10:501, 1967.

35. Kiel, F. W.: Chloroquine suicide. J.A.M.A. 190:398, 1964.

36. Prouty, R. W., and Kuroda, K.: Spectrophotometric determination and distribution of chloroquine in human tissues. J. Lab. Clin. Med. 52:477, 1958.

37. French, J. K., Hurst, N. P., O'Donnell, M. L., and Betts, W. H.: Uptake of chloroquine and hydroxychloroquine by human blood leucocytes in vitro: Relation to cellular concentrations during antirheumatic therapy. Ann. Rheum. Dis. 46:42, 1987.

38. Vargo, F.: Intracellular localization of chloroquine in the liver and kidney of the rat. Acta Physiol. Acad. Sci. Hung. 34:327, 1968.

39. Bernstein, H., Zvaifler, N., Rubin, M., and Mansour, A. M.: The ocular deposition of chloroquine. Invest. Ophthalmol. 2:384, 1963.

40. Sams, W. M.: Chloroquine: Mechanism of action. Mayo Clin. Proc. 42:300, 1967.

41. Matsuzawa, Y., and Hostetler, K. Y.: Inhibition of lysosomal phospholipase A and phospholipase C by chloroquine and 4,4-bis-(diethylaminoethoxy)-α,β-diethyldiphenylethane. J. Biol. Chem. 255:5190, 1980.

42. Wada, A., Saktrai, S., Kobayashi, H., Yanangihara, N., and Izumi, F.: Suppression by phospholipase A$_2$ inhibitors of secretion of catecholamines from isolated medullary cells by suppression of cellular calcium uptake. Biochem. Pharmacol. 32:1175, 1983.

43. Greaves, M. W. S., and McDonald-Gibson, W.: Effect of nonsteroidal antiinflammatory drugs and antipyretic drugs on prostaglandin biosynthesis by human skin. J. Invest. Dermatol. 61:127, 1973.

44. Kench, J. G., Seale, J. P., Temple, D. M., and Tennant, C.: The effects of nonsteroidal inhibitors of phospholipase A$_2$ on leukotriene and histamine release from human and guinea-pig lung. Prostaglandins 30:199, 1985.

45. Weissman, G.: Labilization and stabilization of lysosomes. Fed. Proc. 23:1038, 1984.

46. Ohkuma, S., and Poole, B.: Cytoplasmic vacuolation of mouse peritoneal macrophages and the uptake into lysosomes of weakly basic substances. J. Cell. Biol. 90:656, 1981.

47. Poole, B., and Ohkuma, S.: Effect of weak bases on the intralysosomal pH in mouse peritoneal macrophages. J. Cell. Biol. 90:665, 1981.

48. Jones, C. P., and Jayson, M. I. V.: Chloroquine: Its effect on leukocyte auto- and heterophagocytosis. Ann. Rheum. Dis. 43:205, 1984.

49. Gonzalez-Noriega, A., Grubb, J. H., Talkad, V., and Sly, W. S.: Chloroquine inhibits lysosomal enzyme pinocytosis and enhances lysosomal enzyme secretion by impairing receptor recycling. J. Cell. Biol. 85:839, 1980.

50. Tietse, C., Schlessinger, P., and Stahl, P.: Chloroquine and ammonium can inhibit receptor-mediated endocytosis of mannose-glycoconjugates by macrophages; apparent inhibition of receptor recycling. Biochem. Biophys. Res. Commun. 93:1, 1980.

51. Oda, K., Koriyama, Y., Yamada, E., and Ikehara, Y.: Effects of weakly basic amines on proteolytic processing and terminal glycosylation of secretory proteins in cultured rat hepatocytes. Biochem. J. 240:739, 1986.

52. McChesney, E. W., Nachod, F. C., and Tainter, M. L.: Rationale for treatment of lupus erythematosus with antimalarials. J. Invest. Dermatol. 29:97, 1957.

53. Lester, R. S., Burnham, T. K., Fine, G., et al.: Immunologic concepts of light reactions in lupus erythematosus and polymorphous light eruptions. Arch. Dermatol. 96:1, 1967.

54. Cahn, M. M., Levy, E. J., and Shaffer, B.: Polymorphous light eruption: Effect of chloroquine phosphate in modifying reactions to ultraviolet light. J. Invest. Dermatol. 26:201, 1956.

55. Shaffer, B., Cahn, M. M., and Levy, E. J.: Absorption of antimalarial drugs in human skin: Spectroscopic and chemical analysis in epidermis and corium. J. Invest. Dermatol. 30:341, 1958.

56. Thompson, G. R., and Bartholomew, L. E.: The effect of chloroquine on antibody formation. Univ. Mich. Med. Cent. J. 30:227, 1964.

57. Kalmonson, G. M., and Gage, I. G.: Effects of hydroxychloroquine on immune mechanisms. Clin. Res. 11:106, 1963.

58. Szilagyi, T., and Kavai, M.: The effect of chloroquine on the antigen-antibody reaction. Acta Physiol. Acad. Sci. Hung. 38:411, 1970.

59. Holtz, G., Mantel, W., and Buck, W.: The inhibition of antigen-antibodies reactions by chloroquine and its mechanism of action. A. Immunitaetsforsch. 146:145, 1973.

60. Segal-Eiras, A., Segura, G. M., Babini, J. C., Arturi, A. S., Fraguela, M. J., and Marcos, J. C.: Effect of antimalarial treatment on circulating immune complexes in rheumatoid arthritis. J. Rhematol. 12:87, 1985.

61. Hurvitz, D., and Hirschhorn, K.: Suppression of "in vitro" lymphocyte responses by chloroquine. N. Engl. J. Med. 273:23, 1965.

62. Panayi, G. S., Neill, W. A., Duthie, J., Jr., and McCormick, J. N.: Action of chloroquine phosphate in rheumatoid arthritis. I. Immunosuppresive effect. Ann. Rheum. Dis. 32:316, 1973.

63. Ausiello, C., Sorrentino, V., Ruggiero, V., and Rossi, G. B.: Action of lysosomotropic amines on spontaneous and interferon-enhanced NK and CTL cytolysis. Immunol. Lett. 8:11, 1984.

64. Ausiello, C. M., Barbieri, P., Spagnoli, G. C., Ciompi, M. L., and Casciani, C. U.: In vivo effects of chloroquine treatment on spontaneous and interferon-induced natural killer activities in rheumatoid arthritis patients. Clin. Exp. Rheumatol. 1:255, 1986.

65. Salmeron, G., and Lipsky, P. E.: Immunosuppressive potential of antimalarials. Am. J. Med. 75(Suppl. July 18):19, 1983.

66. Baker, D. G., Baumgarten, D. F., and Dwyer, J. P.: Chloroquine inhibits the production of a mononuclear cell factor by inhibition of lectin binding. Arthritis Rheum. 27:888, 1984.

67. Rainsford, K. D.: Effects of anti-inflammatory drugs on catabalin-induced cartilage destruction in vitro. Int. J. Tissue React. 7:123, 1985.

68. Cohen, S. N., and Yielding, K. L.: Spectrophotometric studies of the interaction of chloroquine and deoxyribonucleic acid. J. Biol. Chem. 240:3123, 1965.

69. Kurnick, N. B., and Radcliffe, I. E.: Reactions between DNA and quinacrine and other antimalarials. J. Lab. Clin. Med. 60:669, 1962.

70. Cohen, S. N., and Yielding, K. L.: Inhibition of DNA and RNA polymerase reactions by chloroquine. Proc. Natl. Acad. Sci. U.S.A. 54:521, 1965.

71. Ciak, J., and Hahn, F. E.: Chloroquine: Mode of action. Science 151:347, 1966.

72. Stoller, D., and Levine, L.: Antibodies to denatured DNA in lupus erythematosus serum. V. Mechanism of DNA–anti-DNA inhibition by chloroquine. Arch. Biochem. 101:355, 1963.

73. Dubois, E. L.: Effect of quinacrine (Atabrine) upon lupus erythematosus phenomenon. Arch. Dermatol. 71:570, 1955.
74. Dubois, E.: Antimalarials in the management of discoid and systemic lupus erythematosus. Semin. Arthritis Rheum. 8:33, 1978.
75. Mullins, J. F., Watts, F. L., and Wilson, C. J.: Plaquenil in the treatment of lupus erythematosus. J.A.M.A. 161:879, 1956.
76. Crissey, J. T., and Murray, P. F.: A comparison of chloroquine and gold in the treatment of lupus erythematosus. Arch. Dermatol. 74:69, 1956.
77. Kraak, J. H., vanKetel, W. G., Prakken, J. R., and vanZwet, W. R.: The value of hydroxychloroquine (Plaquenil) for the treatment of chronic discoid lupus erythematosus: A double-blind trial. Dermatologica 130:293, 1965.
78. Winkelman, R. K., Merwin, C. F., and Brunsting, L. A.: Antimalarial therapy of lupus erythematosus. Ann. Intern. Med. 55:772, 1961.
79. Goldman, L., Cole, D. P., and Preston, R. H.: Chloroquine diphosphate in the treatment of discoid lupus erythematosus. J.A.M.A. 152:1428, 1953.
80. Rogers, J., and Finn, O. A.: Synthetic antimalarial drugs in chronic discoid lupus erythematosus and light eruptions. Arch. Dermatol. Syph. 70:61, 1954.
81. Rudnicki, R. D., Gresham, G. E., and Rothfield, N. F.: The efficacy of antimalarials in systemic lupus erythematosus. J. Rheumatol. 2:323, 1975.
82. The Canadian Hydroxychloroquine Study Group: A randomized study of the effect of withdrawing hydroxychloroquine sulfate in systemic lupus erythematosus. N. Engl. J. Med. 324:150, 1991.
83. Dubois, E. L.: Quinacrine (Atabrine) in treatment of systemic and discoid lupus erythematosus. Arch. Intern. Med. 94:131, 1954.
84. Ziff, M., Esserman, P., and McEwen, C.: Observations on the course and treatment of systemic lupus erythematosus. Arthritis Rheum. 1:332, 1956.
85. Conte, J. J., Mignon-Conte, M. A., and Fournie, G. J.: Lupus nephritis: Treatment with indomethacin-hydroxychloroquine combination and comparison with corticosteroid treatment. Nouv. Presse Med. 4:91, 1975.
86. Adams, E. M., Yocum, D. E., and Bell, C. L.: Hydroxychloroquine in the treatment of rheumatoid arthritis. Am. J. Med. 75:321, 1983.
87. Felson, D. T., Anderson, J. J., and Meenan, R. F.: The comparative efficacy and toxicity of second-line drugs in rheumatoid arthritis. Arthritis Rheum. Vol 33(10):1990.
88. Cohen, A. S., and Calkins, E.: A controlled study of chloroquine as an antirheumatic agent. Arthritis Rheum. 1:297, 1958.
89. Popert, A. J., Meijers, K. A. E., Sharp, J., and Bier, F.: Chloroquine diphosphate in rheumatoid arthritis. A controlled study. Ann. Rheum. Dis. 20:18, 1961.
90. Freedman, A.: Chloroquine and rheumatoid arthritis. Short-term controlled trial. Ann. Rheum. Dis. 15:251, 1965.
91. Rinehart, R. E., Rosenbaum, E. E., and Hopkins, C. E.: Chloroquine therapy in rheumatoid arthritis. Northwest. Med. 56:703, 1957.
92. Freedman, A., and Steinberg, V. L.: Chloroquine in rheumatoid arthritis, a double-blindfold trial of treatment for one year. Ann. Rheum. Dis. 19:243, 1960.
93. Hamilton, E. B. D., and Scott, J. T.: Hydroxychloroquine sulfate (Plaquenil) in treatment of rheumatoid arthritis. Arthritis Rheum. 5:502, 1962.
94. Mainland, D., and Sutcliffe, M. I.: Hydroxychloroquine sulfate in rheumatoid arthritis, a six-month, double-blind trial. Bull. Rheum. Dis. 13:287, 1957.
95. Davis, M. J., Dawes, P. T., Fowler, P. D., Clarke, S., Fisher, J., and Shadforth, M. F.: Should disease-modifying agents be used in mild rheumatoid arthritis? Br. J. Rheumatol. 30:451, 1991.
96. Bunch, T. W., O'Duffy, J. D., Tompkins, R. B., and O'Fallon, W. M.: Controlled trial of hydroxychloroquine and D-penicillamine singly and in combination in the treatment of rheumatoid arthritis. Arthritis Rheum. 27:267, 1984.
97. Nuver-Zwart, I. H., VanRiel, P. L. C. M., VanDePutte, L. V. A., and Gribnau, F. W. J.: A double-blind comparative study of sulphasalazine and hydroxychloroquine in rheumatoid arthritis: evidence of an earlier effect of sulphasalazine. Ann. Rheum. Dis. 48:389, 1989.
98. Richter, J. A., Runge, L. A., Pinals, R. S., and Oates, R. P.: Analysis of treatment termination with gold and antimalarial compounds in rheumatoid arthritis. J. Rheum. 7:153, 1980.
99. Husain, Z., and Runge, L. A.: Treatment complications of rheumatoid arthritis with gold, hydroxychloroquine, D-penicillamine, and levamisole. J. Rheumatol. 7:825, 1980.
100. Dwosh, I. L., Stein, H. B., Urowitz, M. B., Smythe, H. A., Hunter, T., and Ogryzlo, M. A.: Azathioprine in early rheumatoid arthritis: Comparison with gold and chloroquine. Arthritis Rheum 20:685, 1977.
100a. Bird, H. A., LeGallez, P., Dixon, J. S., et al.: A single-blind comparative study of auranofin and hydroxychloroquine in patients with rheumatoid arthritis. Clin. Rheumatol. 3(Suppl. 1):57, 1984.
101. Gibson, T., Emery, P., Armstrong, R. D., Crisp, A. J., and Panayi, G. S.: Combined D-penicillamine and chloroquine treatment of rheumatoid arthritis: a comparative study. Br. J. Rheumatol. 26:279, 1987.
101a. Fowler, P. D., Shadforth, M. F., Crook, P. R., and Lawton, A.: Report on chloroquine and dapsone in the treatment of rheumatoid arthritis: A 6-month comparative study. Ann. Rheum. Dis. 43:200, 1984.
102. VanderHeijde, D. M., VanRiel, P. L., Zuver-Zwart, I. H., Gribnau, F. W., and VanDePutte, L. B.: Effects of hydroxychloroquine and sulphasalazine on progression of joint damage in rheumatoid arthritis. Lancet 1:1036, 1989.
103. VanderHeijde, D. M., VanRiel, P. L., Nuver-Zwart, I. H., VanDePutte L. B.: Sulphasalazine versus hydroxychloroquine in rheumatoid arthritis: 3-year follow-up. Lancet 335:539, 1990.
104. Kremer, J. M., and Lee, J. K.: The safety and efficacy of the use of methotrexate in long-term therapy for rheumatoid arthritis. Arthritis Rheum. 29:822, 1986.
105. Wilske, K. R., and Healey, L. A.: Remodeling the pyramid—a concept whose time has come. J. Rheumatol. 16:565, 1989.
106. Sievers, K., and Hurri, L.: Combined therapy of rheumatoid arthritis with gold and chloroquine. I. Evaluation of therapeutic effect. Acta Rheumatol. Scand. 9:48, 1963.
107. Sievers, K., Hurri, L., and Sievers, U. M.: Combined therapy of rheumatoid arthritis with gold and chloroquine. II. Evaluation of side effects. Acta Rheumatol. Scand. 9:56, 1963.
108. Scott, D. L., Dawes, P. T., Tunn, E., Fowler, P. D., Shadforth, M. F., Fisher, J., Clarke, S., Collins, M., Jones, P., Popert, A. J., and Bacon, P. A.: Combination therapy with gold and hydroxychloroquine in rheumatoid arthritis: a prospective, randomized, placebo-controlled study. Br. J. Rheumatol. 28:128, 1989.
109. Luthra, H. S., the Midwest Cooperative Rheumatic Disease Study Group: Double-blind study comparing auranofin (AU) and hydroxychloroquine (HCQ) alone or in combination (AU + HCQ) in rheumatoid arthritis. Arthritis Rheum. 33(Suppl.):S25, 1990.
110. Csuka, M. D., Carrera, G. M., and McCarty, D. J.: Treatment of intractable rheumatoid arthritis with combined cyclophosphamide, azathioprine, and hydroxychloroquine. J.A.M.A. 255:2315, 1986.
111. Fries, J. R., Gurkirpal, S., Lenert, L., and Furst, D. E.: Aspirin, hydroxychloroquine and hepatic enzyme abnormalities with methotrexate in rheumatoid arthritis. Arthritis Rheum. 33:1611, 1990.
112. Wallace, D. J., Metzger, A. L., Stecher, V. J., Turnbull, B. A., and Kern, P. A.: Cholesterol-lowering effect of hydroxychloroquine (Plaquenil) in rheumatic disease patients. Reversal of deleterious effects of steroids on lipids. Am. J. Med. 89:322, 1990.
113. Kammer, G. M., Soter, N. A., Gibson, D. J., and Schur, P. H.: Psoriatic arthritis: A clinical, immunologic, and HLA study of 100 patients. Semin. Arthritis Rheum. 9:75, 1979.
114. Cornbleet, T.: Action of synthetic antimalarial drugs on psoriasis. J. Invest. Dermatol. 26:435, 1956.
115. Kvien, T. K., Hoyeraal, H. M., and Sandstad, B.: Slow-acting antirheumatic drugs in patients with juvenile rheumatoid arthritis evaluated in a randomized, parallel 50-week clinical trial. J. Rheumatol. 12:533, 1985.
116. Manners, P. J., and Ansell, B. M.: Slow-acting antirheumatic drug use in systemic onset juvenile chronic arthritis. Pediatrics 77:99, 1986.
117. Brewer, E. J., Giannini, E. H., Kuzima, N., and Alekseev, L.: Penicillamine and hydroxychloroquine in the treatment of severe juvenile rheumatoid arthritis. N. Engl. J. Med. 315:1269, 1986.
118. Fox, R. I., Chan, E., Benton, L., Fong, S., Friedlaender, M., and Howel, F. V.: Treatment of primary Sjögren's syndrome with hydroxychloroquine. Am. J. Med. 85:62, 1988.
119. Auvergne, B., Liote, R., Roucoules, J., and Kuntz, D.: Pyrazinamide, hyperuricemie et arthrite goutteuse. Rev. Rhum. 55:797, 1988.
120. Reed, W. B.: Psoriatic arthritis. A complete study of 86 patients. Acta Dermatol. Venereol. 41:396, 1961.
121. Juozevicius, J. L., and Rynes, R. I.: Treatment of psoriatic arthritis with hydroxychloroquine: Favorable response but increased dermatologic toxicity (abstract). Arthritis Rheum. 28(Suppl.):S98, 1985.
122. Berliner, R. W., Earle, D. P., Jr., Taggert, J. V., Zubrod, C. G., Welch, W. J., Conan, N. J., Bauman, E., Scuddar, S. T., and Schannon, J. A.: Studies on the chemotherapy of human malarias. VI. The physiological deposition, antimalarial activity and toxicity of several derivatives of 4-aminoquinolines. J. Clin. Invest. 27(Suppl.):98, 1948.
123. Alving, A. S., Eichelberger, C. B., Jr., Jones, J. R., Wharton, C. M., and Pullman, T. N.: Studies on the chronic toxicity of chloroquine (SN-7618). J. Clin. Invest. (Suppl.) 27:60, 1948.
124. Estes, M. L., Ewing-Wilson, D., Chou, S. M., Mitsumoto, H., Hanson, M., Shirey, E., and Ratliff, N. B.: Chloroquine neuromyotoxicity, clinical and pathologic perspective. Am. J. Med. 82:447, 1987.
125. Whisnant, J. P., Espinosa, R. E., Kierland, R. R., and Lambert, E. H.: Chloroquine neuropathy. Proc. Mayo Clin. 38:501, 1963.
126. Hicklin, J. A.: Chloroquine neuromyopathy. Ann. Phys. Med. 9:189, 1968.
127. Pearson, C. M., and Yamazaki, J. N.: Vacuolar myopathy in systemic lupus erythematosus. Am. J. Clin. Pathol. 29:455, 1958.
128. Ratliff, N. B., Estes, M. L., Myles, J. L., Shirey, E. K., and McMahon, J. T.: Diagnosis of chloroquine cardiomyopathy by endomyocardial biopsy. N. Engl. J. Med. 316:191, 1987.

129. Rubin, M. L., Thomas, W. C., Jr.: Diplopia and loss of accommodation due to chloroquine. Arthritis Rheum. 13:75, 1970.
130. Hobbs, H. E., and Calnan, C. D.: The ocular complications of chloroquine therapy. Lancet 1:1207, 1958.
131. Bernstein, H. N.: Ocular safety of hydroxychloroquine. Ann. Ophthalmol. 23:292, 1991.
132. Rynes, R. I., Krohel, G., Falbo, A., Reinecke, R. D., Wolfe, B., and Bartholomew, L. E.: Ophthalmologic safety of long-term hydroxychloroquine treatment. Arthritis Rheum. 22:832, 1979.
133. Arden, G. B., and Kolb, H.: Antimalarial therapy and early retinal changes in patients with rheumatoid arthritis. Br. Med. J. 1:270, 1966.
134. Okun, G., Gouras, P., Bernstein, H., and VonSallmann, L.: Chloroquine retinopathy. Arch. Ophthalmol. 69:59, 1963.
135. Nylander, U.: Ocular damage in chloroquine therapy. Acta Ophthalmol. 44:335, 1966.
136. Burns, R. P.: Delayed onset of chloroquine retinopathy. N. Engl. J. Med. 275:6983, 1966.
137. Bernstein, H. N., and Ginsberg, J.: The pathology of chloroquine retinopathy. Arch. Ophthalmol. 71:238, 1964.
138. Easterbrook, M.: The use of Amsler grids in early chloroquine retinopathy. Ophthalmology 91:1368, 1984.
139. Easterbrook, M.: Dose relationships in patients with early chloroquine retinopathy. J. Rheumatol. 14:472, 1987.
140. Laaksonen, A. L., Koshiahyde, V., and Juva, K.: Dosage of antimalarial drugs for children with juvenile rheumatoid arthritis and systemic lupus erythematosus. Scand. J. Rheumatol. 3:103, 1974.
141. Cann, H. M., and Verhulst, H. L.: Fatal acute chloroquine poisoning in children. Pediatrics 27:95, 1961.
142. Hart, C. W., and Naunton, R. F.: The ototoxicity of chloroquine phosphate. Arch. Otolaryngol. 80:407, 1964.
143. Parke, A. L.: Antimalarial drugs, systemic lupus erythematosus, and pregnancy. J. Rheumatol. 15:607, 1988.
144. Torrey, E. F.: Chloroquine seizures. J.A.M.A. 204:867, 1968.
145. Umez-Eronimi, E. M., and Eronimi, E. A.: Chloroquine-induced involuntary movements. Br. Med. J. 1:945, 1977.
146. Dewar, W. A., and Mann, H. M.: Chloroquine in lupus erythematosus (letter). Lancet 1:780, 1954.
147. Mukherjee, D. K.: Chloroquine ototoxicity—a reversible phenomenon? J. Laryngol. Otol. 93:809, 1979.
148. Burrell, Z. L., and Marintez, A. C.: Chloroquine and hydroxychloroquine in the treatment of arrhythmias. N. Engl. J. Med. 258:798, 1958.
149. Rab, S. M.: Two cases of chloroquine psychoses. Br. Med. J. 1:275, 1963.
150. Percival, S. P. B., and Behrman, J.: Ophthalmological safety of chloroquine. Br. J. Ophthalmol. 53:101, 1969.
151. Henkind, P., and Rothfield, N. F.: Ocular abnormalities in patients treated with synthetic antimalarial drugs. N. Engl. J. Med. 269:433, 1963.
152. Hart, C. W., and Naunton, R. F.: The ototoxicity of chloroquine phosphate. Arch. Otolaryngol. 80:407, 1964.
153. Polano, M. K., Cats, A., and vanOlder, G. A. J.: Agranulocytosis following treatment with hydroxychloroquine sulphate. Lancet 1:1275, 1965.
154. Propp, R. P., and Stillman, J. S.: Correspondence: Report of a non-fatal case of agranulocytosis on hydroxychloroquine therapy. N. Engl. J. Med. 277:492, 1967.
155. Nagaratnam, N., Chetiyawardana, A. N., and Rajiyah, S.: Aplasia and leukemia following chloroquine therapy. Postgrad. Med. J. 54:108, 1978.
156. Neill, W. A., Panayi, G. S., Duthie, J., Jr., and Prescott, R. J.: Action of chloroquine phosphate in rheumatoid arthritis. II. Chromosome-damaging effect. Ann. Rheum. Dis. 32:547, 1973.
157. Magnussen, I., and deFine Olivamus, B.: Cardiomyopathy after chloroquine treatment. Acta Med. Scand. 202:429, 1977.
158. Baler, C. R.: Porphyria precipitated by hydroxychloroquine treatment of systemic lupus erythematosus. Cutis 17:96, 1976.

Chapter 45

Duncan A. Gordon

Gold Compounds in the Rheumatic Diseases

Gold has been advocated for the treatment of many human diseases for centuries. It was not until 1890, however, when Koch reported the in vitro inhibition of tubercle bacilli by gold cyanide, that gold compounds were used for treating tuberculous disorders.[1, 2] Forestier in 1929[3] pioneered the use of gold compounds for the treatment of rheumatoid arthritis (RA), assuming that both conditions might have a common infectious cause. He reported in 1935 his experience with gold thiopropanol sodium sulfanate (Allochrysine) in more than 550 cases, with improvement in 70 to 80 percent. Subsequently, Hartfall et al.[4] confirmed "apparent cure or striking improvement" in 80 percent of 900 British cases of RA. Later, a few randomized, controlled trials confirmed the value of parenteral gold in RA.[5–8]

Gold treatment is also recommended for selected patients with psoriatic arthritis or ankylosing spondylitis affecting peripheral joints and for patients with juvenile rheumatoid arthritis (JRA). It has also been prescribed for palindromic rheumatism (sometimes a forerunner of RA) and for disorders such as pemphigus and bronchial asthma. An orally administered gold compound, auranofin (Ridaura), was the first slow-acting antirheumatic drug developed specifically for RA.[9] Although oral gold may be less effective than parenteral forms, it causes fewer serious side effects.[10]

PHARMACOLOGY OF GOLD

Gold Preparations

Numerous gold-containing compounds have been used to treat RA in the past 50 years. Of the several oxidation states for gold compounds, only complex gold compounds are used therapeutically. Gold sodium thiomalate (GSTM), gold sodium thioglucose (GSTG), and gold thioglycoanilid are administered by intramuscular injection only; gold sodium thiosulfate also may be given intravenously. The orally ingested absorbable compound known as auranofin (triethyl phosphine gold thioglucosetetra-acetate) has become generally available. Previous oral preparations were absorbed poorly.

GSTM and GSTG are the most widely used

compounds in the United States; their structural formulas are shown in Figure 45–1. They are water-soluble preparations and contain a sulfur moiety attached to the gold. GSTM, GSTG, and gold thioglycoanilid are about 50 percent gold by weight; gold sodium thiosulfate is 37 percent gold.

Although both GSTM and GSTG are effective, GSTG may be preferred because of lesser toxicity. GSTM is associated with postinjection reactions rarely seen with GSTG. A higher incidence of adverse reactions is seen with aqueous preparations of GSTM

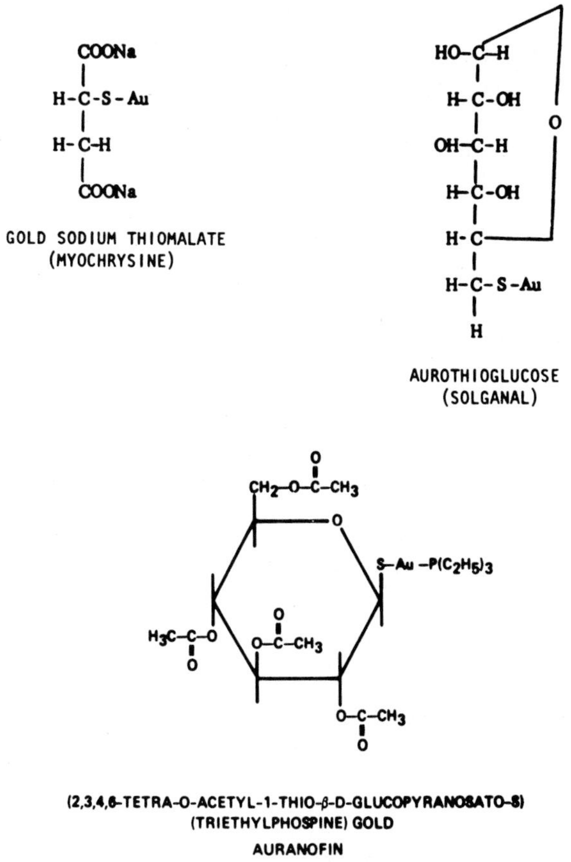

Figure 45–1. Gold sodium thiomalate and aurothioglucose, the two intramuscular gold preparations most widely used in the United States, are aurous salts, contain 50 percent gold by weight, and are attached to a sulfur moiety. Auranofin, a conjugated gold compound with two ligands, contains sulfur and is 29 percent gold by weight.

(30 percent) than oily suspensions with GSTG (9 percent). GSTG shows poor miscibility because of sesame oil vehicle; if the vial is not thoroughly shaken, dosage may be inexact. GSTG may cause intramuscular lumps at injection sites, and the long large-bore needle (1.5 inch, 20 gauge) required for injection of the viscous materal may cause pain.

Auranofin, a triethylphosphine gold compound that contains 29 percent gold by weight, is distinctly different physicochemically from the parenteral compounds. Some of its unique characteristics include absorption after oral administration (about 25 percent of the administered dose), a monomeric form, lipid solubility, nonconductivity, and weak reactivity with sulfhydryl groups.

Gold Distribution

Gold concentrations have been measured in animal and human tissue using colorimetric methods, atomic absorption, spectroscopy, neutron activation analysis, radionuclide, and radiographic fluorescence analysis. In general, the kidneys, adrenals, and reticuloendothelial system organs achieve highest gold concentrations. Intracellularly, gold localizes in the nuclear, mitochondrial, and lysosomal fractions, attached to organelle membranes.

In patients with RA, gold is widely distributed throughout the tissues (Table 45–1). During a standard course of chrysotherapy, blood and urine gold levels generally average 300 to 400 μg per dl and 30 to 60 μg per dl when measured 1 week after administration. Synovial fluid gold levels are about 50 percent of serum concentrations, but gold preferentially localizes in the synovial membrane during active chrysotherapy.

Pharmacokinetics

Pharmacokinetic studies elucidate the metabolism, excretion, and distribution of gold within the

Table 45–1. DISTRIBUTION OF GOLD IN BODY TISSUES*

Tissue	Gold Content (mg Gold)	Percent Total Gold Retained
Bone marrow	159	26
Liver	148	24
Skin	117	19
Bone	110	18
Muscle	33	5
Spleen	19	3
Other	33	5
Total	619	100

*Based on tissues assayed; some organ weights used in determining gold content were estimated.

Adapted from Gottlieb, N. L., et al.: Tissue gold concentration in a rheumatoid arthritic receiving chrysotherapy. Arthritis Rheum. 15:16, 1972.

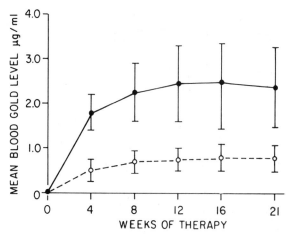

Figure 45–2. Mean whole blood gold concentrations in 59 auranofin-treated patients (O—O) and 51 gold sodium thiomalate-treated patients (●—●) after 21 weeks of therapy. Higher blood gold concentrations are achieved with conventional doses of gold sodium thiomalate than with auranofin (triethylphosphine gold). Gold levels reach a plateau after 6 to 8 weeks of injectable treatment and after 12 weeks of auranofin, reflecting the longer half-life of the oral compound. Bars show standard deviations. (Adapted from Dahl, S. L., et al.: Lack of correlation between blood gold concentrations and clinical response in patients with definite or classic RA receiving auranofin or gold sodium thiomalate. Arthritis Rheum. 28:1211, 1985.)

intravascular, serum protein, synovial fluid, tissue, and intracellular compartments with details outlined previously.[1]

Blood Gold

Serum contains less than 0.5 ng per dl of gold before therapy. Gold levels gradually rise with treatment; a plateau is reached after 6 to 8 weeks (Fig. 45–2). Serum gold concentrations correlate with the dose of gold. With maintenance doses, concentrations range from 75 to 125 μg per dl when 50 mg of gold is given every 3 to 4 weeks. After administration of oral gold (auranofin, 6 mg per day), serum levels gradually increase during 3 months and plateau.

Gold Excretion

About 40 percent of the dose of intramuscular gold is eliminated, 70 percent in the urine and 30 percent in the feces.

Gold Retention

Body gold retention (Fig. 45–3) has been measured after intravenous 195 Au-GSTM, with a whole body radiation counting chamber. After 20 weekly injections of 50 mg, about 300 mg of elemental gold is retained. After 20 weeks of oral gold doses of 6 mg per day, about 73 mg of gold is retained.

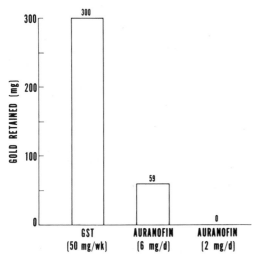

GOLD RETENTION AFTER SIX MONTHS OF CHRYSOTHERAPY

Figure 45–3. The quantity of gold retained in body tissues is much greater with injectable than with oral gold and is related to the dose of auranofin administered. (Adapted from Gottlieb, N. L.: Comparative pharmacokinetics of parenteral and oral gold compounds. J. Rheumatol. 9[Suppl. 8]:99, 1982.)

Mechanisms of Action

The use of gold in the treatment of RA remains empirical. Despite better knowledge of the properties of gold and the pathogenesis of RA, it is not understood exactly how gold works.

Microbial Agents

Infectious agents, especially viruses, have long been incriminated in the pathogenesis of RA. Rationale for the use of gold has stemmed in part from the fact that in vitro gold compounds inhibit the growth of various microorganisms.[1]

Humoral Immunity

Remissions induced by chrysotherapy may be associated with improvement in hematologic and immunologic indices. Decrease in serum and synovial fluid, gamma immunoglobulin G (IgG), IgA, and IgM may be associated with a selective effect on rheumatoid factor (RF) production (Fig. 45–4). In some studies, reductions of IgM and IgG-RF occurred only in patients with RA who improved after gold injections, but in vitro production of IgM-RF corrected with disease severity, whether or not patients were taking gold.[11]

Hypogammaglobulinemia after gold treatment has also been associated with selective IgG or IgA deficiency.[12] Gold treatment is also associated with decreased mitogen-induced in vitro synthesis of IgM and IgM-RF.[13]

Gold compounds affect the classic and alternative complement systems in vitro. GSTM, gold sodium thiosulfate, and gold chloride partially inacti-vate the first component (C1) of the complement system in serum and synovial fluid, in concentrations achieved during chrysotherapy. An example of the GSTM on C1, C4, and C2 in rheumatoid synovial fluid is shown in Figure 45–5.

Lymphocytes and Monocytes

Clinical improvement in RA after lymphapheresis highlights the importance of the lymphocyte in the pathogenesis of RA. Immunologic examination of RA synovium from seven patients, before and 6 months after parenteral gold treatment, showed reduction in infiltrating T and B cells.[14]

The in vitro effects of gold on lymphocytes and monocytes have been reported. GSTM inhibits antigen-triggered and mitogen-triggered human lymphocyte DNA synthesis in vitro.[15] Preincubation of purified monocytes with gold renders them deficient in their ability to support mitogen-induced T lymphocyte proliferation on subsequent culture. These and other observations suggest that gold blocks thymus-derived lymphocyte activation by interfering with monocyte function. GSTM and gold sodium thiosulfate inhibit transformation of human lymphocytes stimulated by other lymphocytes in the mixed lymphocyte culture, purified protein derivative, phytohemagglutinin, concanavalin A, and pokeweed mitogen in vitro.[16]

Similar effects are found in peripheral blood lymphocytes inhibited by auranofin.[17] Gold may also affect immunoregulation in mice, as measured by plaque-forming cells, rosette-forming cells, and serum antibody assays.[18]

Parenteral gold suppresses adjuvant-induced arthritis of rats. After passive transfer of arthritis, spleen cells from the gold-treated donor rats appeared to inhibit the development of arthritis in the recipient animals.[19] In these studies, gold could have reduced the number of specific lymphocytes or macrophages responsible for the transfer of adjuvant induced arthritis.

Monocyte/Macrophage Function

The macrophage participates in the pathogenesis of RA because of its role in antigen presentation and release of mediators such as interleukin-1 (IL-1). Micromolar concentrations of gold inhibit peptide-stimulated chemotactic responsiveness of human blood monocytes, but not polymorphonuclear leukocytes.[20]

It has been postulated that extravasated macrophages in rheumatoid synovium elaborate IL-1 and stimulate fibroblast proliferation within rheumatoid pannus. Low doses of GSTM or auranofin in vitro, however, inhibited IL-1–induced fibroblast proliferation without having effect on IL-1 production by macrophages.[21] The effect of IL-1 production, however, may be dose-dependent because low concentrations of GSTG or auranofin may potentiate IL-1

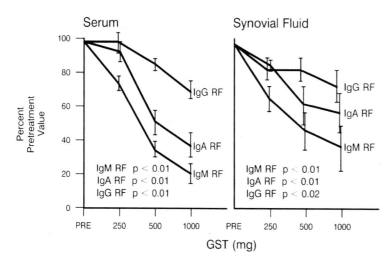

Figure 45–4. Comparison of changes in serum and synovial fluid IgM rheumatoid factor (IgM RF), IgA RF, and IgG RF levels after administration of gold sodium thiomalate (GST). Results are expressed as a percentage of the pretreatment values, mean ± SEM. (Adapted by Gottlieb, N. L.: Pharmacology of auranofin. Scand. J. Rheumatol. Suppl. 63:19, 1986, from Hanly, J. G., et al.: Effects of gold therapy on the synthesis and quantity of serum and synovial fluid IgM, IgG, and IgA rheumatoid factors in rheumatoid arthritis patients. Arthritis Rheum. 29:480, 1986.)

production, whereas higher concentrations inhibit it.[22]

In the adjuvant arthritic rat model, GSTM and auranofin also were both associated with a decrease in splenic IL-1 activity, whereas chloroquine and penicillamine were not.[23] Further, indomethacin had no effect in decreasing IL-1 activity in the same model.[24]

The capacity of blood monocytes to generate superoxide anion in vitro after stimulation was studied before and after GSTM treatment in 12 patients with RA.[25] Increased rates of superoxide anion were seen with successful treatment, whereas lesser increases were seen in treatment failures.

Neutrophil Functions

It has been shown that GSTM inhibits neutrophil chemotaxis and random migration in vitro in normal subjects and in gold-responsive patients with RA but not in gold-resistant patients.[26]

The phagocytic activity of certain inflammatory cells is enhanced in patients with RA. Intramuscular gold compounds inhibit macrophage and polymorphonuclear leukocyte phagocytic activity at inflammatory sites in vitro, using a *skin window* technique.[27]

Blood neutrophils (or monocytes) when stimulated generate reactive oxygen species shown by a chemiluminescent response. This response is enhanced in cells from patients with RA. Leukocytes eluted from RA synovial tissue had in vitro decreased chemiluminescent responses with auranofin but not GSTM.[28]

Inflammation in RA is associated with activated phagocytes that produce superoxide anion oxidizable to singlet oxygen; gold compounds are effective deactivators of singlet oxygen.[29]

Leukocyte adhesion receptors on endothelial cells appear to promote rheumatoid synovitis by recruitment of leukocytes to sites of inflammation. Serial synovial biopsy data in patients with RA after gold therapy showed a decrease in the expression of

endothelial leukocyte adhesion molecule 1 (ELAM-1) in keeping with another mechanism for the downregulation of acute synovitis in RA by gold.[30]

Enzyme Inhibition

GSTM inhibits acid phosphatase, beta (β) glucuronidase, and malic dehydrogenase in guinea pig peritoneal macrophages; acid phosphatase, β glucuronidase, and cathepsin in human synovial fluid cells; and several human epidermal enzymes.[31] This suggests that gold may ameliorate rheumatoid inflammation by inhibiting lysosomal enzyme release or production. The release of hydrolases from lysosomes, however, is unaffected by gold compounds.[32]

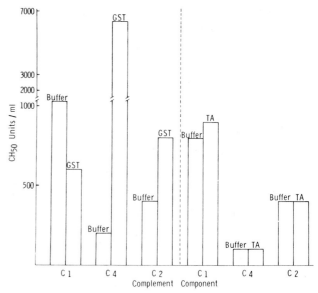

Figure 45–5. Gold sodium thiomalate (GST) (3.1 μg per ml) partially inactivates the functional hemolytic activity of C1 and protects against C4 and C2 destruction, the natural substrates of C1, in vitro. Thiomalic acid (TA) has no effect on C1. (Courtesy of Duane Schultz, Ph.D.)

CLINICAL APPLICATIONS

Patient Selection

Gold is used primarily for progressive polyarticular RA. Thus, the use of gold should be based on a firm diagnosis of RA. The institution of effective control measures, however, depends on reliable rheumatologic assessments. This provides a baseline for measuring response to therapy. Initially, the patient with RA requires a comprehensive treatment plan that includes rest, physical therapy, nonsteroidal anti-inflammatory drugs (NSAIDs), and occasional intra-articular glucocorticoids. If after a few weeks of such a program the patient is not coping with daily activities, referral to a rheumatologist is recommended. Such an approach leads to a prompter recognition of progressive disease and the earlier addition of a disease-modifying agent (Fig. 45–6).

Unfortunately, in the earliest stages of RA, we lack sufficiently good markers to identify progressive disease. Thus, in many instances, disease-modifying therapy cannot be instituted before active disease can be arrested and long-term disability prevented. Further, after 5 years, a majority of patients given slow activity drugs such as gold are no longer taking them because of either side effects or inefficacy. The result is that too frequently medical management of RA fails to control progressive disease. For this reason, early aggressive therapy with combinations of agents rather than a single one has been advocated.[33] It has been suggested that the treatment of RA should be analogous to that of tuberculosis or cancer. Because the toxicity of combination therapy does not appear excessive once a second agent has been added, it is likely to be continued if improvement has been observed. Unfortunately, there are few controlled trials comparing multiple drugs versus single events, and most of these studies have been inconclusive.[34]

Gold compounds form the backbone of remission-inducing therapy for RA because traditionally most rheumatologists practicing in North America have advocated an initial trial of chrysotherapy over other disease-modifying drugs. Some studies have shown that gold therapy is most effective in early, nonerosive RA,[5, 6] and others have demonstrated its value in active disease of long duration despite joint damage.[7] Gold is not indicated for advanced RA without evidence of active synovitis, but we have found it effective in controlling monoarticular or pauciarticular RA. If patients have responded poorly to gold in the past, they are less likely to respond to a second course.[35] Even previous responders fare worse.

Factors that do not apparently influence the response to chrysotherapy include patient age, sex, race, extra-articular features of RA, erythrocyte sedimentation rate (ESR), and presence or absence of RF.[1]

Low-dose prednisone, 5 to 7.5 mg per day in the morning, has been recommended as a temporary bridge for several weeks until gold takes effect. Steroids may be tapered gradually once clinical improvement is evident.

Gold compounds may be employed in patients with RA who have Felty's or Sjögren's syndrome, pre-existing neutropenia, or eosinophilia.[1, 36] Available evidence suggests that with gold, neutropenia and splenomegaly improve without undue toxicity.

Chronic anemia is also a feature of RA that may improve with gold. Despite earlier admonitions against gold in RA-associated Sjögren's syndrome, it is generally well tolerated.[37] Similarly, nonprogressive proteinuria or benign hematuria without renal insufficiency does not preclude gold treatment. Nevertheless, pre-existing proteinuria and dermatitis are relative contraindications to the use of gold because they could mimic toxic effects of the drug.

Pregnancy is well known to improve rheumatoid disease activity. Parenteral therapy does not appear to affect babies born to mothers treated with gold. Nevertheless, any newborn exposed to maternal gold during pregnancy or lactation should be monitored closely.[38] Auranofin is not recommended for pregnant or nursing mothers.

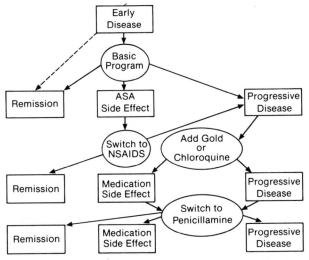

Figure 45–6. Flow chart depicting the relationship of the clinical state of the patient (rectangles) and various treatment options (ovals) available; highlighting the place of gold in the treatment of progressive disease. (Adapted from Gordon, D. A.: Rheumatoid Arthritis. New York, Medical Examination Publishing Co., 1985, p. 233. Reprinted by permission of the publisher. Copyright 1985 by Elsevier Science Publishing Co., Inc.)

Efficacy

The benefit of gold treatment in RA has been well documented over the past 50 years.[1] Although most studies were descriptive and would not meet contemporary standards, they represent milestones in the evolution of better treatment for RA. Moreover, these uncontrolled trials anticipated more con-

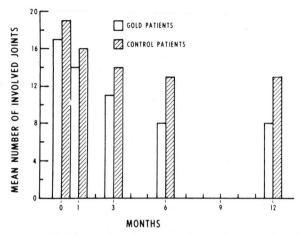

Figure 45–7. Mean number of involved joints declined significantly in gold-treated rheumatoid arthritis patients, but not in control subjects. (Adapted from the Empire Rheumatism Council Study: Gold therapy in rheumatoid arthritis. Ann. Rheum. Dis. 19:95, 1960.)

vincing ones. For example, the first antirheumatic drug ever tested in a controlled trial was gold.[39]

Further review of clinical trials comparing injectable gold with placebo shows that there are few studies published in English that include criteria such as random allocation of patients, administration of placebo injections, and double-blind evaluation with complete account of all clinical outcomes.

The first double-blind study to meet these criteria was that of the Empire Rheumatism Council.[5, 6] It provided strong impetus for the use of chrysotherapy in RA. This multicenter study involved nearly 200 patients with disease duration mostly less than 3 years and none more than 5. Half received a cumulative dose of 1000 mg of GSTM and the remainder (controls) a total dose of 0.01 mg over a 6-month period; a maintenance gold schedule was not provided. After 3 months of therapy, the gold-treated group improved more than the controls subjectively and objectively. The reduction in number of involved joints is illustrated in Figure 45–7.

A similar trial was undertaken by the Cooperating Clinics Committee (CCC) in the United States, but only 68 patients with RA were recruited.[7] Possibly because of the small number of patients studied, the only variable that changed significantly was the ESR.

In 1974, a 30-month, double-blind study compared a standard course of GSTM with placebo followed by a comparison of maintenance gold against placebo.[8] Twenty-seven patients with RA for less than 5 years were randomly assigned to treatment or placebo groups. Improvement required at least 3 months of treatment and sometimes took 9 months. Good effects were maintained for a mean of 28 months. The increase of grip strength in the treated versus the placebo group over 24 months is illustrated in Figure 45–8. Despite the small number of cases, serial radiographs of the hands and wrists

revealed fewer bone erosions in the gold-treated group. These findings were first to document that gold compounds favorably alter the natural history of RA by reducing bone and cartilage destruction. A methodologic analysis of 60 studies also examined the effect of drug therapy on radiographic deterioration in RA.[40] The authors concluded that the 1974 study cited here provided the strongest support that parenteral gold could retard radiographic progression of RA.

Roentgenographic progression was correlated with clinical disease activity in a 2-year GSTM trial involving 73 patients with RA.[41] Patients whose synovitis was suppressed the most developed the fewest hand and wrist erosions and least joint space narrowing.

There have also been a number of comparative studies involving other antirheumatic agents. GSTM and D-penicillamine were compared in a 6-month controlled study of 89 patients with RA.[42] Both agents were similarly effective. The previous use of gold does not preclude the likelihood of response to penicillamine. Its use after an episode of gold toxicity such as proteinuria, however, is likely to be associated with similar toxicity.

GSTM, azathioprine, 2.5 mg per kilogram per day, and cyclophosphamide, 1.5 mg per kilogram per day, were compared in an 18-month, double-blind trial of 121 patients with early RA (mean duration of disease, 5 years).[43] Improvement in clinical variables and reduction in ESR and RF titer were comparable in all patient groups. Roentgenographic joint deterioration was least and steroid sparing effect greatest with cyclophosphamide.

GSTM, 50 mg per week intramuscularly; azathioprine, 1.0 to 2.0 mg per kilogram per day orally;

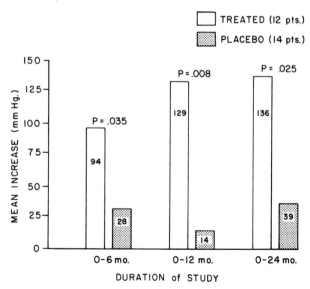

Figure 45–8. Mean grip strength at 6, 12, and 24 months compared with pretreatment values. (Adapted and reproduced, with permission, from Sigler, J. W., et al.: Gold salts in the treatment of rheumatoid arthritis. Ann. Intern. Med. 80:21, 1974.)

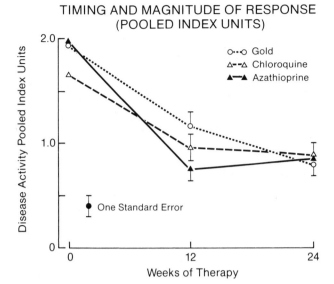

Figure 45–9. The initial disease activity was similar for all three agents in pooled index units (derived by using a combination of articular index, joint count, grip strength, morning stiffness, and erythrocyte sedimentation rate). At 12 weeks, total disease activity was significantly improved in all three groups (p < 0.5). At 24 weeks, disease activity was still significantly decreased in all three groups (p < 0.001). (Adapted from Dwosh, I. L., et al.: Azathioprine in early RA. Arthritis Rheum. 20:685, 1977.)

or chloroquine, 250 mg per day orally, was given to 33 patients with early RA (duration, about 2 years) in a nonblinded, randomly assigned 24 week study. Azathioprine groups were faring marginally better than the chloroquine group at the final evaluation (Fig. 45–9).

Two 6-month controlled trials compared sulfasalazine with GSTM and placebo. Results in 90 patients with active RA showed equal benefit for these agents.[44] Results of a CCC trial in 187 patients with RA were similar.[45] The main side effects from sulfasalazine were gastrointestinal.

Interest in pulse methotrexate (MTX) as a second-line agent has led to its comparison with gold in a few controlled trials. A 26-week trial in 40 patients with RA compared parenteral MTX, 10 mg weekly, with GSTM, 50 mg weekly.[46] Similar efficacy was shown, but MTX side effects (20 percent) were much less than gold toxicity (50 percent). Similar results were obtained in another trial with 35 patients with RA in whom oral MTX, 12.5 mg weekly, was compared with GSTM, 50 mg weekly.[47] A 1-year controlled trial of 102 patients with RA compared parenteral MTX, 15 mg weekly, with GSTM weekly.[48] Efficacy was similar, but side effects were greater with gold patients (20 of 51) compared with MTX patients (11 of 51). The high frequency of gold toxicity, however, may have related to a weekly dosage of gold for 1 year.

The efficacy of auranofin has been tested worldwide in many thousands of patients with RA.[9] Oral gold has been compared with placebo, GSTG, GSTM, gold sodium thiopropanosulphonate, penicillamine,

and hydroxychloroquine. Although some were well-designed trials, others were not. A short-term, 21-week trial completed by the CCC involved 209 patients with RA who received GSTM (n = 82), auranofin (n = 77), or placebo (n = 50).[11] There were no striking differences between intramuscular and oral gold for any clinical variables (Fig. 45–10). Certain laboratory tests (hemoglobin and platelet count) improved more with GSTM, but serum RF titer and ESR declined similarly. Both compounds were better than placebo. Many of these patients (147) then entered a 1-year, open-label study taking auranofin, 6 mg daily.[49] Initial response to GSTM was maintained, but by the end of the year, half of the patients had stopped taking auranofin. When patients 65 years of age or older were compared with their younger counterparts in this and two other comparable trials, there were no age-based differences in efficacy or adverse drug reactions.[50]

In a study of similar design, 90 patients with RA were randomly allocated to receive auranofin, placebo, or GSTM.[51] Follow-up over 3 years showed clinical improvement in both gold-treated groups. All groups, however, showed radiographic deterioration. About half the auranofin patients dropped out because of inefficacy, but there were no long-term differences between oral or injectable responders. In a 1-year comparative study of GSTM and auranofin in 120 patients with RA, lack of effect dropouts were twice as common in the auranofin group, whereas dropouts from toxicity were twice as common in the GSTM group.[52]

In 340 patients with RA followed for 6 months, auranofin was superior to placebo; 67 and 43 percent of patients showed moderate or marked improve-

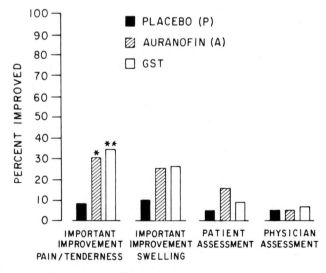

Figure 45–10. Proportion of patients who obtained important improvement of selected measurements by treatment group (193 patients). GST, Gold sodium thiomalate. (Adapted from Ward, J. R., et al.: Comparison of auranofin, gold sodium thiomalate, and placebo in the treatment of RA. Arthritis Rheum. 26:1303, 1983.)

ment, and 9 and 29 percent were withdrawn for lack of efficacy.[53] Radiographic follow-up of hands and wrists of patients from this randomized study followed for a year were scored by two independent readers.[54] A reduction of advancement of erosive disease was seen in the auranofin-treated group.

A 6-month, randomized, double-blinded study involved 303 patients with RA from 14 centers; auranofin, 3 mg twice daily, was compared with placebo.[55] Outcome assessments were expanded to include some 20 nontraditional measures of the patient's quality of life as well as the standard clinical indices. Results confirmed a modest effect of auranofin on synovitis, but greater improvement was noted in the patients' quality of life. Only 10 percent of auranofin patients withdrew from the study because of adverse effects.

A 24-month, randomized, double-blind study from Scandinavia involved 132 patients with early (less than 2 years) RA and showed a more favorable effect than the previous study.[56] This was attributed to the shorter disease duration of patients studied. Only 35 of 67 patients completed the 2 years of study, and dropouts were more related to cutaneous and gastrointestinal side effects than inefficacy. An analysis of 268 patients with RA taking auranofin enrolled in the ARAMIS databank examined differences between half of the patients who responded and those who did not.[57] Responders were younger, with early severe disease. They had never tried other second-line therapies.

It is uncertain whether auranofin can sustain remission after good response to parenteral treatment. A 12-month controlled trial of 22 patients with RA well maintained on parenteral gold were randomized into no change in parenteral gold or were switched to auranofin, 6 mg daily.[58] The parenteral group remained unchanged, whereas ten of 14 auranofin patients were withdrawn because of drug side effects or exacerbation of arthritis. In another study, 15 of 20 patients with RA on maintenance gold injections were switched to oral gold.[59] Again ten of 15 auranofin patients were withdrawn with side effects or arthritis flare over 8 months. In the foregoing studies, a switch back to parenteral gold usually recaptured remission. When serious side effects develop from parenteral gold, a switch to oral gold may be safely accomplished.[60] This rechallenge, however, should be carefully monitored.

The possibility of switching patients from oral gold after remission to parenteral doses has been suggested as a cost-saving measure. When parenteral gold was tried in a few nonresponders to auranofin, there was no improvement.[61]

Auranofin has not been as well studied as other second-line agents. Ninety patients with RA were evaluated in a 12-month controlled trial comparing auranofin, 6 mg daily, with penicillamine, 750 mg daily.[62] Results showed fewer side effects from auranofin but greater efficacy with penicillamine.

A 36-week, double-blind, multicenter, controlled trial with 281 patients with active RA made comparison between daily auranofin and weekly oral MTX.[63] Both groups showed improvement, but MTX response was earlier, with fewer side effects.

The influence of parenteral gold treatment in psoriatic arthritis was contrasted in patients with RA.[64] The patients with psoriatic arthritis experienced better functional activity and fewer severe toxic reactions. A 6-month, multicenter, double-blind trial involving 238 patients with psoriatic arthritis showed only a moderate advantage of auranofin over NSAID: Psoriatic rash was unaffected by auranofin.[65] Another 6-month, multicenter, controlled trial involving 82 patients compared auranofin, GSTM, and placebo.[66] Parenteral gold was safe and more effective than auranofin.

Auranofin has been found safe as a treatment for JRA. A USA–USSR double-blind, placebo-controlled trial involved 231 children with 80 percent showing polyarticular disease.[67] Although the auranofin group showed a trend toward improvement, individualized intergroup differences were not significant.

The advantage of combining study results was shown in two meta-analyses that examined comparable controlled studies.[68, 69] Both analyses confirmed a favorable magnitude of efficacy for parenteral gold. One study compared various commonly used second-line drugs and showed that auranofin tended to be weaker than parenteral gold and other agents.[69] In both meta-analyses, treatment duration were short-term studies of 2 months or less. Long-term controlled efficacy studies beyond 1 year are limited because they are expensive and difficult to perform. One approach is the utilization of life-table analysis of treatment terminations. In one study, 80% of patients after 5 years were no longer using second-line medications,[70] and in another study most patients discontinued their slow-acting medication in less than 2 years.[71]

With the advent of new, supposedly less toxic agents, however, the result of these studies may be a reflection of an easy willingness to switch patients from gold to an apparently less toxic, equally effective oral agent. When faced with a skin rash, physicians may be too easily inclined to switch from gold rather than attempt to individualize gold dosages.

In another report, 30 percent of patients taking gold continued to show benefit after 5 years.[72] A retrospective analysis also showed a long-term survival benefit for patients taking gold.[73] This study from Finland reported on the deaths of 251 of 573 patients with RA who died over a 25-year period. The mortality rate in those taking gold was only 25 percent compared with 70 percent of those not taking gold.

Most rheumatologists would subscribe to the results of a retrospective review that emphasized the value of protracted chrysotherapy;[74] 73 percent of 39 patients who received gold for 3 or more years entered a remission, in contrast to only 6 percent of

36 patients who discontinued treatment during the first 18 months. Most clinicians believe that gold compounds are capable of increasing the likelihood of a permanent remission in a minority of patients with RA.

Thus, although gold constitutes a mainstay in the treatment of RA, its role in altering the long-term course of RA remains controversial. Despite the success of short-term clinical trials with gold, concern has been expressed about the disappointing long-term outcomes cited previously. This concern has led to interest in the use of combinations of second-line agents for the treatment of RA. A formal overview of the topic compared the benefits and risks of combinations of agents with the same drugs used singly.[34] Only three trials met criteria for analysis. One of these compared a combination of parenteral gold and hydroxychloroquine (52 patients) in gold and placebo (49 patients).[75] The combination group showed more rapid improvement and better overall reduction of disease activity after 12 months. Withdrawals from the study because of toxicity were greater in the combination group (18 versus 10).

Three studies have examined combination of auranofin with either MTX or hydroxychloroquine. A 48-week, double-blind, randomized trial compared auranofin, 6 mg per day, MTX 7.5 mg per week, and the combination of both.[76] All three treatment groups were similar in efficacy. Although there were more withdrawals for adverse drug reactions in the combined group, there were fewer withdrawals for lack of response. A longer-term study evaluated the same combination over a longer period.[77] A total of 267 patients received the combination of auranofin and MTX over 6 months followed by a double-blinded phase. Successfully treated patients continued the combination or took auranofin alone. Benefits were better maintained in the combination group (66 of 89) than the auranofin group (43 of 85). Another 24-week, double-blind study used 229 patients with RA divided into three groups taking auranofin, hydroxychloroquine, or a combination of both.[78] In this study, combined therapy offered at best only marginal improvement. Although these three studies suggest interesting possibilities, they reflect the short-term benefits seen in earlier controlled, single-drug comparisons. We have no idea what the effect of these combinations might have on the long-term outcome of RA.

Despite reports that the efficacy of gold treatment does not correlate with gold toxicity, we have often seen an association between treatment response and a skin rash.[79] Immunogenetic data also suggest that patients with RA possessing human leukocyte antigen (HLA)-DR3 may be more responsive to gold treatment than patients with RA who possess HLA-DR4 without DR3.[80] The fact that responsiveness or side effects may be unrelated to HLA typing is illustrated by a family study in which two pairs of siblings with RA responded in a similar way to parenteral gold.[81] Both pairs were HLA identical. Although one pair possessed HLA antigen B8 and DR3, the other did not possess either of these antigens.

As noted, 6 months may be insufficient to obtain maximum benefit from chrysotherapy; treatment should be extended to 18 or more months before termination for lack of improvement.[8, 74] Although loss of efficacy may occur after long-term maintenance therapy,[70, 71] patients whose disease exacerbates while receiving monthly maintenance gold injections frequently benefit from a return to weekly treatment.[82] Lastly, the beneficial effects of gold compounds may persist for months or even years after treatment has been abandoned, presumably reflecting tissue gold stores.[83]

Decisions regarding duration of gold therapy are largely empirical. In our view, however, gold therapy should be continued indefinitely after an acceptable response. Adoption of this recommendation implies commitment on the part of the patient and physician to periodic evaluation and long-term monitoring.

Dosage Schedules

The usual intramuscular gold dosage schedule was derived empirically from clinical experience. At present, the standard gold schedule for adults with RA consists of test doses of 10 mg and 25 mg given 1 week apart, followed by 50 mg weekly, until the cumulative dose totals 1 g, or toxicity or major clinical improvement supervenes.

There are numerous variations in the aforementioned schedule, such as weekly injections of 25 mg rather than 50 mg of gold compound; others recommend 50 mg until 500 to 700 mg is attained, at which time the dose is reduced to 25 mg weekly.

One multicenter study compared the results of administering 1000 mg or 2500 mg of GSTG in 21 weeks, followed by maintenance therapy, to more than 200 patients with RA.[84] The "low" dose group received 25 mg twice weekly for 11 weeks followed by 50 mg once weekly, whereas the "high" dose group received 100 mg twice weekly for 11 weeks and then 50 mg weekly for 10 weeks. The efficacy of both dosage regimens was similar; however, the frequency of toxicity was significantly greater with the high dose (58 percent) than with the low dose (24 percent) group (Table 45–2). Although few variable dosage regimens have been reported, a high-dose, low-frequency schedule was effective in 20 of 30 patients with RA.[85] Patients received 200 mg of GSTG every 4 weeks, with improvement about 18 weeks after onset. Side effects resembled other series.

Many clinicians stop therapy after 1000 mg in unresponsive cases, whereas others administer an additional 10 to 20 injections of 50 mg, hoping that higher cumulative doses will prove beneficial. Maintenance gold therapy, which generally consists of 25 to 50 mg of compound every 2 to 4 weeks, is advocated after completion of the initial course. Ter-

Table 45–2. OVERALL TOXICITY/PROTEINURIA WITH PARENTERAL GOLD

Investigator[1]	Conventional Gold Dose[1] (50 mg/week)			Alternative Gold Dose*		
	No. of Cases	Toxicity (%)	Proteinuria (%)	No. of Cases	Toxicity (%)	Proteinuria (%)
Griffin et al., 1983	20	80	10	21	62*a	14
Sharp et al., 1977	38	13	16	37	11*b	24
Rothermich et al., 1976	55	18	4	42	21*c	0
Furst et al., 1977	23	13	26	24	67*d	38
Cats et al., 1976	119	24	3	111	58*e	9

*Alternative dosage schedules: *a = 10 mg/week; *b = 25 mg/week; *c = 1 mg/kg/week; *d = 150 mg/kg/week; *e = 200 mg/week.

mination of gold after remission increases the probability that a second course will be ineffective.[35] Thus, we recommend indefinite maintenance of gold once remission has been achieved.

The recommended auranofin schedule derives from several studies of dosage range. Although 3 mg twice daily appears optimal for the majority of adults with RA, some improve with 1 mg daily, and others require 9 mg daily. Diarrhea and abdominal cramps are the most common limiting factors to achieving high daily dosage. For JRA, 0.1 to 0.2 mg per kg per day has been recommended.[67]

Pharmacologic Correlates

Investigators have been unable to correlate the response to chrysotherapy with the pharmacokinetics of gold. A comparison of oral and parenteral treatment showed no correlation between whole blood gold concentration and clinical outcomes (Fig. 45–11). Results of a study using atomic absorption spectrometry, however, showed that toxicity correlated with an increase in free gold over total gold levels.[88] Moreover, the frequency of severe toxicity is increased twofold to fivefold when high-dose treatment schedules (150 to 200 mg per week) are employed (see Table 45–2).

Cost of Gold Treatment

Administration and monitoring of the initial phase (20 weeks) of intramuscular gold treatment is expensive. A survey conducted in 1976 indicated a variable cost depending on the number of laboratory tests and physician (versus allied health assistant) visits.[89]

When cost-effectiveness analysis was applied to a comparison of auranofin versus placebo, benefits of disease modification outweighed adverse effects with additional medical costs for auranofin of about $800 per year.[90] Strategies to reduce costs include fewer and less frequent laboratory tests and administration of gold at home by a family member or nurse.[89] The cost of parenteral gold versus auranofin suggests that induction of disease remission with GSTM or GSTG weekly for 20 weeks followed biweekly for a further 20 weeks costs about $700.[91–93]

On the other hand, monthly maintenance costs for parenteral gold average about $50, whereas monthly auranofin costs average about $80.

Selection of Gold Compound

If a patient with RA is doing poorly and gold treatment is a consideration, referral to a rheumatologist is recommended. Although the ultimate place of auranofin vis-a-vis the intramuscular compounds in the therapeutic hierarchy of RA is not established, it appears most promising for use in milder forms and earlier phases of RA.

TOXICITY OF GOLD

Adverse Effects

When a patient with RA does poorly despite treatment, a number of complications should be

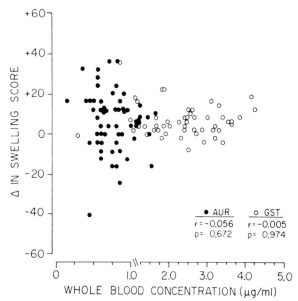

Figure 45–11. Changes in joint swelling scores versus whole blood gold concentrations for 59 auranofin (AUR)–treated patients and 51 gold sodium thiomalate (GST)–treated patients, assessed at week 21 of treatment. There were no significant correlations for either treatment group. (Adapted from Dahl, S. L., et al.: Lack of correlation between blood gold concentrations and clinical response in patients with definite or classic RA receiving auranofin or gold sodium thiomalate. Arthritis Rheum. 28:1211, 1985.)

Table 45–3. TOXICITY PROFILE WITH GOLD COMPOUNDS

Adverse Effects	Aurothiomalate	Aurothioglucose	Auranofin
Postinjection Reactions			
Vasomotor (nitritoid)	Uncommon*	Rare	Rare*
Anaphylaxis/syncope	Rare	Unknown	Unknown
Myalgias/arthralgias	Common	Rare	Unknown
Mucocutaneous Effects			
Dermatitis/stomatitis	Common†	Less common	Common
Pruritus	Common	Less common	Common
Alopecia	Rare	Rare	Rare
Urticaria	Rare	Rare	Uncommon
Trophic nails	Rare	Rare	Unknown
Chrysiasis/pigmentation	Rare	Rare	Unknown
Photosensitivity	Rare	Rare	Unknown
Kidney			
Proteinuria	Common‡	Less common	Rare
Hematuria	Uncommon	Less common	Rare
Nephrotic syndrome	Rare	Rare	Rare
Renal insufficiency	Rare	Rare	Unknown
Blood			
Eosinophilia	Common	Common	Rare
Thrombocytopenia	Rare‡	Rare	Rare
Granulocytopenia	Rare	Rare	Rarer
Lymphocytopenia	Uncommon	Rare	Rare
Hypogammaglobulinemia	Rare	Rare	Unknown
Aplastic anemia	Rare	Rare	Unknown
Pulmonary Complications			
Diffuse infiltrates	Rare	Rare	Rare
Intestinal Effects			
Upper gastrointestinal symptoms	Rare	Rare	Uncommon
Mild enterocolitis	Rare	Rare	Common
Severe enterocolitis	Rare	Rare	Rare
Liver			
Cholestatic jaundice	Rare	Rare	Unknown
Hepatocellular effects	Rare	Rare	Uncommon
Pancreas			
Pancreatitis	Rare	Rare	Rare
Nervous System			
Peripheral/cranial			
Neuropathies	Rare	Rare	Rare
Encephalopathy	Rare	Rare	Rare
Eye			
Corneal or lens chrysiasis	Common	Common	Unknown
Conjunctivitis	Rare	Rare	Uncommon
Iritis/corneal ulcer	Rare	Rare	Unknown
Miscellaneous			
Metallic taste	Common	Common	Common
Headaches	Rare	Rare	Rare

*Reported in hypertensives on angiotensin converting enzyme inhibitors.
†HLA-DR3: possible relationship.
‡HLA-DR3: relationship proved.

considered. Unexpected symptoms may be related to the disease itself or to side effects from antirheumatic medications such as gold.

Parenteral Gold

Adverse reactions develop in about one third of patients with RA treated with intramuscular gold, varying from 5 to 80 percent (Table 45–3). Most complications are trivial, consisting primarily of localized dermatitis, stomatitis, transient hematuria, or mild proteinuria. More serious reactions involve the hematopoietic system, kidneys, liver, or other vital organs.

Oral Gold

Complications with auranofin differ importantly from characteristics of complications of the injectable gold compounds (see Table 45–3). Mucocutaneous lesions and serious complications occur less commonly with auranofin than with the intramuscular preparations.[10] About four times as many patients are withdrawn from intramuscular gold treatment (20 percent) because of drug intolerance as from oral gold (5 percent).

Immunogenetic Aspects

Gold-induced proteinuria and thrombocytopenia, representing immune-mediated reactions, occur many times more frequently than anticipated (increased relative risk is 32 times for proteinuria and nine times for thrombocytopenia) in RA patients possessing HLA-DR3 and DR3.[94]

Postinjection Reactions

Reactions may be rapid-onset vasomotor type or the slower-onset nonvasomotor type. Vasomotor (nitritoid) reactions, characterized by weakness, dizziness, nausea, vomiting, sweating, and facial flushing, may follow GSTM injections. The prevalence of this reaction has varied to as high as 34 percent. Peripheral vasodilation may cause hypotension from the action on arteriolar smooth muscle. Rarely this can result in myocardial infarction or central nervous system injury, especially in the elderly. Hypertensive patients with RA who take angiotensin converting enzyme (ACE) inhibitors such as captopril or analogues may be at risk for nitritoid reactions after taking oral gold or GSTM injections.[95] Switching to another antihypertensive or GSTG may prevent these episodes.

Non-vasomotor postinjection reactions, with transient arthralgias, joint swelling, fatigability, and malaise, developed in 15 percent of patients treated with GSTM. The reaction comes on about 6 to 24 hours after injection but can appear within an hour or last as long as a few days. Postinjection reactions are not a reason to abandon gold treatment because a switch to GSTG, or auranofin, can obviate them.

Mucocutaneous Effects

Dermatitis and stomatitis account for 60 to 80 percent of all adverse gold reactions. The clinical and histologic appearance of gold rash is highly variable and may mimic many other skin conditions. Most gold rashes last 1 or 2 months, are discrete, and are confined to the limbs or trunk. About 85 percent of eruptions are pruritic. Trophic nail changes may be seen with or without dermatitis. Eosinophilia, metallic taste, or proteinuria often accompanies dermatitis.

Skin punch biopsy may allow exclusion of other skin disorders, such as rheumatoid vasculitis. Immunofluorescent studies are of little value in differentiating gold rash from other conditions.[96] Immunochemical and electron microscopic findings in 13 patients with gold dermatitis showed an increased number of macrophages and activated Langerhan's cells in keeping with the presence of immunologic activity.[97]

An interesting relationship has been shown between adverse mucocutaneous reactions to gold and the presence of anti-aurothiomalate IgE antibodies.[98] Twenty-three of 34 patients (68 percent) who had toxic reactions showed anti-aurothiomalate IgE antibodies, whereas only seven of 37 patients (21 percent) without reactions showed antibodies.

A rash during chrysotherapy, especially with pruritus, strongly suggests gold dermatitis. Chrysotherapy should be stopped pending evaluation for a few weeks of observation until the skin lesions resolve. Treatment then may be reinstituted, using a reduced dosage schedule of 5 to 10 mg of gold weekly, with 5 to 10 mg increments every 1 to 4 weeks if toxicity does not recur. Reinstitution of chrysotherapy rarely results in exfoliative dermatitis.

It is interesting that contact allergy to gold jewelry may develop after parenteral gold,[99] and previous contact hypersensitivity to nickel may be provoked by gold injection.[100]

Rarely, gray or blue discoloration of the skin develops with protracted chrysotherapy. This condition, known as chrysiasis, is asymptomatic and may be associated with hyperpigmentation,[101] but without other side effects, its distinction from silver or mercury impregnation may be made by transmission electron microscopy.[102]

Kidney

Transient proteinuria, microscopic hematuria, and nephrotic syndrome are well-described complications of gold therapy. The frequency of proteinuria increases with higher gold doses (see Table 48–2).[84] Proteinuria has also been described in about 3 percent of patients with RA never treated with gold, an effect of hypertension, diverse urinary tract disorders, or various medications. Urinary protein may resolve spontaneously despite continuation of chrysotherapy. Nephrotic syndrome is the most frequent serious renal abnormality associated with gold therapy. Seventy-five percent of cases develop during the first year of treatment; HLA-B8/DR3 alloantigens are present in more than half the cases.[103]

The prognosis for gold-associated nephrotic syndrome is generally favorable; renal insufficiency is rare, with 70 percent of patients fully recovering within months to years (Fig. 45–12). Renal complications are extremely rare with auranofin. Therefore, oral gold may be preferable to other agents, such as GSTM or penicillamine, in chronic renal failure patients who develop active RA.[1]

Blood

Hematologic disorders resulting from chrysotherapy include eosinophilia, leukopenia or agranulocytosis, thrombocytopenia, anemia, pancytopenia, and aplastic anemia. Eosinophilia occurs in about 5

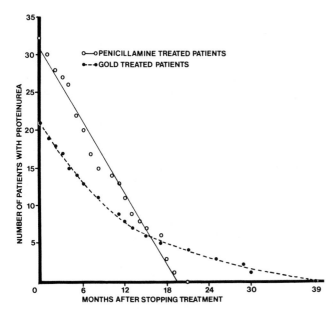

Figure 45–12. Resolution of proteinuria after stopping treatment. (From Hall, C. L.: The natural course of gold and penicillamine nephropathy: a long-term study of 54 patients. Adv. Exp. Med. Biol. 252:247, 1989. Used with permission.)

percent of gold-treated patients but varies up to 40 percent.[52] Eosinophilia has correlated with serum IgE levels and gold toxicity, although others have not confirmed this finding.[96]

Thrombocytopenia is a rare (1 to 3 percent) complication of gold treatment that may be serious or life-threatening.[104] It may develop shortly after gold is begun or as long as 18 months after cessation of therapy. The initial manifestations may be easy bruisability or spontaneous petechiae or purpura affecting the skin or mucous membranes. Less commonly, epistaxis or gingival, gastrointestinal, or genitourinary hemorrhage leads to the diagnosis of thrombocytopenia.

Although gold-induced thrombocytopenia may result from marrow suppression, an active marrow is usual, with peripheral destruction of platelets and platelet-associated IgG.[104] To date, 85 percent of reported patients with gold-induced thrombocytopenia possess HLA-DR3, whereas its general frequency is 30 percent in patients with RA. It is noteworthy that patients who develop thrombocytopenia after parenteral gold may develop thrombocytopenia again after taking other second-line agents.[105] Thrombocytopenia may also develop after oral gold.[106]

Leukopenia may develop during parenteral or oral gold treatment owing to granulocytopenia or agranulocytosis. The prevalence of leukopenia is low, and the extent and duration of white cell reductions are variable. Lymphocytopenia associated with GSTM has not been a forerunner of any serious hematologic complications.

The most feared complication of chrysotherapy is severe pancytopenia or bone marrow aplasia.[107] The incidence of the latter is low, with a prevalence

of less than 0.5 percent. In the past, the mortality rate has been high, with more than 60 percent of affected individuals succumbing to infection, bleeding, or other complications. More recently, prognosis has been improved by aggressive therapy, including bone marrow transplantation and the use of antithymocyte globulin.[107] Pure red cell aplasia has also been a rare but serious complication of parenteral gold.[108] In one instance, treatment with prednisone and N-acetylcysteine infusion was associated with a prompt and complete hematologic recovery.[108]

Gold therapy has also been associated with generalized hypogammaglobulinemia. This may affect patients of any age and has been associated with recurrent bacterial infections and pulmonary manifestations.[109] It may be reversible after cessation of gold treatment.[110] Adult acquired combined immune deficiency has also been reported as a complication of GSTM therapy.[111]

Organ systems rarely affected by gold treatment include the lungs, gut, liver, and nervous system.

Pulmonary Complications

Acute respiratory distress associated with diffuse pulmonary infiltration characteristically causes cough productive of small amounts of sputum, shortness of breath, pleuritic chest pain, and pulmonary crackles.[112] The clinical picture develops after about 500 mg of parenteral gold. Radiographs show patchy areas of pulmonary consolidation, and pulmonary function tests are consistent with restrictive lung disease. Bronchoalveolar lavage may show a predominance of lymphocytes suggesting a hypersensitivity reaction. Dramatic improvement follows withdrawal of chrysotherapy and administration of systemic glucocorticoids.

Intestinal Effects

Enterocolitis is an uncommon but serious complication of parenteral gold, occurring primarily in middle-aged women after small total doses of gold.[113] Symptoms may include abdominal pain, bloody or nonbloody diarrhea, nausea, vomiting, and fever. Despite supportive treatment, the mortality rate approaches 50 percent.

About 85 percent of the total dose of auranofin is eliminated in the feces. It is therefore not surprising that patients with RA taking auranofin have twice the frequency of diarrhea as patients taking parenteral gold. Most side effects are mild and transient, affect the lower gastrointestinal tract, and are dose related. Fewer than 5 percent of patients have to stop taking auranofin because of diarrhea.

Liver

Cholestatic jaundice, with hyperbilirubinemia, elevated transaminases, and high alkaline phosphatase levels, has been ascribed to gold treatment. Liver biopsy may show bile stasis and thrombi in the biliary tree or ballooning hepatocytes with sinusoidal compression and minimal cholestasis. Hepatotoxicity usually develops early (less than 200 mg of compound), often with eosinophilia, and recedes rapidly with cessation of gold therapy. A positive lymphocyte transformation test may indicate cell-mediated hypersensivity to gold.[114] Hepatic necrosis after gold may rarely have fatal consequences.[115] Pancreatitis may also be a rare benign complication of oral or injectable gold.[116]

Nervous System

Neurologic complications of chrysotherapy are rare but reversible and include peripheral neuropathy, a Guillain-Barré–type syndrome, cranial nerve palsies including ophthalmoplegia, and encephalopathy.[117] It usually arises after 3 months of weekly injections, and myokymia is a characteristic clinical sign. Recognition of the neuropathy may be difficult because it can resemble some features of RA itself. Sural nerve biopsy, however, shows both axonal degeneration and segmental demyelination, and computed tomographic brain scan may show evidence of cerebral demyelination. Auranofin has also been incriminated in the onset of encephalopathy and motor neuropathy.[118]

Eye

Corneal and lens chrysiasis is benign and directly related to cumulative dose, occurring in 75 percent of patients receiving more than 1500 mg of intramuscular gold.

Treatment Monitoring

Efforts to reduce untoward gold reactions have been fairly successful. The mortality rate has fallen from an estimated 4 percent in the early years of chrysotherapy to less than 0.05 percent at present. Improved medical care and lower gold doses appear to account for the declining mortality rate. Precautionary measures do not prevent gold complications; they merely permit their recognition. Fortunately, immediate cessation of gold, coupled with appropriate treatment, can prevent severe target-organ damage in most cases.

Monitoring chrysotherapy requires history about drug reactions, rash, renal disease, or proteinuria. Examination includes looking for psoriasis, fungal infection, leukoplakia, palatal mucosal ulceration, or dental inflammation. A complete blood count with differential, platelet count, urinalysis, and biochemical profile is obtained. It is useful to have the patient keep a diary of blood counts and urinalyses as a double check to the danger signals of cytopenias or proteinuria. Blood work and urinalyses for protein are obtained every 1 to 3 weeks.

Chrysotherapy is terminated promptly should any of the aforementioned symptoms or significant eosinophilia, leukopenia, anemia, thrombocytopenia, microscopic hematuria, or proteinuria develop. Other causes than gold toxicity, such as laboratory error, incidental skin or mucous membrane lesions, side effects from other medications, or extra-articular features of RA should be considered. If no other explanation is found, presumably the reaction is gold related, and treatment is held depending on the type and severity of the reaction.

Gold compounds should never be administered to patients with a history of severe gold toxicity (e.g., exfoliative dermatitis, significant depression of any blood cell type, heavy proteinuria, or chronic renal failure). Because vasomotor reactions occur within several minutes after injection, it is wise to give GSTM with the patient recumbent. As noted earlier, hypertensive patients taking ACE inhibitors such as captopril may be at risk for this type of reaction. Ordinarily, gold is not recommended for pregnant or lactating women because the safety for the fetus or newborn infant has not been established. Women of childbearing age in whom chrysotherapy is contemplated are advised to use contraceptive measures; treatment is stopped if pregnancy develops.

Treatment of Gold Toxicity

Most adverse gold reactions resolve spontaneously weeks or months after cessation of gold therapy. Most patients with symptomatic gold dermatitis benefit from antihistamines, topical corticosteroids, or other local measures. Sun and soap should be avoided. Generalized pruritic eruptions may improve with systemic glucocorticoids. Stomatitis, glossitis, cheilitis, and gingivitis may require no treatment or avoidance of spicy foods. Stronger measures include alkaline mouthwashes or the application of lidocaine (Xylocaine Viscous) or triamcinolone (Kenalog in Orabase). We have found betamethasone (Betnasol) pellets sucked three or four times a day to be useful.

Moderate to high dose glucocorticoid therapy (20 to 60 mg daily in divided doses) may be beneficial in gold-induced nephrotic syndrome, thrombocytopenia, and less often, other hematologic disorders, enterocolitis, and pulmonary infiltrates.

Dimercaprol, penicillamine, N-acetylcysteine, and other chelating agents have been employed in severe reactions unresponsive to glucocorticoid therapy or in conjunction with steroids.[1] Patients with severe thrombocytopenia associated with hemorrhage may require volume repletion and platelet transfusions. Vincristine, other potent chemotherapeutic agents, splenectomy, and more recently intravenous gamma globulin have been used.[104] Those suffering from significant granulocytopenia or agranulocytosis often improved spontaneously within 2 weeks. In unresponsive cases and in those with bone marrow aplasia, supportive measures, including androgenic hormones, bone marrow transplantation, and peritoneal dialysis, also have been used. Antithymocyte globulin has been recommended as initial treatment for gold-induced aplastic anemia.[107]

References

1. Gordon, D. A.: Gold compounds. *In* Kelley, W. N., Harris, E. D., Ruddy S., and Sledge C. B. (eds.): Textbook of Rheumatology. 3rd ed. Philadelphia, W. B. Saunders, 1989, pp. 804–823.
2. Kean, W. F., Forestier, F., Kassam, Y., Buchanan, W. W., and Rooney, P. J.: The history of gold therapy in rheumatoid disease. Sémin. Arthritis Rheum. 14:180, 1985.
3. Forestier, J.: Rheumatoid arthritis and its treatment by gold salts. J. Lab. Clin. Med. 20:827, 1935.
4. Hartfall, S. J., Garland, H. G., and Goldie, W.: Gold treatment of arthritis: A review of 900 cases. Lancet 233:838, 1937.
5. Empire Rheumatism Council: Gold therapy in rheumatoid arthritis. Ann. Rheum. Dis. 19:95, 1960.
6. Empire Rheumatism Council: Gold therapy in rheumatoid arthritis: Final report of a multicentre controlled trial. Ann. Rheum. Dis. 20:315, 1961.
7. The Cooperative Clinics Committee of the ARA: A controlled trial of gold salt therapy in rheumatoid arthritis. Arthritis Rheum. 16:353, 1973.
8. Sigler, J. W., Bluhm, G. B., Duncan, H., et al.: Gold salts in the treatment of rheumatoid arthritis: A double-blind study. Ann. Intern. Med. 80:21, 1974.
9. Abruzzo, J. L.: Auranofin: A new drug for rheumatoid arthritis. Ann. Intern. Med. 105:274, 1986.
10. Ward, J. R., Williams, H. J., Egger, M. J., Reading, J. C., Boyce, E., Altz-Smith, M., Samuelson, C. O., Jr., Willkens, R. F., Solsky, M. A., Hayes, S. P., et al.: Comparison of auranofin, gold sodium thiomalate, and placebo in the treatment of rheumatoid arthritis. A controlled clinical trial. Arthritis Rheum. 26:1303, 1983.
11. Olsen, N. J., Callahan, L. F., and Pincus, T.: In vitro rheumatoid factor synthesis in patients taking second-line drugs for rheumatoid arthritis. Independent associations with disease activity. Arthritis Rheum. 31:1090, 1988.
12. Guillemin, F., Bene, M-C., Aussedat, R., et al.: Hypogammaglobulinemia associated with gold therapy: Evidence for a partial maturation blockade of B cells. J. Rheumatol. 14:1034, 1987.
13. Olsen, N. J., and Jasin, H. E.: Decreased pokeweed mitogen-induced IgM and IgM rheumatoid factor synthesis in rheumatoid arthritis patients treated with gold sodium thiomalate or penicillamine. Arthritis Rheum. 27:985, 1984.
14. Rooney M., Whelan, A., Feighery, C., and Bresnihan, B.: Changes in lymphocyte infiltration of the synovial membrane and the clinical course of rheumatoid arthritis. Arthritis Rheum. 32:361, 1989.
15. Lipsky, P. E., and Ziff, M.: Inhibition of antigen- and mitogen-induced human lymphocyte proliferation by gold compounds. J. Clin. Invest. 59:455, 1977.
16. Lies, R. B., Cardin, C., and Paulus, H. E.: Inhibition by gold of human lymphocyte stimulation. Ann. Rheum. Dis. 36:216, 1977.
17. Griswold, D. E., Lee, J. C., Poste, G., et al.: Modulation of macrophage-lymphocyte interactions by the antiarthritic gold compound auranofin. J. Rheumatol. 12:490, 1985.
18. Measel, J. W., Jr.: Effect of gold on the immune response of mice. Infect. Immun. 11:350, 1975.
19. Cannon, G. W., and McCall, S.: Inhibition of the passive transfer of adjuvant induced arthritis by gold sodium thiomalate. J. Rheumatol. 17:436, 1990.
20. Ho, P. P. K., Young A. L., and Southard, G. L.: Methyl ester of N-formylmethionyl-leucyl-phenylalanine. Chemotactic responses of human blood monocytes and inhibition of gold compounds. Arthritis Rheum. 21:133, 1978.
21. Matsubara, T., and Hirohata, K.: Low dosage of gold compounds inhibit interleukin-1–induced fibroblast proliferation but unaffect IL-2 secretion by macrophage (Abstract). Arthritis Rheum. 30:S57, 1987.
22. Danis, V. A., Kulesz, A. J., Nelson, D. S., and Brooks, P. M.: The effect of gold sodium thiomalate and auranofin on lipopolysaccharide-induced interleukin-1 production by blood monocytes in vitro: Variation in healthy subjects and patients with arthritis. Clin. Exp. Immunol. 79:335, 1990.
23. Connolly, K. M., Stecher, V. J., Danis, E., Pruden, D. J., and LaBrie, T.: Alteration of interleukin-1 activity and the acute phase response in adjuvant arthritic rats treated with disease modifying antirheumatic drugs. Agents Actions 25:94, 1988.
24. Lee, J. C., Dimartino, M. J., Votta, B. J., and Hanna, N.: Effect of auranofin treatment on aberrant splenic interleukin production in adjuvant arthritic rats. J. Immunol. 139:3268, 1987.
25. Hurst, N. P., Bell, A. P., and Nuki, G.: Studies of the effect of d-penicillamine and sodium aurothiomalate therapy on superoxide anion production by monocytes from patients with rheumatoid arthritis: evidence for in vitro stimulation of monocytes. Ann. Rheum. Dis. 45:37, 1986.
26. Mowat, A. G.: Neutrophil chemotaxis in rheumatoid arthritis. Ann. Rheum. Dis. 37:1, 1978.
27. Jessop, J. D., Vernon-Roberts, B., and Harris, J.: Effects of gold salts and prednisolone on inflammatory cells. Ann. Rheum. Dis. 32:294, 1973.
28. Harth, M., McCain, G. A., and Orange, J. F.: The effects of auranofin and gold sodium aurothiomalate on the chemiluminescent response of stimulated synovial tissue cells from patients with rheumatoid arthritis. J. Rheumatol. 12:881, 1985.
29. Corey, E. J., Mehrotra, M. M., and Kahn, A. U.: Antiarthritic gold compounds effectively quench electronically excited singlet oxygen. Science 236:68, 1987.
30. Corkill, M. M., Kirkham, B. W., Haskard, D. O., Barbatis, C., Gibson, T., and Panayi, G. S.: Gold treatment of rheumatoid arthritis decreases synovial expression of the endothelial leukocyte adhesion receptor ELAM-1. J. Rheumatol. 18:1453, 1991.
31. Penneys, N. S., Ziboh, V., Gottlieb, N. L., et al.: Inhibition of prostaglandin synthesis and human epidermal enzymes by aurothiomalate in vitro: Possible actions of gold in pemphigus. J. Invest. Dermatol. 63:356, 1974.
32. Ennis, R. S., Granda, J. L., and Posner, A. S.: Effect of gold salts and other drugs on the release and activity of lysosomal hydrolases. Arthritis Rheum. 11:756, 1968.
33. Paulus, H. E.: The use of combinations of disease-modifying antirheumatic agents in rheumatic arthritis. Arthritis Rheum. 33:113, 1990.
34. Boers, M., and Ramsden, M.: Longacting drug combinations in rheumatoid arthritis. A formal overview. J. Rheumatol. 18:316, 1991.
35. Evers, A. E., and Sundstrom, W. R.: Second course gold therapy in the treatment of rheumatoid arthritis. Arthritis Rheum. 26:1071, 1983.
36. Dillon, A. M., Luthra, H. S., Conn, D. L., and Ferguson, R. H.: Parenteral gold therapy in the Felty syndrome. Experience with 20 patients. Medicine (Baltimore) 65:107, 1986.
37. Gordon, M. H., Tiger, L. H., and Ehrlich, G. E.: Gold reactions are *not* more common in Sjögren's syndrome. Ann. Intern. Med. 82:47, 1975.
38. Bennett, P. N., Humphries, S. J., Osborne, J. P., Clarke, A. K., and Taylor, A.: Use of sodium aurothiomalate during lactation. Br. J. Clin. Pharmacol. 29:777, 1990.
39. Fraser, T. N.: Gold treatment in rheumatoid arthritis. Ann. Rheum. Dis. 4:71, 1945.
40. Iannuzzi, L., Dawson, N., Zein, N., and Kushner, I.: Does drug therapy slow radiographic deterioration in rheumatoid arthritis? N. Engl. J. Med. 309:1023, 1983.
41. Sharp, J. T., Lipsky, M. D., and Duffy, J.: Clinical responses during gold therapy for rheumatoid arthritis: Changes in synovitis, radiologically detectable erosive lesions, serum proteins, and serologic abnormalities. Arthritis Rheum. 25:540, 1982.
42. Huskisson, E. C., Gibson, T. J., and Balme, H. W.: Trial comparing D-penicillamine and gold in rheumatoid arthritis. Ann. Rheum. Dis. 33:532, 1974.
43. Currey, H. L. F., Harris, J., and Mason, R. M.: Comparison of azathioprine, cyclophosphamide, and gold in treatment of rheumatoid arthritis. Br. Med. J. 3:763, 1974.
44. Pullar, T., Hunter, J. A., and Capell, A. J.: Sulphasalazine in rheumatoid arthritis: A double-blind comparison of sulphasalazine with placebo and sodium aurothiomalate. Br. Med. J. 287:1102, 1982.
45. William, H. J., Ward, J. R., Dahl, S. L., Clegg, D. O., Willkens, R. F., Oglesby, T., Weisman, M. H., Schlegel, S., Michaels, R. M., Luggen, M. E., et al.: A controlled trial comparing sulfasalazine, gold sodium thiomalate, and placebo in rheumatoid arthritis. Arthritis Rheum. 31:702, 1988.
46. Suarez-Almazor, M. E., Fitzgerald, A., Grace, M., and Russell, A. S.: A randomized controlled trial of parenteral methotrexate compared with sodium aurothiomalate (Myochrysine) in the treatment of rheumatoid arthritis. J. Rheumatol. 15:753, 1988.
47. Morassut, P., Goldstein, R., Cyr, M., Karsh, J., and McKendry, R. J.: Gold sodium thiomalate compared to low dose methotrexate in the treatment of rheumatoid arthritis—a randomized, double-blind 26 week trial. J. Rheumatol. 16:302, 1989.
48. Rau, R., Herborn, G., Menninger, H., Stryz, M., Karger, T., and Elhardt, D.: One year randomized double-blind study of methotrexate (MTX) and gold sodium thiomalate (GST) in early erosive rheumatoid arthritis (RA). Arthritis Rheum. 33:S39, 1990.
49. Williams, H. J., Dahl, S. L., Ward, J. R., Karg, M., Willkens, R. F., Meenan, R. F., Altz-Smith, M., Clegg, D. O., Mikkelsen, W. M., Kay, D. R., et al.: One-year experience in patients treated with auranofin

following completion of a parallel, controlled trial comparing auranofin, gold sodium thiomalate, and placebo. Arthritis Rheum. 31:9, 1988.

50. Dahl, S. L., Samuelson, C. O., Williams, H. J., Ward, J. R., and Karg, M.: Second-line antirheumatic drugs in the elderly with rheumatoid arthritis: A post hoc analysis of three controlled trials. Pharmacotherapy 19:79, 1990.

51. Capell, H. A., Lewis, D., and Carey, J.: A three year follow up of patients allocated to placebo, or oral or injectable gold therapy for rheumatoid arthritis. Ann. Rheum. Dis. 9:705, 1987.

52. Davis, P., Menard, H., Thompson, J., Harth, M., and Beaudet, F.: One-year comparative study of gold sodium thiomalate and auranofin in the treatment of rheumatoid arthritis. J. Rheumatol. 12:60, 1985.

53. Wenger, M. E., Alexander, S., Bland, J. H., and Blechman, W. J.: Auranofin versus placebo in the treatment of rheumatoid arthritis. Am. J. Med. 75:123, 1983.

54. Gofton, J. P., O'Brien, W. M., Hurley, J. N., and Scheffer, B. J.: Radiographic evaluation of erosion in rheumatoid arthritis. Double-blind study of auranofin vs. placebo. J. Rheumatol. 11:768, 1984.

55. Bombardier, C., Ware, J., Russell, I. J., Larson, M., Chalmers, A., and Read, J. L.: Auranofin therapy and quality of life in patients with rheumatoid arthritis. Results of a multicenter trial. Am. J. Med. 81:565, 1986.

56. Borg, G., Allander, E., Lund, B., Berg, E., Brodin, U., Pettersson, H., and Trang, L.: Auranofin improves outcome in early rheumatoid arthritis. Results from a 2-year double-blind, placebo controlled study. J. Rheumatol. 15:1747, 1988.

57. Singh, G., Fries, J. F., Leigh, J. P., Bloch, D. A., and Williams, A.: From experiment to experience: the effectiveness of auranofin in clinical practice (Abstract). Arthritis Rheum. 33:S82, 1990.

58. Zane, J., Bulanowski, M., and Prete, T.: Oral versus parenteral gold for maintenance of RA patients in remission: 1 year follow-up (Abstract). Arthritis Rheum. 30:S59, 1987.

59. Blackburn, W. D.: Auranofin: Its use in rheumatoid arthritis patients maintained on parenteral chrysotherapy. J. Rheumatol. 14:863, 1987.

60. Davis, P., and Landon, M.: Treatment with auranofin in patients with rheumatoid arthritis, previously experiencing drug related side effects to sodium aurothiomalate (Letter). J. Rheumatol. 12:622, 1985.

61. Wessel, J., and Davis, P.: The efficacy of parenteral gold after auranofin failure in rheumatoid arthritis. J. Rheumatol. 10:664, 1983.

62. Hochberg, M. C.: Auranofin or d-penicillamine in the treatment of rheumatoid arthritis. Ann. Intern. Med. 195:528, 1986.

63. Weinblatt, M. E., Kaplan, H., Germain, B. F., Merriman, R. C., Solomon, S. D., Wall, B., Anderson, L., Block., S., Irby, R., Wolfe, F., et al.: Low dose methotrexate compared with auranofin in adult rheumatoid arthritis. A thirty-six-week, double-blind trial. Arthritis Rheum. 33:330, 1990.

64. Dorwart, B. B., Gall, E. P., Schumacher, H. R., et al.: Chrysotherapy in psoriatic arthritis. Arthritis Rheum. 21:513, 1978.

65. Carette, S., Calin, A., McCafferty, J. P., Wallin, B. A., and the Auranofin Cooperating Group: A double-blind placebo-controlled study of auranofin in patients with psoriatic arthritis. Arthritis Rheum. 32:158, 1989.

66. Palit, J., Hill, J., Capell, H. A., Carey, T., Daunt, S., Cawley, I. D., Bird, H. A., and Muki, G.: A multi-centre double-blind comparison of auranofin intramuscular gold thiomalate and placebo in patients with psoriatic arthritis. Br. J. Rheumatol. 29:280, 1990.

67. Giannini, E. H., Brewer, E. J., Jr., Kuzmina, N., Shaikov, A., and Wallin, B.: Auranofin in the treatment of juvenile rheumatoid arthritis. Results of the USA-USSR double-blind, placebo-controlled trial. The USA Pediatric Rheumatology Collaborative Study Group. The USSR Cooperative Children's Study Group. Arthritis Rheum. 33:466, 1990.

68. Clark, P., Tugwell, P., Bennett, K., and Bombardier, C.: Meta-analysis of injectable gold in rheumatoid arthritis. J. Rheumatol. 16:442, 1989.

69. Felson, D. T., Anderson, J. J., and Meenan, R. F.: The comparative efficacy and toxicity of second-line drugs in rheumatoid arthritis. Arthritis Rheum. 33:1449, 1990.

70. Situnayake, R. D., Grindulis, K. A., and McConkey, B.: Long term treatment of rheumatoid arthritis with sulphasalazine, gold, or penicillamine: A comparison using life-table methods. Ann. Rheum. Dis. 46:177, 1987.

71. Wolfe, F., Hawley, D. J., and Cathey, M-A.: Termination of slow acting antirheumatic therapy in rheumatoid arthritis: A 14-year prospective evaluation of 1017 consecutive starts. J. Rheumatol. 17:994, 1990.

72. Ferraccioli, G., Salaffi, F., Nervetti, A., and Cavalieri, F.: Slow acting drugs—outcome no different than 15 years ago (Letter). J. Rheumatol. 17:1249, 1990.

73. Lehtinen, K., and Isomaki, H.: Intramuscular gold therapy prevents premature death in patients with rheumatoid arthritis. J. Rheumatol. 18:524, 1991.

74. Srinivasa, N. R., Miller, B. L., and Paulus, H. E.: Long term chrysotherapy in rheumatoid arthritis. Arthritis Rheum. 22:105, 1979.

75. Scott, D. L., Dawes, P. T., Tunn, E., Fowler, P. D., Shadforth, M. F., Fisher, J., Clarke, S., Collins, M., Jones, P., Popert, A. J., et al.:

76. Williams, H. J., Ward, J. R., and Reading, J. C.: Comparison of auranofin, methotrexate, and the combination of both in the treatment of rheumatoid arthritis (Abstract). Arthritis Rheum. 33:S10, 1990.

77. Kantor, S. M., Wallin, B. A., Grier, C. G., McCafferty, J. P., Wetherington, J. D., Fox, M. J., and The Auranofin Cooperating Group: A combination of auranofin and methotrexate as initial DMARD therapy in rheumatoid arthritis (Abstract). Arthritis Rheum. 33:S60, 1990.

78. Luthra, H. S., et al.: Double-blind study comparing auranofin (AU) and hydroxychloroquine (HCQ) alone or in combination (AU-HCQ) in rheumatoid arthritis (Abstract). Arthritis Rheum. 33:S25, 1990.

79. Fremont-Smith, P., and Fremont-Smith, K.: Association between gold induced skin rash and remission in patients with rheumatoid arthritis (Letter). Ann. Rheum. Dis. 49:271, 1990.

80. Speerstra, F., Van Riel, P. L. C. M., Reekers, P., Van de Putte, L. B. A., Vanderbrouke, J. R., and collaborating clinics: The influence of HLA phenotypes on the response to parenteral gold in rheumatoid arthritis. Tissue Antigens 28:1, 1987.

81. Van de Putte, L. B. A., Speerstra, F., Van Riel, P. L. C. M., Boerbooms, A. M. T. H., Van pad Bosch, P. J. I., and Reekers, P.: Remarkably similar responses to gold therapy in HLA identical sibs with rheumatoid arthritis. Ann. Rheum. Dis. 45:1004, 1986.

82. Sagransky, D. M., and Greenwald, R. A.: Efficacy and toxicity of retreatment with gold salts: A retrospective view of 25 cases. J. Rheumatol. 7:474, 1980.

83. Van der Leeden, H., Dijkmans, B. A., Hermans, J., and Cats, A.: A double-blind study on the effect of discontinuation of gold therapy in patients with rheumatoid arthritis. Clin. Rheumatol. 5:56, 1986.

84. Cats, A.: A multicenter controlled trial of the effects of different dosage of gold therapy, followed by maintenance dosage. Agents Actions 6:355, 1976.

85. Norton, W. L., and Donnelly, R. J.: High dose, low frequency parenteral gold administration. J. Rheumatol. 10:454, 1983.

86. Hanson, V.: Dosage of gold salts in treatment of juvenile rheumatoid arthritis. Arthritis Rheum. 20(Suppl. 2):548, 1977.

87. Ansell, B. M.: The management of juvenile chronic polyarthritis (Still's disease). Practitioner 208(1243):91, 1972.

88. Heath, M. J.: Measurement of "free" gold in patients receiving disodium aurothiomalate and the association of high free to total gold levels with toxicity. Ann. Rheum. Dis. 47:18, 1988.

89. Liang, M. H., and Fries, J. F.: Containing costs in chronic disease: Monitoring strategies in the gold therapy of rheumatoid arthritis. J. Rheumatol. 5:241, 1978.

90. Thompson, M. S., Read, J. L., Hutchings, H. C., and Harris, E. D.: The cost-effectiveness of auranofin: Results of a randomized clinical trial. J. Rheumatol. 15:35, 1988.

91. Godfrey, N., and Lorber, A.: Long term auranofin treatment in rheumatoid arthritis. J. Rheumatol. 12:620, 1985.

92. Block, S. R.: The cost of parenteral gold vs oral gold in the long term treatment of rheumatoid arthritis (Letter). J. Rheumatol. 13:663, 1986.

93. Davis, P.: Cost of gold (Letter). J. Rheumatol. 13:664, 1986.

94. Wooley, P. H., Griffin, J., Panayi, G. S., Batchelor, J. R., Welsh, K. I., and Gibson, T. J.: HLA-DR antigens and toxic reaction to sodium thiomalate and D-penicillamine in patients with rheumatoid arthritis. N. Engl. J. Med. 303:300, 1980.

95. Healey, L. A., and Backes, M. B.: Nitritoid reactions and angiotensin-converting-enzyme inhibitors (Letter). N. Engl. J. Med. 321:763, 1989.

96. Iveson, J. M., Scott, D. G., Perera, W. D. H., et al.: Immunofluorescence of the skin in gold rashes-with particular reference to IgE. Ann. Rheum. Dis. 36:520, 1977.

97. Ranki, A., Niemi, K. M., and Kanerva, L.: Clinical, immunohistochemical, and electron-microscopic finds in gold dermatitis. Am. J. Dermatopathol. 11:22, 1989.

98. Bretza, J., Wells, I., and Novey, H. S.: Association of IgE antibodies to sodium aurothiomalate and adverse reactions to chrysotherapy for rheumatoid arthritis. Am. J. Med. 74:945, 1983.

99. Wicks, I. P., Wong, D., McCullagh, R. B., and Fleming, A.: Contact allergy to gold after systemic administration of gold for rheumatoid arthritis. Ann. Rheum. Dis. 47:421, 1988.

100. Wijnands, M. J., Perret, C. M., van den Hoogen, F. H., van de Putte, L. B., and van Riel, P. L.: Chrysotherapy provoking exacerbation of contact hypersensitivity to nickel (Letter). Lancet 335:867, 1990.

101. Leonard, P. A., Moatamed, F., Ward, J. R., Piepkorn, M. W., Adams, E. J., and Knibbe, W. P.: Chrysiasis: The role of sun exposure in dermal hyperpigmentation secondary to gold therapy. J. Rheumatol. 13:58, 1986.

102. Millard, P. R., Chaplin, A. J., Venning, V. A., Wilson, C., and Wallach, R.: Chrysiasis: Transmission electron microscopy, laser microprobe mass spectrometry and epipolarized light as adjuncts to diagnosis. Histopathology 13:281, 1988.

103. Hall, C. L.: The natural course of gold and penicillamine nephropathy: A long term study of 54 patients. Adv. Exp. Med. Biol. 252:247, 1989.

104. Adachi, J. D., Bensen, W. G., Kassam, Y., et al.: Gold-induced thrombocytopenia: 12 cases and a review of the literature. Semin. Arthritis Rheum. 16:287, 1987.

105. Wijnands, M. J., Allebes, W. A., Boerbooms, A. M., van de Putte, L. B., and van Riel, P. L.: Thrombocytopenia due to aurothioglucose, sulphasalazine and hydroxycholoroquine. Ann. Rheum. Dis. 49:798, 1990.

106. Cicuttini, F. M., Wiley, J. S., and Fraser, K. J.: Immune thrombocytopenia in association with oral gold treatment. Arthritis Rheum. 31:299, 1988.

107. Yan, A., and Davis, P.: Gold induced marrow suppression: A review of 10 cases. J. Rheumatol. 17:47, 1990.

108. Hansen, R. M., Varmas, R. R., and Hanson, G. A.: Gold-induced hepatitis and pure red cell aplasia complete recovery following corticosteroid and N-acetylcysteine therapy. J. Rheumatol. 18:1251, 1991.

109. Stuckey, B. G. A., Hanrahan, P. S., Zilco, T. J., and Owen, E. T.: Hypogammaglobulinemia and lung infiltrates after gold therapy. J. Rheumatol. 13:468, 1986.

110. Olson, J. C., Lovell, D. J., and Levinson, J. E.: Hypogammaglobulinemia associated with gold therapy in a patient with juvenile rheumatoid arthritis. J. Rheumatol. 13:224, 1986.

111. Haskard, D. O., and Macfarlane, D.: Adult acquired combined immune deficiency in a patient with rheumatoid arthritis on gold. J. R. Soc. Med. 81:548, 1988.

112. Gordon, D. A., Hyland, R. H., and Broder, I.: Rheumatoid arthritis. *In* Cannon, G. W., and Zimmerman, G. A. (eds.): The Lung in Rheumatic Diseases. New York, Marcel Dekker, 1990, pp. 229–259.

113. Fam, A. G., Paton, T. W., Shamess, C. J., and Lewis, A. J.: Fulminant colitis complicating gold therapy. J. Rheumatol. 7:479, 1986.

114. Edelman, J., Donnelly, R., Graham, D. N., and Percy, J. S.: Liver dysfunction associated with gold therapy for rheumatoid arthritis. J. Rheumatol. 10:510, 1983.

115. Watkins, P. B., Schade, R., Mills, A. S., Carithers, R. L., Jr., and Van Thiel, D. H.: Fatal hepatic necrosis associated with parenteral gold therapy. Dig. Dis. Sci. 33:1025, 1988.

116. Eisemann, A. D., Backer, N. J., Miner, P. B., Jr., and Fleming, J.: Pancreatitis and gold treatment of rheumatoid arthritis (Letter). Ann. Intern. Med. 111:860, 1989.

117. Fam, A. G., Gordon, D. A., Sarkozi, J., Blair, G. R., Cooper, P. W., Harth, M., and Lewis, A. J.: Neurologic complications associated with gold therapy for rheumatoid arthritis. J. Rheumatol. 11:700, 1984.

118. Gambari, P., Ostuni, P., Lazzarin, P., Tavolato, B., and Todesco, S.: Neurotoxicity following a very high dose of oral gold (auranofin) (Letter). Arthritis Rheum. 11:1316, 1984.

Penicillamine

D-Penicillamine (DP) is a component of the penicillin molecule that may be obtained from it by acid hydrolysis. In rheumatology, it is approved for the treatment of rheumatoid arthritis (RA). It is also used, although not labeled, for the treatment of systemic sclerosis (see Section X).

CHEMISTRY

The structural formula for DP is shown in Figure 46–1. It is a sulfhydryl (SH) amino acid that differs from the naturally occurring cysteine because of the two methyl groups that replace hydrogen in the beta (β)-carbon position. It may be made from penicillin by a semisynthetic process, or it may be made entirely synthetically. All of the DP in clinical use is the D-isomer.

METABOLISM

DP is well absorbed from the upper gastrointestinal tract when given in the postabsorptive state. Approximately half of an orally administered dose can be accounted for in urine and feces. Using radiolabeled (^{14}C) DP, 85 percent of the radioactivity is recovered in 24 hours. There is little free DP in the urine, most of the drug being eliminated in the oxidized form as the internal disulfide (penicillamine–penicillamine), the mixed disulfide (penicillamine–cysteine), or S-methyl-penicillamine.[1]

When DP administration is discontinued, free DP rapidly disappears from the urine, but the two disulfides can be recovered for more than 3 months. This suggests a release from tissue stores (in the oxidized form), which might explain the persistence of both efficacy and toxicity after termination.[2] In plasma, binding is greatest to albumin, (α)-globulin, and ceruloplasmin. In tissues, radioactive DP is found in greatest amount in collagen-containing structures, skin and tendon.

BIOCHEMICAL AND CLINICAL PHARMACOLOGY

The biochemical and pharmacologic properties of DP in humans form the basis for certain of its clinical applications.[3] *Chelation* of divalent cations such as copper and trace metals accounts for its usefulness in the treatment of Wilson's disease and heavy metal poisoning. It forms a *thiazolidine* with pyridoxal phosphate, which may result in antagonism to vitamin B$_6$, although it is much weaker in this regard than L-penicillamine.[4] A thiazolidine bond may also be formed between DP and the aldehyde groups of collagen, thereby inhibiting collagen cross-linking (dermolathyrism).[5] This is the biochemical basis for its application to the treatment of systemic sclerosis. The *SH–SS interchange* reaction with amino acids is the mechanism by which avid binding to intravascular and extravascular proteins is achieved and accounts for the in vivo formation of penicillamine–cysteine mixed disulfide with cystine. This is the molecular basis for the use of DP in cystinuria, for the mixed disulfide is highly soluble, thereby preventing formation of new cystine calculi. Which, if any, of these actions is responsible for the efficacy of DP in RA is not known (see later).

DP is available as a 250- or 125-mg capsule or as a 250-mg scored tablet. Various dosage regimens have been studied in RA, and it is recommended that treatment be initiated with 125 or 250 mg per day for 4 to 8 weeks. The dosage may then be raised by a similar increment until improvement commences or a maximum of 1.0 g has been achieved. Although total daily dosages as high as 2.0 g may sometimes be required, the current trend is to employ an average dose not greater than 500 mg per day.

Absorption of DP is hindered by food, antacids, and oral iron; hence, it is optimal in the postabsorptive state.[3] It usually may be given in a single daily dose, 1 to 2 hours apart from food or other medicines. Both indomethacin and chloroquine have been shown to raise blood levels of DP.[6] The mechanism of this interaction has not been elucidated, and it is possible that similar effects with other drugs might also exist. These findings might explain apparent discrepancies with regard to both efficacy and toxicity

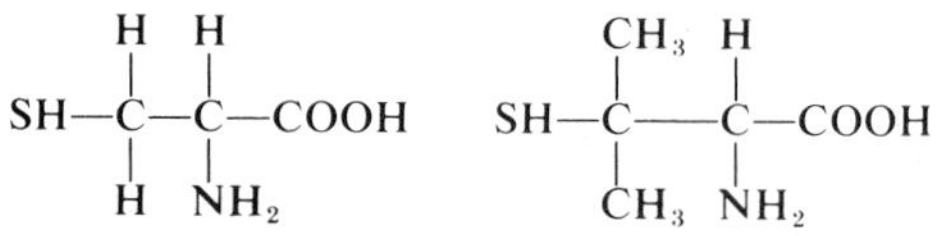

Figure 46–1. The chemical structure of penicillamine. The drug is an analogue of the naturally occurring amino acid cysteine, with CH$_3$ groups replacing H + at the B carbon position.

in various trials, when no information is given about concomitant medications and the timing of the dose in relation to DP.

INDICATIONS AND POSITIONING

DP is indicated for the treatment of active RA (seropositive or seronegative) and in selected patients with juvenile RA. The efficacy of DP for RA was first established by the United Kingdom MultiCenter Trial.[7] Subsequent studies showed it to be as effective as azathioprine, intramuscular gold, and antimalarial drugs and more effective than oral gold.[8] It has been particularly useful in some patients with RA with extra-articular manifestations, such as vasculitis, Felty's syndrome, amyloidosis, and rheumatoid lung disease.[9] It is not of value in the seronegative spondyloarthropathies,[10] psoriatic arthritis, and other types of inflammatory connective tissue disease.

In the treatment of uncomplicated RA, the use of DP is generally considered after the failure of at least one other slow-acting agent. Newer practice patterns, particularly in the United States, would position the use of DP after a trial of methotrexate had failed, either because of toxicity or lack of efficacy. The reasons for this are the advantages of methotrexate with regard to more rapid onset of therapeutic effect, higher response rate, and greater safety. In younger patients in the reproductive age group, this latter sequence might be reversed, because the long-term safety of methotrexate has not yet been defined.

CONTRAINDICATIONS AND PRECAUTIONS

DP is contraindicated in pregnancy, although there are reports of successful pregnancies when the drug has been continued throughout gestation.[11] If a patient with RA becomes pregnant while receiving DP, the drug should be stopped, but termination of the pregnancy is not indicated. A history of a previous allergic or hypersensitivity reaction to penicillin is *not* a contraindication to the use of DP, and no additional precautions are required.[12] DP does not interfere with wound healing, and it does not need to be terminated before elective surgery.[13]

Because of the potential for the precipitate onset of certain of the toxic reactions, particularly hematologic, prescriptions for DP should be written for a limited time and clearly labeled *nonrefillable*. Previous failure to respond or the development of an adverse reaction to gold does not preclude a favorable outcome with DP.[14, 15] Nevertheless, patients who have experienced major side effects with gold are more likely to experience toxicity with DP than those who have not.[16]

RESPONSE PATTERN

The pattern of improvement in a DP-responsive patient is similar to that observed during a successful course of chrysotherapy. There is a gradual decrease in the duration of morning stiffness and the severity of joint pain. Objective signs of a decrease in synovitis may be found by 6 months. Laboratory studies show a gradual improvement in the sedimentation rate and the C-reactive protein, and a rise in hemoglobin. A reduction in the titer of serum rheumatoid factor is a consistent finding, and it usually correlates with clinical improvement.[17]

Because of the latent period of 8 to 12 weeks before improvement is evident, administration of analgesic and anti-inflammatory drugs must be maintained. As the response evolves, they may be reduced and often eliminated completely. The ability to dispense with symptomatic therapies, particularly glucocorticoids, may be used as a measure of the response to DP. Exacerbations in disease activity may be observed throughout the course of treatment. They are usually self-limited but may require an increase in the maintenance dose to regain control. As with most drugs of this class, secondary failures are seen, and this late escape from control usually does not respond to higher doses. It has been shown that antibodies to DP may develop during treatment, and this may be an explanation for the loss of efficacy in some patients over time.[18]

ADVERSE EFFECTS AND TOXICITY

The adverse effects that may result from DP administration have been the major factor limiting its usefulness. Certain of these effects can be favorably influenced by the "go low, go slow" graduated dosage regimens, but others can occur regardless of the maximum maintenance dose or the duration of treatment. Most of the side effects are encountered during the first 18 months of therapy (Fig. 46–2; see color section at front of this volume); however, careful surveillance must be maintained throughout the treatment period.[19]

Various factors have been studied in an attempt to find a predictive marker for development of DP toxicity. It was first shown that there was an association between HLA-B8 and DR3 and toxic reactions to both gold salts and DP, particularly with respect to nephropathy.[20, 21] This finding was given further impetus from a study in Japan, in which only four cases of nephropathy were encountered in 5124 patients given a course of DP.[22] Both HLA-B8 and DR3 are extremely rare in Japanese persons. Sulfoxidation status (the ability to oxidize carbocysteine) was studied in relation to DP toxicity. Patients who had poor sulfoxidation status were almost four times more likely to develop side effects to DP than those who had good sulfoxidation status.[23] The sulfoxidation status and HLA were independent predictors. Of

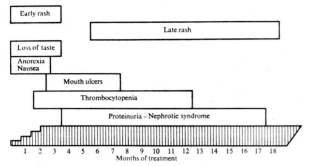

Figure 46–2. The chronopharmacology of penicillamine. This depicts the peak incidence of some of the more common side effects of penicillamine during a course of therapy with a maintenance dose of 1 g per day. Most of the serious reactions will have developed during the first 18 months of treatment. Aplastic anemia was not included in this illustration, but it may occur at any time, particularly after an increment in dosage. (After Balme, H. W., and Huskisson, E. C.: Chronopharmacology of penicillamine and gold. Scand. J. Rheumatol. 4[Suppl. 8]:21, 1975. Used by permission.)

interest was the observation that the group with RA had a higher percentage of patients with poor sulfoxidation status than did the control group, and this might explain the apparent higher increase of DP toxicity in patients with RA than in those with Wilson's disease.

Other studies showed that SSA (Sjögren's syndrome antibody [Ro]) and cryoglobulins predisposed to development of DP toxicity in Greek patients.[24] It has been noted anecdotally that RA patients with Sjögren's syndrome are more prone to DP toxicity than are RA patients without this feature. Antibodies to DP also are associated with a higher incidence of adverse reactions,[18] and this also is an independent variable.

Although these observations are of extreme interest, a prospective study showed that HLA typing was not useful in predicting either the therapeutic outcome or the development of toxicity in DP-treated RA patients.[21, 21a] Furthermore, in view of the high percentage of RA patients with poor sulfoxidation status, this status would not be a useful pretreatment screening test. These tests are costly, are not generally available, and do not offer absolute predictability for development of toxicity, and it is not justified to withhold a trial of DP based on these findings.

Hematologic toxicity is certainly the most serious of the adverse reactions. Leukopenia, thrombocytopenia, and aplastic anemia have been observed. Thrombocytopenia may be dose related, with normal numbers of megakaryocytes, and treatment can be continued, or it may be idiosyncratic and a harbinger of marrow aplasia when the megakaryocyte numbers are decreased.

Complete blood counts with platelets should be done every 2 weeks for the first 6 months and monthly thereafter. A white blood cell count below 3000 cells per mm³ or a platelet count below 100,000 cells per mm³ requires that the DP therapy be dis-

continued until the nature of the reaction can be better defined. It is emphasized again that *prescriptions for DP should never be labeled refillable.* In DP aplastic anemia, high-dose glucocorticoids, granulocyte transfusions, and bone marrow grafts have not helped and perhaps have been detrimental.

Nephropathy is most often of the membranous type, secondary to immune complex deposition.[25] Proteinuria may be asymptomatic or may be associated with signs of nephrotic syndrome. Urinalysis should be performed at the same time as the hematologic studies. Twenty-four–hour determinations of urinary protein are of value, and up to 2.0 g per 24 hours is considered acceptable in the absence of clinical signs of nephrotic syndrome. Two groups of RA patients with DP nephropathy were compared with regard to renal function and continued DP therapy. In one group, DP administration was stopped after proteinuria developed, and in the other, DP therapy was continued. At the end of 1 year, renal function was the same in both groups.[26]

Microscopic hematuria is usually benign and does not require discontinuation of treatment.[27] Gross hematuria should be evaluated with regard to possible causes. If none are found, it is probably a result of the DP, and the drug should be stopped. Rapidly progressive (crescentic) glomerulonephritis is a rare occurrence, but it may require short-term dialysis and immunosuppressive therapy.[28] Crescentic nephritis with pulmonary infiltrates and hemoptysis resembles Goodpasture's syndrome (see later), but the basement membrane stains in a granular manner, and there is no anti–glomerular basement membrane antibody.

Dermatologic reactions—pruritus and a variety of early and late rashes—are the most common side effects of the drug. Simple pruritus can often be managed by a temporary interruption of DP therapy and the addition of an antihistamine. Aphthous ulcers and stomatitis may occur, but they often resolve with a modest reduction in dosage. The appearance of a bullous dermatitis might herald the development of DP-induced pemphigus (Fig. 46–3). Administration of the drug must be stopped, and immunosuppressive therapy may be required.

Gastrointestinal symptoms due to penicillamine are usually not serious. Anorexia and nausea may be dose limiting but usually disappear with time. Although DP is best absorbed when given before a meal, administering the dose after food sometimes reduces nausea even though a higher dose may be required. There have been infrequent reports of cholestatic jaundice, but serious hepatotoxicity is extremely rare.[29]

Pulmonary complications are also rare. A Goodpasture-like syndrome has already been described. There have been reports of DP-associated bronchiolitis obliterans. Obliterative bronchiolitis is a serious, often irreversible, disorder that may be fatal.[30] It can occur as part of the spectrum of rheumatoid lung disease, independent of any drug, or in association

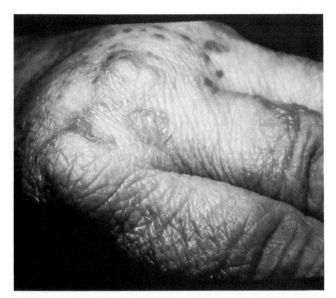

Figure 46–3. This photograph shows bullous lesions in the skin of a DP-treated patient with RA. The clinical and histologic findings are those of pemphigus. The DP was stopped, and glucocorticoids were required; the lesions gradually resolved.

with gold or DP. The role of DP in development of this entity is not clear, but the appearance of dyspnea associated with midinspiratory rhonchi should alert the physician to this possibility.

Neuromuscular disorders may infrequently be caused by DP. Myasthenia gravis is the most common in this category, and it is virtually identical to the spontaneously occurring disease. There are antibodies to the acetylcholine receptor, and the patients respond to anticholesterase drugs. Ocular myasthenia is invariably part of the DP-induced disease.[31] The myasthenia is reversible after DP withdrawal, but months may be required before dependence on anticholinesterase drugs ends. Whereas spontaneous myasthenia is associated with HLA-DR3 and B1, DP-induced myasthenia is almost always associated with HLA-DR1 and Bw35.[32, 32a] Polymyositis and dermatomyositis also can be produced by DP. Clinically, by biopsy, and by electromyographic studies, these cases are indistinguishable from the spontaneously occurring disease, except that they remit after withdrawal of the DP.

Autoimmune syndromes have already been discussed under the various organ systems. They have been described in the other diseases for which DP is given, such as Wilson's disease and cystinuria, indicating that they are a feature of the drug rather than an altered immune responsiveness in patients with RA. Certain of the hematologic reactions and renal toxicities appear to be immunologically mediated. Myasthenia gravis, pemphigus, and polymyositis are clearly in this category. Autoantibodies to insulin and the insulin receptor have been described.[33] DP-induced lupus has been well recognized, and these patients differ from other examples of drug-induced lupus in that they have antibody to native, double-stranded DNA rather than to single-stranded DNA.[34, 34a] No other drug has the unique proclivity for induction of autoimmune phenomena that DP does, and this may relate to its mechanism of action.[35]

Miscellaneous side effects are usually self-limited and may not require cessation of therapy. Hypogeusia or dysgeusia—blunting or alteration in taste perception—is common. Although it is most often encountered early in treatment, it may develop at any time. Drug fever, often associated with a morbilliform rash, usually develops shortly after treatment is begun and recurs on rechallenge. A benign enlargement of the breasts, mammary gigantism, has been described that may require danazol therapy, although no hormonal abnormalities have been described.[36]

MECHANISM OF ACTION

The mechanism of action of DP in RA, like that of the other noncytotoxic agents (gold, hydroxychloroquine, and sulfasalazine), is unknown. The DP molecule is so highly reactive that the demonstration of an effect in an in vitro test system cannot necessarily be extrapolated to explain its mode of action in RA. Laboratory and animal experiments that have yielded negative results should be given at least equal weight in trying to clarify this issue. In test systems, DP is neither anti-inflammatory nor immunosuppressive, and it has no effect on animal models of arthritis.[37] It does not inhibit the function of macrophages, B lymphocytes, or the suppressor (CD8) subset of T lymphocytes. It does, however, inhibit selectively the function of the T helper cell (CD4).[37]

This observation may have relevance in view of the role of the CD4 cell in rheumatoid synovitis. After DP treatment of RA, there was a significant reduction in T lymphocytes and a disproportionate fall in the helper/inducer subset in the synovial tissue.[38] These observations suggest a highly specific and selective type of immunosuppression directed against the CD4 subset.

Some clinical observations made in the treatment of RA with DP might provide direction in the attempt to elucidate the mechanism. The specificity of DP for only RA is unique among the antirheumatic drugs. As indicated earlier, DP is of no benefit in any other type of inflammatory joint disease.[10] This drug–disease specificity suggests that DP acts on a pathogenetic mechanism present only in RA. If RA is ultimately proved to depend on the CD4 cell for its expression, in contrast with other arthritides, the specificity of DP for RA could be explained by the remarkably selective inhibitory effect of DP on that cell type.

Another observation that helps elucidate the site of action of DP is the consistent reduction of rheumatoid factor titer and immune complexes with DP treatment (Figs. 46–4 and 46–5). These immunoglob-

an autoimmune disease (RA) with improvement in its *immunologic,* as well as clinical, manifestations. These observations suggest a role in immune regulation and dysregulation.

Alternative explanations to that of a primary action of DP on the immune system have been suggested. In vitro, it was found that DP (with copper) produced a marked suppression of human fibroblast proliferation.[39] It was suggested that this could inhibit pannus formation in RA, and collagen production in scleroderma. A suppression of human endothelial production in vitro and neovascularization in vivo by DP was reported.[40] This antiangiogenic effect, it was suggested, could reduce the number of small blood vessels available for egress of inflammatory cells and thereby reduce synovial proliferation. Non-SH angiotensin-converting enzyme (ACE) inhibitors were given to patients with RA to determine whether ACE inhibition or the thiol group was responsible for the beneficial effects. The non-SH ACE inhibitors were ineffective,[41] and it was concluded that the SH group was essential for a DP-like drug effect in RA.[42]

OUTCOME STUDIES

After 5 years, only about 25 percent of patients given DP were able to continue with a satisfactory result.[43] Withdrawals were due largely to adverse reactions and, to a lesser degree, to loss of efficacy. Progression of radiologic damage did not differ between patients treated with DP for 5 years and those receiving any other treatment.[44] In an 18-month trial with DP, radiologic progression was not halted.[45] In a comparison study of radiologic progression with DP and hydroxychloroquine, initial radiologic damage was less with DP; by 2 years, however, no difference was noted between the drugs.[46] The fail-

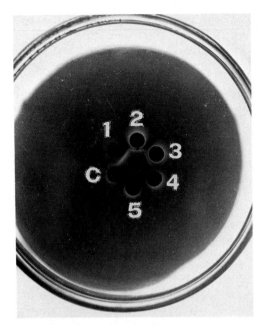

Figure 46–4. The effect of penicillamine therapy on complexes as measured by precipitation with a purified IgM rheumatoid factor. Well No. 1 contains synovial fluid, and well No. 2 contains serum from the same patient prior to treatment. Well No. 3 shows a decrease in the amount of complexes after 6 weeks on the drug. Wells No. 4 and No. 5 show the absence of serum complexes at 3 and 6 months, respectively. Well C is normal serum. A serial examination of synovial fluid was not possible, as the effusion had reabsorbed. (Courtesy of Dr. Robert Winchester.)

ulins and complexes are the product of synthesis by B lymphocytes. Because DP has no direct inhibitory effect on B cell function, it is reasonable to assume that its inhibition is exerted *before* the step of antibody synthesis by B cells. It is probable also that a drug that has such a dramatic effect on the immune system, resulting in the induction of such a wide spectrum of autoimmune diseases, is acting at a fundamental level. At the same time, it ameliorates

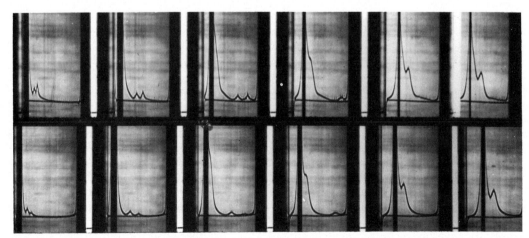

Figure 46–5. The ultracentrifugal pattern of serum proteins before treatment (top) and after 3 months on the drug (bottom). (Kindly performed by Dr. Henry Kunkel.) Serum was diluted 1:1 with saline. Centrifugation was at 52,640 rpm and proceeds from left to right. Pictures were taken at 16, 32, 48, 64, 80, and 90 minutes. The post-treatment pattern shows a reduction in the 22S complex, 19S macroglobulin, and the intermediate gamma globulin complexes.

ure of DP to influence radiologic progression is similar to that reported for most of the second-line drugs.

OTHER SULFHYDRYL COMPOUNDS

Numerous attempts have been made to find an SH compound with a DP-like beneficial effect in RA but with greater safety. 5-Thiopyridoxine, pyrithioxine (pyritinol), thiopronine (α-mercaptopropionyl glycine), and captopril have been studied. All were effective, although captopril was the weakest. Unfortunately, they all displayed a similar and characteristic spectrum of adverse effects, including induction of autoimmune disease.[47, 47a, 47b] In Europe, both pyritinol and thiopronine are being used for RA, since a failure with DP does not preclude a good response to one of the others. Similarly, an adverse reaction to DP is not necessarily replicated by one of the alternative SH-containing drugs in an individual patient.[48]

References

1. Joyce, D. A.: D-Penicillamine pharmacokinetics and pharmacodynamics in man. Pharmacol. Ther. 42:405, 1989.
2. Wei, P., and Sass-Kortsak, A.: Urinary excretion and renal clearances of D-penicillamine in humans and the dog. Gastroenterology 58:288, 1970.
3. Lock, H. E., Lock, C. J., Mewa, A., and Kean, W. F.: D-Penicillamine chemistry and clinical use in rheumatic disease. Semin. Arthritis Rheum. 15:261, 1986.
4. Jaffe, I. A., and Merryman, P.: The antipyridoxine effect of penicillamine in man. J. Clin. Invest. 43:1869, 1964.
5. Nimni, M. E., and Bavetta, L. A.: Collagen defect induced by penicillamine. Science 150:905, 1965.
6. Seidman, P., and Lindström, B.: Pharmacokinetic interactions of penicillamine in rheumatoid arthritis. J. Rheumatol. 16:473, 1989.
7. Multi-Center Trial Group: Controlled trial of D-penicillamine in severe rheumatoid arthritis. Lancet 1:275, 1973.
8. Felson, D. T., Anderson, J. J., and Meenan, R. F.: The comparative efficacy and toxicity of second-line drugs in rheumatoid arthritis. Arthritis Rheum. 33:1449, 1990.
9. Jones, J. S.: Rheumatoid lung cavitation and response to penicillamine. Thorax 42:988, 1987.
10. Steven, M. M., Morrison, M., and Sturrock, R. D.: Penicillamine in ankylosing spondylitis. J. Rheumatol. 12:735, 1985.
11. Scheinberg, I. H., and Sternlieb, I.: Pregnancy in penicillamine-treated patients with Wilson's disease. N. Engl. J. Med. 293:1300, 1975.
12. Bell, C. L., and Graziano, F. M.: The safety of administration of penicillamine to penicillin-sensitive subjects. Arthritis Rheum. 26:801, 1983.
13. Ansell, B. M., Moran, H., and Arden, G. P.: Penicillamine and wound healing in rheumatoid arthritis. Proc. R. Soc. Med. 70(Suppl. 3):75, 1977.
14. Webley, M., and Coomes, E.: An assessment of penicillamine therapy in rheumatoid arthritis and the influence of previous gold therapy. J. Rheumatol. 6:20, 1979.
15. Steven, M. M., Hunter, J. A., Murdoch, R. M., and Capell, H. A.: Does the order of second-line treatment in rheumatoid arthritis matter? Br. Med. J. 1:79, 1982.
16. Kean, W. F., Lock, C. J. L., Howard-Lock, H. E., and Buchanan, W. W.: Prior gold therapy does not influence the adverse effects of penicillamine in rheumatoid arthritis. Arthritis Rheum. 25:1975, 1982.
17. Thoen, J., Helgetveit, O., Forre, Y. H., and Kass, E.: Effects of piroxicam on T lymphocyte subpopulations, natural killer cells, and rheumatoid factor production in rheumatoid arthritis. Scand. J. Rheumatol. 17:91, 1988.
18. Storch, W. B.: Clinical significance of penicillamine antibodies. Lancet 2:214, 1988.
19. Cooperative Systematic Studies of Rheumatic Disease Group: Toxicity

20. of low-dose D-penicillamine therapy in rheumatoid arthritis. J. Rheumatol. 14:67, 1987.
20. Panayi, G. S., Wooley, P., and Batchelor, J. R.: Genetic basis of rheumatoid disease: HLA antigens, disease manifestations, and toxic reactions to drugs. Br. Med. J. 2:1326, 1978.
21. Bernelot Moens, H. J., Ament, B. J. W., Feltkamp, B. W., and van der Korst, J. K.: Long-term follow-up of treatment with D-penicillamine for rheumatoid arthritis: Effectivity and toxicity in relation to HLA antigens. J. Rheumatol. 14:1115, 1987.
21a. Clarkson, R. W. E., Sanders, P. A., and Grennan, C. M.: Complement C4 null alleles as a marker of gold or D-penicillamine toxicity in the treatment of rheumatoid arthritis. Br. J. Rheumatol. 31:53, 1992.
22. Kashiwazaki, S.: Current status of D-penicillamine therapy in Japan. Z. Rheumatol. 47(Suppl. 1):38, 1988.
23. Madhok, R., Zoma, A., Torley, H. I., Capell, H. A., Waring, R., and Hunter, J. A.: The relationship of sulfoxidation status to efficacy and toxicity of penicillamine in the treatment of rheumatoid arthritis. Arthritis Rheum. 33:574, 1990.
24. Vlachoyiannopoulis, P. G., Zerva, L. V., Skopouli, F. N., Drosos, A. A., and Moutsopoulos, H. M.: D-Penicillamine toxicity in Greek rheumatoid arthritis patients: anti-RO(SSA) antibodies and cryoglobulinemia are predicting factors. J. Rheumatol. 18:44, 1991.
25. Bacon, P. A., Tribe, C. R., MacKenzie, J. C., Verrier Jones, J., Cumming, R. H., and Amer, B.: Penicillamine nephropathy in rheumatoid arthritis: A clinical, pathological, and immunological study. Q. J. Med. 45:661, 1976.
26. Hall, C. L., and Tighe, R.: The effect of continuing penicillamine and gold treatment on the course of penicillamine and gold nephropathy. Br. J. Rheumatol. 28:53, 1989.
27. Leonard, P. A., Bienz, S. R., Clegg, D. O., and Ward, J. R.: Hematuria in patients receiving gold and D-penicillamine. J. Rheumatol. 14:55, 1987.
28. Devogelaer, J.-P., Pirson, Y., Vandenbroucke, J.-M., Cosyns, J.-P., Brichard, S., and Nagant de Deuxchaisnes, C.: D-Penicillamine–induced crescentic glomerulonephritis: Report and review of the literature. J. Rheumatol. 14:1036, 1987.
29. Langan, M. N., and Thomas, P.: Penicillamine-induced liver disease. Am. J. Gastroenterol. 82:1318, 1987.
30. Obliterative bronchiolitis (Editorial). Lancet 1:603, 1982.
31. Katz, L. J., Lesser, R. L., Merikangas, J. R., and Silverman, J. P.: Ocular myasthenia gravis after D-penicillamine administration. Br. J. Ophthalmol. 73:1015, 1989.
32. Garlepp, M. J., Dawkins, R. L., and Christiansen, F.: HLA antigens and acetylcholine receptor antibodies in penicillamine-induced myasthenia gravis. Br. Med. J. 286:338, 1983.
32a. Morel, E., Feuillet-Fieux, M. N., Vernet-der Garabedian, B., Raimond, F., D'Angelejan, J., Bataille, R., Sany, H., and Bach, J. F.: D-Penicillamine–induced myasthenia gravis: a comparison with idiopathic myasthenia and rheumatoid arthritis. Clin. Immunol. Immunopathol. 58:318, 1991.
33. Benson, E. A., Healey, L. A., and Barron, E. J.: Insulin antibodies in patients receiving penicillamine. Am. J. Med. 78:857, 1985.
34. Enzenauer, R. J., Sterling, G. W., and Rubin, R. L.: D-Penicillamine–induced lupus erythematosus. Arthritis Rheum. 33:1582, 1990.
34a. Chin, G. L., Kong, N. C. T., Lee, B. C., and Rose, I. M.: Penicillamine-induced lupus syndrome in a patient with classical rheumatoid arthritis. J. Rheumatol. 18:947, 1991.
35. Jaffe, I. A.: Induction of auto-immune syndromes by penicillamine therapy in rheumatoid arthritis and other diseases. Semin. Immunopathol. 4:193, 1981.
36. Craig, H. R.: Penicillamine-induced mammary hyperplasia: Report of a case and review of the literature. J. Rheumatol. 15:1294, 1988.
37. Lipsky, P. E., and Ziff, M.: Inhibition of human helper T cell function in vitro by D-penicillamine and $CuSO_4$. J. Clin. Invest. 65:1069, 1980.
38. Walters, M. T., Smith, J. L., Moore, K., Evans, P. R., and Cawley, M. I. D.: An investigation of the action of disease modifying antirheumatic drugs on the rheumatoid synovial membrane: Reduction in T lymphocyte subpopulations and HLA-DP and DQ antigen expression after gold or penicillamine therapy. Ann. Rheum. Dis. 46:7, 1987.
39. Matsubara, T., and Hirohata, K.: Suppression of human fibroblast proliferation by D-penicillamine and copper sulfate in vitro. Arthritis Rheum. 31:964, 1988.
40. Tsukasa, M., Saura, R., Hirohata, K., and Ziff, M.: Inhibition of human endothelial cell proliferation in vitro and neovascularization in vivo by D-penicillamine. J. Clin. Invest. 83:158, 1989.
41. Jaffe, I. A.: Angiotensin-converting enzyme inhibitor in rheumatoid arthritis. Arthritis Rheum. 27:840, 1984.
42. Bird, H. A., Le Gallez, P., Dixon, J. S., Catalano, M., Traficante, A., Liauw, L., Sussman, H., Rotman, H., and Wright, V.: A clinical and biochemical assessment of a nonthiol ACE inhibitor (pentopril; CGS-13945) in active rheumatoid arthritis. J. Rheumatol. 17:603, 1990.
43. Proceedings of the VIIIth French Conference of Rheumatology, Paris, 1985. Rev. Rhum. 53:1, 1986.
44. Multi-Center Trial Group: A prospective five-year comparison of treat-

ment that included penicillamine with that excluding penicillamine in early rheumatoid arthritis. Br. J. Rheumatol. 25:184, 1986.

45. Scott, D. L., Greenwood, A., Bryans, R., and Huskisson, E. C.: Progressive joint damage during penicillamine therapy for rheumatoid arthritis. Rheumatol. Int. 8:135, 1988.

46. Scott, D. L., Greenwood, A., Davies, J., Maddison, P. J., Maddison, M. C., and Hall, N. D.: Radiological progression in rheumatoid arthritis: Do D-penicillamine and hydroxychloroquine have different effects? Br. J. Rheumatol. 29:126, 1990.

47. Jaffe, I. A.: Adverse effects profile of sulfhydryl compounds in man. Am. J. Med. 80:471, 1986.

47a. Ehrhart, A., Chicault, P., Fauquert, P., and LeGoff, P.: Effets secondaires dus au traitement par la tiopronine de 74 polyarthrites rhumatoïdes. Rev. Rhum. Mal. Osteoartic. 58:193, 1991.

47b. Lindell, A., Denneberg, T., Eneström, S., Fich, C., and Skogh, T.: Membranous glomerulonephritis induced by 2-mercaptopropionyl glycine (2-MPG). Clin. Nephrol. 34:108, 1990.

48. Sigaud, M., Maugars, Y., Maisonneuve, H., and Prost, A.: Tiopronine dans 69 cas de polyarthrite rheumatoïde traités antérieurement par la D-penicillamine. Rev. Rhum. 55:467, 1988.

Chapter 47

Michael E. Weinblatt

Methotrexate

Methotrexate has become an established treatment for rheumatoid arthritis. Low-dose weekly methotrexate was approved by the United States Food and Drug Administration in 1988 as a therapy for active rheumatoid arthritis. There is also significant interest in low-dose methotrexate as a therapy for a variety of other autoimmune, inflammatory, and rheumatologic conditions.

CHEMICAL STRUCTURE

Methotrexate is an antimetabolite and is a structural analogue of folic acid. The structure of folic acid (pteroylglutamic acid) consists of three elements: a multiring pteridine group linked to a para-aminobenzoic acid that is connected to a terminal glutamic acid residue (Fig. 47–1). Methotrexate differs from folic acid in that an amino group substitutes for a hydroxyl group in position 4 of the pteridine portion of the molecule and by the addition of a methyl group in position 10 of the 4 amino–benzoic acid structure (see Fig. 47–1).

BIOCHEMICAL PHARMACOLOGY

Dietary folic acid is reduced enzymatically by the enzyme dihydrofolate reductase to both dihydrofolate and tetrahydrofolate, which are metabolically active reduced folates. These reduced folates are essential in the conversion of homocysteine to methionine, in the metabolism of histidine, in the synthesis of purines, and in the biosynthesis of thymidylate, which is required for DNA synthesis. Methotrexate, an antimetabolite, binds and inactivates the enzyme dihydrofolate reductase, resulting in the depletion of metabolically active intracellular folates with subsequent inhibition of the synthesis of thymidylate and inosinic acid (Fig. 47–2). Additionally, methotrexate affects protein synthesis by preventing the conversion of glycine to serine and homocysteine to methionine. Methotrexate exerts its maximum inhibitory effect on cells that are actively undergoing DNA synthesis, particularly those cells in the S phase of the cell cycle. Cells undergoing rapid cellular turnover such as in the epidermis and gastrointestinal tract are the most susceptible to the effects of the drug. Folinic acid (leucovorin), a fully reduced metabolically active folate coenzyme, func-

tions without the need for reduction by the enzyme dihydrofolate reductase. Folinic acid (leucovorin) is used to "rescue" normal cells from the toxicity induced by methotrexate. Folinic acid is used as a "rescue" agent in cancer chemotherapy and as a treatment for acute methotrexate overdose and hematologic toxicity.

Folates in the blood have a single terminal glutamate structure. Most intracellular folates are metabolized to a polyglutamated compound. These polyglutamates have longer cellular retention and are more efficient cofactors than the monoglutamate compound. Similar to the folate cofactors, methotrexate also is metabolized from a monoglutamate to a polyglutamated derivative. Methotrexate polyglutamates have stronger cellular retention, remain within the cell in the absence of extracellular drugs, and are more potent than the monoglutamate structure.[1] The synthesis of the methotrexate polyglutamates increases with the duration of therapy. The polyglutamated derivatives predominate in hepatic tissue, which may be a factor in toxicity. The concentration of hepatic methotrexate polyglutamates decreases after folinic acid therapy.[2]

The mechanism of action of low-dose methotrexate in rheumatoid arthritis is not known. Whether its therapeutic effect is due to its antifolate activity, immunomodulating properties, immunosuppressive properties, or anti-inflammatory effects is under study. It is most likely that a combination of these factors accounts for its therapeutic profile in rheumatoid arthritis. High-dose methotrexate at doses used for cancer therapy has immunosuppressive properties including suppression of antibody formation and suppression of primary and secondary immune response.[3] In rheumatoid arthritis, however, a profound immunosuppressive effect has not been documented with low-dose methotrexate. Neither a global suppression of T cell function nor changes in T cell subsets were reported in short-term studies in rheumatoid arthritis.[4, 5] After 2 years of therapy, however, a significant increase in the percentage of T3 and T4 cells and an increase in thymidine incorporation responses to selected mitogens and antigens were noted.[6] These changes may have reflected the reduction in prednisone dose and overall improvement in disease activity that occurred after 2 years of drug administration rather than a selective effect of the drug.

The effect of methotrexate on in vivo gamma M immunoglobulin (IgM) rheumatoid factor production

767

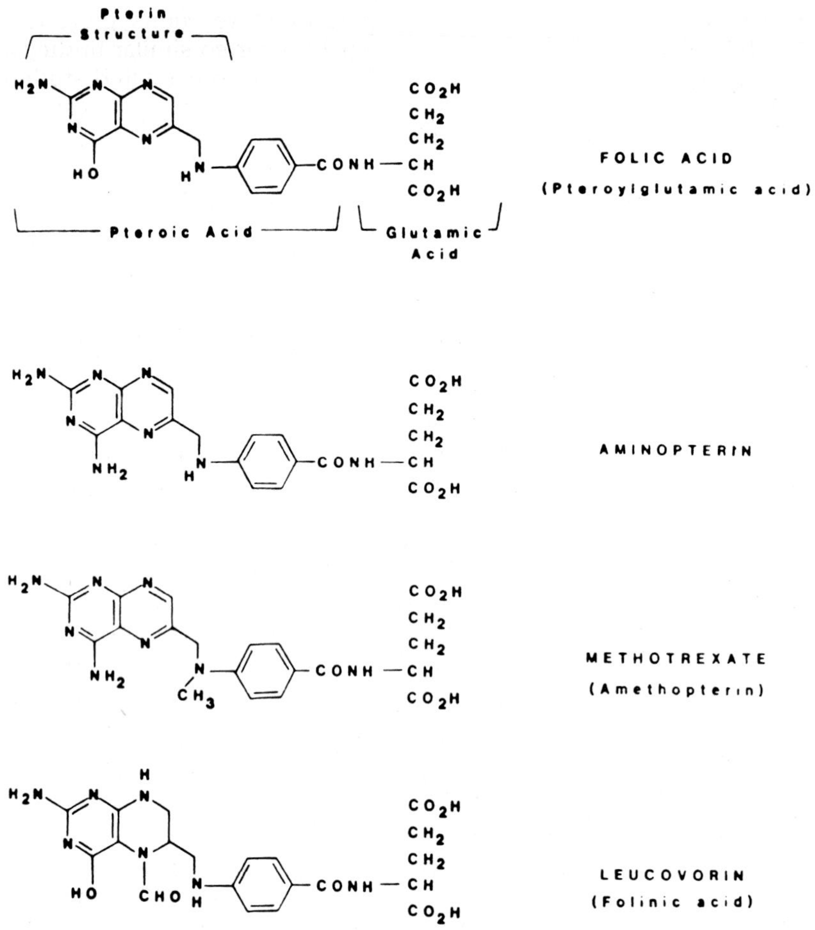

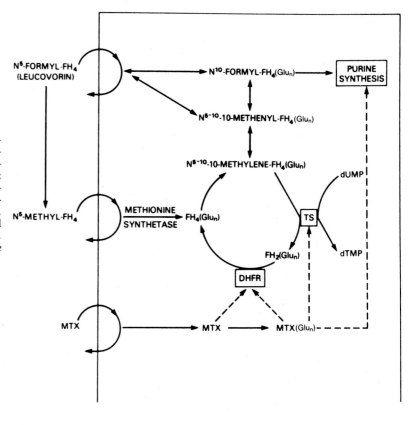

Figure 47–1. Structure of folic acid, aminopterin, methotrexate, and leucovorin.

Figure 47–2. Mechanism of action of methotrexate. MTX, Methotrexate; DHFR, dihydrofolate reductase; TS, thymidylate synthetase; FH_4, tertrahydrofolate; FH_2 dihydrofolate; Glu, glutamyl; dTMP, thymidylate; dUMP, dioxyuridylate. Broken lines indicate enzyme inhibition. (From Jolivet, J., Cowan, K. H., Curt, G. A., Clendeninn, N. J., and Chabner, B. A.: The pharmacology and clinical use of methotrexate. N. Engl. J. Med. 309:1095, 1983. Reprinted by permission of the New England Journal of Medicine.)

as measured by agglutination assays has been variable.[4, 5, 7] A suppression of IgA rheumatoid factor and IgM rheumatoid factor as measured by an enzyme-linked immunosorbent assay (ELISA), however, was observed in vivo in patients enrolled in multicenter trials of methotrexate.[8] A suppression of in vitro rheumatoid factor production has also been observed.[9] Inhibition of selected interleukin-1 (IL-1) activity has been reported in vitro, but the in vivo data are inconclusive.[10] Methotrexate exerts an antiproliferative effect on peripheral blood mononuclear cells in vitro,[11] inhibits in vitro vascular epithelial cell proliferation and in vivo neovascularization, and may affect adenosine release.[12, 12a]

An anti-inflammatory effect with methotrexate has been suggested by its rapid onset of action and the flare after drug discontinuation. In an air sac model of inflammation, pretreatment of mice with low-dose methotrexate inhibited neutrophil migration that was induced by both C5a and leukotriene B_4.[13] In vivo chemotaxis after stimulation with C5a and leukotriene B_4 was blocked in psoriasis patients after methotrexate administration.[14, 15] Suppression of leukotriene B_4 ex vivo was observed with methotrexate in rheumatoid arthritis patients.[16]

Low-dose methotrexate inhibited adjuvant induced and streptococcal cell wall induced arthritis.[17] In adjuvant arthritis, methotrexate inhibited macrophage activation, inhibited neutrophil migration, and prevented the induction of an IL-2 deficiency in animals.[17]

PHARMACOKINETICS

Methotrexate at low doses can be administered by either an oral or parenteral route. The bioavailability of low-dose oral methotrexate is relatively high, but there is individual patient variability. In 41 rheumatoid patients who received 10 mg per m^2 of oral methotrexate, a mean bioavailability of 0.7 with a range of 0.4 to 1.0 was reported.[18] Patients not responding on oral methotrexate should be given a trial of parenteral methotrexate to ensure complete bioavailability. Intramuscular and subcutaneous methotrexate are rapidly absorbed; the maximum serum concentration is attained within 2 hours of injection. The pharmacokinetics of subcutaneous methotrexate is the same as intramuscular methotrexate in rheumatoid arthritis.[19] Methotrexate diffuses into synovial fluid at concentrations equal to serum levels.[18]

Methotrexate distributes throughout the body, with higher concentrations found in intestinal epithelium and hepatic cells. Methotrexate is only 50 to 60 percent bound to plasma proteins. An increase in free methotrexate owing to its displacement from albumin by more highly protein bound drugs such as aspirin, nonsteroidal anti-inflammatory drugs, and sulfonamides can occur. This displacement appears to be of limited clinical significance with low meth-

otrexate doses because the increase in free methotrexate may only be modest. Methotrexate may undergo hepatic metabolism by the enzyme aldehyde oxidase to 7-hydroxymethotrexate. Excretion of methotrexate and its metabolites is by the kidney by both glomerular filtration and proximal tubular secretion. Organic acids such as phenylbutazone, penicillin, sulfonamides, salicylates, and probenecid competitively inhibit tubular secretion, which may affect methotrexate clearance. The plasma half-life of methotrexate is less than 10 hours but increases in the presence of renal insufficiency. The toxic effect of methotrexate on normal tissue is generally related to the duration of exposure rather than the peak level of the drug.

Several kinetic studies have failed to note a significant interaction between low-dose methotrexate and a variety of nonsteroidal anti-inflammatory drugs.[20, 21] With high doses of methotrexate, coadministration of nonsteroidal anti-inflammatory drugs or aspirin may be toxic and must be avoided. Drugs that affect renal function, such as probenecid, or drugs with antifolate activity, such as trimethoprim/sulfamethoxazole, should be used with great caution owing to an increased risk for toxicity.

RHEUMATOID ARTHRITIS

Because aminopterin was a potent inhibitor of connective tissue proliferation, Gubner et al.[22] in 1951 administered this drug to six patients with rheumatoid arthritis. A rapid improvement in the arthritis symptoms occurred in five of the six patients, but exacerbations followed drug discontinuation. In 1972, Hoffmeister[23] reported the beneficial effect of low-dose intramuscular methotrexate in 29 patients. Hoffmeister expanded his series to include 78 patients with a treatment follow-up as long as 15 years.[24] Forty-five patients (58 percent) had a "marked" improvement, including 28 patients who were judged to be in "complete remission." Seven patients discontinued therapy owing to adverse reactions, including elevation in liver blood tests, stomatitis, headaches, nausea, or increasing fatigue.

In another open study, 67 patients received low-dose oral weekly methotrexate for a treatment period that ranged from 3 months to 10 years.[25] A "one-step" response was noted in 33 (49 percent) and a "two-step" response was noted in 18 (27 percent) of the patients. Thirty-four patients discontinued therapy, including 11 because of nausea or gastrointestinal intolerance.

There was significant improvement in a 21-patient open study of 38 weeks' duration. The methotrexate dose ranged from 7.5 to 25.0 mg per week.[26] Eleven (52 percent) of the patients had an "unequivocal" response, five (24 percent) had an "equivocal" response, and two patients were unresponsive to therapy. Three patients discontinued methotrexate: two because of noncompliance and fear of toxicity

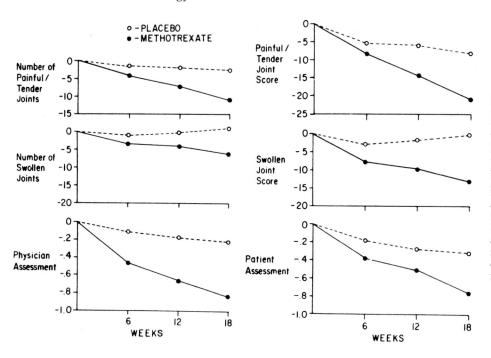

Figure 47–3. Mean change in selected clinical variables by treatment (placebo vs. methotrexate) at 6, 12, and 18 weeks of therapy. (From Williams, H. J., Willkens, R. F., Samuelson, C. O., Jr., et al.: Comparison of low-dose oral pulse methotrexate and placebo in the treatment of rheumatoid arthritis: A controlled clinical trial. Arthritis Rheum. 28:276, 1985. Reprinted from Arthritis and Rheumatism Journal, copyright 1985. Used by permission of the American College of Rheumatology.)

and one because of a hypersensitivity reaction that included fever and hepatitis. In a follow-up of these 18 patients, there was sustained clinical response after a mean of 42 months of treatment.[27] Three patients withdrew from this long-term study: two because of gastrointestinal toxicity and one because of a planned pregnancy.

In another study, intravenous methotrexate at a dose as high as 50 mg per week was effective in 11 of 14 patients, with improvement occurring within 4 weeks of drug initiation.[28] Twelve of these 14 patients, however, developed toxicity, primarily nausea and stomatitis, that led to drug discontinuation in three patients.

The positive results from these uncontrolled studies led to four placebo-controlled trials in patients who had failed prior second-line therapies, including gold salts. In an 18-week randomized multicenter study, 189 patients received either oral methotrexate (7.5 mg to 15.0 mg per week) or placebo.[7] There was a significant improvement in all clinical variables (Fig. 47–3) as well as the erythrocyte sedimentation rate in the methotrexate group. Thirty patients on methotrexate withdrew owing to adverse reactions that included elevated liver blood tests in 18, stomatitis in five, gastrointestinal toxicity in three, pancytopenia in two, and leukopenia in two. All the adverse reactions resolved with drug discontinuation.

A significant improvement in efficacy parameters was also reported in a 35-patient, 24-week, double-blind crossover trial of low-dose weekly methotrexate versus placebo.[4] An improvement in clinical parameters began within 3 weeks after methotrexate initiation. Individual patient response defined as a greater than 50 percent improvement in the joint pain or tenderness index or joint swelling index occurred in 54 percent and 34 percent of the metho-

trexate patients (Fig. 47–4). During the crossover period, an increase in disease activity occurred within 3 weeks after methotrexate discontinuation. One patient withdrew owing to drug toxicity that caused severe diarrhea that resolved with drug discontinuation.

Two other randomized trials, including a 6-week parallel study[29] and a 24-week crossover study,[5] noted similar improvement with methotrexate therapy. A meta-analysis of the four randomized trials noted a significant improvement with methotrexate in all parameters except the 50-foot walk time.[30] There was a 46 percent reduction in the duration of morning stiffness, a 27 percent reduction in the number of painful joints, and a 26 percent reduction in the number of swollen joints in the methotrexate-treated patients.

Two short-term crossover studies[4, 5] and two longer-term studies[31, 32] reported a flare of arthritis activity following methotrexate discontinuation. In one study, ten patients who had previously received 36 months of methotrexate were now randomized to receive placebo or methotrexate.[31] A flare of arthritis activity occurred in all the patients randomized to the placebo group. This flare occurred within 4 weeks of discontinuing methotrexate.

There have been several studies comparing methotrexate with other second-line therapies. In patients with advanced disease who had received prior therapy with either gold salts or D-penicillamine, methotrexate was compared with azathioprine. Forty-two patients entered a 24-week randomized trial of methotrexate versus azathioprine, and both treatment groups improved on therapy.[33] There was no significant difference between the response in the two groups. In a 53-patient study, both treatment groups improved and there was no difference be-

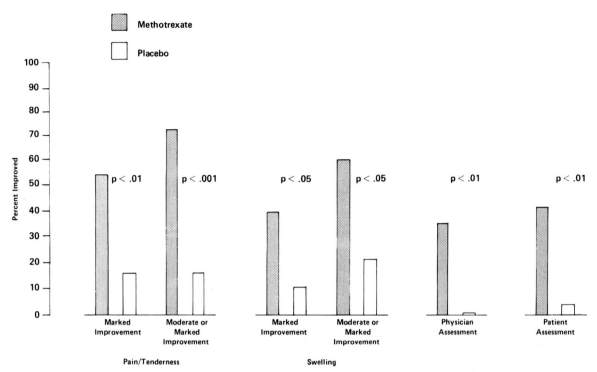

Figure 47–4. Individual patient response in a 35-patient, 24-week crossover trial. Marked improvement in the joint pain/tenderness and swelling index defined as a decrease of 50 percent or more in their value; moderate improvement defined as a decrease of 30 to 49 percent in these indexes. Improvement in physician and patient assessments represented at least a 2-point change in a 5-point scale.

tween groups in the clinical response.[34] Fifty percent of the patients withdrew from the study owing to either toxicity or a lack of drug efficacy. Owing to the small study populations, a type II statistical error likely occurred, so conclusion from these trials about relative drug efficacy is not possible.

Gold therapy, both parenteral and oral, has been compared with methotrexate. These studies enrolled patients with earlier and milder disease in contrast to all the other studies of methotrexate. In studies of 35 and 40 patients who had never received other second-line therapies, intramuscular gold therapy and methotrexate induced similar improvements in disease activity, but gold salts were more toxic.[35, 36] In a 9-month, 282-patient trial comparing methotrexate with auranofin, there was an improvement in disease parameters with both drugs.[37] Methotrexate was superior to auranofin in improving disease activity parameters and individual patient response (Fig. 47–5). Auranofin was also more toxic than methotrexate in this study.

There have been several long-term studies of methotrexate in rheumatoid arthritis. Twenty-nine patients were treated in an open study of methotrexate for a mean of 29 months.[38] There was a significant improvement, with the maximum beneficial effect being achieved by month 6. This beneficial response was maintained through the study period. There was also a significant reduction in prednisone dose. The

maximum dose of methotrexate was 25.0 mg per week. Two patients withdrew owing to toxicity that included pneumonitis and gastrointestinal toxicity. There was a sustained clinical improvement after 54 months of therapy in the 25 patients who remained in the study.[39] The mean dose of methotrexate increased from 12.4 to 14.6 mg per week. Adverse events were frequent but were generally mild.

Similar efficacy results were seen in another long-term prospective study. Twenty-six patients who completed a 24-week crossover trial[4] enrolled in an open study of methotrexate.[6] In this study, the maximum dose of oral methotrexate was 15.0 mg per week. Sixteen patients received 36 months of therapy. There was a significant improvement in disease activity, with the maximum beneficial effect being seen by 6 months (Fig. 47–6). The prednisone dose was significantly reduced. Adverse events were frequent but were generally mild. Only one patient withdrew owing to a lack of efficacy.

Intramuscular methotrexate at a dose of 5.0 to 25.0 mg per week was administered to 128 patients.[40] Forty-nine patients received 3 years of therapy. The clinical variables improved with treatment. Forty-three patients withdrew from the study, including 23 because of toxicity and 15 because of a lack of drug efficacy.

A total of 123 patients who had successfully completed a 9-month randomized trial comparing

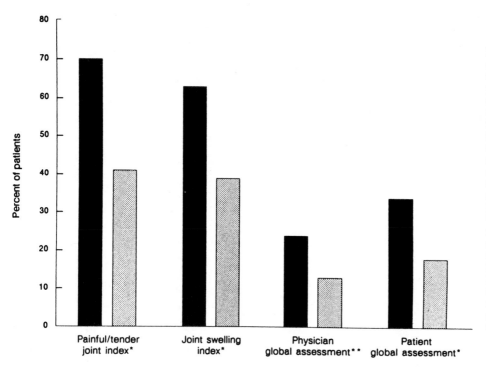

Figure 47–5. Individual patient response, methotrexate versus auranofin study. Percentage of patients with marked improvement in four clinical measures of rheumatoid arthritis activity, by treatment group. Solid column indicates methotrexate group; shaded column indicates auranofin group. The significance of differences between groups was calculated by the Mantel-Haenszel chi-square text. (*) indicates $P < 0.01$; ** $P = 0.03$. (From Weinblatt, M., et al.: Low-dose methotrexate compared with auranofin in adult rheumatoid arthritis. A 36-week, double-blind trial. Arthritis Rheum. 33:330, 1990. Reprinted from Arthritis and Rheumatism Journal, copyright, 1992. Used by permission of the American College of Rheumatology.)

methotrexate with auranofin[37] enrolled in a long-term open study of oral methotrexate.[41] The maximum dose of methotrexate in this study was 20.0 mg per week. Thirty-two patients received at least 36 months of therapy. The standard parameters of rheumatoid arthritis activity significantly improved. The mean number of painful joints and swollen joints decreased by 80 percent. There was no significant difference between the improvement seen at month 6 and that seen at month 36. A significant reduction in prednisone dose was achieved. Adverse events occurred frequently but were generally mild. Twenty-seven patients (22 percent) withdrew, including four (3 percent) because of a lack of efficacy and six (5 percent) because of clinical and laboratory adverse experiences. The overall probability of remaining on therapy for 48 months was projected at 72 percent.

Several retrospective studies reported that a significant percentage of patients initiating methotrexate could be maintained on long-term therapy. In a review of 124 patients treated with methotrexate, 60 patients (48 percent) continued to receive methotrexate for 2 years with a sustained clinical benefit.[42] Adverse drug reactions were the major reason for patient withdrawal. In a study of 152 rheumatoid patients, the probability of continuing methotrexate at 1 year was 71 percent and at 6 years was projected at 49 percent.[43] The major reason for withdrawal was drug toxicity. Of 230 patients enrolled in ongoing long-term prospective studies of methotrexate, 174 (75 percent) still remain on methotrexate.[44] Fifty-one patients (23 percent) have received more than 4 years of treatment. It was projected that 63 percent of the patients would remain on drug therapy for at least 6 years.

The effects of methotrexate on radiographic changes are variable. A halting of radiographic progression has not yet been demonstrated. One study reported a healing of erosions within the first 29 months of methotrexate therapy;[38] however, after a mean of 54 months of therapy, new erosions were noted.[39] In another study, after a mean of 28 months of treatment worsening of the radiographs was noted in six of 14 patients.[6] An improvement in the number and size of the erosions was seen in five of the 14 patients, but a marked narrowing of the joint space was observed in these five patients. Three of these five patients had the most "substantial" clinical response on methotrexate. In a study of 18 patients who experienced significant improvement on methotrexate, radiographic progression continued despite 30 months of treatment.[45] In the two patients who achieved a clinical remission, there was no evidence of radiographic progression. Two other studies suggested slowing of radiologic progression in a subset of patients.[40, 46] Methodologic differences, lack of an appropriate control group, and a limited treatment duration hinder interpretation of all of these studies.

Methotrexate has been used in combination with several other second-line therapies. A randomized trial of methotrexate in combination with auranofin noted no difference in either efficacy or toxicity with the combination compared with solo therapy.[47] An improvement without greater toxicity was noted with the combination of methotrexate and intramuscular gold,[48] methotrexate and sulfasalazine,[49] and methotrexate and azathioprine.[50] Several of these combinations are being studied in randomized trials.

OTHER DISEASES

After the initial report[22] of the beneficial effects of aminopterin in psoriasis and psoriatic arthritis,

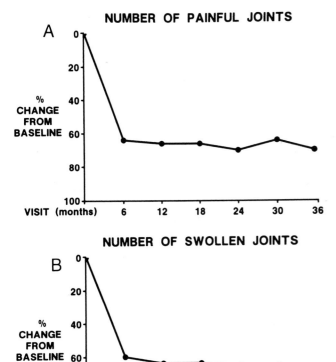

NUMBER OF PAINFUL JOINTS

A

NUMBER OF SWOLLEN JOINTS

B

Figure 47–6. Long-term response in patients receiving methotrexate. Mean percentage of change from baseline (A) and number of painful joints and number of swollen joints (B). Number of patients at each visit was as follows: 12 months, 19 patients; 24 months, 18 patients; 36 months, 16 patients. (From Weinblatt, M. E., et al.: Long-term prospective trial of low-dose methotrexate in rheumatoid arthritis. Arthritis Rheum. 31:167, 1988. Reprinted from Arthritis and Rheumatism Journal, copyright 1992. Used by permission of the American College of Rheumatology.)

extensive studies with methotrexate in psoriasis were performed. An important risk factor for toxicity was the frequency of methotrexate dosing. Weekly administration was less toxic than daily administration of the drug. An oral regimen based on skin kinetics was developed in which methotrexate was administered at 12-hour intervals for three doses once a week.[51] This regimen produced less toxicity than daily therapy and was as effective and no more toxic than weekly parenteral therapy.

Methotrexate is also effective for psoriatic arthritis and Reiter's syndrome at doses of 7.5 to 30.0 mg per week. In a review of 21 patients with Reiter's syndrome, there was improvement in the mucocutaneous disease in 90 percent and an improvement in the arthritis in 75 percent of patients.[52] Three patients discontinued therapy owing to toxicity that included stomatitis, anemia, and abnormal liver blood tests.

In Felty's syndrome, the leukocyte count improved with low-dose methotrexate.[53] The leukopenia, however, returned with drug discontinuation.

Open studies in glucocorticoid-resistant polymyalgia rheumatica and giant cell arteritis,[54] systemic lupus erythematosus,[55] and cutaneous vasculitis of rheumatoid arthritis[56] all reported improvement with low-dose methotrexate. Preliminary open studies suggested some effect with methotrexate in scleroderma.[57, 58] Efficacy with methotrexate was reported in juvenile rheumatoid arthritis.[59, 60] A preliminary analysis of an international study of methotrexate in juvenile rheumatoid arthritis noted that methotrexate at a dose of 10 mg per m^2 per week was more effective than placebo.[61] Methotrexate at doses of 30 to 50 mg per week was also effective in glucocorticoid-resistant polymyositis and dermatomyositis.[62]

Open studies in sarcoidosis,[63] sclerosing cholangitis,[64] primary biliary cirrhosis,[65] and inflammatory bowel disease[66] all suggested efficacy with low-dose methotrexate. Short-term randomized trials[67, 68] and a longer-term study[69] reported efficacy with low-dose methotrexate in glucocorticoid-dependent asthma. Studies of methotrexate are continuing in these diseases as well as in multiple sclerosis, uveitis, and recent-onset diabetes.

DOSE AND DRUG ADMINISTRATION

Methotrexate is given only on a *weekly basis* because more frequent administration is associated with a greater incidence of acute and chronic toxicity. Methotrexate is administered either orally or by parenteral injection. Oral methotrexate can be taken as one dose, or it can be cycled over a 24-hour period. The initial dose of methotrexate is generally 7.5 mg per week, but a lower dose may be used in patients for whom toxicity is a particular concern. If a positive response has not been noted within 4 to 8 weeks after methotrexate initiation and there has been no toxicity, the dose may be increased. Even though the optimal dose in rheumatoid arthritis is unknown, most studies used doses of 7.5 to 20.0 mg per week. In the randomized trial comparing auranofin with methotrexate, 43 percent of the methotrexate patients increased their methotrexate dose from 7.5 to 15.0 mg per week for greater efficacy.[37] A dose response study suggested a linear dose response between placebo at 5 mg per m^2 and at 10 mg per m^2.[70] Once a satisfactory clinical response occurs, the dose of methotrexate may be slowly reduced. Some patients may require higher doses over time to maintain a beneficial response. Doses above 20 mg per week should be administered parenterally owing to decreased oral bioavailability at these higher doses. Doses above 30 mg per week have been associated with greater toxicity. One study of 10 patients, however, reported efficacy and tolerability with intravenous therapy at an initial dose of 40 mg per m^2 and a final dose of 26 mg per m^2.[71] A pilot study of five patients with refractory disease reported efficacy and good tolerability with high-dose intravenous methotrexate (500 mg per m^2) and leucovorin (50 mg per m^2) administered biweekly for 8 weeks.[72] The clinical response lasted 6 to 14 weeks after the infusions were completed. Further studies with high-dose therapy are in progress.

A depletion in the serum folate concentration and an alteration in a folate-dependent enzyme system (the C_1 index) developed with methotrexate therapy.[73] Supplemental folic acid at a dose of 1 mg per day did not reduce the efficacy of methotrexate in a 24-week, placebo-controlled trial.[74] There was a suggestion of less toxicity in the folic acid–treated group. Folinic acid (leucovorin) administered midway between methotrexate doses did not influence either the efficacy or the toxicity of methotrexate in a 13-patient randomized trial.[75] In another study, seven patients received folinic acid (15 mg) starting 4 to 6 hours after the methotrexate dose for 3 consecutive days.[76] Each patient received a total of 45 mg per week of folinic acid for 4 weeks. Nausea that was present before the study resolved on folinic acid therapy. A flare of arthritis, however, occurred on folinic acid therapy and resolved with folinic acid discontinuation. Folinic acid at a dose that was equal to the methotrexate dose (5 to 15 mg) was administered 4 hours after the methotrexate in another 20-patient randomized trial.[77] There was no decrease in the efficacy of methotrexate; there was less stomatitis and nausea in the folinic acid–treated group. Additional studies of folinic acid and methotrexate are in progress.

Despite an initial report of efficacy with intra-articular methotrexate,[78] subsequent trials have not demonstrated any improvement with intra-articular methotrexate when compared with saline or glucocorticoid injections.[79, 80]

TOXICITY

Adverse reactions with low-dose weekly methotrexate have been frequently reported in clinical trials. Despite the high frequency of adverse reactions, serious toxicity has been rare. The most common adverse event with methotrexate is gastrointestinal toxicity, including anorexia, nausea, vomiting, diarrhea, and weight loss.[81] In most patients, this toxicity is generally mild and generally occurs shortly after drug administration. This toxicity may improve with dose reduction or cycled oral or parenteral therapy and may diminish with long-term exposure. In a review of 587 patients receiving therapy, gastrointestinal toxicity was noted in 10 percent; 2.5 percent of the patients had a moderate to severe reaction that led to drug withdrawal.[81] Stomatitis consisting of erythema, painful ulcers, or erosions may also occur and varies in severity. Folinic acid therapy may improve the nausea and stomatitis.[77]

Alopecia, reactivation of ultraviolet light–induced erythema, urticaria, and cutaneous vasculitis may occur with low doses of the drug.[81, 82] Despite an improvement in articular disease, an increase in the number and the size of rheumatoid nodules has been observed.[6, 83]

Hematologic toxicity including leukopenia, thrombocytopenia, megaloblastic anemia, and pancytopenia is rare, occurring in less than 5 percent of patients.[81] Risk factors for this toxicity include renal insufficiency, folic acid deficiency, acute infections including viral illnesses, and concomitant use of selected drugs including probenecid and trimethoprim/sulfamethoxazole.[84, 85] An elevation in the mean corpuscular volume might be a predictor of impending hematologic toxicity.[86] Folinic acid (leucovorin) should be administered immediately for a suspected methotrexate overdose or for hematologic toxicity. Folinic acid is generally most effective when administered within 24 to 48 hours of the dose of methotrexate. In the setting of renal insufficiency, however, folinic acid may still be effective even if administered after this time period. Folinic acid should be administered at a dose that is equal to the methotrexate dose every 4 to 6 hours until there is no longer a detectable serum level of methotrexate.

There are no reports of renal toxicity from low-dose weekly methotrexate. Owing to the excretion of the drug, however, renal insufficiency from any cause can lead to sustained and toxic levels of methotrexate. Regular monitoring of renal function is essential. High doses of methotrexate, however, may crystallize in the renal tubules, resulting in renal failure.

Transient but reversible oligospermia has been reported with high-dose methotrexate for cancer chemotherapy[87] and low-dose therapy for psoriasis.[88] Ovarian dysfunction has not been reported with the drug.[87] Methotrexate is, however, a definite teratogenic agent. Aminopterin was used as an abortifacient, and its use has been associated with specific fetal abnormalities described as the *aminopterin syndrome*.[89] These defects include multiple skeletal abnormalities, hydrocephalus, cleft palate, ear abnormalities, and anencephaly. Methotrexate should not be administered to women of childbearing age unless adequate birth control measures are used. Women should discontinue therapy at least one ovulatory cycle, and men at least 90 days before attempting conception.

Methotrexate has not yet been identified as a carcinogenic agent despite concerns that relate to in vitro studies in which lymphocytes deprived of folic acid developed fragile sites.[90] Studies in animals have not demonstrated a carcinogenic effect.[91] Patients receiving high-dose methotrexate for choriocarcinoma did not have an increased risk of a second malignancy.[92] A carcinogenic effect was not reported in studies of psoriasis patients receiving low-dose weekly methotrexate.[93, 94]

Pulmonary toxicity, both acute and chronic, has been reported with methotrexate therapy. This toxicity has been reported in patients receiving methotrexate for malignancy, polymyositis, psoriasis, and rheumatoid arthritis.[95–99] Pulmonary reactions with methotrexate appear to be more common in rheumatoid arthritis than in other diseases, with a reported frequency of 3 to 5 percent.[98, 99] There is no association between this toxicity and age, sex, dose, duration of therapy, or route of administration. Underlying pulmonary disease, particularly interstitial fibrosis, has been suggested as a risk factor.[100] Headaches and malaise are early symptoms followed by a nonproductive cough, dyspnea, and fever. The clinical symptoms may precede the radiographic evidence of lung disease by several weeks. Bilateral interstitial infiltrates generally develop. Alveolar infiltrates, diffuse nodular infiltrates, hilar adenopathy, and pleural effusions have been observed.[95] The lung pathology is consistent with a hypersensitivity reaction with inflammatory infiltrates consisting primarily of mononuclear cells, giant cells, granuloma formation, and varying degrees of bronchiolitis and fibrosis. The pathology may be indistinguishable from rheumatoid lung disease. Rarely the fibrosis may progress, and extensive scarring of the lung with honeycomb changes may develop.[101] The pathogenesis of this reaction is unknown. Treatment has included discontinuation of methotrexate, respiratory support, and administration of glucocorticoids. Infections with opportunistic organisms including *Pneumocystis carinii* and fungi may occur, so infection must be excluded.[102, 103] The outcome is variable. Most patients have recovered, but chronic dyspnea and mortality have been reported.

Hepatic fibrosis was reported shortly after the introduction of antifolate drugs for childhood leukemia and psoriasis. In 88 psoriatic patients from Scandinavia, cirrhosis was noted in 6 percent after a mean cumulative dose of 1.7 g of methotrexate.[104] In 68 patients who received methotrexate for 5 years, with a mean cumulative dose of 3.9 g, fibrosis was seen in 24 percent and cirrhosis in 21 percent of the patients. This suggested that cumulative dose was a risk factor for toxicity.[105] These results contrast with the experience from the United States, in which a lower incidence of hepatic toxicity has been noted.[106] The greater incidence of hepatic abnormalities reported from Scandinavia may relate to greater alcohol consumption and a longer duration of therapy. Histologic abnormalities may occur in psoriasis patients independent of drug exposure, so pretreatment biopsies have been advocated. Suggested risk factors for methotrexate-associated liver toxicity in psoriatic patients include prior arsenic therapy, insulin-dependent diabetes, renal insufficiency, morbid obesity, alcohol consumption, daily or several methotrexate doses per week, and the cumulative dose of methotrexate.[106] The natural history of methotrexate-associated liver disease in psoriasis is unknown. It has been suggested that it will not progress once the drug is discontinued. Twenty-five psoriatic patients who developed cirrhosis on methotrexate were maintained on methotrexate.[107] Repetitive biopsies failed to demonstrate a progression in the liver pathology;

Table 47–1. CLASSIFICATION OF LIVER BIOPSY FINDINGS

Grade I:	Normal: fatty infiltration; mild: nuclear variability, mild; portal inflammation, mild
Grade II:	Fatty infiltration, moderate–severe; nuclear variability, moderate–severe; portal tract expansion, portal tract inflammation, and necrosis, moderate–severe
Grade III:	A. Fibrosis, mild. Portal fibrosis here denotes formation of fibrotic septa extending into the lobules. Slight enlargement of portal tracts without disruption of limiting plates or septum formation does not put the biopsy in grade III. This distinction requires a connective tissue stain or reticular preparation B. Fibrosis, moderate–severe
Grade IV:	Cirrhosis

this may have been due to the sampling error associated with the biopsy rather than histologic stabilization.

The characteristic hepatic pathology associated with methotrexate is fibrosis or cirrhosis. A grading system developed by dermatologists to describe the histopathology is also being used by rheumatologists (Table 47–1).[106] Therapy should be discontinued for marked fibrosis (IIIB) or cirrhosis (IV).

Studies to date in rheumatoid arthritis are encouraging. Of 217 rheumatoid patients who underwent a liver biopsy before methotrexate therapy, fibrosis was noted in only 2 (0.9 percent) of the patients.[108] Of 714 patients who underwent a liver biopsy after approximately 1.5 g of methotrexate therapy, mild fibrosis was noted in 8 percent of the patients.[108] Fibrosis was seen primarily only with the more sensitive trichrome stain. Moderate fibrosis was noted in 4 (0.5 percent) of the patients. In a prospective liver biopsy study after a mean of 52 months of therapy, mild fibrosis was noted in 52 percent of 27 patients.[109] Eighteen of these patients have continued to undergo liver biopsies. After a mean of 81 months of therapy and a mean cumulative dose of 5.0 g, mild fibrosis was noted in seven (38 percent) of the 18 patients.[110] In 23 rheumatoid patients who received methotrexate for more than 10 years, there were no cases of cirrhosis.[111] There are, however, isolated reports of cirrhosis[112, 113] and acute decompensated liver disease with chronic active hepatitis[114, 115] in rheumatoid patients receiving methotrexate therapy. The risk of liver disease from methotrexate in rheumatoid arthritis is unknown, but studies examining this question are in progress.

Isolated elevations in serum transaminases occur frequently. These elevations are usually one to four times the normal range and usually resolve within 1 to 3 weeks after temporary drug discontinuation. The significance of these enzyme elevations is uncertain, but one study reported that enzyme elevations correlated with a change in liver pathology grade.[109] Normal enzyme levels may not exclude pathology, and a decreasing serum albumin may be predictive of hepatic pathology.

A baseline liver biopsy in rheumatoid arthritis is not indicated unless there is a history of alcoholism, underlying liver disease, positive hepatitis B serologies, or extreme morbid obesity. Within the first several years of methotrexate therapy, the reported incidence of liver toxicity appears to be low. There is a paucity of biopsy data after 3 to 4 years of treatment. Owing to this lack of long-term data, recommendations regarding routine liver biopsies have not been made. Some rheumatologists are recommending biopsies after 4 to 5 years of therapy until sufficient longer-term biopsy data are available. The risk of the biopsy must be considered, and an informed discussion between the patient and the rheumatologist is essential.

Other adverse experiences noted with low-dose methotrexate include headaches, weight loss, fatigue, fever, polyarthralgias, mood alterations, and dizziness.[116] Infections, including herpes zoster both localized and disseminated and other opportunistic organisms such as *Pneumocystis carinii* and fungi, have been reported.[102, 103] Localized osteoporosis, severe bone pain, and nontraumatic fractures have been noted in patients receiving high-dose methotrexate for acute leukemia.[117] The symptoms and radiographic abnormalities resolved with drug discontinuation. The relevance of these observations for adult and juvenile rheumatoid arthritis is unknown.

MONITORING

Patients with active rheumatoid arthritis that has not responded to nonsteroidal anti-inflammatory drugs and usually one other second-line agent are potential candidates for methotrexate therapy. Women contemplating childbearing and patients with renal insufficiency, untreated folate deficiency, active liver disease, excessive alcohol consumption, serious concomitant medical illnesses, or a history of noncompliance should be excluded from receiving therapy. Baseline laboratory parameters should include a complete blood count, platelet count, serum creatinine, liver blood tests, chest radiograph, and when indicated a creatinine clearance. After initiation of therapy, a complete blood count should be monitored at least monthly, and serum creatinine and liver blood tests should be monitored on a regular basis. Decisions about the need for liver biopsy should be discussed between the rheumatologist and the patient. Methotrexate should be temporarily discontinued during acute infections and for major surgical procedures. The risk of continuing methotrexate during the immediate postoperative period for total joint arthroplasty is unknown. Owing to subtle reductions in renal function in the immediate postoperative period, however, it is prudent to discontinue methotrexate for the immediate perioperative and postoperative period. Appropriate patient selection, patient education, and rigorous monitoring

are required with methotrexate to reduce the potential for adverse reactions.

The position of methotrexate in the hierarchy of second-line therapy for rheumatoid arthritis continues to evolve. The information obtained from studies on methotrexate in rheumatoid arthritis has been critical in generating interest in studying methotrexate in other rheumatic and nonrheumatic diseases. New applications for methotrexate promise to be exciting areas of investigation.

References

1. Jolivet, J., Cowan, K. H., Curt, G. A., et al.: The pharmacology and clinical use of methotrexate. N. Engl. J. Med. 309:1094, 198.
2. Kremer, J. M., Galivan, J., Streckfuss, A., et al.: Methotrexate metabolism analysis in blood and liver of rheumatoid arthritis patients. Association with hepatic folate deficiency and formation of polyglutamates. Arthritis Rheum. 29:832, 1986.
3. Mitchell, M. S., Wade, M. E., DeConti, R. C., et al.: Immunosuppressive effects of cytosine arabinoside and methotrexate in man. Ann. Intern. Med. 70:535, 1969.
4. Weinblatt, M. E., Coblyn, J. S., Fox, D. A., et al.: Efficacy of low-dose methotrexate in rheumatoid arthritis. N. Engl. J. Med. 312:818, 1985.
5. Andersen, P. A., West, S. G., O'Dell, J. R., et al.: Weekly pulse methotrexate in rheumatoid arthritis. Clinical and immunologic effects in a randomized, double-blind study. Ann. Intern. Med. 103:489, 1985.
6. Weinblatt, M. E., Trentham, D. E., Fraser, P. A., et al.: Long-term prospective trial of low-dose methotrexate in rheumatoid arthritis. Arthritis Rheum. 31:167, 1988.
7. Williams, H. J., Willkens, R. F., Samuelson, C. O., Jr., et al.: Comparison of low-dose oral pulse methotrexate and placebo in the treatment of rheumatoid arthritis. A controlled clinical trial. Arthritis Rheum. 28:721, 1985.
8. Alarcón, G. S., Schrohenloher, R. E., Bartolucci, A. A., et al.: Suppression of rheumatoid factor production by methotrexate in patients with rheumatoid arthritis: Evidence for differential influences of therapy and clinical status on IgM and IgA rheumatoid factor expression. Arthritis Rheum. 33:1156, 1990.
9. Olsen, N. J., Callahan, L. F., and Pincus, T.: Immunologic studies of rheumatoid arthritis patients treated with methotrexate. Arthritis Rheum. 30:481, 1987.
10. Segal, R., Mozes, E., Yaron, M., et al.: The effects of methotrexate on the production and activity of interleukin-1. Arthritis Rheum. 32:370, 1989.
11. Olsen, N. J., and Murray, L. M.: Antiproliferative effects of methotrexate on peripheral blood mononuclear cells. Arthritis Rheum. 32:378, 1989.
12. Hirata, S., Matsubara, T., Saura, R., et al.: Inhibition of in vitro vascular endothelial cell proliferation and in vivo neovascularization by low-dose methotrexate. Arthritis Rheum. 32:1065, 1989.
12a. Cronstein, B. N., Eberle, M. A., Gruber, H. E., and Levin, R. I.: Methotrexate inhibits neutrophil function by stimulating adenosine release from connective tissue cells. Proc. Natl. Acad. Sci. U.S.A. 88:2441, 1991.
13. Suarez, C. R., Pickett, W. C., Bell, D. H., et al.: Effect of low dose methotrexate on neutrophil chemotaxis induced by leukotriene B4 and complement C5a. J. Rheumatol. 14:9, 1987.
14. van de Kerkhof, P. C., Bauer, F. W., and Maassen-de Grood, R. M.: Methotrexate inhibits the leukotriene B4 induced intraepidermal accumulation of polymorphonuclear leukocytes. Br. J. Dermatol. 113:251a, 1985.
15. Ternowitz, T., Bjerring, P., Andersen, P. H., et al.: Methotrexate inhibits the human C5a-induced skin response in patients with psoriasis. J. Invest. Dermatol. 89:192, 1987.
16. Sperling, R. I., Coblyn, J. S., Larkin, J. K., et al.: Inhibition of leukotriene B₄ synthesis in neutrophils from patients with rheumatoid arthritis by a single oral dose of methotrexate. Arthritis Rheum. 33:1149, 1990.
17. Kerwar, S. S., and Oronsky, A. L.: Methotrexate in rheumatoid arthritis: Studies with animal models. Adv. Enzyme Regul. 29:247, 1989.
18. Herman, R. A., Veng-Pedersen, P., Hoffman, J., et al.: Pharmacokinetics of low-dose methotrexate in rheumatoid arthritis patients. J. Pharm. Sci. 78:165, 1989.
19. Brooks, P. J., Spruill, W. J., Parish, R. C., et al.: Pharmacokinetics of methotrexate administered by intramuscular and subcutaneous injec-

tions in patients with rheumatoid arthritis. Arthritis Rheum. 33:91, 1990.

20. Stewart, C. F., Fleming, R. A., Arkin, C. R., et al.: Coadministration of naproxen and low-dose methotrexate in patients with rheumatoid arthritis. Clin. Pharmacol. Ther. 47:540, 1990.

21. Ahern, M., Booth, J., Loxton, A., et al.: Methotrexate kinetics in rheumatoid arthritis: Is there an interaction with nonsteroidal antiinflammatory drugs? J. Rheumatol. 15:1356, 1988.

22. Gubner, R., August, S., and Ginsberg, V.: Therapeutic suppression of tissue reactivity. II. Effect of aminopterin in rheumatoid arthritis and psoriasis. Am. J. Med. Sci. 22:176, 1951.

23. Hoffmeister, R. T.: Methotrexate in rheumatoid arthritis (Abstract). Arthritis Rheum. 15:114, 1972.

24. Hoffmeister, R. T.: Methotrexate therapy in rheumatoid arthritis: 15 years experience. Am. J. Med. 75:69, 1983.

25. Willkens, R. F., and Watson, M. A.: Methotrexate: A perspective of its use in the treatment of rheumatic diseases. J. Lab. Clin. Med. 100:314, 1982.

26. Steinsson, K., Weinstein, A., Korn, J., et al.: Low dose methotrexate in rheumatoid arthritis. J. Rheumatol. 9:860, 1982.

27. Weinstein, A., Marlowe, S., Korn, J., et al.: Low-dose methotrexate treatment of rheumatoid arthritis. Long-term observations. Am. J. Med. 79:331, 1985.

28. Michaels, R. M., Nashel, D. J., Leonard, A., et al.: Weekly intravenous methotrexate in the treatment of rheumatoid arthritis. Arthritis Rheum. 25:339, 1982.

29. Thompson, R. N., Watts, C., Edelman, J., et al.: A controlled two-centre trial of parenteral methotrexate therapy for refractory rheumatoid arthritis. J. Rheumatol. 11:760, 1984.

30. Tugwell, P., Bennett, K., and Gent, M.: Methotrexate in rheumatoid arthritis. Indications, contraindications, efficacy, and safety. Ann. Intern. Med. 107:358, 1987.

31. Kremer, J. M., Rynes, R. I., and Bartholomew, L. E.: Severe flare of rheumatoid arthritis after discontinuation of long-term methotrexate therapy. Double-blind study. Am. J. Med. 82:781, 1987.

32. Szanto, E.: Low-dose methotrexate in rheumatoid arthritis: Effect and tolerance. An open trial and a double-blind randomized study. Scand. J. Rheumatol. 15:97, 1986.

33. Hamdy, H., McKendry, R. J., Mierins, E., et al.: Low-dose methotrexate compared with azathioprine in the treatment of rheumatoid arthritis. A twenty-four–week controlled clinical trial. Arthritis Rheum. 30:361, 1987.

34. Arnold M. H., O'Callaghan J., McCredie M., et al.: Comparative controlled trial of low-dose weekly methotrexate versus azathioprine in rheumatoid arthritis: 3-year prospective study. Br. J. Rheumatol. 29:120, 1990.

34a. Jeurissen, M. E. C., Boerbooms, A. M. T., van de Putte, L. B. A., et al.: Methotrexate versus azathioprine in the treatment of rheumatoid arthritis: A 48-week randomized, double-blind trial. Arthritis Rheum. 34:961, 1991.

35. Morassut, P., Goldstein, R., Cyr, M., et al.: Gold sodium thiomalate compared to low dose methotrexate in the treatment of rheumatoid arthritis—a randomized, double-blind 26-week trial. J. Rheumatol. 16:302, 1989.

36. Suarez-Almazor, M. E., Fitzgerald, A., Grace, M., et al.: A randomized controlled trial of parenteral methotrexate compared with sodium aurothiomalate (Myochrysine) in the treatment of rheumatoid arthritis. J. Rheumatol. 15:753, 1988.

36a. Rau, R., Herborn, G., Karger, T., Menninger, H., Elhardt, D., and Schmitt, J.: A double-blind randomized parallel trial of intramuscular methotrexate and gold sodium thiomalate in early erosive rheumatoid arthritis. J. Rheumatol. 18:328, 1991.

37. Weinblatt, M. E., Kaplan, H., Germain, B. F., et al.: Low-dose methotrexate compared with auranofin in adult rheumatoid arthritis. A thirty-six–week, double-blind trial. Arthritis Rheum. 33:330, 1990.

38. Kremer, J. M., and Lee, J. K.: The safety and efficacy of the use of methotrexate in long-term therapy for rheumatoid arthritis. Arthritis Rheum. 29:822, 1986.

39. Kremer, J. M., and Lee, J. K.: A long-term prospective study of the use of methotrexate in rheumatoid arthritis. Update after a mean of fifty-three months. Arthritis Rheum. 31:577, 1988.

39a. Kremer, J. M., and Phelps, C. T.: Long-term prospective study of the use of methotrexate in rheumatoid arthritis: Update after a mean of 90 months. Arthritis Rheum. 35:138, 1992.

39b. Weinblatt, M. E., Weissman, B. N., Holdsworth, D. E., et al.: Long-term prospective study of methotrexate in the treatment of rheumatoid arthritis: 84-month update. Arthritis Rheum. 35:129, 1992.

40. Hanrahan, P. S., Scrivens, G. A., and Russell, A. S.: Prospective long term follow-up of methotrexate therapy in rheumatoid arthritis: Toxicity, efficacy and radiological progression. Br. J. Rheumatol. 28:147, 1989.

41. Weinblatt, M. E., Kaplan, H., Germain, B. F., et al.: Methotrexate in rheumatoid arthritis: Effects on disease activity in a multicenter prospective study. J. Rheumatol. 18:334, 1991.

42. Fehlauer, C. S., Carson, C. W., Cannon, G. W., et al.: Methotrexate therapy in rheumatoid arthritis: 2-year retrospective followup study. J. Rheumatol. 16:307, 1989.

43. Alarcon, G. S., Tracy, I. C., and Blackburn, W. D., Jr.: Methotrexate in rheumatoid arthritis. Toxic effects as the major factor in limiting long-term treatment. Arthritis Rheum. 32:671, 1989.

43a. Wolfe, F., and Cathey, M. A.: Analysis of methotrexate treatment effect in a longitudinal observational study: Utility of cluster analysis. J. Rheumatol. 18:672, 1991.

44. Weinblatt, M. E., and Maier, A. L.: Longterm experience with low dose weekly methotrexate in rheumatoid arthritis. J. Rheumatol. (Suppl.) 22:33, 1990.

45. Nordstrom, D. M., West, S. G., Andersen, P. A., et al.: Pulse methotrexate therapy in rheumatoid arthritis. A controlled prospective roentgenographic study. Ann. Intern. Med. 107:797, 1987.

46. Reykdal, S., Steinsson, K., Sigurjonsson, K., et al.: Methotrexate treatment of rheumatoid arthritis: Effects on radiological progression. Scand. J. Rheumatol. 18:221, 1989.

47. Williams, H. J., Ward, J. R., Reading, J. C., et al.: Comparison of auranofin, methotrexate, and the combination of both in the treatment of rheumatoid arthritis: A controlled clinical trial. Arthritis Rheum. 35:259, 1992.

48. Karger, T., and Rau, R.: Treatment of chronic polyarthritis with low-dose methotrexate. Dtsch. Med. Wochenschr. 113:839, 1988.

49. Shiroky, J. B., Watts, C. S., and Neville, C.: Combination methotrexate and sulfasalazine in the management of rheumatoid arthritis: Case observations. Arthritis Rheum. 32:1160, 1989.

50. Biro, J. A., Segal, A., MacKenzie, A. H., et al.: The combination of methotrexate and azathioprine for resistant rheumatoid arthritis (Abstract). Arthritis Rheum 30(Suppl. 4):S18, 1987.

51. Weinstein, G. D., and Frost, P.: Methotrexate for psoriasis. A new therapeutic schedule. Arch. Dermatol. 103:33, 1971.

52. Lally, E. V., and Ho, G., Jr.: A review of methotrexate therapy in Reiter syndrome. Semin. Arthritis Rheum. 15:139, 1985.

53. Fiechtner, J. J., Miller, D. R., and Starkebaum, G.: Reversal of neutropenia with methotrexate treatment in patients with Felty's syndrome. Correlation of response with neutrophil-reactive IgG. Arthritis Rheum. 32:194, 1989.

54. Krall, P. L., Mazanec, D. J., and Wilke, W. S.: Methotrexate for corticosteroid-resistant polymyalgia rheumatica and giant cell arteritis. Cleve. Clin. J. Med. 56:253, 1989.

55. Rothenberg, R. J., Graziano, F. M., Grandone, J. T., et al.: The use of methotrexate in steroid-resistant systemic lupus erythematosus. Arthritis Rheum. 31:612, 1988.

56. Espinoza, L. R., Espinoza, C. G., Vasey, F. B., et al.: Oral methotrexate therapy for chronic rheumatoid arthritis ulcerations. J. Am. Acad. Dermatol. 15:508, 1986.

57. Bode, B. Y., Yocum, D. E., Gall, E. P., et al.: Methotrexate (MTX) in scleroderma: Experience in ten patients (Abstract). Arthritis Rheum. 33:S66, 1990.

58. van den Hoogen, F., Boerbooms, A., Rasker, J., et al.: Treatment of systemic sclerosis with methotrexate: Results of a one-year open study (Abstract). Arthritis Rheum. 33:S66, 1990.

59. Truckenbrodt, H., and Hafner, R.: Methotrexate therapy in juvenile rheumatoid arthritis: A retrospective study. Arthritis Rheum. 29:801, 1986.

60. Wallace, C. A., Bleyer, W. A., Sherry, D. D., et al.: Toxicity and serum levels of methotrexate in children with juvenile rheumatoid arthritis. Arthritis Rheum. 32:677, 1989.

61. Giannini, E. H., Brewer, E. J., Kuzmina, N., et al.: Methotrexate in resistant juvenile rheumatoid arthritis—results of the U.S.A.–U.S.S.R. double-blind, placebo-controlled trial. N. Engl. J. Med. 326:1043, 1992.

62. Arnett, F. C., Whelton, J. C., Zizic, T. M., et al.: Methotrexate therapy in polymyositis. Ann. Rheum. Dis. 32:536, 1973.

63. Toews, G. B., and Lynch, J. P., III: Methotrexate in sarcoidosis. Am. J. Med. Sci. 300:33, 1990.

64. Kaplan, M. M., Arora, S., and Pincus, S. H.: Primary sclerosing cholangitis and low-dose oral pulse methotrexate therapy. Clinical and histologic response. Ann. Intern. Med. 106:231, 1987.

65. Kaplan, M. M., Knox, T. A., and Arora, S. A.: Primary biliary cirrhosis treated with low-dose oral pulse methotrexate. Ann. Intern. Med. 109:429, 1988.

66. Kozarek, R. A., Patterson, D. J., Gelfand, M. D., et al.: Methotrexate induces clinical and histologic remission in patients with refractory inflammatory bowel disease. Ann. Intern. Med. 110:353, 1989.

67. Mullarkey, M. F., Blumenstein, B. A., Andrade, W. P., et al.: Methotrexate in the treatment of corticosteroid-dependent asthma. A double-blind crossover study. N. Engl. J. Med. 318:603, 1988.

68. Shiner, R. J., Nunn, A. J., Chung, K. F., et al.: Randomised, double-blind, placebo-controlled trial of methotrexate in steroid-dependent asthma. Lancet 336:137, 1990.

69. Mullarkey, M. F., Lammert, J. K., and Blumenstein, B. A.: Long-term methotrexate treatment in corticosteroid-dependent asthma. Ann. Intern. Med. 112:577, 1990.

70. Furst, D. E., Koehnke, R., Burmeister, L. F., et al.: Increasing methotrexate effect with increasing dose in the treatment of resistant rheumatoid arthritis. J. Rheumatol. 16:313, 1989.
71. Gabriel, S., Creagan, E., O'Fallon, W. M., et al.: Treatment of rheumatoid arthritis with higher dose intravenous methotrexate. J. Rheumatol. 17:460, 1990.
72. Shiroky, J., Allegra, C., Inghirami, G., et al.: High dose intravenous methotrexate with leucovorin rescue in rheumatoid arthritis. J. Rheumatol. 15:251, 1988.
73. Morgan, S. L., Baggott, J. E., and Altz-Smith, M.: Folate status of rheumatoid arthritis patients receiving long-term, low-dose methotrexate therapy. Arthritis Rheum. 30:1348, 1987.
74. Morgan, S. L., Baggott, J. E., Vaughn, W. H., et al.: The effect of folic acid supplementation on the toxicity of low-dose methotrexate in patients with rheumatoid arthritis. Arthritis Rheum. 33:9, 1990.
75. Hanrahan, P. S., and Russell, A. S.: Concurrent use of folinic acid and methotrexate in rheumatoid arthritis. J. Rheumatol. 15:1078, 1988.
76. Tishler, M., Caspi, D., Fishel, B., et al.: The effects of leucovorin (folinic acid) on methotrexate therapy in rheumatoid arthritis patients. Arthritis Rheum. 31:906, 1988.
77. Buckley, L. M., Vacek, P. M., and Cooper, S. M.: Administration of folinic acid after low dose methotrexate in patients with rheumatoid arthritis. J. Rheumatol. 17:1158, 1990.
78. Hall, G. H., Jones, B. J., Head, A. C., et al.: Intra-articular methotrexate. Clinical and laboratory study in rheumatoid and psoriatic arthritis. Ann. Rheum. Dis. 37:351, 1978.
79. Marks, J. S., Stewart, I. M., and Hunter, J. A.: Intra-articular methotrexate in rheumatoid arthritis (letter). Lancet 2:857, 1976.
80. Bird, H. A., Ring, E. F., Daniel, R., et al.: Comparison of intra-articular methotrexate with intra-articular triamcinolone hexacetonide by thermography. Curr. Med. Res. Opin. 5:141, 1977.
81. Weinblatt, M. E.: Toxicity of low dose methotrexate in rheumatoid arthritis. J. Rheumatol. (Suppl.) 12:35, 1985.
82. Marks, C. R., Willkens, R. F., Wilske, K. R., et al.: Small-vessel vasculitis and methotrexate (letter). Ann. Intern. Med. 100:916, 1984.
83. Segal, R., Caspi, D., Tishler, M., et al.: Accelerated nodulosis and vasculitis during methotrexate therapy for rheumatoid arthritis. Arthritis Rheum. 31:1182, 1988.
84. MacKinnon, S. K., Starkebaum, G., and Willkens, R. F.: Pancytopenia associated with low dose pulse methotrexate in the treatment of rheumatoid arthritis. Semin. Arthritis Rheum. 15:119, 1985.
85. Maricic, M., Davis, M., and Gall, E. P.: Megaloblastic pancytopenia in a patient receiving concurrent methotrexate and trimethoprim-sulfamethoxazole treatment. Arthritis Rheum. 29:133, 1986.
86. Weinblatt, M. E., and Fraser, P.: Elevated mean corpuscular volume as a predictor of hematologic toxicity due to methotrexate therapy. (MTX) (Abstract). Arthritis Rheum. 32:1592, 1989.
87. Shamberger, R. C., Rosenberg, S. A., Seipp, C. A., et al.: Effects of high-dose methotrexate and vincristine on ovarian and testicular functions in patients undergoing postoperative adjuvant treatment of osteosarcoma. Cancer Treat. Rep. 65:739, 1981.
88. Sussman, A., and Leonard, J. M.: Psoriasis, methotrexate, and oligospermia. Arch. Dermatol. 116:215, 1980.
89. Milunsky, A., Graef, J. W., and Gaynor, M. F., Jr.: Methotrexate-induced congenital malformations. J. Pediatr. 72:790, 1968.
90. Jensen, M. K., and Nyfors, A.: Cytogenetic effects of methotrexate on human cells in vivo: Comparison between results obtained by chromosome studies on bone-marrow cells and blood lymphocytes and by the micronucleus test. Mutat. Res. 64:339, 1979.
91. Rustia, M., and Shubik, P.: Life-span carcinogenicity tests with 4-amino-N10-methylpteroylglutamic acid (methotrexate) in Swiss mice and Syrian golden hamsters. Toxicol. Appl. Pharmacol. 26:329, 1973.
92. Rustin, G. J., Rustin, F., Dent, J., et al.: No increase in second tumors after cytotoxic chemotherapy for gestational trophoblastic tumors. N. Engl. J. Med. 308:473, 1983.
93. Bailin, P. L., Tindall, J. P., Roenigk, H. H., Jr., et al.: Is methotrexate therapy for psoriasis carcinogenic? A modified retrospective-prospective analysis. J.A.M.A. 232:359, 1975.
94. Stern, R. S., Zierler, S., and Parrish, J. A.: Methotrexate used for psoriasis and the risk of noncutaneous or cutaneous malignancy. Cancer 50:869, 1982.
95. Sostman, H. D., Matthay, R. A., Putman, C. E., et al.: Methotrexate-induced pneumonitis. Medicine (Baltimore) 55:371, 1976.
96. Engelbrecht, J. A., Calhoon, S. L., and Scherrer, J. J.: Methotrexate pneumonitis after low-dose therapy for rheumatoid arthritis. Arthritis Rheum. 26:1275, 1983.
97. Cannon, G. W., Ward, J. R., Clegg, D. O., et al.: Acute lung disease associated with low-dose pulse methotrexate therapy in patients with rheumatoid arthritis. Arthritis Rheum. 26:1269, 1983.
98. St. Clair, E. W., Rice, J. R., and Snyderman, R.: Pneumonitis complicating low-dose methotrexate therapy in rheumatoid arthritis. Arch. Intern. Med. 145:2035, 1985.
99. Carson, C. W., Cannon, G. W., Egger, M. J., et al.: Pulmonary disease during the treatment of rheumatoid arthritis with low dose pulse methotrexate. Semin. Arthritis Rheum. 16:186, 1987.
100. Searles, G., and McKendry, R. J.: Methotrexate pneumonitis in rheumatoid arthritis: Potential risk factors. Four case reports and a review of the literature. J. Rheumatol. 14:1164, 1987.
101. Kaplan, R. L., and Waite, D. H.: Progressive interstitial lung disease from prolonged methotrexate therapy. Arch. Dermatol. 114:1800, 1978.
102. Perruquet, J. L., Harrington, T. M., and Davis, D. E.: *Pneumocystis carinii* pneumonia following methotrexate therapy for rheumatoid arthritis (letter). Arthritis Rheum. 26:1291, 1983.
103. Altz-Smith, M., Kendall, L. G., Jr., and Stamm, A. M.: Cryptococcosis associated with low-dose methotrexate for arthritis. Am. J. Med. 83:179, 1987.
104. Nyfors, A., and Poulsen, H.: Liver biopsies from psoriatics related to methotrexate therapy. 2. Findings before and after methotrexate therapy in 88 patients. A blind study. Acta Pathol. Microbiol. Scand. [A] 84:262, 1976.
105. Nyfors, A.: Liver biopsies from psoriatics related to methotrexate therapy. 3. Findings in post-methotrexate liver biopsies from 160 psoriatics. Acta Pathol. Microbiol. Scand. [A] 85:511, 1977.
106. Roenigk, H. H., Jr., Auerbach, R., Maibach, H. I., et al.: Methotrexate in psoriasis: Revised guidelines. J. Am. Acad. Dermatol. 19:145, 1988.
107. Zachariae, H., and Sogaard, H.: Methotrexate-induced liver cirrhosis. A follow-up. Dermatologica 175:178, 1987.
108. Weinblatt, M. E., and Kremer, J. M.: Methotrexate in rheumatoid arthritis. J. Am. Acad. Dermatol. 19:126, 1988.
109. Kremer, J. M., Lee, R. G., and Tolman, K. G.: Liver histology in rheumatoid arthritis patients receiving long-term methotrexate therapy. A prospective study with baseline and sequential biopsy samples. Arthritis Rheum. 32:121, 1989.
110. Kremer, J. M.: Long-term prospective sequential liver biopsies (Bxs) in patients with rheumatoid arthritis (RA) on weekly oral methotrexate (MTX) (Abstract). Arthritis Rheum. 33:S40, 1990.
111. Aponte, J., and Petrelli, M.: Histopathologic findings in the liver of rheumatoid arthritis patients treated with long-term bolus methotrexate. Arthritis Rheum. 31:1457, 1988.
112. Phillips, C., Cera, P., Mangan, T., et al.: Liver disease in rheumatoid arthritis (RA) patients on methotrexate (MTX) (Abstract). Arthritis Rheum. 33:S60, 1990.
113. Augur, N. A., Anderson, L. C., Cogen, L., et al.: Prospective study of hepatotoxicity in patients receiving methotrexate for rheumatoid arthritis (Abstract). Arthritis Rheum. 33:S60, 1990.
114. Clegg, D. O., Furst, D. E., Tolman, K. G., et al.: Acute, reversible hepatic failure associated with methotrexate treatment of rheumatoid arthritis. J. Rheumatol. 16:1123, 1989.
115. Kujala, G. A., Shamma'a, J. M., Chang, W. L., et al.: Hepatitis with bridging fibrosis and reversible hepatic insufficiency in a woman with rheumatoid arthritis taking methotrexate. Arthritis Rheum. 33:1037, 1990.
116. Wernick, R., and Smith, D. L.: Central nervous system toxicity associated with weekly low-dose methotrexate treatment. Arthritis Rheum. 32:770, 1989.
117. O'Regan, S., Melhorn, D. K., and Newman, A. J.: Methotrexate-induced bone pain in childhood leukemia. Am. J. Dis. Child. 126:489, 1973.

Glucocorticoids

INTRODUCTION

The history of glucocorticoid therapy and the history of rheumatology are inseparable. From the beginning, during the initial studies of the effects of cortisone on patients with rheumatoid arthritis (RA), it was apparent that the dramatic anti-inflammatory effects of glucocorticoids are frequently accompanied by the unwelcome manifestations of Cushing's syndrome.[1] This chapter examines the risks associated with the use of glucocorticoids as anti-inflammatory and immunosuppressive agents and provides guidelines for the long-term systemic use of these commonly prescribed substances. The indications for the use of glucocorticoids in the rheumatic disorders are discussed in the chapters of this book that consider the several rheumatic diseases for which these agents are sometimes indicated. This chapter is concerned primarily with the general principles of glucocorticoid therapy.

STRUCTURE OF COMMONLY USED GLUCOCORTICOIDS

Glucocorticoids are 21-carbon steroid molecules with numerous metabolic and physiologic effects. Figure 48–1 reveals the structures of several commonly used glucocorticoids.[2] Cortisol (hydrocortisone) is the principal circulating glucocorticoid in humans.

The existence of glucocorticoid activity depends on the presence of a hydroxyl group at carbon number 11 of the steroid molecule. Thus, cortisone and prednisone, which are 11-keto compounds, lack glucocorticoid activity until converted in vivo to cortisol and prednisolone, the corresponding 11-beta (β)-hydroxyl compounds.[3, 4] This transformation occurs predominantly in the liver.[5, 6] Cortisone and prednisone are available only for systemic therapy. All glucocorticoid preparations marketed for topical or local use are 11-β-hydroxyl compounds, thus eliminating the need for biotransformation.

PHYSIOLOGY: THE REGULATION OF CORTISOL SECRETION

The production of cortisol by the adrenal cortex is regulated directly by the anterior pituitary gland and indirectly by the hypothalamus. Under normal circumstances, adrenocorticotropic hormone (ACTH) is released from the anterior pituitary gland in a pulsatile fashion.[7] Although plasma ACTH levels are thus subject to minute-to-minute variation, these levels are higher on the average in the early morning hours than later in the day; that is, there is a diurnal rhythm of ACTH release. ACTH is itself subject to release by corticotropin-releasing hormone (CRH), a substance synthesized in the hypothalamus and carried directly to the anterior pituitary gland by a local circulation, the hypophyseal–portal system. Stressful stimuli originating at a suprahypothalamic level lead to an augmented release of CRH from the hypothalamus. This substance in turn provokes the discharge of ACTH from the anterior pituitary gland.

This sequence is subject to negative feedback inhibition. Increasing levels of cortisol or a synthetic glucocorticoid result in decreasing secretion of ACTH. This feedback regulation has both fast and delayed components and includes inhibitory effects on the synthesis and release of both CRH and ACTH.[8, 9] In normal persons, stressful stimuli can overcome the effect of this feedback inhibition.[10]

Interleukin-1 (IL-1) stimulates the release of ACTH and glucocorticoids, whereas glucocorticoids inhibit the production and action of IL-1.[11, 12] Thus, an IL-1–mediated increase in glucocorticoid secretion may be part of a normal host response to environmental antigenic stimuli, and this process may be subject to feedback inhibition by glucocorticoids.

PHARMACODYNAMICS

Our understanding of the pharmacology of glucocorticoids has improved in recent years as a consequence of improved techniques for the measurement of these substances in the circulation.[13–15]

Half-Life, Potency, and Duration of Action. The important differences among the available glucocorticoid compounds are in duration of action, relative glucocorticoid potency, and relative mineralocorticoid potency[2] (Table 48–1). Commonly used glucocorticoids are categorized as short, intermediate, and long acting on the basis of the duration of ACTH suppression after a single dose, equivalent in anti-inflammatory activity to 50 mg of prednisone.[16] The values provided for relative glucocorticoid potency are approximations derived from several sources.[17–26]

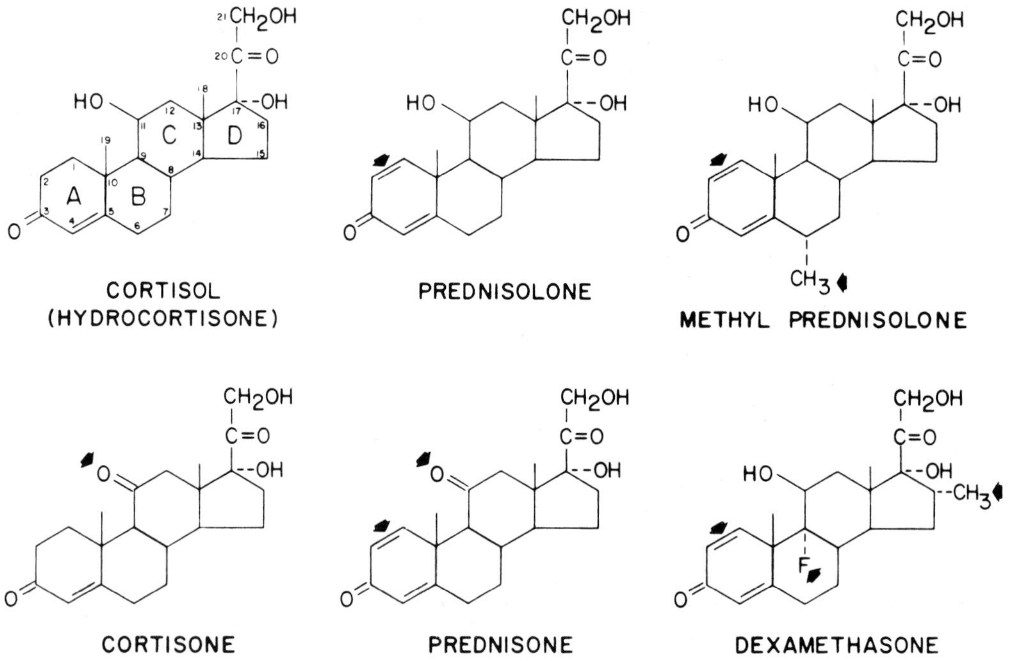

Figure 48–1. Commonly used glucocorticoids. In the representation of cortisol, the 21 carbon atoms of the glucocorticoid skeleton are designated by numbers, and the four rings are designated by letters. The arrows indicate the structural differences between cortisol and each of the other molecules. (From Axelrod, L.: Glucocorticoid therapy. Medicine 55:39, 1976. © by Williams & Wilkins, 1979.)

The relative potencies of the glucocorticoids correlate with their affinity for the cytoplasmic glucocorticoid receptor.[27, 28] However, the observed potency of a glucocorticoid is a measure not only of the intrinsic biologic potency but also of the duration of action.[26, 27] Consequently, the relative potency of two glucocorticoids varies as a function of the time interval between the administration of the two steroids and the determination of the potency. In particular, failure to account for the duration of action may lead to a marked underestimation of the potency of dexamethasone.[26]

The half-life of cortisol in the circulation is in the range of 80 to 115 minutes.[2] Values for other commonly used agents are as follows: cortisone, 0.5 hour; prednisone, 3.4 to 3.8 hours; prednisolone, 2.1 to 3.5 hours; methylprednisolone, 1.3 to 3.1 hours; and dexamethasone, 1.8 to 4.7 hours.[2, 26, 29] The variability in the reported values for the half-life of an individual glucocorticoid may be a consequence in part of the pharmacokinetic characteristics of the glucocorticoid being dose dependent. With increasing intravenous doses of prednisolone, there is an increase in the volume of distribution and an increase in the clearance of this steroid.[13, 15, 29, 30] The dose-dependent kinetic behavior of prednisolone may be due to the

Table 48–1. COMMONLY USED GLUCOCORTICOIDS

Duration of Action*	Glucocorticoid Potency†	Equivalent Glucocorticoid Dose (mg)	Mineralocorticoid Activity
Short-acting			
Cortisol (hydrocortisone)	1	20.0	Yes‡
Cortisone	0.8	25.0	Yes‡
Prednisone	4	5.0	No
Prednisolone	4	5.0	No
Methylprednisolone	5	4.0	No
Intermediate-acting			
Triamcinolone	5	4.0	No
Long-acting			
Betamethasone	25	0.6	No
Dexamethasone	30	0.75	No

From Axelrod, L.: Glucocorticoid therapy. Medicine 55:39, 1976; © by Williams & Wilkins, 1979; and Axelrod, L.: Adrenal corticosteroids. In Miller, R. R., and Greenblatt, D. J. (eds.): Handbook of Drug Therapy. New York, Elsevier North-Holland, 1979, p. 809. Used by permission.

*The classification by duration of action is based on the work of Harter.[16]

†The values given for glucocorticoid potency are relative. Cortisol is arbitrarily assigned a value of one. These values are approximations derived from several sources.[17-26]

‡Mineralocorticoid effects are dose related. At doses close to or within the basal physiologic range for glucocorticoid activity, no such effect may be detectable.

nonlinear binding of prednisolone to plasma proteins; with an increase in dose, there is an increase in the percentage of the steroid that is unbound.[13, 15, 29, 30]

The relation between the circulating half-life of a glucocorticoid and its potency is not strict. Prednisolone and dexamethasone have comparable circulating half-lives, but dexamethasone is clearly more potent. Similarly, the correlation between the circulating half-life of a glucocorticoid and its duration of action is imprecise. The many actions of glucocorticoids do not have an equal duration, and the duration of action may be a function of the dose.[16, 31–33]

Harter studied the duration of one effect of glucocorticoids—the length of time after a single dose during which ACTH remains suppressed.[16] He did this by administering metyrapone to a normal person and measuring the urinary 17-ketogenic steroids during 6-hour periods as an index of ACTH secretion. He divided glucocorticoids into three groups based on the duration of ACTH suppression after a single dose of a glucocorticoid, equivalent in anti-inflammatory activity to 50 mg of prednisone. The first group, the short-acting steroids, is characterized by a return of ACTH activity within 24 to 36 hours. This group includes cortisone, hydrocortisone, prednisone, prednisolone, and methylprednisolone. The second group, the intermediate-acting steroids, consists of compounds that suppress ACTH for 48 hours. This group includes triamcinolone and paramethasone. The third group, the long-acting glucocorticoids, consists of substances that suppress ACTH for well over 48 hours. This class includes dexamethasone and betamethasone. This formulation is based on studies in a single patient. It does not provide information about variations from individual to individual, about prolonged therapy, or about persons who have not received metyrapone.

Because these variations in the duration of ACTH suppression are achieved by doses of glucocorticoids with comparable anti-inflammatory activity, the duration of ACTH suppression is not simply a function of the level of anti-inflammatory activity. The duration of ACTH suppression produced by an individual glucocorticoid is probably dose related, however.[16, 33] Long-acting conjugates of the glucocorticoids given as intramuscular injections may be released slowly and exert an effect for much more prolonged periods, often several weeks.

The slight differences in the circulating half-lives of the glucocorticoids contrast with the marked differences between them in potency and in the duration of ACTH suppression. In addition, the duration of ACTH suppression exceeds the half-life by more than the five-fold factor that would be expected if the duration of effect were a function of the circulating level of the steroid. Such data suggest that the duration of action of a glucocorticoid is not determined by its presence in the circulation, which is consistent with our understanding of the mechanism of action of steroid hormones. A steroid molecule passes through the cell membrane and enters the cytoplasm, where it binds to a specific cytoplasmic receptor protein.[34] This complex enters the nucleus, where it modifies the process of transcription, whereby RNA is synthesized (or transcribed) from the DNA template. The consequence is an alteration in the rate of synthesis of specific proteins. In this manner, the steroid modifies the phenotypic expression of the genetic information. Thus, the glucocorticoid continues to act within the cell after it has disappeared from the circulation. In addition, the series of events initiated by the glucocorticoids may continue to occur, or a product of this sequence (such as a specific protein) may be present after the disappearance of the glucocorticoid.

Bioavailability, Absorption, and Biotransformation. In normal persons, plasma cortisol levels after oral administration of cortisone are much lower than after equal doses of cortisol.[35] This suggests that, although oral cortisone administration may be adequate replacement therapy in chronic adrenal insufficiency, it is unwise to use this agent orally when pharmacologic effects are sought. In contrast, comparable plasma prednisolone levels are achieved in normal persons after equivalent oral doses of prednisone and prednisolone.[29] Wide variation exists in the prednisolone concentration after both drugs, which may reflect variability in absorption.[29]

Plasma cortisol levels after an intramuscular injection of cortisone acetate rise little or not at all, in contrast to the marked rises that follow the intramuscular injection of hydrocortisone.[36–42] Although intramuscular cortisone acetate was once used for perioperative management, it does not provide adequate plasma cortisol levels and offers no advantage over hydrocortisone by the same route.

Plasma Transport Proteins. Under normal physiologic conditions, cortisol and, to a lesser extent, its synthetic derivatives are bound primarily to corticosteroid-binding globulin (CBG; transcortin), an alpha (α)globulin, in the plasma. CBG is a vehicle for the transportation of the steroid; the bound steroid is not active. Albumin binds most of the remaining glucocorticoid (10 to 15 percent) not complexed with CBG, leaving only a small portion of the steroid unbound and free to exert its physiologic and pharmacologic actions. Circadian fluctuations occur in the capacity of CBG to bind cortisol and prednisolone in normal subjects.[43] In contrast, patients who have been given prolonged treatment with prednisone have no diurnal variation in the binding capacity of CBG for cortisol or prednisolone, and both capacities are reduced in comparison with normal subjects.[43] Thus, long-term glucocorticoid therapy alters not only the endogenous secretion of steroids but also the transport of some glucocorticoids in the circulation. This may explain the observation that the disappearance of prednisolone is more rapid in those who have previously received glucocorticoids than in those who have not.[44, 45]

Glucocorticoid Therapy in the Presence of Liver

Disease. Plasma cortisol levels are normal in patients with liver disease.[46] Although cortisol clearance is reduced in cirrhotic patients, the hypothalamic–pituitary–adrenal (HPA) homeostatic mechanism appears to be intact. Thus, a decreased rate of metabolism is accompanied by decreased synthesis of cortisol.[46]

In patients with active liver disease, the conversion of prednisone to prednisolone is impaired.[45, 47, 48] This is offset in good measure by a decreased rate of elimination of prednisolone from the plasma in patients with active liver disease or cirrhosis.[48–50] In patients with liver disease, the plasma availability of prednisolone may be variable after oral doses of either prednisone or prednisolone.[48] The conversion of cortisone to cortisol has been studied in only one patient with hepatic disease and was normal.[35] The situation is further complicated by the fact that a lower percentage of circulating prednisolone is bound to protein in patients with active liver disease than in normal subjects[45, 47]; the unbound fraction is inversely related to the serum albumin concentration.[47] An increased frequency of prednisone side effects is observed at low serum albumin levels[51]; possibly both findings reflect impaired hepatic function. Because the impairment of conversion of prednisone to prednisolone in the presence of liver disease is quantitatively small and is offset by a decreased rate of clearance of prednisolone, and because of the marked variability in plasma prednisolone levels after administration of either steroid, there is no clear mandate to use prednisolone rather than prednisone in a patient with active liver disease or cirrhosis.[15, 29] Whichever agent is used, a somewhat lower dose than would otherwise be used should be employed if the serum albumin level is low.

Glucocorticoid Therapy and the Nephrotic Syndrome. When hypoalbuminemia is due to the nephrotic syndrome, the fraction of prednisolone that is protein bound is decreased. The unbound fraction is related inversely to the serum albumin concentration. Nevertheless, the unbound prednisolone concentration remains normal.[52, 53] Because the unbound concentration determines the pharmacologic effect, altered prednisolone kinetics in patients with hypoalbuminemia do not explain the increased frequency of prednisolone-related side effects in these patients.

Glucocorticoid Therapy and Hyperthyroidism. The systemic bioavailability of prednisolone after an oral dose of prednisone is reduced in patients with hyperthyroidism.[54] This is attributable to decreased absorption of prednisone and increased hepatic clearance of prednisolone.[54]

Glucocorticoids During Pregnancy. Glucocorticoid therapy appears to be well tolerated in pregnancy.[55] Although glucocorticoids cross the placenta, there is no convincing evidence that this produces clinically significant HPA suppression or Cushing's syndrome in the neonate,[55] although subnormal responsiveness to exogenous ACTH may occur.[56, 57] Nor is there evidence that glucocorticoids increase the incidence of congenital defects in humans.[55] Glucocorticoids appear to decrease the birthweight of full-term infants[58]; the long-term consequences of this effect are unknown. Because of low concentrations of prednisone and prednisolone in breast milk, the administration of these drugs to the mother of a nursing infant is unlikely to produce deleterious effects.[59, 60]

Drug Interactions. The concomitant use of other drugs can alter the effectiveness of the glucocorticoids.[13, 15]

The metabolism of glucocorticoids is accelerated by compounds that induce hepatic microsomal enzyme activity, such as phenytoin,[61–65] barbiturates,[63, 65–67] carbamazepine,[65] and rifampin.[68–70] Administration of these compounds can increase the steroid requirement of a patient with adrenal insufficiency[68] or can lead to deterioration in the condition of a patient whose underlying disorder is well controlled by glucocorticoid therapy.[66, 67, 69, 71] These substances should be avoided if possible in patients receiving steroids. Diazepam does not alter the metabolism of glucocorticoids and is preferable to barbiturates.[63] If an inducer of hepatic microsomal enzyme activity must be used in a patient receiving steroids, an increase in the required dosage of the steroid should be anticipated.

Conversely, ketoconazole increases the bioavailability of large doses of prednisolone (0.8 mg per kg) by inhibiting hepatic microsomal enzyme activity.[72] Ketoconazole does not have this effect on lower doses of prednisolone.[73]

The bioavailability of prednisone is decreased by antacid doses comparable to those used clinically,[74] but it is not altered by sucralfate,[75] by H_2-receptor blockade,[76, 77] or by cholestyramine.[78]

Glucocorticoids can alter the effectiveness of other medications. The concurrent administration of a glucocorticoid and salicylate may reduce serum salicylate levels; conversely, reduction of the steroid dose during administration of a fixed dose of salicylate may lead to higher and possibly toxic serum salicylate levels.[79–81] This interaction may reflect the induction of salicylate metabolism by glucocorticoids.[80]

Glucocorticoids may increase requirements for insulin or oral hypoglycemic agents, antihypertensive drugs, or glaucoma medications. They may also alter the requirement for sedative–hypnotic or antidepressant therapy. Digitalis toxicity can result from hypokalemia induced by glucocorticoids, as from hypokalemia of any cause. Glucocorticoids may reverse the neuromuscular blockade induced by pancuronium.[82, 83] The mechanism is not known.

CONSIDERATIONS BEFORE THE USE OF GLUCOCORTICOIDS AS PHARMACOLOGIC AGENTS

Cushing's syndrome is a serious disorder. The 5-year mortality rate was over 50 percent in a series

Table 48–2. CONSIDERATIONS BEFORE THE USE OF GLUCOCORTICOIDS AS PHARMACOLOGIC AGENTS

How serious is the underlying disorder?
How long will therapy be required?
What is the anticipated effective steroid dose?
Is the patient predisposed to any of the known hazards of glucocorticoid therapy?
    Diabetes mellitus
    Osteoporosis
    Peptic ulcer, gastritis, or esophagitis
    Tuberculosis or other chronic infections
    Hypertension and cardiovascular disease
    Psychological difficulties
Which glucocorticoid preparation should be used?
Have other modes of therapy been used to minimize the glucocorticoid dosage and to minimize the side effects of glucocorticoid therapy?
Is an alternate-day regimen indicated?

Modified from Thorn, G. W.: Clinical considerations in the use of corticosteroids. N. Engl. J. Med. 274:775, 1966. Reprinted by permission of *The New England Journal of Medicine.*

of patients studied at the beginning of the era of glucocorticoid and ACTH therapy.[84] Infection and cardiovascular complications are frequent causes of death in this disorder. High-dose exogenous glucocorticoid therapy is similarly hazardous.

Table 48–2 summarizes the important questions to consider before initiating glucocorticoid therapy.[85] These enable the physician to assess the potential risks that must be weighed against the potential benefits of treatment. The more severe the underlying disorder, the more readily glucocorticoid therapy can be justified. Thus, steroid therapy is usually employed in patients with some severe forms of systemic lupus erythematosus, active vasculitis, asthma, severe chronic active hepatitis, transplantation rejection, severe pemphigus, or diseases of comparable severity. Systemic glucocorticoids generally should not be administered to patients with RA or mild bronchial asthma; they should receive more conservative therapy first.

The anticipated dose and duration of glucocorticoid therapy is another critical variable. In general, the incidence of side effects is a function of the total dose and duration of treatment.[86, 87] The use of glucocorticoids for 1 to 2 weeks for a condition such as poison ivy or allergic rhinitis is unlikely to be associated with serious side effects if there is no contraindication to their use. An exception to this rule is a steroid-induced psychosis, which may occur after only a few days of high-dose glucocorticoid therapy, even in patients with no history of psychiatric disease.[87, 88] Because so many complications are dose and time related, the smallest possible dose should be prescribed for the shortest possible period. If hypoalbuminemia is present, the dose should be appropriately reduced.[29, 47, 51] If long-term treatment is indicated, consideration should be given to the use of an alternate-day schedule.

Whenever possible, a local steroid preparation should be used, since systemic effects are minimal when these substances are properly administered.

Examples are topical therapy in dermatologic disorders, steroid enemas in ulcerative proctitis, steroid aerosols in bronchial asthma and allergic rhinitis, and intra-articular steroids.[89, 90]

Agents with minimal or no mineralocorticoid activity should be used when a glucocorticoid is prescribed for pharmacologic purposes. If the dose is to be tapered over a few days, a long-acting agent may be undesirable. For alternate-day therapy, a short-acting agent that generally does not cause sodium retention (e.g., prednisone, prednisolone, or methylprednisolone) should be used. There is no indication for the systemic administration of glucocorticoid conjugates that are designed to achieve a prolonged duration of action (several days or several weeks) after a single intramuscular injection. The absorption and bioavailability of such agents cannot be regulated precisely, the duration of action cannot be estimated reliably, and it is not possible to taper the dose rapidly in the event of an adverse reaction such as a steroid-induced psychosis. The use of such preparations may produce HPA suppression more often than the use of comparable doses of the same glucocorticoid given orally.[91] The use of supplementary agents to minimize the steroid dose and to minimize the side effects of systemic glucocorticoids should always be considered.

EFFECTS OF EXOGENOUS GLUCOCORTICOIDS

Anti-inflammatory and Immunosuppressive Effects. One of the important physiologic functions of glucocorticoids is to protect the organism from damage caused by its own defense reactions and the products of these reactions during stress.[92] Consequently, the use of glucocorticoids as anti-inflammatory and immunosuppressive agents represents an application of the physiologic effects of glucocorticoids to the treatment of disease.[92] The effects of glucocorticoids on inflammatory and immune responses are exceedingly complex. This complexity derives from the complexity of the inflammatory and immune processes themselves and from the ability of glucocorticoids to modify these processes in numerous ways.[93–98] Studies performed in steroid-sensitive species, such as mice, rats, and rabbits, may not apply to steroid-resistant species such as guinea pigs, monkeys, and humans.[93, 94] In addition, many studies in in vitro systems use concentrations of glucocorticoids that are unattainable in humans.[97, 98]

It is not yet possible to identify a single mechanism of action underlying the numerous effects of glucocorticoids on inflammatory and immune responses. As noted, glucocorticoid hormones (like other steroid hormones) act by binding to a specific cytoplasmic receptor protein. The steroid–receptor complex then enters the nucleus, where it modifies the transcription of RNA from the DNA template. This results in an alteration of the rate of synthesis of specific proteins. It is tempting to try to relate this receptor-mediated mechanism of action to the numerous effects of glucocorticoids on inflammation and immunity. In fact, glucocorticoid receptors have been demonstrated in normal human lymphocytes, monocytes, neutrophils, and eosinophils and in human neoplastic cells.[98] Although the number of cytoplasmic glucocorticoid receptors correlates with a clinical response to glucocorticoid therapy in some patients with lymphoid tumors, the presence of receptors in malignant tissue does not guarantee responsiveness.[98] Variations in corticosteroid receptor density, affinity, or binding constants do not correlate with the range of responses of immunoreactive cells to glucocorticoids.[98]

Glucocorticoid effects on inflammatory and immune phenomena include effects on leukocyte movement, leukocyte function, and humoral factors (Table 48–3). In general, glucocorticoids have a greater effect (1) on leukocyte traffic than on function and (2) on cellular than humoral processes.[97] Probably the most important anti-inflammatory effect of glucocorticoids is their ability to inhibit recruitment of neutrophils and monocyte–macrophages to an inflammatory site.[97]

Glucocorticoids alter the traffic of all the major leukocyte populations within the circulation. The administration of a single dose of a glucocorticoid produces a neutrophilic leukocytosis; peak levels occur 4 to 6 hours after the steroid is given.[95, 99] This leukocytosis is the consequence of an accelerated release of mature neutrophils from the bone marrow,[100] an increase in the circulating half-life of the neutrophils,[101] and decreased egress of neutrophils from the circulation to an inflammatory site.[100, 102] The administration of a single dose of a glucocorticoid to normal human subjects produces a marked but transient lymphocytopenia; the nadir is reached 4 to 6 hours after administration (Fig. 48–2).[95, 103–107] This lymphocytopenia involves all lymphocyte subpopulations. It is also selective, since thymus-derived lymphocytes are decreased to a greater degree than bone marrow–derived lymphocytes,[95, 103, 104, 107] and within the total T lymphocyte population, certain subsets are decreased to a greater extent than others.[98]

The mechanism of the lymphocytopenia in humans involves the redistribution of lymphocytes out of the circulation.[95, 97] In general, there are two distinct populations of lymphocytes in the circulation. The first population, the recirculating lymphocytes, freely migrates into and out of the intravascular space in equilibrium with the much larger total body pool of recirculating lymphocytes. The second population, the nonrecirculating lymphocytes, remains in the intravascular space. Glucocorticoids cause the recirculating lymphocyte to leave the intravascular space, but they do not affect the nonrecirculating lymphocyte.[108] This alteration of the normal lymphocyte traffic may be due to suppression of entry of lymphocytes into the circulation.[109] Glucocorticoids also

Table 48–3. EFFECTS OF GLUCOCORTICOIDS ON INFLAMMATORY AND IMMUNE RESPONSES IN HUMANS

Effects on Leukocyte Movement
Lymphocytes
  Circulating lymphocytopenia 4 to 6 hours after drug administration, secondary to redistribution of cells to other lymphoid compartments
  Depletion of recirculating lymphocytes
  Selective depletion of T lymphocytes more than of B lymphocytes
Monocyte–macrophages
  Circulating monocytopenia 4 to 6 hours after drug administration, probably secondary to redistribution
  Inhibition of accumulation of monocyte–macrophages at inflammatory sites
Neutrophils
  Circulating neutrophilia
  Accelerated release of neutrophils from the bone marrow
  Blockade of accumulation of neutrophils at inflammatory sites
Eosinophils
  Circulating eosinopenia, probably secondary to redistribution
  Decreased migration of eosinophils into immediate hypersensitivity skin test sites

Effects on Leukocyte Function
Lymphocytes
  Suppression of delayed hypersensitivity skin testing by inhibition of recruitment of monocyte–macrophages
  Suppression of lymphocyte proliferation to antigens more easily than proliferation to mitogens
  Suppression of mixed leukocyte reaction proliferation
  Suppression of T lymphocyte–mediated cytotoxicity (at high concentrations in vitro)
  No effect on antibody-dependent, cell-mediated cytotoxicity
  Suppression of spontaneous (natural) cytotoxicity
  Regulatory effects on helper and suppressor cell populations
Monocyte–macrophages
  Suppression of cutaneous delayed hypersensitivity by inhibition of lymphokine effect on the macrophage
  Blockade of Fc-receptor binding and function
  Depression of bactericidal activity
  Possible decrease in monocyte chemotaxis
  Inhibition of interleukin-1 production
Neutrophils
  Possibly no effect on phagocytic and bactericidal capability (controversial)
  Increase in antibody-dependent cellular cytotoxicity
  Probable decrease in lysosomal release but little effect on lysosomal membrane stabilization at pharmacologic concentrations
  Inhibition of chemotaxis only by suprapharmacologic doses

Effects on Humoral Factors
  Mild decrease in immunoglobulin levels but no decrease in specific antibody production
  Probably no effect on complement metabolism
  Decreased reticuloendothelial clearance of antibody-coated cells
  Decreased synthesis of prostaglandins and leukotrienes
  Effects on kinins controversial
  Inhibition of plasminogen activator release
  Potentiation of the actions of catecholamines
  Antagonism of histamine-induced vasodilation

Adapted from Parrillo, J. E., and Fauci, A. S.: Mechanisms of glucocorticoid action on immune processes. Annu. Rev. Pharmacol. Toxicol. 19:179, 1979. Reproduced, with permission, from the Annual Review of Pharmacology and Toxicology, © 1979 by Annual Reviews, Inc.

cause a profound monocytopenia and eosinopenia; the time courses after a single steroid dose are similar to that of the lymphocytopenia.

The mechanism of the decrease in the accumulation of inflammatory cells at an inflammatory site caused by glucocorticoids is not fully understood. Glucocorticoids modify the increased capillary and membrane permeability that occurs at an inflammatory site.[110] By decreasing the dilation of the microvasculature and the increased capillary permeability that occur during the inflammatory response, exu-

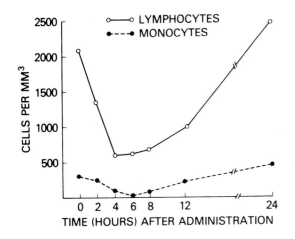

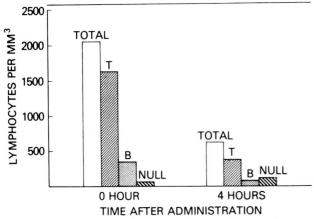

Figure 48–2. The effect of hydrocortisone administration on circulating lymphocytes and monocytes. Hydrocortisone, 400 mg, was administered intravenously in a single dose to a normal volunteer. The upper panel shows the effect on the total lymphocyte and monocyte counts. The lower panel shows the effect on circulating thymus-derived (T) and bone marrow–derived (B) lymphocytes, as well as lymphocytes without detectable surface markers (null cells), 4 hours after drug administration. T lymphocytes were measured by the sheep erythrocyte rosette assay, and B lymphocytes were measured by the complement receptor assay. (Reproduced, with permission, from Fauci, A. S., Dale, D. C., and Balow, J. E.: Glucocorticosteroid therapy: Mechanisms of action and clinical considerations. Ann. Intern. Med. 84:304, 1976.)

dation of fluid and the formation of edema may be reduced, and the migration of leukocytes may be impaired.[96, 97, 110, 111] The decrease in accumulation of inflammatory cells may be due also to decreased adherence of the inflammatory cells to the vascular endothelium.[112–114] It is not possible to determine the relative contributions of a direct vascular effect, of an effect on inflammatory cell adherence to the vascular wall, or of an effect on chemotaxis to the reduction in the inflammatory response caused by glucocorticoids.

Glucocorticoids have numerous effects on leukocyte function. Steroid therapy suppresses cutaneous delayed hypersensitivity responses. This occurs after approximately 14 days of glucocorticoid therapy and disappears approximately 6 days after treatment is withdrawn; these rates vary considerably

from patient to patient.[115] This suppression is a consequence of decreased recruitment of macrophages necessary for the expression of hypersensitivity and is not due to suppression of the sensitized lymphocyte.[115–119] Steroids antagonize the effects of migration inhibition factor on the macrophage.[119, 120] Although human lymphoid tissue is generally resistant to the lytic effect of glucocorticoids, certain activated lymphocyte subsets may be sensitive to the lytic effect of steroids. Other effects of glucocorticoids on lymphocyte function are summarized in Table 48–3.

Monocyte–macrophage traffic and function are relatively sensitive to glucocorticoids. Glucocorticoids administered in divided daily doses depress the bactericidal activity of monocytes.[121, 122] Because the monocyte is thought to be the principal cell involved in granuloma formation, the sensitivity of monocytes to glucocorticoids may explain the effectiveness of glucocorticoids in many granulomatous diseases.[97]

Although neutrophil traffic is sensitive to glucocorticoids, neutrophil function appears to be relatively resistant to these agents.[97] While most in vivo studies of neutrophil phagocytosis have found no evidence for impairment of phagocytosis or bacterial killing,[97] other data are consistent with the view that glucocorticoids induce a generalized phagocytic defect, affecting granulocytes as well as monocytes.[123]

Glucocorticoid therapy retards the disappearance of sensitized erythrocytes, platelets, and artificial particles from the circulation.[97, 123, 124] This may explain the efficacy of glucocorticoids in the treatment of idiopathic thrombocytopenic purpura and autoimmune hemolytic anemia.

Glucocorticoids are potent inhibitors of prostaglandin synthesis.[125–129] This is of particular interest in view of the evidence for synthesis of prostaglandin E_2 (PGE_2) by rheumatoid synovia[130] and the possibility that the bone resorption–stimulating activity of this prostaglandin accounts for the bone destruction in RA.[130] Glucocorticoids inhibit prostaglandin synthesis by inhibition of arachidonic acid release from phospholipids in some tissues.[128, 129] This is distinct from the mechanism of action of the nonsteroid anti-inflammatory drugs (NSAIDs), such as salicylates and indomethacin, which inhibit the cyclooxygenase that converts arachidonic acid to the cyclic endoperoxide intermediates in the prostaglandin synthetic pathway. Thus, the glucocorticoids and the nonsteroid anti-inflammatory agents act at two distinct but adjacent loci in the synthetic pathway of a substance with known bone resorption–stimulating activity that is synthesized by rheumatoid synovia.

Glucocorticoids and NSAIDs have different spectra of anti-inflammatory effects. Some of the therapeutic effects of steroids that are not produced by the nonsteroidal agents may be due to inhibition of leukotriene formation.[131] Leukotrienes are a class of substances originally found in leukocytes, which share a conjugated triene as a common structural feature. Leukotriene B_4 causes adhesion and chemotactic movement of leukocytes. Leukotrienes C_4, D_4, and E_4 (the constituents of the slow-reacting substance of anaphylaxis) increase vascular permeability. These leukotrienes (B_4, C_4, D_4, and E_4) may act synergistically with the vasodilator substances PGE_2 and PGI_2 to mediate inflammation. The glucocorticoid-mediated inhibition of arachidonic acid release prevents formation not only of prostaglandins and thromboxanes (as do the nonsteroidal anti-inflammatory agents) but also of leukotrienes and other oxygenated derivatives. Consequently, some of the therapeutic effects of steroids that are not shared by the nonsteroidal agents may be due to inhibition of leukotriene formation.

Glucocorticoids also inhibit the production of many other mediators of the immune response, such as IL-1.[12, 132, 133]

Side Effects. Adverse reactions to glucocorticoids include the diverse manifestations of Cushing's syndrome and HPA suppression[9, 21, 134] (Table 48–4). Iatrogenic Cushing's syndrome differs from spontaneous Cushing's syndrome in several respects[135, 136]

Table 48–4. ADVERSE REACTIONS TO GLUCOCORTICOIDS

Ophthalmic
  Posterior subcapsular cataracts, increased intraocular pressure
    and glaucoma, exophthalmos
Cardiovascular
  Hypertension
  Congestive heart failure in predisposed patients
Gastrointestinal
  Peptic ulcer disease, pancreatitis
Endocrine–metabolic
  Truncal obesity, moon facies, supraclavicular fat deposition,
    posterior cervical fat deposition (buffalo hump), mediastinal
    widening (lipomatosis), hepatomegaly due to fatty liver
    (rare)
  Acne, hirsutism or virilism, impotence, menstrual irregularities
  Suppression of growth in children
  Hyperglycemia; diabetic ketoacidosis; hyperosmolar,
    nonketotic diabetic coma; hyperlipoproteinemia
  Negative balance of nitrogen, potassium, and calcium
  Sodium retention, hypokalemia, metabolic alkalosis
  Secondary adrenal insufficiency
Musculoskeletal
  Myopathy
  Osteoporosis, vertebral compression fractures, spontaneous
    fractures
  Avascular necrosis of femoral and humeral heads and other
    bones
Neuropsychiatric
  Convulsions
  Benign intracranial hypertension (pseudotumor cerebri)
  Alterations in mood or personality
  Psychosis
Dermatologic
  Facial erythema, thin fragile skin, petechiae and ecchymoses,
    violaceous striae, impaired wound healing
Immune, infectious
  Suppression of delayed hypersensitivity
  Neutrophilia, monocytopenia, lymphocytopenia, decreased
    inflammatory responses
  Susceptibility to infections

From Axelrod, L.: Adrenal corticosteroids. *In* Miller, R. R., and Greenblatt, D. J. (eds.): Handbook of Drug Therapy. New York, Elsevier North-Holland, 1979, p. 809. Used by permission.

Table 48–5. NATURAL VERSUS IATROGENIC CUSHING'S SYNDROME

More common in natural Cushing's syndrome
  Hypertension
  Acne
  Menstrual disturbances
  Hirsutism or virilism
  Impotence in men
  Striae
  Purpura
  Plethora
Virtually unique to iatrogenic Cushing's syndrome
  Benign intracranial hypertension
  Glaucoma
  Posterior subcapsular cataract
  Pancreatitis
  Avascular necrosis of bone
Nearly equal frequency in both syndromes
  Obesity
  Psychiatric symptoms
  Edema*
  Poor wound healing

Adapted from Ragan, C.: Corticotropin, cortisone and related steroids in clincial medicine: Practical considerations. Bull. N. Y. Acad. Med. 29:355, 1953; and Christy, N. P.: Iatrogenic Cushing's syndrome. *In* Christy, N. P. (ed.): The Human Adrenal Cortex. New York, Harper & Row, 1971, p. 395. Used by permission.
*The incidence of edema in iatrogenic Cushing's syndrome may depend on the glucocorticoid employed. Ragan used cortisone.[136]

(Table 48–5). These differences may be explained in part by the fact that in iatrogenic Cushing's syndrome caused by exogenous glucocorticoids, ACTH is suppressed, whereas in spontaneous, ACTH-dependent Cushing's syndrome, the elevated ACTH output results in bilateral adrenal hyperplasia. In the former circumstance, the secretion of adrenocortical androgens and mineralocorticoids is not increased. When ACTH output is elevated, the secretion of adrenal androgens and mineralocorticoids may be increased.[2, 137] The augmented secretion of adrenal androgens may account for the higher incidence of virilism, acne, and menstrual irregularities reported in patients with the spontaneous form of Cushing's syndrome, and the enhanced production of mineralocorticoids may explain the higher incidence of hypertension.[2]

The complications that are virtually unique to iatrogenic Cushing's syndrome arise after prolonged use or large doses of glucocorticoids. This is the case with benign intracranial hypertension,[138, 139] posterior subcapsular cataract,[140–142] and avascular necrosis of bone.[143–149]

The occurrence of avascular necrosis (aseptic necrosis, osteonecrosis) as a consequence of glucocorticoid therapy is a matter of great concern to the physician because of the morbidity associated with this complication and, unfortunately, because of fear engendered by large awards in malpractice litigation. It is difficult to determine the relation between the dose and duration of glucocorticoid therapy and the likelihood of developing avascular necrosis. This is because avascular necrosis occurs in the absence of glucocorticoid therapy; because it occurs as a consequence of other conditions; because it may be related, at least in part, to the primary disease under treatment with glucocorticoids; because of variability in the criteria used to make the diagnosis of avascular necrosis; and because of the typically long interval between the initiation of glucocorticoid therapy and the appearance of signs and symptoms of avascular necrosis.[147] In general, avascular necrosis occurs only in patients who have received glucocorticoid therapy for at least 1 month at pharmacologic doses. The risk of avascular necrosis may be related to the highest dose used, to the total dose, or to the total duration of treatment.[143–149]

Although the association of glucocorticoid therapy and peptic ulcer disease is controversial,[150–156] it appears that glucocorticoids increase the risk of peptic ulcer disease and gastrointestinal hemorrhage.[154, 155] The magnitude of the association between glucocorticoid therapy and these complications is small and is related to the total dose and duration of therapy.[151, 154]

Glucocorticoid therapy, especially daily therapy, may suppress the immune response to skin tests for tuberculosis.[115] When possible, tuberculin skin testing is advisable before glucocorticoid therapy is initiated. Routine isoniazid prophylaxis for corticosteroid-treated patients, even those with positive tuberculin skin test results, is probably not indicated.[157]

Some patients respond to glucocorticoids and develop side effects more readily than others at equivalent doses. Of course, variations in responsiveness to glucocorticoids may result from drug interactions (see earlier discussion) or from variations in the severity of the underlying disease. Alterations in the bioavailability of administered glucocorticoids probably do not account for the variations in therapeutic response in most patients.[28] In patients who experience side effects, the metabolic clearance rate of prednisolone and the volume of distribution are lower[44] and the circulating half-life is longer[44] than in those who do not. Impairment of renal function may decrease the clearance of prednisolone and thereby increase the prevalence of side effects.[158] Patients who develop a cushingoid habitus on prednisone have higher endogenous plasma cortisol levels than those who do not, perhaps because of a resistance of the HPA axis to suppression by exogenous glucocorticoids.[159]

Variations in the effectiveness of steroids may be due to altered cellular responsiveness to steroids.[28, 160–163] In patients with primary open-angle glaucoma, glucocorticoids produce a greater rise of intraocular pressure,[160] greater suppression of the 8:00 A.M. plasma cortisol level (when dexamethasone, 0.25 mg, is administered the previous evening at 11:00 P.M.),[162] and greater suppression of phytohemagglutinin-induced transformation of lymphocytes than in normal subjects.[161, 163] Because primary open-angle glaucoma is not uncommon, these findings suggest that a distinct subpopulation of patients is hyper-responsive to glucocorticoids and that this sensitivity is genetically determined.

Withdrawal from Glucocorticoids. The symptoms associated with glucocorticoid withdrawal include arthralgia, myalgia, anorexia, nausea, emesis, lethargy, headache, fever, desquamation, weight loss, and postural hypotension. Many of these symptoms can occur with normal plasma levels of glucocorticoids[164] and in patients with normal responsiveness to conventional tests of the HPA system.[165, 166] These patients may have an abnormal response to a more sensitive test using 1 μg of α-1-24 ACTH rather than the conventional 250-μg dose.[167] The steroid-withdrawal syndrome may contribute to psychologic dependence on glucocorticoid treatment and to one's difficulties in withdrawing such therapy.

SUPPRESSION OF THE HYPOTHALAMIC–PITUITARY–ADRENAL SYSTEM

Development of Hypothalamic–Pituitary–Adrenal Suppression. There are few well-documented cases of acute adrenocortical insufficiency after chronic glucocorticoid therapy and no such cases after ACTH therapy.[2] Therefore, the minimal duration of glucocorticoid therapy that can produce HPA suppression must be ascertained from studies of adrenocortical weight and adrenocortical responsiveness to provocative tests.[2, 135, 168] Adrenocortical atrophy is detectable 5 days after the onset of glucocorticoid therapy.[169] Abnormalities in responsiveness to ACTH and to metyrapone are observed in some patients within 3 days of initiation of treatment with glucocorticoids.[2, 135, 168] Abnormalities in responsiveness to ACTH and to insulin-induced hypoglycemia occur after the administration of prednisone, 25 mg twice daily for 5 days.[170] Abnormalities in response to insulin-induced hypoglycemia occur with a similar time course after comparable doses in children.[171] It must be emphasized that there is considerable variation from patient to patient[172] and from study to study.[135] These figures define the earliest time at which abnormalities are observed in some but not all patients. Because assessment of the onset of HPA suppression depends on anatomic and biochemical (but not clinical) evidence, and because the biochemical abnormalities observed are sometimes mild, it is not possible to identify definitively the shortest interval or the smallest dose at which suppression may occur. On the basis of the available evidence, any patient who has received a glucocorticoid in doses equivalent to 20 to 30 mg of prednisone per day for more than 5 days should be suspected of having HPA suppression.[2] If the doses are closer to but above the physiologic range, 1 month is probably the minimal interval.[2] When such suspicions are entertained, there are two alternatives—perform an ACTH test or treat the patient as though adrenocortical insufficiency were present.

The adrenocortical response to an ACTH test is

Table 48–6. ASSESSMENT OF HYPOTHALAMIC–PITUITARY–ADRENAL FUNCTION IN PATIENTS TREATED WITH GLUCOCORTICOIDS

Method
　　Withhold exogenous steroids for 24 hours
　　Give cosyntropin (synthetic alpha 1-24 ACTH) 250 μg (25
　　　　units) as intravenous bolus or intramuscular injection
　　Obtain plasma cortisol level 30 or 60 minutes after
　　　　administration of ACTH
　　Note: Performance of the test in the morning is customary but
　　　　not essential

Interpretation
　　Normal response: Plasma cortisol level above 18 μg/dl at 30 or
　　　　60 minutes after ACTH administration
　　Note: Traditional recommendations also specify an increment
　　　　above baseline of 7 μg/dl at 30 minutes or 11 μg/dl at 60
　　　　minutes and a doubling of the baseline value at 60 minutes.
　　　　These parameters are valid in normal, unstressed subjects
　　　　but are frequently misleading in ill patients with a normal
　　　　hypothalamic–pituitary–adrenal axis, in whom stress may
　　　　raise the baseline plasma cortisol level by an increase in
　　　　endogenous ACTH levels.[173]

ACTH = adrenocorticotropic hormone.

a useful guide to the presence or absence of suppression in glucocorticoid-treated patients[173] (Table 48–6). The maximal response of the plasma cortisol level to ACTH corresponds to the maximal plasma cortisol level observed during the induction of general anesthesia and surgery in patients who have received glucocorticoid therapy.[174–177] A normal response to ACTH preoperatively is unlikely to be followed by markedly impaired secretion of cortisol during anesthesia and surgery in steroid-treated patients. In general, other tests of the HPA system, such as insulin-induced hypoglycemia and the metyrapone test, are not indicated in the evaluation of the steroid-treated patient for possible HPA axis suppression.

The stress of general anesthesia and surgery is not hazardous to patients who have received only replacement doses (no more than 25 mg of hydrocortisone, 5 mg of prednisone, 4 mg of triamcinolone, or 0.75 mg of dexamethasone),[178] if the steroid is given early in the day.[179] If doses of this size are given late in the day, suppression may occur as a result of inhibition of the diurnal release of ACTH.[179, 180]

ACTH and the Hypothalamic–Pituitary–Adrenal System. Pharmacologic doses of ACTH produce supranormal cortisol secretory rates and elevated plasma cortisol levels. One might expect such elevated levels to suppress ACTH release. In fact, there is no evidence of clinically significant hypothalamic–pituitary suppression in patients who have received ACTH therapy.[2] The failure of ACTH to cause suppression of HPA function is not explained by the dose of ACTH employed, the frequency of injections, the time of administration, or the plasma cortisol pattern after ACTH administration.[181] Another possible explanation is that the hyperplastic and overactive adrenal cortex that results from ACTH therapy might compensate for hypothalamic or pituitary

suppression.[182] Although threshold adrenocortical sensitivity to ACTH is not changed in patients who have received daily ACTH therapy,[181] the possibility remains that there is altered adrenocortical responsiveness to ACTH in the physiologic range. In addition, evidence exists that the preservation of the normal response of the plasma cortisol level in patients treated with ACTH is due, at least in part, to the fact that ACTH treatment reduces the rate of ACTH secretion but not the total amount secreted, whereas glucocorticoids reduce both the rate of secretion and the total amount secreted.[183]

Recovery from Hypothalamic–Pituitary–Adrenal Suppression. During recovery from HPA suppression, hypothalamic–pituitary function returns before adrenocortical function.[184] Twelve months must elapse after withdrawal of large doses of glucocorticoids given for a prolonged period before homeostatic function, including responsiveness to stress, returns to normal.[2, 184, 185] In contrast, recovery from HPA suppression induced by a brief course of steroids (i.e., prednisone, 25 mg twice daily for 5 days, or prednisone, 20 mg twice daily for 3 weeks) occurs within 5 days.[170, 186] Recovery from HPA suppression induced by a comparable 5-day course of steroids occurs at about the same rate in children.[171] As a group, patients with mild suppression of the HPA axis (i.e., normal basal plasma and urine steroid levels but diminished responses to ACTH and insulin-induced hypoglycemia) resume normal functional capacity more rapidly than those with severe depression of the HPA axis (i.e., low basal plasma and urine steroid levels and diminished responses to ACTH and insulin-induced hypoglycemia).[187] The time course of recovery correlates with the total duration of previous glucocorticoid therapy and the total previous steroid dose.[187–189] Nevertheless, it is not possible in an individual patient to predict the time course of recovery from a course of glucocorticoid therapy at supraphysiologic doses lasting more than a few weeks, so persistence of HPA suppression should be suspected for 12 months after such a course of treatment. The course of recovery from suppression of the contralateral adrenal cortex by the products of an adrenocortical tumor may exceed 12 months.[185, 190] Recovery from suppression induced by exogenous glucocorticoids may be more rapid in children than in adults.[191]

WITHDRAWAL OF PATIENTS FROM GLUCOCORTICOIDS

Risks of Withdrawal. The decision to discontinue glucocorticoid therapy provokes apprehension among physicians. The untoward consequences of such an action include precipitation of adrenocortical insufficiency, the steroid withdrawal syndrome, and an exacerbation of the underlying disease.

Adrenocortical insufficiency after the withdrawal of glucocorticoids is justly feared. The likelihood of precipitating the underlying disease almost certainly depends on the activity and natural history of the illness in question. When there is any possibility that the underlying illness may flare up, the glucocorticoid should be withdrawn gradually, over an interval of weeks to months, with frequent reassessment of the patient.

Management of the Patient with Hypothalamic–Pituitary–Adrenal Suppression. There is no proved means of hastening a return to normal HPA function after inhibition has resulted from glucocorticoid therapy. The use of ACTH does not appear to prevent or reverse the development of glucocorticoid-induced adrenal insufficiency.[166, 192–194] Conversion to an alternate-day schedule permits but does not accelerate recovery.[195, 196] In children, alternate-day glucocorticoid therapy may delay recovery.[197]

Recovery from steroid-induced adrenal insufficiency is time dependent and spontaneous. During this interval, small doses of hydrocortisone (10 to 20 mg) or prednisone (2.5 to 5 mg) in the morning may alleviate withdrawal symptoms. Recovery of HPA function does occur during the administration of small doses of glucocorticoids in the morning; the rate of recovery is determined not only by the doses given when the steroids are being tapered but also by the dose administered during the initial phase of treatment, before tapering is commenced.[187–189] The available studies do not exclude the possibility that small doses of glucocorticoids in the morning retard the rate of recovery from HPA suppression, even though they do not prevent recovery. This requires further investigation.

ALTERNATE-DAY GLUCOCORTICOID THERAPY

Alternate-day glucocorticoid therapy is defined as the administration of a short-acting glucocorticoid with no appreciable mineralocorticoid effect (such as prednisone, prednisolone, or methylprednisolone) once every 48 hours in the morning, at about 8:00 A.M. The objective is to minimize the adverse effects of glucocorticoids while retaining therapeutic effectiveness. The original basis for this approach was the hypothesis that the anti-inflammatory effects of glucocorticoids persist longer than the undesirable metabolic effects.[198–202] If so, it should be possible to find a schedule that allows rest periods between doses during which the patient is not exposed to the side effects of glucocorticoids while the desired anti-inflammatory action persists.[199, 200] This hypothesis is not supported by observations of the duration of steroid effects (see earlier discussion).

A second hypothesis emphasizes that intermittent rather than continuous administration produces a cyclic, though not diurnal, pattern of glucocorticoid levels in the circulation and within the target cells that simulates the normal diurnal cycle. This might prevent the development of Cushing's syndrome and

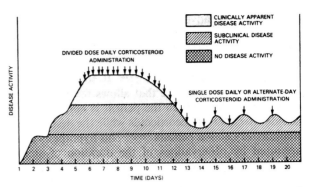

Figure 48–3. The effect of glucocorticoid administration on the activity of the underlying disease. Full-blown disease activity may require the use of a divided daily dose schedule. When the disease is controlled, or from the start of therapy in certain diseases, alternate-day therapy may be effective. (Reproduced, with permission, from Fauci, A. S., Dale, D. C., and Balow, J. E.: Glucocorticosteroid therapy: Mechanisms of action and clinical considerations. Ann. Intern. Med. 84:304, 1976.)

HPA suppression but provide therapeutic benefit. Because the full expression of a disease frequently occurs only when the inflammatory activity continues over a protracted period, the intermittent administration of a glucocorticoid may be sufficient to shorten the interval during which the disorder develops without interruption, thereby preventing the level of disease activity from becoming clinically apparent (Fig. 48–3).[95] The duration of action of the glucocorticoids is important in this context. The selection of prednisone, prednisolone, and methylprednisolone as the agents of choice for alternate-day therapy and 48 hours as the appropriate interval between doses has an empiric basis. Harter and associates found that intervals of 36, 24, and 12 hours were accompanied by adrenal suppression, and that an interval of 72 hours was therapeutically ineffective when prednisone (and, in some cases, triamcinolone) was employed. An interval of 48 hours was found to be optimal.[200]

Alternatively, the effects of alternate-day therapy may reflect decreased total exposure to prednisolone as a consequence of the dose-dependent systemic availability of prednisolone (see above) after oral prednisone or prednisolone.[203] That is, the bioavailability of prednisolone is lower when the same total amount of prednisone or prednisolone is given as a single oral dose rather than as several small doses.[203] While the dose-dependent bioavailability of prednisone and prednisolone may explain in part the reduction in side effects that is observed during alternate-day therapy, it cannot be the only explanation for the effectiveness of alternate-day therapy because it implies that alternate-day therapy reduces the benefits of glucocorticoid therapy as well as the side effects,[15, 203] contrary to the findings described below.

Alternate-Day Glucocorticoids and Cushing's Syndrome. An alternate-day regimen can prevent or ameliorate the manifestations of Cushing's syndrome, including not only the somatic and psychologic manifestations but also quantifiable end-points such as high blood pressure, retarded linear growth rate in children, altered leukocyte kinetics, impaired responsiveness to skin testing for delayed hypersensitivity, impaired monocyte cellular function, elevated urinary excretion rates of nitrogen and potassium, impaired intestinal absorption of calcium, reduced serum 25-hydroxyvitamin D levels, and elevated serum cholesterol and triglyceride levels.[2, 204–206]

Despite the beneficial effects of alternate-day therapy on intestinal calcium absorption and serum 25-hydroxyvitamin D levels, this therapeutic approach does not prevent loss of bone, especially trabecular bone, in humans.[207–209] Although this suggests that an alternate-day regimen may not prevent fractures of vertebrae and other bones, this question has not been studied.

The susceptibility to infections that characterizes Cushing's syndrome[84, 210–212] may be alleviated by an alternate-day program. The available reports strongly suggest that alternate-day therapy is associated with a lower incidence of infections than daily medication but do not firmly establish this point.[2] Intermittently normal leukocyte kinetics, preservation of delayed hypersensitivity, and preservation of monocyte cellular function may explain the apparently reduced susceptibility to infections of patients on alternate-day therapy.[2]

Effects of Alternate-Day Glucocorticoid Therapy on Hypothalamic–Pituitary–Adrenal Responsiveness. Patients on alternate-day glucocorticoid therapy may have some suppression of basal steroid levels, but they have normal to nearly normal responsiveness to provocative tests such as the corticotropin-releasing hormone stimulation test, ACTH stimulation tests, insulin-induced hypoglycemia, and the metyrapone test.[2, 213] They also have less suppression of HPA function than patients on daily therapy.[2]

Effects of Alternate-Day Therapy on the Underlying Disease. Alternate-day glucocorticoid therapy is as effective or nearly as effective in controlling a diverse group of diseases as daily therapy in divided doses. This approach has been used with apparent benefit in patients with childhood nephrotic syndrome, adult nephrotic syndrome, membranous nephropathy, renal transplantation, membranoproliferative glomerulonephritis, lupus nephritis, ulcerative colitis, RA, acute rheumatic fever, myasthenia gravis, Duchenne's muscular dystrophy, dermatomyositis, idiopathic polyneuropathy, asthma, sarcoidosis, cystic fibrosis, alopecia areata and other chronic dermatoses, and pemphigus vulgaris.[2] In one study, alternate-day therapy was not as effective as daily therapy in reducing the sedimentation rate in giant cell arteritis.[214] However, patients were transferred abruptly from daily therapy with divided doses to alternate-day therapy. In addition, there were few adverse effects of steroids and no evidence of progression of the arteritis on the alternate-day regimen, so there may be a role for this approach in

giant cell arteritis.[215] In another study, 18 of 27 patients with giant cell arteritis were treated successfully with an alternate-day regimen after a gradual transition from daily single-dose therapy.[216] Prospective controlled studies demonstrate the efficacy of alternate-day therapy in membranous nephropathy[217] and renal transplantation.[218, 219]

Use of Alternate-Day Therapy. Because alternate-day therapy can prevent or ameliorate the manifestations of Cushing's syndrome, can avert or permit recovery from HPA suppression, and is as effective (or nearly as effective) as continuous therapy, whenever possible a patient for whom chronic glucocorticoid administration is indicated should be placed on such a program. Yet, some physicians are reluctant to use alternate-day schedules, often because of an unsuccessful experience. Many efforts fail because of lack of familiarity with the indications for, and use of, such therapy.

The benefits of alternate-day glucocorticoid therapy are demonstrable only when steroids are used for a prolonged period. There is no reason to use an alternate-day schedule when the anticipated duration of therapy is no longer than several weeks.

Alternate-day therapy may not be necessary or appropriate during the initial stages of therapy or during exacerbation of the underlying disease. Nevertheless, patients with childhood and adult nephrotic syndrome, membranous nephropathy, lupus nephritis, RA, myasthenia gravis, dermatomyositis, asthma, sarcoidosis, rheumatic fever, pemphigus vulgaris, a variety of ocular diseases, and several other disorders have been treated with an alternate-day regimen as initial therapy with apparent benefit.[2] It appears to be easier to establish treatment with alternate-day steroids than to convert from daily therapy in patients with RA.[195, 220] Studies in recipients of renal transplants have initially used daily therapy and then converted to an alternate-day schedule. Thus, an alternate-day schedule as initial therapy may be beneficial in some disorders but ineffective in others.

Alternate-day therapy may be hazardous in the presence of adrenocortical insufficiency of any cause because the patient is unprotected against glucocorticoid insufficiency during the last 12 hours of the 48-hour cycle.[195, 200, 221] In a patient who has been on glucocorticoids for more than a brief period, or who may have adrenal insufficiency on another basis, adequacy of HPA function should be determined before the initiation of an alternate-day program. It may be possible to surmount this obstacle by giving a small dose of a short-acting glucocorticoid (i.e., 10 mg of hydrocortisone) in the afternoon of the second day; this approach has not been studied.

Alternate-day glucocorticoid therapy may fail to prevent or ameliorate the manifestations of Cushing's syndrome or HPA suppression if a short-acting glucocorticoid is not used, or if it is used incorrectly.[16, 222–224] For example, the use of prednisone four times per day on alternate days may be less successful than the use of the same total dose once every 48 hours.

An abrupt alteration from daily to alternate-day therapy should be avoided because the prolonged use of daily-dose glucocorticoids may have resulted in HPA suppression. In addition, patients with normal function of the HPA axis may experience withdrawal symptoms in these circumstances and have an exacerbation of the underlying disease.[225]

No program of conversion from continuous therapy to alternate-day therapy has been proved to be optimal. One approach is to reduce the frequency of drug administration each day, until the total dose for each day is given in the morning, and then gradually to increase the dose on the first day of each 2-day period and to decrease the dose on the second day. Another approach is to double the dose on the first day of each 2-day cycle, and to give this as a single morning dose, if possible, and then to taper gradually the dose on the second day.[226] It is not clear how often such changes should be made with any approach. This probably depends on the underlying disease involved, the duration of previous glucocorticoid therapy, the personality of the patient, and the physician's ability to use adjunctive therapy. In any event, the conversion should be made as quickly as the patient will tolerate it. If the patient develops evidence of adrenal insufficiency, of the steroid withdrawal syndrome, or of an exacerbation of the underlying disease, the previously effective regimen should be reinstituted and then tapered more gradually. Occasionally, it will be necessary to resume full daily doses temporarily. Changes in the dose should be approximately 10 mg of prednisone (or equivalent) at total daily doses of more than 30 mg, 5 mg at total doses of more than 20 mg, and 2.5 mg at lower doses. At small total daily doses, an absolute change of dose represents a larger percentage change in dose than at large total daily doses. The interval between changes in dose may be as short as 1 day or as long as many weeks.

In addition, optimal results from alternate-day glucocorticoid therapy may not be achieved because of failure to use supplemental therapy for the underlying disorder. Conservative (nonglucocorticoid) therapy is often used until a glucocorticoid is initiated, at which time these less toxic therapeutic measures are ignored. Use of adjunctive therapy may facilitate the use of the lowest possible dose of glucocorticoids. On alternate-day therapy, these measures should be used especially during the end of the second day, when symptoms may be prominent. The potential benefits of NSAIDs in the rheumatic diseases should not be neglected. Supplemental therapy may be especially helpful in disorders in which the patient may experience symptoms of the disease on the day off therapy, such as asthma and RA. In illnesses in which disabling symptoms are less likely to appear on the alternate day, such as the childhood nephrotic syndrome, less difficulty may be encountered.

Alternate-day therapy may fail because of failure to inform the patient about the purposes of this regimen. Because glucocorticoids may induce euphoria, a patient may be reluctant to accept modification of a schedule of frequent doses. Careful explanation about the risks of glucocorticoid excess, attuned to the patient's intellectual and emotional ability to comprehend, maximizes the likelihood of success. Close communication between patient and physician is indispensable.

DAILY SINGLE-DOSE GLUCOCORTICOID THERAPY

In some situations, alternate-day therapy fails because the patient experiences symptoms of the underlying disease during the last few hours of the second day. In these cases, single-dose glucocorticoid therapy may be of value. This regimen appears to be as effective as divided daily doses in controlling such underlying diseases as RA, systemic lupus erythematosus, polyarteritis, and proctocolitis.[227–230] In giant cell arteritis, a daily dose in the morning is nearly as effective as daily therapy in divided doses.[214] Daily single-dose therapy appears to reduce the likelihood that a patient will develop HPA suppression.[33, 229, 231, 232] On the other hand, the manifestations of Cushing's syndrome are probably not prevented or ameliorated by a daily single-dose regimen.[227, 228]

GLUCOCORTICOIDS OR ADRENOCORTICOTROPIC HORMONE?

Disorders that respond to glucocorticoid therapy also respond to ACTH therapy if the adrenal cortex is normal. However, there is no evidence that ACTH is superior to glucocorticoids for the treatment of any disorder when comparable doses are used.[2, 21, 233] In fact, hydrocortisone and ACTH, when given intravenously in pharmacologically equivalent dosage (determined by plasma cortisol levels and urinary steroid excretion rates) are equally effective in the treatment of inflammatory bowel disease.[234] Because ACTH does not appear to offer any therapeutic advantage, glucocorticoids are preferable for therapeutic purposes[2]; they can be administered orally, the dose can be regulated precisely, the effectiveness does not depend on adrenocortical responsiveness (an important consideration in patients who have been treated with glucocorticoids), and they produce a lower incidence of certain side effects, such as acne, hypertension, and increased pigmentation.[235] When one is unable to use alternate-day therapy, ACTH might appear to be preferable because it does not suppress the HPA axis. This benefit is usually outweighed by the advantages of glucocorticoids enumerated earlier and by the fact that daily injections of ACTH are not superior to single daily doses of short-acting glucocorticoids; in both cases, HPA suppression is unlikely to result, but Cushing's syndrome is not prevented. In life-threatening situations, glucocorticoids are indicated because maximal blood levels are obtained immediately after intravenous administration, whereas with ACTH infusion, the plasma cortisol level rises to a plateau over several hours. The principal indication for ACTH continues to be the assessment of adrenocortical reserve.

References

1. Polley, H. F., and Slocumb, C. H.: Behind the scenes with cortisone and ACTH. Mayo Clin. Proc. 51:471, 1976.
2. Axelrod, L.: Glucocorticoid therapy. Medicine 55:39, 1976.
3. Hollander, J. L., Brown, E. M., Jr., Jessar, R. A., and Brown, C. Y.: Hydrocortisone and cortisone injected into arthritic joints. J.A.M.A. 147:1629, 1951.
4. Robinson, R. C. V., and Robinson, H. M., Jr.: Topical treatment of dermatoses with steroids. South. Med. J. 49: 260, 1956.
5. Jenkins, J. S.: The metabolism of cortisol by human extrahepatic tissues. J. Endocrinol. 34:51, 1966.
6. Schalm, S. W., Summerskill, W. H. J., and Go, V. L. W.: Development of radioimmunoassays for prednisone and prednisolone: Application to studies of hepatic metabolism of prednisone. Mayo Clin. Proc. 51:761, 1976.
7. Krieger, D. T., Allen, W., Rizzo, F., and Krieger, H. P.: Characterization of the normal temporal pattern of plasma corticosteroid levels. J. Clin. Endocrinol. Metab. 32:266, 1971.
8. Keller-Wood, M. E., and Dallman, M. F.: Corticosteroid inhibition of ACTH secretion. Endocr. Rev. 5:1, 1984.
9. Axelrod, L.: Side effects of glucocorticoid therapy. In Schleimer, R. P., Claman, H. N., and Oronsky, A. (eds.): Anti-inflammatory Steroid Action: Basic and Clinical Aspects. San Diego, Academic Press, 1989, p. 377.
10. Estep, H. L., Island, D. P., Ney, R. L., and Liddle, G. W.: Pituitary adrenal dynamics during surgical stress. J. Clin. Endocrinol. Metab. 23:419, 1963.
11. Woloski, B. M., Smith, E. M., Meyer, W. J., III, Fuller, G. M., and Blalock, J. E.: Corticotropin-releasing activity of monokines. Science 230:1035, 1985.
12. Besedovsky, H., Del Rey, A., Sorkin, E., and Dinarello, C. A.: Immunoregulatory feedback between interleukin-1 and glucocorticoid hormones. Science 233:652, 1986.
13. Frey, F. J.: Kinetics and dynamics of prednisolone. Endocr. Rev. 8:453, 1987.
14. Szefler, S. J.: General pharmacology of glucocorticoids. In Schleimer, R. P., Claman, H. N., and Oronsky, A. (eds.): Anti-inflammatory Steroid Action: Basic and Clinical Aspects. San Diego, Academic Press, 1989, p. 353.
15. Frey, B. M., and Frey, F. J.: Clinical pharmacokinetics of prednisone and prednisolone. Clin. Pharmacokinet. 19:126, 1990.
16. Harter, J. G.: Corticosteroids: Their physiologic use in allergic diseases. N. Y. State J. Med. 66:827, 1966.
17. Boland, E. W.: 16-α-Methyl corticosteroids. Calif. Med. 88:417, 1958.
18. Boland, E. W., and Liddle, G. W.: Metabolic and antirheumatic activities of 6-methylprednisolone (Medrol). Ann. Rheum. Dis. 16:297, 1957.
19. Bondy, P. K.: The adrenal cortex. In Bondy, P. K., and Rosenberg, L. E. (eds.): Duncan's Diseases of Metabolism. 7th ed. Philadelphia, W. B. Saunders Company, 1974, p. 1105.
20. Bunim, J. J., Black, R. L., Lutwak, L., Peterson, R. E., and Whedon, G. D.: Studies on dexamethasone, a new synthetic steroid, in rheumatoid arthritis: A preliminary report. Arthritis Rheum. 1:313, 1958.
21. Cope, C. L.: Adrenal Steroids and Disease. 2nd ed. London, Pitman Medical, 1972.
22. Kleeman, C. R., Koplowitz, J., and Maxwell, M. H.: Metabolic effects of two newer adrenal analogs, 6-methylprednisolone (Medrol) and 6-methyl-9α-fluoro-21-desoxyprednisolone (9α-fluoro-21-desoxymedrol). Metabolism 7:425, 1958.
23. Liddle, G. W.: Studies of structure-function relationships of steroids. II. The 6-α-methylcorticosteroids. Metabolism 7:405, 1958.
24. Liddle, G. W.: Clinical pharmacology of the anti-inflammatory agents. Clin. Pharmacol. Ther. 2:615, 1961.
25. Liddle, G. W.: The adrenal cortex. In Williams, R. H. (ed.): Textbook of Endocrinology. 5th ed. Philadelphia, W. B. Saunders Company, 1974, p. 233.
26. Meikle, A. W., and Tyler, F. H.: Potency and duration of action of glucocorticoids: Effects of hydrocortisone, prednisone and dexamethasone on human pituitary-adrenal function. Am. J. Med. 63:200, 1977.
27. Ballard, P. L., Carter J. P., Graham, B. S., and Baxter, J. D.: A radioreceptor assay for evaluation of the plasma glucocorticoid activity of natural and synthetic steroids in man. J. Clin. Endocrinol. Metab. 41:290, 1975.
28. Morris, H. G.: Factors that influence clinical responses to administered corticosteroids. J. Allergy Clin. Immunol. 66:343, 1980.
29. Pickup, M. E.: Clinical pharmacokinetics of prednisone and prednisolone. Clin. Pharmacokinet. 4:111, 1979.
30. Pickup, M. E., Lowe, J. R., Leatham, P. A., Rhind, V. M., Wright, V., and Downie, W. W.: Dose-dependent pharmacokinetics of prednisolone. Eur. J. Clin. Pharmacol. 12:213, 1977.
31. Walton, J., Watson, B. S., and Ney, R. L.: Alternate-day vs. shorter-interval steroid administration. Arch. Intern. Med. 126:601, 1970.
32. Ellul-Micallef, R., Borthwick, R. C., and McHardy, G. J. R.: The time course of response to prednisolone in chronic bronchial asthma. Clin. Sci. 47:105, 1974.
33. Grant, S. D., Forsham, P. H., and DiRaimondo, V. C.: Suppression of 17-hydroxycorticosteroids in plasma and urine by single and divided doses of triamcinolone. N. Engl. J. Med. 273:1115, 1965.
34. LaPointe, M. C., and Baxter, J. D.: Molecular biology of glucocorticoid hormone action. In Schleimer, R. P., Claman, H. N. and Oronsky, A. (eds.): Anti-inflammatory Steroid Action: Basic and Clinical Aspects. San Diego, Academic Press, 1989, p. 3.
35. Jenkins, J. S., and Sampson, P. A.: Conversion of cortisone to cortisol and prednisone to prednisolone. Br. Med. J. 2:205, 1967.
36. Nelson, D H., Sandberg, A. A., Palmer, J. G., and Tyler, F. H.: Blood levels of 17-hydroxycorticosteroids following the administration of adrenal steroids and their relation to levels of circulating leukocytes. J. Clin. Invest. 31:843, 1952.
37. Gemzell, C. A., and Franksson, C.: Blood levels of 17-hydroxycorticosteroids in normal and adrenalectomized men following administration of cortisone acetate. Acta Endocrinol. 12:218, 1953.
38. Plumpton, F. S., Besser, G. M., and Cole, P. V.: Corticosteroid treatment and surgery. 2. The management of steroid cover. Anaesthesia 24:12, 1969.
39. Banks, P.: The adreno-cortical response to oral surgery. Br. J. Oral Surg. 8:32, 1970.
40. Kehlet, H., Nistrup Madsen, S., and Binder, C.: Cortisol and cortisone acetate in parenteral glucocorticoid therapy? Acta Med. Scand. 195:421, 1974.
41. Kehlet, H.: A rational approach to dosage and preparation of parenteral glucocorticoid substitution therapy during surgical procedures: A short review. Acta Anaesth. Scand. 19:260, 1975.
42. Fariss, B. L., Hane, S., Shinsako, J., and Forsham, P. H.: Comparison of absorption of cortisone acetate and hydrocortisone hemisuccinate. J. Clin. Endocrinol. Metab. 47:1137, 1978.
43. Angeli, A., Frajria, R., DePaoli, R., Fonzo, D., and Ceresa, F.: Diurnal variation of prednisolone binding to serum corticosteroid-binding globulin in man. Clin. Pharmacol. Ther. 23:47, 1978.
44. Kozower, M., Veatch, L., and Kaplan, M. M.: Decreased clearance of prednisolone, a factor in the development of corticosteroid side effects. J. Clin. Endocrinol. Metab. 38:407, 1974.
45. Schalm, S. W., Summerskill, W. H. J., and Go, V. L. W.: Prednisone for chronic active liver disease: Pharmacokinetics, including conversion to prednisolone. Gastroenterology 72:910, 1977.
46. Peterson, R. E.: Adrenocortical steroid metabolism and adrenal cortical function in liver disease. J. Clin. Invest. 39:320, 1960.
47. Powell, L. W., and Axelsen, E.: Corticosteroids in liver disease: Studies on the biological conversion of prednisone to prednisolone and plasma protein binding. Gut 13:690, 1972.
48. Davis, M., Williams, R., Chakraborty, J., English, J., Marks, V., Ideo, G., and Tempini, S.: Prednisone or prednisolone for the treatment of chronic active hepatitis? A comparison of plasma availability. Br. J. Clin. Pharmacol. 5:501, 1978.
49. Araki, Y., Yokota, O., Tatsuo, K., Kashima, M., and Miyazaki, T.: Dynamics of synthetic corticosteroids in man. In Pincus, G., Nakao, T., and Tait, J. F. (eds.): Steroid Dynamics. New York, Academic Press, 1966, p. 463.
50. Renner, E., Horber, F. F., Jost, G., Frey, B. M., and Frey, F. J.: Effect of liver function on the metabolism of prednisone and prednisolone in humans. Gastroenterology 90:819, 1986.
51. Lewis, G. P., Jusko, W. J., Burke, C. W., Graves, L., and the Boston Collaborative Drug Surveillance Program: Prednisone side-effects and serum-protein levels, a collaborative study. Lancet 2:778, 1971.
52. Frey, F. J., and Frey, B. M.: Altered prednisolone kinetics in patients with the nephrotic syndrome. Nephron 32:45, 1982.
53. Gatti, G., Perucca, E, Frigo, G. M., Notarangelo, L. D., Barberis, L., and Martini, A.: Pharmacokinetics of prednisone and its metabolite prednisolone in children with nephrotic syndrome during the active phase and in remission. Br. J. Clin. Pharmacol. 17:423, 1984.
54. Frey, F. J., Horber, F. F., and Frey, B. M.: Altered metabolism and decreased efficacy of prednisolone and prednisone in patients with hyperthyroidism. Clin. Pharmacol. Ther. 44:510, 1988.
55. Schatz, M., Patterson, R., Zeitz, S., O'Rourke, J., and Melam, H.: Corticosteroid therapy for the pregnant asthmatic patient. J.A.M.A. 233:804, 1975.

56. Ohrlander, S., Gennser, G., Nilsson, K. O., and Eneroth, P.: ACTH test to neonates after administration of corticosteroids during gestation. Obstet. Gynecol. 49:691, 1977.

57. Grajwer, L. A., Lilien, L. D., and Pildes, R. S.: Neonatal subclinical adrenal insufficiency: Result of maternal steroid therapy. J.A.M.A. 238:1279, 1977.

58. Reinisch, J. M., Simon, N. G., Karow, W. G., and Gandelman, R.: Prenatal exposure to prednisone in humans and animals retards intrauterine growth. Science 202:436, 1978.

59. Katz, F. H., and Duncan, B. R.: Entry of prednisone into human milk (Letter). N. Engl. J. Med. 293:1154, 1975.

60. McKenzie, S. A., Selley, J. A., and Agnew, J. E.: Secretion of prednisolone into breast milk. Arch. Dis. Child. 50:894, 1975.

61. Choi, Y., Thrasher, K., Werk, E. E., Jr., Sholiton, L. J., and Olinger, C.: Effect of diphenylhydantoin on cortisol kinetics in humans. J. Pharmacol. Exp. Ther. 176:27, 1971.

62. Haque, N., Thrasher, K., Werk, E. E., Jr., Knowles, H. C., Jr., and Sholiton, L. J.: Studies on dexamethasone metabolism in man: Effect of diphenylhydantoin. J. Clin. Endocrinol. Metab. 34:44, 1972.

63. Stjernholm, M. R., and Katz, F. H.: Effects of diphenylhydantoin, phenobarbital, and diazepam on the metabolism of methylprednisolone and its sodium succinate. J. Clin. Endocrinol. Metab. 41:887, 1975.

64. Petereit, L. B., and Meikle, A. W.: Effectiveness of prednisolone during phenytoin therapy. Clin. Pharmacol. Ther. 22:912, 1977.

65. Bartoszek, M., Brenner, A. M., and Szefler, S. J.: Prednisolone and methylprednisolone kinetics in children receiving anticonvulsant therapy. Clin. Pharmacol. Ther. 42:424, 1987.

66. Brooks, S. M., Werk, E. E., Ackerman, S. J., Sullivan, I., and Thrasher, K.: Adverse effects of phenobarbital on corticosteroid metabolism in patients with bronchial asthma. N. Engl. J. Med. 286:1125, 1972.

67. Brooks, P. M., Buchanan, W. W., Grove, M., and Downie, W. W.: Effects of enzyme induction on metabolism of prednisolone: Clinical and laboratory study. Ann. Rheum. Dis. 35:339, 1976.

68. Edwards, O. M., Courtenay-Evans, R. J., Galley, J. M., Hunter, J., and Tait, A. D.: Changes in cortisol metabolism following rifampicin therapy. Lancet 2:549, 1974.

69. Buffington, G. A., Dominguez, J. H., Piering, W. F., Hebert, L. A., Kauffman, H. M., Jr., and Lemann, J., Jr.: Interaction of rifampin and glucocorticoids. Adverse effect on renal allograft function. J.A.M.A. 236:1958, 1976.

70. Bergrem H., and Refvem, O. K.: Altered prednisolone pharmacokinetics in patients treated with rifampicin. Acta Med. Scand. 213:339, 1983.

71. Hendrickse, W., McKiernan, J., Pickup, M., and Lowe, J.: Rifampicin-induced non-responsiveness to corticosteroid treatment in nephrotic syndrome. Br. Med. J. 1:306, 1979.

72. Zürcher, R. M., Frey, B. M., and Frey, F. J.: Impact of ketoconazole on the metabolism of prednisolone. Clin. Pharmacol. Ther. 45:366, 1989.

73. Yamashita, S. K., Ludwig, E. A., Middleton, E., Jr., and Jusko, W. J.: Lack of pharmacokinetic and pharmacodynamic interactions between ketoconazole and prednisolone. Clin. Pharmacol. Ther. 49:558, 1991.

74. Uribe, M., Casian, C., Rojas, S., Sierra, J. G., and Go, V. L. W.: Decreased bioavailability of prednisone due to antacids in patients with chronic active liver disease and in healthy volunteers. Gastroenterology 80:661, 1981.

75. Gambertoglio, J. G., Romac, D. R., Yong, C.-L., Birnbaum, J., Lizak, P., and Amend, W. J. C., Jr.: Lack of effect of sucralfate on prednisone bioavailability. Am. J. Gastroenterol. 82:42, 1987.

76. Morrison, P. J., Rogers, H. J., Bradbrook, I. D., and Parsons, C.: Concurrent administration of cimetidine and enteric-coated prednisolone: Effects on plasma levels of prednisolone. Br. J. Clin. Pharmacol. 10:87, 1980.

77. Sirgo, M. A., Rocci, M. L., Ferguson, R. K., Eskelman, F. N., and Veanes, P. H.: Effects of cimetidine and ranitidine on the conversion of prednisone to prednisolone. Clin. Pharmacol. Ther. 37:534, 1985.

78. Audétat, V., and Bircher, J.: Bioavailability of prednisolone during simultaneous treatment with cholestyramine. Gastroenterology 71:1110, 1976.

79. Klinenberg, J. R., and Miller, F.: Effect of corticosteroids on blood salicylate concentration. J.A.M.A. 194:131, 1965.

80. Graham, G. G., Champion, G. D., Day, R. O., and Paull, P. D.: Patterns of plasma concentrations and urinary excretion of salicylate in rheumatoid arthritis. Clin. Pharmacol. Ther. 22:410, 1977.

81. Bardare, M., Cislaghi, G. U., Mandelli, M., and Sereni, F.: Value of monitoring plasma salicylate levels in treating juvenile rheumatoid arthritis. Arch. Dis. Child. 53:381, 1978.

82. Meyers, E. F.: Partial recovery from pancuronium neuromuscular blockade following hydrocortisone administration. Anesthesiology 46:148, 1977.

83. Laflin, M. J.: Interaction of pancuronium and corticosteroids. Anesthesiology 47:471, 1977.

84. Plotz, C. M., Knowlton, A. I., and Ragan, C.: The natural history of Cushing's syndrome. Am. J. Med. 13:597, 1952.

85. Thorn, G. W.: Clinical considerations in the use of corticosteroids. N. Engl. J. Med. 274:775, 1966.

86. Singleton, J. W., Law, D. H., Kelley, M. L., Jr., Mekhjian, H. S., and Sturdevant, R. A. L.: National cooperative Crohn's disease study: Adverse reactions to study drugs. Gastroenterology 77:870, 1979.

87. Boston Collaborative Drug Surveillance Program: Acute adverse reactions to prednisone in relation to dosage. Clin. Pharmacol. Ther. 13:694, 1972.

88. Hall, R. C. W., Popkin, M. K., Stickney, S. K., and Gardner, E. R.: Presentation of the steroid psychoses. J. Nerv. Ment. Dis. 167:229, 1979.

89. Fitzgerald, R. H., Jr.: Intrasynovial injection of steroids: Uses and abuses. Mayo Clin. Proc. 51:655, 1976.

90. Balch, H. W., Gibson, J. M. C., El-Ghobarey, A. F., Bain, L. S., and Lynch, M. P.: Repeated corticosteroid injections into knee joints. Rheumatol. Rehab. 16:137, 1977.

91. Carson, T. E., Daane, T. A., and Weinstein, R. L.: Long-term intramuscular administration of triamcinolone acetonide: Effect on the hypothalamic-pituitary-adrenal axis. Arch. Dermatol. 111:1585, 1975.

92. Munck, A., and Guyre, P. M.: Glucocorticoid physiology and homeostasis in relation to anti-inflammatory actions. In Schleimer, R. P., Claman, H. N., and Oronsky, A. (eds.): Anti-inflammatory Steroid Action: Basic and Clinical Aspects. San Diego, Academic Press, 1989, p. 30.

93. Claman, H. N.: Corticosteroids and lymphoid cells. N. Engl. J. Med. 287:388, 1972.

94. Claman, H. N.: How corticosteroids work. J. Allergy Clin. Immunol. 55:145, 1975.

95. Fauci, A. S., Dale, D. C., and Balow, J. E.: Glucocorticosteroid therapy: Mechanisms of action and clinical considerations. Ann. Intern. Med. 84:304, 1976.

96. Schreiber, A. D.: Clinical immunology of the corticosteroids. Prog. Clin. Immunol. 3:103, 1977.

97. Parrillo, J. E., and Fauci, A. S.: Mechanisms of glucocorticoid action on immune processes. Annu. Rev. Pharmacol. Toxicol. 19:179, 1979.

98. Cupps, T. R., and Fauci, A. S.: Corticosteroid-mediated immunoregulation in man. Immunol. Rev. 65:133, 1982.

99. Dale, D. C., Fauci, A. S., Guerry, D., IV, and Wolff, S. M.: Comparison of agents producing neutrophilic leukocytosis in man: Hydrocortisone, prednisone, endotoxin, and etiocholanolone. J. Clin. Invest. 56:808, 1975.

100. Bishop, C. R. Athens, J. W., Boggs, D. R., Warner, H. R., Cartwright, G. E., and Wintrobe, M. M.: Leukokinetic studies. XIII. A non-steadystate kinetic evaluation of the mechanism of cortisone-induced granulocytosis. J. Clin. Invest. 47:249, 1968.

101. Athens, J. W., Haab, O. P., Raab, S. O., Mauer, A. M., Ashenbrucker, H., Cartwright, G. E., and Wintrobe, M. M.: Leukokinetic studies. IV. The total blood, circulating and marginal granulocyte pools and the granulocyte turnover rate in normal subjects. J. Clin. Invest. 40:989, 1961.

102. Boggs, D. R., Athens, J. W., Cartwright, G. E., and Wintrobe, M. M.: The effect of adrenal glucocorticosteroids upon the cellular composition of inflammatory exudates. Am. J. Pathol. 44:763, 1964.

103. Fauci, A. S., and Dale, D. C.: The effect of in vivo hydrocortisone on subpopulations of human lymphocytes. J. Clin. Invest. 53:240, 1974.

104. Yu, D. T. Y., Clements, P. J., Paulus, H. E., Peter, J. B., Levy, J., and Barnett, E. V.: Human lymphocyte subpopulations: Effect of corticosteroids. J. Clin. Invest. 53:565, 1974.

105. Clarke, J. R., Gagnon, R. F., Gotch, F. M., Heyworth, M. R. MacLennan, I. C. M., Truelove, S. C., and Waller, C. A.: The effect of prednisolone on leucocyte function in man: A double-blind controlled study. Clin. Exp. Immunol. 28:292, 1977.

106. Cooper, D. A., Petts, V., Luckhurst, E., and Penny, R.: The effect of acute and prolonged administration of prednisolone and ACTH on lymphocyte subpopulations. Clin. Exp. Immunol. 28:467, 1977.

107. Cook, J. D., Trotter, J. L., Engel, W. K., and Sciabbarrasi, J. S.: The effects of single-dose alternate-day prednisone therapy on the immunological status of patients with neuromuscular disease. Ann. Neurol. 3:166, 1978.

108. Fauci, A. S., and Dale, D. C.: The effect of hydrocortisone on the kinetics of normal human lymphocytes. Blood 46:235, 1975.

109. Yu, D. T. Y., Clements, P. J., and Pearson, C. M.: Effect of corticosteroids on exercise-induced lymphocytosis. Clin. Exp. Immunol. 28:326, 1977.

110. Ebert, R. H., and Barclay, W. R.: Changes in connective tissue reaction induced by cortisone. Ann. Intern. Med. 37:506, 1952.

111. Zweifach, B. W., Shorr, E., and Black, M. M.: The influence of the adrenal cortex on behavior of terminal vascular bed. Ann. N. Y. Acad. Sci. 56:626, 1953.

112. MacGregor, R. R., Spagnuolo, P. J., and Lentnek, A. L.: Inhibition of granulocyte adherence by ethanol, prednisone, and aspirin, measured with an assay system. N. Engl. J. Med. 291:642, 1974.

113. MacGregor, R. R.: The effect of anti-inflammatory agents and inflammation on granulocyte adherence: Evidence for regulation by plasma factors. Am. J. Med. 61:597, 1976.

114. MacGregor, R. R.: Granulocyte adherence changes induced by hemodialysis, endotoxin, epinephrine, and glucocorticoids. Ann. Intern. Med. 86:35, 1977.

115. Bovornkitti, S., Kangsadal, P., Sathirapat, P., and Oonsombatti, P.: Reversion and reconversion rate of tuberculin skin reactions in correlation with the use of prednisone. Dis. Chest 38:51, 1960.

116. Cummings, M. M., and Hudgins, P. C.: The influence of cortisone on the passive transfer of tuberculin hypersensitivity in the guinea pig. J. Immunol. 69:331, 1952.

117. Seebohm, P. M., Tremaine, M. M., and Jeter, W. S.: The effect of cortisone and adrenocorticotropic hormone on passively transferred delayed hypersensitivity to 2, 4-dinitrochlorobenzene in guinea pigs. J. Immunol. 73:44, 1954.

118. Weston, W. L., Mandel, M. J., Yeckley, J. A., Krueger, G. G., and Claman, H. N.: Mechanism of cortisol inhibition of adoptive transfer of tuberculin sensitivity. J. Lab. Clin. Med. 82:366, 1973.

119. Guyre, P. M., and Munck, A.: Glucocorticoid actions on monocytes and macrophages. In Schleimer, R. P., Claman, H. N., and Oronsky, A. (eds.): Anti-inflammatory Steroid Action: Basic and Clinical Aspects. San Diego, Academic Press, 1989, p. 199.

120. Balow, J. E., and Rosenthal, A. S.: Glucocorticoid suppression of macrophage migration inhibitory factor. J. Exp. Med. 137:1031, 1973.

121. Rinehart, J. J., Balcerzak, S. P., Sagone, A. L., and LoBuglio, A. F.: Effects of corticosteroids on human monocyte function. J. Clin. Invest. 54:1337, 1974.

122. Rinehart, J. J., Sagone, A. L., Balcerzak, S. P., Ackerman, G. A., and LoBuglio, A. F.: Effects of corticosteroid therapy on human monocyte function. N. Engl. J. Med. 292:236, 1975.

123. Handin, R. I., and Stossel, T. P.: Effect of corticosteroid therapy on the phagocytosis of antibody-coated platelets by human leukocytes. Blood 51:771, 1978.

124. Frank, M. M., Schreiber, A. D., Atkinson, J. P., and Jaffe, C. J.: Pathophysiology of immune hemolytic anemia. Ann. Intern. Med. 87:210, 1977.

125. Lewis, G. P., and Piper, P. J.: Inhibition of release of prostaglandins as an explanation of some of the actions of anti-inflammatory corticosteroids. Nature 254:308, 1975.

126. Kantrowitz, F., Robinson, D. R., McGuire, M. B., and Levine, L.: Corticosteroids inhibit prostaglandin production by rheumatoid synovia. Nature 258:737, 1975.

127. Tashjian, A. H., Jr., Voelkel, E. F., McDonough, J., and Levine L.: Hydrocortisone inhibits prostaglandin production by mouse fibrosarcoma cells. Nature 258:739, 1975.

128. Gryglewski, R. J.: Steroid hormones, anti-inflammatory steroids and prostaglandins. Pharmacol. Res. Commun. 8:337, 1976.

129. Hong, S.-C. L., and Levine, L.: Inhibition of arachidonic acid release from cells as the biochemical action of anti-inflammatory corticosteroids. Proc. Natl. Acad. Sci. U. S. A. 73:1730, 1976.

130. Robinson, D. R., Tashjian, A. H., Jr., and Levine, L.: Prostaglandin-stimulated bone resorption by rheumatoid synovia: A possible mechanism for bone destruction in rheumatoid arthritis. J. Clin. Invest. 56:1181, 1975.

131. Samuelsson, B.: Leukotrienes: Mediators of immediate hypersensitivity reactions and inflammation. Science 220:568, 1983.

132. Snyder, D. S., and Unanue, E. R.: Corticosteroids inhibit murine macrophage Ia expression and interleukin-1 production. J. Immunol. 129:1803, 1982.

133. Morris, H. G.: Mechanisms of glucocorticoid action in pulmonary disease. Chest 88:133S, 1985.

134. Janoski, A. H., Shaver, J. C., Christy, N. P., and Rosner, W.: On the pharmacologic actions of 21-carbon hormonal steroids (glucocorticoids) of the adrenal cortex in mammals. In Deane, H. W., and Rubin, B. L. (eds.): Handbuch der Experimentellen Pharmakologie. Vol. XIV, Part 3 (The Adrenocortical Hormones). Berlin, Springer-Verlag, 1968, p. 256.

135. Christy, N. P.: Iatrogenic Cushing's syndrome. In Christy, N. P. (ed.): The Human Adrenal Cortex. New York, Harper & Row, 1971, p. 395.

136. Ragan, C.: Corticotropin, cortisone and related steroids in clinical medicine: Practical considerations. Bull. N.Y. Acad. Med. 29:355, 1953.

137. Seely, E. W., Conlin, P. R., Brent, G. A., and Dluhy, R. G.: Adrenocorticotropin stimulation of aldosterone: Prolonged continuous versus pulsatile infusion. J. Clin. Endocrinol. Metab. 69:1028, 1989.

138. Intracranial hypertension and steroids. Lancet 2:1052, 1964.

139. Walker, A. E., and Adamkiewicz, J. J.: Pseudotumor cerebri associated with prolonged corticosteroid therapy. J.A.M.A. 188:779, 1964.

140. David, D. S., and Berkowitz, J. S.: Ocular effects of topical and systemic corticosteroids. Lancet 2:149, 1969.

141. Lubkin, V. L.: Steroid cataract: a review and a conclusion. J. Asthma Res. 14:55, 1977.

142. Pavlin, C. R., DeVeber, G. A., Cook, G. T., and Chisholm, L. D. J.: Ocular complications in renal transplant recipients. Can. Med. Assoc. J. 117:360, 1977.

143. Heimann, W. G., and Freiberger, R. H.: Avascular necrosis of the femoral and humeral heads after high-dosage corticosteroid therapy. N. Engl. J. Med. 263:672, 1960.

144. Velayos, E. E., Leidholt, J. D., Smyth, C. J., and Priest, R.: Arthropathy associated with steroid therapy. Ann. Intern. Med. 64:759, 1966.

145. Harrington, K. D., Murray, W. R., Kountz, S. L., and Belzer, F. O.: Avascular necrosis of bone after renal transplantation. J. Bone Joint Surg. 53A:203, 1971.

146. Fisher, D. E., and Bickel, W. H.: Corticosteroid-induced aseptic necrosis: A clinical study of seventy-seven patients. J. Bone Joint Surg. 53A:859, 1971.

147. Park, W. M.: Spontaneous and drug-induced aseptic necrosis. In Davidson, J. K. (ed.): Aseptic Necrosis of Bone. Amsterdam, Excerpta Medica, 1976, P. 213.

148. Cruess, R. L.: Cortisone-induced avascular necrosis of the femoral head. J. Bone Joint Surg. 59B:308, 1977.

149. Abeles, M., Urman, J. D., and Rothfield, N. F.: Aseptic necrosis of bone in systemic lupus erythematosus. Arch. Intern. Med. 138:750, 1978.

150. Fenster, L. F.: The ulcerogenic potential of glucocorticoids and possible prophylactic measures. In Azarnoff, D. L. (ed.): Steroid Therapy. Philadelphia, W. B. Saunders Company, 1975, p. 42.

151. Conn, H. O., and Blitzer, B. L.: Nonassociation of adrenocorticosteroid therapy and peptic ulcer. N. Engl. J. Med. 294:473, 1976.

152. Langman, M. J. S., and Cooke, A. R.: Gastric and duodenal ulcer and their associated diseases. Lancet 1:680, 1976.

153. Jick, H., and Porter, J.: Drug-induced gastrointestinal bleeding. Lancet 2:87, 1978.

154. Messer, J., Reitman, D., Sacks, H. S., Smith, H., Jr., and Chalmers, T. C.: Association of adrenocorticosteroid therapy and peptic-ulcer disease. N. Engl. J. Med. 309:21, 1983.

155. Spiro, H. M.: Is the steroid ulcer a myth? N. Engl. J. Med. 309:45, 1983.

156. Conn, H. O., and Poynard, T.: Adrenocorticosteroid administration and peptic ulcer: A critical analysis. J. Chronic Dis. 38:457, 1985.

157. Schatz, M., Patterson, R., Kloner, R., and Falk, J.: The prevalence of tuberculosis and positive tuberculin skin tests in a steroid-treated asthmatic population. Ann. Intern. Med. 84:261, 1976.

158. Bergrem, H., Jervell, J., and Flatmark, A.: Prednisolone pharmacokinetics in cushingoid and non-cushingoid kidney transplant patients. Kidney Int. 27:459, 1985.

159. Frey, F. J., Amend, W. J. C., Jr., Lozada, F., Frey, B. M., and Benet, L. Z.: Endogenous hydrocortisone, a possible factor contributing to the genesis of cushingoid habitus in patients on prednisone. J. Clin. Endocrinol. Metab. 53:1076, 1981.

160. Becker, B.: Intraocular pressure response to topical corticosteroids. Invest. Ophthalmol. 4:198, 1965.

161. Bigger, J. F., Palmberg, P. F., and Becker, B.: Increased cellular sensitivity to glucocorticoids in primary open angle glaucoma. Invest. Ophthalmol. 11:832, 1972.

162. Becker, B., Podos, S. M., Asseff, C. F., and Cooper, D. G.: Plasma cortisol suppression in glaucoma. Am. J. Ophthalmol. 75:73, 1973.

163. Becker, B., Shin, D. H., Palmberg, P. F., and Waltman, S. R.: HLA antigens and corticosteroid response. Science 194:1427, 1976.

164. Good, T. A., Benton, J. W., and Kelley, V. C.: Symptomatology resulting from withdrawal of steroid hormone therapy. Arthritis Rheum. 2:299, 1959.

165. Amatruda, T. T., Jr., Hollingsworth, D. R., D'Esopo, N. D., Upton, G. V., and Bondy, P. K.: A study of the mechanism of the steroid withdrawal syndrome: Evidence for integrity of the hypothalamic-pituitary-adrenal system. J. Clin. Endocrinol. Metab. 20:339, 1960.

166. Amatruda, T. T., Jr., Hurst, M. M., and D'Esopo, N. D.: Certain endocrine and metabolic facets of the steroid withdrawal syndrome. J. Clin. Endocrinol. Metab. 25:1207, 1965.

167. Dickstein, G., Shechner, C., Nicholson, W. E., Rosner, I., Shen-Orr, Z., Adawi, F., and Lahav, M.: Adrenocorticotropin stimulation test: Effects of basal cortisol level, time of day, and suggested new sensitive low-dose test. J. Clin. Endocrinol. Metab. 72:773, 1991.

168. Paris, J.: Pituitary-adrenal suppression after protracted administration of adrenal cortical hormones. Proc. Mayo Clin. 36:305, 1961.

169. Salassa, R. M., Bennett, W. A., Keating, F. R., and Sprague, R. G.: Postoperative adrenal cortical insufficiency: Occurrence in patients previously treated with cortisone. J.A.M.A. 152:1509, 1953.

170. Streck, W. F., and Lockwood, D. H.: Pituitary adrenal recovery following short-term suppression with corticosteroids. Am. J. Med. 66:910, 1979.

171. Zora, J. A., Zimmerman, D., Carey, T. L., O'Connell, E. J., and Yunginger, J. W.: Hypothalamic-pituitary-adrenal axis suppression after short-term, high-dose glucocorticoid therapy in children with asthma. J. Allergy Clin. Immunol. 77:9, 1986.

172. Christy, N. P., Wallace, E. Z., and Jailer, J. W.: Comparative effects of prednisone and of cortisone in suppressing the response of the adrenal cortex to exogenous adrenocorticotropin. J. Clin. Endocrinol. Metab. 16:1059, 1956.

173. May, M. E., and Carey, R. M.: Rapid adrenocorticotropic hormone test in practice: Retrospective review. Am. J. Med. 79:679, 1985.

174. Jasani, M. K., Freeman, P. A., Boyle, J. A., Reid, A. M., Diver, M. J.,

and Buchanan, W. W.: Studies of the rise in plasma 11-hydroxycorticosteroids (11-OHCS) in corticosteroid-treated patients with rheumatoid arthritis during surgery: Correlations with the functional integrity of the hypothalamic-pituitary-adrenal axis. Q. J. Med. 37:407, 1968.

175. Kehlet, H., and Binder, C.: Value of an ACTH test in assessing hypothalamic-pituitary-adrenocortical function in glucocorticoid-treated patients. Br. Med. J. 2:147, 1973.

176. Marks, L. J., Donovan, M. J., Duncan, F. J., and Karger, R.: Adrenocortical response to surgical operations in patients treated with corticosteroids or corticotropin prior to surgery. J. Clin. Endocrinol. Metab. 19:1458, 1959.

177. Sampson, P. A., Winstone, N. F., and Brooke, B. N.: Adrenal function in surgical patients after steroid therapy. Lancet 2:322, 1962.

178. Danowski, T. S., Bonessi, J. V., Sabeh, G., Sutton, R. D., Webster, M. W., Jr., and Sarver, M. E.: Probabilities of pituitary-adrenal responsiveness after steroid therapy. Ann. Intern. Med. 61:11, 1964.

179. Nichols, T., Nugent, C. A., and Tyler, F. H.: Diurnal variation in suppression of adrenal function by glucocorticoids. J. Clin. Endocrinol. Metab. 25:343, 1965.

180. Chamberlain, M. A., and Keenan, J.: The effect of low doses of prednisolone compared with placebo on function and on the hypothalamic pituitary adrenal axis in patients with rheumatoid arthritis. Rheumatol. Rehab. 15:17, 1976.

181. Carter, M. E., and James, V. H. T.: Comparison of effects of corticotrophin and corticosteroids on pituitary-adrenal function. Ann. Rheum. Dis. 30:91, 1971.

182. Daly, J. R., and Glass, D.: Corticosteroid and growth hormone response to hypoglycaemia in patients on long-term treatment with corticotrophin. Lancet 1:476, 1971.

183. Daly, J. R., Fletcher, M. R., Glass, D., Chambers, D. J., Bitensky, L., and Chayen, J.: Comparison of effects of long-term corticotrophin and corticosteroid treatment on responses of plasma growth hormone, ACTH, and corticosteroid to hypoglycaemia. Br. Med. J. 2:521, 1974.

184. Graber, A. L., Ney, R. L., Nicholson, W. E., Island, D. P., and Liddle, G. W.: Natural history of pituitary-adrenal recovery following long-term suppression with corticosteroids. J. Clin. Endocrinol. Metab. 25:11, 1965.

185. Livanou, T., Ferriman, D., and James, V. H. T.: Recovery of hypothalamo-pituitary-adrenal function after corticosteroid therapy. Lancet 2:856, 1967.

186. Webb, J., and Clark, T. J. H.: Recovery of plasma corticotrophin and cortisol levels after a three-week course of prednisolone. Thorax 36:22, 1981.

187. Spitzer, S. A., Kaufman, H., Koplovitz, A., Topilsky, M., and Blum, I.: Beclomethasone dipropionate and chronic asthma: The effect of long-term aerosol administration on the hypothalamic-pituitary-adrenal axis after substitution for oral therapy with corticosteroids. Chest 70:38, 1976.

188. Westerhof, L., Van Ditmars, M. J., DerKinderen, P. J., Thijssen, J. H. H., and Schwarz, F.: Recovery of adrenocortical function during long-term treatment with corticosteroids. Br. Med. J. 4:534, 1970.

189. Westerhof, L., Van Ditmars, M. J., DerKinderen, P. J., Thijssen, J. H. H., and Schwarz, F.: Recovery of adrenocortical function during long-term treatment with corticosteroids. Br. Med. J. 2:195, 1972.

190. Kyle, L. H., Meyer, R. J., and Canary, J. J.: Mechanism of adrenal atrophy in Cushing's syndrome due to adrenal tumor. N. Engl. J. Med. 257:57, 1957.

191. Morris, H. G., and Jorgensen, J. R.: Recovery of endogenous pituitary-adrenal function in corticosteroid-treated children. J. Pediatr. 79:480, 1971.

192. Young, I. I., DeFilippis, V., Meyer, F. L., and Wolfson, W. Q.: Maintenance of adrenal cortical responsiveness during prolonged corticoid therapy. Arch. Intern. Med. 100:1, 1957.

193. Fleischer, N., Abe, K., Liddle, G. W., Orth, D. N., and Nicholson, W. E.: ACTH antibodies in patients receiving depot porcine ACTH to hasten recovery from pituitary-adrenal suppression. J. Clin. Invest. 46:196, 1967.

194. Carter, M. E., and James, V. H. T.: An attempt at combining corticotrophin with long-term corticosteroid therapy: With a view to preserving hypothalamic-pituitary-adrenal function. Ann. Rheum. Dis. 29:409, 1970.

195. Carter, M. E., and James, V. H. T.: Effect of alternate-day, single-dose corticosteroid therapy on pituitary-adrenal function. Ann. Rheum. Dis. 31:379, 1972.

196. Portner, M. M., Thayer, K. H., Harter, J. G., Rayyis, S., Liang, T. C., and Kent, J. R.: Successful initiation of alternate-day prednisone in chronic steroid-dependent asthmatic patients. J. Allergy Clin. Immunol. 49:16, 1972.

197. Morris, H. G., Neuman, I., and Ellis, E. F.: Plasma steroid concentrations during alternate-day treatment with prednisone. J. Allergy Clin. Immunol. 54: 350, 1974.

198. Haugen, H. N., Reddy, W. J., and Harter, J. G.: Intermittent steroid therapy in bronchial asthma. Nord. Med. 63:15, 1960.

199. Reichling, G. H., and Kligman, A. M.: Alternate-day corticosteroid therapy. Arch. Dermatol. 83:980, 1961.

200. Harter, J. G., Reddy, W. J., and Thorn, G. W.: Studies on an intermittent corticosteroid dosage regimen. N. Engl. J. Med. 269:591, 1963.

201. Jacobson, M. E.: The rationale of alternate-day corticosteroid therapy. Postgrad. Med. 49:181, 1971.

202. Soyka, L. F.: Alternate-day corticosteroid therapy. Adv. Pediatr. 19:47, 1972.

203. Frey, F. J., Rüegsegger, M. K., and Frey, B. M.: The dose-dependent systemic availability of prednisone: One reason for the reduced biological effect of alternate-day prednisone. Br. J. Clin. Pharmacol. 21:183, 1986.

204. Klein, R. G., Arnaud, S. B., Gallagher, J. C., DeLuca, H. F., and Riggs, B. L.: Intestinal calcium absorption in exogenous hypercortisonism: Role of 25-hydroxyvitamin D and corticosteroid dose. J. Clin. Invest. 60:253, 1977.

205. Norris, D. A., Fine, R., Weston, W. L., and Spector, S.: Monocyte cellular function in asthmatic patients on alternate-day steroid therapy. J. Allergy Clin. Immunol. 61:255, 1978.

206. Curtis, J. J., Galla, J. H., Woodford, S. Y., Lucas, B. A., and Luke, R. G.: Effect of alternate-day prednisone on plasma lipids in renal transplant recipients. Kidney Int. 22:42, 1982.

207. Chesney, R. W., Mazess, R. B., Rose, P., and Jax, D. K.: Effect of prednisone on growth and bone mineral content in childhood glomerular disease. Am. J. Dis. Child. 132:768, 1978.

208. Gluck, O. S., Murphy, W. A., Hahn, T. J., and Hahn, B.: Bone loss in adults receiving alternate-day glucocorticoid therapy: A comparison with daily therapy. Arthritis Rheum. 24:892, 1981.

209. Ruegsegger, P., Medici, T. C., and Anliker, M.: Corticosteroid-induced bone loss: A longitudinal study of alternate-day therapy in patients with bronchial asthma using quantitative computed tomography. Eur. J. Clin. Pharmacol. 25:615, 1983.

210. Kass, E. H., and Finland, M.: Adrenocortical hormones in infection and immunity. Annu. Rev. Microbiol. 7:361, 1953.

211. Thomas, L.: Cortisone and infection. Ann. N. Y. Acad. Sci. 56:799, 1953.

212. Dale, D. C., and Petersdorf, R. G.: Corticosteroids and infectious diseases. In Azarnoff, D. L. (ed.): Steroid Therapy. Philadelphia, W. B. Saunders Company, 1975, p. 209.

213. Schürmeyer, T. H., Tsokos, G. C., Avgerinos, P. C., Balow, J. E., D'Agata, R., Loriaux, D. L., and Chrousos, G. P.: Pituitary-adrenal responsiveness to corticotropin-releasing hormone in patients receiving chronic, alternate-day glucocorticoid therapy. J. Clin. Endocrinol. Metab. 61:22, 1985.

214. Hunder, G. G., Sheps, S. G., Allen, G. L., and Joyce, J. W.: Daily and alternate-day corticosteroid regimens in treatment of giant cell arteritis: Comparison in a prospective study. Ann. Intern. Med. 82:613, 1975.

215. Abruzzo, J. L.: Alternate-day prednisone therapy. Ann. Intern. Med. 82:714, 1975.

216. Bengtsson, B.-A., and Malmvall, B.-E.: An alternate-day corticosteroid regimen in maintenance therapy of giant cell arteritis. Acta Med. Scand. 209:347, 1981.

217. Collaborative Study of the Adult Idiopathic Nephrotic Syndrome: A controlled study of short-term prednisone treatment in adults with membranous nephropathy. N. Engl. J. Med. 301:1301, 1979.

218. McDonald, F. D., Horensten, M. L., Mayor, G. B., Turcotte, J. G., Selezinka, W., and Schork, M. A.: Effect of alternate-day steroids on renal transplant function: A controlled study. Nephron 17:415, 1976.

219. Curtis, J. J., Galla, J. H., Woodford, S. Y., Saykaly, R. J., and Luke, R. G.: Comparison of daily and alternate-day prednisone during chronic maintenance therapy: A controlled crossover study. Am. J. Kidney Dis. 1:166, 1981.

220. Ansell, B. M., and Bywaters, E. G. L.: Alternate-day corticosteroid therapy in juvenile chronic polyarthritis. J. Rheumatol. 1:176, 1974.

221. Reed, W. P., Lucas, Z. J., and Cohn, R.: Alternate-day prednisone therapy after renal transplantation. Lancet 1:747, 1970.

222. Easton, J. G., Busser, R. J., and Heimlich, E. M.: Effect of alternate-day steroid administration on adrenal function in allergic children. J. Allergy Clin. Immunol. 48:355, 1971.

223. Jasani, M. K., Boyle, J. A., Dick, W. C., Williamson, J., Taylor, A. K., and Buchanan, W. W.: Corticosteroid-induced hypothalamo-pituitary-adrenal axis suppression: Prospective study using two regimens of corticosteroid therapy. Ann. Rheum. Dis. 27:352, 1968.

224. Rabhan, N. B.: Pituitary-adrenal suppression and Cushing's syndrome after intermittent dexamethasone therapy. Ann. Intern. Med. 69:1141, 1968.

225. Potter, D. E., Holliday, M. A., Wilson, C. J., Salvatierra, O., Jr., and Belzer, F. O.: Alternate-day steroids in children after renal transplantation. Transplant. Proc. 7:79, 1975.

226. Fauci, A. S.: Alternate-day corticosteroid therapy. Am. J. Med. 64:729, 1978.

227. Dubois, E. L., and Adler, D. C.: Single-daily dose oral administration of corticosteroids in rheumatic disorders: An analysis of its advantages, efficacy and side effects. Curr. Ther. Res. 5:43, 1963.

228. Nugent, C. A., Ward, J., MacDiarmid, W. D., McCall, J. C., Baukol, J., and Tyler, F. H.: Glucocorticoid toxicity: Single contrasted with divided daily doses of prednisolone. J. Chronic Dis. 18:323, 1965.

229. Myles, A. B., Schiller, L. G. F., Glass, D., and Daly, J. R.: Single daily dose corticosteroid treatment. Ann. Rheum. Dis. 35:73, 1976.

230. Powell-Tuck, J., Bown, R. L., and Lennard-Jones, J. E.: A comparison of oral prednisone given as single or multiple daily doses for active proctocolitis. Br. J. Gastroenterol. 13:833, 1978.

231. DiRaimondo, V. C., and Forsham, P. H.: Pharmacophysiologic principles in the use of corticoids and adrenocorticotropin. Metabolism 7:5, 1958.

232. Myles, A. B., Bacon, P. A., and Daly, J. R.: Single daily dose corticosteroid treatment: Effect on adrenal function and therapeutic efficacy in various diseases. Ann. Rheum. Dis. 30:149, 1971.

233. Allander, E.: ACTH or corticosteroids? A critical review of results and possibilities in the treatment of severe chronic disease. Acta Rheumatol. Scand. 15:277, 1969.

234. Kaplan, H. P., Portnoy, B., Binder, H. J., Amatruda, T., and Spiro, H.: A controlled evaluation of intravenous adrenocorticotropic hormone and hydrocortisone in the treatment of acute colitis. Gastroenterology 69:91, 1975.

235. Savage, O., Copeman, W. S. C., Chapman, L., Wells, M. V., and Treadwell, B. L. J.: Pituitary and adrenal hormones in rheumatoid arthritis. Lancet 1:232, 1962.

Chapter 49

Anthony S. Fauci
K. Randall Young, Jr.

Immunoregulatory Agents

Immunoregulation can be broadly defined as the complex process whereby immunologic reactivity, either cellular or humoral, is constantly modulated to result in the net expression of an appropriate or, in certain circumstances, inappropriate immune response.[1] Intensive interest and investigation in immunology, which have led to certain rather striking advances in our understanding of the complexities of immune function and regulation in animal models as well as in humans, together with the observations that many rheumatic diseases are at least associated with aberrancies of immune function including immunoregulation[1-5] form the intellectual basis for the use of immunoregulatory agents in the treatment of certain rheumatic diseases. It should be pointed out, however, that the use of cytotoxic and other immunoregulatory agents in these diseases antedated the most recent advances in our understanding of many of the subtle complexities of immune regulation. This is particularly true of the use of glucocorticoids and cytotoxic agents in diseases whose clinicopathologic manifestations were strongly suggestive of aberrant inflammatory or immune-mediated phenomena. Because the use of these agents generally resulted in suppression of inflammation and immune function, it is not surprising that they have been extensively used in certain rheumatic, connective tissue, and autoimmune diseases.[6-10]

Unfortunately, even though advances in our understanding of immune function and regulation have allowed a greater intellectual understanding of the potential mechanisms of aberrant immune function in the diseases in question, the extraordinary complexity of the immune system, with its various inductive, regulatory, effector, and feedback mechanisms, has made it clear to clinical investigators that perturbation of the system by agents used for therapeutic purposes may have multifaceted effects on the system, some of which might be unpredictable, if not unrecognized. This very complexity of the system in the face of the relatively crude and usually nonspecific modulation effected by most of the therapeutic agents in question may result in only a minor or temporary dampening of the expression of the disease process. On the other hand, the adverse effects associated with perturbation of the immune system in this manner may place the resultant ther-

apeutic efficacy beyond the limits of the price that one is willing to pay for such an effect. Certain immunoregulatory agents have been used and are being used inappropriately in diseases whose severity or projected clinical course clearly does not warrant such an aggressive approach. Nonetheless, despite these general caveats, certain cytotoxic and other immunoregulatory agents have been successfully and appropriately employed in the treatment of a number of rheumatic diseases and in certain situations with rather impressive results.[6, 8-10]

It is the aim of this chapter to consider some of the real and potential mechanisms whereby one can feasibly and successfully modify the expression of aberrant inflammatory and immune responses. This chapter also discusses the mechanisms of action of the various categories of immunoregulatory agents as well as their proved and potential usefulness in the treatment of rheumatic diseases to appreciate better the positive and negative aspects of such a therapeutic approach.

IMMUNE SYSTEM AND ITS REGULATION

A number of models of the immune system and its regulation have been proposed, and each almost invariably has the common denominator of a cellular and humoral network of immune reactivity reflected by different cell types. The dual limbs of the immune response hypothesized years ago[11-14] and now clearly substantiated are the thymus-derived (T) lymphocyte limb and the bone marrow–derived or bursa-equivalent (B) lymphocyte limb, both of which derive from a common stem cell. Other cell types, such as the monocyte-macrophage, play a major role in the inductive, regulatory, and effector phases of the immune response.[15]

A somewhat simplified scheme of the immune system is illustrated in Figure 49–1. Despite its inherent simplification, this figure illustrates the manifold complexity and multiple interrelationships among various immune cells. As has been previously and extensively described, the expression of immune function can be conveniently looked on as a series of phases. Both T and B lymphocytes mediate a number of critical immune functions, and each of these cell types, when given the appropriate signal, passes through phases, from activation or induction through proliferation, differentiation, and ultimately effector

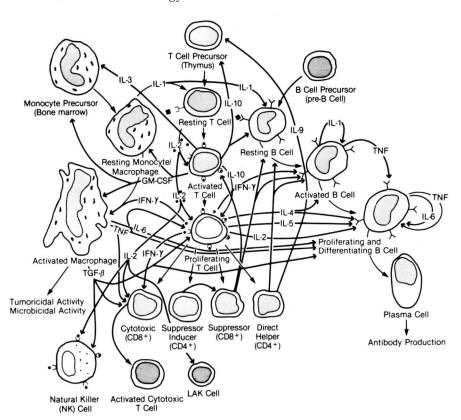

Figure 49–1. Schematic diagram of the human immunoregulatory network. IL, Interleukin; IFN, interferon; LAK, lymphokine-activated killer cell; TGF-β, transforming growth factor-β; TNF, tumor necrosis factor; GM-CSF, granulocyte-macrophage colony-stimulating factor. See text for explanation.

function.[3, 5] The effector function that is expressed may be at the end point of a response, such as secretion of antibody by a differentiated B lymphocyte or plasma cell, or it might serve a regulatory function that modulates other end-stage functions, as is seen with inducer or suppressor T lymphocytes, which modulate the function of B lymphocytes, T lymphocytes, other lymphoid cells, or even certain nonlymphoid cell types. Briefly, in addition to induction and suppression, T lymphocytes mediate a number of other important immune functions, such as specific cell-mediated cytotoxicity, certain types of graft rejection, graft-versus-host phenomena, delayed-type hypersensitivity, and the production and release of a broad range of soluble mediators termed *lymphokines*, which have profound effects on virtually all phases of the immune response. These lymphokines include interleukin 2 (IL-2), interferon gamma (INF-γ), and growth and differentiation factors for B lymphocytes.

On the other hand, B lymphocytes subserve a much more uniform function. They are the precursors of antibody-forming cells, and when appropriately stimulated, they proliferate and differentiate into cells that secrete antibody of the various classes and subclasses. Natural killer (NK) cells are lymphoid cells. They are neither of B lymphocyte nor of T lymphocyte lineage, although they share some, but not all, phenotypic characteristics of T lymphocytes.[16] These cells are believed to be involved in immune

surveillance against neoplastically transformed cells as well as in the elimination of virus-infected target cells.[17]

The monocyte-macrophage system, which is represented by monocytes in the peripheral blood and by macrophages in various tissues, plays a major role in the expression of immune reactivity by mediating a number of important functions, such as the presentation of antigen to lymphocytes and the secretion of factors such as interleukin 1 (IL-1) that are involved in the activation of lymphocytes. In addition, they directly mediate certain effector functions, such as the destruction of antibody-coated bacteria, tumor cells, or even normal cells such as hematologic elements in certain types of autoimmune cytopenias.[15, 18] Furthermore, activated macrophages can directly eliminate various cell types even in the absence of antibody.

Finally, nonlymphoid cells such as neutrophils, eosinophils, and basophils play a major role in the inflammation that results from certain immune-mediated reactions and as such must be considered in the scheme of immune function despite their not being classically viewed as part of the immune system.

The net expression of immune function, be it a specific or nonspecific effector function, is the result of a balance between positive and negative influences mediated by the inducer or suppressor populations of cells alluded to previously.[1, 3, 5] They may exert their influence either directly or via the release of soluble immunoregulatory molecules. In addition to the classic cellular regulation of immune reactivity, the idiotypic network has been proposed as a potentially important mechanism of immunoregulation. Elaborate and complex schemes have been proposed for the mechanisms of such immunoregulation,[19] with secreted idiotype and anti-idiotype antibodies as well as idiotype-bearing and anti-idiotype–bearing cells having been demonstrated as playing a major role in the regulation of immune function in the murine system.[20] The demonstration of regulation of human immune function by idiotype–anti-idiotype reactions has been reported[21] and awaits further delineation before its role in the regulation of normal and abnormal lymphocyte physiology can be appreciated fully. In this regard, evidence suggests that the idiotype network may play a role in the regulation of autoimmune states such as systemic lupus erythematosus (SLE).[22]

ABERRANCIES OF IMMUNE REACTIVITY

The established and potential mechanisms of disease activity in the broad range of rheumatic diseases are discussed in the individual chapters dealing with these disorders. If one considers Figure 49–1 and the preceding discussion, however, it is clear that there are a number of potential mechanisms for the expression of aberrant immune reactivity related to the occurrence of even slight perturbations of the delicate balance in the cellular or humoral immunoregulatory network. This may take the form of a selective deficiency in suppressor cell function or an abnormal heightening of inducer cell activity. In addition to imbalances in immunoregulation, one can have primary hyper-reactivity of certain effector functions such as B lymphocyte reactivity.[1] Under these circumstances, it is conceivable that even a normally functioning helper or suppressor cell network might not successfully dampen the aberrant B lymphocyte hyper-reactivity. Even more likely, there may be a combination of hyperactive effector cell function such as hyper-reactivity at the B lymphocyte level together with abnormalities of immunoregulatory T lymphocyte function. In fact, this is precisely the situation that has been noted in SLE. It is still disputed whether the B lymphocyte hyper-reactivity is a primary state independent of the deficiency of suppressor T lymphocyte function, whether the B lymphocyte hyper-reactivity is secondary to the suppressor cell defect, or whether the abnormalities of immune reactivity actually result from a combination of both of these phenomena together with a number of other recognized as well as ill-defined factors.[1]

In this regard, the net expression of immune function in most of the rheumatic diseases appears to be one of aberrant hyper-reactivity. As such, we generally distinguish these disorders from immunodeficiency diseases in which the net expression of immune function is usually that of hyporeactivity. Given the balance between positive and negative influences in the immune network, however, one can easily appreciate that a deficiency of immune function such as suppressor cell activity (hence strictly speaking an immunodeficiency state) can actually result in hyperactive effector immune function.[1, 23] This point is not trivial and has important implications in appreciating the basis of certain of the therapeutic strategies that are described subsequently. Thus, although we commonly refer to the therapeutic strategy of immunosuppression for diseases of inflammation or immunologic hyper-reactivity, we would more correctly think in terms of therapeutic immunoregulation either by dampening hyperactive responses or by directly or indirectly enhancing defective negative immunoregulatory influences.

POTENTIAL AREAS OF MODIFICATION OF IMMUNE RESPONSES BY THERAPEUTIC AGENTS

Suppression

Abnormally hyperactive immune responses at either the T or B lymphocyte level can be theoretically as well as practically eliminated or at least dampened by nonspecifically suppressing the entire immune system. Clearly, sufficient amounts of cytotoxic agents, irradiation, antilymphocyte sera, and other immunosuppressive agents can be administered to eliminate virtually any immune response. These therapeutic modalities are truly nonspecific in that they do not selectively eliminate abnormally active lymphoid cells, nor do they spare normal lymphoid cells. Thus, although the desired effect can ultimately be obtained, the inevitable toxic side effects render such an approach nonfeasible in the treatment of nonneoplastic diseases. Within the realm of nonspecific suppression of immune function, therapeutic strategies are employed that strike a balance between the desired effect of suppression of aberrant immune reactivity and maintenance of sufficient immune function as well as phagocyte, particularly neutrophil, cell number and function to maintain the integrity of the host defense system as well as the level of inflammatory and immune function required to maintain immunologic homeostasis.

This approach usually takes the form of administration of cytotoxic drugs in dosage regimens that, although still nonspecific, would relatively more selectively dampen the ongoing aberrant immune response. An example is the use of chronically administered cyclophosphamide in doses of 2 mg per kg per day in certain of the severe systemic vasculitis syndromes.[24, 25] These disorders are characterized by hyper-reactivity of B lymphocyte responses with hypergammaglobulinemia, immune complex deposition, and spontaneous secretion of polyclonal immunoglobulin (Ig) by activated B lymphocytes.[26] Administration of cyclophosphamide in the above-mentioned regimen results in a selective suppression of B lymphocyte responses despite the fact that a total lymphocytopenia inevitably results from such long-term therapy.[27] Thus, although all B lymphocyte function is suppressed, rendering such an approach nonspecific, there appears to be a selective suppression of the hyperactive B lymphocyte function more than other lymphoid cell function.[27]

Other nonspecific but less globally immunosuppressive modalities include thoracic duct drainage, plasmapheresis, leukopheresis, the use of antilymphocyte globulin or monoclonal antibodies directed against lymphocyte subsets, irradiation of groups of regional lymph nodes, and the use of agents such as cyclosporin A, which relatively selectively suppresses T lymphocyte function while sparing other lymphoid and nonlymphoid cells. Each of these approaches represents an attempt within the realm of a fundamentally nonspecific immunosuppressive regimen to render the approach somewhat more selective.

Despite these attempts at introducing varying degrees of selectivity into nonspecific immunosuppressive regimens, the extraordinary complexity of the immune system, with its multiple levels of regulation and feedback mechanisms, adds a considerable degree of uncertainty to such approaches. Nonetheless, despite the limitations of such an approach, nonspecific immunosuppression has resulted in favorable therapeutic results in a number of rheumatic diseases. Given the state of the art at present, however, realization of these limitations is essential for proper application of such regimens as well as for providing an impetus to continuing the search for more specific and less toxic forms of immunosuppression.

Enhancement

As already mentioned, even disorders that express a net hyperactive immune response may have components that are hypoactive. In this regard, immune enhancement should theoretically be beneficial, provided that the defective element can be selectively enhanced. Because virtually all of the immune-enhancing drugs or agents that are discussed subsequently are indeed nonspecific, they suffer from the same limitations as immunosuppressive agents in the modulation of aberrant immune reactivity in disease states. Nonetheless, certain drugs that enhance immune responses have been used with limited success in certain immunologically mediated diseases and are mentioned subsequently.

The ultimate enhancement of the immune response would be complete replacement, as with ablation and bone marrow transplantation. Given the nature of the diseases in question together with the logistic constraints on bone marrow transplants, however, such an approach is not feasible at present

for rheumatic diseases. Transfer of mature immune competent lymphoid cells has the theoretic potential of reversing the imbalance of immunoregulatory lymphocyte subsets. Again, logistic constraints, with regard to histocompatibility requirements and restrictions, make such an approach untenable. Of particular interest, however, has been the availability of purified preparations of lymphokines such as IL-2 and the various interferons. These factors, particularly IL-2, are capable of exerting profound enhancing effects on the immune response in vitro,[28] and the therapeutic use of such factors holds at least theoretic potential for the future.

CYTOTOXIC AGENTS

General Considerations

Of all the immunoregulatory agents that are used in the treatment of rheumatic diseases, the cytotoxic drugs pose perhaps the greatest difficulty for the clinician from both theoretical and practical standpoints. This stems largely from the fine line between risk and benefit, which exists for virtually all such agents used in the treatment of these diseases. Unfortunately, the terminology that is frequently employed with regard to the cytotoxic agents is somewhat misleading in that the term *cytotoxic agent* is used synonymously with the term *immunosuppressive agent*. Indeed, cytotoxic agents can be and are frequently immunosuppressive; however, a number of other drugs discussed in this chapter as well as the glucocorticoids (see Chapter 48) can be potent immunosuppressive agents. The cytotoxic agents differ from many of these other agents in that the common denominator of their effect is that they destroy cells, hence the derivation of the term *cytotoxic*, which means simply that the drugs are directly toxic or damaging to cells. It is this ability to kill cells that distinguishes the cytotoxic immunosuppressive agents from the other categories of immunosuppressive drugs and explains their extensive use in the treatment of a variety of neoplastic diseases. Indeed, their use as antineoplastic agents long antedates their use as immunosuppressive agents in non-neoplastic inflammatory and immune-mediated diseases. Only when the profound immunosuppressive effects of these agents as used in the treatment of neoplastic diseases became apparent did clinical investigators conceive of their use in diseases that manifested marked inflammatory responses and apparent immune-mediated mechanisms. Certain of the mechanisms of action of cytotoxic agents on inflammatory and immunologic responses are listed in Table 49–1.

It cannot be emphasized too strongly that the rationale for the use of cytotoxic agents as well as the goals that one wishes to achieve by therapy are for the most part quite different depending on whether one uses these agents in the treatment of non-neoplastic, immune-mediated diseases or neo-

Table 49–1. PRINCIPAL MECHANISMS OF ACTION OF CYTOTOXIC AGENTS ON INFLAMMATORY AND IMMUNOLOGIC REACTIONS

Elimination of sensitized and immunologically committed lymphoid cells
Elimination of nonsensitized lymphoid cells secondarily engaged in aberrant immunologic reactivity
Elimination of nonlymphoid cells engaged in nonspecific inflammatory responses to aberrant immunologic reactions
Suppression of functional capabilities of surviving lymphoid cells

plastic diseases. The rationale and goal for the use of cytotoxic agents in the treatment of neoplastic diseases are simply to eliminate where possible every tumor cell. This approach is almost invariably associated with significant destruction of the normal elements of host defense mechanisms, such that a life-threatening or near life-threatening state exists for variable periods of time during and after chemotherapy until the normal cellular elements can recover. If the tumor is sensitive to the chemotherapeutic agents used, such that a reasonable chance of remission or cure exists, the attendant risks are clearly justifiable, since the malignant neoplasm will otherwise inevitably result in the death of the patient. Under such circumstances, the goals are rather clear-cut, and the options are few.

The situation is quite different when using these agents to treat non-neoplastic diseases. Because there are no recognizable malignant clones in the immune-mediated diseases, the rationale and goal are usually to suppress the aberrant inflammatory and immune-mediated reactions that are responsible for the tissue damage without markedly suppressing the normal host defense mechanisms, which would put the patient at significant risk for either an infection or a neoplasm resulting from the suppression of normal immune surveillance mechanisms.[24, 25] Unfortunately, maintaining this balance between risk and benefit is not an easy task because, as mentioned previously, the agents employed are almost always nonspecific in their suppressive effects, and suppression of normal immune mechanisms will invariably accompany suppression of the aberrant reactions. It is hoped that suppression of these abnormal immune responses will be effected before the point at which such a degree of suppression of normal immune mechanisms occurs, so the patient would not be at a significant risk.

Of equal if not greater importance than the suppression of normal immunologic mechanisms is the suppression of normal nonspecific mechanisms of host defenses in the form of the circulating polymorphonuclear neutrophils. Owing to the relatively rapid turnover of the neutrophil series in the bone marrow, cytotoxic agents are particularly effective in causing a neutropenia, which becomes one of the major limiting factors in the use of these agents. In this regard, another important difference in the use of these agents in neoplastic versus non-neoplastic diseases is that in non-neoplastic diseases the drugs are usually administered chronically over extended periods of time, ranging from months to years, and so the risk of a host defense defect is a relatively persistent problem as opposed to the relatively brief (albeit usually more severe) periods of defect seen following the intermittent courses of chemotherapy usually administered for neoplastic diseases.

Finally, the major difference in the use of these agents in the treatment of neoplastic versus non-neoplastic diseases lies in the exercise of clinical judgment as to when to employ such an aggressive chemotherapeutic approach in a non-neoplastic disease that might not be invariably fatal. The clinical course of most neoplastic diseases that are left untreated or that are not aggressively treated is usually rather clear, which makes the decision to initiate aggressive therapy relatively easy. In contrast, many of the rheumatic diseases, such as SLE, rheumatoid arthritis, the systemic vasculitides, scleroderma, and dermatomyositis/polymyositis, as well as several of the organ-specific autoimmune diseases in which cytotoxic agents have been used have variable clinical courses. Only when the disease seems to be progressing with irreversible organ system dysfunction that is not responsive to more conventional therapy, such as nonsteroidal anti-inflammatory agents (NSAIDs) or glucocorticoids, does one consider employing a cytotoxic agent. This is often a difficult decision because the efficacy of these agents in many of these diseases has not been conclusively proved by appropriately controlled studies. Furthermore, the chronicity of most of these diseases dictates that even though a cytotoxic agent may be effective in suppressing disease activity, the agent cannot be used indefinitely. Thus, it is essential to set reasonable goals for the use of cytotoxic agents in the treatment of rheumatic diseases.

Therapeutic Goals

Few situations exist in which the use of cytotoxic agents can be expected to effect a true and long-term "cure" of a non-neoplastic disease. One such situation is the use of these agents, particularly cyclophosphamide, in the treatment of certain vasculitic syndromes. Paramount among these syndromes is Wegener's granulomatosis in which long-term remissions, which can indeed be called "cures," have been effected in as many as 90 percent of patients treated with cyclophosphamide, 2 mg per kg per day, together with prednisone, 1 mg per kg per day, administered first daily and then on an alternate-day schedule.[24, 25] Similar results have been obtained with other vasculitic syndromes, particularly the polyarteritis nodosa group of the systemic necrotizing vasculitides.[29] Before the institution of this therapy, virtually all patients with Wegener's granulomatosis died of the disease, as did most patients with the polyarteritis nodosa type of systemic necrotizing vasculitis.[24, 25] It is conceivable that the drug does not in fact "cure" the disease but merely suppresses the inflammatory and aberrant immune-mediated mechanisms long enough for the disease to run its course spontaneously and remit permanently. Therefore, given these reported therapeutic results, a reasonable goal for the use of cytotoxic agents (in this case cyclophosphamide) in these vasculitic syndromes is a true permanent remission or cure. One can hope that a single course of therapy, which is usually administered for over a year, will result in a situation in which the drug would not have to be used again in the patient. At worst, it may be necessary to treat a minor relapse with an additional brief course of therapy.

The goals for the use of cytotoxic agents in most of the other immune-mediated rheumatic diseases, particularly the classic connective tissue diseases, are somewhat different from those of the vasculitic syndromes. Because the connective tissue diseases usually run waxing and waning courses, which are characterized by exacerbations and remissions, the use of cytotoxic agents should be reserved for treatment of flares of disease in which there is a clear-cut danger of irreversible organ system dysfunction. Even though cytotoxic agents have been used for several years in the treatment of the severe manifestations of the connective tissue and other rheumatic diseases, there are unfortunately few controlled studies that definitively document the efficacy of such an approach.[6, 8, 9] A few controlled trials of cytotoxic agents have been carried out, and they have documented short-term benefits in flares of disease activity. In this regard, Austin et al.[30] compared intravenous cyclophosphamide plus low-dose prednisone with prednisone alone in the treatment of lupus nephritis and concluded that cyclophosphamide, when used in this manner, reduced the risk of end-stage renal disease. There is, however, still little information available regarding long-term effects of these agents on the ultimate course of the disease. Thus, given the present state of knowledge in this area, a reasonable goal for the use of cytotoxic agents in the connective tissue diseases would be to suppress flares of disease activity that are serious enough to be organ system–threatening or life-threatening until such a point that the disease goes into remission and the drug can be withdrawn. Under such circumstances, the drug can be used again for a limited course should another relapse occur.

If it is necessary to continue the cytotoxic agent indefinitely to effect a sustained remission or even a partial remission, one must carefully examine the risks of such long-term treatment with a drug whose potential adverse side effects are so substantial.[10, 31, 32] A classic example of this latter point would be the use of chronic cytotoxic therapy in a patient with rheumatoid arthritis. Given the normal life expectancy in patients with rheumatoid arthritis (see Chapters 51 and 53), it may be inappropriate to risk a serious and even fatal complication of therapy to suppress disease activity that is rarely life-threatening. On the other hand, the patient's life situation may be such that he or she feels that the risk is worth the benefit of suppressing certain unacceptable manifestations of disease activity. Thus, the goals may differ depending on the individual patient.

Individual Cytotoxic Agents

Although a wide variety of cytotoxic agents of various classes have been used in the chemotherapy of neoplastic diseases, only a limited number of these have been regularly employed in the treatment of non-neoplastic, inflammatory, and immune-mediated diseases. The three major categories of cytotoxic drugs employed in the latter disease are the alkylating agents and two groups of antimetabolites, the purine analogues, and the folic acid antagonists. The mechanisms of action of these cytotoxic agents are outlined in Table 49–2, and their structures are illustrated in Figure 49–2. Other cytotoxic agents that are used almost exclusively in the treatment of neoplastic diseases are covered in detail elsewhere[33] and include other antimetabolites such as the pyrimidine

Table 49–2. MECHANISMS OF ACTION OF CLASSES OF CYTOTOXIC AGENTS COMMONLY EMPLOYED IN TREATMENT OF INFLAMMATORY AND IMMUNE-MEDIATED NON-NEOPLASTIC DISEASES

Class	Typical Agent	Mechanisms of Action
Alkylating agents	Nitrogen mustard Cyclophosphamide Chlorambucil	Under physiologic conditions the drug reacts chemically with biologically vital macromolecules such as DNA by contributing alkyl groups to the molecule, resulting in cross-linkage
Purine analogues	6-Mercaptopurine Thioguanine Azathioprine	Although incorporation of the analogue into cellular DNA with subsequent inhibition of nucleic acid synthesis is generally considered the basic mechanism of action of these agents, they likely exert their cytotoxic effects by one or more of multiple mechanisms, including effects on purine nucleotide synthesis and metabolism as well as alterations in the synthesis and function of RNA and DNA
Folic acid antagonists	Methotrexate	Binds with high affinity to dihydrofolate reductase, preventing the formation of tetrahydrofolate and thus causing an acute intracellular deficiency of folate coenzymes. Consequently, one-carbon transfer reactions critical for de novo synthesis of purine nucleotides and thymidylate cease, with resulting interruption of the synthesis of DNA and RNA

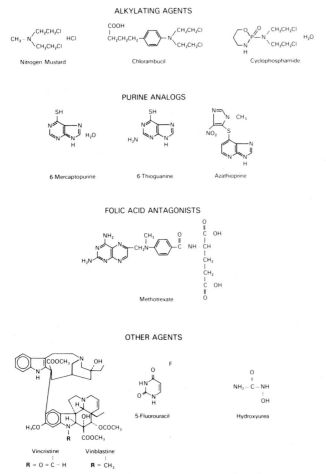

Figure 49–2. Structure of cytotoxic agents used in the treatment of certain rheumatic diseases.

analogues in the form of 5-fluorouracil, cytosine arabinoside, and triacetyl-6-azauridine. In addition, natural products used in the treatment of neoplastic diseases include the vinca alkaloids (vinblastine and vincristine) and antibiotics (actinomycin D, daunomycin, rubidomycin, adrioblastina, bleomycin, mithramycin, and mitomycin C). Finally, miscellaneous cytotoxic agents include cisplatin, hydroxyurea, procarbazine, and mitotane. The list is surely not complete, as newer agents are constantly being developed. Within this group of agents used predominantly in neoplastic processes are some that have also been used in certain non-neoplastic diseases. For example, as is discussed subsequently, vincristine has been successfully employed as a therapeutic modality in idiopathic thrombocytopenic purpura,[34] and hydroxyurea has been employed in the treatment of the idiopathic hypereosinophilic syndrome.[35]

Alkylating Agents

Alkylating agents are chemicals that can substitute alkyl radicals into other molecules. Biologically effective alkylating agents are usually bifunctional or polyfunctional in that each molecule has two or more

alkylating groups.[33] Thus, each molecule of the alkylating agent can covalently bind with two or more molecules of other substances. In this manner, two or more molecules may be linked to each other, i.e., in cross-linkage. By virtue of the induction of these structural changes at the molecular level, alkylating agents can potentially alter the function of proteins and nucleic acids. For example, when the DNA of a cell such as a lymphocyte is cross-linked by the agent, replication of its strands is blocked, and the cell cannot divide properly, leading ultimately to cell death.[36]

Nitrogen Mustard. Mechlorethamine was the first of the nitrogen mustards to be used clinically. The drug is administered intravenously, and its clearance from the blood is extremely rapid. Following administration, the drug rapidly undergoes chemical transformation and combines with either water or reactive compounds of cells such that the drug is no longer present in its active form after only a few minutes.[33] Nitrogen mustard has been virtually replaced by cyclophosphamide as the alkylating agent of choice in the treatment of non-neoplastic diseases. The former has the disadvantage of requiring intravenous administration, it has significant potential toxic side effects, and its therapeutic index in experimental animals has been shown to be much lower than that of cyclophosphamide with respect to immunosuppressive effects. Historically, however, nitrogen mustard is an important agent, which led the way for the use of cyclophosphamide in the treatment of immune-mediated diseases. For example, the early success in treatment of a patient with Wegener's granulomatosis with nitrogen mustard in 1954[37] laid the rational basis for the use of cyclophosphamide in the successful induction of remission in large numbers of patients with that disease.[25]

Cyclophosphamide. Cyclophosphamide is well absorbed orally and so has the advantage of administration by either the oral or the intravenous route. The drug is inert and is activated by metabolism in the liver by the mixed-function oxidase system of the smooth endoplasmic reticulum.[38] The plasma half-life of cyclophosphamide is 6 to 7 hours; this may be significantly prolonged by prior treatment with allopurinol.[39] Maximal concentrations are reached in plasma 1 hour after administration and urinary recovery of unmetabolized drug is approximately 14 percent with negligible fecal recovery after intravenous administration.[33] Because approximately 60 percent of the drug is excreted through the kidney in the form of active metabolites, renal failure may result in impaired excretion of these active metabolites, with a resulting relative increase in immunosuppressive effect as well as in toxicity of a given dose of drug. Because certain enzymes of the mixed-function oxidase system can be induced by drugs such as barbiturates and glucocorticoids, these agents can influence the metabolism of cyclophosphamide from its inert to its active form.[40] The biologic actions of cyclophosphamide, however, seem to be more

Table 49–3. IMMUNOSUPPRESSIVE EFFECTS OF CHRONICALLY ADMINISTERED CYCLOPHOSPHAMIDE THERAPY IN HUMANS

Absolute lymphocytopenia of both T and B lymphocytes, with early preferential depletion of B lymphocytes

Significant suppression of in vitro lymphocyte blastogenic responses to specific antigenic stimuli, with only mild suppression of responses to mitogenic stimuli

Suppression of antibody response and cutaneous delayed hypersensitivity to a new antigen, with relative sparing of established cutaneous delayed hypersensitivity

Reduction of elevated serum immunoglobulin levels as well as occurrence of hypogammaglobulinemia in patients treated for extended periods of time (years)

Selective suppression of in vitro B lymphocyte function, with diminution of increased spontaneous immunoglobulin production of individual B lymphocytes as well as suppression of mitogen-induced immunoglobulin production

substantially affected by alterations in the rates of detoxification and elimination than by changes in the rate of generation of the active metabolites.[33] Indeed, the antitumor and therapeutic index of cyclophosphamide was shown not to be significantly modified by pretreatment of animals with phenobarbital.[41]

Although cyclophosphamide acts primarily during the S phase of the cell cycle and so has a profound effect on rapidly dividing cells, it also affects cells at all phases of the cell cycle including resting (G_0) cells.[8] A large amount of literature has accumulated, particularly using the mouse and other animal models, demonstrating the effects of cyclophosphamide on virtually all components of the cellular and humoral immune responses.[42, 43] Of particular note is the ability of cyclophosphamide to inhibit antibody production. Although this has been shown to occur most dramatically when the drug is administered before the antigen,[43, 44] for practical purposes, cyclophosphamide inhibits antibody production when given at the same time or even after the antigen. Cyclophosphamide has been shown to inhibit suppressor T lymphocytes selectively as opposed to inducer or helper T lymphocytes.[45, 46] In the therapeutic protocols in which cyclophosphamide is administered to patients with rheumatic diseases, however, a more global rather than a selective suppression of T lymphocyte function is seen. The immunosuppressive effects of chronically administered cyclophosphamide therapy in humans[27, 47–49] are summarized in Table 49–3. The most consistent finding in cyclophosphamide-treated patients is a lymphocytopenia of both T and B lymphocytes. B lymphocyte function is clearly more profoundly suppressed than T lymphocyte function, and this is reflected at the cellular level as well as in the suppression of Ig production and serum levels of Ig in patients treated chronically with cyclophosphamide.

Cyclophosphamide is generally administered to patients with non-neoplastic diseases in a dosage regimen of 2 mg per kg per day orally. Immunosuppressive and clinical effects are usually seen within 2 to 3 weeks after initiation of therapy. An alternative

regimen is the administration of single large intravenous bolus doses of 750 to 1000 mg per m^2. This latter regimen is usually reserved for patients with neoplastic diseases but has been used for the treatment of rheumatic diseases such as SLE. In a study by Austin et al.[30] bolus cyclophosphamide combined with oral prednisone was determined to be effective in reducing the incidence of end-stage renal disease in patients with SLE and nephritis. Hoffman et al.[50] examined the use of intermittent high-dose intravenous cyclophosphamide in the treatment of 14 patients with Wegener's granulomatosis. Initial response rates were high, but responses were not maintained or patients failed to tolerate continued treatment, leading the authors to conclude that daily low-dose cyclophosphamide remains the treatment of choice for this disorder. As with the use of any cytotoxic and potentially myelosuppressive agent, the dosage must be modified throughout the therapeutic course in accordance with the degree of myelosuppression that occurs (see later).

Although cyclophosphamide has proved to be an extremely effective immunosuppressive agent in the treatment of non-neoplastic diseases, its potential toxic side effects are considerable, and the physician must be aware of them whenever he or she undertakes the treatment of a patient with this agent[31, 32] (Table 49–4). Although suppression of all marrow elements is seen with cyclophosphamide therapy, neutropenia is clearly the most important hematologic effect of the drug with regard to factors limiting its use. It should be appreciated that chronically administered cyclophosphamide will have a cumulative effect on the bone marrow reserve such that a dose that is well tolerated at one point in time may produce significant neutropenia after 1 or more years of therapy. This will necessitate frequent monitoring of the white blood cell count (WBC) and appropriate adjustment of dosage. Gonadal suppression is an almost invariable effect of long-term administration of cyclophosphamide and is due to the damaging effects of the drug on the germinal epithelium.[51, 52] The oligospermia and azoospermia in males[53] and oligomenorrhea and amenorrhea in premenopausal women[51] may be permanent if treatment is continued for a year or longer. Although prepubertal testes are damaged, return of spermatogenesis after drug with-

Table 49–4. TOXIC SIDE EFFECTS OF CHRONICALLY ADMINISTERED LOW-DOSE* CYCLOPHOSPHAMIDE THERAPY

Marrow suppression—predominantly neutropenia
Gonadal suppression—oligospermia, ovarian dysfunction
Alopecia
Gastrointestinal intolerance
Hemorrhagic cystitis
Hypogammaglobulinemia after extended use
Pulmonary interstitial fibrosis
Oncogenesis

*2 mg per kg per day.

drawal occurs more frequently in this younger age bracket.[54]

Although significant alopecia occurs quite frequently after high doses of cyclophosphamide, only minor degrees occur during long-term low-dose therapy; in both cases, it is reversible on cessation of the drug. Gastrointestinal intolerance is unpredictable and can be quite severe in certain patients. Although nausea and vomiting can usually be successfully treated with antiemetics, gastric discomfort may be refractory to the usual therapeutic modalities. The latter complication not infrequently disappears on continuation of the drug.

Hemorrhagic cystitis is seen in from 15 to 30 percent of patients and can be a most difficult complication.[25] Although the cystitis usually clears on cessation of the drug, bladder fibrosis, intractable hemorrhage, and bladder carcinoma have been reported.[55] Under most circumstances, the onset of hemorrhagic cystitis is an absolute indication for discontinuation of the drug. If the cystitis is severe, the drug must be stopped regardless of the circumstances. If lack of an adequate substitute makes it necessary to continue the drug in a patient with only mild cystitis, however, the dosage should be decreased and the patient followed with urinary cytologic studies and intermittent cystoscopies. If the cystitis persists or worsens on the lower dose, the drug must be discontinued even though the alternative drug for the disease in question is inferior to cyclophosphamide.

The authors have noted a few patients who have developed hypogammaglobulinemia during chronically administered cyclophosphamide therapy. This is of potential importance because of the synergistic host defense defects created by neutropenia and hypogammaglobulinemia. Although pulmonary and cardiac toxicity are generally seen only at high doses of the drug,[56, 57] interstitial pulmonary fibrosis can occur with chronically administered low-dose cyclophosphamide, and the physician should be alert to this possibility. In addition, an antidiuretic hormone effect has been reported with large doses of cyclophosphamide but not with lower doses.[58, 59] Finally, neoplastic diseases, particularly lymphomas and leukemias, may occur as a result of cyclophosphamide therapy.[60]

Chlorambucil. Chlorambucil is available for oral administration, and absorption is adequate and reliable. The drug is related to nitrogen mustard in that the methyl group of the mustard is replaced by phenylbutyric acid. The drug is metabolized by beta oxidation of the butyric acid.[61] The drug is almost completely metabolized and has a plasma half-life of approximately 90 minutes. At recommended doses, chlorambucil is the slowest acting nitrogen mustard in clinical use.[33]

The mechanism of action of chlorambucil is similar to that of the other alkylating agents. At high doses, it suppresses all myeloid elements, and the therapeutic strategy is to suppress immune function in the form of lymphocytes before the suppression of other bone marrow elements. In this regard, it has been reported that at lower doses, chlorambucil exerts a more selective effect on lymphopoiesis than on granulopoiesis. Clearly, chlorambucil has not been as extensively studied as cyclophosphamide with regard to its immunosuppressive effects. It is generally believed, however, that it is not as potent an immunosuppressive agent as cyclophosphamide, and although its toxic side effects may be somewhat less than those of cyclophosphamide, its efficacy in suppressing disease activity in the non-neoplastic diseases is probably less than that of cyclophosphamide. An example of this is the greater efficacy of cyclophosphamide than of chlorambucil in suppressing disease activity in generalized Wegener's granulomatosis.[63] Nonetheless, chlorambucil has been used with some success in certain of the connective tissue diseases.[8]

Chlorambucil is generally administered to patients with non-neoplastic diseases in a dosage regimen of 0.1 or 0.2 mg per kg per day orally. The dose is adjusted according to the degree of nonlymphocytic myelosuppression that is encountered, i.e., neutropenia and thrombocytopenia. When severe myelosuppression occurs, the drug should be discontinued. Marrow function usually recovers rapidly; however, irreversible marrow failure has been reported in a number of patients treated with chlorambucil for non-neoplastic diseases.[64] Such complications highlight the inherent danger in the treatment of non-neoplastic diseases with cytotoxic agents of any class. Other side effects include gastrointestinal discomfort with nausea and vomiting, hepatotoxicity, dermatitis, and infertility.[33] Oncogenesis is a particularly disturbing potential complication of chlorambucil therapy, and a marked increase in the incidence of leukemia and other tumors has been associated with the use of this agent.[65, 66]

Purine Analogues

The two major purine analogues that have been used clinically are 6-mercaptopurine (6-MP) and azathioprine, which is the purine analogue currently used almost exclusively. 6-MP is an analogue of hypoxanthine in which the 6-OH radical is replaced by a thiol group. When an imidazole group is attached to the S of 6-MP, azathioprine is formed. In vivo, azathioprine is metabolized to 6-MP, which is the active drug. The ultimate mechanism of action of 6-MP is the inhibition of nucleic acid synthesis. Despite extensive studies in this area, however, the precise mechanism of action whereby these purine analogues cause cell death or cytotoxicity remains unclear. Certain potential mechanisms of action have been proposed, including the conversion of 6-MP to its ribonucleotide, which inhibits the enzymes necessary for the conversion of inosinic acid to xanthylic acid as well as the conversion of adenylosuccinic acid to adenylic acid, leading to the inhibition of DNA synthesis.[67] In addition, feedback inhibition of 5-phosphoribosylamine occurs with reduction of de novo purine biosynthesis and resulting inhibition of DNA synthesis and cell death.

Azathioprine and 6-MP are available for oral administration, and absorption is quite good. Because azathioprine is converted in vivo to 6-MP, which is the active drug, their pharmacokinetics can be considered together. About one half of an oral dose of drug is found excreted in the urine within the first 24 hours.[33] After an intravenous dose, the half-life of the drug is 60 to 90 minutes, with clearance from the blood resulting from uptake by cells, renal excretion, and metabolic degradation. There are two major pathways for the metabolism of 6-MP. The first is the methylation of the sulfhydryl group and oxidation of the methylated derivatives. The second is the oxidation of 6-MP to 6-thiouric acid by the enzyme xanthine oxidase.[33] Because allopurinol inhibits xanthine oxidase, this drug decreases the metabolism of 6-MP and so accounts for the increase in toxicity of azathioprine and 6-MP when allopurinol is simultaneously administered.

Azathioprine and 6-MP inhibit both cell-mediated and humoral immunity. Because of the diversity of studies that have been carried out in animal models and humans, there have been certain disagreements with regard to the type and extent of immunosuppression that occurs during azathioprine and 6-MP therapy.[42, 67] Despite this, there have been some rather consistent findings with regard to the effects of azathioprine and 6-MP on immune and inflammatory responses. Azathioprine and 6-MP cause a total lymphocytopenia of both T and B lymphocytes.[68] Gamma globulin synthesis is suppressed by azathioprine therapy,[69] as is the antibody response (particularly the secondary response) to vaccination.[70] In addition, B lymphocyte proliferation is suppressed by azathioprine.[71] There has been some controversy with regard to the effects of these agents on T lymphocytes, including inhibition of sheep red blood cell rosette formation.[72] Other studies, however, claim no selective effect on T lymphocytes and in fact demonstrate that treatment with azathioprine has little suppressive effect on mitogen-induced blastogenesis of human T lymphocytes.[73, 74] In this regard, there seems to be little question that azathioprine is not as effective as cyclophosphamide in the suppression of lymphocyte function. Azathioprine and 6-MP can suppress the induction of de novo delayed hypersensitivity; however, it is generally agreed that established delayed hypersensitivity remains intact during drug therapy.[70, 74] Azathioprine has potent anti-inflammatory effects, which are probably related to its ability to reduce the number of monocytes in an inflammatory site by inhibition of monocyte production.[75] This suppression of monocyte function may also explain the effects of these drugs on the induction of delayed hypersensitivity.[76]

Azathioprine and 6-MP are generally administered in doses of approximately 2 mg per kg per day.

Table 49–5. TOXIC SIDE EFFECTS OF CHRONICALLY ADMINISTERED AZATHIOPRINE AND 6-MERCAPTOPURINE THERAPY

Marrow suppression—predominantly neutropenia
Hepatotoxicity—probably on an allergic basis
Infectious disease complications—not necessarily correlated with neutropenia
Gastrointestinal intolerance
Oncogenesis—particularly lymphoid malignancies

As with the other cytotoxic agents, the dosage must be adjusted according to the degree of resulting myelosuppression. Immunosuppressive and clinical effects are usually seen within 3 or 4 weeks after initiation of therapy. Patients with impaired renal function may have reduced clearance of the drug and its metabolites, with a resulting cumulative effect and increased toxicity unless the dosage is appropriately adjusted downward.

The major toxicity of both 6-MP and azathioprine is bone marrow suppression, with leukopenia rather than thrombocytopenia and anemia being the major manifestations. The major toxic side effects of chronically administered azathioprine or 6-MP therapy[77] are listed in Table 49–5. Of note with regard to the neutropenia associated with these agents is the fact that a rapid fall in WBC within a week of starting therapy has been reported and resembles an idiosyncratic reaction. In addition, the peripheral WBC cannot always be an accurate measure of the host defense defect, since infections may occur in individuals with normal neutrophil counts, suggesting a functional impairment of immune-competent cells involved in host defense, most likely at the T lymphocyte–monocyte axis. The suppression of delayed hypersensitivity by these agents[75, 76] as well as the fact that neutrophil function is generally normal in individuals receiving azathioprine[78] adds credence to this hypothesis. This point should be fully appreciated, since infectious disease complications cannot be totally predicted regardless of the level of the WBC. Finally, although the effects on gonadal function have not been fully evaluated with regard to azathioprine, it is clear that sterility is not the invariable rule, since several normal pregnancies have been reported in patients who had been receiving azathioprine. Fetal abnormalities do not appear to be a problem.[32]

Other Agents

Methotrexate. Methotrexate is discussed in detail in Chapter 41.[79]

Vinca **Alkaloids.** The commonly used *Vinca* alkaloids, vincristine and vinblastine, are cell cycle–specific agents that block mitosis by interfering with protein assembly of the mitotic spindle, leading to metaphase arrest.[33] Vincristine is administered intravenously in doses of 2 mg per m² of body surface area weekly. After intravenous injection, vincristine is cleared almost entirely from the blood in approximately 30 minutes. The drug is excreted primarily by the liver into the bile, with less than 5 percent of the drug appearing in the urine.

Immunosuppression with these compounds has been negligible, and antibody formation in rabbits was shown not to be significantly affected by administration of *Vinca* alkaloids.[42] Vinblastine has been employed in a unique immunosuppression protocol in the treatment of idiopathic thrombocytopenia in which the drug was bound to platelets for the purposes of delivering the toxic drug directly and selectively to the cells that were removing and killing the platelets.[80]

The major toxic side effect of the *Vinca* alkaloids is neurotoxicity. This is usually manifested by peripheral neuropathy in the form of paresthesias, loss of deep tendon reflexes, neuritic pain, muscle weakness, and wasting. Other toxicities include hoarseness owing to vocal cord paralysis, diplopia, severe constipation, bladder atony, alopecia, cytopenias, pyuria, dysuria, fever, gastrointestinal symptoms, mutagenicity, local inflammation at sites of venous extravasation, and inappropriate secretion of antidiuretic hormone.

5-Fluorouracil. 5-Fluorouracil (5-FU) is a pyrimidine analogue that competes with uracil in various metabolic pathways but cannot be converted to thymidine. Thus, it ultimately blocks DNA synthesis. In addition, it inhibits enzymes such as thymidylate synthetase required for the synthesis of ribonucleotides and deoxyribonucleotides. The drug has been used predominantly in the treatment of neoplastic diseases, and its precise immunosuppressive properties are not well studied in humans.[33] The drug works throughout the cell cycle, and it is metabolized almost exclusively in the liver. It is usually administered intravenously, since absorption after oral ingestion is unpredictable and incomplete. The major toxic side effects result from the inevitable myelosuppression, particularly leukopenia. Other side effects include nausea and vomiting, alopecia, dermatitis, nail changes, atrophy of the skin, ulcerative stomatitis and gastroenteritis, and neurologic manifestations such as cerebellar ataxia.[33]

Hydroxyurea. Hydroxyurea inhibits the enzyme ribonucleotide diphosphate reductase, which catalyzes the reductive conversion of ribonucleotides to deoxyribonucleotides and which is a crucial step in the synthesis of DNA. The drug is specific for the S phase of the cell cycle.[33] It is readily absorbed from the gastrointestinal tract, and peak plasma concentrations are reached within 2 hours of administration of an oral dose. Within 24 hours, it is undetectable in the blood, with approximately 80 percent of the drug recovered in the urine within 12 hours of oral or intravenous administration. The drug is administered orally in doses of 20 to 30 mg per kg per day as a single dose. Although the drug has been used predominantly in the management of chronic myelogenous leukemia, it has also been used in the

treatment of the idiopathic hypereosinophilic syndrome.[35] Toxic side effects include myelosuppression, nausea and vomiting, gastrointestinal ulcerations, and mild skin rashes.

THEORETIC AND PRACTICAL CONSIDERATIONS IN THE USE OF CYTOTOXIC AGENTS FOR TREATMENT OF NON-NEOPLASTIC DISEASES

As already mentioned, one of the major goals in the use of cytotoxic agents for the treatment of non-neoplastic diseases is to achieve a degree of immunosuppression that results in suppression of the aberrant inflammatory and immune reactivity in a disease state without seriously compromising host defense mechanisms, which would lead to an increased incidence of infectious disease complications. For reasons that are not entirely clear, in those inflammatory and immune-mediated diseases for which cytotoxic agents have proved to be beneficial, it appears that disease activity can indeed be suppressed without the invariable occurrence of a serious defect in clinically relevant host defense mechanisms.

Although the cytotoxic agents have a number of immediate and long-term toxic side effects that must be considered in the decision to employ such agents in a given patient, once the decision has been made to use a cytotoxic agent, awareness and recognition of these side effects become of paramount importance in the successful management of the patient. In this regard, although the different classes of cytotoxic agents used in the treatment of non-neoplastic diseases differ somewhat in their mechanisms of action, the major immediate limiting side effect common to virtually all of them is myelosuppression, particularly neutropenia and to a lesser extent thrombocytopenia and anemia.

When the physician undertakes the treatment of non-neoplastic diseases with these agents, it is essential to appreciate the necessity for careful and continuous monitoring of the WBC, with appropriate modification of the dosage regimen to maintain the WBC above the neutropenic range. It has been consistently observed that if the WBC is maintained above 3000 to 3500 cells per mm^3, which usually results in a neutrophil count of 1000 to 1500 per mm^3, there is little chance of opportunistic infections as a result of drug-induced host defense defects, particularly when the agent employed is an alkylating agent such as cyclophosphamide or chlorambucil. For example, this has clearly been shown to be the case with the use of cyclophosphamide in the treatment of Wegener's granulomatosis[25] and other of the severe systemic vasculitic syndromes.[24, 26] This observation holds true provided that there is not a concomitant and synergistic cause of host defense defects, such as daily glucocorticoid therapy. For this reason, it is suggested that glucocorticoids be administered on an alternate-day basis, when possible, in patients receiving cytotoxic agents together with glucocorticoids for the treatment of non-neoplastic diseases.[24–26] Using such a regimen of chronically administered cyclophosphamide at a dose of 2 mg per kg per day, with frequent adjustments of dosage to maintain the WBC above 3000 per mm³, together with prednisone, 60 mg per day or less with conversion to alternate-day prednisone within 1 to 2 months of initiating therapy and maintenance of alternate-day prednisone together with the cyclophosphamide, there has been virtually no increased incidence of opportunistic infections in a large series of patients.[25] The exception to this was an increased incidence of herpes zoster infections in patients receiving long-term cyclophosphamide therapy.[81] The zoster did not disseminate viscerally in any patient, and there were no serious sequelae of the infection.

Maintaining the WBC above the neutropenic level while effecting remission of disease activity requires continuous monitoring of the WBC as well as appreciation that as patients receive a cytotoxic agent for extended periods of time, their tolerance for a given dose will decrease, necessitating downward adjustment of the dose. It should also be pointed out that an appreciation of the *slope of the curve* of the WBC is important, in that the effect of a given dose of drug on one day may be reflected several days later. Therefore, one should not wait until the patient is already seriously neutropenic before decreasing the dose of cytotoxic agent but should decrease the dose based on the projection of the downward slope of the WBC curve. In this way, a smooth plateauing of the WBC can be maintained and infectious disease complications largely avoided. This phenomenon is illustrated in Figure 49–3.

The preceding principles of the relationship between neutropenia and infection generally hold true except under certain circumstances, such as the concomitant use of other agents, which cause a host defense defect but do not cause neutropenia. As mentioned, this is the case with the use of daily glucocorticoids, which negates the ability to use the WBC as an accurate gauge of the degree of host defense defect. Further, agents such as azathioprine can result in an increased incidence of infectious disease complications even without neutropenia. When using such agents, it is still important to monitor the WBC; however, the danger of the occurrence of unpredicted infectious disease complications must be appreciated. In addition, the gradual dropping of the WBC on a constant dose of cytotoxic agent is the rule, but certain drugs such as azathioprine can give an idiosyncratic, precipitous drop in WBC. All of these possibilities must be taken into consideration in the use of these agents.

It should be pointed out that under certain circumstances the bone marrow reserve of a given patient may be suppressed to a point at which the dosage of cyclophosphamide must be reduced even though the disease is still active. In these situations, the addition of or increase in the dose of alternate-day prednisone may allow one to administer higher doses of cyclophosphamide with a lesser degree of leukopenia. It is thought that the mechanism of this marrow sparing effect of glucocorticoid in patients treated with cyclophosphamide is the result of a beneficial effect on marrow regeneration, most likely caused by an altering of cell cycle characteristics of granulocyte progenitor cells.[25]

Once disease remission has been achieved and maintained for an adequate period of time with the use of cytotoxic agents, it is important to attempt to taper the dosage of drug continually with the ultimate goal of discontinuation. The time for maintenance of remission on cytotoxic agents varies with each disease. The general principle, however, stands that the physician should always have the ultimate discontinuation of the cytotoxic agent as a goal of the regimen.

Finally, a thorough familiarization with all of the other immediate as well as long-term potential side effects of these agents should be undertaken by the physician who prescribes them, and careful following of the patient during and after use of these agents is essential to detect the onset of these complications as early as possible.

THERAPEUTIC APHERESIS

The word *apheresis* is a Greek derivative meaning withdrawal. Therapeutic apheresis implies withdrawal of a substance from a patient, ultimately leading to clinical improvement in a disease state. Although the original aphereses were solely confined to the removal of plasma for hyperviscosity states such as Waldenström's macroglobulinemia, the development of sophisticated equipment for removal of plasma as well as selected cellular components has led to an acceleration of the use of apheresis in a number of different disease states, including hematologic, connective tissue, neurologic, and even neoplastic disorders.[82] Plasmapheresis is the removal of plasma without significant removal of cellular elements. Cytapheresis is the removal of cells without significant removal of noncellular elements such as plasma. For example, lymphocytapheresis is the selective removal of mononuclear cells, especially lymphocytes, without significant removal of either plasma or nonlymphoid cellular elements. Selective lymphocyte removal can be accomplished either by thoracic duct drainage (which strictly speaking is lymphocytapheresis) or by continuous flow cell separators via venous access. Lymphoplasmapheresis is the removal of both plasma and lymphocytes with sparing of nonlymphoid cellular elements.

In addition to the removal of the hyperviscous macroglobulin in Waldenström's macroglobulinemia, plasmapheresis has the theoretic and practical effect of removing pathogenic autoantibodies in diseases such as Goodpasture's syndrome, immune thrombocytopenia, autoimmune hemolytic anemia, myas-

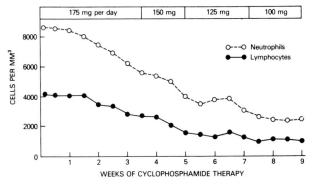

Figure 47–3. Schematic diagram of the use and modification of cyclophosphamide therapy according to the white blood cell count in a patient with Wegener's granulomatosis. The major goal in the treatment of non-neoplastic diseases with cytotoxic agents such as cyclophosphamide is the suppression of disease activity and avoidance of toxic side effects such as significant neutropenia. As shown with the patient indicated in this figure, the dose of drug must be continually modified in accordance with the white blood cell count so as to allow the total white blood cell count to remain above 3000 to 3500 cells per mm³, which generally results in a neutrophil count above 1000 to 1500 cells per mm³. It is essential to realize that the dosage must be decreased as the slope of the white blood cell count declines, since a given dose of drug will be reflected by the white blood cell count several days later. One must anticipate this and modify the dosage so as to arrive smoothly at a maintenance dose of cyclophosphamide, which is almost always lower than the initial induction dose. Once the maintenance dose is reached, the patient will usually be able to tolerate it for several months. However, usually even this dose must ultimately be decreased, as the bone marrow is less able to tolerate the drug over a period of time. Again, this requires frequent and consistent monitoring of the counts throughout the period of drug administration.

thenia gravis, and severe Rh disease.[82–86] Plasmapheresis has been used in the treatment of connective tissue diseases, particularly rheumatoid arthritis and SLE, and to a lesser degree in the treatment of certain of the vasculitic syndromes.[86–90] Given the evidence that lymphocytes appear to be involved in both the initiation and the propagation of the inflammatory responses in rheumatoid arthritis, lymphocytapheresis and lymphoplasmapheresis have been performed in the treatment of this disease.[91, 92] Finally, evidence has indicated that a form of plasmapheresis in which plasma is perfused over immobilized protein A may be effective in inducing tumor rejection in patients with malignant neoplasms by removing serum factors that inhibit rejection.[93] In this regard, the area of selective removal of potentially harmful components of plasma by extracorporeal modification of plasma either by selective absorption, cryogelation, and membrane filtration or by chemical and physical precipitation is under intensive study.[94, 95]

The major rationale for the use of plasmapheresis in the treatment of immune complex–mediated disease such as SLE is the physical removal of the immune complexes from the circulation, making them unavailable for deposition in tissue. A further rationale, however, may relate to abnormalities in reticuloendothelial system (RES) function seen in certain immune complex–mediated diseases such as

SLE.[96] A study has demonstrated that plasmapheresis re-established previously abnormal splenic RES function, and this did not necessarily correlate with immune complex levels.[89] In addition, studies have demonstrated that defective monocyte function improved following plasmapheresis.[97] Hence, the therapeutic efficacy of plasmapheresis may well extend beyond the mere removal of a substance that is directly toxic to tissues.

Plasmapheresis carries with it the potential problem of a rebound in production of antibodies to higher levels than pretreatment by removal of either feedback inhibitory mechanisms or actual suppressor factors.[83] This difficulty, however, is generally obviated because most protocols employing plasmapheresis also call for the simultaneous administration of immunosuppressive agents, which not only synergize with the effects of the plasmapheresis, but also blunt any potential rebound phenomena that might occur.[98]

Plasmapheresis protocols vary considerably in the specific details of the procedure. Current uses of plasmapheresis, however, are usually true plasma exchanges in that large amounts of plasma are removed and replaced by various types of replacement fluids. A commonly used protocol is the performance of plasma exchanges three times per week over a 2- to 6-week period. Each procedure usually lasts from 2 to 4 hours. At each procedure, variable amounts of plasma may be removed, but a relatively standard amount is 40 ml of plasma per kg of body weight or up to 3 liters per exchange. Plasma volume is usually replaced by a combination of albumin and normal saline with or without other fluids such as acid citrate dextrose.[87] Replacement of plasma volume and oncotic pressure are accomplished by these materials.

Theoretically, however, one must at least consider the replacement of other factors, such as Ig, clotting factors, and other proteins. It has been reported that a prolongation of prothrombin, partial thromboplastin, and thrombin times as well as a reduction in fibrinogen, clotting factors, and platelet counts occurred 4 hours after plasmapheresis; however, these all cleared up by 24 hours.[99] The effect of plasmapheresis with albumin replacement on normal plasma constituents was also studied.[100] All plasma constituents were shown to have recovered within 48 hours except fibrinogen, C3, cholesterol, IgG, and IgM. Although fresh frozen plasma is the most physiologic replacement fluid available, as it supplies Ig, coagulation factors, complement, and possibly other factors that might be beneficial to and lacking in the patient, it does carry the risk of transmission of viral disease. Thus, albumin and normal saline remain the standard replacement fluids.

Sakamoto et al.[101] examined the effects of apheresis on a small number of patients with rheumatoid vasculitis and found beneficial responses in a majority of individuals.

Lymphapheresis, like plasmapheresis, has been carried out under a variety of protocols. In one study, lymphapheresis was carried out in a group of patients with rheumatoid arthritis, and each procedure was repeated two to three times per week for a total of 13 to 16 procedures over a 5-week period.[91] A mean of 13.7×10^{10} lymphocytes were removed per patient during the study, and every patient became lymphopenic. Although short periods of lymphapheresis resulted in equal losses of T and B lymphocytes, this extended 5-week course resulted in a disproportionate fall in circulating T lymphocytes by 26 to 58 percent. In addition, serum IgM fell by 30 percent. Clearly significant lymphodepletion with resulting immunosuppression can be achieved with repeated lymphocytapheresis using continuous flow centrifugation.[102] In a double-blind controlled trial of lymphoplasmapheresis versus sham apheresis in patients with rheumatoid arthritis, by the ninth treatment, treated patients had significant reductions in absolute lymphocyte counts; total serum protein; alpha, beta, and gamma globulins; IgG, IgM, IgA; C3; and circulating immune complexes; there were no significant changes in WBC, serum sodium, potassium, or albumin.[92] Of note is the fact that Westergren sedimentation rates fell significantly, as did rheumatoid factor (RF) titers.

Lymphapheresis has for the most part replaced thoracic duct drainage as a modality for removing lymphocytes largely because of the ease, convenience, and relative lack of complications of the former. Significantly favorable and sometimes dramatic clinical responses, however, have been reported in a study of the effects of long-term thoracic duct drainage in a group of patients with autoimmune diseases.[103] Significant degrees of immunosuppression, particularly of T lymphocyte–mediated responses, were noted in the treated patients,[103, 104] and disease was transiently exacerbated in three patients in whom autologous lymphocytes were reinfused.[104]

Detrimental side effects and complications of apheresis include depletion of platelets as well as important components of plasma, such as clotting factors, with resulting bleeding diatheses, hypotension, fluid and electrolyte imbalance, and complications relating to access sites. The potential long-term complications of these procedures are unclear at present.

The long-term therapeutic benefits from apheresis are uncertain, and a number of controlled and uncontrolled studies are being conducted to determine the precise immediate and long-term benefits of this approach in several rheumatic diseases. Several studies have indicated at least a significant short-term clinical improvement in patients with rheumatoid arthritis treated with various apheresis protocols.[82, 91, 92, 101] The situation is less clear in SLE, and a review of the available data indicates no significant benefit of plasmapheresis in the treatment of SLE.[88]

IONIZING RADIATION

Ionizing radiation exerts its effects on tissues by inducing the ionization of atoms, leading to the formation of highly reactive free radicals. These free radicals interact with biologically relevant macromolecules such as DNA.[105] Rapidly dividing cells such as bone marrow, intestinal epithelium, and certain types of lymphocytes appear to be selectively affected by irradiation. However, irradiation may also impair cell function and viability by mechanisms unrelated to the mitotic event.[105]

Ionizing radiation can have profound effects on lymphoid cells, including those involved in the initiation and propagation of immune-mediated connective tissue diseases. The ultimate effect of irradiation on the immune system of the host is highly dependent on the dose delivered. Although this may vary according to the protocol employed, there is generally a gradation of sensitivity of lymphoid subsets as well as lymphoid cells at various stages of differentiation to increasing doses of irradiation.[106] Precursor cells are usually exquisitely sensitive to irradiation. Low doses of irradiation may selectively kill certain subpopulations of T and B lymphocytes while sparing others. Resting or undifferentiated B lymphocytes are quite sensitive to irradiation, whereas fully differentiated plasma cells are rather resistant to the effects of radiation.[107] Among immunoregulatory T lymphocyte subsets, suppressor T lymphocytes are generally more sensitive to irradiation than are helper T lymphocytes.[107] It should be pointed out that the net effect of irradiation on lymphocyte subpopulations in particular and on immune function in general is usually highly dependent on the total dosage and the dosage schedule employed. For example, total body irradiation is profoundly immunosuppressive and is designed to eliminate as extensively as possible the immune competence of the host. The side effects of this modality are extreme and may be fatal. Therefore, this type of radiation protocol is reserved for special clinical circumstances such as preparation for bone marrow transplantation. For this reason, we do not discuss this modality in the present setting.

Total Lymph Node Irradiation

A potentially important advance in the use of radiation therapy for non-neoplastic diseases has been made with the introduction of the use of fractionated total lymph node irradiation in the treatment of rheumatoid arthritis. The rationale for this approach is similar to that described for the use of lymphapheresis in that evidence indicates that lymphocytes, particularly T lymphocytes, appear to be involved in the immunopathogenic expression of rheumatoid arthritis. Total lymph node irradiation has been used for the past 25 years in the treatment of Hodgkin's disease and non-Hodgkin's lymphoma.[108, 109] Of note is the fact that there have been no serious long-term sequelae such as leukemia, second tumors, or serious host defense defects leading to infectious disease complications. Nonetheless, cell-mediated immunity was shown to be suppressed for several years following treatment. Thus, this approach has been employed in the treatment of intractable rheumatoid arthritis as an alternative to the use of cytotoxic agents such as cyclophosphamide and azathioprine.

The results of several studies, including randomized double-blind trials, have demonstrated substantial efficacy in patients with rheumatoid arthritis, employing doses ranging between 750 and 3000 cGy administered over 1 to 4 months.[111-118] Significant side effects were noted, however, especially at higher doses; these adverse effects included viral and bacterial infections, cytopenias, xerostomia, hypothyroidism, cutaneous vasculitis, and pericarditis. Controlled comparisons of irradiation with immunosuppressive therapy are needed to define better the precise role this modality should play in the treatment of advanced rheumatoid arthritis.

Although the usefulness of total lymphoid irradiation in treating other autoimmune disorders has been less well studied, Strober et al.[119] reported improvement in each of ten patients who received irradiation for the treatment of intractable lupus nephritis.

ANTILYMPHOCYTE ANTIBODIES

Standard Antisera

Heterologous antilymphocyte serum (ALS) refers to antiserum raised in one species against lymphocytes to another species. Because such antisera generally contain antibodies directed against cell types other than lymphoid cells, absorption of the serum with nonlymphoid cells is required to make the serum relatively specific for lymphocyte antigens. The serum may then be fractionated to obtain the IgG fraction with antilymphocyte activity; this is referred to as antilymphocyte globulin (ALG). This latter manipulation removes a number of serum factors that might be immunogenic and cause hypersensitivity reactions such as serum sickness.

Because the ultimate target of the ALS is usually T lymphocytes, it would be preferable to have the antiserum react only with T lymphocytes while sparing B lymphocytes. In this regard, further absorptions of the ALS with B lymphocytes may yield an antiserum that is relatively specific for T lymphocytes, i.e., anti–T lymphocyte serum (ATS).

The common denominator of the mechanism of immunosuppression of ALS is a lymphocytopenia. Although ALS bound to lymphocytes in the presence of complement in vitro can cause cytotoxicity[120] and ultimately cell death, the major mechanism of lymphocytopenia in vivo is the selective depletion of circulating T lymphocytes by opsonization and clearance via the RES, predominantly of the liver.[121] It should be pointed out that in the absence of complement, ALS may bind to the lymphocyte and induce blast transformation, and so modulation of lympho-

cyte function can potentially occur, although the net effect is almost invariably the removal of cells from the recirculating pool. The potency of the immunosuppressive effects of a given batch of ALS depends on the relative ability of the antiserum to bind to and induce the clearance of lymphocytes.

ALS has been used extensively in humans as an immunosuppressive agent in recipients of renal allografts with rather impressive results.[122, 123] With regard to the use of ALS in immune-mediated diseases, a number of investigators have employed this agent in uncontrolled trials of the treatment of diseases such as autoimmune hemolytic anemia, myasthenia gravis, multiple sclerosis, and a variety of connective tissue diseases.[120] Although several reports indicated favorable results, the use of ALS in connective tissue diseases has not been extensive, owing to the lack of convincing controlled trials demonstrating its efficacy.

The toxic side effects of ALS preparations have been markedly decreased by the use of meticulous absorption procedures that remove non-Ig proteins, which might increase the incidence of serum sickness, as well as antibodies to a variety of nonlymphoid cells, particularly platelets and erythrocytes. Nonetheless, one must be aware of the considerable potential toxic side effects of the use of ALS. These include fever, chills, arthralgias, and back pain as well as serum sickness and anaphylaxis.[124]

Infectious complications of the immunosuppression include herpes zoster; nephrotoxic nephritis caused by antiglomerular antibodies in the ALS preparation has been reported. Further, the long-range toxic side effects of ALS are unclear at this point, which adds to the reluctance to use these agents widely in the treatment of connective tissue diseases.

Monoclonal Antibodies

Immunologic research was virtually revolutionized by the demonstration by Kohler and Milstein in 1975[125] that somatic cell hybridization could be employed in the immortalization of B lymphocyte lines, producing monoclonal antibody (mAb). This new dimension in immunobiologic analysis witnessed immediate application in immunodiagnosis.[126] The potential for therapeutic use of monoclonal antibodies, however, is clear, and a number of studies are being conducted for the use of these agents in the treatment of certain neoplastic diseases.

Murine monoclonal antibodies against the CD3 pan–T cell determinant have been approved for clinical use in the suppression of acute renal allograft rejection and have been studied in other transplant settings.[127-132] This approach has been shown to be effective for short periods of time, but the development of host antibodies against the murine proteins and the temporary antigenic modulation of the CD3 antigen off the T cell surface have presented obstacles to long-term use of this antibody. Genetically engineered antibodies, created using recombinant DNA techniques to splice murine variable region genes to human constant region genes, may provide a means of avoiding host responses to the foreign antibody. These chimeric or "exon-shuffled" antibodies may also obviate a current problem that murine antibodies are poor activators of human effector mechanisms.[133, 134]

With regard to the use of monoclonal antibodies in the treatment of autoimmune diseases, experimental data have indicated at least the feasibility of employing this approach in animal models of diseases such as experimental allergic encephalitis and myasthenia gravis. Studies are currently under way examining the efficacy of monoclonal antibodies directed against the CD4 lymphocyte determinant in the treatment of rheumatoid arthritis.

In addition to antibodies directed against specific T cell subsets, antibodies directed against other antigens on the surfaces of immune cells make possible additional therapeutic strategies. An example of such an approach is the use of antibodies against the IL-2 receptor in organ transplant recipients.[135–138] Antibodies against human leukocyte antigen (HLA) antigens on the surface of lymphocytes and monocytes also may serve to interrupt the generation of immune responses.[139] Antibodies or cytokines conjugated to cellular toxins such as ricin or diphtheria toxin may lead to specific destruction of those cells bearing the antibody's target molecule or the receptor for the specific cytokine. Toxin-conjugated IL-2 and anti–IL-2 receptor antibodies are currently in clinical trials in patients with rheumatoid arthritis, and over the next several years we will likely see numerous such therapies employed in the treatment of inflammatory disorders.

STEROID HORMONES

Glucocorticoids

Glucocorticoids are used extensively in the treatment of rheumatic diseases. These agents manifest both anti-inflammatory and immunosuppressive effects.[7] Although virtually any function of an inflammatory or immune-competent cell can be suppressed by a high enough concentration of glucocorticoid in vitro, in the dosages of drug that are generally employed in the treatment of rheumatic diseases, the effects of the drug are somewhat selective for one or another of the components of the inflammatory or immune response.[7, 140] For example, the inductive phase of the immune response is clearly more sensitive to the immunosuppressive effects of glucocorticoids than is the effector phase.[7] Further, the T lymphocyte or cell-mediated limb of immunity is clearly more sensitive to glucocorticoids than is the B lymphocyte or humoral limb. In addition, within the T lymphocyte fraction, certain subsets are selectively more sensitive to the drug than are others.[142]

Of particular importance in the understanding of the effects of glucocorticoids on inflammatory and immune competent cells is an appreciation that the drugs can affect the inflammatory and immune response by a number of mechanisms. For example, administration of glucocorticoids may affect the circulatory kinetics of a given cell type such as a neutrophil, monocyte, or lymphocyte subset and thus block the availability of these cells to the inflammatory site without directly suppressing the functional capability of the cell. On the other hand, the drug may directly affect the functional capability of a cell in a situation in which circulatory kinetics are not relevant.[7] In general, lower concentrations of the drug are required to affect circulatory kinetics, whereas higher concentrations are needed to suppress directly a functional capability of a cell.[7] Finally, the effects of glucocorticoids on a given cell type may vary, depending on the state of activation of the cell in question. Understanding these concepts is important in the proper design of therapeutic protocols for the use of glucocorticoids in the treatment of non-neoplastic diseases. A detailed discussion of the use of glucocorticoid therapy is contained in Chapter 48. Nonglucocorticoid hormones, including androgens, estrogens, growth hormone, thyroxine, and insulin, may also exert potent effects on immunoregulation.[143]

CYCLOSPORIN A AND FK506

The fungal products cyclosporin A and FK506 have received considerable attention as immunosuppressive agents for use in preventing and treating rejection in transplant recipients and for the treatment of autoimmune disease. As noted subsequently, these two compounds, although differing in structure, share similarities in their mechanism of action and thus are considered together. The structures of these two molecules are illustrated in Figure 49–4.

Cyclosporin A

Cyclosporin A was discovered in 1972 during a search for biologically produced antifungal agents. It is a 1200-dalton fungal metabolite, which proved to be only mildly active as an antifungal agent but did manifest certain profound effects on the immune response. Cyclosporin A is a cyclic endecapeptide of original chemical structure in which some amino acids are unconventional or modified (N-methylated).[144] This latter property is responsible for the drug's effectiveness by oral administration in that pH and enzymes of the gastrointestinal tract do not seem to inactivate it. It can be administered by both parenteral and oral routes; it exhibits poor water solubility; and it does not need to be activated in vivo, as witnessed by the fact that it is directly active in vitro. The drug has been employed extensively as

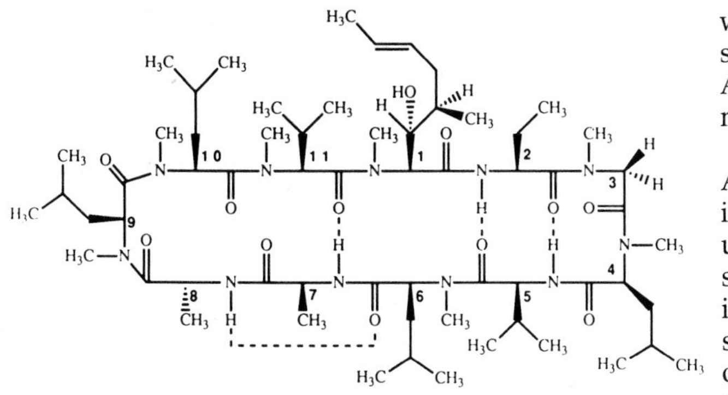

Cyclosporin A

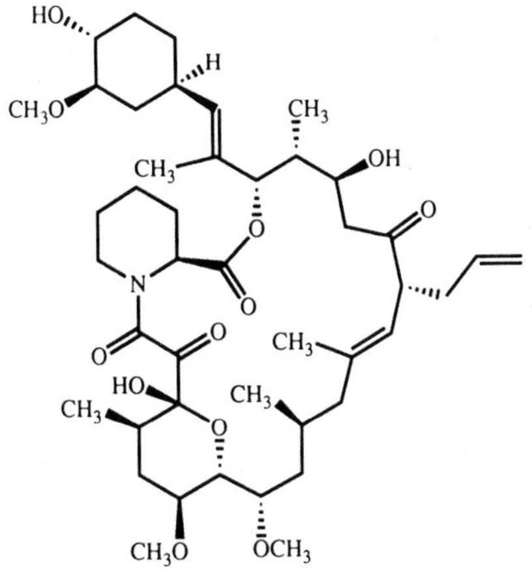

FK 506

Figure 49–4. Structures of the immunosuppressant molecules cyclosporin A and FK506. (Adapted from Sigal, N. H., Siekierka, J. J., and Dumont, F. J.: Observations on the mechanism of action of FK 506. Biochem. Pharmacol. 40:2201, 1990, with permission. Copyright 1990, Pergamon Press Ltd.)

an immunosuppressive agent for organ transplantation.[145] It is administered either as the sole immunosuppressive agent or together with glucocorticoids and other compounds. The optimal dose with regard to efficacy balanced against toxic side effects has not been precisely determined. Studies in patients receiving cadaveric renal transplants, however, have arrived at a dosage of 17 mg per kg per day with gradual tapering by about 2 mg per kg per day decrements at monthly intervals until a maintenance dose of 6 to 8 mg per kg per day is reached. In most protocols, blood levels of cyclosporin A are closely monitored. Because of its nephrotoxicity, cyclosporin is being used in some transplant protocols mainly in the induction phase and to treat acute rejection, whereas conventional immunosuppressive therapy is employed in long-term maintenance.[145–148]

The availability of cyclosporin and the consequent ability of transplant protocols to rely less heavily on other immunosuppressive drugs have virtually revolutionized the field of organ transplantation. The implications of this experience are extraordinary for the use of organ transplantation in a wide variety of clinical situations. In this regard, studies have demonstrated the efficacy of cyclosporin A in suppressing graft-versus-host reactions in bone marrow transplants.[145, 149]

The major constraint in the use of cyclosporin A, as with other immunosuppressive agents, lies in its toxicity. Although it has few myelotoxic effects, use of the agent is not without risks. By far the most serious toxic side effect of the drug is its nephrotoxicity.[145, 150–153] This toxic side effect is particularly serious in a renal transplantation program, since it is often unclear whether a deterioration in renal function is due to insufficient drug, allowing rejection to occur, or to too much cyclosporin A, causing nephrotoxicity. Other toxic side effects include abnormalities of liver function test results, transient hirsutism, and gum hypertrophy. Bacterial infection has not been a problem with the use of this drug. Reactivation of certain viral infections, however, particularly Epstein-Barr virus, has occurred sporadically. Of note is the fact that lymphomas have occurred in patients treated with cyclosporin A and were believed to result from the immunosuppressive effects rather than from any carcinogenicity of the drug.[154]

Of particular interest for the present discussion is the potential for the use of cyclosporin A in the treatment of rheumatic diseases characterized by hyper-reactivity or aberrant immune function at the T lymphocyte level. A number of studies have extended the potential role of cyclosporin to the treatment of autoimmune diseases. Nussenblatt et al.[155–157] have been successful in treating uveitis with cyclosporin in patients whose ocular disease had been resistant to glucocorticoids and cytotoxic agents. Van Rijthoven et al.[158] examined the effect of cyclosporin in 36 patients with rheumatoid arthritis in a double-blind, placebo-controlled trial. They noted that treated patients experienced significant improvement in joint disease compared with their condition on entering the study and in comparison to the placebo group. In subsequent studies, Dougados and Amor[159] and Weinblatt et al.[160] confirmed the efficacy of cyclosporin in refractory rheumatoid arthritis. In all of these investigations, use of the drug was frequently limited by toxicity.

Additionally, more limited investigations have suggested that cyclosporin may be useful in the treatment of diverse immune-mediated disorders such as autoimmune chronic active hepatitis,[161] pulmonary sarcoidosis,[162] inflammatory bowel disease,[163–165] bullous pemphigoid,[166] psoriasis,[167, 168] ichthyosis,[169] Graves' ophthalmopathy,[170] and primary biliary cirrhosis.[171] Significant interest has focused on the use of cyclosporin in the treatment of type 1 diabetes mellitus, in which an autoimmune component is frequently present.[172]

Although the need for additional carefully controlled trials of cyclosporin in the treatment of inflammatory disorders is clear, it is evident that this potent drug will likely prove to be extremely useful in patients with rheumatic and autoimmune diseases.

FK506

FK506 is a macrolide produced by the fungus *Streptomyces tukubaensis*.[173, 174] In vitro and in vivo studies have suggested that FK506 has immunosuppressant effects comparable to those of cyclosporin but at doses 10 to 100 times lower.[175] Studies of organ transplantation in a variety of animal models have demonstrated that this compound is extremely effective in preventing rejection, although these studies have been hampered by the development of toxicities that may be unique to the species studied, including the interesting finding in dogs of arteritis and lymphocytic infiltration of organs.[176] These toxicities have not been observed in primates or in human studies.

Clinical studies of FK506 in human liver transplantation were begun in 1989, and the Pittsburgh group has reported remarkable success in their early trials.[177] Additional trials are ongoing at a number of medical centers around the world.

Toxicities of FK506 in human transplant recipients have been remarkably few. In one study of 31 liver transplant recipients, 87 percent of patients reported no side effects.[178] Some individuals experienced headache and insomnia. Other investigators, however, have noted the occurrence of nephrotoxicity and hyperglycemia[179] in individuals receiving FK506.

Information has begun to appear in the literature regarding the potential efficacy of FK506 in inflammatory disorders. In animal studies, the compound has proved effective in treating collagen-induced arthritis,[180] nephrotoxic serum glomerulonephritis,[181] autoimmune uveoretinitis,[182] autoimmune encephalomyelitis,[183] and autoimmune disease in MRL/lpr and (NZB × NZW) F1 mice.[184]

Data on the use of FK506 in the treatment of human autoimmune disease are more limited, but case reports suggesting efficacy in the treatment of cyclosporin-induced hemolytic uremic syndrome following organ transplantation[185] and in steroid-resistant focal sclerosing glomerulonephritis[186] have been published.

Molecular Mechanism of Action of Cyclosporin A and FK506

These two compounds and related ones such as rapamycin appear to function via binding to novel cellular proteins with specific binding properties.[187] The binding proteins, termed *immunophilins,* have been described, and insights into the biology of these proteins and their ligands have significantly advanced our understanding of the activation of immune cells.

The major cyclosporin A binding protein cyclophilin and the predominant FK506 binding protein (FKBP) are enzymes with peptidyl-prolyl isomerase activity, important in catalyzing the interconversion of cis-rotamers and trans-rotamers of amide bonds in cellular peptides and proteins.[187]

Cyclosporin A and FK506 share the feature of being potent inhibitors of T cell activation, and in particular they inhibit the transcription of early T cell activation genes.[188, 189] These genes include IL-2, IL-3, IL-4, granulocyte-macrophage colony-stimulating factor (GM-CSF), tumor necrosis factor alpha (TNF-α), and interferon gamma (γ). The mechanism of this action appears to be interference of the binding of the nuclear regulatory factor NF-AT to its target region in the enhancer region of these inducible genes.[188, 189] Binding of other nuclear factors may be similarly affected.

The immunologic effects of cyclosporin A and FK506 are complex but appear to be specific for lymphocytes. Numerous studies have demonstrated the ability of cyclosporin A to block the activation of T lymphocytes,[190] and effects on B cells are also likely.[191]

OTHER AGENTS

Levamisole

Levamisole is a three-ring molecule with the extremely low molecular weight of 241. It was introduced into veterinary practice in 1966 as a nematocidal agent and was subsequently used in humans. It is highly active against a wide range of nematodes and is particularly effective in ascariasis. It has, however, received attention as an immunoenhancing agent in humans. Levamisole is absorbed rapidly from the gastrointestinal tract. Following administration of a 150-mg dose in humans, peak blood levels of 5 μg per ml are reached at 2 hours.[192] The plasma half-life is approximately 4 hours, and the drug is metabolized predominantly in the liver, with excretion of the breakdown products via the kidney and to a lesser extent in the feces.

The mechanism of action of levamisole remains in doubt, but it has a number of well-recognized immunologic effects. These include correction of chemotactic defects of monocytes[193] and neutrophils[194] from patients with viral infections or the hyperimmunoglobulin E syndrome,[195] enhancement of delayed-type hypersensitivity,[196] and enhancement of a variety of lymphocyte functions.[197]

Levamisole has been used in malignant diseases as an adjuvant agent, most notably gastrointestinal carcinomas,[198] and it has been approved by the Food and Drug Administration for this purpose; it has also been used in a number of nonmalignant diseases. Of particular interest has been its use in the treatment of rheumatoid arthritis in which rather favorable clinical responses have been reported.[199, 200] The drug is generally administered in doses of 150 mg orally on a daily basis for periods up to 16 weeks. The major constraint of its use clinically is the incidence and severity of the toxic side effects. Side effects of the drug have included gastrointestinal disturbances, fatigue, fever, and skin rash. The most severe and limiting toxic side effect, however, is granulocytopenia, which seems to be disproportionately more frequent in patients with rheumatic diseases. It is of particular interest that agranulocytosis owing to levamisole is particularly common in patients with HLA-B27.[201, 202] In a study of the treatment of 20 rheumatoid arthritis patients with levamisole, agranulocytosis or neutropenia occurred at some time in four patients. Despite the favorable clinical results with regard to the activity of rheumatoid arthritis in that study, the toxicity clearly renders the drug unacceptable for routine use in rheumatoid arthritis.

Other Immune Enhancers and Adjuvants

Clearly the most extensively employed adjuvant in experimental animals is complete Freund's adjuvant (CFA), which is composed of paraffin oil and an emulsifying agent to which killed mycobacteria have been added. Injection of emulsions of antigens in CFA into experimental animals results in markedly augmented antibody responses as well as delayed hypersensitivity.[203] Unfortunately, the severe local and systemic toxic side effects of CFA render it unacceptable for use in humans. Preparations of adjuvants such as the synthetic N-acetylmuramyl-L-alanyl-D-isoglutamine have been shown to be effective enhancers of antibody production without appreciable toxic side effects.[204] Such studies may prove extremely fruitful in the ultimate development of a clinically acceptable adjuvant, which could be used in the enhancement of immune function in the absence of significant toxic side effects.

Dapsone

Dapsone is a sulfone (4,4'-diaminodiphenyl sulfone) and first gained attention as an agent effective in the treatment of *Mycobacterium leprae*. It has been recognized as an effective agent in the treatment of dermatitis herpetiformis[205] and erythema elevatum diutinum[206] as well as the bullous eruptions of SLE.[207] Dapsone is available for oral administration and is slowly and nearly completely absorbed from the gastrointestinal tract. Peak concentrations of dapsone are reached in plasma 1 to 3 hours after oral administration, and its half-life ranges from 10 to 50 hours, with a mean of 28 hours.[208] Twenty-four hours after an oral dose of 100 mg, plasma concentrations range from 0.4 to 1.2 μg per ml. The sulfones are distributed throughout the total body water and are present in all tissues. They tend to be retained in skin, muscle, liver, and kidney, with traces of the drug present in these organs up to 3 weeks after cessation of administration. Dapsone is acetylated in the liver, and about 70 to 80 percent of a dose is excreted in the urine.

The drug is administered orally in doses of 50 to 100 mg per day. The effect is seen within days, and particularly with erythema elevatum diutinum, relapses occur almost immediately after cessation of the drug,[206] which is somewhat paradoxical given that the drug is present in organs for weeks after cessation of therapy. The sudden relapses following cessation might be explained by a need for a critical concentration of drug in plasma below which a dramatic deterioration in clinical condition is seen.

The limiting factor in the use of dapsone is its toxicity, which includes hemolysis and methemoglobinemia and which occurs relatively frequently. Other side effects include anorexia, nausea, and vomiting. Rarely, headache, nervousness, insomnia, and peripheral neuropathy have been reported.

Interferons

The interferons are relatively small glycoproteins that inhibit the multiplication of certain viruses. They first attracted significant attention because of their potential antiviral activities. They are elaborated from virus-infected cells and protect noninfected cells from viral infection.[209] They induce a transient state of refractoriness to viral infection by altering nucleotide metabolism and cytoplasmic enzyme induction.[209] It soon became clear, however, that in addition to their antiviral properties, interferons had significant effects on cell differentiation, cell growth, expression of surface antigens, cellular morphology, and, most importantly for the purposes of this discussion, immunoregulation.[209, 210]

In general, interferon γ is much more potent in its immunoregulatory effects than are the other interferons. It should be pointed out that in the evaluation of the effects of interferon on the immune system, one must be aware that the type and degree of effect may be heavily dependent on the time and dose of interferon used in both in vivo and in vitro studies.[211]

The relatively recent availability of recombinant interferons has made possible the study of the potential therapeutic efficacy of these compounds in disorders of immunoregulation. Interferon γ has been used successfully to abrogate the defective bactericidal activity of cells from patients with chronic granulomatous disease, a congenital disorder of oxidative metabolism.[212, 213] The mechanism of its effect in this setting is not clear, but studies suggest that both oxidative and nonoxidative killing mechanisms are stimulated by interferon γ administration.[212]

An interesting study by Kahan et al.[214] suggests that recombinant interferon γ may have a beneficial effect on the cutaneous fibrotic abnormalities in patients with systemic sclerosis. These investigators demonstrated a significant improvement in overall skin thickening, maximal oral opening, joint range of motion, creatinine clearance, and other parameters after 6 months of daily intramuscular treatment with

Table 49–6. PHARMACOLOGIC PROPERTIES OF IMMUNOREGULATORY AGENTS

Agent	Administration	Dosage	Gastrointestinal Absorption	Plasma Half-life	Major Side Effects
Cytotoxic Agents					
Nitrogen mustard	IV	0.4 mg/kg q 3–4 weeks	—	Few minutes	Leukopenia, thrombocytopenia, nausea, vomiting, local reactions at injection site
Cyclophosphamide	IV or oral	2 mg/kg/day orally or IV; 750 mg/m² IV bolus	Excellent	6–7 hours	Neutropenia, gonadal suppression, cystitis, alopecia, oncogenesis, pulmonary fibrosis, gastrointestinal intolerance
Chlorambucil	IV or oral	0.1–0.2 mg/kg/day orally	Good	90 minutes	Leukopenia, thrombocytopenia, oncogenesis, gonadal suppression, gastrointestinal intolerance, hepatotoxicity, dermatitis
Azathioprine and 6-mercaptopurine	IV or oral	2 mg/kg/day orally	Excellent	60–90 minutes	Leukopenia, hepatotoxicity, gastrointestinal intolerance, oncogenesis, host defense defect
Methotrexate	IV or oral	5–50 mg/week as single IV dose or orally in 3 divided doses (q 12 hours) or orally daily for 5 days of the week	Intermittent to good	2 hours	Leukopenia, thrombocytopenia, oral mucositis, gastrointestinal intolerance, hepatotoxicity, fetal intolerance in first trimester of pregnancy
Vinca alkaloids (vincristine and vinblastine)	IV	2 mg/m²	—	Less than 30 minutes	Neurotoxicity
5-Fluorouracil	IV	12 mg/kg/day for 4 days followed by 6 mg/kg on alternate days for 2–4 doses; repeat monthly with adjustment of dose according to response	Unpredictable	10–20 minutes	Leukopenia, gastrointestinal intolerance, alopecia, dermatitis, mucositis
Hydroxyurea	IV or oral	20–30 mg/kg/day orally	Good	6–8 hours	Myelosuppression, gastrointestinal intolerance and ulcerations, mild skin rashes
Other Agents					
Levamisole	Oral	Up to 150 mg/day	Excellent	4 hours	Granulocytopenia, gastrointestinal intolerance, fever, skin rash, fatigue
Cyclosporin A	IV or oral	17 mg/kg/day with monthly tapering until maintenance dose of 6–8 mg/kg/day is reached	Fair to good	2–24 hours	Nephrotoxicity, hepatotoxicity, reactivation of viral infections, oncogenesis, transient hirsutism, gum hypertrophy
FK506	IV, SC, oral	~0.3 mg/kg/day	Good		Headache, insomnia, nephrotoxicity, hyperglycemia
Interferons					
IFN-α	SC or IM	10–100 g/day	—		Fever, fatigue, others to be determined
IFN-γ	IM	Variable	—		Fever, nausea, vomiting, diarrhea, leukopenia, myocardial infarction, others to be determined
Dapsone	Oral	50–100 mg/day	Good	10–50 hours	Hemolysis, methemoglobinemia, gastrointestinal intolerance

interferon γ. Although provocative, these observations need to be confirmed in randomized, blinded, controlled trials incorporating larger numbers of patients. A double-blind, placebo-controlled trial showed no significant benefit in the treatment of 105 patients with rheumatoid arthritis,[215] despite animal studies in collagen-induced arthritis in which some benefit was found.[216]

Interferon γ has also been used for monocyte activation in the acquired immunodeficiency syndrome.[217]

Administration of interferon α has been shown to be of some therapeutic value in certain viral infections, including those due to herpes zoster and hepatitis B virus,[209, 218, 219] and in chronic non-A, non-B hepatitis.[220] It has also been shown to be efficacious in the treatment of neoplasms such as hairy cell leukemia, in which it has been extremely effective, and Kaposi's sarcoma in the setting of the acquired immunodeficiency syndrome.[223–225]

Interleukin-2

The availability of recombinant IL-2 has led to wider investigation of use of this T cell–derived lymphokine as an immunostimulatory agent in the treatment of neoplasms and immunodeficiencies. To date, IL-2 has not found application in the treatment of rheumatic disorders.

Transforming Growth Factor-beta and Retinoids

Transforming growth factor-beta (TGF-β) is a homodimeric 25-kilodalton peptide with several molecular forms and a variety of actions, including both promotion and inhibition of growth and differentiation, in different systems.[226] Among its many biologic actions are potent immunosuppressive properties, leading to the possibility that it may be a useful clinical immunosuppressant in the near future. The retinoids are a group of small molecules, related to vitamin A, with immunosuppressive properties. Several lines of evidence suggest that their immunomodulatory actions may be mediated via the action of TGF-β,[226] and they may become important therapeutic agents in the near future.

A summary of certain of the pharmacologic properties of several of the immunoregulatory agents discussed in this chapter is given in Table 49–6.

CONCLUSIONS

The use of cytotoxic and immunoregulatory agents has played a major role in the treatment of non-neoplastic, immune-mediated disease. Most of these agents are nonspecific, however, and are invariably associated with a variety of toxic side effects. Because most of the rheumatic diseases in which

these agents are used are chronic in nature and are rarely curable, the physician must establish the clear-cut goals of a given therapeutic regimen and must be aware of the actual as well as the potential and the immediate as well as the long-term toxic side effects of these agents. Insightful use of these agents under appropriate clinical circumstances can often lead to dramatic improvements in the clinical course as well as gratifying improvements in lifestyle. Under other circumstances, the effects may even be life-saving. Use of these agents, however, should be avoided in circumstances in which a less aggressive approach would be more appropriate given the nature of the illness and the projected balance between clinical results and toxic side effects. The treating physician should be acquainted as much as possible with the established results of controlled trials as they appear in the literature and should critically evaluate uncontrolled trials, which may represent a true advance in therapy but which may also give a false sense of security that a particular agent will be beneficial. All things considered, sound clinical judgment applied to each individual patient with regard to the choice and actual usage of an immunoregulatory agent is indispensable.

References

1. Fauci, A. S.: Immunoregulation in autoimmunity. J. Allergy Clin. Immunol. 66:5, 1980.
2. NIAID Group: New Initiatives in Immunology Report. Bethesda, MD, National Institute of Allergy and Infectious Diseases. DHHS Publication No. (NIH) 81–2215:1, 1981.
3. Paul, W. E.: The immune system: An introduction. In Paul W. E. (ed.): Fundamental Immunology. 2nd ed. New York, Raven Press, 1989.
4. Fauci, A. S.: The revolution in clinical immunology. J.A.M.A. 246:2567, 1981.
5. Fauci, A. S., Lane, H. C., and Volkman, D. J.: Activation and regulation of human immune responses: Implications in normal and disease states. Ann. Intern. Med. 98:76, 1983.
6. Steinberg, A. D., Plotz, P. H., Wolff, S. M., Wong, V. G., Agus, S. G., and Decker, J. L.: Cytotoxic drugs in treatment of nonmalignant diseases. Ann. Intern. Med. 76:619, 1972.
7. Fauci, A. S., Dale, D. C., and Balow, J. E.: Glucocorticosteroid therapy: Mechanisms of action and clinical considerations. Ann. Intern. Med. 84:304, 1976.
8. Gerber, N. L., and Steinberg, A. D.: Clinical use of immunosuppressive drugs. Part I. Drugs 11:36, 1976.
9. Gerber, N. L., and Steinberg, A. D.: Clinical use of immunosuppressive drugs. Part II. Drugs 11:90, 1976.
10. Handschumacher, R. E.: Immunosuppressive agents. In Gilman A. G., Rall, T. W., Nies, A. S., and Taylor, P. (eds.): Goodman and Gilman's The Pharmacologic Basis of Therapeutics. 8th ed. New York, Pergamon Press, 1990.
11. Cooper, M. D., Peterson, R. D. A., South, M. A., and Good, R. A.: Delineation of the thymus system and the bursa system in the chicken. Nature 205:143, 1965.
12. Cooper, M. D., Peterson, R. D. A., South, M. A., and Good, R. A.: The functions of the thymus system and the bursa system in the chicken. J. Exp. Med. 123:75, 1966.
13. Claman, H. N., Chaperon, E. A., and Triplett, R. F.: Thymus-marrow cell combinations. Synergism in antibody production. Proc. Soc. Exp. Biol. Med. 12:1167, 1966.
14. Miller, J. F. A. P., and Mitchell, G. F.: Cell-cell interactions in immune response. I. Hemolysin-forming cells in neonatally thymectomized mice reconstituted with thymus or thoracic duct lymphocytes. J. Exp. Med. 128:801, 1968.
15. Unanue, E. R.: Macrophages, antigen-presenting cells, and the phenomena of antigen handling and presentation. In Paul W. E. (ed.): Fundamental Immunology. 2nd ed. New York, Raven Press, 1989.
16. Möller, G. (ed.): Natural killer cells. Immunol. Rev. 44:1, 1979.

17. Herberman, R. B., and Ortaldo, J. R.: Natural killer cells: Their role in defenses against disease. Science 214:24, 1981.
18. Gallin, J. I., and Fauci, A. S. (eds.): Advances in Host Defense Mechanisms. Vol. 1. New York, Raven Press, 1982.
19. Jerne, N. K.: Towards a network theory of the immune system. Ann. Immunol. (Inst. Pasteur) 125:373, 1974.
20. Möller, G. (ed.): Idiotypes on T and B cells. Immunol. Rev. 34:1, 1977.
21. Geha, R. S.: Presence of auto-anti-idiotypic antibody during the normal human immune response to tetanus toxoid antigen. J. Immunol. 129:139, 1982.
22. Abdou, N. I., Wall, H., Lindsley, H. B., Halsey, J. F., and Suzuki, T.: Network theory in autoimmunity. In vitro suppression of serum anti-DNA antibody binding to DNA by anti-idiotypic antibody in systemic lupus erythematosus. J. Clin. Invest. 67:1297, 1981.
23. Hodes, R. J.: T-cell–mediated regulation: Help and suppression. In Paul, W. E. (ed.): Fundamental Immunology. 2nd ed. New York, Raven Press, 1989.
24. Fauci, A. S., Haynes, B. F., and Katz, P.: The spectrum of vasculitis: Clinical, pathologic, immunologic, and therapeutic considerations. Ann. Intern. Med. 89:660, 1978.
25. Fauci, A. S., Haynes, B. F., Katz, P., and Wolff, S. M.: Wegener's granulomatosis: Prospective clinical and therapeutic experience with 85 patients over 21 years. Ann. Intern. Med. 98:76, 1983.
26. Cupps, T. R., and Fauci, A. S.: The vasculitides. In Smith, L. H. (ed.): Major Problems in Internal Medicine. Vol. XXI. Philadelphia, W. B. Saunders Company, 1981.
27. Cupps, T. R., Edgar, L. C., and Fauci, A. S.: Suppression of human B lymphocyte function by cyclophosphamide. J. Immunol. 128:2453, 1982.
28. Farrar, J. J., Benjamin, W. R., Hilfiker, M. L., Howard, M., Farrar, W. L., and Fuller-Farrar, J.: The biochemistry, biology, and role of interleukin-2 in the induction of cytotoxic T cell and antibody-forming B cell responses. Immunol. Rev. 63:129, 1982.
29. Fauci, A. S., Katz, P., Haynes, B. F., and Wolff, S. M.: Cyclophosphamide therapy of severe necrotizing vasculitis. N. Engl. J. Med. 301:235, 1979.
30. Austin, H. A., III, Klippel, H. H., Balow, J. E., le Riche, N. G., and Steinberg, A. D.: Therapy of lupus nephritis: Controlled trial of prednisone and cytotoxic drugs. N. Engl. J. Med. 314:614, 1986.
31. Decker, J. L.: Toxicity of immunosuppressive drugs in man. Arthritis Rheum. 16:89, 1973.
32. Schein, P. S., and Winokur, S. T.: Immunosuppressive and cytotoxic chemotherapy: Long-term complications. Ann. Intern. Med. 82:84, 1975.
33. Calabresi, P., Chabner, B. A.: Antineoplastic agents. In Gilman, A. G., Rall, T. W., Nies, A. S., and Taylor, P. (eds.): Goodman and Gilman's The Pharmacologic Basis of Therapeutics. 8th ed. New York, Pergamon Press, 1990.
34. Ahn, Y. S., Harrington, W. J., Seelman, R. C., and Eytel, C. S.: Vincristine therapy of idiopathic and secondary thrombocytopenias. N. Engl. J. Med. 291:376, 1974.
35. Fauci, A. S., Harley, J. B., Roberts, W. C., Ferrans, V. J., Gralnick, H. R., and Bjornson, B. J.: The idiopathic hypereosinophilic syndrome: Clinical, pathologic and therapeutic considerations. Ann. Intern. Med. 97:78, 1982.
36. Roberts, J. J., Brent, T. P., and Crathorn, A. R.: Evidence for the inactivation and repair of the mammalian DNA template after alkylation by mustard gas and half mustard gas. Eur. J. Cancer 7:515, 1971.
37. Fahey, J. L., Leonard, E., Churg, J., and Godman, G.: Wegener's granulomatosis. Am. J. Med. 17:168, 1954.
38. Brock, N.: Pharmacologic characterization of cyclophosphamide (NSC-26271) and cyclophosphamide metabolites. Cancer Chemother. Rep. 51:315, 1967.
39. Bagley, C. M., Bostick, F. W., and DeVita, V. T., Jr.: Clinical pharmacology of cyclophosphamide. Cancer Res. 33:226, 1973.
40. Gershwin, M. E., Goetzel, E. J., and Steinberg, A. D.: Cyclophosphamide: Use in practice. Ann. Intern. Med. 80:531, 1974.
41. Sladek, N. E.: Therapeutic efficacy of cyclophosphamide as a function of its metabolism. Cancer Res. 32:535, 1972.
42. Makinodan, T., Santos, G. W., and Quinn, R. P.: Immunosuppressive drugs. Pharmacol. Rev. 22:189, 1970.
43. Shand, F. L.: The immunopharmacology of cyclophosphamide. Int. J. Pharmacol. 1:165, 1979.
44. Berenbaum, M. C., and Brown, I. N.: Dose-response relationships for agents inhibiting the immune response. Immunology 7:65, 1964.
45. Askenase, P. W., Hayden, B. J., and Gershon, R. K.: Augmentation of delayed-type hypersensitivity by doses of cyclophosphamide which do not effect antibody responses. J. Exp. Med. 141:697, 1965.
46. Sy, M. S., Miller, S. D., and Claman, H. N.: Immune suppression with supraoptimal doses of antigen in contact sensitivity. I. Demonstration of suppressor cells and their sensitivity to cyclophosphamide. J. Immunol. 119:240, 1977.
47. Fauci, A. S., Wolff, S. M., and Johnson, J. S.: Effect of cyclophosphamide upon the immune response in Wegener's granulomatosis. N. Engl. J. Med. 285:1493, 1972.

48. Fauci, A. S., Dale, D. C., and Wolff, S. M.: Cyclophosphamide and lymphocyte subpopulations in Wegener's granulomatosis. Arthritis Rheum. 17:355, 1974.
49. Dale, D. C., Fauci, A. S., and Wolff, S. M.: The effect of cyclophosphamide on leukocyte kinetics and susceptibility to infection in patients with Wegener's granulomatosis. Arthritis Rheum. 16:657, 1973.
50. Hoffman, G. S., Leavitt, R. Y., Fleisher, T. A., Minor, J. R., and Fauci, A. S.: Treatment of Wegener's granulomatosis with intermittent high-dose intravenous cyclophosphamide. Am. J. Med. 89:403, 1990.
51. Warne, G. L., Fairley, K. F., Hobbs, J. B., and Martin, F. I. R.: Cyclophosphamide-induced ovarian failure. N. Engl. J. Med. 289:1159, 1973.
52. Schilsky, R. L., Lewis, B. J., Sherins, R. J., and Young, R. C.: Gonadal dysfunction in patients receiving chemotherapy for cancer. Ann. Intern. Med. 93:109, 1980.
53. Trompeter, R. S., Evans, P. R., and Barratt, T. M.: Gonadal function in boys with steroid-responsive nephrotic syndrome treated with cyclophosphamide for short periods. Lancet 1:1177, 1981.
54. Fairley, K. F., Barrie, J. U., and Johnson, W.: Sterility and testicular atrophy related to cyclophosphamide therapy. Lancet 1:568, 1972.
55. Plotz, P. H., Klippel, J. H., Decker, J. L., et al.: Bladder complications in patients receiving cyclophosphamide for systemic lupus erythematosus or rheumatoid arthritis. Ann. Intern. Med. 91:221, 1979.
56. Cooper, J. A. D., Jr., White, D. A., and Matthay, R. A.: State of the art: Drug-induced pulmonary disease. Am. Rev. Respir. Dis. 133:321, 1986.
57. Appelbaum, F. R., Strauchen, J. A., Graw, R. G., Jr., et al.: Acute lethal carditis caused by high-dose combination chemotherapy. A unique clinical and pathological entity. Lancet 1:58, 1976.
58. De Fronzo, R. A., Braine, H., Colvin, O. M., and Davis, P. J.: Water intoxication in man after cyclophosphamide therapy. Time course and relation to drug activation. Ann. Intern. Med. 78:861, 1973.
59. Bressler, R. B., and Huston, D. T.: Water intoxication following moderate-dose intravenous cyclophosphamide. Arch. Intern. Med. 145:548, 1985.
60. Penn, I.: Depressed immunity and the development of cancer. Clin. Exp. Immunol. 45:459, 1981.
61. McLean, A., Newell, J., and Baker, G.: The metabolism of chlorambucil. Biochem. Pharmacol. 25:2331, 1976.
62. Stukov, A. N.: Experimental study of the combined effect of leukoran, degranol, and prednisolone. Neoplasma 22:181, 1976.
63. Israel, H., and Patchefsky, A. S.: Treatment of Wegener's granulomatosis of lung. Am. J. Med. 58:671, 1975.
64. Rudd, P., Fried, J. F., and Epstein, W. V.: Irreversible bone marrow failure with chlorambucil. J. Rheumatol. 2:421, 1975.
65. Cameron, S.: Chlorambucil and leukemia. N. Engl. J. Med. 296:1065, 1977.
66. Lerner, H. J.: Acute myelogenous leukemia in patients receiving chlorambucil as long-term adjuvant chemotherapy for Stage II breast cancer. Cancer Treat. Rep. 60:1431, 1978.
67. Gabrielsen, A. E., and Good, R. A.: Chemical suppression of adaptive immunity. Adv. Immunol. 6:91, 1967.
68. Yu, D. T., Clements, P. J., Peter, J. B., Levy, J., Paulus, H. E., and Barnett, E. V.: Lymphocyte characteristics in rheumatic patients and the effect of azathioprine therapy. Arthritis Rheum. 17:37, 1974.
69. Levy, J., Barnett, E. V., MacDonald, N. S., Klinenberg, J. R., and Pearson, C. M.: The effect of azathioprine on gammaglobulin synthesis in man. J. Clin. Invest. 51:2233, 1972.
70. Maibach, H. I., and Epstein, W. L.: Immunologic responses of healthy volunteers receiving azathioprine (Imuran). Int. Arch. Allergy 27:102, 1965.
71. Abdou, N. I., Zweiman, B., and Casella, S. R.: Effects of azathioprine therapy on bone marrow-dependent and thymus-dependent cells in man. Clin. Exp. Immunol. 13:55, 1973.
72. Fournier, C., Bach, M. A., Dardenne, M., and Bach, J. F.: Selective action of azathioprine on T cells. Transplant. Proc. 5:523, 1973.
73. Campbell, A. C., Skinner, J. M., Hersey, P., Roberts-Thompson, P., MacLennan, I. C. M., and Truelove, S. C.: Immunosuppression in the treatment of inflammatory bowel disease. I. Changes in lymphoid subpopulations in the blood and rectal mucosa following cessation of treatment with azathioprine. Clin. Exp. Immunol. 16:521, 1974.
74. Sharbaugh, R. J., Ainsworth, S. K., and Fitts, C. T.: Lack of effect of azathioprine on phytohemagglutinin-induced lymphocyte transformation and established delayed cutaneous hypersensitivity. Int. Arch. Allergy Appl. Immunol. 51:681, 1976.
75. Gassman, A. E., and van Furth, R.: The effect of azathioprine (Imuran) on the kinetics of monocytes and macrophages during the normal steady state and an acute inflammatory reaction. Blood 46:51, 1975.
76. Phillips, S. M., and Zweiman, B.: Mechanisms in the suppression of delayed hypersensitivity in the guinea pig by 6-mercaptopurine. J. Exp. Med. 137:1494, 1973.
77. Rosman, M., and Bertino, J. R.: Azathioprine. Ann. Intern. Med. 79:694, 1973.
78. Losito, A., Williams, D. G., and Harris, L.: The effects on polymor-

phonuclear leukocyte function of prednisolone and azathioprine in vivo and prednisolone, azathioprine and 6-mercaptopurine in vitro. Clin. Exp. Immunol. 32:423, 1978.

79. Henderson, F. S., Adamson, R. H., and Oliverio, V. T.: The metabolic rate of tritiated methotrexate. II. Absorption and excretion in man. Cancer Res. 25:1018, 1965.

80. Ahn, Y. S., Byrnes, J. J., Harrington, W. J., et al.: The treatment of idiopathic thrombocytopenia with vinblastine-loaded platelets. N. Engl. J. Med. 298:1101, 1978.

81. Cupps, T. R., Silverman, G. J., and Fauci, A. S.: Herpes zoster in patients with treated Wegener's granulomatosis. A possible role for cyclophosphamide. Am. J. Med. 69:881, 1980.

82. Tindall, R. S. A. (ed.): Therapeutic Apheresis and Plasma Perfusion. New York, A. R. Liss, Inc., 1980.

83. Branda, R. F., Molodow, C. F., McCollough, J. J., and Jacob, H. S.: Plasma exchange in the treatment of immune disease. Transfusion 5:570, 1975.

84. Lockwood, C. M., Pearson, T. A., Rees, A. J., Evans, D. J., Peters, D. K., and Wilson, C. B.: Immunosuppression and plasma exchange in the treatment of Goodpasture's syndrome. Lancet 1:711, 1976.

85. Pinching, A. J., Peters, D. K., and Newsom Davis, J.: Remission of myasthenia gravis following plasma-exchange. Lancet 2:1373, 1976.

86. Vogler, W. R.: Therapeutic apheresis: Where we've been and where we are going. In Tindall, R. S. A. (ed.): Therapeutic Apheresis and Plasma Perfusion. New York, A. R. Liss, Inc., 1980.

87. Wallace, D. J., Goldfinger, D., Gatti, R., et al.: Plasmapheresis and lymphoplasmapheresis in the management of rheumatoid arthritis. Arthritis Rheum. 22:703, 1979.

88. Balow, J. E., and Tsokos, G. C.: Plasmapheresis in systemic lupus erythematosus: Facts and perspectives. Int. J. Artif. Organs 5:286, 1982.

89. Lockwood, C. M., Worlledge, S., Nicholas, A., Cotton, D., and Peters, D. K.: Reversal of impaired splenic function in patients with nephritis or vasculitis (or both) by plasma exchange. N. Engl. J. Med. 300:524, 1979.

90. Kauffmann, R. H., and Houwert, D. A.: Plasmapheresis in rapidly progressive Henoch-Schoenlein glomerulonephritis and the effect on circulating IgA immune complexes. Clin. Nephrol. 16:155, 1982.

91. Karsh, J., Klippel, J. H., Plotz, P. H., Decker, J. L., Wright, D. G., and Flye, M. W.: Lymphapheresis in rheumatoid arthritis. A randomized trial. Arthritis Rheum. 24:867, 1981.

92. Wallace, D., Goldfinger, D., Lowe, C., et al.: A double-blind controlled study of lymphoplasmapheresis versus sham apheresis in rheumatoid arthritis. N. Engl. J. Med. 306:1406, 1982.

93. Terman, D. S., Young, J. B., Shearer, W. T., et al.: Preliminary observations of the effects on breast adenocarcinoma of plasma perfused over immobilized protein A. N. Engl. J. Med. 305:1195, 1981.

94. Saal, S. D., and Gordon, B. R.: Extracorporeal modification of plasma and whole blood. In Tindall, R. S. A. (ed.): Therapeutic Apheresis and Plasma Perfusion. New York, A. R. Liss, Inc., 1980.

95. Pineda, A. A.: Methods for selective removal of plasma constituents. In Tindall, R. S. A. (ed.): Therapeutic Apheresis and Plasma Perfusion. New York, A. R. Liss, Inc., 1980.

96. Hamburger, M. I., Lawley, T. J., Kimberly, R. P., Plotz, P. H., and Frank, M. M.: A serial study of splenic reticuloendothelial system Fc receptor functional activity in systemic lupus erythematosus. Arthritis Rheum. 25:48, 1982.

97. Steven, M. M., Tanner, A. R., Holdstock, T. J., and Wright, R.: Effect of plasma exchange on the in vitro monocyte function of patients with immune complex diseases. Clin. Exp. Immunol. 45:240, 1981.

98. Lockwood, C. M., Rees, A. J., Pearson, T. A., Evans, D. J., Peters, D. K., and Wilson, C. B.: Immunosuppression and plasma exchange in the treatment of Goodpasture's syndrome. Lancet 1:711, 1976.

99. Flaum, M. A., Cuneo, R. A., Appelbaum, F. A., Deisseroth, A. B., Engel, W. K., and Gralnick, H. R.: The hemostatic imbalance of plasma-exchange transfusion. Blood 54:694, 1979.

100. Orlin, J. B., and Berkman, E. M.: Partial plasma exchange using albumin replacement: Removal and recovery of normal constituents. Blood 56:1055, 1980.

101. Sakamoto, H., Takaoka, T., Usami, M., et al.: Apheresis: Clinical response of patients unresponsive to conventional therapy. Trans. Am. Soc. Artif. Intern. Organs 31:704, 1985.

102. Wright, D. G., Karsh, J., Fauci, A. S., et al.: Lymphocyte depletion and immunosuppression with repeated leukapheresis by continuous flow centrifugation. Blood 58:451, 1981.

103. Machleder, H. I., and Paulus, H.: Clinical and immunological alterations observed in patients undergoing long-term thoracic duct drainage. Surgery 84:157, 1978.

104. Paulus, H. E., Machleder, H. I., Levine, S., Yu, D. T. Y., and Macdonald, N. S.: Lymphocyte involvement in rheumatoid arthritis. Studies during thoracic duct drainage. Arthritis Rheum. 20:1249, 1977.

105. Hutchinson, F.: The molecular basis for radiation effects on cells. Cancer Res. 26:2045, 1966.

106. Anderson, R. E., and Warner, N. L.: Ionizing radiation and the immune response. Adv. Immunol. 24:215, 1976.

107. Fauci, A. S., Pratt, K. R., and Whalen, G.: Activation of human B lymphocytes. VIII. Differential radiosensitivity of subpopulations of lymphoid cells involved in the polyclonally induced PFC responses of peripheral blood B lymphocytes. Immunology 35:715, 1978.

108. Kaplan, H. S.: Hodgkin's Disease. 2nd ed. Cambridge, Harvard University Press, 1980.

109. Hellman, S., Mauch, P., Goodman, R. L., Rosenthal, D. S., and Moloney, W. C.: The place of radiation in the treatment of Hodgkin's disease. Cancer 42:971, 1978.

110. Fuks, Z., Strober, S., Bobrove, A. M., Sasazuki, T., McMichael, A., and Kaplan, H. S.: Long-term effects of radiation on T and B lymphocytes in peripheral blood of patients with Hodgkin's disease. J. Clin. Invest. 58:803, 1976.

111. Kotzin, B. L., Strober, S., Engleman, E. G., et al.: Treatment of intractable rheumatoid arthritis with total lymphoid irradiation. N. Engl. J. Med. 305:969, 1981.

112. Trentham, D. E., Belli, J. A., Anderson, R. J., et al.: Clinical and immunologic effects of fractionated total lymphoid irradiation in refractory rheumatoid arthritis. N. Engl. J. Med. 305:976, 1981.

113. Strober, S., Slavin, S., Gottlieb, M., et al.: Allograft tolerance after total lymphoid irradiation (TLI). Immunol. Rev. 46:87, 1979.

114. Strober, S., Tanay, A., Field, E., et al.: Efficacy of total lymphoid irradiation in intractable rheumatoid arthritis: A double-blind, randomized trial. Ann. Intern. Med. 102:441, 1985.

115. Hanly, J. G., Hassan, J., Moriatry, M., et al.: Lymphoid irradiation in intractable rheumatoid arthritis. A double-blind, randomized study comparing 750-rad treatment with 2,000-rad treatment. Arthritis Rheum. 29:16, 1986.

116. Brahn, E., Helfgott, S. M., Belli, J. A., et al.: Total lymphoid irradiation therapy in refractory rheumatoid arthritis. Fifteen- to forty-month follow-up. Arthritis Rheum. 27:481, 1984.

117. Nusslein, H. G., Herbst, M., Manger, B. J., et al.: Total lymphoid irradiation in patients with refractory rheumatoid arthritis. Arthritis Rheum. 28:1205, 1985.

118. Tanay, A., Field, E. H., Hoppe, R. T., and Strober, S.: Long-term followup of rheumatoid arthritis patients treated with total lymphoid irradiation. Arthritis Rheum. 30:1, 1987.

119. Strober, S., Field, E., Hoppe, R. T., et al.: Treatment of intractable lupus nephritis with total lymphoid irradiation. Ann. Intern. Med. 102:450, 1985.

120. Taub, R. N., and Deutsch, V.: Antilymphocytic serum. Pharmacol. Ther. 2:89, 1977.

121. Harris, N. S., Merino, G., and Najarian, J. S.: Mode of action of antilymphocyte sera (ALS). Transplant. Proc. 3:797, 1971.

122. Starzl, T. E., Marchioro, T. L., Hutchinson, D. E., Porter, K. A., Cerilli, G. J., and Brettschneider, L.: The clinical use of antilymphocyte globulin in renal homotransplantation. Transplantation (Suppl.) 5:1100, 1967.

123. Sheil, A. G. R., Mears, D., Kelly, G. E., et al.: Controlled clinical trial of antilymphocyte globulin in patients with renal allografts from cadaver donors. Lancet 1:359, 1971.

124. Lawley, T. J., Bielory, L., Gascon, P., Yancey, K. B., Young, N. S., and Frank, M. M.: A prospective clinical and immunologic analysis of patients with serum sickness. N. Engl. J. Med. 311:1407, 1984.

125. Kohler, G., and Milstein, C.: Continuous cultures of fused cells secreting antibody of predefined specificity. Nature 256:495, 1975.

126. Kennett, R. H., McKearn, T. J., and Bechtol, K. B. (eds.): Monoclonal Antibodies and Hybridomas: A New Dimension in Biologic Analyses. New York, Plenum Press, 1980.

127. Ortho Multicenter Transplant Study Group: A randomized clinical trial of OKT3 monoclonal antibody for acute rejection of cadaveric renal transplants. N. Engl. J. Med. 313:337, 1985.

128. Renlund, D. G., O'Connell, J. B., Gilbert, E. M., et al.: A prospective comparison of murine monoclonal CD3 (OKT3) antibody-based and equine antithymocyte globulin-based rejection prophylaxis in cardiac transplantation. Transplantation 47:599, 1989.

129. Millis, J. M., McDiarmid, S. V., Hiatt, J. R., et al.: Randomized prospective trial of OKT3 for early prophylaxis of rejection after liver transplantation. Transplantation 47:82, 1989.

130. Gilbert, E. M., De Witt, C. W., Eiswirth, C. C., et al.: Treatment of refractory cardiac allograft rejection with OKT3 monoclonal antibody. Am. J. Med. 82:202, 1987.

131. Bach, J-F., and Chatenoud, L.: Immunologic problems and perspectives in the therapeutic use of monoclonal antibodies in nephrology. Adv. Nephrol. 15:365, 1984.

132. Kreis, H., Chkoff, N., Vigeral, P., et al.: Therapeutic use of monoclonal antibodies in kidney transplantation. Adv. Nephrol. 14:389, 1984.

133. Morrison, S. L., Johnson, M. J., Herzenberg, L. A., and Oi, V. T.: Chimeric human antibody molecules: Mouse antigen-binding domains with human constant region domains. Proc. Natl. Acad. Sci. U.S.A. 81:6851, 1984.

134. Fauci, A. S., Rosenberg, S. A., Sherwin, S. A., Dinarello, C. A., Longo, D. L., and Lane, H. C.: Immunomodulators in clinical medicine. Ann. Intern. Med. 106:421, 1987.

135. Soulillou, J.-P., and Jacques, Y.: Monoclonal anti-IL-2-receptor in organ transplantation. Transplant. Int. 2:46, 1989.
136. Soulillou, J.-P., Cantarovich, D., Le Mauff, B., et al.: Randomized controlled trial of a monoclonal antibody against the interleukin-2 receptor (33B3.1) as compared with rabbit antithymocyte globulin for prophylaxis against rejection of renal allografts. N. Engl. J. Med. 322:1175, 1990.
137. Cantarovich, D., Le Mauff, B., Hourmant, M., et al.: Anti-interleukin 2 receptor monoclonal antibody in the treatment of ongoing acute rejection episodes of human kidney graft—a pilot study. Transplantation 47:454, 1989.
138. Ramos, E. L., Milford, E. L., Kirkman, R. I., et al.: Differential IL-2 receptor expression in renal allograft recipients treated with an anti-IL-2 receptor antibody. Transplantation 48:415, 1989.
139. Steinman, L., Rosenbaum, J. T., Sriram, S., and McDevitt, H. O.: In vivo effects of antibodies to immune response gene products: Prevention of experimental allergic encephalitis. Proc. Natl. Acad. Sci. U.S.A. 78:7111, 1981.
140. Cupps, T. R., and Fauci, A. S.: Corticosteroid-mediated immunoregulation in man. Immunol. Rev. 65:133, 1982.
141. Fauci, A. S., and Dale, D. C.: The effect of in vivo hydrocortisone on subpopulations of human lymphocytes. J. Clin. Invest. 53:240, 1974.
142. Haynes, B. F., and Fauci, A. S.: The differential effect of in vivo hydrocortisone on kinetics of subpopulations of human peripheral blood thymus-derived lymphocytes. J. Clin. Invest. 61:703, 1978.
143. Stevenson, H. C., and Fauci, A. S.: The effect of glucocorticosteroids and other hormones on inflammatory and immune responses. In Oppenheim, J. J., Rosenstreich, D. L., and Potter, M. (eds.): Cellular Functions in Immunity and Inflammation. New York, Elsevier/North Holland, 1981.
144. Borel, J. F., Feurer, C., Gubler, H. U., and Stahelin, H.: Biological effects of cyclosporin A: A new antilymphocytic agent. Agents Actions 6:468, 1976.
145. Cohen, D. J., Loertscher, R., Rubin, M. F., Tilney, N. L., Carpenter, C. B., and Strom, T. B.: Cyclosporine: A new immunosuppressive agent for organ transplantation. Ann. Intern. Med. 101:667, 1984.
146. Preliminary Results of a European Trial: Cyclosporin A as a sole immunosuppressive agent in recipients of kidney allografts from cadaver donors. Lancet 2:57, 1982.
147. Starzl, T. E., Klintmalm, G. B. G., Weil, R., III, et al.: Cyclosporin A and steroid therapy in sixty-six cadaver kidney recipients. Surg. Gynecol. Obstet. 153:486, 1982.
148. Morris, P. J., Chapman, J. R., Allen, R. D., et al.: Cyclosporin conversion versus conventional immunosuppressive agents for organ transplantation. Ann. Intern. Med. 101:667, 1984.
149. Powles, R. L., Clink, H. M., Spence, D., et al.: Cyclosporin A to prevent graft-versus-host disease in man after allogenic bone-marrow transplantation. Lancet 1:327, 1980.
150. Palestine, A. G., Austin, H. A., III, Balow, J. E., et al.: Renal histopathologic alterations in patients treated with cyclosporine for uveitis. N. Engl. J. Med. 314:1293, 1986.
151. Palestine, A. G., Austin, H. A., III, and Nussenblatt, R. B.: Renal tubular function in cyclosporine-treated patients. Am. J. Med. 81:419, 1986.
152. Dijkmans, B. A., van Rijthoven, A. W., Goei The, H. S., Montnor-Beckers, Z. L., Jacobs, P. C., and Cats, A.: Effect of cyclosporin on serum creatinine in patients with rheumatoid arthritis. Eur. J. Clin. Pharmacol. 31:541, 1987.
153. Kolkin, S., Nahman, N. S., Jr., and Mendell, J. R.: Chronic nephrotoxicity complicating cyclosporine treatment of chronic inflammatory demyelinating polyradiculoneuropathy. Neurology 37:147, 1987.
154. Beveridge, T., Krupp, P., and McKibbin, C.: Lymphoma and lymphoproliferative lesions developing under cyclosporin therapy. Lancet 1:788, 1984.
155. Nussenblatt, R. B., Palestine, A. G., Chan, C. C., Mochizuki, M., and Yancey, K.: Effectiveness of cyclosporin therapy for Behcet's disease. Arthritis Rheum. 28:671, 1985.
156. Nussenblatt, R. B., Palestine, A. G., Rook, A. H., Scher, I., Wacker, W. C., and Gery, I.: Treatment of intraocular inflammatory disease with cyclosporin A. Lancet 2:235, 1983.
157. Nussenblatt, R. B., Palestine, A. G., and Chan, C. C.: Cyclosporin A in the treatment of intraocular inflammatory disease resistant to systemic corticosteroids and cytotoxic agents. Am. J. Ophthalmol. 96:275, 1983.
158. van Rijthoven, A. W., Dijkmans, B. A., Goei The, H. S., et al.: Cyclosporin treatment for rheumatoid arthritis: A placebo-controlled, double-blind, multicentre study. Ann. Rheum. Dis. 45:726, 1986.
159. Dougados, M., and Amor, B.: Cyclosporin A in rheumatoid arthritis: Preliminary clinical results of an open trial. Arthritis Rheum. 30:83, 1987.
160. Weinblatt, M. E., Coblyn, J. S., Fraser, P. A., et al.: Cyclosporin A treatment of refractory rheumatoid arthritis. Arthritis Rheum. 30:11, 1987.
161. Mistilis, S. P., Vickers, C. R., Darroch, M. H., and McCarthy, S. W.:
Cyclosporin, a new treatment for autoimmune chronic active hepatitis. Med. J. Aust. 143:463, 1985.
162. Rebuck, A. S., Stiller, C. R., Braude, A. C., Laupacis, A., Cohen, R. D., and Chapman, K. R.: Cyclosporin for pulmonary sarcoidosis. Lancet 1:1174, 1984.
163. Allison, M. C., and Pounder, R. E.: Cyclosporin for Crohn's disease. Lancet 1:902, 1984.
164. Bianchi, P. A., Mondelli, M., Quarto-di-Palo, R., and Ranzi, T.: Cyclosporin for Crohn's disease. Lancet 1:1242, 1984.
165. Gupta, S., Keshavarzian, A., and Hodgson, H. J. F.: Cyclosporin in ulcerative colitis. Lancet 2:1277, 1984.
166. Thivolet, J., Barthelmy, H., Rigot-Muller, G., and Bendelac, A.: Effects of cyclosporin on bullous pemphigoid and pemphigus. Lancet 1:334, 1985.
167. Mueller, W., and Hermann, B.: Cyclosporin A for psoriasis. N. Engl. J. Med. 301:555, 1984.
168. Harper, J. I., Keat, A. C. S., and Staughton, R. C. D.: Cyclosporin for psoriasis. Lancet 2:981, 1984.
169. Velthius, P. J., and Jesserun, R. F. M.: Improvement of ichthyosis by cyclosporin. Lancet 1:335, 1985.
170. Weetman, A. P., McGregor, A. M., Ludgate, M., et al.: Cyclosporin improves Graves' ophthalmopathy. Lancet 2:486, 1983.
171. Routhier, G., Epskin, O., Janossy, G., et al.: Effects of cyclosporin A on suppressor and inducer T lymphocytes in primary biliary cirrhosis. Lancet 2:1223, 1980.
172. Cyclosporin in autoimmune disease. Lancet 1:909, 1985.
173. Kino, T., Hatanaka, H., Hashimoto, M., et al.: FK506, a novel immunosuppressant isolated from a Streptomyces. I. Fermentation, isolation, and physicochemical and biological characteristics. J. Antibiot. (Tokyo) 40:1249, 1987.
174. Kino, T., Hatanaka, H., Miyata, S., et al.: FK506, a novel immunosuppressant isolated from a Streptomyces. II. Immunosuppressive effect of FK506 in vitro. J. Antibiot. (Tokyo) 41:1256, 1988.
175. Thomson, A. W.: FK-506—how much potential? Immunol. Today 10:6, 1989.
176. Collier, D. StJ., Calne, R. Y., Thiru, S., Friend, P. J., Lim, S. M. L., and White, D. J. G.: FR-900506 (FK 506) in experimental renal allografts in dogs and primates. Transplant. Proc. 20:226, 1988.
177. Starzl, T. E., Todo, S., and Fung, J.: FK 506 for liver, kidney, and pancreas transplantation. Lancet 2:1000, 1989.
178. Shapiro, R., Fung, J. J., and Jain, A.: The side effects of FK 506 in humans. Transplant. Proc. 22:35, 1990.
179. White, D. J. G.: FK506: The promise and the paradox. Clin. Exp. Immunol. 83:1, 1991.
180. Arita, C., Hotokebuchi, T., Miyahara, H., Arai, K., Sugioka, Y., and Kaibara, N.: Inhibition by FK 506 of established lesions of collagen-induced arthritis in rats. Clin. Exp. Immunol. 82:456, 1990.
181. Hara, S., Fukatsu, A., Suzuki, N., Sakamoto, N., and Matsuo, S.: The effects of a new immunosuppressive agent, FK506, on the glomerular injury in rats with accelerated nephrotoxic serum glomerulonephritis. Clin. Immunol. 57:351, 1990.
182. Kawashima, H., Fujino, Y., and Mochizuki, M.: Effects of a new immunosuppressive agent, FK-506, on experimental autoimmune uveoretinitis in rats. Invest. Ophthalmol. Vis. Sci. 29:1265, 1988.
183. Inamura, N., Hashimoto, H., Nakahara, K., et al.: Immunosuppressive effect of FK-506 on experimental allergic encephalomyelitis in rats. Int. J. Immunopharmacol. 10:991, 1988.
184. Takabayashi, K., Koike, T., Kurasawa, K., et al.: Effect of FK-506, a novel immunosuppressive drug on murine systemic lupus erythematosus. Clin. Immunol. Immunopathol. 51:110, 1989.
185. McCauley, J., Bronsther, O., Fung, J., Todo, S., and Starzl, T. E.: Treatment of cyclosporin-induced haemolytic uraemic syndrome with FK 506. Lancet 2:1516, 1989.
186. McCauley, J., Tzakis, A. G., Fung, J. J., Todo, S., and Starzl, T. E.: FK 506 in steroid-resistant focal sclerosing glomerulonephritis in childhood. Lancet 1:674, 1990.
187. Schreiber, S. L.: Chemistry and biology of the immunophilins and their immunosuppressive ligands. Science 251:283, 1991.
188. Tocci, M. J., Matkovich, D. A., Collier, K. A., et al.: The immunosuppressant FK-506 selectively inhibits expression of early T cell activation genes. J. Immunol. 143:718, 1989.
189. Emmel, E. A., Verweij, C. L., Durand, D. B., Higgins, K. M., Lacy, E., and Crabtree, G. R.: Cyclosporin-A specifically inhibits function of nuclear proteins involved in T-cell activation. Science 246:1617, 1989.
190. Shevach, E. M.: The effects of cyclosporin A on the immune system. Annu. Rev. Immunol. 3:397, 1985.
191. Muraguchi, A., Butler, J. L., Kehrl, J. H., Falkoff, R. J. M., and Fauci, A. S.: Selective suppression of an early step in human B-cell activation by cyclosporin A. J. Exp. Med. 158:690, 1983.
192. Symoens, J., and Rosenthal, M.: Levamisone in the modulation of the immune response: The current experimental and clinical state. J. Reticuloendothel. Soc. 21:175, 1977.
193. Snyderman, R., and Pike, M. C.: Pathophysiologic aspects of leukocyte chemotaxis: Identification of a specific chemotactic factor binding site

on human granulocytes and defects of macrophage function associated with neoplasia. *In* Gallin, J. I., and Quie, P. G. (eds.): Leukocyte Chemotaxis: Methods, Physiology and Clinical Implications. New York, Raven Press, 1978.

194. Rabson, A. R., Whiting, D. A., Anderson, R., Glover, A., and Koornhof, H. J.: Depressed neutrophil motility in patients with recurrent herpes simplex virus infections: In vitro restoration with levamisole. J. Infect. Dis. 135:113, 1977.

195. Wright, D. G., Kirkpatrick, C. H., and Gallin, J. I.: Effects of levamisole on normal and abnormal leukocyte locomotion. J. Clin. Invest. 59:941, 1977.

196. Tripodi, D., Parks, L. C., and Brugmans, J.: Drug-induced restoration of cutaneous delayed hypersensitivity in anergic patients with cancer. N. Engl. J. Med. 289:354, 1973.

197. Sampson, D., and Lui, A.: The effect of levamisole on cell-mediated immunity and suppressor cell function. Cancer Res. 36:952, 1976.

198. Moertel, C. G., Fleming, T. R., Macdonald, J. S., et al.: Levamisole and fluorouracil for adjuvant therapy of resected colon carcinoma. N. Engl. J. Med. 322:352, 1990.

199. Miller, B., DeMerieux, P., Srinivasan, R., et al.: Double-blind placebo-controlled crossover evaluation of levamisole in rheumatoid arthritis. Arthritis Rheum. 23:172, 1980.

200. Runge, L. A., Pinals, R. S., Lourie, S. H., and Tomar, R. H.: Treatment of rheumatoid arthritis with levamisole. A controlled trial. Arthritis Rheum. 20:1445, 1977.

201. Schmidt, K. L., and Mueller-Eckhardt, C.: Agranulocytosis, levamisole and HLA-B27. Lancet 2:85, 1977.

202. Veys, E. M., Mielants, H., and Verbruggen, G.: Levamisole-induced adverse reactions in HLA-B27-positive rheumatoid arthritis. Lancet 1:148, 1978.

203. Freund, J.: Some aspects of active immunization. Annu. Rev. Microbiol. 1:291, 1947.

204. Chedid, L., Audibert, F., LeFrancier, P., Chory, J., and Lederer, E.: Modulation of the immune response by a synthetic adjuvant and analogs. Proc. Natl. Acad. Sci. U.S.A. 73:2472, 1976.

205. Katz, S. I., Hall, R. P., Lawley, T. J., and Strober, W.: Dermatitis herpetiformis: The skin and the gut. Ann. Intern. Med. 93:857, 1980.

206. Katz, S. I., Gallin, J. I., Hertz, K. C., Fauci, A. S., and Lawley, T. J.: Erythema elevatum diutinum: Skin and systemic manifestations, immunologic studies and successful treatment with dapsone. Medicine 56:443, 1977.

207. Hall, R. P., Lawley, T. J., Smith, H. R., and Katz, S. I.: Bullous eruption of systemic lupus erythematosus. Ann. Intern. Med. 97:165, 1982.

208. Mandell, G. L., and Sande, M. A.: Drugs used in the chemotherapy of tuberculosis and leprosy. *In* Gilman, A. G., Rall, T. W., Nies, A. S., and Taylor, P. (eds.): Goodman and Gilman's The Pharmacologic Basis of Therapeutics. 8th ed. New York, Pergamon Press, 1990.

209. Stiehm, E. R., Kronenberg, L. H., Rosenblatt, H. M., Bryson, Y., and Merigan, T. C.: Interferon: Immunobiology and clinical significance. Ann. Intern. Med. 96:80, 1982.

210. Bloom, B. R.: Interferons and the immune system. Nature 284:593, 1980.

211. Mannering, G. J., and Deloria, L. B.: The pharmacology and toxicology of the interferons: An overview. Annu. Rev. Pharmacol. Toxicol. 26:455, 1986.

212. Gallin, J. I., Sechler, J. M. G., and Malech, H. L.: Reconstitution of defective phagocyte function in chronic granulomatous disease of childhood with recombinant human interferon-γ. Trans. Assoc. Am. Physicians 101:12, 1988.

213. Ezekowitz, R. A. B., Orkin, S. H., and Newberger, P. E.: Recombinant interferon-gamma augments phagocyte superoxide production and X-chronic granulomatous gene expression in X-linked variant chronic granulomatous disease. J. Clin. Invest. 80:1009, 1987.

214. Kahan, A., Amor, B., Menkes, C. J., and Strauch, G.: Recombinant interferon-γ in the treatment of systemic sclerosis. Am. J. Med. 87:273, 1989.

215. Cannon, G. W., Pincus, S. H., Emkey, R. D., et al.: Double-blind trial of recombinant γ-interferon versus placebo in the treatment of rheumatoid arthritis. Arthritis Rheum. 32:964, 1989.

216. Nakajima, H., Takamori, H., Hiyama, Y., and Tsukada, W.: The effect of treatment with interferon-gamma on type II collagen-induced arthritis. Clin. Exp. Immunol. 81:441, 1990.

217. Murray, H. W.: Interferon-gamma therapy in AIDS for mononuclear phagocyte activation. Biotherapy 2:149, 1990.

218. Ringenberg, Q. S., and Anderson, P. C.: Interferons in the treatment of skin disease. Int. J. Dermatol. 25:273, 1986.

219. Stanton, G. J., Weigent, D. A., Fleischmann, W. R., Dianzani, F, and Baron, S.: Interferon review. Invest. Radiol. 22:259, 1987.

220. Hoofnagle, J. H., Mullen, K. D., Jones, D. B., et al.: Treatment of chronic non-A, non-B hepatitis with recombinant human alpha interferon. A preliminary report. N. Engl. J. Med. 315:1575, 1986.

221. Quesada, J. R., Reuben, J., Manning, J. T., Hersh, E. M., and Gutterman, J. U.: Alpha interferon for reinduction of remission in hairy-cell leukemia. N. Engl. J. Med. 310:15, 1984.

222. Foon, K. A., Maluish, A. E., Abrams, P. G., et al.: Recombinant leukocyte A interferon therapy for advanced hairy cell leukemia: therapeutic and immunologic results. Am. J. Med. 80:351, 1986.

223. Krown, S. E., Real, F. X., Cunningham-Rundles, S., et al.: Preliminary observations on the effect of recombinant leukocyte A interferon in homosexual men with Kaposi's sarcoma. N. Engl. J. Med. 308:1071, 1983.

224. Lane, H. C., Davey, V., Kovacs, J. A., et al.: Interferon-α in patients with asymptomatic human immunodeficiency virus (HIV) infection. A randomized placebo-controlled trial. Ann. Intern. Med. 112:805, 1990.

225. Krown, S. E., Gold, J. W., Niedzwiecki, D., et al.: Interferon-α with zidovudine: Safety, tolerance, and clinical and virologic effects in patients with Kaposi sarcoma associated with acquired immunodeficiency syndrome (AIDS). Ann. Intern. Med. 112:812; 1990.

226. Roberts, A. B., and Sporn, M. B.: The transforming growth factor-βs. *In* Sporn, M. B., and Roberts, A. B. (eds.): Peptide Growth Factors and Their Receptors. Vol. 1. Heidelberg, Springer-Verlag, 1990.

Chapter 50

Irving H. Fox

Antihyperuricemic Drugs

INTRODUCTION

The existence of hyperuricemia, a common biochemical abnormality, requires investigation to discern the cause. Treatment is usually appropriate only for symptomatic hyperuricemia, including gout, renal calculi associated with hyperuricemia or hyperuricaciduria, and for the prevention of acute uric acid nephropathy.

There are two major causes of hyperuricemia—increased production of uric acid and decreased excretion of uric acid. The two major therapeutic approaches to antihyperuricemic therapy oppose these mechanisms of hyperuricemia. One approach involves the inhibition of urate synthesis with allopurinol. The other therapeutic approach is to increase the excretion of urate through the use of uricosuric drugs such as sulfinpyrazone and probenecid. A third approach to the treatment of hyperuricemia involves increasing the destruction of urate by the use of an enzyme, uricase, that destroys urate. Uricase is being used experimentally, but it is practical and may be available in the future.

On rare occasions, when one therapy is not effective alone, combinations of these therapies are used. Most commonly, a combination of inhibition of urate synthesis and stimulation of uric acid excretion has been used. However, this is only rarely necessary.

INHIBITION OF URATE SYNTHESIS

Allopurinol

Allopurinol is a drug commonly used for the treatment of gout.

Mechanism of Action

In the final steps of urate synthesis, hypoxanthine is oxidized to xanthine and xanthine is oxidized to uric acid. This reaction is catalyzed by a single enzyme, xanthine dehydrogenase.

Allopurinol decreases urate synthesis by inhibiting xanthine dehydrogenase (Fig. 50–1). Allopurinol is itself a substrate for xanthine dehydrogenase and is oxidized to oxipurinol. In fact, 6 hours after a single dose of allopurinol, it is no longer detectable

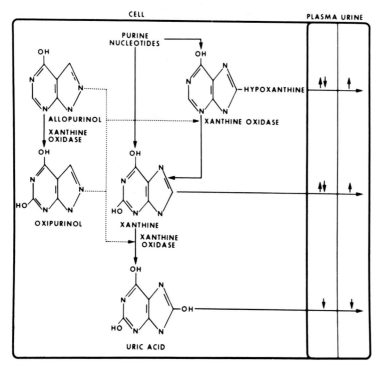

Figure 50–1. Effect of allopurinol on uric acid formation in human beings. Purine nucleotides are eventually degraded to hypoxanthine, xanthine, and uric acid. Final steps are catalyzed by xanthine oxidase. Allopurinol is converted to oxipurinol by this enzyme. Both compounds inhibit xanthine oxidase. Effects on plasma and urinary concentrations are indicated as increase, decrease, or no substantial change.

in the plasma and only oxipurinol is present.[1] Oxipurinol actively inhibits xanthine dehydrogenase.

Allopurinol [4-hydroxypyrazolo (3,4-*d*) pyrimidine] and its major metabolic product oxipurinol [4,6-dihydroxypyrazolo (3,4-*d*) pyrimidine] are analogues of hypoxanthine and xanthine, respectively. Both are potent inhibitors of xanthine dehydrogenase.[2–4] The Michaelis constant of allopurinol for this enzyme is one twentieth the Michaelis constant of xanthine. In contrast, oxipurinol and xanthine have similar Michaelis constants. Allopurinol is a competitive inhibitor of xanthine dehydrogenase. Both allopurinol and oxipurinol produce pseudoirreversible inactivation of

xanthine dehydrogenase. Inactivation results from the incubation of allopurinol and enzyme without substrate. Oxipurinol inactivates the enzyme with the addition of xanthine and molecular oxygen as the hydrogen acceptor.

Allopurinol and its derivatives have additional actions on purine and pyrimidine metabolism that are explained by its own complex metabolism (Fig. 50–2).[5, 6] As a result of inhibition of xanthine dehydrogenase, there is a buildup of hypoxanthine and xanthine in body fluids. Xanthinuria results from this activity. Orotic aciduria and orotidinuria also occur during allopurinol therapy. This is related to inhibi-

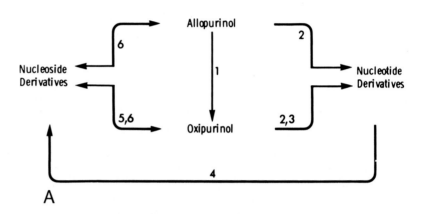

Figure 50–2. Allopurinol metabolism in humans. *A*, Allopurinol undergoes a complex series of metabolic alterations. Allopurinol is oxidized to oxipurinol. Small quantities of these compounds are converted to the nucleoside and nucleotide derivatives. The reactions are catalyzed by the enzymes indicated: 1 = xanthine dehydrogenase; 2 = hypoxanthine-guanine phosphoribosyltransferase; 3 = orotate phosphoribosyltransferase; 4 = 5'-nucleotidase; 5 = pyrimidine nucleoside phosphorylase; 6 = purine nucleoside phosphorylase. *B*, The structures of the allopurinol metabolites are outlined. Oxipurinol has two types of derivatives, the 7-N or 1-N, depending on whether metabolism occurred by orotate phosphoribosyltransferase or hypoxanthine-guanine phosphoribosyltransferase, respectively.

tion of de novo pyrimidine synthesis at orotidylic decarboxylase by allopurinol ribonucleotide and oxipurinol ribonucleotide.

Allopurinol therapy also decreases total urinary purine excretion. This decrease in total urinary purine excretion requires hypoxanthine-guanine phosphoribosyltransferase and is not observed with a deficiency of this enzyme.[5] The decreased urinary purine excretion is associated with inhibition of de novo purine synthesis. This inhibition results from nucleotide derivatives of allopurinol and oxipurinol[5, 6] or from enhanced reutilization of hypoxanthine.[7]

Metabolism and Pharmacokinetics

By virtue of its being a structural analogue of hypoxanthine, allopurinol [4-hydroxypyrazolo (3,4-d) pyrimidine] undergoes complex interconversions (see Fig. 50–2).[5, 6] There are three pathways of metabolism. Allopurinol can be converted to a nucleoside 5'-monophosphate derivative [1-N(5'-ribosyl)allopurinol]. This can be dephosphorylated to a nucleoside derivative [1-N(5'-ribosyl)allopurinol]. The latter compound can also be formed directly from allopurinol by the reaction of purine nucleoside phosphorylase. The major pathway of allopurinol metabolism is oxidation to oxipurinol.

Oxipurinol is a structural analogue of xanthine and has four distinct pathways of metabolism. In parallel to allopurinol xanthine is a substrate for hypoxanthine-guanine phosphoribosyltransferase and purine nucleoside phosphorylase. The purine nucleotide and nucleoside derivatives are similarly formed. In contrast to allopurinol, oxipurinol is also a substrate for orotate phosphoribosyltransferase and pyrimidine nucleoside phosphorylase. The compounds formed are 7-N(5'-phosphoribosyl)-oxipurinol and 7-N(5'-ribosyl) oxipurinol derivatives.

Allopurinol is completely absorbed from the gastrointestinal tract. Parenteral and rectal administration may be used for patients unable to ingest oral medication. However, drug absorption is limited by poor solubility.[1] A prodrug approach has been recommended to overcome this problem, including the use of N_1 acyclomethyl derivatives of allopurinol.[8] Allopurinol has a half-life in vivo of 39 to 180 minutes. Forty-five to 65 percent of allopurinol is rapidly oxidized to oxipurinol in vivo. Allopurinol is cleared by the kidney at a rate of 14 to 20 ml per minute.[2, 4, 9]

Oxipurinol is only poorly absorbed from the gastrointestinal tract.[2, 10] It is excreted by a monoexponential decay with a half-life ranging from 12 to 17 hours.[11] The half-life can be markedly increased to 50 hours with a low-protein diet.[11] Therefore, in protein-malnourished patients, the dose of allopurinol should be reduced. Oxipurinol is cleared by the kidney at a rate of 23 to 31 ml per minute.

There are important therapeutic implications for the metabolism and excretion of allopurinol and oxipurinol.[2] Because of its prolonged half-life, oxipurinol is primarily responsible for xanthine dehydrogenase inhibition in vivo when allopurinol is administered. In addition, factors that change uric acid excretion generally alter oxipurinol excretion in a similar direction.[12] For example, uricosuric agents increase the renal excretion of oxipurinol and uric acid, and renal insufficiency reduces the excretion of both compounds. Therefore, dose adjustments are required to compensate for these clinical considerations.

Because allopurinol and uricosuric drugs are occasionally used together, their interaction needs to be considered. Allopurinol lengthens the biologic half-life of probenecid and thus potentiates its uricosuric effect. On the other hand, uricosuric drugs increase the clearance of oxipurinol in humans[12] and thus diminish the degree of xanthine dehydrogenase inhibition. The net effect of these drug interactions suggests that lower than usual doses of probenecid and greater than usual doses of allopurinol would be indicated when the drugs are used concurrently. Clinically, however, the drugs are tolerated so well that they can be used together without altering the usual dosages of either.

Therapeutic Actions

The administration of allopurinol to patients with normal renal function is followed by a decrease in serum and urinary uric acid values within 24 to 48 hours. Maximum reductions are achieved in 4 to 14 days. Serum urate values then remain relatively constant over prolonged periods[2, 4] (Fig. 50–3). Withdrawal of allopurinol usually results in a return to pretreatment serum urate levels within a few days. After 3 to 6 months of normouricemia, a reduction in the frequency of gouty attacks may be expected.

Allopurinol has proved to be a highly effective drug for the treatment of hyperuricemia and gout after use for more than 25 years.[13] Normal serum urate values can be achieved in most patients with normal renal function using a dose of 300 mg per day.[14] The optimal end-point of antihyperuricemic therapy is to reduce the serum urate concentration to a level at which the urate concentration is no longer saturating (i.e., less than 6 mg per 100 ml). A single 300-mg tablet may be used once each day because of the long biologic half-life of oxipurinol. Rarely is a dose higher than 300 mg per day needed.

In some patients with frequent episodes of gout, beginning with a low dose may decrease the probability of precipitating a series of incapacitating attacks. In all patients being treated with allopurinol or any antihyperuricemic agent, the drug dosage should be adjusted to the individual's need through monitoring the serum urate concentration. In individuals with reduced glomerular filtration rates, it may be advisable to reduce the maintenance dose of allopurinol because of the prolonged half-life of oxipurinol in patients with renal failure. In patients

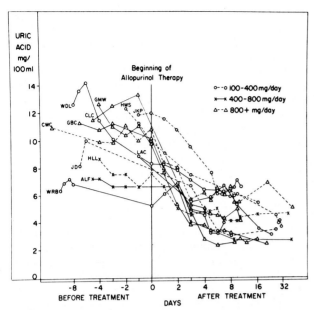

Figure 50-3. Effect of allopurinol on serum uric acid in 12 patients with gout.

with renal impairment, the creatinine clearance is highly correlated to the plasma oxipurinol concentrations.[12, 15] Table 50-1 lists suggested doses for allopurinol in patients with different glomerular filtration rates. Parenteral and rectal administration may be tried for patients unable to ingest oral medication.

Tophi resolve in 6 to 12 months with maintenance of normal serum urate levels.[2] Destructive arthritis improves in most patients. In an occasional patient with rapid resolution of tophi, bony lesions do not heal and telescoped digits may result.[16] Slower improvement can be anticipated in patients with renal insufficiency. However, the progression of gouty nephropathy appears to halt in most patients.

Once antihyperuricemic therapy is instituted for firm medical indications, it should be continued indefinitely if possible. Intermittent administration of allopurinol is less effective than continuous therapy in controlling the symptoms of gout.[17] If allopurinol is stopped after a few years of control of hyperuricemia, the patient may re-enter an asymptomatic phase.[18] Ultimately, acute attacks then recur.

Uricosuric agents are occasionally used together

Table 50-1. RECOMMENDED MAINTENANCE DOSE OF ALLOPURINOL BASED ON THE GLOMERULAR FILTRATION RATE (GFR)

GFR (ml/min)	Dose (mg)
100	300
80	250
60	200
40	150
20	100
10	100 q2d
0	100 q3d

with allopurinol to hasten mobilization of urate deposits in tophaceous gout.[2, 3] The administration of allopurinol and a uricosuric agent to a patient with good renal function usually increases urinary uric acid excretion and further decreases the serum urate level.

Despite the availability of allopurinol for many years, the clinical use of the drug is not always appropriate. In a recent study, less than 20 percent of physicians diagnosed gout definitely before prescribing allopurinol.[19] In another study, many physicians did not cover the introduction of allopurinol with anti-inflammatory agents, titrate the dose against the uric acid, or adjust the dose according to the serum creatinine level.[15, 20]

Tolerability and Adverse Reactions

Acute Attacks of Gout. There is a relatively high frequency of gouty attacks on initiation of therapy.[21] Typical attacks have occurred with serum urate levels as low as 2 mg per 100 ml and comparably low urinary urate excretions. Daily colchicine should be given during at least the first 6 to 12 months of therapy with allopurinol to minimize the likelihood of recurrent acute attacks.

Xanthine Stones. The urinary excretion of xanthine, a poorly soluble compound, increases during full-dose allopurinol therapy to the level of xanthine excretion observed in hereditary xanthinuria.[2, 3] In this disorder associated with deficient xanthine oxidase activity, the major disorder is the formation of urinary calculi composed of xanthine. Thus far, development of xanthine crystalluria or lithiasis as a complication of allopurinol therapy has been observed rarely during the treatment of gout or uric acid stones,[2] usually in patients with partial deficiency of hypoxanthine-guanine phosphoribosyltransferase.[2]

In addition, xanthine stone formation induced by allopurinol therapy has been reported in children with Lesch-Nyhan syndrome[22] and patients with lymphosarcoma or Burkitt's lymphoma.[23] Allopurinol should be given cautiously and in minimal doses to patients with extraordinarily great uric acid excretion values, particularly those with an inability to reutilize hypoxanthine and xanthine because of hypoxanthine-guanine phosphoribosyltransferase deficiency.

Acute xanthine nephropathy has been observed in the acute tumor lysis syndrome during allopurinol therapy.[24] The mechanism for this is the same as for xanthine calculi.

Formation of oxipurinol sludge and stones in the urinary tract has been reported rarely.

Toxicity. Serious toxicity of allopurinol therapy occurs but is unusual. Some adverse reactions to allopurinol may be mediated by lymphocyte reactivity to oxipurinol.[25] These adverse reactions to allopurinol may represent delayed-type hypersensitivity to oxipurinol.

About 5 percent of patients find it necessary to

discontinue therapy with the drug. Allopurinol may lead to the development of gastrointestinal intolerance, skin rashes (sometimes with fever), occasionally toxic epidermal necrolysis, alopecia, bone marrow suppression with leukopenia and thrombocytopenia, agranulocytosis, aplastic anemia,[26] granulomatous hepatitis, severe jaundice, sarcoid-like reaction, and vasculitis.[2, 26] The incidence of side effects of all kinds may be about 20 percent.[2, 3]

Skin rashes occur in about 2 percent of patients receiving allopurinol. This increases ten-fold in patients receiving allopurinol and ampicillin.[27] The occurrence of skin rash in a patient receiving allopurinol does not necessarily require that the drug be discontinued. The rash of allopurinol often involves the hands and feet alone, or at least chiefly. There may be swelling and intense itching, and the body and face may be involved. Provided there is no laryngeal edema, it may suffice to administer large doses of diphenhydramine or other antihistaminic agent to control the itching. A minimal amount of swelling of the hands and feet then is often well tolerated. After a few weeks, it may be possible to stop the antihistamine without recurrence of the rash. Reduction of the dose of allopurinol may also be helpful in reducing the severity of the skin lesions, especially in patients with renal insufficiency. Desensitization has apparently been effective in patients allergic to allopurinol by initiating therapy with a very low dose of allopurinol (0.05 mg per day) and gradually increasing the amount given over a period of 30 days.[28, 29]

Toxic effects tend to occur more often in the presence of renal insufficiency and thiazide therapy. The allopurinol hypersensitivity syndrome consists of a constellation of findings, including fever, skin rash, progressive renal insufficiency, eosinophilia, and hepatitis. In a group of 78 patients with this putative syndrome, the following abnormalities were noted: skin rash, 92 percent; fever, 87 percent; worsening renal function, 85 percent; eosinophilia, 73 percent; hepatitis, 68 percent; and leukocytosis, 39 percent.[30] Twenty-one percent of these patients died. Diffuse vasculitis involving multiple organ systems was observed at postmortem examination. The median dose of allopurinol was 300 mg per day, and the mean duration of therapy was 3 weeks. Prior renal insufficiency was recorded in 81 percent of these patients, and 49 percent received concomitant diuretic therapy.[31] Despite its rarity, the potential severity of allopurinol hypersensitivity syndrome emphasizes (1) the need for restricting allopurinol therapy to those hyperuricemic patients who have specific indications for antihyperuricemic therapy and (2) the need to reduce the dose of allopurinol in patients with renal insufficiency (see Table 50–1).

Interactions With Other Drugs

Several drug–drug interactions involving allopurinol are important clinically. The use of allopurinol and a uricosuric drug together was described earlier. The effects of compounds that are inactivated by xanthine dehydrogenase, such as 6-mercaptopurine and azathioprine, are potentiated by allopurinol administration. An increased incidence of bone marrow suppression has been observed in patients taking allopurinol who are also receiving cyclophosphamide.[5, 32] Allopurinol has been shown to reduce the activity of hepatic microsomal drug-metabolizing enzymes and thus to prolong the half-lives of antipyrine, aminophenazene, dicumarol, warfarin sodium, and theophylline.[33]

Oxipurinol

The therapeutic effects of allopurinol are mediated by its metabolic product oxipurinol, whose half-life is about eight times longer than that of allopurinol. A direct comparison of the two agents given orally indicates that allopurinol is the more effective because of the relatively poor absorption of oxipurinol from the gastrointestinal tract.[2] Nevertheless, oxipurinol has been effectively used therapeutically in some patients who are sensitive to allopurinol. In most patients allergic to allopurinol, hyperuricemia may be controlled with oxipurinol without evidence of toxicity.[28, 29] However, toxic reactions identical to those observed with allopurinol were observed in 30 percent of the patients treated with oxipurinol. Cross-sensitivity to the two drugs is expected on the basis of their structural similarities. Oxipurinol is not marketed in the United States but is available in Europe and Japan.

ENHANCEMENT OF URIC ACID EXCRETION

Uricosuric Drugs and Mechanism of Action

Uricosuric therapy has been used to treat hyperuricemia and gout for about 40 years. A uricosuric drug increases the rate of excretion of uric acid.[34] Uric acid is normally handled in the human kidney by filtration at the glomerulus and by secretion and reabsorption mechanisms in the renal tubules. Uricosuric drugs modify the tubular transport mechanisms of uric acid and have their pharmacologic activity in the renal tubule. Uric acid and other drugs handled by these transport mechanisms are organic anions.

There are separate transport systems for the secretion and reabsorption of organic anions, including uric acid.[34] Because urate is reabsorbed by a renal tubular brush border transporter, this reabsorption of urate can be inhibited when uricosuric drugs such as probenecid are present in the lumen and compete with urate for the brush border transporter. In this way, uricosuric drugs inhibit urate reabsorption. The secretory transport system is quantitatively much smaller than reabsorption and is located at the basolateral membrane of the renal tubule. When uri-

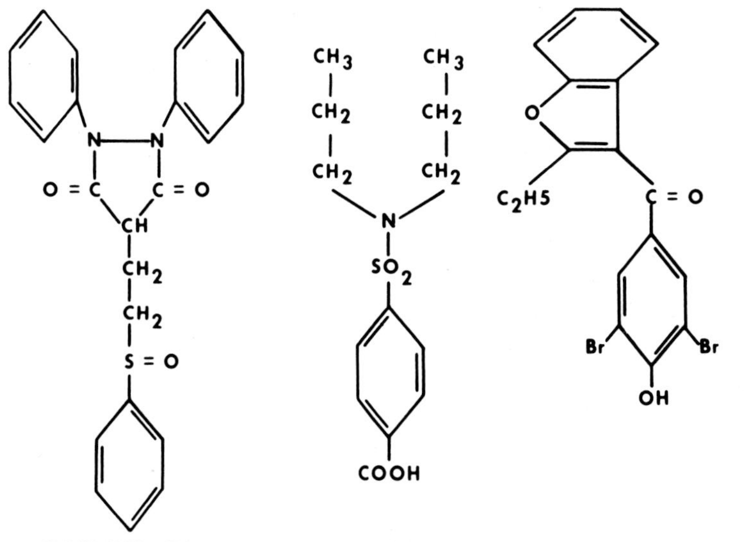

Figure 50–4. Structure of sulfinpyrazone, probenecid, and benzbromarone.

cosuric drugs are given in very low doses, they actually decrease the renal excretion of uric acid by inhibiting this secretory transport system. Decreased excretion usually occurs at low dose, and increased excretion is observed at a higher dose of uricosuric drugs, with inhibition of the reabsorptive anion transporter. This higher dose is usually the dose recommended for uricosuric therapy.

The fact that uric acid and other organic anions are secreted in the tubule is of importance clinically, because it may lead to interactions between uricosuric drugs and other organic anionic drugs secreted in the tubule. This is responsible for some of the interactions of uricosuric drugs with other drugs that are described later.

Thus, the pharmacologic action of uricosuric drugs such as probenecid is to inhibit the transport of organic acids across epithelial barriers.[35, 36] Uric acid is the only important endogenous compound whose excretion is known to be increased by probenecid. This results from inhibition of uric acid resorption. Probenecid and sulfinpyrazone (Fig. 50–4) are most widely used for this purpose in the United States. In Europe, benzbromarone and zoxazolamine are used as well.

The uricosuric action of probenecid and sulfinpyrazine is blunted by the concomitant administration of salicylate, which is an organic anion. Probenecid inhibits the tubular secretion of a number of other drugs (Table 50–2). In addition, probenecid inhibits the transport of 5-hydroxyindoleacetic acid and other acid metabolites of cerebral monoamines from the subarachnoid space to the plasma. Furthermore, probenecid is secreted into the bile and depresses the biliary secretion of other compounds. This ability to inhibit biliary secretion allows probenecid to increase plasma levels of rifampin during the treatment of tuberculosis.

Many drugs with diverse chemical structures decrease the serum urate concentration in humans by enhancing the renal excretion of uric acid (see Table 50–2).[2]

Metabolism and Pharmacokinetics

Probenecid

Probenecid is readily absorbed from the gastrointestinal tract. The half-life of probenecid in plasma is dose dependent[37] and ranges from 6 to 12 hours. This may be prolonged by the concomitant administration of allopurinol. Probenecid is extensively bound to plasma proteins (89 to 94 percent of drug)

Table 50–2. DRUGS SHOWN TO BE URICOSURIC IN HUMANS

Acetoheximide	Glycopyrrolate
ACTH	Halofenate (MK 185)
Amflutizole	Iodopyracet
Ascorbic acid	Iopanoic acid
Azapropazone	Meclofenamic acid
Azauridine	Meglumine iodipamide
Benzbromarone	Mersalyl
Benziodarone	Metiazininic acid
Calcitonin	Niridazole
Calcium ipodate	Orotic acid
Carinamide	Outdated tetracyclines
Chlorprothixene	Phenolsulfonphthalein
Cinchophen	Phenylbutazone
Citrate	Phenylindandione
Dicumarol	Phenoxyisobutyric acid
Diflumidone	Probenecid and metabolites
Diflunisal	Salicylates
Estrogens	Sodium diatrizoate
Ethyl biscoumacetate	Sulfaethylthiadiazole
Ethyl p-chlorophenoxyisobutyric acid	Sulfinpyrazone
Glyceryl guaiacholate	Ticrynafen
Glycine	W 2354 (5-chlorosalicylic acid)
	Zoxazolamine

and is largely confined to the extracellular fluid. The maintenance dose of probenecid ranges from 500 mg per day to 3 g per day given in three or four divided doses.[2, 3]

Probenecid is rapidly metabolized in vivo. Less than 5 percent of the administered dose is recovered in the urine within 24 hours. The major urinary metabolite, probenecid acyl monoglucuronide, accounts for 41 percent of the administered compound within 48 hours. The rest of the metabolites result from oxidation of the *n*-propyl side-chain.[2] These side-chain metabolites possess uricosuric activity in animals.[38]

Sulfinpyrazone

Sulfinpyrazone is rapidly and completely adsorbed from the gastrointestinal tract.[2] The peak concentration is reached in the serum 1 hour after its oral administration and the half-life is 1 to 3 hours. The drug is bound to plasma proteins and as a result it is largely confined to the extracellular fluid. Most of the drug is excreted in the urine as the parahydroxyl metabolite, which is also uricosuric in humans. Some 20 to 45 percent of the drug is excreted unchanged in 24 hours.

Sulfinpyrazone is three to six times more potent than probenecid on a weight basis.[36] The usual daily dose is 300 to 400 mg per day given in three or four divided doses.

Benziodarone and Benzbromarone

Benziodarone and benzbromarone are potent uricosuric agents in humans.[2, 3] Benziodarone contains iodine, and benzbromarone contains bromide (see Fig. 50–4). The former compound has found limited clinical use, in part because of its effect on thyroid function. The latter drug has been well tolerated during clinical uses.[38]

Benzbromarone is bound to plasma proteins. It undergoes successive oxidation of the ethyl side-chain and one- and two-fold hydroxylation of the benzofuran ring followed by methylation of one of the hydroxyl groups.[40, 41]

Therapeutic Action

Therapy with uricosuric drugs is started at a low dose to minimize the risk of renal calculi associated with the transient increase in uric acid excretion. In patients with normal renal function, a full therapeutic dose of probenecid may cause a brisk and pronounced uricosuria (Fig. 50–5). Because uric acid is relatively insoluble, especially in acid urine, this sudden increase in uric acid excretion can lead to the precipitation of uric acid crystals in the collecting ducts of the kidney or ureters or, more commonly, to the development of uric acid stones in 9 percent of the patients treated.[42]

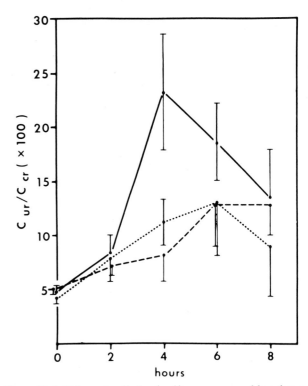

Figure 50–5. Uricosuric effects of sulfinpyrazone and benzbromarone. Sulfinpyrazone, 300 mg (....), benzbromarone 160 mg (—), or both drugs together (------) were given to four, six, and four patients, respectively. Each point represents the mean percentage of Curate: Creatinine plus or minus the standard error of the means. Sulfinpyrazone had its peak effect at 4 to 6 hours, while benzbromarone had its peak effect at 2 to 4 hours but continued its uricosuria beyond 8 hours, up to 24 hours. With sulfinpyrazone, the mean serum urate diminished from a control value of 7.0 to 6.0 after 8 hours and to 6.6 mg per dl after 24 hours. With benzbromarone, the mean serum urate decreased from a control value of 7.8 to 6.1 after 8 hours and to 4.3 mg per dl after 24 hours. Administration of both drugs resembled the sulfinpyrazone effect for the first 6 hours. (From Sinclair, D. S., and Fox, I. H.: The pharmacology of hypouricemic effect of benzbromarone. J. Rheumatol. 2:437, 1975.)

Uric acid precipitation with initiation of uricosuric therapy is unusual in the normal producer of uric acid. The maintenance of adequate urine flow and alkalinization of the urine with oral sodium bicarbonate (2 to 6 g per day) or sodium citrate (Scholl's solution, 20 to 60 ml per day) further diminish the possibility of uric acid stone formation, but use of these drugs is probably unnecessary in most patients.

Sulfinpyrazone administration is started at a dose of 50 mg twice per day, increasing in a few days to 100 mg three or four times each day. The maximum effective dose is 800 mg per day. Probenecid therapy is started at a dose of 250 mg twice per day, increasing after several weeks to 500 to 1000 mg two or three times each day. The maximum effective dose is 3 g per day.

Probenecid and sulfinpyrazone are effective for most gouty patients. Some 75 to 80 percent of patients with tophaceous gout have demonstrated improvement. In the remaining 20 percent of patients whose conditions are not brought under ideal control, failure is a result of drug intolerance, concomitant salicylate ingestion, or impaired renal function. Salicylate ingestion at any dose blocks the uricosuric effect of probenecid and sulfinpyrazone. When the glomerular filtration rate is below 20 to 30 ml per minute, most uricosuric drugs are ineffective.

An extensive clinical experience attests to the usefulness of sulfinpyrazone.[2] Tolerance for sulfinpyrazone is somewhat better than that for probenecid.[42, 43] Nevertheless, almost one quarter of patients stop the drug for one reason or another. The leading causes of failure of control, as with probenecid, are concomitant salicylate ingestion and renal insufficiency.

Benzbromarone is a potent uricosuric drug during clinical use. It is more effective than other uricosuric agents in patients with renal insufficiency.

Tolerability and Adverse Reactions

The major side effects of uricosuric drugs include skin rash, precipitation of acute gouty arthritis, gastrointestinal intolerance, and uric acid calculus formation. Probenecid has a calciuric action in gouty patients.[2, 3] The complication of urinary uric acid crystal or stone formation is preventable by forcing fluids and urinary alkalinization as described earlier. This complication of probenecid therapy reinforces the contraindication for use in gouty patients with nephrolithiasis or with overproduction of uric acid. In addition, probenecid should not be used in hyperuricemic cystinuric patients because of increased cystine, and decreased cysteine–penicillamine mixed disulfide and penicillamine disulfide metabolites.[2, 3]

A potential complication of all forms of antihyperuricemic drug therapy is the precipitation of an attack of acute gouty arthritis during the initial days or weeks of therapy, at a time when serum urate levels are being lowered. This complication occurs in 10 to 20 percent of patients started on probenecid therapy alone.[42] The incidence can be greatly reduced by concomitant administration of colchicine or indomethacin.

Toxicity. The frequency of side effects of probenecid has been extensively documented[45] as follows: hypersensitivity reactions, 0.3 percent; drug fever, 0.4 percent; skin rash, 1.4 percent; and gastrointestinal disturbances, 3.1 percent. In longer-term studies of gouty patients, there was an 8 to 18 percent incidence of gastrointestinal complaints and a 5 percent incidence of hypersensitivity and rash.[46]

Serious toxicity of probenecid is rare. Hepatic necrosis has been reported in one patient and the nephrotic syndrome in at least two.[2] Autoimmune hemolytic anemia is reported with probenecid therapy.[47] About one third of patients eventually became intolerant of probenecid and discontinued its use.[48] The experience with sulfinpyrazone is similar.

Table 50–3. EFFECTS OF PROBENECID ON METABOLISM OF OTHER DRUGS

Decreased Renal Excretion
p-Aminohippuric acid
Phenolsulfonphthalein
Salicylic acid and its acyl and phenolic glucuronides
Phlorizin and its glucuronide
Acetazolamide
Dapsone and its metabolites
Sulfinpyrazone and its parahydroxyl metabolite
Indomethacin
Ampicillin
Penicillin
Cephradine
Reduced Volume of Distribution
Ampicillin
Ancillin
Nafcillin
Cephaloridine
Impairment of Hepatic Uptake
Bromsulfonphthalein
Indocyanin green
Rifampicin
Delayed Metabolism
Heparin

Interaction with Other Drugs

Uricosuric drugs alter the transport of other organic acids across cell membranes, resulting in numerous drug interactions (Table 50–3).[2, 3, 34]

Because of these interactions, certain drugs should be used with caution in patients receiving probenecid. Dapsone and indomethacin, for example, should be used at a lower dose in patients receiving probenecid.[2] Not only does probenecid delay the renal excretion of salicylic acid and many of its glucuronide derivatives, but acetylsalicylate completely blocks the uricosuric effect of probenecid and most other uricosuric agents. Diuretics, on the other hand, do not block the uricosuric effect of probenecid. Subtherapeutic doses of heparin may have profound anticoagulant effects in patients receiving probenecid.[49]

The effect of probenecid on the metabolism of some drugs has been used to enhance their clinical activity. The renal excretion of penicillin and ampicillin is decreased by probenecid, and thus the half-life of these antibiotics is prolonged. Therefore, probenecid has been used, for example, to enhance the blood levels of ampicillin and penicillin. In addition, the half-life of rifampin is also prolonged because the hepatic uptake of rifampin is impaired by probenecid. The prolonged half-lives of rifampin[50] and cephradine[51] in the presence of probenecid may be therapeutically useful. Probenecid reduces the volume of distribution of several antibiotics, including ampicillin, ancillin, nafcillin, and cephaloridine.[51] If the concentration of these antibiotics is significantly reduced in body fluids in the presence of probenecid, the net effect could be detrimental.

The interaction of uricosuric drugs with allopurinol was described earlier.

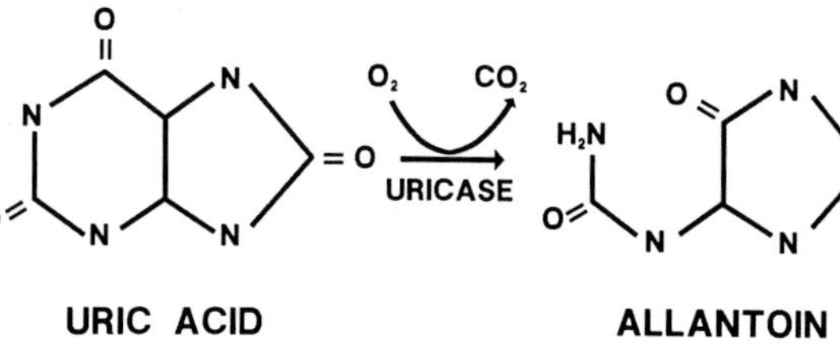

Figure 50–6. Uricase degrades uric acid to allantoin.

DESTRUCTION OF URATE

The enzymatic destruction of urate provides a novel experimental approach to treat hyperuricemia and the related disorders. Urate oxidase degrades uric acid to allantoin and carbon dioxide (Fig. 50–6). The administration of urate oxidase is especially promising in prophylaxis against acute uric acid nephropathy.[5, 52, 53] Polyethylene glycol–conjugated uricase may be particularly useful, since it has a prolonged half-life and appears to be non-antigenic.[52] After intermuscular injection of uricase, activity appears in the plasma rapidly, peaks within 24 hours, and persists for about 5 days.[54]

In patients with non-Hodgkin's lymphoma, uricase at 3 units per kg of body weight administered during the first 30 hours lowered the serum urate concentration from 15.3 to 3.2 mg per dl.[54] A dose of 2 units per kg every 5 to 6 days maintained the serum urate level at 9 mg per dl or lower.

I wish to thank Ed Yanisch for his excellent typing of this manuscript.

References

1. Appelbaum, S. J., Mayersohn, M., Dorr, R. T., and Perrier, D.: Allopurinol kinetics and bioavailability: Intravenous, oral and rectal administration. Cancer Chemother. Pharmacol. 8:93, 1982.
2. Kelley, W. N., and Fox, I. H.: Antihyperuricemic drugs. In Kelley, W. N., Harris, E. D., Jr., Ruddy, S., and Sledge, C. B. (eds.): Textbook of Rheumatology. 3rd ed. Philadelphia, W. B. Saunders Company, 1989, p. 889.
3. Palella, T. D., and Fox, I. H.: Hyperuricemia and gout. In Scriver, C. R., Beaudet, A. L., Sly, W. S., and Valle, D. (eds.): The Metabolic Basis of Inherited Disease. 6th ed. New York, McGraw-Hill, 1989, p. 965.
4. Rundles, R. W., Wyngaarden, J. B., and Hitchings, G. H.: Drugs and uric acid. Annu. Rev. Pharmacol. 9:345, 1969.
5. Wyngaarden, J. B., Kelley, W. N.: Gout. In Stanbury, J. B., Wyngaarden, J. B., Fredrickson, D. S., Goldstein, J. L., and Brown, M. S. (eds.): The Metabolic Basis of Inherited Disease. 5th ed. New York, McGraw-Hill, 1983, p. 1043.
6. Rundles, R. W.: The development of allopurinol. Arch. Intern. Med. 145:1492, 1985.
7. Edwards, N. L., Recker, D., Airozo, D., and Fox, I. H.: Enhanced purine salvage during allopurinol therapy: An important pharmacologic property in humans. J. Lab. Clin. Med. 98:673, 1981.
8. Bundgaard, H., and Falch, E.: Improved rectal and parenteral delivery of allopurinol using the prodrug approach. Arch. Pharm. Chem. Sci. Ed. 13:39, 1985.
9. Hande, K., Reed, E., and Chabner, B.: Allopurinol kinetics. Clin. Pharmacol. Ther. 23:598, 1978.
10. Chalmers, R. A., Kromer, H., and Scott, J. T.: A comparative study of the xanthine oxidase inhibitors, allopurinol and oxipurinol in man. Clin. Sci. 35:353, 1968.
11. Berlinger, W. G., Park, G. D., and Spector, R.: The effect of dietary

protein on the clearance of allopurinol and oxypurinol. N. Engl. J. Med. 313:771, 1985.
12. Elion, G. B., Yu, T. F., and Gutman, A. B.: Renal clearance of oxipurinol, the chief metabolite of allopurinol. Am. J. Med. 45:69, 1968.
13. Rundles, R. W.: The development of allopurinol. Arch. Intern. Med. 145:1492, 1985.
14. Yu, T. F.: The effect of allopurinol in primary and secondary gout. Arthritis Rheum. 8:907, 1965.
15. Day, R. O., Miners, J. O., and Birkett, D. J.: Allopurinol dosage selection: Relationships between dose and plasma oxipurinol and urate concentrations and urinary urate excretion. Br. J. Clin. Pharmacol. 26:423, 1988.
16. Gottlieb, N. L., and Gray, R. G.: Allopurinol-associated hand and foot deformities in chronic tophaceous gout. J.A.M.A. 238:1663, 1977.
17. Bull, P. W., and Scott, J. T.: Intermittent control of hyperuricemia in the treatment of gout. J. Rheumatol. 16:1246, 1989.
18. Loebl, W. Y., and Scott, J. T.: Withdrawal of allopurinol in patients with gout. Ann. Rheum. Dis. 33:304, 1974.
19. Zell, S. C., and Carmichael, J. M.: Evaluation of allopurinol use in patients with gout. Am. J. Hosp. Pharm. 46:1813, 1989.
20. Bellamy, N., Gilbert, J. R., and Brooks, P. M.: A survey of current prescribing practices of antiinflammatory and urate lowering drugs in gouty arthritis in the province of Ontario. J. Rheumatol. 15:1841, 1988.
21. Yu, T. F., and Gutman, A. B.: Effects of allopurinol [4-hydroxypyrazolo (3,4-d) pyrimidine] on serum and urinary uric acid in primary and secondary gout. Am. J. Med. 37:885, 1964.
22. Greene, M. L., Fujimoto, W. Y., and Seegmiller, J. E.: Urinary xanthine stones: A rare complication of allopurinol therapy. N. Engl. J. Med. 280:426, 1969.
23. Band, P. R., Silverberg, D. S., and Henderson, J. F.: Xanthine nephropathy in a patient with lymphosanoma treated with allopurinol. N. Engl. J. Med. 283:254, 1970.
24. Hande, K. R., Hixson, C. B., and Chabner, B. A.: Postchemotherapy purine excretion in lymphoma patients receiving allopurinol. Cancer Res. 41:2273, 1981.
25. Emmerson, B. T., Hazelton, R. A., and Frazer, I. H.: Some adverse reactions to allopurinol may be mediated by lymphocyte reactivity to oxypurinol. Arthritis Rheum. 31:3, 1988, 436.
26. Okafuji, K., and Shinohara, K.: Aplastic anemia probably induced by allopurinol in a patient with renal insufficiency. Rinsho Ketsueki 31:89, 1990.
27. Boston Collaborative Drug Surveillance Program: Excess of ampicillin rashes associated with allopurinol or hyperuricemia. N. Engl. J. Med. 286:505, 1972.
28. Fam, A. G., Paton, T. W., and Chaiton, A.: Reinstitution of allopurinol therapy for gouty arthritis after cutaneous reactions. Can. Med. Assoc. J. 123:128, 1980.
29. Meyrier, A.: Desensitization in a patient with chronic renal disease and severe allergy to allopurinol. Br. Med. J. 2:458, 1976.
30. Hande, K. R., Noone, R. M., and Stone, W. J.: Severe allopurinol toxicity: Description and guidelines for prevention in patients with renal insufficiency. Am. J. Med. 76:47, 1984.
31. Singer, J. Z., and Wallace, S. L.: The allopurinol hypersensitivity syndrome. Unnecessary morbidity and mortality. Arthritis Rheum. 29:82, 1986.
32. Fox, I. H., and Kelly, W. N.: Management of gout. J.A.M.A. 242:361, 1979.
33. Barry, M., and Feely, J.: Allopurinol influences aminophenazone elimination. Clin. Pharmacokin et. 19:167, 1990.
34. Weiner, and I. M., Mudge, G. H.: Inhibitors of tubular transport of organic compounds. In Gilman, A. G., Rall, T. W., Nies, A. S., and Taylor, P. (eds.): The Pharmacologic Basis of Therapeutics. 8th ed. New York, Pergamon Press, 1990, p. 920.
35. Diamond, H. S.: Uricosuric drugs. In Kelley, W. N., Weiner, I. M. (eds.): Uric Acid. Berlin, Springer-Verlag, 1978, p. 459.
36. Weiner, I. M., Blanchard, K. C., and Mudge, G. H.: Factors influencing renal excretion of foreign organic acids. Am. J. Physiol. 207:953, 1964.
37. Dayton, P. G., Yu, T. F., and Chen, W.: The physiological disposition of probenecid, including renal clearance in man, studied by an improved method for its estimation in biological material. J. Pharmacol. Exp. Ther. 140:278, 1963.
38. Israeli, Z. A., Perel, J. M., and Cunningham, R. F.: Metabolites of probenecid: Chemical, physical and pharmacological studies. J. Med. Chem. 15:709, 1972.
39. de Gery, A., Auscher, C., and Saporta, L.: Treatment of gout and hyperuricemia by benzbromarone, ethyl 2 (dibromo-3,5-hydroxy-4-benzoyl)-3 benzofuran. In Sperling, O., de Vries, A., Wyngaarden, J. B. (eds.): Purine Metabolism in Man. New York, Plenum Press, 1974, p. 683.
40. Maurer, H., and Wollenberg, P.: Urinary metabolites of benzbromarone in man. Arzneimittelforschung 40:460, 1990.
41. Walter-Sack, I., de Vries, J. X., and Ittensohn, A.: Benzbromarone disposition and uricosuric action; evidence for hydroxylation instead of debromination to benzarone. Klin. Wochenschr. 66:160, 1988.

42. Gutman, A. B.: Treatment of primary gout: The present status. Arthritis Rheum. 8:911, 1965.
43. Persellin, R. H., and Schmid, F. R.: The use of sulfinpyrazone in the treatment of gout reduces serum uric acid levels and diminishes severity of arthritis attacks, with freedom from significant toxicity. J.A.M.A. 175:971, 1961.
44. Emmerson, B. T.: A comparison of uricosuric agents in gout, with special reference to sulphinpyrazone. Med. J. Aust. 1:839, 1963.
45. Boger, W. P., and Strickland, S. C.: Probenecid (Benemid): Its use and side-effects in 2502 patients. Arch. Intern. Med. 95:83, 1955.
46. Gutman, A. B., Yu, T. F.: Protracted uricosuric therapy in tophaceous gout. Lancet 2:1258, 1957.
47. Kickler, T. S., Buck, S., Ness, P., Shirley, R. S., and Sholar, P. W.: Probenecid-induced immune hemolytic anemia. J. Rheumatol. 13:208, 1986.
48. de Seze, S., Ryckewaert, A., and d'Anglejan, G.: The treatment of gout by probenecid (a study based on 156 cases, 68 of which were treated from 1 to 9 years). Rev. Rhum. Mal. Osteoartic. 30:93, 1963.
49. Sanchez, G.: Enhancement of heparin effect by probenecid. N. Engl. J. Med. 292:48, 1975.
50. Kenwright, S., and Levi, A. J.: Impairment of hepatic uptake of rifamycin antibiotics by probenecid, and its therapeutic implications. Lancet 2:1401, 1973.
51. Gibaldi, M., and Schwartz, M. A.: Apparent effect of probenecid on distribution of penicillin in man. Clin. Pharmacol. Ther. 9:345, 1968.
52. Davis, S., and Park, Y. K.: Hypouricaemic effect of polyethyleneglycol modified urate oxidase. Lancet 1:281, 1981.
53. Masera, G., Jankovic, M., Zurlo, M. G., Locasciulli, A., Rossi, M. R., Uderzo, C., and Recchia, M.: Urate-oxidase prophylaxis of uric acid–induced renal damage in childhood leukemia. J. Pediatr. 100:152, 1982.
54. Chua, C. C., Greenberg, M. L., and Viau, A. T.: Use of polyethylene glycol-modified uricase (PEG-uricase) to treat hyperuricemia in a patient with non-Hodgkin lymphoma. Ann. Intern. Med. 109:114, 1988.

Section VI
Rheumatoid Arthritis

Chapter 51   Edward D. Harris, Jr.

Etiology and Pathogenesis of Rheumatoid Arthritis

INTRODUCTION

Rheumatoid arthritis (RA) is a common chronic disease. It affects about 1 percent of the general population worldwide[1] and has served to spur on much research that has elucidated mechanisms of normal immune responses as well as of disease. A major unknown in the pathogenesis of RA is the reason that inflammation begins and continues within joints, often without specific involvement of other organ systems. Conversely, we have little explanation of why extra-articular manifestations and positive tests for rheumatoid factor develop in some patients with RA but not all. Keys to understanding these phenomena lie in comprehension of arthrotropism of antigens and inflammatory cells for joints and in learning what specific receptors and chemotactic gradients exist to focus the inflammation within joints.

To explain the tissue specificity, a number of hypotheses abound. Several relate to the unique anatomy of the diarthrodial joint. Joints move, but paralyzed limbs usually manifest less inflammation in joints in patients with RA. Does motion itself make the joints susceptible to the particular causative agent in this disease? Another difference between joint and other spaces in the body is that the joint has no epithelial tissue. The synovial lining cells are mesenchymal in origin; thus, the only basement membrane separating the components of blood from the joint spaces is that in the synovial capillary wall. Whether or not these obvious differences between joints and other organs have relevance to why the chronic inflammation of RA occurs in joints is not known, but these differences must be encompassed in any set of hypotheses that "explain" RA.

The first criteria for classification (not diagnosis) of RA were published in 1958. These were used heavily, but criticized, for 30 years[2] and were revised in 1988.[3] The new criteria are:

1. Morning stiffness in and around joints lasting at least 1 hour before maximal improvement.
2. Soft tissue swelling (arthritis) of three or more joint areas observed by a physician.
3. Swelling (arthritis) of the proximal interphalangeal, metacarpophalangeal, or wrist joints.
4. Symmetric arthritis.
5. Subcutaneous nodules.
6. Positive test for rheumatoid factor (RF).
7. Radiographic erosions or periarticular osteopenia in hand or wrist joints.

To make a diagnosis of RA, criteria 1 through 4 must have been present for at least 6 weeks; 4 or more criteria must be present. The new criteria demonstrate 91 to 94 percent sensitivity and 89 percent specificity for RA when compared with non-RA rheumatic disease control subjects.[3] The diagnosis of RA should not be made by criteria alone if another systemic disease associated with arthritis is definitely present; conditions most likely to be confused with early-onset RA include systemic lupus erythematosus (SLE), psoriatic arthritis and other seronegative spondyloarthropathies, mixed connective tissue disease, Reiter's syndrome, polymyalgia rheumatica, and Sjögren's syndrome with polyarthritis. Not included in the new criteria are the distinctions among "classic," "definite," and "probable" RA; doing away with the "probable" criterion both enhances specificity of the criterion and minimizes overestimates of prevalence of RA.

Rheumatologists in previous decades have defined very well the clinical manifestations of RA. In contrast, it is in the areas of pathogenesis, prognosis, and treatment that a wealth of new knowledge has become available in the past 10 years. RA can now be appreciated as a process determined by immunogenetics of the class II major histocompatibility (MHC) loci, precipitated by unknown antigens (possibly infectious in nature) and resulting in poorly restrained proliferation of macrophages, T and B lymphocytes, and their products, cytokines and immunoglobulins. The inflammation that these cells and their gene products evoke leads to proliferation and activation of synovial cells, and these, behaving much as a localized malignancy, invade and destroy articular cartilage, subchondral bone, tendons, and ligaments (Fig. 51–1). New appreciation of these pathogenic mechanisms has increased awareness that irreversible loss of articular cartilage begins relatively early in the course of RA and that therapies to suppress the synovitis must be effective early if joint destruction is to be avoided.

To treat patients with RA better, it is essential to realize at what pathogenetic stage of disease a patient is in during different clinical phases. The following sections will correlate pathobiologic, clinical, diagnostic, and therapeutic stages of the disease. The stages of RA that have diagnostic or therapeutic

Table 51–1. IMMUNOGENETICS AND RHEUMATOID ARTHRITIS

Increased risk of RA[26]
*DR4 (Dw4, Dw14)
DR1
Decreased risk of RA[30]
DR2
DR2, DR3
DR3, DR7
Increased severity of RA[29]
DQw7

*Also known as DRB1*0404.

relevance are listed in Table 51–1 and are correlated with symptoms, physical signs, and radiographic or imaging abnormalities. It should be noted from Table 51–1 that when the disease has progressed to stage 4 or 5, it is unlikely that therapy can reverse or retard destruction of articular cartilage; it follows that effective therapy must be instituted during stages 2 and 3 if irreversible loss of articular cartilage is to be prevented.

SUSCEPTIBILITY TO DEVELOPMENT OF RHEUMATOID ARTHRITIS

It is becoming apparent that many host influences are major determinants in the development of this disease. Although immunogenetics may be the most dominant of these, the most powerful additional factor recognized in the host is the sex of the patient.

Sex

RA is one of many autoimmune diseases that predominate in females. The ratio of female to male patients (2:1 to 4:1) is significant, yet not nearly as high as that found in Hashimoto's thyroiditis (25:1 to 50:1), SLE (9:1), or even autoimmune diabetes mellitus (type I, 5:1).[4] Estrogens have multiple effects on T lymphocytes and may inhibit neutrophil activation as well.[5]

Still incompletely understood are the mechanisms underlying the effect of pregnancy on RA. Pregnancy usually is associated with remission of the disease in the last trimester, with subsequent relapses after delivery.[6, 7] More than 75 percent of pregnant patients with RA improve, starting in the first or second trimester, but 90 percent of these will have a flare of disease in the weeks or months after delivery. Hazes[8] has summarized the epidemiologic data on pregnancy as follows:

1. Pregnancy has an ameliorating effect on RA.
2. Patients with RA were more often nulliparous before disease onset than controls.
3. Perhaps a first pregnancy at a young age decreases the risk of developing RA.

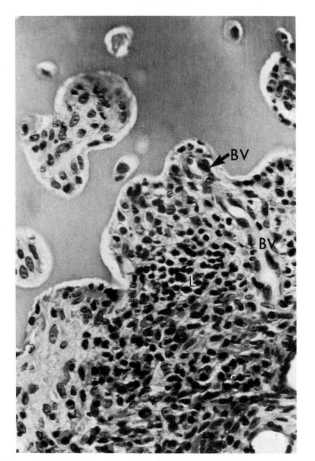

Figure 51–1. High-power light microscopy at the pannus-synovium junction. The space between them is shrinkage artifact. Tongues of proliferating tissue have invaded the residual cartilage shown at the upper left. Small blood vessels (*BV*) are seen just below the cartilage-pannus junction. Small, darkly staining cells, probably lymphocytes (*L*), are just below the invading surface.

Attempts have been made to relate disease suppression during pregnancy to serum concentration of pregnancy alpha$_2$ (α_2) glycoprotein (PAG), although it is not known what biologic role this protein has in vivo.[9] In one study, pregnancy-related changes were not found in the numbers of T, B, or null cells nor in changes in response to mitogens; however, significant reversible depression of the purified tuberculin (purified protein derivative [PPD]) response was noted in the second half of pregnancy.[10]

Consonant with the relief of RA during pregnancy are the data indicating a decreased risk of RA in women who had been pregnant;[11] in this study, the relative risk was 0.49 compared with that of women never pregnant and was a factor independent of oral contraceptive use, measurable immunogenetic factors, or family history of RA. These data are at odds with an earlier study suggesting that pregnancy might increase the risk of RA;[12] additional studies are needed to settle the debate.

In 1978, it was reported that oral contraceptives protected against the development of RA.[13] A similar negative association was found between the onset of RA and the previous use of noncontraceptive hormones; this negative association persisted with univariant and multivariant control of potentially confounding variables as well as with the subgroup analysis.[14] A decrease in the incidence of RA noted in Rochester, Minnesota, after 1960 was ascribed to the availability of oral contraceptives and postmenopausal estrogens.[15] Two subsequent case studies by the Mayo Clinic group in this same population, however, failed to confirm any protection from RA of prior or current oral contraceptive use.[16, 17] A subsequent study of 121 consecutive patients with definite RA indicated that the use of oral contraceptives prior to the onset of RA was associated only with a reduction in the incidence of severe, not mild or moderate, RA.[17a] This may explain the divergence of conclusions using data gathered in different areas and countries.

A possible link between the protective effect of both fecundity and oral contraceptives may be induction of similar hormonal changes by both phenomena that could generate arthritis-protective T cell clones or reduce arthritogenic clones or have another suppressive effect upon joint inflammation.[19]

The possible relationship between alleviation of RA symptoms during the last trimester of pregnancy and immunogenetics may be indicated by the observation that alloantibodies in the maternal circulation are developed during pregnancy against paternal human leukocyte antigen (HLA) antigens.[20] Indeed, placenta-eluted gamma globulins have been used in France for 10 years to treat classic, severe, and active RA successfully.[20, 21] Data have demonstrated the presence of alloantibodies directed against class II (DR) HLA in these eluted antibodies. Thus, the hypothesis must be tested that blocking function of the HLA-DR epitopes associated with RA could therapeutically down-regulate and effectively treat this disease.

New data from the Netherlands lead to the possible conclusion that cigarette smoking and alcohol consumption both exert a protective effect from RA in young women.[18]

Immunogenetic and Other Heritable Predisposing Factors in Rheumatoid Arthritis

Evidence is accumulating that the structure of class II surface molecules on antigen-presenting cells is of equal or even more importance than the nature of the antigen presented to the T lymphocyte at the initiation of immune response in RA. Chapter 6 presents a detailed discussion of class I and class II MHC antigens and of the insights provided by intensive study of the molecular genetics of RA. As Winchester has emphasized,[22]

Whereas in principle the clonal repertoires of B and T cell antigen receptors are immense and present in each person . . . an entirely different strategy is followed by the MHC system. Here it is the species that has the repertoire for all varieties of MHC molecules, with each person having only a small proportion of all potentially reactive polymorphic receptors.

This means that whether or not certain T cell immune responses occur is because of the presence or absence of particular MHC (in this case, DR) allelic products. The MHC also determine the T cell repertoire in a given individual; those T cells that cannot recognize the MHC antigens around them are eliminated in fetal development through thymic selection. At the same time, auto-reactive T cells are eliminated. The end result is a fine balance in discrimination between self and nonself; it is not surprising that autoantibodies occur to various antigens and to a variable extent in all of us.

In the 1970s, Stastny[23] provided evidence that RA was associated with an antigen of the HLA-D locus. The T cell receptor–HLA-DR interaction, rather than TCR-peptide interactions, is believed to be determined by the allelic variations in HLA-DR expression.[23a] HLA-Dw4, identified by the mixed lymphocyte reaction, was shown to be the D locus antigen associated with RA as well as with more severe forms of the disease.[24] The finding of B cell alloantigens closely related to HLA-D enabled investigators to demonstrate that the B lymphocyte alloantigen HLA-DR4 occurred in 70 percent of patients compared with 28 percent of controls, giving a relative risk of having RA to those with HLA-DR4 of approximately 4 to 5.[25]

Careful study of the MHC using cDNA probes directed against specific alpha (α) and beta (β) chains of the DR loci has revealed *susceptibility cassettes* or shared epitopes on the β chains of DR that predispose to development of RA. HLA-DR4 can be divided into at least five subtypes: Dw4, Dw10, Dw13, Dw14, and Dw15. The susceptibility to developing RA is associated with the third hypervariable region of DR β chains, from amino acid 70 through 74.[26, 27] The susceptibility epitope is glutamine-leucine-arginine-alanine-alanine (QKRAA) or ones with minor substitutions that do not affect polarity of the cassette. This sequence is found in Dw4 and Dw14 (in which RA is more prevalent) and in DR1β chains as well[26] (see Table 51–1). DRβ chains with other substitutions in this region (e.g., Dw10) have no susceptibility to RA. This epitope may also code for the severity of RA once it is established.[28, 28a] Patients who are homozygous for disease-associated alleles of the HLA-DRB1 gene are more likely than others with only one disease-associated allele to have severe erosive RA with nodules and extra-articular manifestations of disease.[28a]

Another genetic factor that may influence severity, if not susceptibility, to RA is the DQ system. The homologous duplicated genes of the class II region of the MHC are grouped into three subregions: DP, DQ, and DR. It has been reported that a DR4-associated allele DQw7 was found to be significantly increased only in patients with severe RA, whereas DR1 was readily increased only with mild RA often controlled by nonsteroidal anti-inflammatory drugs.[29]

Protective HLA-DR phenotypes can be identified as well. Data suggest that four phenotypes with half or less of the expected frequency of RA are DR1, DR5; DR2; DR2, DR3; and DR3, DR7.[30]

In summary, although it is likely that every person who develops RA will share an important common epitope on DRβ chains, only a small percentage of these "susceptible" individuals will, in turn, develop RA.

In the humoral immune system, a certain immunoglobulin *kappa* (κ) genotype appears to confer risk of RA.[31, 32]

Although it cannot be considered an immunogenetic determinant, strictly speaking, information is accumulating that deficient galactosylation of immunoglobulin may be a risk factor for development of autoimmune diseases, including RA.[33] The IgG glycosylation defect has been demonstrated to exist before the onset of RA.[34]

Another genetic possibility, intriguing but unproved, is that certain individuals have a deficient hypothalamic response to acute inflammation. Experiments showed that in contrast to rats resistant to arthritis, a strain that was susceptible to streptococcal cell wall arthritis had markedly impaired plasma corticotropin and corticosterone responses to streptococcal cell walls or to other phlogistic compounds and that corticotropin-releasing hormone mRNA was not generated in the hypothalamus in these animals.[35, 36] It is intriguing to develop the hypothesis that a genetic impairment in hypothalamic-pituitary-adrenal responsiveness to inflammation would be sufficient to permit symmetric synovitis to develop and proliferate and eventually to become a self-sustaining process that we diagnose as RA.

POSSIBLE DIRECT CAUSES OF RHEUMATOID ARTHRITIS

As reviewed earlier, one or multiple genetic factors may predispose an individual to develop RA. Just as it is unlikely that all common viruses or bacteria could stimulate genesis of a polyarticular synovitis, it is unlikely that only one environmental (infectious or noninfectious) agent could trigger the disease. A guess, based on available data, is that several environmental stimuli, probably viruses, infect an individual and through some mechanism the inflammatory response is focused in joints. After gaining a toehold there, the synovitis will persist even in the absence of the offending agent because of autoimmunity and the cyclic automaticity that enables the disease to become self-perpetuating.

Infectious Agents

Bacteria, Viruses, and Their Components

There is no good evidence that a pyogenic bacterium or mycobacterium is causative in RA, and although mycoplasma have been put forth as a possible cause, there is no evidence yet to support claims that these agents are involved etiologically in RA. The striking similarity of histopathologic changes in RA and in joints of occasional patients with Lyme disease caused by the spirochete *Borrelia burgdorferi* leaves open the possibility that an as yet unappreciated or unknown organism is causative. Lyme disease is different from RA in its immunogenetic background. When HLA-DR4–positive patients were excluded from consideration, a secondary association with HLA-DR2 was noted to be an independent, dominant marker for Lyme disease.[37] As mentioned earlier, DR2 is apparently protective against RA.

Epstein-Barr Virus

In 1975, Alspaugh and Tan[38] described an antibody in the sera of patients with RA that reacted with an antigen extracted from a lymphoblastic cell line carrying the Epstein-Barr virus (EBV). Alspaugh et al.[39] went on to demonstrate that the antibodies, named rheumatoid arthritis precipitin (RAP), were indeed directed against EBV-specific antigens. Although it was demonstrated that there was an abnormally elevated frequency of EBV-infected B cells in blood of patients with RA,[40] it also was shown that in patients with early RA, titers of antibody to EBV-associated nuclear antigen or to viral capsid antigen were not elevated, suggesting that EBV infection was a sequel to and not the cause of RA.[41] Sophisticated techniques to look for EBV genome in rheumatoid synovial tissue have been unsuccessful.[42, 43]

Despite these data, there are still many reasons

to implicate EBV in the pathogenesis, if not the etiology, of RA. The EBV receptor on human B lymphocytes is actually a complement receptor type 2 (CR2),[44] and the virus gains access to the cell at this site. The EBV is a polyclonal activator of B lymphocytes, and as is reiterated later in more detail, rheumatoid macrophages and T cells combine to generate a defect in suppression of EBV proliferation in human B cells. Rheumatoid patients appear to have higher levels of EBV shedding in throat washings, an increased number of virus-infected B cells in the circulating blood, higher levels of antibodies to the EBV antigens, and abnormal EBV-specific cytotoxic T cell responsiveness compared with controls.[45, 46]

There is a fascinating molecular link between RA and HLA-DR4 and DR1: It is the EBV glycoprotein gp110. Patients with serologic evidence of a previous infection with EBV have been shown to have antibodies against the epitope (Gln-leu-arg-ala-ala) that is the *susceptibility cassette* on β chains of certain subgroups of HLA-DR4 and on DR1.[47, 48] An inference from these data can be that T cell recognition of EBV epitopes in some patients with HLA-Dw4, HLA-Dw14, or HLA-DR1 may lead to RA, whereas in those with other class II MHC alleles, no cross-reactivity with EBV proteins would exist.

Parvovirus and Rheumatoid Arthritis

A small particle resembling parvoviruses in morphologic and physical chemical properties has been derived from rheumatoid synovial tissue.[49] Polyclonal antibodies developed against this putative virus were able to detect reactive antigen and synovial cells from different rheumatoid arthritis patients but not from individuals with osteoarthritis. It must be concluded that the virus was in the synovium, but did it initiate the arthritis? Supporting the possibility are reports that two patients with early RA had evidence of a recent infection with human parvovirus B19.[50] Anti–human parvovirus immunoglobulin G (IgG) levels declined but were still present 8 months or more after the onset of symptoms. Despite these cases, however, it is important to point out that very few rheumatoid patients have evidence of such a coincident infection; in a total of 69 patients with RA, only four acquired the parvovirus infection near the time of onset of their RA.[50]

Other Viruses

Lentiviruses are a subfamily of retroviruses and derive their name from the slow time course of the infections they cause in humans and animals. The human immunodeficiency virus (HIV) is one of these. Pathologic changes in lentivirus infections are, for the most part, indirectly mediated by the immune and inflammatory responses of the host. Finding cells infected by virus is extremely difficult. A deforming arthritis in goats and sheep is caused by lentiviruses, which are difficult to find although

known to be the cause of the disease.[51] In some experimental animals, a "Trojan horse" mechanism can be invoked; the viral genome can be concealed within monocytes and transported without detection to other sites; perhaps the synovium could be one of these. Restricted gene expression[51] is the underlying mechanism in the persistence and spread of lentiviruses and the slow evolution of the disease that they produce. The arthritogenicity of such infections might be related to the fact that synovial lymphocytes appear to respond quantitatively much more to certain viruses (i.e., adenovirus, mumps, and cytomegalovirus) than do peripheral blood lymphocytes.

Because rubella virus and the rubella vaccine have caused a synovitis in humans, there is interest in this virus as a triggering agent. In one series, 21 instances were reported in which live rubella virus was isolated from synovial fluid obtained from six patients with inflammatory oligoarthritis or polyarthritis over a period of 2 years in the absence of firm clinical evidence of rubella.[52] None of these patients, however, had the classic polyarticular involvement seen so often in RA; most had an oligoarthritis involving large joints.

Transgenic mice have been produced that carry the genome for human T cell leukemia virus type I (HLTV-1).[53] In 10 to 30 percent of females in the transgenic lines, synovial inflammation and an erosive pannus developed at 2 to 3 months of age in multiple joints. HTLV-I mRNA expression in affected joints was five to ten times higher than that in control transgenic mice. *Tax*, a transcriptional activator coded in the virus that is a potent inducer of cellular genes, was also markedly expressed in the affected joints. It is possible that *Tax* could induce inflammatory and proliferative changes in the joints. These data set up the testable hypothesis that HTLV-I is a primary cause of RA.

In summary, the hypothesis that one or more viral infections may serve as a triggering agent in the genetically susceptible host is appealing. Qualities of candidate viruses should be similar to those of the lentivirus, which has a restricted expression within cells and can remain hidden from defense mechanisms in the host. It is possible that just a small alteration in T cell reactivity or responsiveness induced by a viral infection or generation of a neoantigen by insertion of a viral genome into the host itself could be sufficient to trigger the disease. It is also possible that subsequent to this event, infection by a ubiquitous second virus (such as EBV) capable of generating polyclonal B cell stimulation would be sufficient to amplify the immune response and in the immunogenetically appropriate host, enable it to become self-perpetuating through cross-reactivity of epitopes.

Heat Shock Proteins—Omnipresent and Cross-Reactive

There is a link between heat shock proteins (HSP) and RA. The HSP are a family of medium-

Table 51–2. MOLECULAR MIMICRY AND
RHEUMATOID ARTHRITIS

Epstein-Barr virus glycoprotein (gp110) and HLA-DR4 and DR1
β chains share common epitope:

  Glutamine-leucine-arginine-alanine-alanine,[47, 48] or QKRAA

Bacterial heat shock proteins have significant sequence homology
to human heat shock proteins[54]

---

sized (60 to 90 kDa) proteins produced by cells of all
species in response to stress. These proteins have
conserved amino acid sequences; for example, certain
HSP of *Mycobacterium tuberculosis* have a 65 percent
sequence homology with HSP of humans.[54] The HSP
may facilitate intracellular folding and translocation
of proteins as they serve as protection from insults
induced by heat, bacteria, host cell attack (in the case
of bacteria), oxygen radicals, and nutrient depletion,
but they may have additional functions as well. T
lymphocytes from animals with adjuvant arthritis
recognize an epitope of mycobacteria HSP 65 (amino
acids 180 to 188); T cells from rat streptococcal cell
wall arthritis recognize this antigen also. Both forms
of experimental arthritis can be transferred to naïve
animals by such reactive T cells.[55, 56] Protection from
both forms of arthritis is conferred on rats by immunization with mycobacterial HSP. Some patients
with RA have elevated levels of antibodies to mycobacterial HSP,[57] particularly in synovial fluid.[58] The
majority of T cell clones isolated from RA synovial
fluid with specificity to mycobacterial components
are γδ cells that express neither CD4 nor CD8 surface
antigens. The γδ cells recognize small peptide epitopes in a manner similar to the more common cells
that bear the αβ T cell receptor.[59]

How could HSP be related to the cause of RA?
The possibility exists of cross-reactive epitopes; HSP
from bacteria have *molecular mimicry* (i.e., similar
amino acid sequences) with numerous human proteins (Table 51–2). More interesting, yet more complex, is the hypothesis that antibodies and T cells
exist that recognize epitopes shared by HSP of both
infectious agents and host cells; in inflammation of
the joints, synovial cells would express HSP, and
these would be recognized by cross-reactive T cells
and antibodies. Thus, it would not matter which
microbe in the environment appeared in a particular
patient, but rather whether the immunogenes would
facilitate cross-reactivity of lymphocytes with HSP of
host cells. The HSP may be functioning as a superantigen, triggering reactive T cells in virtually all
species and tissues. In that context, it is of interest
that staphylococcal enterotoxin B superantigen has
caused arthritis in susceptible mice.[60]

Another hypothesis deserving of testing is related to the amelioration of RA during pregnancy.
Since some HSP are overexpressed during pregnancy, if, indeed, HSP are related to RA, it is possible
that HSP overexpression would induce a state of

immunotolerance to non–MHC-dependent triggering
of T cell clones directed against HSP.[60a]

Arthritis Induced by Collagen—Is There Relevance for Rheumatoid Arthritis?

The discoveries that type II collagen can cause
arthritis in rats and mice and that the disease and
some of its manifestations can be passively transferred by IgG fractions containing anticollagen
antibodies[61] or by transfer of lymphocytes from affected animals[67] have spawned extensive experiments
that illustrate the antigenicity of collagen, the arthro-
tropic nature of the disease produced, and the dependence of experimental animals on immune response genes for reactivity. In these rodents, it is
clear that functional T cells are necessary to initiate
a collagen-induced arthritis;[63] that a lymphokine produced by T cells may cause synovitis, binds to type
II collagen, and is found in animals after type II
immunization;[64] and that a major immunogenic and
arthritogenic epitope on type II collagen resides in a
restricted area of the type II collagen chains.[65] One
provocative study demonstrated that if spleen cells
from mice immunized with immune complexes contained both native type II collagen and a monoclonal
anticollagen type II antibody, lymphocyte clones
could be isolated that produced two monoclonal IgG
rheumatoid factors, one of which also appeared to
be an anti-idiotype of anticollagen II antibodies.[66]

Most data in humans are consistent with the
hypothesis that RA is not caused by development of
antibodies to type II collagen but that the inflammatory response is amplified by production of these
antibodies. Monoclonal antibodies to native type II
collagen have been shown to react with cells within
the invasive synovium at the pannus-cartilage junction in material taken from rheumatoid joints.[67] Using
an enzyme-linked immunosorbent assay (ELISA),
these antibodies were shown to be directed against
type II collagen only and were not found in cartilage
of patients with osteoarthritis.[68] Sera from patients
with RA contained antibody titers to denatured bovine type II collagen that were significantly higher
than those found in control sera;[69] however, there
was no difference in antibody titers to native collagen, suggesting that the denatured form generated
after breakdown of connective tissue had served as
the immunogen. It has been suggested that antibodies that do form against collagen have pathogenic
capability.[70] It was shown that the major subclass of
anti–type II collagen antibodies was IgG3. It was also
demonstrated that the anticollagen antibodies purified from the sera of patients with RA had the
capability to activate complement, generating, among
other products, C5a when these antibodies became
bound to cartilage.[70] This has relevance to the observations by Jasin that anticollagen antibodies can be
eluted from rheumatoid articular cartilage.[71] Some of
the biologic details relating to collagen as an immu-

nogen are included in Chapter 2. It is of interest that sera from RA and from polychondritis differ in their reactivity with peptides of collagen, suggesting recruitment of a different T cell group in each disease.[68]

Rheumatoid Factor: Cause or Effect in Rheumatoid Arthritis?

The evidence is strong that RF contributes to amplification of the rheumatoid synovitis through activation of complement and formation of immune complexes that are phagocytosed by polymorphonuclear neutrophils (PMNs) in synovial fluid. Is it possible, however, that RF has a primary role in etiology, that a T cell–mediated immune response develops against IgG, and that no exogenous infectious agent or other antigenic stimulation is necessary to trigger RA?

The chemistry and biology of RFs are discussed in detail in Chapter 8, as is their clinical relevance in Chapter 52. As reviewed in these chapters, it has been shown by use of stored blood samples that, although some patients have RF present in their sera before the onset of any symptoms of arthritis, this does not usually occur. However, the report 18 years ago of cross-reactive idiotypes among monoclonal IgM proteins with anti-IgG activity[72] and the possible implications of expression of this germ line by so many individuals has continued to stimulate interest in the possibility that antibodies against IgG are the triggering event. As detailed and referenced in Chapter 8, amino acid sequences of several RF light chains are remarkably similar. One mouse monoclonal antibody reacts with isolated light chains of approximately 50 percent of RFs from unrelated individuals.[73] Additional investigations have been consistent with the conclusion that the variable region amino acid sequences of the RF light chains were homologous and were probably the product of a single V gene, conserved through multiple generations. This gene has been isolated, cloned, and sequenced.[74] Unlike in Sjögren's syndrome and mixed cryoglobulinemia, however, in which there is a restricted expression of RFs suggestive of autonomous proliferation of B lymphocytes, the wider distribution of RFs among κ variable region subgroups of light chains and the fact that RF response is distributed among IgM and IgG as well as IgA classes suggest that in RA this autoantibody response is antigen driven and T lymphocyte dependent and not a monoclonal proliferation.[75]

Data from several laboratories have indicated that patients who are seronegative but otherwise have a clinical diagnosis consistent with RA have "hidden" RFs in their 19S or 7S serum fractions and that these can be identified by antibody specific for the major RF cross-reactive idiotype.[76] A potentially important observation about RF concerns the data that implicate a decreased galactosylation of IgG in patients with RA[77] caused by a reduced B cell galac-

tosyltransferase activity in RA. This galactosylation defect, found in certain rheumatoid patients before they developed manifestations of RA,[34] could generate IgG that more easily could become an autoantigen and amplify a nonspecific inflammation into a full-blown rheumatoid process.

INITIATION OF THE INFLAMMATORY AND IMMUNE RESPONSE IN RHEUMATOID ARTHRITIS

Several pieces of evidence point rather directly to the fact that T lymphocytes, particularly the CD4+ helper/inducer cells, are a crucial early component of the rheumatoid response: (1) Patients with RA who develop acquired immunodeficiency syndrome (AIDS) have a sustained remission of their disease. (2) Antibodies against CD4[78, 78a] and interleukin-2 (IL-2) fused to diphtheria toxin[79] both have beneficial effects when used in therapeutic trials in RA.

Antigen Presentation to T Lymphocytes

In the subsynovial areas around the small capillaries and what will become, after initiation of the immune response, high endothelial venules in synovium, tissue macrophages are available to process and present antigen to T lymphocytes (Fig. 51–2). Many different types of cells in chronically inflamed tissues, including rheumatoid synovium, may bear HLA-DR antigens on their surfaces, but this does not necessarily correlate with antigen-presenting function. Although normal synovial lining cells can mediate T lymphocyte proliferation, their activating ability appears to be lower than that of epidermal Langerhans' cells, which stand as barriers to entrance of antigen through the skin. In contrast, rheumatoid synovial macrophage-like/dendritic cells are extremely efficient in allogeneic T cell activation.[80] The microheterogeneity of the rheumatoid synovial tissue, with different densities of different types of cells at various areas, probably ensures not only microheterogeneity of function within the synovium (i.e., some areas would be involved in active T cell activation, other areas would not), but also that the proper ratio of antigen-presenting cell, T lymphocyte, and other accessory cells and factors necessary for amplification of the immune response would be present in some areas but not in others. At many locations in the synovium, therefore, the histopathologic findings resemble those of a classic delayed type hypersensitivity reaction.[81] Large, strongly HLA-DR positive, macrophage-like cells express a dendritic appearance and form close contact with cells bearing CD4 markers that, presumably, will function as helper cells in the immune response.[80, 82] Chapter 7 outlines the details of how antigen is internalized and processed by the mature macrophage in preparation for presentation to lymphocytes

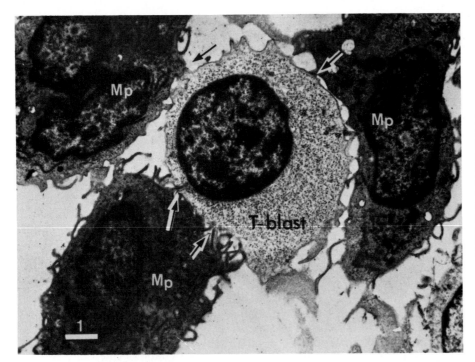

Figure 51–2. T lymphoblast in rheumatoid synovial tissue surrounded by three macrophages (*Mp*). The arrows point to probable intercellular bridging. This may be the morphologic manifestation of presentation of antigen to the helper T cell by the antigen-presenting cells. (Photograph provided by Hitoshi Ishikawa and Morris Ziff, University of Texas Southwestern Medical Center, Dallas, Texas.)

as peptides lying in the groove of class II antigens. Antigen appears to enter an acid prelysosomal compartment, where it is denatured and partially fragmented. This endosomal vesicle may contain newly synthesized or recycled DR molecules with which it interacts, and the complex is then transported to the plasma membrane for presentation to helper T cells.

Many data suggest that IL-1 has a role in T cell activation following recognition of DR molecules and antigen. When antigen, DR molecules, and IL-1 are available, the CD4+ T cell generates a cascade of activation steps that includes secretion of products such as interferon-γ that act on the mononuclear phagocyte system.[83] Human B lymphocytes have antigen-presenting function and, as well, produce IL-1–like activity.[84]

Angiogenesis in Rheumatoid Arthritis: Basis for Synovitis

From the vantage of the proliferation of new blood vessels in the synovium, synovitis in RA resembles both tumor growth and wound healing (Table 51–3). The importance of luxurious new capillary growth early in the development of synovitis was emphasized by Kulka et al. many years ago[85] (Fig. 51–3). Decades later, Folkman and colleagues demonstrated the first soluble factors responsible for inducing an endothelial cell with the capability to proliferate and develop new capillaries. In rheumatoid patients, it is likely that heparin binding growth factor (HBGF-1), the precursor of acidic fibroblast growth factor (FGF), is a major mitogen for many cell types and stimulates angiogenesis.[86, 87] Immuno-

staining of rheumatoid synovial tissue has revealed HBGF-1, and mRNA for HBGF-1 is present in the same tissue samples in rough proportion to the mononuclear cell infiltrate within the tissues.[88] In animal models of arthritis, the apparent persistence of HBGF-1, like the disease itself, was T cell dependent.[87]

FGF induced capillary endothelial cells to invade a three-dimensional collagen matrix, organizing themselves to form characteristic tubules that resemble blood capillaries.[89] This invasive quality of endo-

Table 51–3. ANGIOGENESIS AND CELL MIGRATION IN RHEUMATOID SYNOVIUM

Angiogenesis
Stimulation
  Heparin-binding growth factor (precursor of fibroblast growth factor)[86]
Inhibition
  Platelet factor-4[90]
  TGF β[104]
Cell Adhesion and Migration
Enhancement of endothelial expression of adhesive glycoprotein(s) CD18[94]
  Chemotactic peptides
  Leukotriene B₄
  Platelet activating factor
Enhancement of lymphocyte homing receptors[95–97]
  Interferon-γ
  Interleukin-1
  Tumor necrosis factor α
Inhibition of lymphocyte/PMN adherence (perhaps facilitating migration through vessels to subsynovial space)
  Soluble homing receptors[100]
  Interleukin-8[103]

TGF β, Transforming growth factor-beta; PMN, polymorphonuclear neutrophils.

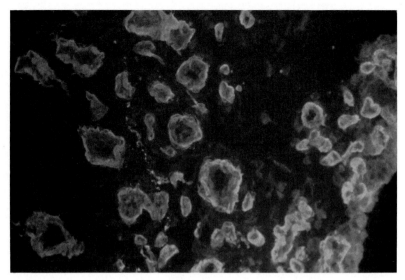

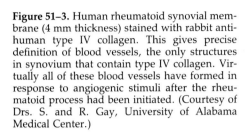

Figure 51–3. Human rheumatoid synovial membrane (4 mm thickness) stained with rabbit anti-human type IV collagen. This gives precise definition of blood vessels, the only structures in synovium that contain type IV collagen. Virtually all of these blood vessels have formed in response to angiogenic stimuli after the rheumatoid process had been initiated. (Courtesy of Drs. S. and R. Gay, University of Alabama Medical Center.)

thelial cells is mediated by their capacity to produce plasminogen activator and metalloproteinases as well as inhibitors of these proteinases[90] in response to angiogenic stimuli. These are the same enzymes that are involved subsequently in destruction of cartilage, tendon, ligament, and bone. A number of specific and nonspecific inhibitors of angiogenesis have been found, including recombinant platelet factor-4.[91]

Homing Receptors and Adhesion Proteins

Formation of new capillaries is only a portion of the involvement of blood vessels in the rheumatoid process. The endothelial cells must be activated to express adhesion proteins (addressins) that bind homing receptors on lymphocytes and PMN leukocytes from the circulation and facilitate their transfer through into the subsynovial tissue (see Chapter 12.) When activated, these endothelial cells take on a tall, plump appearance and in the aggregate are referred to as high endothelial venules (HEV). The structure of addressins from HEV in rheumatoid synovial membrane differs from those in other lymphoid-rich organs (e.g., gut or lymph nodes), indicating a specificity for deposits of lymphoid cells.[92, 93] A number of factors found in rheumatoid inflammation enhance neutrophil adherence to microvascular endothelial cells. Chemotactic peptides, leukotriene B$_4$, and platelet activating factor (PAF) enhance PMN binding through an increase in expression of the CD18 antigen (Mac-1 plus LFA-1 plus p150, 95 glycoproteins).[94] Other cytokines, such as interferon gamma (IFN-γ),[95] IL-1,[96] and tumor necrosis factor (TNF),[97] stimulate expression of specific homing receptors on lymphocytes. One has been cloned, sequenced, and its structure analyzed in the mouse.[98] Interesting features of this protein (designated gp90) include a carbohydrate binding (lectin) domain, a transmembrane domain, an epidermal growth factor (EGF)–

like domain, and a portion with a motif seen in complement regulatory proteins; some or all may be involved in the binding of lymphocytes to HEV. A similar structure has been determined for endothelial leukocyte adhesion molecule-1 (ELAM-1), a cell surface glycoprotein expressed by cytokine-activated endothelium.[99]

Intuitively one expects that a process such as binding of homing receptors to addressins must have regulatory indicators and inhibitors, or else cells would bind to HEV and stick there indefinitely. Accordingly, it is of interest that homing receptor proteins shed from inflammatory cells may inhibit lymphocyte-HEV binding, allowing extravasation of cells into the subsurface interstices of synovium.[100, 101] Similarly, IL-8[102] (described first as neutrophil-activating peptide) also inhibits neutrophil-endothelial cell interactions,[103] and transforming growth factor-beta (TGF-β) inhibits endothelial cell proliferation.[104] Sodium salicylate, in low concentrations, inhibits neutrophil adherence to endothelial cells.[105] The immunomodulating agent lobenzarit disodium inhibits both endothelial cell proliferation and T cell adherence to endothelial cells.[106]

T Lymphocyte Activation in Rheumatoid Arthritis

It is likely that symptoms begin in the rheumatoid patient near the time that T cell activation becomes prominent in the synovial lining. Coincident with the emigration of mononuclear cells through subsynovial capillaries is the accumulation of edema fluid and formation of new blood vessels. T cell activation becomes the first major amplification step in the pathogenesis of this disease. Clonal expansion of T cells in response to one or several antigens will subsequently drive B lymphocyte proliferation and production of antibodies, including RF. T lymphocytes and their function and cell-surface markers have been examined in blood, synovial fluid, and the synovium itself. Those from the synovium, more difficult to collect because of the rare availability of tissue, are the most important to study. Nevertheless, interesting data have been derived from examination of peripheral blood as well as synovial fluid lymphocytes.

There is also evidence that T cell function is deranged in a qualitative and a quantitative fashion in RA. Patients with RA have problems with the control and elimination of EBV-transformed lymphocytes;[107] this has helped fuel speculation that a lymphocyte defect is the principal triggering event in this disease.

There are many reasons other than the association of certain class II MHC antigens with RA to conclude that T lymphocytes have an important function in generating RA. One piece of indirect evidence, documented in 1957, is that RA and agammaglobulinemia caused by inactive B lymphocytes occurred simultaneously in a number of patients.[108] Thus, B cells are not essential in development of RA. More direct evidence for T cell involvement is derived from experimental therapeutics. Fistula of the thoracic duct that removes T lymphocytes from the body was shown in 1970 to be an effective (albeit complicated) treatment for RA,[109] and leukapheresis has been associated with brief but substantial improvement associated with the return toward normal of in vitro anergy of peripheral blood mononuclear cells.[110] The hypothesis to explain this latter observation is that leukapheresis interrupted cell traffic by removing activated T lymphocytes from the circulation, attenuating their movement into the synovium, and producing the observed reductions of articular inflammation. The decline in the number of activated circulating cells would permit, it was postulated, nonactivated T cells to be recruited to the synovium, where a delayed type of hypersensitivity reaction was in progress.[110]

Confirmatory evidence for a primary role of lymphocytes in RA is the tragic epidemic of AIDS; patients with RA who develop AIDS have remission of their joint symptoms as their CD4+ cells disappear.

The questions to be answered about lymphocytes in RA include: What is the level of activation of these cells? Is there oligoclonal proliferation of lymphocytes? Are there common epitopes recognized by different patients?

Peripheral Blood T Lymphocytes in Rheumatoid Arthritis

RA is a disease of activated immunologic response. In peripheral blood mononuclear cells (PBMCs), it has been demonstrated that both T and B cells are activated in peripheral blood.[110] This activated state is not specific for RA; PBMCs in patients with dermatitis herpetiformis and in those with glu-

ten-sensitive enteropathy as well as in presumed healthy persons with HLA-B8 antigen also are activated to variable degrees. It may be that the HLA-B8-DR3 haplotype is associated with increased numbers of HLA-DR+ T cells rather than correlated with rheumatoid disease per se.[112]

Most data show that the number of cytotoxic (CD8) lymphocytes is decreased relative to helper-inducer (CD4) cells in patients with active RA, resulting in a higher helper to suppressor T lymphocyte ratio.[113–115] A significant inverse correlation was observed between disease activity and the percentage of suppressor T cells in peripheral blood of the RA patients studied.[115]

The lymphocyte profile at any given time suggests prior activation of T cells with persistent MHC class II expression, down-regulation of the T cell receptor,[115] and IL-2 receptor expression.[116] Elevated levels of soluble IL-2 receptors are found both in sera and synovial fluid of rheumatoid patients, and sequential serum levels of IL-2 are being assessed as a way to follow activity of RA.[117]

Synovial Fluid Lymphocytes in Rheumatoid Arthritis

Cells in synovial fluid differ from those in peripheral blood; because they are not separated by any basement membrane from the tissue, they may be more relevant to study than PBMCs. Fox et al.[118] found that synovial fluid contained significantly more activated T cells (based on the presence of DR antigens) and noted a CD4 to CD8 ratio on cells of 1.1 compared with 2.4 found in peripheral blood. It could be inferred from these data that the CD4+ cells were homing to synovial tissues, where they became activated and were in equilibrium with cells in synovial fluid, yielding relatively more CD8+ cells in the fluid. It has been demonstrated that a very late activation antigen, VLA-1, an antigen associated with the late stages of T cell activation, is expressed on synovial fluid cells from patients with RA but not on peripheral blood lymphocytes from either rheumatoid or control patients.[119] IL-2 receptors were not present on these cells, perhaps because of a failure of the synovial tissue to produce adequate amounts of IL-2. Of CD4+ cells in rheumatoid synovial fluid, most bear the helper/inducer phenotype (CD4+, 4B4+), whereas there are relatively few suppressor/inducer cells (CD4+, 2H4+),[120, 121] in contrast to peripheral blood from the same patients.

As already mentioned, there is another population of lymphocytes in rheumatoid synovial fluid that may contribute to the synovitis.[122] These are the *double negative* γδ cells without CD4 or CD8 surface proteins and T cell receptors distinct from the αβ bearing cells. These γδ cells are not MHC restricted and therefore may respond by proliferation to many antigens, including superantigens such as heat shock proteins.

Lymphocyte Infiltration Within the Synovial Membrane

In patients proved later to have RA, lymphocytes are the predominant infiltrating cell in the sublining layer in the earliest stages of disease.[123] A definite organization of the lymphoid tissue in rheumatoid synovium can be seen.[124] The lymphocytes accumulate around blood vessels in large numbers. Peripheral to these foci is a transitional zone, where there are a large mixture of cells, including lymphocytes, undifferentiated blast cells, plasmablasts, plasma cells, and macrophages. It is likely that much intercellular communication by mediators takes place here, and it has been shown that activated, not naïve, T cells bind to synovial cells in vitro, a process mediated by their lymphocyte function–associated antigen, a phenomenon certain to enhance "cytokine talk" among these cells.[125] Immunoelectron microscopic study of the distribution of T cell subsets has shown that the majority of lymphocytes present in the lymphocyte rich areas near blood vessels have CD4 surface proteins, indicating that they are helper/inducer cells. The transitional areas of cellular heterogeneity show a mixture of both CD4+ and CD8+ cells amidst the macrophages.[126] The higher numbers of CD8+ cells in the transitional areas may represent a host attempt to modulate the immune response taking place there as antigen-presenting cells interact with helper T cells.

Overall, within the synovium, T cells predominate over B cells.[127, 128] B lymphocytes are located primarily within reactive lymphoid centers, whereas plasma cells are often found outside these centers, as are macrophages. This arrangement is consistent with T-dependent B cell activation; plasma cells, the immunoglobulin producers, migrate away from the germinal centers after differentiation.[129] CD4+ cells in RA synovium have been found to be intimately related to B lymphocytes and to HLA-DR positive cells,[130, 131] which resemble morphologically the interdigitating cells of lymph nodes. They are presumed to be antigen-presenting cells.[130]

In striking contrast to peripheral blood in RA, synovial lymphocytes bear an activated phenotype with fewer CD3+ cells and high expression of DR antigens similar to synovial fluid (Table 51–4); suppressor/inducer cells are reduced and helper/inducer cells increased[132]. Synovial lymphocytes also bear adhesion molecules of the VLA and LFA super-family of integrins, which may enable the inflammatory response to localize and persist within the synovium.[133] It is not surprising that helper/inducer T lymphocytes adhere better to endothelial proteins than do the suppressor/inducer cells and thus gain access more easily to the extracellular matrix within the synovial membrane.

One study has shown that in patients who benefit clinically from total lymphoid irradiation there has been a marked decrease in both the number and the function of peripheral blood helper/inducer cells;[134] by extrapolation (without proof), it may be inferred that the same occurred within the synovium.

Table 51–4. LYMPHOCYTE PHENOTYPES IN RHEUMATOID ARTHRITIS: ACTIVATED, ADHESIVE, HELPER CELLS

| | Peripheral Blood | | Synovium | |
	RA	Control	RA	Control
Activation Antigens				
HLA-DR	760	326	1804	326
IL-2 receptor	212	91	100	91
Adhesion Antigens				
LFA-1	2332	1680	3220	1681
VLA-1	383	62	1217	64
T cell differentiation Antigens				
CD3	4077	7367	3642	7367
CD4	1941	2459	1578	2459
CD8	3321	4121	2290	4121

LFA, Leukocyte function antigen; VLA, very late activation antigen.
Data from Cush, J. J., and Lipsky, P. E.: Arthritis Rheum. 31:1230–1238, 1988.

There have been several studies suggesting that the T helper cells induced to proliferate in rheumatoid synovium originate from few rather than many clones. If true, it would make feasible, by structure analysis of the T cell receptors, determination of the immunogenic epitope that activates the cells. More recently oligoclonal T cells were observed in RA using fresh synovial cells not yet expanded in vitro.[135] In previous studies using Southern blot analysis of T cell receptor β-chain genes, it was found that each culture from rheumatoid synovium, but not from peripheral blood of the same patients, had a limited number of clones.[136] Data from Denver have provided evidence for both oligoclonal proliferation of T cells and for involvement of a superantigen in RA.[137]

A striking T cell reactivity toward chondrocyte membranes has been found in both blood and synovial tissue of patients with RA and appears to be an antigen-driven process.[137a] This reactivity could explain in part the proclivity of the rheumatoid pannus to invade articular cartilage.

Large granular lymphocytes frequently are present in large numbers in peripheral blood in RA. They have been demonstrated to be cytotoxic. These cells produce a 70,000 molecular weight protein that is a membrane component, has a capability in isolation to be cytotoxic, and has an immunochemical relationship to the ninth component of complement.[138] The protein appears to work, as does the attack complex of complement, by forming functional transmembrane channels in the target cell membrane. The large granular lymphocyte may be an important producer of lymphokines, including IFN-γ, IL-2, B cell growth factor, and colony-stimulating factor (CSF). It has been shown that human peripheral blood contains CD8+ granular lymphocytes that are transformed into large granular lymphocytes under the influence of a factor that apparently is different from the interferons, IL-1, or IL-2.[139] It has been observed that there is an association of an expanded population of granular lymphocytes in patients with neutropenia and polyarthritis.[140] Using the monoclonal antibody CD11 that recognizes the CR3 complement receptor on large granular lymphocytes, it was shown that some patients with RA have increased numbers of these cells and that there may be a correlation between disease activity and the numbers of CD11+ cells, but that neutropenia need not be present.[141]

CYTOKINES AND IMMUNOREGULATORY DEFECTS IN RHEUMATOID ARTHRITIS

In 1981, suggestions of an interesting immunoregulatory dysfunction in RA were noted.[142, 143] It was observed that the outgrowth of EBV-infected B lymphocytes was inadequately suppressed by lymphoid cells from rheumatoid patients. It was demonstrated that this was related to a defect in suppressor T cell function. This deficient T cell response could be correlated somewhat with activity of the disease, but it was noted also that the abnormality was present in T cells of patients with inflammatory arthropathies other than RA.[144] It was subsequently observed that a defect in rheumatoid synovial cells in producing nonspecific cytotoxicity could be reversed by incubating the lymphocytes with IL-2.[145] In addition, peripheral blood T lymphocytes from rheumatoid patients demonstrated defective IL-2 production.[146] Indomethacin could partially reverse this defect in the presence of mononuclear cells, and it was suggested that an increased sensitivity to prostaglandins by the rheumatoid T cells might be the basis for this deficient IL-2 production. Similarly, the amount of IL-2 produced by synovial fluid lymphocytes was significantly less than that produced by the corresponding blood cells,[147] and this was not due to production of a suppressor substance in the heterogeneous mixed lymphocyte cultures. In addition, rheumatoid synovial fluid cells appeared to be particularly unresponsive to activation by a cellular antigen such as PPD.[148, 149] This is especially interesting in light of the clinical evidence that patients whose lymphocytes were anergic to soluble recall antigens were more likely to have synovial biopsies showing a high intensity of inflammation and proliferation.[149] When these patients were given a brief course of leukapheresis without lymphopenia being induced, the anergic T cell response to soluble recall antigens rose to a normal level. It was hypothesized that physical depletion of the activated cells unresponsive to exogenous stimuli from the circulation results in their replacement by naïve, reactive cells recruited from the marrow.[150]

A possible mechanism that ties all these observations together surfaced with the data that synovial fluid mononuclear cells from rheumatoid patients produce a potent IL-1 inhibitor.[150] Although this particular inhibitor was not characterized further, an IL-1 receptor antagonist produced by macrophages has been purified, its gene cloned and expressed in large quantity.[151–153] Because there is evidence that IL-1 has a crucial role in enhancing and facilitating MHC antigen activation of T lymphocytes and that an inhibitor of IL-1 would impair T lymphocyte activation (perhaps particularly the suppressor/inducer subset of T lymphocytes), this would result in a diminished secretion of IL-2 by this pool of cells. This might further decrease the expected amplification of suppressor cell proliferation, leading to unrestricted polyclonal B cell proliferation and diminished NK cell and LAK cell activity.[150] Unlike lymphocytes from control patients, recombinant IL-2 had minimal effect on IFN-γ production by peripheral blood lymphocytes from patients with active RA.[154]

This hypothesis is not inconsistent with the appearance of large granular lymphocytes with possible cytotoxic activity in RA. It is also consistent with the evidence that these large granular lymphocytes are transformed by a factor different from IL-1, IL-2, or IFN-γ.[139] As noted earlier, this hypothesis presupposes a particular specificity for the cells that induce suppressor cells and the suppressor cells themselves.

Whatever the direct cause, there is increasing evidence that cytokines produced by lymphocytes are diminished in RA, whereas those generated by mononuclear phagocyte/macrophages and by synovial fibroblasts are increased (Table 51–5).[155–157] These studies used in situ hybridization on dispersed synovial cells from patients with RA. It also has been shown that IL-2, IL-3, IFN-γ, and IL-4 are present in very low levels in synovial fluids from RA.[156, 157] In addition, peripheral blood monocytes from patients with RA have a defect of failing to have HLA-DR and HLA-DQ induced as effectively by IFN-γ compared with normal cells.[158]

In Table 51–6, the effects of different soluble mediators are recorded on the target cells against which they have been tested. As with other similar sources of information, there is really no significant technique to test effects of one factor in combination with many others so the net effect on the organism of these factors is known. In addition, there is no way to measure the concentrations of each autacoid at its receptors on cell surfaces, although studies using in situ hybridization perhaps come close to giving these data. It should also be noted that vitamin D is the exception to the principle that these factors are generally produced locally. Vitamin D has a hormonal effect, but it acts in a manner extremely similar to the autacoids produced locally. It is also appropriate to note that responses of dermal fibroblasts to many of these agents appear to be different from those of synovial fibroblasts, because one assay or another may have been tried in one but not in the other (e.g., antiviral activity assays).

Macrophages are the most vigorous producers of intercellular mediators. These cells, which are

Table 51–5. LEVEL OF PRODUCTION OF SYNOVIAL CYTOKINES IN RHEUMATOID ARTHRITIS ACCORDING TO CELLULAR SOURCE

Cellular Source	Level of Production in Rheumatoid Arthritis Synovium
T cells	
Interleukin-2	−
Interleukin-3	−
Interleukin-4	−
Interleukin-6	−
Interferon-γ	−
TNF-α	−
TNF-β	−
GM-CSF	−
Macrophages*	
Interleukin-1	+ + +
Interleukin-6	+
Interleukin-8	+ +
TNF-α	+ +
M-CSF (CSF-1)	+
GM-CSF	+
TGF-β	+ +
Interferon-α	±
Fibroblasts†	
Interleukin-6	+ + +
GM-CSD	+
Fibroblast growth factor	+

*Tissue macrophages or type A synoviocytes.
†Tissue fibroblasts or type B synoviocytes.
−, Less than normal; +, greater than "normal;" M-CSF, macrophage colony-stimulating factor.
Adapted from Firestein, G. S., and Zvaifler, N. J.: Down-regulation of human monocyte differentiation antigens by interferon gamma. Arthritis Rheum. 33:768, 1990; with permission.

present in small numbers in normal synovium, increase in number by migration from extrasynovial sites after inflammation begins. Their responses include secretion of more than 100 substances (see Chapter 16) and cover a biologic array of activity from induction of cell growth to cell death.[159]

Interferon Gamma (IFN-γ)

IFN-γ is believed to be the primary inducer of MHC class II antigen mononuclear cells. It concurrently activates synthetic and secretory activity in the monocytes/macrophages. After incubation with IFN-γ, monocytes show morphologic, metabolic, and phenotypic changes consistent with activation to vigorous macrophages; they also begin to express class II MHC antigens and Fc receptors.[160] Endothelial cells similarly express class II MHC antigens after stimulation with IFN-γ.[161] It is important to remember, however, that although multiple cell types in RA can be demonstrated to express class II antigens on their surface membranes, this is not synonymous with their being able to act as antigen-presenting cells. Similarly, there is evidence that in RA, monocytes/macrophages are present in synovial fluid and probably represent cells that have emigrated there after originating in bone marrow and have egressed from the circulation and into the superficial synovial

layers.[162] The low levels of IFN-γ in both rheumatoid synovial fluid and tissue suggest that it is not the primary macrophage activating factor.[163]

One of the most important functions for IFN-γ, and one that may be used therapeutically in the future, is its capacity to inhibit collagen synthesis. These experiments have been carried out both in vitro[164] and in vivo.[165] In examining the histology of rheumatoid synovitis, this observation may explain in part the polarized histologic findings of enormous proliferation of collagen in the subcapsular and capsular areas but little collagen proliferation in the synovial lining itself, the area containing lymphocytes that generate IFN-γ. This cytokine has been shown to decrease levels of type I and type III procollagen mRNAs in rheumatoid synovial fibroblast-like cells in culture.[166]

Studies using IFN-γ have documented the antagonistic and competitive effects of different cytokines. For example, TNF-α inhibits IFN-γ mediated expression of class II MHC antigens (e.g., HLA-DR on synovial cells in culture), whereas IFN-γ inhibits the proliferative stimulus and collagenase-inductive effects that TNF-α exerts on these cells.[167] It could be argued that since IFN-γ is relatively diminished in RA, the proliferative effects of TNF-α would be magnified in this disease.

Interleukin-1

IL-1 is a ubiquitous family of polypeptides with a wide range of biologic activity. Its actions make it a candidate for the major amplification factor and translator of the inflammatory response of RA into a proliferative one. IL-1, including its properties and its actions in comparison with those of other active factors, is discussed in Chapter 13. Indirect evidence for the importance of this mediator is its existence in many tissues and the production by many cells of fairly specific IL-1 inhibitors. The potential for a major role for IL-1 in the initiation of inflammatory and proliferative responses is great. It has been demonstrated, for example, that recombinant IL-1β injected into rabbit knee joints induces the accumulation of polymorphonuclear and mononuclear leukocytes in the joint space and the loss of proteoglycan from articular cartilage.[168] Leukocytes alone did not explain the depletion of proteoglycans, and there was no measurable increase of production of prostaglandins or leukotrienes in this process. It was inferred that IL-1 was inducing chondrocytes or synovial cells, or both, to generate enzymes that degrade proteoglycans in this relatively simple model. IL-1 activity produced by peripheral blood mononuclear cells that are adherent to surfaces and have macrophage function was much greater when cells were collected from rheumatoid patients who had recent onset of disease or an exacerbation of disease than from patients with stable arthritis or from controls.[169] IL-1 activity sufficient to stimulate collagenase and pros-

Table 51–6. EFFECTS OF SOLUBLE MEDIATORS ON NON–B CELL FUNCTIONS IN VITRO*

	Endothelial Cell	T Lymphocyte	Monocyte/ Macrophage	Synovial Fibroblast	Dermal Fibroblast	Bone
Interleukin-1 (IL-1)	↑ Proliferation ↑ PGE₂ and prostacyclin production ↑ Neutrophil adherence ↑ Procoagulant activity	↑ Proliferation in the presence of lectin or antigen (↑ IL-2 and IL-2 receptors)		↑ PGE₂, collagenase, types I and III collagens, fironectin, plasminogen activator ↓ Proliferation as a result of ↑ PGE₂ ↑ Proliferation with indomethacin ↓ cAMP response to PGE₂	↑ Same as synovial fibroblasts	↑ Bone resorption
Interleukin-2 (IL-2)		↑ Proliferation of activated cells ↑ IFN-γ ↑ IL-2				
Tumor necrosis factor α (TNF-α)	↑ Procoagulant activity ↑ Adherence of neutrophils ↑ IL-1 ↓ Proliferation	Proliferation (species-specific)	↑ IL-1	↑ GM-CSF ↑ PGE₂, collagenase, types I and III collagens	↑ Antiviral activity ↑ MHC class I antigen	↑ Bone resorption
Tumor necrosis factor β (TNF-β) (lymphotoxin)	↑ Neutrophil adherence	Proliferation (species-specific)		↑ PGE2, collagenase, types I and III collagens	↑ Antiviral activity	↑ Bone resorption
Interferon-γ (IFN-γ)	↓ Proliferation ↑ MHC class I and II antigens ↑ Adherence for lymphocytes		↑ MHC class I and II antigens ↑ IL-1, + TNF-α ↑ Fc receptors ↑ oxidative burst ↑ Monocyte surface antigens	↑ MHC class I and II antigens ↓ Collagen synthesis ↑ GM-CSF	+ Antiviral activity (weak)	Inhibits bone formation; ↓ IL-1 and TNF-α–induced bone resorption
Vitamin D		↓ IL-2 ↓ IFN-γ ↓ Transferrin receptors ↓ CD4 surface antigen	↑ Macrophage phenotype and function ↑ Monocyte/ macrophage surface antigen ↑ Fc receptor ↓ CD4 ↑ Phagocytosis ↑ Oxidative burst ↑ IL-1	↓ Proliferation	↓ Proliferation	↓ Type I collagen synthesis ↑ Osteoclast number
Transforming growth factor β (TGF-β)	↓ Proliferation	↓ Proliferation ↓ Natural killer (NK) cell function		↑ Collagen and fibronectin synthesis ↑ or ↓ Proliferation, depending on growth conditions and other soluble factors ↑ Glucose, amino acid transport, and glycolysis ↓ Collagenase enzyme activity	↑ Collagen and fibronectin synthesis ↑ or ↓ Proliferation, depending on growth conditions and other soluble factors ↑ Glucose, amino acid transport, and glycolysis ↓ Collagenase enzyme activity	↑ Bone resorption ↑ PGE₂

*Information in this table was kindly provided by Dr. Ed Amento of Genentech Corporation.
GM-CSF, Colony-stimulating factor for granulocytes and macrophages.

taglandin E_2 (PGE$_2$) production from synovial lining fibroblasts has been shown to be generated by monocytes/macrophages isolated from synovial fluid of patients with RA.[170] High-affinity receptors for IL-1α and IL-1β have been identified on cultured human rheumatoid synovial cells.[171] Even PMNs stimulated by phagocytosis or by other activating substances produce IL-1.[172] Thus, the macrophages, synovial fibroblasts, PMNs, and endothelial cells[173] can be induced to generate this powerful mediator. IL-1 activity has been detected in culture supernatants of rheumatoid synovial biopsy specimens, and in one study, the amount produced correlated with joint degradation found on roentgenograms.[174]

What induces production of IL-1? Early studies by Dayer et al[175] showed that production of mononuclear cell factor (later shown to be identical to IL-1) was produced by mononuclear cells with help from T lymphocytes. This has been confirmed in many subsequent studies.[176] IFN-γ enhances the production of IL-1 by endothelial cells that have been activated.[173] In contrast, the human monocyte cell line U937 requires a lymphokine induction signal that is distinct from other IL-2 or interferons.[177] A broad range of substances are capable of inducing IL-1 production; for example, immunoglobulin Fc fragments and to a lesser extent immune complexes can generate IL-1 production by rheumatoid synovial monocytes/macrophages.[178] Collagen fragments can induce IL-1 production, and it is intriguing that type IX collagen, which has been found only in articular cartilage and localized into intersections of collagen fibrils,[179] is a potent inducer of IL-1 by human monocytes/macrophages.[180]

Within the rheumatoid joint, IL-1 has activities other than inducing prostaglandin and collagenase formation. It sets off fibroblast proliferation, stimulates biosynthesis of IL-6 by synovial cells, enhances collagen production, and thus contributes to the proliferation of cells in this process and in so doing antagonizes the inhibitory effects of IFN-γ on cell proliferation and collagen production.[181] IL-1 stimulates glycosaminoglycan (GAG) production in human synovial fibroblast cultures,[182] although the effect of IL-1 on production of intact proteoglycan molecules by articular cartilage in some models seems to be decreased,[183] indicating that production of components of the GAG complex by IL-1 may be altered. Additionally, IL-1 stimulates human synovial cells to increase both cell-associated and extracellular plasminogen activator activity,[184] and it has been demonstrated that the cytokine osteoclast-activating factor (OAF) capable of stimulating bone resorption is identical to IL-1β.[185] Another activity of IL-1, that of chemotactic activity for B and T cells, can be found in rheumatoid synovial fluids; a substantial proportion of the chemotactic activity can be removed by specific antibody to IL-1.[186]

Interleukin-6

IL-6 is a cloned, IL-1–inducible protein produced by T cells, monocytes, and fibroblasts. It can induce immunoglobulin synthesis in B cell lines, is involved in differentiation of cytotoxic T lymphocytes,[187] and is the major factor in regulation of acute-phase response proteins by the liver.[188] In patients with RA, a striking correlation between serum IL-6 activity and serum levels of C-reactive protein, α$_1$-antitrypsin, fibrinogen, and haptoglobin was found.[189] Very high levels of IL-6 are present in RA synovial fluid, and synovial cells in culture from diverse inflammatory arthropathies produce IL-6.[190]

Tumor Necrosis Factor

This activity was named for the capability of a purified polypeptide to cause necrosis in tumors. Extensive purification and cloning of the factor have revealed that there are two forms, TNF-α, derived from monocytes, and TNF-β (previously called lymphotoxin), that have similar cytotoxic effects on neoplastic cell lines. TNF-α has been detected in rheumatoid synovial fluid and serum, but not TNF-β.[191] Interestingly, levels of TNF-α correlated with erythrocyte sedimentation rates and synovial fluid leukocyte counts.[191] Except for the failure of TNF to facilitate T cell activation by antigen or mitogen, IL-1 and TNF have similar activities (see Chapter 13); in some systems, the effects of these two agents in the same system are more than additive, suggesting synergism. If this were true, inhibition of one might drastically minimize the effects of the other and provide a useful therapy. TNF-α stimulates collagenase and PGE$_2$ production by human synovial cells and dermal fibroblasts,[192] induces bone resorption, inhibits bone formation in vitro,[193] and stimulates resorption of proteoglycan and inhibits its biosynthesis in explants of cartilage.[194] Thus, TNF-α is a second macrophage-derived cytokine whose production in RA could contribute to tissue destruction.

Neuropeptides

Evidence is accumulating to relate neuropeptides, substance P in particular, to the pathogenesis of RA. Pain is a common symptom of RA. As reviewed by Levine et al.,[195] kinins, prostaglandins, and leukotrienes lower the activation threshold of peripheral unmyelinated afferent fibers. These same fibers generate inflammatory mediators when the neurons are activated, thus contributing to inflammation. Substance P, the best studied of these, is an undecapeptide that can release other mediators such as leukotrienes, stimulate lymphocyte proliferation, support proliferation of synovial cells, induce the biosynthesis of matrix metalloproteinases by these cells,[112] and induce release of IL-1, TNF-α, and IL-6 from monocytes.[196] Elevated synovial fluid levels of substance P are found in RA as well as in other forms of inflammatory, traumatic, and degenerative arthritis. It is intriguing to postulate that centrally directed release of neuropeptides at terminal efferent nerve endings in joints may explain the symmetry of RA.

Granulocyte-Macrophage Colony-Stimulating Factor

The first evidence for granulocyte-macrophage colony-stimulating factor (GM-CSF) at a site of disease activity was its demonstration by radioimmunoassay in rheumatoid synovial effusions.[197] This cytokine, used as a recombinant preparation therapeutically to encourage marrow rebound after suppression and in other hematologic diseases, stimulates mature neutrophils and macrophages and can enhance antigen presentation by accessory cells.[198] Rheumatoid synovial cells in culture as well as endothelial cells and lymphocytes synthesize GM-CSF. In RA, this potent cytokine may act to enhance the inflammatory potential of neutrophils, and it may be the principal early inducer of HLA-DR expression human monocytes, helping to initiate the primary immune response in RA.

Transforming Growth Factor

There are a number of mediators, less well characterized than IL-1 or TNF, that have subtle and unusual effects in vitro and conceivably could have an important role in rheumatoid synovitis. TGF is a family of polypeptides that stimulate cells to lose contact inhibition. Two types have been isolated and characterized, TGF-α and TGF-β. TGF-α has sequence and activity homology to EGF and binds to the same receptor. TGF-α stimulates bone resorption in vitro by prostaglandin-mediated events.[199] It also inhibits bone formation through effects on collagen synthesis, stimulates the formation of osteoclast-like cells in human marrow cultures, and has inhibitory effects on collagen synthesis.[200] TGF-β is widely distributed in different tissues and cells, including T cells, monocytes, and platelets. Its effects in cell cultures are dependent on other factors. For example, although TGF-β alone has little effect on the expression of genes for collagenase and collagenase inhibitor, in the presence of other growth factors (such as EGF) it represses the production of collagenase (in contrast to IL-1 or TNF, which stimulate it) but can superinduce expression of tissue inhibitor of metalloproteinases.[201] TGF-β accelerates healing of incisional wounds,[202] and this is consistent with its capability of inducing both fibrosis and angiogenesis in vivo in experimental animals.[203] It would appear, therefore, that TGF-β is an important mediator of tissue repair. Although it has not been demonstrated that TGF-β itself has any direct effect on the proliferation of capillary endothelial cells, its adjunct role, perhaps related to its source in platelets, may be to help induce new blood vessel formation within the inflamed and proliferating synovial tissue in RA.

Connective Tissue Activating Peptides

One set of factors with clear anabolic capability and a potential for involvement in synovial inflammation are the connective tissue-activating peptides (CTAP). Synovial cells in culture are activated by CTAP I from lymphoid cells, CTAP III and IV from human platelets, and CTAP V from endothelial cells. The actions on these cells include increased glucose transport, glycolysis, PGE_2 formation, cyclic adenosine monophosphate (cAMP) accumulation, increased hyaluronic acid and proteoglycan synthesis, and, in some instances, mitogenesis.[204] CTAP III has common antigenic determinants with platelet factor IV and β-thromboglobulin.[204] Amino terminal sequence data suggest that CTAP III, platelet factor IV, and β-thromboglobulin have remarkable sequence homology. What remains to be determined is how these peptides interact with other factors mentioned earlier within inflamed connective tissue.

Platelet-Derived Growth Factor

One of the most potent growth factors yet isolated is platelet-derived growth factor (PDGF). It has generated particular interest since evidence was presented that a transforming protein of a primate sarcoma virus and PDGF are derived from the same or closely related cellular oncogenes.[205] PDGF is both chemoattractant and mitogenic for fibroblasts and induces collagenase expression.[206] With the presence of new blood vessels and the frequency of formation of microthrombi in them in RA, it is logical to attribute to PDGF a major role in generating proliferation of these synovial cells as the progression of rheumatoid synovitis continues in a given individual.[207, 208]

In a study of comparative effects of numerous cytokines (e.g., PDGF, FGF, EGF, TGF-β, IL-1, TNF-α, and IFN-α), PDGF was clearly the most potent stimulant of long-term growth of synovial cells in culture.[209] In these experiments, the strong mitogenic activity of rheumatoid synovial fluids was inhibited by an anti-PDGF antibody; as predicted, TGF-β antagonized these proliferative effects of PDGF.

Vitamin D

The role of vitamin D and its metabolites in the regulation of cell growth and differentiation is a complex one. As noted in Table 51–6, vitamin D has definite effects on the immune response. It also appears to affect interaction of cells with components of the extracellular matrix. It appears specifically to regulate collagen binding to monocyte precursors[210] and has a direct dose-dependent effect on production of osteopontin, a cell attachment glycoprotein produced by osteoblasts.[211] Perhaps vitamin D may enable osteoblasts to assume a three-dimensional conformation essential for production of a matrix suitable for mineralization, and it is probable (although not proved) that it has some effects on osteoclast development as well.

Other Cytokines

There is at least one activity related to factors produced by mononuclear cells that has not been well defined. It is the factor that generates formation of multinucleate giant cells from human monocyte precursors and appears to be produced by antigen-stimulated or mitogen-stimulated lymphocytes.[212] Such a factor could be important in pannus development because giant cells are seen frequently in rheumatoid synovium and because experimental evidence suggests they are virtual factories for proteolytic enzymes and can have a major role in cartilage and soft tissue destruction.

An enzyme inhibitor, α_1-antitrypsin (α_1-AT), appears to do more than inhibit serine proteinases. Deficiencies of α_1-AT have been associated with RA and multiple diseases other than emphysema. The inhibitor α_1-AT may diminish activation of helper T cells and B cell proliferation as well as help downregulate inflammatory cascades such as that observed in complement activation.

B CELL ACTIVATION AND RHEUMATOID FACTOR

Activated B lymphocytes are present in peripheral blood as well as in the rheumatoid synovium. Using computer-assisted flow cytometry, it has been demonstrated that many patients with RA with normal circulating numbers of lymphocytes show an abnormal κ chain to λ chain analysis compared with controls. This implies oligoclonal B cell proliferation.[213] It is not known whether this reflects expansion of the restricted number of clones capable of producing RF or whether the inciting antigen is something other than IgG and related specifically to RA.

PBMCs demonstrate spontaneous production of immunoglobulins. The highest levels of spontaneous IgM RF production are by PBMCs from patients with severe disease; these have been defined as a subset demonstrating depressed proliferative responses to soluble antigens, clinical improvement after short-term leukapheresis, and synovial biopsy showing high-intensity helper T lymphocyte and plasma cell infiltration.[214] Thus, the degree of T cell activation affects B cell activation and supports the hypothesis that the immune response in RA is T cell dependent.

The process of B cell activation and the mediators controlling it is detailed in Chapter 7 and in a review by Lipsky,[215] but it is useful to review this in the context of RA. As with other activation systems in this disease (as well as in normal physiology), it is

cytokines and their binding to specific receptors that generate antibody production. The B cell subset that is enriched in autoantibody production is characterized by a surface determinant CD25,[216, 217] and it will be of special interest to sort out which cytokines regulate its activation. In humans, IL-2 plays a leading role in inducing all immunoglobulin isotypes; although other cells can enhance this response, none affects lymphocyte responses of activation, proliferation, or differentiation in the absence of IL-2.[215] Despite the diminished amount of IL-2 found in joints, it is likely that there is sufficient IL-2 to process all of the lymphocytes in synovial tissue. IL-4 has growth-promoting effects on human B cells[218] and, similar to IFN-γ, can help induce class II MHC expression on cells. IL-4 directly enhances both T cell proliferation and IL-2 production.[219]

The immunochemical nature of RF and the definition of genes responsible for the cross-reactive idiotypes on RF that are responsible for the partially restricted RF repertoire are reviewed in Chapter 8. It is apparent that the expression of any particular idiotype on RFs (or other immunoglobulins, for that matter) is under genetic control. This limited response is related to restriction of the number of relevant or expressible V genes available in the germ line.[220–222]

Persons with a certain polymorphic part of the gene expressing a constant region of the κ light chains of IgG have a relative risk for development of RA that is 2.8 times control populations. This has been interpreted to suggest that immunogenetic susceptibility to RA may include genetic factors outside the MHC.[31, 32]

Studies of RF in synovial membrane cultures have indicated that only cells from patients with seropositive RA synthesize RF spontaneously.[223] IgM RF represented 7.3 percent of total IgM produced by cells from 12 patients, and IgG RF represented 2.6 percent of IgG synthesized in those cultures. Significantly, no IgG or IgM RF was detectable in seronegative patients, accentuating even more the growing appreciation that seronegative RA is more often than not a different disease from that of its seropositive counterpart.

Although no data clearly implicate RF as a principal causative agent in RA, the role of antiglobulins in the amplification and perpetuation of the process is well supported:

1. Although some patients with virtually no circulating IgG develop RA,[108] it is known that patients with a positive test for RF in blood have more severe clinical disease and complications[224] than do seronegative patients.

2. Polyclonal IgM RF is able to fix and activate complement by the classic pathway.[225]

3. Using a cell assay for anti-IgG (RF) plaque-forming cells, it was noted that the appearance of these cells coincided with flares of clinical activity of the disease.[226] Anti-IgG plaque-forming cells were more concentrated in bone marrow and synovial fluid than in peripheral blood.

4. IgG RF produced in large quantity in rheumatoid synovial tissue can form large complexes of itself through self-association[227] because these molecules have a much higher frequency of double valent Fc binding regions than do most normal IgG molecules. It appears that these large complexes fix complement and can bind to IgM RF.

5. Immune complexes containing RF have been localized within synovial tissues by immunofluorescent techniques.[228, 229] A hyperviscosity syndrome that affects the central nervous system (producing headache, tinnitus, vertigo, and seizures) and that causes striking retinal pathologic changes and diffuse hemorrhages has been reported in RA;[230, 231] circulating intermediate-sized immune complexes have been demonstrated in some of these patients.

6. Increased levels of IgG RF have been associated with a high frequency of subcutaneous nodules, vasculitis, elevated erythrocyte sedimentation rate, decreased complement levels, and increased number of involved joints.[232, 233]

7. In experiments performed in patients with RA, a marked inflammatory response was elicited when RF from the patient was injected into a joint but not when normal IgG was given.[234] RF becomes involved in pathogenesis when it forms immune complexes sufficiently large to activate complement[234] or be phagocytized by macrophages or PMNs.

Several hypotheses have been advanced to explain how IgG could become immunogenic:

1. New determinants on IgG may be exposed following polymerization among molecules to form aggregates or as IgG complexes with specific non-IgG antigens.[236]

2. A structural anomaly in the IgG of rheumatoid patients may render it immunogenic. Studies using circular dichroism spectropolarimetry have suggested that there may be a defect in the hinge region of rheumatoid IgG that could increase the binding affinity to membrane Fc receptors on B lymphocytes.[237]

3. Depletion of suppressor T lymphocytes might allow B lymphocytes to produce autoantibodies against certain determinants on IgG.[238]

4. Autoantigenic reactivity of IgG could be related to demonstrated changes in the relative extent of galactosylation. A deficiency of the galactosylation enzyme machinery may increase the relative risk of developing RA.[33, 85]

In addition to RFs of the mu (μ) and gamma (γ) isotypes in RA, epsilon (ϵ) isotypes also have been demonstrated in certain patients.[239, 240] Of 13 sera containing IgE immune complexes, 11 were from patients with extra-articular manifestations.[240] It has been suggested that IgE RF could complex with aggregated (self-associating) IgG in synovial tissue and that the IgG–IgE complexes could then activate mast cells and basophils in the synovium.[239] This is of particular interest in light of reports that there are numerous mast cells in rheumatoid synovium and that these may release factors capable of stimulating collagenase production by synovial cells.[241]

Considering the restricted number of idiotypes of RF, it is interesting that the four major classes of immunoglobulins (IgM, IgG, IgA, and IgE) are all produced in RA. It has been shown that, although only 73 percent of patients with RA were seropositive by standard tests for RF, 92 percent were positive for IgM RF using ELISA.[242] In the same group, 65 percent, 68 percent, and 66 percent were positive for IgA, IgE, and IgG RF. Disease activity correlated with IgM RF and IgA RF, as did levels of circulating immune complexes. Extra-articular features correlated positively with levels of IgA and IgE RF. In another study, a double-binding ELISA developed to bind a cross-reactive determinant shared on human and sheep IgG has been found to be extremely specific for RA.[242a]

Although enhanced helper T cell function for the spontaneous production of RF has been demonstrated only for IgM, it is likely that the same applies to the other isotypes as well.[243]

IMMUNE COMPLEXES: THEIR SIGNIFICANCE IN THE CIRCULATION, SYNOVIAL FLUID, AND CARTILAGE

The significance of complexes of gamma globulin circulating in blood and in synovial fluid was appreciated several decades ago (see review by Winchester et al.).[244] It was not until more reliable assays for immune complexes were available, however, that broad studies correlating disease activity and immune complexes could be generated.

As with studies of lymphocytes, studies of synovial fluid have generated data more relevant to the pathophysiology of the disease than the same studies in blood of the same patients because the disease process is initiated and perpetuated in the synovium. Findings in blood may reflect only what "spills out" from the synovial fluid and synovial tissue. Levels of IgM-containing circulating immune complexes are elevated in both RA and SLE, although levels of IgG immune complexes are not.[245] In all assays for circulating immune complexes, the possibility of in vitro formation of IgM and IgG complexes giving false-positive tests must be constantly controlled for.[246] Assays such as the C1q binding assay overestimate the concentration of immune complexes. False-positive results are also found in the Raji cell test. In studies designed to identify the components of immune complexes in the circulation of rheumatoid patients, most data have found no specific antigen other than IgG complexed with RF. Using more sensitive techniques, it has been found that circulating immune complexes in RA are composed of as many as 20 polypeptides, including albumin, immunoglobulin, complement, and acute phase reactants. In one study, a polypeptide of molecular weight 48,000 has remained unidentified and is an intriguing candidate for an extrinsic antigen in this disease.[247]

Most relevant to the pathogenesis of joint destruction in RA has been the identification of immunoglobulins and complement in articular collagenous tissues from RA. Ninety-two percent of cartilage and meniscal samples from 42 rheumatoid patients had evidence of these components in the avascular connective tissue.[248] Electron microscopic morphology of immunoglobulin aggregates showed that there were pathologic changes in the matrix of cartilage in the microenvironment of the aggregates themselves.[249] Immune complexes were absent under areas in cartilage invaded actively by synovial pannus, suggesting that phagocytic cells in the invasive synovium had perhaps ingested the immune complexes,[250] lending credence to the possibility that immune complexes deposited in the avascular superficial layers of cartilage in the joint may serve as chemoattractants for the pannus and be an explanation for the centripetal orientation of the rheumatoid lesion. Jasin[71] has extracted immune complexes from cartilage of rheumatoid and osteoarthritic patients. Rheumatoid cartilage contained 37 times more IgM and 14 times more IgG than did normal cartilage extracts. IgM RF was found in 13 of 16 rheumatoid cartilage extracts and in none of 11 osteoarthritic or six normal control extracts. In addition, more than 60 percent of the rheumatoid cartilage extracts were positive for native and denatured collagen type II antibody, as were osteoarthritic specimens. These deposits seldom are deeper than 20 μm from the surface of cartilage,[251] suggesting that the deposits are sequestered there. To link these hypotheses, it is essential to demonstrate by some experimental system that cartilage containing these superficial deposits of immune complexes indeed can attract invasive synovial tissue.

These observations help support the hypothesis that the presence of cartilage itself, and perhaps these complexes, is responsible for the chronicity and persistence of rheumatoid inflammation. Orthopedic surgeons have noted many times that joints from which all cartilage is removed do not participate in general flares of rheumatoid disease following surgery. "Burnt out" RA may mean that with the combination of loss of motion and loss of cartilage in a joint, there is nothing to sustain continued inflammation.

SYNOVIAL FLUID IN RHEUMATOID ARTHRITIS

Although it would be advisable to examine synovial tissue from each patient with RA to compare histologic changes with those from previous specimens and assay for T cell subsets and enzyme production by synovial cells, this is impractical. As stressed earlier, blood is one step removed from the site of disease and the focus of inflammatory activity. On the other hand, synovial fluid is a good compromise; by examination of its characteristics, one can gain a good appreciation for the extent of inflammation, and by using synovial fluid investigators can learn much about events within the synovium itself. Chapter 36 describes techniques for analysis of synovial fluid. Components of the inflammatory and proliferative response that can be dissected by examination of synovial fluid from patients are discussed subsequently.

Polymorphonuclear Leukocytes

The number of PMNs remains one of the most accurate indices of inflammation within a particular joint. These are cells that truly amplify inflammatory responses, and although it is unlikely that they destroy much cartilage directly, their role in amplification and thereby perpetuation of the inflammation within joints is probably significant.

Hollingsworth et al.[252] determined that the joint space serves as a depository for PMNs; they enter the synovial fluid by direct passage from postcapillary venules in the synovial lining. As mentioned earlier, without appearance on endothelial cells in the HEV of adhesive proteins, neutrophils would pass through the synovial vessels without adhering to endothelium. Once adherent, however, agents such as IL-8 produced by endothelium and fibroblasts may facilitate egress through the capillaries into the chemoattractant gradients of the synovium. In the joint space, they have no means of egress. Thus, considering the survival time of PMNs in synovial fluid, it has been estimated that the breakdown with an average (30 ml) rheumatoid effusion containing 25,000 PMNs per mm^3 may well exceed a billion cells each day[252] (Fig. 51–4).

The physiology of granulocytes is discussed in detail in Chapter 15. As detailed there, the strong attraction of chemotactic agents within the synovial fluid in RA is responsible for the large number of cells found there (occasionally up to 100,000 per mm^3). Few PMNs are seen in the pannus itself and subsynovial tissue; once in the synovium they move rapidly to the synovial fluid, drawn by the activated component of cleavage of the fifth component of complement (C5a), leukotriene B$_4$ (LTB$_4$), and platelet-activating factor (PAF acether). In the synovial fluid, PMNs come in contact with immune complexes and particulate material (i.e., fibrin, cell membranes, cartilage fragments). Phagocytosis occurs, particularly on particles coated with IgG. After phagocytosis begins, the PMN is activated. Through a complex set of changes in the membrane potential of the cell involving calcium flux and both phospholipid metabolism and cyclic nucleotide activation, the neutrophil begins to degranulate, to generate products of oxygen metabolism, to metabolize arachidonic acid (AA), and to develop the capacity for aggregation.[253] In

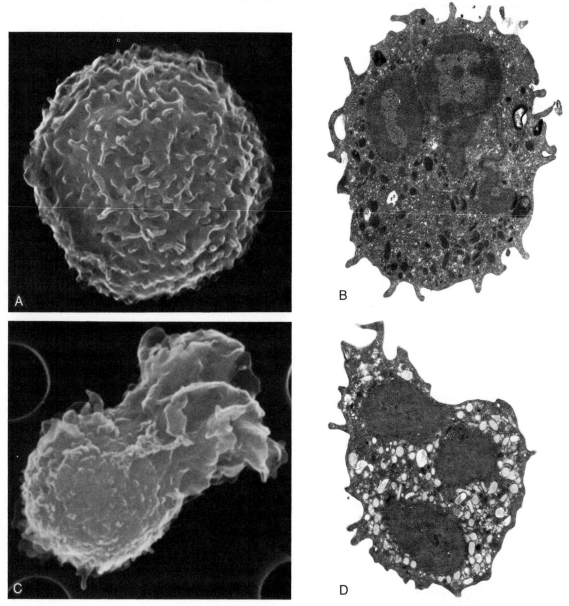

Figure 51–4. Normal and rheumatoid arthritis peripheral blood polymorphonuclear neutrophils (PMNs). *A,* Scanning electron micrograph (SEM) of a PMN from peripheral blood of a normal 73-year-old man (30,000 ×). It is characteristically apolar and spherical with surfaces completely covered by plasma membrane elaborated into irregular ridges or small ruffles. *B,* Transmission electron micrograph (TEM) of PMN from a normal man. The apolar cell has few phagocytic vacuoles but many undischarged electron-dense granules (19,800 ×). *C,* SEM of a PMN from peripheral blood of a 78-year-old woman with RA. This striking polarized appearance is much more common in rheumatoids than in normal individuals and suggests that the cells have been activated (19,200 ×). *D,* TEM of a PMN from peripheral blood of a 59-year-old woman with RA. This cell has many phagocytic vacuoles but relatively few undischarged electron-dense granules (17,500 ×). (From McCarthy, D. A., et al.: Scanning electron microscopy of rheumatoid arthritis peripheral blood polymorphonuclear leucocytes. Ann. Rheum. Dis. 45:899, 1986. Courtesy of the publisher and the authors.)

addition, PMNs from synovial fluid in RA release de novo synthesized proteins, including fibronectin,[254] neutral proteinases, and IL-1.[255]

Oxygen Free Radicals in Rheumatoid Arthritis

Because of the chemoattractant agents in synovial fluid, the polymorphonuclear leukocytes accumulate there rather than in the synovium itself.

Among the other consequences of phagocytosis by these cells and their subsequent activation is production of free radicals of oxygen, including hypochlorite (OCl), superoxide anion, hydroxyl radical, and chloramines (see review by Weiss).[256, 257] Phagocytosis triggers a *respiratory burst* characterized by increased oxygen consumption, increased anaerobic glycolysis, and the generation of these oxygen radicals. Using chemiluminescence assays, it has been demonstrated that activation of the neutrophil myeloperoxidase-H_2O_2 system takes place at a vigorous rate in synovial fluids from patients with RA.[258] This oxidant stress may contribute to the cyclic, self-perpetuating nature of rheumatoid inflammation.

As already mentioned, it is important to remember that the predominant reaction in RA is one of enormous cellular proliferation. Cytotoxicity, unless it is directed against specific and isolated cell types, is not obvious in the net weight of synovium. Luxuriant growth of cells, not necrosis, is the rule. Nevertheless, there could well be an important role for the oxygen radicals, especially when considering possible alterations in matrix and the enzymes that degrade it. It has been demonstrated that enzymatically generated superoxide radicals, reacting with hydrogen peroxide in vitro to produce hypochlorite (i.e., bleach), can depolymerize purified hyaluronic acid[259] and damage protease inhibitors, allowing certain proteinases to act unabated.[256, 260]

Some investigators have focused attention on *redox stress* in rheumatoid inflammation. Their data support the hypothesis that free radicals from oxygen metabolism destroy antioxidant systems (e.g., ascorbic acid and serum sulfhydryl groups).[261] Using an assay to test the resistance of serum to attach by peroxyl radicals, they have implicated serum urate as an antioxidant, a concept that could explain the infrequent occurrence of both active RA and gout in the same patient.[262]

The role of iron in enhancing production of free radicals may be significant (see discussion of synovium later). There are a number of conditions in inflamed joints that predispose to iron's becoming available and facilitating production of hydroxyl radicals from hydrogen peroxide. If the pH around activated phagocytes is less than 6.0, iron becomes detached from transferrin, its major transport protein. Iron from hemoglobin in lysed erythrocytes can exacerbate inflammation[263] (Fig. 51-5.) Hydrogen peroxide generated in the early phases of a respiratory burst can facilitate iron release from free hemoglobin; the released iron may stimulate radical reactions.[264]

There are many checks and balances in a system in which such potentially toxic elements are released in sites of inflammation. Oxygen radical scavengers should be protective in inflammation. Superoxide dismutase is a ubiquitous and important intracellular enzyme induced by high oxygen tension. It is protective against oxygen radical–mediated damage. It appears identical to orgotein, an anti-inflammatory protein isolated from liver and touted in Europe as therapy for arthritis. Catalase, found in the cytoplasm of cells, reduces H_2O_2 to water. Glutathione peroxidase also detoxifies H_2O_2. Ceruloplasmin, a major copper-containing protein in serum, chemically scavenges superoxide radicals;[265] an acute phase reactant, it is found in elevated levels in RA. As mentioned earlier, sodium urate may have significant antioxidant properties. Copper-penicillamine complexes can

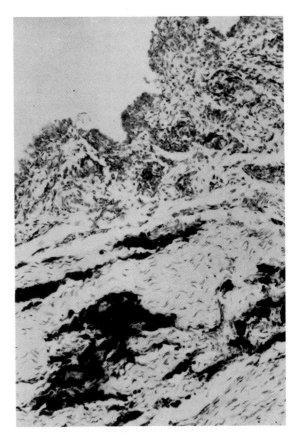

Figure 51–5. In this section of rheumatoid synovium prepared with Prussian blue stain, large collections of iron, the product of many microhemorrhages, are found deep in the subsynovial tissue (315 ×). (Courtesy of K. Muirden, M.D.)

reduce superoxide concentrations, and vitamin E can terminate free radical lipid peroxidative reactions affecting cell membranes.

Arachidonate Metabolites in Rheumatoid Arthritis

Accompanying activation of PMNs is the increased mobilization of membrane phospholipids in these cells to AA and its subsequent oxidation by cyclo-oxygenase to prostaglandins (PGs) and thromboxanes, or by lipoxygenases to leukotrienes. Although the stable PGs do produce vasodilation, cause increased vascular permeability, and are involved centrally in fever production, there is increasing evidence that they have significant anti-inflammatory activities as well. For example, stable PG can retard development of adjuvant arthritis,[266] and the drug misoprostol, a PG analogue, may have significant anti-inflammatory or immunomodulatory effects.[267]

As detailed in Chapter 11, LTB_4, rather than the PGs, is receiving the most attention as a proinflammatory product of neutrophil activation. It is chemotactic for neutrophils, eosinophils, and macrophages; it promotes neutrophil aggregation; it enhances neutrophil adherence to endothelium; and it enhances NK cell cytotoxic activity. As mentioned earlier, neutrophils become necrotic in the abyss of synovial fluid, having no means of easy exit from the joint. Metabolism of AA into the pathway mediated by lipoxygenase is directly proportional to breakdown of these cells in the joint cavity; cell breakdown facilitates access of AA to lipoxygenase from the cytosol.[268] It is of interest that peripheral blood PMNs from rheumatoid patients have an enhanced capacity for production of LTB_4 compared with similar cells from control groups.[269] No mechanism for this has been elucidated, and it is not known whether synovial fluid leukocytes have the same enhanced capacity for LTB_4 release.

Therapeutic studies have given indirect support for the role of AA metabolites in promoting the inflammation in RA. In a joint study from Boston and London, 12 patients with active RA supplemented their usual diet with 20 g of eicosapentaenoic acid (EPA) and docosahexaenoic acid, both found in fish oils.[270] Following this supplementation, the ratio of AA to eicosapentaenoic acid in the patients' neutrophil cellular lipids decreased from 8:1 to 3:1, and the capacity of these cells to generate LTB_4 declined by one third. In addition, there was a significant decline in PAF acether generation by mononuclear cells. Of interest, chemotactic response of the rheumatoid patients' neutrophils to agents such as LTB_4 was diminished before the study. It increased substantially during dietary supplementation with fish oil.

Much of the data being generated about the effect of nonsteroidal anti-inflammatory drugs (NSAIDs) on AA metabolism and neutrophil function suggest that, in agreement with Abramson et al.[271] the principal mode of action of these drugs may be to inhibit neutrophil function through an effect on early events critical to activation of PMNs.

Complement in Rheumatoid Arthritis

The components and pathways involved in complement activation are described in Chapter 10. As in studies of lymphocyte function and in measures of inflammation, synovial fluid serves as a better index of complement metabolism in RA than does peripheral blood. Despite local production of complement components, the activities of C4, C2, and C3 and total hemolytic complement in rheumatoid (seropositive) synovial effusions are lower than in synovial fluids from patients with other joint diseases.[272–276]

Using a sensitive solid phase radioimmunoassay to quantitate the activation of the classic pathway of complement by RF, it has been demonstrated that IgM RF is a much more important determinant of complement activation than is IgG RF in both sera and synovial fluids.[277] Combined with other data showing that there is an accelerated catabolism of C4

in RA and that the presence of C4 fragments[278] in the plasma of rheumatoid patients correlates with titers of IgM RF, the weight of evidence indicates a role in vivo for IgM RF in complement activation.

The biologically active products of complement activation are probably the most important consequence of intra-articular complement consumption. Like proteinases from PMNs, these inflammatory components may build up in synovial fluid during acute inflammation. The potential for interaction between PMNs and the complement system is substantial. Neutrophil lysosomal lysates contain enzymatic activity capable of generating chemotactic activity (probably C5a) from fresh serum.[279, 280] C5a, in addition to being a principal chemotactic factor in inflammatory effusions, is capable of mediating lysosomal release from human PMNs.[279] This sets up one of many amplification loops in inflammatory synovial fluid.

Another amplification loop in synovial inflammation may involve complement activation by C-reactive protein (CRP). As reviewed in Chapter 40, CRP concentrations increase markedly following an inflammatory stimulus. CRP may combine with phospholipid constituents of necrotic cell membranes at inflammatory sites or with the first complement components.[281, 282]

In most rheumatoid patients, levels of C3 and C4 in plasma are normal. Measurements of inactivation fragment C3dg and the terminal complement complex, however, show parallel increases in rheumatoid synovial fluids, indicating that the whole complement cascade is involved in RA.[283] No good correlation between these components in synovial fluid and in plasma has been noted, emphasizing again the importance of synovial fluid assays; levels in plasma may be related more to biosynthesis of complement components as a part of an acute phase reactivity. In a prospective study of plasma levels of C3 anaphylatoxin (C3a), the mean level of this activated component in 37 plasma specimens was twice as high as that in samples obtained from normal volunteers.[284] Clinical measurements of disease activity correlated well with plasma C3a level as well as with other laboratory test results such as serum C-reactive protein and erythrocyte sedimentation rate.[284] Future studies of both C3a and C3dg (which has a longer half-life than C3a) in samples from the same patients may yield helpful data that correlate with joint inflammation.

Other Synovial Fluid Manifestations of Rheumatoid Inflammation

A number of diverse biologic activities and proteins have been assayed in rheumatoid synovial fluid.

Enzymes

Both polymorphonuclear leukocytes and synovial lining cells contribute to the proteolytic activity found in synovial fluid. Neutral proteinases, collagenase, and elastase are present.[285–288] As with other active substances, there is an equilibrium between enzymes and their inhibitors. The net effect biologically or pathologically is the sum of these. For instance, it has been demonstrated that in rheumatoid synovial fluid, free collagenolytic activity is not generally measurable unless the PMN count is greater than 50,000 cells per mm^3. This is probably related to the fact that in the higher cell counts seen in severe rheumatoid disease, inflammation from sepsis, or crystal synovitis, the protease inhibitors in synovial fluid (principally α_2-macroglobulin) are saturated and free enzyme activity can act on articular connective tissue.[285, 289, 290] The direct effect of these enzymes on articular cartilage may be substantial and may augment the proteoglycan depletion in cartilage that is manifested early in rheumatoid inflammation (see Chapter 14).

Coagulation and Kinin System Activation

The role of the clotting system in fibrinolysis is discussed later, but it is important to remember the inter-relationships among the soluble mediators in synovial infusions (see Chapter 18). For example, activation of Hageman's factor can be an initial step in kinin formation. RF-IgG complexes activate kininogens, although RF and unaltered, nonassociated IgG do not.[291] Kallikrein activator and kininase are both present in human granulocytes, and kallikrein itself is a potent and versatile proteinase that can activate plasminogen to plasma, precursor to active Hageman's factor, and latent to active synovial collagenase.

The end point of activation of the clotting sequence is the formation of fibrin. The accumulation of fibrin is one of the most striking pathologic features of rheumatoid synovitis. Fibrin accumulates on the synovial surface, on cartilage surfaces, in areas of subsynovial hemorrhage or infarction, and as particulate aggregates in synovial fluid. At the final stages of fibrin formation, fibrinopeptides are formed (released from fibrinogen by the action of thrombin during clotting), which may have the capacity to increase vascular permeability. What initiates the clotting sequence? It has not been demonstrated that immune complexes of RF and IgG can do this,[292] but plasmin (activated by plasminogen activator from plasminogen) has the capability, as (possibly) does collagen. Production of a procoagulant by mononuclear cells in culture is stimulated by immune complexes.[293]

The presence of fibrin on synovium and cartilage may impede normal nutrition to these tissues and may amplify conditions that lead to hypoxia and acidosis in synovial fluid. In addition, homologous fibrin appears to generate a chronic immunologic response in experimental animals.[294] It is possible that, in addition to being entrapped in the collagen matrix, immune complexes may be caught up in fibrin clots within the joint space, a phenomenon that would perpetuate the inflammatory and proliferative disease. Like the build-up of other components of the inflammatory reaction, the accumulation of fibrin in joints reflects an imbalance caused by the inadequacy of the joint lining to clear the large quantities of by-products of inflammation. In some rheumatoid joints, a strong inhibition of fibrinolysis by plasmin has been observed as well as diminished activity of plasminogen activator.[295]

ABNORMAL PHYSIOLOGY OF BLOOD FLOW IN RHEUMATOID SYNOVITIS: AN IMPORTANT CONTRIBUTOR TO THE RHEUMATOID LESION

There is a state of relative hypoxia within synovial tissue that is reflected in synovial fluid. Oxygen tensions can be remarkably low, lactate measurements are frequently high, and pH as low as 6.8 has been found.[296] Mean rheumatoid synovial fluid pO_2 in 85 samples from rheumatoid knees was 27 mm Hg,[297] and in a subsequent study, a pO2 of less than 15 mm Hg was measured in a quarter of fluids examined;[298] this is profound hypoxia. Another cause of diminished blood flow may be the increased positive pressure exerted by synovial effusions within the joint, a process that could effectively obliterate capillary flow and exacerbate the decrease in oxygen availability to these tissues,[299–301] producing hypoxic-reperfusion injury in the joint. Physiologic determinations by Wallis et al.[302] have supported this; clearance values generated by kinetics of iodine(^{123}I) removal from synovial fluid have shown that small solute clearance from rheumatoid synovial effusions is less than in normal individuals or in patients with other rheumatic diseases.[302] Patients with the lowest synovial iodide clearance have the lowest synovial fluid pH, the lowest synovial fluid to serum glucose ratios, the lowest synovial fluid temperatures, the highest synovial fluid lactate levels, and the highest numbers of synovial fluid neutrophils. Thus, the most seriously affected rheumatoid joints may be both hypoperfused and ischemic. Diminished blood flow relative to need may be decreased further by high intrasynovial pressure from effusions[300] as well as the existence of abnormal microvascular structures.[123, 303]

Altered vascular flow may not be the only cause of hypoxia in joints. It has been estimated that the oxygen consumption of the rheumatoid synovium (per unit of tissue) is 20 times normal.[304, 305]

The dynamics of protein concentrations within rheumatoid synovial fluid are interesting as well. It has been known for many years that there was an inverse relationship between the molecular weight of proteins and their concentrations in minimally inflamed synovial fluid and serum, that high molecular weight proteins gained access more easily to synovial fluid in inflamed joints, and that the relatively high concentration of IgG in RA synovial fluid was good evidence for local (synovial) synthesis of IgG.[306, 307] In studies, "protein traffic" in human synovial effusion has been measured by determining clearance of albumin and other proteins from synovial fluid. This gives a useful measure of affected synovial lymph flow. An increased "permeance" of proteins in rheumatoid patients was found to be more than seven times greater than that suggested by synovial fluid to serum ratios and underscores the severity of the microvascular lesion in rheumatoid synovitis.[308]

SYNOVIUM IN RHEUMATOID ARTHRITIS: A HETEROGENEOUS MIXTURE OF CELLS AND MATRIX

Along with lymphocytes and plasma cells in RA synovium, there are large numbers of plump luxuriant cells that may be up to 100 layers thick and that are formed in response to the proliferative factors described earlier generated by the activated immune response. It is logical to assume that PDGF TNF-α and IL-1 produced by many different cells combine with products of AA metabolism to generate proliferation of these cells presumed to be synovial fibroblasts. The problem with this hypothesis is that studies to demonstrate active cell division in the rheumatoid synovium rarely show mitotic figures, and thymidine studies show uptake in only 4 percent of synovial cells.[309] Using a monoclonal antibody that recognizes dividing cells, an even lower rate of cell division (approximately 0.05 percent) was found.[310] There are several explanations for this: Either at a certain point hyperplasia levels off to keep synovial cell volume at a steady state, or else synovial hyperplasia in RA really represents colonization by marrow-derived macrophages. Advocates for the latter interpretation[311] point to monoclonal antibody studies that indicate that most synovial lining cells in rheumatoid joints bear markers for blood monocytes[312] and thus must be macrophages. In marked contrast to these data, studies using immunolocalization of metalloproteinases have shown that approximately 60 percent of synovial lining cells have morphologic and immunostaining characteristics of synovioblasts or B cells, whereas the remainder were cells that did not stain for metalloproteinases and had the election micrograph appearance of macrophages.[313]

One other interpretation of these apparently discordant results about the lineage of cells lining synovium in RA is that the majority are indeed mesenchymal (fibroblastic, type B) in origin but, in response to onslaught from multiple cytokines, develop macrophage markers as well as the expression of proteinase biosynthesis. Synovial cells from RA do develop anchorage-independent growth when cultured in agar with PDGF; this change to a phenotype characteristic of transformed cells was readily inhibited by TGF-β.[314] The concentration of both TGF-β and PDGF in rheumatoid synovial fluid is well above that needed for synovial cell stimulation or repression.[315] The reasonable hypothesis has been put forth that the biologic effect of a certain cytokine on rheumatoid cells depends partially on their activation or differentiated state at the time of cytokine contact as well as intrinsic properties of the cytokine itself.

Using enzymatically dissociated rheumatoid cells, it is generally agreed that nonlymphocyte cells from rheumatoid synovial tissue can be divided into three types by use of monoclonal antibodies.[316] Type I cells are macrophage-like; they have DR antigens, Fc receptors, and monocyte lineage differentiation antigens and are capable of phagocytosis. A second distinctive cell population (type II) is nonphagocytic, is occasionally binucleate, and has abundant DR antigens but lacks IgG Fc receptors, monocyte lineage antigens, or fibroblast-associated antigens. Many cells in this group have a dendritic or stellate morphology (Fig. 51–6). Another population (type III) contains all the remaining cells and is defined by the presence of antigens expressed primarily on fibroblasts and by the absence of phagocytic capability, demonstrable DR antigens, or antigens of the monocytic lineage. A successful attempt to clone dissociated rheumatoid synovial cells and place them in long-term culture has supported this classification.[317] Each type of cell could be cloned, but the type I and II cells grew slowly, with a doubling time of 5 to 7 days. The type III cells have a doubling time of 1 to 2 days. Fibroblast-like cells (type III cells) generated a dendritic appearance when they were incubated with PGE$_2$.[318] After removal of the PG, the cells reverted to normal appearance, unlike the type II cells that maintained the dendritic or stellate appearance through their slow doubling times. A study on cloned synovial cells[317] indicated that the dendritic-like cells produced significant amounts of Il-1, greater than the activity produced by type I or type III cells. What remains to be determined is whether the dendritic type II cells, with a significant ability to produce IL-1 and prominent response to activation, are the same cells that have been shown by immunohistochemistry to produce large amounts of collagenase, or whether the collagenase-producing cells are type III fibroblast-like cells induced to produce proteins by IL-1 and given a stellate appearance by PGs or other substances. In studies of cloned cells from synovial fluid in rheumatoid patients, morphology is variable, and functional studies matched with cell surface antigen expression have not been carried out.[319] It has been suggested that because the human synovial stellate cells that are PG responsive and form stellate cells (type III) may lose their characteristic morphology on culture and because they appear to lack Ia antigens in the unstimulated state, they are more closely related to fibroblasts than to macrophages.[320]

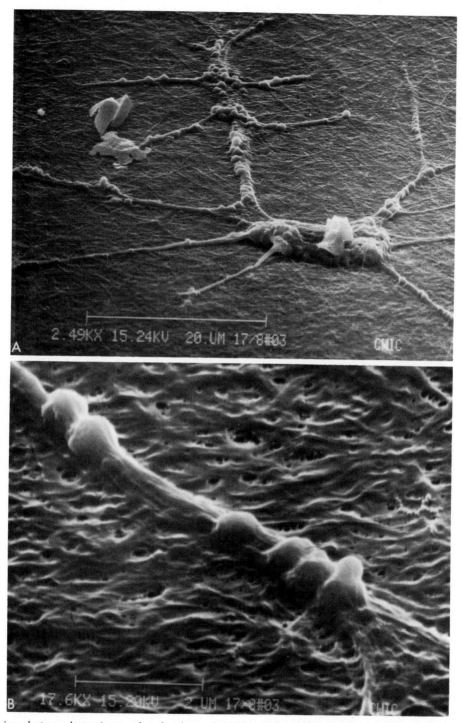

Figure 51–6. Scanning electron photomicrographs of a classic dendritic cell from rheumatoid synovium. Cells were dissociated from matrix and grown in monolayer culture on a thin film of collagen. Individual collagen fibrils are seen, presenting a matte-like surface. Knobby inclusions within the cell processes are as yet undefined, although transmission electron microscopic studies show that they are not mitochondria. In *B,* a thin linear "ribbing" is seen below the plasma membrane and is stretched over the knobby inclusions. Magnification: *A,* 2490 ×; *B,* 17,600 ×. The bar in *A* is 20 μm; in *B* it is 2 μm.

As mentioned earlier, there are many ways to link mitogenic and proliferative factors released by macrophages and lymphocytes and the profusion of synovial cells that develop in this disease. It is also worth observing, however, that the arthritis that develops in MRL/1 mice, even though caused by a specific defect in T lymphocytes, is associated with a synovial pannus tissue that consists largely of transformed mesenchymal cells and few immunocytes.[321, 322]

SYNOVIAL PATHOLOGY

There are many dimensions to RA. Gross changes have been correlated with disease activity, as have the findings at microscopic and electron microscopic levels, but geographic differences of disease within individual joints are of major importance as well.

Gross Pathologic Changes

In considering gross pathologic findings, one must account for the change from the relatively acellular lining of mesenchymal cells (two to five layers thick with relatively few blood vessels) to the bulky, hyperplastic, hypervascular, proliferative lesion resembling a tumor. All of the synovium in a normal knee joint may weigh less than 5 g; synovial tissue taken from a rheumatoid knee joint can weigh up to 500 g or more.

The built-in redundancy of the joint space permits this proliferative growth; there is room for tissue accumulation within diarthrodial joints without immediate increase in pressure or displacement of other tissue. Nowhere else in the body can such proliferation take place without encroachment on a vital function. The geometry of synovial proliferation enables an enormous surface area of cells to maintain contact with synovial fluid. Synovium does not proliferate as a tumorous mass would enlarge within a capsule. There is an intricate system of villous fronds that proliferate as would branches of ferns from a common stalk. At times, distal portions of villi become necrotic, as blood supply cannot keep pace with cellular proliferation. These dead areas may consolidate into acellular fibrinous masses, be auto-amputated, and accumulate in the synovial fluid. The loss of the terminal vasculature can produce arteriovenous shunting and synovial hypoxia, as discussed earlier.

What are the associations between gross pathologic changes and invasiveness between rheumatoid synovium? There appears to be some correlation between the location of synovial involvement and joint destruction. A detailed study using double-contrast arthrography in 131 patients with classic RA has provided geographic patterns of synovium within rheumatoid knee joints.[323, 324] Panarticular disease involved all the surfaces of the joint space, including the suprapatellar pouch. Joint destruction was rapid and severe in these patients, a not surprising finding. Interestingly, highly proliferative synovium confined to the suprapatellar pouch was not destructive, nor was disease localized in the posterior pouches of the knee. "Burnt-out" disease characterized by fibrotic and relatively avascular synovium was not observed in patients who have any remaining cartilage.

The increasing use of arthroscopy has enabled investigators to look for correlations of joint destruc-tion with the appearance of synovium.[325] One series of observations[326] of 51 knees in 32 patients has identified four distinct stages of disease progression, as follows.

Stage I. Visible evidence of joint pathologic changes was restricted to the synovial lining, and although villus proliferation had taken place, there was no invasion of meniscal or articular cartilage. Radiographic examination was normal in most of these patients.

Stage II. Proliferative pannus extended over meniscal surfaces, and erosions and fissuring of the menisci were visible, but articular cartilage appeared normal by observation and radiographs.

Stage III. Full-thickness meniscal tears and free-floating debris were observed, as was articular cartilage erosion associated with invasive, full-thickness craters containing proliferative tissue. Radiographic appearance was normal in 75 percent of these patients, and in the remaining 25 percent there was minimal joint-line narrowing.

Stage IV. Only when articular cartilage was severely eroded and menisci were often missing in their entirety were significant numbers of patients shown to have radiographic defects.

The importance of this classification is that invasion of meniscal cartilage appears to occur earlier than that of articular cartilage. It is now recognized that magnetic resonance imaging can provide early evidence of meniscal cartilage disease and therefore give a fair warning before articular cartilage invasion by synovitis begins[326] and, in some instances, visualize pannus as it begins to spread over or into articular cartilage (Fig. 51–7).

Microscopic Pathologic Changes

Examination of synovial tissue obtained from biopsies of patients with early synovitis who were proved later to have RA reveals a variable intensity of lining cell proliferation, moderate numbers of lymphocytes in the perivascular areas, and prominent new vessel formation with some thrombosis and evidence of vasculitis.[123] These are not specific findings, but they underscore the importance of angiogenesis in providing a scaffold around which the inflammation and proliferative cellular response can be built.

Modern investigators tend to study cells and subcellular organelles rather than tissues. Thus, it is not surprising that assays of cells from different samples of the same synovium may give different qualitative data because the cell population may be so different from 1 mm of synovium to the next.[327, 328] This has generated the question of whether histologic correlations with disease activity or prognosis can be generated. In one study, six histologic features in synovitis were chosen[329] and scored. They were:

1. Synoviocyte hyperplasia.

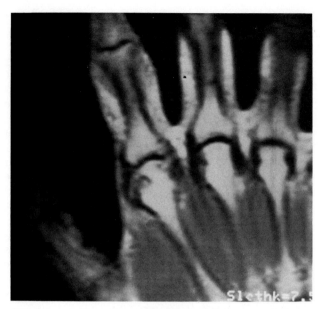

Figure 51–7. The mottled gray areas on the radial side of the second metacarpal head of a 38-year-old woman with RA represent synovial proliferation beginning to overlie articular cartilage and bone. These changes precede evidence of erosions or joint space narrowing seen on conventional radiographs. T$_2$ weighted (TR 2000 m; TE 34 ms). (Courtesy of Drs. James Seibold and Reuben Mezrich, UMDNJ-Robert Wood Johnson Medical School.)

2. Fibrosis in subsynovial layer.
3. Proliferating blood vessels (per high-power field).
4. Perivascular infiltrates of lymphocytes.
5. Focal aggregates of lymphocytes.
6. Diffuse infiltrates of lymphocytes.

In 29 patients with early, progressive disease not yet treated with disease-modifying drugs, multiple closed synovial needle biopsies were obtained. A remarkable histologic homogeneity was found, and there were significant correlations between clinical disease activity and synovial hyperplasia, vessel proliferation, and lymphoid infiltrates and aggregates. Fibrosis correlated negatively with synovial proliferation.

As mentioned earlier, rheumatoid synovial cells are derived from many origins. They are the products of the inflammatory response that drive proliferation of the synovial cells; they increase in number to extraordinary proportions[330] and behave abnormally in culture with increased rates of glucose uptake, hyaluronic acid synthesis, lactate formation, and growth rates.[331–333] Histologically synovium is characterized primarily by heterogeneity. Previous discussions have emphasized the different types of synovial cells and their membrane antigens, the presence of new blood vessels, the diverse types of lymphocytes and their microscopic distribution, and the relative paucity of polymorphonuclear leukocytes in the synovial lesion. Indeed, although PMNs have been described in the pannus, existing either as small microabscesses or as isolated cells,[334] there are re-

markably few PMNs in the synovium when one considers the enormous numbers that are frequently present in synovial fluid and that they must have traversed the synovium en route to the joint space.

The *mast cells* have great interest to those who study rheumatoid synovium because they are present in the synovial membranes of patients with RA[335] and may be localized in some patients at sites of cartilage erosion.[336] In one study, rheumatoid synovial membranes contained a mean of 48.5 mast cells per 20 high-power fields compared with 3.9 mast cells per 20 high-power fields in control synovial samples from patients undergoing surgery for meniscectomy. Patients with high numbers of mast cells had more intense clinical synovitis in the affected joints.[335] Mast cells also have been prominent in intraosseous invasive tissue. Mast cells can be found in a majority of synovial fluid specimens from inflammatory synovitis, and there is measurable histamine content in these synovial fluids.[337] Rheumatoid synovial fluids contained higher levels of histamine than did corresponding plasma samples.[338]

A detailed analysis of several indicators of proliferation and the enumeration of synovial mast cells[339] has demonstrated strong positive correlations between the number of mast cells per cubic millimeter of synovial tissue and the degree of lymphocyte infiltration (the number of helper T lymphocytes and plasma cells). A negative correlation was found between the synovial mast cell count and fibrin deposition within the synovium. Glucocorticoid injections into joints decreased by 70 to 90 percent the number of synovial tissue mast cells.

What could be the contribution of mast cells to rheumatoid synovitis? On the one hand, they could be responding to lymphokines that stimulate mast cell growth and chemotaxis. On the other hand, a mast cell–derived lymphocyte chemotactic factor has been described in animals.[340] Thus, once recruited to the synovium, the mast cell could help recruit lymphocytes to the synovium. Extracts of mast cells can induce adherent rheumatoid synovial cells to increase production of PGE$_2$ and collagenase; the stimulatory factor was neither histamine nor heparin.[341] Heparin, however, does have significant effects on connective tissue. In particular, it may modulate the effects of bone hormones on osseous cells and thereby alter the balance of bone synthesis toward degradation. Heparin increases basal cAMP levels in both bone cells and adherent rheumatoid synovial cells; the significance of these changes to cartilage or bone destruction must be determined.[342]

Another factor with potential for involvement in acceleration of joint destruction in rheumatoid arthritis is *iron* (see Fig. 51–5). Since the earliest associations of iron in rheumatoid synovitis, there have been speculations as to its role in this disease.[343] Other diseases, namely hemophilia and villonodular synovitis, are associated both with tissue destruction and with excessive iron in macrophages and hyperplastic synovial cells. It appears to be the breakdown

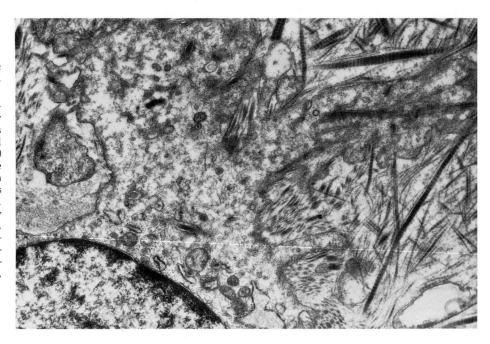

Figure 51–8. The leading edge of a pannus cell extends diffusely into cartilage. Collagen fibers, characterized by 69 nm periodicity, can be seen about to be or actually engulfed by the cell. This close contact of synovium and cartilage is found in less than 10 percent of patients but is the type of process associated with phagocytosis of collagen by this leading edge of cells (30,000 ×). (Electron photomicrograph by Andrey M. Glauert. From Harris, E. D., Jr., et al.: Intracellular collagen fibers at the pannus-cartilage junction in rheumatoid arthritis. Arthritis Rheum. 20:657, 1977.)

of red blood cells that stimulates synovial cells in hemophilia to produce significant amounts of proteolytic enzymes.[344] Iron is also known to enhance the toxicity of oxygen free radicals. It facilitates production of the toxic hydroxyl radical in the presence of hydrogen peroxide and superoxide. In rheumatoid patients, levels of the iron-binding protein ferritin are much higher in synovial fluid than in serum.[345] Ferritin-bound iron concentrations in rheumatoid synovial tissue are quite high and are adequate to stimulate hydroxyl radical formation. Decreased tissue pH associated with rapid rate of glycolysis in these tissues and inadequate blood supply (see earlier) could lead to release of iron from ferritin and stimulate hydroxyl ion formation.[346]

Cartilage is destroyed in RA by both enzymatic and mechanical processes (Fig. 51–8). The enzymes induced by factors such as IL-1, TNF, phagocytosis of debris by synovial cells, and both free and bound iron cause the joint destruction. Early in synovitis, proteoglycans are depleted from the tissue, and this leads to mechanical weakening of cartilage. As proteoglycans are depleted from cartilage (Fig. 51–9), it loses the capability to rebound from a deforming load and thereby becomes susceptible to mechanical fragmentation and fibrillation and eventually loss of functional integrity concurrent with its complete dissolution by collagenase and stromelysin.[347]

As in osteoarthritis, cartilage destruction in patients with RA is marked by a compensatory increase in proteoglycan synthesis, but in the absence of a true remission of the disease, once started, cartilage erosion continues and progresses. One of the first useful descriptions of the pannus-cartilage junction was provided by Kingsley-Mills in 1970.[348] These observations, made from tissue removed at early synovectomy, showed cellular fingers composed of mesenchymal cells and small blood vessels penetrating cartilage at the synovium-cartilage junction near the cartilage-bone junction where synovium originates. These findings were consistent with the concept that cartilage was not destroyed by diffuse loss of tissue but rather that degradation was related to the release of enzymes at a tight junction between invasive cell and the cartilage.[349]

Subsequent studies have focused on this pannus-cartilage junction as well as on the possibility that diffuse enzyme release from polymorphonuclear leukocytes in synovial fluid could have an effect on loss of cartilage. Consistent with the findings of immune complexes in superficial layers of cartilage, electron microscopic examinations of articular cartilage in RA have revealed amorphous-appearing material and evidence of breakdown of collagen and proteoglycan consistent with superficial diffuse activity of joint fluid enzymes[248] (Fig. 51–10).

Pannus-Cartilage Junction

Multiple different types of histopathologic findings have been seen at the pannus-cartilage junction (Fig. 51–11):

1. Numerous areas are seen in which *aggressive cell clusters* of mesenchymal cells, both macrophage-like and fibroblast-like, appear to have a leading edge of penetration of cartilage matrix far from blood vessels of lymphocytes.[350, 351]

2. Some areas show relatively acellular pannus tissue, suggesting that there is little if any enzyme action in these areas.[352]

3. Other sections show microfoci of one particular cell type, including microabscesses of polymor-

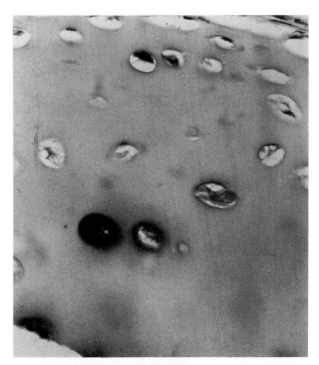

Figure 51–9. Human articular cartilage from active rheumatoid arthritis removed at joint arthroplasty and stained for metachromasia. The only dark metachromatic stain surrounds a few chondrocytes, which, presumably, are actively making proteoglycan only to have it broken down by proteinases derived from synovial fluid, chondrocytes, or synovial tissue. The form of this depleted cartilage is normal; however, its functional capacity to rebound from a deforming load is seriously impaired.

phonuclear leukocytes, mast cells, or dendritic or "stellate" cells. Macrophagic and fibroblastic foci were three to five times more common than those containing mast cells or PMNs.[353]

4. Rarely proliferating small blood vessels surrounded by cellular infiltrates penetrate deeply into the cartilage.[354]

5. Multinucleate giant cells are particularly common at the erosive front when penetration is from the subchondral side of cartilage. Both osteoclasts and large giant cells named chondroclasts have been observed degrading bone and mineralized cartilage as well as areas of unmineralized (hyaline) articular cartilage.[355] These multinucleate cells stain brightly for acid phosphatase. It should be remembered that experimental production of multinucleate cells in cultures of synovial fibroblasts is associated with an enormous increase in production in these cultures of collagenase and, presumably, other matrix metalloproteinases.[356] It may be that bradykinin released by the proliferating cells has a significant effect on bone resorption at the pannus-cartilage junctions; it appears to stimulate osteoclast-mediated bone degradation by a process that is dependent on endogenous PG formation.[357]

There may be consistent variations in the histopathology of the cartilage-pannus junction between different joints. It was observed that an invasive pannus was more commonly found in sections from involved metatarsophalangeal joints as compared with hip and knee joints[358] in which a layer of resting fibroblasts appeared to separate pannus from cartilage. It was hypothesized that this could explain the fact that erosions are seen more often around small

joints such as metatarsophalangeal joints, whereas joint space narrowing without erosions is more common in knees.

The rapidity with which resorption of joint structures occurs may be determined by the type of cellular response and therefore the morphologic findings at the pannus-cartilage junction. In most cases of RA, electron micrographic studies show an area of amorphous degraded connective tissue in a zone a few microns wide between cell processes and relatively intact cartilage collagen fibrils. Occasionally, however, perhaps associated with aggressive disease, intracellular collagen fibers in various stages of degradation can be found within cells that have processes tightly linked to and penetrating the cartilage[359] (see Fig. 51–8).

In summary, there are many different types of cells that can be involved in loss of cartilage. It is likely that in response to new blood vessel formation and growth factors there is a great deal of proliferation of macrophage-like and fibroblast-like cells within the synovium infiltrated intermittently with mast cells and multinucleate cells and occasional polymorphonuclear leukocytes. In response to as yet unknown autocoids, in addition to the presence of immune complexes in the superficial layers of cartilage, the proliferative synovial tissue that appears to overlie cartilage begins to penetrate and degrade the cartilage. Multinucleate cells and stellate cells are markers for rapid resorption. Quiescent fibroblast-like cells with few new blood vessels in the vicinity are not likely to be in the process of active resorption. It is probable that the activity of new blood vessel formation dictates rates of synovial cell proliferation at a microgeographic level and that this may vary

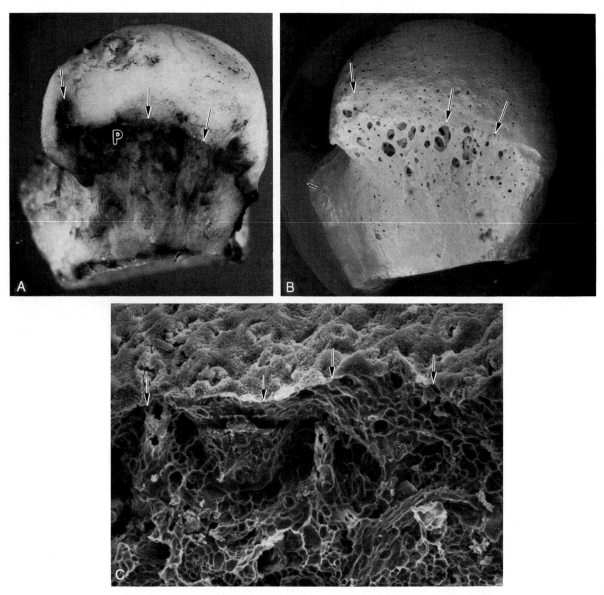

Figure 51–10. *A,* Gross view of the volar (palmar) surface of a left, third finger metacarpal head. The eroding front (*arrows*) of the pannus (*P*) stained with India ink is shown (8 ×). *B,* Gross view of the volar surface of the same left, third finger metacarpal head after chemical maceration. The eroding front adjacent to the pannus is delineated (*arrows*). Various-sized holes, which differ from penetrations through the subchondral plate, are seen in the bony surface originally covered by the pannus (8 ×). *C,* The eroding front (*arrows*) at the junction of pannus with the layer of calcified cartilage and subchondral bone is obvious in the macerated sample viewed with the scanning electron microscope at a higher magnification. The calcified cartilage and subchondral bone originally covered by the pannus show confluent lacunae typical of the pattern of osteoclastic resorption (270 ×). (Photographs provided by J. C. C. Leisen, M.D. and Howard Duncan, M.D. at Henry Ford Hospital.)

along the synovium-pannus junction from micron to micron.

There is often little difference in the rates of bone and cartilage degradation, and the cellular front directed against each of these tissues is similar, including the presence of large multinucleate cells with prominent stains for acid hydrolases. It is important to remember that, although multinucleate cells and dendritic cells may be high producers of degradative enzymes, their existence is dependent on stimulation by cytokines (PDGF, IL-1, TNF-α) (discussed earlier) associated with the inflammatory

and immune response. Thus, well behind the invasive front are the foci of helper T cells, immunoglobulin-bearing cells, and HLA-DR–expressing cells that are generating the immune response and the proliferative reaction that evolves from it.[328]

The rate-limiting step in cartilage loss is degradation of collagen because PGs are degraded very soon after inflammation begins. Metalloproteinases, released into the extracellular space and active at neutral pH, are probably responsible for the majority of effective proteolysis of articular cartilage proteins, but other classes of enzymes may play a role in joint

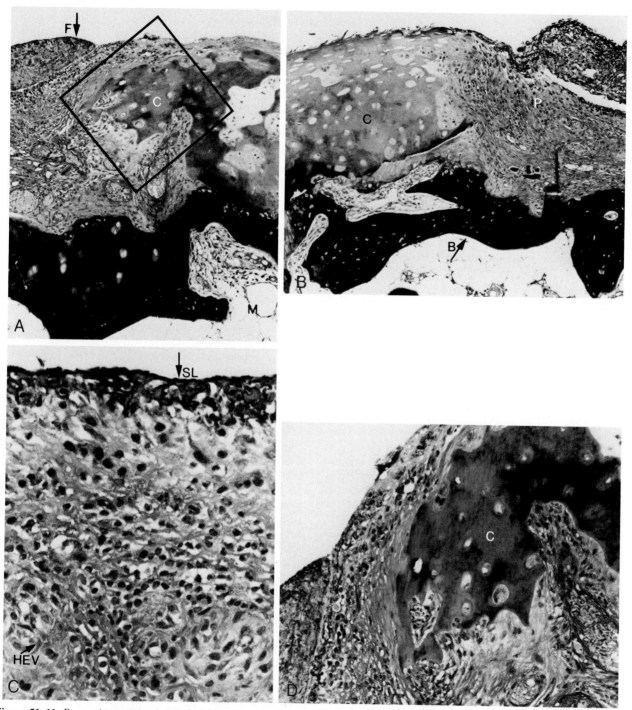

Figure 51–11. Four microscopic views of a rheumatoid metatarsal head removed at time of arthroplasty and stained as a tri-chrome preparation. In *A* and *B*, the black areas represent subchondral bone. *M*, Marrow; *P*, pannus; *C*, cartilage; *D*, the square from *A* enlarged. *A*, The heterogeneity of the invasive pannus is shown here. Whorls of proliferative synovial tissue become relatively avascular as they abut against the remaining cartilage, destroying it by proteases. The rheumatoid process in the marrow is capable of destroying bone as well. *B*, A similar picture to *A*. In the invasive pannus, there are numerous lymphocytes (left of *P*), but these are relatively rare at the invasive front. Several large lacunae are seen in the cartilage, probably representing tongues of invasive pannus, but other areas show enlarged areas without matrix surrounding individual chondrocytes that have been activated to produce proteases by cytokines. *C*, A section through synovial tissue near the invasive front. The synovial cells on the surface, *SL*, in continuity with synovial fluid, always develop a distinct morphology from sub-lining cells, even though they are, presumably, the same cell (macrophage or fibroblast). One small capillary, *HEV*, shows plump, tall endothelium. Lymphocytes here are not organized into a follicular pattern but distribute irregularly throughout the synovium. *D*, Different patterns of cells surrounding cartilage being destroyed. (Photomicrographs courtesy of Donald Regula, M.D., Department of Pathology, Stanford University Medical Center. Tissue samples provided from surgery by Gordon Brody, M.D.)

destruction. Lysosomal enzymes such as cathepsins B, G, and H may play a role within and outside of cells in degrading noncollagenous matrix proteins. Serine proteinases (e.g., elastin and plasmin) are doubtless similarly involved.

Mediators of Metalloproteinase Induction in Synovial Cells

Many factors have the capability to induce biosynthesis of metalloproteinases. Some appear to work directly after receptor binding to induce transcription of mRNA for the enzymes. Others induce synthesis of direct mediators, and still others modulate effects of direct mediators. PDGF has a direct effect (see subsequently) on induction of proteinases in mesenchymal cells as well as being both a chemoattractant and a mitogen for these cells.[206] It is likely that PDGF is released into rheumatoid tissues in large quantities as platelet activation in the presence of angiogenesis and clot formation occurs. IL-1 is produced by many cells; in the joint in RA, IL-1 is probably generated by activated macrophages and synovial cells.[175] Cloned, adherent synovial cells from rheumatoid synovitis also produce cytokine(s) with IL-1 activity; stellate cells (i.e., those similar to ones that produce large amounts of metalloproteinases) produce more than macrophage-like cells or fibroblasts. The cytokine that induces osteoclast formation and named osteoclast activating factor has been identified as IL-1β.[185] It is not yet known whether IL-6 induces metalloproteinase production by synovial cells. In models in vitro, it has been shown that, although culture medium from rheumatoid synovium stimulates cartilage degradation, this can be inhibited by an antibody against IL-1; these data implicate rheumatoid synovium as a source of IL-1 that activates chondrocytes to produce proteases.[360] TNF-α stimulates collagenase and PGE₂ production by human synovial cells.[192] This cytokine, produced by macrophages, is synergistic with IL-1.

In contrast to these cytokines that induce production of enzymes that degrade connective tissue, there are several that inhibit biosynthesis of proteolytic enzymes. One of these (TGF-β) inhibits collagenase synthesis in vitro and enhances production of tissue inhibitor of metalloproteinases (TIMP).[201]

Substances other than cytokines are capable of inducing synovial cells to produce metalloproteinases in vitro, and it is probable that many have a role in vivo as well. It is not known for many whether their effects are mediated through cytokines such as PDGF. Proteinases,[361] phagocytosable debris,[362] soluble iron,[363] collagens,[364, 365] crystals of monosodium urate monohydrate,[366] and various calcium crystals[367] are all found in joints at one time or another, and all stimulate collagenase biosynthesis. The crystals and perhaps other substances in this group stimulate metalloproteinase production by triggering IL-1 (and possibly other cytokine) production. These factors operate, it is presumed, by activating receptors that, in turn, enhance expression of transacting factors that bind to cis-element in the 5′ flanking region of the metalloproteinase genes. One of these, AP-1, is probably a complex of proteins expressed by the cellular jun and fos proto-oncogenes (Jun and Fos, respectively) that may be held together by a leucine "zipper," in which residues of leucine in a portion of the protein that is an α-helix project out and interact with homologous residues on another protein. This combination of Jun and Fos might somehow juxtapose the DNA-binding domains of Jun and Fos and enable them to attach (as AP-1) to specific cis-elements on the DNA, enhancing expression of metalloproteinase mRNA.[368-371]

Collagenase (matrix metalloproteinase 1 [MMP1]) and stromelysin (MMP3) have, between them, the capability to degrade all the important structural proteins in the extracellular tissues within joints. Collagenase was first found in culture medium of explants of rheumatoid synovium in 1967.[372] The rheumatoid synovial collagenase is a metalloproteinase with maximal activity in a range between pH 7.0 and 8.0; in pure form, the collagenase has very little activity against substrates other than collagen, including denatured collagen (i.e., gelatin).[373] It cleaves through the triple helical collagen molecule at a single glycine-isoleucine bond approximately ¾ distance from the amino terminus of the 300 nm protein. This enzyme has the capability to degrade only the interstitial helical collagens (e.g., types I, II, III, and X collagens); it has little or no activity against types IV, V, IX, and other nonhelical collagens. The process of degradation is slow; kinetics for the human skin enzyme (which is very similar if not identical to the synovial collagenase) indicated that only 25 molecules of collagen are cleaved per molecule of enzyme per hour at 37°C.[374] The temperature of the interaction between collagenase and collagen is a crucial determinant of rate of lysis; an increase of only a few degrees (as one would expect within an inflamed joint) may increase the rate of collagenolysis by manyfold, a fact that has led some investigators to question the benefit of applying deep heat (e.g., microwave) to inflamed arthritic joints.

Stromelysin (MMP3) was described first from rheumatoid synovial cells in 1986[375] as a metalloproteinase of similar molecular weight to collagenase and having the same pH range for activity. It has no activity against interstitial collagens but effectively degrades type IV collagen, fibronectin, laminin, proteoglycan core protein, and type IX collagen.[376] Stromelysin removes the NH2-terminal propeptides from type I procollagen, producing products similar to those produced by procollagen N-proteinase, the enzyme believed responsible in vivo for performing this function. Stromelysin is integrally involved in activation of procollagenase.

Most data indicate that there is a cascade of activation of the matrix metalloproteinases. Prostromelysin is activated, and the presence of stromelysin is essential for subsequent activation of procollagenase. Prostromelysin from human synovial cells can be activated by other proteases, including trypsin, chymotrypsin, plasma kallikrein, plasmin, and thermosysin,[377] and by mast cell tryptase.[378]

A leading candidate for a protease that initiates the collagenolytic process in RA would be plasmin because rheumatoid synovial cells produce plasminogen activator.[379] In addition to demonstration of plasminogen activator production in vitro in cell culture, fragments of plasminogen with "mini-plasminogen" activity have been demonstrated in inflammatory synovial fluids from rheumatoid joints.[380]

Inhibition of Metalloproteinase Activity

It was demonstrated more than 10 years ago that α_2-macroglobulin (α_2M) accounted for more than 95% of collagenase inhibitory capacity in serum.[381] The mechanism of inhibition by α_2M involves hydrolysis by the proteinase of a susceptible region in one of the four polypeptide chains of α_2M with subsequent trapping of the proteins within the interstices of the α_2M.

The first inhibitor of mammalian collagenase to be isolated and purified from human tissues was a protein of 25,000 Mr produced by cells in explants of human tendons. This tendon inhibitor inhibited trypsin-activated rheumatoid synovial collagenase as well as the collagenase obtained from polymorphonuclear leukocytes.[382] The same protein was subsequently purified from skin; the primary structure has been determined, cDNA clones have been prepared,[383] and the protein is known as TIMP. Immunohistochemical studies[384] have localized the inhibitor in hyperplastic synovial lining cells in rheumatoid synovium but not in the cells of normal synovium. The same cells that express TIMP express collagenase. The almost ubiquitous finding of functional TIMP in tissues suggests that this protein plays an important role in regulation of connective tissue remodeling and destruction. It follows that any substance that would increase expression of TIMP while diminishing or repressing expression of metalloproteinase secretion might decrease degradation of connective tissue in pathologic states. TGF-β may be such a substance; exposure of quiescent cells to growth factors in the presence of TGF-β resulted in inhibition by transcriptional mechanisms of collagenase induction and a synergistic increase in TIMP expression.[201]

Extra-articular Pathology in Rheumatoid Arthritis

The specific clinical syndromes associated with extra-articular disease in RA are outlined in Chapter 52. Because it is not known what factors determine "arthrotropism" in RA, it cannot be determined what produces extra-articular manifestations in the systemic circulation. The principal factors would appear to be immune complexes that generate vasculitis and growth factors that are associated with mesenchymal proliferation.

Two representative and generic extra-articular manifestations are considered here: rheumatoid nodules and vasculitis.

Rheumatoid Nodules

Rheumatoid nodules have been well characterized morphologically.[385, 386] These nodules are most often found subcutaneously over pressure points and represent a proliferative diathesis of mesenchymal tissue. In response to minimal trauma, there is an intriguing combination of tissue destruction following proliferation and vasculitis to give the final result. Anatomically there is a central necrotic zone surrounded at a fairly sharp border by a highly cellular area of radially arranged cells amid strands of collagen. The intense cellularity gives way at the periphery to more densely packed connective tissue. Mononuclear cells infiltrate around blood vessels in this capsular zone. Electron microscopic studies of the central necrotic areas have shown a mixture of collagen fibers in varying stages of degradation, noncollagenous filamentous material, granular debris, cell membranes, and fat globules.[387] Palmer et al.[388] have presented convincing immunohistologic evidence that monocytes continue to be recruited to these nodules and migrate from the outer vascular zone toward the palisade and central necrotic area. This observation suggests that there is a potent chemoattractant for monocytes being emitted from the interior of the rheumatoid nodule. Data show that the majority of cells in the palisading layer express epitopes found exclusively on mononuclear phagocytes including HLA-DR.[389]

Study of nodules shortly after they have developed has revealed inflammation of venules with deposition of fibrin within vessel walls and in surrounding tissue. Intense proliferation of monocytes and fibroblasts in these early lesions is often found. The intense exudation from small blood vessels accounts for the space-occupying qualities of these nodules and explains how they can appear in less than 24 hours. The cellular proliferation is induced somehow by the vascular inflammation and gives structure to the nodule. Central necrosis is probably a result of two processes: the microinfarctions caused by thrombosis of terminal vessels and the enormous quantities of collagenase and other proteinases produced by the cellular palisading area.[390]

Vasculitis

The most prominent of extra-articular pathologic change in RA is vasculitis. It may present clinically as a variety of syndromes and may be associated with involvement of medium-sized arteries, small arteries, and venules. All layers of the vessel wall are infiltrated by lymphocytes.[391] Intimal proliferation and thrombosis occasionally are found, particularly in digital arteries. Deposits of IgG, IgM, and C3 have been noted in the walls of involved arteries,[392] notably in those patients with severe disease, high titers of RF, low serum levels of C3, and clinical features such as peripheral neuropathy, digital gangrene, nail fold infarcts, and cutaneous ulcers.

In some patients, involvement of medium-sized rather than small arteries with necrosis, fibrinoid changes, PMN infiltration, and disruption of the internal elastic lamina may resemble closely the pathologic changes of polyarteritis nodosa.[393] Palpable purpura, reflecting involvement of venules in a leukocytoclastic vasculitis, is the third pattern of involvement. Immunofluorescence sometimes reveals the presence of immunoglobulins and complement in and around the venules,[394] although studies of cutaneous vessel immune deposits have been positive in more than 50 percent of seropositive RA patients whether or not they have clinical vasculitis.[395] The persistence of fibrin in chronic lesions of vasculitis involving small arteries has led to the speculation that fibrin may play an active role in the genesis of these chronic and occlusive arterial lesions.[396]

References

1. Wolfe, A. M.: The epidemiology of rheumatoid arthritis: A review. Bull. Rheum. Dis. 19:518, 1968.
2. Mitchell, D. M., and Fries, J. F.: An analysis of the American Rheumatism Association criteria for rheumatoid arthritis. Arthritis Rheum. 25:481, 1982.
3. Arnett, F. C., and Committee: The American Rheumatism Association 1987 revised criteria for the classification of rheumatoid arthritis. Arthritis Rheum. 31:315, 1988.
4. Ahmed, S. A., Penhale, W. J., and Talal, N.: Sex hormones, immune responses, and autoimmune diseases. Am. J. Pathol. 121:431, 1985.
5. Buyon, J. P., Korchak, H. M., Rutherford, L. E., Ganguly, M., and Weissmann, G.: Female hormones reduce neutrophil responsiveness in vitro. Arthritis Rheum. 27:623, 1984.
6. Persellin, R. H.: The effect of pregnancy on rheumatoid arthritis. Bull. Rheum. Dis. 27:922, 1977.
7. Hench, P. S.: The ameliorating effect of pregnancy on chronic atrophic (infectious rheumatoid) arthritis, fibrositis, and intermittent hydrarthosis. Mayo Clin. Proc. 13:161, 1938.
8. Hazes, J. M. W.: Pregnancy and its effect on the risk of developing rheumatoid arthritis. Ann. Rheum. Dis. 50:71, 1991.
9. Ungar, A., Kay, C. R., Griffin, A. J., and Panayi, G. S.: Disease activity in rheumatoid arthritis during pregnancy. Br. Med. J. 286:750, 1983.
10. Thomson, A. W., and Horne, C. H. W.: Biological and clinical significance of pregnancy associated α2 glycoprotein (PAG). Invest. Cell Pathol. 3:295, 1980.
11. Birkeland, S. A., and Kristoffersen, K.: Cellular immunity in pregnancy: Blast transformation and rosette formation of maternal T and B lymphocytes. A cross-section analysis. Clin. Exp. Immunol. 30:408, 1977.
12. Oka, M.: Effect of pregnancy on the onset and course of rheumatoid arthritis. Ann. Rheum. Dis. 12:227, 1953.
13. Wingrave, S. J., and Kay, C. R.: Reduction in incidence of rheumatoid arthritis associated with oral contraceptives. Lancet 1:569, 1978.
14. Vandenbroucke, J. P., Witteman, J. C. M., Valkenburg, H. A., Boersma, J. W., Cats, A., Festen, J. J. M., Hartman, A. P., Huber-Bruning, O., Rasker, J. J., and Weber, J.: Noncontraceptive hormones and rheumatoid arthritis in perimenopausal and postmenopausal women. J.A.M.A. 255:1299, 1986.
15. Linos, A., Worthington, J. W., O'Fallon, W. M., and Kurland, L. T.: The epidemiology of rheumatoid arthritis in Rochester, Minnesota: A study of incidence, prevalence, and mortality. Am. J. Epidemiol. 111:87, 1980.
16. Linos, A., Worthington, J. W., O'Fallon, W. M., and Kurland, L. T.: Case-control study of rheumatoid arthritis and prior use of oral contraceptives. Lancet 1:1299, 1983.
17. del Junco, D. J., Annegers, J. F., Luthra, H. S., Coulam, C. B., and Kurland, L. T.: Do oral contraceptives prevent rheumatoid arthritis? J.A.M.A. 254:1938, 1985.
17a. Van Zeben, D., Hazes, J. M. W., Vandenbroucke, J. P., Dijkmans, B. A., and Cats, A.: Diminished incidence of severe rheumatoid arthritis associated with oral contraceptive use. Arthritis Rheum. 33:1462, 1990.
18. Hazes, J. M. W., Dijkmans, B. A. C., Vandenbroucke, J. P., de Vries, R. R. P., and Cats, A.: Lifestyle and the risk of rheumatoid arthritis: Cigarette smoking and alcohol consumption. Ann. Rheum. Dis. 49:980, 1990.
19. Beer, A. E., and Billingham, R. E.: Immunoregulatory aspects of pregnancy. Fed. Proc. 37:2374, 1978.
20. Combe, B., Cosso, B., Clot, J., Bonneau, M., and Sany, J.: Human placenta-eluted gamma globulins in immunomodulating treatment of rheumatoid arthritis. Am. J. Med. 78:920, 1985.
21. Moynier, M., Cosso, B., Brochier, J., and Clot, J.: Identification of class II HLA alloantibodies in placenta-eluted gamma globulins used for treating rheumatoid arthritis. Arthritis Rheum. 30:375, 1987.
22. Winchester, R.: Immunogenetics. In Kelley, W. N., (ed.): Textbook of Internal Medicine. 2nd ed. Philadelphia, J. B. Lippincott, 1992.
23. Stastny, P.: Mixed lymphocyte cultures in rheumatoid arthritis. J. Clin. Invest. 57:1148, 1976.
23a. Goronzy, J. J., Xie, C., Hu, W., van Kenlen, V. G., and Weyland, C. M.: HLA epitopes associated with rheumatoid arthritis determine the interaction with the T cell receptor. Clin. Res. 40:198A, 1992.
24. McMichael, A. J., Sasazuki, T., McDevitt, H. O., and Payne, R. O.: Increased frequency of HLA-Cw3 and HLA-Dw4 in rheumatoid arthritis. Arthritis Rheum. 30:1037, 1977.
25. Stastny, P.: Association of the B-cell alloantigen DRw4 with rheumatoid arthritis. N. Engl. J. Med. 298:869, 1978.
26. Gregersen, P. K., Shen, M., Song, Q. L., et al.: Molecular diversity of HLA-DR4 haplotypes. Proc. Natl. Acad. Sci. U.S.A. 83:2642, 1986.
27. Nepom, G. T., Byers, P., Seyfried, C., et al.: HLA genes associated with rheumatoid arthritis: Identification of susceptibility alleles using specific oligonucleotide probes. Arthritis Rheum. 32:15, 1989.
28. Calin, A., Elswood, J., and Klouda, P. T.: Destructive arthritis, rheumatoid factor, and HLA-DR4: Susceptibility versus severity, a case-control study. Arthritis Rheum. 32:1221, 1989.
28a. Weyland, C. M., and Goronzy, J. J.: Allelic combinations at the HLA-DRB1 locus are characteristic for disease patterns in rheumatoid arthritis. Clin. Res. 40:297A, 1992.
29. McCusker, C. T., Reid, B., Green, D., Gladman, D. D., Buchanan, W. W., and Singal, D. P.: HLA-D region antigens in patients with rheumatoid arthritis. Arthritis Rheum. 34:192, 1991.
30. Larsen, B. A., Alderdice, C. A., Hawkins, D., Martin, J. R., Mitchell, D. M., and Sheridan, D. P.: Protective HLA-DR phenotypes in rheumatoid arthritis. J. Rheumatol. 16:4, 1989.
31. Moxley, G.: DNA polymorphism of immunoglobulin kappa confers risk of rheumatoid arthritis. Arthritis Rheum. 32:634, 1989.
32. Moxley, G.: Immunoglobulin kappa genotype confers risk of rheumatoid arthritis among HLA-DR4 negative individuals. Arthritis Rheum. 32:1365, 1989.
33. Parekh, R. B., Dwek, R. A., Sutton, B. J., Fernandes, D. L., Leung, A., Stanworth, D., and Rodemacher, T. W.: Association of rheumatoid arthritis and primary osteoarthritis with changes in the glycosylation pattern of total serum IgG. Nature 316:452, 1985.
34. Schrohenloher, R. E., Tomana, M., Koopman, W. J., del Puente, A., and Bennett, P. H.: Occurrence of IgG galactosylation deficiency prior to the onset of rheumatoid arthritis. Abstracts for South East region, American College of Rheumatology, April 1991.
35. Sternberg, E. M., Hill, J. M., Chrousos, G. P., Kamilaris, T., Listwak, S. J., Gold, P. W., and Wilder, R. L.: Inflammatory mediator-induced hypothalamic-pituitary-adrenal axis activation is defective in streptococcal cell wall arthritis-susceptible Lewis rats. Proc. Natl. Acad. Sci. U.S.A. 86:2374, 1989.
36. Sternberg, E. M., Young, W. S., III, Bernardini, R., Calogero, A. E., Chrousos, G. P., Gold, P. W., and Wilder, R. L.: A central nervous system defect in biosynthesis of corticotropin-releasing hormone is associated with susceptibility to streptococcal cell wall-induced arthritis in Lewis rats. Proc. Natl. Acad. Sci. U.S.A. 86:4771, 1989.
37. Steere, A. C., Dwyer, E., and Winchester, R.: Association of chronic Lyme arthritis with HLA-DR4 and HLA-DR2 alleles. N. Engl. J. Med. 323:219, 1990.
38. Alspaugh, M. A., and Tan, E. M.: Antibodies to cellular antigens in Sjögren's syndrome. J. Clin. Invest. 55:1067, 1975.
39. Alspaugh, M. A., Henle, G., Lennette, E. T., and Henle, W.: Elevated levels of antibodies to Epstein-Barr virus antigens in sera and synovial fluids of patients with rheumatoid arthritis. J. Clin. Invest. 67:1134, 1981.
40. Tosato, G., Steinberg, A. D., Yarchoan, R., Heilman, C. A., Pike, S.

E., De Seau, V., and Blaese, R. M.: Abnormally elevated frequency of Epstein-Barr virus-infected B cells in the blood of patients with rheumatoid arthritis. J. Clin. Invest. 73:1789, 1984.

41. Silverman, S. L., and Schumacher, H. R.: Antibodies to Epstein-Barr viral antigens in early rheumatoid arthritis. Arthritis Rheum. 24:1465, 1981.

42. Alspaugh, M. A., Shoji, H., and Nonoyama, M.: A search for rheumatoid arthritis–associated nuclear antigen and Epstein-Barr virus specific antigens or genomes in tissues and cells from patients with rheumatoid arthritis. Arthritis Rheum. 26:712, 1983.

43. Fox, R. I., Chilton, T., Rhodes, G., and Vaughan, J. H.: Lack of reactivity of rheumatoid arthritis synovial membrane DNA with cloned Epstein-Barr virus DNA probes. J. Immunol. 137:498, 1986.

44. Fingeroth, J. D., Weis, J. J., Tedder, T. F., Strominger, J. L., Biro, P. A., and Fearon, D. T.: Epstein-Barr virus receptor of human B lymphocytes is the C3d receptor CR2. Proc. Natl. Acad. Sci. U.S.A. 81:4510, 1984.

45. Yaq, Q. Y., Rickinson, A. B., Gaston, J. S. H., and Epstein, M. A.: Disturbance of the Epstein-Barr virus-host balance in rheumatoid arthritis patients: A quantitative study. Clin. Exp. Immunol. 64:302, 1986.

46. Depper, J. M., and Zvaifler, N. J.: Epstien-Barr virus. Its relationship to the pathogenesis of rheumatoid arthritis. Arthritis Rheum. 24:755, 1981.

47. Roudier, J., Rhodes, G., Petersen, J., Vaughan, J. H., and Carson, D. A.: The Epstein-Barr virus glycoprotein gp110, a molecular link between HLA DR4, HLA DR1, and rheumatoid arthritis. Scand. J. Immunol. 27:367, 1988.

48. Roudier, J., Petersen, J., Rhodes, G. H., et al.: Susceptibility to rheumatoid arthritis maps to a T-cell epitope shared by the HLA-Dw4 DR beta-1 chain and the Epstein-Barr virus glycoprotein gp110. Proc. Natl. Acad. Sci. U.S.A. 86:5104, 1989.

49. Simpson, R. W., McGinty, L., Simon, L., Smith, C. A., Godzeski, C. W., and Boyd, R. J.: Association of parvoviruses with rheumatoid arthritis of humans. Science 223:1425, 1984.

50. Cohen, B. J., Buckley, M. M., Clewley, J. P., Jones, V. E., Puttick, A. H., and Jacoby, R. K.: Human parvovirus infection in early rheumatoid and inflammatory arthritis. Ann. Rheum. Dis. 45:832, 1986.

51. Haase, A. T.: Pathogenesis of lentivirus infections. Nature 322:130, 1986.

52. Grahame, R., Armstrong, R., Simmons, N., Wilton, J. M. A., Dyson, M., Laurent, R., Millis, R., and Mims, C. A.: Chronic arthritis associated with the presence of intrasynovial rubella virus. Ann. Rheum. Dis. 42:2, 1983.

53. Iwakura, Y., Tosu, M., Yoshida, E., et al.: Induction of inflammatory arthropathy resembling rheumatoid arthritis in mice transgenic for HTLV-1. Science 253:1026, 1991.

54. Kaufmann, S. H. E.: Heat-shock proteins: A link between rheumatoid arthritis and infection? Curr. Opin. Rheumatol. 2:420, 1990.

55. DeJoy, S. Q., Ferguson, K. M., Sapp, T. M., et al.: Streptococcal cell wall arthritis: Passive transfer of disease with a T cell line and crossreactivity of streptococcal cell wall antigens with *Mycobacterium tuberculosis*. J. Exp. Med. 170:369, 1989.

56. van Eden, W., Thole, J. E., van der Zee, R., et al.: Cloning of the mycobacterial epitope recognized by T lymphocytes in adjuvant arthritis. Nature 331:171, 1988.

57. Tsoulfa, G., Rook, G. A., Van-Embden, J. D., et al.: Raised serum IgG and IgA antibodies to mycobacterial antigens in rheumatoid arthritis. Ann. Rheum. Dis. 48:118, 1989.

58. Gaston, J. S. H., Life, P. F., Bailey, L. C., Bacon, P. A.: In vitro responses to a 65-kilodalton mycobacterial protein by synovial T cells from inflammatory arthritis patients. J. Immunol. 143:2494, 1989.

59. Born, W., Hall, L., Dallas, A., et al.: Recognition of a peptide antigen by heat shock-reactive γδ T lymphocytes. Science 249:67, 1990.

60. Moentz, J. D., Zhou, T., Gay, R. E., Gay, S., Blüthmann, H., and Edwards, C. K.: A superantigen model for arthritis in Vβ8 TCR transgenic *lpr/lpr* mice. ACR Southeast region scientific program, April 1991.

60a. daSilva, J. A.: Heat shock proteins: the missing link between hormonal and reproductive factors and rheumatoid arthritis? Ann. Rheum. Dis. 50:735, 1991.

61. Stuart, J. M., Cremer, M. A., Townes, A. S., and Kang, A. H.: Type II collagen-induced arthritis in rats: Transfer with serum. J. Exp. Med. 155:1, 1982.

62. Trentham, D. E., Dynesius, R. A., and David, J. R.: Passive transfer by cells of type II collagen-induced arthritis in rats. J. Clin. Invest. 62:359, 1978.

63. Klareskog, L., Holmdahl, R., Larsson, E., and Wigzell, H.: Role of T lymphocytes in collagen II induced arthritis in rats. Clin. Exp. Immunol. 51:117, 1983.

64. Helfgott, S. M., Dynesius-Trentham, R., Brahn, E., and Trentham, D. E.: An arthritogenic lymphokine in the rat. J. Exp. Med. 162:1531, 1985.

65. Terato, K., Hasty, K. A., Cremer, M. A., Stuart, J. M., Townes, A. S., and Kang, A. H.: Collagen-induced arthritis in mice: Localization of an arthritogenic determinant to a fragment of the type II collagen molecule. J. Exp. Med. 162:637, 1985.

66. Holmdahl, R., Nordling, C., Rubin, K., Tarkowski, A., and Klareskog, L.: Generation of monoclonal rheumatoid factors after immunization with collagen II-anti-collagen immune complexes: An anti-idiotype antibody to anti-collagen II is also a rheumatoid factor. Scand. J. Immunol. 24:197, 1986.

67. Klareskog, L., Johnell, O., Hulth, A., Holmdahl, R., and Rubin, K.: Reactivity of monoclonal anti-type II collagen antibodies with cartilage and synovial tissue in rheumatoid arthritis and osteoarthritis. Arthritis Rheum. 29:1, 1986.

68. Terato, K., Shimozuru, Y., Katayama, K., Takemitsu, Y., Yamashita, I., Miyatsu, M., Fujii, K., Sagara, M., Kobayashi, S., Goto, M., Nishioka, K., Miyasaka, N., and Nagai, Y.: Specificity of antibodies to type II collagen in rheumatoid arthritis. Arthritis Rheum. 33:1493, 1990.

69. Rowley, M., Tait, B., Mackay, I. R., Cunningham, T., and Phillips, B.: Collagen antibodies in rheumatoid arthritis. Significance of antibodies to denatured collagen and their association with HLA-DR4. Arthritis Rheum. 29:174, 1986.

70. Watson, W. C., Cremer, M. A., Wooley, P. H., and Townes, A. S.: Assessment of the potential pathogenicity of type II collagen autoantibodies in patients with rheumatoid arthritis. Arthritis Rheum. 29:1316, 1986.

71. Jasin, H. E.: Autoantibody specificities of immune complexes sequestered in articular cartilage of patients with rheumatoid arthritis and osteoarthritis. Arthritis Rheum. 28:241, 1985.

72. Kunkel, H. G., Agnello, V., Jaslin, F. G., Winchester, R. J., and Capra, J. D.: Cross-idiotypic specificity among monoclonal IgM proteins with anti-IgG activity. J. Exp. Med. 137:331, 1973.

73. Carson, D. A., and Fong, S.: A common idiotope on human rheumatoid factors identified by a hybridoma antibody. Mol. Immunol. 20:1081, 1983.

74. Radoux, V., Chen, P. P., Sorge, J. A., and Carson, D. A.: A conserved human germline V_k directly encodes rheumatoid factor light chains. J. Exp. Med. 164:2119, 1986.

75. Carson, D. A., Chen, P. P., Kipps, T. J., Radoux, V., Jirik, F. R., Goldfien, R. D., Fox, R. I., Silverman, G. J., and Fong, S.: Idiotypic and genetic studies of human rheumatoid factors. Arthritis Rheum. 30:1321, 1987.

76. Bonagura, V. R., Wedgwood, J. F., Agostino, N., Hatam, L., Mendez, L., Jaffe, I., and Pernis, B.: Seronegative rheumatoid arthritis, rheumatoid factor cross reactive idiotype expression, and hidden rheumatoid factors. Ann. Rheum. Dis. 48:488, 1989.

77. Axford, J. S., Lydyard, P. M., Isenberg, D. A., Mackenzie, L., Hay, F. C., and Roitt, I. M.: Reduced B-cell galactosyltransferase activity in rheumatoid arthritis. Lancet 2:1486, 1987.

78. Horneff, G., Burmester, G. R., Emmrich, F., and Kalden, J. R.: Treatment of rheumatoid arthritis with an anti-CD4 monoclonal antibody. Arthritis Rheum. 34:129, 1991.

78a. Wendling, D., Wijdenes, J., Racadot, E., and Morel-Fourrier, B.: Therapeutic use of monoclonal anti-CD4 antibody in rheumatoid arthritis. J. Rheumatol. 18:325, 1991.

79. Sewell, K. L., and Trentham, D. E.: Rapid improvement in refractory rheumatoid arthritis by an interleukin-2 receptor targeted immunotherapy. Clin. Res. 39:314A, 1991.

80. Poulter, L. W., and Janossy, G.: The involvement of dendritic cells in chronic inflammatory disease. Scand. J. Immunol. 21:401, 1985.

81. Klareskog, L., Forsum, U., Scheynius, A., Kabelitz, D., and Wigzell, H.: Evidence in support of a self-perpetuating HLA-DR-dependent delayed-type cell reaction in rheumatoid arthritis. Proc. Natl. Acad. Sci. U.S.A. 79:3632, 1982.

82. Janossy, G., Panayi, G. S., Duke, O., Bofill, M., Poulter, L. W., and Goldstein, G.: Rheumatoid arthritis: A disease of T-lymphocyte/macrophage immunoregulation. Lancet 1:839, 1981.

83. Unanue, E. R., and Allen, P. M.: The basis for the immunoregulatory role of macrophages and other accessory cells. Science 236:551, 1987.

84. Scala, G., Kuang, Y. D., Hall, R. E., Muchmore, A. V., and Oppenheim, J. J.: Accessory cell function of human B cells. I. Production of both interleukin 1-like activity and an interleukin-1 inhibitory factor by an EBV-transformed human B cell line. J. Exp. Med. 159:1637, 1984.

85. Kulka, J. P., Blocking, D., Ropes, M. W., and Bauer, W.: Early joint lesions of rheumatoid arthritis. Arch. Pathol. 59:129, 1955.

86. Folkman, J., and Klagsbrun, M.: Angiogenic factors. Science 235:442, 1987.

87. Thompson, J. A., Anderson, K. D., DiPietro, J. M., Zwiebel, J. A., Zametta, M., Anderson, W. F., and Maciag, T.: Site-directed neovessel formation in vivo. Science 241:1349, 1988.

88. Sano, H., Forough, R., Maier, J. A. M., Case, J. P., Jackson, A., Engleka, K., Maciag, T., and Wilder, R. L.: Detection of high levels of heparin binding growth factor-1 (acidic fibroblast growth factor) in inflammatory arthritic joints. J. Cell Biol. 110:1417, 1990.

89. Montesano, R., Vassalli, J.-D., Baird, A., Guillemin, R., and Orci, L.:

Basic fibroblast growth factor induces angiogenesis in vitro. Proc. Natl. Acad. Sci. U.S.A. 83:7297, 1986.

90. Herron, G. S., Banda, M. J., Clark, E. J., Gavrilovic, J., and Werb, Z.: Secretion of metalloproteinases by stimulated capillary endothelial cells. II. Expression of collagenase and stromelysin activities is regulated by endogenous inhibitors. J. Biol. Chem. 261:2814, 1986.

91. Maione, T. E., Gray, G. S., Petro, J., Hunt, A. J., Donner, A. L., Bauer, S. I., Carson, H. F., and Sharpe, R. J.: Inhibition of angiogenesis by recombinant human platelet factor-4 and related peptides. Science 247:77, 1990.

92. Jalkanen, S., Steere, A. C., Fox, R. I., and Butcher, E. C.: A distinct endothelial cell recognition system that controls lymphocyte traffic into inflamed synovium. Science 233:556, 1986.

93. Pitzalis, C., Kingsley, G., Haskard, D., and Panayi, G.: The preferential accumulation of helper-inducer T lymphocytes in inflammatory lesions: Evidence for regulation by selective endothelial and homotypic adhesion. Eur. J. Immunol. 18:1397, 1988.

94. Tonnesen, M. G., Anderson, D. C., Springer, T. A., Knedler, A., Avdi, N., and Henson, P. M.: Adherence of neutrophils to cultured human microvascular endothelial cells: Stimulation by chemotactic peptides and lipid mediators and dependence upon the Mac-1, LFA-1, p1150,95 glycoprotein family. J. Clin. Invest. 83:637, 1989.

95. Yu, C.-L., Haskard, D., Cavender, D., Johnson, A. R., and Ziff, M.: Human gamma interferon increases the binding of T lymphocytes to endothelial cells. Clin. Exp. Immunol. 62:554, 1985.

96. Cavender, D. E., Haskard, D., Joseph, S., and Ziff, M.: Interleukin-1 increases the binding of human B and T lymphocytes to endothelial cell monolayers. J. Immunol. 136:203, 1986.

97. Cavender, D. E., Saegusa, Y., and Ziff, M.: Treatment of endothelial cells with recombinant human tumour necrosis factor (TNF) increases their adhesiveness for lymphocytes. Fed. Proc. 46:405, 1987.

98. Siegelman, M. H., van de Rijn, M., and Weissman, I. L.: Mouse lymph node homing receptor cDNA clone encodes a glycoprotein revealing tandem interaction domains. Science 243:1165, 1989.

99. Bevilacqua, M. P., Stengelin, S., Gimbrone, M. A., Jr., and Seed, B.: Endothelial leukocyte adhesion molecule 1: An inducible receptor for neutrophils related to complement regulatory proteins and lectins. Science 243:1160, 1989.

100. Gamble, J. R., Skinner, M. P., Berndt, M. C., and Vadas, M. A.: Prevention of activated neutrophil adhesion to endothelium by soluble adhesion protein GMP140. Science 249:414, 1990.

101. Kishimoto, T. K., Jutila, M. A., Berg, E. L., and Butcher, E. C.: Neutrophil Mac-1 and MEL-14 adhesion proteins inversely regulated by chemotactic factors. Science 245:1238, 1989.

102. Baggiolini, M., Walz, A., and Kunkel, S. L.: Neutrophil-activating peptide-1/Interleukin 8, a novel cytokine that activates neutrophils. J. Clin. Invest. 84:1045, 1989.

103. Gimbrone, M. A., Jr., Obin, M. S., Brock, A. F., Luis, E. A., Hass, P. E., Hébert, C. A., Yip, Y. K., Leung, D. W., Lowe, D. G., Kohr, W. J., Darbonne, W. C., Bechtol, K. B., and Baker, J. B.: Endothelial Interleukin-8: A novel inhibitor of leukocyte-endothelial interactions. Science 246:1601, 1989.

104. Heimark, R. L., Twardzik, D. R., and Schwartz, S. M.: Inhibition of endothelial regeneration by type-beta transforming growth factor from platelets. Science 233:1078, 1986.

105. Cronstein, B. N., Kimmel, S. C., Van de Stouwe, M. H., Levin, R. I., and Weissmann, G.: A final common pathway for antiinflammatory agents: inhibition of leukocyte-endothelial interactions. Clin. Research 39:285A, 1991.

106. Kawakami, A., Eguchi, K., Ueki, Y., Migita, K., Ida, H., Nakao, H., Kurata, A., Fukuda, T., Ishimaru, T., Kurouji, K., Fujita, N., and Nagataki, S.: Effects of lobenzarit disodium on human endothelial cells: Lobenzarit disodium inhibits proliferative response, HLA-DR antigen expression, and T cell adherence toward endothelial cells. Arthritis Rheum. 34:296, 1991.

107. Slaughter, L., Carson, D. A., Jensen, F. C., Holbrook, T. L., and Vaughan, J. H.: In vitro effects of Epstein-Barr virus on peripheral blood mononuclear cells from patients with rheumatoid arthritis and normal subjects. J. Exp. Med. 148:1429, 1978.

108. Good, R. A., Rotstein, J., and Mazzitello, W. F.: The simultaneous occurrence of rheumatoid arthritis and agammaglobulinemia. J. Lab. Clin. Med. 49:343, 1957.

109. Wegelius, O., Laine, V., Lindstrom, B., and Klockars, M.: Fistula of the thoracic duct as immunosuppressive treatment in rheumatoid arthritis. Acta Med. Scand. 187:539, 1970.

110. Wahl, S. M., Wilder, R. L., Katona, I. M., Wahl, L. M., Allen, J. B., Scher, I., and Decker, J. L.: Leukapheresis in rheumatoid arthritis. Association of clinical improvement with reversal of anergy. Arthritis Rheum. 26:1076, 1983.

111. Carter, S. D., Bacon, P. B., and Hall, N. D.: Characterization of activated lymphocytes in the peripheral blood of patients with rheumatoid arthritis. Ann. Rheum. Dis. 40:293, 1981.

112. Clegg, D. O., Pincus, S. H., Zone, J. J., and Ward, J. R.: Circulating HLA-DR bearing T cell: Correlation with genetic rather than clinical variables. J. Rheumatol. 13:870, 1986.

113. Luyten, F., Suykens, S., Veys, E. M., Van Lerberghe, J., Ackerman, C., Mielants, H., and Verbruggen, G.: Peripheral blood T lymphocyte subpopulations determined by monoclonal antibodies in active rheumatoid arthritis. J. Rheumatol. 13:864, 1986.

114. Goto, M., Miyamoto, T., Nishioka, K., and Okumura, K. O.: Selective loss of suppressor T cells in rheumatoid arthritis patients: Analysis of peripheral blood lymphocytes by 2-dimensional flow cytometry. J. Rheumatol. 13:853, 1986.

115. Smith, M. D., and Roberts-Thomson, P. J.: Lymphocyte surface marker expression in rheumatic diseases: Evidence for prior activation of lymphocytes in vivo. Ann. Rheum. Dis. 49:81, 1990.

116. Smith, M. D., and Roberts-Thomson, P. J.: Interleukin 2 and interleukin 2 inhibitors in human serum and synovial fluid. 2. Mitogenic stimulation, interleukin 2 production and interleukin 2 receptor expression in rheumatoid arthritis, psoriatic arthritis and Reiter's syndrome. J. Rheumatol. 16:897, 1989.

117. Keystone, E. C., Snow, K. M., Bombardier, C., Chang, C.-H., Nelson, D. L., and Rubin, L. A.: Elevated soluble interleukin-2 receptor levels in the sera and synovial fluids of patients with rheumatoid arthritis. Arthritis Rheum. 31:844, 1988.

118. Fox, R. I., Fong, S., Sabharwal, N., Carstens, S. A., Kung, P. C., and Vaughan, J. H.: Synovial fluid lymphocytes differ from peripheral blood lymphocytes in patients with rheumatoid arthritis. J. Immunol. 128:351, 1982.

119. Hemler, M. E., Glass, D., Coblyn, J. S., and Jacobsen, J. G.: Very late activation antigens on rheumatoid synovial fluid T lymphocytes. Association with stages of T cell activation. J. Clin. Invest. 78:696, 1986.

120. Lasky, H. P., Bauer, K., and Pope, R. M.: Increased helper inducer and decreased suppressor inducer phenotypes in the rheumatoid joint. Arthritis Rheum. 31:52, 1988.

121. Pitzalis, C., Kingsley, G., Murphy, J., and Panayi, G.: Abnormal distribution of the helper-inducer and suppressor-inducer T-lymphocyte subsets in the rheumatoid joint. Clin. Immunol. Immunopathol. 45:252, 1987.

122. Holoshitz, J., Koning, F., Coligan, J. E., DeBruyn, J., Strober, S.: Isolation of CD4-CD8- mycobacteria-reactive T lymphocyte clones from rheumatoid arthritis synovial fluid. Nature 339:226, 1989.

123. Schumacher, H. R., and Kitridou, R. C.: Synovitis of recent onset. A clinicopathological study during the first month of disease. Arthritis Rheum. 15:465, 1972.

124. Ziff, M.: Relation of cellular infiltration of rheumatoid synovial membrane to its immune response. Arthritis Rheum. 17:313, 1974.

125. Haynes, B. F., Grover, B. J., Whichard, L. P., Hale, L. P., Nunley, J. A., McCollum, D. E., and Singer, K. H.: Synovial microenvironment–T cell interactions: Human T cells bind to fibroblast-like synovial cells in vitro. Arthritis Rheum. 31:947, 1988.

126. Kurosaka, M., and Ziff, M.: Immunoelectron microscopic study of the distribution of T cell subsets in rheumatoid synovium. J. Exp. Med. 158:1191, 1983.

127. Bankhurst, A. D., Husby, G., and Williams, R. C., Jr.: Predominance of T cells in the lymphocytic infiltrates of synovial tissues in rheumatoid arthritis. Arthritis Rheum. 19:555, 1976.

128. van Boxel, J. J., and Paget, S. A.: Predominantly T-cell infiltrate in rheumatoid synovial membranes. N. Engl. J. Med. 293:517, 1975.

129. Konttinen, Y. T., Reitamo, S., Ranki, A., Hayry, P., Kankaanpaa, U., and Wegelius, O.: Characterization of the immunocompetent cells of rheumatoid synovium from tissue sections and eluates. Arthritis Rheum. 24:71, 1981.

130. Duke, O., Panayi, G. S., Janossy, G., and Poulter, L. W.: An immunohistological analysis of lymphocyte subpopulations and their microenvironment in the synovial membranes of patients with rheumatoid arthritis using monoclonal antibodies. Clin. Exp. Immunol. 49:22, 1982.

131. Poulter, L. W., Duke, O., Panayi, G. S., Hobbs, S., Raftery, M. J., and Janossy, G.: Activated T lymphocytes of the synovial membrane in rheumatoid arthritis and other arthropathies. Scand. J. Immunol. 22:683, 1985.

132. Nakao, H., Eguchi, K., Kawakami, A., Migita, K., Otsubo, T., Ueki, Y., Shimomura, C, Tezuka, H., Matsunaga, M., Maeda, K., and Nagataki, S.: Phenotypic characterization of lymphocytes infiltrating synovial tissue from patients with rheumatoid arthritis: Analysis of lymphocytes isolated from minced synovial tissue by dual immunofluorescent staining. J. Rheumatol. 17:142, 1990.

133. Cush, J. J., and Lipsky, P. E.: Phenotypic analysis of synovial tissue and peripheral blood lymphocytes isolated from patients with rheumatoid arthritis. Arthritis Rheum. 31:1230, 1988.

134. Gaston, J. S. H., Strober, S., Solovera, J. J., Gandour, D., Lane, N., Schurman, D., Hoppe, R. T., Chin, R. C., Eugui, E. M., Vaughan, J. H., and Allison, A. C.: Dissection of the mechanisms of immune injury in rheumatoid arthritis, using total lymphoid irradiation. Arthritis Rheum. 31:21, 1988.

135. Chatila, M. K., Pandolfi, F., Stamenkovich, I., and Kurnick, J. T.: Clonal dominance among synovial tissue-infiltrating lymphocytes in arthritis. Hum. Immunol. 28:252, 1990.

136. Stamenkovic, I., Stegaguo, M., Wright, K. A., Krane, S. M., Amento, E. P., Colvin, R. B., Duqusnoy, R. J., and Kurnick, J. T.: Clonal dominance among T-lymphocyte infiltrates in arthritis. Proc. Natl. Acad. Sci. U.S.A. 85:1179, 1988.

137. Pallard, X., West, S. G., Lafferty, J. A., et al.: Evidence for the effects of a superantigen in rheumatoid arthritis. Science 253:325, 1991.

137a. Alsalameh, S., Mollenhauer, J., Hain, N., Stock, K.-P., Kalden, J. R., and Burmester, G. R.: Cellular immune response toward human articular chondrocytes. Arthritis Rheum. 33:1477, 1990.

138. Zalman, L. S., Brothers, M. A., Chiu, F. J., and Muller-Eberhard, H. J.: Mechanism of cytotoxicity of human large granular lymphocytes: Relationship of the cytotoxic lymphocyte protein to the ninth component (C9) of human complement. Proc. Natl. Acad. Sci. U.S.A. 83:5262, 1986.

139. Timonen, T. T., and Pakkanen, R.: Induction of large granular lymphocyte morphology in human peripheral blood mononuclear cells. J. Immunol. 138:2837, 1987.

140. Barton, J. C., Prasthofer, E. F., Egan, M. L., Heck, L. W., Jr., Koopman, W. J., and Grassi, C. E.: Rheumatoid arthritis associated with expanded populations of granular lymphocytes. Ann. Intern. Med. 104:314, 1986.

141. Cooper, S. M., Roessner, K., Ferriss, J. A., Baigent, G., and Bakke, A. C.: Increase in OKM1+ granular lymphocytes in patients with rheumatoid arthritis. Arthritis Rheum. 30:1089, 1987.

142. Tosato, G., Steinberg, A. D., and Blaese, R. M.: Defective EBV-specific suppressor T-cell function in rheumatoid arthritis. N. Engl. J. Med. 305:1238, 1981.

143. Depper, J. M., Bluestein, H. G., and Zvaifler, N. J.: Impaired regulation of Epstein-Barr virus-induced lymphocyte proliferation in rheumatoid arthritis is due to a T cell defect. J. Immunol. 127:1899, 1981.

144. Gaston, J. S. H., Rickinson, A. B., Yao, Q. Y., and Epstein, M. A.: The abnormal cytotoxic T cell response to Epstein-Barr virus in rheumatoid arthritis is correlated with disease activity and occurs in other arthropathies. Ann. Rheum. Dis. 45:932, 1986.

145. Goto, M., and Zvaifler, N. J.: Impaired killer cell generation in the autologous mixed leukocyte reaction by rheumatoid arthritis lymphocytes. Arthritis Rheum. 28:731, 1985.

146. Combe, B., Pope, R. M., Fischbach, M., Darnell, B., Baron, S., and Talal, N.: Interleukin 2 in rheumatoid arthritis: Production of and response to interleukin 2 in rheumatoid synovial fluid, synovial tissue, and peripheral blood. Clin. Exp. Immunol. 59:520, 1985.

147. Nouri, A. M. E., and Panayi, G. S.: Cytokines and the chronic inflammation of rheumatic disease. III. Deficient interleukin-2 production in rheumatoid arthritis is not due to suppressor mechanisms. J. Rheumatol. 14:902, 1987.

148. Kingsley, G. H., Pitzalis, C., and Panayi, G. S.: Abnormal lymphocyte reactivity to self—major histocompatibility antigens in rheumatoid arthritis. J. Rheumatol. 14:667, 1987.

149. Decker, J. L., Malone, D. G., Haraoui, B., Wahl, S. M., Schrieber, L., Klippel, J. H., Steinberg, A. D., and Wilder, R. L.: Rheumatoid arthritis: Evolving concepts of pathogenesis and treatment. Ann. Intern. Med. 101:810, 1984.

150. Lotz, M., Tsoukas, C. D., Robinson, C. A., Dinarello, C. A., Carson, D. A., and Vaughan, J. H.: Basis for defective responses of rheumatoid arthritis synovial fluid lymphocytes to anti-CD3 (T3) antibodies. J. Clin. Invest. 78:713, 1986.

151. Hannum, C. H., Wilcox, C. J., Arend, W. P., Joslin, F. G., Dripps, D. J., Heimdal, P. L., Armes, L. G., Sommer, A., Eisenberg, S. P., and Thompson, R. C.: Interleukin-1 receptor antagonist activity of a human interleukin-1 inhibitor. Nature 343:336, 1990.

152. Eisenberg, S. P., Evans, R. J., Arend, W. P., Verderber, E., Brewer, M. T., Hannum, C. H., and Thompson, R. C.: Primary structure and functional expression from complementary DNA of a human interleukin-1 receptor antagonist. Nature 343:341, 1990.

153. Arend, W. P., Welgus, H. G., Thompson, R. C., and Eisenberg, S. P.: Biological properties of recombinant human monocyte-derived interleukin 1 receptor antagonist. J. Clin. Invest. 85:1694, 1990.

154. Hasler, F., and Dayer, J.-M.: Diminished IL-2-induced gamma-interferon production by unstimulated peripheral-blood lymphocytes in rheumatoid arthritis. Br. J. Rheumatol. 27:15, 1988.

155. Geppert, T. D., and Lipsky, P. E.: Dissection of defective antigen presentation by interferon-γ-treated fibroblasts. J. Immunol. 138:385, 1987.

156. Miossec, P., Naviliat, M., Dupuy D'Angeac, A., Sany, J., and Banchereau, J.: Low levels of interleukin-4 and high levels of transforming growth factor beta in rheumatoid arthritis. Arthritis Rheum. 145:2514, 1990.

157. Firestein, G. S., Xu, W.-D., Townsend, K., Broide, D., Alvaro-Gracia, J., Glasebrook, A., and Zvaifler, N. J.: Cytokines in chronic inflammatory arthritis. I. Failure to detect T cell lymphokines (interleukin 2 and interleukin 3) and presence of macrophage colony-stimulating factor (CSF-1) and a novel mast cell growth factor in rheumatoid synovitis. J. Exp. Med. 168:1573, 1988.

158. Bergroth, V., Zvaifler, N. J., and Firestein, G. S.: Cytokines in chronic inflammatory arthritis. III. Rheumatoid arthritis monocytes are not unusually sensitive to γ-interferon, but have defective γ-interferon-mediated HLA-DQ and HLA-DR induction. Arthritis Rheum. 32:1074, 1989.

159. Nathan, C. F.: Secretory products of macrophages. J. Clin. Invest. 79:319, 1987.

160. Firestein, G. S., and Zvaifler, N. J.: Down regulation of human monocyte differentiation antigens by gamma interferon. Cell Immunol. 104:343, 1987.

161. Pober, J. S., Gimbrone, M. A., Cotran, R. S., et al.: Ia expression by vascular endothelium is inducible by activated T cells and by human interferon. J. Exp. Med. 157:1339, 1983.

162. Hagg, N., Palmer, D. G., and Revell, P. A.: Mononuclear phagocytes of normal and rheumatoid synovial membrane identified by monoclonal antibodies. Immunology 56:673, 1985.

163. Firestein, G. S., and Zvaifler, N. J.: Peripheral blood and synovial fluid monocyte activation in inflammatory arthritis. II. Low levels of synovial fluid and synovial tissue interferon suggest that γ-interferon is not the primary macrophage activating factor. Arthritis Rheum. 30:864, 1987.

164. Duncan, M. R., and Berman, B.: γ Interferon is the lymphokine and β interferon the monokine responsible for inhibition of fibroblast collagen production and late but not early fibroblast proliferation. J. Exp. Med. 162:516, 1985.

165. Granstein, R. D., Murphy, G. F., Margolis, R. J., Byrne, M. H., and Amento, E. P.: Gamma-interferon inhibits collagen synthesis in vivo in the mouse. J. Clin. Invest. 79:1254, 1987.

166. Stephenson, M. L., Krane, S. M., Amento, E. P., McCroskery, P. A., and Byrne, M.: Immune interferon inhibits collagen synthesis by rheumatoid synovial cells associated with decreased levels of the procollagen mRNAs. FEBS Lett. 180:43, 1985.

167. Alvaro-Gracia, J. M., Zvaifler, N. J., and Firestein, G. S.: Cytokines in chronic inflammatory arthritis. V. Mutual antagonism between interferon-gamma and tumor necrosis factor-alpha on HLA-DR expression, proliferation, collagenase production, and granulocyte macrophage colony-stimulating factor production by rheumatoid arthritis synoviocytes. J. Clin. Invest. 86:1790, 1990.

168. Pettipher, E. R., Higgs, G. A., and Henderson, B.: Interleukin 1 induces leukocyte infiltration and cartilage proteoglycan degradation in the synovial joint. Proc. Natl. Acad. Sci. U.S.A. 83:8749, 1986.

169. Shore, A., Jaglal, S., and Keystone, E. C.: Enhanced interleukin 1 generation by monocytes in vitro is temporally linked to an early event in the onset or exacerbation of rheumatoid arthritis. Clin. Exp. Immunol. 65:293, 1986.

170. Poubelle, P., Damon, M., Blotman, F., and Dayer, J.-M.: Production of mononuclear cell factor by mononuclear phagocytes from rheumatoid synovial fluid. J. Rheumatol. 12:412, 1985.

171. Chin, J., Rupp, E., Cameron, P. M., MacNaul, K. L., Lotke, P. A., Tocci, M. J., Schmidt, J. A., and Bayne, E. K.: Identification of a high-affinity receptor for interleukin 1α and interleukin 1β on cultured human rheumatoid synovial cells. J. Clin. Invest. 82:420, 1988.

172. Tiku, K, Tiku, M. S., and Skosey, J. L.: Interleukin 1 production by human polymorphonuclear neutrophils. J. Immunol. 136:3677, 1986.

173. Miossec, P., and Ziff, M.: Immune interferon enhances the production of interleukin 1 by human endothelial cells stimulated with lipopolysaccharide. J. Immunol. 137:2848, 1986.

174. Miyasaka, N., Sato, K., Goto, M., Sasano, M., Natsuyama, M., Inoue, K., and Nishioka, K.: Augmented interleukin-1 production and HLA-DR expression in the synovium of rheumatoid arthritis patients: Possible involvement in joint destruction. Arthritis Rheum. 31:480, 1988.

175. Dayer, J.-M., Goldring, S. R., Robinson, D. R., et al.: Cell-cell interactions and collagenase production. In Wooley, D. E., and Evanson, J. M. (eds.): Collagenase in Normal and Pathological Connective Tissues. New York, John Wiley & Sons, 1980, pp. 873–1104.

176. Wood, D. D., Ihrie, E. J., and Hamerman, D.: Release of interleukin-1 from human synovial tissue in vitro. Arthritis Rheum. 28:853, 1985.

177. Amento, E. P., Kurnick, J. T., and Krane, S. M.: Interleukin 1 production by the human monocyte cell line U937 requires a lymphokine induction signal distinct from interleukin 2 or interferons. J. Immunol. 134:350, 1985.

178. Dayer, J.-M., Passwell, H. J., Schneeberger, E. E., and Krane, S. M.: Interactions among rheumatoid synovial cells and monocyte-macrophages: Production of collagenase-stimulating factor by human monocytes exposed to concanavalin A or immunoglobulin Fc fragments. J. Immunol. 124:1712, 1980.

179. Muller-Glauser, W., Humbel, W., Glatt, M., Strauli, P., Winterhalter, K. H., and Bruckner, P.: On the role of type IX collagen in the extracellular matrix of cartilage: Type IX collagen is localized to intersections of collagen fibrils. J. Cell Biol. 1092:1931, 1986.

180. Dayer, J.-M., Ricard-Blum, S., Kaufman, M.-T., and Herbage, D.: Type IX collagen is a potent inducer of PGE₂ and interleukin 1 production by human monocyte macrophages. FEBS Lett. 198:208, 1986.

181. Postlethwaite, A. E., Lachman, L. B., and Kang, A. H.: Induction of fibroblast proliferation by interleukin-1 derived from human monocytic leukemia cells. Arthritis Rheum. 27:995, 1984.

182. Yaron, I., Meyer, F. A., Dayer, J.-M., and Yaron, M.: Human recombinant interleukin-1β stimulates glycosaminoglycan production in human synovial fibroblast cultures. Arthritis Rheum. 30:424, 1987.

183. Tyler, J. A.: Articular cartilage cultured with catabolin (pig interleukin 1) synthesizes a decreased number of normal proteoglycan molecules. Biochem. J. 227:869, 1985.

184. Mochan, E., Uhl, J., and Newton, R.: Interleukin 1 stimulation of synovial cell plasminogen activator production. J. Rheumatol. 13:15, 1986.

185. Dewhirst, F. E., Stashenko, P. P., Mole, J. E., and Tsurumachi, T.: Purification and particle sequence of human osteoclast-activating factor: Identity with interleukin 1β. J. Immunol. 135:2562, 1985.

186. Miossec, P., Dinarello, C. A., and Ziff, M.: Interleukin-1 lymphocyte chemotactic activity in rheumatoid arthritis synovial fluid. Arthritis Rheum. 29:461, 1986.

187. Takai, Y., Wong, G. G., Clark, S. C., Burakoff, S. J., and Herrman, S. H.: B cell stimulatory factor-2 is involved in the differentiation of cytotoxic T lymphocytes. J. Immunol. 140:508, 1988.

188. Gauldie, J., Richards, C., Harnish, D., Landsdorp, P., and Baumann, H.: Interferon β₂/BSF-2 shares identity with monocyte derived hepatocyte stimulating factor (HSF) and regulates the major acute phase protein response in liver cells. Proc. Natl. Acad. Sci. U.S.A. 84:7251, 1987.

189. Houssiau, F. A., Devogelaer, J.-P., van Damme, J., Nagant de Deuxchaisnes, C., and van Snick, J.: Interleukin-6 in synovial fluid and serum of patients with rheumatoid arthritis and other inflammatory arthritides. Arthritis Rheum. 31:784, 1988.

190. Guerne, P.-A., Zuraw, B. L., Vaughan, J. H., Carson, D. A., and Lotz, M.: Synovium as a source of interleukin 6 in vitro: Contribution to local and systemic manifestations of arthritis. J. Clin. Invest. 83:585, 1989.

191. Saxne, T., Palladino, M. A., Jr., Heinegård, D., Talal, N., and Wollheim, F. A.: Detection of tumor necrosis factor α but not tumor necrosis factor β in rheumatoid arthritis synovial fluid and serum. Arthritis Rheum. 31:1041, 1988.

192. Dayer, J.-M., Beutler, B., and Cerami, A.: Cachectin/tumor necrosis factor stimulates collagenase and prostaglandin E₂ production by human synovial cells and dermal fibroblasts. J. Exp. Med. 162:2163, 1985.

193. Bertolini, D. R., Nedwin, G. E., Bringman, T. S., Smith, D. D., and Mundy, G. R.: Stimulation of bone resorption and inhibition of bone formation in vitro by human tumour necrosis factors. Nature 319:516, 1986.

194. Saklatvala, J.: Tumour necrosis factor α stimulates resorption and inhibits synthesis of proteoglycan in cartilage. Nature 322:547, 1986.

195. Levine, J. D., Goetzl, E. J., and Basbaum, A. I.: Contribution of the nervous system to the pathophysiology of rheumatoid arthritis and other polyarthritides. Rheum. Dis. Clin. North Am. 13:369, 1987.

196. Lotz, M., Vaughan, J. H., and Carson, D. A.: Effect of neuropeptides on production of inflammatory cytokines by human monocytes. Science 241:1218, 1988.

197. Xu, W. D., Firestein, G. S., Taetle, R., Kaushansky, K., and Zvaifler, N. J.: Cytokines in chronic inflammatory arthritis. II. Granulocyte-macrophage colony-stimulating factor in rheumatoid synovial effusions. J. Clin. Invest. 83:876, 1989.

198. Morrissey, P. J., Bressler, L., Park, L. S., Alpert, A., and Gillis, S.: Granulocyte-macrophage colony-stimulating factor augments the primary antibody response by enhancing the function of antigen-presenting cells. J. Immunol. 139:1113, 1987.

199. Ibbotson, K. J., Harrod, J., Gowens, M., D'Souza, S. D., Smith, D. D., Winkler, M. E., Derynck, R., and Mundy, G. R.: Human recombinant transforming growth factor α stimulates bone resorption and inhibits formation in vitro. Proc. Natl. Acad. Sci. U.S.A. 83:2228, 1986.

200. Takahashi, N., MacDonald, B. R., Hon, J., Winkler, M. E., Derynck, R., Mundy, G. R., and Roodman, G. D.: Recombinant human transforming growth factor-alpha stimulates the formation of osteoclast-like cells in long-term human marrow cultures. J. Clin. Invest. 78:894, 1986.

201. Edwards, D. R., Murphy, G., Reynolds, J. J., Whitham, S. E., Docherty, A. J. P., Angel, P., and Heath, J. K.: Transforming growth factor beta modulates the expression of collagenase and metalloproteinase inhibitor. EMBO J. 6:1899, 1987.

202. Mustoe, T. A., Pierce, G. F., Thomason, A., Gramates, P., Sporn, M. B., and Deuel, T. F.: Accelerated healing of incisional wounds in rats induced by transforming growth factor-β. Science 237:1333, 1987.

203. Roberts, A. B., Sporn, M. B., Assoian, R. K., Smith, J. M., Roche, N. S., Wakefield, L. M., Heine, U. I., Liotta, L. A., Falanga, V., Kehrl, J. H., and Fauci, A. S.: Transforming growth factor type β: Rapid induction of fibrosis and angiogenesis in vivo and stimulation of collagen formation in vitro. Proc. Natl. Acad. Sci. U.S.A. 83:4167, 1986.

204. Castor, C. W., Miller, J. W., and Waltz, D. A.: Structural and biological characteristics of connective tissue activating peptide (CTAP-III), a major human platelet-derived growth factor. Proc. Natl. Acad. Sci. U.S.A. 80:765, 1983.

205. Doolittle, R. F., Hunkapiller, M. W., Hood, L. E., Devare, S. G., Robbins, S. A., and Antoniades, H. N.: Simian sarcoma virus oncogene, v-sis, is derived from the gene (or genes) encoding a platelet-derived growth factor. Science 221:275, 1983.

206. Bauer, E. A., Cooper, T. W., Huang, J. S., Altman, J., and Deuel, T. F.: Stimulation of in vitro human skin collagenase expression by platelet-derived growth factor. Proc. Natl. Acad. Sci. U.S.A. 82:4132, 1985.

207. Deuel, T. F., and Huang, J. S.: Platelet-derived growth factor. Structure, function, and roles in normal and transformed cells. J. Clin. Invest. 74:669, 1984.

208. Rose, R., Raines, E. W., and Bowen-Pope, D. F.: The biology of platelet-derived growth factor. Cell 48:155, 1986.

209. Remmers, E. F., Lafyatis, R., Kumkumian, G. K., Case, J. P., Roberts, A. B., Sporn, M. B., and Wilder, R. L.: Cytokines and growth regulation of synoviocytes from patients with rheumatoid arthritis and rats with streptococcal cell wall arthritis. Growth Factors 2:179, 1990.

210. Polla, B. S., Healy, A. M., Byrne, M., and Krane, S. M.: 1,25-Dihydroxyvitamin D₃ induces collagen binding to the human monocyte line U937. J. Clin. Invest. 80:962, 1987.

211. Prince, C. W., and Butler, W. T.: 1,25-Dihydroxyvitamin D₃ regulates the biosynthesis of osteopontin, a bone-derived cell attachment protein, in clonal osteoblast-like osteosarcoma cells. Collagen Rel. Res. 7:305, 1987.

212. Postlethwaite, A. E., Jackson, B. K., Beachey, E. H., and Kang, A. H.: Formation of multinucleated giant cells from human monocyte precursors. J. Exp. Med. 155:168, 1982.

213. Fox, D. A., and Smith, B. R.: Evidence for oligoclonal B cell expansion in the peripheral blood of patients with rheumatoid arthritis. Ann. Rheum. Dis. 45:991, 1986.

214. Boling, E. P., Ohishi, T., Wahl, S. M., Misiti, J., Wistar, R., Jr., and Wilder, R. L.: Humoral immune function in severe, active rheumatoid arthritis. Clin. Immunol. Pathol. 43:185, 1987.

215. Lipsky, P. E.: The control of antibody production by immunomodulatory molecules. Arthritis Rheum. 32:1345, 1989.

216. Burastero, S. E., Casali, P., Wilder, R. L., and Notkins, A. L.: Monoreactive high affinity and polyreactive low affinity rheumatoid factors are produced by CD5+ B cells from patients with rheumatoid arthritis. J. Exp. Med. 168:1979, 1988.

217. Hardy, R. R., Hayakawa, K., Shimizu, M., Yamasaki, K., and Kishimoto, T.: Rheumatoid factor secretion from human Leu-1+ B cells. Science 236:81, 1987.

218. Paul, W. E.: Interleukin 4/B cell stimulatory factor 1: One lymphokine, many functions. FASEB J. 1:456, 1987.

219. Mitchell, L., C., Davis, L. S., Lipsky, P. E.: Promotion of human T lymphocyte proliferation by IL-4. J. Immunol. 142:1548, 1989.

220. Bonagura, V. R., Mendez, L., Agostino, N., and Pernis, B.: Monomeric (7S) IgM found in the serum of rheumatoid arthritis patients share idiotypes with pentameric (19S) monoclonal rheumatoid factors. J. Clin. Invest. 79:813, 1987.

221. Fong, S., Chen, P. P., Gilbertson, T. A., Weber, J. R., Fox, R. I., and Carson, D. A.: Expression of three cross-reactive idiotypes on rheumatoid factor autoantibodies from patients with autoimmune diseases and seropositive adults. J. Immunol. 137:122, 1986.

222. Bouvet, J.-P., Xin, W. J., and Pillot, J.: Restricted heterogeneity of polyclonal rheumatoid factor. Arthritis Rheum. 30:998, 1987.

223. Wernick, R. M., Lipsky, P. E., Marban-Arcos, E., Maliakkal, J. J., Edelbaum, D., and Ziff, M.: IgG and IgM rheumatoid factor synthesis in rheumatoid synovial membrane cell cultures. Arthritis Rheum. 28:742, 1985.

224. Cats, A., and Hazevoet, H. M.: Significance of positive tests for rheumatoid factor in the prognosis of rheumatoid arthritis. Ann. Rheum. Dis. 29:254, 1970.

225. Vaughan, J. H.: Lymphocyte function in rheumatic disorders. Arch. Intern. Med. 135:1324, 1975.

226. Tanimoto, K., Cooper, N. R., Johnson, J. S., and Vaughan, J. H.: Complement fixation by rheumatoid factor. J. Clin. Invest. 55:437, 1975.

227. Pope, R. M., Teller, D. C., and Mannik, M.: The molecular basis of self-association of antibodies to IgG (rheumatoid factor) in rheumatoid arthritis. Proc. Natl. Acad. Sci. U.S.A. 71:517, 1974.

228. Rodman, W. S., Williams, R. C., Jr., Bilka, P. J., and Muller-Eberhard, H. J.: Immunofluorescent localization of the third and fourth component of complement in synovial tissues from patients with rheumatoid arthritis. J. Lab. Clin. Med. 69:141, 1967.

229. Zvaifler, N. J.: Immunopathology of joint inflammation in rheumatoid arthritis. Immunology 16:265, 1973.

230. Pope, R. M.: Rheumatoid arthritis associated with hyperviscosity syndrome and intermediate complex formation. Arch. Intern. Med. 135:281, 1975.

231. Jasin, H. E., LoSpalluto, J. J., and Ziff, M.: Rheumatoid hyperviscosity syndrome. Am. J. Med. 49:484, 1970.

232. Theofilopoulos, A. N., Burtonboy, G., LoSpalluto, J. J., and Ziff, M.: IgM rheumatoid factor and low molecular weight IgM: An association with vasculitis. Arthritis Rheum. 17:272, 1977.

233. Allen, C., Elson, C. J., Scott, D. G. I., Bacon, P. A., and Bucknall, R. C.: IgG antiglobulins in rheumatoid arthritis and other arthritides: Relationship with clinical features and other parameters. Ann. Rheum. Dis. 40:127, 1981.

234. Rawson, A. J., Hollander, J. L., Quismorio, F. P., and Abelson, N. M.: Experimental arthritis in man and rabbit dependent upon serum anti-immunoglobulin factors. Ann. N.Y. Acad. Sci. 168:188, 1969.

235. Kaplan, R. A., DeHeer, D. H., Carson, D. A., Pangburn, M. K., Muller-Eberhard, H. J., and Vaughan, J. H.: Metabolism of C4 and factor b in rheumatoid arthritis: Relation to rheumatoid factor. Arthritis Rheum. 34:911, 1980.

236. Henney, G. S., Stanworth, D. R., and Gell, P. G. H.: Demonstration of the exposure of new antigenic determinants following antigen-antibody combination. Nature 205:1079, 1965.

237. Johnson, P. M., Watkins, J., Scopes, P. M., and Tracey, B. M.: Differences in serum IgG structures in health and rheumatoid disease. Ann. Rheum. Dis. 33:366, 1974.

238. Allison, A. C. L.: Heberden Oration. Mechanism of tolerance and autoimmunity. Ann. Rheum. Dis. 32:283, 1973.

239. Zuran, B. L., O'Hair, C. H., Vaughan, J. H., Mathison, D. A., Curd, J. G., and Katz, D. H.: Immunoglobulin E-rheumatoid factor in the serum of patients with rheumatoid arthritis, asthma, and other diseases. J. Clin. Invest. 68:1610, 1981.

240. Metetey, K., Falus, A., Erhardt, C. C., and Maini, R. N.: IgE and IgE-rheumatoid factors in circulating immune complexes in rheumatoid arthritis. Ann. Rheum. Dis. 41:405, 1982.

241. Crisp, A. J., Chapman, C. M., Kirkhan, S., Schiller, A. L., and Krane, S. M.: Synovial mastocytosis in adult rheumatoid arthritis. Arthritis Rheum. 26:552, 1983.

242. Paquet-Gioud, M., Auvinet, M., Raffin, T., Girard, P., Bouvier, M., Lejeune, E., and Monier, J. C.: IgG rheumatoid factor (RF), IgA RF, IgE RF, and IgG RF detected by ELISA in rheumatoid arthritis. Ann. Rheum. Dis. 46:65, 1987.

242a. Noritake, D. T., Colburn, K. K., Chan, G., and Weisbart, R. H.: Rheumatoid factors specific for active rheumatoid arthritis. Ann. Rheum. Dis. 49:910, 1990.

243. Patel, V., and Panayi, G. S.: Enhanced T helper cell function for the spontaneous production of IgM rheumatoid factor in vitro in rheumatoid arthritis. Clin. Exp. Immunol. 57:584, 1984.

244. Winchester, R. J., Agnello, V., and Kunkel, H. G.: Gamma globulin complexes in synovial fluids of patients with rheumatoid arthritis. Clin. Exp. Immunol. 6:689, 1970.

245. Panush, R. S., Katz, P., Longley, S., and Yonker, R. A.: Detection and quantitation of circulating immune complexes in arterial blood of patients with rheumatic disease. Clin. Immunol. Pathol. 36:217, 1985.

246. Faaber, P., Truus, P. M., Schilder, R., Capel, P. J. A., and Koene, R. A. P.: Circulating immune complexes and rheumatoid arthritis. J. Rheumatol. 12:849, 1985.

247. Melsom, R. D., Smith, P. R., and Maini, R. N.: Demonstration of an unidentified 48 kD polypeptide in circulating immune complexes in rheumatoid arthritis. Ann. Rheum. Dis. 46:104, 1987.

248. Cooke, T. D., Hurd, E. R., Jasin, H. E., Bienenstock, J., and Ziff, M.: Identification of immunoglobulins and complement in rheumatoid articular collagenous tissues. Arthritis Rheum. 18:541, 1975.

249. Ohno, O., and Cooke, T. D.: Electron microscopic morphology of immunoglobulin aggregates and their interactions in rheumatoid articular collagenous tissues. Arthritis Rheum. 21:516, 1978.

250. Shiozawa, S., Jasin, H. E., and Ziff, M.: Absence of immunoglobulins in rheumatoid cartilage-pannus junctions. Arthritis Rheum. 23:816, 1980.

251. Ishikawa, H., Smiley, J. D., and Ziff, M.: Electron microscopic demonstration of immunoglobulin deposition in rheumatoid cartilage. Arthritis Rheum. 18:563, 1975.

252. Hollingsworth, J. W., Siegel, E. R., and Creasey, W. A.: Granulocyte survival in synovial exudate of patients with rheumatoid arthritis and other inflammatory joint diseases. Yale J. Biol. Med. 39:289, 1967.

253. Korchak, H. M., Vienne, K., Rutherford, L. E., and Weissmann, G.: Neutrophil stimulation: Receptor, membrane, and metabolic events. Fed. Proc. 43:2749, 1984.

254. Beaulieu, A. D., Lang, F., Belles-Isles, M., and Poubelle, P.: Protein biosynthetic activity of polymorphonuclear leukocytes in inflammatory arthropathies. Increased synthesis and release of fibronectin. J. Rheumatol. 14:656, 1987.

255. Tiku, K., Tiku, M. L., and Skosey, J. L.: Interleukin 1 production by human polymorphonuclear neutrophils. J. Immunol. 136:3677, 1986.

256. Weiss, S. J.: Tissue destruction by neutrophils. N. Engl. J. Med. 320:365, 1989.

257. Merry, P., Winyard, P. G., Morris, C. J., Grootveld, M., and Blake, D. R.: Oxygen free radicals, inflammation and synovitis: The current status. Ann. Rheum. Dis. 48:864, 1989.

258. Nurcombe, H. L., Bucknall, R. C., and Edwards, S. W.: Activation of the neutrophil myeloperoxidase-H$_2$O$_2$ system by synovial fluid isolated from patients with rheumatoid arthritis. Ann. Rheum. Dis. 50:237, 1991.

259. McCord, J. M.: Free radicals and inflammation: Protection of synovial fluid by superoxide dismutase. Science 185:529, 1974.

260. Davis, P., Johnston, C., Bertouch, J., and Starkebaum, G.: Depressed superoxide radical generation by neutrophils from patients with rheumatoid arthritis and neutropenia: Correlation with neutrophil reactive IgG. Ann. Rheum. Dis. 45:51, 1987.

261. Situnayake, R. D., Thurnham, D. I., Kootathep, S., Chirico, S., Lunec, J., Davis, M., and McConkey, B.: Chain breaking antioxidant status in rheumatoid arthritis: Clinical and laboratory correlates. Ann. Rheum. Dis. 50:81, 1991.

262. Agudelo, C. A., Turner, R., A., Panetti, M., and Pisko, E.: Does hyperuricaemia protect from rheumatoid inflammation? A clinical study. Arthritis Rheum. 27:443, 1984.

263. Yoshino, S., Blake, D. R., Hewitt, S., Morris, C., and Bacon, P. A.: Effect of blood on the activity and persistence of antigen-induced inflammation in the rat air pouch. Ann. Rheum. Dis. 44:485, 1985.

264. Cross, C. E., Halliwell, B., Borish, E. T., Pryor, W. A., Ames, B. N., Saul, R. L., McCord, J. M., and Harman, D.: Oxygen radicals and human disease. Ann. Rheum. Dis. 107:526, 1987.

265. Goldstein, I., Edelson, H. S., Kaplan, M. B., and Weissman, G.: Ceruloplasmin: A scavenger of superoxide union radicals. J. Biol. Chem. 254:4040, 1979.

266. Zurier, R. B., and Quagliata, F.: Effect of prostaglandin E$_1$ on adjuvant arthritis. Nature 234:304, 1971.

267. Nicholson, P. A.: Recent advances in defining the role of misoprostol in rheumatology. J. Rheumatol. 17:50, 1990.

268. McGuire, J., McGee, J., Crittenden, N., and Fitzpatrick, F.: Cell damage unmasks 15-lipoxygenase activity in human neutrophils. J. Biol. Chem. 260:8316, 1985.

269. Elmgreen, J., Haagen, N., and Ahnfelt-Ronne, I.: Enhanced capacity for release of leucotriene B$_4$ by neutrophils in rheumatoid arthritis. Ann. Rheum. Dis. 46:501, 1987.

270. Sperling, R. I., Weinblatt, M., Robin, J.-L., Ravalese, J., III, Hoover, R. L., House, F., Coblyn, J. S., Fraser P. A., Spur, B. W., Robinson, D. R., Lewis, R. A., and Austen, K. F.: Effects of dietary supplementation with marine fish oil on leukocyte lipid mediator generation and function in rheumatoid arthritis. Arthritis Rheum. 30:988, 1987.

271. Abramson, S., Korchak, J., Ludewig, R., et al.: The modes of action of aspirin-like drugs. Proc. Natl. Acad. Sci. U.S.A. 82:7227, 1985.

272. Ruddy, S., Britton, M. C., Schur, P. H., and Austen, K. F.: Complement components in synovial fluid: Activation and fixation in seropositive rheumatoid arthritis. Ann. N.Y. Acad. Sci. 168:161, 1969.

273. Kaplan, R. A., Curd, J. G., DeHeer, D. H., Carson, D. A., Pangburn, M. K., Muller-Eberhard, H. J., and Vaughan, J. H.: Metabolism of C4 and factor B in rheumatoid arthritis: Relation to rheumatoid factor. Arthritis Rheum. 23:911, 1980.

274. Ruddy, S., and Colten, H. R.: Biosynthesis of complement proteins by synovial tissues. N. Engl. J. Med. 290:1284, 1974.

275. Ruddy, S., and Austen, K. F.: The complement system in rheumatoid synovitis. I. An analysis of complement component activities in rheumatoid synovial fluids. Arthritis Rheum. 13:713, 1970.

276. Pekin, T. J., Jr., and Zvaifler, N. J.: Hemolytic complement in synovial fluid. J. Clin. Invest. 43:1372, 1964.

277. Sabharwal, U. K., Vaughan, J. H., Fong, S., Bennett, P. H., Carson, D. A., and Curd, J. G.: Activation of the classical pathway of complement by rheumatoid factors. Assessment by radioimmunoassay for C4. Arthritis Rheum. 25:161, 1982.

278. Elmgren, J., and Hansen, T. M.: Subnormal sensitivity of neutrophils to complement split-product C5a in rheumatoid arthritis: Relation to complement catabolism and disease extent. Ann. Rheum. Dis. 44:514, 1985.

279. Goldstein, I. M., and Weissmann, G.: Generation of C5-derived lysosomal enzyme-releasing activity (C5a) by lysates of leukocyte lysosomes. J. Immunol. 113:1583, 1974.

280. Borel, J. F., Keller, H. U., and Sorkin, E.: Studies on chemotaxis. XI. Effect on neutrophils of lysosomal and other subcellular fractions from leukocytes. Int. Arch. Allergy Appl. Immunol. 35:194, 1969.

281. Kaplan, M. H., and Volanakis, J. E.: Interaction of C-reactive protein complexes with the complement system. I. Consumption of human complement associated with the reaction of C-reactive protein with pneumococcal C-polysaccharide and with the choline phosphatides, lecithin and sphingomyelin. J. Immunol. 112:2135, 1974.

282. Kushner, I., Rakitu, L., and Kaplan, M. H.: Studies of acute phase protein. II. Localization of C-reactive protein in heart in induced myocardial infarction in rabbits. J. Clin. Invest. 42:286, 1963.

283. Mollnes, T. E., Lea, T., Mellbye, O. J., Pahle, J., Grand, O., and Harboe, M.: Complement activation in rheumatoid arthritis evaluated by C3dg and the terminal complement complex. Arthritis Rheum. 29:715, 1986.

284. Moxley, G., and Ruddy, S.: Elevated plasma C3 anaphylatoxin levels in rheumatoid arthritis patients. Arthritis Rheum. 30:1097, 1987.

285. Harris, E. D., Jr., Faulkner, C. S., II, and Brown, F. E.: Collagenolytic systems in rheumatoid arthritis. Clin. Orthop. 110:303, 1975.
286. Gysen, P., Malaise, M., Gaspar, S., and Franchimont, P.: Measurement of proteoglycans, elastase, collagenase and protein in synovial fluid in inflammatory and degenerative arthropathies. Clin. Rheumatol. 4:39, 1985.
287. Al-Haik, N., Lewis, D. A., and Struthers, G.: Neutral protease, collagenase and elastase activities in synovial fluid in inflammatory and degenerative arthropathies. Clin. Rheumatol. 4:39, 1985.
288. Hibbs, M. S., Hasty, K. A., Kang, A. H., and Mainardi, C. L.: Secretion of collagenolytic enzymes by human polymorphonuclear leukocytes. Collagen Rel. Res. 4:467, 1984.
289. Harris, E. D., Jr., DiBona, D. R., and Krane, S. M.: Collagenases in human synovial fluid. J. Clin. Invest. 48:2104, 1969.
290. Krane, S. M.: Aspects of the cell biology of the rheumatoid synovial lesion. Ann. Rheum. Dis. 40:433, 1981.
291. Melmon, K. L., and Cline, M. J.: Kallikrein activator and kininase in human granulocytes: A model of inflammation. In Rocha, E., and Silva, M. (eds.): Symposium on Vasoactive Polypeptides: Bradykinin and Related Kinins. Oxford, Pergamon Press, 1967.
292. Cochrane, C. G., et al.: The interaction of Hageman factor and immune complexes. J. Clin. Invest. 51:2736, 1972.
293. Rothberger, H., Zimmerman, T. S., Spiegelberg, H. L., and Vaughan, J. H.: Leucocyte procoagulant activity: Enhancement of production in vitro by IgG and antigen-antibody complexes. J. Clin. Invest. 59:549, 1977.
294. Glynn, L. E.: Heberden Oration. The chronicity of inflammation and its significance in rheumatoid arthritis. Ann. Rheum. Dis. 27:105, 1968.
295. Van de Putte, L. B. A., Hegt, V. N., and Overbeek, T. E.: Activators and inhibitors of fibrinolysis in rheumatoid and non-rheumatoid synovial membranes. Arthritis Rheum. 20:671, 1977.
296. Falchuk, H., Goetzl, J., and Kulka, P.: Respiratory gases of synovial fluids. Am. J. Med. 49:223, 1970.
297. Lund-Olesen, K.: Oxygen tension in synovial fluids. Arthritis Rheum. 13:769, 1970.
298. Treuhaft, P. S., and McCarty, D. J.: Synovial fluid pH, lactate, oxygen and carbon dioxide partial pressures in various joint diseases. Arthritis Rheum. 14:475, 1971.
299. Jayson, M. I. V., and Dixon, A. St. J.: Intra-articular pressure in rheumatoid arthritis of the knee. Ann. Rheum. Dis. 29:261, 1970.
300. Jayson, M. I. V., and Dixon, A. St. J.: Intra-articular pressure in rheumatoid arthritis of the knee. II. Effect of intra-articular pressure on blood circulation to the synovium. Ann. Rheum. Dis. 29:266, 1970.
301. Blake, D. R., Merry, P., Unsworth, J., et al.: Hypoxic-reperfusion injury in the inflamed human joint. Lancet 1:289, 1989.
302. Wallis, W. J., Simkin, P. A., and Nelp, W. B.: Low synovial clearance of iodide provides evidence of hypoperfusion in chronic rheumatoid synovitis. Arthritis Rheum. 28:1096, 1985.
303. Kulka, J. P.: Vascular derangement in rheumatoid arthritis. In Hill, A. G. S. (ed.): Modern Trends in Rheumatology. London, Butterworths, 1961, pp. 49–69.
304. Dingle, J. T. M., Page-Thomas, D. P.: In vitro studies in human synovial membrane. A metabolic comparison of normal and rheumatoid disease. Br. J. Exp. Pathol. 37:318, 1956.
305. Roberts, J. E., McLees, B. D., and Kerby, G. P.: Pathways of glucose metabolism in rheumatoid and non-rheumatoid synovium. J. Lab. Clin. Med. 70:503, 1967.
306. Kushner, I., and Somerville, J. A.: Permeability of human synovial membrane to plasma proteins: Relationship to molecular size and inflammation. Arthritis Rheum. 14:560, 1971.
307. Cecere, F., Lessard, J., McDuffy, S., and Pope, R. M.: Evidence for the local production and utilization of immune reactants in rheumatoid arthritis. Arthritis Rheum. 25:1307, 1982.
308. Wallis, W. J., Simkin, P. A., and Nelp, W. B.: Protein traffic in human synovial effusions. Arthritis Rheum. 30:57, 1987.
309. Nykanen, P., Helve, T., Kankaanpaa, U., and Larsen, A.: Characterisation of the DNA-synthesizing cells in rheumatoid synovial tissue. Scand. J. Rheumatol. 7:118, 1978.
310. Revell, P. A., Mapp, P. I., Lalor, P. A., and Hall, P. A.: Proliferative activity of cells in the synovium as demonstrated by a monoclonal antibody, Ki67. Rheumatol. Int. 7:183, 1987.
311. Henderson, B., Revell, P. A., and Edwards, J. C. W.: Synovial lining cell hyperplasia in rheumatoid arthritis: dogma and fact. Ann. Rheum. Dis. 47:348, 1988.
312. Hogg, N., Palmer, D. G., and Revell, P. A.: Mononuclear phagocytes of normal and rheumatoid synovial membrane identified by monoclonal antibodies. Immunology 56:673, 1985.
313. Okada, Y., Takeuchi, N., Tomita, K., Nakanishi, I., and Nagase, H.: Immunolocalisation of matrix metalloproteinase 3 (stromelysin) in rheumatoid synovioblasts (B cells): Correlation with rheumatoid arthritis. Ann. Rheum. Dis. 48:645, 1989.
314. Lafyatis, R., Remmers, E. F., Roberts, A. B., Yocum, D. E., Sporn, M. B., and Wilder, R. L.: Anchorage-independent growth of synoviocytes from arthritic and normal joints: Stimulation by exogenous platelet-derived growth factor and inhibition by transforming growth factor-beta and retinoids. J. Clin. Invest. 83:1267, 1989.
315. Lafyatis, R., Thompson, N., Remmers, E., Flanders, K., Roberts, A., Sporn, M., and Wilder, R.: Demonstration of local production of PDGF and TGF-beta by synovial tissue from patients with rheumatoid arthritis. Arthritis Rheum. 31:S62, 1988.
316. Burmester, G. R., Dimitriu-Bona, A., Waters, S. J., and Winchester, R. J.: Identification of three major synovial lining cell populations by monoclonal antibodies directed to Ia antigens and antigens associated with monocytes/macrophages and fibroblasts. Scand. J. Immunol. 17:69, 1983.
317. Goto, M., Sasano, M., Yamanaka, H., Miyasaka, N., Kamatani, N., Inove, K., Nishka, K., and Miyamoto, T.: Spontaneous production of an interleukin 1–like factor by cloned rheumatoid synovial cells in long-term culture. J. Clin. Invest. 80:786, 1987.
318. Baker, D. G., Dayer, J.-M., Roelke, M., Schumacher, H. R., and Krane, S. M.: Rheumatoid synovial cell morphologic changes induced by a mononuclear cell factor in culture. Arthritis Rheum. 26:8, 1983.
319. Andreasen, A., Jensen, P. K. A., and Jakobsen, E.: Cloning of cells from synovial membrane for the investigation of rheumatoid arthritis. Exp. Cell Biol. 54:220, 1986.
320. Hendler, P. L., Lavoie, P. E., Werb, Z., Chan, J., and Seaman, W. E.: Human synovial dendritic cells. Direct observation of transition to fibroblasts. J. Rheumatol. 12:660, 1985.
321. Tarkowski, A., Johnsson, R., Holmdahl, R., and Klareskog, L.: Immunohistochemical characterization of synovial cells in arthritis in MRL-lpr/lpr mice. Arthritis Rheum. 30:75, 1987.
322. Gay, R. E., Snider, C., Gay, S., et al.: Cellular composition of proliferating synovial tissue involved in the destructive arthritis of MRL/l mice. Coll. Res. 33:788, 1985.
323. Fujikawa, K.: Arthrographic study of the rheumatoid knee. Part 1. Synovial proliferation. Ann. Rheum. Dis. 40:332, 1981.
324. Fujikawa, K., Tanaka, Y., Matsubayashi, T., and Iseki, F.: Arthrographic study of the rheumatoid knee. Part 2. Articular cartilage and menisci. Ann. Rheum. Dis. 40:344, 1981.
325. Yates, D. B., and Scott, J. T.: Rheumatoid synovitis and joint disease. Ann. Rheum. Dis. 34:1, 1975.
326. Salisbury, M. D., and Nottage, W. M.: A new evaluation of gross pathologic changes and concepts of rheumatoid articular cartilage degeneration. Clin. Orthop. Rel. Res. 199:243, 1985.
327. Henderson, D. R. F., Jayson, M. I. V., and Tribe, C. R.: Lack of correlation of synovial histology with joint damage in rheumatoid arthritis. Ann. Rheum. Dis. 34:7, 1975.
328. Lindblad, S., and Hedfors, E.: Intraarticular variation in synovitis: Local macroscopic and microscopic signs of inflammatory activity are significantly correlated. Arthritis Rheum. 28:977, 1985.
329. Rooney, M., Condell, D., Quinlan, W., Daly, L., Whelan, A., Feighery, C., and Bresnihan, B.: Analysis of the histologic variation of synovitis in rheumatoid arthritis. Arthritis Rheum. 31:956, 1988.
330. Wahl, S. M. Malone, D. G., and Wilder, R. L.: Spontaneous production of fibroblast-activating factor(s) by synovial inflammatory cells. J. Exp. Med. 161:210, 1985.
331. Thomas, D. P., and Dingle, J. T.: Studies on human synovial membrane in vitro. Biochem. J. 68:231, 1957.
332. Castor, C. W.: Connective tissue activation. II. Abnormalities of cultured rheumatoid synovial cells. Arthritis Rheum. 14:55, 1971.
333. Anastassiades, T. P., Ley, J., Wood, A., and Irwin, D.: The growth kinetics of synovial fibroblastic cells from inflammatory and noninflammatory arthropathies. Arthritis Rheum. 21:461, 1978.
334. Mohr, W., and Wessinghage, D.: The relationship between polymorphonuclear granulocytes and cartilage destruction in rheumatoid arthritis. J. Rheumatol. 37:81, 1978.
335. Crisp, A. J., Chapman, C. M., Kirkham, S. E., Schiller, A. L., and Krane, S. M.: Articular mastocytosis in rheumatoid arthritis. Arthritis Rheum. 27:845, 1984.
336. Bromley, M., Fisher, W. D., and Woolley, D. E.: Mast cells at sites of cartilage erosion in the rheumatoid joint. Ann. Rheum. Dis. 43:76, 1984.
337. Malone, D. G., Irani, A.-M., Schwartz, L. B., Barrett, K. E., and Metcalfe, D. D.: Mast cell numbers and histamine levels in synovial fluids from patients with diverse arthritides. Arthritis Rheum. 29:956, 1986.
338. Frewin, D. B., Cleland, L. G., Johnsons, J. R., and Robertson, P. W.: Histamine levels in human synovial fluid. J. Rheumatol. 13:13, 1986.
339. Malone, D. G., Wilder, R. L., Saavedra-Delgado, A. M., and Metcalfe, D. D.: Mast cell numbers in rheumatoid synovial tissues. Arthritis Rheum. 30:130, 1987.
340. Center, D. M.: Identification of rat mast cell-derived chemoattractant factors for lymphocytes. J. Allergy Clin. Immunol. 71:29, 1983.
341. Yoffe, J. R., Taylor, D. J., and Woolley, D. E.: Mast cell products stimulate collagenase and prostaglandin E production by cultures of adherent rheumatoid synovial cells. Biochim. Biophys. Res. Commun. 122:270, 1984.
342. Crisp, A. J., Roelke, M. S., Goldring, S. R., and Krane, S. M.: Heparin

modulates intracellular cyclic AMP in human trabecular bone cells and adherent rheumatoid synovial cells. Ann. Rheum. Dis. 43:628, 1984.

343. Muirden, K. D.: The anaemia of rheumatoid arthritis: The significance of iron deposits in the synovial membrane. Aust. Ann. Med. 2:97, 1970.

344. Mainardi, C. L., Levine, P. H., Werb, Z., and Harris, E. D., Jr.: Proliferative synovitis in hemophilia. Arthritis Rheum. 21:137, 1978.

345. Biemond, P., Swaak, A. J. G., van Eijk, H. G., and Koster, J. F.: Intraarticular ferritin-bound iron in rheumatoid arthritis. Arthritis Rheum. 29:1187, 1986.

346. Blake, D. R., Hall, N. D., Dieppe, P. A., Halliwell, B., and Gutteridge, J. M.: The importance of iron in rheumatoid disease. Lancet 2:1142, 1981.

347. Harris, E. D., Jr., Parker, H. G., Radin, E. L., and Krane, S. M.: Effects of proteolytic enzymes on structural and mechanical properties of cartilage. Arthritis Rheum. 15:497, 1972.

348. Kingsley-Mills, W. M.: Pathology of the knee joint in rheumatoid arthritis. J. Bone Joint Surg. 52:746, 1970.

349. Harris, E. D., Jr., DiBona, D. R., and Krane, S. M.: A mechanism for cartilage destruction in rheumatoid arthritis. Trans. Assoc. Am. Physicians 83:267, 1970.

350. Annefeld, M.: The potential aggressiveness of synovial tissue in rheumatoid arthritis. J. Pathol. 139:399, 1983.

351. Harris, E. D., Jr., Evanson, J. M., DiBona, D. R., et al.: Collagenase and rheumatoid arthritis. Arthritis Rheum. 13:83, 1970.

352. Shiozawa, S., Shiozawa, K., and Fujita, T.: Morphologic observations in the early phase of the cartilage-pannus junction. Arthritis Rheum. 26:472, 1983.

353. Bromley, M., and Woolley, D. E.: Histopathology of the rheumatoid lesion. Arthritis Rheum. 27:857, 1984.

354. Kobayashi, I., and Ziff, M.: Electron microscopic studies of the cartilage-pannus junction in rheumatoid arthritis. Arthritis Rheum. 18:475, 1975.

355. Bromley, M., and Woolley, D. E.: Chondroclasts and osteoclasts at subchondral sites of erosion in the rheumatoid joint. Arthritis Rheum. 27:968, 1984.

356. Brinckerhoff, C. E., and Harris, E. D., Jr.: Collagenase production by cultures containing multinucleated cells derived from synovial fibroblasts. Arthritis Rheum. 21:745, 1978.

357. Lerner, U. H., Jones, I. L., and Gustafson, G. T.: Bradykinin, a new potential mediator of inflammation-induced bone resorption. Arthritis Rheum. 30:530, 1987.

358. Allard, S. A., Muirden, K. D., and Maini, R. N.: Correlation of histopathological features of pannus with patterns of damage in different joints in rheumatoid arthritis. Ann. Rheum. Dis. 50:278, 1991.

359. Harris, E. D., Jr., Glauert, A. M., and Murley, A. H. G.: Intracellular collagen fibers at the pannus-cartilage junction in rheumatoid arthritis. Arthritis Rheum. 20:657, 1977.

360. Yodlowski, M. L., Hubbard, J. R., Kispert, J., Keller, K., Sledge, C. B., and Steinberg, J. J.: Antibody to interleukin 1 inhibits the cartilage degradative and thymocyte proliferative actions of rheumatoid synovial culture medium. J. Rheumatol. 17:1600, 1990.

361. Werb, Z., and Aggeler, J.: Proteases induce secretion of collagenase and plasminogen activator by fibroblasts. Proc. Natl. Acad. Sci. U.S.A. 75:1839, 1978.

362. Werb, Z., and Reynolds, J. J.: Stimulation by endocytosis of the secretion of collagenase and neutral proteinase from rabbit synovial fibroblasts. J. Exp. Med. 140:1482, 1974.

363. Okazaki, I., Brinckerhoff, C. E., Sinclaire, J. F., Sinclaire, P. R., Bonkowsky, H. L., and Harris, E. D., Jr.: Iron increases collagenase production by rabbit synovial fibroblasts. J. Lab. Clin. Med. 97:396, 1981.

364. Biswas, C., and Dayer, J.-M.: Stimulation of collagenase production by collagen in mammalian cell cultures. Cell 18:1035, 1980.

365. Fisher, W. D., Golds, E. E., van der Rest, M., Cooke, T. D., Lyons, H. E., and Poole, A. R.: Stimulation of collagenase secretion from rheumatoid synovial tissue by human collagen peptides. J. Bone Joint Surg. 64:546, 1982.

366. Hasselbacher, P., McMillan, R. M., Vater, C. A., Hahn, J., and Harris, E. D., Jr.: Stimulation of secretion of collagenase and prostaglandin E_2 by synovial fibroblasts in response to crystals of monosodium urate monohydrate: A model for joint destruction in gout. Trans. Assoc. Am. Phys. 94:243, 1981.

367. Cheung, H. S., Halverson, P. B., and McCarty, D. J.: Release of collagenase, neutral proteinase, and prostaglandins from cultured mammalian synovial cells by hydroxyapatite and calcium pyrophosphate dihydrate crystals. Arthritis Rheum. 24:1338, 1981.

368. Bohmann, D., Bos, T. J., Admon, A., Nishimura, T., Vogt, P. K., and Tjian, R.: Human proto-oncogene c-jun encodes a DNA binding protein with structural and functional properties of transcription factor AP-1. Science 238:1386, 1987.

369. Rauscher, F. J., III, Cohen, D. R., Bos, T. J., Vogt, P. K., Bohmann, D., Tjian, R., and Franza, B. R., Jr.: Fos-associated protein p39 is the product of the jun proto-oncogene. Science 240:1010, 1988.

370. Chiu, R., Boyle, W. J., Meek, J., Smeal, T., Hunter, T., and Karin, M.: The c-Fos protein interacts with c-Jun/AP-1 to stimulate transcription of AP-1 responsive genes. Cell 54:541, 1988.

371. Curran, T., and Franza, B. R., Jr.: Fos and Jun: The AP-1 connection. Cell 55:395, 1988.

372. Evanson, J. M., Jeffrey, J. J., and Krane, S. M.: Human collagenase: Identification and characterization of an enzyme from rheumatoid synovium in culture. Science 158:499, 1967.

373. McCroskery, P. A., Wood, S., Jr., and Harris, E. D., Jr.: Gelatin: A poor substrate for a mammalian collagenase. Science 182:70, 1973.

374. Welgus, H. G., Jeffrey, J. J., Stricklin, G. P., Roswit, W. T., and Eisen, A. Z.: Characteristics of the action of human skin fibroblast collagenase on fibrillar collagen. J. Biol. Chem. 255:6806, 1980.

375. Okada, Y., Nagase, H., and Harris, E. D., Jr.: A metalloproteinase from human rheumatoid synovial fibroblasts that digests connective tissue matrix components: Purification and characterization. J. Biol. Chem. 261:14245, 1986.

376. Okada, Y., Konomi, H., Yada, T., Kimata, K., and Nagase, H.: Degradation of type IX collagen by matrix metalloproteinase (stromelysin) from human rheumatoid synovial cells. FEBS Lett. 244:473, 1989.

377. Okada, Y., Harris, E. D., Jr., and Nagase, H.: The precursor of a metalloendopeptidase from human rheumatoid synovial fibroblasts: Purification and mechanisms of activation by endopeptidases and 4-aminophenylmercuric acetate. Biochem. J. 254:731, 1988.

378. Gruber, B. L., Marchese, M. J., Suzuki, K., Schwartz, L. B., Okada, Y., Nagase, H., and Ramamurthy, N. S.: Synovial procollagenase activation by human mast cell tryptase: Dependence upon matrix metalloproteinase 3 activation. J. Clin. Invest. 84:1657, 1989.

379. Werb, Z., Mainardi, C. L., Vater, C. A., and Harris, E. D., Jr.: Endogenous activation of latent collagenase by rheumatoid synovial cells: Evidence for a role of plasminogen activator. N. Engl. J. Med. 296:1017, 1977.

380. Moroz, L. A., Wing, S., and Liote, F.: Mini-plasminogen-like fragments of plasminogen in synovial fluid in acute inflammatory arthritis. Thromb. Res. 43:417, 1986.

381. Eisen, A. A., Bauer, E. A., Stricklin, G. P., Seltzer, J. L., Koob, T. J., and Jeffrey, J. J.: Control of human skin collagenase activity. In McCabe, B., F., Sade, J., and Abramson, M. (eds.): Cholesteatoma. First International Conference. Birmingham, Aesculapius Publishing Co., 1977, p. 115.

382. Vater, C. A., Mainardi, C. L., and Harris, E. D., Jr.: An inhibitor of mammalian collagenases from cultures in vitro of human tendon. J. Biol. Chem. 254:3045, 1979.

383. Carmichael, D. F., Sommer, A., Thompson, R. C., Anderson, D. C., Smith, C. G., Welgus, H. G., and Stricklin, G. P.: Primary structure and cDNA cloning of human fibroblast collagenase inhibitor. Proc. Natl. Acad. Sci. U.S.A. 83:2407, 1986.

384. Okada, Y., Gonoji, Y., Nakanishi, I., Nagase, H., and Hayakawa, T.: Immunohistochemical demonstration of simultaneous production of collagenase and tissue inhibitor of metalloproteinases (TIMP) by synovial lining cells in rheumatoid synovium. Virchows Arch. [B] Cell Pathol. 59:305, 1990.

385. Collins, D. H.: The subcutaneous nodule of rheumatoid arthritis. J. Pathol. Bacteriol. 45:97, 1985.

386. Bennett, G. A., Zeller, J. W., and Bauer, W.: Subcutaneous nodules of rheumatoid arthritis and rheumatic fever. A pathologic study. Arch. Pathol. 30:70, 1970.

387. Cochrane, W., Davies, D. V., Dorleng, J., and Bywater, E. G. L.: Ultramicroscopic structures of the rheumatoid nodule. Ann. Rheum. Dis. 23:345, 1964.

388. Palmer, D. G., Hogg, N., Highton, J., Hessian, P. A., and Denholm, I.: Macrophage migration and maturation within rheumatoid nodules. Arthritis Rheum. 30:729, 1987.

389. Athanasou, N. A., Quinn, J., Woods, C. G., and McGee, J. O'D.: Immunohistology of rheumatoid nodules and rheumatoid synovium. Ann. Rheum. Dis. 47:398, 1988.

390. Harris, E. D., Jr.: A collagenolytic system produced by primary cultures of rheumatoid nodule tissue. J. Clin. Invest. 51:2973, 1972.

391. Sokoloff, L., Wilikens, S. L., and Bunim, J. J.: Arteritis of striated muscle in rheumatoid arthritis. Am. J. Pathol. 27:157, 1951.

392. Conn, D. L., McDuffie, F. C., and Dyck, P. J.: Immunopathologic study of sural nerves in rheumatoid arthritis. Arthritis Rheum. 15:135, 1972.

393. Sokoloff, L., and Bunim, J. J.: Vascular lesions in rheumatoid arthritis. J. Chronic Dis. 5:668, 1957.

394. Glass, D., Soter, N. A., and Schur, P. H.: Rheumatoid vasculitis. Arthritis Rheum. 19:950, 1976.

395. Conn, D. L., Schroeter, A. L., and McDuffie, F. C.: Cutaneous vessel immune deposits in rheumatoid arthritis. Arthritis Rheum. 19:15, 1976.

396. Conn, D. L., and McDuffie, F. C.: The pathogenesis of rheumatoid neuropathy. In Eberl, R., and Rosenthal, M. (eds.): Organic Manifestations and Complications in Rheumatoid Arthritis. New York, F. K. Schattaner Verlag, 1975, pp. 295–306.

Clinical Features of Rheumatoid Arthritis

INTRODUCTION

Medical historians disagree about the first references to rheumatoid arthritis (RA) in lay and medical writings.[1–6] Some have concluded that RA developed only recently as a clear-cut entity, but others interpret writings of Soranus in the second century as referring to a patient with RA.

Regardless of history, RA has become an important cause of disability and morbidity and a drain on human and monetary resources. In 1985, the average annual cost for inpatient and outpatient care of a patient with RA seen only by a rheumatologist was over $2000[7]; by 1990, this had increased to $2500. RA is a chronic and progressive disease, and it is likely that once it is active and chronic in a given individual it will become progressively worse. It is probable that if active disease has been present for 1 year in a particular joint, cartilage loss will be irreversible.

CRITERIA FOR DIAGNOSIS

The diagnosis of RA is based primarily on clinical grounds. Despite the usefulness of tests for rheumatoid factor (RF) in both diagnosis and understanding of the pathophysiology of the disease, neither the presence of anti-immunoglobulin G (IgG) nor any other laboratory variable is specific for RA. For epidemiologic studies, several sets of criteria have been developed for classification of adult RA by the American Rheumatism Association (ARA). The most recent of these was published in 1988[8] and has replaced criteria published in 1958.[9] In the earlier criteria, distinction was made among "classic," "definite," and "probable" RA. Over the years, it has become apparent to most clinicians that there is little to be gained by distinguishing classic from definite RA and that probable RA often, in fact, is another disease entity. The 1988 criteria were constructed using data from 262 patients with RA and 262 control patients representing a cross section of rheumatic diseases. Table 52–1 lists the 1988 ARA criteria. These perform better than the 1958 ARA criteria, and fewer extensive, costly investigations are needed for their rigorous application. A major problem with the 1958 criteria was mirrored in marked discrepancies among various series in the ratios of probable to definite RA, in the ratios of female to male cases,[10] and in the large number of patients who meet criteria for diagnosis of probable RA but who evolve either to a healthy state or into another process.[11]

Another set of criteria was proposed at the Third

Table 52–1. 1988 REVISED ARA CRITERIA FOR CLASSIFICATION OF RHEUMATOID ARTHRITIS (RA)*

Criteria	Definition
Morning stiffness	Morning stiffness in and around the joints lasting at least 1 hour before maximal improvement
Arthritis of three or more joint areas	At least three joint areas have simultaneously had soft tissue swelling or fluid (not bony overgrowth alone) observed by a physician. The 14 possible joint areas are (right or left) PIP, MCP, wrist, elbow, knee, ankle, and MTP joints
Arthritis of hand joints	At least one joint area swollen as above in wrist, MCP, or PIP joint
Symmetric arthritis	Simultaneous involvement of the same joint areas (as in 2) on both sides of the body (bilateral involvement of PIP, MCP, or MTP joints is acceptable without absolute symmetry)
Rheumatoid nodules	Subcutaneous nodules, over bony prominences, or extensor surfaces, or in juxta-articular regions, observed by a physician
Serum rheumatoid factor	Demonstration of abnormal amounts of serum rheumatoid factor by any method that has been positive in less than 5% of normal control subjects
Radiographic changes	Radiographic changes typical of RA on posteroanterior hand and wrist radiographs, which must include erosions or unequivocal bony decalcification localized to or most marked adjacent to the involved joints (osteoarthritis changes alone do not qualify)

PIP = proximal interphalangeal; MCP = metacarpophalangeal; MTP = metatarsophalangeal.

*For classification purposes, a patient is said to have RA if he or she has satisfied at least four of the above seven criteria. Criteria 1 through 4 must be present for at least 6 weeks. Patients with two clinical diagnoses are not excluded. Designation as classic, definite, or probable rheumatoid arthritis is *not* to be made.

Table 52–2. NEW YORK CRITERIA FOR THE DIAGNOSIS OF RHEUMATOID ARTHRITIS

RA is present if criteria 1 and 2 plus either 3 or 4 are met:
1. History of an episode of three painful limb joints. Each group of joints (e.g., proximal interphalangeal joint) is counted as one joint, scoring each side separately
2. Swelling, limitation of motion, subluxation, or ankylosis of three limb joints. *Necessary inclusions:* (1) at least one hand, wrist, or foot; (2) symmetry of one joint pair. *Exclusions:* (1) distal interphalangeal joints; (2) fifth proximal interphalangeal joints; (3) first metatarsophalangeal joints; (4) hips
3. Radiographic changes (erosions)
4. Serum positive for rheumatoid factors

International Symposium of Population Studies of the Rheumatic Diseases in New York City in 1967 (Table 52–2).[12] Meeting these criteria is a more difficult task and clearly would exclude monoarticular or diarticular disease, seronegative arthritis, and mild, nondeforming disease. The 1988 ARA criteria resemble these New York criteria more than the 1958 ARA criteria, and this is helpful in specificity of diagnosis. For example, an interesting comparison of the 1958 ARA and New York criteria was carried out by O'Sullivan and Cathcart in Sudbury, Massachusetts.[13] In 1964, of 4522 persons examined, 17 appeared to have RA according to the New York criteria, and 118 had either probable or definite RA by the 1958 ARA criteria. Five years later, only a handful of those classified as having RA by the ARA criteria still met criteria for the diagnosis. These data indicate that the New York criteria identify persons whose disease remains clinically meaningful and establish the prevalence of RA as 0.5 percent in women and 0.1 percent in men. The data did not define the nature of the disease manifested in the 88 patients who initially met the 1958 ARA criteria for RA and who failed to meet the criteria on later examination. However, early RA (probable or definite by 1958 ARA criteria) is a relatively benign process with a high probability for undergoing remission within several years or being recognized as another entity (e.g., Lyme disease or spondyloarthropathy).

EPIDEMIOLOGY

Wolfe[14] summarized the results of 14 studies of population samples, including the National Health Survey,[15] the survey of Tecumseh, Michigan,[16] various Native American groups,[17] and representative atomic bomb survivors from Hiroshima and Nagasaki.[18] Using 1958 ARA criteria for definite RA, the prevalence rate varied from 0.3 to 1.5 percent. It is reasonable to estimate that there were 5 million cases of RA in the United States in 1991; an estimate of prevalence of 1 percent in the adult population is appropriate. A conservative estimate would be that 150,000 new cases of definite or classic RA developed

in the United States in 1990. The lifetime costs of RA, including medical expenses as well as costs associated with illness-related work loss, can be estimated to be more than $29,000 per case in 1990 dollars, as great as that for stroke and coronary artery disease.[19]

Regional variations from these incidence and prevalence data are unusual, indicating that specific genetic and environmental influences on the development of RA, if significant, are widespread in the world. However, a few subpopulations with an apparent excessive predisposition to development of RA exist. A frequency of definite RA of 3.4 percent in Yakima Indian women aged 18 to 79 years has been found; this is compared with a prevalence of 1.4 percent in the general population.[20] In a geographically and socially isolated band of 227 Chippewa Indians, the minimum prevalence of RA was found to be 5.3 percent. The prevalence of HLA-DR4 was 68 percent, significantly higher than in most general populations, and all of the 12 with RA expressed HLA-DR4.[21]

Black Africans may have an unusually high incidence of severe erosive disease with high titers of RF.[22, 23] There is a striking increase in prevalence of RA in urban South African blacks (3.3 percent) compared with rural blacks (0.87 percent).[24, 25]

Definite RA is two to three times more common in women than in men, although if groups with early probable RA are considered, the male-to-female ratio may approach 1. In Italy, a country with less DR4 positivity than the United States, deforming RA with nodule formation is believed to be less common than in the United States.

In Rochester, Minnesota, there has been a decline in the incidence of RA in the female population since 1960.[26] However, a case-control study of this population showed no association between RA and the use of oral contraceptives or the use of estrogens for menopause-related or postmenopausal symptoms. These data contradict those from England[27] reporting that patients with RA were found to have used oral contraceptives only half as much as did control subjects. (See Chapter 51 for a more detailed analysis of a possible link between RA and oral contraceptives.)

There is a higher prevalence of RA and greater mortality from the disease in patients of either sex who have had less than 5 years of education and in those with lower yearly incomes.[28–31] The correlation of less formal education and increased morbidity and mortality of RA has been extended by a study showing that formal education levels are inversely correlated with markers of clinical status in RA.[32]

Since 1948, when the studies of Rose and colleagues[33] confirmed the findings of Waaler,[34] linking a factor in sera of patients with RA to agglutination of normal and sensitized sheep erythrocytes, the presence or absence of RF in serum has occupied attention of epidemiologists in this field. RF is found more frequently (3 to 5 percent) than is RA in population studies; in the general population, the prevalence of seropositivity is about equal in men and women.[35, 36] Several studies have yielded conflicting results in examining whether HLA-DR4, the histocompatibility antigen associated with RA, is associated independently with the presence of RF.[37, 38] Frequently, patients appear to have RA yet are seronegative.[39] These individuals probably have a distinct disease.[40] The assay for RF itself may explain false positives, because when an enzyme-linked immunoabsorbent assay (ELISA) was used instead of the usual agglutination tests, almost complete specificity for RA (99%) has been demonstrated.[41]

Evidence that genetic factors are permissive for RA using twin studies are variable. The data have ranged from evidence for discordance[42] to, in one study, almost 50 percent concordance.[43] In another study, the risk of erosive arthritis in monozygotic co-twins was about 30 times that in the reference population, whereas the risk in dizygotic co-twins and in nontwin siblings was about six times that of control groups.[44, 45] Relative risk in a nationwide Finnish study was less impressive,[46] a series of 4137 monozygotic and 9162 dizygotic twins showing a relative risk of 8.2 for monozygotic and 3.4 for dizygotic twins. Functionally incapacitating (grade 3 or 4) RA has been found to occur at four times the expected rate in first-degree relatives of probands with seropositive disease; erosive radiographic changes were found at three times the expected rate. Serologic study in first-degree relatives of patients with RA has revealed no higher frequency of RF than in relatives of matched controls.[47]

A number of other observations suggest certain associations with RA. Some of these are listed below, but none has been substantiated by independent studies.

1. RA was less common in schizophrenics than in a control population.[48]
2. In studies of identical twins discordant for RA, a history of psychologic stress was more common in the affected twin.[42]
3. Occupations involving heavy outdoor labor or work in health fields were associated with RA.[49]
4. Rheumatoid patients had an increased frequency of exposure to sick pets (e.g., dogs, cats, birds, or other sick animals) in the 5 years before developing their disease than did a control group.[50]

Still inadequately understood is the apparent negative association between gout and RA. In 1979, it was estimated that there should be a thousand cases of coexistent gout and RA in the United States rather than the seven reported cases.[51] In a subsequent study, 12 of 160 seropositive patients with RA were found to have hyperuricemia. Eleven of the 12 had quiet disease; indeed, the onset of hyperuricemia and improvement of RA appeared to coincide. In patients with fluctuations in uric acid levels, there was a statistically significant correlation ($r = -0.66$,

$P \leq 0.01$) of an increase in serum uric acid concentration and improvement in disease activity.[52] Thus, the hypothesis stands: the hyperuricemic state may be anti-inflammatory.

CLINICAL SYNDROME OF EARLY RHEUMATOID ARTHRITIS

In the northern hemisphere, the onset of RA is more frequent in winter than in summer. In several series the onset of RA from October to March is twice as frequent as in the other 6 months,[53, 54] and exacerbations of the disease are more common in winter.[55] Comparable data from the southern hemisphere are not available.

Recent data suggest that the appearance of RF may precede symptoms of arthritis in more patients than was previously recognized. Of 30 patients from whom frozen sera were available from a time before symptoms of RA began, half had positive latex fixation test results.[56] The number of men with positive results was eight times that of women.

Much more diffuse, subjective, and difficult to study are *precipitating factors* of arthritis. There is no evidence that any have a direct cause-and-effect relation. Trauma is one of the most common preludes to arthritis; this can include surgery. Other stimuli, including infections, vaccine inoculations, and emotional trauma, have been implicated by many patients as the cause of their problems.

Patterns of Onset (Table 52–3)

Insidious Onset. RA usually has an insidious, slow onset over weeks to months. Fifty-five to 70 percent of cases begin this way.[53, 57] The initial symptoms may be systematic or articular. In some patients, fatigue, malaise, or diffuse musculoskeletal pain may be the first nonspecific complaint, with joints becoming involved later. Although symmetric involvement is common, asymmetric presentation (often developing more symmetry later in the course of disease)

Table 52–3. ONSET OF RHEUMATOID ARTHRITIS IN 300 PATIENTS WITH DEFINITE OR CLASSIC DISEASE

Characteristic		Percentage
Mode of onset	Rapid* (days or weeks)	46
	Insidious	54
Site of onset	Small joints	32
	Medium-sized joints	16
	Large joints	29
	Combined	26
Pattern of onset	Monarticular	21
	Oligoarticular	44
	Polyarticular	35

*This time frame includes patients described in other studies as having intermediate onset.
(From Fallahi, S., Halla, J. T., and Hardin, J. G.: Clin. Res. 31:650A, 1983, with permission.)

is not unusual. The reason for symmetry of joint involvement may be related to release of phlogistic neuropeptides at terminal nerve endings in joints (see Chapter 51).

Morning stiffness may be the first symptom, appearing even before pain. This phenomenon is probably related to accumulation of edema fluid within the inflamed tissue during sleep, and it clears as edema and products of inflammation are absorbed by lymphatics and venules and returned to the circulation by motion accompanying use of muscles. Pain and stiffness may develop in other joints, but it is rare for symptoms to remit completely in one set of joints while developing in another. This lack of a migratory quality of arthritis sets RA apart from rheumatic fever, in which a true migratory pattern of arthritis is common.

A subtle, early change in RA is development of muscle atrophy around affected joints. This decreases efficiency and strength, and the patient develops weakness that is out of proportion to pain. Opening doors, climbing stairs, and doing repetitive work become more demanding. A low-grade fever without chills is not uncommon. Depression, anxiety, and fear of the future affect the patient and accentuate symptoms. Weight loss is common, and anorexia contributes to this.

Acute Onset. Eight to 15 percent of patients have an acute onset of symptoms within a few days. Rarely, a patient pinpoints onset of disease to a specific time or activity, such as opening a door or driving a golf ball. Symptoms mount, with pain developing in other joints, often in a less symmetric pattern than in patients who have an insidious type of onset. Pain in muscles can be severe and mimic that accompanying muscle necrosis from ischemia. Diagnosis of RA when it presents acutely is difficult to make, and sepsis or vasculitis must be ruled out first.

Intermediate Onset. Fifteen to 20 percent of patients have an intermediate type of onset. Symptoms develop over days or weeks. Systemic complaints are more noticeable than in the insidious type of onset.

Joint Involvement in Early Rheumatoid Arthritis

The joints most commonly involved first in RA are the metacarpophalangeal (MCP) joints, proximal interphalangeal (PIP) joints, and wrists.[58] Combined data from two series are listed in Table 52–4. Larger joints generally become symptomatic after small joints. This raises the question of whether early disease in large joints remains asymptomatic for a longer time. The answer was sought in one study by performing xenon clearances on clinically normal knees of patients with early RA.[59] Seven of 22 had abnormally high perfusion, supporting this hypothesis. A recent anatomic study has correlated the area in square centimeters of synovial membrane with that of hyaline cartilage in each joint. The joints with the highest ratio of synovium to articular cartilage correlated positively with the joints most frequently involved in the disease.[60]

Unusual Patterns of Early Disease

Adult-Onset Still's Disease. This disease appears in adults, usually in the third or fourth decade, as a syndrome similar to that seen in children with the acute, febrile onset of juvenile arthritis. That the syndrome can occur in adults supports those who hold that Still's disease is distinct from RA, rather than its being a different presentation of the same process. It was first described by Bywaters in 14 patients.[61] Women are more commonly affected than are men. Results from serologic studies (RF and antinuclear antibody [ANA]) are normal, and patients do not have subcutaneous nodules.[62] Most are febrile. Fever patterns in these patients are usually quotidian (i.e., reaching normal levels at least once each day). They often have the appearance of salmon-colored or pink macules that are evanescent and that become more prominent when patients are febrile. The cervical spine is involved, and loss of neck motion may be striking. Pericarditis and pleural effusions and severe abdominal pain (possibly mesenteric adenitis) may be present and may confound attempts at diagnosis.[63] Unlike systemic lupus erythematosus (SLE), serum complement level is normal or high.[64]

In a more recent series, 11 patients (all of whom were white women) followed up for a mean of 20.2 years after disease onset had the following characteristics[65]: (1) Ten had a polycyclic pattern (characterized by remissions and exacerbations). (2) Patterns of exacerbations were similar to but less severe than the original presentations. (3) Loss of wrist extension was the most common clinical abnormality, and carpal ankylosis was present in 10 patients. (4) Five of 11 patients developed distal interphalangeal (DIP) joint involvement. (5) Biopsy

Table 52–4. JOINTS INVOLVED IN RHEUMATOID ARTHRITIS*

	Percentage Initially Involved[406]			Percentage Ultimately Involved[384]
	Right	*Left*	*Bilateral*	
Metacarpophalangeal	65	58	52	87
Wrist	60	57	48	82
Proximal interphalangeal	63	53	45	63
Metatarso-phalangeal	48	47	43	48
Shoulder	37	42	30	47
Knee	35	30	24	56
Ankle	25	23	18	53
Elbow	20	15	14	21

*Other joints (e.g., distal interphalangeal joints) are not tabulated here.

of the characteristic skin rash of Still's and juvenile RA (JRA) showed perivascular infiltrate of neutrophils in the superficial dermis.

In another series, retrospective classification of 21 patients into four groups was made: I, monocyclic systemic; II, polycyclic systemic; III, chronic articular or monocyclic systemic; and IV, chronic articular or polycyclic systemic.[66] Groups I and II had joint involvement only during initial and subsequent flares of the disease. Groups III and IV had significant morbidity. Of the total group, 20 percent showed significant functional deterioration from erosive joint disease. Functional class III and IV (Steinbrocker's classification) was usually related to hip disease. Adult Still's disease can be recurrent after apparent remissions (55 percent in one Japanese study).[67] In this later study, it is of interest that an increased level of serum ferritin was an important diagnostic marker for the disease.[67] As in classic RA in adults, polyarticular disease was more often associated with a poor functional outcome than was oligoarticular disease. Individuals with monocyclic or polycyclic systemic disease, no arthritis at presentation, or oligoarticular presentation and progression tended to have a considerably better functional outcome. The occurrence of amyloidosis may be as high as 30 percent within 10 years of onset of the illness.[67]

Palindromic Pattern of Onset. Palindromic rheumatism was described by Hench and Rosenberg in 1941.[68] Like many other clinical complexes in rheumatology, it should be considered a syndrome that can be the initial manifestation of many different organic processes or one that never evolves into anything more. The syndrome is more like gout than anything else. Pain usually begins in one joint; symptoms worsen for several hours and are associated with swelling and erythema. An intercritical period, as in gout, is asymptomatic. It is likely that 30 to 50 percent of patients with palindromic rheumatism go on to develop RA, particularly those with HLA-DR4. In these, multiple joints become involved, swelling does not subside completely between attacks, and tests become positive for RF. Neither the characteristics of joint fluid nor the pathologic findings of synovial biopsies allows the prediction that RA will evolve from the palindromic rheumatism.[69]

Effects of Age on Onset. RA developing in older men (60 years of age and older) is often dominated by stiffness, limb girdle pain, and diffuse boggy swelling of the hands, wrists, and forearms. One study emphasized that an initial clinical onset resembling polymyalgia rheumatica occurs four times more frequently in the elderly than in younger patients.[70] Those with onset at age 60 or more are less likely to have subcutaneous nodules or RF at the onset of disease, despite the high prevalence of RF in the general population in this age group. In general, elderly individuals who develop RA tend to have a more benign course than do younger patients. In those who develop RA after age 60, there is a lower frequency of positive tests for RF, but there is a strong association with HLA-DR4.[71] Onset is slow, but the stiffness is often incapacitating. In other respects, the disease is similar to other forms of adult RA, but the therapy is not the same. Nonsteroidal anti-inflammatory drugs (NSAIDs) are rarely effective, but low-dose glucocorticoids (less than 7.5 mg of prednisone per day) may be helpful in reducing edema and increasing motion and function.

Rheumatoid Arthritis and Paralysis: Asymmetric Disease. Being relatively common, RA is likely to occur with many other types of chronic disease. A striking asymmetry of even unilateral involvement has been described in patients with poliomyelitis, meningioma, encephalitis, neurovascular syphilis, strokes, and cerebral palsy.[72, 73] Joints are spared on the paralyzed side, and the degree of protection demonstrates a rough correlation with the extent of paralysis.[74] Protective effect is less if a neurologic deficit develops in a patient who already had RA.[75]

Arthritis Robustus. Arthritis robustus is not so much an unusual presentation of disease as it is an unusual reaction of patients to the disease.[76, 77] Men usually form this group. Their disease is characterized by proliferative synovitis that appears to cause little pain. Patients are athletic and invariably keep working (often at physical labor). Osteopenia is less severe, and new bone proliferation at joint margins is common. Bulky subcutaneous nodules develop. Subchondral cysts develop, presumably from the excessive pressure developed from synovial fluid within a thick joint capsule during muscular effort.

COURSE

Intermittent Course. The intermittent course is marked by partial to complete remissions without need for continuous therapy. This type of disease is usually mild. Initially, only a few joints are usually involved. Insidious return of disease is often marked by involvement of more joints than during the first episode. Fifteen to 20 percent of patients with RA enjoy these periods of remission.[78, 79] Within this group, it is reported that about half had remissions that lasted more than a year, and in the entire group remissions lasted longer than exacerbations.

Long Clinical Remissions. In one study of 250 patients receiving only simple medical and orthopedic treatment, almost 10 percent were in clinical remission for 12 to 31 years (mean, 22 years).[80] Although most of these patients had RA for less than 6 months at the time of inclusion, 40 percent had remained in remission. Many of these patients had an acute onset of symptoms with marked fever and severe joint pain and inflammation, raising the question (in retrospect) of whether they indeed had RA. Nevertheless, some sign of disease activity (e.g., an elevated erythrocyte sedimentation rate [ESR]) persisted in many throughout the clinical remission, and occasional patients had brief but true flares of disease in one or a few joints.

Progressive Disease. Patients with progressive disease may have a rapid or slow course, but the end-point is the same—disabling, destructive disease.

Although each physician readily believes that his or her management of RA results in substantial benefit for individual patients, substantiating data are difficult to find. In fact, it is probable that inexorable progression, albeit at a variable rate, is the outcome for those who have established disease of a year or more with signs of continuously active proliferative disease. This may occur, in part, because cartilage partially damaged by synovitis cannot withstand normal impact loading. In one study of 75 patients with RA examined after 9 years, almost all had significantly lower functional capacity and an increase in mortality.[81] This outcome was despite aggressive therapy begun shortly after the initial examination.

In assessing symptoms in RA, both patients and their physicians must be aware of environmental factors that may accentuate symptoms. One of these, the weather, has a strong base in folklore as a major determinant of symptom severity in RA and other rheumatic diseases. A number of studies have attempted scientific inquiry into this perception. Using a climate-controlled chamber for patients, early data suggested that symptoms worsened if humidity was raised and barometric pressure lowered simultaneously.[82] In a more recent study of RA and osteoarthritis, 62 percent of patients believed that changes in weather aggravated their symptoms, but this could not be confirmed by standard assessments of symptoms using visual analogue scores.[83] In contrast, another study showed that pain in patients with RA increased significantly as temperature and vapor pressure increased.[84] The folklore may be accurate: a consistent dry and temperate climate may alleviate symptoms in RA.

DIAGNOSIS

Diagnosis of RA must be by established criteria that are based on effective clinical history and examination, laboratory tests, and diagnoses that exclude it (see earlier discussion). There is no single feature that makes a definite diagnosis. Diagnosis is made by a synthesis of all information available. The ARA criteria for classification need not be used in individual cases for diagnosis; however, the requirement that objective evidence for synovitis must be present for at least 6 weeks is an important one. On one hand, a physician should not make a premature diagnosis of RA in a patient who may have a self-limited synovitis; on the other hand, to prevent irreversible damage to joints, the diagnosis of RA should be ruled in or out within 2 months after the onset of synovitis. Before discussion of the exclusions (i.e., the findings that point to the presence of

another disease process), diagnosis will be addressed positively, listing factors typical of the disease.

The characteristic patient with RA complains of pain and stiffness in multiple joints. The joint swelling is boggy and includes both soft tissue and synovial fluid. These joints are tender to touch, especially the small joints of the hands and feet. Often palmar erythema and prominent veins on the dorsum of the hand indicate an increase in blood flow to the joint areas. DIP joints are involved rarely. Temperature over the involved joints (except the hip) is elevated, but the joints are not usually red. Range of motion is limited, and muscle strength and function around inflamed joints are diminished. Soft, poorly delineated subcutaneous nodules are often found in the extensor surface of the forearm. Findings on general physical examination are normal, except for a possible lowgrade fever (38°C); soft, small lymph nodes occasionally are found in epitracheal, axillary, and cervical areas. Movement is guarded, and apprehension often dominates facial expression. Initial laboratory tests often show the following: (1) a slight leukocytosis with normal differential leukocyte count; (2) thrombocytosis; (3) a slight anemia (10 gm or more of hemoglobin per dl), normochromic and either normocytic or microcytic; (4) normal urinalysis; (5) ESR (Westergren's method) of 30 mm or more per hour; (6) normal renal, hepatic, and metabolic function; (7) a normal serum uric acid level (before initiation of salicylate therapy); (8) positive RF test and negative ANA test; (9) elevated levels of alpha$_2$ (α_2)-globulins and α_1-globulins; and (10) normal or elevated serum complement level.

A typical arthrocentesis (see Chapter 36) reveals the following. Joint fluid is straw-colored and slightly cloudy and contains many flecks of fibrin. Within the fluid, a clot forms on standing at room temperature. There are 5000 to 25,000 leukocytes per mm^3, and at least 85 percent of these are polymorphonuclear leukocytes (PMNs). Occasional large PMNs with granules staining positively for IgG, IgM, and C3 are found. No crystals are present. The mucin clot is fair. C4 and C2 levels are slightly depressed, but C3 is normal. IgG in synovial fluid may approach serum concentrations. Synovial fluid glucose level is depressed, occasionally to less than 25 mg per dl. Cultures are negative.

Differential Diagnosis

It is important to exclude many other diseases before making a diagnosis of RA.[85] The relative frequency of the entities discussed in this section is recorded as common, uncommon, or rare; they are listed in alphabetical order.

Amyloidosis (Rare). Deposits of the glycoprotein amyloid can be found in synovial and periarticular tissues[105] and are, presumably, responsible for the joint complaints that patients with amyloidosis often have (see Chapter 82). The synovial fluid in amyloid arthropathy is noninflammatory, and, on occasion, particulate material with apple-green fluorescence after Congo red staining may be found in the fluid. Amyloid formed of β_2-microglobulin is found in joints of patients with chronic renal failure.

Angioimmunoblastic Lymphadenopathy (Rare). Nonerosive, symmetric, seronegative polyarthritis involving large joints can be an initial complaint in angioimmunoblastic lymphadenopathy, an unusual disease.[86] Typical clinical features are lymphadenopathy, hepatosplenomegaly, rash, and hypergammaglobulinemia. It can resemble Still's disease in adults if the arthritis precedes other manifestations. Diagnosis is made by the characteristic appearance of a lymph node or skin biopsy specimen—effacement of lymph node architecture, proliferation of small vessels, and a cellular infiltrate (immunoblasts, plasma cells, T lymphocytes, and histiocytes) within amorphous acidophilic interstitial material. It is believed that symptoms may be related to excessive production of interleukin-2 (IL-2) by T-helper cells in this process.

Ankylosing Spondylitis, Seronegative Spondyloarthropathy, and Reactive Arthritis (Common). These are often referred to as the B27-associated diseases. The problem in differentiating them from RA arises when the patient (particularly a woman) has minimal back pain and definite peripheral joint involvement. Suspicion that this is not RA is generated when small joints are not involved, when joint disease is asymmetric, and when the lumbar spine is involved (see Chapter 56).

In some cases, the conclusion is inescapable that RA and ankylosing spondylitis are present in the same patient. In one series, nine patients with RF in their sera had spinal ankylosis and symmetric erosive polyarthritis; eight of the nine carried HLA-B27.[87] If one assumes that these two diseases occur completely independently, simultaneous occurrence in the same patient should occur once in every 50,000 to 200,000 of the adult population.

In distinguishing patients with *Reiter's syndrome* from those with RA, a careful search for heel pain or tenderness and ocular or urethral symptoms is of great importance. Polyarthritis persists chronically in over 80 percent of patients with Reiter's syndrome (see Chapter 57). The characteristics of enthesopathy in patients with Reiter's syndrome (i.e., sausage digits indicating periarticular soft tissue inflammation), insertional tendinitis, periostitis, and peri-insertional osteoporosis or erosions may point to the diagnosis.

The differential diagnosis between RA with psoriasis and psoriatic arthritis may be artificial (see Chapter 58). Some patients with DIP joint involvement and severe skin involvement obviously have a disease that is not RA. Others, however, have a seropositive symmetric polyarthritis that appears to be RA, but they also have psoriasis. These patients can be treated with the same disease-modifying drugs as those with progressive RA.

A syndrome described extensively in the French literature, *acne-pustulosis-hyperostosis-osteitis*,[88] may resemble psoriatic arthritis and, occasionally, when peripheral arthritis is present, RA. As implied in the name, these patients variably express severe acne, palmar, and plantar pustules, hyperostotic reactions (particularly in the clavicles and sternum), sacroilitis, and peripheral inflammatory arthritis.

Inflammatory bowel disease (IBD; ulcerative colitis and Crohn's disease) is associated with arthritis in 20 percent of cases[89] (see Chapter 59). Peripheral arthritis occurs more commonly than spondylitis in many series.[90] Ankles, knees, and elbows are the most often involved of peripheral joints, PIP joints and wrists being next in frequency. Joint symptoms can precede diagnosis of bowel disease. Simultaneous attacks of arthritis and development of erythema nodosum are not uncommon. Attacks of joint pain begin more rapidly than usually occurs in RA, and most often only two or three joints are affected at once. Involvement is usually asymmetric, and erosions are uncommon. The occurrence of peripheral arthritis in IBD is not related to HLA-B27.

Behçet's syndrome (see Chapter 64) is marked by an asymmetric polyarthritis in 50 to 60 percent of cases.[91] In more than in half of the cases, the attacks of arthritis are monarticular.[92] Knees, ankles, and wrists are affected most often; synovial fluid usually contains less than 5000 but more than 30,000 leukocytes per mm³. Joint deformity is unusual. The painful oral and genital ulcers and central nervous system involvement are unusual in RA. Uveal tract involvement seen in Behçet's syndrome must be differentiated from the scleritis characteristic of RA in patients with ocular and joint disease. Spondylitis, as in the other disorders classified here, is found in Behçet's syndrome, mainly when HLA-B27 is present.

Enteric infections are complicated occasionally by inflammatory joint disease resembling RA (see Chapter 59). The joint disease associated with infections with *Yersinia enterocolitica* occurs several weeks after the gastrointestinal illness.[93] Knees and ankles are the joints most commonly involved, and most patients (even those with peripheral arthritis and no spondylitis) have HLA-B27.[94] Reactive arthritis also has been reported after *Salmonella*, *Shigella*, and *Campylobacter (Helicobacter) jejuni*.

Arthropathy may precede other findings of *Whipple's disease* (see Chapter 59). The pattern is that of a migratory polyarthritis or oligoarthritis involving ankles, knees, shoulders, elbows, and fingers, as with IBD. Remission may occur when diarrhea begins. As with the arthritis of IBD, joint destruction is rare,[95] presumably because the synovitis lacks sustained chronicity.

Arthritis Associated with Oral Contraceptives (Uncommon). A syndrome of persistent arthralgias, myalgias, and morning stiffness with occasional development of polyarticular synovitis has been described in women, usually in their 20s, who have been taking oral contraceptives (estrogens and progestins).[96] Positive tests for ANA are common, and several patients have had circulating RF. Symptoms resolve after the contraceptive is discontinued.

Arthritis of Thyroid Disease (Uncommon). In hypothyroidism, synovial effusions and synovial thickening simulating RA have been described (see Chapter 92).[97] The ESR may be elevated because of hypergammaglobulinemia. Joint fluid is noninflammatory and may have an increased viscosity. Knees, wrists, hands, and feet are involved most often, and not infrequently coexisting calcium pyrophosphate dehydrate (CPPD) deposition disease is found.

The syndrome of thyroid acropachy complicates less than 1 percent of cases of hyperthyroidism.[98] This represents periosteal new bone formation, which may be associated with a low-grade synovitis similar to hypertrophic osteoarthropathy. Although impossible to quantitate, patients with coexisting RA and hyperthyroidism have pain from their arthritis that appears to exceed that expected from the degree of inflammation.

Bacterial Endocarditis (Uncommon). Arthralgias, arthritis, and myalgias occur in about 30 percent of patients with subacute bacterial endocarditis.[99] The joint symptoms are usually in one or several joints, usually large proximal ones. It is probable that this synovitis is caused by circulating immune complexes.[100] Fever out of proportion to joint findings in the setting of leukocytosis should lead to consideration of infective endocarditis as a diagnostic possibility, even in the absence of a significant heart murmur. It is wise to obtain blood cultures in all patients with polyarthritis and significant fever. Embolic phenomena with constitutional symptoms, including arthralgias, can be presenting symptoms of atrial myxoma, but this process usually mimics systemic vasculitis or subacute bacterial endocarditis more than it does RA.[101]

Calcific Periarthritis (Uncommon). Although usually involving single joints, calcific periarthritis can be confused occasionally with polyarthritis.[106] The skin is red over and around the affected joints and the tissues are boggy and tender, but no joint effusion is present. Passive motion is easier than active motion. Periarticular calcification is visible on radiographs. Unless the periarthritis can be differentiated from true arthritis the findings may mimic palindromic rheumatism or early monarticular RA.

Calcium Pyrophosphate Dihydrate Deposition Disease (Common). CPPD disease is a crystal-induced synovitis that has many different forms (see Chapter 77), ranging from a syndrome of indolent osteoarthrosis to that of an acute, hot joint. About 5 percent of patients have a chronic polyarthritis (sometimes referred to as pseudo-RA) associated with proliferative erosions at subchondral bone.[102] Although radiographs are of great help when chondrocalcinosis is present, CPPD deposition may be present in the absence of calcification on radiographs.[103] Diagnosis then can be made only by ar-

throcentesis. One of the radiographic signs of CPPD deposition that helps differentiate it from RA is the presence of unicompartmental disease in the wrists.

Chronic Fatigue Syndrome (Common). Although numerous physicians prefer to separate chronic fatigue syndrome from fibromyalgia because of the possibility that it is caused by a slow virus infection (e.g., Epstein-Barr virus), there is such a great overlap between the two that the best approach is to consider both as forms of generalized rheumatism and to approach management in the same way. The finding of true synovitis essentially rules out the diagnosis of either chronic fatigue syndrome (perhaps caused by hypomagnesemia) or fibromyalgia (see Chapter 29).

Congenital Camptodactyly and Arthropathy (Rare).[107] Congenital deformities that begin in utero, and camptodactyly and arthropathy produce synovial cell hypertrophy and hyperplasia without inflammatory cells. Clinical manifestations include contractures of the fingers, flattening of the metacarpals, and short, thick femoral necks. This can present as oligoarticular seronegative RA.

Diffuse Connective Tissue Disease: Systemic Lupus Erythematosus, Scleroderma, Dermatomyositis and Polymyositis, Vasculitis, Mixed Connective Tissue Disease (Common). These entities, all discussed in depth in other chapters, may begin with a syndrome of mild systemic symptoms and minimal polyarthritis involving the PIP and MCP joints. It is not uncommon for one of these illnesses, diagnosed at one point in time, to evolve into another as years go by. The following list contains rules of thumb for characterizing joint disease of the various entities:

1. In SLE (see Chapter 61), an organized synovitis that causes erosion is rare. Soft tissue and muscle inflammation may lead to dislocation of normal tendon alignment, resulting in ulnar deviation similar to Jaccoud's arthropathy.

2. Limitation of joint motion in scleroderma (see Chapter 66) is almost always due to taut skin bound to underlying fascia. The same considerations hold for dermatomyositis and polymyositis; proliferative synovitis is rarely sustained in these processes.

3. In reports of mixed connective tissue disease (MCTD; i.e., patients with arthralgias, arthritis, hand swelling, sclerodactyly, Raynaud's phenomenon, esophageal hypomotility, and myositis with circulating antibody to ribonucleoprotein), 60 to 70 percent have arthritis (see Chapter 63). Few have significant titers in serum of RF. Many are given an initial diagnosis of RA. Numerous studies of MCTD have shown deforming, erosive arthritis. In one series, for example, eight of 17 patients had presentation similar to that of RA.[104] Articular and periarticular osteopenia alone was found in eight. Six had loss of joint space, and five had erosions typical of RA.

Familial Mediterranean Fever (Uncommon). The articular syndrome in familial Mediterranean fever is an episodic monarthritis or oligoarthritis of the large joints that appears in childhood or adolescence, mimicking oligoarthritic forms of JRA.[108] Episodes of arthritis come on acutely with fever and all cardinal signs of inflammation and can precede other manifestations of the disease. Although usually self-limited (days to weeks), attacks occasionally last for months and are associated with radiographic changes of periarticular osteopenia without erosions. The abdominal pain these patients experience can be a key to diagnosis.

Fibromyalgia (Common). Fibromyalgia (fibrositis) should not be confused with RA because in fibromyalgia there is rarely evidence of synovitis (see Chapter 29). Although no specific diagnostic tests define fibrositis, certain recurrent nonarticular locations for pain are seen in different patients (see Chapter 29). In an analysis of the pain properties[109] compared with those of RA, patients with fibromyalgia used diverse modifiers to describe their pain, the most common being pricking, pressing, shooting, gnawing, cramping, splitting, and crushing. Most patients in both groups defined the pain as aching and exhausting. Evidence is accumulating that patients with RA may develop a superimposed fibromyalgia. Rheumatoid patients have fewer psychologic disturbances than patients with primary fibrositis, but patients with both syndromes score higher on testing scales for hypochondriasis, depression, and hysteria than those with RA who do not have fibrositis. Disease severity in patients with RA and in those with both fibrositis and RA is similar.[110]

Glucocorticoid Withdrawal Syndrome (Common). Often confused with RA are the symptoms of glucocorticoid withdrawal. These patients, treated for nonrheumatic diseases, may have diffuse polyarticular pain, particularly in the hands, if the glucocorticoid dose is tapered too rapidly. Although glucocorticoids suppress inflammation and pain, there is an arthropathy associated with their use[111] that resembles avascular necrosis.

Gout (Common). Before a diagnosis of chronic erosive RA is made, chronic tophaceous gout must be ruled out (see Chapter 76). The reverse applies as well. Features of gouty arthritis that mimic those of RA include polyarthritis, symmetric involvement, fusiform swelling of joints, subcutaneous nodules, and subacute presentation of attacks. Conversely, certain aspects of RA that suggest gouty arthritis include hyperuricemia (after treatment with low doses of aspirin), periarticular nodules, and seronegative disease (particularly in men).[112] Radiographic findings may be similar, with appearance of the subcortical erosion of RA resembling small osseous tophi in gout.[113] Although large asymmetric erosions with ballooning of the cortex are more likely to be gout than RA, this is not always the case.[114] Serologic test results may be misleading as well; RF has been found in as many as 30 percent of patients with chronic tophaceous gout,[115] and these patients have had no clinical or radiographic signs of RA.

The coexistence of RA and gout is rare and curiously so. Only ten cases of gout coexisting with RA have been reported in the medical literature since 1881, even though more than 10,000 cases could have been anticipated considering the combined prevalence of the two diseases. Wallace and associates have calculated that, considering the prevalence of the two diseases, gout and RA should be anticipated to coexist in 10,617 persons in the United States.[116] In several patients with definite RA and persistent hyperuricemia, flares of the rheumatoid process coincided with normalization of the uric acid level.[117] Several other case reports have noted this, and, as mentioned earlier in the chapter, the possibility that the hyperuricemic state is anti-inflammatory must be investigated further.

Hemochromatosis (Uncommon). The characteristic feature of hemochromatosis that is almost diagnostic is firm bony enlargement of the MCP joints, particularly the second and third, with associated cystic degenerative disease on radiographs and, not infrequently, chondrocalcinosis (see Chapter 84).[118] Marginal erosions, juxta-articular osteoporosis, synovial proliferation, and ulnar deviation are not seen in the arthropathy of hemochromatosis but are common in RA. Wrists, shoulders, elbows, hips, and knees are involved less often than are the MCP joints. More than a third of patients with this iron overload syndrome have arthropathies.[119]

Hemoglobinopathies (Uncommon). In homozygous (SS) sickle cell disease, the most common arthropathy is associated with crises and is believed to be a result of microvascular occlusion in articular tissues or to gout (see Chapter 91).[120] However, in some cases, a destructive arthritis with loss of articular cartilage has been defined,[121] and this resembles severe RA. In most patients with sickle cell disease and joint complaints, periosteal elevation, bone infarcts, fishmouth vertebrae, and avascular necrosis can be found on radiographs.[120] In a series of 37 patients with SS disease from which those with gout or avascular necrosis of the femoral head were excluded, 12 complained of monarthritis or oligoarthritis associated with painful crises; tenderness was most marked over the epiphyses rather than the joint space, and synovial fluid was noninflammatory. Another 12 patients had arthritis of the ankle associated with a malleolar ulcer; this arthritis was chronic and resolved with improvement of the leg ulcer.[122] Episodic polyarthritis and noninflammatory synovial effusions are also found in sickle cell or β-thalassemia.[123]

Hemophilic Arthropathy (Uncommon). A deficiency of factor VIII or, less frequently, factor IX sufficient to produce clinical bleeding frequently results in hemarthroses. The iron overload in the joint generates a proliferative synovitis that often leads to joint destruction. The clotting abnormality rarely is overlooked, however, and it is unlikely that a diagnosis of RA would be made in the setting of hemophilia A or B (see Chapter 90).

Hyperlipoproteinemia (Uncommon). Achilles

tendinitis and tenosynovitis in familial hyperlipoproteinemia can be presenting symptoms in this affliction and may be accompanied by arthritis.[124] Synovial fluid findings may resemble those of mild RA, and the tendon xanthomas may be mistaken for rheumatoid nodules or gouty tophi. Similarly, bilateral pseudoxanthomatous rheumatoid nodules have been described.[125] Asymmetric and oligoarticular synovitis has been described in type IV hyperlipoproteinemia.[126] The absence of morning stiffness in the presence of noninflammatory synovial effusion helps rule out RA. The treatment of hyperlipoproteinemia with clofibrate may cause an acute muscular syndrome[127] that resembles myositis or polymyalgia rheumatica more than it does RA.

Hypertrophic Osteoarthropathy (Uncommon). Hypertrophic osteoarthropathy may present as oligoarthritis involving knees, ankles, or wrists (see Chapter 93). The synovial inflammation accompanies periosteal new bone formation that can be seen on radiographs. Correction of the inciting factor (e.g., cure of pneumonia in a child with cystic fibrosis) usually alleviates the synovitis. The synovium is characterized primarily by an increased blood supply and synovial cell proliferation. Little infiltration by mononuclear cells is seen.[128] Pain, which increases when extremities are dependent, is characteristic, although not always present. If clubbing is not present or is not noticed, this entity is easily confused with RA.

Infectious Arthritis (Common). Bacterial sepsis may be superimposed on RA (see later discussion). Viral infections, however, may present as arthritis, with many characteristics of RA (see Chapters 86 to 89). Rubella arthritis occurs more often in adults than in children and often affects small joints of the hands.[129] Lymphocytes predominate in synovial effusions. Synovitis (pain greater than swelling) has occurred after vaccination with rubella vaccine, particularly with canine kidney preparations, which are no longer used.[130]

Arthritis often precedes viral hepatitis and is associated with the presence of circulating hepatitis B surface antigen (HBsAg) and hypocomplementemia.[131] HBsAg has been found in synovial tissues by direct immunofluorescence, supporting the concept that this synovitis is mediated by immune complexes.[132] A relatively acute onset of diffuse polyarthritis with small joint effusions and minimal synovial swelling should prompt the physician to obtain liver function tests in patients with histories of exposure to hepatitis. With the onset of icterus, the arthritis usually resolves, leaving no trace.

Fever, sore throat, and cervical adenopathy followed by symmetric polyarthritis are compatible with infection due to hepatitis B, rubella, adenovirus type 7, echovirus type 9, *Mycoplasma pneumoniae*, or Epstein-Barr virus[133] as well as acute rheumatic fever or adult-onset Still's disease.

Parvovirus infections can resemble RA and are reviewed in Chapter 89 because a chronic polyarthritis resembling RA has been described following serologic proof of parvovirus infection. Usually, the process is self-limited and does not progress to a destructive synovitis.

Intermittent Hydrarthrosis (Common). Intermittent hydrarthrosis is a syndrome of periodic attacks of benign synovitis in one or few joints, usually the knee, beginning in adolescence.[134] The difference between this and oligoarticular JRA or RA is one of degree, not kind. In contrast to palindromic rheumatism, in which acute synovitis often may occur in different joints during successive attacks,[135] the same joint or joints are affected during each attack in intermittent hydrarthrosis.[136] Joint destruction does not occur because there is no proliferative synovitis.

Lyme Disease. Lyme disease can closely simulate RA in adults or children by having an intermittent course with development in chronic synovitis (see Chapter 88).[137] A proliferative, erosive synovitis necessitating synovectomy has evolved in several cases. The proliferative synovium is not different from that of RA.

Malignancy. Direct involvement by cancer of synovium usually presents as a monarthritis (see Chapter 94).[138] However, non-Hodgkin's lymphoma can occur as seronegative polyarthritis without hepatomegaly or lymphadenopathy.[139] In children, acute lymphocytic leukemia can present as a polyarticular arthritis.[140]

Multicentric Reticulohistiocytosis (Rare). Multicentric reticulohistiocytosis (MR) is particularly interesting because it causes severe arthritis mutilans with an opera glass hand (*main en lorgnette*; see Chapter 85).[141] Other causes of arthritis mutilans are RA, psoriatic arthritis, erosive osteoarthritis treated with glucocorticoids and gout (after treatment with allopurinol). The cell that effects damage to tissues is the multinucleate lipid-laden histiocyte, which appears to release degradative enzymes sufficient to destroy connective tissue. Differential characteristics from RA include the following[142]:

1. *Skin manifestations.* In MR, nodules are often widely disseminated and the histology findings are entirely different in rheumatoid nodules.
2. *Joint manifestations.* In MR, DIP joints are frequently and extensively involved.
3. *Radiographic manifestations.* In MR, the joint spaces appear to widen as destruction of subchondral bone occurs faster than cartilage is lost.
4. *Laboratory test results.* In MR, the ESR is often normal despite severe resorptive disease, and RF is not present.

Osteoarthritis (Common). Although osteoarthritis begins as a degeneration of articular cartilage (see Chapter 79) and RA begins as inflammation in the synovium the processes approach each other as the disease progresses. In osteoarthritis, as cartilage deteriorates and joint congruence is altered and stressed, a reactive synovitis often develops. Conversely, as the rheumatoid pannus erodes cartilage,

Table 52–5. FACTORS USEFUL FOR DIFFERENTIATING EARLY RHEUMATOID ARTHRITIS FROM OSTEOARTHROSIS (OSTEOARTHRITIS)

	Rheumatoid Arthritis	Osteoarthritis
Age at onset	Childhood and adults; peak incidence in 6th decade	Increases with age
Predisposing factors	HLA-DR4, DR1	Trauma, congenital abnormalities (e.g., shallow acetabulum)
Symptoms, early	Morning stiffness	Pain increases through the day and with use
Joints involved	MCP joints, wrists, PIP joints most often; DIP joints almost never	DIP joints (Heberden's nodes), weight-bearing joints (hips, knees)
Physical findings	Soft tissue swelling, warmth	Bony osteophytes, minimal soft tissue swelling early
Radiologic findings	Periarticular osteopenia, marginal erosions	Subchondral sclerosis, osteophytes
Laboratory findings	Increased ESR; rheumatoid factor, anemia, leukocytosis	Normal

MCP = metacarpophalangeal; PIP = proximal interphalangeal; DIP = distal interphalangeal; ESR = erythrocyte sedimentation rate.

secondary degenerative changes in bone and cartilage develop. In end stages of both degenerative joint disease and RA, the involved joints appear the same. To differentiate clearly between the two, therefore, the physician must delve into the early history and functional abnormalities of the disease. Factors useful in separating the two processes are listed in Table 52–5.

One overlap condition exists—erosive osteoarthritis. This occurs in middle-aged women (more frequently than in men) and is characterized by inflammatory changes in PIP joints with destruction and functional ankylosis of the joints. The PIP joints can appear red and hot, yet there is almost no synovial proliferation or effusion. Joint swelling is hard, bony tissue, not synovium. The ESR may be slightly elevated, but RF is not found.[143]

Parkinson's Disease (Common). Although the tremor and rigidity of Parkinson's disease are rarely confused with symptoms of RA, patients with Parkinson's disease have a predilection for developing swan-neck deformities of the hands (Fig. 52–1), a phenomenon generally unappreciated by rheumatologists. This abnormality, the pathogenesis of which still is unknown, was first described in 1864.[144]

Pigmented Villondular Synovitis (Rare). Pigmented villondular synovitis is a nonmalignant but proliferative disease of synovial tissue that has many functional characteristics similar to those of RA and usually involves only one joint. The histopathology is characterized by proliferation of histiocytes, multinucleate giant cells, and hemosiderin- and lipid-laden macrophages. Clinically, this is a relatively painless chronic synovitis (most often of the knee), with joint effusions and greatly thickened synovium.[145] Subchondral bone cysts and cartilage erosion may be associated with the bulky tissue. It is not clear whether this should be classified as an inflammation or neoplasm of synovium (see Chapter 98).

Polychondritis (Uncommon). Polychondritis can mimic infectious processes, vasculitis, granulomatous disease, or RA (see Chapter 81). Patients with RA and ocular inflammation (e.g., scleritis) usually have active joint disease before ocular problems develop; the reverse is true in polychondritis. In addition, polychondritis is not associated with RF. The joint disease is usually episodic. Nevertheless, erosions can develop that are similar to those of RA.

Polymyalgia Rheumatica and Giant Cell Arteritis (Common). Although joint radionuclide imaging studies have indicated increased vascular flow in synovium of patients with classic polymyalgia rheumatica, it remains appropriate to exclude polymyalgia rheumatica as a diagnosis if significant synovitis (soft tissue proliferation or effusions) can be detected (see

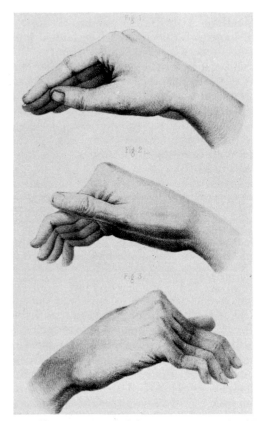

Figure 52–1. These swan-neck deformities are a result of Parkinson's disease, not rheumatoid arthritis. (From Ordenstein, L.: Sur la Paralysie Agitante et la Sclerose en Plaques Generalisee. Paris, Imprimerie de E. Martinet, 1864.)

Chapter 65). Otherwise, many patients who actually have RA would be diagnosed as having polymyalgia rheumatica and treated with potentially harmful doses of glucocorticoids. A careful history usually differentiates shoulder or hip girdle muscle pain from shoulder or hip joint pain. Examination of synovial biopsy specimens from patients with polymyalgia rheumatica indicates that the synovitis is more mild than that found in RA.[146] It is probable that RA and polymyalgia rheumatica coexist in numerous patients, but careful descriptions of such patients are rare.

Several patients have been described whose initial symptom of giant cell arteritis was a peripheral polyarthritis clinically indistinguishable from RA.[147] In 19 such patients found in a group of 522 with biopsy-proven giant cell arteritis, only three were positive for RF. The interval between onset of each set of symptoms was 3 years or less in 15 of the 19, which also suggests a relation between the two.

Rheumatic Fever (Uncommon). Rheumatic fever is much less common than it was previously but still must be considered in adults with polyarthritis (see Chapter 71). In adults, the arthritis is the most prominent clinical finding of rheumatic fever, carditis is less frequent than it is in children, and erythema marginatum, subcutaneous nodules, and chorea are rare.[148, 149] The presentation is often that of an additive, symmetric, large joint polyarthritis (involving lower extremities in 85 percent of patients) developing within a week and associated with a severe tenosynovitis.[148] This extremely painful process is dramatically responsive to salicylates.[148, 150] Unlike Still's disease in the adult, rheumatic fever generally has no remittent or quotidian fevers, has a less protracted course, and shows evidence of antecedent streptococcal infection. There are many similarities between rheumatic fever in adults and "reactive" postinfectious synovitis that develops from infections with *Shigella, Salmonella, Brucella, Neisseria,* or *Yersinia.* These latter processes do not respond well to salicylates, however. As rheumatic fever becomes less frequent, and as penicillin prophylaxis effectively prevents recurrences of the disease, Jaccoud's arthritis (chronic postrheumatic fever arthritis) is becoming rare. This entity, described first by Bywaters in 1950,[151] resulted from severe and repeated bouts of rheumatic fever and synovitis, which stretched joint capsules and produced ulnar deformity of the hands without erosions.[152] The same deformity can develop in SLE characterized by recurrent synovitis and soft tissue inflammation or in Parkinson's disease (see Fig. 52–1). Differentiating rheumatic fever from RA is particularly difficult when subcutaneous nodules associated with rheumatic fever are present.[153]

Sarcoidosis (Uncommon). The two most frequent forms of sarcoid arthritis are usually easily differentiated from RA (see Chapter 83). In the acute form with erythema nodosum and hilar adenopathy, the articular complaints usually are related to periarthritis that affects large joints of the lower extremities. Differential diagnosis may be confused because many of these patients have RF in their sera.[154] Joint erosions and proliferative synovitis do not occur in this form of sarcoidosis.

In chronic sarcoidosis, cystlike areas of bone destruction, mottled rarefaction of bone, and a reticular pattern of bone destruction giving a lacelike appearance on radiographs may simulate destructive RA. This form of sarcoid is often polyarticular, and biopsy of bone or synovium for diagnosis may be essential, particularly because there is often no correlation between joint disease and clinical evidence for sarcoid involvement of other organ systems.[155] It is likely that Poncet's disease, or tuberculous rheumatism,[156] actually represents granulomatous idiopathic arthritis (i.e., sarcoidosis).

Sweet's Syndrome (Rare). Sweet's syndrome, or acute febrile neutrophilic dermatosis,[157, 158] has been described in adults, often after influenza-like illness. The three major features are an acute illness with fever, leukocytosis, and raised painful plaques on the skin that show neutrophilic infiltration of the dermis on biopsy. Joint disease occurs in 20 to 25 percent of cases and is characterized by acute, self-limited polyarthritis. Because of the skin lesions, Sweet's syndrome is confused with SLE, erythema nodosum, and erythema elevatum diutinum more often than with RA. It has been treated effectively with indomethacin[158] and glucocorticoids.

Thiemann's Disease (Rare). Thiemann's disease is a rare form of idiopathic vascular necrosis of the PIP joints of the hands, with occasional involvement of other joints.[159, 160] Bony enlargement begins relatively painlessly, and the digits (one or more may be involved) become fixed in flexion. The primary lesion is in the region of the epiphysis, and the lesion begins most often before puberty, distinguishing it from erosive osteoarthritis, which it resembles radiographically. It is clearly a heritable disease, but the genetic factors have not been defined.

COURSE AND COMPLICATIONS OF ESTABLISHED RHEUMATOID ARTHRITIS

Involvement of Specific Joints: Effects of Disease on Form and Function

When rheumatoid synovitis is established in joints by the sequences outlined in Chapter 51, the effects that the process has on joints are a complex function of the intensity of the underlying disease, its chronicity, and the stress put on individual involved joints by the patient.

Cervical Spine. Unlike other nonsynovial joints, such as the sternomanubrial joint or symphysis pubis, the discovertebral joints in the cervical spine often manifest osteochondral destruction in RA[161, 162] and on lateral radiographs may be found narrowed to less than 5 mm. There is significant pain, but passive range of motion, in the absence of muscle spasm, may be normal. There are two possible mechanisms for this process: (1) extension of the inflammatory process from adjacent neurocentral joints, the joints of Luschka, which are lined by synovium, into the discovertebral area,[161, 162] and (2) chronic cervical instability initiated by apophyseal joint destruction leading to vertebral malalignment or subluxation.[163] This may produce microfractures of the vertebral end-plates, disc herniation, and degeneration of disc cartilage.

The atlantoaxial joint is prone to subluxation in several directions: (1) The atlas moves *anteriorly* on the axis (most common). This results from laxity of the ligaments induced by proliferative synovial tissue developing in adjacent synovial bursa or from fracture or erosion of the odontoid process. (2) The atlas moves *posteriorly* on the axis. This can occur only if the odontoid peg has been fractured from the axis or destroyed. (3) The *vertical* subluxation of the atlas is in relation to the axis (least common). This results from destruction of the lateral atlantoaxial joints or of bone around the foramen magnum. One patient with RA has been described with superior, posterior, and lateral displacement of C1.[164]

The earliest and most common symptom of cervical subluxation is pain radiating up into the occiput.[165] Two other less common clinical patterns include slowly progressive spastic quadriparesis, frequently with painless sensory loss of the hands, and transient episodes of medullary dysfunction associated with vertical penetration of the dens and probable vertebral artery compression.[166] Paresthesias in the shoulders or arms may occur during movement of the head.

Physical findings suggestive of atlantoaxial subluxation include loss of occipitocervical lordosis, resistance to passive spine motion, and abnormal protrusion of the axial arch, felt by the examining finger on the posterior pharyngeal wall. Radiographic views (lateral, with the neck in flexion) should reveal more than 3 mm of separation between the odontoid peg and the axial arch.[166, 167] In symptomatic patients, the films in flexion should be taken only after radiographs (including an open-mouth posteroanterior view) have ruled out an odontoid fracture or severe atlantoaxial subluxation. Studies have indicated that computed tomography (CT) is useful for demonstrating spinal cord compression by loss of posterior subarachnoid space in patients with C1-2 subluxation.[168] Magnetic resonance imaging (MRI) is also valuable in determining pathologic anatomy in this syndrome.[169]

Neurologic symptoms often have little relation to the degree of subluxation and may be related to individual variations in diameter of the spinal canal. Symptoms of spinal cord compression that demand intervention include (1) a sensation of the head falling forward on flexion of the cervical spine; (2) changes in levels of consciousness; (3) "drop" attacks; (4) loss of sphincter control; (5) dysphagia, vertigo, convulsions, hemiplegia, dysarthia, or nystagmus; and (6) peripheral paresthesias without evidence of peripheral nerve disease or compression.[170] Some of these symptoms may be related to compression of the vertebral arteries, which must wind through foramina in the transverse process of C-1 and C-2, rather than to compression of the spinal cord.

The progression of peripheral joint erosions parallels cervical spine disease in RA. The two coincide in severity and timing; development of cervical subluxation is more likely in patients with erosion of the hands and feet.[171]

Is mortality increased in patients with atlantoaxial subluxation? It has been shown in a 5-year follow-up that neurologic signs do not develop inevitably in patients with large subluxations.[172] On the other hand, when signs of cervical cord compression do appear, myelopathy progresses rapidly and half the patients die within a year.[173, 174] In one series of 104 consecutive autopsies of patients with RA, 11 cases of severe dislocation were found.[175] In all 11 cases, the odontoid protruded posterosuperiorly and impinged on the medulla within the foramen magnum. In five, spinal cord compression was determined to be the only cause of death. These patients are at risk during even small falls, whiplash injuries, and general anesthesia with intubation. Cervical collars should be prescribed for stability. Operative stabilization may be considered if symptoms are progressive. In a series of 84 patients with some form of subluxation but without cord or brainstem lesions, one fourth worsened and one fourth improved without surgery over 5 to 14 years of follow-up.[176] Using survival tables, it was concluded that nonsymptomatic cervical luxations do not significantly shorten life in patients with RA. In most series, fewer than 20 percent of patients with RA exhibited C1-2 disease.

Vertical atlantoaxial subluxation is important, although less common. It was noted in one study in 13 of 476 (3.7 percent) hospitalized patients with RA.[177] Symptoms associated with this collapse of the lateral support system of the atlas occur in patients with severe erosive disease. Neurologic findings have included decreased sensation in the distribution of cranial nerve V and sensory loss in the C2 area, nystagmus, and pyramidal lesions. Vertical subluxations are believed to have a worse prognosis than the other varieties.[178]

Bywaters has demonstrated bursal spaces between the cervical interspinous processes in autopsies of patients without joint disease; in patients with rheumatoid disease, bursal proliferation led in several cases to radiographically demonstrated destruction of the spinous processes.[179]

MRI is particularly valuable in assessment of cervical spine disease in RA because the spinal cord as well as bone can be visualized. Breedveld and coworkers showed that soft tissue swelling around the odontoid and loss of subarachnoid space are demonstrated particularly well by MRI.[169] Symptoms and signs consistent with cervical cord compression were confirmed by MRI. It is probable that MRI will make myelography unnecessary and redundant in this clinical situation, even when surgery is being planned.

Thoracic, Lumbar, and Sacral Spine. The thoracic, lumbar, and sacral portions of the spine usually are spared in RA, and symptoms there rarely can be traced to a rheumatoid process. The exceptions are the apophyseal joints; rarely, synovial cysts at the apophyseal joint can impinge as an epidural mass on the spinal cord causing pain or neurologic deficits.[180]

Temporomandibular Joints. The temporomandibular joints (TMJs) are commonly involved in RA. Careful history revealed that 55 percent of patients had jaw symptoms at some time during the course of their disease.[181] Radiographic examination revealed structural alterations in 78 percent of the joints examined. An overbite may develop[182] as the mandibular condyle and the corresponding surface of the temporal bone, the eminentia articularis, are eroded. Physical examination of the patient with rheumatoid disease should include palpation for tenderness and auscultation for crepitus. Occasional patients have acute pain and are unable to close the mouth, necessitating intra-articular glucocorticoids to suppress the acute process. It is important to remember that TMJ abnormalities are common in nonrheumatoid populations. The only specific findings for RA in the TMJ are erosions and cysts of the mandibular condyle detected by CT, and there is no correlation between clinical and CT findings of TMJ in RA.[183]

Cricoarytenoid Joints. The cricoarytenoid joints are small diarthrodial joints that have an important function; they rotate with the vocal cords as they abduct and adduct to vary pitch and tone of the voice. Careful history may reveal hoarseness in up to 30 percent of patients with rheumatoid disease.[184] This is not disabling in itself, but there is a danger that the cricoarytenoid joints may become inflamed and immobilized, with the vocal cords adducted to the midline, causing inspiratory stridor.[185] Autopsy examinations have demonstrated cricoarytenoid arthritis in almost half the patients with RA, suggesting that much significant disease of the larynx may be asymptomatic.[186] This is borne out by the finding that, although CT scans detected laryngeal abnormalities in 54 percent of patients with moderately severe RA, no symptoms predicted these abnormalities.[187] In contrast, findings with indirect laryngoscopy, which detected mucosal and gross functional abnormalities, were abnormal in 32 percent of the same patients and correlated with symptoms of sore throat and difficulty during inspiration. It follows that indirect laryngoscopy should be performed in patients with RA who are chronically hoarse or have intermittent stridor. It should be noted also that symptomatic rheumatoid nodules within the vocal cord itself, mimicking laryngeal carcinoma, have been described. Asymptomatic cricoarytenoid synovitis may occasionally lead to aspiration of pharyngeal contents, particularly at night.

Ossicles of the Ear. Many patients with rheumatoid disease experience a decrease in hearing. In general, this has been ascribed to salicylate toxicity, and it is believed to be reversible when the drug is discontinued (see Chapter 41). On the other hand, conductive hearing loss in patients not taking salicylates was reported by Copeman.[188] Studies using otoadmittance measurements have been carried out in patients with RA in an attempt to determine whether the interossicle joints were involved.[189] The data showed that 38 percent of "rheumatoid ears" and 8 percent of controls demonstrated a pattern characteristic of an increase in the flacidity of a clinically normal tympanic membrane. This is consistent with erosions and shortening of the ossicles produced by the erosive synovitis, not with ankylosis.

Sternoclavicular and Manubriosternal Joints. The sternoclavicular and manubriosternal joints, both possessing synovium and a large cartilaginous disc, are often involved in RA.[190] Because of their relative immobility, there are few symptoms. Patients occasionally complain of pain in sternoclavicular joints while lying on their sides in bed. When symptoms do occur, the physician must be concerned about superimposed sepsis. CT may be a useful technique for careful delineation of the sternoclavicular joint. Manubriosternal involvement is almost never clinically important, although by tomographic criteria it is common in RA.[191] Some patients develop manubriosternal joint subluxation. This deformity may be associated with cervical spine disease; in one study of ten patients with manubriosternal subluxation, eight had radiographic evidence of significant atlantoaxial subluxation.[192]

Shoulder. RA of the shoulder not only affects synovium within the glenohumeral joint but also involves the distal third of the clavicle, various bursae and the rotator cuff, and multiple muscles around the neck and chest wall.

One of the most important principles of rehabilitation (see Chapter 105) is that joint pain causes decreased mobility of joints and that decreased mobility quickly leads to muscle weakness and atrophy. Rheumatoid involvement of the shoulder often can be detected by an examination that demands effort from various muscle groups.

In recent years, it has been appreciated that involvement of the rotator cuff in RA is a principal cause of morbidity. The function of the rotator cuff is to stabilize the humeral head in the glenoid. Weakness of the cuff results in superior subluxation. Rotator cuff tears or insufficiency for other reasons can be demonstrated by shoulder arthrogram. In a series of 200 consecutive patients with RA studied by arthrography, 42 (21 percent) had rotator cuff tears and an additional 48 (24 percent) had evidence of fraying of tendons.[193] One likely mechanism for tears is that the rotator cuff tendon insertion into the greater tuberosity is vulnerable to erosion by the proliferative synovitis that develops there.[194] Previous injury and aging may predispose to the development of tears.[195] Sudden tears may be accompanied by pain and inflammation so great as to suggest sepsis.

Standard radiographic examinations of the shoulder in RA reveal erosions (69 percent) and superior subluxation (31 percent).[196] In addition to showing tears of the rotator cuff, arthrograms can demonstrate (1) diffuse nodular filling defects, (2) irregular capsular attachment, (3) bursal filling defects, (4) adhesive capsulitis, and (5) dilation of the biceps tendon sheath (perhaps unique to RA).[197] High-resolution CT may provide much of this information without invasive techniques, and MRI should provide even more precision in delineating abnormalities of the soft tissues. Marked soft tissue swelling of the anterolateral aspect of the shoulders in RA may be caused by chronic subacromial bursitis rather than by glenohumeral joint effusions.[198] In contrast to rotator cuff tears, bursal swelling is not necessarily associated with decreased range of motion or pain. Synovial proliferation within the subdeltoid bursa may explain resorption of the undersurface of the distal clavicle seen in this disease.[199] Rarely, the shoulder joint may rupture, causing symptoms that resemble those of obstruction of venous return from the arm.[200]

Elbow. Perhaps because it is a stable hinge joint, severe pain in the elbow rarely is manifest in RA. Nevertheless, involvement of the elbow is common, and if lateral stability at the elbow is lost as the disease progresses, disability can be severe.

The frequency of elbow involvement varies from 20 to 65 percent, depending on the severity of disease in the patient populations studied. The relatively low prevalence shown in Table 52–4 is in contrast with the 67 percent involvement found in another study.[201] One of the earliest findings, often unnoticed by the patient, is loss of full extension. Because the elbow is primarily a connecting joint between the hand and trunk, the shoulder and wrists can compensate for the loss of elbow motion.[202] For example, pronation of the arm normally mediated at the radioulnar joint at the elbow can be assisted 45 to 50 degrees by abducting the shoulder, and shoulder elevation and wrist flexion can be substituted for flexion at the elbow.

Wrist and Hand. The wrist and hand should be considered together because they form a functional unit. There are data, for example, linking disease of the wrist to ulnar deviation of the MCP joints[203, 204]; the hypothesis is that weakening of the extensor carpi ulnaris muscle leads to radial deviation of the wrist as the carpal bones rotate (the proximal row in an ulnar direction, the distal ones in a radial direction).[203] Ulnar deviation of the fingers (a zigzag deformity) occurs in response to this to keep the tendons to the phalanges in a normal line with the radius. (Fig. 52–2). Other factors, including the tendency for power grasp to pull the fingers into an ulnar attitude[205] and inappropriate intrinsic muscle action,[206] are probably involved as well[207–211] (Fig. 52–3). Erosion of bone or articular cartilage is not essential for development of ulnar deviation. Significant although reducible ulnar deviation can result from repeated synovitis or muscle weakness in the hands (e.g., in SLE).

Dorsal swelling on the wrist within the tendon sheaths of the extensor muscles is one of the earliest signs of disease. Typically, the extensor carpi ulnaris and extensor digitorum communis sheaths are involved. Rarely, cystic structures resembling ganglia are early findings of RA.[212, 213]

As the synovial proliferation develops within the wrist, pressure increases within the relatively nondistensible joint spaces. Proliferative synovium develops enzymatic machinery sufficient to destroy ligaments, tendons, and the articular disc distal to the ulnar head. Pressure and enzymes combine to produce communications among radiocarpal, radioulnar, and midcarpal joints in about 70 percent of

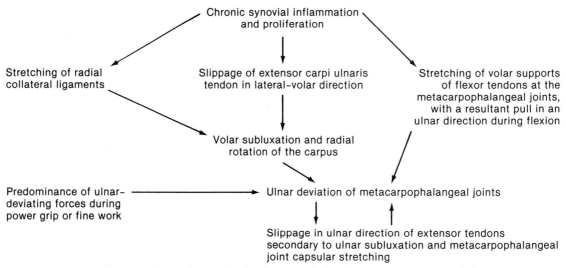

Figure 52–2. A sequence of pathology in the development of ulnar deviation at metacarpophalangeal joints.

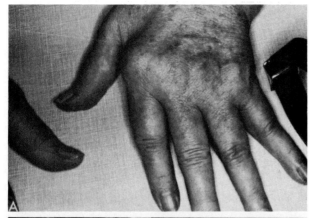

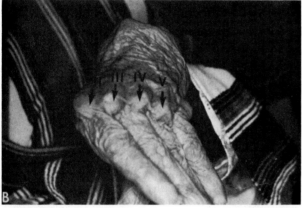

Figure 52–3. *A,* Early ulnar deviation of the metacarpophalangeal joints without subluxation. Extensor tendons have slipped to the ulnar side. The fifth finger, in particular, is compromised with weak flexion, causing loss of power grip. *B,* Complete subluxation with marked ulnar deviation at the metacarpophalangeal joints of a 90-year-old woman with RA. Arrows mark the heads of the metacarpals, now in direct contact with the joint capsule instead of the proximal phalanges. (Courtesy of James L. McGuire, M. D.)

patients with RA compared with 15 percent of control persons.[214] Integrity of the distal radioulnar joint is lost; the ulnar collateral ligament, stretched by the proliferative synovium of the radioulnar joint, finally either ruptures or is destroyed; and the ulnar head springs up into dorsal prominence, where it floats and can easily be depressed by the examiner's fingers.

On the volar side of the wrist, synovial protrusion cysts develop; they can be palpated, and their origins can be confirmed by arthrography.[215] The thick transverse carpal ligament prevents significant resistance to decompression, however, and compression of the median nerve by hyperplastic synovium can cause carpal tunnel syndrome (see Chapter 101).

A common site for bone erosion by proliferative synovitis in the wrist is at the periphery of the joint where no protective cartilage is found.[216] Enzymes and pressure may be synergistic in producing fracture, and osseous and cartilaginous debris may accumulate in the joint spaces.[217] Irregular bone edges from which fragments have been separated may

serve as weapons to erode tendons already weakened and attenuated by action of proteinases.

Progression of disease in the wrist is characterized by loss of joint space and loss of bone. This foreshortening of the carpus has been quantitated as a carpal to metacarpal (C:MC) ratio (length of the carpus divided by that of the third metacarpal). There is a linear decrease in the C:MC ratio with progressive disease[218] (Fig. 52–4). This is caused by compaction of bone at the radiolunate, lunate–capitate, and capitate–third metacarpal joints, which usually accompanies severe disease. One study has confirmed the usefulness of the C:MC ratio for quantitating joint destruction and making correlations with anatomic progression over time.[219] Early detection of carpal bone involvement by RA is possible using magnetic resonance imaging. Although too expensive for routine use, MRI has been found to be superior to standard radiographs in two respects: (1) synovial proliferation can be demonstrated, and (2) carpal bone erosions are detectable earlier.[220]

The hand often has many joints involved in RA. A sensitive index of hand involvement is grip strength. The act of squeezing brings stress on all hand joints. Muscular contraction causes ligamentous tightening around joints, compressing inflamed synovium. The immediate result is weakness, with or without pain; the reflex inhibition of muscular contraction due to pain may be a primary factor in this weakness. Quantitative radiographic scores for joint space narrowing, erosion, and malalignment correlate well with loss of motion but do not correlate with joint count tenderness scores[221]; these data support the concept that inflammatory synovitis and the erosive and destructive potential of proliferative synovitis in RA are not one and the same, but rather reflect different aspects of the same disease.

The *swan-neck deformity* is one of flexion of the DIP and MCP joints, with hyperextension of the PIP joint. The lesion probably begins with shortening of the interosseous muscles and tendons. Shortening of the intrinsic muscles exerts tension on the dorsal tendon sheath, leading to hyperextension of the PIP joint[222] (Fig. 52–5). Deep tendon contracture or, rarely, DIP joint involvement with RA leads to the DIP joint flexion.[223] Rupture of the sublimis tendon, which would reduce capacity to flex the PIP joint, can lead to the same deformity.[224]

If, during chronic inflammation of a PIP joint, the extensor hood stretches or is avulsed, the PIP joint may pop up in flexion, producing *a boutonnière deformity* (Fig. 52–6).[208, 224] The DIP joint remains in hyperextension. Without either of these deformities, limitation of movement develops at the PIP and DIP joints. Limitation of full flexion of the DIP joint is common in RA and represents incomplete profundus contraction. Similarly, tight intrinsic muscles may prevent full flexion of PIP joints when the MCP joints are in full extension.

The most serious result of rheumatoid involvement of the hand is resorptive arthropathy, defined

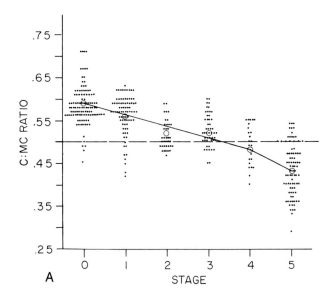

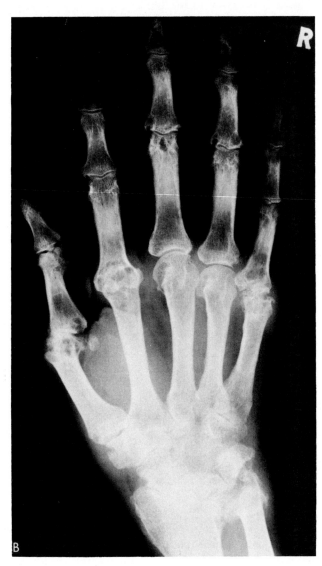

Figure 52–4. *A,* The carpal:metacarpal ratio in relation to radiographic state of disease in 390 hand films of 73 female RA patients. (From Trentham, D. E., and Masi, A. T.: Carpo:metacarpal ratio. A new quantitative measure of radiologic progression of wrist involvement in rheumatoid arthritis. Arthritis Rheum. 19:939, 1976.) *B,* Radiograph of the right wrist of a 42-year-old woman with RA. The carpal-metacarpal index (see text) is 4.28, significantly below the lower limit of normal, consistent with destructive synovitis in the wrist, particularly in the radiocarpal joint. Despite severe disease this patient has developed no ulnar deviation at the metacarpophalangeal joints.

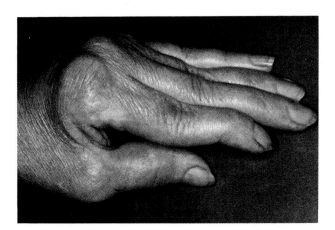

Figure 52–5. Early swan-neck deformity in rheumatoid arthritis. Synovial proliferation and early subluxation of the metacarpophalangeal joints are present as well. (Courtesy of G. Uribarri and the Ministerio de Sanidad y Consuma, Madrid, Spain.)

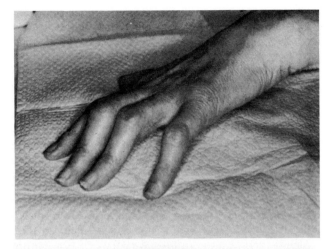

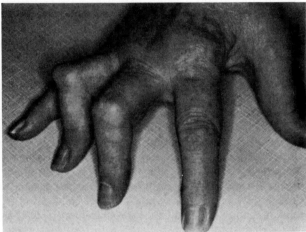

Figure 52–6. Early (*Top*) and late (*Bottom*) "boutonnière" deformity of the phalanges in RA. *Bottom,* Moderate soft tissue swellings at the second and third MCP joints are visible.

as severe resorption of bone that begins at the articular cartilage and spreads along the diaphysis of the involved phalanges. Digits appear shortened, excess skin folds are present, and phalanges can be retracted (telescoped) into one another and then pulled out into abnormally long extension, often without pain. In one study of more than 250 patients, resorptive arthropathy confirmed by radiographs was present in 5.1 percent of patients.[225]

Nalebuff's classification of thumb disease in RA gives a sequence of functional problems with this joint.[226] Three types of deformity have been described. In type I, MCP inflammation leads to stretching of the joint capsule and a boutonnière-like deformity. In type II, inflammation of the carpometacarpal joint leads to volar subluxation during contracture of the adductor hallucis. In type III, after prolonged disease of both MCP joints, exaggerated adduction of the first metacarpus, flexion of the MCP joint, and hyperextension of the DIP joint result from the patient's need to provide a means to pinch.

One of the most common manifestations of RA in hands is tenosynovitis in flexor tendon sheaths.

This is manifested on the volar surfaces of the phalanges as diffuse swelling between joints or a palpable grating within flexor tendon sheaths in the palm. In one series, hand flexor tenosynovitis was observed in 55 of 100 patients with RA,[227] a higher frequency than found in other studies and probably related more to careful examination than to any difference in population or disease. Although hand flexor tenosynovitis was not associated with more prolonged or severe disease, there was an association with a number of para-articular manifestations (distinct from extra-articular manifestations).[228] It is particularly important to diagnose *de Quervain's tenosynovitis* because it causes severe discomfort and yet is relatively easily treated; it represents tenosynovitis in the extensors of the thumb. Pain originating from these sheaths can be demonstrated by Finklestein's test: ulnar flexion at the wrist after the thumb is maximally flexed and adducted. Many factors may lead to loss of hand strength in patients with RA (Table 52–6). Tenosynovitis, rather than articular synovitis, is probably the most significant of these.[229]

Not infrequently, rheumatoid nodules develop on the tendons that may lock the finger painfully into flexion, necessitating surgical excision or glucocorticoid injections when they become chronic and recurrent. If flexor tenosynovitis reduces active motion, peritendinous and pericapsular adhesions result and limit PIP joint motion.[229]

Hands can be painful in RA without much evidence of inflammation. It has been suggested that ischemia caused by vascular spasm from excess sympathetic tone may contribute to hand pain, particularly during grasp motion.[230]

The DIP joints have less synovial membrane than the PIP joints; perhaps because of this and of lower intra-articular temperatures protecting them, DIP joints are less often involved in the RA. However, in one study using DIP joints as a primary focus, radiographic abnormalities (surface erosions and joint space narrowing) were observed in 23 (37 percent) of 62 RA patients and only in 9 (14 percent) of control patients. The DIP joint changes were not related to duration or overall severity of the RA.[231]

Hip. The hip is less frequently involved early in adult forms of RA than in JRA. Hip joint involvement must be ascertained by a careful clinical examination. Pain on the lateral aspect of the hip is often a

Table 52–6. FACTORS DIMINISHING HAND GRASP STRENGTH IN RHEUMATOID ARTHRITIS

Synovitis in joints
Reflex inhibition of muscular contraction secondary to pain
Altered kinesiology; distorted relation of joint, bones, and tendons during motion
Flexor tenosynovitis, with or without rheumatoid nodules on tendons
Vascular ischemia leading to pain; from altered sympathetic tone
Edema of all structures, from inflammation and perhaps altered lymphatic drainage
Intrinsic muscle atrophy or fibrosis

Table 52–7. DIFFERENTIAL DIAGNOSIS OF
POPLITEAL CYSTS

Lipoma	Hemangioma
Xanthoma	Lymphadenopathy
Fibrosarcoma	Charcot joint
Vascular tumor	Thrombophlebitis
Varicose veins	

manifestation of trochanteric bursitis rather than of synovitis. True hip joint involvement usually produces pain or tenderness in the groin or the lower buttock.

About half of the patients with established RA have radiographic evidence of hip disease.[232] The femoral head may collapse and be reabsorbed, while the acetabulum often remodels as it is pushed medially, leading to protrusio acetabuli. Significant protrusion occurs in about 5 percent of all patients with RA.[233] Loss of internal rotation on physical examination correlates best with radiographic findings. Similar to the situation in other weight-bearing joints, the femoral head may develop cystic lesions. Communication of these with the joint space can often be demonstrated on surgically resected femoral heads.[234]

Synovial cysts can develop around the hip joint. Communication between the iliopsoas bursa and the hip joint can facilitate formation of a cyst that appears within the pelvis and that can be large enough to obstruct venous return from the extremity.[235]

Knees. In contrast with the hips, synovial inflammation and proliferation in the knees are readily demonstrated. Synovial fluid in excess of 5 ml may be demonstrated by the bulge sign—milking fluid from the lateral superior recess of the joint across to the medial side and producing a fluid wave across the normally concave area inferomedial to the patella.[236] Early in knee disease, often within a week after onset of symptoms, quadriceps atrophy is noticeable and leads to the application of more force than usual through the patella to the femoral surface. Another early manifestation of knee disease in RA is loss of full extension, a functional loss that can become a fixed flexion contracture unless corrective measures are undertaken.[237]

Flexion of the knee markedly increases the intra-articular pressure (see Chapter 54) and may produce an outpouching of posterior components of the joint space, a popliteal or Baker's cyst. Jayson and Dixon have demonstrated that fluid from the anterior compartments of the knee may enter the popliteal portion but does not readily return.[238] This one-way valve may produce pressures so high in the popliteal space that it may rupture down into the calf or, rarely, superiorly into the posterior thigh. Rupture occurs posteriorly between the medial head of the gastrocnemius and the tendinous insertion of the biceps. Clinically, popliteal cysts and complications of them have several manifestations (Table 52–7). The intact popliteal cyst may compress superficial venous flow to the upper part of the leg, producing dilation of superficial veins or edema.[239] Rupture of the joint posteriorly with dissection of joint fluid into the calf may resemble acute thrombophlebitis with swelling and tenderness, as well as systemic signs of fever and leukocytosis.[240, 241] One helpful sign in identifying joint rupture may be the appearance of a crescentic hematoma beneath one of the malleoli.[242] Part of the examination of patients with rheumatoid disease should be observation from the rear while the patient stands. Although arthrography clearly defines the abnormal anatomy of a Baker's cyst, this invasive procedure has been replaced by ultrasound[243] and, when necessary, MRI.

It has been well documented that high-resolution MRI accurately portrays the gross state of articular cartilage in the knee, including its precise thickness, erosions or thinning, and irregularities.[244] Were it not prohibitively expensive, MRI could provide an objective, quantitative, and noninvasive assessment in vivo of the state of cartilage in patients with rheumatoid disease.

Ankle and Foot. The ankle rarely is involved in mild or oligoarticular RA but often is damaged in severe progressive forms of the disease. Clinical evidence for ankle involvement is a cystic swelling anterior and posterior to the malleoli. Much of the stability of the ankle depends on the integrity of the ligaments holding the fibula to the tibia and these two bones of the talus. In RA, inflammatory and proliferative disease may loosen these connections by stretching and eroding the collagenous ligaments. The result is incongruity, which, once initiated, progresses to pronation deformities and eversion of the foot (Fig. 52–7).

The Achilles tendon is a major structural component and kinetic force in the foot and ankle. Rheumatoid nodules develop in this collagenous structure, and spontaneous rupture of the tendon has been reported when diffuse granulomatous inflammation is present.[245] The subtalar joint controls eversion and inversion of the foot on the talus; patients with RA invariably have more pain while walking on uneven ground, and this is related to the relatively common subtalar joint involvement in RA.[246]

Computed tomography is particularly useful for definition of hindfoot abnormalities in RA. Use of this technique allows depiction of the structures in the coronal plane. In particular, an increased heel valgus angulation, flattening of the sustentaculum tali, and medial or downward slippage of the talar head have been noted.[247]

More than one third of patients with RA have significant disease in the feet.[248] Metatarsophalangeal (MTP) joints are involved often, and gait is altered as pain develops during push-off in striding. It is of interest that downward subluxation of the metatarsal heads occurs soon after the MTP joints become involved, producing cock-up toe deformities. Hallux valgus and bunion or callus formation occurs if disease continues. Cystic collections representing

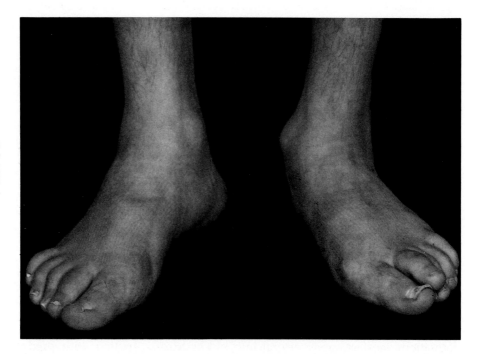

Figure 52–7. Valgus of ankle, pes planus, and forefoot varus deformity of the left foot related to painful synovitis of the ankle, forefoot, and metatarsophalangeal joint in a 24-year-old man with severe RA.

outpouchings of flexor tendon sheaths often develop under the MTP joints.[249] Patients with subluxation of metatarsal heads to the subcutaneous area may develop pressure necrosis. Alternatively, patients who have subluxation of MTP joints often develop pressure necrosis over the PIP joints that protrude dorsally (hammer toes).

The sequence of changes as disease progresses in the foot is as follows[250, 251]: (1) intermetatarsal joint ligaments stretch; (2) spread of the forefoot occurs; (3) the fibrofatty cushion on the plantar surface migrates anteriorly; (4) there is subluxation of toes dorsally, and extensor tendons shorten; (5) subluxation of metatarsal heads to a subcutaneous site on the plantar surface occurs; and (6) development of hallux valgus often results in stacking of the second and third toes on top of the great toe. DIP joints of the foot rarely are affected in RA.

Another cause of foot pain in patients with rheumatoid disease is the tarsal tunnel syndrome. In a group of 30 patients with RA, radiographically demonstrated erosions in the feet, and foot pain, four (13 percent) were shown by electrodiagnostic techniques to have slowing of medial or lateral plantar nerve latency.[252] Clinically, these patients are difficult to distinguish from those with foot pain but without compression neuropathy (see Chapter 101).

Involvement of the Skeleton

The skeleton has two anatomically and functionally separate components—cortical and trabecular bone—that respond differently to systemic and local diseases and to drugs (see Chapters 4 and 92). There are three questions about bones that are of great interest to those studying and caring for patients with rheumatoid arthritis: Does RA produce a generalized osteopenia? What are the influences of sex and age on the skeleton in patients with RA? What are the effects of low-dose glucocorticoids on bone in RA and, if deleterious, can they be prevented or treated?

Two patterns of osteopenia are observed in RA— periarticular and diffuse. There is abundant evidence that the periarticular (juxta-articular) resorption reflects local production of prostaglandins of the E series, induced by tumor necrosis factor (TNF), and interleukin 1 (IL-1), that stimulate local bone resorption[253] (these are discussed in Chapter 51).

Patients with RA who never have had steroid treatment differ from control populations in having biochemical evidence for an increase in the metabolic activity of bone. This is especially true in postmenopausal women with RA who have higher serum phosphorus, alkaline phosphatase, osteocalcin, and urinary hydroxyproline[254] levels and a reduced peripheral bone mineral content at the radius.[255] Postmenopausal patients with RA have more significantly reduced levels of estrone and testosterone as well as femoral bone mineral density than do postmenopausal control patients.[256]

This diffuse loss of bone leads to the high incidence of stress fractures of long bones in RA.[257, 258] The fibula is the most common fracture site. Acute leg pain in the thin, elderly, rheumatoid patient, even without a history of trauma, should generate suspicion of a stress fracture. Geodes (i.e., subchondral cysts developed by synovial penetration of the cortex or subchondral plate and subsequent proliferation) produce weak bone and can predispose to fracture, even in phalanges.[259]

Most reports of osteoporotic fracture incidence in RA have been anecdotal. One study using a control population compared the estimated incidence of osteoporotic fractures among RA patients with that in the general population[260]: 388 female patients in Rochester, Minnesota, who developed RA between 1950 and 1974 were observed for 4902 person-years. Relative risks for fracture at various sites were pelvis, 2.6; proximal femur, 1.51; and proximal humerus and distal forearm, not statistically significantly different from controls. Vertebral fracture incidence in the control population could not be estimated accurately in this study. These authors concluded that, given the higher risk of fractures associated with increased age, disability and impaired ambulation, and thinness, RA itself need not be involved as an independent variable with power to generate fractures. Danish investigators reached similar conclusions in a study of more than 100 patients with RA not treated with glucocorticoids.[261] In addition to measuring bone mineral content using single-photon absorptiometry, these investigators looked at serum alkaline phosphatase and serum bone gamma-carboxyglutamic acid–containing protein as indicators of bone formation, and fasting urinary calcium and hydroxyproline as markers of bone resorption. Their data showed a correlation among increased bone turnover, decreased bone mineral content, and the degree of functional impairment (rather than the duration of disease) of patients with RA.

The histologic type of bone disease in RA is almost always osteoporosis (a decrease in bone mass with normal mineralization) rather than osteomalacia (decreased mineralization of matrix). In a study of 45 patients with RA and 41 with osteoarthritis who had had bone biopsies, about a quarter of all patients showed osteoporosis but only one (a patient with osteoarthritis) had evidence of osteomalacia.[262] It is probable that previous reports of vitamin D deficiency and osteopenia in some RA patients[257] and of hypercalcemia in others[263] were related to abnormal nutrition in patients selected and not to generalizable abnormalities in the rheumatoid population worldwide.

Radiographic studies of axial bone mass must be discounted as insensitive; results vary widely depending on technique. The same criticism can be applied to single-photon absorptiometry. Direct measurement of bone density at axial sites is possibly only by CT or dual-photon absorptiometry. Using the latter technique as a measure of bone mineral density in 104 controls and 111 patients with RA had revealed decreases of bone mass in both the lumbar spine and the femoral neck of patients with RA. Physical activity and multiparity protected against bone loss in women of all ages with RA. Interestingly, glucocorticoid therapy (up to 8 mg of prednisolone equivalents per day) in women was *not* associated with accelerated bone loss, although the male patients taking glucocorticoids (more than 10 mg of prednisolone equivalents per day) had significantly less bone mineral density than did male patients not taking glucocorticoids.[264]

Studies of the interrelations of glucocorticoid therapy and the premenopausal and postmenopausal state in RA patients have revealed contrasts in data. A Danish study incorporating dual-photon absorptiometry found significantly lower bone mineral content and total body bone mineral in premenopausal glucocorticoid-treated women compared with penicillamine-treated women, but it found no difference between the same treatment groups in postmenopausal women.[265] In contrast, Nagant de Deuxchaisnes and associates used single-photon absorptiometry and found decreased radial bone mineral density in postmenopausal but not in premenopausal women taking low-dose glucocorticoids.[266]

Data also are contradictory about whether low-dose glucocorticoid treatment predisposes patients with RA to develop fracture. In one study, although there were insignificant differences in bone mineral content of spines of glucocorticoid-treated and untreated patients with RA, there was a significantly higher incidence of fracture in the steroid-treated patients.[267] In another, 44 rheumatoid patients treated with prednisone (mean dose, 8.0 ± 0.5 mg per day) for 9 to 12 months were compared with 40 similar patients with RA not given glucocorticoids.[268] There were no significant differences between the two groups in either bone mineral density or the radiologic evidence of vertebral fractures.

In summary, there have been so many different methods to study the effect of RA and glucocorticoids on bone, and so many influences on bone other than these two variables (e.g., age, disease duration, disability, and sex hormone status), that the degree to which low-dose glucocorticoids adversely affect the skeleton in RA is not definitely known. It seems wise to encourage optimal nutrition in these patients and maximal activity levels. If low doses of glucocorticoids can help patients walk more and stay in bed less, the deleterious effects on bone of these low doses probably are cancelled out by the beneficial effects of activity on bone structure. Structural modifications of prednisolone, such as deflazacort, that have fewer effects on calcium absorption or bone metabolism than the parent compound should be considered in patients at higher risk for fracture and osteoporosis.[269] Calcium and vitamin D supplements and a liberal and timely use of estrogen replacement in menopausal rheumatoid patients are indicated as well.

Muscle Involvement

Clinical weakness is common in RA, but is it caused by muscle involvement in the rheumatoid inflammation or is it a reflex weakness response to pain? Most rheumatoid patients have muscle weakness, but few have muscle tenderness. An exception to this is the occasional patient with a severe flare of activity disease; such a patient may cry out in severe pain, unable to move either muscles or joints. These symptoms resemble those of vascular insufficiency (ischemic pain) in their intensity.

In an early autopsy series, focal accumulations of lymphocytes and plasma cells with some contiguous degeneration of muscle fibers was found in all rheumatoid patients and named *nodular myositis*.[270] More recent studies have pointed to at least five different stages of muscle disease in RA[271, 272]: (1) diminution of muscle bulk with atrophy of type II fibers; (2) peripheral neuromyopathy, usually due to mononeuritis multiplex; (3) steroid myopathy; (4) active myositis and muscle necrosis with foci of endomysial mononuclear cell infiltration; and (5) chronic myopathy resembling a dystrophic process, probably the end stage of inflammatory myositis. Atrophy of type II fibers is most common. Active myositis and focal necrosis is not seen in patients with inactive disease but is commonly noted on biopsy specimens of patients with active disease, particularly in an interesting subset with mild synovitis and a disproportionately high ESR.[272] To emphasize the systemic nature of RA, the lymphocytes in muscle biopsy specimens have been shown in some patients to synthesize IgM rheumatic factor. Thus, the nodules of myositis contain plasma cells as well as lymphocytes. Unlike polymyositis or dermatomyositis, myositis in RA is patchy, and the weakness experienced by these patients responds readily to low-dose prednisone.

EXTRA-ARTICULAR COMPLICATIONS OF RHEUMATOID ARTHRITIS

The complications of RA may be fatal. In general, the number and severity of extra-articular features vary with the duration and severity[273, 274] of the disease.

Ocular and dermatologic complications are not considered in detail here; they are presented in the context of other manifestations in those organ systems in Chapters 32 and 33, respectively. Nerve compression syndromes commonly seen in RA are outlined in Chapter 101.

Rheumatoid Nodules

The pathologic findings in rheumatoid nodules are well documented.[275, 276] In the well-formed nodule, there is a central area of necrosis rimmed by a corona of palisading fibroblasts that is surrounded by a collagenous capsule with perivascular collections of chronic inflammatory cells (see Chapter 51).

Careful histologic study of early lesions[277] has suggested that development of the nodule is mediated through affected small arterioles and the terminal vascular bed of tissues; small vessels proliferate, and this is associated with proliferation of resident histiocytes and fibroblasts, as well as an influx of macrophages from circulation. Palmer and

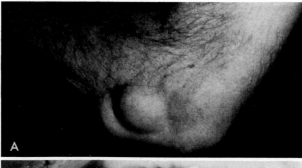
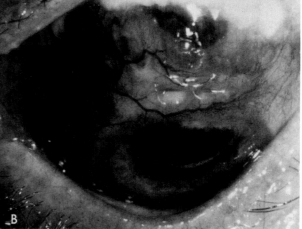

Figure 52–8. Manifestations of increased reactivity of mesenchymal tissue in rheumatoid arthritis appearing (*A*) as nodules on the elbow and (*B*) within the sclera of the eye. The eye lesion represents scleral perforation associated with a granulomatous scleral reaction. Treatment was placement of a scleral patch graft. Note the increase in vascularity of the sclera. The dark areas represent scleral thinning with exposure of uveal pigment. (Patient of Drs. S. Arthur Bouchoff and G. N. Fouhls. Photograph courtesy of Marty Schener.)

colleagues, using monoclonal antibodies against receptors for C3b and C3bi, monocytes, activated macrophages, and HLA-DR molecules, have presented data to suggest that mononuclear phagocytes constantly being recruited into the peripheral layers then migrate into the palisade layer and make up most of the cell population in this area.[278] The nodule tissue in organ culture has the capacity to produce collagenase and protease in large quantity, similar to synovial tissue.[279] It has been suggested that these enzymes released by the palisading layer of cells may be sufficient to result in destruction of the extracellular matrix collagen around the cells, leading to their death and a centrifugally expanding central necrosis commonly found in these nodules.

Occurring in 20 to 35 percent of patients with definite or classic RA, nodules are found most easily on extensor surfaces such as the olecranon process and the proximal ulna (Fig. 52–8*A*). They are subcutaneous and vary in consistency from a soft, amorphous, entirely mobile mass to firm rubber masses attached firmly to periosteum.

Rheumatoid factor is almost always found in the serum of patients with rheumatoid nodules. Rarely, such nodules are present without obvious arthritis.[280] Multiple nodules on the hands and a positive test for RF associated with episodes of acute intermittent synovitis and subchondral cystic lesions of small bones of the hands and feet has been called *rheumatoid nodulosis*.[281, 282]

The *differential diagnosis* of rheumatoid nodules includes the following:

1. *Benign nodules*. These usually are found in healthy children without RF or arthritis. They are nontender; appear often on the pretibial regions, feet, and scalp; increase rapidly in size; and are histologically identical to rheumatoid nodules.[283] They usually resolve spontaneously, although in one case classic RA developed 50 years after the first appearance of benign olecranon nodules.[284]

2. *Granuloma annulare*. These nodules are intracutaneous but histologically identical to rheumatoid nodules. They slowly resolve and are not associated with other disease.[285]

3. *Xanthomatosis*. These nodules usually have a yellow tinge, and patients have abnormally high plasma lipoprotein and cholesterol levels. There is no underlying bone involvement.[286]

4. *Tophi*. These collections of monosodium urate crystals in patients with gout are associated with small, punched-out bone lesions and are rarely found in patients with a normal serum urate concentration. A search for crystals with a polarizing microscope reveals the classic needle-shaped, negatively birefringent crystals.

5. *Miscellaneous nodules*. The nodules of multicentric reticulohistiocytosis were described earlier. Numerous proliferative disorders affecting cutaneous tissue—including erythema elevatum diutinum, acrodermatitis chronica atrophicans, bejel, yaws, pinta, and leprosy—can resemble rheumatoid nodules. A rheumatoid nodule, particularly when it occurs on the face, may simulate basal cell carcinoma.[287]

Appearance of nodules in unusual sites may lead to confusion in diagnosis. Sacral nodules may be mistaken for bedsores if the overlying skin breaks down.[288] Occipital nodules also occur in bedridden patients. In the larynx, rheumatoid nodules on the vocal cords may cause progressive hoarseness.[289] Nodules found in the heart and lungs are discussed later. A nodule in the eye is shown in Figure 52–8B. There have been at least 14 reports of rheumatoid nodule formation within the CNS,[290] involving leptomeninges more than parenchyma. Occasional patients develop rheumatoid nodules within vertebral bodies, resulting in bone destruction and signs of myelopathy.[291]

Fistula Development

Cutaneous sinuses near joints develop rarely in seropositive patients with long-standing disease and positive tests for RF.[292] These fistulas can be either sterile or septic and connect the skin surface with a joint, with a para-articular cyst in bone or soft tissues,[293] or with a bursa.[294] The pathogenesis of fistulas without a septic origin is particularly difficult to understand, because the rheumatoid process usually is so clearly centripetal in nature (i.e., progressing toward the center of the joint), rather than having a centrifugal orientation.

Infection

Neither before nor after onset of joint disease has a higher frequency of genitourinary or bronchopulmonary infections been reported in rheumatoid patients than in osteoarthritic patients.[295] Thus, the increased mortality in RA from infection appears related to factors that evolve during the course (and treatment) of the disease and not to any predisposition to infection. Incidence of infections as a complication of RA has paralleled the use of glucocorticoids and immunosuppressive agents.[296] Pulmonary infections, skin sepsis, and pyarthrosis are most common.[297, 298] In addition to the presence of drugs that suppress host resistance, the phagocytic capacity of leukocytes in RA may be less than normal.[299] Difficulty in diagnosis is accentuated by the similarity of aggressive RA to infection, particularly in joints.

Hematologic Abnormalities

Most patients with RA have mild normocytic hypochromic anemia that correlates with the ESR elevation and with activity of the disease.[300, 301]

Anemia is often of mixed causes in RA. One deficiency may mask evidence for others, resulting in ineffective therapy. In a recent European series of 25 patients, iron deficiency (assessed by bone marrow iron content) was present in 52 percent, vitamin B_{12} deficiency in 29 percent, and folate deficiency in 21 percent.[302] All are likely to have had anemia of chronic disease. The following guidelines may be helpful in sorting out anemia in rheumatoid patients:

1. Anemia of chronic disease has significantly higher serum ferritin concentration than does iron deficiency.

2. Folate and vitamin B_{12} deficiency may mask iron deficiency by increasing the mean cell volume and mean cell hemoglobin of erythrocytes.

3. The ESR correlates inversely with hemoglobin in RA, as expected in anemia of chronic disease.[303]

4. Erythropoietin levels are elevated more in patients with iron deficiency anemia than in those with the anemia of chronic disease who also have a diminished response to erythropoietin.[302]

In patients with the anemia of chronic disease, total erythroid heme turnover is slightly reduced, and ineffective erythropoiesis accounts for a much higher than normal percentage of total heme turnover.[304-306] These patients also may demonstrate a diminished ability to absorb iron through the gastrointestinal tract, usually related to the irritative presence of one or another anti-inflammatory medications.[307] In contrast with anemia associated with blood loss, the ineffective erythropoiesis returns to normal if remission can be induced in RA.[308] Red blood cell aplasia, immunologically mediated, is a rare finding in RA. However, because erythropoiesis in animals has been shown to depend on T lymphocytes, it is logical to search for immunologic factors that can induce anemia in RA. Serum from RA patients profoundly suppresses erythroid colony formation,[309] but T lymphocytes from bone marrow of patients with rheumatoid disease have not been shown to inhibit erythroid development in vitro as do T cells from certain patients with aplastic anemia or pure red blood cell aplasia.[310]

Eosinophilia and *thrombocytosis* are often associated with RA. Eosinophilia (at least 5 percent of total leukocytes) was observed in 40 percent of patients with severe seropositive disease.[311] Similarly, a significant relation exists between thrombocytosis and extra-articular manifestations of rheumatoid disease[312] and disease activity.[313]

An interesting subset of patients with RA have increased numbers of large granular lymphocytes in the peripheral blood, bone marrow, and liver. The lymphocytes contain many azurophilic granules in the cytoplasm and may account for more than 90 percent of mononuclear cells in blood. The cells are E-rosette positive, are Fc-receptor positive, do not produce IL-2, respond poorly to mitogens, and have antibody-dependent cell-mediated cytotoxicity activity but little or no natural killer cell activity.[314] Of previously described patients with large granular lymphocyte proliferation, almost one quarter have had RA.

Vasculitis

In one sense, it is redundant to think of vasculitis as a complication of RA, since the initial pathologic change in RA is believed to rest in small blood vessels (see Chapters 51 and 64). However, it is useful to use the term *vasculitis* to group those extra-articular complications related not to proliferative granulomas but rather to inflammatory vascular disease.

Clinical vasculitis usually takes one of the following forms: (1) distal arteritis (ranging from splinter hemorrhages to gangrene); (2) cutaneous ulceration (including pyoderma gangrenosum); (3) peripheral neuropathy; (4) pericarditis; (5) arteritis of viscera, including heart, lungs, bowel, kidney, liver, spleen, pancreas, lymph nodes, and testis; (6) acro-osteolysis; or (7) palpable purpura.

The pathologic findings in rheumatoid vasculitis is that of panarteritis. All layers of the vessel wall are infiltrated with mononuclear cells. Fibrinoid necrosis is seen in active lesions. Intimal proliferation may predispose to thrombosis. Obliterative endarteritis of the finger is one of the most frequent manifestations of vasculitis, and immune complex deposits have been demonstrated in those vessels.[315, 316] When larger vessels are involved, the pathologic changes resemble those of polyarteritis nodosa.[317] In addition, a venulitis associated with RA has been described.[318, 319] In patients with hypocomplementemia, the cellular infiltrate around the vessels contains neutrophils; in normocomplementemic patients, lymphocytes predominate. Uninvolved skin from rheumatoid patients is positive for IgG and complement when sections for histopathology are stained with fluorescein-labeled antibodies to these components. The presence of IgG correlates directly with circulating immune complexes, vasculitic skin lesions, subcutaneous nodules, and a high titer of RF.[320]

It is unusual for vasculitis to be active in any but the sickest patients—those with severe deforming arthritis and high titers of RF; this subgroup represents less than 1 percent of patients with RA. Although RA is more common in women than in men, vasculitis is seen more often in men with RA. Supporting the hypothesis that vascular injury is mediated by deposition of circulating immune complexes are (1) depressed levels of C2 and C4[321]; (2) hypercatabolism of C3[322]; (3) deposition of IgG, IgM, and C3 in involved arteries[323]; and (4) the presence of large amounts of cryoimmunoglobulin in the sera of patients with vasculitis.[324]

Neurovascular disease may be the only manifestation of vasculitis. The two common clinical patterns are a mild distal sensory neuropathy and a severe sensorimotor neuropathy (mononeuritis multiplex).[325] The latter form is characterized by severe arterial damage on nerve biopsy specimens. Symptoms of the milder form may be paresthesias, or "burning feet," in association with decreased touch and pain sensation distally. Patients with mononeuritis multiplex have weakness (e.g., foot drop) in addition to sensory abnormalities. Symptoms and signs are identical to those found in polyarteritis. Rheumatoid pachymeningitis is a rare complication of RA. Confined to the dura and pia mater, this process may be limited to certain areas (e.g., lumbar cord or cisternae).[326] Elevated levels of IgG (including IgM and IgG RF and low-molecular-weight IgM) and immune complexes are found in the cerebrospinal fluid. Although there is a possible negative association between psychosis and RA, organic brain syndromes may be related to RA in patients not taking glucocorticoids or indomethacin,[327] and it is presumed that these manifestations are caused by small-vessel disease.

Visceral lesions occur generally as claudication or infarction of the organ supplied by the involved arteries. Intestinal involvement with vasculitis presents as abdominal pain, at first intermittent, progressing often to continuous pain and a tender, quiet belly on examination. If infarction develops, resection must be accomplished promptly.[328] A sudden reduction or cessation of glucocorticoid therapy also has been implicated as a causative factor in vasculitis[329]; a large study done subsequently, however, showed no relation between steroid dose and vasculitis.[330] The presence of gangrene of digits and extremities, the development of intestinal lesions with bleeding or perforation, cardiac or renal involvement, and mononeuritis multiplex indicate extensive vasculitis and are associated with a poor prognosis.[331, 332]

Renal Disease

The kidney is an example of an organ that is rarely involved directly in RA but often is compromised indirectly. Amyloidosis (see Chapter 82) is a complication of chronic RA and particularly of Still's disease. Another indirect cause of renal disease is toxicity from therapy. Phenacetin abuse causes renal papillary necrosis, and salicylates and other NSAIDs may cause abnormalities as well.[333] A membranous nephropathy is the pathologic lesion related to therapy with gold salts and D-penicillamine, but a long-term study has suggested that perhaps membranous nephropathy is related to the underlying disease and that gold treatment may exacerbate the underlying process.[334] Rarely, a focal necrotizing glomerulitis is seen in patients dying with disseminated vasculitis.[335] Hematuria has been evaluated in 24 patients with RA.[336] Three had local urologic problems, but 14 had a mild mesangial glomerulonephritis. Fortunately, this lesion does not appear to be a cause of impaired glomerular function. Its true prevalence is not known.

Pulmonary Disease

There are at least six forms of lung disease in RA: (1) pleural disease, (2) interstitial fibrosis, (3) nodular lung disease, (4) pneumonitis, (5) arteritis, and (6) airways disease.

Pleural Disease. Pleuritis is commonly found at autopsy of patients with RA, but clinical disease during life is seen less frequently.[337] Characteristics of the rheumatoid effusions are as follows: glucose, 10 to 50 mg per dl; protein, more than 4 g per dl; cells, 100 to 3500 (mononuclear) per mm^3; elevated lactic dehydrogenase; and depressed CH_{50}. The low glucose concentrations are of interest. Sepsis (particularly tuberculosis) is the only other condition that commonly has such a low pleural fluid glucose level. Impaired transport of glucose into the pleural space appears to be the cause.[338]

Interstitial Fibrosis. The increased reactivity of mesenchymal cells in RA is believed to be the cause of pulmonary fibrosis in interstitial fibrosis. Similar to findings in scleroderma, physical findings are of fine, diffuse, dry rales. Radiographs show a diffuse reticular (interstitial) or reticulonodular pattern in both lung fields[339, 340]; these progress to a honeycomb appearance on plain radiographs and a characteristic lattice net shown on high-resolution CT. The pathologic findings are those of diffuse fibrosis in the midst of a mononuclear cell infiltrate.[339] The principal functional defect is impairment of alveolocapillary gas exchange with decreased diffusion capacity, best measured using single-breath carbon monoxide diffusion capacities.[341, 342] It is likely that patients with RA who smoke are at a higher risk for fibrotic complications in the lungs than are those in the general population. It has been reported that bronchoalveolar lavage may reveal increased numbers of lymphocytes, even in those with only mildly abnormal chest radiographs and normal pulmonary function test results.[343]

Nodular Lung Disease. Pulmonary nodules may appear singly or in clusters that coalesce. Single ones appear as a coin lesion and, when significant peripheral arthritis and nodules are present, can be diagnosed by needle biopsy without thoracotomy. Caplan's syndrome,[344] in which pneumoconiosis and RA are synergistic and produce a violent fibroblastic reaction with obliterative granulomatous fibrosis, is a rare occurrence since the respiratory environment in mining operations has improved. Nodules may cavitate and create a bronchopleural fistula[345] and may precede arthritis.[346] In several cases, solitary pulmonary nodules in patients with RA have proved to be rheumatoid nodules and a coexistent bronchogenic carcinoma,[347] a finding that suggests caution in interpreting benign results from fine-needle aspiration biopsy in such patients.

Pneumonitis. A rare finding is an interstitial pneumonitis that progresses to alveolar involvement, respiratory insufficiency, and death. Pathologic studies show a cellular loose fibrosis and proteinaceous exudate in alveoli (Fig. 52–9).

Arteritis. Pulmonary hypertension from arteritis of the pulmonary vasculature is rare and is occasionally associated with digital arteritis.[348]

Airways Disease. Defined by a reduced maximal midexpiratory flow rate and maximal expiratory flow rate at 50 percent of functional vital capacity, small-airways disease was observed in 15 (50 percent) of 30 RA patients, compared with 22 percent of a control population.[349] The study was adjusted for pulmonary infections, α_1-antitrypsin deficiency, penicillamine treatment, environmental pollution, and smoking. Other investigations have not found small-airways dysfunction in RA and have suggested that, if it is present, it probably is related to factors other than RA.[350] If real, this phenomenon may be part of a generalized exocrinopathic process in the disease, expressed most flagrantly, of course, in Sjögren's syndrome.

Cardiac Complications

Cardiac disease in RA can take many forms related to granulomatous proliferation or vasculitis.

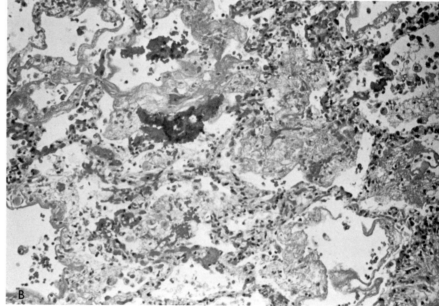

Figure 52–9. Severe, subacute interstitial pneumonitis in RA. This complication proved fatal in 5 weeks in this 66-year-old woman with severe, active seropositive RA. *A,* The gross photograph of the left lung shows dense interalveolar thickening by a fibrofibrinous exudate. Air sacs are becoming obliterated. Lungs were heavy and incompressible, but there was only a trace of excess fluid. *B,* Microscopic sections showed thickened alveo lar septa with a rich fibrinous exudate present. (Courtesy of Charles Faulkner, III, M. D.)

Involvement can be classified as follows: (1) pericarditis, (2) myocarditis (rheumatoid carditis), (3) endocardial (valve) inflammation, (4) conduction defects, (5) coronary arteritis, and (6) granulomatous aortitis. Advances in echocardiography have made diagnosis of pericarditis and endocardial inflammation easier and more specific.[351] Myocardial biopsy through vascular catheters has facilitated diagnosis and classification of myocarditis.

Pericarditis. Infrequently diagnosed by history and physical examination in RA, pericarditis is present in up to half of patients at autopsy.[352, 353] In one study, 31 percent of patients with RA had echocardiographic evidence of pericardial effusion. The same study revealed only rare evidence of impaired left ventricular function in prospectively studied outpatients with RA.[354] Although unusual, cardiac tamponade with constrictive pericarditis develops in RA and may require pericardectomy.[355, 356] Most patients test positively for RF, and half have nodules.

Myocarditis. Myocarditis can take the form of either granulomatous disease or interstitial myocarditis. The granulomatous process resembles subcutaneous nodules and could be considered specific for the disease. Diffuse infiltration of the myocardium by mononuclear cells, on the other hand, may involve the entire myocardium and yet have no clinical manifestations.[353]

Endocardial Inflammation. Echocardiographic studies have reported evidence of previously unrecognized mitral valve disease diagnosed by a reduced E to F slope of the anterior leaflet of the mitral valve.[357, 358] Although aortic valve disease and arthritis are generally associated through ankylosing spondylitis, a number of granulomatous nodules in the valve have been reported.[359]

Conduction Defects. Atrioventricular block is unusual in RA but is probably related to direct granulomatous involvement. Pathologic examination may reveal proliferative lesions[360, 361] or healed scars.[362] Complete heart block has been described in more than 30 patients with RA. It generally occurs in patients with established erosive nodular disease.[362] It usually is permanent and is caused by rheumatoid granulomas in or near the atrioventricular node or bundle of His. Rarely, amyloidosis is responsible for heart block.

Coronary Arteritis. Patients with severe RA and active vasculitis who develop a myocardial infarction are likely to have coronary arteritis as a basis for the process.[363]

Granulomatous Aortitis. In severe rheumatoid heart disease, granulomatous disease can spread to involve even the base of the aorta.[364]

PROGNOSIS

Natural History

Epidemiologists have pointed out the multiple difficulties in attempting to establish change in patterns of RA in different time periods or different communities. The best data suggest that patients admitted to the hospital for RA today are likely to have fewer joint contractures and less ankylosis of peripheral joints at admission than did patients admitted 20 years ago, whereas the prevalence of RF and subcutaneous nodules, and the mean number of affected joints have, if anything, increased slightly.[365] These and other findings suggest that the disease is not changing, but that earlier, more effective treatment has perhaps diminished the morbidity. As with other chronic diseases, both physicians and patients are eager to know the chances for remission and are anxious about the threat of severe morbidity or death.

There are now well-tested criteria for a clinical remission.[366] Six have yielded optimal discrimination (see Table 52–8). Few patients achieve five of these six criteria. Most fail to achieve a true remission. Using these criteria in an analysis of 450 patients with RA observed prospectively for 6 years, 81 (18 percent) had at least one remission.[367] In the aggregate, the remission periods occupied 35 percent of the duration of follow-up of those entering remission; the mean length of the remission was 10 months. Being male or developing RA after age 60 years increased chances of remission. Early development of erosions decreased chances for remission. Not definitively determined by this study is whether drug treatment increases the likelihood of developing remission.

In well-established RA, however, median life expectancy is less than in control populations.[368] In one study, a 25-year prospective follow-up of 208 patients, median life expectancy was shortened by 7 years in males and 3 years in females.[369] Infection, renal disease, and respiratory failure are the primary contributory factors to excess mortality in RA patients.[370] A more recent study revealed that in 100 patients with RA observed for 25 years, 63 had died—an excess mortality of approximately 40 percent.[371]

The challenge to rheumatologists is to predict which patients will do well and which will not. In an attempt to identify initial factors that might predict subsequent disability, 39 potentially predictive vari-

Table 52–8. CRITERIA FOR COMPLETE CLINICAL REMISSION IN RHEUMATOID ARTHRITIS (RA)

A minimum of five of the following requirements must be fulfilled for at least 2 consecutive months in a patient with definite or classic RA*:
1. Morning stiffness not to exceed 15 minutes
2. No fatigue
3. No joint pain
4. No joint tenderness or pain on motion
5. No soft tissue swelling in joints or tendon sheaths
6. Erythrocyte sedimentation rate (Westergren's) less than 30 mm/hr (females) or 20 mm/hr (males)

Exclusions: Clinical manifestations of active vasculitis, pericarditis, pleuritis, myositis, or unexplained recent weight loss or fever secondary to RA prohibit a designation of complete clinical remission.

Data from Pinals, R. S., Masi, A. F., et al.: Preliminary criteria for clinical remission in rheumatoid arthritis. Arthritis Rheum. 24:1308, 1981.

ables were studied over 11.9 years in 681 consecutive patients[372] who had been diagnosed as having definite or classic RA. Initially, 48 percent were without disability; at the end of the study, this had declined to 17 percent. Similarly, although only 3 percent were completely disabled at onset of the study, this number had increased to 16 percent by the conclusion. Disability developed most rapidly during the first 2 years of the disease and progressed slowly in subsequent years, especially in older women with decreased function. Absent from the list of valuable predictors were factors previously thought to correlate with disease outcome; thus, there was no evidence that disease with an acute, explosive onset had a better prognosis.[372, 373] The reason that patients with large proximal joint involvement do worse than those with disease limited to hands[58] may be related to the larger area of these involved joints; the correlation of surface area of involved joints with the C-reactive protein and of C-reactive protein with joint destruction may give a basis for this observation.

Death associated with RA generally is due to the complications (both articular and extra-articular) of RA and to side effects of therapy. The probability of death varies directly with the severity of complications. Such potentially morbid articular complications include the various forms of atlantoaxial subluxation, cricoarytenoid synovitis, and sepsis of involved joints. Extra-articular complications directly causing a higher mortality include Felty's syndrome, Sjögren's syndrome, cardiopulmonary complications, diffuse vasculitis, gastrointestinal complications of therapy, amyloidosis, and infection.[374–376]

One of the largest and best documented studies of survival, prognosis, and causes of death in patients with RA was published by Mitchell and associates.[377] In this prospective study in which 805 patients completed 12 years of observation, 233 died during the course of the study; survivorship was only half that in population controls. As reinforced by other studies,[378] the increased mortality associated with RA is impressive and equals that of all patients with Hodgkin's disease, diabetes mellitus, and stroke (when age adjusted). In another group of 107 patients observed for 8 years, each of whom had extra-articular disease or who needed hospitalization for some aspect of their disease,[379] those with cutaneous ulcers, vasculitic rash, neuropathy and scleritis had a higher mortality than those whose disease was confined to joints. Of great concern to all health care workers is the correlation of lack of formal education with increased mortality in RA.[378, 380] Total mortality from cancer does not appear to differ between patients with RA and control patients, although more patients with RA die of lymphoma than do control patients.[381]

Variables Related to Prognosis

Rheumatoid Factor. Many studies have confirmed that seropositivity is associated with a poorer prognosis in RA. One series of 60 patients with active disease showed this association.[382] Patients with RF have more involved joints when they visit a physician for the first time and develop more erosions and ligamentous instability.[383, 384] As mentioned, increasing numbers of individuals with the diagnosis of seronegative RA[385] are being recognized as having other classifiable entities.

Of all the RF isotypes, IgA RF correlates best with ESR and grip strength, and its presence may indicate patients likely to develop aggressive, erosive disease.[386]

Rheumatoid Nodules. Rheumatoid nodules occur almost always in patients with RF, although without correlation with titer of RF.[374, 383, 384] Therefore, similar to those patients with RF alone, patients with subcutaneous nodules have a poorer outcome and more frequent bone erosions.[374, 387, 388]

Sex. In young adults who develop RA, women generally have a worse outcome with more swollen and tender joints and erosions than do men.[383]

Synovial Histopathology. Although it is generally agreed that persistence and intensity of synovial inflammation are related to joint destruction, no single feature or group of features demonstrable by routine histopathologic examinations of synovium have been correlated with destructive lesions in RA.[389, 390] In part, this may be related to the major histologic variations found from area to area within the synovium.[391] A finding of cartilage erosion associated with synovial lining cell proliferation and few subsynovial lymphocytes[392] has not been confirmed.[389, 390] The finding of meniscal cartilage erosions using MRI may be the earliest sign of potentially destructive disease of articular cartilage of the knee (see Chapter 37).

Synovial Fluid Analysis. Chemotactic factors in synovial fluid in RA attract PMNs, which accumulate and eventually are lysed within the joint space (see Chapter 36). It has been demonstrated that, when the joint fluid leukocyte count exceeds 50,000 to 60,000 per mm³, protease inhibitors in the fluid can be saturated or inhibitors can be damaged or rendered effete, so that protease activity is manifest.[393] It is probable that at times such as these, proteases (e.g., collagenase and stromelysin) act unopposed on cartilage components. Acidosis of synovial fluid correlates with leukocyte counts in synovial fluid[394] and with radiographic evidence for joint destruction.[395] Depression of glucose and complement components in synovial fluid can be roughly correlated with the intensity of inflammation in the fluid and levels of IgG with the degree of subsynovial lymphocyte accumulation.[396]

Other Laboratory Data. A number of laboratory tests in addition to those for RF have prognostic significance (Table 52–9).

CLASSIFICATION AND ASSESSMENT

The inflammatory lesion in RA is reflected reasonably well by heat, pain, welling, and tenderness.

Table 52–9. LABORATORY TESTS THAT CORRELATE WITH ACTIVE RHEUMATOID ARTHRITIS (RA)
OR A POOR PROGNOSIS

Test	Special Features
Blood IgA rheumatoid factor[386]	Correlates well with grip strength, ESR, and erosive disease
Acidosis of synovial fluid[394, 413]	Correlates with leukocyte count and intensity of synovial inflammation; an insufficient nutritional supply is inferred
IgA-containing immune complexes[386]	Correlates with development of hand and foot erosions
Eosinophilia[311]	Correlates with extra-articular manifestations
Thrombocytosis[312]	Correlates with disease severity and extra-articular manifestations
CRP[414, 415]	Correlates with ESR, erosive disease and joint counts
C1q levels[416]	Increased levels correlated with extent of proliferative synovitis, erosive disease and CRP
NH₂-terminal peptide of type III procollagen in blood[417]	This fragment is cleaved off during fibrillogenesis of collagen; correlated with active and erosive disease
Cryoglobulins elevated in serum[379]	Correlates with extra-articular disease and increased mortality
Precipitating antibodies to soluble cellular antigens[418]	Correlates with extra-articular disease
Serum phospholipase A₂[419] (this enzyme acts upon membrane phospholipids to release arachidonic acid)	Correlates with disease activity using clinical and other laboratory criteria
ESR[414, 415]	Fibrinogen, ceruloplasmin, complement components C3 and C4, α₁-acid glycoprotein, haptoglobin, serum amyloid protein and CRP are the best-studied acute phase reactants and are induced primarily by IL-6
Anti-RA33[418]	RA-33 is a protein antigen from nuclear extracts of HeLa cells and is highly specific for RA, though not sensitive
Synovial fluid: neopterin (a product of guanosine triphosphate metabolism in macrophages)[420]	Increased synovial fluid levels correlated with systemic activity of disease
Urine: hydroxypyridinium cross-links of collagen in urine[421]	Increased urinary excretion in RA patients correlating with ESR, CRP, and the reciprocal of grip strength

ESR = erythrocyte sedimentation rate; CRP = C-reactive protein.

Joint destruction can occur with minimal inflammation, however, and means to assess cartilage destruction are limited to radiographic determination of apparent joint space narrowing and erosions. MRI may, as it evolves, provide a way to visualize pannus development and loss of cartilage (Fig. 52–10), but this procedure is too expensive for routine use.

Whereas the Steinbrocker criteria appear to correlate hand radiographs poorly with functional health status of rheumatoid patients,[397] the more recently developed Larsen grading system[398] appears to be a more sensitive and reproducible index of disease progression.[399] To emphasize that there are differences between the inflammatory and the proliferative and destructive components of RA, Sharp makes a good case for having radiographic assessment incor-

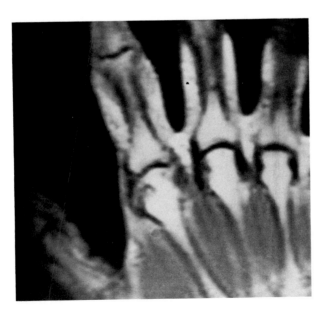

Figure 52–10. Magnetic resonance (MR) image of the right hand of a 35-year-old woman with a 6-year history of RA. Physical examination revealed soft tissue swelling of the metacarpophalangeal joint. Radiographs showed some narrowing of the second metacarpophalangeal joint, without bone erosions. The MR image shows bone in white, articular capsule in black, and pannus as gray mottled areas on the medial portion of the second and third metacarpal heads. (These T₂-weighted [T_R2000 m; T_E34 ms] images are provided courtesy of Reuben Mesrich, M. D., and James Seibold, M. D.)

Table 52–10. ARTICULAR INDICES

Ritchie Articular Index[406]
  (This sums grades of tenderness.)
  Single joints
    Elbows
    Wrists
    Hips
    Knees
    Ankles
    Talocalcaneal joints
    Midtarsal joints
  Units
    Temporomandibular joint
    Cervical spine (assayed by passive motion)
    Sternoclavicular joint
    Acromioclavicular joint
    MCP joint
    PIP joint
    MTP joint
American Rheumatism Association Index[407]
  Clinically active joints are defined as tenderness *and/or* pain, *and/or* soft tissue swelling, of the following joints examined individually or bilaterally:
    Temporomandibular joint
    Sternoclavicular joint
    Acromioclavicular joint
    Shoulder
    IP of the thumb
    Hip
    Knee
    Ankle (mortise)
    Tarsus
    IP of great toe
  And of the following joints as units and bilaterally:

Wrist	1 unit
MCP joints	5 units
PIP and DIP joints of fingers	8 units
MTP joints	5 units
PIP and DIP joints of toes	4 units

Lansbury Articular Index[408–410]
  "Severity of inflammation" for each joint is weighted for joint surface area. Joints examined bilaterally are the same as the ARA index, but the following joints are examined separately:
    Carpometacarpal
    Transverse carpal
    PIP and DIP of toes
    Transverse intertarsal
    Tarsometatarsal
    Talonavicular–calcaneocuboid
    Talocalcaneal

MCP = metacarpophalangeal; PIP = proximal interphalangeal; MTP = metatarsophalangeal; IP = interphalangeal; DIP = distal interphalangeal.

porated into clinical trials of all new drugs developed for treatment of RA.[400]

The availability of computer technology for comparison of articular indices in RA has made objective assessment of these indexes possible. Traditionally, three indices have been used in most studies (Table 52–10).

For office practice, clinical studies, and epidemiologic surveys, a *reduced joint survey* (RJS)[401] was developed as a compromise between laborious redundancy and superficial evaluation. The RJS indexes were developed using statistical and clinical approaches. The data suggested that five chief groupings of joints improved or deteriorated together— MCP joints of hands, interphalangeal joints of the hand, MTP joints of feet, interphalangeal joints of feet, and large joints. The data suggested that RJS indexes can be used reasonably by both the clinician and the researcher in quantifying the status of joint disease in RA.

Computer technology has opened possibilities of comparing great numbers of indexes. The problem has been, however, to determine what standard to measure indexes against. Radiographic and functional indexes over time are affected by factors other than joint inflammation. Thompson and associates make a case for measuring effectiveness of indexes against levels of C-reactive protein,[402] which shows a fast response, short half-life, large incremental change, and a constant catabolic rate (see Chapter 40), and which has been shown to have predictive value for development of erosion. Thompson and coworkers studied 66 combinations of indexes, including the Ritchie, ARA, and Lansbury (see Table 52–9), and found the best correlations with C-reactive protein in an index that is relatively simple to perform. It links joint surface area to joints with *simultaneous* tenderness and swelling that can readily be assessed with three changes from previous indexes:

1. Weighting of the index for surface area of the joint (e.g., PIP = X; wrist = 6X; elbow = 10X; knee = 19X)

2. Requiring that joints identified as inflamed exhibit *simultaneous* tenderness and swelling, not one *or* the other

3. Exclusion of joints difficult to examine for true synovitis (i.e., TMJ, cervical spine, shoulders, and hips)

A sample of this system is shown as Table 52–11. Until better information is available, this method for scoring activity of RA should be considered first for use by clinicians, as well as those planning controlled therapeutic trials.

Classification of RA also can be achieved by functional analysis (Table 52–12).[403] It also is appropriate to correlate functional class with an anatomic radiographic staging system. Functional assays determined by self-report questionnaires issued to patients appear to be cost-effective in assessing and monitoring the status of RA in an individual patient.[404] In evaluating the status of a particular patient, the physician can use, as a rough guide, the radiographic staging system as an index of whether the functional status of that individual is appropriate. For instance, if a functional grade III patient has only grade II radiographic changes, it is likely that aggressive physical therapy and attention to care of nonarticular complications of the disease may improve functional status.

Patients can take an active role in assessing disease activity. A pain scale (see Table 52–12) based on activities of daily living and a visual analogue scale required less than 5 minutes to complete and was simple for patients to fill out.[405] The results correlated moderately well with joint counts and

Table 52–11. WEIGHTED AND SELECTIVE INDEX FOR ACTIVITY OF SYNOVITIS

Joint	Weighted Factor (Related to Joint Surface Area)	Degree of Tenderness *and* Swelling (Scale: 0–3)	Joint Score
Elbow			
R	48	————	————
L	48	————	————
Wrist			
R	32	————	————
L	32	————	————
MCP (separately)			
R	5	————	————
L	5	————	————
PIP (separately)			
R	5	————	————
L	5	————	————
Knee			
R	95	————	————
L	95	————	————
Ankle (mortise)			
R	32	————	————
L	32	————	————
1st MTP			
R	8	————	————
L	8	————	————
2nd to 5th MTP (separately)			
R	5	————	————
L	5	————	————
		TOTAL	————————

MCP = metacarpophalangeal; PIP = proximal interphalangeal; MTP = metatarsophalangeal.
From Thompson, P. W., Silman, A. J., Kirwan, J. R., and Currey, H. L. F.: Articular indices of joint inflammation in rheumatoid arthritis: Correlation with the acute phase response. Arthritis Rheum. 30:618, 1987.

Table 52–12. ACTIVITIES OF DAILY LIVING AND VISUAL ANALOGUE QUESTIONNAIRE

How often is it painful for you to:	Never	Sometimes	Most of the Time	Always
Dress yourself?	————	————	————	————
Get in and out of bed?	————	————	————	————
Lift a cup or glass to your lips?	————	————	————	————
Walk outdoors on flat ground?	————	————	————	————
Wash and dry your entire body?	————	————	————	————
Bend down to pick up clothing from the floor?	————	————	————	————
Turn faucets on or off?	————	————	————	————
Get in and out of a car?	————	————	————	————

How much pain have you had in the past week (mark the scale)?

No pain ————————————————————————————— Pain as bad as it could be
　　　　0　　　　　　　　　　　　　　　　　　　　　　　　　100

From Callahan, L. F., Brooks, R. H., Summey, J. A., and Pincus, T.: Quantitative pain assessment for routine care of rheumatoid arthritis patients, using a pain scale based on activities of daily living and a visual analog pain scale. Arthritis Rheum. 30:630, 1987.

some other objective measurements of disease activity.

Care of the patient with rheumatoid disease should include a careful record of the physical examination and functional and radiographic assessment. This permits care of patients in a prospective fashion and provides a systematic assessment of disease activity. With proper assessment, effective therapy (as outlined in Chapter 53) can be started, evaluated, and changed if necessary.

References

1. Snorrason, E.: Landre-Beauvais and his goutte asthenique primitive. Acta Med. Scand. 142 (Suppl. 266):115, 1952.
2. Boyle, J. A., and Buchanan, W. W.: Clinical Rheumatology. Philadelphia, F. A. Davis Company, 1971, pp. 71–72.
3. Short, C. L.: The antiquity of rheumatoid arthritis. Arthritis Rheum. 17:193, 1974.
4. Copeman, W. S. C.: A Short History of the Gout and the Rheumatic Diseases. Berkeley, University of California Press, 1964.
5. Soranus of Ephesus: On Acute Diseases and on Chronic Diseases. (Translated into Latin by Caelius Aurelianus [5th century]. English translation by I. E. Drabkin.) Chicago, University of Chicago Press, 1950, pp. 923–929.
6. Ruffer, M. A., and Rietti, A.: On osseous lesions in ancient Egyptians. J. Pathol. Bacteriol. 16:439, 1912.
7. Lubeck, D. P., Spitz, P. W., Fries, J. F., Wolfe, F., Mitchell, D. M., and Roth, S. H.: A multicenter study of annual health service utilization and costs in rheumatoid arthritis. Arthritis Rheum. 29:488, 1986.
8. Arnett, F. C., et al.: The 1987 revised ARA criteria for classification of rheumatoid arthritis. Arthritis Rheum. 31:315, 1988.
9. Ropes, M. W., Bennett, E. A., Cobb, S., Jacox, R., and Jessar, R.: 1958 revision of diagnostic criteria for rheumatoid arthritis. Bull. Rheum. Dis. 9:175, 1958.
10. Wood, P. H. N.: Epidemiology of rheumatic disorders: Problems in classification. Proc. R. Soc. Med. 63:189, 1970.
11. Schumacher, H. R., and Kitridou, R. C.: Synovitis of recent onset: A clinicopathologic study during the first month of disease. Arthritis Rheum. 15:465, 1972.
12. Bennett, P. H., and Burch, T. A.: New York symposium on population studies in the rheumatic diseases: New diagnostic criteria. Bull. Rheum. Dis. 17:453, 1967.
13. O'Sullivan, J. B., and Cathcart, E. S.: The prevalence of rheumatoid arthritis: Follow-up evaluation of the effect of criteria on rates in Sudbury, Massachusetts. Ann. Intern. Med. 76:573, 1972.
14. Wolfe, A. M.: The epidemiology of rheumatoid arthritis: A review. Bull. Rheum. Dis. 19:518, 1968.
15. Engel, A., Roberts, J., and Burch, T. A.: Rheumatoid arthritis in adults in the United States 1960–1962. In Vital and Health Statistics, Series 11, Data from the National Health Survey, Number 17. Washington, D. C., National Center for Health Statistics, 1966.
16. Mikkelsen, W. M., Dodge, H. J., Duff, I. F., and Kato, I. H.: Estimates of the prevalence of rheumatic disease in the population of Tecumseh, Michigan, 1959–1960. J. Chronic Dis. 20:351, 1967.
17. O'Brien, W. M., Bennett, P. H., Burch, T. A., et al.: A genetic study of rheumatoid arthritis and rheumatoid factor in Blackfeet and Pima Indians. Arthritis Rheum. 10:163, 1967.
18. Wood, W. J., Kato, H., Johnson, K. G., et al.: Rheumatoid arthritis in Hiroshima and Nagasaki, Japan. Arthritis Rheum. 10:21, 1967.
19. Stone, C. E.: The lifetime economic costs of rheumatoid arthritis. J. Rheumatol. 11:819, 1984.
20. Beasley, R. P., Willkens, R. F., and Bennett, P. H.: High prevalence of rheumatoid arthritis in Yakima Indians. Arthritis Rheum. 16:743, 1973.
21. Harvey, J., Lotze, M., Arnett, F. C., et al.: Rheumatoid arthritis in a Chippewa band. II. Field study with clinical serologic and HLA-D correlations. J. Rheumatol. 10:28, 1983.
22. Moolenburgh, J. D., Moore, S., Valkenburgh H. A., and Erasmus, M. G.: Rheumatoid arthritis in Lesotho. Ann. Rheum. Dis. 43:40, 1984.
23. Beighton, P., Solomon, L., and Valkenburg, H. A.: Rheumatoid arthritis in a rural South African Negro population. Ann. Rheum. Dis. 34:136, 1975.
24. Solomon, L., Robin, G., and Valkenburg, H. A.: Rheumatoid arthritis in an urban South African Negro population. Ann. Rheum. Dis. 34:128, 1975.
25. Lawrence, J. S.: Prevalence of rheumatoid arthritis. Ann. Rheum. Dis. 20:11, 1961.
26. Linos, A., Worthington, J. W., O'Fallon, W. M., and Kurland, L. T.: The epidemiology of rheumatoid arthritis in Rochester, Minnesota: A study of incidence, prevalence and mortality. Am. J. Epidemiol. 11:87, 1980.
27. Wingrave, S., and Kay, C. R.: Reduction in incidence of rheumatoid arthritis associated with oral contraceptives. Lancet 1:569, 1978.
28. Cobb, S., Kasl, S. V., Chen, E., and Christenfeld, R.: Some psychological and social characteristics of patients hospitalized for rheumatoid arthritis, hypertension, and duodenal ulcer. J. Chronic Dis. 18:1259, 1965.
29. Wolfe, A. M.: The epidemiology of rheumatoid arthritis: A review. I. Surveys. Bull. Rheum. Dis. 19:518, 1968.
30. Pincus, T., Callahan, L. F.: Taking mortality in rheumatoid arthritis seriously: Predictive markers, socioeconomic status and comorbidity. J. Rheumatol. 13:841, 1986.
31. Mitchell, J. M., Burkhauser, R. V., Pincus, T.: The importance of age, education, and comorbidity in the substantial earnings losses of individuals with symmetric polyarthritis. Arthritis Rheum. 31:348, 1988.
32. Callahan, L. F., and Pincus, T.: Formal education level as a significant marker of clinical status in rheumatoid arthritis. Arthritis Rheum. 31:1346, 1988.
33. Rose, H. M., Ragan, C., Pearce, E., and Lipman, M. O.: Differential agglutination of normal and sensitized sheep erythrocytes by sera of patients with rheumatoid arthritis. Proc. Soc. Exp. Biol. Med. 68:1, 1948.
34. Waaler, E.: On the occurrence of a factor in human serum activating the specific agglutination of sheep blood corpuscles. Acta Pathol. Microbiol. Scand. 17:172, 1940.
35. Lawrence, J. S.: Prevalence of rheumatoid arthritis. Ann. Rheum. Dis. 20:11, 1961.
36. Lawrence, J. S., Laine, V. A. I., and DeGraaff, R.: The epidemiology of rheumatoid arthritis in northern Europe. Proc. R. Soc. Med. 54:454, 1961.
37. Engleman, E. G., Sponzilli, E. E., Batey, M. E., Rancharan, S., and McDevitt, H. O.: Mixed lymphocyte reaction in healthy women with rheumatoid factor. Arthritis Rheum. 21:690, 1978.
38. Nunez, G., Moore, S. E., Ball, G. V., et al.: Study of HLA antigens in ten multiple-case rheumatoid arthritis families. J. Rheumatol. 11:129, 1984.
39. Plotz, C. M., and Singer, J. M.: The latex fixation test. II. Results in rheumatoid arthritis. Am. J. Med. 21:893, 1956.
40. Alarcon, G. S., Koopman, W. J., Acton, R. T., and Barger, B. O.: Seronegative rheumatoid arthritis: A distinct immunogenetic disease? Arthritis Rheum. 25:502, 1982.
41. Noritake, D. T., Colburn, K. K., Chan, G., and Weisbart, R. H.: Rheumatoid factors specific for active rheumatoid arthritis. Ann. Rheum. Dis. 49:910, 1990.
42. Myerowitz, S., Jacox, R. F., and Hers, D. W.: Monozygotic twins discordant for rheumatoid arthritis. Arthritis Rheum. 11:1, 1968.
43. Harvald, B., and Hauge, M.: In Genetics and the Epidemiology of Chronic Diseases. Washington, D. C., U. S. Government Printing Office, 1965, p. 61.
44. Lawrence, J. S.: Genetics of rheumatoid factor and rheumatoid arthritis. Clin. Exp. Immunol. S2:769, 1967
45. Lawrence, J. S.: Rheumatoid arthritis—nature or nurture? Ann. Rheum. Dis. 29:357, 1970.
46. Ahok, M., Koskenvuo, M., Tuominen, J., and Kaprio, J.: Occurrence of rheumatoid arthritis in a nation-wide series of twins. J. Rheumatol. 13:899, 1986.
47. Siegel, M., Lee, S. L., Widelock, D., Gwon, N. V., and Kravitz, H: A comparative family study of rheumatoid arthritis and systemic lupus erythematosus. N. Engl. J. Med. 273:893, 1965.
48. Mellsop, G. W., Koadlow, L., Syme, J., et al.: Absence of rheumatoid arthritis in schizophrenia. Aust. N. Z. J. Med. 4:247, 1974.
49. Hellgren, L.: The prevalence of rheumatoid arthritis in occupational groups. Acta Rheumatol. Scand. 16:106, 1970.
50. Gottlieb, N. L., Dichek, N., Poiley, J., and Kiem, I. M.: Pets and rheumatoid arthritis. An epidemiologic survey. Arthritis Rheum. 17:229, 1974.
51. Wallace, D. J., Klinenberg, J. R., Morhaim, D., Berlanstein, B., Biren, P. C., and Callis, G.: Coexistent gout and rheumatoid arthritis. Arthritis Rheum. 22:81, 1979.
52. Agudelo, C. A., Turner, R. A., Panetti, M., and Pisko, E.: Does hyperuricemia protect from rheumatoid inflammation? Arthritis Rheum. 27:443, 1984.
53. Jacoby, R. K., Jayson, M. I. V., and Cosh, J. A.: Onset, early stages and prognosis of rheumatoid arthritis: A clinical study of 100 patients with 11 year follow-up. Br. Med. J. 2:96, 1973.
54. Lawrence, J. S.: Surveys of rheumatoid complaints in the population. In Dixon, A. St. J. (ed.): Progress in Clinical Rheumatology. London, Churchill Livingstone, 1965, p. 1.
55. Short, C. L., and Bauer, W.: The course of rheumatoid arthritis in patients receiving simple medical and orthopedic measures. N. Engl. J. Med. 238:142, 1948.

56. Aho, A., Palosuo, T., Raunio, V., et al.: When does rheumatoid disease start? Arthritis Rheum. 28:485, 1985.

57. Fleming, A., Crown, J. M., and Corbett, M.: Early rheumatoid disease. 1. Onset. Ann. Rheum. Dis. 35:357, 1976.

58. Fleming, A., Benn, R. T., Corbett, M., and Wood, P. H. N.: Early rheumatoid disease. II. Patterns of joint involvement. Ann. Rheum. Dis. 35:361, 1976.

59. Dick, W. C., Grayson, M. F., Woodburn, A., Nuki, G., and Buchanan, W. W.: Indices of inflammatory activity: Relationship between isotope studies and clinical methods. Ann. Rheum. Dis. 29:643, 1971.

60. Mens, J. M. A.: Correlation of joint involvement in rheumatoid arthritis and in ankylosing spondylitis with the synovial:cartilagenous surface ratio of various joints. Arthritis Rheum. 30:359, 1987.

61. Bywaters, E. G. L.: Still's disease in the adult. Ann. Rheum. Dis. 30:121, 1971.

62. Gupta, R. C., and Mills, D. M.: Still's disease in an adult: A link between juvenile and adult rheumatoid arthritis. Am. J. Med. Sci. 269:137, 1975.

63. Aptekar, R. G., Decker, J. L., Bujak, J. S., Wolff, S. M.: Adult onset of juvenile rheumatoid arthritis. Arthritis Rheum. 16:715, 1973.

64. Strampl, I. J., and Lozar, J. D.: Adult-onset Still's disease: Variant of rheumatoid arthritis. Postgrad. Med. 58:175, 1975.

65. Elkon, K. B., Hughes, G. R. V., Bywaters, E. G. L., et al.: Adult-onset Still's disease: Twenty-year follow-up and further studies of patients with active disease. Arthritis Rheum. 25:647, 1982.

66. Cush, J. J., Medsger, T. A., Jr., Christy, W. C., Hubert, D. C., and Cooperstein, L. A.: Adult-onset Still's disease. Arthritis Rheum. 30:186, 1987.

67. Ohta, A., Yamaguchi, T., Tsunematsu, T., et al.: Adult Still's disease: A multicenter survey of Japanese patients. J. Rheumatol. 17:1058, 1990.

68. Hench, P. S., and Rosenberg, E. F.: Palindromic rheumatism: New oft-recurring disease of joints (arthritis, periarthritis, para-arthritis) apparently producing no articular residues; report of 34 cases. Proc. Mayo Clin. 16:808, 1942.

69. Schumacher, H. R.: Palindromic onset of rheumatoid arthritis. Arthritis Rheum. 25:361, 1982.

70. Deal, C. L., Meenan, R. F., Goldenberg, D. L., et al.: The clinical features of elderly-onset rheumatoid arthritis. Arthritis Rheum. 28:987, 1985.

71. Terkeltaub, R., D'Ecary, F., and Esdaile, J.: An immunogenetic study of older age onset rheumatoid arthritis. J. Rheumatol. 11:147, 1984.

72. Yoghami, I., Rookolamini, S. M., and Faunce, H. F.: Unilateral rheumatoid arthritis: Protective effects of neurologic deficits. Am. J. Roentgenol. 128:299, 1977.

73. Bland, J., and Eddy, W.: Hemiplegia and rheumatoid hemiarthritis. Arthritis Rheum. 11:72, 1968.

74. Glick, E. N.: Asymmetrical rheumatoid arthritis after poliomyelitis. Br. Med. J. 3:26, 1967.

75. Thompson, M., and Bywaters, E. G. L.: Unilateral rheumatoid arthritis following hemiplegia. Ann. Rheum. Dis. 21:370, 1961.

76. Bywaters, E. G. L.: The hand. In Radiological Aspects of Rheumatoid Arthritis: International Congress Series. Amsterdam, Excerpta Medica Foundation, No. 64, 1964, p. 43.

77. de Haas, W. H. D., de Boer, W., Griftioen, F., and Oostenelst, P.: Rheumatoid arthritis of the robust reaction type. Ann. Rheum. Dis. 31:81, 1974.

78. Short, C. L., Bauer, W., and Reynolds, W. E.: Rheumatoid Arthritis: A Definition of the Disease and a Clinical Description Based on a Numerical Study of 293 Patients and Controls. Cambridge, Massachusetts, Harvard University Press, 1957.

79. Short, C. L.: Rheumatoid arthritis: Types of course and prognosis. Med. Clin. North Am. 52:549, 1968.

80. Short, C. L., and Bauer, W.: The course of rheumatoid arthritis in patients receiving simple medical and orthopedic measures. N. Engl. J. Med. 238:142, 1948.

81. Pincus, T., Callahan, L. F., Sale, W. G., Brooks, A. L., Payne, L. E., and Vaughn, W. K.: Severe functional declines, work disability, and increased mortality in 75 RA patients studied over 9 years. Arthritis Rheum. 27:864, 1984.

82. Hollander, J. L., and Yeostros, S. J.: The effects of simultaneous variations of humidity and barometric pressure on arthritis. Bull. Am. Meteorol. Soc. 44:389, 1963.

83. Sibley, J. T.: Weather and arthritis symptoms. J. Rheumatol. 12:707, 1985.

84. Patberg, W. R., Nienhuis, R. L. F., and Veringa, F.: Relation between meteorological factors and pain in rheumatoid arthritis in a marine climate. J. Rheumatol. 12:711, 1985.

85. Hoffman, G. S.: Polyarthritis: The differential diagnosis of rheumatoid arthritis. Semin. Arthritis Rheum. 8:115, 1978.

86. Davies, P. G., and Fordham, J. N.: Arthritis and angioimmunoblastic lymphadenopathy. Ann. Rheum. Dis. 42:516, 1983.

87. Fallet, G. H., Mason, M., Berry, H., Mowat, A. G., Bonssina, I., and Gerster, J-C.: Rheumatoid arthritis and ankylosing spondylitis occurring together. Br. Med. J. 1:604, 1976.

88. Chamot, A. M., Benhamou, C. L., Kahn, M. F., Beraneck, L., Kaplan, G., and Prost, A.: Le syndrome acne pustulose hyperostose osteite (SAPHO)—85 observations. Rev. Rhum. 54:187, 1987.

89. Morris, R. I., Metzger, A. L., Bluestone, R., et al.: HLA B27: A useful discriminator in arthropathies of inflammatory bowel disease. N. Engl. J. Med. 290:1117, 1974.

90. McEwen, C., Lingg, C., and Kirsner, J. B.: Arthritis accompanying ulcerative colitis. Am. J. Med. 33:923, 1962.

91. Zizic, T. M., and Stevens, M. B.: The arthropathy of Behçet's disease. Johns Hopkins Med. J. 136:243, 1975.

92. Yurdakul, S., Yazici, H., Tuzuir, Y., Pazarli, H., Yalcin, B., Altoc, M., Ozuazgen, Y., Tuziinez, N., and Muftuoglus, A.: The arthritis of Behçet's disease: A prospective study. Ann. Rheum. Dis. 42:505, 1983.

93. Ahvonen, P., Sievers, K., and Ano, K.: Arthritis associated with Yersinia enterocolitica infection. Acta Rheumatol. Scand. 15:232, 1969.

94. Ano, K., Ahvonen, P., Lassus, A., Sievers, K., and Tulisinen, A.: HLA-B27 in reactive arthritis: A study of Yersinia arthritis and Reiter's disease. Arthritis Rheum. 17:521, 1974.

95. Hawkins, C. F., Farr, M., Morris, C. J., House, A. M., and Williamson, N.: Detection by electron microscope of rod-shaped organisms in synovial membrane from a patient with the arthritis of Whipple's disease. Ann. Rheum. Dis. 35:502, 1976.

96. Bole, G. G., Friedlaender, M. H., and Smith, C. K.: Rheumatic symptoms and serological abnormalities induced by oral contraceptives. Lancet 1:323, 1969.

97. Bland, J. H., and Frymoyer, J. W.: Rheumatic syndromes of myxedema. N. Engl. J. Med. 282:1171, 1970.

98. Gimlette, T. M. D.: Thyroid acropathy. Lancet 1:22, 1960.

99. Churchill, M. D., Geraci, J. E., and Hunder, G. G.: Musculoskeletal manifestations of bacterial endocarditis. Ann. Intern. Med. 87:754, 1977.

100. Bayer, A. S., Theofilopoulos, A. N., Eisenberg, R., Dixon, F. J., and Guze, L. B.: Circulating immune complexes in infective endocarditis. N. Engl. J. Med. 295:1500, 1976.

101. Bulkley, B. H., and Hutchins, G. M.: Atrial myxomas: A fifty-year review. Am. Heart J. 97:639, 1979.

102. McCarty, D. J.: Diagnostic mimicry in arthritis: Patterns of joint involvement associated with calcium pyrophosphate dihydrate crystal deposits. Bull. Rheum. Dis. 25:804, 1975.

103. Utsinger, P. D., Zvaifler, N. J., and Resnick, D.: Calcium pyrophosphate dihydrate deposition disease without chondrocalcinosis. J. Rheumatol. 2:258, 1975.

104. Halla, J. T., and Hardin, J. G.: Clinical features of the arthritis of mixed connective tissue disease. Arthritis Rheum. 21:497, 1978.

105. Gordon, D. A., Pruzanski, W., Ogryzlo, M. A., and Little, H. A.: Amyloid arthritis simulating rheumatoid disease in five patients with multiple myeloma. Am. J. Med. 55:142, 1973.

106. Pinals, R. S., and Short, C.: Calcific periarthritis involving multiple sites. Arthritis Rheum. 9:566, 1966.

107. Martin, J. R., Huang, S.-N., Lacron, A., et al.: Congenital contractural deformities of the fingers and arthropathy. Ann. Rheum. Dis. 44:826, 1985.

108. Heller, H. Gafni, J., Michaeli, D., et al.: Arthritis of familial Mediterranean fever (FMF). Arthritis Rheum. 9:1, 1966.

109. Wolfe, F., Cathey, M. A., Kleinkeksel, S. M., et al.: Psychological status in primary fibrositis and fibrositis associated with rheumatoid arthritis. J. Rheumatol. 11:500, 1984.

110. Wolfe, F., Cathey, M. A., and Kleinkeksel, S. M.: Fibrositis (fibromyalgia) in rheumatoid arthritis. J. Rheumatol. 11:814, 1984.

111. Velayos, E. E., Leidholt, J. D., Smyth, C. J., and Priest, R.: Arthropathy associated with steroid therapy. Ann. Intern. Med. 64:759, 1966.

112. Talbott, J. H., Altman, R. D., and Yu, T.-F.: Gouty arthritis masquerading as rheumatoid arthritis or vice versa. Semin. Arthritis Rheum. 8:77, 1978.

113. Resnick, D.: Gout-like lesions in rheumatoid arthritis. Am. J. Roentgenol. 127:1062, 1976.

114. Rappoport, A. S., Sosman, J. L., and Weissman, B. N.: Lesions resembling gout in patients with rheumatoid arthritis. Am. J. Roentgenol. 126:41, 1976.

115. Kozin, F., and McCarty, D. J.: Rheumatoid factor in the serum of gouty patients. Arthritis Rheum. 20:1559, 1977.

116. Wallace, D. J., Klinenberg, J. R., Morbaim, D., Berlanstein, B., Biren, P. C., and Callis, G.: Coexistent gout and rheumatoid arthritis: Case report and literature review. Arthritis Rheum. 22:81, 1979.

117. Agudelo, C. A., Turner, R. A., Panetti, M., and Pisko, E.: Does hyperuricemia protect from rheumatoid inflammation? A clinical study. Arthritis Rheum. 27:443, 1984.

118. Hisch, J. H., Killien, F. C., and Troupin, R. H.: The arthropathy of hemochromatosis. Diagn. Radiol. 118:591, 1976.

119. Dymock, I. W., Hamilton, E. B. D., Laws, J. W., and Williams, R.: Arthropathy of hemochromatosis. Ann. Rheum. Dis. 29:469, 1970.

120. Schumacher, H. R., Andrews, R., and McLaughlin, G.: Arthropathy in sickle cell disease. Ann. Intern. Med. 78:203, 1973.

121. Schumacher, H. R., Dorwart, B. B., Boud, J., Alavi, A., and Miller,

W.: Chronic synovitis with early cartilage destruction in sickle cell disease. Ann. Rheum. Dis. 36:413, 1977.

122. deCeulaer, K., Forbes, M., Roper, D., et al.: Non-gouty arthritis in sickle cell disease: Report of 37 consecutive cases. Ann. Rheum. Dis. 43:599, 1984.

123. Crout, J. E., McKenna, C. H., and Petitt, R. M.: Symptomatic joint effusions in sickle cell–β-thalassemia disease. J. A. M. A. 235:1878, 1976.

124. Glueck, C. J., Levy, R. I., and Fredickson, D. S.: Acute tendinitis and arthritis: A presenting symptom of familial type II hyperlipoproteinemia. J. A. M. A. 206:2895, 1968.

125. Watt, T. L., and Baumann, R. R.: Pseudoxanthomatous rheumatoid nodules. Arch. Dermatol. 95:156, 1967.

126. Buckingham, R. B., Bole, G. G., and Bassett, D. R.: Polyarthritis associated with type IV hyperlipoproteinemia. Arch. Intern. Med. 135:286, 1975.

127. Langer, T., and Levy, R. I.: Acute muscular syndrome associated with administration of clofibrate. N. Engl. J. Med. 279:856, 1968.

128. Schumacher, H. R.: Articular manifestations of hypertropic pulmonary osteoarthropathy in bronchogenic carcinoma. Arthritis Rheum. 19:629, 1976.

129. Yanez, J. E., Thompson, G. R., Mikkelsen, W. M., and Bartholomew, L. E.: Rubella arthritis. Ann. Intern. Med. 64:772, 1966.

130. Spruance, S. L., and Smith, C. B.: Joint complications associated with derivatives of HPV-77 rubella virus vaccine. Am. J. Dis. Child. 122:105, 1971.

131. Alpert, E., Isselbacher, K. J., and Aschur, P. H.: The pathogenesis of arthritis associated with viral hepatitis. Complement component studies. N. Engl. J. Med. 285:185, 1971.

132. Schumacher, H. R., and Gall, E. P.: Arthritis in acute hepatitis and chronic active hepatitis: Pathology of the synovial membrane with evidence for the presence of Australia antigen in synovial membranes. Am. J. Med. 57:655, 1974.

133. Sigal, L. H., Steere, A. C., and Niederman, J. C.: Symmetric polyarthritis associated with heterophile-negative infectious mononucleosis. Arthritis Rheum. 26:553, 1983.

134. Weiner, A. D., and Ghormley, R. K.: Periodic benign synovitis: Idiopathic intermittent hydrarthrosis. J. Bone Joint Surg. 38A:1039, 1956.

135. Williams, M. H., Sheldon, P. J. H. S., Torrigiani, G., and Mattingly, S.: Palindromic rheumatism: Clinical and immunological studies. Ann. Rheum. Dis. 30:375, 1971.

136. Ehrlich, G. E.: Intermittent and periodic rheumatic syndromes. Bull. Rheum. Dis. 24:746, 1974.

137. Steere, A. C., Malawista, S. E., Hardin, J. A., Ruddy, S., Askenasy, W., and Andiman, W. A.: Erythema chronicum migrans and Lyme arthritis: The enlarging clinical spectrum. Ann. Intern. Med. 86:685, 1977.

138. Moulsopoulos, H. M., Fye, K. H., Pugay, P. I., and Shearn, M. D.: Monarthritic arthritis caused by metastatic breast carcinoma. J. A. M. A. 234:75, 1975.

139. Dorfman, H. D., Siegel, H. L., Perry, M. C., and Oxenhandler, R.: Non-Hodgkin's lymphoma of the synovium simulating rheumatoid arthritis. Arthritis Rheum. 30:155, 1987.

140. Emkey, R. D., Ragsdale, B. D., Ropes, M. W., and Miller, W.: A case of lymphoproliferative disease presenting as juvenile rheumatoid arthritis. Am. J. Med. 54:825, 1972.

141. Gold, R. H., Metzger, A. L., Mina, J. M., Weinberger, H. J., and Killebrew, K.: Multicentric reticulohistiocytosis (lipoid dermato-arthritis). Am. J. Roentgenol. 124:610, 1975.

142. Orkin, M., Goltz, R. W., Good, R. A., Michael, A., and Fisher, I.: A study of multicentric reticulohistiocytosis. Arch. Dermatol. 89:641, 1964.

143. Ehrlich, G. E.: Inflammatory osteoarthritis. I. The clinical syndrome. J. Chronic Dis. 25:317, 1972.

144. Ordenstein, L: Sur la Paralysie Agitante et la Sclerose en Plaques Generalisee Paris. Imprimerie de E. Martinet, 1864 (original in the Library of the New York Academy of Medicine).

145. Granowitz, S. P., and Mankin, H. J.: Localized pigmented villonodular synovitis of knee. J. Bone Joint Surg. 49A:122, 1967.

146. Chon, C-T., and Schumacher, H. R., Jr.: Clinical and pathological studies of synovitis in polymyalgia rheumatica. Arthritis Rheum. 27:1107, 1984.

147. Ginsburg, W. W., Cohen, M. D., Hall, S. B., et al.: Seronegative polyarthritis in giant cell arteritis. Arthritis Rheum. 28:1362, 1985.

148. McDanold, E. C., and Weissman, M. H.: Articular manifestations of rheumatic fever in adults. Ann. Intern. Med. 89:917, 1978.

149. Barnett, A. L., Terry, E. E., and Persellin, R. H.: Acute rheumatic fever in adults. J. A. M. A. 232:925, 1975.

150. Stollerman, G. H., Markowitz, M., Tarania, A., Wannamaker, L. W., and Whittemore, R.: Jones' criteria (revised) for guidance in the diagnosis of rheumatic fever. Circulation 32:664, 1965.

151. Bywaters, E. G. L.: Relation between heart and joint disease including "rheumatoid heart disease" and chronic post-rheumatic arthritis (type Jaccoud). Br. Heart J. 12:101, 1950.

152. Zvaifler, N. J.: Chronic postrheumatic-fever (Jaccoud's) arthritis. N. Engl. J. Med. 267:10, 1962.

153. Ruderman, J. E., and Abruzzo, J. L.: Chronic post rheumatic-fever arthritis (Jaccoud's): Report of a case with subcutaneous nodules. Arthritis Rheum. 9:640, 1966.

154. Spilberg, I., Siltzbach, L. E., and McEwen, C. E.: The arthritis of sarcoidosis. Arthritis Rheum. 12:126, 1969.

155. Kaplan, H.: Sarcoid arthritis: A review. Arch. Intern. Med. 112:162, 1963.

156. Poncet, A.: Address to the Congress Français de Chirurgie, 1897. Bull. Acad. Med. Paris 46:194, 1901.

157. Krauser, R. E., and Schumacher, H. R.: The arthritis of Sweet's syndrome. Arthritis Rheum. 18:35, 1975.

158. Hoffman, G. S.: Treatment of Sweet's syndrome (acute febrile neutrophilic dermatosis) with indomethacin. J. Rheumatol. 4:201, 1977.

159. Thiemann, H.: Juvenile epiphysenstorungen. Fortschr. Geb. Rontgenstr. Nuklearmed. 14:79, 1909–1910.

160. Rubenstein, H. M.: Thiemann's disease: A brief reminder. Arthritis Rheum. 18:357, 1975.

161. Bland, J.: Rheumatoid arthritis of the cervical spine. J. Rheumatol. 1:319, 1974.

162. Ball, J.: Enthesopathy of rheumatoid and ankylosing spondylitis. Ann. Rheum. Dis. 30:213, 1971.

163. Martel, W.: Pathogenesis of cervical discovertebral destruction in rheumatoid arthritis. Arthritis Rheum. 20:1217, 1977.

164. Weiner, S., Bassett, L., and Spiegel, T.: Superior, posterior, and lateral displacement of C1 in rheumatoid arthritis. Arthritis Rheum. 25:1378, 1982.

165. Stevens, J. C., Cartilage, N. E. F., Saunders, M., Appleby, A., Hall, M., and Shaw, D. A.: Atlantoaxial subluxation and cervical myelopathy in rheumatoid arthritis. Q. J. Med. 40:391, 1971.

166. Nakano, K. K., Schoene, W. C., Baker, R. A., and Dawson, D. U.: The cervical myelopathy associated with rheumatoid arthritis: Analysis of patients with 2 postmortem cases. Ann. Neurol. 3:144, 1978.

167. Martel, W.: The occipito-atlanto-axial joints in rheumatoid arthritis and ankylosing spondylitis. Am. J. Roentgenol. 86:223, 1961.

168. Raskin, R. J., Schnapf, D. J., Wolf, C. R., Killian, P. J., and Lawless, O. J.: Computerized tomography in evaluation of atlantoaxial subluxation in rheumatoid arthritis. J. Rheumatol. 10:32, 1983.

169. Breedveld, F. C., Algra, P. R., Veilvoye, C. J., and Cats, A.: Magnetic resonance imaging in the evaluation of patients with rheumatoid arthritis and subluxations of the cervical spine. Arthritis Rheum. 30:624, 1987.

170. Mayer, J. W., Messner, R. P., and Kaplan, R. J.: Brain stem compression in rheumatoid arthritis. J. A. M. A. 236:2094, 1976.

171. Winfield, J., Young, A., Williams, P., et al.: Prospective study of the radiological changes in hands, feet, and cervical spine in adult rheumatoid disease. Ann. Rheum. Dis. 42:613, 1983.

172. Pellicci, P. M., Ranawat, C. S., Tsairis, P., and Bryan, W. J.: A prospective study of the progression of rheumatoid arthritis in the cervical spine. J. Bone Joint Surg. 65A:342, 1981.

173. Meyers, K. A. E., Cats, A., Kremer, H. P. H., Lujendijk, W., Onulee, G. J., and Thomeer, R. T. W. M.: Cervical myelopathy in rheumatoid arthritis. Clin. Exp. Rheumatol. 2:239, 1984.

174. Davidson, R. C., Horn, J. R., Hernton, J. H., and Oliver, G. D.: Brainstem compression in rheumatoid arthritis. J. A. M. A. 238:2633, 1977.

175. Mikulowski, P., Wollheim, F. A., Rotmil, P., and Olsen, J.: Sudden death in rheumatoid arthritis with atlanto-axial dislocation. Acta Med. Scand. 198:445, 1975.

176. Smith, P. H., Benn, R. T., and Sharp, J.: Natural history of rheumatoid cervical luxations. Ann. Rheum. Dis. 31:431, 1972.

177. Henderson, D. R. F.: Vertical atlanto-axial subluxation in rheumatoid arthritis. Rheumatol. Rehab. 14:31, 1975.

178. Davidson, R. C., Horn, J. R., Hernton, J. H., and Oliver, G. D.: Brainstem compression in rheumatoid arthritis. J. A. M. A. 238:2633, 1977.

179. Bywaters, E. G. L.: Rheumatoid and other diseases of the cervical interspinous bursae, and changes in the spinous process. Ann. Rheum. Dis. 41:360, 1982.

180. Jacob, J. R., Weisman, M. H., Murk, J. H., et al.: Reversible cause of back pain and sciatica in rheumatoid arthritis: An apophyseal joint cyst. Arthritis Rheum. 29:431, 1986.

181. Ericson, S., and Lundberg, M.: Alterations in the temporomandibular joints at various stages of rheumatoid arthritis. Acta Rheum Scand. 13:257, 1967.

182. Marbach, J. J., and Spiera, H.: Rheumatoid arthritis of the temporomandibular joints. Ann. Rheum. Dis. 26:538, 1967.

183. Goupille, P., Fouquet, B., Cotty, P., Goga, D., Mateu, J., and Valat, J-P.: The temporomandibular joint in rheumatoid arthritis: Correlations between clinical and computed tomography features. J. Rheumatol. 17:1285, 1990.

184. Lofgren, R. H., and Montgomery, W. W.: Incidence of laryngeal involvement in rheumatoid arthritis. N. Engl. J. Med. 267:193, 1962.

185. Polisar, I. A., Burbank, B., Levitt, L. M., Katz, H. M., and Morrione, T. G.: Bilateral midline fixation of cricoarytenoid joints as serious medical emergency. J. A. M. A. 172:901, 1960.
186. Bienenstock, H., Ehrich, G. E., and Freyberg, R. H.: Rheumatoid arthritis of the cricoarytenoid joint: A clinicopathologic study. Arthritis Rheum. 6:48, 1963.
187. Lawry, G. V., Finerman, M. L., Hanafee, W. N., Mancuso, A. A., Fan, P. T., and Bluestone, R.: Laryngeal involvement in rheumatoid arthritis. Arthritis Rheum. 27:873, 1984.
188. Copeman, W. S. C.: Rheumatoid oto-arthritis. Br. Med. J. 2:1536, 1963.
189. Moffat, D. A., Ramsden, R. T., Rosenberg, J. N., Booth, J. B., and Gibson, W. P. R.: Otoadmittance measurements in patients with rheumatoid arthritis. J. Laryngol. Otol. 91:917, 1977.
190. Kalliomaki, J. L., Viitanen, S-M., and Virtama, P.: Radiological findings of sternoclavicular joints in rheumatoid arthritis. Acta Rheumatol. Scand. 14:233, 1968.
191. Kormano, M.: A microradiographic and histological study of the manubriosternal joint in rheumatoid arthritis. Acta Rheumatol. Scand. 14:233, 1968.
192. Khong, T. K., and Rooney, P. J.: Manubriosternal joint subluxation in rheumatoid arthritis. J. Rheumatol. 9:712, 1982.
193. Ennevaara, K.: Painful shoulder joint in rheumatoid arthritis. Acta Rheumatol. Scand. Suppl. 11, 1967.
194. Weiss, J. J., Thompson, G. R., Doust, V., and Burgener, F.: Rotator cuff tears in rheumatoid arthritis. Arch. Intern. Med. 135:521, 1975.
195. Mosley, H. F.: Ruptures of the Rotator Cuff: Shoulder Lesions. 3rd ed. Edinburgh, E & S Livingston Ltd., 1969, p. 73.
196. Edeiken, J., and Hodes, P. J.: Roentgen Diagnosis of Disease of Bone. 2nd ed. Baltimore, Williams & Wilkins, 1978, pp. 690–709.
197. DeSmet, A. A., Ting, Y. M., and Weiss, J. J.: Shoulder arthrography in rheumatoid arthritis. Diagn. Radiol. 116:601, 1975.
198. Huston, K. A., Nelson, A. M., and Hunder, G. G.: Shoulder swelling in rheumatoid arthritis secondary to subacromial bursitis. Arthritis Rheum. 21:145, 1978.
199. Resnick, D., and Niwayama, G.: Resorption of the undersurface of the distal clavicle in rheumatoid arthritis. Diagn. Radiol. 120:75, 1976.
200. deJager, J. P., and Fleming, A.: Shoulder joint rupture and pseudo-thrombosis in rheumatoid arthritis. Ann. Rheum. Dis. 43:503, 1984.
201. Laine, V., and Vainio, K.: The elbow in rheumatoid arthritis. In Hymans, W., Paul, W. D., and Herschel, H.: Early Synovectomy in Rheumatoid Arthritis. Amsterdam, Excerpta Medica, 1969, p. 112.
202. Peterson, L. F. A., and James, J. M.: Surgery of the rheumatoid elbow. Orthop. Clin. North Am. 2:667, 1971.
203. Shapiro, J. S.: A new factor in the etiology of ulnar drift. Clin. Orthop. 68:32, 1970.
204. Hastings, D. E., and Evans, J. A.: Rheumatoid wrist deformities and their relation to ulnar drift. J. Bone Joint Surg. 57A:930, 1975.
205. Inglis, A. E.: Rheumatoid arthritis in the hand. Am. J. Surg. 109:368, 1965.
206. Swezey, R. L., and Fiegenberg, D. S.: Inappropriate intrinsic muscle action in the rheumatoid hand. Ann. Rheum. Dis. 30:619, 1972.
207. Fearnley, G. R.: Ulnar deviation of the fingers. Ann. Rheum. Dis. 10:126, 1951.
208. Flatt, A. E.: Surgical rehabilitation of the arthritic hand. Arthritis Rheum. 11:278, 1959.
209. Hakstian, R. W., and Tubiana, R.: Ulnar deviation of the fingers. J. Bone Joint Surg. 49A:299, 1967.
210. Snorrason, E.: The problem of ulnar deviation of the fingers in rheumatoid arthritis. Acta Med. Scand. 140:359, 1951.
211. Vainio, K., and Oka, M.: Ulnar deviation of the fingers. Ann. Rheum. Dis. 12:122, 1953.
212. Martin, L., and Benson, W. G.: An unusual synovial cyst in rheumatoid arthritis. J. Rheumatol. 14:139, 1987.
213. Croft, J. D., and Jacox, R. F.: Rheumatoid "ganglion" as an unusual presenting sign of rheumatoid arthritis. J. A. M. A. 203:144, 1968.
214. Harrison, M. D., Freiberger, R. H., and Ranawat, C. S.: Arthrography of the rheumatoid wrist joint. Am. J. Roentgenol. 112:480, 1971.
215. Iveson, J. M. I., Hill, A. G. S., and Wright, V.: Wrist cysts and fistulae: An arthrographic study of the rheumatoid wrist. Ann. Rheum. Dis. 34:388, 1975.
216. Martel, W., Hayes, J. T., and Duff, I. F.: The pattern of bone erosion in the hand and wrist in rheumatoid arthritis. Radiology 84:204, 1965.
217. Resnick, D., and Gmelich, J. T.: Bone fragmentation in the rheumatoid wrist: Radiographic and pathologic considerations. Diagn. Radiol. 114:315, 1975.
218. Trentham, D. E., and Masi, A. T.: Carpo:metacarpal ratio: A new quantitative measure of radiologic progression of wrist involvement in rheumatoid arthritis. Arthritis Rheum. 191:939, 1976.
219. Alarcon, G. S., and Koopman, W. J.: The carpometacarpal ratio: A useful method for assessing disease progression in rheumatoid arthritis. J. Rheumatol. 12:846, 1985.
220. Gilkeson, G., Polisson, R., Sinclair, H., Vogler, J., Rice, J., Caldwell, D., Spritzer, C., and Martinez, S.: Early detection of carpal erosions in patients with rheumatoid arthritis: A pilot study of magnetic resonance imaging. J. Rheumatol. 15:1361, 1988.

221. Fuchs, H. A., Callahan, L. F., Kaye, J. J., Brooks, R. H., Nance, E. P., and Pincus, T.: Radiographic and joint count findings of the hand in rheumatoid arthritis. Arthritis Rheum. 31:44, 1988.
222. Brewerton, D. A.: Hand deformities in rheumatoid disease. Ann. Rheum. Dis. 16:183, 1957.
223. McCarty, D. J., and Gatter, R. A.: A study of distal interphalangeal joint tenderness in rheumatoid arthritis. Arthritis Rheum. 9:325, 1966.
224. Vaughan-Jackson, O. J.: Rheumatoid hand deformities considered in the light of tendon imbalance. J. Bone Joint Surg. 44B:764, 1962.
225. Mody, G. M., and Meyers, O. L.: Resorptive arthropathy in rheumatoid arthritis. J. Rheumatol. 15:1075, 1988.
226. Nalebuff, E. A.: Diagnosis, classification, and management of rheumatoid thumb deformities. Bull. Hosp. Joint Dis. 24:119, 1968.
227. Kellgren, J. H., and Ball, J.: Tendon lesions in rheumatoid arthritis: A clinicopathological study. Ann. Rheum. Dis. 9:48, 1950.
228. Gray, R. G., and Gottlieb, N. L.: Hand flexor tenosynovitis in rheumatoid arthritis. Arthritis Rheum. 20:1003, 1977.
229. Millis, M. B., Millender, L. H., and Nalebuff, E. A.: Stiffness of the proximal interphalangeal joints in rheumatoid arthritis. J. Bone Joint Surg. 58A:801, 1976.
230. Vyden, J. K., Callis, G., Groseth-Dittrich, M. F., Laks, M. M., and Weinberger, H.: Peripheral hemodynamics in rheumatoid arthritis (abstract). Arthritis Rheum. 14:419, 1971.
231. Jacob, J., Sartoris, D., Kursunoglu, S., et al.: Distal interphalangeal joint involvement in rheumatoid arthritis. Arthritis Rheum. 29:10, 1986.
232. Duthie, R., and Harris, C.: A radiographic and clinical survey of the hip joints in sero-positive rheumatoid arthritis. Acta Orthop. Scand. 40:346, 1969.
233. Hastings, D. E., and Parker, S. M.: Protrusio acetabuli in rheumatoid arthritis. Clin. Orthop. 108:76, 1975.
234. Colton, C., and Darby, A.: Giant granulomatous lesions of the femoral head and neck in rheumatoid arthritis. Ann. Rheum. Dis. 29:626, 1970.
235. Levy, R. N., Hermann, G., Haimov, M., et al.: Rheumatoid synovial cyst of the hip. Arthritis Rheum. 25:1382, 1982.
236. Cary, G. R.: Methods for determining the presence of subtle knee joint effusion. J. Louisiana State Med. Soc. 118:147, 1966.
237. Gupta, P. J.: Physical examination of the arthritis patient. Bull. Rheum. Dis. 20:596, 1970.
238. Jayson, M. I. V., and Dixon, A. St. J.: Valvular mechanisms in juxta-articular cysts. Ann. Rheum. Dis. 29:415, 1970.
239. Hench, P. K., Reid, R. T., and Reames, P. M.: Dissecting popliteal cyst stimulating thrombophlebitis. Ann. Intern. Med. 64:1259, 1966.
240. Hall, A. P., and Scott, J. T.: Synovial cysts and rupture of the knee joint in rheumatoid arthritis. Ann. Rheum. Dis. 25:32, 1966.
241. Tait, G. B. W., Bach, F., and Dixon, A. St. J.: Acute synovial rupture. Ann. Rheum. Dis. 24:273, 1965.
242. Kraag, G., Thevathasan, E. M., Gordon, D. A., and Walker, I. H.: The hemorrhage crescent sign of acute synovial rupture. Ann. Intern. Med. 85:477, 1976.
243. Gordon, G. V., and Edell, S.: Ultrasound evaluation of popliteal cysts. Arch. Intern. Med. 140:1453, 1980.
244. Karvonen, R. L., Negendank, W. G., Fraser, S. M., Mayes, M. D., An, T., Fernandez-Madrid, F.: Articular cartilage defects of the knee: Correlation between magnetic resonance imaging and gross pathology. Ann. Rheum. Dis. 49:672, 1990.
245. Rask, M. R.: Achilles tendon rupture owing to rheumatoid disease. J. A. M. A. 239:435, 1978.
246. Dixon, A. St. J.: The rheumatoid foot. In Hill, A. G. S. (ed.): Modern Trends in Rheumatology. Vol. 2. London, Butterworths, 1971, pp. 158–173.
247. Seltzer, S. E., Weissman, B. N., Braunstein, E. M., et al.: Computed tomography of the hind foot with rheumatoid arthritis. Arthritis Rheum. 28:1234, 1985.
248. Vidigal, E., Jacoby, R., Dixon, A. St. J., Rattiff, A. H., and Kirkup, J.: The foot in chronic rheumatoid arthritis. Ann. Rheum. Dis. 34:292, 1975.
249. Bienenstock, H.: Rheumatoid plantar synovial cysts. Ann. Rheum. Dis. 34:98, 1975.
250. Dixon, A. St. J.: The rheumatoid foot. In Hill, A. G. S. (ed.): Modern Trends in Rheumatology. Vol. 2. London, Butterworths, 1971, pp. 158–173.
251. Calabro, J. J.: A critical evaluation of the diagnostic features of the feet in rheumatoid arthritis. Arthritis Rheum. 5:19, 1962.
252. McGuigan, L., Burke, D., and Fleming, A.: Tarsal tunnel syndrome and peripheral neuropathy in rheumatoid disease. Ann. Rheum. Dis. 42:128, 1983.
253. Shimizu, S., Shiozawa, S., Shiozawa, K., Imura, S., and Fujita, T.: Quantitative histologic studies on the pathogenesis of periarticular osteoporosis in rheumatoid arthritis. Arthritis Rheum. 28:25, 1985.
254. Dequeker, J., and Geusens, P.: Osteoporosis and arthritis. Ann. Rheum. Dis. 49:276, 1990.
255. Verstraeten, A., and Dequeker, J.: Vertebral and peripheral bone mineral content and fracture incidence in postmenopausal patients

with rheumatoid arthritis: Effect of low dose corticosteroids. Ann. Rheum. Dis. 45:852, 1986.

256. Sambrook, P. N., Eisman, J. A., Champion, G. D., and Pocock, N. A.: Sex hormone status and osteoporosis in postmenopausal women with rheumatoid arthritis. Arthritis Rheum. 31:973, 1988.

257. Maddison, P. J., and Bacon, P. A.: Vitamin D deficiency, spontaneous fractures and osteopenia in rheumatoid arthritis. Br. Med. J. 2:433, 1974.

258. Schneider, R., and Kaye, J. J.: Insufficiency and stress fractures of the long bones occurring in patients with rheumatoid arthritis. Diagn. Radiol. 116:595, 1975.

259. Lowthian, P. J., and Calin, A.: Geode development and multiple fractures in rheumatoid arthritis. Ann. Rheum. Dis. 44:130, 1985.

260. Hoayman, J. R., Melton, L. J., III, Nelson, A. M., O'Fallon, W. M., and Riggs, B. L.: Fractures after rheumatoid arthritis: A population-based study. Arthritis Rheum. 27:1353, 1984.

261. Als, O. S., Gotfredsen, A., Rus, B. J., and Christiansen, C.: Are disease duration and degree of functional impairment determinants of bone loss in rheumatoid arthritis? Ann. Rheum. Dis. 44:406, 1985.

262. Ng, K. C., Revell, P. A., Beer, M., Boucher, B. J., Cohen, R. D., and Currey, H. L. F.: Incidence of metabolic bone disease in rheumatoid arthritis and osteoarthritis. Ann. Rheum. Dis. 43:370, 1984.

263. Kennedy, A. C., Allarn, B. F., Rooney, P. J., et al.: Hypercalcaemia in rheumatoid arthritis: Investigation of its causes and implications. Ann. Rheum. Dis. 38:401, 1979.

264. Sambrook, P. N., Eisman, J. A., Champion, G. D., Yeates, M. G., Pocock, N. A., and Eberl, S.: Determinants of axial bone loss in rheumatoid arthritis. Arthritis Rheum. 30:721, 1987.

265. Als, O. S., Gotfredsen, A., and Christiansen, C.: The effect of gluco-corticoids on bone mass in rheumatoid arthritis patients. Arthritis Rheum. 28:369, 1985.

266. Nagant de Deuxchaisnes, C., Devogelaer, J. P., Esselinckx, W., Bouchez, B., Defnesseux, G., Rombouts-Lindemans, C., and Huaux, J. P.: The effect of low dosage glucocorticoids on bone mass in rheumatoid arthritis: A cross-sectional and a longitudinal study using single photon absorptiometry. Adv. Exp. Med. Biol. 171:209, 1984.

267. Verstraeten, A., and Dequeker, J.: Vertebral and peripheral bone mineral content and fracture incidence in post menopausal patients with rheumatoid arthritis: Effect of low dose corticosteroids. Ann. Rheum. Dis. 45:852, 1986.

268. Sambrook, P. N., Eisman, J. A., Yeates, M. G., Pocock, N. A., Eberl, S., and Champion, G. D.: Osteoporosis in rheumatoid arthritis: Safety of low dose corticosteroids. Ann. Rheum. Dis. 45:950, 1986.

269. Gray, R. E. S., Doherty, S. M., Galloway, J., Coulton, L., de Broe, M., and Kanis, J. A.: A double-blind study of deflazacort and prednisone in patients with chronic inflammatory disorders. Arthritis Rheum. 34:287, 1991.

270. Steiner, G., Freund, H. A., Leichtentritt, B., and Maun, M. E.: Lesion of skeletal muscles in rheumatoid arthritis. Am. J. Pathol. 22:103, 1946.

271. Haslock, D. I., Wright, V., and Harriman, D. G. F.: Neuromuscular disorders in rheumatoid arthritis: A motor-point muscle biopsy study. Q. J. Med. 39:335, 1970.

272. Halla, J. T., Koopman, W. J., Fallahi, S., et al.: Rheumatoid myositis. Clinical and histologic features and possible pathogenesis. Arthritis Rheum. 27:737, 1984.

273. Hurd, E. R.: Extra-articular manifestations of rheumatoid arthritis. Semin. Rheum. Dis. 8:151, 1979.

274. Hart, F. D.: Rheumatoid arthritis: Extra-articular manifestations. Br. Med. J. 3:131, 1969.

275. Collins, D. H.: The subcutaneous nodule of rheumatoid arthritis. J. Pathol. Bacteriol. 45:97, 1937.

276. Bennett, G. A., Zeller, J. W., and Bauer, W.: Subcutaneous nodules of rheumatoid arthritis and rheumatic fever: A pathologic study. Arch. Pathol. 30:70, 1940.

277. Sokoloff, L.: The pathophysiology of peripheral blood vessels in collagen diseases. In Orbison J. L., and Smith, D. E. (eds.): The Peripheral Blood Vessels. Baltimore, Williams & Wilkins, 1963, p. 297.

278. Palmer, D. G., Hogg, N., Highton, J., Heissian, P. A., and Denholm, I.: Macrophage migration and maturation within rheumatoid nodules. Arthritis Rheum. 30:729, 1987.

279. Harris, E. D., Jr.: A collagenolytic system produced by primary cultures of rheumatoid nodule tissue. J. Clin. Invest. 51:2973, 1972.

280. Ganda, O. P., and Caplan, H. I.: Rheumatoid disease without joint involvement. J. A. M. A. 228:338, 1974.

281. Ginsberg, M. H., Genant, H. K., Yu, T. F., and McCarty, D. J.: Rheumatoid nodulosis: An unusual variant of rheumatoid disease. Arthritis Rheum. 18:49, 1975.

282. Brower, A. C., NaPombejara, C., Stechschulte, D. J., Mantz, F., and Ketchum, L.: Rheumatoid nodulosis: Another cause of juxta-articular nodules. Diagn. Radiol. 125:669, 1977.

283. Simons, F. E. R., and Schaller, J. G.: Benign rheumatoid nodules. Pediatrics 56:29, 1975.

284. Olive, A., Maymo, J., Lloreta, J.: Evaluation of benign rheumatoid nodules into rheumatoid arthritis after 50 years. Ann. Rheum. Dis. 46:624, 1987.

285. Wood, M. G., and Beerman, H.: Necrobiosis lipoidica, granuloma annulare: Report of a case with lesions in the galea aponeurotica of a child. Am. J. Dis. Child. 96:720, 1958.

286. Watt, T. L., and Baumann, R. R.: Pseudoxanthomatous rheumatoid nodules. Arch. Dermatol. 95:156, 1967.

287. Healey, L. A., Wilske, K. R., and Sagebiel, R. W.: Rheumatoid nodules simulating basal-cell carcinoma. N. Engl. J. Med. 277:7, 1967.

288. Sturrock, R. D., Cowden, E. A., Howie, E., Grennan, D. M., and Buchanan, W. W.: The forgotten nodule: Complications of sacral nodules in rheumatoid arthritis. Br. Med. J. 2:92, 1975.

289. Friedman, B. A., and Rice, D. H.: Rheumatoid nodules of the larynx. Arch. Otolaryngol. 101:361, 1975.

290. Jackson, C. G., Chess, R. L., and Ward, J. R.: A case of rheumatoid nodule formation within the central nervous system and review of the literature. J. Rheumatol. 11:237, 1984.

291. Pearson, M. E., Kosco, M., Huffer, W., Winter, W., Engelbrecht, J. A., and Steigerwald, J. C.: Rheumatoid nodules of the spine: Case report and review of the literature. Arthritis Rheum. 30:709, 1987.

292. Bywaters, E. G. L.: Fistulous rheumatism: A manifestation of rheumatoid arthritis. Ann. Rheum. Dis. 12:114, 1953.

293. Shapiro, R. F., Resnick, D., Castles, J. J., D'Ambrosia, R., Lipscomb, P. R., and Niwayama, G.: Fistulization of rheumatoid joints: Spectrum of identifiable syndromes. Ann. Rheum. Dis. 34:489, 1975.

294. Bassett, L. W., Gold, R. H., and Mirra, J. M.: Rheumatoid bursitis extending into the clavicle and to the skin surface. Ann. Rheum. Dis. 44:336, 1985.

295. Vandenbroucke, J. P., Kaaks, R., Valkenburg, H. A., et al.: Frequency of infections among rheumatoid arthritis patients, before and after disease onset. Arthritis Rheum. 30:810, 1987.

296. Baum, J.: Infection in rheumatoid arthritis. Arthritis Rheum. 14:135, 1971.

297. Gaulhofer de Klerch, E. H., and Van Dam, G.: Septic complications in rheumatoid arthritis. Acta Rheumatol. Scand. 9:254, 1963.

298. Huskisson, E. C., and Hart, F. D.: Severe, unusual and recurrent infections in rheumatoid arthritis. Ann. Rheum. Dis. 31:118, 1972.

299. Bodel, P. T., and Hollingsworth, J. W.: Comparative morphology, respiration, and phagocytic function of leukocytes from blood and joint fluid in rheumatoid arthritis. J. Clin. Invest. 45:580, 1966.

300. Mowat, A. G.: Hematologic abnormalities in RA. Semin. Arthritis Rheum. 1:195, 1971.

301. Engstedt, L., and Strandberg, O.: Haematological data and clinical activity of the rheumatoid diseases. Acta Med. Scand. 180:13, 1966.

302. Vreugdenhil, G., Wognum, A. W., van Eijk, H. G., and Swaak, A. J. G.: Anaemia in rheumatoid arthritis: The role of iron, vitamin B_{12}, and folic acid deficiency, and erythropoietin responsiveness. Ann. Rheum. Dis. 49:93, 1990.

303. Beck, R. L., French, B., Brinck-Johnsen, T., Cornwell, G. G., and Rawnsley, H. M.: Multivariate approach to predictive diagnosis of bone-marrow iron stores. Am. J. Pathol. 70:665, 1978.

304. Samson, D., Holliday, D., and Gumpel, J. M.: Role of ineffective erythropoiesis in the anaemia of rheumatoid arthritis. Ann. Rheum. Dis. 36:181, 1977.

305. Cartwright, G. E.: The anemia of chronic disorders. Semin. Hematol. 3:351, 1966.

306. Raymond, F. D., Bowie, M. A., and Dugan, A.: Iron metabolism in rheumatoid arthritis. Arthritis Rheum. 8:233, 1965.

307. Ridolfo, A. S., Rubin, A., Crabtree, R. E., and Gruber, C. M.: Effects of fenoprofen and aspirin on gastrointestinal microbleeding in man. Clin. Pharmacol. Ther. 14:226, 1973.

308. Williams, R. A., Samson, D., Tikerpae, J., Crowne, J., and Gumpel, J. M.: In-vitro studies of ineffective erythropoiesis in rheumatoid arthritis. Am. J. Rheum. Dis. 41:502, 1982.

309. Reid, C. D. L., Prouse, P. J., Baptista, L. C., et al.: The mechanisms of anaemia in rheumatoid arthritis: Effects of bone marrow adherent cells and of serum on in vivo erythropoiesis. Br. J. Haematol. 58:607, 1984.

310. Prouse, P. J., Bonner, B., Gumpel, J. M., et al.: Stimulation of bone marrow erythropoiesis by T lymphocytes of anaemic patients with rheumatoid arthritis. Ann. Rheum. Dis. 44:220, 1985.

311. Winchester, R. J., Litwin, S. D., Koffler, D., and Kunkel, H. G.: Observations on the eosinophilia of certain patients with rheumatoid arthritis. Arthritis Rheum. 14:650, 1971.

312. Hutchinson, R. M., Davis, P., and Jayson, M. I. V.: Thrombocytosis in rheumatoid arthritis. Ann. Rheum. Dis. 35:138, 1976.

313. Farr, M., Scott, D. L., Constable, T. J., Hawker, R. L., Hawkins, C. F., and Stuart, J.: Thrombocytosis of active rheumatoid disease. Ann. Rheum. Dis. 42:545, 1983.

314. Combe, B., Andary, M., Caraux, J., et al.: Characterization of an expanded subpopulation of large granular lymphocytes in a patient with rheumatoid arthritis. Arthritis Rheum. 29:675, 1986.

315. Wittenborg, A., Gille, J., Ostertag, H., et al.: Die Dugitalartritis bei chronischer Polyarthritis. Folia Angiol. 22:409, 1974.

316. Fischer, M., Mielke, H., Glaefke, S., and Deicher, H.: Generalized vasculopathy and finger blood flow abnormalities in rheumatoid arthritis. J. Rheumatol. 11:33, 1984.

317. Sokoloff, L., and Bunin, J. J.: Vascular lesions in rheumatoid arthritis. J. Chronic Dis. 5:668, 1957.
318. Kulka, J. P., Bocking, D., Ropes, M. W., and Bauer, W.: Early joint lesions of rheumatoid arthritis: Report of 8 cases with knee biopsies of less than one year's duration. Arch. Pathol. 59:129, 1955.
319. Soter, N. A., Mihm, M. C., Gigli, I., and Dvorak, H. F.: Two distinct cellular patterns in cutaneous necrotizing angiitis. J. Invest. Dermatol. 66:344, 1976.
320. Rapaport, R. J., Kozin, F., Mackel, S. E., and Jordon, R. E.: Cutaneous vascular immunofluorescence in rheumatoid arthritis. Am. J. Med. 68:344, 1976.
321. Mongam, E. S., Cass, R. M., Jacox, R. F., and Vaughan, J. H.: A study of the relation of seronegative and seropositive rheumatoid arthritis to each other and to necrotizing vasculitis. Am. J. Med. 47:23, 1969.
322. Weinstein, A., Peters, K., Brown, D., and Bluestone, R.: Metabolism of the third component of complement (C3) in patients with rheumatoid arthritis. Arthritis Rheum. 15:49, 1972.
323. Conn, D. L., McDuffie, F. C., and Dyck, P. J.: Immunopathologic study of sural nerves in rheumatoid arthritis. Arthritis Rheum. 15:135, 1972.
324. Weisman, M., and Zvaifler, N.: Cryoimmunoglobulinemia in rheumatoid arthritis. J. Clin. Invest. 56:725, 1975.
325. Schmid, F. R., Cooper, N. S., Ziff, M., and McEwen, C.: Arteritis in rheumatoid arthritis. Am. J. Med. 30:56, 1961.
326. Markenson, J. A., McDougal, J. S., Tsairis, P., et al.: Rheumatoid meningitis: A localized immune process. Ann. Intern. Med. 119:359, 1967.
327. Siomopoulos, V., and Shah, N.: Acute organic brain syndrome associated with rheumatoid arthritis. J. Clin. Psychol. 40:46, 1979.
328. Bienenstock, H., Minick, R., and Rogoff, B.: Mesenteric arteritis and intestinal infarction in rheumatoid disease. Arch. Intern. Med. 119:359, 1967.
329. Hart, F. D., Golding, J. R., and MacKenzie, D. H.: Neuropathy in rheumatoid disease. Ann. Rheum. Dis. 16:471, 1957.
330. Gordon, D. A., Stein, J. L., and Brody, I.: The extra-articular features of rheumatoid arthritis: A systematic analysis of 127 cases. Am. J. Med. 54:445, 1973.
331. Geirsson, A. J., Sturfelt, G., and Truedsson, L.: Clinical and serological features of severe vasculitis in rheumatoid arthritis: Prognostic implications. Ann. Rheum. Dis. 46:727, 1987.
332. Scott, D. G., Baron, P. A., Elliott P. J., et al.: Systemic vasculitis in a district general hospital 1972–80. Q. J. Med. 51:292, 1982.
333. Lawson, A. A. H., and MacLean, N.: Renal disease and drug therapy in rheumatoid arthritis. Ann. Rheum. Dis. 25:441, 1966.
334. Samuels, B., Lee, J. C., Engleman, E. P., and Hooper, J., Jr.: Membranous nephropathy in patients with rheumatoid arthritis: Relationship to gold therapy. Medicine 57:319, 1977.
335. Via, C. S., Hasbargen, J. A., Moore, J., et al.: Rheumatoid arthritis and membranous glomerulonephritis: A role for immune complex dissociative techniques. J. Rheumatol. 11:342, 1984.
336. Hardon, L. D., Sellars, L., Morley, A. R., Wilkinson, R., Thompson, M., and Griffiths, I. D.: Hematuria in rheumatoid arthritis: An association with mesangial glomerulonephritis. Ann. Rheum. Dis. 43:440, 1984.
337. Walker, W. C., and Wright, V.: Pulmonary lesions and rheumatoid arthritis. Medicine 47:501, 1968.
338. Dodson, W. H., and Hollingsworth, J. W.: Pleural effusion in rheumatoid arthritis: Impaired transport of glucose. N. Engl. J. Med. 275:1337, 1966.
339. Walker, W. C., and Wright, V.: Diffuse interstitial pulmonary fibrosis and rheumatoid arthritis. Ann. Rheum. Dis. 28:252, 1969.
340. Dixon, A. St. J., and Ball, J.: Honeycomb lung and chronic rheumatoid arthritis: A case report. Ann. Rheum. Dis. 16:241, 1957.
341. Stack, B. H. R., and Grant, I. W. B.: Rheumatoid interstitial lung disease. Br. J. Dis. Chest 59:202, 1965.
342. Frank, S. T., Weg, J. G., Harkleroad, L. E., and Fitch, R. F.: Pulmonary dysfunction in rheumatoid disease. Chest 63:27, 1973.
343. Tiskler, M., Grief, J., Fireman, E., et al.: Bronchoalveolar lavage: A sensitive tool for early diagnosis of pulmonary involvement in rheumatoid arthritis. J. Rheumatol. 13:547, 1986.
344. Caplan, A.: Certain unusual radiographic appearances in the chest of coal miners suffering from RA. Thorax 8:29, 1953.
345. Portner, M. M., and Gracie, W. A.: Rheumatoid lung disease with cavitary nodules, pneumothorax and eosinophilia. N. Engl. J. Med. 275:697, 1966.
346. Hull, S., and Mathews, J. A.: Pulmonary necrobiotic nodules as a presenting feature of rheumatoid arthritis. Ann. Rheum. 41:21, 1982.
347. Shenberger, K. N., Schned, A. R., and Taylor, T. H.: Rheumatoid disease and bronchogenic carcinoma: Case report and review of the literature. J. Rheumatol. 11:226, 1984.
348. Gardner, D. L., Duthie, J. R., MacLeod, J., and Allan, W. S. H.: Pulmonary hypertension in RA: Report of a case study with intimal sclerosis of pulmonary and digital arteries. Scott. Med. J. 2:183, 1957.

349. Radoux, V., Menard, H. A., Begin, R., Decary, F., and Koopman, W. J.: Airways disease in rheumatoid arthritis patients: One element of a general exocrine dysfunction. Arthritis Rheum. 30:249, 1987.
350. Sassoon, C. S. H., McAlpine, S. W., Tashkin, D. P., Baydur, A., Quismorio, F. P., and Mongan, E. S.: Small airways function in non-smokers with rheumatoid arthritis. Arthritis Rheum. 27:1218, 1984.
351. Popp, R. L.: Medical Progress: Echocardiography (first of two parts). N. Engl. J. Med. 323:101, 1990.
352. Bonfiglio, T., and Atwater, E.: Heart disease in patients with seropositive rheumatoid arthritis: A controlled autopsy study and review. Arch. Intern. Med. 127:714, 1969.
353. Lebowitz, W. B.: The heart in rheumatoid arthritis: A clinical and pathological study of 62 cases. Ann. Intern. Med. 58:102, 1963.
354. MacDonald, W. J., Jr., Crawford, M. H., Klippel, J. H., Zvaifler, N. J., and O'Rourke, R. A.: Echocardiographic assessment of cardiac structure and function in patients with rheumatoid arthritis. Am. J. Med. 63:890, 1977.
355. Lange, R. K., Weiss, T. E., and Ochsner, J. L.: Rheumatoid arthritis and constrictive pericarditis: A patient benefited by pericardectomy. Arthritis Rheum. 8:403, 1965.
356. Thadini, V., Iveson, J. M. I., and Wright, V.: Cardiac tamponade, constrictive pericarditis and pericardial resection in rheumatoid arthritis. Medicine 54:261, 1975.
357. Prakash, R., Atassi, A., Poske, R., and Rosen, K. M.: Prevalence of pericardial effusion and mitral-valve involvement in patients with rheumatoid arthritis without cardiac symptoms. N. Engl. J. Med. 289:597, 1975.
358. Weintraub, A. M., and Zvaifler, N. J.: The occurrence of valvular and myocardial disease in patients with chronic joint disease. Am. J. Med. 35:145, 1963.
359. Iveson, J. M. I., Thadani, V., Ionescu, M., and Wright, V.: Aortic valve incompetence and replacement in rheumatoid arthritis. Ann. Rheum. Dis. 34:312, 1975.
360. Gowans, J. D. C.: Complete heart block with Stokes-Adams syndrome due to rheumatoid heart disease. N. Engl. J. Med. 262:1012, 1960.
361. Lev, M., Bharati, S., Hoffman, F. G., and Leight, L.: The conduction system in rheumatoid arthritis with complete atrioventricular block. Am. Heart J. 90:78, 1975.
362. Ahern, M., Lever, J. V., and Cash, J.: Complete heart block in rheumatoid arthritis. Ann. Rheum. Dis. 42:389, 1983.
363. Swezey, R. L.: Myocardial infarction due to rheumatoid arthritis. J. A. M. A. 199:191, 1967.
364. Reimer, K. A., Rodgers, R. F., and Oyasu, R.: Rheumatoid arthritis with rheumatoid heart disease and granulomatous aortitis. J. A. M. A. 235:2510, 1976.
365. Valkenburg, H. A.: Pattern of rheumatoid disease in society: Change or disappearance? Scand. J. Rheumatol. 5 (Suppl. 12):89, 1975.
366. Pinals, R. S., Masi, A. F., Larsen, R. A., et al.: Preliminary criteria for clinical remission in rheumatoid arthritis. Arthritis Rheum. 24:1308, 1981.
367. Wolfe, F., and Hawley, D. J.: Remission in rheumatoid arthritis. J. Rheumatol. 12:245, 1985.
368. Pinals, R. S.: Survival in rheumatoid arthritis. Arthritis Rheum. 30:473, 1987.
369. Vandenbrouche, J. P., Hazevoct, H. M., and Cats, A.: Survival and cause of death in rheumatoid arthritis: A 25-year prospective follow-up. J. Rheumatol. 11:158, 1984.
370. Harris, E. D., Jr.: The challenge of therapy for rheumatoid arthritis. Eur. J. Int. Med. 1:325, 1990.
371. Reilly, P. A., Cosh, J. A., Maddison, P. J., Rasker, J. J., Silman, A. J.: Mortality and survival in rheumatoid arthritis: A 25 year prospective study of 100 patients. Ann. Rheum. Dis. 49:363, 1990.
372. Sherrer, Y. S., Block, D. A., Mitchell, D. M., Young, D. Y., and Fries, J. F.: The development of disability in rheumatoid arthritis. Arthritis Rheum. 29:494, 1986.
373. Luukkainen, R., Isomaki, H., and Kajander, A.: Prognostic value of the type of onset of rheumatoid arthritis. Ann. Rheum. Dis. 42:274, 1983.
374. Sharp, J. T., Calkins, E., Cohen, A. S., Schubart, A. F., and Calabro, J. J.: Observations on the clinical, chemical, and serological manifestations of rheumatoid arthritis, based on the course of 154 cases. Medicine 43:41, 1964.
375. Cobb, S., Anderson, F., and Baurer, W.: Length of life and cause of death in rheumatoid arthritis. N. Engl. J. Med. 249:553, 1953.
376. Baum, J.: Infection in rheumatoid arthritis. Arthritis Rheum. 14:135, 1971.
377. Mitchell, D. M., Spitz, P. W., Young, D. Y., Block, D. A., McShane, D. J., and Fries, J. F.: Survival, prognosis, and causes of death in rheumatoid arthritis. Arthritis Rheum. 29:706, 1986.
378. Pincus, T., Callahan, L. F., Sale, W. G., Brooks, A. L., Payne, L. E., and Vaughn, W. K.: Severe functional declines, work disability, and increased mortality in 75 RA patients studied over 9 years. Arthritis Rheum. 27:864, 1984.
379. Erhardt, C. C., Mumford, P. A., Venables, P. J. W., et al.: Factors

predicting a poor life prognosis in rheumatoid arthritis: An eight-year prospective study. Ann. Rheum. Dis. 48:7, 1989.

380. Pincus, T., and Callahan, L. F.: Taking mortality in RA seriously: Predictive markers, socioeconomic status and comorbidity. J. Rheumatol. 13:841, 1986.

381. Laakso, M., Mutru, O., Isomaki, H., and Koota, K.: Cancer mortality in patients with rheumatoid arthritis. J. Rheumatol. 13:522, 1986.

382. Kellgren, J. H., and O'Brien, W. M.: On the natural history of rheumatoid arthritis in relation to the sheep cell agglutination test (SCAT). Arthritis Rheum. 5:115, 1962.

383. Masi, A. T., Maldonado-Cocco, J. A., Kaplan, S. B., Feigenbaum, S. L., and Chandler, R. W.: Prospective study of the early course of rheumatoid arthritis in young adults: Comparison of patients with and without rheumatoid factor positivity at entry and identification of variables correlating with outcome. Semin. Arthritis Rheum. 5:299, 1976.

384. Jacoby, R. K., Jayson, M. I. V., and Cosh, J. A.: Onset, early stages and prognosis of rheumatoid arthritis: A clinical study of 100 patients with 11-year follow-up. Br. Med. J. 2:96, 1973.

385. Dixon, A. St. J.: "Rheumatoid arthritis" with negative serological reaction. Ann. Rheum. Dis. 19:209, 1960.

386. Withrington, R. H., Teitsson, I., Valdimarsson, H., et al.: Prospective study of early rheumatoid arthritis, II. Association of rheumatoid factor isotypes with fluctuations in disease activity. Ann. Rheum. Dis. 43:679, 1984.

387. Duthie, J. J. R., Brown, P. E., Truelove, L. H., Barago, E., and Lawrie, A. J.: Course and prognosis in rheumatoid arthritis: A further report. Ann. Rheum. Dis. 23:193, 1964.

388. Ragan, C., and Farrington, E.: The clinical features of rheumatoid arthritis. J. A. M. A. 181:663, 1962.

389. Henderson, D. R. F., Jayson, M. I. V., and Tribe, C. B.: Lack of correlation of synovial histology with joint damage in rheumatoid arthritis. Ann. Rheum. Dis. 34:7, 1975.

390. Yates, D. B., and Scott, J. T.: Rheumatoid synovitis and joint disease: Relationship between arthroscopic and histological changes. Ann. Rheum. Dis. 34:1, 1975.

391. Cruickshank, B.: Interpretation of multiple biopsies of synovial tissue in rheumatic diseases. Ann. Rheum. Dis. 11:137, 1952.

392. Muirden, K. D., and Mills, K. W.: Do lymphocytes protect the rheumatoid joint? Br. Med. J. 4:219, 1971.

393. Harris, E. D., Jr., Faulkner, C. S., II, and Brown, F. E.: Collagenolytic systems in rheumatoid arthritis. Clin. Orthop. 140:303, 1975.

394. Ward, T. T., and Steigbigel, R. T.: Acidosis of synovial fluid correlates with synovial fluid leukocytosis. Am. J. Med. 64:933, 1978.

395. Geborek, P., Saxne, T., Pettersson, H., et al.: Synovial fluid acidosis correlates with radiological joint destruction in rheumatoid arthritis knee joints. J. Rheumatol. 16:468, 1989.

396. Ruddy, S.: Synovial fluid: Mirror of the inflammatory lesion in rheumatoid arthritis. In Harris, E. D., Jr. (ed.): Rheumatoid Arthritis. New York, Medcom Press, 1974.

397. Regan-Smith, M. G., O'Connor, G. T., Kwoh, C. K., Brown, L. A., Olmstead, E. M., and Burnett, J. B.: Lack of correlation between the Steinbrocker staging of hand radiographs and the functional health status of individuals with rheumatoid arthritis. Arthritis Rheum. 32:128, 1989.

398. Larsen, A., Dale, K., Eek, M.: Radiographic evaluation of rheumatoid arthritis and related conditions by standard reference films. Acta Radiol. 18:481, 1977.

399. O'Sullivan, M. M., Lewis, P. A., Newcombe, R. G., Broderick, N. J., Robinson, D. A., Coles, E. C., and Jessop, J. D.: Precision of Larsen grading of radiographs in assessing progression of rheumatoid arthritis in individual patients. Ann. Rheum. Dis. 49:286, 1990.

400. Sharp, J. T.: Radiologic assessment as an outcome measurement in rheumatoid arthritis. Arthritis Rheum. 32:221, 1989.

401. Egger, M. J., Huth, D. A., Ward, J. R., Reading, J. C., and Williams, H. J.: Reduced joint count indices in the evaluation of rheumatoid arthritis. Arthritis Rheum. 28:613, 1985.

402. Thompson, P. W., Silman, A. J., Kirwan, J. R., and Currey, H. L. F.: Articular indices of joint inflammation in rheumatoid arthritis: Correlation with the acute phase response. Arthritis Rheum. 30:618, 1987.

403. Steinbrocker, O., Traeger, C. H., and Batterman, R. C.: Therapeutic criteria in rheumatoid arthritis. J. A. M. A. 140:659, 1949.

404. Pincus, T., Callahan, L. F., Brooks, R. H., Fuchs, H. A., Olsen, N. J., and Kaye, J. J.: Self-report questionnaire scores in rheumatoid arthritis compared with traditional, physical, radiographic, and laboratory measures. Ann. Intern. Med. 110:259, 1989.

405. Callahan, L. F., Brooks, R. H., Summey, J. A., and Pincus, T.: Quantitative pain assessment for routine care of rheumatoid arthritis patients, using a pain scale based on activities of daily living and a visual analog pain scale. Arthritis Rheum. 30:630, 1987.

406. Ritchie, D. M., Boyle, J. A., McInness, J. M., Jasani, M. K., Dalakos, T. G., Grieveson, P., and Buchanan, W. W.: Clinical studies with an articular index for the assessment of joint tenderness in patients with rheumatoid arthritis. Q. J. Med. 37:393, 1968.

407. The Cooperating Clinics Committee of the ARA: A seven-day variability study of 499 patients with peripheral rheumatoid arthritis. Arthritis Rheum. 8:302, 1965.

408. Lansbury, J.: Report of a three-year study on the systemic and articular indexes in rheumatoid arthritis: Theoretic and clinical considerations. Arthritis Rheum. 1:505, 1958.

409. Lansbury, J., and Haut, D. D.: Quantitation of the manifestations of rheumatoid arthritis: Area of joint surfaces as an index to total joint inflammation and deformity. Am. J. Med. Sci. 232:150, 1956.

410. Lansbury, J.: Quantitation of activity of rheumatoid arthritis: Method for summation of systemic indices of rheumatoid activity. Am. J. Med. Sci. 232:300, 1956.

411. Thompson, P. W., Silman, A. J., Kirwan, J. R., and Currey, H. L. F.: Articular indices of joint inflammation in rheumatoid arthritis: Correlation with the acute phase response. Arthritis Rheum. 30:618, 1987.

412. Callahan, L. F., Brooks, R. H., Summey, J. A., and Pincus, T.: Quantitative pain assessment for routine care of rheumatoid arthritis patients, using a pain scale based on activities of daily living and a visual analog pain scale. Arthritis Rheum. 30:630, 1987.

413. Geborek, P., Saxne, T., Pettersson, H., et al.: Synovial fluid acidosis correlates with radiological joint destruction in rheumatoid arthritis knee joints. J. Rheum. 16:468, 1989.

414. Amos, R. S., Constable, T. J., Crockson, R. A., et al.: Rheumatoid arthritis: Relation of serum C-reactive protein and erythrocyte sedimentation rates to radiographic changes. Br. Med. J. 1:195, 1977.

415. Mallya, R. K., deBeer, F. C., Berry, H., et al.: Correlation of clinical parameters of disease activity in rheumatoid arthritis with serum concentration of C-reactive protein and erythrocyte sedimentation rate. J. Rheumatol. 9:224, 1982.

416. Ochi, T., Yonemasu, K., Iwase, R., et al.: Serum C1q levels as a prognostic guide to articular erosions in patients with rheumatoid arthritis. Arthritis Rheum. 27:883, 1984.

417. Hørslev-Peterson, K., Bentsen, K. D., Junker, P., et al.: Serum aminoterminal type III procollagen peptide in rheumatoid arthritis. Arthritis Rheum. 29:592, 1986.

418. Hassfeld, W., Steiner, G., Hartmuth, K. Kolarz, G., Scherak, O., Graninger, W., Thumb, N., and Smolen, J. S.: Demonstration of a new antinuclear antibody (anti-RA33) that is highly specific for rheumatoid arthritis. Arthritis Rheum. 32:1515, 1989.

419. Pruzanski, W., Keystone, E. C., Sternby, B., et al.: Serum phospholipase A_2 correlates with disease activity in rheumatoid arthritis. J. Rheumatol. 15:1351, 1988.

420. Krause, A., Protz, H., Goebel, K. M.: Correlation between synovial neopterin and inflammatory activity in rheumatoid arthritis. Ann. Rheum. Dis. 48:636, 1989.

421. Blach, D., Marabani, M., Sturrock, R. D., et al.: Urinary excretion of the hydroxypyridinium cross-links of collagen in patients with rheumatoid arthritis. Ann. Rheum. Dis. 48:641, 1989.

422. Ordenstein, L.: Sur la Paralysie Agitante et la Sclerose en Plaques Generalisee. Paris, Imprimerie de E. Martinet, 1864 (original in the Library of the New York Academy of Medicine).

Treatment of Rheumatoid Arthritis

A definite trend exists to treat rheumatoid arthritis (RA) more aggressively and earlier in the course of disease. The reasons for this are several. First, as summarized in detail in Chapter 52, it is now appreciated that RA is not a benign disease; there is a significant increase in mortality in rheumatoid patients. Second, there is little evidence that current approaches to therapy alter the rate of progression of disease or decrease morbidity. The long-term data on prognosis of rheumatoid patients are discouraging to the physician who believes that joint loss can be retarded, if not prevented. Mean radiographic scores, for example, when plotted against years after diagnosis of RA, show no deviation from the straight line determined by a regression equation, implying that when RA is firmly established, progression of joint destruction is inexorable and inevitable.[1] In another study, 50 patients with RA were followed for a minimum of 10 years.[2] In 48 patients, the total joint score deteriorated regardless of treatment. During 10 years, most progression occurred in the wrists, knees, and metacarpophalangeal (MCP) joints, but also there was a highly significant (r = 0.79) correlation between scores in these joints and those in all other joints. More discussion of prognosis is included in Chapter 52.

In another review, it was concluded that the rate of deterioration of function in patients with RA appears not to have changed significantly over the past 15 years.[3] The long-term deterioration occurs in spite of the success of many short-term clinical trials that fill the medical journals. An important reason for this dichotomy probably lies not in delayed diagnosis but in therapy that neither is sufficiently focused on crucial amplification switches in the inflammatory and proliferative circuits in the disease (reviewed in Chapter 51) nor is administered early enough in the process to make a difference. The reasons governing delayed therapy are appropriate: There are insufficient measures of disease progression in place to predict which patient will suffer progressive disease, and the toxicity of many of the broad-spectrum disease-modifying drugs that we use is great enough to delay our early prescription of these compounds.

In the future, rheumatologists must develop better ways of sorting patients early in their disease into subsets with good, less good, and poor prognoses so those destined to have more rapid destructive disease can be identified. At present, the patients more likely to have crippling disease can be defined as those with polyarticular synovitis, significant titers of rheumatoid factor, an elevated C-reactive protein (CRP) and erythrocyte sedimentation rate (ESR), and substantial disability assayed by validated health assessment questionnaires.[4, 5] In controlled studies of advanced therapies, it will be appropriate to identify within this group a smaller cohort who bear the RA susceptibility sequence QKRAA/QRRAA (determined by use of the polymerase chain reaction to amplify DNA from small numbers of cells from peripheral blood) on beta (β) chains of class II major histocompatibility complex (MHC) antigens (see Chapter 51).[6–12] For the present, however, such sophisticated screening is impossible because of its high cost.

STAGED THERAPY FOR RHEUMATOID ARTHRITIS

Phase I

In Chapter 51, the pathogenesis of RA is reviewed. It is likely that many events outlined there occur before the patient experiences significant symptoms. Most individuals, except for those who ignore symptomatic complaints or who have no access to medical care, will seek aid after joint inflammation begins but before synovial tissue has proliferated significantly. The interval between the beginning of the disease and diagnosis can be considered a time for nonspecific intervention.

Even though no specific diagnosis can be made, this period can be used both to rule out other serious or treatable causes of synovitis (e.g., Lyme disease, systemic lupus erythematosus [SLE], polyarticular gout, low-grade sepsis) and to begin anti-inflammatory drug therapy, physical therapy, and instruction in protection of joints during activities of daily living (Fig. 53–1A). After the diagnosis of RA is made, the physician's initial task is to educate the patient about RA while treating pain and early inflammation and alleviating anxiety, frustration, and depression.

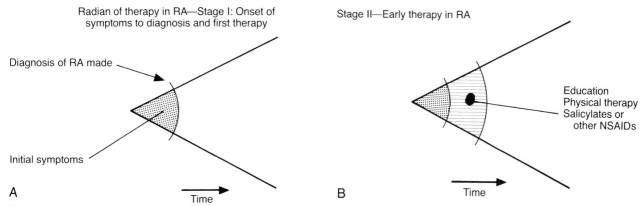

Figure 53–1. *A,* Rheumatoid arthritis begins before the diagnosis is made. In the interval between onset of the disease and diagnosis, a variable amount of both reversible and irreversible damage occurs in each patient. In this figure and subsequent ones, RA is beginning at the intersection of the two lines. With time, and at a variable rate that is unique to each patient, the disease progresses. Schematically, patients with primarily systemic involvement will be progressing along the upper line, and those with disease marked primarily by joint destruction along the lower line. *B,* Phase I of therapy is nonspecific. It would be appropriate for any form of inflammatory arthritis. Education must be emphasized; without it, the patient's attitudes about himself or herself and the disease will be inadequate, and the compliance with therapy will be variable. Now, not later, is the time to emphasize principles of joint protection and exercise.

Psychologic Aspects of Rheumatoid Arthritis and Their Relevance to Therapy

There is no *rheumatoid personality,* a collection of traits that are found more in individuals predisposed to developing arthritis. Rather, the data suggest that the pain and disability of this chronic disease bring out in patients a sense of helplessness, depression, lower levels of self-esteem, and adaptive mechanisms that may either help or hinder ability to cope with the disease.[13]

The outcome of the relationship between physician and patient, as well as the patient's subsequent compliance with therapeutic regimens, may depend on the initial adaptation to the disease. There seems little question that the physician can modify and help determine the degree and type of adaptation. Recognition by the patient that the outcome of the disease may possibly depend on education and awareness of the facts about RA is an important component of therapy. Many patients never adapt effectively to RA. The model of *learned helplessness* may be particularly relevant.[14, 15] In its simplest dimensions, this model, which applies to other illnesses as well as RA, states that the patient comes to believe that pain, disability, and all other consequences of RA cannot be controlled by him or her or the physician because the cause of the disease is unknown, it behaves unpredictably, and there is no known cure. Thus, as the disease evolves, patients react in a helpless manner to situations they once would have been able to control. The helpless state is marked by three deficits: (1) emotional deficits, including development of anxiety, depression, fears of altered appearance, and loss of self-esteem; (2) motivational deficits, including diminished attempts to engage in activities of daily living; and (3) cognitive deficits, that is, new coping behavior. The result of these deficits is a patient who is not compliant, relies on spurious remedies, and may excessively use the resources of the health care system. If the patient is aware of the trap of learned helplessness, he or she may avoid it.

Little can substitute for the sustaining and buoying support of a caring, wise physician. This is an essential ingredient of treatment that cannot be replaced by efforts of nonphysician members of the health care team. The restrictions of time on the physician, however, dilute his or her effectiveness. To extend and amplify beneficial therapy of RA, both physician and patient need physical therapists, occupational therapists, nurses, and social workers trained in their own fields as well as in health education. Data are now accumulating to indicate that early education for RA patients can positively affect the outcome. The most convincing has been the use of the Arthritis Self-Management Program (ASMP) developed, implemented, and tested by Lorig and colleagues.[16, 17] The ASMP educates and, equally important, enables the patient to get involved in the therapy and to learn healthy attitudes toward accepted modes of therapy. All of the currently available health status instruments have been reviewed recently.[17a]

Physical and Occupational Therapy

Specific modalities within the domain of occupational and physical therapy are discussed in detail in Chapter 102. The physician, therapist, and patient must be aware that the physical component of therapy is going to demand re-evaluation as the disease evolves, ebbs, and flares up. Close interaction between the prescribing physician and both physical and occupational therapists is essential.

Nutrition and Diet in Rheumatoid Arthritis

Nutritional status in RA is often inadequately evaluated. In a study in which no control subjects had evidence of malnutrition, 26 percent of rheumatoid patients were malnourished.[18] Of measured variables in 50 control subjects and 50 RA patients, significant differences in body mass index; triceps skin fold thickness; and levels of serum albumin, transferrin, zinc, retinol-binding protein, thyroxine-binding prealbumin, and folic acid were found. Among the rheumatoid patients, the malnourished patients had higher ESRs and levels of CRP.

No disease has generated as many fad diets to cure it as has RA. Characteristic of each has been a failure to measure its effects objectively. One exception to this was a study that attempted to evaluate omission of meat from the diet.[19] No overall benefit was demonstrated; for a few patients, however, the absence of meat consistently correlated with clinical improvement.

More scientifically based has been the logic that if precursors of arachidonic acid (AA) can be eliminated from the diet, the phlogistic prostaglandins and leukotrienes might be diminished. The strategy for accomplishing this has been supplementing diets with eicosapentaenoic acid (EPA), one of the omega-3 (ω-3) fatty acids that are polyunsaturated and abundant in fish. In one study of 17 patients given EPA and 20 control subjects on a regular diet, modest clinical improvement in the EPA-supplemented patients was demonstrated, improvement that regressed when EPA was stopped.[20] A subsequent double-blind, placebo-controlled, crossover trial (14 weeks each) of 40 RA patients given 2.7 g of EPA and 1.8 g of docosahexaenoic acid (DHA) as 15 MaxEPA capsules each day showed an improvement in the treated group in time to onset of fatigue and tender joints.[21] In a study using fractionated fish oils compared with a coconut oil placebo in 16 patients, joint swelling and morning stiffness were statistically improved, but the response resembled an anti-inflammatory rather than a disease-modifying effect.[22] Omega-3 fatty acid supplementation leads to inhibition of platelet-derived growth factor–like protein by endothelial cells,[23] suppression of interleukin-1 and tumor necrosis factor production by mononuclear cells,[24] suppression of human synovial cell proliferation,[25] and a decrease in neutrophil leukotriene B_4 production.[21]

Aspirin and Nonsteroidal Anti-inflammatory Drugs

Traditionally, the outcome variables that are most sensitive and reliable in assessment of disease activity in RA are (1) physician's global evaluation of disease activity, (2) patient's global evaluation of disease activity, (3) swollen and tender joint count, and (4) patient's assessment of pain. It has been shown that aspirin and other nonsteroidal anti-inflammatory drugs (NSAIDs) can lead to improvement in each of these variables.

Salicylates. These drugs are potentially toxic and often maligned. Yet they remain useful in RA for patients who can tolerate them. Aspirin has been in use since the 18th century[26] and is a reasonable initial choice of therapy for the patient with early disease. There are several reasons: Compliance in therapy can be measured objectively (i.e., salicylate levels in serum), aspirin is inexpensive, and serum salicylate levels correlate well with reversible toxic symptoms (e.g., tinnitus) (Fig. 53–1B).

The interaction between patient and physician as the side effects and dosage schedule are discussed and monitoring of toxicity is carried out can be crucial to the patient–physician bond that must develop if long-term management is to be cohesive and effective. For a patient with early RA without allergy to salicylates, without recent history of atopy, and with no history of peptic ulcer, recent gastritis, or bleeding disorder, aspirin is a good choice of therapy. The pharmacodynamics of salicylates are discussed in Chapter 41 in detail. It is useful to begin, in the adult, with 3.6 g per day in four divided doses. If this is tolerated but symptoms are not relieved after 5 to 7 days, an increase to 4.2 g is appropriate. After that, increase in dosage should be no more than 0.3 g per week because the normal pathways for metabolizing the drug to salicylic acid or the glucuronide become saturated at higher doses.

Nonacetylated salicylates have less gastrointestinal toxicity than aspirin, and salicylate levels still can be used to monitor compliance. They include sodium salicylate, 1.8 to 2.4 g per day (three or four doses); choline salicylate, 5 ml three or four times daily; salicylsalicylic acid, 2 to 3 g per day (in two or three divided doses); and choline magnesium trisalicylate, 1.0 to 1.5 g twice daily. Unlike aspirin, these drugs do not acetylate proteins. Thus, any effect on platelet function or cyclo-oxygenase is short-lived (2 to 3 days) when contrasted with that of aspirin (2 weeks or more). As a group, these aspirin alternatives have a more reasonable dosage schedule, less gastrointestinal toxicity, and a higher cost than aspirin. Perhaps the most effective NSAID in patients with aspirin-induced gastrointestinal toxicity is enteric-coated aspirin. Modern preparations are absorbed efficiently.[27]

Elderly patients may be particularly intolerant of salicylates. Tinnitus occurs at lower blood levels, and bleeding from gastritis or colonic diverticuli may occur without warning. Renal excretion of the drugs may fluctuate in response to drugs (e.g., glucocorticoids), dehydration, or disease, causing abrupt fluctuations in blood levels. This difference in salicylate dynamics in the elderly (i.e., an increased toxicity with a lower dose) has been documented in a study using the American College of Rheumatology Medical Information System.[28]

Sustained-release aspirin (although expensive) is available and is particularly effective in patients who refuse to be compliant with the frequent dosage schedule required for aspirin and in patients who particularly need residual anti-inflammatory activity in the early morning.

Nonsalicylate NSAIDs. The pharmacology and impressive toxicity of these drugs are detailed in Chapter 43. There are many of these compounds, and their similarities of action and side effects are greater than their differences.

Although data are scant that NSAIDs can alter the course of RA, one study has identified clinical responders and nonresponders in a cohort of rheumatoid patients receiving fiurbiprofen or ibuprofen. The responders demonstrated significant reductions in levels of gamma M immunoglobulin (IgM) rheumatoid factor and CRP, parameters that have previously been shown to improve when disease-modifying antirheumatic drugs (DMARDs) are used effectively.[29] The NSAIDs do more than inhibit prostaglandins. They inhibit many cell membrane–associated processes,[30] suppress activation of neutrophils,[31] and prevent oxidant injury.[32]

There are several situations in which use of a nonsalicylate NSAID concurrently with aspirin is appropriate. Some patients get relief from aspirin yet develop tinnitus at blood levels inadequate for full anti-inflammatory activity (i.e., below 18 mg per dl). For these, giving the tolerated salicylate dose with meals during the day and a long-acting NSAID (e.g., piroxicam, 10 mg, or naproxen, 750 mg, or indomethacin SR, 75 mg) before bed may relieve morning stiffness.

Giving full doses of both a salicylate and an NSAID around the clock has been inadequately evaluated; one study, however, demonstrated no significant efficacy in combining a full dose of naproxen and a full dose of choline magnesium trisalicylate in the same patient. The cost of medications, of course, was significantly higher.[33] There is no good indication for prescribing more than one nonsalicylate NSAID concurrently.

Use of full dose of one nonsalicylate NSAID in patients not tolerant of salicylates or their dosage schedules is common. It is difficult to predict which drug will be most effective in individual patients. If one is not useful, it should be replaced by another (usually from a different chemical class) after a 2- or 3-week trial at full dosage. Choice should be based on potential toxicity. For example, the physician should not choose indomethacin for a patient with chronic severe headaches or depression, or meclofenamate in patients with colitis. Each of the NSAIDs has special toxicities, but the gastrointestinal and renal side effects are the most common and troublesome.[34]

A major problem in all phases of therapy of RA is patient compliance: Is the patient taking the medication as prescribed? This early phase of treatment gives an opportunity to assess this, for without a cooperative and compliant patient, long-term therapy is doomed to failure.

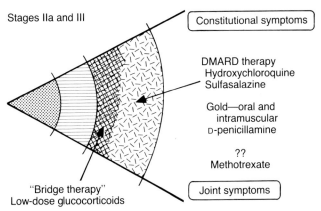

Figure 53–2. Phases I and II of therapy. "Bridge therapy" of glucocorticoids may not be necessary if the decision to initiate therapy with second-line drugs is made relatively early so their effect begins before a phase of intolerable pain or functional impairment. As shown in the figure by the shaded area within DMARD therapy, glucocorticoid bridge therapy may have to be continued longer in patients with more constitutional symptoms than in those primarily with joint symptoms. More and more, methotrexate is being used as a second-line drug; in some instances, it may be justified to use it before, or instead of, gold and/or D-penicillamine.

Glucocorticoids as Bridge Therapy

Low-dose oral prednisone should be reserved for "bridge" therapy between the time when the decision is made to start a DMARD (e.g., gold) and when the drug becomes effective. Implicit in this statement is the reality that if the DMARD does not work, longer therapy with the glucocorticoid probably will be essential (Fig. 53–2).

The major case for low-dose glucocorticoid therapy in RA is that the benefits far outweigh the costs. If prednisone is used and the daily dose kept faithfully to less than 7.5 mg per day, complications from this drug are minimal. It is true, conversely, that benefit from this low dose is small. There are data to show that RA patients given 7.5 mg or less of prednisone per day for up to 40 months have no significant change in mean basal or peak levels of plasma cortisol or in mean peak levels of growth hormone in response to insulin challenge.[35] Interestingly, active rheumatoid inflammation is sufficient in itself to reduce or obliterate the normal circadian rhythm of cortisol secretion by the adrenals in patients who never have had treatment with glucocorticoids.[36]

A principal concern about using even low-dose glucocorticoid therapy for long periods of time is the risk of accelerated osteopenia. Part of the controversy in interpreting data on this issue stems from incomplete understanding of the effects of RA itself on bone structure and function (see Chapters 51 and 52).

Pathogenesis and management of glucocorticoid-induced osteoporosis has been reviewed in detail.[37] Two controlled studies illustrate trends in these evaluations; both used dual photon absorptiometry to measure lumbar spine bone mineral content. One study of postmenopausal women included 28 RA patients given glucocorticoid therapy, 36 RA patients without glucocorticoid therapy, and 43 controls. There was a significant decrease in bone mineral content in the treated RA compared with untreated RA patients but no difference between treated RA patients and controls. The percentage of RA patients who sustained fractures of the vertebrae or femoral neck owing to minimal trauma was 16.3 percent in the glucocorticoid group and only 3.6 percent in the untreated RA group. The treated group had been given a mean prednisone dose of 8.9 mg per day for 4.7 years.[38] In another study, women treated with glucocorticoids (mean dose, 8.0 mg per day of prednisone for 90 months) had significantly lower lumbar bone mineral density than normal individuals but not significantly less than age-matched patients with RA not treated with glucocorticoids.[39] Other studies of patients treated for up to 2 years with a mean dose of 6.6 mg prednisone per day reinforce the data that rheumatoid patients not treated with glucocorticoids may suffer losses in bone mineral density equivalent to treated rheumatoids.[40]

Thus, both the postmenopausal condition and coexisting RA lead to osteopenia that can be clinically significant. Low-dose glucocorticoids probably increase the risk of symptomatic osteopenia in this subset of individuals, but the magnitude of this increase is small. It is probable that if patients become slightly more active (e.g., if they walk more) when given low-dose glucocorticoids, bone density will change little; however, if prednisone is given to a chair-bound or bed-bound patient, incremental bone loss would be expected. Human growth hormone prevents the protein catabolic side effects of prednisone in humans, but its therapeutic use may be limited by the additive effects on glucose metabolism of both of each of these substances.[41] Measures recommended to retard loss of bone in any patient may be effective in glucocorticoid-treated as well as non–glucocorticoid-treated RA patients. Among these regimens, supplemental vitamin D and calcium salts have been shown to have a positive effect.[42] Using dual photon absorptiometry in patients treated this way, recovery from steroid-induced osteoporosis has been demonstrated.[43] A new third-generation glucocorticoid, deflazacort, appears to cause less osteoporosis and fewer derangements of carbohydrate, lipid, or calcium metabolism.[43a]

How is it appropriate to use the low dose of prednisone? This dose (5 to 7.5 mg per day) has no immediate subjective or objective effects on patients, in contrast with the immediate benefit and surge of well-being felt by those given 15 mg per day or more. When it is apparent that more suppression of disease is needed than that provided by NSAIDs alone and help is needed before the slow-acting DMARDs begin to take effect, prednisone can be added to the NSAIDs as a single morning dose. Alternate-day therapy is not helpful at these low doses. A single dose in the evening rather than in the morning may alleviate morning stiffness, but it has not been determined whether this "unphysiologic" dosage schedule puts the patient at greater risk for suppression of the hypothalamic-adrenal-pituitary axis.

Any dose of any drug that is so free of side effects is suspected of not having any pharmacologic benefit. This has been disproved by abrupt discontinuation of prednisone in patients taking 5 mg per day for more than 4 months. The resulting flare of arthritis in almost all patients was persistent for longer than 8 weeks.[44] Unproved by this or other studies is whether prednisone in doses that are not demonstrably anti-inflammatory can suppress production of destructive enzymes by the proliferative synovial tissue.

Pulse therapy with intravenous glucocorticoids is used on occasion in severely ill patients to maximize benefits while minimizing risks. The "standard" dose (1000 mg) is both potentially toxic and very expensive. One study in 36 patients with acute flares of arthritis showed no statistical difference in their striking, prompt, and sustained clinical improvements whether they were given 1000 mg or 100 mg methylprednisolone intravenously.[45] There are suggestive but not definitive data to support the hypothesis that pulsed glucocorticoids may be additive in benefit but not in toxicity with simultaneous gold therapy.[46]

Phase II: Disease-Modifying Drugs

A major decision for the physician treating RA is when to begin therapy with second-line or slow-acting DMARDs. There are no clearly defined rules because there are only inadequate ways of measuring progression of synovitis and destruction of cartilage. In general, physicians err by underestimating the amount of joint destruction, and therefore a case can be made for starting disease-modifying drugs earlier than is usually done (see Fig. 53–2).

Guidelines for Therapy of the Patient with Progressive Disease

The search for the ideal panel of clinical and laboratory parameters that will identify the rate of progression of disease is still ongoing. The need is for a uniform measure of disease assessment.[46a]

Impressions of the Patient. The rheumatoid patient with active, progressive disease almost always admits to being tired and easily fatigued and to losing functional capacity. When the patient gives up previously pleasurable activities, no matter what the excuse, disease is usually active. Patients with active disease sleep poorly and may even develop symptoms consistent with a fibromyalgia syndrome, augmented perhaps by sleep deprivation. These individuals are more likely to have progressive disease than those without systemic symptoms.

Examination of the Patient. Joint destruction rarely occurs in the absence of significant soft tissue swelling in joints. Careful examination can distinguish synovial proliferation from effusions in the joint spaces. Joint counts for simultaneous swelling and tenderness are useful quantitative measures, as is grip strength. A sign of synovitis in a joint or set of joints not previously involved is a certain sign of progressive disease, as is development of or enlargement of already existing nodules. Rarely, symptoms or signs of rheumatoid vasculitis involving skin, peripheral nerves, or the gut may be evident relatively early in the disease and are prognostically ominous findings.[47] Warm joints and prominence of superficial veins over involved joints are confirmation of continued, aggressive synovitis.

Radiographic Findings. Periarticular osteopenia can develop before joint space narrowing or erosions in subchondral intracapsular bone and reflects active inflammation and release by synovial cells of cytokines that mediate bone loss. Which joints should be examined for earliest signs of disease? Interestingly, in patients with polyarticular disease, the metatarsophalangeal (MTP) joints and hallux interphalangeal joints show the earliest signs of involvement on radiographs.[48, 49] Better as a general measure of activity are radiographs of the hands and wrists; these show the best correlation with damage in other joints.[49] Radiographic changes are more likely to develop in the dominant hand or wrist.[50]

Laboratory Tests. Despite the needs of physicians to have objective criteria for starting DMARD therapy in RA, none exist. Laboratory test results must confirm opinions made on clinical grounds about the need for additional therapy. With these disclaimers, the following laboratory tests are useful predictors of progressive disease.

Patients with positive (and high) titers of IgM *rheumatoid factor* have a higher mortality and fewer remissions.[51] *Acute phase reactants* can be useful. The ESR is easy to perform, inexpensive, and available in all hospital laboratories and many offices. Sequential measurements of ESR in a given patient can provide a useful index of disease intensity. Quantitation of CRP is both more expensive and more complicated but, in combination with ESR, may correlate with development of erosive disease.[52, 53]

Other routine laboratory tests are of value. Mirroring increased activity of disease, although difficult to prove because of other confounding variables that affect the results in patients with RA, are a falling hemoglobin, thrombocytosis, and eosinophilia. Other tests, not available routinely, are discussed in Chapter 52.

Synovial fluid analysis is useful. Although polymorphonuclear leukocytes (PMNs) probably cause little direct destruction of articular cartilage or bone, their presence in synovial fluid reflects generation of chemoattractants by the synovial inflammation. Their numbers correlate reasonably well with the activity of proteases released by synovial cells in vitro. A joint fluid leukocyte count greater than 50,000 cells per mm^3 in RA almost always indicates a joint at risk for rapid destruction. More specialized tests on synovial fluids that correlate with disease activity include measurement of products of complement activation and active metalloproteinases.

Because blood is more accessible than synovial fluid, hopes remain high for finding a sensitive and specific *blood test* that is predictive of destructive synovitis. Many different tests for total circulating immune complexes have been generated, but few correlate with disease activity.[54, 55] An exception to this is a report of 57 seropositive patients studied longitudinally[56]; only the levels of IgA immune complexes at initial assessments were predictive of an increase in radiologic lesions after 1 year (r = 0.72; p < 0.001).

Summary. Initiation of more complex therapy in RA is indicated when a patient complains of fatigue, continuing joint symptoms, and loss of expected function. Data supporting such a therapeutic decision include the earliest changes in the hand or wrist radiographs, continued elevation in levels of acute phase reactants, and, when available, synovial fluid analysis consistent with active acute inflammation. Because data from various sources suggest that if disease is active and progressive for 2 years or more from onset, no therapy is likely to retard joint destruction significantly, it is appropriate that second-line drugs begin relatively early, certainly before 6 months of active disease not controlled by phase I drugs have elapsed.

Specific Treatment with Second-Line Drugs

The most commonly used second-line drugs for RA are antimalarial drugs, injectable and oral gold salts, sulfasalazine, D-penicillamine, and methotrexate (MTX). One study has compared efficacy and toxicity of these treatments using meta-analyses.[57] The results can be summarized as follows:

1. Auranofin (oral gold) was weaker than other drugs.

2. Patients treated with chloroquine did better than those treated with hydroxychloroquine.

3. Little difference in efficacy among MTX, injectable gold, D-penicillamine, and sulfasalazine was found.

4. Injectable gold had higher toxicity and dropout rates than the other drugs.

Several guidelines are useful for the physician who plans second-line (DMARD) therapy:

1. It is wise to begin with drugs that have the least toxicity. *Hydroxychloroquine* (see Chapter 44) or *sulfasalazine* (see Chapter 42) are the best examples. Although fewer patients will derive unequivocal benefit from these compounds compared with gold salts, the toxicity is less, and patient dropout because of adverse side effects is less common.[58] An advantage

of sulfasalazine (or sulfapyridine, its probable active metabolite) is that blood levels are available at reasonable cost and access. One study claims that, over a 2-year period, patients treated with sulfasalazine had less progression of erosions than patients treated otherwise.[59]

2. It is important not to decrease or stop administration of NSAIDs when starting second-line drugs (DMARDs). Side effects increase, of course, when additional drugs are given, but there are few well-documented examples of synergistic toxicity between an NSAID and a DMARD.

3. The physician or other arthritis health care professional must dedicate sufficient time to patient education during the induction phase of DMARD therapy. In particular, the patient must not have false expectations about a rapid response. Up to 6 months may be needed before a response to gold salts is manifest, and glucocorticoid therapy may provide an important bridging function.

4. If hydroxychloroquine or sulfasalazine is not effective, a *gold* preparation is the logical choice (see Chapter 45). Auranofin has less toxicity than injectable preparations, but both short-term and long-term efficacy are less as well.[57, 60, 61] The side effect of loose bowels from auranofin may be skirted by beginning therapy at 3 mg per 24 hours and increasing to 6 mg per 24 hours after a month or more. If a patient taking auranofin goes into a relative remission, it may be less expensive and just as effective to maintain this by giving the patient monthly (or biweekly, to start) injectable gold salts rather than continuing the more expensive oral program. The hope that patients achieving remission on injectable gold could be switched to auranofin and maintain remission has not been realized. There seem to be no differences in either efficacy or toxicity of injectable gold compounds administered to older patients (older than 60 years) compared with younger patients.[62]

5. Because of its varied and unpredictable toxicity, D-*penicillamine* should probably not be used until a trial of gold has failed or when, for other reasons, gold salts are not appropriate therapy (see Chapter 46). In one study, patients receiving placebo or different doses of D-penicillamine were followed for 36 weeks.[63] Although 500 mg per day was deemed more efficacious than lower doses, clinical improvement was marginal with any dose. The study was continued for an additional year on an open basis.[64] Of 144 patients taking labeled D-penicillamine, 27 patients withdrew because of adverse reactions, including seven from proteinuria, three from myasthenia, and one from myositis. Rash that did not lead to withdrawal occurred in 25 percent of patients; pruritus, altered taste, stomatitis, gastrointestinal distress, and abdominal pain were annoying side effects in more than 100 cases. The message is clear: Few patients are likely to be maintained on long-term D-penicillamine therapy, and continual monitoring for toxicity is essential during long-term therapy. On the other hand, D-penicillamine is probably more efficacious (although more toxic) than auranofin in RA[65] and should be considered as beneficial as injectable gold. There may be significant differences in susceptibilities of different populations around the world to D-penicillamine. In India, for example, few side effects are seen and efficacy is reported to be high.

6. *Methotrexate*, in a weekly pulse of a low dose, is being considered for use earlier than cytotoxic drugs such as azathioprine and cyclophosphamide. The reasons are that clinical impressions and double-blind studies support its efficacy and reasonable risk of toxicity.

One review[66] supports the claim that efficacy of low-dose weekly MTX can be sustained up to 5 years or more. Of 230 patients enrolled in prospective studies, only 8 percent stopped therapy owing to toxicity and 3 percent owing to lack of efficacy. Some rheumatologists use MTX early, after gold has failed and before D-penicillamine. Others use it instead of gold in patients with proteinuria or thrombocytopenia. The true place of therapy of MTX is uncertain and is the subject of many studies and much interest. In the doses used (5 to 15 mg by mouth or by intramuscular injection once weekly), it is not certain that its effects as a folic acid antagonist are the mechanism of action in RA. Folic acid supplementation during low-dose MTX therapy significantly lowered toxicity scores without affecting efficacy[67]; interestingly, low-normal initial plasma and red blood cell folate levels were predictive of future toxicity with MTX therapy. The onset of action of the drug appears to occur earlier than that noted when gold salts or D-penicillamine is used, often within 3 to 4 weeks after beginning therapy. The principal toxicity[68, 69] is gastrointestinal distress, with stomatitis, nausea, and pain leading the list. Concern about long-term hepatic toxicity persists; however, using the low-dose pulse schedule of therapy, cirrhosis is not being discovered, despite intermittent elevation of serum levels of transaminases of hepatic origin and evidence for a progressive increase in liver collagen.[69a] A hypersensitivity reaction in the lung occurs rarely with this low-dose therapy, but deaths have been reported.[70] Varying degrees of pulmonary fibrosis and bronchiolitis obliterans may develop. Vigilance and being prepared to stop the drug or to admit the patient to the hospital for possible glucocorticoid treatment are essential. In a study sponsored by the Clinical Efficacy Project of the American College of Physicians, MTX-treated patients had a 26 percent greater improvement in joint symptoms and a 39 percent greater improvement in relief of pain than did controls.[71] In other work, patients with RA treated with low-dose MTX showed significantly less radiologic progression than did those treated with azathioprine.

The mechanism of action of low-dose weekly MTX is unknown, although numerous effects in in vitro immune reactions have been noted, and MTX has been observed to inhibit endothelial cell proliferation in vitro and angiogenesis in vivo.[72]

Use of Combinations of Second-Line Drugs in Rheumatoid Arthritis

In practice, up to 45 percent of rheumatologists in Canada use combinations of DMARDs, although proof of efficacy is not available.[73] Similar data for rheumatologists in the United States are not available, but the rationale for combination therapy is clear: to suppress activity of RA to a degree sufficient to prevent joint destruction.[74] Oncologists have used combination therapy for years. Would combination therapy be better than sequential therapy with different drugs in RA? If one excludes combinations using cyclophosphamide (because of fear of lymphomas or other malignancies being spawned), therapies with hydroxychloroquine, azathioprine, and MTX,[75] gold salts plus antimalarials[76]; and gold salts plus D-penicillamine[77] are reported to be efficacious. Trial analysis of combination therapy, however, must await good controlled studies that report toxicity as well as efficacy.[78]

TREATMENT OF PROGRESSIVE AND RESISTANT RHEUMATOID ARTHRITIS

At this point in the course of disease, both patient and physician are often frustrated and discouraged. Disease remains active; joint deformities are progressing; and the gold, D-penicillamine, or MTX (or some combination) has failed.

Despite restrictions and limitations imposed by governmental regulations or Physicians Review Organization guidelines for hospital admission, an effort must be made to admit these patients to the hospital or rheumatic disease unit for several days to a week. The following objectives can be reached:

1. The patient can be given systematic rest matched with appropriate physical therapy (see Chapter 102).

2. Activities of daily living can be assessed, and occupational therapists can recommend appliances, splints, and home care aids (see Chapter 102).

3. Long-acting glucocorticoids can be injected into joints that are inflamed out of proportion to others (see Chapter 35). Indeed, this form of therapy may be appropriate earlier in the course if it is not abused. There should be 3 to 4 months between injections into one joint, and a single joint should not have more than three or four injections before more definitive therapy (e.g., synovectomy by arthroscopy, arthrotomy, or joint replacement).

4. An orthopedic surgeon with a demonstrated interest in RA should evaluate the patient, even if no surgery is planned.

5. A review of the patient's compliance to therapy and psychologic adjustment to the disease should be carried out by members of the arthritis care team.

6. An attempt to rebuild the drug therapy, based on the past history of the particular patient, is useful. Sometimes it can be recognized in retrospect that a particular drug discarded early was indeed effective.

7. Trials of immunoregulatory drugs should be considered. MTX should be used first unless it had failed previously. Experimental therapies should next be considered in refractory cases.

EXPERIMENTAL TREATMENT AND THERAPY OF THE FUTURE

Experimental Therapy

Because RA is a disease that will, in a few patients, enter remission spontaneously and because it has such complex, interlocking cycles of pathogenesis, it is logical to predict that, by use of selective therapies focused at one or a few crucial nodes in the pathogenetic processes, we should be successful in down-regulating the process, leading to sequential switching off of the inflammatory and proliferative components.

Some approaches to this concept of therapy have failed, some are promising, and others have yet to be tried. Examples follow:

Total Lymphoid Irradiation

Driven by the increasing evidence that RA is initially a T cell–mediated immune process, total lymphoid irradiation was given therapeutic trials, with conflicting results.[79, 80] Treated patients show a marked decrease in the number and function of peripheral blood helper/inducer T lymphocytes, interleukin-1 (IL-1) secretion by synovial biopsy specimens, and in activity of joint disease. In contrast, levels of immunoglobulins or C3 in blood or synovial fluid did not change,[81] and exacerbations of active disease recur with predictable consistency.

Cyclosporin A

This drug is a fungal peptide with potent and selective inhibitory activity on T helper (CD4) lymphocyte activation. It is not cytotoxic and acts by blocking IL-2 and other lymphokine production. Its use in preventing rejection of allograft transplants has been of great help. The first reports of double-blind, controlled studies of cyclosporin A in RA have been reported. In a study at the National Institutes of Health,[82] patients were randomized to either 10 mg per kg or 1 mg per kg. Of the patients on high dose cyclosporin A (especially those who were anergic), 67 percent had a beneficial clinical response maintained through 12 months. Similar results in France[83, 84] confirmed the efficacy of cyclosporin A. The problem, however, is nephrotoxicity of cyclosporin A; measurements of both glomerular filtration and renal plasma flow decreased in almost all treated patients. Unless ways can be found to enhance the therapeutic potential at low doses (< 2.5 mg per kg) of cyclosporin A, it is unlikely to be useful for long-term therapy of RA. In this context, it is intriguing that 1,25-dihydroxyvitamin D_3 potentiates the inhibitory effects in vitro of cyclosporin A on T lymphocytes from patients with RA.[85] In addition, there are data to indicate that the prostaglandin analogue misoprostol substantially increases the immunomodulation effects of both cyclosporin A and glucocorticoids.[86, 87] In double-blind, controlled studies, cyclosporin A emerged as an alternative to both D-penicillamine and azathioprine, but again, renal toxicity has been of concern.[87a, 87b]

Specific Antibody Therapy

Following up on the clinical observations that pregnancy induces remissions in RA, one group of investigators carried out a trial treatment of a group of patients with IgG eluted from placentae.[88] The hypothesis was that clinical improvement (64 percent) was due to anti-human leukocyte antigen (HLA) DR activity in the administered IgG. Subsequently, class II HLA alloantibodies were found in these preparations,[89] although the IgG administered to patients contained antibodies with specificities for more than DR antigens. Nevertheless, the data are provocative and the concept useful, although controlled studies of these monoclonal antibodies are woefully lacking.

Three patients with RA have been treated (two with clinical benefit) by rat monoclonal antibodies against the IL-2 receptor given intravenously over 10 days.[90] Because of the inevitable sensitization that would develop to rat proteins, the therapy could not be repeated.

In Switzerland, seven rheumatoid patients have been given mouse monoclonal anti-CD4 antibodies for 7 days.[91] Clinical improvement lasted for a mean of 11 weeks. Few changes in immunologic parameters were noted; in particular, after therapy in vivo, anti-CD4 antibody coated CD4+ cells could be induced to proliferate by anti-CD3 antibody in vitro, suggesting that the anti-CD4 had not transmitted a negative signal to CD4+ cells. An alternative, not tried as yet in RA, would be antibodies directed at the IL-2 receptor on lymphocytes in an attempt to inhibit clonal proliferation of T cells in the synovium. A subsequent study in Germany using mouse monoclonal anti-CD4 showed similar clinical responses and a drop in circulating CD4+ cells that persisted for 3 to 4 weeks.[92]

Three patients with refractory RA have been treated with abbreviated courses (10 mg per kg, intravenously for 4, 6, and 8 days) of antithymocyte globulin (ATGAM). The short courses given were dictated by complications of fever, urticaria, thrombocytopenia, and vasculitis, responsive to short-term glucocorticoid therapy. Beneficial clinical responses have been maintained up to 1 year.[93] Another approach could be directing monoclonal antibody therapy against B cell surface Ig, especially the cross-reactive idiotypes on rheumatoid factor.

Cytokines and Anticytokines as Therapy

Because interferon-gamma (IFNγ) has been found in diminished quantities in rheumatoid fluids and tissues, recombinant IFN-γ has been given as therapy in RA, with limited enthusiasm for the results.[94] The rationale for use of IL-2 in RA is that there may be a deficiency of a subset of T lymphocytes (e.g., suppressor inducer cells) that, if stimulated to proliferate, might down-regulate the immunoproliferation of RA. It is likely that clinical trials in patients with acquired immunodeficiency syndrome (AIDS) will generate data on the feasibility of IL-2 for RA.

Perhaps a more logical form of cytokine therapy would be trials of a substance known to have the capacity to down-regulate inflammatory and proliferative pathways that are activated in RA. Transforming growth factor beta (TGFβ) may be one of these; in broad terms, it prevents induction of genes that lead to cell transformation or matrix destruction. It represses production of collagenase,[95] enhances biosynthesis of reparative matrix proteins,[96] can be immunosuppressive,[97] and is a strong inhibitor of inflammatory cell adhesion to endothelial cells.[98]

A rationale for trials of interleukin-1 receptor antagonist has been clearly defined,[98a] and controlled studies using this bioproduct would be appropriate.

Radiation Synovectomy

Although rarely used in the United States because of possible radiation exposure to tissues outside of the joints, intra-articular injection of radioisotopes to kill off proliferative synovial tissue is common in Europe. Injection of dysprosium[165]–ferric hydroxide macroaggregates into knees of rheumatoid patients, however, appears to achieve similar therapeutic benefit without leakage of isotope.[99] The short half-life (139 minutes) is a mixed blessing; the isotope is present for only a short time, but the physician and patient must be together near the equipment for producing the isotope. The advantage over surgical synovectomy is that this isotope-aggregate can be used effectively more than once in the same joint.[98]

Miscellaneous Drugs

Several other compounds used effectively in other diseases have been reported to be efficacious in RA. *Phenytoin* (a hydantoin anticonvulsant) can produce selective IgA deficiency, induce suppressor T cell activity, and inhibit collagenase production. An advantage of phenytoin is that drug levels in serum can be assayed easily. In two reported trials, side effects have been mild, efficacy was significant, and good effects have persisted after the drug was stopped.[100, 101] Drug levels were lower than expected, and in future studies the competition for plasma protein-binding sites between NSAIDs and phenytoin must be considered.

Based on the growing data that substance P released by peripheral nerve endings might potentiate synovitis in arthritis, regional intravenous infusions of *guanethidine* have been used in a clinical study.[102] Over a 14-day observation period following therapy, pain and pinch strength improved compared with those in the placebo-treated group. With increased interest developing in the role of the nervous system in inflammation and the immune response, study of neuroactive drugs in arthritis may flourish.

For many years, several investigators have claimed that *tetracycline* and its derivatives can be useful therapy in RA. Although a *Mycoplasma* etiology certainly is unproved, data showing that minocycline inhibits collagenase activity in synovial fluid and synovial biopsies[103] have refueled interest in therapeutic trials of tetracyclines in arthritis. One open study of 10 patients treated with *minocycline* (400 mg/day) for 16 weeks has been reported.[104] Although vestibular side effects caused dropout of seven patients, efficacy variables improved significantly. Controlled studies of the tetracycline derivatives are essential.

References

1. Sharp, J. T., Wolfe, F., Mitchell, D. M., and Bloch, D. A.: The progression of erosion and joint space narrowing scores in rheumatoid arthritis during the first 25 years of disease. Arthritis Rheum. 34:660, 1991.
2. Scott, D. L., Coulton, B. L., and Popert, A. J.: Long term progression of joint damage in rheumatoid arthritis. Ann. Rheum. Dis. 45:373, 1986.
3. Pincus, T.: Rheumatoid arthritis: Disappointing long-term outcomes despite successful short-term clinical trials. J. Clin. Epidemiol. 41:1037, 1988.
4. Meenan, R. F., Gertman, P. M., Mason, J. H., et al.: The arthritis impact measurement scales: Further investigation of a healthy status measure. Arthritis Rheum. 25:1048, 1982.
5. Fries, J. F., Spritz, P. W., and Young, D. Y.: The dimensions of health outcomes: The health assessment questionnaire. Disability and pain scales. J. Rheumatol. 9:789, 1982.
6. Gregersen, P. K., Silver, J., and Winchester, R. J.: The shared epitope hypothesis: An approach to understanding the molecular genetics of susceptibility to rheumatoid arthritis. Arthritis Rheum. 30:1205, 1987.
7. Winchester, R. J., and Gregersen, P. K.: The molecular basis of susceptibility to rheumatoid arthritis: The conformational equivalence hypothesis. Springer Semin. Immunopathol. 10:119, 1988.
8. Gregersen, P. K., Shen, M., Song, Q., et al.: Molecular diversity of HLA-DR4 haplotypes. Proc. Natl. Acad. Sci. U.S.A. 83:2642–2646, 1986.
9. Nepom, G. T., Byers, P., Seyfried, C., et al.: HLA genes associated with rheumatoid arthritis: Identification of susceptibility alleles using specific oligonucleotide probes. Arthritis Rheum. 32:15, 1989.
10. Zoschke, D., and Segall, M.: Dw subtypes of DR4 in rheumatoid arthritis: Evidence for a preferential association with Dw4. Human Immunol. 15:118, 1986.
11. Mengl-Gaw, L., Conner, S., McDevitt, H. O., et al.: Gene conversion between murine class II MHC loci: Functional and molecular evidence from the bm12 mutant. J. Exp. Med. 160:1184, 1984.
12. Merryman, P. F., Crapper, R. M., Lee, S., et al.: Class II major histocompatibility complex gene sequences in rheumatoid arthritis: The third diversity regions of both $DR\beta_1$ genes in two DR1, DRw10-positive individuals specify the same inferred amino acid sequence as the $DR\beta_1$ and $DR\beta_2$ genes of a DR 4 (Dw14) haplotype. Arthritis Rheum. 32:251, 1989.
13. Pincus, T., Callahan, L. F., Bradley, L. A., Vaughn, W. K., and Wolfe, F.: Elevated MMPI scores for hypochondriasis, depression, and hysteria in patients with rheumatoid arthritis reflect disease rather than psychological status. Arthritis Rheum. 291:456, 1986.
14. Bradley, L. A.: Psychological aspects of arthritis. Bull. Rheum. Dis. 35(4):1, 1985.
15. Bradley, L. A., Young, L. D., Anderson, K. O., McDaniel, L. K., Turner, R. A., and Agudelo, C. A.: Psychological approaches to the management of arthritis pain. Soc. Sci. Med. 19:1353, 1984.
16. Lorig, K. R., Lubeck, D., Kraines, R. G., Scleznick, M., and Holman, H. R.: Outcomes of self-help education for patients with arthritis. Arthritis Rheum. 28:680, 1985.
17. Lorig, K.: Development and dissemination of an arthritis patient education course. Fam. Commun. Health 9:23, 1986.
17a. Bell, M. J., Bombardier, C., and Tugwell, P.: Measurement of functional status, quality of life, and utility in rheumatoid arthritis. Arthritis Rheum. 33:591, 1990.
18. Helliwell, M., Coombes, E. J., Moody, B. J., Batstone, G. F., and Robertson, J. C.: Nutritional status in patients with rheumatoid arthritis. Ann. Rheum. Dis. 43:386, 1987.
19. Panush, R. S., Carter, R. L., Katz, P., Lowsari, B., Longley, S., and Finnie, S.: Diet therapy for rheumatoid arthritis. Arthritis Rheum. 26:462, 1983.
20. Kremer, J. M., Michalek, A. V., Lininges, L., Huyck, C., Bigariotte, J., Timchalk, M. A., Rynes, R. I., Zieminski, J., and Bartholomew, L. E.: Effects of manipulation of dietary fatty acids on clinical manifestations of rheumatoid arthritis. Lancet 1:184, 1985.
21. Kremer, J. M., Jubiz, W., Michalek, A., Rynes, R. I., Bartholomew, L. E., Bigouette, J., Timchalk, M., Beeler, D., and Linninger, L.: Fish-oil fatty acid supplementation in active rheumatoid arthritis. A double-blinded, controlled, crossover study. Ann. Intern. Med. 106:497, 1987.
22. van der Tempel, H., Tulleken, J. E., Limburg, P. C., Muskiet, F. A. J., and van Rijswijk, M. H.: Effects of fish oil supplementation in rheumatoid arthritis. Ann. Rheum. Dis. 49:76, 1990.
23. Fox, P. L., and DiCorleto, P. E.: Fish oils inhibit endothelial cell production of platelet-derived growth factor-like protein. Science 241:453, 1988.
24. Endres, S., Ghorbani, R., Kelley, V. E., Georgilis, K., Lonnemann, G., van der Meer, J. W. M., Cannon, J. G., Rogers, T. S., Klempner, M. S., Weber, P. C., Schaefer, E. J., Wolff, S. M., and Dinarello, C. A.: The effect of dietary supplementation with ω-3 polyunsaturated fatty acids on the synthesis of interleukin-1 and tumor necrosis factor by mononuclear cells. N. Engl. J. Med. 320:265, 1989.
25. Baker, D. G., Krakauer, K. A., Tate, G., Laposata, M., and Zurier, R. B.: Suppression of human synovial cell proliferation by dihomo-γ-linolenic acid. Arthritis Rheum. 32:1273, 1989.
26. Gross, M., and Greenberg, L. A.: The Salicylates: A Critical Bibliographic Review. New Haven, Hillhouse Press, 1948.
27. Orozco-Alcala, J. J., and Baum, J.: Regular and enteric coated aspirin: A re-evaluation. Arthritis Rheum. 22:1034, 1979.
28. Grigor, R. R., Spitz, P. W., and Furst, D. E.: Salicylate toxicity in elderly patients with rheumatoid arthritis. J. Rheumatol. 14:60, 1987.
29. Cush, J. J., Lipsky, P. E., Postlethwaite, A. E., Schroehenloher, R. E., Saway, A., and Koopman, W. J.: Correlation of serologic indicators of inflammation with effectiveness of nonsteroidal antiinflammatory drug therapy in rheumatoid arthritis. Arthritis Rheum. 33:19, 1990.
30. Abramson, S. B., and Weissmann, G.: The mechanisms of action of nonsteroidal anti-inflammatory drugs. Arthritis Rheum. 32:1, 1989.
31. Abramson, S. B.: Therapy and mechanisms of nonsteroidal anti-inflammatory drugs. Curr. Opinion Rheumatol. 1:61, 1989.
32. Kennedy, T. P., Rao, N. V., Noah, W., Michael, J. R., Jafri, M. H., Jr., Burtner, G. H., and Hoidal, J. R.: Ibuprofen prevents oxidant lung injury and in vitro lipid peroxidation by chelating iron. J. Clin. Invest. 85:1565, 1990.
33. Furst, D. E., Blocka, K., Cassell, S., Harris, R. E., Hirschberg, J. M., Josephson, N., Lachenbruch, P. A., Trimble, R. B., and Paulus, H. E.: A controlled study of concurrent therapy with a nonacetylated salicylate and naproxen in rheumatoid arthritis. Arthritis Rheum. 30:146, 1987.
34. Simon, L. S.: Toxicity of nonsteroidal anti-inflammatory drugs. Curr. Opinion Rheumatol. 1:68, 1989.
35. Myles, A. B., Schiller, L. F. G., Glass, D., and Daly, J. R.: Single daily dose corticosteroid treatment. Ann. Rheum. Dis. 35:73, 1976.
36. Neeck, G., Federlin, K., Graef, V., Rusch, D., and Schmidt, K. L.: Adrenal secretion of cortisol in patients with rheumatoid arthritis. J. Rheumatol. 17:24, 1990.
37. Lukert, B. P., and Raisz, L. G.: Glucocorticoid-induced osteoporosis: Pathogenesis and management. Ann. Intern. Med. 112:352, 1990.
38. Verstraeten, A., and Dequeker, J.: Vertebral and peripheral bone mineral content and fracture incidence in postmenopausal patients with rheumatoid arthritis: Effect of low dose corticosteroids. Ann. Rheum. Dis. 45:852, 1986.
39. Sambrook, P. N., Eisman, J. A., Yeates, M. G., Pocock, N. A., Eberl, S., and Champion, G. D.: Osteoporosis in rheumatoid arthritis: Safety of low dose corticosteroids. Ann. Rheum. Dis. 45:950, 1986.

40. Sambrook, P. N., Cohen, M. L., Eisman, J. A., Pocock, N. A., Champion, G. D., and Yeates, M. G.: Effects of low dose corticosteroids on bone mass in rheumatoid arthritis: A longitudinal study. Ann. Rheum. Dis. 48:535, 1989.
41. Horber, F. F., and Haymond, M. W.: Human growth hormone prevents the protein catabolic side effects of prednisone in humans. J. Clin. Invest. 86:265, 1990.
42. Adachi, J. D., Bensen, W. G., Craig, G. L., Prayer, K., Pack, W. W., Guyatt, G. H., Hirsch, J., and Tugwell, P. X.: A randomized control trial of vitamin D and calcium in steroid-induced osteoporosis. Arthritis Rheum. 30:528, 1987.
43. Pocock, N. A., Eisman, J. A., Dunstan, C. R., Evans, R. A., Thomas, D. H., and Huq, N. L.: Recovery from steroid-induced osteoporosis. Ann. Intern. Med. 107:319, 1987.
43a. Gray, R. E. S., Doherty, S. M., Galloway, J., et al.: A double-blind study of deflazacort and prednisone in patients with chronic inflammatory disorders. Arthritis Rheum. 34:287, 1991.
44. Harris, E. D., Jr., Emkey, R. D., Nichols, J. E., and Newbury, A.: Low dose prednisone therapy in rheumatoid arthritis: A double blind study. J. Rheum. 10:713, 1983.
45. Inglehart, I. W., III, Sutton, J. D., Bender, J. C., Shaw, R. A., Ziminski, C. M., Holt, P. A., Hochberg, M. C., Zizic, T. M., Engle, E. W., and Stevens, M. B.: Intravenous pulsed steroids in rheumatoid arthritis: A comparative dose study. J. Rheumatol. 17:159, 1990.
46. Wong, C. S., Champion, G., Smith, M. D., Soden, M., Wetherall, M., Geddes, R. A., Hill, W. R., Ahern, M. J., and Roberts-Thomson, P. J.: Does steroid pulsing influence the efficacy and toxicity of chrysotherapy? A double blind, placebo controlled study. Ann. Rheum. Dis. 49:370, 1990.
46a. Panush, R. S., Kramer, N., and Rosenstein, E. D.: Assessment and prognosis of rheumatoid arthritis. Curr. Opin. Rheum. 4:355, 1992.
47. Lakhanpal, S., Conn, D. L., and Lie, J. T.: Clinical and prognostic significance of vasculitis as an early manifestation of connective tissue disease syndromes. Ann. Intern. Med. 101:743, 1984.
48. Brook, A., Fleming, A., and Corbett, M.: Relationship of radiological changes to clinical outcome in rheumatoid arthritis. Ann. Rheum. Dis. 36:274, 1977.
49. Scott, D. L., Coulton, B. L., and Popert, A. J.: Long term progression of joint damage in rheumatoid arthritis. Ann. Rheum. Dis. 45:373, 1986.
50. Owsianik, W. D. J., Kandi, A., Whitehead, N., Kraag, G. R., and Goldsmith, C.: Radiological articular involvement in the dominant hand in rheumatoid arthritis. Ann. Rheum. Dis. 39:508, 1980.
51. Kellgren, J. H., and O'Brien, W. M.: On the natural history of rheumatoid arthritis in relation to the sheep cell agglutination test (SCAT). Arthritis Rheum. 5:115, 1962.
52. Amos, R. S., Constable, T. J., Crockson, R. A., Crockson, A. P., and McConkey, B.: Rheumatoid arthritis: Relation of serum C-reactive protein and erythrocyte sedimentation rates to radiographic changes. Br. Med. J. 1:195, 1977.
53. Malkya, R. K., deBeer, F. C., Berry, H., Hamilton, E. D. B., Mace, B. E. W., and Pepys, M. B.: Correlation of clinical parameters of disease activity in rheumatoid arthritis with serum concentration of C reactive protein and erythrocyte sedimentation rate. J. Rheumatol. 9:224, 1982.
54. Lessard, J., Nummery, E., Cecere, F., McDuffy, S., and Pope, R. M.: Relationship between the articular manifestations of rheumatoid arthritis and circulating immune complexes detected by three methods and specific classes of rheumatoid factors. J. Rheumatol. 10:411, 1983.
55. McDougal, J. S., Hubbard, M., McDuffie, F. C., et al.: Comparison of five assays for immune complexes in rheumatoid arthritis. Arthritis Rheum. 25:1156, 1982.
56. Westedt, M.-L., Daha, M. R., Baldwin, W. M., Stijnen, T., and Cats, A.: Serum immune complexes containing IgA appear to predict erosive arthritis in a longitudinal study in rheumatoid arthritis. Ann. Rheum. Dis. 45:809, 1986.
57. Felson, D. T., Anderson, J. J., and Meenan, R. F.: The comparative efficacy and toxicity of second-line drugs in rheumatoid arthritis: Results of two metaanalyses. Arthritis Rheum. 33:1449, 1990.
58. Box, D. E., and Amos, R. S.: Sulphasalazine: A safe effective agent for prolonged control of arthritis. A comparison with sodium aurothiomalate. Ann. Rheum. Dis. 44:194, 1985.
59. Pullar, T., Hunter, J. A., and Capell, H. A.: Effect of sulphasalazine on the radiological progression of rheumatoid arthritis. Ann. Rheum. Dis. 46:398, 1987.
60. Ward, H. R., Williams, H. J., Egger, M. H., et al.: Comparison of auranofin, gold sodium thiomalate, and placebo in the treatment of rheumatoid arthritis. Arthritis Rheum. 26:1303, 1983.
61. Capell, H. A., Lewis, D., and Casey, J.: A three year follow-up of patients allocated to placebo, or oral or injectable gold therapy for rheumatoid arthritis. Ann. Rheum. Dis. 45:705, 1986.
62. Kean, W. F., Bellamy, N., and Brooks, P. M.: Gold therapy in the elderly rheumatoid arthritis patient. Arthritis Rheum. 26:705, 1983.
63. Williams, H. J., Ward, J. R., Reading, J. C., et al.: Low-dose D-penicillamine therapy in rheumatoid arthritis. A controlled, double-blind clinical trial. Arthritis Rheum. 26:581, 1983.
64. Williams, H. J., and the Cooperative Systematic Studies of Rheumatic Diseases Group: Toxicity of longterm low dose D-penicillamine therapy in rheumatoid arthritis. J. Rheumatol. 14:67, 1987.
65. Hochberg, M. C.: Auranofin or D-penicillamine in the treatment of rheumatoid arthritis. Ann. Intern. Med. 105:528, 1986.
66. Weinblatt, M. E., and Maier, A. L.: Long-term experience with low-dose weekly methotrexate in rheumatoid arthritis. J. Rheumatol. 17(suppl. 22):33, 1990.
67. Morgan, S. L., Baggott, J. E., Vaughn, W. H., Young, P. K., Austin, J. V., Krumdieck, C. L., and Alarcón, G. S.: The effect of folic acid supplementation on the toxicity of low-dose methotrexate in patients with rheumatoid arthritis. Arthritis Rheum. 33:9, 1990.
68. Gispen, J. G., Alarcón, G. S., Johnson, J. J., Acton, R. T., Barger, B. O., and Koopman, W. J.: Toxicity to methotrexate in rheumatoid arthritis. J. Rheumatol. 14:74, 1987.
69. Weinblatt, M. E.: Toxicity of low-dose methotrexate in rheumatoid arthritis. J. Rheumatol. 12(suppl. 12):35, 1985.
69a. Ahern, M. J., Kevat, S., Hill, W., et al.: Hepatic methotrexate content and progression of hepatic fibrosis: preliminary findings. Ann. Rheum. Dis. 50:477, 1991.
70. St. Clair, E. W., Rice, J. R., and Snyderman, R.: Severe pneumonitis complicating oral methotrexate in rheumatoid arthritis. Arthritis Rheum. 27:560, 1984.
71. Tugwell, P., Bennett, K., and Gent, M.: Methotrexate in rheumatoid arthritis. Ann. Intern. Med. 107:358, 1987.
72. Hirata, S., Matsubara, T., Saura, R., Tateishi, H., and Hirohata, K.: Inhibition of in vitro vascular endothelial cell proliferation and in vivo neovascularization by low-dose methotrexate. Arthritis Rheum. 32:1065, 1989.
73. Bellamy, N., and Brook, P. M.: Current practice in antimalarial prescribing in rheumatoid arthritis. J. Rheumatol. 13:551, 1986.
74. Ssuka, M., Carrera, G. F., and McCarty, D. J.: Treatment of intractable rheumatoid arthritis with combined cyclophosphamide, azathioprine and hydroxychloroquine. A follow-up study. J.A.M.A. 255:2315, 1986.
75. Wilke, W. S., Scherrer, Y. R., and Clough, J. D.: Combination chemotherapy for severe rheumatoid arthritis. Intern. Med. Specialist 10:59, 1989.
76. Scott, D. L., Dawes, P. T., Tunn, E., Fowler, P. D., Shadforth, M. F., Fisher, J., Clarke, S., Collins, M., Jones, P., Popert, A. J., and Bacon, P. A.: Combination therapy with gold and hydroxychloroquine in rheumatoid arthritis: A prospective, randomized, placebo-controlled study. Br. J. Rheumatol. 28:128, 1989.
77. Bitter, T.: Combined disease-modifying chemotherapy for intractable rheumatoid arthritis. Clin. Rheum. Dis. 10:413, 1984.
78. Paulus, H. E.: The use of combinations of disease-modifying antirheumatic agents in rheumatoid arthritis. Arthritis Rheum. 33:113, 1990.
79. Harris, E. D., Jr.: Management of Rheumatoid Arthritis. In Kelley, W. N., Harris, E. D., Jr., Ruddy, S., and Sledge, C. B. (eds.): Textbook of Rheumatology. 3rd ed. Philadelphia, W. B. Saunders Company, 1989, pp. 982–992.
80. Klippel, J. H., Strober, S., and Wofsy, D.: New therapies for the rheumatic diseases. Bull. Rheum. Dis. 38:1, 1989.
81. Gatson, J. S. H., Strober, S., Solovera, J. J., et al.: Dissection of the mechanisms of immune injury in rheumatoid arthritis, using total lymphoid irradiation. Arthritis Rheum. 31:21, 1988.
82. Yocum, D. E., Klippel, J. H., Wilder, R. L., et al.: Cyclosporin A in severe, treatment-refractory rheumatoid arthritis: A randomized study. Ann. Intern. Med. 109:863, 1988.
83. Dougados, M., Awada, H., and Amor, B.: Cyclosporin in rheumatoid arthritis: A double-blind, placebo-controlled study in 52 patients. Ann. Rheum. Dis. 47:127, 1988.
84. Dougados, M., Duchesne, L., Awada, H., et al.: Assessment of efficacy and acceptability of low-dose cyclosporin in patients with rheumatoid arthritis. Ann. Rheum. Dis. 48:550, 1989.
85. Gepner, P., Amor, B., and Fournier, C.: 1,25-Dihydroxyvitamin D_3 potentiates the in vitro inhibitory effects of cyclosporin A on T cells from rheumatoid arthritis patients. Arthritis Rheum. 32:31, 1989.
86. Moran, M., Mozes, M. F., Maddux, M. S., Veremis, S., Bartkus, C., Ketel, B., Pollak, R., Wallemark, C., and Jonasson, O.: Prevention of acute graft rejection by the prostaglandin E_1 analogue misoprostol in renal-transplant recipients treated with cyclosporine and prednisone. N. Engl. J. Med. 322:1183, 1990.
87. Nicholson, P. A.: Recent advances in defining the role of misoprostol in rheumatology. J. Rheumatol. 27(suppl 20):50, 1990.
87a. van Rijthoven, A. W. A. M., Dijkmans, B. A. C., Thè, H. S. G., Meijers, K. A. E., et al.: Comparison of cyclosporine and D-penicillamine for rheumatoid arthritis: a randomized, double-blind, multicentre study. J. Rheumatol. 18:815, 1991.
87b. Ahern, M. J., Harrison, W., Hollingsworth, P., et al.: A randomized, double-blind trial of cyclosporin and azathioprine in refractory rheumatoid arthritis. Aust. N.Z. J. Med. 24:844, 1991.
88. Sany, J., Clot, J., Borneau, M., et al.: Immunomodulating effect of human placenta-eluted gamma globulins in rheumatoid arthritis. Arthritis Rheum. 25:17, 1982.

89. Moynier, M., Cosso, B., Brochier, J., and Clot, J.: Identification of class II HLA alloantibodies in placenta-eluted gamma globulins used for treating rheumatoid arthritis. Arthritis Rheum. 30:375, 1987.

90. Kyle, V., Coughlan, J., Tighe, H., et al.: Beneficial effect of monoclonal antibody to interleukin-2 receptor on activated T cells in rheumatoid arthritis. Ann. Rheum. Dis. 48:428, 1989.

91. Herzog, C., Walker, C., and Pichler, W. J.: New therapeutic approaches in rheumatoid arthritis. Concepts Immunopathol. 7:79, 1989.

92. Horneff, G., Burmester, G. R., Emmrich, F., and Kalden, J. R.: Treatment of rheumatoid arthritis with an anti-CD4 monoclonal antibody. Arthritis Rheum. 34:129, 1991.

93. Shmerling, R. H., and Trentham, D. E.: Prolonged improvement in refractory rheumatoid arthritis after brief antithymocyte globulin therapy of brief duration. Arthritis Rheum. 32:1495, 1989.

94. Wolfe, F., Cathey, M. A., Hawley, D. J., et al.: Clinical trial with r-IFN-gamma in rheumatoid arthritis. In Biologically Based Immunomodulators in the Therapy of Rheumatic Diseases. Amsterdam, Elsevier, 1985, p 379.

95. Edwards, D. R., Murphy, G., Reynolds, J. J., et al.: Transforming growth factor beta modulates the expression of collagenase and metalloproteinase inhibitor. EMBO J. 6:1899, 1987.

96. Ignotz, R. A., and Massagué, J.: Transforming growth factor-beta stimulates the expression of fibronectin and collagen and their incorporation into the extracellular matrix. J. Biol. Chem. 251:4337, 1986.

97. Wahl, S. M., Hunt, D. A., Wong, H. L., et al.: Transforming growth factor-β is a potent immunosuppressive agent that inhibits IL-1–dependent lymphocyte proliferation. J. Immunol. 140:3026, 1988.

98. Gamble, J. R., and Vadas, M. A.: Endothelial adhesiveness for blood neutrophils is inhibited by transforming growth factor-β. Science 242:97, 1988.

98a. Dinarello, C. A.: Interleukin-1 and interleukin-1 antagonism. Blood 97:1627, 1991.

99. Vella, M., Zuckerman, J. D., Shortkroff, S., Venkatesan, P., and Sledge, C. B.: Repeat radiation synovectomy with dysprosium 165-ferric hydroxide macroaggregates in rheumatoid knees unresponsive to initial injection. Arthritis Rheum. 31:789, 1988.

100. Grindalis, K., Nichol, F. E., and Oldham, R.: Phenytoin in rheumatoid arthritis. J. Rheumatol. 13:1035, 1986.

101. MacFarlane, D. G., Clarke, B., and Panayi, G.: Pilot study of phenytoin in rheumatoid arthritis. Ann. Rheum. Dis. 45:954, 1986.

102. Levine, J. D., Frye, K., Heller, P., Basbaum, A. I., and Whiting-O'Keefe, Q.: Clinical response to regional intravenous guanethidine in patients with rheumatoid arthritis. J. Rheumatol. 13:1040, 1986.

103. Greenwald, R. A., Golub, L., Lavietes, B., Ramamurthy, N. S., Gruber, B., Laskin, R. S., and McNamara, T. F.: Tetracyclines inhibit synovial collagenase in vivo and in vitro. J. Rheumatol. 14:28, 1987.

104. Breedveld, F. C., Dijkmans, B. A. C., and Mattie, H.: Minocycline treatment for rheumatoid arthritis: An open dose finding study. J. Rheumatol. 17:43, 1990.

Chapter 54
Robert S. Pinals
Felty's Syndrome

In 1924, Felty[1] described five patients with chronic arthritis, splenomegaly, and leukopenia and proposed that this association represented a distinct clinical entity. Felty's syndrome represents one of many systemic complications of seropositive rheumatoid arthritis occurring in a group of patients with unusually severe articular disease and immunologic abnormalities. The term *hypersplenism* was derived from the observation that splenectomy usually results in partial or complete resolution of the granulocytopenia, but the role of the spleen in pathogenesis has been a subject of considerable controversy for many years. There is evidence for its participation both in the removal of granulocytes from the circulating pool and in the suppression of granulopoiesis.

With a complex pathogenesis that varies from case to case, Felty's syndrome must be still defined in descriptive terms as a variant of seropositive rheumatoid arthritis with splenomegaly and granulocytopenia (<2000 cells per mm[3]). Although the complete triad is required for a diagnosis of Felty's syndrome, some rheumatoid arthritis patients may be encountered at a time when only granulocytopenia is present. Such individuals resemble full-blown Felty's syndrome patients in most clinical and serologic features. The true prevalence of Felty's syndrome is unknown, but it is probably found in less than 1 percent of patients with rheumatoid arthritis. Splenomegaly alone is more common, identified by palpation in 6.5 percent in one large series[3] and even more frequently by radioactive scanning. The majority of these patients never develop neutropenia and follow a clinical course compatible with chronic rheumatoid arthritis rather than Felty's syndrome.

DIFFERENTIAL DIAGNOSIS

Patients with rheumatoid arthritis may also develop superimposed illnesses that may result in splenomegaly or granulocytopenia. Drug reactions, myeloproliferative disorders, reticuloendothelial malignancies, hepatic cirrhosis, amyloidosis, sarcoidosis, tuberculosis, and other chronic infections must be considered and excluded with reasonable clinical certainty before the diagnosis of Felty's syndrome is accepted. In recent years, a syndrome of neutropenia and large granular lymphocytosis (LGL) has been associated with rheumatoid arthritis (Fig. 54–1).[4, 5, 5a] Most cells with natural-killer and antibody-dependent, cell-mediated cytotoxic activity are found in this population. Among patients with an abnormal proliferation of these cells in peripheral blood and bone marrow, neutropenia, splenomegaly, and susceptibility to infections are common findings. In some

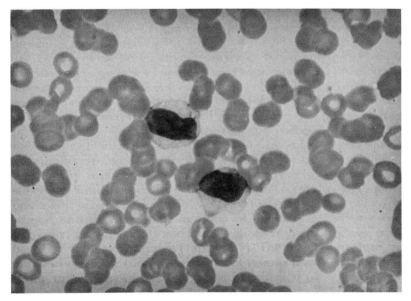

Figure 54–1. Peripheral blood smear with large granular lymphocytes.

cases, there is a progressive course of malignant proliferation, but most are stable over a period of several years. Chronic inflammatory arthritis, usually seropositive and often fulfilling criteria for rheumatoid arthritis, is also commonly associated with LGL. In one series, 23 percent of patients with LGL identified in a large referral center over a 10-year period had rheumatoid arthritis, and most would have been classified as having Felty's syndrome if not for the discovery of typical cells in the bone marrow or peripheral blood.[4] In this report, the prevalence of true Felty's syndrome was twice that of LGL in rheumatoid arthritis patients with neutropenia. The simultaneous appearance of arthritis and neutropenia, the absence of deformity, and the finding of lymphocytosis on peripheral blood smears may provide clues to the presence of LGL. This condition is often relatively benign and may require no specific therapy. Splenectomy, which corrects neutropenia in most Felty's syndrome patients, however, is generally unsuccessful and may even exacerbate the proliferation of large granular lymphocytes.

CLINICAL FEATURES

About two thirds of patients with Felty's syndrome are women. Human leukocyte antigen (HLA) DRw4 is found in 95 percent of patients with Felty's syndrome, compared with 69 to 73 percent in other rheumatoid arthritis patients and 31 to 37 percent in controls.[2] This may account for the rarity of Felty's syndrome in blacks, who are known to have a low frequency of DRw4.[7] The condition is usually recognized in the fifth through the seventh decades of life in patients who have had rheumatoid arthritis for 10 years or more. Juvenile onset has been noted occasionally.[8] Because Felty's syndrome is most often discovered by a routine blood count, the frequency of medical observation is an important factor in early recognition. Splenomegaly and granulocytopenia may be present before symptoms or signs of arthritis in rare instances.[9] The articular disease is usually more severe than in the average case of rheumatoid arthritis, with greater deformity and erosion,[10, 11, 11a] but there are many examples of mild involvement.[9, 12] About one third of the patients have relatively inactive synovitis, as judged by signs and symptoms, but even these patients continue to have an elevated erythrocyte sedimentation rate (ESR). In one large series, the mean ESR was 85 mm per hour.[11]

The spleen size is variable. In 5 to 10 per cent of patients, it is not large enough to be palpable, but occasionally there is massive splenomegaly.[13] The median splenic weight in Felty's syndrome is about four times normal.[13] There is no correlation between spleen size and the degree of granulocytopenia.[10, 11, 14]

Patients with Felty's syndrome tend to have more extra-articular manifestations than others with rheumatoid arthritis[14a] (Table 54–1). Weight loss was mentioned by Felty and has been emphasized by

Table 54–1. FREQUENCY OF EXTRA-ARTICULAR MANIFESTATIONS IN FELTY'S SYNDROME*

Rheumatoid nodules	76%
Weight loss	68%
Sjögren's syndrome†	56%
Lymphadenopathy	34%
Leg ulcers	25%
Pleuritis	19%
Skin pigmentation	17%
Neuropathy	17%
Episcleritis	8%

*From a review of 10 reports since 1962.
†Determined by positive Schirmer's test.

later authors. It may be striking and unexplained, often occurring for several months before the diagnosis of Felty's syndrome is made. Felty also mentioned brown pigmentation over exposed surfaces of the extremities, especially over the tibia. Although noted by others,[2, 10] it is not specific for Felty's syndrome and may be related to stasis and to extravasation of red blood cells secondary to disease of small vessels. Leg ulcers are frequent but do not seem to differ from those in other rheumatoid arthritis patients in terms of chronicity, recurrence, and presumed relationship to vasculitis.

Although about 60 percent of patients with Felty's syndrome are described as having one or more infections that may be attributable to the granulocytopenia, the literature is difficult to interpret because nonleukopenic rheumatoid arthritis patients may also be more susceptible to infection.[2, 15] In one report, Felty's syndrome patients had a 20-fold increase in frequency of infections compared with matched rheumatoid arthritis controls.[2] The degree of granulocytopenia correlates poorly with the number and severity of infections until the granulocyte count falls below 1000 per mm[3]. Other risk factors for infection include skin ulcers, glucocorticoids, severity of the underlying rheumatoid process, and resulting disability.[15, 16] Sepsis is the principal factor in the reduced survival of Felty's syndrome patients compared with rheumatoid arthritis controls.[2] Most of the infections are caused by common bacteria, such as *Staphylococcus*, *Streptococcus*, and gram-negative bacilli,[11] and involve common sites, particularly the skin and respiratory tract (Table 54–2). In spite of the granulocytopenia, pus may accumulate in an appropriate fashion, suggesting that the site of infec-

Table 54–2. PERCENTAGE OF FELTY'S SYNDROME PATIENTS WITH VARIOUS TYPES OF INFECTION*

Skin (abscess, cellulitis, furunculosis)	26%
Pneumonia	24%
Urinary tract	9%
Oral ulcers	4%
Sinusitis and otitis	4%
Septic arthritis	2%

*Taken from four reports[10, 11, 13, 14] in which sufficient information was available on a total of 90 patients.

tion is capable of competing successfully with the spleen for available granulocytes. The response to antibiotic therapy is usually adequate.[11]

Mild hepatomegaly is common in Felty's syndrome as are liver function abnormalities, particularly elevations of alkaline phosphatase and the transaminases, which are described in about a quarter of the patients.[2, 11] An unusual type of liver involvement may be associated with Felty's syndrome but occurs rarely in other rheumatoid arthritis patients.[17, 17a] Histologically, the picture is described as nodular regenerative hyperplasia.[18] Although there is mild portal fibrosis or infiltration with lymphocytes and plasma cells, the appearance is not characteristic of cirrhosis. Obliteration of portal venules may compromise portal blood flow, leading to atrophy and regenerative nodule formation, portal hypertension, and gastrointestinal hemorrhage. It has been suggested that immune complex–mediated platelet activation may be the mechanism of venular injury and occlusion.[18] Other primary disorders may be associated with nodular regenerative hyperplasia, but about a third of the patients have had Felty's syndrome.[17, 18]

HEMATOLOGIC FEATURES

The leukopenia in Felty's syndrome is both relative and absolute granulocytopenia. This is in contrast to systemic lupus erythematosus (SLE), in which lymphopenia is a more prominent feature. Few patients have blood counts often enough to determine the rate at which granulocytopenia develops at the onset of Felty's syndrome, but in some cases only weeks have elapsed between normal and grossly abnormal white blood cell counts. There is often considerable spontaneous variation in the granulocyte count. Patients with mild lowering may return to the normal range, but this is rarely seen when depression is severe. Thus, spontaneous remissions have been observed[2, 10, 19] but are uncommon. During infections or other stressful episodes, the granulocyte count often returns to the normal range but is seldom elevated. This may conceal the diagnosis temporarily because blood counts may be ordered in some patients, mainly in the setting of an infection or other acute illness.

The bone marrow may show no abnormality in some cases, but in most there is a myeloid hyperplasia, with a relative excess of immature forms, often described as *maturation arrest*. Although this might reflect an impaired myelopoietic response, early release of mature forms would result in the same appearance.[10, 11, 14] Rarely the marrow suggests a depression in myeloid activity[14] or shows an increased lymphocytic infiltration.[14]

A mild to moderate anemia is found in most patients, representing the anemia of chronic disease with an additional component of shortened red blood cell survival, which is corrected by splenectomy.

Reticulocyte count elevations are common.[11] Thrombocytopenia (platelet count <150,000 per mm^3) occurs in 38 percent but is seldom severe enough to cause purpura.

SEROLOGIC FEATURES

The alterations in immune response commonly found in rheumatoid arthritis are amplified in patients with Felty's syndrome, in keeping with the general picture of unusually severe articular and systemic disease. Rheumatoid factor has been present in 98 percent of the patients, generally in high titer.[11] Positive LE cell tests are found in one third and antinuclear antibodies (ANA) in two thirds of the patients, with wide differences in frequency (47 to 100 percent), probably reflecting the variable sensitivity of the latter test. Patients with Felty's syndrome also have granulocyte-specific ANA more often than do rheumatoid arthritis patients without neutropenia.[20] Anti-nDNA is elevated occasionally.[2] Antihistone antibodies are present in 83 percent, often in high titer.[22] Immunoglobulin levels are higher than in other rheumatoid arthritis patients;[10, 11] complement levels are lower,[11, 21] although most patients have levels within the normal range. Immune complexes have been detected by various techniques in the majority of Felty's syndrome patients, always in much higher frequency than in rheumatoid controls. These complexes may contain gamma immunoglobulin G (IgG), IgM, IgE, and complement.[21, 23–25] A granulocyte reactive ANA is also selectively concentrated in the cryoprecipitate in some sera,[21] suggesting the possibility that this antibody might be available to act on nuclear antigen following ingestion of the immune complexes by granulocytes.

PATHOGENESIS

Although the spleen certainly plays a key role in the pathogenesis of granulocytopenia, little insight has been gained by routine examinations of surgical specimens because they show only the predictable immune hyperactivity (increased plasma cells, immunoblasts, and germinal center hyperplasia) and inconstant evidence of phagocytic hyperfunction.[11, 13]

The hematologic improvement resulting from splenectomy led some to postulate that the spleen had been producing a humoral inhibitor of granulocyte production[26] and others to support splenic sequestration and destruction of granulocytes as the principal mechanism.[27] The debate appeared to be settled in favor of the latter proposal when granulocyte counts were shown to be lower in the splenic vein than in the artery.[27] Other studies, however, have suggested that the two viewpoints are not mutually exclusive and that a number of factors may contribute to the development of granulocytopenia (Fig. 54–2).

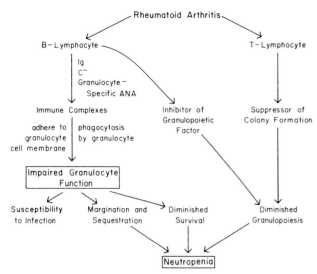

Figure 54–2. Pathogenesis of Felty's syndrome.

Increased Removal of Granulocytes

Granulocyte sequestration and reduced survival might certainly result from impaired motility of cells laden with immune complexes and difficulty in negotiating channels in the splenic pulp. Many granulocytes with large cytoplasmic inclusions containing immunoglobulins and complement were identified in the spleens of patients with Felty's syndrome.[28]

Neutrophil function and survival may also be compromised by the adherence of antibodies and immune complexes to the cell surface. The presence of granulocyte antibodies was suggested by early transfusion experiments in which plasma from a patient with Felty's syndrome produced transient granulocytopenia.[29] A characterization of serum granulocyte binding activity in Felty's syndrome revealed that IgG was the principal immunoglobulin involved, and that both soluble immune complexes and specific antibodies to granulocytes participated.[30] Granulocyte-binding globulins have been demonstrated by various techniques, but recent work suggests that they probably represent immune complexes rather than neutrophil-specific antibodies.[31] The surface immunoglobulins include granulocyte-specific ANA, which may be capable of fixing complement[20] and contributing to cell injury.

Granulocyte kinetic studies have been performed in Felty's syndrome, but technical problems and variations in these studies have led to disputed interpretations.[32] In more recent studies, excessive margination or sequestration was thought to represent a more significant defect than diminished granulocyte survival. The marginated pool consists of neutrophils adherent to the walls of venules in the spleen, lungs, and elsewhere. Thus, neutrophils coated with immune complexes had shifted from the circulating to the marginated pool because of an increased tendency to aggregate and adhere to endothelial cells.[34]

Impaired Production of Granulocytes

Bone marrow granulocyte precursor cells form colonies when grown in vitro in semisolid agar; the number of colonies gives an indication of the proliferative state of the marrow. A glycoprotein colony-stimulating factor normally found in serum and urine is required for this growth. Colony-stimulating activity was found to be lower in Felty's syndrome than in other neutropenic disorders.[15, 35] In one report, eight of 19 Felty's syndrome patients were found to have a heat-stable, nondialyzable serum factor capable of inhibiting colony formation by human marrow granulocyte precursors.[36]

Mononuclear cells have also been shown to induce suppression of colony formation in normal human marrow cultures. Their depletion by E-rosetting in Felty's syndrome marrow cultures augments colony formation, suggesting that the responsible cells are T lymphocytes.[37–39] The observation that occasional patients who have lymphocytic infiltration in the marrow respond poorly to splenectomy lends support to this mechanism.[14]

Immunogenetics

The familial occurrence of Felty's syndrome suggests that immunogenetic factors are operative.[40] Several reports have confirmed a stronger association with HLA DR4 than in rheumatoid arthritis patients in general.[2, 6, 41, 41a] There also appears to be a DQ beta-linked susceptibility gene[2, 41] and a C4B-null allele,[42] which increase the risk of Felty's syndrome in DR4-positive rheumatoid arthritis patients.

Summary

The granulocytopenia in Felty's syndrome appears to be multifactorial in origin[15, 37] (see Fig. 54–2). Ingestion and surface-coating of immune complexes leads to impaired granulocyte functions and facilitates their removal by the reticuloendothelial system. Specific antibodies directed against granulocyte cell surface antigens may also be involved. Sequestration of granulocytes in the spleen and venules results in a diminished circulating pool, either with or without actual premature destruction of granulocytes. In some patients, the marrow does not respond appropriately to granulocytopenia, apparently because of the action of an unidentified humoral inhibitor or mononuclear cells that suppress myelopoiesis. There may be different subsets of Felty's syndrome, as illustrated by one report in which both humoral and cell-mediated mechanisms were investigated. About two thirds of the patients had high levels of neutrophil-bound IgG. In the remaining patients, peripheral blood mononuclear cells inhibited colony growth in normal marrow.[43] In another study, T cell marrow suppression was found to be a more frequent mechanism than serum antiprecursor cell activity.[37] More than one mechanism may account for neutropenia in an individual patient.

The increased susceptibility to infection is probably related to several factors in addition to granulocytopenia. Granulocyte reserves are diminished, and defective function of granulocytes in phagocytosis,[44] chemotaxis,[45] and superoxide production[46] has been demonstrated. Hypocomplementemia may also play a role in some patients.[21, 25]

MANAGEMENT

Splenectomy

Because splenectomy usually reverses the hematologic abnormalities in Felty's syndrome, it was advocated in the past as the treatment of choice, either in all cases[47] or in those patients with very low granulocyte counts or serious infections.[13, 15] No prospective randomized studies of splenectomy have been performed, and the value of the procedure in preventing serious infection and prolonging survival is not entirely clear.[2, 15, 16] There is no dispute, however, about the prompt hematologic response, which is observed within minutes or hours after splenectomy in most patients; 88 percent have a good short-term hematologic response to splenectomy.[15] Granulocytopenia recurs, however, and persists in 24 percent of patients available for follow-up examinations. The absolute granulocyte level in these cases was generally higher than it had been before splenectomy. Continuing immune-mediated granulocyte sequestration may be responsible for these secondary failures.[48] Recurrent or persistent infection was noted in only 26 percent in one large series[13] but in 60 percent in four others.[15] Patients who did not experience infection before splenectomy usually continued to be free of infection afterward, whereas those with the most severe infections had variable and inconsistent responses to splenectomy, suggesting that functional defects in granulocytes and disease severity variables may be as important as granulocytopenia in determining susceptibility to infection.[15, 16, 49]

Thrombocytopenia usually improves after splenectomy, as does anemia, to the extent that it is due to a hemolytic component. Although dramatic improvement in synovitis has been mentioned in several reports,[50] it is apparently not observed in most cases and is often temporary. Leg ulcers may also respond, even those that are not significantly infected,[13] but their variability in etiology and natural course makes these reports difficult to interpret.

Granulocytopenia has been shown to respond to various nonsurgical measures. Splenectomy should probably be reserved for patients who are unresponsive to these therapies (Fig. 54–3).

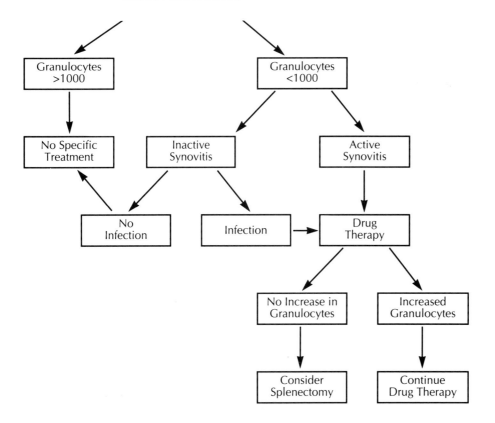

FELTY'S SYNDROME

Figure 54–3. Approach to the management of Felty's syndrome.

Other Treatments

Rheumatoid arthritis should be treated in the same manner as it would in the absence of Felty's syndrome. Frequently granulocytopenia may improve during treatment with second-line antirheumatic drugs.[15] Gold salt injections resulted in a complete hematologic response in 60 percent and partial response in 20 percent in the largest reported series.[50] There is less experience with auranofin, but in one report, all five patients treated had elevations in the neutrophil count.[52] Penicillamine appeared to be both less efficacious than gold and more likely to produce serious toxicity.[53] Limited experience with methotrexate suggests that it is also effective.[54, 56] Low doses of glucocorticoids do not produce consistent improvement in granulocytopenia and also predispose to infection.[10, 11] The mechanisms whereby these second-line agents raise granulocyte counts are undetermined, as are their response rates and relative efficacy. In one reported series, most patients failed to increase neutrophil counts by 50 percent on second-line drug treatment, and several untreated patients improved spontaneously.[2] Therefore, these agents may not be justified in patients without synovitis unless serious infections have occurred.

Other therapies may be directed specifically at the granulocytopenia, but benefits have been limited. High-dose parenteral testosterone may stimulate granulopoiesis and is also reported to reduce the infection rate in a small number of patients[57] but is not suitable for females. Lithium salts also increase granulopoiesis by augmenting colony-stimulating activity, but long-term benefit has not yet been demonstrated, and the treatment has been unsuccessful in the experience of some investigators.[2, 58] Recombinant granulocyte-macrophage colony-stimulating factor raises granulocyte counts, but its use is limited by cost, adverse reactions, and exacerbation of arthritis.[59] Recombinant granulocyte colony-stimulating factor may be a promising alternative as suggested by reports of successful use and good tolerance in patients with cyclic and idiopathic neutropenia.[60, 61]

References

1. Felty, A. R.: Chronic arthritis in the adult, associated with splenomegaly and leucopenia. Johns Hopkins Hosp. Bull. 35:16, 1924.
2. Campion, G., Maddison, P. J., Goulding, N., et al.: The Felty syndrome: A case-matched study of clinical manifestations and outcome, serologic features, and immunogenetic association. Medicine 69:69, 1990.
3. Isomaki, H., and Koivisto, O.: Splenomegaly in rheumatoid arthritis. Acta Rheumatol. Scand. 17:23, 1971.
4. Saway, P. A., Prasthofer, E. F., and Barton, J. C.: Prevalence of granular lymphocyte proliferation in patients with rheumatoid arthritis and neutropenia. Am. J. Med. 86:303, 1989.
5. Wallis, W. J., Loughran, T. P., Jr., Kadin, M. E., et al.: Polyarthritis and neutropenia associated with circulatory large granular lymphocytes. Ann. Intern. Med. 103:357, 1985.
5a. Rosenstein, E. D., and Kramer, N.: Felty's and Pseudo-Felty's syndromes. Semin. Arthritis Rheum. 21:129, 1991.
6. Dinant, H. J., Muller, W. H., van den Berg-Loonen, E. M., Nijenhuis, and Engelfriet, C. P.: HLA DRw4 in Felty's syndrome. Arthritis Rheum. 23:1336, 1980.
7. Termini, T. E., Biundo, J. J., and Ziff, M.: The rarity of Felty's syndrome in blacks. Arthritis Rheum. 22:999, 1979.
8. Toomey, K., and Hepburn, B.: Felty's syndrome in juvenile arthritis. J. Pediatr. 106:254, 1985.
9. Bradley, J. D., and Pinals, R. S.: Felty's syndrome presenting without arthritis. Clin. Exp. Rheumatol. 1:257, 1983.
10. Ruderman, M., Miller, L. M., and Pinals, R. S.: Clinical and serologic observations on 27 patients with Felty's syndrome. Arthritis Rheum. 11:377, 1968.
11. Sienknecht, C. W., Urowitz, M. B., Pruzanski, W., and Stein, H. G.: Felty's syndrome. Clinical and serological analysis of 34 cases. Ann. Rheum. Dis. 36:500, 1977.
11a. McMahon, M. J., Hollis, S., Sanders, P. A., and Grennan, D. M.: Articular disease severity in rheumatoid subjects with and without Felty's syndrome. Br. J. Rheumatol. 30:217, 1991.
12. Davies, P. G., and Thompson, P. W.: Palindromic rheumatism and Felty's syndrome. Ann. Rheum. Dis. 44:640, 1985.
13. Laszlo, J., Jones, R., Silberman, H. R., and Banks, P. M.: Splenectomy for Felty's syndrome: Clinicopathological study of 27 patients. Arch. Intern. Med. 138:597, 1978.
14. Moore, R. A., Brunner, C. M., Sandusky, W. R., and Leavell, B. S.: Felty's syndrome: Long-term follow-up after splenectomy. Ann. Intern. Med. 75:381, 1971.
14a. Sibley, J. T., Haga, M., Visram, D. A., and Mitchell, D. M.: The clinical course of Felty's syndrome compared to matched controls. J. Rheumatol. 18:1163, 1991.
15. Breedveld, F. C., Fibbe, W. E., and Cats, A.: Neutropenia and infections in Felty's syndrome. Br. J. Rheumatol. 27:191, 1988.
16. Breedveld, F. C., Fibbe, W. E., Hermans, J., et al.: Factors influencing the incidence of infections in Felty's syndrome. Arch. Intern. Med. 147:915, 1987.
17. Thorne, C., Urowitz, M. B., Wanless, I., Roberts, E., and Blendis, L. M.: Liver disease in Felty's syndrome. Am. J. Med. 73:35, 1982.
17a. Ruiz, F. P., Martinez, J. J. O., Mendoza, A. C. Z., delArbol, L. R., and Caparros, A. M.: Nodular regenerative hyperplasia of the liver in rheumatic diseases: Report of seven cases and review of the literature. Semin. Arthritis Rheum. 21:47, 1991.
18. Wanless, I. R., Godwin, T. A., Allen, F., and Feder, A.: Nodular regenerative hyperplasia of the liver in hematologic disorders: A possible response to obliterative portal venopathy. Medicine 59:367, 1980.
19. Luthra, H. S., and Hunder, G. G.: Spontaneous remission of Felty's syndrome. Arthritis Rheum. 18:515, 1975.
20. Rustagi, P. K., Currie, M. S., and Logue, G. L.: Activation of human complement by immunoglobulin G antigranulocyte antibody. J. Clin. Invest. 70:1137, 1982.
21. Weisman, M., and Zvaifler, N. J.: Cryoimmuno-globulinemia in Felty's syndrome. Arthritis Rheum. 19:103, 1976.
22. Cohen, M. G., and Webb, J.: Antihistone antibodies in rheumatoid arthritis and Felty's syndrome. Arthritis Rheum. 32:1319, 1989.
23. Andreis, M., Hurd, E. R., Lospalluto, J., and Ziff, M.: Comparison of the presence of immune complexes in Felty's syndrome and rheumatoid arthritis. Arthritis Rheum. 21:310, 1978.
24. Meretey, K., Falus, A., Bohm, U., Permin, H., and Wiik, A.: IgE class immune complexes in Felty's syndrome. Ann. Rheum. Dis. 43:246, 1984.
25. Hurd, E. R., Chubick, A., Jasin, H. E., and Ziff, M.: Increased C1q binding immune complexes in Felty's syndrome. Arthritis Rheum. 22:697, 1979.
26. Dameshek, W.: Hypersplenism. Bull. N.Y. Acad. Sci. 31:113, 1955.
27. Wright, C. S., Doan, C. A., Bouroncle, B. A., and Zollinger, R. M.: Direct splenic arterial and venous blood studies in the hypersplenic syndromes before and after epinephrine. Blood 6:195, 1951.
28. Hurd, E. R.: Presence of leucocyte inclusions in spleen and bone marrow of patients with Felty's syndrome. J. Rheumatol. 5:26, 1978.
29. Calabresi, P., Edwards, E. A., and Schilling, R. F.: Fluorescent antiglobulin studies in leucopenic and related disorders. J. Clin. Invest. 38:2091, 1959.
30. Starkebaum, G., Arend, W. P., Nardella, F. A., and Gavin, S. E.: Characterization of immune complexes and immunoglobulin G antibodies reactive with neutrophils in the sera of patients with Felty's syndrome. J. Lab. Clin. Med. 96:238, 1980.
31. Goldschmeding, R., Breedveld, F. C., Engelfriet, C. P., et al.: Lack of evidence for the presence of neutrophil autoantibodies in the serum of patients with Felty's syndrome. Br. J. Haematol. 68:37, 1988.
32. Bishop, C. R.: The neutropenia of Felty's syndrome. Am. J. Hematol. 2:203, 1977.
33. Breedveld, F. C., Lafeber, G. J. M., de Vries, E., van Krieken, J. H. J. M., and Cats, A.: Immune complexes and the pathogenesis of neutropenia in Felty's syndrome. Ann. Rheum. Dis. 45:696, 1986.
34. Hashimoto, Y., Ziff, M., and Hurd, E. R.: Increased endothelial cell adherence, aggregation, and superoxide generation by neutrophils incubated in systemic lupus erythematosus and Felty's syndrome sera. Arthritis Rheum. 12:1409, 1982.
35. Gupta, R., Robinson, W. A., and Albrecht, D.: Granulopoietic activity in Felty's syndrome. Ann. Rheum. Dis. 34:156, 1975.

36. Goldberg, L. S., Bacon, P. A., Bucknall, R. C., Fitchen, J., and Cline, M. J.: Inhibition of human bone marrow-granulocyte precursors by serum from patients with Felty's syndrome. J. Rheumatol. 7:275, 1980.

37. Abdou, N. L.: Heterogeneity of bone marrow-directed immune mechanisms in the pathogenesis of neutropenia of Felty's syndrome. Arthritis Rheum. 26:947, 1983.

38. Bagby, G. C., Jr., and Gabourel, J. D.: Neutropenia in three patients with rheumatic disorders: Suppression of granulocytes by cortisol-sensitive thymus-dependent lymphocytes. J. Clin. Invest. 64:72, 1979.

39. Slavin, S., and Liang, M. H.: Cell-mediated autoimmune granulocytopenia in a case of Felty's syndrome. Ann. Rheum. Dis. 39:399, 1980.

40. Runge, L. A., Davey, F. R., Goldberg, J., Boyd, P. R.: The inheritance of Felty's syndrome in a family with several affected members. J. Rheumatol. 13:39, 1986.

41. Thomson, W., Sanders, P. A., Davis, M., et al.: Complement C4B-null alleles in Felty's syndrome. Arthritis Rheum. 31:984, 1988.

41a. Wallin, J., Hillert, J., Olerup, O., Carlsson, B., and Strom, H.: Association of rheumatoid arthritis with a dominant DR1/Dw4/Dw14 sequence motif, but not with T cell receptor beta chain gene alleles or haplotypes. Arthritis Rheum. 34:1416, 1991.

42. So, A. K. L., Warner, C. A., Sansom, D., Walport, M. J.: DQ B polymorphism and genetic susceptibility to Felty's syndrome. Arthritis Rheum. 31:990, 1988.

43. Starkebaum, G., Singer, J. W., and Arend, W. P.: Humoral and cellular immune mechanisms of neutropenia in patients with Felty's syndrome. Clin. Exp. Immunol. 39:307, 1980.

44. Breedveld, F. C., van den Barselaar, M. T., Leijh, P. C. J., Cats, A., and van Furth, R.: Phagocytosis and intracellular killing by polymorphonuclear cells from patients with rheumatoid arthritis and Felty's syndrome. Arthritis Rheum. 28:395, 1985.

45. Howe, G. B., Fordham, J. N., Brown, K. A., and Currey, H. L. F.: Polymorphonuclear cell function in rheumatoid arthritis and in Felty's syndrome. Ann. Rheum. Dis. 40:370, 1981.

46. Davis, P., Johnston, C., Bertouch, J., and Starkebaum, G.: Depressed superoxide radical generation by neutrophils from patients with rheumatoid arthritis and neutropenia: Correlation with neutrophil reactive IgG. Ann. Rheum. Dis. 46:51, 1987.

47. Green, R. A., and Fromke, V. L.: Splenectomy in Felty's syndrome. Ann. Intern. Med. 64:1265, 1966.

48. Logue, G. L., Huang, A. T., and Shimm, D. S.: Failure of splenectomy in Felty's syndrome. The role of antibodies supporting granulocyte lysis by lymphocytes. N. Engl. J. Med. 304:580, 1981.

49. Thorne, C., and Urowitz, M. B.: Long-term outcome in Felty's syndrome. Ann. Rheum. Dis. 41:486, 1982.

50. Khan, M. A., and Kushner, I.: Improvement in rheumatoid arthritis following splenectomy for Felty's syndrome. J.A.M.A. 237:1116, 1977.

51. Dillon, A. M., Luthra, H. S., Conn, D. L., and Ferguson, R. H.: Parenteral gold therapy in the Felty syndrome. Medicine 65:107, 1986.

52. Bellelli, A., Veneziani, M., and Tumiati, B.: Felty's syndrome: Long-term followup after treatment with auranofin. Arthritis Rheum. 30:1057, 1987.

53. Lakhanpal, S., and Luthra, H. A.: D-penicillamine in Felty's syndrome. J. Rheumatol. 12:703, 1985.

54. Allen, L. S., and Groff, G.: Treatment of Felty's syndrome with low-dose oral methotrexate. Arthritis Rheum. 29:902, 1986.

55. Fiechtner, J. J., Miller, D. R., and Starkebaum, G.: Reversal of neutropenia with methotrexate treatment in patients with Felty's syndrome. Arthritis Rheum. 32:194, 1989.

56. Isasi, C., Lopez-Martin, J. A., Trujillo, M. A., et al.: Felty's syndrome: Response to low dose oral methotrexate. J. Rheumatol. 16:983, 1989.

57. Wimer, B. M., and Sloan, M. W.: Remission of Felty's syndrome with long-term testosterone therapy. J. A. M. A. 223:671, 1973.

58. Mant, M. J., Akabutu, J. J., and Herbert, F. A.: Lithium carbonate therapy in severe Felty's syndrome: benefits, toxicity, and granulocyte function. Arch. Intern. Med. 146:277, 1986.

59. Hazenberg, B. P. C., VanLeewen, M. A., Van Rijswijk, M. H., et al.: Correction of granulocytopenia in Felty's syndrome by granulocyte-macrophage colony-stimulating factor. Simultaneous induction of interleukin-6 release and flare-up of the arthritis. Blood 74:2769, 1989.

60. Hammond, W. P. IV, Price T. H., Souza, L. M., and Dale, D. C.: Treatment of cyclic neutropenia with granulocyte colony-stimulating factor. N. Engl. J. Med. 320:1306, 1989.

61. Jakubowski, A. A., Souza, L., Kelly, F., et al.: Effects of human granulocyte colony-stimulating factor in a patient with idiopathic neutropenia. N. Engl. J. Med. 320:38, 1989.

Chapter 55
Sjögren's Syndrome

Robert I. Fox
Ho-Il Kang

Sjögren's syndrome (SS) is a chronic inflammatory disorder characterized by lymphocytic infiltration of lacrimal and salivary glands, which results in dry eyes and dry mouth. SS may exist as a primary condition or as a secondary condition in association with rheumatoid arthritis (RA), systemic lupus erythematosus (SLE), or progressive systemic sclerosis (PSS). In some primary SS patients, there may be involvement of the extraglandular organs, including skin, kidney, liver, lung, and nervous system. Further, these patients may develop a lymphoproliferative syndrome that includes lymphadenopathy and increased risk of lymphoma. This chapter concentrates on the differential diagnosis and treatment of primary SS.

There has been considerable debate about the criteria for diagnosis of definite SS. We favor stringent criteria, including (1) objective evidence of keratoconjunctivitis sicca (KCS), (2) objective evidence of decreased salivary gland flow, and (3) presence of autoantibodies such as rheumatoid factor or antinuclear antibody. In many patients, a minor salivary gland biopsy is helpful to confirm the diagnosis. Patients with sarcoidosis, pre-existing lymphoma, or human immunodeficiency virus (HIV) are excluded.

Treatment of primary SS depends on the extent of disease. All SS patients should receive careful instruction for treatment of dry eyes and dry mouth. Increasing mouth and tongue pain in the patient may be caused by oral candidiasis superinfection. Chronic sinusitis is common and frequently exacerbates the dry mouth problems because it forces mouth breathing. When fatigue is a prominent complaint, the role of active systemic autoimmune disease in causing these symptoms can be estimated by evaluating erythrocyte sedimentation rate (ESR) and other acute phase reactants. Other common causes of fatigue in SS patients include hypothyroidism and disordered sleep patterns. In patients with arthralgias, limited bone scans are useful in objectively assessing the symptoms. Antimalarial medications are helpful in many patients with elevated ESR and positive bone scans. When vasculitis or visceral manifestations (i.e., nervous system, lung, kidney) are present, treatment with glucocorticoids or immunosuppressive agents is required, as in SLE patients.

This is Publication No. 6683-IMM from the Research Institute of Scripps Clinic. Supported in part by research grants from the National Institutes of Health AR33983 and M01RR00833, the Hennings Foundation, and the Scripps-Stedham Charitable Trust. H. K. is the recipient of the Eiken Chemical Postdoctoral Fellowship.

BACKGROUND

In 1888, Johann van Mikulicz Radecki described a 42-year-old Prussian farmer with enlargement of lacrimal and salivary glands "consisting of small round cells."[1] In 1933, Henrik Sjögren described the association of KCS, dry mouth (xerostomia), and RA.[2] Although this association of symptoms is generally known as Sjögren's syndrome, it is occasionally referred to as *Gougerout-Sjögren syndrome* to acknowledge the earlier report by Gougerout in 1925.[3] In 1953, Morgan and Castleman[4] demonstrated that a histologically similar infiltrate was present in both SS and Mikulicz's disease. Block et al.[5] suggested that SS be subdivided into primary SS and secondary SS. Secondary SS was defined as that occurring in patients with sicca symptoms in association with particular diseases such as RA, SLE, PSS, and dermatomyositis, whereas primary SS patients lacked these particular diseases. A wide spectrum of extraglandular features, including pulmonary, lung, renal, and neurologic involvement, have been reported in primary SS patients.

EPIDEMIOLOGY

The frequency of primary SS in the general population has been an issue of considerable debate. The specific criteria for inclusion will obviously dictate the frequency. The referral pattern to a specific medical center of a patient with an "unusual" condition will further influence estimates of disease prevalence. One approach to this problem was the evaluation of consecutive blood donor samples for the presence of anti-SS-B antibody in random female blood donors,[6] yielding a frequency of approximately one in 2500. Retrospective studies have shown a high association of anti-SS-B antibody with clinical sicca symptoms and positive minor salivary gland biopsies.[7] As antibodies against SS-B have been found in about 40 to 50 percent of primary SS patients meeting strict criteria for diagnosis,[8] an estimate of primary SS in about one in 1250 females may serve as an approximation. When patients with RA and secondary SS are considered, a much higher prevalence may be present, and these would not be included in the aforementioned estimate because secondary SS patients with RA frequently lack anti-SS-B antibody.

931

Table 55–1. CRITERIA FOR DIAGNOSIS OF PRIMARY AND SECONDARY SJÖGREN'S SYNDROME

Primary SS
  Symptoms and objective signs of ocular dryness
    Schirmer's test less than 8 mm wetting per 5 minutes
    Positive rose bengal or fluorescein staining of cornea and
      conjunctiva to demonstrate keratoconjunctivitis sicca
  Symptoms and objective signs of dry mouth
    Decreased parotid flow rate using Lashley cups or other
      methods
    Abnormal biopsy of minor salivary gland (focus score of ≥2
      based on average of 4 evaluable lobules)
  Evidence of a systemic autoimmune disorder
    Elevated rheumatoid factor >1:160
    Elevated antinuclear antibody >1:160
    Presence of anti–SS-A (Ro) or anti–SS-B (La) antibodies
Secondary SS
  Characteristic signs and symptoms of SS (described above)
    plus clinical features sufficient to allow a diagnosis of RA,
    SLE, polymyositis, or scleroderma.
Exclusions: sarcoidosis, pre-existent lymphoma, acquired
  immunodeficiency disease, and other known causes of
  keratitis sicca or salivary gland enlargement

RA, rheumatoid arthritis; SLE, systemic lupus erythematosus
From Fox, R. I., Robinson, C., Curd, J., et al.: First international symposium on Sjögren's syndrome: Suggested criteria for classification. Scand. J. Rheumatol. 562:28, 1986.

PROBLEM OF DEFINITION OF SJÖGREN'S SYNDROME

One major problem in describing the clinical spectrum of SS is that there is no uniformly accepted definition for this syndrome.[8, 9] This has resulted in confusion in clinical practice as well as in research publications. Three types of patients with "dry eyes and dry mouth" are described here: (1) patients fulfilling strict criteria for SS, (2) elderly patients with low titer antinuclear antibodies but without other evidence of a systemic autoimmune disorder, and (3) patients with widespread systemic vasculitis from whom an abnormal minor salivary gland biopsy is obtained.

At the Second International Symposium on SS, the diagnostic criteria listed in Table 55–1[9] were presented. The patients should have symptoms and objective signs of KCS. These findings can be easily measured by the physician using the Schirmer's test (a strip of filter paper inserted under the eyelid for 5 minutes), where normal wetting is greater than 8 mm per 5 minutes. A modification of this method was suggested by Tsubota,[10] who measured Schirmer's test after stimulation of nasolacrimal gland reflex by inserting a cotton-tipped applicator into the nose. The keratoconjunctivitis can be visualized by instilling a drop of rose bengal dye into the eye and observing the increased uptake in devitalized areas in the interpalpebral region of the conjunctiva and cornea (Fig. 55–1). Although the latter method is best done with a slit lamp, significant changes can easily be detected by the rheumatologist using a simple ophthalmoscope.

The second criterion for diagnosis is the presence of symptomatic and objective xerostomia. Measurement of saliva from the parotid glands can be performed using a Lashley cup that fits over the opening of Stensen's duct.[11] Another easy method to quantitate total salivary flow is to place a cotton sponge under the tongue for 3 minutes and compare the dry weight to the "wet" weight.[12] Perhaps the simplest method to quantify saliva flow is to determine the decrease in weight of a sugarless candy after sucking for 3 minutes. Because there are many causes of decreased salivary flow, a minor salivary gland biopsy may be obtained to confirm the presence of lymphocytic infiltrate.[13] Although these biopsies will be interpreted by the pathologist, it is important for the rheumatologist to be able to verify the adequacy of the biopsy and to confirm the diagnosis. Figure 55–2 shows examples of a minor salivary gland biopsy from a primary SS patient (A) and from a normal individual (B). The site of the biopsy (through histologically normal oral mucosa) and the size of the biopsy (at least four evaluable salivary gland lobules) are important for the results to be interpretable. Several different methods for evaluating biopsies have been proposed. We use the system of Daniels,[13] in which the average number of lymphocytic foci (a focus is defined as a cluster of 50 or more lymphocytes) per 4 mm² is determined. The *focus*

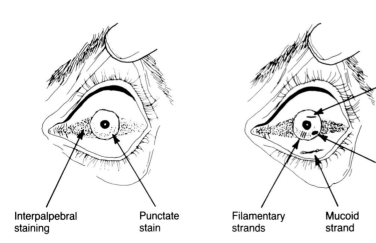

Interpalpebral   Punctate   Filamentary   Mucoid
staining   stain   strands   strand

Corneal abrasion

Coalescent erosion

Figure 55–1. Schematic illustration of increased interpalpebral staining with rose bengal. Since eyelids normally retard evaporation, disruption in the epithelial lining and tear film is most marked in the interpalpebral region (A), leading to increased risk of corneal abrasions (B).

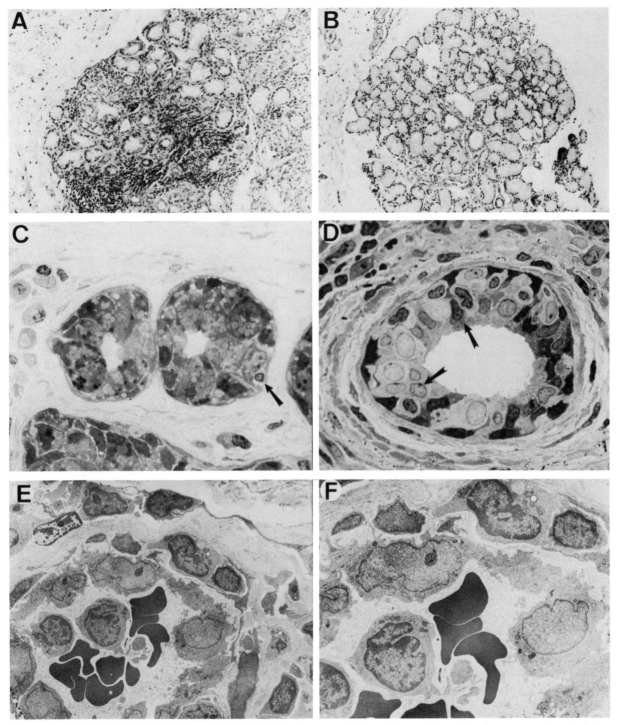

Figure 55–2. Sjögren's syndrome salivary gland biopsies. *A* and *B* show biopsies from a SS patient and from a normal individual. The initial appearance of lymphocytic infiltrates in the central portion of the salivary gland (*A*) is similar to that noted in the minor salivary gland biopsies of SS patients described above. Under higher magnification, the location of lymphocytes adjacent to salivary gland epithelial cells (i.e., beneath the basement membrane enclosing acini and ducts) can be seen. Under electron microscopy (*C* and *D*), the appearance of high endothelial venules (containing RBC and lymphocytes adherent to the vascular endothelium) can be noted as well as the absence of electron-dense immune complexes near the basement membrane (*E* and *F*).

score for the entire biopsy is expressed based on the average of at least four evaluable salivary gland lobules. For example, Figure 55–2*A* shows a 4 mm² portion of the minor salivary gland biopsy with a focus score of 4. Incorrect methods of biopsy (espe-

cially biopsy through an area of oral mucositis) and failure to record the *average* focus score are common causes of incorrect diagnosis of SS.

The third criterion for diagnosis (see Table 55–1) is laboratory evidence suggesting a systemic autoimmune disease, i.e., the presence of rheumatoid factor or antinuclear antibody (titer greater than 1:160). The majority of primary SS patients have antibodies against the ribonuclear proteins SS-A (Ro) and SS-B (La).[14] Although some patients have objective signs of sicca complex and lack autoantibodies, the absence of autoantibodies suggests that we look for other causes, such as sarcoidosis, lymphoma, or retroviral infections. Shah et al.[15] found that sicca symptoms and history of glandular enlargement were not statistically associated with positive findings on lip biopsy. Features predictive of a positive lip biopsy, however, included elevated autoantibody titer and associated objective findings of KCS.

The differential diagnosis of primary SS is often difficult, particularly in the older patient,[16] in whom dry eyes and dry mouth are common. Atrophy and sclerosis of the salivary glands have been detected in a high proportion of biopsies performed during consecutive autopsies of elderly patients with no history of autoimmune disease.[16, 17] Thus, dryness in many older patients is probably a consequence of aging rather than the result of a systemic autoimmune process. An additional group of patients in the differential diagnosis of SS includes individuals with poorly defined "connective tissue disease" and autoantibodies against SS-A/SS-B but who lack significant dry eyes or dry mouth. Salivary gland biopsy of these patients may reveal focal perivascular lymphocytic infiltrates.[18] Because perivascular infiltrates are the hallmark of systemic vasculitis and the salivary gland is a vascular organ, it is possible that the salivary gland simply represented a convenient place to demonstrate this process. We do not label such patients "SS" if they exhibit normal salivary and lacrimal gland function because the definition of SS should include significant eye or mouth problems. These patients certainly must be closely observed for development of SS, but we have followed several SLE patients for more than 10 years after a "positive lip biopsy" was obtained (as part of an earlier research study at our institution) without subsequent development of sicca complaints. Finally, patients with HIV infection may develop parotid swelling and sicca symptoms. Itescu et al.[19] have demonstrated that these patients rarely have antibodies to SS-A/SS-B and have a genetic predisposition that is different from other primary SS patients. Further, the immunohistologic pattern of their lip biopsies differs from other primary SS patients.[8]

OCULAR MANIFESTATIONS OF SJÖGREN'S SYNDROME

Patients with the ocular manifestations of SS, i.e., KCS, suffer from a decrease in the aqueous component of tears. This results from destruction of the serous glands and from interruption of their neurovascular innervation.[8b] The imbalance in aqueous and mucinous tear secretions leads to a relative increase in tenacious secretions, which are clinically noted as long mucinous threads that can be extracted from the patient's eyes. The decrease in aqueous tear flow leads to decreased tear film stability, manifested by a rapid tear breakup time and increased debris in the tear film. As a result, defects in visual acuity and discomfort may occur. The most characteristic symptom is a burning sensation that increases as the day progresses and that is relieved by instillation of artificial tears. Severe eye dryness leads to filamentary keratitis (fine filaments on the anterior surface of the cornea) in SS patients. They are composed primarily of mucus (mucoproteins and mucopolysaccharides) that binds to the cornea and conjunctiva. It is likely that the mucoproteins bind to specific receptors on the epithelium that have been exposed by a deficiency in the tear film. These filaments cause a severe foreign body sensation and may be associated with photophobia and blepharospasm. Corneal edema and conjunctivitis may also occur. These changes are not specific for SS and may be seen in wearers of contact lenses, in patients after intraocular surgery, and in patients with diabetes, ectodermal dysplasia, neurotrophic keratitis, trachoma, ocular pemphigoid, and sarcoidosis.

Other ocular symptoms in SS patients include an increased frequency of inflammation of the eyelids (blepharitis), owing in part to abnormalities affecting the meibomian glands. Irritating side effects from the preservatives in artificial tears and obstruction of the glands by ocular lubricants (discussed later), however, contribute to some cases of ocular irritation and blepharitis.

Among patients meeting stringent criteria for SS, a variety of ocular symptoms were present (Table 55–2). The most characteristic complaint was a *foreign body sensation* that often became more severe as the day progressed. Although patients also complained of a *dry eye, red eye, or painful eye*, these manifestations also were prevalent in the general population.[11, 20] Photosensitivity was not a common complaint unless the keratoconjunctivitis was quite severe.[20b] The presence of this symptom should suggest anterior uveitis rather than SS. Causes of keratitis other than SS, listed in Table 55–3, include pemphigoid, sarcoidosis, trauma infection, vitamin deficiency, neuropathy, and allergy.

It is worth emphasizing that only a small proportion of patients with "painful" eyes have SS. Even the majority of those patients with the tear film abnormalities of KCS are unlikely to have any other manifestations of a systemic autoimmune disease such as SS, and they need to be reassured in this regard.[21] Decreases in ocular tear production occur as a consequence of aging, as do decreases in saliva production. This decrease in tearing with aging appears to occur more frequently in women and to intensify after menopause. It may manifest suddenly in patients who receive medications with anticholinergic side effects, such as antidepressants, cold remedies, and certain cardiac medications.

Table 55-2. CLINICAL FEATURES OF KERATOCONJUNCTIVITIS SICCA

Clinical Features	Sjögren's Syndrome Patients (%)	Control Patients (%)
Symptoms		
Foreign-body sensation that is worse in the evening	85	6
"Dry eye" or "painful eye"	98	22
Dry eye feeling that improves after use of artificial tears	75	7
Itching of the eyes	27	19
Signs		
Dilatation of the bulbar conjunctival vessels (usually interpalpebral)	31	7
Dullness of the conjunctiva and/or cornea	27	0
Schirmer's test ≤9 mm/5 min	95	10
Abnormal rose bengal and/or fluorescein	100	5

ORAL FEATURES

Various methods are used to evaluate salivary gland function and size. In addition to simple measurement of salivary flow rates, salivary gland scintiagraphy using technetium pertechnetate have been employed.[22] Although this latter method provided quantitative measurements, it provided less specific information than the minor salivary gland biopsy.[13] Sialograms using oil-based contrast materials introduced through Stensen's or Wharton's duct have been reported, but this procedure was discontinued

Table 55-3. CAUSES OF KERATITIS AND SALIVARY GLAND ENLARGEMENT OTHER THAN SJÖGREN'S SYNDROME

Keratitis
  Mucous membrane pemphigoid
  Sarcoidosis
  Infections: virus (adenovirus, herpes, vaccinia), bacteria, or Chlamydia (i.e., trachoma)
  Trauma (i.e., from contact lens) and environmental irritants, including chemical burns, exposure to ultraviolet lights, or roentgenograms
  Neuropathy, including neurotropic keratitis (i.e., damage to fifth cranial nerve and familial dysautonomia (Riley-Day syndrome)
  Hypovitaminosis A
  Erythema multiforme (Stevens-Johnson syndrome)
Salivary gland enlargement
  Sarcoidosis, amyloidosis
  Bacterial (including gonococci and syphilis) and viral infections (i.e., infectious mononucleosis, mumps)
  Tuberculosis, actinomycosis, histoplasmosis, trachoma, leprosy
  Iodide, lead, or copper hypersensitivity
  Hyperlipemic states, especially types IV and V
  Tumors (usually unilateral), including cysts (Warthin's tumor), epithelial (adenoma, adenocarcinoma), lymphoma, and mixed salivary gland tumors
  Excessive alcohol consumption
  Human immunodeficiency virus

because of the risk of inflammatory reactions provoked by the viscous contrast materials. Ultrasound evaluation[23, 24] provides a precise size measurement of the salivary gland, and magnetic resonance imaging (MRI) provides detailed evaluations of the glands and surrounding lymph nodes.

Salivary gland enlargement can occur in diseases other than SS (see Table 55-3). Diseases such as sarcoidosis, amyloidosis, and infection (including bacterial, fungal, and viral) or the presence of a tumor must be considered. The finding of an elevated angiotensin converting enzyme (ACE) is a helpful indication of sarcoidosis, since this enzyme is rarely elevated in glandular swelling owing to SS. An unusual presentation of sarcoidosis is *uveoparotid fever* (Heerfordt's disease), in which patients exhibit parotid enlargement and ocular symptoms but lack other features of sarcoidosis (hilar lymphadenopathy, diffuse lung infiltrates, skin sarcoid, or hepatosplenomegaly). A sudden increase in salivary gland pain or size should suggest the possibility of infection, which is more frequent in SS patients owing to inadequate salivary flow rate. The most frequent offending organisms are *Staphylococcus*, *Streptococcus viridans*, *Streptococcus hemolyticus*, and *Pneumococcus*, all normal flora of the oral cavity. Cultures must be taken of the pus escaping from the Stensen or Wharton duct. Salivary gland infections must be treated promptly to prevent formation of abscesses.

INVOLVEMENT OF EXTRAGLANDULAR SITES

Pulmonary Sites

Involvement of exocrine glands in the upper respiratory tract frequently leads to dryness of the nasal passages and bronchi. Hunninghake and Fauci[25] emphasized the high incidence of pulmonary abnormalities in patients with SS, including pleurisy with and without effusion, interstitial fibrosis, dessication of tracheobroncheal mucous membrane, and lymphoid interstitial disease (Table 55-4). In our clinic, the development of respiratory problems associated with mucus plug inspissation is a relatively common problem. This often occurs in the setting of an upper respiratory tract infection, resulting in increased tenacious secretions that cannot be adequately mobilized from the small airways.[26] This problem may be confounded further by the patient taking cold remedies containing compounds with anticholinergic side effects. It may also occur in the postoperative setting when the anesthesiologist gives the SS patient an anticholinergic drug to control upper respiratory tract secretions during surgery, resulting in the inspissation of the patient's secretions. These problems can be minimized by the use of smaller doses of anticholinergic medicines, the use of humidified oxygen in the operating room, and attention to respiratory therapy during the postoperative period.

Table 55–4. EXTRAGLANDULAR MANIFESTATIONS IN PATIENTS WITH PRIMARY SJÖGREN'S SYNDROME

Respiratory
  Chronic bronchitis secondary to dryness of upper and lower
    airway with mucous plugging
  Lymphocytic interstitial pneumonitis
  Pseudolymphoma with nodular infiltrates
  Lymphoma
  Pleural effusions
  Pulmonary hypertension, especially with associated
    scleroderma
Gastrointestinal
  Dysphagia associated with xerostomia
  Atrophic gastritis
  Liver disease, including biliary cirrhosis and sclerosing
    cholangitis
Skin
  Vaginal dryness
  Hyperglobulinemic purpura—nonthrombocytopenic
  Raynaud's phenomena
  Vasculitis
Endocrine, neurologic, and muscular
  Thyroiditis
  Peripheral neuropathy—symmetric involvement of hands and/
    or feet
  Mononeuritis multiplex
  Myalgias
Hematologic
  Neutropenia, anemia, thrombocytopenia
  Pseudolymphoma
  Angioblastic lymphadenopathy
  Lymphoma and myeloma
Renal
  Tubulointerstitial nephritis
  Glomerulonephritis—in absence of antibodies to DNA
  Mixed cryoglobulinemia
  Amyloidosis
  Obstructive nephropathy due to enlarged periaortic lymph
    nodes
  Lymphoma
  Renal artery vasculitis

Clinical studies of pulmonary function in primary SS patients have yielded conflicting results. Newball and Brahim[27] and Siegal et al.[28] found evidence of mild to moderate obstructive airway disease in almost 50 per cent of their primary SS patients. In another study, Oxholm et al.[29] did not find obstructive changes in any of 43 patients with primary SS but did note decreased diffusing capacity and suggested that interstitial pneumonitis was relatively common. During a 7-year follow-up study, these SS patients did not undergo significant deterioration of their diffusing capacity.[30]

Gastrointestinal Sites

Difficulty in swallowing is a frequent occurrence in primary SS patients, owing primarily to decreased saliva production.[31] The patient describes difficulty in deglutition (i.e., food gets stuck at the upper throat) as opposed to subjective feelings of obstruction at the substernal level that occurs in scleroderma patients. Abnormal esophageal motility (particularly in the upper one third of the esophagus) may also

contribute to dysphagia in some primary SS patients.[32] Increased symptoms of "heartburn" and discomfort in distal esophageal structures may be due in part to reflux of gastric acid into the esophagus, where it is not adequately neutralized by the diminished amount of saliva. Gastric biopsy specimens show increased frequency of chronic atrophic gastritis[33] and lymphocytic infiltrates.[34] Patients with marked gastric involvement can be recognized by their decreased serum pepsinogen levels[35] and increased gastrin levels.[33] Investigation of pancreatic function has shown impaired response to secretin and pancreozymin, suggesting subclinical pancreatic disease.[36, 37] Overt pancreatic insufficiency manifesting as diabetes mellitus or malabsorption, however, does not appear to be significantly increased in frequency. Antibodies against pancreatic duct antigen were found in some patients, but antibodies to pancreatic islet cells were not detected.[38]

Clinical or biochemical evidence of liver disease is found in 5 to 10 percent of primary SS patients.[39, 40] The elevations in liver function tests are generally mild (less than twice normal) and without clinical significance. When higher levels are noted, possibilities such as viral hepatitis and drug toxicity (including nonsteroidal anti-inflammatory drugs and aspirin) should be evaluated. In a small proportion of SS patients, the presence of antimitchondrial antibodies indicates co-existent primary biliary cirrhosis (PBC). It is relatively common for PBC patients to develop sicca symptoms late in their disease. Salivary gland biopsy specimens from these patients show lymphoid infiltrates. These findings suggest that a similar pathogenic process may be responsible for salivary gland destruction and damage to the exocrine hepatic apparatus. It is uncommon, however, for PBC patients to exhibit antibodies against SS-B antigen,[41] and thus the PBC-associated sicca complex probably represents a form of secondary SS.

Cutaneous Sites

Dryness of the skin has been attributed to a decrease in the secretory capacity of the sebaceous glands in some patients. Oral candidiasis, particularly angular cheilitis, is extremely common in these patients and is a common contributing factor in their increased mouth pain and decreased sensation of taste. It is particularly common in SS patients who are receiving glucocorticoids, and the onset of symptoms can frequently be traced to the use of antibiotics for another reason.

Vasculitis in SS patients may take multiple forms. The most common "vasculitis" in our clinic is *hypergammaglobulinemic purpura* that occurs symmetrically in the lower extremities.[42] This is found in patients with gammaimmunoglobulin G (IgG) greater than 2000 mg per deciliter, and the earliest stage of the rash exhibits multiple nonpalpable 2- to 3-mm petechial lesions. As these acute lesions fade, they are replaced by hyperpigmentation that may persist from months to years. In addition to nonpalpable purpura, SS patients may develop palpable purpura owing to leukocytoclastic vasculitis and skin lesions of erythema multiforma.[43, 44] Periungual telangiectasis may be detected in these patients, but their presence in large numbers suggests an increased chance of later development of scleroderma.

Endocrine Sites

Clinically apparent hypothyroidism has been reported in 10 to 15 percent of SS patients[45–47] and occurred in a similar proportion of our patients.[11] Antibody to thyroglobulin and thyroid microsomal antigen levels may be elevated in an additional 4 to 5 percent of patients,[46] suggesting that subclinical thyroid damage may be relatively common in SS patients. Thus, endocrine as well as exocrine glandular cells may be targets for immune attack in primary SS. Insulin-dependent diabetes mellitus[45] and pernicious anemia[46] occur with a similar frequency in primary SS as they do in the general population.

Renal Manifestations

Renal tubular function is not a routine clinical measurement, and the renal functional evaluation of most patients with SS remains incomplete, with the available data perhaps not truly representative. The most common functional renal abnormality noted in SS patients is the inability to acidify the urine in response to an administered acid load, such as ammonium chloride.[48–53] This is generally believed to be due to dysfunction of the distal nephron and may be present in 20 to 40 per cent of SS patients in a latent form.[49, 52] Talal et al.[54] demonstrated impairment of urinary acidification in six of 12 patients with SS who also had marked hypergammaglobulinemia. This defect may lead to a higher frequency of nephrocalcinosis.[50, 52]

Proteinuria is uncommon in patients with SS. Only two of 36 patients in one series had proteinuria greater than 3.5 g.[51] Glomerulonephritis in primary SS is unusual,[54–57] and its occurrence suggests an associated disease process, such as SLE, amyloidosis, vasculitis, and mixed cryoglobulinemia.[58–60] Membranoproliferative and membranous forms of glomerulonephritis have been described, and the immunopathologic studies suggest that the glomerular lesions are associated with accumulation of immune complex material.

In considering SS as part of the differential diagnosis of interstitial nephritis, it must be remembered that a wide group of diseases may affect the interstitium and tubules while sparing the glomeruli.[61] The renal abnormalities of interstitial nephritis can occur in virtually any autoimmune disease and are most frequently found in association with hypergammaglobulinemia.[62–65] Of particular importance are the side effects of drugs (antibiotics, nonsteroidal anti-inflammatory drugs) associated with nephropathy, since SS patients frequently receive these medications.

Hematologic Abnormalities

Leukopenia (total white blood cell [WBC] count <4,000 cells per mm³) was present in 20 percent of our SS patients; previous reports have noted leukopenia in 6 to 33 percent of their patients.[5, 46] The mechanism of this leukopenia remains unclear but may involve antibodies to leukocytes, splenic sequestration, or abnormal bone marrow maturation of leukocytes in certain patients.[66]

SS patients have increased frequency of serum and urinary paraproteins.[67, 68] They exhibit increased levels of cryoglobulins, particularly in association with hypergammaglobulinemic purpura.[42] The cryoglobulin is frequently a type II mixed cryoglobulin containing an IgM-kappa monoclonal rheumatoid factor similar to that found in Waldenström's macroglobulinemia.[67] Among Japanese SS patients, an increased incidence of non-IgM paraproteins has been reported.[69]

The relative risk for primary SS patients of developing lymphoma has been estimated to be approximately 40-fold higher than age-matched, sex-matched control subjects by investigators at the National Institutes of Health.[70] Whaley et al.[46] in Glasgow, however, did not find such an increased prevalence. These discrepancies may be attributed to several factors, including the relatively small number of patients reported with lymphoma and ascertainment bias in patient referral patterns. These differences, however, also may reflect the difficulty in distinguishing lymphoma from extensive infiltrates owing to "benign" SS or pseudolymphoma (Fig. 55–3).[71] The lymphomas are predominantly non-Hodgkin's B cell (IgM-kappa) tumors that arise in the salivary gland and cervical lymph nodes. Although the finding of myoepithelial islands (i.e., a degenerating tubule surrounded by lymphocytes) is often interpreted as an indication that the tumor is "benign," malignant lymphomas can be found in the same biopsy specimen that contains myoepithelial islands.[72] The distinction between malignant lymphoma and pseudolymphoma in SS patients is often quite difficult, even when recombinant DNA methods are used.[73–75, 75b] Other forms of nonmalignant lymphoid proliferation in primary SS patients include thymoma[45] and angioimmunoblastic lymphadenopathy.[76] In both pseudolymphoma and angioblastic lymphadenopathy, there appears to be a high frequency of progression to frank lymphoma.[70, 77]

Neurologic Manifestations

SS patients may exhibit both central and peripheral nervous system manifestations. The frequency

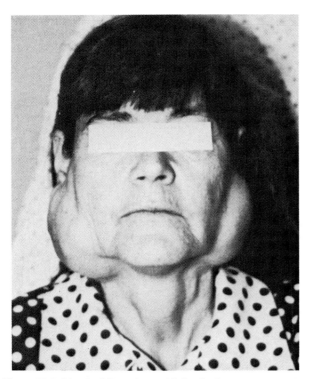

Figure 55–3. Massive bilateral parotid gland enlargement in patient I.R. with pseudolymphoma and SS. Clinical and histologic features of this patient and three additional pseudolymphoma are presented in reference 71. (From Fox, R. I., Adamson, T. C., III, Fong, S., et al.: Lymphocyte phenotype and function of pseudolymphomas associated with Sjögren's syndrome. J. Clin. Invest. 72:52, 1983. Reproduced from the *Journal of Clinical Investigation*, by copyright permission of the American Society for Clinical Investigation.)

of these complications varies in different reported series. Alexander et al.[78] have found central nervous system abnormalities in approximately 20 percent of their primary SS patients. In particular, they have found a multiple sclerosis–like symptom with abnormal cerebrospinal fluid analysis and MRI of the brain.[79] The central nervous system symptoms were associated with cutaneous vasculitis.[43] In comparison, Metz et al.[80] and Sandberg-Wollheim et al.[80b] did not find increased frequency of autoantibodies or abnormal labial biopsies among patients with multiple sclerosis; an increased frequency of sicca symptoms was noted among the multiple sclerosis patients but was attributed to anticholinergic side effects of medicines and perhaps to underlying neurologic dysfunction. Peripheral neuropathies among primary SS include symmetric peripheral neuropathies and mononeuritis multiplex. The symmetric neuropathies frequently present as a sensory neuropathy involving the feet in patients with hypergammaglobulinemic purpura. Mononeuritis multiplex with sensory and motor components occurs less frequently and is often associated with leukocytoclastic vasculitis among our patients.[11]

PATHOGENESIS

The specific etiology of SS remains unknown. It is likely that it involves both genetic and environmental features. Theories of pathogenesis should include the following features: (1) the lacrimal and salivary glands become infiltrated with CD4+ T cells and to a lesser extent with B cells;[81, 82] (2) the salivary epithelial cells express high levels of HLA-DR in comparison to normal salivary gland epithelial cells;[83, 84] (3) antibodies made within the gland are directed against rheumatoid factor (Fc region of IgG)[67] and antinuclear antigens (SS-A, SS-B),[14] which are not specific to salivary or lacrimal glands; (4) although antibodies against salivary ductal antigens are occasionally detected, they are relatively uncommon and unlikely to play a primary role in pathogenesis;[85] (5) genetic predisposition in Caucasians is linked to HLA-DR3[86] and to heterozygosity of HLA-DQ,[87, 87b] whereas different genetic markers appear important in other ethnic groups; and (6) SS patients have increased risk of lymphoma owing to IgM-kappa B cells, and these lymphomas generally originate in the lacrimal/salivary glands or cervical lymph nodes.

At the DNA level, expansion of one or more B cell clones within salivary gland biopsies of SS patients has been demonstrated by Southern blot methods.[73, 75] Because these salivary gland biopsy specimens did not fulfill histologic criteria for malignancy, this suggested that proliferation of certain "autoimmune" clones was responsible for the observed *clonal expansion* of cells corresponding to the 5 to 10 percent of B cells within the biopsy specimen. It is likely that such clonal expansions of B cells are the source of oligoclonal proteins frequently demonstrated in the sera or urine of these patients.[68]

The initial inciting lesion in SS remains unknown. One candidate is Epstein-Barr virus (EBV).[88] In normal individuals, primary infection with EBV (infectious mononucleosis) involves the salivary glands, and EBV has a normal site of latency and reactivation in the salivary gland.[89, 90] Further, EBV can stimulate production of polyclonal antibodies and autoantibodies such as rheumatoid factor.[91] In biopsies from SS patients, an increased frequency of salivary gland epithelial cells expressing EBV-associated antigens and EBV DNA can be detected.[88] Increased EBV DNA can also be detected in SS biopsies by polymerase chain reaction[92] and by in situ hybridization methods.[93] Increased antibody responses to EBV early antigens can be detected in SS patients.[94] Taken together, these findings suggest a potential role for EBV in the pathogenesis of SS. The antibody titers, however, become progressively elevated late in the course of SS and suggest that viral reactivation could occur as a consequence of immune dysregulation in the salivary gland.[95] Because EBV is a strong stimulator of immune T cell responses,[96] reactivation of EBV within the SS salivary gland may serve as a perpetuating factor in salivary gland destruction.

Retroviruses have been suggested as a candidate in some SS patients. Talal et al.[97] found increased reactivity with retroviral protein p24 in a majority of SS sera, and a type A intracisternal particle was subsequently isolated from two salivary gland biopsies by Garry et al.[98] Further studies are required to extend and confirm these interesting results.

CLINICAL MANAGEMENT OF THE PATIENT WITH SJÖGREN'S SYNDROME

The goals of SS treatment are to decrease symptoms and to prevent progression. Many SS patients will have only mild, stable symptoms of dryness of their eyes and mouth, whereas other patients will have systemic manifestations including arthritis, myositis, nephritis, and vasculitis. Therefore, careful diagnosis of the "extent" and activity of the systemic autoimmune component of SS is crucial. In this regard, the overall diagnostic and therapeutic approach to the SS patient must be similar to the SLE or scleroderma patient. In addition, the rheumatologist must coordinate the clinical management of the SS patient with other specialists, including dentists, ophthalmologists, and anesthesiologists to prevent medical complications owing to their sicca symptoms.

Treatment of Dry Eyes

There are a wide variety of commercially available artificial tears differing in their preservatives and their viscosity. In evaluating the response to an artificial tear preparation, the key questions to the patient are (1) how often is it administered? (2) does it "burn" immediately after instillation into the eyes? and (3) how long does relief last?

In some patients, the use of a particular artificial tear may lead to a burning sensation in the eye. This may be due to topical irritation resulting from the preservative in the artificial tear.[99] Thus, all preparations of artificial tears are not identical and are *not* interchangeable. The recognition of this problem can lead to the choice of another artificial tear preparation with a different preservative. Also, several types of preservative-free artificial tears have been developed. If an artificial tear is helpful but relief does not last long enough (i.e., drops must be instilled every hour), an artificial tear preparation with greater viscosity might be introduced. In some patients, *punctal occlusion* might be employed by the ophthalmologist. Punctal occlusion can be temporarily tried by using a variety of different types of "plugs" to determine whether permanent punctal occlusion would be beneficial.

It is worth emphasizing that SS patients are at increased risk for corneal abrasions during anesthesia, owing to the use of anticholinergic agents and the low humidity of the operating room. Therefore, we recommend the use of ocular lubricants in all SS patients during surgery and in the postoperative recovery room. The use of humidifiers is helpful. In areas where the water is hard, distilled water should be used to prevent aerosolization of excessive minerals that may prove irritating to eyes and upper airways.

Treatment of Dry Mouth

Special toothpastes and oral gels have been introduced for the patient with dry mouth and have proved helpful. In parts of the United States where the water supply is not fluoridated, the topical use of a neutral fluoride may help strengthen dental enamel and retard dental deterioration. A common problem in the SS patient is oral candidiasis, which may contribute to symptoms of painful mouth and decreased sense of taste. Treatment with topical nystatin or clotrimazole for 4 to 6 weeks may be required to alleviate symptoms and prevent recurrences. The onset of oral candidiasis often occurs during treatment with antibiotics for another indication. Angular cheilitis, also owing to *Candida*, must be treated with a topical antifungal agent to prevent recurrence.

Myalgias and Fatigue in the Sjögren's Syndrome Patient

It is always important to rule out hypothyroidism (which is a relatively common occurrence in this population)[11] and to look for disordered sleep patterns, especially when the patient arises from bed in the morning with significant fatigue. Such sleep disorders may be due to polydipsia/polyuria (described earlier) or nocturnal myoclonus. The component of fatigue caused by active autoimmune disease is often difficult to assess. The elevation of ESR and total IgG, however, both provide an index of the activity of the disease process. In patients with objective evidence of a systemic inflammatory process (i.e., elevated acute phase reactants) and subjective symptoms of arthralgias and myalgias, we have used hydroxychloroquine at a dose of 5 to 6 mg per kg.[100] Treated patients exhibited decreased acute phase reactants, decreased symptoms, and little toxicity.

For arthralgias, nonsteroidal anti-inflammatory drugs may be used with particular caution, since they may precipitate renal or liver abnormalities. In addition, these agents may provoke esophageal injury[101] because they may adhere to the dryer walls of the esophagus in the absence of the normal salivary flow. To minimize this problem, all medicines should be taken with a large amount of water while sitting upright.

Other Systemic Manifestations

Systemic steroids are generally reserved for life-threatening vasculitis, hemolytic anemia, and pleuropericarditis resistant to nonsteroidal anti-inflammatory drugs. As in SLE patients, other drugs may be used to help lower the dosage of steroids, including hydroxychloroquine (5 to 7 mg per kg per day) and azathioprine (50 to 150 mg per day). In some patients, chlorambucil (4 to 8 mg per day) has proved helpful. We have tried to avoid daily cyclophosphamide in SS patients because of its potential risk of carcinogenesis. When the use of cyclophosphamide is necessary for the treatment of vasculitis, we have administered this medication as an intravenous pulse (250 to 750 mg) at 1 to 3 month intervals.

SUMMARY

SS is a systemic autoimmune disease characterized by lymphocytic infiltrations of lacrimal and salivary glands. Extraglandular organs including skin, nerve, lung, and kidney may be involved. These patients produce a variety of autoantibodies, including rheumatoid factor and antinuclear antibodies. In particular, they produce autoantibodies against ribonuclear proteins SS-A (Ro) and SS-B (La), which are involved in the transport and post-transcriptional modification of mRNA. Genetic factors, including HLA-DR3 and HLA-DQ, predispose to SS.

The precipitating cause of SS remains unknown, although viruses have been suggested as a potential cofactor in pathogenesis. The salivary gland and lacrimal gland are infiltrated by CD4+ T cells. The ductal epithelial cells express HLA-DR+ and DQ+ antigens, thus permitting these epithelial cells to interact with CD4+ T cells. The infiltrating T-cells release cytokines that can perpetuate the immune process by altering blood vessels to become high endothelial venules, stimulating B cells to produce autoantibodies and promoting further influx of T cells.

At the present time, there remains a great deal of confusion regarding the precise definition of SS. As a result, both patients and clinicians frequently have a difficult time in making a specific diagnosis and instituting a specific plan of therapy. Regardless of the diagnostic label, all patients with significant eye and mouth dryness should receive conservative therapy of tear replacement and intensive oral hygiene. Based on the evidence of systemic autoimmunity, additional therapies may prove beneficial in controlling the symptoms and progression of SS.

References

1. Mikulicz, J. H.: Uber eine eigenartige symmetrische Erkrankung der Tranen- und Mundspeicheldrusen. Billroth GT: Beitr. Chir. Fortschr., Stuttgart, 1892.
2. Sjögren, H. S.: Zur kenntnis der keratoconjunctivitis sicca (Keratitis folliformis bei hypofunktion der tranendrusen). Acta Ophthalmol. (Copenh.) 2:1, 1933.
3. Gougerout, A.: Insuffisance progressive et atrophie des glandes salivaires et muqueuses de la bouche, des conjonctives (et parfois des muqueuses, nasale, laryngee, vulvarie). "Secheresse" de la bouche, des conjonctives, etc. Bull. Soc. Fr. Derm. Syph. 32:376, 1925.
4. Morgan, W., and Castleman, B.: A clinicopathologic study of Mikulicz's disease. Am. J. Pathol. 29:471, 1953.
5. Block, K. J., Buchanan, W. W., Woho, M. J., et al.: Sjögren's syndrome: A clinical, pathological and serological study of 62 cases. Medicine (Baltimore) 44:187, 1956.
6. Fritzler, M. J., Pauls, J. D., Kinsella, T. D., et al.: Antinuclear, anticytoplasmic, and anti-Sjögren's syndrome antigen A (SS-A/Ro) antibodies in female blood donors. Clin. Immunol. Immunopathol. 36:120, 1985.
7. Martinez-Lavin, M., Vaughan, J., and Tan, E.: Autoantibodies and the spectrum of Sjögren's syndrome. Ann. Intern. Med. 91:185, 1979.
8. Fox, R. I., Robinson, C. A., Curd, J. C., et al.: Sjögren's syndrome: Proposed criteria for classification. Arthritis Rheum. 29:577, 1986.
8b. Kontinen, Y., Sorsa, T., Hukkanen, M., Sergenberg, M., et al.: Topology of innervation of labial salivary glands. J. Rheumatol. 19:30, 1991.
9. Fox, R. I., Robinson, C., Curd, J., et al.: First international symposium on Sjögren's syndrome: Suggested criteria for classification. Scand. J. Rheumatol. 562:28, 1986.
10. Tsubota, K.: The importance of Schirmer test with nasal stimulation. Am. J. Ophthalmol. 11:106, 1991.
11. Fox, R. I., Howell, F. V., Bone, R. C., et al.: Primary Sjögren's syndrome: Clinical and immunopathologic features. Semin. Arthritis Rheum. 14:77, 1984.
12. Stevens, W. J., Swartele, F. E., Empsten, F. A., et al.: Use of the Saxon test as a measure of saliva production in a reference population of schoolchildren. Am. J. Dis. Child. 144:570, 1990.
13. Daniels, T. E.: Labial salivary gland biopsy in Sjögren's syndrome. Arthritis Rheum. 27:147, 1984.
14. Tan, E. M.: Antinuclear antibodies. Diagnostic markers for autoimmune diseases and probes for cell biology. Adv. Immunol. 44:93, 1989.
15. Shah, F., Rapini, R. P., Arnett, F. C., et al.: Association of labial salivary gland histopathology with clinical and serologic features of connective tissue diseases. Arthritis Rheum. 33:1682, 1990.
16. Whaley, K., Williamson, J., Wilson, T., et al.: Sjögren's syndrome and autoimmunity in a geriatric population. Age Aging 1:197, 1972.
17. Chisholm, D., Waterhouse, J., and Mason, D.: Lymphocytic sialadenitis in the major and minor glands: A correlation in postmortum subjects. J. Clin. Pathol. 23:690, 1970.
18. Rankow, R. M., and Polayes, I. M.: Inflammatory conditions of the salivary gland. In Rankow, R. M., and Polayes, I. M. (eds.): Diseases of the Salivary Glands. Philadelphia, W. B. Saunders Company, 1976, p. 147.
19. Itescu, S., Brancato, L. J., Buxbaum, J., et al.: A diffuse infiltrative CD8 lymphocytosis syndrome in human immunodeficiency virus (HIV) infection: A host immune response associated with HLA-DR5. Ann. Intern. Med. 112:3, 1990.
20. Whaley, K., Williamson, J., Chisholm, D., et al.: Sjögren's syndrome. I. Sicca components. Quart. J. Med. 66:279, 1973.
20b. Bridges, A., and Burns, R.: Acute iritis associated with Sjögren's syndrome. Arthritis Rheum. 35:560, 1992.
21. Lemp, M. A.: Lacrimal hyposecretions. In Fraunfelder, F. T., and Roy, F. H. (eds.): Current Ocular Therapy 2. Philadelphia, W. B. Saunders Company, 1985.
22. Daniels, T. E., Powell, M. R., Sylvester, R. A., et al.: An evaluation of salivary scintigraphy in Sjögren's syndrome. Arthritis Rheum. 22:809, 1979.
23. De Clerck, L. S., Corthouts, R., Francx, L., et al.: Ultrasonography and computer tomography of the salivary glands in the evaluation of Sjögren's syndrome. Comparison with parotid sialography. J. Rheumatol. 15:1777, 1988.
24. Kawamura, J., Taniguchi, N., Itoh, K., et al.: Salivary gland echography in patients with Sjögren's syndrome. Arthritis Rheum. 33:505, 1990.
25. Hunninghake, G., and Fauci, A.: Pulmonary involvement in the collagen vascular diseases. Am. Rev. Respir. Dis. 119:471, 1979.
26. Fairfax, A., Haslam, P., Pavia, D., et al.: Pulmonary disorders associated with Sjögren's syndrome. Q. J. Med. 50:279, 1981.
27. Newball, H., and Brahim, S.: Chronic obstructive airway disease in patients with Sjögren's syndrome. Am. Rev. Respir. Dis. 115:295, 1977.
28. Siegal, I., Fink, G., Machtey, I., et al.: Pulmonary abnormalities in Sjögren's syndrome. Thorax 36:286, 1981.
29. Oxholm, P., Bundgaard, A., Madsen, E., et al.: Pulmonary function in patients with primary Sjögren's syndrome. Rheum. Int. 2:179, 1982.
30. Linstow, M., Kriegbaum, N. J., Backer, V., et al.: A follow-up study of pulmonary function in patients with primary Sjögren's syndrome. Rheumatol. Int. 10:47, 1990.
31. Kjellén, G., Fransson, S. G., Lindström, F., et al.: Esophageal function, radiography, and dysphagia in Sjögren's syndrome. Dig. Dis. Sci. 31:225, 1986.
32. Ramirez-Mata, M., Pena-Acir, F., and Alarcon-Segovia, D.: Abnormal esophageal motility in Sjögren's syndrome. J. Rheumatol. 3:63, 1976.
33. Maury, C. P. J., Törnroth, T., and Teppo, A. -M.: Arthropic gastritis in Sjögren's syndrome. Arthritis Rheum. 28:388, 1985.
34. Jebavy, M., Hradsky, M., and Herout, V.: Gastric biopsy in patients with Sjögren's syndrome. Zschr. Med. 16:930, 1961.

35. Maury, C., Rasaneu, V., Teppo, A., et al.: Serum pepsinogen I in rheumatic diseases. Reduced levels in Sjögren's syndrome. Arthritis Rheum. 25:1059, 1982.
36. Fenster, L., Buchanan, W., Laster, L., et al.: Studies of pancreative function in Sjögren's syndrome. Ann. Intern. Med. 61:498, 1964.
37. Hradsky, M., Bartos, V., and Keller, O.: Pancreatic function in Sjögren's syndrome. Gastroenterologia 108:252, 1962.
38. Sundkvist, G., Lindahl, G., Koskinen, P., et al.: Pancreatic autoantibodies and pancreatic function in Sjögren's syndrome. J. Intern. Med. 229:61, 1991.
39. Whaley, K., Williamson, J., Dick, W., et al.: Liver disease in Sjögren's syndrome. Lancet 1:861, 1970.
40. Webb, J., Whaley, K., MacSween, R., et al.: Liver disease in rheumatoid arthritis and Sjögren's syndrome. Ann. Rheum. Dis. 34:70, 1975.
41. Fujikura, S., Davis, P. A., Fox, R., et al.: Autoantibodies to purified mitochondrial 2 OXO acid dehydrogenases in patients with Sjögren's syndrome. J. Rheumatol. 17:1453, 1990.
42. Kyle, R., Gleich, G., Baynd, E., et al.: Benign hyperglobulinemic purpura of Waldenström. Medicine (Baltimore) 50:113, 1971.
43. Alexander, E., and Provost, T. T.: Sjögren's syndrome. Association of cutaneous vasculitis with central nervous system disease. Arch. Dermatol. 123:801, 1987.
44. Alexander, E. L., Arnett, F. C., Provost, T. T., et al.: Sjögren's syndrome: Association of anti-Ro(SS-A) antibodies with vasculitis, hematologic abnormalities, and serologic hyperactivity. Ann. Intern. Med. 98:155, 1983.
45. Alspaugh, M., and Whaley, K.: Sjögren's syndrome. In Kelley, A., Harris, E., Ruddy, S., and Sledge, C. B. (eds.): Textbook of Rheumatology. Philadelphia, W. B. Saunders, 1982.
46. Whaley, K., Webb, J., McAvoy, B., et al.: Sjögren's syndrome. 2. Clinical associations and immunological phenomena. Q. J. Med. 66:513, 1973.
47. Karsh, J., Paulidis, N., Weintraub, B., et al.: Thyroid disease in Sjögren's syndrome. Arthritis Rheum. 23:1326, 1980.
48. Bailey, R. R., and Swainson, C. P.: Renal involvement in Sjögren's syndrome. N. Z. Med. J. 99:579, 1986.
49. Kahnm, M., Merritt, A., and Orloff, J.: Renal concentrating defect in Sjögren's syndrome. Ann. Int. Med. 56:883, 1962.
50. Shioji, R., Furuyama, T., Onodera, S., et al.: Sjögren's syndrome and renal tubular acidosis. Am. J. Med. 48:456, 1970.
51. Siamopoulos, K. C., Mavridis, A. K., Elisaf, M., et al.: Kidney involvement in primary Sjögren's syndrome. Scand. J. Rheumatol. Suppl. 43:156, 1986.
52. Tu, W., and Shearn, M.: Interstitial nephritis in Sjögren's syndrome. Ann. Intern. Med. 69:1163, 1968.
53. Winer, R. L., Cohen, A. H., Sawhney, A. S., et al.: Sjögren's syndrome with immune-complex tubulointerstitial renal disease. Clin. Immunol. Immunopathol. 8:494, 1977.
54. Talal, N., Zisman, E., and Schur, P.: Renal tubular acidosis, glomerulonephritis and immunologic factors in Sjögren's syndrome. Arthritis Rheum. 11:774, 1968.
55. Kahn, M. A., Akhtar, M., and Taher, S. M.: Membranoproliferative glomerulonephritis in a patient with primary Sjögren's syndrome. Report of a case with review of the literature. Am. J. Nephrol. 8:235, 1988.
56. Moutsopoulos, H. M., Balow, J. E., Lawley, T. J., et al.: Immune complex glomerulonephritis in sicca syndrome. Am. J. Med. 64:955, 1978.
57. Moutsopoulos, H. M., and Fauci, A. S.: Immunoregulation in Sjögren's syndrome. J. Clin. Invest. 65:519, 1980.
58. Aizawa, Y., Zawadzki, Z. A., Micolonghi, T. S., et al.: Vasculitis and Sjögren's syndrome with IgA-IgG cryoglobulinemia terminating in immunoblastic sarcoma. Am. J. Med. 67:160, 1979.
59. Palcoux, J. B., Janin-Mercier, A., Campagne, D., et al.: Sjögren's syndrome and lupus erythematosus nephritis. Arch. Dis. Child. 59:175, 1984.
60. Schwartzberg, M., Burnstein, S. L., Calabro, J. J., et al.: The development of membranous glomerulonephritis in a patient with rheumatoid arthritis and Sjögren's syndrome. J. Rheumatol. 6:65, 1979.
61. Harrington, T. M., Bunch, T. W., and Van Den Berg, C. J.: Renal tubular acidosis. A new look at treatment of musculoskeletal and renal disease. Mayo Clin. Proc. 58:354, 1983.
62. McCurdy, R. C., Cornwell, G. G., III, and DePratti, V. J.: Hyperglobulinemic renal tubular acidosis. Ann. Intern. Med. 67:110, 1967.
63. Morris, R. C., and Fudenberg, H. H.: Impaired renal acidification in patients with hypergammaglobulinemia. Medicine 46:57, 1967.
64. Runeberg, L., Lahdevirta, J., Collan, Y., et al.: Renal tubular dysfunction and hypergammaglobulinaemia. Electrolyte balance, electron microscopic and immunohistochemical studies. Acta Med. Scand. 189:341, 1971.
65. Wilson, I. D., Williams, R. C., and Tobian, L., Jr.: Renal tubular acidosis. Three cases with immunoglobulin abnormalities in the patients and their kindreds. Am. J. Med. 43:356, 1967.
66. Starkebaum, G., Dancey, J., and Arend, W.: Chronic neutropenia: Possible association with Sjögren's syndrome. J. Rheumatol. 8:679, 1982.
67. Fox, R. I., Chen, P. P., Carson, D. A., et al.: Expression of a cross-reactive idiotype on rheumatoid factor in patients with Sjögren's syndrome. J. Immunol. 136:477, 1986.
68. Moutsopoulos, H. M., Costel, R., Drosos, A. A., et al.: Demonstration and identification of monoclonal proteins in the urine of patients with Sjögren's syndrome. Ann. Rheum. Dis. 44:109, 1985.
69. Sugai, T., Konda, T., Shirasaka, T., et al.: Non-IgM monoclonal gammopathy in patients with Sjögren's syndrome. Am. J. Med. 68:861, 1980.
70. Kassan, S. S., Thomas, T. L., Moutsopoulos, H. M., et al.: Increased risk of lymphoma in sicca syndrome. Ann. Intern. Med. 89:888, 1978.
71. Fox, R. I., Adamson, T. C., III, Fong, S., et al.: Lymphocyte phenotype and function of pseudolymphomas associated with Sjögren's syndrome. J. Clin. Invest. 72:52, 1983.
72. Schmid, U., Helbron, D., and Lennert, K.: Development of malignant lymphoma in myoepithelial sialadenitis (Sjögren's syndrome). Virchows Arch. 395:11, 1982.
73. Fishleder, A., Tubbs, R., Hesse, B., et al.: Immunoglobulin-gene rearrangement in benign lymphoepithelial lesions. N. Engl. J. Med. 316:1118, 1987.
74. Freimark, B., and Fox, R. I.: Immunoglobulin gene rearrangements in Sjögren's syndrome. Letter. N. Engl. J. Med. 317:1158, 1987.
75. Freimark, B., Fantozzi, R., Bone, R., et al.: Detection of clonally expanded salivary gland lymphocytes in Sjögren's syndrome. Arthritis Rheum. 32:859, 1989.
75b. Pisa, E., Pisa, P., Kang, H., and Fox, R.: High frequency of t(14;18) translocation in salivary gland lymphomas from Sjögren's syndrome patients. J. Exp. Med. 174:1245, 1991.
76. Pierce, P., Stern, R., Jaffe, R., et al.: Immunoblastic sarcoma with features of Sjögren's syndrome and SLE in a patient with immunoblastic lymphadenopathy. Arthritis Rheum. 22:911, 1979.
77. Lukes, R., and Tindle, B.: Immunoblastic lymphadenopathy. A hyperimmune entity resembling Hodgkin's disease. N. Engl. J. Med. 292:1, 1975.
78. Alexander, E. L., Malinow, K., Lejewski, J. E., et al.: Primary Sjögren's syndrome with central nervous system disease mimicking multiple sclerosis. Ann. Intern. Med. 104:323, 1986.
79. Alexander, E. L., Beall, S. S., Gordon, B., et al.: Magnetic resonance imaging of cerebral lesions in patients with the Sjögren's syndrome. Ann. Intern. Med. 108:815, 1988.
80. Metz, L. M., Seland, T. P., and Fritzler, M. J.: An analysis of the frequency of Sjögren's syndrome in a population of multiple sclerosis patients. J. Clin. Lab. Immunol. 30:121, 1989.
80b. Sandberg-Wollheim, M., Axell, T., Hansen, B., Henrickson, V., et al.: Primary Sjögren's syndrome in patients with multiple sclerosis. Neurology 42:845, 1992.
81. Adamson, T. C., III, Fox, R. I., Frisman, D. M., et al.: Immunohistologic analysis of lymphoid infiltrates in primary Sjögren's syndrome using monoclonal antibodies. J. Immunol. 130:203, 1983.
82. Fox, R. I., Hugli, T. E., Lanier, L. L., et al.: Salivary gland lymphocytes in primary Sjögren's syndrome lack lymphocyte subsets defined by Leu 7 and Leu 11 antigens. J. Immunol. 135:207, 1985.
83. Fox, R. I., Bumol, T., Fantozzi, R., et al.: Expression of histocompatibility antigen HLA-DR by salivary gland epithelial cells in Sjögren's syndrome. Arthritis Rheum. 29:1105, 1986.
84. Lindahl, G., Hedfors, E., Kloreskog, L., et al.: Epithelial HLA-DR expression and T-cell subsets in salivary glands in Sjögren's syndrome. Clin. Exp. Immunol. 61:475, 1985.
85. Macsween, R. N. M., Goudie, R. B., Anderson, J. R., et al.: Occurrence of antibody to salivary duct epithelium in Sjögren's disease, rheumatoid arthritis, and other arthritides. Ann. Rheum. Dis. 26:402, 1967.
86. Mann, D., and Moutsopoulos, H.: HLA-DR alloantigens in different subsets of patients with Sjögren's syndrome and in family members. Ann. Rheum. Dis. 42:533, 1983.
87. Harley, J., Reichlin, M., Arnett, F., et al.: Gene interaction at HLA-DQ enhances autoantibody production in primary Sjögren's syndrome. Science 232:1145, 1986.
87b. Fei, H., Kang, H., Erlich, H., and Fox, R.: Specific HLA-DQA1 and HLA-DQB1 alleles confer susceptibility to Sjögren's syndrome. J. Clin. Lab. Anal. 5:338, 1991.
88. Fox, R. I., Pearson, G., and Vaughan, J. H.: Detection of Epstein-Barr virus–associated antigens and DNA in salivary gland biopsies from patients with Sjögren's syndrome. J. Immunol. 137:3162, 1986.
89. Zur Hausen, H.: Biochemical detection of the virus genome. In Epstein, M., and Achong, B. (eds.): The Epstein-Barr Virus. New York, Springer-Verlag, 1979.
90. Miller, G.: Biology of Epstein-Barr virus. In Klein G. (ed.): Viral Oncology. New York, Raven Press, 1980.
91. Slaughter, L., Carson, D. A., Jensen, F., et al.: In vitro effects of Epstein-Barr virus on peripheral blood mononuclear cells from patients with rheumatoid arthritis and normal subjects. J. Exp. Med. 148:1429, 1978.

92. Saito, I., Servenius, B., Compton, T., et al.: Detection of Epstein-Barr virus DNA by polymerase chain reaction in blood and tissue biopsies from patients with Sjögren's syndrome. J. Exp. Med. 169:2191, 1989.

93. Mariette, X., Gozlan, J., Clerc, D., et al.: Detection of Epstein-Barr virus DNA by in situ hybridization and polymerase chain reaction in salivary gland biopsy specimens from patients with Sjögren's syndrome. Am. J. Med. 90:286, 1991.

94. Fox, R. I., Scott, S., Houghton, R., et al.: Synthetic peptide derived from the Epstein-Barr virus encoded early diffuse antigen (EA-D) reactive with human antibodies. J. Clin. Lab. Anal. 1:140, 1987.

95. Fox, R. I.: Epstein-Barr virus and human autoimmune diseases: Possibilities and pitfalls. J. Virol. Methods 241:1218, 1988.

96. Rickinson, A., Moss, D., and Wallace, L.: Long-term T-cell–mediated immunity to EBV. Cancer Res. 41:4216, 1981.

97. Talal, N., Dauphinée, M. J., Dang, H., et al.: Detection of serum antibodies to retroviral proteins in patients with primary Sjögren's syndrome (autoimmune exocrinopathy). Arthritis Rheum. 33:774, 1990.

98. Garry, R. F., Fermin, C. D., Hart, D. J., et al: Detection of a human intracisternal A-type retroviral particle antigenically related to HIV. Science 250:1127, 1990.

99. Fox, R. I., Chan, R., Michelson, J. B., et al.: Beneficial effect of artificial tears made with autologous serum in patients with keratoconjunctivitis sicca. Arthritis Rheum. 27:459, 1984.

100. Fox, R. I., Chan, E., Benton, L., et al.: Treatment of primary Sjögren's syndrome with hydroxychloroquine. Am. J. Med. 85:62, 1988.

101. El-Mallakh, R. S., Bryan, R. K., Masi, A. T., et al.: Long-term low-dose glucocorticoid therapy associated with remission of overt renal tubular acidosis in Sjögren's syndrome. Am. J. Med. 79:509, 1985.

Section VII

Spondyloarthropathies

Chapter 56

Frank A. Wollheim

Ankylosing Spondylitis

Ankylosing spondylitis (AS) means inflamed spine growing together or getting crooked, and this term is used to designate a disease that has been known under a number of names, among them the American *rheumatoid spondylitis*, the French *spondylarthrite rhizomegalique* and the Scandinavian *Pelvospondylitis ossificans*. It has also been named by the eponyms Marie's, von Bechterew's, or Strümpell's disease after physicians who in the late 19th century contributed to clinical descriptions of AS.[1]

AS is the main representative of the family of spondyloarthropathies, which have a number of common clinical features (Table 56–1) and may relate pathogenetically.[2] AS became recognized as a major cause of disability in young men during compulsory military draft in World War II and thereafter. Academic interest in AS and related diseases was greatly stimulated by the discovery in 1973 of its relation to human leukocyte antigen (HLA) B27[3, 4] and has remained extremely high, not least because of unique opportunities to study interactions of genetic and environmental factors in causing disease.

HISTORY

AS has been assumed to occur in ancient Egypt, although some alleged descriptions may in fact have been cases of diffuse idiopathic skeletal hyperostosis (DISH). The first documented case was the classic skeleton unearthed by the Irish medical student Bernard Connor in Paris in 1691[5] and later reported in a letter to the Royal Society in London. Detailed case reports appeared in the second half of the 19th century. The history of AS has been reviewed.[6]

DEFINITION AND CRITERIA FOR ANKYLOSING SPONDYLITIS

AS is a chronic inflammatory joint disease of axial joints and in particular both sacroiliac joints. It is more common in men, and its peak age of onset is around puberty. In addition, AS is characterized by a number of extra-articular manifestations, such as enthesopathy and anterior uveitis, and is closely linked to HLA-B27. To standardize clinical materials and allow epidemiologic studies, criteria for AS have been proposed. The first two of these are called the Rome criteria of 1961[7] and the New York criteria of 1966[8] (Table 56–2).[9] They have been tested and discussed in a number of studies.[9–12] The Rome criteria give a high sensitivity but low specificity. The New York criteria, on the other hand, require radiologic evidence of unequivocal sacroiliitis and are more specific but less sensitive. Based on Dutch data, the New York criteria were modified[13] (see Table 56–2) to improve sensitivity and yet retain specificity.

CRITERIA FOR SPONDYLOARTHROPATHIES

A difficulty in attempts to classify AS with help of criteria is its associations and overlaps with other spondyloarthropathies such as psoriatic arthritis and Reiter's syndrome. A European spondyloarthropathy study group has undertaken to develop classification criteria for spondyloarthropathy in general[14] (Table 56–3).[9] They deal with a heterogeneous group of patients that at present cannot be classified into any of the defined entities—AS, psoriatic arthritis, reac-

Table 56–1. CLINICAL AND LABORATORY FEATURES OF THE SPONDYLOARTHROPATHIES

Spinal including sacroiliac involvement
Enthesopathy
Asymmetric peripheral arthritis of lower limbs
Familial occurrence
Extra-articular manifestations of skin, gut, urogenitals, eyes
Negative rheumatoid factor
HLA-B27 association

Table 56–2. CRITERIA FOR ANKYLOSING
SPONDYLITIS

ROME, 1961

Clinical criteria
  Low back pain and stiffness for more than 3 months, not
    relieved by rest
  Pain and stiffness in thoracic region
  Limited motion in lumbar spine
  Limited chest expansion
  History or evidence of iritis or its sequelae
Radiologic criterion
  Roentgenogram showing bilateral sacroiliac changes
    characteristic of ankylosing spondylitis (this would exclude
    bilateral osteoarthritis of the sacroiliac joints)
Definite ankylosing spondylitis
  Grade 3 to 4 bilateral sacroiliitis with at least one clinical
    criterion
  At least 4 clinical criteria

NEW YORK, 1966

Clinical criteria
  Limitation of motion of lumbar spine in all 3 planes: anterior
    flexion, lateral flexion, and extension
  Pain at dorsolumbar junction or in lumbar spine
  Limitation of chest expansion to 2.5 cm or less measured at
    the level of the fourth intercostal space
Grading of radiograph
  Normal, 0; suspicious, 1; minimal sacroiliitis, 2; moderate
    sacroiliitis, 3; ankylosis, 4
Definite ankylosing spondylitis
  Grade 3 to 4 bilateral sacroiliitis with at least 1 clinical criterion
  Grade 3 to 4 unilateral or grade 2 bilateral sacroiliitis with
    clinical criterion 1 or with both clinical criteria 2 and 3
Probable ankylosing spondylitis
  Grade 3 to 4 bilateral sacroiliitis with no clinical criteria

MODIFIED NEW YORK CRITERIA, 1984

  Low back pain at least 3 months' duration improved by
    exercise and not relieved by rest
  Limitation of motion of lumbar spine in sagittal and frontal
    planes
  Chest expansion decreased relative to normal values for age
    and sex
  Bilateral sacroiliitis grade 2 to 4
  Unilateral sacroiliitis grade 3 to 4
Definite ankylosing spondylitis
  Unilateral grade 3 or 4 or bilateral grade 2 to 4 sacroiliitis and
    at least one of the 3 clinical criteria

From Kahn, M. A., van der Linden, S. M.: Ankylosing spondylitis and
other spondyloarthropathies. Rheum. Dis. Clin. North Am. 16(3):551, 1990.
Used by permission.

EPIDEMIOLOGY

AS has been the subject of numerous epidemiologic studies in various populations. A strong familial aggregation was reported in 1957,[20] and in 1961, de Blecourt[21] in a classic study compared AS and rheumatoid arthritis (RA), giving a 23 times higher prevalence of AS among relatives of probands, whereas RA occurred two to three times more often among RA relatives. Prevalence figures, on the other hand, were 0.08 percent for AS and 2.3 percent for RA. Kellgren[22] in 1964 estimated AS prevalence to

0.1 percent in control subjects and 4 percent in relatives. One review[9] lists prevalence figures in white populations in Europe and the United States varying between 0.05 and 0.23 percent in studies published before 1980.

After the discovery of a close link between HLA-B27 and AS,[3, 4] worldwide investigations showed marked differences in HLA-B27 prevalence between populations, with highest figures among whites, some Asians, and, in particular, some North American Indian tribes.[23] Among Haida Indians in British Columbia, 50 percent are HLA-B27 positive, and 10 percent of adult men have radiologic evidence of sacroiliitis.[24] In contrast, South American Indians, Australian Aborigines, Japanese, and African blacks have extremely low prevalence of HLA-B27.[23] In general, there is a strong association between AS or other spondyloarthropathies and HLA-B27 in the different populations, but there are also some quantitative variations in correlation. For example, although prevalence of HLA-B27 in Japan is less than 1 percent, AS occurs with a prevalence of 25 to 50 percent of that in whites.[25] There are also some intriguing differences in the spectrum of clinical manifestations between otherwise closely related populations. Thus, AS dominates in one, Reiter's syndrome in another, and undifferentiated spondyloarthropathy in a third environment.[26, 27] This presumably may be attributed to differences in triggering factors. Prevalence studies based on hospital records are likely to be biased and underestimate milder cases and total prevalence. This is well illustrated in a population survey performed in Tromsö in northern Norway.[28] Investigating a population of some 20,000 people aged 20 to 50 years, Gram and associates found a prevalence of 0.4 percent from hospital records. A total prevalence of 1.1 to 1.4 percent was

Table 56–3. ESSG PRELIMINARY CRITERIA FOR
CLASSIFICATION OF SPONDYLOARTHROPATHY

Inflammatory spinal pain
or synovitis
  Asymmetric
  Predominantly in the lower limbs

and any one of the following
  Positive family history
  Psoriasis
  Inflammatory bowel disease
  Alternate buttock pain
  Enthesopathy

  Sensitivity 77%*
  Specificity 89%*

Adding
  Sacroiliitis

  Sensitivity 86%†
  Specificity 87%†

*Based on 403 patients and 674 controls.
†Based on 361 patients and 455 controls.
From Kahn, M. A., and van der Linden, S. M.: A wider spectrum of
spondyloarthropathies. Semin. Arthritis Rheum. 20:107, 1990. Used by
permission.

tive arthritis, or enteropathic arthritis—and that may be common in certain populations[15–18] and may have been underestimated in the past.[19]

found, however, when a questionnaire was used and a representative sample of individuals with back pain of duration longer than 3 months was examined clinically and radiologically. Most "epidemiologic" cases had been in contact with physicians previously without obtaining a correct diagnosis. Ninety-one percent of all cases were HLA-B27 positive. The population prevalence of HLA-B27 in the area, however, was as high as 15.9 percent,[29] presumably owing to Lappish influence.

HLA-B27 AS A RISK FACTOR

In most series of patients with AS, 90 percent or more carry the B27 gene, regardless of whether the population prevalence of HLA-B27 is high or low.[9] Lower figures, between 22 and 57 percent, are found in South African blacks and blacks in the United States.[30] The risk for HLA-B27–positive individuals in the general population to develop AS is 1 to 2 percent. Ten times higher figures prevail among HLA-B27–positive relatives of AS patients.[31, 32]

It is not known whether the additional risk in family members is of genetic or environmental nature. The B27 antigen occurs in at least seven variants, but disease susceptibility is not restricted to any of these and thus may rest with common and conserved HLA-B27 structures.[33, 34] A B27-dependent non-genetic factor probably accounts for the higher risk in relatives. Environmental factors are also suggested by the discordance of occurrence and disease severity in monozygous twins.[35]

The close association between AS and HLA-B27 has both pathogenetic and etiologic implications and, although still enigmatic, is one of the more fascinating interfaces between clinical rheumatology and molecular biology. Some aspects have been reviewed.[36] A basic question is whether HLA-B27, in itself, is responsible for susceptibility to AS or is closely linked to an AS gene.

A direct demonstration of the pathogenic role of HLA-B27 in spondyloarthropathies in humans derives from the use of transgenic rats expressing human HLA-B27 and beta$_2$-microglobulin.[37] The transfected rats show many features of human spondyloarthropathy (Table 56–4). In addition to supporting a pathogenic role of HLA-B27, a new and

MODELS FOR ONE-GENE THEORY

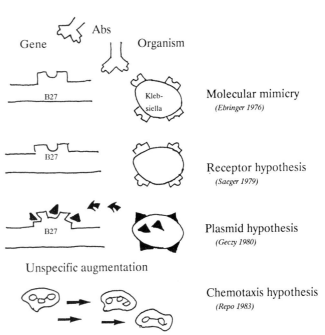

Figure 56–1. Specific and unspecific models for possible relations between HLA-B27 and ankylosing spondylitis.

relevant animal model for the investigation of HLA-B27–related diseases is now at hand. Germ-free transgenic B27 rats have not yet been successfully established, and thus the role of microbials in this model is unknown.

MICROBIOLOGIC FACTORS

In view of the well-established link between certain enteric or urogenital infections and HLA-B27–related reactive arthritis (see Chapter 4), it was not far-fetched to look for microorganisms in AS. A certain strain of *Klebsiella pneumoniae* K43 was found in fecal cultures from AS patients and related to disease activity.[38, 39] According to the *cross-tolerance* or simple molecular mimicry hypothesis, an antigenic similarity exists between bacterial and B27 structures, and immune response to *Klebsiella* therefore could cause autoimmune disease[40] (Fig. 56–1). Although attractive, the connection between immune response to fecal *Klebsiella* and AS is far from simple. In one Scottish study, serum γ-immunoglobulin A (IgA) antibodies to *K. pneumoniae* K43 were moderately elevated in AS but also in Crohn's disease and in RA, and the interpretation was that the results may be unspecific and perhaps secondary to increased gut permeability.[41]

The other hypothesis rests on the observation by Geczy's group that antisera raised against *K. pneumoniae* K43 lyse lymphocytes from HLA-B27–positive AS patients but not healthy B27 individ-

Table 56–4. FEATURES OF SPONDYLOARTHROPATHY IN RATS TRANSFECTED WITH HUMAN BETA$_2$-MICROGLOBULIN AND HLA-B27

Gut inflammation	Male predominance
Normal fecal microorganisms	Orchitis
Hind joint synovitis	Myocarditis
Spondylitis	Uveitis

Data from Hammer, R. E., Maika, S. D., Richardson, J. A., et al.: Spontaneous inflammatory disease in transgenic rats expressing HLA-B27 and human β$_2$m: An animal model of HLA-B27–associated human disorders. Cell 63:1099, 1990.

uals.[42, 43] Further, incubation of lymphocytes from the control subjects with *K. pneumonia* K43 organisms rendered them later lysable when exposed to the *Klebsiella* antiserum.

It was inferred from these data that a modifying factor or plasmid is secreted by the *Klebsiella* organism and interacts with host cells to render them targets for autoimmune reactions and induction of cytotoxic T cells[43] (see Fig. 56–1). Many attempts to confirm Geczy's results have failed, including those of a Dutch group that initially had reported production of an antiserum that could discriminate HLA-B27 + AS + from HLA-B27 + AS − cells.[44]

The elucidation of the three-dimensional structure of class I molecules[45, 46] stimulated the search for pathogenic peptides mimicking exposed parts of the B27 groove. In 1987, a 6 amino acid homology between HLA-B27 and *K. pneumoniae* nitrogenase was described.[47] Using rat antisera raised against the *K. pneumoniae* nitrogenase amino acid hexamer as well as reagents reacting with the HLA-B27.1 hypervariable region, a study found strongly expressed crossreacting epitopes in synovial tissue derived from patients with AS and reactive arthritis. Antibodies to the epitope were also present in sera from the patients.[48, 49]

Following another approach, plasmids were isolated from arthritogenic and monarthritogenic strains of *Shigella flexneri*.[50] A 2-MD plasmid was identified in four arthritogenic strains with DNA sequence homologies to the variable alpha (α)1-domain of HLA-B27 corresponding to the amino acids 71 through 75. Antibodies to both B27 and plasmid correlated highly, supporting the mimicry theory.[51, 51a] Other work, however, has not supported a pathogenic role for antibodies to HLA-B27 homologic microbial peptides, casting doubts on the issue of molecular mimicry.[52–54]

Enhanced neutrophil chemotaxis has been found in HLA-B27 individuals both with and without AS and reactive arthritis and may contribute some to susceptibility to spondyloarthropathy.[55–57]

PROTEOGLYCANS AS AUTOANTIGENS IN ANKYLOSING SPONDYLITIS

Following observations of arthritis in rabbits[58] and dogs[59] after immunization with cartilage proteoglycan antigen, a model for AS was developed in Balb/c mice immunized with human fetal cartilage proteoglycan. The disease starts with polyarthritis including spondylitis, and spinal stiffness and erosions develop with time. The disease is strain specific and is associated with cellular and humoral immunity to proteoglycan.[60] In human studies, the same group has found cellular immunity to proteoglycan antigens in AS but not in RA.[170] In further analyses with monoclonal antibodies, the binding of antibodies to cartilage proteins and release from cartilage of proteoglycan seemed involved in the pathogenesis.[61]

PATHOLOGY

AS is a chronic destructive and deforming joint disease[62] that affects both axial and peripheral joints and is characterized by lesions described as enthesopathies in a classic Heberden oration[63] (Fig. 56–2). The peripheral joint manifestations of synovial hyperplasia with infiltration with lymphocytes, vascular lesions, and fibrosis[64] differ from those of RA in their distribution and in the absence of rheumatoid factor but are otherwise similar.

The columnal changes characteristically first affect the sacroiliac joints and may be unilateral initially but soon become symmetric. Advanced cases have been examined in post mortem studies for 300 years,[5] but early lesions have for natural reasons only rarely been examined.[65, 66] An investigation of sacroilial biopsy specimens from five Japanese men with AS for 1 to 2 years, however, revealed the presence of subchondral granulation tissue, replacement of cartilage with fibrous tissue as well as new cartilage, and bone formation. Similar changes were found at the site of enthesitis of the ischial tuberosity. Mast cells were identified on electron microscopy.[66a]

Squaring of the vertebral bodies (Fig. 56–3) is a characteristic sign of early AS, and a post mortem report of a 25-year-old man with a 7-year history of AS describes in detail the histology of the twelfth thoracic vertebral body.[62, 67] Acute and chronic spondylitis with destruction and rebuilding of cortical bone were present as well as an aseptic inflammation of the marrow.

Enthesopathy, the inflammation of ligamentous insertions, characteristically involves the vertebrae in an ascending manner. Syndesmophytes are arising from enthesitis of the vertebral bodies.[65] Other common sites are the spinal processes, the pelvis, shoulders, and Achilles tendons.[63] It is not known why AS and other spondyloarthropathies localize to the entheses.

EARLY SPINAL DISEASE

AS typically starts in adolescent men, with insidious onset of low back pain and stiffness. Because low back pain is common and usually has causes other than AS, it is important to identify distinguishing features. In a large population survey identifying 27 individuals with back pain and definite AS as well as more than 300 individuals with back pain without spondylitis, characteristics of back pain were tested and the results expressed by the Youden index, that is, sensitivity + specificity − 100. Table 56–5 shows that the most discriminating screening question was whether the subject had to leave bed at night because of pain.[68] A set of five anamnestic features derived from investigating patients with mechanical and inflammatory back pain[69] were positive in only 23 percent of these cases. Other features that are of some use in identifying early AS are improvement on

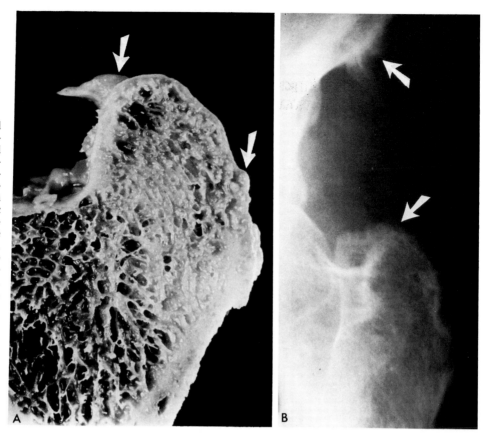

Figure 56–2. Entheses: General radiologic and pathologic abnormalities. Femoral trochanter and sacroiliac joint. *A,* Coronal section through the greater trochanter reveals mild osseous excrescences *(arrows)* related to an enthesopathy. *B,* Radiographic findings include irregular hyperostosis of the trochanter and the iliac crest arrows. (From Resnick, D., and Niwayama, G. [eds]: Diagnosis of Bone and Joint Disorders. 2nd ed. Philadelphia, W. B. Saunders Company, 1988. Used by permission.)

exercise and worsening during rest, for instance, while sitting in a chair. Diffuse radiation of pain to buttocks and thorax and the absence of sensory and motor symptoms were also helpful. Chest pain may cause sleep disturbance in some patients.[69]

PERIPHERAL JOINT SYMPTOMS

Twenty percent of AS is said to start with extraspinal arthritis, more often in the lower extremities. A history of knee effusion in childhood could be a

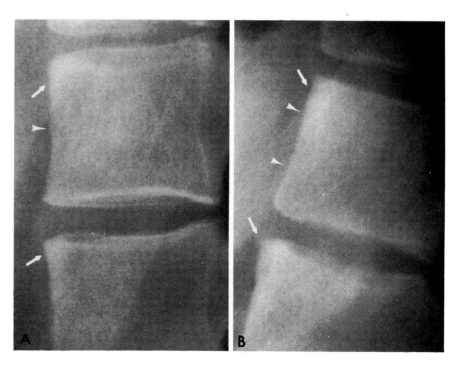

Figure 56–3. Osteitis: radiographic abnormalities (three different patients). *A,* Osseous erosion and sclerosis have produced whitening of the corners and margins along the anterior surfaces of the vertebrae *(arrows)*. Note the straightening of the vertebral surface *(arrowhead)*. *B,* Considerable straightening *(arrowheads)* and bone formation *(arrows)* along the anterior vertebral surface are observed. (From Resnick, D., and Niwayama, G. [eds]: Diagnosis of Bone and Joint Disorders. 2nd ed. Philadelphia, W. B. Saunders Company, 1988. Used by permission.)

Table 56–5. FEATURES OF BACK PAIN IN THE DIAGNOSIS OF ANKYLOSING SPONDYLITIS

	Sensitivity (%)	Specificity (%)	Youden Index (%)
Must leave bed during night	65.2	79.2	44.2
Pain not relieved by lying down	80.0	48.7	28.7
Duration >3 months	71.4	53.6	25.0
Back pain at night	70.8	53.2	24.0
Morning stiffness >30 minutes	64.0	58.8	22.8
Age at onset <35 years	91.7	30.0	21.7
Insidious onset	52.6	50.7	3.3

Data from Gran, J. T.: An epidemiological survey of the signs and symptoms of ankylosing spondylitis. Clin. Rheumatol. 4:161, 1985.

prodromal sign of AS. Any joint may, however, be involved. In one study, 10 percent of patients had temporomandibular involvement.[70] Peripheral arthritis occurs in at least one third of all AS cases and may start many years after spinal disease.[71] Enthesopathy is widespread and common. Heel pain indicative of plantar fasciitis or Achilles tendinitis was present in 20 per cent in a study of early AS.[72]

LATER SPINAL DISEASE

AS may come to rest at an early stage without causing much disability but often follows a chronic progressive course with extra-articular features. Such patients also are liable to a number of complications that may or may not be severe.

Progressive ascending involvement of lumbar, thoracic, and cervical vertebrae leading to complete ankylosis and kyphosis is the extreme form of AS and occurs only in a minority of all cases. In general, more severe cases accumulate at referral centers. The extent of sacroiliac changes or HLA-B27 positivity, however, does not differ between "hospital" and epidemiologic cases.[73] Involvement of the apophyseal joints contributes largely to the spinal immobility in AS, as was realized in 1958[74] and confirmed by computed tomography (CT) examination.[75] Loss of motion in this latter study did not correlate to sacroiliac involvement but was closely linked to changes in the apophyseal joints.

Fixed forward flexion is another hallmark of progression in AS. Loss of extension precedes loss of flexion[76] and is more pronounced in mild and severe cases in both men and women.[77] The facet joints are subject to loading in the erect position of the columna, and in the presence of synovitis, this may elicit pain, which is relieved by forward flexion. In one study, spinal immobility measured with Schober's test correlated well with scored CT injury

to the L4–L5 and L5–SI apophyseal joints.[78] It is likely that similar mechanisms are in operation in higher parts of the columna as well.

OCULAR INVOLVEMENT

Acute anterior uveitis (AAU) occurs in 20 to 40 percent of AS[78a]; AAU is often recognized before AS[79] and is helpful in the early diagnosis of AS. Of all cases of nontraumatic AAU, 25 percent or more are associated with spondyloarthropathies.[80] The association of AAU with HLA-B27 also is strong, although it is less than that with AS; 50 percent or more of AAU patients carry the antigen, giving a relative risk of 10.[81, 82] Of interest, *Yersinia* antibodies were present in 12 of 28 consecutive cases of AAU, eight of which had IgM antibodies, indicating recent infection.[82a]

In a Swiss study, first-degree relatives *with* AS had AAU 10 times more often than B27-positive relatives *without* AS, indicating a real link with AS rather than coincidence.[83] AAU in AS is usually unilateral but often recurrent on either side.[78a] It is more prevalent in men and seems not to be associated with disease severity of AS.[84] The long-term prognosis of AAU in AS is good.

CARDIAC INVOLVEMENT

Aortic regurgitation is a well-established extra-articular manifestation of AS, with reported prevalence figures of up to 90 percent.[85] Although occasionally severe, aortic disease is often asymptomatic.[86] Aortitis is associated with more severe AS.[84] Thickening of the valve cusps and fibrosis of the aorta are seen.[85, 85a] Fibrosis also extends to the interventricular septum and causes conduction defects and arrhythmias in men with AS[87, 88]; complete heart block[87] or milder forms of atrioventricular conduction abnormalities occur in 5 to 10 percent of men with AS. More recently, subtle abnormalities of early diastolic function were found to be frequent.[89, 89a]

RENAL INVOLVEMENT

Amyloidosis does occur in AS but with low frequency.[90–91a] In our unit, where 50 patients attend an amyloidosis clinic, five had amyloidosis of the AA type secondary to AS. All had widespread active disease with peripheral joint involvement and high erythrocyte sedimentation rates (ESR) and C-reactive protein (CRP) levels. IgA nephritis has been reported in at least 15 cases, and in some of these, both diseases became symptomatic simultaneously.[92] Earlier reports failed to produce evidence for a specific renal involvement in AS.[93]

PULMONARY INVOLVEMENT

Chest pain and restricted costovertebral mobility is a prominent feature of AS[94] and has even been reported in HLA-B27–positive, first-degree relatives with increased frequency.[95] Spirometry shows restrictive changes, with decreased vital capacity but normal forced 1-second expiratory volume.[96, 97] Vital capacity may be useful in monitoring functional changes.[96]

Another rare condition associated with severe AS is apical lobe fibrosis,[98] which has been found primarily in men. It starts insidiously, usually after several years of illness. The apical lesions may shrink and cause basal emphysema and, most important, become cavitated and infected with fungi or mycobacteria.[99] It is suspected that smoking and alcohol abuse may contribute to the pathogenesis.

NEUROLOGIC INVOLVEMENT

Multiple sclerosis has been reported in AS.[100–103] Multiple sclerosis is associated with the haplotype HLA-A3, B7, DR3[104] and not with HLA-B27. It is unlikely that a close genetic link exists between the conditions, and their co-occurrence may be coincidental.

The cauda equina syndrome is a rare neurologic complication of longstanding AS first described in 1961.[105, 106] Fifty cases have been reviewed.[107, 108] The condition starts after decades of AS, and the most common symptoms are listed in Table 56–6. The pathophysiology is poorly understood. The condition is characterized by enlargement of the caudal sac and dorsal arachnoid diverticula. It is best diagnosed by magnetic resonance imaging (MRI), but may also be seen on myelography or CT scan[107–109] (Fig. 56–4). The course is either stationary or progressive, and no medical or surgical treatment is effective.

Chronic otitis was found in 12 of 42 consecutive cases of classic AS.[109a]

Table 56–6. INITIAL AND LATER SYMPTOMS OF CAUDA EQUINA SYNDROME IN ANKYLOSING SPONDYLITIS

	Initial No. of Patients	Overall No. of Patients.
Sensory disturbance	16	47
Urinary or rectal sphincter disturbance	14	44
Lower extremity/peripheral pain	10	23
Weakness of lower limbs	3	27
Combinations	5	

Data from Tullous, M. W., Skerhult, H. E. I., Story, J. L., et al.: Cauda equina syndrome of long-standing ankylosing spondylitis. Case report and review of the literature. J. Neurosurg. 73:441, 1990.

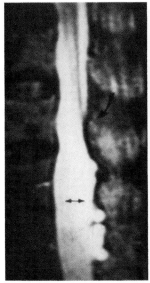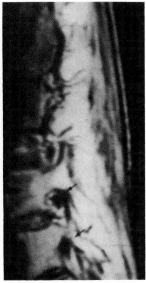

Figure 56–4. *Left*, Sagittal T$_2$-weighted magnetic resonance imaging (MRI) scan revealing increased anteroposterior diameter of the lumbar spinal canal *(double-ended arrow)*, dorsal thecal diverticula lying within areas of erosion of the L-3 and L-4 vertebrae, and clumped nerve roots of the cauda equina, which are adherent to the dorsal theca rostral to the L-3 diverticula *(curved arrow)*. *Right*, Sagittal T$_1$-weighted MRI scan at the level of the neural foramina showing dilatation of lower lumbar and sacral nerve-root sleeves *(arrows)*. (From Tullous, M. W., Skerhut, H. E., Story J. L., et al.: Cauda equina syndrome of long-standing ankylosing spondylitis. Case report and review of the literature. J. Neurosurg. 73:441, 1990. Used by permission.)

ANKYLOSING SPONDYLITIS IN WOMEN

AS is one of the few inflammatory joint diseases with a higher prevalence among men. Figures of 10:1 in male favor were generally accepted, but more recent data indicate a male preponderance of only 4 to 6:1.[110] Contrary to earlier belief, the onset of the disease, peripheral joint involvement, occurrence of AAU, and other extra-articular manifestations do not differ between men and women. Both genders have the same HLA-B27 prevalence. Spinal involvement and sacroiliac joint changes, however, are more common in men.[28, 111–113]

Pregnancies usually are uneventful in women with AS, and the offspring are healthy.[114] Disease remission occurs only in 25 percent of pregnancies, whereas in the remaining, the disease is either unimproved or deteriorating. AS does not, however, contraindicate pregnancy.

CLINICAL EXAMINATION

History

History gives often the most important clues toward the diagnosis of AS. This is highlighted by the population study in Tromsö,[68] where apparently most cases were identified using a simple questionnaire. The most discriminating features are low back pain waking the patient during the night, morning stiffness of more than 30 minutes duration, improvement by mild exercise, age under 35 years, and chronicity. A family history of spondyloarthropathy has only limited additional value in practice. A history of acute uveitis adds considerably to the likelihood of AS and was present before diagnosis in 33 percent of women and 15 percent of men in one study.[115]

Physical Examination

Stiffness and stooped posture are characteristic enough, even in moderately advanced AS, to raise diagnostic suspicion. Signs of enthesitis, often asymmetric, may be found (e.g., in the back, pelvis, shoulders, and feet). Sacroiliitis is the hallmark of AS, and numerous tests have been devised for its clinical diagnosis. None are satisfactory. A knee to shoulder stress movement in supine position related best to current symptoms.[116] Direct tenderness located in the sacroiliac region is not a reliable sign of sacroiliitis. Indirect pain elicited by compression or forced movement is, however, a useful sign of active sacroiliitis.

Measuring spinal movement is important in the diagnosis and essential in the management of AS. Spondylometry is precise and useful in investigative work, and diminished extension is particularly prevalent in early disease[117] (Fig. 56–5). The convenient classic Schober's test[118] can be improved by using 15 cm and not 10 cm as initial erect measure. Women have physiologically a less mobile lumbar spine, and an age-related diminution is seen in both sexes.[119] A further refinement, Smythe's test, sums changes in extension and flexion in three 10-cm segments.[120] Lateral movement is another useful measure, which has been standardized and is approximately 10 percent of body height in normal young men.[121]

Pile et al.[122] tested 22 clinical measures for reliability and sensitivity. The most useful were cervical rotation measured with a protractor, cervical flexion measured with a goniometer, thoracolumbar flexion distention from C-7 to the iliac crest measured with a tape measure, Schober's test, and lateral flexion measured as fingertip-floor distance. Chest expansion did not perform well.

Questionnaires

The health assessment questionnaire of Fries has been modified for AS by adding two subscales dealing with carrying, sitting, working at a desk, and driving a car in reverse. This improved sensitivity and correlated well with anthropomorphic measurements.[123] This questionnaire may be useful in investigative as well as clinical work. Another questionnaire consisting of 20 items was designed for AS and

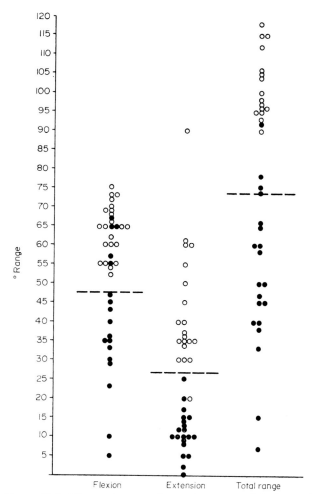

Figure 56–5. The scattergram shows the range of flexion and extension in a control group of 20 normal subjects matched for age and sex with the measurements of 20 spondylitis patients at presentation. The dotted lines represent the overall mean for each parameter of movements in the normal male population. ○, Normal; ●, ankylosing spondylitis. (From Sturrock, R. D., Wojtulewski, J. A., and Hart, F. D.: Spondylometry in a normal population and in ankylosing spondylitis. Rheumatol. Phys. Med. 12:135, 1973. Used by permission.)

correlated with an articular index and was changed in a short-term therapeutic trial.[124]

LABORATORY INVESTIGATIONS

Biochemical signs of inflammatory activity are less prevalent in AS than in RA[125, 126] but reflect similar hepatic cytokine-induced synthesis, as judged from the glucosylation pattern of orosomucoid.[127] Circulating granulocyte-derived elastase in complex with its inhibitor, α_1-antitrypsin, is elevated in active RA, but normal in AS, indicating another biochemical difference between these conditions.[128] Elevated IgA levels are seen in active AS,[127] as are IgA antibodies to *Klebsiella*.[41, 128a]

The value of testing for HLA-B27 in diagnosing AS is limited by low specificity and occurrence of

HLA-B27–negative cases of AS.[129, 130] In patients with back pain suspected of being inflammatory and absent radiographic signs, however, it may be useful to know the HLA status.[131, 132]

RADIOGRAPHY AND OTHER IMAGING

The radiographic changes in AS and their relation to clinical disease and pathology have been extensively reviewed and illustrated.[62] Scintigraphy has been attractive in attempts to diagnose early sacroiliitis, but this technique remains a research tool owing to problems with standardization and lack of distinct differences between normal and abnormal.[133–135] Conventional radiography retains its dominance as a diagnostic and monitoring tool in AS. The initial abnormalities are seen most often in the sacroiliac joints and in the thoracolumbar and lumbosacral junctions. With advancing disease, all parts of the axial skeleton as well as sites of enthesopathy may develop characteristic abnormalities.

The involvement of the sacroiliac joints is of key importance. The anatomy of this joint poses difficulties for good exposure, and its proximity to the gonads puts limits to its radiographic investigation. The New York criteria distinguish a 0 to 4 scale of changes (Fig. 56–6), and it is notable that only the moderate and advanced changes are reliable in a clinical setting.[136] CT scanning allows a detailed imaging of the sacroiliac joints, both in the sagittal and in the axial planes, and should replace conventional tomography when available (Figs. 56–7 and 56–8). The sacroiliitis of AS may start unilaterally but, within years, becomes symmetric. Symmetric sacroiliitis is rarely seen in RA.[137] Other differential diagnoses include hyperparathyroidism, osteitis condensans ilii, gouty arthritis, and degenerative joint disease.[62]

Spinal changes may be seen early in AS and occasionally without signs of sacroiliitis,[138] and this entity may be a mild subset of AS. The characteristic spinal changes of AS involve squaring (see Fig. 56–3) and formation of syndesmophytes (Fig. 56–9) and, in some cases, advanced ankylotic bamboo spine. The symphysis pubis is also commonly affected (Fig. 56–10).

In the diagnosis of the rare cauda equina syndrome MRI is the method of choice and often eliminates the need for myelography[107, 139] (see Fig. 56–4). Another indication for MRI is investigation of the cervical neck, allowing direct demonstration of medulla compression in atlantoaxial instability.[140] MRI and CT are also helpful in imaging discovertebral destruction.[141]

CT has proved to be superior to conventional tomography in visualizing pseudoarthritis[142] and as well is suited to diagnose apophyseal arthritis.[143]

MRI, CT, and conventional radiography were evaluated in a study of 27 patients with suspected sacroiliitis. Although MRI was not superior in sensitivity, it conveyed new information regarding subchondral bone pathology not visualized by other techniques.[144]

SPINAL COMPLICATIONS

In a minority of AS patients, spinal disease progresses to complete or nearly complete stiffness; concomitantly pain diminishes or disappears. The fused spine, however, is particularly fragile and sensitive to trauma. Fractures may occur even after minor trauma such as a fall to the floor[145] or a minor rear-end automobile collision. The majority of fractures are cervical, and in addition to severe pain, they can cause spinal cord injury with neurologic lesions.[146] Radiology may fail to visualize a fracture and should be supplemented by bone scintigraphy. Immediate diagnosis and immobilization are essential. Laminectomy and surgical fusion may be necessary if the neurologic symptoms are progressive.

Thoracic and lumbar fractures occur less frequently, causing sharp pain of sudden onset. Neurologic symptoms of cord injury are seen only in one in four of such patients.[147]

Sudden onset of pain in a spinal segment without known trauma may be caused by spondylodiscitis or Andersson's lesion[149] (a destructive lesion with or without instability and with increased uptake of bone-seeking radionuclide). It is important to separate sterile spondylodiscitis from septic spondylitis and fracture. Immobilization may enable healing to occur.[150] Finally, osteoporotic compression fractures are often found when sought. They may cause less dramatic symptoms and contribute to deformity in some patients.[151]

SUBSETS OF ANKYLOSING SPONDYLITIS

Variations in clinical course, location, and severity of AS are marked and have generated attempts to distinguish homogeneous subsets. AS sparing the sacroiliac joints was found in six men and one woman in a population survey dealing with some 21,000 inhabitants in northern Norway. The patients had milder spinal restriction on spondylometry than the remaining cases, three of seven were HLA-B27 negative, and morning stiffness was absent in four of seven. Disease duration was 12 years or more in six of seven cases.[138] Similar cases of mild disease have been described earlier.[152, 153]

A French group described 10 men with HLA-B27–related disease with minimal involvement of the axial skeleton, onset after age 50 years, oligoarthritis of the lower limbs, and pronounced signs of systemic inflammation. Four of the patients later developed typical AS with symmetric sacroiliitis. This report also illustrates the diagnostic difficulties arising from atypical initial courses of AS.[154] Delay in diagnosis remains an important problem in AS.[155, 156]

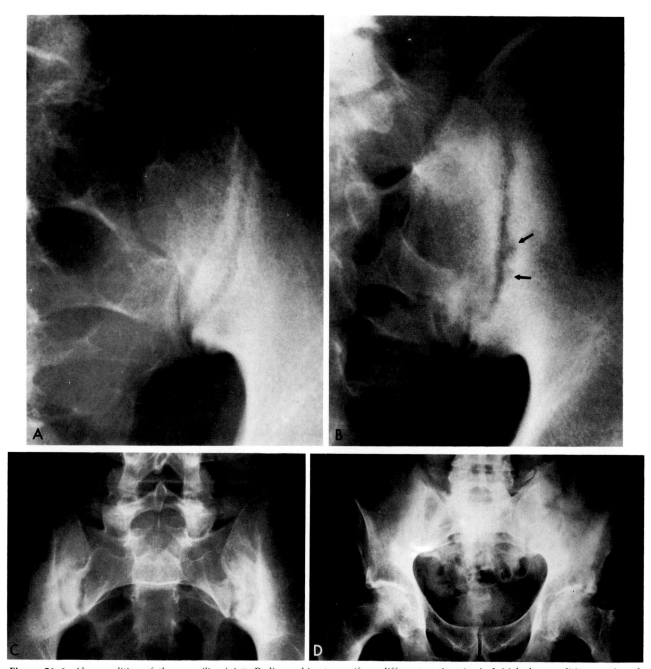

Figure 56–6. Abnormalities of the sacroiliac joint. Radiographic stages (four different patients). *A,* Initial abnormalities consist of superficial bone erosion and eburnation, predominantly on the ilium. *B,* At a slightly later stage, note larger erosions *(arrows),* progressive sclerosis, and focal narrowing of the articular space. *C,* At a more advanced stage, bilateral symmetric changes consist of extensive sclerosis and focal ankylosis. *D,* Eventually, complete ankylosis of the synovial and ligamentous portions of the sacroiliac space on both sides is evident. Sclerosis has largely disappeared. (From Resnick, D., and Niwayama, G. [eds]: Diagnosis of Bone and Joint Disorders. 2nd ed. Philadelphia, W. B. Saunders Company, 1988. Used by permission.)

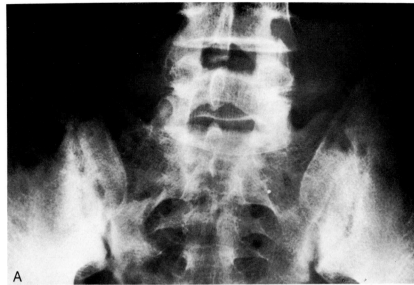

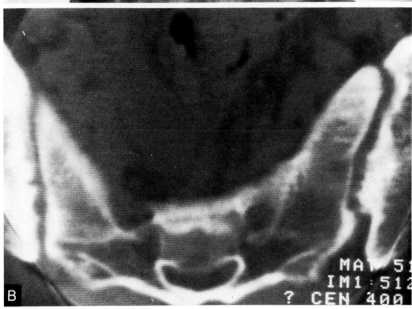

Figure 56–7. Abnormalities of the sacroiliac joint: Use of computed tomography (CT). *A,* The routine radiograph documents bilateral, symmetric abnormalities consisting of bone erosion and sclerosis. *B,* With CT, a transverse section of the lower portion of the synovium-lined area of the joint confirms the bilateral alterations and the predominant involvement of the ilium. (From Resnick, D., and Niwayama, G., [eds.]: Diagnosis of Bone and Joint Disorders. 2nd ed. Philadelphia, W. B. Saunders Company, 1988. Used by permission.)

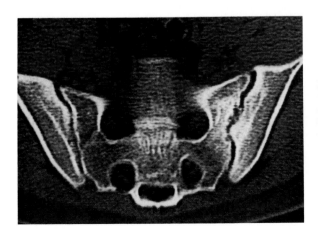

Figure 56–8. CT in ankylosing spondylitis. Sacroiliitis: An axial image through the lower portion of the sacroiliac joint shows bilateral articular abnormalities, greater on the left side, consisting of joint surface irregularity and erosion in both the ilium and the sacrum, with associated new bone formation. (From Resnick, D., and Niwayama, G. [eds.]: Diagnosis of Bone and Joint Disorders. 2nd ed. Philadelphia, W. B. Saunders Company, 1988. Used by permission.)

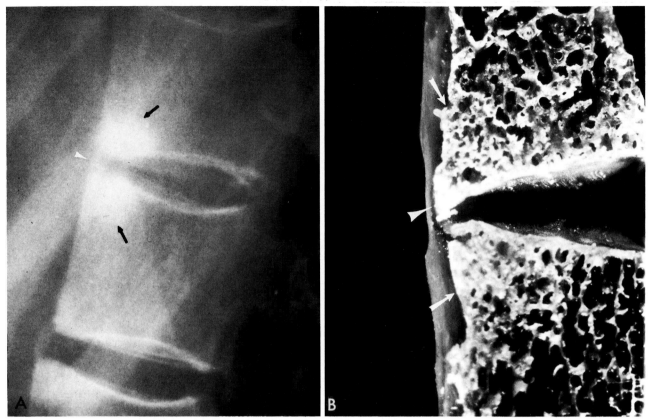

Figure 56–9. Osteitis and syndesmophytosis: Radiographic and pathologic abnormalities. *A*, In association with osteitis of the corners of the vertebral bodies *(arrows)*, early syndesmophyte formation has produced blurring of the margin of the intervertebral disc *(arrowhead)*. *B*, A photograph of a sagittal section of two vertebral bodies reveals osteitis *(arrows)* and syndesmophytosis *(arrowhead)*, representing ossification of the intervertebral disc. (From Resnick, D., and Niwayama, G. [eds.]: Diagnosis of Bone and Joint Disorders. 2nd. ed. Philadelphia, W. B. Saunders Company, 1988. Used by permission.)

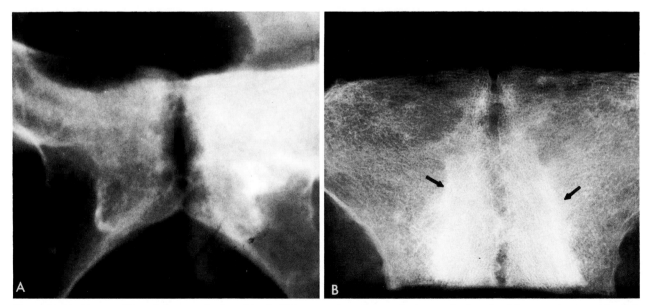

Figure 56–10. Abnormalities of the symphysis pubis. *A*, Note narrowing, osseous fusion, and sclerosis of the symphysis pubis. *B*, In a spondylitic cadaver, a radiograph of a coronal section through the symphysis pubis demonstrates focal bony ankylosis with surrounding eburnation *(arrows)*. (From Resnick, D., and Niwayama, G. [eds.]: Diagnosis of Bone and Joint Disorders. 2nd ed. Philadelphia, W. B. Saunders Company, 1988. Used by permission.)

JUVENILE-ONSET SPONDYLOARTHROPATHY

Juvenile AS, Reiter's disease, psoriatic arthritis with sacroiliitis, and inflammatory bowel disease–associated sacroiliitis are well-recognized spondyloarthropathies occurring in children.[157] Although in most respects they are similar to the corresponding adult diseases, some distinguishing features are noteworthy.

Enthesitis is a prominent and early sign, and a special syndrome of seronegativity, enthesopathy, and arthropathy (SEA) has been described in children.[158] The sites of enthesitis commonly involve heels, crista iliaca, tibial tuberosity, the lateral epicondyles of the humerus, and acromion.[159] In a Mexican study,[160] SEA progressed to juvenile AS in 11 of 12 cases. The arthritis is most prevalent in the legs, and hip involvement is common, whereas sacroiliitis may be absent.[161] SEA, like juvenile AS, is three to ten times more common in boys.[159, 161]

The occurrence of acute iritis or conjunctivitis in children is distinct from the more severe chronic iridocyclitis of juvenile chronic arthritis. Reduced axial motion and sacroiliitis were absent in 65 percent initially,[162] but on later follow-up, many cases had typical AS of the columna and sacroiliac joints. The knee joint is the most common presenting peripheral joint involved, followed by the ankle and the foot.[162] In a follow-up study comparing juvenile-onset with adult-onset AS, hip arthroplasty was performed four times more often in the former.[163] Children with spondyloarthropathies often have a family history of similar disease, and the HLA-B27 association is as pronounced as it is in adults. The intriguing question of why their disease starts in childhood is not solved. Homozygosity for B27 was present in only one of eight patients in one study[164] and does not explain early onset.

ANKYLOSING SPONDYLITIS AND DISH

Diffuse idiopathic skeletal hyperostosis (DISH) is a noninflammatory disease occurring predominantly in middle-aged and elderly men characterized by spinal immobility and flexion, moderate pain, and characteristic axial and peripheral hyperostosis.[165] The disease is not associated with sacroiliitis or HLA-B27. It is occasionally confused with AS radiographically[166, 167] and may occasionally coexist with AS.[168] The flowing osteophytes in DISH are joined primarily on the right side.

RELAPSING POLYCHONDRITIS AND SPONDYLOARTHROPATHY

Three cases of relapsing polychondritis and spondyloarthropathy were described, two with AS and one with Reiter's disease. Two of the patients were HLA-B27 negative. It is not clear from what population the cases were derived, and it is not possible to differentiate between coincidence and association.[169] It is of interest that autoimmunity to proteoglycans has been suggested as a cause of both conditions.[170, 171]

FAMILIAL MEDITERRANEAN FEVER AND ANKYLOSING SPONDYLITIS

A number of case reports have appeared describing spinal abnormalities, including sacroiliac joint fusion, in Familial Mediterranean Fever in HLA-B27–negative or HLA-untyped individuals.[172–174] No histologic evidence of AS has been documented.

PROGNOSIS

Long-term follow-up studies of AS show a higher than expected mortality.[175, 176] The disease-related mortality is relevant to cervical spinal subluxation, aortic regurgitation, respiratory failure, and amyloidosis.[177] A further cause of premature death is the occurrence of malignancies secondary to radiation therapy.[178, 179] Trauma immediately preceding accelerated destructive peripheral arthritis has attracted some attention.[179a] It is not possible to distinguish between fortuitous or causal relation between the events.

Although progressive impairment of spinal mobility occurs in half the cases or more, functional outcome is often satisfactory.[177] The early presence of peripheral joint disease, iritis, pulmonary fibrosis, and persistently high sedimentation rate is indicative of a poor prognosis. Among approximately 50 patients with secondary AA amyloidosis, five were AS patients, and all five had histories of peripheral joint involvement and persistent acute phase reaction.[180] Long-term disability and sick leave are, not surprisingly, higher in patients with work exposure to cold conditions and prolonged standing.[181] Data do not support a changing disease pattern or age at onset for AS.[156]

MANAGEMENT

AS is a chronic disease with a variable, often benign outcome but with a risk of both handicap and life-threatening complications. The goal of optimal management is to facilitate a normal, fulfilled, and independent life.

Patient education should start with diagnosis. Teaching about the disease should motivate the patients for active physical therapy but avoidance of harmful activities and injuries.[182] Vocational guidance may be an important ingredient. Group therapy and information in patient organizations may also be helpful.

Physical therapy should be lifelong; it usually is

initiated by the physiotherapist. The goals are the relief of pain and a maintainance of functional capacity. The means are a daily exercise program adapted to individual needs and abilities. Exercises in a warm pool and some periods in a spa-like environment with more intensive active physiotherapy may be useful. The immediate reward of physiotherapy is improved well-being.

Nonsteroidal anti-inflammatory drug (NSAID) treatment reduces pain, is often a prerequisite for active physiotherapy, and may diminish stiffness. Indomethacin is probably unsurpassed in effectiveness but, if not tolerated, can be substituted by one of the newer NSAIDs. Some patients still prefer salicylate as the only NSAID, or to supplement other NSAIDs.[183]

The place of glucocorticoid therapy in AS is unsettled. Glucocorticoids may have short-term benefits when administered by the intravenous route in high dose in severe cases.[184, 185] Synovitis of peripheral joints responds well to intra-articular injections of triamcinolone hexacetonide.

Following its successful performance in RA, sulfasalazine has been tested in six independent, placebo-controlled studies published between 1986 and 1990 from France, Sweden, Finland, England, and Scotland and involving 292 patients.[186–191] All but one report[191] conclude that sulfasalazine was of significant, although not impressive, benefit. Divergent results may relate to patient selection.[192] The majority of patients in the negative study had radiologically late disease. It is not established whether sulfasalazine is disease modifying in long-term use. Its mode of action is also not known and could well be anti-inflammatory.[193, 194] The use of sulfasalazine is also limited by gastrointestinal and bone marrow toxicity and negative effects on spermiogenesis.[195, 196] Methotrexate may be another candidate for early drug intervention in AS.[197]

Although generalized radiotherapy for AS was abandoned for good reasons in the 1960s,[179] local radiation for intractable chronic enthesopathy of the feet was reported successful in four anecdotal cases when ten times 100 cGy was administered.[198]

Surgical intervention is essential for selected cases. Peripheral joint replacement, most often of the hip, is generally successful, although heterotopic bone formation occasionally occurs.[199, 200] NSAID administration may diminish this risk without jeopardizing results of hip replacement.[200, 201]

As mentioned, the cervical spine is the site of fractures complicated by neurologic symptoms and surgical fixation may be required.[202, 203] Finally, there is occasionally a need for surgical correction of flexion deformity of the spine. The procedure is risky and should be performed only in centers where a great deal of experience has been accumulated.[204, 205]

References

1. Spencer, D. G., Sturrock, R. D., and Buchanan, W. W.: Ankylosing spondylitis: Yesterday and today. Med. Hist. 24:60, 1980.
2. Moll, J. M. H., Haslock, I., Macrae, I. F., and Wright, V.: Associations between ankylosing spondylitis, psoriatic arthritis, Reiter's disease, the intestinal arthropathies and Behçet's syndrome. Medicine 53:343, 1974.
3. Brewerton, D. A., Caffrey, M., Hart, F. D., et al.: Ankylosing spondylitis and HL-A 27. Lancet 1:904, 1973.
4. Schlosstein, L., Terasaki, P. I., Bluestone, R., et al.: High association of an HL-A antigen, W27, with ankylosing spondylitis. N. Engl. J. Med. 288:704, 1973.
5. Connor, B.: Sur la continuité de plusieurs os, à l'occasion d'un tronc de squelette humain, où les côtes, l'os sacrum, et les os des iles, qui naturellements sont distincts et separés, ne font qu'un seul os continu et inséparable. Rheims 1691.
6. Bywaters, E. G. L.: Historical introduction. In Moll, J. M. H. (ed.): Ankylosing Spondylitis. Edinburgh, Churchill Livingstone, 1980, p. 1.
7. Kellgren, J. H., Jeffrey, M. R., and Ball, J.: The Epidemiology of Chronic Rheumatism. Oxford, Blackwell, 1963, p. 236.
8. Bennet, P. H., and Wood, P. H. N.: Population studies in the rheumatic diseases. Amsterdam, Excerpta Medica, 1968, p. 456.
9. Khan, M. A., and van der Linden, S. M.: Ankylosing spondylitis and other spondyloarthropathies. Rheum. Dis. Clin. North Am. 16(3):551, 1990.
10. Moll, J. M. H., and Wright, V.: New York criteria for ankylosing spondylitis. A statistical evaluation. Ann. Rheum. Dis. 32:354, 1973.
11. van der Linden, S. M., Valkenburg, H. A., and Cats, A.: Evaluation of diagnostic criteria for ankylosing spondylitis. A proposal for modification of the New York criteria. Arthritis Rheum. 27:361, 1984.
12. Ahearn, J. M., and Hochberg, M. C.: Epidemiology and genetics of ankylosing spondylitis. J. Rheumatol. 15(Suppl. 16):22, 1988.
13. The, H. S. G., Steven, M. M., van der Linden, S. M., and Cats, A.: Evaluation of diagnostic criteria for ankylosing spondylitis: A comparison of the Rome, New York, and modified New York criteria in patients with a positive clinical history screening test for ankylosing spondylitis. Br. J. Rheumatol. 24:242, 1985.
14. Kahn, M. A., and van der Linden, S. M.: A wider spectrum of spondyloarthropathies. Semin. Arthritis Rheum. 20:107, 1990.
15. Bardin, T., and Lathrop, M.: HLA-B27 and Reiter's syndrome in the Inuit of Greenland. Arthritis Rheum. 30(Suppl. 4):s75, 1987.
16. Boyer, G. S., Lanier, A. P., and Templin, D. W.: Prevalence rates of spondyloarthropathies, rheumatoid arthritis, and other rheumatic disorders in an Alaskan Inupiat Eskimo population. J. Rheumatol. 15:678, 1988.
17. Boyer, G. S., Lanier, A. P., Templin, D. W., et al.: Spondyloarthropathy and rheumatoid arthritis in Alaskan Yupik Eskimos. J. Rheumatol. 17:489, 1990.
18. Oen, K., Postl, B., and Chalmers, I. M.: Rheumatic diseases in an Inuit population. Arthritis Rheum. 29:65, 1986.
19. Kahn, M. A., and van der Linden, S. M.: A wider spectrum of spondyloarthropathies. Semin. Arthritis Rheum. 20:107, 1990.
20. Graham, W., and Uchida, I. A.: Heredity in ankylosing spondylitis. Ann. Rheum. Dis. 16:334, 1957.
21. de Blecourt, J. J., Polman, A., and de Blecourt-Meindersma, T.: Hereditary factors in rheumatoid arthritis and ankylosing spondylitis. Ann. Rheum. Dis. 20:215, 1961.
22. Kellgren, J. H.: The epidemiology of rheumatic diseases. Ann. Rheum. Dis. 23:109, 1964.
23. Khan, M. A.: Spondyloarthropathies in non-Caucasian populations of the world. In Ziff, M., and Cohen, S. B. (eds.): Advances in Inflammation Research. Vol. 9. New York, Raven Press, 1985, p. 91.
24. Gofton, J. P., Chalmers, A., Price, G. E., et al.: HL-A27 and ankylosing spondylitis in B. C. Indians. J. Rheumatol. 2:318, 1975.
25. Tsujimoto, M.: Epidemiological research on the prevalence of ankylosing spondylitis. Med. J. Osaka Univ. 28:363, 1978.
26. Rate, R. G., Morse, H. G., Bonnell, M. D., and Kuberski, T. T.: Navajo arthritis reconsidered. Relationship to HLA-B27. Arthritis Rheum. 23:1299, 1980.
27. Muggia, A. L., Bennaham, D. A., and Williams, R. C. Jr.: Navajo arthritis—an unusual acute self-limited disease. Arthritis Rheum. 14:348, 1971.
28. Gran, J. T., Husby, G., and Hordvik, M.: Prevalence of ankylosing spondylitis in males and females in a young middle-aged population of Tromsö, northern Norway. Ann. Rheum. Dis. 44:359, 1985.
29. Gran, J. T., Mellby, A. S., and Husby, G.: The prevalence of HLA-B27 in northern Norway. Scand. J. Rheumatol. 13:173, 1984.
30. Khan, M. A., Braun, W. E., Kushner, I., et al.: HLA-B27 in ankylosing spondylitis. Differences in frequency and relative risk in American blacks and Caucasians. J. Rheumatol. 4(Suppl. 3):39, 1977.
31. Calin, A., Marder, A., Becks, E., et al.: Genetic differences between B27-positive patients with ankylosing spondylitis and B27-positive healthy controls. Arthritis Rheum. 26:140, 1983.
32. van der Linden, S. M., Valkenburg, H. A., de Jong, B. M., et al.: The risk of developing ankylosing spondylitis in HLA-B27–positive individuals: A comparison of relatives of spondylitis patients with the general population. Arthritis Rheum. 27:241, 1984.

33. van Bohemen, C. G., Grumet, F. C., and Zanen, H. C.: HLA-B27 M1 and M2 cross-reactive enterobacterial antigens. *In* Ziff, M., and Cohen, S. B. (eds.): The Spondyloarthropathies. Advance in Inflammation Research, Vol. 9. New York, Raven Press, 1985, p. 157.

34. Breur-Vriesendorp, B. S., Dekker-Saeys, A. J., and Ivanyi, P.: Distribution of HLA-B27 subtypes in patients with ankylosing spondylitis: The disease is associated with a common determinant of the various B27 molecules. Ann. Rheum. Dis. 46:353, 1987.

35. Eastmond, C. J., and Woodrow, J. C.: Discordance for ankylosing spondylitis in monozygotic twins. Ann. Rheum. Dis. 36:360, 1977.

36. Benjamin, R., and Parham, P.: HLA-B27 and disease: A consequence of inadvertent antigen presentation? Rheum. Dis. Clin. North Am. 18:11, 1992.

37. Hammer, R. E., Maika, S. D., Richardson, J. A., et al.: Spontaneous inflammatory disease in transgenic rats expressing HLA-B27 and human β_2m: An animal model of HLA-B27–associated human disorders. Cell 63:1099, 1990.

38. Ebringer, R. W., Cawdell, D. R., and Ebringer, A.: Sequential studies in ankylosing spondylitis. Association of *Klebsiella pneumoniae* with active disease. Ann. Rheum. Dis. 37:146, 1978.

39. Calguneri, M., Swinburne, L., Shinebaum, R., et al.: Secretory IgA: Immune defence pattern in ankylosing spondylitis and *Klebsiella*. Ann. Rheum. Dis. 40:600, 1981.

40. Ebringer, A., Cox, N. L., and Abuljadayel, I.: *Klebsiella* antibodies in ankylosing spondylitis and *Proteus* antibodies in rheumatoid arthritis. Br. J. Rheumatol. 27(Suppl. 2):72, 1988.

41. Cooper, R., Fraser, S. M., Sturrock, R. D., et al.: Raised titres of anti-*Klebsiella* IgA in ankylosing spondylitis, rheumatoid arthritis, and inflammatory bowel disease. Br. Med. J. 296:1432, 1988.

42. Geczy, A. F., Alexander, K., and Bashir, H. V.: A factor(s) in *Klebsiella* filtrates specifically modifies an HLA-B27–associated cell-surface component. Nature 283:782, 1980.

43. Geczy, A. F., Alexander, K., Bashir, H. V., et al.: *Klebsiella* and ankylosing spondylitis: Biological and chemical studies. Immunol. Rev. 70:23, 1983.

44. Benkelman, C. J., et al.: Scand. J. Rheumatol. 87(Suppl.):74, 1990.

45. Bjorkman, P. J., Saper, M. A., Samraoui, B., et al.: Structure of the human class I histocompatibility antigen HLA-A2. Nature 329:506, 1987.

46. Bjorkman, P. J., Saper, M. A., Samraoui, B., et al.: The foreign antigen binding site and T-cell recognition regions of class I histocompatibility antigens. Nature 329:512, 1987.

47. Schwimmbeck, P. L., Yu, D. T. Y., and Oldstone, M. B. A.: Autoantibodies to HLA-B27 in the sera of HLA-B27 patients with ankylosing spondylitis and Reiter's syndrome: Molecular mimicry with *Klebsiella pneumoniae* as potential mechanism of autoimmune disease. J. Exp. Med. 166:173, 1987.

48. Husby, G., Tsuchiya, N., Schwimmbeck, P. L., et al.: Cross-reactive epitope with *Klebsiella pneumoniae* nitrogenase in articular tissue of HLA-B27–positive patients with ankylosing spondylitis. Arthritis Rheum. 32:437, 1989.

49. Tsuchiya, N., Husby, G., and Williams, R. C. Jr.: Studies of humoral and cell-mediated immunity to peptides shared by HLA-B27.1 and *Klebsiella pneumoniae* nitrogenase in ankylosing spondylitis. Clin. Exp. Immunol. 76:354, 1989.

50. Stieglitz, H., Fosmire, S., and Lipsky, P.: Identification of a 2-Md plasmid from *Shigella flexneri* associated with reactive arthritis. Arthritis Rheum. 32:937, 1989.

51. Tsuchiya, N., Husby, G., Williams, R. C., Jr., et al.: Autoantibodies to the HLA-B27 sequence cross-react with the hypothetical peptide from the arthritis-associated *Shigella* plasmid. J. Clin. Invest. 86:1320, 1990.

51a. Williams, R. C., Jr., Tsuchiya, N., and Husby, G.: Molecular mimicry, ankylosing spondylitis, and reactive arthritis—something missing? Scand. J. Rheumatol. 21:105, 1992.

52. Cavender, D. E., and Ziff, M.: Absence of anti-Enterobacteriaceae and anti–HLA-B27 antibodies in mitogen-stimulated cultures of lymphocytes from patients with Reiter's syndrome and ankylosing spondylitis. J. Rheumatol. 15:315, 1988.

53. de Vries, D. D., Dekker-Saeys, A. J., Gyodi, E., and Ivanyi, P.: Failure to detect cross-reacting antibodies to HLA-B27.5 and *Klebsiella pneumoniae* nitrogenase in sera from patients with ankylosing spondylitis and Reiter's syndrome. Scand. J. Rheumatol. Suppl 87:72, 1990.

54. Lahesmaa, R., Skurnik, M., Vaara, M., et al.: Amino acid sequences shared by HLA-B27 and arthritis triggering microbes are not recognized by the human immune system (abstract). Clin. Rheumatol. 9:586, 1990.

55. Leirisalo, M., Repo, H., Tiilikainen, A., et al.: Chemotaxis in *Yersinia* arthritis: HLlLA-B27–positive neutrophils show high stimulated motility in vitro. Arthritis Rheum. 23:1036, 1980.

56. Pease, C. T., Fordham, J. N., and Currey, H. L. F.: Polymorphonuclear cell motility, ankylosing spondylitis, and HLA-B27. Ann. Rheum. Dis. 43:279, 1984.

57. Pease, C. T., Fennell, M., Brewerton, D. A., et al.: Polymorphonuclear leucocyte motility in men with ankylosing spondylitis. Ann. Rheum. Dis. 48:35, 1989.

58. Glant, T. T., and Olàh, I.: Experimental arthritis produced by proteoglycan antigens in rabbits. Scand. J. Rheumatol. 9:271, 1980.

59. Glant, T. T.: Induction of cartilage degradation in experimental arthritis produced by allogeneic and xenogeneic proteoglycan antigens. Connect. Tissue Res. 9:137, 1982.

60. Glant, T. T., Mikecz, K., Arzoumanian, A., and Poole, A. R.: Proteoglycan-induced arthritis in BALB/c mice: Clinical features and histopathology. Arthritis Rheum. 30:201, 1987.

61. Dayer, E., Mathai, L., Glant, T. T., et al.: Cartilage proteoglycan-induced arthritis in BALB/c mice. Arthritis Rheum. 33:1394, 1990.

62. Resnick, D., and Niwayama, G.: Ankylosing spondylitis. *In* Resnick, D., and Niwayama, G. (eds.): Diagnosis of Bone and Joint Disorders. Philadelphia, W. B. Saunders Company, 1988, p. 1103.

63. Ball, J.: Enthesopathy of rheumatoid and ankylosing spondylitis. Ann. Rheum. Dis. 30:213, 1971.

64. Revell, P. A., and Mayston, V.: Histopathology of the synovial membrane of peripheral joints in ankylosing spondylitis. Ann. Rheum. Dis. 41:579, 1982.

65. Bywaters, E. G. L.: Pathologic specificity of ankylosing spondylitis: Is it yet established? *In* Ziff, M., and Cohen, S. B. (eds.): Advances in Inflammation Research. Vol. 9: The Spondyloarthropathies. New York, Raven Press, 1985, p. 1.

66. Sutherland, R. I. L., and Mahteson, D.: Inflammatory involvement of vertebrae in ankylosing spondylitis. J. Rheumatol. 2:296, 1975.

66a. Shichikawa, K., Tsujimoto, M., Nishioka, J., et al.: Histopathology of early sacroiliitis and enthesitis in ankylosing spondylitis. *In* Ziff, M., and Cohen, S. B. (eds.): Advances in Inflammation Research. Vol. 9: The Spondyloarthropathies. New York, Raven Press, 1985, p. 15.

67. Aufdermaur, M.: Pathogenesis of square bodies in ankylosing spondylitis. Ann. Rheum. Dis. 48:628, 1989.

68. Gran, J. T.: An epidemiological survey of the signs and symptoms of ankylosing spondylitis. Clin. Rheumatol. 4:161, 1985.

69. Calin, A., Porta, J., and Fries, J. F. F.: The clinical history as a screening test for ankylosing spondylitis. J.A.M.A. 237:2613, 1977.

70. Davidson, C., Wojtulewski, J. A., Bacon, P. A., et al.: Temporomandibular joint disease in ankylosing spondylitis. Ann. Rheum. Dis. 34:87, 1975.

71. Cohen, M. D., and Ginsburg, W. W.: Late-onset peripheral joint disease in ankylosing spondylitis. Ann. Rheum. Dis. 41:574, 1982.

72. Mau, W., Zeidler, H., Mau, R., et al.: Clinical features and prognosis of patients with possible ankylosing spondylitis. Results of a 10-year follow-up. J. Rheumatol. 15:1109, 1988.

73. Gran, J. T., and Husby, G.: Ankylosing spondylitis: A comparative study of patients in an epidemiological survey, and those admitted to a department of rheumatology. J. Rheumatol. 11:788, 1984.

74. Wilkinson, M., and Bywaters, E. G. L.: Clinical features and course of ankylosing spondylitis. Ann. Rheum. Dis. 17:209, 1958.

75. Russel, A. S. and Jackson, F.: Computer-assisted tomography of the apophyseal changes in patients with ankylosing spondylitis. J. Rheumatol. 13:581, 1986.

76. Hart, F. D., Robinson, K. C., Allchin, F. M., et al.: Ankylosing spondylitis. Q. J. Med. 18:217, 1949.

77. Gran, J. T., Husby, G., Hordvik, M., et al.: Radiological changes in men and women with ankylosing spondylitis. Ann. Rheum. Dis. 43:570, 1984.

78. Simkin, P. A., Downey, D. J., and Kilcoyne, R. F.: Apophyseal arthritis limits lumbar motion in patients with ankylosing spondylitis. Arthritis Rheum. 31:798, 1988.

78a. Edmunds, L., Elswood, J., and Calin, A.: New light on uveitis in ankylosing spondylitis. J. Rheumatol. 18:50, 1991.

79. Rosenbaum, J. T.: Acute anterior uveitis and spondyloarthropathies. Rheum. Dis. Clin. North Am. 18:143, 1992.

80. Sparling, M., Dillon, A., Maguire, L., et al.: Association of uveitis with systemic or rheumatic diseases in a community-based population (abstract). Arthritis Rheum. 32:38, 1989.

81. Brewerton, D. A., Nicholls, A., Walters, D., et al.: Acute anterior uveitis and HLA-B27. Lancet 2:994, 1973.

82. Ryder, L. P., Andersen, E., and Svejgaard, A.: HLA and Disease Registry, Third Report. Copenhagen, Munksgaard, 1979.

82a. Wakefield, D., Stahlberg, T. H., Toivanen, A., et al.: Serologic evidence of *Yersinia* infection in patients with anterior uveitis. Arch. Ophthalmol. 108:219, 1990.

83. van der Linden, S. M., Rentsch, H. V., Gerber N., et al.: The association between ankylosing spondylitis, acute anterior uveitis and HLA-B27: The results of a Swiss family study. Br. J. Rheumatol. 27 (Suppl. II):39, 1988.

84. Youssef, W., and Russel, A. S.: Cardiac, ocular, and renal manifestations of seronegative spondyloarthropathies. Curr. Opin. Rheumatol. 2:582, 1990.

85. Bulkley, B. H., and Roberts, W. C.: Ankylosing spondylitis and aortic regurgitation. Description of the characteristic cardiovascular lesions from a study of eight necropsy patients. Circulation 18:1014, 1973.

85a. O'Neill, T. W., King, G., Graham, I. M., Molony, J., and Bresnihan, B.: Echocardiographic abnormalities in ankylosing spondylitis. Ann. Rheum. Dis. 51:652, 1992.

86. Tucker, C. R., Fowles, R. E., Calin, A., et al.: Aortitis in ankylosing spondylitis: Early detection of aortic root abnormalities with two-dimensional echocardiography. Am. J. Cardiol. 9:680, 1982.

87. Bergfeldt, L., and Moller, E.: Pacemaker treated women with heart block have no increase in the frequency of HLA-B27 and associated rheumatic disorders in contrast to men—a sex-linked difference in disease susceptibility. J. Rheumatol. 13:941, 1986.

88. Bergfeldt, L.: HLA-B27–associated rheumatic diseases with severe cardiac bradyarrhythmias. Clinical features and prevalence in 223 men with permanent pacemakers. Am. J. Med. 75:210, 1983.

89. Brewerton, D. A., Gibson, D. G., Goddard, D. H., et al.: The myocardium in ankylosing spondylitis. Lancet 1:995, 1987.

89a. Gould, B. A, Turner, J., Keeling, D. H., Hickling, P., and Marshall, A. J.: Myocardial dysfunction in ankylosing spondylitis. Ann. Rheum. Dis. 51:227, 1971.

90. Jayson, M. I. V., Salmon, P. R., and Harrison, W.: Amyloidosis in ankylosing spondylitis. Rheum. Phys. Med. 1:78, 1971.

91. Cruickshank, B.: Pathology of ankylosing spondylitis. Bull. Rheum. Dis. 10:211, 1960.

91a. Lance, N. J., and Curran, J. J.: Amyloidosis in a case of ankylosing spondylitis with a review of the literature. J. Rheumatol. 18:100, 1991.

92. Bruneau, D., Villiaumey, J., Avouac, B., et al.: Seronegative spondyloarthropathies and IgA glomerulonephritis: A report of four cases and a review of the literature. Semin. Arthritis Rheum. 15:179, 1986.

93. Calin, A.: Renal glomerular function in ankylosing spondylitis. Scand. J. Rheumatol. 4:241, 1975.

94. Dawnes, P. T., Sheeran, T. P., and Hothersall, T. E.: Chest pain—a common feature of ankylosing spondylitis. Postgrad. Med. J. 64:27, 1988.

95. van der Linden, S. M., Khan, M. A., Rentsch, H. -U., et al.: Chest pain without radiographic sacroiliitis in relatives of patients with ankylosing spondylitis. J. Rheumatol. 15:836, 1988.

96. Franssen, M. J. A. M., van Herwaarden, C. I. A., van de Putte, L. B. A., and Gribnau, F. W. J.: Lung function in patients with ankylosing spondylitis. A study of the influence of disease activity and treatment with nonsteroidal antiinflammatory drugs. J. Rheumatol. 13:936, 1986.

97. Travis, D. M., Cook, C. B., Julian, D. G., et al.: The lungs in rheumatoid spondylitis. Am. J. Med. 29:623, 1960.

98. Hamilton, K. A.: Pulmonary disease manifestations of ankylosing spondylarthritis. Ann. Intern. Med. 31:216, 1949.

99. Boushea, D. K., and Sundstrom, W. R.: The pleuropulmonary manifestations of ankylosing spondylitis. Semin. Arthritis Rheum. 18:277, 1989.

100. Thomas, D. J., Kendall, M. J., and Whitfield, A. G. W.: Nervous system involvement in ankylosing spondylitis. Br. Med. J. 1:148, 1974.

101. Kahn, M. A., and Kushner, I.: Ankylosing spondylitis and multiple sclerosis: A possible association. Arthritis Rheum. 22:784, 1979.

102. Wordsworth, B. P., and Mowat, A. G.: A review of 100 patients with ankylosing spondylitis with particular reference to socio-economic effects. Br. J. Rheumatol. 25:175, 1986.

103. Whitman, G. J., and Kahn, M. A.: Unusual occurrence of ankylosing spondylitis and multiple sclerosis in a black patient. Cleve. Clin. J. Med. 56:819, 1989.

104. Kolstad, A., Hannestad, K., Vandvik, B., et al.: Multiple sclerosis patients have a high frequency of an HLA-DQβ epitope defined by a human-human hybridoma antibody. Tissue Antigens 33:546, 1989.

105. Bowie, E. A., and Glasgow, G. L.: Cauda equina lesions associated with ankylosing spondylitis: Report of three cases. Br. Med. J. 2:24, 1961.

106. Hauge, T.: Chronic rheumatoid spondylitis and spondyloarthritis associated with neurological symptoms and signs occasionally simulating an intraspinal expansive process. Acta Chir. Scand. 120:395, 1961.

107. Tullous, M. W., Skerhult, H. E. I., Story, J. L., et al.: Cauda equina syndrome of long-standing ankylosing spondylitis. Case report and review of the literature. J. Neurosurg. 73:441, 1990.

108. Mitchell, M. J., Sartoris, D. J., Moody, D., and Resnick, D.: Cauda equina syndrome complicating ankylosing spondylitis. Radiology 175:521, 1990.

109. Sparling, M. J., Bartelson, J. D., McLeod, R. A., et al.: Magnetic resonance imaging of arachnoid diverticula associated with cauda equina syndrome in ankylosing spondylitis. J. Rheumatol. 16:1335, 1989.

109a. Camilleri, A. E., Swan, I. R. C., Murphy, E., and Sturrock, R. D.: Chronic otitis media: a new extra-articular manifestation in ankylosing spondylitis? Ann. Rheum. Dis. 51:655, 1992.

110. Gran, J. T., and Husby, G.: Ankylosing spondylitis in women. Semin. Arthritis Rheum. 19:303, 1990.

111. Kidd, B., Mullee, M., Frank, A., and Cawley, M.: Disease expression of ankylosing spondylitis in males and females. J. Rheumatol. 15:1407, 1988.

112. Resnick, D., Dwosh, I. L., Goergen, T. G., et al.: Clinical and radiographic abnormalities in ankylosing spondylitis: A comparison between men and women. Radiology 119:293, 1976.

113. Will, R., Edmunds, L., Elswood, J., and Calin, A.: Is there sexual inequality in ankylosing spondylitis? A study of 498 women and 1202 men. J. Rheumatol. 17:1649, 1990.

114. Östensen, M., and Husby, G.: A prospective clinical study of the effect of pregnancy on rheumatoid arthritis and ankylosing spondylitis. Arthritis Rheum. 26:1155, 1983.

115. Ringsdal, V. S., and Andreasen, J. J.: Ankylosing spondylitis—experience with a self-administered questionnaire: An analytic study. Ann. Rheum. Dis. 48:924, 1989.

116. Rudge, S. R., Swannel, A. J., Rose, D. H., et al.: The clinical assessment of sacro-iliac joint involvement in ankylosing spondylitis. Rheumatol. Rehab. 21:15, 1982.

117. Sturrock, R. D., Wojtulewski, J. A., and Hart, F. D.: Spondylometry in a normal population and in ankylosing spondylitis. Rheumatol. Rehab. 12:135, 1973.

118. Schober, P.: Lendenwirbelsäule und Kreuzschmerzen. Münch. Med. Wochenschr. 84:336, 1937.

119. Macrae, I. F., and Wright, V.: Measurement of back movement. Ann. Rheum. Dis. 28:584, 1969.

120. Miller, M. H., Lee, P., Smythe, H. A., et al.: Measurement of spinal mobility in the sagittal plane: New skin contraction technique compared with established methods. J. Rheumatol. 11:507, 1985.

121. Domjan, L., Nemes, T., Bàlint, G. P., et al.: A simple method for measuring lateral flexion of the dorsolumbar spine. J. Rheumatol. 17:663, 1990.

122. Pile, K. D., Laurent, M. R., Salmond, C. E., et al.: Clinical assessment of ankylosing spondylitis: A study of observer variation in spinal measurements. Br. J. Rheumatol. 30:29, 1991.

123. Daltroy, L. H., Larson, M. G., Roberts, W. N., Liang, M. H.: A modification of the health assessment questionnaire for the spondyloarthropathies. J. Rheumatol. 17:946, 1990.

124. Dougados, M., Gueguen, A., Nakache, J. -P., et al.: Evaluation of a functional index and an articular index in ankylosing spondylitis. J. Rheumatol. 15:302, 1988.

125. Nashel, D. J., Petrone, D. L., Ulmer, C. C., and Sliwinski, A. J.: C-reactive protein: A marker for disease activity in ankylosing spondylitis and Reiter's syndrome. J. Rheumatol. 13:364, 1986.

126. Sanders, K. M., Hertzman, A., Escobar, M. R., and Littman, B. H.: Correlation of immunoglobulin and C-reactive protein levels in ankylosing spondylitis and rheumatoid arthritis. Ann. Rheum. Dis. 46:273, 1987.

127. Mackiewicz, A., Khan, M. A., Reynolds, T. L., et al.: Serum IgA acute phase proteins, and glycosylation of alpha^1-acid glycoprotein in ankylosing spondylitis. Ann. Rheum. Dis. 48:99, 1989.

128. Feltelius, N., and Hällgren, R.: Circulating inhibitor bound elastase in patients with ankylosing spondylitis and rheumatoid arthritis and the influence of sulphasalazine treatment. Ann. Rheum. Dis. 47:10, 1988.

128a. Shodjai-Moradi, F., Ebringer, A., and Abuljadayel, I.: IgA antibody response to Klebsiella in ankylosing spondylitis measured by immunoblotting. Ann. Rheum. Dis. 51:233, 1992.

129. Calin, A.: HLA-B27 in 1982. Reappraisal of a clinical test. Ann. Intern. Med. 96:114, 1982.

130. Baron, M., and Zendel, I.: HLA-B27 testing in ankylosing spondylitis: An analysis of the presenting assumptions. J. Rheumatol. 16:631, 1989.

131. Woodrow, J. C.: Clinical conundrum. Br. J. Rheumatol. 27:461, 1988.

132. Khan, M. A., and Khan, M. K.: HLA-B27 as an aid to diagnosis of ankylosing spondylitis. Spine 4:617, 1990.

133. Russel, A. S., Lentle, B. C., and Percy, J. S.: Investigation of sacroiliac disease: Comparative evaluation of radiological and radionuclide techniques. J. Rheumatol. 2:45, 1975.

134. Szanto, E., and Ruden, B. -I.: ^{99m}Tc in evaluation of sacroiliac arthritis. Scand. J. Rheumatol. 5:11, 1976.

135. Dunn, E. C., Ebringer, R. W., and Ell, R. J.: Quantitative scintigraphy in the early diagnosis of sacroiliitis. Rheumatol. Rehab. 19:69, 1980.

136. Hollingsworth, P. N., Cheah, P. S., Dawkins, R. L., et al.: Observer variation in grading sacroiliac radiographs in HLA-B27–positive individuals. J. Rheumatol. 10:247, 1983.

137. DeCarvalho, A., and Graudal, H.: Sacroiliac joint involvement in classical or definite rheumatoid arthritis. Acta Radiol. (Diagn.) 21:417, 1980.

138. Gran, J. T., Husby, G., and Hordvik, M.: Spinal ankylosing spondylitis: A variant form of ankylosing spondylitis or a distinct disease entity? Ann. Rheum. Dis. 44:368, 1985.

139. Rubenstein, D. J., Alvarez, O., Gelman, B., et al.: Cauda equina syndrome complicating ankylosing spondylitis: MR features. J. Comput. Assist. Tomogr. 13:511, 1989.

140. Zygmont, S., Säveland, H., Brattström, H., Ljunggren, B., Larsson, E. M., and Wollheim, F.: Reduction of rheumatoid periodontoid pannus following posterior occipitocervical fusion visualized by magnetic resonance imaging. Br. J. Neurosurg. 2:315, 1988.

141. Kenny, J. B., Hughes, P. L., and Whitehouse, G. H.: Discovertebral destruction in ankylosing spondylitis: The role of computed tomography and magnetic resonance imaging. Br. J. Radiol. 63:448, 1990.

142. Chan, F. L., Ho, E. K. W., and Chau, E. M. T.: Spinal pseudoarthrosis complicating ankylosing spondylitis: Comparison of CT and conventional tomography. Am. J. Radiol. 150:611, 1988.

143. Downey, D. J., and Kilcoyne, R. F.: Apophyseal arthritis limits lumbar motion in patients with ankylosing spondylitis. Arthritis Rheum. 31:798, 1988.
144. Ahlström, H., Feltelius, N., Nyman, R., and Hällgren, R.: Magnetic resonance imaging of sacroiliac joint inflammation. Arthritis Rheum. 33:1763, 1990.
145. Hunter, T., and Dubo, H. I. C.: Spinal fractures complicating ankylosing spondylitis. A long-term follow-up study. Arthritis Rheum. 26:751, 1983.
146. Murray, G. C., and Persellin, R. H.: Cervical fracture complicating ankylosing spondylitis. A report of eight cases and review of the literature. Am. J. Med. 70:1033, 1981.
147. Thorngren, K. G., Liedberg, E., and Aspelin, P.: Fractures of the thoracic and lumbar spine in ankylosing spondylitis. Acta Orthop. Traumat. Surg. 98:101, 1981.
148. Gelineck, J., and DeCarvalho, A.: Fractures of the spine in ankylosing spondylitis. Fortschr. Röntgenstr. 152:307, 1990.
149. Dihlmann, W., and Delling, G.: Discovertebral destructive lesions (so-called Andersson lesions) associated with ankylosing spondylitis. Skel. Radiol. 3:10, 1983.
150. Dunn, N., Preston, B., and Jones, K. L.: Unexplained acute backache in longstanding spondylitis. Br. Med. J. 291:1632, 1985.
151. Ralston, S. H., Urquhart, G. D. K., Brzeski, M., and Sturrock, R. D.: Prevalence of vertebral compression fractures due to osteoporosis in ankylosing spondylitis. Br. Med. J. 300:563, 1990.
152. Calin, A.: Ankylosing spondylitis sine sacroiliitis. Arthritis Rheum. 22:303, 1979.
153. Courtois, C., Fallet, G. H., Vischer, T. L., and Wettstein, P.: Erosive spondylopathy. Ann. Rheum. Dis. 39:462, 1980.
154. Dubost, J. J., and Sauvezie, B.: Late-onset peripheral spondyloarthropathy. J. Rheumatol. 16:1214, 1989.
155. Kidd, B. L., and Cawley, M. I.: Delay in diagnosis of spondylarthritis. Br. J. Rheumatol. 27:230, 1988.
156. Fries, J. F., Singh, G., Bloch, D. A., and Calin, A.: The natural history of ankylosing spondylitis: Is the disease really changing? (Editorial). J. Rheumatol. 16:860, 1988.
157. Petty, R. E.: HLA-B27 and rheumatic diseases of childhood. J. Rheumatol. 17(Suppl. 26):7, 1990.
158. Rosenberg, A. M., and Petty, R. E.: A syndrome of seronegative enthesopathy and arthropathy in children. Arthritis Rheum. 25:1041, 1982.
159. Hussein, A., Abdul-Khalig, H., and van der Hardt, H.: Atypical spondyloarthritis in children: Proposed diagnostic criteria. Eur. J. Pediatr. 148:513, 1989.
160. Burgos-Vargas, R., and Clark, P.: Axial involvement in the seronegative enthesopathy and arthropathy syndrome and its progression to ankylosing spondylitis. J. Rheumatol. 16:192, 1989.
161. Prieur, A. M.: HLA-B27–associated chronic arthritis in children: Review of 65 cases. Scand. J. Rheumatol. Suppl. 66:51, 1987.
162. Sheerin, K. A., Giannini, E. H., Brewer, E. J., et al.: HLA-B27–associated arthropathy in childhood: Long-term clinical and diagnostic outcome. Arthritis Rheum. 31:1165, 1988.
163. Calin, A., and Elswood, J.: The natural history of juvenile-onset ankylosing spondylitis: A 24-year retrospective case-control study. Br. J. Rheumatol. 27:91, 1988.
164. Kvien, T. K., Möller, P., and Dale, K.: Juvenile ankylosing spondylitis and HLA-B27 homozygocity. Scand. J. Rheumatol. 14:47, 1985.
165. Resnick, D., Shaul, S. R., and Robins, J. M.: Diffuse idiopathic skeletal hyperostosis (DISH): Forestier's disease with extraspinal manifestations. Radiology 115:513, 1975.
166. Johnsson, K. E., Petersson, H., Wollheim, F. A., et al.: Diffuse idiopathic skeletal hyperostosis (DISH) causing spinal stenosis and sudden paraplegia. J. Rheumatol. 10:784, 1983.
167. Yagan, R., and Kahn, M. S.: Confusion of roentgenographic differential diagnosis between ankylosing hyperostosis (Forestier's disease) and ankylosing spondylitis. Clin. Rheumatol. 2:285, 1983.
168. Rillo, O. L., Scheines, E. J., Moreno, C., et al.: Coexistence of diffuse idiopathic skeletal hyperostosis and ankylosing spondylitis. Clin. Rheumatol. 8:499, 1989.
169. Pazirandeh, M., Ziran, B. H., Khandenwal, B. K., Reynolds, T. L., and Kahn, M. A.: Relapsing polychondritis and spondylarthropathies. J. Rheumatol. 15:630, 1988.
170. Golds, E. E., Stephen, I. B. M., Esdaile, J. M., Strawczynski, H., and Poole, A. R.: Lymphocyte transformation to connective tissue antigens in adult and juvenile rheumatoid arthritis, osteoarthritis, ankylosing spondylitis, systemic lupus erythematosus, and a nonarthritic control population. Cell Immunol. 82:196, 1983.
171. Herman, J. H., and Dennis, M. V.: Immunopathologic studies in relapsing polychondritis. J. Clin. Invest. 52:549, 1973.
172. Brodey, P. A., and Wolff, S. M.: Radiographic changes in the sacroiliac joints in familial Mediterranean fever. Radiology 114:331, 1975.
173. Lehman, T. J., Hansen, V., Konreich, H., et al.: HLA-B27–negative sacroiliitis: A manifestation of familial Mediterranean fever in childhood. Pediatrics 61:423, 1979.
174. Knockaert, D. C., Malysse, I. G., and Peetermans, W. E.: Ankylosing spondylitis. An unusual manifestation of familial Mediterranean fever. Report of a case complicated by amyloidosis and polyneuropathy. Clin. Rheumatol. 8:408, 1989.
175. Khan, M. A., Khan, M. K., and Kushner, I.: Evidence of decreased survival in ankylosing spondylitis by life-table analysis. Arthritis Rheum. 22:365, 1979.
176. Radford, E. P., Doll, R., and Smith, P. G.: Mortality among patients with ankylosing spondylitis not given x-ray therapy. N. Engl. J. Med. 297:572, 1977.
177. Carette, S., Graham, D., Little, H., et al.: The natural course of ankylosing spondylitis. Arthritis Rheum. 26:186, 1983.
178. Smith, P. G., and Doll, R.: Mortality among patients with ankylosing spondylitis after a single treatment course with x-rays. Br. Med. J. 284:449, 1982.
179. Darby, S. C., Doll, R., Gill, S. K., and Smith, P. G.: Long-term mortality after a single treatment course with x-rays in patients treated for ankylosing spondylitis. Br. J. Cancer 55:179, 1987.
179a. Olivieri, I., Gherardi, S., Bini, C., et al.: Trauma and seronegative spondyloarthropathy: Rapid joint destruction in peripheral arthritis triggered by physical injury. Ann. Rheum. Dis. 47:73, 1988.
180. Hultquist, R.: Personal communication.
181. Guillemin, F., Briancon, S., Pourel, J., and Gaucher, A.: Long-term disability and prolonged sick leaves as outcome measurements in ankylosing spondylitis. Possible predictive factors. Arthritis Rheum. 33:1001, 1990.
182. Kraag, G., Stokes, B., Groh, J., et al.: The effect of comprehensive home physiotherapy and supervision on patients with ankylosing spondylitis: A randomized, controlled trial. J. Rheumatol. 17:228, 1990.
183. Khan, M. A.: Medical and surgical treatment of seronegative spondyloarthropathy. Curr. Opin. Rheumatol. 2:592, 1990.
184. Mintz, G., Enriques, H. M., Mercado, U., et al.: Intravenous methylprednisolone pulse therapy in severe ankylosing spondylitis. Arthritis Rheum. 24:734, 1981.
185. Richter, M. B., Woo, P., Panayi, G. S., et al.: The effects of intravenous pulse methylprednisolone on immunological and inflammatory processes in ankylosing spondylitis. Clin. Exp. Immunol. 53:51, 1983.
186. Dougados, M., Boumier, P., and Amor, B.: Sulphasalazine in ankylosing spondylitis: A double-blind, controlled study in 60 patients. Br. Med. J. 293:911, 1986.
187. Feltelius, N., and Hällgren, R.: Sulphasalazine in ankylosing spondylitis. Ann. Rheum. Dis. 45:396, 1986.
188. Nissilä, M., Lehtinen, K., Leirisalo-Repo, M., et al.: Sulfasalazine in the treatment of ankylosing spondylitis. A twenty-six–week placebo-controlled clinical trial. Arthritis Rheum. 31:1111, 1988.
189. Davis, M. J., Dawes, P. T., Beswick, E., et al.: Sulphasalazine therapy in ankylosing spondylitis: Its effects on disease activity, immunoglobulin A, and the complex immunoglobulin A–alpha₁-antitrypsin. Br. J. Rheumatol. 28:410, 1989.
190. Fraser, S. M., and Sturrock, R. D.: Evaluation of sulphasalazine in ankylosing spondylitis—an interventional study. Br. J. Rheumatol. 29:37, 1990.
191. Corkill, M. M., Jobanputra, P., Gibson, T., and MacFarlane, D. G.: A controlled trial of sulphasalazine treatment of chronic ankylosing spondylitis: Failure to demonstrate clinical effect. Br. J. Rheumatol. 29:41, 1990.
192. McConkey, B.: Sulphasalazine and ankylosing spondylitis (editorial). Br. J. Rheumatol. 29:2, 1990.
193. Molin, L., and Stendal, O.: The effect of sulfasalazine and its active components in human polymorphonuclear leukocyte function in relation to ulcerative colitis. Acta Med. Scand. 206:451, 1979.
194. Miyachi, Y., Yoshioka, A., Imamura, S., et al.: Effect of sulfasalazine and its metabolites on the generation of reactive oxygen species. Gut 28:190, 1987.
195. Guillemin, F., Aussedat, R., Guerci, A., et al.: Fatal agranulocytosis in sulfasalazine-treated rheumatoid arthritis. J. Rheumatol. 16:1166, 1989.
196. Zelissen, P. M. J., van Hattum, J., Poen, H., et al.: Influence of salazosulphapyridine and 5-aminosalicylic acid on seminal qualities and male sex hormones. Scand. J. Gastroenterol. 23:1100, 1988.
197. Handler, R. P.: Favourable results using methotrexate in the treatment of patients with ankylosing spondylitis (letter). Arthritis Rheum. 32:234, 1989.
198. Grill, V., Smith, M., Ahaern, M., and Littlejohn, G.: Local radiotherapy for pedal manifestations of HLA-B27–related arthropathy. Br. J. Rheumatol. 27:390, 1988.
199. Kilgus, D. J., Namba, R. S., Gorek, J. E., et al.: Total hip replacement for patients who have ankylosing spondylitis. The importance of the formation of heterotopic bone and of the durability of fixation of cemented components. J. Bone Joint Surg. 72A:834, 1990.
200. Calin, A., and Elswood, J.: The outcome of 138 total hip replacements and 12 revisions in ankylosing spondylitis: High success rate after a mean follow-up of 7.5 years. J. Rheumatol. 16:955, 1989.
201. Trancik, T. M., and Mills, W.: The effects of several nonsteroidal

antiinflammatory medications on bone in growth into a porous coated implant. Trans. Orthop. Res. Soc. 14:338, 1989.

202. Baldursson, H., Brattström, H., and Olsson, T. H.: Total hip replacement in ankylosing spondylitis. Acta Orthop. Scand. 48:499, 1977.

203. Detwiler, K. N., Loftus, C. M., Godersky, J. C., et al.: Management of cervical spine injuries in patients with ankylosing spondylitis. J. Neurosurg. 72:210, 1990.

204. Camargo, F. P., Cordiero, E. N., and Napoli, M. M. M.: Corrective osteotomy of the spine in ankylosing spondylitis. Experience with 66 cases. Clin. Orthop. 208:157, 1986.

205. Böhm, H., Hehne, H. -J., and Zielke, K.: Die Korrektur der Bechterew-Kyphose. Orthopäde 18:142, 1989.

Chapter 57
Reiter's Syndrome

Peng Thim Fan
David T. Y. Yu

INTRODUCTION

The clinical triad of arthritis, nongonoccocal urethritis, and conjunctivitis, first reported by Reiter in 1916,[1] was described formally as a syndrome by Bauer and Engelman in 1942.[2] The strong association of Reiter's syndrome with the histocompatibility antigen, HLA-B27, was established in 1973.[3] This association allowed Arnett et al.[4] to classify 13 patients with asymmetric oligoarthritis of the lower extremities and positive HLA-B27 but without conjunctivitis or urethritis in a category of *incomplete Reiter's syndrome*. The clinical course of incomplete Reiter's syndrome was identical to the full syndrome, and it became evident that they represented subsets of the same disease. Wright and Moll[5] popularized the concept of *seronegative spondyloarthropathies* to emphasize the many similar clinical features shared by ankylosing spondylitis, Reiter's syndrome, psoriatic arthritis, and arthritis of inflammatory bowel disease. The extensive overlap of clinical features within these diseases prompted a committee of the American Rheumatism Association to evaluate criteria for a definite diagnosis of Reiter's syndrome in 1981.[6] They studied 83 patients and compared them with 166 patients with other diseases, and their conclusion was that Reiter's syndrome was best defined as "an episode of peripheral arthritis of more than 1 month duration occurring in association with urethritis and/or cervicitis." They acknowledged that these criteria would not distinguish Reiter's syndrome from certain cases of ankylosing spondylitis or psoriatic arthritis. Subsequent population studies have identified many patients with either isolated extra-articular features such as uveitis without any associated arthritis or an *undifferentiated spondyloarthropathy* that cannot be classified into the categories of ankylosing spondylitis or Reiter's syndrome.[7, 8, 88]

Another term frequently associated with Reiter's syndrome is *reactive arthritis*. This was introduced in 1969 by Ahvonen et al.[9] to describe an acute arthritis that developed soon after or during an infection elsewhere in the body but in which the microorganism did not enter the joint. More recent studies have proved the presence of noninfectious components of the infective organism within the synovial tissue or fluid,[10–12] and it would be more accurate now to define a reactive arthritis as one in which the infectious organism cannot be cultured from the joint fluid or synovium.

It is now clear that Reiter's syndrome is only one clinical manifestation of reactive arthritis. Besides its distinctive arthropathy, reactive arthritis is occasionally accompanied by a variety of extra-articular symptoms such as uveitis, bowel inflammation, carditis, and nephritis, which may occur in the setting of classic Reiter's syndrome[13] or in a more limited spectrum, sometimes even as an isolated event (e.g., isolated uveitis[14] or carditis).[15] Many of the extra-articular features as well as the severity and chronicity of the arthritis are related to the presence of the histocompatibility antigen, HLA-B27.[13] A study has demonstrated that a 3-month course of tetracycline is effective in reducing the chronicity and severity of *Chlamydia*-induced reactive arthritis.[16] It is therefore important to stress the "reactive" nature of the arthritis and to look diligently for the infectious organism in all such cases. Perhaps it is time to consider retiring *Reiter's syndrome* to a historical role (just as we now avoid the term *rheumatoid variant*) because it has no privileged etiologic identity and to adopt the broader concept of reactive arthritis in all our descriptions of these clinical entities. As currently defined, *reactive arthritis* is restricted to the conditions frequently associated with HLA-B27 and does not include rheumatic fever, Lyme arthritis, arthritis associated with ulcerative colitis or regional enteritis, Whipple's disease, parasitic infections, and postviral arthritides.

ETIOLOGY AND PATHOGENESIS

In considering the pathogenesis of Reiter's syndrome, two factors are important. The first is genetic predisposition. The second is the observation that some cases of arthritis are induced by infections.

Genetic Predisposition

Of all the possible genetic factors that might predispose to Reiter's syndrome, HLA-B27 is clearly one of them. This is an allele of the B locus of the class I major histocompatibility complex. At least 906 white patients have been reported and compared with 13,477 control subjects. Eighty percent of the patients are HLA-B27 positive compared with 9 percent of the control subjects. This difference is highly significant. The relative risk is 37.13.[17] The biologic significance of HLA-B27 is even clearer with another spondyloarthropathy, ankylosing spondylitis, in which more than 90 percent of the patients are HLA-B27 positive. With this high correlation, it is extremely likely that the HLA-B27 genes are the disease-causing genes. An even more dramatic demonstration of the pathogenic importance of HLA-B27 is the finding that generation of a line of HLA-B27 transgenic Lewis rats designated as 21-4H leads to spontaneous development of peripheral and axial arthritis in 10 of 14 male rats.[18] The HLA-B27 genes have at least six suballeles.[19] There is no clear evidence that Reiter's syndrome or ankylosing spondylitis is linked to only one of these.

It is suspected that HLA-B27 is not the only genetic factor that predisposes to Reiter's syndrome because blacks in the United States with the disease have a much lower incidence of HLA-B27. More compelling are the statistics from some epidemics of bacterial infections that are followed by outbreaks of reactive arthritis. For example, after one such epidemic of dysentery in 1984 in Canada involving 423 subjects, 25 patients developed reactive arthritis, and only five were positive for HLA-B27.[20] If there are non–HLA-B27 genetic factors that predispose to Reiter's syndrome, however, they have not yet been identified. Genes located between the HLA-B and the class III loci are suspected.

Identification of Arthritis-Causing Bacteria and Study of Immune Responses

A considerable number of bacteria species are commonly accepted to be the cause of arthritis. Those that reside in the gastrointestinal tracts are the *Shigella flexneri, Salmonella typhimurium, Salmonella enteritidis, Salmonella heidelberg, Salmonella choleraesuis, Yersinia enterocolitica, Yersinia pseudotuberculosis,* and *Campylobacter jejuni. Chlamydia trachomatis* that resides in the genitourinary tract is also an accepted cause. Reports of other incriminating organisms are more sporadic. In all these cases, infections are diagnosed by serology or more reliably by bacterial culture from the stool or urethra. There has been no consistent success at culturing organisms from the inflamed joints.

The availability of these arthritis-causing bacteria have allowed investigators to study the immune responses.[20a] Even with crude bacterial antigenic preparations, it becomes clear that the synovial compartment is a self-sufficient milieu for specific cell-mediated immunity. Not only are there macrophages armed with such antigens, but also detectable are specific T lymphocytes capable of in vitro proliferative reactivity toward the causative microbes.[21] In contrast, the mononuclear cells from the peripheral blood compartment serves as a negative control in having an impaired response.[22] With the successful generation of T cell clones, the responsible bacterial macromolecules will be identified. Although the heat

shock proteins are suspected, verification and more evaluation are needed.

Equally impressive are results carried out with serum antibacterial antibodies. Serial observations of patients with *Yersinia*-induced arthritis have been compared with control subjects who were infected with the same bacteria. There are more persistent immunoglobulin A (IgA) anti-*Yersinia* serum antibodies in patients with arthritis, and the predominant antigen is the lipopolysaccharide.[23, 24] Similar observations, although to a lesser degree, have also been reported with other arthritis-causing bacteria.[25] The values of these observations are not diagnostic. There is considerable overlapping in values between the arthritis and control subjects. Nor are the antibodies specific for a single, presumably arthritis-causing bacterial macromolecule.

The crux of the problem appears to be the factor that leads to these cell-mediated and humoral responses in arthritis patients. Observation from experimental animals indicates that they might reflect a persistence of the bacteria or bacterial components in the hosts. Thus, the particular strain of rats that is susceptible to *Yersinia*-induced arthritis is also the one that allows persistence of the bacteria.[26] Transgenic mice carrying HLA-B27 antigens are also more susceptible to *Yersinia* infection.[27] Indeed in the synovial tissues of arthritis patients, bacterial antigens have been reported with *Yersinia, Salmonella,* and *Chlamydia.*[10–12] With *Chlamydia,* the bacterial antigens have been recognized both with monoclonal antibodies and with electron microscopy.[28] The monoclonal antibodies used in these studies are directed either against the lipopolysaccharides or, in the case of *Chlamydia,* against a major membrane protein. It would be important to know if viable bacteria are present. Although one group of investigators has detected chlamydial RNA in synovial tissues, it still remains to be demonstrated that the chlamydia can replicate.[28a]

Theories Concerning the Relationship Between HLA-B27 and Arthritis-Causing Bacteria

The physiologic function of the class I major histocompatibility antigens is to present antigenic peptides to cytotoxic T lymphocytes. That HLA-B27 can serve such a purpose has been demonstrated in human as well as in transgenic mice.[29] Hence the logical hypothesis is that this peptide-presenting activity has been subverted to induce arthritis. To test this will require identification of the presumably arthritis-causing antigenic peptides, which are as yet unavailable. With the rapid accumulation of information on the structure of HLA-B27, such identification may be achieved soon.[29a]

Another hypothesis for the role of HLA-B27 is that it serves as a receptor for certain bacterial macromolecules. One group has described a plasmid-encoded *Klebsiella* protein to be capable of complexing with HLA-B27. This plasmid was described as being shared among a variety of bacteria and as being capable of integrating into the genome of the hosts.[30] Multiple attempts at demonstrating this protein by several laboratories, however, have not been uniformly successful. Nevertheless, the receptor hypothesis remains a reasonable possibility.

A third possibility considered is that of mimicry between HLA-B27 and bacterial macromolecules. Two approaches have been adopted to identify such macromolecules. One is to search for bacterial proteins, which have linear amino acid sequences similar to that of the alpha (α) 1 helix domain of HLA-B27. Three proteins have been identified. They are the *Klebsiella* nitrogenase reductase,[31] the *Shigella flexneri* pHS-2 plasmid-encoded protein,[32] and the *Yersinia enterocolitica* plasmid-encoded adhesin (YOP1) protein.[33] The lengths of amino acid sequences that simulate the HLA-B27 are six, five, and four. Especially with the hexamer in *Klebsiella* nitrogenase reductase, the probability of this similarity being a chance occurrence is rather small. One potential problem of using sequence similarity to search for molecular mimicry is that the critical part of the HLA-B27 protein is an α helix. Even though a bacterial protein may have a sequence similar to it, unless the conformation is similar, there may not be serologic cross-reactivity.

An alternative experimental approach is to use monoclonal anti–HLA-B27 antibodies to probe for reactive bacterial proteins. At least two outer membrane proteins have been found to be reactive.[34] Using amino acid or DNA sequencing, one of them has been identified as the OmpA protein.[35] This protein does not share sequence similarity with HLA-B27. The likelihood is that cross-reactivity is through discontinuous epitopes. It is not clear whether the two types of molecular mimicry with HLA-B27 can lead to arthritis. A minority of arthritis patients do carry "autoantibodies" against a synthetic peptide derived from the α1 domain of the HLA-B27.[36] Two epitopes on this sequence are responsible: KAKAQTDR and REDLRTLI.[37] T cell reactivity against this peptide is absent. Possibilities other than autoreactivity also have to be considered. For example, it has been proposed that molecular mimicry would lead to a lack of host response toward certain critical bacterial antigens and perhaps through this tolerance would develop, resulting in persistence of the pathogens. Alternatively, if the bacterial proteins exist in complexes with other bacterial macromolecules such as the lipopolysaccharides, the cross-reactivity with the HLA-B27 antigens would suggest that HLA-B27 could similarly complex with bacterial antigens. This in turn could also lead to the persistence of bacterial antigens in the patients.

These studies with HLA-B27 and bacterial components provide examples of analysis at the molecular level. The treatment of reactive arthritis is rather empirical and not directed toward the pathogenetic mechanisms of arthritis. With rapid understanding of the various factors contributing to the arthritis, a more rational approach may soon be possible.

EPIDEMIOLOGY

It is difficult to perform accurate epidemiologic studies in Reiter's syndrome.[38] There are no definitive diagnostic tests for this disease. Reiter's syndrome commonly occurs in young patients who tend to be mobile and are difficult to follow. The venereal or dysenteric episode may be mild or silent and may have been forgotten. Urethritis cannot be diagnosed in women, and cervicitis may be asymptomatic or dismissed as nonspecific. Some cases of Reiter's syndrome may have been misdiagnosed as *seronegative rheumatoid arthritis*, whereas others as ankylosing spondylitis because of overlapping features. The fragmentation of care among different specialties because of the multisystem complaints adds to the problem.

Michet and co-workers at the Mayo Clinic[39] retrospectively reviewed all cases of Reiter's syndrome, ankylosing spondylitis, sacroiliitis, psoriatic arthritis, gonococcal arthritis, iritis, uveitis, and keratoderma blenorrhagica in Rochester, Minnesota, between 1950 and 1980. They identified only 16 cases of Reiter's syndrome, all male. The age of diagnosis ranged from 18 to 45. This gave an age-adjusted incidence rate for males younger than age 50 of 3.5 per 100,000. They concluded that Reiter's syndrome was as common as definite rheumatoid arthritis but less common than ankylosing spondylitis. Nonetheless, Reiter's syndrome is probably the most common cause of inflammatory arthritis of the lower extremities in a young male.[38]

Studies of reactive arthritis provide more accurate estimates of incidence. One to three percent of unselected individuals develop arthritis following an episode of nonspecific urethritis.[45] *Chlamydia trachomatis* is the offending agent; the role of *Ureaplasma urealyticum* is uncertain. Similarly, 1 to 4 percent of unselected populations develop arthritis following enteric infections with *Shigella*, *Salmonella*, and *Campylobacter*.[13] In a Swedish study, 13 percent of 75 patients hospitalized because of *Yersinia* developed arthritis.[40] In another study, 55 percent of patients had arthritis.[41] In an outbreak of *Yersinia* pseudotuberculosis infection in Finland, 4 of 19 patients (21 percent) developed reactive arthritis.[42] Sievers et al.[43] estimated that the annual prevalence of *Yersinia* arthritis requiring medical care in Finland was between 0.02 and 0.04 percent. The number of subjects susceptible to reactive arthritis in Finland is high because the prevalence of HLA-B27 positivity is 14 percent.[44] This contrasts with 9 percent in the general white population. For unknown reasons, *Yersinia* arthritis has almost never been reported in the United States.

Following an outbreak of *Shigella flexneri* dysentery, 25 percent of HLA-B27–positive patients developed Reiter's syndrome.[46] *Shigella sonnei* was not considered capable of inducing reactive arthritis, but three cases were reported; two of the patients were HLA-B27 positive.[47] Ten cases of *Clostridium difficile*–associated reactive arthritis have been reported; HLA-B27 was determined in eight patients, and five of the patients were HLA-B27 positive.[48] The multitude of enteric pathogens capable of provoking reactive arthritis and the high incidence of arthritis following chlamydial urethritis emphasizes the importance of the gastrointestinal tract and the urethra as portals of entry. A report from Germany, however, in a region where Lyme disease was endemic indicated that 18 percent of patients with reactive arthritis or Reiter's syndrome demonstrated circulating antibodies and proliferative T cell responses to *Borrelia burgdorferi*.[49] If these results can be confirmed, it would appear that a wider range of infectious stimuli could provoke reactive arthritis in the susceptible host.[50]

Reiter's syndrome and reactive arthritis have been reported worldwide. Twenty-two cases were reported from China,[51] and 10 cases from Zimbabwe.[52] The high prevalence of the spondyloarthropathies throughout the world is related to the high frequency of HLA-B27 in different populations. Reactive arthritis is less frequently reported in nonwhite populations, perhaps reflecting the lower incidence of HLA-B27. Reiter's syndrome is rare in blacks. Indeed, when Reiter's syndrome does occur, the patients are frequently HLA-B27 negative. All ten patients with Reiter's syndrome reported from Zimbabwe were HLA-B27 negative.[52]

Reiter's syndrome is rarely recognized in children. Most reported cases are postenteric rather than postvenereal. The clinical spectrum is more restricted in children, severe heel pain with plantar fasciitis and enthesopathy being the common clinical picture.[53, 54] In older children, *Chlamydia*-induced reactive arthritis has been reported following sexual exposure. Most patients are male and HLA-B27 positive. A 15-year-old boy who was HLA-B27 positive developed Reiter's syndrome following acute gangrenous appendicitis, illustrating that reactive arthritis can occur after peritoneal infection.[55]

Most reported cases of Reiter's syndrome are male, and it has been estimated that Reiter's syndrome is 20 times more frequent in men. This sex distribution, however, is probably highly exaggerated because cervicitis is difficult to recognize in women and has not been systematically evaluated.[38] In a carefully performed study of *Chlamydia*-induced reactive arthritis, 6 of 21 patients (21 percent) were women.[16] Postdysenteric reactive arthritis shows an equal sex distribution, reflecting the equal incidence of HLA-B27 in men and women.[13]

CLINICAL FEATURES

The symptoms of reactive arthritis typically develop within 1 to 3 weeks of the inciting episode of urethritis or diarrhea. Constitutional symptoms are usually mild, and fever, if present, is low grade without accompanying chills. Rarely, a patient may appear very toxic with high fever, weight loss, and severe malaise. The initial episode of urethritis in postvenereal reactive arthritis may be mild or unapparent, and yet it is not uncommon for a patient with postdysenteric reactive arthritis to develop a sterile urethritis within 1 to 2 weeks of the initial bout of diarrhea.[13] It is therefore difficult at times to decide whether the reactive arthritis is postdysenteric or postvenereal.[38]

Joints

Joint stiffness, myalgia, and low back pain are prominent early symptoms. The back discomfort is made worse by bed rest and inactivity, and it radiates into the buttocks and thighs. The cause of the back pain is not clear. Radiographs of the spine at this stage are typically normal. Scintiscans performed during acute Reiter's syndrome were abnormal, however, around the sacroiliac joints in 73 percent of a series of 33 patients.[56] The specificity of increased sacroiliac uptake has been called into question, and attempts at standardizing the test by doing quantitative scintigraphy have not been uniformly successful. Computed tomography (CT) scanning may demonstrate occult sacroiliitis not visible on plain radiographs.

The knees, ankles, and feet are most commonly affected in an asymmetric pattern (Fig. 57–1). Typically only a few joints are involved, and occasionally the wrist may be an early target. The inflammation is usually low grade, manifesting more as joint tenderness, stiffness, and restricted range of motion rather than gross swelling. The knee, however, can become markedly swollen with inflammatory synovial fluid, and popliteal cyst dissection and rupture can happen early in the course of the disease.

The distinctive arthropathy of Reiter's syndrome consists of a local enthesopathy: The principal target of inflammation is located at the tendinous insertion into bone rather than the synovium. In the digits, this gives the appearance of a uniformly swollen "sausage" finger or toe (Fig. 57–2; see color section at the front of this volume); this contrasts with rheumatoid arthritis, in which the inflammation is confined to the synovium and the phalangeal shafts are normal. The presence of a sausage digit is of great diagnostic help because only Reiter's syndrome and psoriatic arthritis demonstrate this abnormality. In the ankle, the enthesopathic process causes chronic hindfoot swelling and pain. The Achilles tendon and plantar fascia are inflamed at the site of insertion into the calcaneus, as are the ligaments around the ankle and subtalar joints. Exuberant calcaneal spurs may develop followed by ossification of the tendinous insertions (Fig. 57–3). Reiter's syndrome should always be suspected in a young man

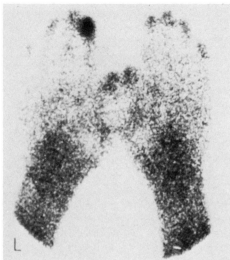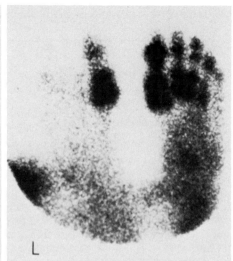

Figure 57–1. Scintiscan in early Reiter's syndrome demonstrating asymmetric synovitis involving the distal interphalangeal joint of the left index finger and several "sausage toes." (Courtesy of Dr. Rodney Bluestone.)

who presents with subacute arthritis of the knees, chronic hindfoot pain, metatarsalgia, and tenderness in the low back over the sacroiliac joints[57] (Table 57–1). Less commonly the shoulder, elbow, hip, symphysis pubis, and manubriosternal joint can be affected. A relatively painless soft tissue and bony enlargement of one of the sternoclavicular joints may occur.

The spine is prominently involved in those patients with severe, chronic, or recurrent disease. Earlier on, the patients complain of pleuritic-type chest pain probably caused by tendinous inflammation at the intercostal muscles, sternum, and costovertebral articulation. Later the patients experience back and neck stiffness and reduced mobility. A few patients with long-standing Reiter's syndrome may develop axial disease indistinguishable from ankylosing spondylitis. Sacroiliitis develops in 20 to 30 percent of patients overall and is related to the presence

of HLA-B27.[38, 58] At 10-year follow-up, 41 percent of patients with *Yersinia* arthritis who were HLA-B27 positive had radiographic sacroiliitis as compared with 7 percent of patients who were HLA-B27 negative.[59] In Good's series, patients with persistent Reiter's syndrome over 2 years had a 57 percent prevalence of radiographic sacroiliitis.[60]

Urogenital Tract

Urethritis may be a principal feature of reactive arthritis and is seen even in some postdysenteric cases. As a precipitating event, it precedes the symptoms of reactive arthritis by 1 to 3 weeks, but urogenital symptoms have been reported in women 5

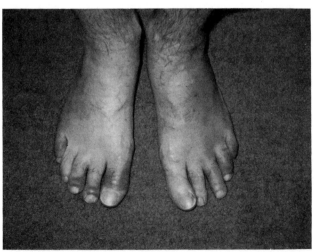

Figure 57–2. Asymmetric polyarthritis of the feet. Note the sausage toes with severe redness and swelling of the phalangeal shafts and the swelling of the tarsus.

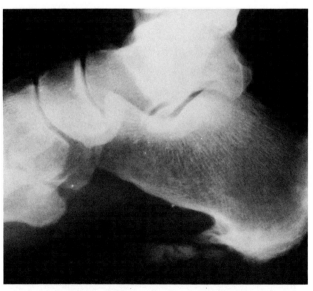

Figure 57–3. Calcaneal spurs at both Achilles tendon and plantar fascial insertions with sclerosis and fluffy indistinct periosteal new bone. Note ossification of the plantar fascia and normal ankle and talonavicular joints.

Table 57–1. CLINICALLY USEFUL FEATURES IN
DIAGNOSING REACTIVE ARTHRITIS

Preceding or current urethritis or diarrhea
Conjunctivitis or unilateral iritis
Asymmetric lower extremity oligoarthritis
Sausage finger or toe
Heel pain and swelling
Low back pain and sacroiliac tenderness
Negative rheumatoid factor
Positive HLA-B27
Radiologic signs of fluffy periostitis, bone spurs, tendinous
    ossification, asymmetric sacroiliitis, and paravertebral comma-
    shaped ossification

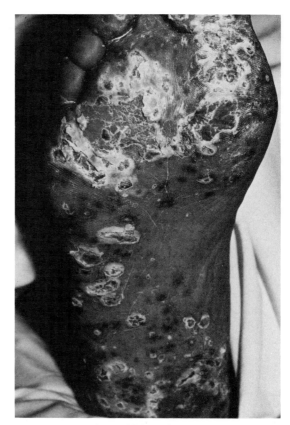

Figure 57–5. Keratoderma blennorrhagica. Hyperkeratotic vesicles, papules, and plaques on the sole. (Courtesy of Dr. Kenneth Landow.)

years before the onset of joint complaints.[13] Males experience frequency and burning during urination. Examination of the penis reveals meatal erythema and edema, and a clear mucoid discharge can be expressed. Pyuria is best detected in a first-void urine.[14] Prostatitis is common and has been reported in as many as 80 percent of patients. Hemorrhagic cystitis may develop, and it may clear spontaneously.[61] Urethral stricture developed in a man with chronic Reiter's syndrome who had 3 years of persistent urethritis.[62] He underwent a complete urethrectomy 10 years after the onset of his disease, and the arthritis, conjunctivitis, and mucocutaneous lesions, which had not been controlled, remitted after urethrectomy. This interesting case suggests that the systemic disease in reactive arthritis can be sustained by the inflammatory reaction within the urethral tract and remits when this focus is removed. In women, a *reactive salpingitis* has been described.[63] This occurs in 22 percent of postvenereal reactive arthritis, and

57 percent of these women were HLA-B27 positive. Vulvovaginitis and aseptic pyuria have also been reported.[13]

Mucous Membrane and Skin

Small shallow painless ulcers of the glans penis and urethral meatus, termed *balanitis circinata*, have been described in 23 percent of patients with post-*Shigella* reactive arthritis and postvenereal arthritis.[58] In uncircumcised patients, the lesions are moist, and they are asymptomatic unless secondarily infected (Fig. 57–4). The foreskin has to be retracted during the physical examination to detect these lesions. On the circumcised penis, the lesions harden to a crust that may scar and cause pain. Fox et al.[64] noted four patients in their series of 131 who developed circinate balanitis 4 years before the onset of other symptoms of reactive arthritis.

Keratoderma blennorrhagica is a hyperkeratotic skin lesion that is seen in 12 to 14 percent of patients.[65] It begins as clear vesicles on erythematous bases and progresses to macules, papules, and nodules. The lesions are frequently found on the soles of the feet (Fig. 57–5), and they may also involve the toes, scrotum, penis, palms, trunk, and scalp. The lesions cannot be distinguished either clinically or

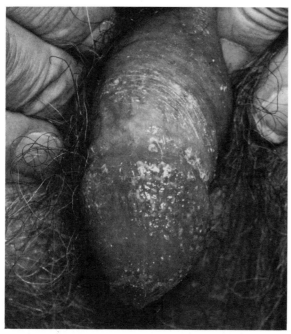

Figure 57–4. Balanitis circinata in an uncircumcised penis. Moist, painless, shallow ulcers are seen at the corona when the foreskin is retracted. (Courtesy of Dr. Kenneth Landow.)

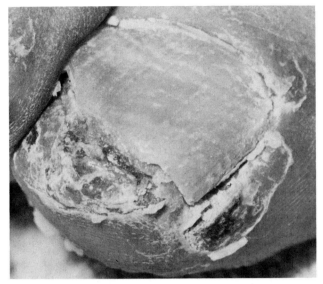

Figure 57–6. The toenail is thickened and ridged. Part of the nail is trimmed to reveal the keratotic deposits, which are lifting the nail from the nail bed. (Courtesy of Dr. Kenneth Landow.)

microscopically from pustular psoriasis, and they do not correlate with the course of the disease. The nails can become thickened and ridged. Keratotic material accumulates under the nail and lifts it from the nail bed (Fig. 57–6). Previous reports of keratoderma have been exclusively confined to postvenereal reactive arthritis, but more recently two cases have been reported in a series of 85 patients with *Yersinia* arthritis.[59]

Superficial oral ulcers are an early and transient feature of the disease. They begin as vesicles and progress to small, shallow, sometimes confluent ulcers. Because they are often painless, they may go unnoticed by the patient. Erythema nodosum is a unique feature of *Yersinia* arthritis. *Yersinia* is the cause of 20 percent of the cases of erythema nodosum in Finland and Sweden.[13] Erythema nodosum occurs typically in women, especially those who are HLA-B27 negative, and its presence correlates with either the absence of arthritis or the milder joint symptoms. It is reported in 10 to 20 percent of post-*Yersinia* reactive arthritis.[13]

Eye

Conjunctivitis is the most common ocular complication of reactive arthritis. It occurs in the majority of patients with *Shigella* infections and is often the initial symptom.[58] It is also commonly seen after *Salmonella* and *Campylobacter* infections, but its prevalence is only 10 percent in *Yersinia* arthritis.[66] About 35 percent of cases of postvenereal reactive arthritis develop conjunctivitis.[58] Patients experience redness, smarting, and tearing, and a few have photophobia, chemosis, and swelling of the lids. The mucopurulent discharge is typically sterile, although rarely *Chla-*

mydia has been cultured from the eye during bouts of inclusion conjunctivitis.[58] Symptoms commonly subside within a week, but they may persist for 7 months.

Uveitis probably occurs as an independent, asynchronous event owing to the shared genetic susceptibility of HLA-B27 positivity.[14] Nevertheless, Reiter's syndrome was found to be the most frequently diagnosed systemic disease (17 cases) in a survey of 236 uveitis patients reviewed at a uveitis clinic at the University of Oregon.[67] The initial attack is always acute and unilateral, but recurrent episodes often affect the other eye. The inflammation is anterior (iritis) and tends to spare the choroid and retina. Patients with iritis complain of photophobia, redness, and pain and occasionally reduced vision and increased tearing. The inflammation tends to resolve completely within 2 to 4 months. Rare complications include keratitis, hypopyon, corneal ulcerations, posterior uveitis, optic neuritis, and intraocular hemorrhage.[58] It has been stated that if blindness occurs in association with a spondyloarthropathy, it is most likely due to Reiter's syndrome.[68]

Gastrointestinal Tract

The precipitating episode of diarrhea is often mild, but occasionally it may be bloody and prolonged. Other signs of reactive arthritis start 1 to 3 weeks later. Patients with *Yersinia* enteritis often have mild recurrent abdominal complaints.[13] In a seminal study, Mielants and co-workers[69] documented the presence of inflammatory lesions in the ileum in 16 of 35 patients with idiopathic reactive arthritis and microscopic inflammation in 33 patients (94 percent). The vast majority of these patients had no gastrointestinal symptoms at the time of ileocolonoscopy. Follow-up reports indicated that the HLA-Bw62 antigen was strongly correlated with the presence of chronic inflammatory gut lesions,[70] and more intriguingly, the severity of the bowel inflammation was temporally related to the activity of the joint disease.[71] During articular clinical remission, the inflammatory gut lesions disappeared, but patients with active joint disease continued to show inflammatory lesions. Treatment with sulfasalazine relieved the joint inflammation, and the bowel histology also became normal.

Heart

Cardiac complications are reported as late sequelae in 10 percent of patients with severe and long-standing disease.[38] The two most common are conduction abnormalities and aortic regurgitation. Conduction defects sometimes occur early, the most common being a prolonged P-R interval.[71a] This is the result of inflammation and fibrosis of the membranous portion of the interventricular septum giving rise to disease in the atrioventricular node.[68] One case each of second-degree atrioventricular block with Wenckebach's phenomenon[72] and complete heart block[73] have been reported, both occurring within weeks of onset of Reiter's syndrome. Aortic regurgitation is the result of inflammation and scarring of the aortic wall and valves.[68] The valvular cusps become fibrotic, thickened, and retracted. It is identical to the lesion seen in cases of ankylosing spondylitis. An echocardiogram may detect aortic root disease before clinical evidence of regurgitation or heart block.[74] Bergfeldt et al.[15] studied 91 patients with aortic regurgitation and found a group of 24 with aortic regurgitation and severe conduction system abnormalities who had no discernible cause for their cardiac disease and no clinical evidence of ankylosing spondylitis or Reiter's syndrome. Twenty-two of these patients underwent HLA-B27 typing, and it was positive in 17 (77 percent). This suggests that cardiac disease can exist as an independent feature of an HLA-B27–associated disease process.

Miscellaneous Complications

Four cases of IgA glomerulonephritis in association with Reiter's syndrome have been reported,[75] and renal amyloidosis may complicate chronic Reiter's syndrome.[76] Other unusual complications include cranial and peripheral neuropathies,[77] thrombophlebitis, purpura, and livedo reticularis.[78]

REITER'S SYNDROME AND HIV DISEASE

The advent of the human immunodeficiency virus (HIV) pandemic has altered our understanding and management of Reiter's syndrome. Reiter's syndrome was the first rheumatic disease to be recognized in association with HIV infection.[79] The clinical features of Reiter's syndrome usually follow the onset of HIV infection, but they may precede any overt signs of HIV disease. The disease spectrum resembles that seen in HIV-negative patients, and the incidence of HLA-B27 is equally high (75 percent).[80] HIV infection does not alter the severity of the arthritis, and there may be no clues to its presence until the patient with Reiter's syndrome is treated with immunosuppressive drugs such as methotrexate or azathioprine.[79] These drugs further suppress the immune response and provoke a full expression of the acquired immunodeficiency syndrome (AIDS). It is claimed that the development of a malar rash in a patient with Reiter's syndrome may be a clue to the presence of HIV.[81]

Two cases of *Yersinia*-reactive arthritis occurring in HIV-positive homosexuals have been described in the United Kingdom, where reports of *Yersinia* arthritis have been rare.[82] Fourteen black Zimbabweans who were HIV positive but HLA-B27 negative developed reactive arthritis.[83] These case reports raise the question of whether HIV itself may provoke a reactive arthritis. The coexistence of Reiter's syndrome and HIV disease suggests that CD4 helper-inducer lymphocytes are not important in the pathogenesis of reactive arthritis.[84]

LABORATORY EVALUATION

The first group of laboratory tests documents the presence of a specific bacterial infection. Because chronic antimicrobial therapy is proved helpful for *Chlamydia*-induced reactive arthritis[16] but not for postdysenteric cases, it is now of critical importance to document the presence or absence of chlamydial infection in every suspected case of reactive arthritis. In a research setting, *Chlamydia* has been cultured from the throat, urethra, and cervix.[16] Several factors make it difficult for culture to be used on a routine clinical basis. *Chlamydia* is an obligate intracellular parasite, and it cannot be grown on artificial media.[85] Although culture is the most sensitive test, it requires a cold chain to protect the viability of the organism. Transport of viable organisms is difficult, and a delay of 24 hours will significantly reduce the yield.

Three sensitive and specific nonculture tests have been introduced that are ideal in the routine clinical environment. The proper collection of the specimen is crucial. Because chlamydiae are intracellular parasites, collection of discharge fluids is inappropriate. The affected mucous membrane should be cleared of discharge and then rubbed briskly with a cotton swab for several seconds. For the cervix, the use of cytobrushes may be more efficient. The two most commonly used nonculture tests are the direct fluorescent antibody test (DFA) and the enzyme-immunoassay (EIA).[85] Both have sensitivity of 75 to 83 percent and specificity of 97 to 98 percent. EIA methods require relatively large amounts of antigen for detection. A recently developed DNA-probe technique may prove to be the best test for *Chlamydia*.[86] It uses the hybridization of labeled DNA probes to chlamydial ribosomal RNA, and it has a sensitivity of 95 percent and a specificity of virtually 100 percent. Positive serology is too delayed in onset to be useful for diagnosing all cases of chlamydial infections, although it is accepted that IgG titers of greater than 128, the presence of specific IgM, or fourfold seroconversion signifies a positive diagnosis.[16] Stool cultures may secure a diagnosis of infection by *Salmonella*, *Shigella*, *Campylobacter*, and *Yersinia* even when bowel symptoms are mild or unapparent.[16] The presence of an appropriate triggering microbe secures the diagnosis of reactive arthritis in an otherwise undefined case of arthritis.

The second group of laboratory tests reflects the presence of inflammation. A moderate neutrophilic leukocytosis is common during the acute illness, and the erythrocyte sedimentation rate (ESR) and C-reactive protein are elevated. As the disease subsides, the ESR returns slowly to normal; its persistence signifies continuing disease activity. A mild normochromic anemia is seen in chronic cases. Antinuclear antibody and rheumatoid factor are absent, and C3 and C4 levels, being acute phase reactants, are elevated. Urine, urethral secretions, and prostatic massage fluids contain abundant pus cells during active urethritis. When cystitis is present, the urine may be grossly hemorrhagic.[61]

Synovial fluid may be mildly to severely inflammatory and may contain large macrophages that have ingested vacuoles, nuclear debris, and whole leukocytes. These are called Reiter's cells, but they are not specific for Reiter's syndrome.[87] Synovial fluid smears and cultures are always negative for infective pathogens. Synovial biopsies show nonspecific inflammatory changes[28] and are useful only for excluding other diagnoses.

HLA-B27 typing is diagnostically helpful in suspected cases of reactive arthritis in which characteristic extra-articular features are absent. A case can be made for performing this test in all cases of reactive arthritis. In recent years, the cost of the test has dropped substantially, and there is increasing evidence that the possession of the HLA-B27 antigen correlates with axial disease[59] and extra-articular manifestations such as carditis[89] and uveitis.[98]

RADIOLOGIC FINDINGS

Joint involvement in Reiter's syndrome is asymmetric, oligoarticular, and more common in the lower extremities. In early disease, soft tissue prominence is frequent around the ankles, digits, and knees as a consequence of intra-articular effusion, periarticular edema, and bursal and tendinous inflammation. The digits give a sausage-like appearance, and inflammation at the retrocalcaneal bursa may obliterate the radiolucent fat-pad above the calcaneus.[90] Juxta-articular osteoporosis may be seen in acute episodes of arthritis, but bone density is surprisingly well preserved in chronic disease in distinct contrast to rheumatoid arthritis.[91] Joint space narrowing is typically seen in the smaller joints of the hand, foot, and wrist rather than the ankle or knee, and it is symmetric and diffuse.

Erosions are detected in the small joints of the foot, hand, and wrist and in the knee and sacroiliac joint. They show indistinct margins and are often surrounded by fluffy periosteal new bone because of the tendency of reactive new bone proliferation at the sites of inflammation. The presence of bone proliferation is seen in Reiter's syndrome, psoriatic arthritis, and ankylosing spondylitis and is the most helpful radiologic feature in distinguishing these diseases from rheumatoid arthritis. Linear periostitis is seen along the metacarpal, metatarsal, and phalangeal shafts, and exuberant periosteal spurs with indistinct margins can be seen along the sites of tendinous insertion into bone such as the calcaneus

(see Fig. 57–3), ischial tuberosity, fibula, tibial tuberosity, and trochanter. Tendons may calcify and ossify. Heel enthesopathy is a prominent feature of juvenile Reiter's syndrome.[53, 54] Bony ankylosis is seen across the small joints of the hands and feet, but this is uncommon and its presence would rather suggest psoriatic arthritis.[91]

Sacroiliitis can be detected in 5 to 10 percent of patients with early disease, but eventually up to 70 percent of chronic Reiter's syndrome patients show sacroiliac abnormalities.[92] Although unilateral sacroiliac changes are seen far more commonly in Reiter's syndrome than in ankylosing spondylitis, these are typically early findings. Bilateral sacroiliitis is more common in chronic disease.[91] Pathologic changes of sacroiliitis cannot be recognized at an earlier stage with the use of magnetic resonance imaging (MRI) than with conventional radiographs or CT, but MRI provides new insight into the pathologic events in sacroiliitis: Early inflammatory changes occur in the subcortical bone, and they appear patchy, with abnormal areas adjacent to normal areas along the sacroiliac joint.[93]

Asymmetric paravertebral comma-shaped ossification is a distinctive finding in Reiter's syndrome and psoriatic arthritis, and it typically involves the lower three thoracic and upper three lumbar vertebrae.[91] This is more common than the thinner syndesmophyte and the diffuse bamboo spine appearance, which is more typical of ankylosing spondylitis. Squaring of the vertebra is uncommon, and atlantoaxial subluxation is unusual.[91] Five cases of atlantoaxial subluxation, however, have been reported.[94–96]

DIFFERENTIAL DIAGNOSIS

Postvenereal cases of reactive arthritis have to be distinguished from gonococcal arthritis. There is a 20 to 50 percent co-positive rate of concurrent *Chlamydia* and *Neisseria gonorrhoeae* infections. The use of DNA-probe techniques is helpful because both organisms can be detected on the same sample.[86] Gonoccocal arthritis is more frequently encountered in women. Psoriatic arthritis may be indistinguishable from Reiter's syndrome. The presence of urethritis and bowel symptoms would favor Reiter's syndrome.

There is a current resurgence of acute rheumatic fever in the United States, and the oligoarthritis and carditis may mimic Reiter's syndrome.[97] Subcutaneous nodules and erythema marginatum would suggest rheumatic fever, but they are rarely present. A positive Streptozyme test, antistreptolysin-O, and anti-DNase B titers help secure the diagnosis.

The arthritis of inflammatory bowel disease is clinically similar to that of reactive arthritis. Bowel symptoms should be more prominent and persistent in inflammatory bowel disease, and they tend to parallel the activity of the peripheral arthritis. In

North America, the presence of erythema nodosum favors inflammatory bowel disease because post-*Yersinia* arthritis is so infrequent. As discussed previously, ileocolonoscopy may not necessarily distinguish between the two entities.[69] The confirmed presence of a triggering microbe is the only sure way to diagnose reactive arthritis in this setting.

HIV infection has to be looked for in all cases of reactive arthritis, particularly when the use of prednisone, methotrexate, and other immunosuppressive drugs is contemplated.

COURSE AND PROGNOSIS

The natural history of Reiter's syndrome is highly variable and probably related to the particular infective organism. Most patients experience hectic and often severely symptomatic episodes of arthritis lasting several weeks to 6 months.[58] A small number of patients may have only a single self-limiting episode of disease, but 15 to 50 percent of patients have recurrent bouts of arthritis. Patients commonly complain of persistent or recurrent arthralgia with oligoarthritis, tendinitis, fasciitis, and low back pain.

Fox et al.[64] found in a community and university based study that polyarthritis persisted in 83 percent of 122 patients located 5.6 years later. Over a quarter of these patients were either unemployed or forced to change their occupation. The presence of heel pain at the time of diagnosis correlated with a poor prognosis. In contrast, even though Butler's study in Canada documented recurrent synovitis in 80 percent of 48 patients followed for a mean of 6.5 years, all the patients were in functional class 1 or 2 between flares of the disease, none were not working, and only one had to change his job as a direct result of the disease.[98] A generally accepted estimate is that 20 percent of patients with Reiter's syndrome develop chronic peripheral arthritis or axial disease.[14]

Several reported series of epidemic Reiter's syndrome have documented a poor prognosis. A 20-year follow-up of Paronen's 1944 study of the Finnish *Shigella* epidemic[99] located 100 of the 344 original patients.[100] Of these patients, 80 had persistent active disease, 32 had ankylosing spondylitis, and 18 had recurrent arthritis. After a shipboard epidemic reported by Noer,[101] four of five patients had active and severe joint symptoms 13 years later.[46] At 1-year follow-up, 7 of 15 patients with post-*Salmonella* reactive arthritis had persistent joint symptoms[20]; at 10-year follow-up of *Yersinia* arthritis, only 5 of 85 patients had persistent joint complaints.[59]

The presence of HLA-B27 has prognostic significance. In a 10-year follow-up of 85 patients with *Yersinia* arthritis, more patients with HLA-B27 had low back pain and sacroiliitis, but there was no association of this genetic factor with the residual symptoms in peripheral joints.[59] In Butler's study, all seven patients who developed acute iritis were HLA-B27 positive.[98]

TREATMENT

The most significant advance in our understanding of Reiter's syndrome has been the demonstration of the persistence of microbial antigens, but not intact infectious bacteria, in the synovial membrane and fluid of patients with reactive arthritis. So far *Chlamydia, Salmonella,* and *Yersinia* antigens have been reported.[10–12, 28] These studies have raised the question as to whether long-term antimicrobial therapy could improve the outcome of reactive arthritis. Uncontrolled studies on the use of antibiotics have been inconclusive.[38] The only controlled study of short-term tetracycline in Reiter's syndrome failed to show any benefit.[102] Lauhio and colleagues[16] performed a double-blind, placebo-controlled study of 3 months of treatment with lymecycline in 40 patients with reactive arthritis. Lymecycline is a lysine conjugate of tetracycline, and it was used because of its tolerability and lack of interaction with milk products. They reported that 50 percent of patients with *Chlamydia*-triggered reactive arthritis recovered within 15 weeks when treated with lymecycline compared with 39.5 weeks in the placebo group ($P = 0.017$). Interestingly patients with post-*Yersinia* and post-*Campylobacter* arthritis failed to show any improvement. These findings, if confirmed, indicate the importance of searching for chlamydial infection in all suspected cases of reactive arthritis and treating all affected patients with a long-term tetracycline group antibiotic such as doxycycline.[102a] Sexual partners should be given 2 weeks of doxycycline. The possibility that early treatment of chlamydial infections may prevent the onset of arthritis, as reported in the Inuit population of Greenland,[103] deserves to be investigated. The next logical step would be to study the effect of long-term treatment of postdysenteric cases of reactive arthritis with an effective antibiotic such as trimethoprim-sulfa or one of the quinolones. The documentation of chlamydial infection during subsequent flares of the disease and the treatment of such episodes with prolonged antibiotics are also deserving of study.

Joint symptoms are best treated with the newer nonsteroidal anti-inflammatory drugs (NSAIDs). They are superior to aspirins and generally better tolerated, but high sustained doses often have to be used. For acute arthritis, indomethacin is often an effective drug. It is started at 25 mg four times per day with food, but the dosage may have to be incrementally raised to 200 mg per day. Strict bed rest is sometimes effective, but prolonged splinting of joints should be avoided because of the tendency toward fibrous ankylosis. Once the symptoms subside, usually within 1 to 2 weeks, range of motion and isometric strengthening exercises are prescribed. The accompanying fever is a good guide to clinical response, but the ESR may stay elevated.[5] Residual pain and tenderness in the plantar fascia or Achilles tendon should be treated with local glucocorticoid injection so the ankle can be mobilized early to avoid heel cord shortening and fibrous ankylosis. Heel and foot pain are a major source of disability in chronic Reiter's syndrome.[64]

Other NSAIDs, including diclofenac, naproxen, and piroxicam, are also effective. Phenylbutazone works in an occasional patient who is refractory to the other NSAIDs. The use of the NSAIDs and their side effects are discussed in detail in another chapter. With any of the NSAIDs, a month's treatment at maximum dosage is usually needed to induce a partial remission. Maintenance dosage is achieved judiciously by phased reduction over many months.

The patient with severe or intractable Reiter's syndrome represents one of the most challenging problems in clinical rheumatology. Systemic glucocorticoids are rarely beneficial, even at moderate doses of 20 to 40 mg per day. Repeated aspiration and injection of chronically inflamed joints with glucocorticoids in combination with a sequence of NSAIDs at full dosage are only occasionally effective.

When NSAIDs fail to control the arthritis, sulfasalazine may be added. In an open study, 16 patients with Reiter's syndrome were treated with sulfasalazine at a daily dosage of 2000 mg.[104] All patients showed a "profound improvement" between week 5 and 15, but 21 percent of patients had to stop the drug because of side effects. A placebo-controlled, double-blind study of sulfasalazine, published as an abstract, showed a beneficial response in reactive arthritis.[105] Mielants et al.[71] showed that with a clinical response to sulfasalazine, there was simultaneous disappearance of inflammatory lesions in the intestinal mucosa. In ulcerative colitis, the 5-aminosalicylic acid component of sulfasalazine is effective,[106] and in rheumatoid arthritis, sulfapyridine is effective.[107] Which of the two components is effective in reactive arthritis remains to be determined.

When the disease is aggressive and unremitting, cytotoxic therapy remains the only alternative. Before such treatment is considered, the patient should undergo HIV antibody testing. If it is positive, cytotoxic drugs are contraindicated. Methotrexate has been shown to be effective in several uncontrolled trials of small numbers of patients.[108–110] It is given weekly by the oral or intramuscular route at dosages of 10 to 50 mg. Once a remission is achieved, maintenance doses of 5 to 15 mg weekly are effective. Azathioprine was effective in a placebo-controlled study at a daily dosage of 1 to 2 mg per kg.[111] A beneficial response was observed within 4 to 8 weeks. Reiter's syndrome frequently pursues a relapsing course, with variable intervals of remission, punctuated by periods of acute exacerbation, so it is difficult to assess the efficacy of any form of therapy. It is a good policy to reduce the dosage of methotrexate or azathioprine as soon as a response is observed and to try to discontinue the drug during periods of quiescence. Gold salts, antimalarials, and penicillamine have not been generally accepted as effective drugs in the management of Reiter's syndrome.[108] Surgical or arthroscopic synovectomy is indicated when chronic effusions and extending popliteal cysts develop in the knee.

Few treatment options are available to the patient with severe Reiter's syndrome who is also HIV infected. Sulfasalazine can be safely used, and it is usually beneficial[79]; prednisone at low dosage may be judiciously prescribed, but prolonged treatment is unwise. A patient with AIDS and a 3-year history of oligoarthropathy, psoriasis, and cutaneous manifestations of Reiter's syndrome responded well to a combination of etretinate and topical fluorinated steroids.[112] The skin lesions cleared, and the arthritis improved.

References

1. Reiter, H.: Ueber eine bisher unerkannte Spirochateninfektion (Spirochaetosis arthritica). Dtsch. Med. Wschr. 42:1535, 1916.
2. Bauer, W., and Engelman, E. P.: Syndrome of unknown aetiology characterized by urethritis, conjunctivitis, and arthritis (so-called Reiter's disease). Trans. Assn. Am. Phy. 57:307, 1942.
3. Brewerton, D. A., Nicholls, A., Oates, J. K., et al.: Reiter's disease and HL-A 27. Lancet 2:996, 1973.
4. Arnett, F. C., McClusky, O. E., Schacter, B. Z., and Lordon, R. E.: Incomplete Reiter's syndrome: Discriminating features and HL-A W27 in diagnosis. Ann. Intern. Med. 84:8, 1976.
5. Wright, V., and Moll, J. M. H.: Seronegative Polyarthritis. Amsterdam, New Holland Biomedical Press, 1976.
6. Willkens, R. F., Arnett, F. C., Bitter, T., Calin, A., Fisher, L., Ford, D. K., Good, A. E., and Masi, A. T.: Reiter's syndrome: Evaluation of preliminary criteria for definite diagnosis. Arthritis Rheum. 24:844, 1981.
7. Boyer, G. S., Lanier, A. P., Templin, D. W., and Bulkow, L.: Spondyloarthropathy and rheumatoid arthritis in Alaskan Yupik Eskimos. J. Rheumatol. 17:489, 1990.
8. Khan, M. A., and van der Linden, S. M.: A wider spectrum of spondyloarthropathies. Sem. Arthritis Rheum. 20:107, 1990.
9. Ahvonen, P., Sievers, K., and Aho, K.: Arthritis associated with *Yersinia enterocolitica* infection. Acta Rheum. Scand. 15:232, 1969.
10. Keat, A., Thomas, B., Dixey, J., Osborn, M., Sonnex, C., and Taylor-Robinson, D.: *Chlamydia trachomatis* and reactive arthritis: The missing link. Lancet 1:72, 1987.
11. Granfors, K., Jalkanen, S., von Essen, R., Lahesmaa-Rantala, R., Isomaki, O., Pekkola-Heino, K., Merilahti-Palo, R., Saario, R., Isomaki, H., and Toivanen, A.: *Yersinia* antigens in synovial fluids cells from patients with reactive arthritis. N. Engl. J. Med. 320:216, 1989.
12. Granfors, K., Jalkanen, S., Lindberg, A. A., Maki-Ikola, O., von Essen, R., Lahesmaa-Rantala, R., Isomaki, H., Saario, R., Arnold, W. J., and Toivanen, A.: *Salmonella* lipopolysaccharide in synovial cells from patients with reactive arthritis. Lancet 335:685, 1990.
13. Lahesmanaa-Rantala, R., and Toivanen, A.: Clinical spectrum of reactive arthritis. *In* Toivanen, A., and Toivanen, P. (eds.): Reactive Arthritis. Boca Raton, FL, CRC Press, 1988, p. 1.
14. Arnett, F. C.: Seronegative spondylarthropathies. Bull. Rheum. Dis. 37:1, 1987.
15. Bergfeldt, L., Insulander, P., Lindblom, D., Moller, E., and Edhag, O.: HLA-B27: An important genetic risk factor for lone aortic regurgitation and severe conduction system abnormalities. Am. J. Med. 85:12, 1988.
16. Lauhio, A., Leirisalo-Repo, M., Lahdevirta, J., Saikku, P., and Repo, H.: Double-blind, placebo-controlled study of three-month treatment with lymecycline in reactive arthritis, with special reference to *Chlamydia* arthritis. Arthritis Rheum. 34:6, 1991.
17. Tiwari, J. L., and Terasaki, P. I.: Ankylosing spondylitis. In HLA and Disease Associations. New York, Springer Verlag, 1985.
18. Hammer, R. E., Maika, S. D., Richardson, J. A., Tang, J.-P., and Taurog, J. D.: Spontaneous inflammatory disease in transgenic rats expressing HLA-B27 and human beta2m: An animal model of HLA-B27–associated human disorder. Cell 63:1099, 1990.
19. Lopez de Castro, J. A.: HLA-B27 and HLA-A2 subtypes: Structure, evolution and function. Immunol. Today 10:239, 1989.
20. Inman, R. D., Johnston, E. A., Hodge, M., Falk, J., and Helewa, A.: Postdysenteric reactive arthritis: A clinical and immunogenetic study following an outbreak of salmonellosis. Arthitis Rheum. 31:1377, 1988.
20a. Kingsley, G., and Panayi, G.: Antigenic responses in reactive arthritis. Rheum. Dis. Clin. North Am. 18:49, 1992.

21. Gaston, J. S., Life, P. F., Bailey, L. C., and Bacon, P. A.: In vitro responses to a 65-kilodalton mycobacterial protein by synovial T cells from inflammatory arthritis patients. J. Immunol. 143:2494, 1989.

22. Inman, R. D., Chiu, B., Johnson, M. E., Vas, S., and Falk, J.: HLA class I-related impairment in IL-2 production and lymphocyte response to microbial antigens in reactive arthritis. J. Immunol. 142:4256, 1989.

23. Granfors, K.: Measurement of immunoglobulin M (IgM), IgG and IgA antibodies against Yersinia enterocolitica by enzyme-linked immunosorbent assay: Persistence of serum antibodies during disease. J. Clin. Microbiol. 9:336, 1979.

24. Granfors, K., Ogasawara, M., Hill, J. L., Lahesmaa-Rantala, R., Toivanen, A., and Yu, D. T. Y.: Analysis of IgA anti-lipolysaccharide antibodies in Yersinia-triggered reactive arthritis. J. Infect. Dis. 159:1142, 1989.

25. Van Bohemen, G. G., Nabbe, A. J. J. M., Landheer, J. E., Grumet, F. G., Mazurkiewicz, E. S., Dinant, H. J., Lionarons, R. J., van Bodegom, P. C., and Zanen, H. C.: HLA-B27M1M2 and high immune responsiveness to Shigella flexneri in post-dysenteric arthritis. Immunol. Lett. 13:71, 1986.

26. Hill, J. L., and Yu, D. T. Y.: Development of an experimental animal model for reactive arthritis induced by Yersinia enterocolitica. Infect. Immun. 55:721, 1987.

27. Nickerson, C. L., Luthra, H. S., Sararirayan, S., and David, C. S.: Susceptibility of HLA-B27 transgenic mice to Yersinia enterocolitica infection. Hum. Immunol. 28:382, 1990.

28. Schumacher, Jr., H. R., Magg, S., Cherian, P. V., Sleckman, J., Rothfuss, S., Claybourne, G., and Sieck, M.: Light and electron microscopic studies on the synovial membrane in Reiter's syndrome: Immunocytochemical identification of chlamydial antigens in patients with early disease. Arthritis Rheum. 31:937, 1988.

28a. Rahman, M. U., Cheema, M. A., Schumacher, H. R., and Hudson, A. P.: Molecular evidence for the presence of Chlamydia in the synovium of patients with Reiter's syndrome. Arthritis Rheum. 35:521, 1992.

29. Kievitis, F., Ivanyi, P., Krimpenfort, P., Berns, A., and Ploegh, H. L.: HLA restricted recognition of viral antigens in HLA transgenic mice. Nature 329:447, 1987.

29a. Madden, D. R., Giorga, J. C., Strominger, J. L., and Wiley, D. C.: The structure of HLA-B27 reveals nonamer self-peptides bound in an extended conformation. Nature 353:321, 1991.

30. Seager, K., Bashir, H. V., Geczy, A. F., Edmonds, J., and de Vere-Tyndall, A.: Evidence for a specific B27-associated cell surface marker on lymphocytes of patients with ankylosing spondylitis. Nature 227:68, 1979.

31. Schwimmbeck, P. L., Yu, D. T. Y., and Oldstone, M. B. A.: Auto-antibodies to HLA-B27 in the sera of HLA-B27 patients with ankylosing spondylitis and Reiter's syndrome: Molecular mimicry with Klebsiella pneumoniae nitrogenase reductase as potential mechanisms of autoimmune disease. J. Exp. Med. 166:173, 1987.

32. Stieglitz, H., Fosmire, S., and Lipsky, P. E.: Identification of a 2-Md plasmid from Shigella flexneri associated with reactive arthritis. Arthritis Rheum. 32:937, 1989.

33. Lahesmaa, R., Skurnik, M., Vaara, M., Leirisalo-Repo, M., Nissila, M., Gransfors, K., and Toivanen, P.: Molecular mimicry between HLA-B27 and Yersinia, Salmonella, Shigella and Klebsiella with the same region of HLA alpha1 helix. Clin. Exp. Immunol. 86(3):399, 1991.

34. Raybourne, R. B., Bunning, V. K., and Williams, K. M.: Reaction of anti–HLA-B monoclonal antibodies with envelope proteins of Shigella species. Evidence for molecular mimicry in the spondyloarthropathies. J. Immunol. 140:3489, 1988.

35. Zhang, J. J., Hamachi, M., Hamachi, T., Zhao, Y., and Yu, D. T. Y.: The bacterial outer membrane protein that reacts with anti–HLA-B27 antibodies is the OmpA protein. J. Immunol. 143:2955, 1989.

36. Tsuchiya, N., Husby, G., Williams, Jr., R. C., Stieglitz, H., Lipsky, P. E., and Inman, R. D.: Autoantibodies to the HLA-B27 sequence cross-reactive with the hypothetical peptide from the arthritis-associated Shigella plasmid. J. Clin. Invest. 86:1193, 1990.

37. Ewing, C., Ebringer, R., Tribbick, G., and Geysen, H. M.: Antibody activity in ankylosing spondylitis sera to two sites on HLA-B27.1 at MHC groove region (within sequence 65–85) and to a Klebsiella pneumoniae nitrogenase reductase peptide (within sequence 181–199). J. Exp. Med. 171:1635, 1990.

38. Calin, A.: Reiter's syndrome. In Kelley, W. N., Harris, E. D., Ruddy, S., and Sledge, C. B. (eds.): Textbook of Rheumatology. 3rd ed. Philadelphia, W. B. Saunders Co., 1989, p. 1038.

39. Michet, C. J., Machado, E. B. V., Ballard, D. J., and McKenna, C. H.: Epidemiology of Reiter's syndrome in Rochester, Minnesota: 1950–1980. Arthritis Rheum. 31:428, 1988.

40. Arvastson, B., Damgaard, K., and Winblad, S.: Clinical symptoms of infection with Yersinia enterocolitica. Scand. J. Infect. Dis. 3:37, 1971.

41. Leino, R., and Kalliomaki, J. L.: Yersiniosis as an internal disease. Ann. Intern. Med. 81:458, 1974.

42. Tertti, R., Granfors, K., Lehtonen, O. P., Mertsola, J., Makela, A. L., Valimaki, I., Hanninen, P., and Toivanen, A.: An outbreak of Yersinia pseudotuberculosis infection. J. Infect. Dis. 149:245, 1984.

43. Sievers, K., Ahvonen, P., and Aho, K.: Epidemiological aspects of Yersinia arthritis. Int. J. Epidemiol. 1:45, 1972.

44. Aho, K., Leirisalo-Repo, M., and Repo, H.: Reactive arthritis. Clin. Rheum. Dis. 11:25, 1985.

45. Keat, A., Maini, R. N., Nkwazi, G. C., Pegrum, G. D., Ridgway, G. L., and Scott, J. T.: Role of Chlamydia trachomatis and HLA-B27 in sexually acquired reactive arthritis. Br. Med. J. 1:605, 1978.

46. Calin, A., and Fries, J. F.: An "experimental" epidemic of Reiter's syndrome revisited: Follow-up evidence on genetic and environmental factors. Ann. Intern. Med. 84:564, 1976.

47. Lauhio, A., Lahdevirta, J., Janes, R., Kontiainen, S., and Repo, H.: Reactive arthritis associated with Shigella sonnei infection. Arthritis Rheum. 31:1190, 1988.

48. Mermel, L. A., and Osborn, T. G.: Clostridium difficile associated reactive arthritis in an HLA-B27–positive female: Report and literature review. J. Rheumatol. 16:133, 1989.

49. Weyand, C. M., and Goronzy, J. J.: Immune responses to Borrelia burgdorferi in patients with reactive arthritis. Arthritis Rheum. 32:1057, 1989.

50. Arnett, F. C.: The Lyme spirochete: Another cause of Reiter's syndrome? Arthritis Rheum. 32:1182, 1989.

51. Xing-hua, C., and Gui-ying, S.: Reiter's syndrome: Clinical analysis of 22 cases. Chin. Med. J. 95:533, 1982.

52. Stein, M., Davis, P., Emmanuel, J., and West, G.: The spondyloarthropathies in Zimbabwe: A clinical and immunogenetic profile. J. Rehumatol. 17:1337, 1990.

53. Rosenberg, A. M., and Petty, R. E.: A syndrome of seronegative enthesopathy and arthropathy in children. Arthritis Rheum. 25:1041, 1982.

54. Gerster, J.-C., and Piccinin, P.: Enthesopathy of the heels in juvenile onset seronegative B-27 positive spondyloarthropathy. J. Rheumatol. 12:310, 1985.

55. Weisman, L. F., Hebert, J. C., and Cooper, S. M.: Reiter's syndrome and recurrent peritonitis after appendectomy. Surgery 101:508, 1987.

56. Russell, A. S., Davis, P., Percy, J. S., and Lentle, B. C.: The sacroiliitis of acute Reiter's syndrome. J. Rheumatol. 4:293, 1977.

57. Bluestone, R.: Practical Rheumatology. Menlo Park, CA, Addison-Wesley, 1980, p. 195.

58. Keat, A.: Reiter's syndrome and reactive arthritis in perspective. N. Engl. J. Med. 309:1606, 1983.

59. Leirisalo-Repo, M., and Suoranta, H.: Ten-year followup study of patients with Yersinia arthritis. Arthritis Rheum. 31:533, 1988.

60. Good, A. E.: Reiter's disease and ankylosing spondylitis. Acta Rheum. Scand. 11:305, 1965.

61. Berg, R. L., Weinberger, H., and Dienes, L.: Acute hemorrhagic cystitis. Am. J. Med. 22:848, 1957.

62. Rubin, R. A., Goldfarb, R. A., Lidsky, M. D., and Abrams, J.: Decreased activity of Reiter's syndrome after urethrectomy. Arthritis Rheum. 33:885, 1990.

63. Yli-Kerttula, U. I., and Vilppula, A. H.: Reactive salpingitis. In Toivanen, A., and Toivanen, P (eds.): Reactive Arthritis. Boca Raton, FL, CRC Press, 1988, p. 125.

64. Fox, R., Calin, A., Gerber, R. C., and Gibson, D.: The chronicity of symptoms and disability in Reiter's syndrome: An analysis of 131 consecutive patients. Ann. Intern. Med. 91:190, 1979.

65. Gutierrez, F. J., and Espinoza, L. R.: Reactive arthritis: Diagnostic considerations. J. Musculoskel. Med. 7:43, 1990.

66. Ahvonen, P.: Human yersiniosis in Finland. II. Clinical features. Ann. Clin. Res. 4:39, 1972.

67. Rosenbaum, J. T.: Characterization of uveitis associated with spondyloarthritis. J. Rheumatol. 16:792, 1989.

68. Youssef, W., and Russell, A. S.: Cardiac, ocular, and renal manifestations of seronegative spondyloarthropathies. Curr. Opinion Rheumatol. 2:582, 1990.

69. Mielants, H., Veys, E. M., Cuvelier, C., De Vos, M., and Botelberghe, L.: HLA-B27 related arthritis and bowel inflammation. Part 2. Ileocolonoscopy and bowel histology in patients with HLA-B27 related arthritis. J. Rheumatol. 12:294, 1985.

70. Mielants, H., Veys, E. M., Joos, R., Noens, L., Cuvelier, C., and De Vos, M.: HLA antigens in seronegative spondyloarthropathies. Reactive arthritis and arthritis in ankylosing spondylitis: Relation to gut inflammation. J. Rheumatol. 14:466, 1987.

71. Mielants, H., Veys, E. M., Joos, R., Cuvelier, C., and De Vos, M.: Repeat ileocolonoscopy in reactive arthritis. J. Rheumatol. 14:456, 1987.

71a. Deer, T., Rosencrance, J. G., and Chillag, S. A.: Cardiac conduction manifestations of Reiter's syndrome. South. Med. J. 84:799, 1991.

72. Haverman, J. F., Van Albada-Kuipers, G. A., Dohmen, H. J., and Dijkmans, B. A.: Atrioventricular conduction disturbance as an early feature of Reiter's syndrome. Ann. Rheum. Dis. 47:1017, 1988.

73. Shetty, H. G., Fraser, A. G., Phillips, D. I., Lazarus, J. H., and Williams, B. D.: Carotid sinus hypersensitivity and complete heart block in Reiter's syndrome. Br. J. Rheumatol. 27:321, 1988.

74. LaBresh, K. A., Lally, E. V., Sharma, S. C., and Ho, G.: Two-dimensional echocardiographic detection of preclinical aortic root abnormalities in rheumatoid variant diseases. Am. J. Med. 78:908, 1985.

75. Bruneau, C., Villiaumey, J., Avouac, B., Martigny, J., Laurent, J., Pichot, A., Belghiti, D., and Lagrue, G.: Seronegative spondyloarthropathies and IgA glomerulonephritis: A report of four cases and a review of the literature. Sem. Arthritis Rheum. 15:179, 1986.

76. Anderson, C. J., Gregory, M. C., Groggeland, G. C., and Clegg, D. O.: Amyloidosis and Reiter's syndrome: Report of a case and review of the literature. Am. J. Kidney Dis. 14:319, 1989.

77. Good, A. E.: Reiter's disease: A review with special attention to cardiovascular and neurologic sequelae. Semin. Arthritis Rheum. 3:253, 1974.

78. Sadana, A., Merrick-Thomas, D., and Scott, D. L.: Vasculitis in Reiter's syndrome. Clin. Rheumatol. 7:114, 1988.

79. Winchester, R., Bernstein, D. H., Fischer, H. D., Enlow, R., and Solomon, G.: The co-occurrence of Reiter's syndrome and acquired immunodeficiency. Ann. Intern. Med. 106:19, 1987.

80. Espinoza, L. R., Aguilar, J. L., Berman, A., Gutierrez, F. J., Vasey, F. B., and Germain, B. F.: Rheumatic manifestations associated with human immunodeficiency virus infection. Arthritis Rheum. 32:1615, 1989.

81. Buskilla, D., Langevitz, P., Tenenbaum, J., and Gladman, D. D.: Malar rash in a patient with Reiter's syndrome—a clue for the diagnosis of human immunodeficiency virus infection. J. Rheumatol. 17:843, 1990.

82. Hughes, R. A., and Keat, A. C. S.: Yersinia reactive arthritis and human immunodeficiency virus infection. Arthritis Rheum. 33:758, 1990.

83. Davis, P., Stein, M., Latif, A., and Emmanuel, J.: Acute arthritis in Zimbabwean patients: Possible relationship to human immunodeficiency virus infection. J. Rheumatol. 16:346, 1989.

84. Winchester, R., Brancato, L., Itescu, S., Skovron, M. L., and Solomon, G.: Implications from the occurrence of Reiter's syndrome and related disorders in association with advanced HIV infection. Scand. J. Rheumatol. (Suppl.) 74:89, 1988.

85. Schachter, J.: Chlamydial infections. West. J. Med. 153:523, 1990.

86. Errs, R. K.: DNA-probes: An overview and comparison with current methods. Lab. Med. 19:295, 1988.

87. Pekin, R. J., Malinin, T. I., and Zvaifler, N. J.: Unusual synovial fluid findings in Reiter's syndrome. Ann. Intern. Med. 66:677, 1967.

88. Thomson, G. T. D., and Inman, R. D.: Diagnostic conundra in the spondyloarthropathies: Towards a base for revised nosology. J. Rheumatol. 17:426, 1990.

89. Bergfeldt, L., Edhag, O., and Rajs, J.: HLA-B27–associated heart disease: Clinicopathologic study of three cases. Am. J. Med. 77:961, 1984.

90. Canoso, J. J., Wohlgethan, J. R., Newberg, A. H., and Goldsmith, M. R.: Aspiration of the retrocalcaneal bursa. Ann. Rheum. Dis. 43:308, 1984.

91. Resnik, D.: Reiter's syndrome. In Resnik, D., and Niwayama, G. (eds.): Diagnosis of Bone and Joint Disorders. Vol 2. 2nd ed. Philadelphia, W. B. Saunders Co., 1988, p. 1199.

92. Wright, V.: Seronegative polyarthritis: A unified concept. Arthritis Rheum. 21:619, 1978.

93. Ahlstrom, H., Feltelius, N., Nyman, R., and Hallgren, R.: Magnetic resonance imaging of sacroiliac joint inflammation. Arthritis Rheum. 33:1763, 1990.

94. Santavirta, S., Slatis, P., Sandelin, J., Lindqvist, C., and Konttinen, Y. T.: Atlanto-axial subluxation in patients with seronegative spondylarthritis. Rheumatol. Int. 7:43, 1987.

95. Kransdorf, M. J., Wehrle, P. A., Moser, R. P., Jr.: Atlantoaxial subluxation in Reiter's syndrome. A report of three cases and review of the literature. Spine 13:12, 1988.

96. Melsom, R. D., Benjamin, J. C., and Barnes, C. G.: Spontaneous atlantoaxial subluxation: An unusual presenting manifestation of Reiter's syndrome. Ann. Rheum. Dis. 48:170, 1989.

97. Veasy, L., Wiedmeier, S., Orsmond, G., Ruttenberg, H., et al.: Resurgence of acute rheumatic fever in the intermountain area of the United States. N. Engl. J. Med. 316:421, 1987.

98. Butler, M. J., Russell, A. S., Percy, J. S., and Lentle, B. C.: A follow-up study of 48 patients with Reiter's syndrome. Am. J. Med. 67:808, 1979.

99. Paronen, I.: Reiter's disease: A study of 344 cases observed in Finland. Acta Med. Scand. (Suppl.) 131:1, 1948.

100. Sairanen, D., Paronen, I., and Mohonen, H.: Reiter's syndrome: A follow-up study. Acta Med. Scand. 185:57, 1969.

101. Noer, H. R.: An "experimental" epidemic of Reiter's syndrome. J.A.M.A. 198:693, 1966.

102. Popert, A. J., Gill, A. J., and Laird, S. M.: A prospective study of Reiter's syndrome: An interim report on the first 82 cases. Br. J. Vener. Dis. 40:160, 1964.

102a. Bardin, T., and Schumacher, H. R.: Should we treat postvenereal Reiter's syndrome by antibiotics? J. Rheumatol. 18:1780, 1991.

103. Bardin, T., Enel, C., Cornelis, F., Salski, C., Jorgensen, C., Ward, R., and Lathrop, G. M.: Antibiotic treatment of venereal disease and Reiter's syndrome in a Greenland population. Arthritis Rheum. 35:190, 1992.

104. Stroehmann, I., Wustenhagen, E., and Martini, M.: Therapy of seronegative oligoarthritis with Salazopyrine. Z. Rheumatol. 46:79, 1987.

105. Peliskova, Z., Pavelka, Jr., K., and Trnavsky, K.: A placebo-controlled, double-blind study of Salazopyrin-EN (SASP) in refractory reactive arthritis (ReA) (Abstract). Scand. J. Rheumatol. (Suppl.) 85:45, 1990.

106. Dew, M., Hughes, P., Harries, A. D., Williams, G., Evans, B. K., and Rhodes, J.: Maintenance of remission in ulcerative colitis with oral preparation of 5-aminosalicylic acid. Br. Med. J. 285:1012, 1982.

107. Pullar, T., Hunter, J. A., and Capell, H. A.: Which component of sulphasalazine is active in rheumatoid arthritis? Br. Med. J. 290:1535, 1985.

108. Editorial: Treating Reiter's syndrome. Lancet 2:1125, 1987.

109. Owen, E. T., and Cohen, M. L.: Methotrexate in Reiter's disease. Ann. Rheum. Dis. 38:48, 1979.

110. Lally, E. V., and Ho, Jr., G.: A review of methotrexate therapy in Reiter's syndrome. Sem. Arthritis Rheum. 15:139, 1985.

111. Calin, A.: A placebo-controlled cross-over study of azathioprine in Reiter's syndrome. Ann. Rheum. Dis. 45:653, 1986.

112. Belz, J., Breneman, D. L., Nordlund, J. J., and Solinger, A.: Successful treatment of a patient with Reiter's syndrome and acquired immunodeficiency syndrome using etretinate. J. Am. Acad. Dermatol. 20:898, 1989.

Chapter 58

Psoriatic Arthritis

Clement J. Michet

INTRODUCTION

The association between psoriasis and arthritis was first observed by the French in the early 19th century. Alibert described the occurrence of psoriasis and arthritis.[1] The term *psoriasis arthritique* was introduced later by Bazin.[2] Earlier in the 20th century, the association between psoriasis and arthritis was supported by a number of case reports. The relationship was established by the work of Wright and Baker based on clinical observation and verified by epidemiologic studies.[3, 4]

Psoriatic arthritis differs from rheumatoid arthritis on the basis of the pattern of arthritic involvement, rheumatoid factor negativity, and roentgenographic features. Because these patients may have sacroiliitis or spondylitis, psoriatic arthritis is classified as a seronegative spondyloarthropathy. The association with HLA-B27, however, is less than that which occurs in idiopathic ankylosing spondylitis or Reiter's syndrome.[5]

EPIDEMIOLOGY

Psoriatic arthritis is an uncommon disease in the community and probably occurs in no more than 5 percent of the general psoriatic population.[6] Cross-sectional surveys or specialty clinic and hospital based psoriatic populations provide widely disparate prevalence estimates for psoriatic arthritis, ranging up to nearly 50 percent, reflecting the bias of studies using highly selected, referred patient populations with disproportionate representation of the more seriously ill. When broader population surveys have addressed the issue, the prevalence of inflammatory arthritis among psoriatics is lower. Lomholt[7] identified only four cases of arthritis among 253 Faroe Island psoriasis patients. Hellgren[6] documented a 5 percent prevalence of inflammatory arthritis, including both psoriatic and rheumatoid arthritis, among psoriatics in a Swedish population survey. The majority of musculoskeletal complaints among psoriatics reflect symptoms related to osteoarthritis and soft tissue rheumatic disease syndromes occurring in no greater frequency than that among the general population.[8]

GENETICS

A genetic predisposition to psoriatic arthritis exists. Psoriasis is four times more common in pa-

tients with seronegative arthritis than in patients with seropositive arthritis.[9] First-degree relatives of arthritic probands may be up to 50 times more likely to develop psoriatic arthritis than the general population.[10] Within a family, there may be some members who develop only the skin disease, and others only seronegative arthritis; further, there may be no consistent pattern of temporal onset of psoriasis and arthritis among relatives.[10, 11] Psoriatic arthritis is thought to be dominantly inherited with variable penetrance.[12, 13] Preliminary DNA probe analysis of the switch region of the immunoglobulin heavy chain genes using restriction fragment length polymorphism (RFLP) analysis has revealed a 2.6 kilobase (kb) band, which may be a marker for susceptibility to peripheral arthritis in psoriasis.[14] A report of discordance for psoriatic arthritis in monozygotic twins indicates that environmental factors also influence disease expression.[15]

HLA typing among patient populations reveals polygenetic influences in psoriasis and psoriatic arthritis. HLA-Cw6 has been most frequently observed to occur in the entire psoriatic population,[16] although in children, HLA-A2 and HLA-B17 are most frequently increased.[17] HLA-B38 or B39, splits of HLA-B16, have been linked to psoriatic arthritis in a number of studies.[18, 19] HLA-B27 is observed in 46 to 78 percent of psoriatic spondylitics. Attempts to correlate specific HLA phenotypes with patterns and severity of peripheral arthritis have generally been unsuccessful. Some authors have reported a relationship between DR4 and rheumatoid-like polyarthritis,[19] DR3 and erosive disease,[20] B27 with distal interphalangeal joint involvement,[19, 21] and DR4, B38 with earlier asymmetric joint disease[22, 23] as well as the B17/Cw6 haplotype for oligoarthritis.[24]

HLA class II allele analysis has demonstrated an association with HLA-DR1 and a HLA-DR7 subtype DR7a, possibly via linkage to HLA-Cw6 in one study, but no association with DR7 in another.[25, 26] No association with HLA-DQ, HLA-DP, or T cell receptor genes has been observed.

ETIOLOGY AND PATHOGENESIS

There are microvascular abnormalities in both normal and involved skin of psoriatic patients, including excessive capillary tortuosity and coiling.[27, 28] These capillaries display a multilayered basement membrane with fenestrations.[29] Nail fold capillary microscopy demonstrates a decrease in the number of vessels with engorged capillary tufts.[30] Study of involved synovium in psoriatic arthritis reveals endothelial cell swelling, thickening of the vessel walls, and an inflammatory cell infiltration.[31]

Psoriatic arthritis may represent a form of reactive arthritis in which the inciting environmental triggers are the streptococci and staphylococci in psoriatic plaques and nails. Psoriatic arthritis patients have higher levels of antistreptococcal DNAase beta (β) and antistaphylococcal alpha (α) toxin as well as antistaphylococcal peptidoglycan antibodies than those persons with uncomplicated psoriasis.[32–34] Microbial antigens could act as superantigens as well, generating T cell cross-reactivity with autoantigens. It has been demonstrated that the epidermis of psoriatic arthritis patients more frequently contains HLA-DR positive keratinocytes than the skin of psoriatic patients without arthritis.[34–36] These cells may activate HLA-DR–positive T lymphocytes in the dermis by processing antigenic bacterial cell wall peptidoglycans.

The major internal protein (P27) of a retrovirus-like particle is expressed by epidermal cells in psoriatic lesions, uninvolved skin, and fewer than 1 percent of peripheral blood lymphocytes in psoriatic patients.[37, 38] This antigen is also expressed on less than 1 percent of mononuclear synovial membrane cells and some synovial blood vessel cell walls from patients with psoriasis, rheumatoid arthritis, and ankylosing spondylitis. Possibly a product of an endogenous retrovirus genome, its antigenic determinants may lead to immune complex formation, contributing to the inflammatory process of both psoriasis and psoriatic arthritis.

The possibility that trauma may precipitate psoriatic arthritis, the *deep Koebner effect,* has been suggested by several case reports. Post-traumatic synovitis as well as acro-osteolysis has been described.[39]

There are multiple immunologic factors observed that potentially perpetuate joint inflammation in psoriasis. Plasma cells contain gamma immunoglobulin G (IgG) and IgA, differing from seropositive rheumatoid arthritis in which IgM and C3 are found in psoriatic synovium in addition to IgA and IgG.[40] Synovial tissue from psoriatic arthritis patients contains T cell lymphocytic infiltration, similar to seropositive rheumatoid arthritis.[41]

Serum rheumatoid factor is found in a small percentage of the subgroup of persons who have the polyarthritis pattern of psoriatic arthritis. Hidden rheumatoid factor, closely bound to IgG, has not been observed.[42] Study of in vitro synthesis of IgM and IgM rheumatoid factor by peripheral blood B cells from psoriatic arthritis patients shows that the IgM rheumatoid factor is not spontaneously formed as it is in seropositive rheumatoid arthritis.[43]

Approximately 60 percent of patients with psoriatic arthritis have circulating immune complexes[44] containing IgG, and most have an elevation of serum IgG and IgA; there is no relationship between the level of circulating immune complexes and disease activity.[45] The IgA complexes are found in all patterns of psoriatic arthritis, but the titers are higher in patients with severe peripheral arthritis. The role of these complexes in disease is not known. Like rheumatoid arthritis, autoantibodies to collagen are also observed in some psoriatic arthritis cases.[46]

There is a suppressor cell defect and a reduction in suppressor cells in psoriasis and psoriatic arthritis.[47, 48] The total T cell population in psoriasis is normal, but the early and late erythrocyte rosettes are diminished. This may be due to the presence of immature T cells, or the sheep red blood cell receptors may be blocked.

PATHOLOGY

The primary pathologic lesion in the peripheral arthritis of psoriasis is a synovitis, which is generally indistinguishable from that of rheumatoid arthritis. Synovium from involved larger joints in psoriatic arthritis such as the knee shows hypertrophic villi, lymphocytes, and lymphocytic germinal centers identical to the findings in rheumatoid arthritis.[49] Other authors report that the psoriatic synovial membrane contains more proliferating fibroblasts, edema, and vessel wall necrosis.[31] Vascular lesions are a dominant feature in the involved psoriatic synovium of large joints. Vascular changes include endothelial cell swelling, thickening of the vessel wall, and an inflammatory cell infiltration. The early lesion in the involved small finger joints includes thickening of the synovial membrane and swelling. Later lesions reveal fibrous reaction, some villous formation, and inflammatory cell infiltration.[50] The c-*myc* proto-oncogene is expressed in psoriatic synovial lining cells and may play a role in the proliferative lesion.[51]

Examination of advanced involvement of the distal finger joints in psoriatic arthritis shows articular destruction, bone reabsorption, and marginal bone overgrowth at the sites of tendon insertion. The widened joint spaces are replaced by a cellular fibrous tissue with no trace of residual synovial membrane.[49, 52]

CLINICAL FEATURES

The onset of psoriatic arthritis is usually insidious, but in approximately one third of the patients it may develop acutely, mimicking gout or septic tenosynovitis or arthritis.[53] The age at onset is similar to that for rheumatoid arthritis, occurring commonly between ages 35 and 45. The sex ratio differs, however; in psoriatic arthritis, the female-to-male ratio is approximately 1:1, similar to the ratio in psoriasis without arthritis.

Several distinct subtypes of psoriatic arthritis have been described.[3, 53, 54, 55a] One pattern may evolve into another, resulting in heterogeneous combinations of joint disease. The dominant distal joint involvement is unique for psoriasis. The oligoarticular form is similar to the peripheral arthritis that complicates other spondyloarthropathies. Both of these patterns clinically distinguish psoriatic arthritis from typical rheumatoid arthritis. Sacroiliitis and spondylitis may be associated with each of the peripheral patterns.[55] One half to two thirds of the patients will present with a monoarticular or oligoarticular arthritis.

Pattern of Joint Involvement

Asymmetric Oligoarticular Arthritis

This is the most common pattern and accounts for more than one half of the patients.[54, 56] The distal interphalangeal joints, proximal interphalangeal joints of the hands and feet, and metatarsophalangeal joints are usually involved first. The knees, hips, ankles, and wrists may also be affected. There may be associated tendon sheath inflammation, giving the involved digit a sausage shape (Fig. 58–1).

Predominantly Distal Interphalangeal Joint Involvement

This classic type of psoriatic arthritis is commonly related to psoriatic nail disease (Fig. 58–2).[39, 54] This pattern usually occurs as an oligoarticular form and is observed in only 5 to 10 percent of patients.

Arthritis Mutilans

In approximately 5 percent of patients, the distal arthritis in one or more joints progresses to osteolysis of the involved phalanges, with resulting severe deformities (Fig. 58–3). The deformities have been described as *telescoping* and *opera-glass*, or *doigt en lorgenette*, deformities.[4] A subset of patients, aged 20 to 40, have mutilans, severe widespread skin disease, and usually associated sacroiliitis.[56]

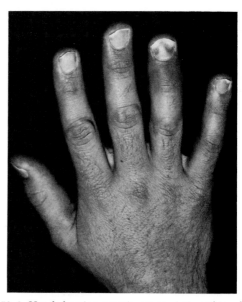

Figure 58–2. Hand showing prominent psoriatic nail involvement of fourth finger and swelling of the fourth distal interphalangeal joint.

Polyarthritis

This group usually represents fewer than 25 percent of patients with psoriatic arthritis.[54] In two university clinic–based studies, however, this pattern represented more than 60 percent of the cases.[55, 55a] Some persons with polyarthritis are seropositive and may represent coincidental rheumatoid arthritis. Others are clinically indistinguishable from rheumatoid arthritis but are seronegative and have a predilection for involvement of the wrists, proximal interphalangeal joints, and distal interphalangeal joints as well as fusion of joints (Fig. 58–4). The arthritis is usually less extensive and deforming than that seen in seropositive rheumatoid arthritis, and half of the cases have asymmetric involvement.[55]

Spinal Involvement

Spinal and sacroiliac disease may occur in all of the seronegative peripheral patterns of arthritis and is often asymptomatic. Sacroiliac joint involvement occurs in 20 to 40 percent of patients with psoriatic arthritis.[57] Spondylitis as manifest by syndesmophytes may be found in as many as 40 percent of the patients with psoriatic arthritis.[58] It may occur without sacroiliitis and can affect any portion of the spine randomly with marginal or submarginal syndesmophytes (Fig. 58–5).[57] The cervical spine may be preferentially involved. One pattern of spondylitis affects males, who have a later onset of psoriasis, associated iritis, infrequent peripheral arthritis, and progression of the spinal involvement from the sacroiliac joints cephalad. This probably represents a coincidental ankylosing spondylitis, and the cases are usually HLA-B27 positive.[58, 59] Another pattern affects both sexes equally, with random occurrence

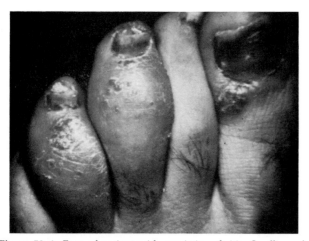

Figure 58–1. Foot of patient with psoriatic arthritis. Swelling of the toes gives them a sausage-shaped appearance.

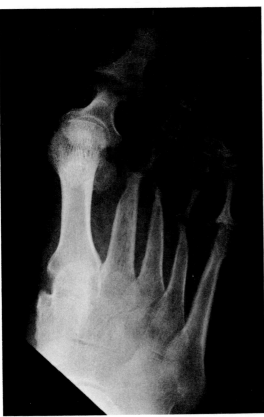

Figure 58–3. Radiograph of foot showing destructive changes of the first interphalangeal joint with widening. Destructive changes of distal ends of second through fifth metatarsals and proximal ends of proximal phalanges with tapering. Note complete osteolysis of the third phalanx.

of the spinal submarginal syndesmophytes, sacroiliac involvement, and peripheral arthritis.[58] This type of spinal involvement seems to be more uniquely associated with psoriasis. HLA-B27 positivity correlates with the sacroiliac involvement.

Unusual Articular Manifestations

Rarely, patients with severe psoriasis develop resorption of the distal phalanx, and acro-osteolysis, without any clinical or radiographic evidence of arthritis.[59] The cervical spine may be involved in a manner similar to rheumatoid arthritis, with resulting C-1–C-2, lateral, and subaxial subluxation.[60–62] The temporomandibular joint can be involved, with destructive changes and, rarely, osteolysis.[63]

Sternocostoclavicular arthro-osteitis associated with pustulosis palmoplantaris (PPP) has been described in Japan as well as in other populations.[64, 65] Characterized by sclerosis and periostitis of the anterior thoracic articulations, this syndrome may also involve the pelvis, lumbar spine, and peripheral joints.[66, 67] Children may present with the syndrome of chronic recurrent multifocal osteomyelitis, accompanied by PPP or the usual psoriatic lesions.[68] There are no associations with HLA-B27 observed in these entities, and the causes are unknown.

Skin Involvement

In most cases, psoriasis precedes the arthritis, often for several years. As many as 15 to 20 percent of patients may develop the psoriasis after arthritis[3, 55] (see Chapter 33). No particular pattern of psoriasis is associated with arthritis, and the involvement may vary from small hidden patches in the scalp or perineum to a generalized exfoliation. Although psoriasis tends to be more extensive in those patients with widespread, deforming arthritis, the majority of arthritis patients do not have extensive skin disease.[69] The frequency of synchronous flares of the skin and joints is debatable and occurs in only a small proportion of patients, possibly in those with no underlying spondylitis.[70]

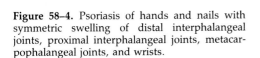

Figure 58–4. Psoriasis of hands and nails with symmetric swelling of distal interphalangeal joints, proximal interphalangeal joints, metacarpophalangeal joints, and wrists.

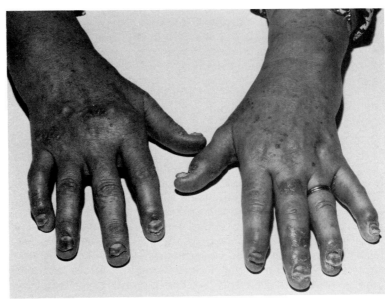

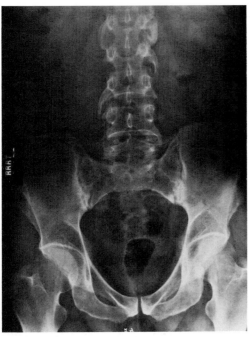

Figure 58–5. Lumbar spine and pelvic radiograph showing asymmetric nonmarginal syndesmophytes and sacroiliitis.

Nail disease is observed in 80 percent of psoriatic arthritis cases, compared with only 15 percent of uncomplicated psoriatics.[3, 71] The clinical signs of psoriatic nail involvement are listed in Table 58–1.[72] The types of nail involvement in the order of frequency are (1) thickening (hyperkeratosis) beginning at the distal nail, (2) separation of the subungual bed, (3) nail ridging and cracking, (4) nail pitting, and (5) spoon-shaped nails secondary to the hyperkeratosis.[3]

There is an association between distal joint arthritis and nail disease. A synchronous flare of the joints and nails occurs more commonly than a flare of the joints and skin.[69] Patients with more severe arthritis tend to have greater nail involvement.[73]

Extra-Articular Features

Extra-articular manifestations characterizing seropositive rheumatoid arthritis do not occur in psoriatic arthritis. Eye inflammation accompanies psoriatic arthritis in approximately 30 percent of patients, with conjunctivitis in about 20 percent and iritis in 7 percent.[74] The iritis is more commonly associated with sacroiliitis or spondylitis. It may be chronic but usually follows a benign course, similar to the iritis associated with idiopathic ankylosing spondylitis. Iritis is more common in the male subset of patients with deforming arthritis. Other uncommon extra-articular manifestations of spondylitis, such as aortic insufficiency and upper lobe pulmonary fibrosis, may also occur in the setting of psoriatic spondylitis. Amyloidosis complicating long-standing psoriasis and arthritis has been observed.[75] A noninflamma-

Table 58–1. CLINICAL SIGNS OF NAIL PSORIASIS

Nail Plate
  Pits
  Furrows or transverse depressions (Beau's lines)
  Crumbling nail plate
  Leukonychia with rough surface

Nail Bed
  Splinter hemorrhages
  Oval, reddish discoloration of entire or partial nail bed
  Horny mass simulating fallen nail plate

Hyponychium
  Accumulated horny debris under nail plate
  Onycholysis often involving nail bed
  Yellowish-green discoloration of material under nail bed in
    onycholytic area

tory myopathy has rarely been reported.[76] Relapsing polychondritis may rarely complicate psoriatic arthritis.[77]

DIAGNOSIS

Psoriatic arthritis is diagnosed by the presence of psoriasis or psoriatic nail disease and a seronegative inflammatory peripheral arthritis, with or without axial skeletal involvement. The pattern of peripheral arthritis may be a monoarthritis, sausage-like swelling of the distal joint, asymmetric oligoarthritis, symmetric rheumatoid-like arthritis, or destructive arthritis of the distal joints.[56]

Occasionally, the pattern of joint involvement will suggest psoriatic arthritis in a person without current skin lesions. Psoriasis must be sought in hidden areas, including the scalp, internatal cleft, perineum, umbilicus, and groin. Psoriasis must be accurately differentiated from other types of skin disease, particularly seborrheic dermatitis (Table 58–2). When psoriatic nail involvement is the only cutaneous manifestation, a fungus infection must be

Table 58–2. CRITERIA FOR BORDERLINE PSORIASIS

Psoriasis in the scalp must be palpable.
Mild psoriasis of the scalp simulating dandruff must show areas of uninvolved skin between patches.
In the presence of eczema, seborrhea corporis, or seborrheic dermatitis anywhere on the body, lesions other than classic plaques on the scalp or elsewhere cannot be accepted as psoriasis.
Toenail lesions alone cannot be accepted as evidence of psoriasis.
Only classic fingernail lesions of psoriasis can be accepted in the absence of unequivocal psoriasis elsewhere or a definite previous history of psoriasis. Culture of the nail should have excluded infection.
Flexural lesions in the absence of psoriasis elsewhere are rare and should be accepted only in the presence of other lesions. They may be accepted if they appear classic. Scrapings must exclude tinea or *Candida* infection.
Pustular dermatosis of the palms and soles cannot be accepted as psoriasis in the absence of unequivocal lesions of the skin elsewhere or nail lesions.

excluded by the appropriate cultures. Isolated nail pitting occurs commonly in nonpsoriatics. It has been estimated that 20 fingernail pits per person suggests psoriasis, and more than 60 is seen only in psoriasis.[78]

Keratoderma blennorrhagicum is clinically and histologically similar to pustular psoriasis. Other lesions, ulcers of the mucous membranes and circinate balanitis, support the diagnosis of Reiter's syndrome.[79] There are some cases of Reiter's syndrome with keratoderma blennorrhagicum, however, that may eventually evolve into typical psoriasis and psoriatic arthritis.[80]

Asymmetric distal and proximal interphalangeal finger joint involvement may resemble inflammatory osteoarthritis. Osteoarthritis is characterized by bone hypertrophy and joint space narrowing, roentgenographically differing from the distal joint space widening in psoriatic arthritis. When monoarticular psoriatic arthritis occurs acutely, gout or infection must also be considered. Synovial fluid should be obtained, analyzed for monosodium urate crystals, and cultured. A symmetric polyarthritis in the setting of psoriasis may represent the chance occurrence of rheumatoid arthritis. If the patient with psoriasis and symmetric polyarthritis remains seronegative and has sacroiliac or spinal involvement, this is most likely psoriatic arthritis.

OUTCOME

As a group, patients with psoriatic arthritis suffer less functional impairment and loss of time from work than rheumatoid patients.[81] Many patients will have relatively asymptomatic periods with episodic flares of synovitis. The oligoarticular form tends to be least aggressive. This is not an entirely benign arthropathy, however, as up to 12 percent of one clinic population were classified as American Rheumatism Association (ARA) functional class III or IV.[82] Although signs of inflammatory synovitis may be controlled, the risk of progressive joint disease exists, with up to 41 percent of the cases having five or more damaged joints after 5 years of follow-up.[82] Specific risk factors for more aggressive disease have not been completely identified, but the mutilans variant tends to occur in patients with more extensive skin and nail disease.[4] The spinal arthritis may progress radiographically, but symptoms and spinal mobility may remain stable, possibly owing to the segmental "skip" lesion tendency in psoriatic spondylitis.[83]

Mortality in psoriatic arthritis is usually due to the presence of an unrelated disease, but fatal complications from treatment with glucocorticoids or cytotoxic drugs may occur.[56] In one study of 16 deaths in patients with psoriatic arthritis, five deaths were due to myocardial infarction, but other common causes of death were attributable to possible glucocorticoid toxicity, including perforated peptic ulcer, staphylococcal septicemia, and accelerated hypertension.

The association of psoriatic arthritis and acquired immunodeficiency syndrome (AIDS) is an interesting one, is obviously linked to a higher mortality in the psoriatic patients, and is reviewed extensively in Chapter 73.

CHILDHOOD PSORIATIC ARTHRITIS

Psoriatic arthritis occurs in a small percentage of patients with psoriasis before the age of 16, more commonly in females. The peak incidence ages may be bimodal, with an early peak in girls less than age four and a later peak near puberty with boys predominating.[84, 85] Psoriasis is observed initially in about half of the cases but may only appear years later in others. Psoriatic nail involvement is as common as in adults. There is a strong history of psoriasis in the families of patients with psoriatic arthritis. The arthritis often develops acutely, initially involving the knee. Although usually monoarticular or oligoarticular in onset, the arthritis frequently progresses to asymmetric polyarticular involvement. Distal and proximal interphalangeal involvement of the small joints of the feet occurs more than in the juvenile rheumatoid arthritis.[86] Sacroiliitis occurs in up to 30 percent of the children. Tenosynovial involvement, dactylitis, may be present in half the patients. Uveitis complicates childhood psoriatic arthritis in 10 to 17 percent of the cases, less frequently than in juvenile rheumatoid arthritis. Antinuclear antibodies are detectable in up to 60 percent of cases but do not predominate in any specific pattern of joint involvement.[85]

The functional outcome is favorable for most children, with the majority maintaining good joint function. A 2-year follow-up study demonstrated that 95 percent of the children were ARA functional class I or II.[17] The disease may, however, follow an intermittent course and persist into adulthood. A small percentage may develop destructive debilitating disease. In two studies, those with antinuclear antibodies seem to have either more difficult to control synovitis or more destructive joint disease.[87] Most patients with childhood psoriatic arthritis can be managed with nonsteroidal anti-inflammatory drugs (NSAIDs). The group developing the progressive polyarthritis, however, will require disease-modifying drugs as are used in adults.

LABORATORY ANALYSIS

There are no characteristic laboratory abnormalities observed in psoriatic arthritis. Analysis of synovial fluid from joints of patients with psoriatic arthritis reveals an inflammatory synovial fluid with predominantly polymorphonuclear neutrophils. The synovial fluid total hemolytic complement is elevated in comparison to normal and is particularly elevated compared with patients with seropositive rheumatoid arthritis.[88] Patients with arthritis are more likely to have an elevated erythrocyte sedimentation rate and anemia than patients with uncomplicated psoriasis. Polyclonal hypergammaglobulinemia may occur.[55] Rheumatoid factor and antinuclear antibodies are not observed any more commonly among adult psoriatic arthritis patients than among control subjects.[55, 89] Documentation of synovial fluid urate in some persons with pre-existing antinuclear antibodies may develop a higher titer during phototherapy for skin disease.[90, 91–93]

RADIOGRAPHIC FINDINGS

In psoriatic arthritis, the distal interphalangeal joints, terminal phalanges, and sacroiliac joints are involved frequently.[94] There are roentgenographic features thought to be characteristic of psoriatic arthritis. Some investigators, however, report similar radiographic findings in patients with seronegative polyarthritis without associated psoriasis.[95] These features include bone ankylosis of the interphalangeal joints of the hands and feet, destruction of the interphalangeal joints with widening of the joint spaces, bone proliferation of the base of the distal phalanx, and resorption of the tufts of the involved distal phalanges (Fig. 58–6).[96] The combination of joint erosion with tapering of a proximal phalanx and bone proliferation of the distal phalanx results

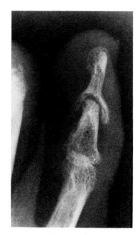

Figure 58–7. Radiograph of finger showing pencil and cup deformity.

in a pencil and cup deformity (Fig. 58–7). Early radiographic findings of bone change in psoriatic arthritis reveal focal discontinuity and irregularity of cortical tuft with erosions in the bare areas of joints. Both psoriasis and osteoarthritis have a propensity to involve the distal interphalangeal joints but may be distinguished radiographically.[97] The erosions in psoriatic arthritis involve the bare areas, giving a "mouse ear" appearance. The erosions in osteoarthritis are subchondral, with a "gull wing" appearance.

Radiographically, sacroiliac involvement may be unilateral. Nonmarginal syndesmophytes occur at several levels asymmetrically and may skip some spinal segments. They may occur only in the cervical spine (Fig. 58–8). Squaring of the vertebra and liga-

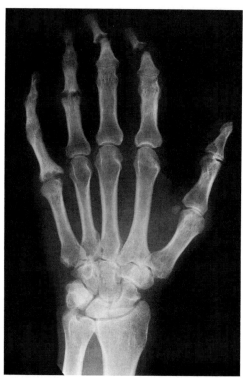

Figure 58–6. Hand radiograph showing widening and destruction of the second and third distal interphalangeal joints, third proximal interphalangeal joint, and fifth metacarpophalangeal joint. Ankylosis of fifth proximal interphalangeal joint and distal interphalangeal joints of fourth and fifth fingers. Bone proliferation of the base of second and third distal phalanges.

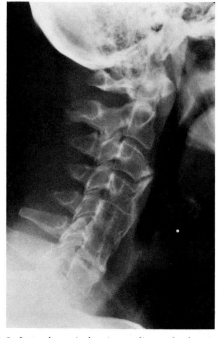

Figure 58–8. Lateral cervical spine radiograph showing anterior syndesmophytes.

mentous calcification are observed less commonly than in idiopathic ankylosing spondylitis.[98, 99]

THERAPY

Nonsteroidal Anti-Inflammatory Drugs

The majority of mildly active peripheral arthritis cases as well as the symptoms of spondylitis are managed by NSAIDs alone. Although many rheumatologists perceive that nonsalicylate anti-inflammatory drugs are more effective in psoriatic arthritis, controlled studies confirming this impression have not been performed.

Arachidonic acid metabolism, especially the leukotrienes, mediates psoriasis via effect on epidermal proliferation and inflammation.[100] Drug-induced cyclo-oxygenase inhibition in the skin with diversion of arachidonate into the lipo-oxygenase pathway may result in amplification of the cutaneous activity. As a consequence, NSAIDs may modify psoriatic lesions. This effect has been observed clinically with indomethacin, phenylbutazone, and oxyphenbutazone inducing psoriatic flare[101] and with benoxaprofen improving skin lesions.[102] A preliminary report suggesting that meclofenamate might alleviate psoriasis has not been confirmed.[103]

Oligoarticular synovitis or tenosynovitis may also be managed with supplemental local glucocorticoid injections. Injections through psoriatic plaques should be avoided; if they cannot be, careful antiseptic skin preparation is mandatory. Systemic glucocorticoids should be used rarely to manage arthritis because of the risk of inducing a rebound flare of psoriasis or potentiating evolution to pustular psoriasis.[104]

When NSAID-resistant or progressive erosive deforming peripheral arthritis develops, disease-modifying agents should be considered. Unfortunately, few well-designed, controlled studies exist to guide the choice of specific agents. Methotrexate, etretinate, sulfasalazine, cyclosporine, and photochemotherapy potentially assist in managing both the joint and the skin disease. To date, no study has shown that any of these drugs or those derived from use in rheumatoid arthritis therapy alter the ultimate course of psoriatic arthritis, and none of these disease-modifying agents have been demonstrated to affect psoriatic spondylitis.

Parenteral gold has been used in psoriatic arthritis for more than 30 years. The composite literature experience is based on few patients in primarily open, small studies. Observed response/remission rates have ranged from 40 to 80 percent, with 20 to 30 percent of the patients discontinuing therapy because of toxicity.[54, 105, 106] The cumulative drug dose response is similar to that observed in rheumatoid arthritis. A controlled, blinded comparison of gold thiomalate versus auranofin and placebo revealed that parenteral gold therapy was more effective than oral gold therapy.[107] A large, double-blind, placebo-controlled study demonstrated only a modest response to auranofin and NSAID combination therapy compared with NSAID alone.[108] The consensus from available trials does not indicate an increased risk of cutaneous flare with parenteral gold and only a 2 percent attributable risk of flare with auranofin.

Experience with penicillamine is only anecdotal, but improvement has been observed, especially in polyarticular cases.[54, 109]

Antimalarial therapy is controversial. In a retrospective review, advocates claim up to 75 percent response rate to hydroxychloroquine (200 to 400 mg per day) within 3 to 4 months of initiating therapy.[54] Concern remains regarding the potential for increased exfoliative reactions in psoriatic patients. Reported experience suggests that hydroxychloroquine may be safer than chloroquine in psoriatic arthritis, with up to a 53 percent rate of adverse cutaneous reactions to chloroquine compared with 19 percent for hydroxychloroquine.[110]

Methotrexate has been used extensively to treat severe resistant psoriasis and was shown to be beneficial against arthritis in a double-blind, placebo parenteral trial.[111] Low-dose oral methotrexate on a daily or intermittent schedule was reported to be efficacious in several small open trials or retrospective reports, with response rates ranging from 43 to 80 percent.[112-114] A 12-week, double-blind, placebo-controlled study using the standard schedule of once weekly dosing with 2.5 to 5 mg every 12 hours for three consecutive doses has been reported.[115] Physician assessment of response favored methotrexate, but the study otherwise lacked statistical power to document objective drug efficacy. Oral hydroxyurea has also been used as an antimetabolite but is thought to be less effective than methotrexate.[116]

Purine analogues, azathioprine, and 6-mercaptopurine have been used in small, controlled and open studies.[117, 118] Their potential toxicities limit their use to severe cases of peripheral arthritis not responsive to more conventional therapies.

Preliminary open trials suggest that the retinoid, etretinate, is beneficial when taken in mean daily maintenance doses of 30 to 50 mg per day.[119-121] A response was seen within 6 weeks to 3 months of therapy. Because of potential teratogenicity, it should not be used in women of child-bearing age. A high frequency of mucocutaneous side effects is observed with etretinate as well as hypertriglyceridemia. Up to 49 percent of patients taking this drug also report proximal arthralgias with myalgias, which respond to dose reduction. The risk for radiographic extraspinal calcification with etretinate may be as high as 50 percent.[122]

Photochemotherapy with methoxypsoralen and long wave ultraviolet-A light (PUVA) will benefit some arthritis patients. A prospective study found that a nonspondylitic subgroup of patients with a high frequency of synchronous skin and joint flares responded to PUVA with a 49 percent improvement in peripheral joint activity.[123] Those patients with spondylitis tended to have discordant skin and joint activity and responded less well to PUVA. More extensive initial skin involvement may also predict less articular improvement with PUVA. A short-term open study of extracorporeal photochemotherapy resulted in only minimal articular improvement and no change in the skin.[124]

Cyclosporin A is effective in clearing psoriasis and has been demonstrated to improve psoriatic arthritis in short-term open studies, within 2 months at a dose of 3.0 to 5 mg per kg per day.[125, 126]

Therapeutic modalities including 1,25-dihydroxyvitamin D_3,[127] sulfasalazine,[128, 129] bromocriptine,[130] total lymphoid irradiation,[131] plasmapheresis,[132] nitrogen mustard, and peptide T,[133, 133a] have all been reported to be potentially effective. Further controlled studies are necessary to establish their therapeutic roles.

When psoriatic patients require total joint arthroplasty, there is concern about the increased risk of deep wound infections, with estimates between 2 and 17 percent, much greater than the expected frequency.[134–136] Staphylococcus aureus is found twice as frequently on the skin of psoriatics compared with normals, with rates up to 44 percent among hospitalized psoriatics.[137, 138] A prolonged preoperative inpatient stay to clear the skin increases the risk of colonization and is not warranted because a standard presurgical preparation can sterilize psoriatic plaques. Psoriatic skin heals normally; a history of Koebner's phenomenon does not strongly predict postoperation incisional psoriasis.[139]

Psoriatic hand implant arthroplasty surgery is less satisfactory than in rheumatoid patients as a result of a greater tendency toward fibrosis and stiffness.[52] In those with aggressive hand arthritis, close, early consultation with a hand surgeon is important because attempts to correct progressively severe "pencil-in-cup" and "opera-glass" deformities surgically becomes technically difficult.[140] Distraction lengthening with osteotomy and bone grafting has been reported as a technique for reconstructing the mutilans hand deformity.[141] Other surgeons, however, recommend prophylactic proximal interphalangeal fusion before the hand deteriorates to a mutilans state.[142]

References

1. Alibert, J. L.: Precis Theorique sur les Maladies de la Peau. Paris, Calille et Ravier 1818, p. 21.
2. Bazin, P.: Lecons Theoriques et Cliniqwues sur les Affections Cutanees de Nature Arthritique et Dartreus. Paris, Delahaye, 1860, p. 154.
3. Wright, V.: Psoriasis and arthritis. Ann. Rheum. Dis. 15:348, 1956.
4. Baker, H., Golding, D. N., and Thompson, M.: Psoriasis and arthritis. Ann. Intern. Med. 58:909, 1963.
5. Moll, J. M. H.: Psoriatic arthritis. Br. J. Rheumatol. 23:241, 1984.
6. Hellgren, L.: Association between rheumatoid arthritis and psoriasis in total populations. Acta Rheumatol. Scand. 15:316, 1969.
7. Lomholt, G.: Psoriasis: Prevalence, spontaneous course and genetics. A census study on the prevalence of skin diseases on the Faroe Islands. Copenhagen, Gad, 1963.
8. van Romunde, L. K. J., Valkenburg, M. A., Swart-Bruinsma, W., Cats, A., and Hermans, J.: Psoriasis and arthritis. I. A population study. Rheumatol. Int. 4:55, 1984.
9. Mongan, E. S., and Atwater, E. C.: A comparison of patients with seropositive and seronegative rheumatoid arthritis. Med. Clin. North Am. 52:533, 1968.
10. Moll, J. M. H., and Wright, V.: Familial occurrence of psoriatic arthritis. Ann. Rheum. Dis. 32:181, 1973.
11. Baker, H., Golding, D. N., and Thompson, M.: Atypical polyarthritis in psoriatic families. Br. Med. J. 2:348, 1963.
12. Espinoza, L. R., Bombardier, C., Gaylord, S. W., Lauter, S., Vasey, F. B., and Osterland, C. K.: Histocompatibility studies in psoriasis vulgaris: Family studies. J. Rheumatol. 7:455, 1980.
13. Marcusson, J.: Psoriasis and arthritic lesions in relation to the inheritance of HLA genotypes. Acta Derm. Venereol. 59:3, 1979.
14. Sakkas, L. I., Demaine, A. G., Panayi, G. S., and Welsh, K. I.: Arthritis in patients with psoriasis is associated with an immunoglobulin gene polymorphism. Arthritis Rheum. 31:276, 1988.
15. Gottlieb, M., Calin, A., and Gale, R. P.: Discordance for psoriatic arthropathy in monozygotic twins. Arthritis Rheum. 22:805, 1979.
16. Murray, C., Mann, D. L., Gerber, L. N., Barth, W. F., Perlman, S. G., Decker, J. L., and Nigra, T. A.: Histocompatibility alloantigens in psoriasis and psoriatic arthritis. Evidence for the influence of multiple genes in the major histocompatibility complex. J. Clin. Invest. 66:670, 1980.
17. Hamilton, M. L., Gladman, D. D., Shore, A., Laxer, R. M., and Silverman, E. D.: Juvenile psoriatic arthritis and HLA antigens. Ann. Rheum. Dis. 49:694, 1990.
18. Beauleiu, A. D., Roy, R., Mathon, G., Morissette, J., Latulippe, L., Lang, J-Y. Mathieu, J-P., Brunet, D., Hebert, J., Archambault, H., and Cloutier, R.: Psoriatic arthritis: Risk factors for patients with psoriasis—a study based on histocompatibility antigens frequencies. J. Rheumatol. 10:633, 1983.
19. Gladman, D., Anhorn, K., Schachter, R., and Mervart, H.: HLA antigens in psoriatic arthritis. J. Rheumatol. 13:586, 1986.
20. Armstrong, R. D., Panayi, G. S., and Welsh, K. I.: Histocompatibility antigens in psoriasis, psoriatic arthropathy and ankylosing spondylitis. Ann. Rheum. Dis. 42:142, 1983.
21. Eastmond, C. J., and Woodrow, J. C.: The HLA system and the arthropathies associated with psoriasis. Ann. Rheum. Dis. 36:112, 1977.
22. Kantor, S. M., Hsu, S. H., Bias, W. B., and Arnett, F. C.: Clinical and immunogenetic subsets of psoriatic arthritis. Clin. Exp. Rheumatol. 2:105, 1984.
23. Salvarani, C., Macchioni, P. L., Zizzi, F., Mantovani, W., Rossi, F., Baricchi, R., Ghirelli, L., Frizziero, L., and Portioli, I.: Clinical subgroups and HLA antigens in Italian patients with psoriatic arthritis. Clin. Exp. Rheumatol. 7:391, 1989.
24. Lopez-Parrea, C., Alonso, J. C. T., Perez, A. R., and Coto, E.: HLA antigens in psoriatic arthritis subtypes of a Spanish population. Ann. Rheum. Dis. 49:318, 1990.
25. Sakkas, L. I., Loqueman, N., Bird, H., Vaughan, R. W., Welsh, K. I., and Panayi, G. S.: HLA class II and T cell receptor gene polymorphisms in psoriatic arthritis and psoriasis. J. Rheumatol. 17:11, 1990.
26. McMenemy, A., and Reveille, J.: MHC-class II heterogeneity by restriction fragment length polymorphism (RFLP) and polymerase chain reaction (PCR) in psoriatic arthritis. Arthritis Rheum. 33:S68, 1990.
27. Ross, J. B.: The psoriatic capillary: Its nature and value in the identification of the unaffected psoriatic. J. Rheumatol. 76:511, 1964.
28. Ryan, T. J.: Microcirculation in psoriasis: Blood vessels, lymphatics, and tissue fluid. Pharmacol. Ther. 10:27, 1980.
29. Bravermann, I. M., and Yen, A.: Ultrastructure of the capillary loop in dermal papillae of psoriasis. J Invest. Dermatol. 68:53, 1977.
30. Zaric, D., Worm, A. M., Stahl, D., and Clemmensen, O. J.: Capillary microscopy of the nailfold in psoriatic and rheumatoid arthritis. Scand. J. Rheumatol. 10:249, 1981.
31. Espinoza, L. R., Vasey, F. B., Espinoza, C. G., Bocanegra, T. S., and Germain, B. F.: Vascular changes in psoriatic synovium: A light and electron microscopic study. Arthritis Rheum. 25:677, 1982.
32. Vasey, F. B., Deitz, C., Fenske, N. A., Germain, B. F., and Espinoza, L. R.: Possible involvement of Group A streptococci in the pathogenesis of psoriatic arthritis. J. Rheumatol. 9:719, 1982.
33. Mustakallio, K. K., and Lassus, A.: Staphylococcal alpha-antitoxin in psoriasis arthropathy. Br. J. Dermatol. 76:544, 1964.
34. Rahman, M. U., Ahmen, S., Schumacher, H. R., and Zeiger, A. R.: High levels of antipeptidoglycan antibodies in psoriatic and other seronegative arthritides. J. Rheumatol. 17:621, 1990.
35. Gottlieb, A. B.: Immunologic mechanisms in psoriasis. J. Am. Acad. Derm. 18:1376, 1988.
36. Gottlieb, A. B., Fu, S. M., Carter, M., and Fotino, M.: Marked increase in the frequency of psoriatic arthritis in psoriasis patients with HLA-DR+ keratinocytes. Arthritis Rheum. 30:901, 1987.
37. Iversen, O. J., and Rodahl, E.: The major internal protein, p27, of a retrovirus-like particle participates in immune complex formation in psoriasis. Arch. Virol. 86:37, 1985.
38. Rodahl, E., and Iversen, O. J.: Antigens related to the major internal protein, p27, of a psoriasis associated retrovirus-like particle are expressed in patients with chronic arthritis. Ann. Rheum. Dis. 44:761, 1985.
39. Moll, J. M. H., and Wright, V.: Psoriatic arthritis. Sem. Arth. Rheum. 3:55, 1973.

40. Fyrand, O., Mellbye, O. J., and Natvig, J. B.: Immunofluorescence studies for immunoglobulins and complement C3 in synovial joint membranes in psoriatic arthritis. Clin. Exp. Immunol. 29:422, 1977.

41. Braathen, L. R., Fyrand, O., and Mellbye, O. J.: Predominance of cells with T-markers in the lymphocytic infiltrates of synovial tissue in psoriatic arthritis. Scand. J. Rheum. 8:75, 1979.

42. Cracchiolo, A., Bluestone, R., and Goldberg, L. S.: Hidden antiglobulins in rheumatic disorders. Clin. Exp. Immunol. 7:651, 1970.

43. Alarcon, G. S., Koopman, W. J., and Schrohenloher, R. E.: In vitro synthesis of IgM and IgG rheumatoid factor in seronegative arthritides. Rheumatol. Int. 4:49, 1984.

44. Hall, R. P., Gerber, L. H., and Lawley, T. J.: IgA containing immune complexes in patients with psoriatic arthritis. Clin. Exp. Rheum. 2:221, 1984.

45. Laurent, M. R., Panayi, G. S., and Shepherd, P.: Circulating immune complexes, serum immunoglobulins, and acute phase proteins in psoriasis and psoriatic arthritis. Ann. Rheum. Dis. 40:66, 1981.

46. Trentham, D. E., Kammer, G. M., McCune, W. J., and David, J. R.: Autoimmunity to collagen: A shared feature of psoriatic and rheumatoid arthritis. Arthritis Rheum. 24:1363, 1981.

47. Gladman, D. D., Keystone, E. C., Russell, M. L., and Schachter, R. K.: Impaired antigen-specific suppressor cell activity in psoriasis and psoriatic arthritis. J. Invest. Dermatol. 77:406, 1981.

48. Gladman, D. D., Keystone, E. C., and Schacter, R. K.: Aberrations in T-cell subpopulations in patients with psoriasis and psoriatic arthritis. J. Invest. Dermatol. 80:286, 1983.

49. Bauer, W., Bennett, G. A., and Zeller, J. W.: The pathology of joint lesions in patients with psoriasis and arthritis. Trans. Assoc. Am. Physicians 56:349, 1941.

50. Fassbender, H. G.: Psoriatic arthritis. In Fassbender, H. G. (ed.): Pathology of Rheumatic Diseases. New York, Springer-Verlag, 1975.

51. Osterland, C. K., Wilkinson, R. D., and St. Louis, E. A.: Expression of c-myc protein in skin and synovium in psoriasis and psoriatic arthritis. Clin. Exp. Rheumatol. 8:145, 1990.

52. Belsky, M. R., Feldon, P., Millender, L. H., Nalebuff, E. A., and Phillips, C.: Hand involvement in psoriatic arthritis. J. Hand Surg. 7:203, 1982.

53. Laurent, M. R.: Psoriatic arthritis. Clin. Rheum. Dis. 11:61, 1985.

54. Kammer, G. M., Soter, N. A., Gibson, D. J., and Schur, P. H.: Psoriatic arthritis: A clinical, immunologic and HLA study of 100 patients. Semin. Arth. Rheum. 9:75, 1979.

55. Gladman, D. D., Shuckett, R., Russell, M. L., Thorne, J. C., and Schachter, R. K.: Psoriatic arthritis (PSA)—an analysis of 220 patients. Q. J. Med. 62:127, 1987.

55a. Helliwell, P., et al.: A re-evaluation of the osteoarticular manifestations of psoriasis. Br. J. Rheumatol. 30:339, 1991.

56. Roberts, M. E. T., Wright, V., Hill, A. G. S., and Mehra, A. C.: Psoriatic arthritis: Follow-up study. Ann. Rheum. Dis. 35:206, 1976.

57. Green, L., Meyers, O. L., Gordon, W., and Briggs, B.: Arthritis in psoriasis. Ann. Rheum. Dis. 40:366, 1981.

58. Lambert, J. R., and Wright, V.: Psoriatic spondylitis: A clinical and radiological description of the spine in psoriatic arthritis. Q. J. Med. 46:411, 1977.

59. Suarez-Almazor, M. E., and Russell, A. S.: Sacroiliitis in psoriasis: Relationship to peripheral arthritis and HLA-B27. J. Rheumatol. 17:804, 1990.

60. Miller, J. L., Soltani, K., and Tourtellotte, C. D.: Psoriatic acro-osteolysis without arthritis. J. Bone Joint Surg. 53A:371, 1971.

61. Yeadon, C., Dumas, J., and Karsh, J.: Lateral subluxation of the cervical spine in psoriatic arthritis: A proposed mechanism. Arthritis Rheum. 26:109, 1983.

62. Salvarini, C., Macchioni, P., et al.: The cervical spine in patients with psoriatic arthritis: a clinical, radiological and immunogenetic study. Ann. Rheum. Dis. 51(1):73, 1992.

63. Kudryk, W. H., Baker, G. L., and Percy, J. S.: Ankylosis of the temporomandibular joints from psoriatic arthritis. J. Otolaryngol. 14:336, 1985.

64. Sonozaki, H., Mitsui, H., Miyanaga, Y., Okitsu, K., Igarashi, M., Hayashi, Y., Matsuura, M., Azuma, A., Okai, K., and Kawashima, M.: Clinical features of 53 cases with pustulotic arthro-osteitis. Ann. Rheum. Dis. 40:547, 1981.

65. Edlund, E., Johnsson, U., Lidgren, L., Pettersson, H., Sturfelt, G., Svensson, B., Theander, J., and Willen, H.: Palmoplantar pustulosis and sternocostoclavicular arthro-osteitis. Ann. Rheum. Dis. 47:809, 1988.

66. Loet, X. L., Bonnet, B., Thomine, E., Louvel, J. P., Mejjad, O., Lauret, P., and Deshayes, P.: Psoriasis (PSO) and palmoplantar pustulosis (PPP) have different osteoarticular manifestations: Aren't they distinct diseases? Arthritis Rheum. 33:S160, 1990.

67. Benhamou, C. L., Chamot, A. M., and Kahn, M. F.: Synovitis-acne-pustulosis hyperostosis-osteomyelitis syndrome (Sapho). A new syndrome among the spondyloarthropathies? Clin. Exp. Rheumatol. 6:109, 1988.

68. Laxer, R. M., Shore, A. D., Manson, D., King, S., Silverman, E. D., and Wilmot, D. M.: Chronic recurrent multifocal osteomyelitis and psoriasis—a report of a new association and review of related disorder. Semin. Arthritis Rheum. 17:260, 1988.

69. Wright, V.: Psoriatic arthritis. Arch. Dermatol. 80:27, 1959.

70. Gerber, L. H., and Espinoza, L. R.: Psoriatic Arthritis. Orlando, FL, Grune & Stratton, 1985.

71. Scarpa, R., Oriente, P., Pucion, A., Torella, M., Vignone, L., Riccio, A., and Oriente, C. B.: Psoriatic arthritis in psoriatic patients. Br. J. Rheum. 23:246, 1984.

72. Zaias, N.: Psoriasis of the nail. Arch. Dermatol. 99:567, 1969.

73. Baker, H., Golding, D. N., and Thompson, M.: The nails in psoriatic arthritis. Br. J. Derm. 76:549, 1964.

74. Lambert, J. R., and Wright, V.: Eye inflammation in psoriatic arthritis. Ann. Rheum. Dis. 35:354, 1976.

75. Abraham, M. D., Weinberger, A., and Feuerman, E. J.: Generalised pustular psoriasis, psoriatic arthritis and nephrotic syndrome associated with systemic amyloidosis. Dermatologica 165:168, 1982.

76. Thomson, G., Johnston, J. L., Baragar, F. D., and Toole, J.: Psoriatic arthritis and myopathy. J. Rheumatol. 17:395, 1990.

77. Hager, M. H., and Moore, M. E.: Relapsing polychondritis syndrome associated with pustular psoriasis, spondylitis and arthritis mutilans. J. Rheumatol. 14:162, 1987.

78. Eastmond, C. J., and Wright, V.: The nail dystrophy of psoriatic arthritis. Ann. Rheum. Dis. 38:226, 1979.

79. Wright, V.: Psoriatic arthropathy and seronegative rheumatoid arthritis with psoriasis: Distinguishing features from Reiter's syndrome. Ann. Rheum. Dis. 38:59, 1979.

80. Perry, H. O., and Mayne, J. G.: Psoriasis and Reiter's syndrome. Arch. Dermatol. 92:129, 1965.

81. Nissila, M., Isomaki, H., Kaarela, K., Kiviniema, P., Martio, J., and Sarna, S.: Prognosis of inflammatory joint diseases. Scand. J. Rheumatol. 12:33, 1983.

82. Gladman, D. D., Stafford-Brady, F., Chang, C-H., Lewandowski, K., and Russell, M. L.: Longitudinal study of clinical and radiological progression in psoriatic arthritis. J. Rheumatol. 17:809, 1990.

83. Hanly, J. G., Russell, M. L., and Gladman, D. D.: Psoriatic spondyloarthropathy: A long term prospective study. Ann. Rheum. Dis. 47:385, 1988.

84. Lambert, J. R., Ansell, B. M., Stephenson, E., and Wright, V.: Psoriatic arthritis in childhood. Clin. Rheum. Dis. 2:339, 1976.

85. Southwood, T. R., Petty, R. E., Malleson, P. N., Delgado, E. A., Hung, D. W. C., Wood, B., and Schroeder, M. L.: Psoriatic arthritis in children. Arthritis Rheum. 332:1007, 1989.

86. Sills, E. M.: Psoriatic arthritis in childhood. Johns Hopkins Med. J. 146:49, 1980.

87. Shore, A., and Ansell, B. M.: Juvenile psoriatic arthritis—an analysis of 60 cases. J. Pediatr. 100:529, 1982.

88. Kim, H. J., McCarty, D. J., Kozin, F., and Koethe, S.: Clinical significance of synovial fluid total hemolytic complement activity. J Rheumatol. 7:143, 1980.

89. Lambert, J. R., Scott, G., and Wright, V.: Psoriatic arthritis and antinuclear factor. Br. J. Dermatol. 96:11, 1977.

90. Leipold, B., Grimm, H., Vogt, H. J., and Remy, W.: Effect of selective ultraviolet phototherapy on DNA and antinuclear antibody titers in psoriatic patients. Arch. Dermatol. Res. 276:297, 1984.

91. Eisen, A. Z., and Seegmiller, J. E.: Uric acid metabolism in psoriasis. J. Clin. Invest. 40:1486, 1961.

92. Fordham, J. N., and Storey, G. O.: Psoriasis and gout. Postgrad. Med. J. 58:477, 1982.

93. Lundquist, C. D., Aronson, I. K., Henderson, T. W., Skosey, J. L., and Solomon, L. M.: Psoriasis and normouricemic gout. Dermtologica 164:104, 1982.

94. Wright, V.: Psoriatic arthritis: A comparative radiographic study of rheumatoid arthritis and arthritis associated with psoriasis. Ann. Rheum. Dis. 20:123, 1961.

95. Burns, T. M., and Calin, A.: The hand radiograph as a diagnostic discriminant between seropositive and seronegative "rheumatoid arthritis": A controlled study. Ann. Rheum. Dis. 42:605, 1983.

96. Wright, V.: Psoriasis and arthritis: A study of the radiographic appearances. Br. J. Radiol. 30:113, 1957.

97. Martel, W., Stuck, K. J., Sworin, A. M., and Hylland, R. G.: Erosive osteoarthritis and psoriatic arthritis: A radiologic comparison in the hand, wrist, and foot. A. J. R. 134:125, 1980.

98. McEwen, C., DiTata, D., Lingg, C., Porini, A., Good, A., and Rankin, T.: Ankylosing spondylitis and spondylitis accompanying ulcerative colitis, regional enteritis, psoriasis and Reiter's disease. Arthritis Rheum. 14:291, 1971.

99. Jajic, I.: Radiological changes in the sacro-iliac joints and spine of patients with psoriatic arthritis and psoriasis. Ann. Rheum. Dis. 27:1, 1968.

100. Voorhees, J. J.: Leukotrienes and other lipoxygenase products in the pathogenesis and therapy of psoriasis and other dermatoses. Arch. Dermatol. 119:541, 1983.

101. Reshad, H., Hargreaves, G. K., and Vickers, C. F. H.: Generalized

pustular psoriasis precipitated by phenylbutazone and oxyphenbutazone. Br. J. Dermatol. 108:111, 1983.

102. Kragbelle, K., and Herlin, T.: Benoxaprofen improves psoriasis. Arch. Dermatol. 119:548, 1983.

103. Ellis, C. N., Goldfarb, M. T., Roenigk, H. H., Rosenbaum, M., Wheeler, S., and Voorhees, J. J.: Effects of oral meclofenamate therapy in psoriasis. J. Am. Acad. Dermatol. 14:49, 1986.

104. Roenick, H. H., Jr., and Maibach, H. I.: Psoriasis. New York, Marcel Dekker, 1985.

105. Dorwart, B. B., Gall, E. P., Schumacher, H. R., and Krauser, R. E.: Chrysotherapy in psoriatic arthritis. Efficacy and toxicity compared to rheumatoid arthritis. Arthritis Rheum. 21:513, 1978.

106. Richter, M. B., Kinsella, P., and Corbett, M.: Gold in psoriatic arthopathy. Ann. Rheum. Dis. 39:279, 1980.

107. Palit, J., Hill, J., Capell, H. A., Carey, J., Daunt, S. O'N., Cawley, M. E. D., Bird, H. A., and Nuki, G.: A multicentre double-blind comparison of auranofin, intramuscular gold thiomalate and placebo in patients with psoriasis arthritis. Br. J. Rheumatol. 29:280, 1990.

108. Carette, S., Calin, A., McCafferty, J. P., and Wallin, B. A.: A double-blind placebo-controlled study of auranofin in patients with psoriatic arthritis. Arthritis Rheum. 32:158, 1989.

109. Price, R., and Gibson, T.: D-Penicillamine and psoriatic arthropathy. Br. J. Rheum. 25:228, 1986.

110. Slagel, G. A., and James, W. D.: Plaquenil-induced erythroderma. J. Am. Acad. Dermatol. 12:857, 1985.

111. Black, R. L., O'Brien, W. M., Van Scott, E. J., Auerbach, R., Eisen, A. Z., and Bunim, J. J.: Methotrexate therapy in psoriatic arthritis. J.A.M.A. 189:743, 1964.

112. Kersley, G. D.: Amethopterin (Methotrexate) in connective tissue disease—psoriasis and polyarthritis. Ann. Rheum. Dis. 27:64, 1968.

113. Chaouat, Y., Kanovitch, B., Faures, B., Grupper, C., and Bourgeois-Spinasse, J.: Le rhumatisme psoriasique traitement par le Methotrexate. Revue du Rhumatisme 38:453, 1971.

114. Kragballe, K., Zachariae, E., and Zachariae, H.: Methotrexate in psoriatic arthritis: A retrospective study. Acta Derm. Venereol. 63:165, 1983.

115. Willkens, R. F., Williams, H. J., Ward, J. R., Egger, M. J., Reading, J. C., Clements, P. J., Cathcart, E. S., Samuelson, C. O., Solsky, M. A., Kaplan, S. B., Guttadauria, M., Halla, J. T., and Weinstein, A.: Randomized, double-blind, placebo controlled trial of low-dose pulse methotrexate in psoriatic arthritis. Arthritis Rheum. 27:376, 1984.

116. Leavell, U. W., and Yarbro, J. W.: Treatment of psoriasis by hydroxyurea. South. Med. J. 64:1253, 1971.

117. Levy, J., Paulus, H. E., Barnett, E. V., Sokoloff, M., Bangert, R., and Pearson, C. M.: A double-blind controlled evaluation of azathioprine treatment in rheumatoid arthritis and psoriatic arthritis. Arthritis Rheum. 15:116, 1972.

118. Baum, J., Hurd, E., Lewis, D., Ferguson, J.L., and Ziff, M.: Treatment of psoriatic arthritis with 6-Mercaptopurine. Arthritis Rheum. 16:139, 1973.

119. Hopkins R., Bird, H. A., Jones, H., Hill, J., Surrall, K. E., Astbury, C., Miller, A., and Wright, V.: A double-blind controlled trial of etretinate (Tigason) and ibuprofen in psoriatic arthritis. Ann. Rheum. Dis. 44:189, 1985.

120. Chieregato, G. C., and Leoni, A.: Treatment of psoriatic arthropathy with etretinate: A two-year follow-up. Acta. Derm. Venereol. 66:321, 1986.

121. Klinkhoff, A. V., Gertner, E., Chalmers, A., Gladman, D. D., Stewart, W. D., Schachter, G. D., and Schachter, R. K.: Pilot study of etretinate in psoriatic arthritis. J. Rheumatol. 16:789, 1989.

122. DiGiovanna, J. J., Helfgott, R. K., Gerber, L. H., and Peck, G. L.: Extraspinal tendon and ligament calcification associated with long-term therapy with etretinate. N. Engl. J. Med. 315:1177, 1986.

123. Perlman, S. G., Gerber, L. H., Roberts, R. M., Nigra, T. P., and Barth, W. F.: Photochemotherapy and psoriatic arthritis. Ann. Int. Med. 91:717, 1979.

124. Wilfert, H., Honigsmann, H., Steiner, G., Smolen, J., and Wolff, K.: Treatment of psoriasis by extracorporeal photochemotherapy. Br. J. Dermatol. 122:225, 1990.

125. Salvarini, C., Macchioni, P., et al.: Low-dose cyclosporin A in psoriatic arthritis: relationship between soluble interleukin-2 receptors and response to therapy. J. Rheumatol. 19(1):74, 1992.

126. Steinsson, K., Jonsdottir, I., and Valdimarsson, H.: Cyclosporin A in psoriatic arthritis: An open study. Ann. Rheum. Dis. 49:603, 1990.

127. Huckins, D., Felson, D. T., and Holick, M.: Treatment of psoriatic arthritis with oral 1,25-dihydroxyvitamin D_3: A pilot study. Arthritis Rheum. 33:1723, 1990.

128. Newman, E. D., Perruquet, J. L., and Harrington, T. M.: Sulfasalazine therapy in psoriatic arthritis: clinical and immunologic response. J. Rheumatol. 18(9):1379, 1991.

129. Farr, M., Kitas, G. D., Waterhouse, L., Jubb, R., Felix-Davies, D., and Bacon, P. A.: Treatment of psoriasis with sulphasalazine: A one year open study. Clin. Rheumatol. 7:372, 1988.

130. Weber, G., and Frey, H.: Treatment of psoriatic arthritis with bromocriptine. J. Am. Acad. Dermatol. 16:388, 1987.

131. Yazici, H., Bilge, N., and Kinay, M.: Total lymphoid irradiation for psoriatic arthritis: Case report. Arthritis Rheum. 26:1052, 1983.

132. Grivet, V., Carli, M., MacDonald, F., Cancelli, M., and Pristera, G.: Plasmapheresis. An additional treatment of psoriasis. Acta Derm. Venereol. 146:130, 1989.

133. Wilke, W. S., Sexton, C., and Steck, W.: Parenteral nitrogen mustard for inflammatory arthritis. Cleve. Clin. J. Med. 57:643, 1990.

133a. Marcusson, J. A., and Wetterberg, L.: Peptide T in the treatment of psoriasis and psoriatic arthritis. Acta Derm. Venereol. 69:86, 1989.

134. Lambert, J. R., and Wright, V.: Surgery in patients with psoriasis and arthritis. Rheumatol. Rehab. 18:35, 1979.

135. Stern, S. H., Insall, J. N., Windsor, R. E., Inglis, A. E., and Dines, D. M.: Total knee arthroplasty in patients with psoriasis. Clin. Orthop. 248:108, 1989.

136. Menon, T. J., and Wroblewski, B. M.: Charley low-friction arthroplasty in patients with psoriasis. Clin. Orthop. 176:127, 1983.

137. Noble, W. C., and Savin, J. A.: Carriage of staphylococcus aureus in psoriasis. Br. Med. J. 1:417, 1968.

138. Aly, R., Maibach, H. I., and Mandel, A.: Bacterial flora in psoriasis. Br. J. Dermatol. 95:603, 1976.

139. Lynfield, Y. L., Ostroff, G., and Abraham, J.: Bacteria, skin sterilization, and wound healing in psoriasis. N.Y. St. J. Med. June 1, 72:1247, 1972.

140. Kapasi, O. A., Ruby, L. K., and Calney, K.: The psoriatic hand. J. Hand Surg. 7:492, 1982.

141. Walton, R. L., Brown, R. E., and Giansiracusa, D. F.: Psoriatic arthritis mutilans: Digital distraction lengthening: Pathophysiologic and current therapeutic review. 13A:510, 1988.

142. Nalebuff, E. A., and Garrett, J.: Opera-glass hand in rheumatoid arthritis. J. Hand Surg. 1:210, 1976.

Chapter 59

Frank A. Wollheim

Enteropathic Arthritis

INTRODUCTION

Enteropathic arthritis can be defined as arthritis induced by or occurring with intestinal disease. The gut as a causative factor in diseases of unknown origin has always fascinated both laymen and physicians. Earlier in this century, such procedures as appendectomy, cholecystectomy, and even partial ileocolectomy were recommended for the treatment and cure of rheumatoid arthritis. Although it has been difficult to support the hypothesis that food antigens might cause arthritis,[1-3] it is known that certain allergens can pass the gut in intact form. This is illustrated in breast-fed babies who develop colic after the mother ingests cow's milk.[4] Increased gut permeability, allowing penetration of harmful products, is of possible pathophysiologic significance in several of the conditions discussed in this chapter.[5] The intestinal mucosal immune system and gut wall peptide hormones are capable of inducing both local and extraintestinal tissue damage. Gut-associated rheumatoid diseases have attracted increasing attention.[5, 5a]

PHYSIOLOGY

The gastrointestinal canal in humans has an estimated surface of 50 to 2000 m^2. It has the dual function of allowing absorption of nutrients and excluding harmful and toxic substances. Gut permeability is potentially of central importance in the pathogenesis of several diseases. Molecules smaller than 5000 daltons can pass through the epithelial membranes of the microvilli, whereas larger molecules may enter Peyer's patches by endocytosis.[5] Gut permeability can be studied by using various probes[5-8] (Table 59–1). Pathogenic microorganisms can both

Table 59–1. PROBES USED TO STUDY INTESTINAL PERMEABILITY

Probe	Reference
Peg 400	5, 7
Peg 280-1000	6
Mannitol	5, 7
Rhamnose	5, 7
Lactulose	5, 7
51CrEDTA	5, 7
Human α-lactalbumin	8

decrease (Rotavirus) and augment (*Yersinia, Salmonella*) permeability.[9]

In normal conditions, peristalsis, low pH, and high redox potential suppress microbial growth in the upper intestinal tract. In the ileum and cecum, however, normally bacterial counts of up to 10^{12} per gram are found. In the large bowel, fastidious anaerobic organisms dominate.

Gut-associated lymphoid tissue, constituting an impressive 25 percent of the mucosa, can be divided into three anatomically, morphologically, and functionally distinct parts.[10]

Peyer's patches are separated from the lumen by membrane (M) cells lacking microvilli but specialized for pinocytosis and antigen presentation to lymphocytes that they partly surround. T lymphocytes and B lymphocytes committed principally to gamma immunoglobulin A (IgA) production have been shown to migrate to sites in the *mucosal lamina propria* and locate near lymph and blood vessels.[11] Seventy to 80 percent of the B lymphocytes/plasma cells in these locations produce IgA; 15 to 20 percent, IgM; and 2 percent, IgE. The T lymphocytes are mostly CD4+. The third locus of lymphoid tissue is intraepithelial, with one T cell per six to ten columnar epithelial cells. Here, CD8+ cells are predominant. In contrast to the other two lymphoid compartments, this one develops even under germ-free conditions. There is evidence for recirculation of lymphocytes to the lamina propria and from Peyer's patches to intraepithelial sites. Intraepithelial lymphocytes are increased in active sprue. Intestinal lymphocyte populations have a close relationship through migration to those in the lung, mammary gland, and female genital tract. Whether gut-derived lymphocytes can reach joint structures is an open question that can be solved only by models to track lymphocyte traffic.

The explosion of knowledge in the field of neuropeptides and gastrointestinal peptide hormones[12] may well become relevant in enteropathic and other forms of arthritis. Substance P, abundant in both myenteric and submucosal intrinsic nerves, activates human synoviocytes in low concentrations (e.g., 10^{-9}m).[13]

INFLAMMATORY BOWEL DISEASE

Although described in 1895,[14] joint manifestations in ulcerative colitis were neither appreciated

Table 59–2. EXTRACOLONIC MANIFESTATIONS IN CROHN'S DISEASE AND ULCERATIVE COLITIS

	Crohn's Disease	Ulcerative Colitis
Peripheral arthritis	20%	9–11%
Septic arthritis	+	?
Sacroiliitis/ankylosing spondylitis	16%/16%	14%/16%
Skin		
Erythema nodosum	0.5–9%	
Erythema multiforme	0.5–9%	
Pyoderma gangrenosum	0.5%	0.3–4%*
Aphthous ulceration	+	8%
Renal lithiasis	15%†	?
Amyloidosis	30 cases published	Rare
Liver disease	3–5%	7%
Uveitis	13%	4%
Clubbing	4–13%	1–5%
Vasculitis	Takayasu	1–5%

*More frequent with severe or extensive disease.
†Oxalate stones most common.

nor systematically studied until much later.[15, 16] Similar observations were made in Crohn's disease,[17–19] leading to the concept of seronegative spondyloarthropathy. Articular manifestations with ulcerative colitis and Crohn's disease show many similarities, but there are differences (Table 59–2). Crohn's disease–like lesions are frequently present in children[20] and adult patients with seronegative oligoarthritis in the absence of intestinal symptoms.[21–23, 44]

HLA-B27, when present in individuals who develop inflammatory bowel disease (IBD), substantially increases the risk for ankylosing spondylitis, compared with the risk for HLA-B27 carriers without bowel disease. The overall prevalence of HLA-B27 in ankylosing spondylitis associated with IBD is, however, lower than that in ankylosing spondylitis in general,[24] indicating the presence of a pathogenetic factor independent of HLA-B27. Isolated sacroiliitis in IBD is unrelated to the presence of HLA-B27 and is evenly distributed among men and women.[58, 72, 73]

Evidence is gathering that HLA-B alleles different from B27 may contribute to susceptibility to spondyloarthropathy in both HLA-B27–positive and HLA-B27–negative individuals.[59, 60]

Ulcerative Colitis

Ulcerative colitis occurs in 50 to 100 per 100,000 individuals in England[25] and Scandinavia[26] but may be less prevalent in other geographic locations.[27] Immune mechanisms are strongly suggested by histologic as well as clinical features. Antibodies with specificity for mucopolysaccharides in colon epithelial cells have been identified.[28, 29] Antibodies to *Escherichia coli* polysaccharide with cross-reaction to colon antigens have been described in patients and relatives.[30] The link of these antibodies to disease is

weak, however, and lends only anecdotal support for a hypothesis of autoimmunity based on molecular mimicry. Lymphocytotoxic antibodies have also been described in patients and families.[31]

Disease-related autoimmunity has been supported by the isolation from the colon of patients with ulcerative colitis of tissue-bound IgG reactive with a 40-kD organ-specific protein.[32] This protein antigen has been found in all colon specimens, including some from germ-free rats. In contrast, patients with Crohn's disease have serum antibodies to different glycoproteins identified only in the small and large bowel from patients with this disease.[33] These observations may provide leads toward understanding the pathogenesis of IBD.

Peripheral Arthritis

Peripheral arthritis of ulcerative colitis is seronegative, usually beginning after the intestinal disease has become manifest and most often affecting large joints (Fig. 59–1). The total prevalence is close to 10 percent,[34, 35] and the sex distribution is equal. The prevalence and distribution are about the same in children,[36, 37] in whom arthritis is the most common extracolonic manifestation. In children, however, arthritis may precede diarrhea.[38] In adults, arthritis is more prevalent when the disease is complicated by peritoneal abscess formation, pseudomembranous polyposis,[16] erythema nodosum, aphthous stomatitis,[35] uveitis, or pyoderma gangrenosum (Fig. 59–2).

Sudden onset of migrating oligoarthritis involving no more than four to ten joints and lasting 1 or several months or years is a characteristic feature.[40, 41] Most attacks occur during the first years of the disease coincident with flares of bowel disease and may remit after colectomy. Rarely is there evidence for cartilage destruction or erosion of bone.

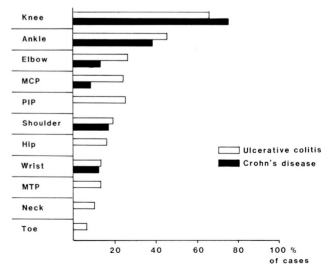

Figure 59–1. Distribution of peripheral joint involvement in ulcerative colitis (Wright and Watkinson)[43] and Crohn's disease (Haslock and Wright).[57]

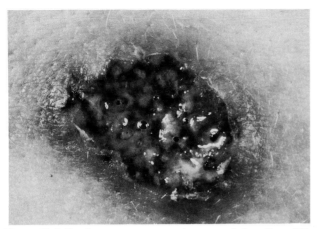

Figure 59–2. Pyoderma gangrenosum in a case of ulcerative colitis. (Courtesy of Professor Hans Rorsman, Lund, Sweden.)

Spinal Involvement

In contrast to peripheral arthritis, spondylitis often is present years before the onset of colitis.[18, 42] In the study performed on an unselected group of 234 patients in Leeds, England, 6.4 percent had frank ankylosing spondylitis, but in addition, 14 percent had asymptomatic sacroiliitis.[43] To complicate matters further, it was found that silent colitis may occur in ankylosing spondylitis.[44] The intestinal and joint symptoms often fail to fluctuate in parallel. The female-to-male ratio is 0.57,[46] but in other respects the spinal disease is clinically indistinguishable from idiopathic ankylosing spondylitis.

Radiology. The radiologic findings are identical with those of classic ankylosing spondylitis.[47] In peripheral arthritis, one observes nonspecific soft tissue swelling and periarticular osteoporosis. Rarely, joint space narrowing, erosions, and periostitis are seen. In the spine, the whole spectrum from squaring and mild sacroiliitis to ankylosed sacroiliac joints and "bamboo" spine may be seen.

Treatment. Symptomatic treatment with local glucocorticoid injections is often effective in peripheral arthritis. In spinal disease, daily exercises are as important as they are in classic ankylosing spondylitis. In addition, nonsteroidal anti-inflammatory drugs (NSAIDs) are often required but should be administered with awareness of possible gastrointestinal intolerance. Sulfasalazine is well documented to be effective in early spinal disease, and the recommended dosage is 2 or 3 g daily.[45]

Crohn's Disease

The prevalence of Crohn's disease equals or exceeds that of ulcerative colitis.[27] According to North American, British, and Swedish reports, the disease has become more frequent in recent years.[48, 49] Between 1958 and 1973, the incidence in Malmö, Sweden, increased from 3.5 to 6.0 per 100,000, and the prevalence in 1973 was 75 per 100,000.[50] The highest mortality figures were published from Denmark and West Germany.[51]

Immunologic studies have demonstrated circulating antibodies to synthetic double-stranded RNA and lymphotoxic antibodies.[31] In both Crohn's disease and ulcerative colitis, increased number of mucosal B lymphocytes bearing surface IgG are prevalent.[52, 53] In the blood, IgG_2 dominates in contrast to ulcerative colitis, in which IgG_1 and IgG_3 are most increased.[54, 55] This might indicate immune response to different antigens in the two conditions. Cell-mediated immune response has been more difficult to study.[10]

Genetic studies have shown a relationship to ulcerative colitis[48, 56] and increased occurrence of sacroiliitis among relatives.[57]

Peripheral Arthritis

Peripheral arthritis is the most frequent extraintestinal manifestation and occurs in 10 to 20 percent in most series[19, 57, 58] of Crohn's disease patients. It has a distribution similar to that of ulcerative colitis (see Fig. 59–1).[19, 57] Patients with large bowel lesions are more prone to developing peripheral arthritis.[35, 48, 61, 62] Fistula formation or malabsorption does not increase the frequency.[57] The sex distribution is even, and children are affected with the same frequency as adults.[36, 37] There is a higher incidence of peripheral arthritis in patients with other extraintestinal manifestations, such as erythema nodosum, stomatitis, uveitis, and pyoderma gangrenosum.[35, 39] Clinical features are closely similar to those of ulcerative colitis. The condition is marked by large joint oligoarthritis that resolves within a few weeks or months in the majority of cases.[40, 57, 58]

A limited number of histologic examinations of joint specimens have been performed,[15, 63] showing nonspecific synovitis. Among ten patients with recurrent arthralgias of the knees examined by arthroscopy, inflammation was found in only one patient, whereas four had deposition of "glittering crystals," and four others had positively birefringent crystals with the appearance of calcium pyrophosphate dihydrate.[64] Crystal arthropathy is suggested by this report, but it needs confirmation. Granulomatous nonerosive synovitis was described in a case of prolonged ankle swelling[65] and in one wrist at synovectomy after 1 year's duration.[66] Subsequently, a few cases of erosive large joint arthritis have been reported.[67–69, 71] Synovial granulomas in the knee have repeatedly been found without definitive relation to duration or severity of the arthritis.[36, 66, 70, 71]

Spinal Involvement

Ankylosing spondylitis has been reported in up to 25 percent of cases.[41] When strict diagnostic criteria are used, the usual figure is around 5 percent.[28, 57, 63, 72] Radiologic evidence of sacroiliitis is three times more common and often clinically silent.[58, 72] The ankylosing spondylitis may precede, coincide with, or start after the intestinal disease, a phenomenon that has caused speculation regarding a "secondary" form of ankylosing spondylitis.[72] No consistent relationship has been found between flares of spondylitis and the intestinal disease, although in a few studies the extent of gut involvement has correlated with that of spinal disease.[34, 58] The radiologic changes are indistinguishable from those of classic ankylosing spondylitis.[34, 47]

Other Manifestations

Clubbing of fingers was present in 40 percent of patients in one report,[74] but most observers find lower figures.[46] Clubbing is related to proximal intestinal involvement and also to fibrotic lesions in resected gut specimens; it may regress after effective surgery.[75] New bone formation reminiscent of hypertrophic osteoarthropathy has been described and may involve periosteal granulomas.[76] Septic arthritis of the hip is an important but rare complication that has been described in connection with psoas or retroperitoneal abscess formation.[77–79] Early diagnosis is of the utmost importance for a favorable outcome.

Treatment. No specific treatment is available, and the same principles apply as for ulcerative colitis. It is usually possible to control joint symptoms by means of local glucocorticoid injections or NSAIDs. Sulfasalazine may be helpful in early disease.[45] Physiotherapy is important in preventing deforming ankylosis in some patients with peripheral joint disease, notably children, and is mandatory in patients with spinal disease.

Pyoderma Gangrenosum

Pyoderma gangrenosum is a painful and ulcerating skin disease that is frequently associated with systemic diseases (see Fig. 59–2).[80, 81] In a review of 86 consecutive patients seen at the Mayo Clinic from 1970 to 1983, all but 19 had no associated disease. Arthritis occurred in 32 and inflammatory bowel disease in 31. Thirteen of the arthritis patients had bowel disease and oligoarticular large joint synovitis. Nine other patients had similar joint disease but no signs of intestinal involvement, although endoscopy, which might have uncovered asymptomatic cases,[82] was not performed. One half of 1 percent of ulcerative colitis patients and 0.33 percent of Crohn's disease patients develop pyoderma (see Table 59–2). The condition is also described in children.[83] Minor trauma or insect bites may precipitate the condition in these patients. Healing of pyoderma and arthritis has been observed following "complete" resection of the affected bowel.

Pathogenesis. Altered immune reactivity[81] and defective granulocyte[84] and monocyte[85] function have been observed in Crohn's disease. An association

with monoclonal gammopathy, usually of the IgA type, has been reported in several cases.[81, 85–87] Pyoderma gangrenosum has been successfully treated by elimination of E. coli and skin antigens. Anecdotal effects with clofazimine[84] and sulfamethoxypyridazine[89] as well as dramatic remission with thalidomide[89, 90] have been reported. A case of Sjögren's syndrome in a patient with Crohn's disease was observed.[91] Presence of DR4 and absence of antibodies to SSA/Ro or SSB/La and DR3 argued that the Sjögren's syndrome was of the secondary rheumatoid-related variety.

POSTENTERITIC REACTIVE ARTHRITIS

Terminology

Aho et al.[92] introduced the term *reactive arthritis* in 1973[112] for arthritic conditions following infection in other organs in which no microbial antigens could be isolated from the joint. Reiter's syndrome is one clinical form of reactive arthritis, and rheumatic fever is another. In contrast, "postinfective" arthritis, by definition, denotes conditions in which traces of microbial material but no viable organisms can be found in the joint lesions.[93] This has been best described in connection with several viral diseases such as Ross River virus disease and parvovirus infections.[94] The issue has changed, however, by the finding of antigenic material from *Chlamydia, Yersinia,* and *Salmonella* organisms in specimens from joints,[84, 95, 96] indicating that antigen presence is not a basic difference between reactive and postinfective arthritis and lending support to previous hypotheses.[104]

History

Sydenham in 1672 reported dysenteric arthritis, a condition that was also well known in the nineteenth century.[105] Poor hygienic conditions during World War I with epidemic *Shigella* outbreaks led to the classic observations of Reiter,[106] Fiessinger and Leroy,[107] and others. In an extensive paper published in 1918, more than 50 cases were analyzed, of which one third had shigellosis; one third, enteritis; and one third, no enteric symptoms but an identical type of joint affection.[108] In 1948, Paronen[109] wrote his famous thesis on a large epidemic of *Shigella flexneri* with 344 cases of Reiter's syndrome in the Finnish army. Later, *Salmonella,*[110, 111] *Yersinia enterocolitica,*[112] and *Campylobacter*[113, 114] were identified as arthritogenic agents.

Pathogenesis

Postentertic reactive arthritis is triggered by a limited number of organisms and shows strong predilection for HLA-B27–positive individuals. The exact nature of the "reactive" process, however, remains obscure. HLA-B27 is no absolute requirement, and the number of triggering organisms may still be incomplete because no organism can as yet be implicated in 25 percent of cases.[115, 148] Elucidation of the three-dimensional structure of the HLA-A2 molecule[116] accelerated the search for molecular mechanisms linking the triggering organisms to HLA-B27 (see chapter on ankylosing spondylitis). The role of HLA-B27 has been explored in experimental models employing transgenic animals.[117] Claims that HLA-B27 transgenic mice are more susceptible to the development of paraspinal abscesses and have a higher mortality after intravenous injection of live Yersinia organisms[118] have not been confirmed.[119]

Presence of bacterial antigens in synovial biopsy and synovial fluid has been confirmed for Y. enterocolitica,[96, 97] Salmonella enteritides and Salmonella typhimurium,[98] and Chlamydia trachomatis.[95, 99, 100, 100a] Immunohistology using polyclonal and monoclonal antisera and immunoblotting was employed in these experiments. Efforts to show presence of microbial DNA using the polymerase chain reaction, however, have been unsuccessful.[101] Synovial fluid but not blood lymphocytes do recognize the triggering agents[102, 103] supporting local presence of microbial antigenic material.

Molecular mimicry has been an attractive hypothesis advanced by several authors.[121–124, 127] Antimicrobial antibodies with reactivity for HLA-B27[122] and homologies between exposed regions of the HLA-B27 molecule and arthritogenic Shigella flexneri plasmids have been found,[125] but at present a direct role for molecular mimicry in the pathogenesis of reactive arthritis is unlikely.[126]

Enhanced antibody response and persistence of specific IgA antibodies is characteristic of Yersinia arthritis[166] and Salmonella arthritis.[167] An unspecifically enhanced polymorphonuclear neutrophil (PMN) chemotaxis in patients with reactive arthritis who are HLA-B27 positive has been documented,[145] but the differences are small and of uncertain significance.

Etiologic Agents

It is striking that only a limited number of microorganisms are commonly implicated in postenteric reactive arthritis (Table 59–3). No obvious biologic differences can be defined between arthritogenic and nonarthritogenic species.[115] Differences in cell adhesion do not seem important.[128, 129] Claims for less common etiologic agents are accumulating. These include Shigella sonnei,[130] Y. enterocolitica 08,[131] Salmonella muenchen,[143] Salmonella heidelberg,[144] Salmonella hadar,[146] Salmonella saint paul, Salmonella montevideo, Salmonella agona,[147] and Clostridium difficile.[132, 133] A word of caution should be added, since the link to the agent is often based only on serology or enzyme-linked immunosorbent assay (ELISA) anti-

Table 59–3. ETIOLOGIC AGENTS IN POSTENTERIC REACTIVE ARTHRITIS

Common	Unusual
Shigella dysenteriae	Shigella sonnei
Shigella flexneri	
Salmonella typhimurium	Salmonella paratyphi B
Salmonella enteritidis	Salmonella paratyphi C
Yersinia enterocolitica 03	Yersinia enterocolitica 08
Yersinia enterocolitica 09	
Yersinia pseudotuberculosis	
Campylobacter jejuni	

body positivity in these cases. Anecdotal evidence further implicates Staphylococcus epidermidis,[135] Streptococcus,[136] Giardia lamblia,[137, 138] Leptospira icterohaemorrhagiae,[140] Borrelia burgdorferi,[139] and Brucella abortus.[142, 143] The presence of septic arthritis cannot be excluded, however, in some of these reports.

Clinical Features

Postenteritic arthritis has many characteristics in common with Reiter's syndrome (see Chapter 60). These include an abrupt onset of oligoarthritis, principally in knees and ankles.[149] Wrists, fingers, and toes come next in frequency.[150–152] Fever is common. Skin symptoms usually are not prominent, although erythema nodosum sometimes is observed in yersiniosis, and balanitis circinata often is present in Shigella arthritis (Table 59–4).

The symptoms of enteritis are often mild and may even be absent.[108, 154] The interval between the start of enteric and arthritic symptoms varies from days to weeks. Most patients present in the autumn in the Northern Hemisphere. The sex distribution is even except for Shigella arthritis. The high prevalence in men with Shigella arthritis, however, is mainly based on the 344 reported cases from the epidemic in the Finnish army.[109] The mean age is close to 30 years in most reports.[149] Reactive arthritis has only rarely been reported in children.

Peripheral joint involvement may cause significant disability for many months; healing eventually occurs. Recurrences are rare but do occur perhaps after reinfection. The duration of the initial episode of arthritis is on average 20 weeks, varying from 2 weeks to more than 12 months. HLA-B27 is strongly associated with all these forms of reactive arthritis, and the duration and severity of symptoms are longer among HLA-B27–positive individuals. The relative risk for developing reactive arthritis is 50 times higher in HLA-B27–positive individuals. On the other hand, in Yersinia arthritis, erythema nodosum presents primarily among HLA-B27–negative individuals.[115] Back pain occurs in 30 percent of patients in the acute stage, and 20 percent or more develop radiologic sacroiliitis within 5 years,[152, 157] a feature shared with Reiter's syndrome.[159]

Estimates from epidemic outbreaks indicate that

Table 59–4. FEATURES OF REACTIVE ARTHRITIS ACCORDING TO CAUSATIVE AGENT

	Shigella	*Salmonella*	*Campylobacter*	*Yersinia*	SARA*
Number of patients	371	46	21	329	557
Prevalence of arthritis	1–3%	1–3%	1–3%	10–20%	1%
Sex ratio M:F	9	1.6	1.3	0.9	28
Prevalence of HLA-B27	79%	84%	72%	75%	80%
Genital inflammation	70%	15%	24%	13%	100%
Circinate balanitis	24%	—	—	—	23%
Keratoderma blennorrhagicum	—	—	—	—	12%
Reiter's syndrome	85%	12%	10%	10%	35%
Symptoms lasting >1 yr	18%	—	5%	10%	17%
Erythema nodosum	—	—	—	5%	—
Enthesopathy	8%	13%	5%	11%	22%

*SARA, Sexually acquired reactive arthritis.
— = Data not available, probably negative.
Data from Keat, A.: N. Engl. J. Med. 309:1606, 1983.

up to 20 percent of *Yersinia*-infected individuals[154] and 7.5 percent of *Salmonella enteritis* cases develop reactive arthritis,[155] although most reports indicate figures between 1 and 2 percent of all infected individuals.[149]

Immunopathology

As pointed out by Aho,[115] *Salmonella, Yersinia,* and *Campylobacter* share the invasive behavior of spreading into lymph nodes and blood with enteric *E. coli*, which, however, is an agent not known to cause reactive arthritis. *Shigella*, on the other hand, is arthritogenic without invading lymph nodes or blood. Thus, bacteremia does not seem essential in the triggering of arthritis.

After *Yersinia* infection, polyclonal hypergammaglobulinemia[164] is present in both arthritis and enteritis cases. Specific humoral immunity is, however, more intense and of longer duration in patients who develop arthritis.[165] ELISA tests show higher and more prolonged circulating levels of IgA and IgG anti-*Yersinia* antibodies[166] and are useful in the differential diagnosis of seronegative rheumatoid arthritis.[168] The most significant discriminatory feature in *Yersinia* arthritis has been specific IgA antibodies of the secretory type indicating that they arose from local stimulation in the intestinal tract lymphoid system.[169] Interestingly, rheumatoid factors are not found in any stage of reactive arthritis.[170] Nonspecific circulating immune complexes have been detected in a high proportion of both arthritis and enteritis cases.[171] More recently, *Yersinia*-specific immune complexes containing secretory IgA were detected both in the circulation and in the synovial fluid several months after onset of arthritis, showing persistence of the antigen for prolonged periods in arthritis and uncomplicated enteritis.[172] IgA-containing circulating complexes were more prevalent in arthritis cases.[173] These complexes were only slightly larger than the corresponding immunoglobulins, suggesting that the *Yersinia*-derived component is small.[174] Such immune complexes have also been demonstrated in synovial fluid.[175] Likewise in *Salmonella*-triggered reactive arthritis, antibodies with specificity for lipopolysaccharide, in particular of the IgA class, were found to persist in the circulation. *Yersinia* antigens have been demonstrated at the basement membrane of the capillary loops and in the mesangium by immunofluorescence in a high proportion of cases of glomerulonephritis, many of which showed serologic signs only of *Yersinia* infection.[176] Persistent antigen presence in synovial tissue and synovial fluid has already been discussed above,[95, 97, 98] and may explain the prolonged humoral immune response.

Cellular immunity in reactive arthritis has been studied with crude antigen mixtures of *Yersinia* organism.[146] High levels of lymphoblastic stimulation in response to these antigens have been found even in cells of patients without serum antibodies to *Yersinia*.[177] In another report, however, depressed cellular immunity was found in patients with *Yersinia* arthritis.[178] In yet another study, synovial fluid, but not peripheral blood lymphocytes, was stimulated by the triggering bacterium.[179] The observation of severe Reiter's syndrome in patients with acquired immunodeficiency syndrome (AIDS) indicates that helper T cell function may not be essential in the pathogenesis of reactive arthritis.[180] Further work is needed before a clear-cut picture evolves.

Clinical Features

Prognosis is generally good, compared with that in sexually acquired Reiter's syndrome; one reason for this may be that there are fewer reinfections than in sexually acquired disease.[149, 156] Long-term follow-up studies in *Yersinia*[144, 152] and *Shigella* arthritis[157] have, however, demonstrated development of sacroiliitis in at least 20 percent of cases after 5 to 10 years and chronic disease in some *Salmonella*-triggered cases.[155, 158] Further, a large proportion of the patients had continued pain in entheses and initially affected joints, although this did not significantly influence working capacity.[152] Ankylosing spondylitis

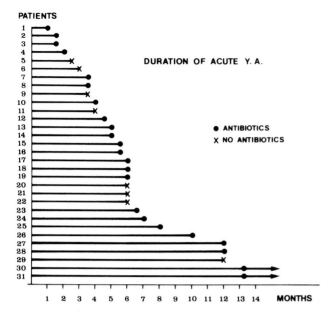

PATIENTS

DURATION OF ACUTE Y. A.

● ANTIBIOTICS

X NO ANTIBIOTICS

MONTHS

Figure 59–3. Duration of acute symptoms in relation to antibiotic treatment. (From Marsal, L., Winblad, S., and Wollheim, F. A.: *Yersinia enterocolitica* arthritis in southern Sweden: a four-year follow-up study. Br. Med. J. 283:101, 1981. Used by permission.)

will develop in a small proportion of patients, but it is not clear whether reactive arthritis actually increases the risk. *Salmonella*-triggered reactive arthritis occurring in two patients with ankylosing spondylitis did not seem to modify this disease.[153] Rheumatoid arthritis occasionally has developed after *Yersinia* arthritis,[115, 144, 152] but this probably represents coincidence of two common diseases. The idea that *Yersinia* infection may trigger rheumatoid arthritis[160] has not been supported.[161] HLA-B27 positivity is not a prerequisite for the development of reactive arthritis but predisposes for more widespread and longer lasting joint disease[144] as well as more spinal disease. This may in part be based on an exaggerated inflammatory response conferred by the presence of the HLA-B27 antigen.[145]

Treatment

Postenteritic reactive arthritis is often a self-limiting disease, requiring only symptomatic supportive treatment with NSAIDs and cautious use of local glucocorticoid injections. Aspirin is not useful in postenteritic arthritis.[108] Effectiveness of antibiotic therapy seemed unlikely in retrospective studies[152, 162] (Fig. 59–3). A prospective, placebo-controlled study in 40 consecutive patients confirmed that short-term antibiotic therapy was of no benefit.[163] There are as yet no data supporting effectiveness of slow-acting drugs such as sulfasalazine, antimalarials, or methotrexate in chronic cases of reactive arthritis.

BYPASS ARTHRITIS-DERMATITIS SYNDROME

Intestinal bypass as therapy for obesity was introduced in 1952.[181] Eleven years later, it was shown that the procedure, although often achieving the desired weight reduction, also caused frequent complications, including malabsorption and joint symptoms.[182] The prevalence of this clearly enteropathic form of arthritis is now low, since bypass surgery was abandoned in the mid-1980s.[183] The condition, however, deserves attention as a model disease for systemic complications of intestinal bacterial overgrowth.

Clinical Features

Incidence figures from 8 to 52 percent have been observed.[184–187] The arthritis usually develops within 1 year after the bypass procedure[188] and may last from a week to several months or years.[189] It is three times more prone to occur in women.[186] Knees, ankles, fingers, wrists, and shoulders are the most common locations.[184, 185, 188] The arthritis is intensely painful, but objective signs are discrete and erosive changes are rare.[187] Back pain is frequent, and sacroiliac joint radiographs have shown subchondral sclerosis but no sacroiliitis.[186] Tenosynovitis is not unusual.[186, 187]

In 80 percent of the patients, cutaneous macular, papular, postular, urticarial, or erythema nodosum–like lesions are present along with the arthritis (Fig. 59–4; see color section at the front of this volume). Skin biopsy shows microvascular inflammation of the dermis with mild vasculitis. Raynaud's phenomenon is present in up to one third of patients,[186] fever is less common.

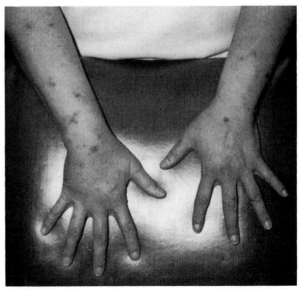

Figure 59–4. Recurrent pustular rash in a case of bypass arthritis-dermatitis.

Laboratory Findings

Elevated erythrocyte sedimentation rate, cryo-globulinemia, elevated acute phase reactants, and immunoglobulins are common. Neither positive rheumatoid factor nor antinuclear antibodies are present. Immune complexes containing bacterial components from *E. coli* and *Bacteroides fragilis* as well as C1q, C3, and C4 are present in serum levels and correlate with symptoms of arthritis.[190] There is no HLA-B27 association.[186]

Pathogenesis

Bacterial overgrowth in the blind loop is the basis for the syndrome.[183] IgG, IgA, and complement deposition was induced by intradermal histamine injection in two of two patients but in none of eight control patients.[191] The predominant production and absorption of complexes containing secretory IgA and intestinal bacterial products have been found in an experimental blind-loop model.[192] The increased IgA production could be suppressed by antibiotic treatment. Circulating IgG-sIgA complexes were found in 13 patients, six of whom had arthritis. Such complexes are not present normally.[193] Evidence is thus accumulating to implicate gut-derived immune complexes in the pathogenesis of the condition.

Treatment

Antibiotics and NSAIDs are effective against gastrointestinal and locomotor symptoms but less successful in controlling recurrent skin manifestations. Reanastomosis of the bypassed bowel segments may be the most effective treatment in the rare severe cases. An unusual case, in which a blind-loop syndrome with severe arthritis and dermatitis developed after a Billroth I gastrectomy, responded well to surgical removal of two strictures.[194]

GLUTEN-SENSITIVE ENTEROPATHY

Case reports describe arthropathy in three cases of gluten-sensitive enteropathy.[233–235] Effusive arthritis was present in knees and ankles and responded promptly to gluten-free diet. The arthropathy may precede symptomatic enteropathy by years. It is assumed that bacterial products contribute to pathogenesis. On the other hand, arthralgias, sclerodactyly, and finger contractures presented after relapse, 10 years after the initial diagnosis of celiac disease, in a 60-year-old man.[236]

WHIPPLE'S DISEASE

In 1907, Whipple described a case of diarrhea, wasting, and joint inflammation with widespread intestinal fat infiltration as "intestinal lipodystrophy."[195] The characteristic PAS staining of the lesions strongly suggests but does not prove the diagnosis.[196] It is a rare disease that can appear under many guises, in which joint symptoms are present in the vast majority of cases and in which early diagnosis may save a life and decrease morbidity.

Prevalence

The disease is most common in middle-aged men.[197] Familial cases have been observed.[198] Whipple's disease has been described mostly among whites, and the incidence of HLA-B27 is 10 (30 percent) of 33 typed cases.[198]

Systemic Manifestations

Most organ systems can become involved. Prolonged diarrhea, weight loss, steatorrhea, and, rarely, melena are typical intestinal symptoms. Diarrhea may also be spurious or totally absent. Pronounced signs of malabsorption are sometimes present. Chest pain with pleuritis and pneumonias may be prominent, with a relapse prevalence of 30 percent.[199] Sudden death as a result of heart involvement occurs in 20 percent of cases.[199] Endocarditis, aortic insufficiency, thyroiditis, lymphadenopathy, interstitial nephritis, liver damage,[200] uveitis,[201] hyperpigmentation, rash, subcutaneous nodules,[202] and clubbing are other established extraintestinal manifestations. Common central nervous system signs are loss of memory, confusion, apathy, and progressive pseudodementia.[203]

Arthritis

Seronegative oligoarthritis or polyarthritis is the presenting symptom in 60 percent and is present in 90 percent of all patients.[204, 205] It can occasionally be erosive[206] and may precede other disease manifestations by decades.[204, 207] The disease has been diagnosed at hip arthroplasty for avascular necrosis in a 34-year-old man after 6 years of arthritis in the ankles, knees, and wrists. The arthritis was seronegative and unresponsive to treatment with gold, penicillamine, and dapsone.[208] The arthritis is often of migratory type, and its intensity fluctuates independently of intestinal symptoms. Sacroiliitis is present in 7 percent and ankylosing spondylitis in 4 percent of cases.[209] Based on this and the increased prevalence of HLA-B27, Whipple's disease is classified as a spondyloarthropathy.

Diagnosis

Joint fluid examination[205, 210, 214] may show PAS-positive material, and similar findings can be present in the gut, lymph nodes, pericardium, myocardium, liver, spleen, kidney, and brain. Abundance of macrophages filled with PAS-positive material in the lamina propria of the small intestine is, however, the most characteristic finding. Presence of bacterial cell remnants on electron microscopy of intestinal wall, lymph nodes, subcutaneous nodules, synovial membrane,[210] brain, or other tissues is final proof of the diagnosis. Whipple's disease can be confused with sarcoidosis when PAS-positive material is lacking.[211, 212] Ultrasound examination of the heart may reveal retroperitoneal lymph node abnormalities.[213] Joint fluid cultures are sterile.

Therapy

Prolonged therapy with penicillin, 0.5 g four times a day; tetracycline, 500 mg four times a day; or erythromycin, 500 mg four times a day, will often result in dramatic improvement of disease manifestations.[196, 215, 216] Relapses occur, however, after discontinuation of antibiotics and sometimes even during ongoing medication.[208] In such instances, a switch to another antimicrobial drug is indicated.

Etiology

Despite the electron microscopic findings and the well-established response to antibiotics, no causative microorganism has been identified. An immune defect of T lymphocytes has been postulated but not established.[217, 218]

COLLAGENOUS COLITIS

This condition was first described in 1976,[219] and of some 100 reported patients, at least 10 percent have had arthritis.[222, 223] The clinical features consist of intermittent or persistent water-like diarrhea without bleeding. In a review of 36 cases,[220] 30 were women. The age ranged from 23 to 86 years, with a mean of 56 years. Thyroid disease, joint disease including rheumatoid arthritis, and antinuclear antibody positivity have been common in several reports,[221, 226, 227] suggesting autoimmune mechanisms.

Diagnosis

The diagnostic findings are linear deposition in the subepithelium of the colon of hyaline material, 1 to 100 μm thick, consisting principally of collagen III (Fig. 59–5; see color section at the front of this volume). Lymphocytes, plasma cells, and a few eosinophils are also found, and sometimes an inflammatory exudate is present.[220] The histologic findings are distinct enough to differentiate the condition from other diseases of the colon.

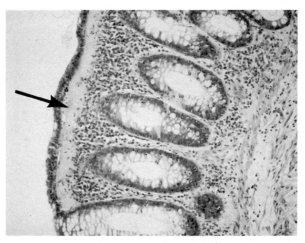

Figure 59–5. Biopsy specimen of colon in a case of collagen colitis. Arrow indicates layer of collagen deposition. Hematoxylin-eosin stain. (Courtesy Dr. C. Lindström.)

Etiology

The etiology is unknown. Increased levels of prostaglandin E_2 have been found in jejunal aspirates[24] and in stools,[228] and a good therapeutic response to NSAIDs has been described.[220] No information is at hand to explain the increased prevalence of arthritis.

Treatment

Treatment is symptomatic. Spontaneous remissions do occur.[229-231] Sulfasalazine has been recommended,[220] but no controlled trials have been performed.

LYMPHOCYTIC COLITIS

A related but distinct entity is lymphocytic or microscopic colitis.[232] In a survey of 18 patients with watery diarrhea, radiologic, endoscopic, and cultural data were unrevealing. Biopsy showed no collagen deposits but abundance of intraepithelial lymphocytes. No female preponderance was seen.

PONCET'S DISEASE

A sterile polyarthritis of insidious onset has been described in a few patients suffering from mostly extrapulmonal tuberculosis, and the term *Poncet's disease* or *tuberculous rheumatism*[237, 238] has been attached to it. Two case reports describe young adults of both sexes with pyrexia, weakness, and arthritis of insidious onset, who later turned out to have caseating tuberculosis of lymph nodes and bone.[239, 240] Antituberculous therapy resulted in slow clearing within months of all joint symptoms. Because the lungs appeared normal, it was assumed that the port of entry of the tuberculosis in these cases was the gut. Allergic or autoimmune pathogenetic mechanisms were suggested based on experimental evidence for cross-reactivity between mycobacteria and cartilage proteoglycan.[241] Although this remains highly speculative, it is important to keep tuberculosis in mind in atypical febrile cases of seronegative joint disease.

References

1. Panush, R. S., Carter, I. I., Katz, P., et al.: Diet therapy for rheumatoid arthritis. Arthritis Rheum. 26:462, 1982.
2. Panush, R. S., Stroud, R. M., and Webster, E. M.: Food-induced (allergic) arthritis. Arthritis Rheum. 29:220, 1986.
3. Ziff, M.: Diet in the treatment of rheumatoid arthritis. Arthritis Rheum. 26:457, 1983.
4. Jakobsson, I., Lindberg, T., Benediktsson, B., et al.: Dietary bovine β-lactoglobulin is transferred to human milk. Acta Pediatr. Scand. 74:342, 1985.
5. Rooney, P. J., Jenkins, R. T., and Buchanan, W. W.: A short review of the relationship between intestinal permeability and inflammatory joint disease. Clin. Exp. Rheumatol. 8:75, 1990.
5a. Gaston, J. S. H.: Enteropathic arthritis. Rheumatol. Rev. 1:107, 1992.
6. Tagesson, C., and Bengtsson, A.: Intestinal permeability to different-sized polyethylene glycol in patients with rheumatoid arthritis. Scand. J. Rheumatol. 12:124, 1983.
7. Maxton, D. G., Bjarnason, I., Reynolds, A. P., et al.: Lactulose, ^{51}CrEDTA, 1-rhamnose and polyethylene glycol 400 as probe markers for assessment in vivo of human intestinal permeability. Clin. Sci. 71:71, 1986.
8. Jakobsson, I., Lindberg, T., Lothe, L., et al.: Human α-lactalbumin as a marker of macromolecular absorption. Gut 27:1029, 1986.
9. Lahesmaa-Rantala, R., Magnusson, K. E., Granfors, K., et al.: Intestinal permeability in patients with Yersinia-triggered reactive arthritis. Ann. Rheum. Dis. 50:91, 1991.
10. Kagnoff, M. F.: Immunology of the immune system. In Johnson, L. (ed.): Physiology of the Gastrointestinal Tract. 2nd ed. New York, Raven Press, 1987, p. 1699.
11. Streeter, P. R., Berg, E. L., Rouse, B. T. N., et al.: A tissue-specific endothelial molecule involved in lymphocyte homing. Nature 331:41, 1988.
12. Polak, J. M.: Regulatory peptides. Basel, Birkhauser Verlag, 1989.
13. Lotz, M., Carson, D. A., and Vaughan, J. H.: Substance P activation of rheumatoid synoviocytes: Neural pathway in pathogenesis of arthritis. Science 235:893, 1987.
14. White, M. H.: Colitis. Lancet 1:583, 1895.
15. Bywaters, E. G. L., and Ansell, B. M.: Arthritis associated with ulcerative colitis. Ann. Rheum. Dis. 17:169, 1958.
16. Wright, V., and Watkinson, G.: Articular complications of ulcerative colitis. Am. J. Proctol. 17:107, 1966.
17. van Patter, W. N., Bargen, J. A., Dockerty, M. B., et al.: Regional enteritis. Gastroenterology 26:347, 1954.
18. Acheson, E. D.: An association between ulcerative colitis, regional enteritis, and ankylosing spondylitis. Q. J. Med. 29:489, 1960.
19. Ansell, B. M., and Wigley, R. A. D.: Arthritis manifestations in regional enteritis. Ann. Rheum. Dis. 23:64, 1964.
20. Mielants, H., Veys, E. M., Joos, R., et al.: Late-onset pauciarticular juvenile chronic arthritis: Relation to gut inflammation. J. Rheumatol. 14:459, 1987.
21. Mielants, H., Veys, E. M., Cuvelier, C., et al.: Subclinical involvement of the gut in undifferentiated spondylarthropathies. Clin. Exp. Rheumatol. 7:499, 1989.
22. De Vos, M., Cuvelier, C., and Mielants, H.: Ileocolonoscopy in seronegative spondylarthropathy. Gastroenterology 96:339, 1989.
23. Mielants, H., and Veys, E. M.: The gut in the spondyloarthropathies. J. Rheumatol. 17:7, 1990.
24. Woodrow, J. C., and Eastmond, C. J.: HLA-B27 and the genetics of ankylosing spondylitis. Ann. Rheum. Dis. 37:504, 1978.
25. Evans, J. G., and Acheson, E. D.: An epidemiological study of ulcerative colitis and regional enteritis in the Oxford area. Gut 6:311, 1965.
26. Bonnevie, O., Riis, P., and Anthonisen, P.: An epidemiological study of ulcerative colitis in Copenhagen County. Scand. J. Gastroenterol. 3:432, 1968.
27. Monk, M., Mendeloff, A. S., Siegal, C. I., and Liebenfieldt, A.: An epidemiological study of ulcerative colitis and regional enteritis among adults in Baltimore. Gastroenterology 53:198, 1967.
28. Broberger, O., and Perlmann, P.: Autoantibodies in human ulcerative colitis. J. Exp. Med. 110:657, 1959.
29. Broberger, O., and Perlmann, P.: Demonstration of an epithelial antigen in colon by means of fluorescent antibodies from children with ulcerative colitis. J. Exp. Med. 115:13, 1962.
30. Lagercrantz, R., Perlmann, P., and Hammarström, S.: Immunological studies in ulcerative colitis. V. Family studies. Gastroenterology 60:381, 1971.
31. Korsmeyer, S. J., Williams, Jr., R. C., Wilson, I. D., and Strickland, R. G.: Lymphocytotoxic and RNA antibodies in inflammatory bowel disease: A comparative study in patients with their families. Ann. N. Y. Acad. Sci. 278:574, 1976.
32. Takahasi, F., and Das, K. M.: Isolation and characterization of a colonic autoantigen, specifically recognized by colon tissue-bound immunoglobulin G from idiopathic ulcerative colitis. J. Clin. Invest. 76:311, 1985.
33. Bagashi, S., Baral, B., and Das, K. M.: Isolation and characterization of Crohn's disease tissue-specific glycoproteins. Gastroenterology 91:326, 1986.
34. Wright, V., and Watkinson, G.: The arthritis of ulcerative colitis. Br. Med. J. 12:670, 1965.
35. Greenstein, A. J., Janowitz, H. D., and Sachar, D. B.: The extraintestinal complications of Crohn's disease and ulcerative colitis: A study of 700 patients. Medicine 55:401, 1976.
36. Lindsley, C. B.: Arthritis in inflammatory bowel disease in children. Arthritis Rheum. 20(Suppl.):411, 1977.
37. Passo, M. H., Fitzgerald, J. F., and Brandt, K. D.: Arthritis associated with inflammatory bowel disease in children. Relationship of joint disease to activity and severity of bowel lesion. Dig. Dis. Sci. 31:492, 1986.
38. Ament, M. E.: Inflammatory diseases of the colon: Ulcerative colitis and Crohn's colitis. J. Pediatr. 86:332, 1975.
39. Wright, V., and Watkinson, G.: The arthritis of ulcerative colitis. Medicine 38:243, 1959.
40. Palumbo, P. J., Ward, L. E., Sauer, W. G., and Scudamore, H. H.: Musculoskeletal manifestations of inflammatory bowel disease: Ulcerative and granulomatous colitis and ulcerative proctitis. Mayo Clin. Proc. 48:411, 1973.
41. McEwen, C.: Arthritis accompanying ulcerative colitis. Clin. Orthop. 57:9, 1968.
42. McBride, J. A., King, M. H., Baikie, A. G., et al.: Ankylosing spondylitis and chronic inflammatory disease of the intestine. Br. Med. J. 2:483, 1963.
43. Wright, V., and Watkinson, G.: Sacroiliitis and ulcerative colitis. Br. Med. J. 2:675, 1965.
44. Jayson, M. I. V., Salmon, P. R., and Harrison, W. J.: Inflammatory bowel disease in ankylosing spondylitis. Gut 11:506, 1970.
45. McConkey, B.: Sulphasalazine and ankylosing spondylitis. Br. J. Rheumatol. 29:2–5, 1990.
46. Wright, V., and Moll, J. M. H.: Seronegative polyarthritis. Amsterdam, North-Holland, 1976.
47. Kerr, R., and Resnick, D.: Radiology of the seronegative spondyloarthropathies. Clin. Rheum. Dis. 11:1, 1985.
48. Moll, J. M. H.: Inflammatory bowel disease. Clin. Rheum. Dis. 11:1, 1985.
49. Sedlack, R. E., Whishant, J., Elveback, L. R., and Kurland, L. T.: Incidence of Crohn's disease in Olmsted County, Minnesota, 1939–1975. Am. J. Epidemiol. 112:759, 1975.
50. Brahme, F., Lindström, C., and Wenckert, A.: Crohn's disease in a defined population. An epidemiological study of incidence, prevalence, mortality and secular trends in the city of Malmö, Sweden. Gastroenterology 69:342, 1975.
51. Mayberry, J. F., and Rhodes, J.: Epidemiological aspects of Crohn's disease. Gut 25:886, 1984.
52. Strickland, R. G., Husby, G., Black, W. C., and Williams, Jr., R. C.: Peripheral blood and intestinal lymphocyte subpopulations in Crohn's disease. Gut 16:847, 1975.
53. Meuwissen, S. G. M., Feltkamp-Vroom, T. M., De La Riviere, A. B., et al.: Analysis of the lympho-plasmacytic infiltrate in Crohn's disease with special reference to identification of lymphocyte-subpopulations. Gut 17:770, 1976.
54. Kett, K., Rognum, T. O., and Brandtzaeg, P.: Mucosal subclass distribution of immunoglobulin G-producing cells in different ulcerative colitis and Crohn's disease of the colon. Gastroenterology 93:919, 1987.
55. MacDermott, R. P., Nash, G. S., Auer, I. O., et al.: Alterations in serum immunoglobulin-G subclasses in patients with ulcerative colitis and Crohn's disease. Gastroenterology 96:764, 1989.
56. Kyle, J.: An epidemiologic study of Crohn's disease in northeast Scotland. Gastroenterology 61:826, 1971.
57. Haslock, I., and Wright, V.: The musculoskeletal complications of Crohn's disease. Medicine 52:217, 1973.

58. Münch, H., Purrman, J., Reis, H. E., et al.: Clinical features of inflammatory joint and spine manifestations in Crohn's disease. Hepatogastroenterology 33:123, 1986.

59. Purrmann, J., Zeidler, H., Bertrams, J., et al.: HLA antigens in ankylosing spondylitis associated with Crohn's disease. Increased frequency of the HLA phenocytype B27, B44. J. Rheumatol. 15:1658, 1988.

60. Kahn, M. A.: HLA-B27 and B12 (B44) in Crohn's disease with ankylosing spondylitis. J. Rheumatol. 16:851, 1989.

61. Rankin, G. B., Watts, H. D., Melnyk, C. S., Kelley, M. L.: National Cooperative Crohn's Disease Study: Extraintestinal manifestations and perianal complications. Gastroenterology 77:914, 1979.

62. Selby, W. S., Kater, R. M., Heap, T. R., and Gallagher, N. D.: Crohn's disease: A review of 122 cases. Aust. N. Z. J. Med. 9:145, 1979.

63. Soren, A.: Joint affections in regional enteritis. Arch. Intern. Med. 117:78, 1966.

64. Heuman, R., Boeryd, B., Billquist, J., et al.: Arthralgia and crystal deposits in Crohn's disease. Scand. J. Rheumatol. 10:313, 1981.

65. Lindström, C., Wramsby, H., and Östberg, G.: Granulomatous arthritis in Crohn's disease. Gut 13:257, 1972.

66. Hermans, P. J., Fievez, M. L., Descamps, C. L., and Aupaiz, M. A.: Granulomatous synovitis and Crohn's disease. J. Rheumatol. 11:710, 1984.

67. Frayha, R., Stevens, M. B., and Bayless, T. M.: Destructive monarthritis and granulomatous synovitis as the presenting manifestation of Crohn's disease. Johns Hopkins Med. J. 137:151, 1975.

68. Tomlingson, I. W., and Jayson, M. I. V.: Erosive Crohn's arthritis. J. Roy. Soc. Med. 74:540, 1981.

69. Clark, R. L., Muhletaler, C. A., and Margulies, S. I.: Colitic arthritis. Clinical and radiographic manifestations. Radiology 101:585, 1971.

70. Alh-Hadidi, S., Khatib, G., Chhatwal, P., and Khatib, R.: Granulomatous arthritis in Crohn's disease. Arthritis Rheum. 27:1061, 1984.

71. Toubert, A., Dougados, M., and Amor, B.: Erosive granulomatous arthritis in Crohn's disease (letter). Arthritis Rheum. 28:958, 1985.

72. Dekker-Saeys, B. J., Meuwissen, S. G. M., van den Berg-Loonen, E. M., et al.: Prevalence of peripheral arthritis, sacoiliitis and ankylosing spondylitis in patients suffering from inflammatory bowel disease. Ann. Rheum. Dis. 37:33, 1978.

73. Hyla, J. F., Frank, W. A., and Davis, J. S.: Lack of association of HLA-B27 with radiographic sacroiliitis in inflammatory bowel disease. J. Rheumatol. 3:196, 1976.

74. Anderson, D. O., Mullinger, M. A., and Bagoch, A.: Regional enteritis involving the duodenum with clubbing of the fingers and steatorrhoea. Gastroenterologý 32:917, 1957.

75. Kitis, G., Thompson, H., and Allan, R. N.: Finger clubbing in inflammatory bowel disease: Its prevalence and pathogenesis. Br. Med. J. 2:825, 1979.

76. Bookman, A. A. M., Gould, M. I., Barrowman, J. A., et al.: Periosteal new bone formation and disseminated granulomatosis in a patient with Crohn's disease. Am. J. Med. 84:330, 1988.

77. Kyle, J.: Psoas abscess in Crohn's disease. Gastroenterology 61:149, 1971.

78. London, D., and Fitton, J. M.: Acute septic arthritis complicating Crohn's disease. Br. J. Surg. 57:536, 1970.

79. Jakobsen, J., and Helleland, H.: Bakteriel coxitis som komplikation til intestinal infektion. Ugeskr. Laeger 148:1766, 1986.

80. Holt, P. J. A., Davies, M. G., Saunders, K. C., and Nuki, G.: Clinical and laboratory findings in 15 patients with special reference to polyarthritis. Medicine 59:114, 1980.

81. Powell, F. C., Schroeter, A. L., Su, W. P. D., and Perry, H. O.: Pyoderma gangrenosum: A review of 86 patients. Q. J. Med. 55:173, 1985.

82. Mielants, H., Veys, E. M., Cuvelier, C., et al.: HLA-B27 related arthritis and bowel inflammation. J. Rheumatol. 12:294, 1985.

83. Powell, F. C., and Perry, H. O.: Pyoderma gangrenosum in childhood. Arch. Dermatol. 120:757, 1984.

84. Brandt, L., Gärtner, I., Nilsson, P. G., et al.: Pyoderma gangrenosum associated with regional enteritis: Improvement in defective granulocyte function and healing of skin lesions during the administration of clofazimine. Acta Med. Scand. 201:141, 1977.

85. Norris, D. A., Weston, W. L., Thorne, G., and Humbert, J. R.: Pyoderma gangrenosum: Abnormal monocyte function corrected in vitro with hydrocortisone. Arch. Dermatol. 114:906, 1978.

86. Sluis, I.: Two cases of pyoderma gangrenosum associated with the presence of an abnormal serum protein (β_2A-paraprotein): With a review of the literature. Dermatologica 132:409, 1966.

87. Möller, H., Waldenström, J. G., Zettervall, O.: Pyoderma gangrenosum (dermatitis ulcerosa) and monoclonal (IgA) globulin healed after melphalon treatment. Acta Med. Scand. 203:293, 1978.

88. Driessen, L. H. H. M., and van Saene, H. K. F.: A novel treatment of pyoderma gangrenosum by intestinal decontamination (abstract). Br. J. Dermatol. 108:108, 1983.

89. Buckley, C., Sarkany, I., and Bayoumi, A. H. M.: Pyoderma gangrenosum with severe pharyngeal ulceration. J. Roy. Soc. Med. 83:590, 1990.

90. Munro, C. S., and Cox, N. H.: Pyoderma gangrenosum associated with Behcet's syndrome—response to thalidomide. Clin. Exp. Dermat. 13:408, 1988.

91. Gainey, R., Ronney, P. J., and Alspaugh, M.: Sjögren's syndrome and Crohn's disease. Clin. Exp. Rheumatol. 3:67, 1985.

92. Aho, K., Ahvonen, P., Lassus, A., et al.: HL-A antigen 27 and reactive arthritis. Lancet 2:157, 1973.

93. Dumonde, D. C.: Principal evidence associating rheumatic diseases with microbial infection. In Dumonde, D. C. (ed.): Infection and Immunology in the Rheumatic Diseases. Oxford, Blackwell Scientific, 1976, p. 97.

94. Fraser, J. R. A.: Epidemic polyarthritis and Ross River virus disease. Clin. Rheum. Dis. 12:2, 1986.

95. Keat, A., Dixey, J., Sonnex, C., et al.: Chlamydia trachomatis and reactive arthritis: The missing link. Lancet 1:72, 1987.

96. Merilahti-Palo, R., Söderström, K.-O., Lahesmaa-Rantala, R., et al.: Bacterial antigens in synovial biopsy specimens in Yersinia-triggered reactive arthritis. Ann. Rheum. Dis. 50:87, 1991.

97. Granfors, K., Jalkanen, S., von Essen, R., et al.: Yersinia antigens in synovial-fluid cells from patients with reactive arthritis. N. Engl. J. Med. 26:320, 1989.

98. Granfors, K., Jalkanen, S., Lindberg, A. A., et al.: Salmonella lipopolysaccharide in synovial cells from patients with reactive arthritis. Lancet 1:685, 1990.

99. Schumacher, H. R., Jr., Magge, S., Cherian, P. V., et al.: Light and electron microscopic studies on the synovial membrane in Reiter's syndrome. Immunocytochemical identification of chlamydial antigen in patients with early disease. Arthritis Rheum. 31:937, 1988.

100. Taylor-Robinson, D., Thomas, B. J., Dixey, J., et al.: Evidence that Chlamydia trachomatis causes seronegative arthritis in women. Ann. Rheum. Dis. 47:295, 1988.

100a. Rahman, M. U., Chooma, M. A., Schumacher, H. R., and Hudson, A. P.: Molecular evidence for the presence of Chlamydia in the synovium of patients with Reiter's syndrome. Arthritis Rheum. 35:521, 1992.

101. Toivanen, P., and Toivanen, A.: Microbial antigens in the synovium in reactive arthritis. In Reactive Arthritis Workshop, Berlin 10–11.6. Berlin, Deutsches RheumaForschungsZentrum, 1990, p. 48.

102. Ford, D. K., da Roza, D. M., and Schulzer, M.: Lymphocytes from the site of disease but not blood lymphocytes indicate the cause of arthritis. Ann. Rheum. Dis. 44:701, 1985.

103. Gaston, J. S. H., Life, P. F., Granfors, K., et al.: Synovial T lymphocyte recognition of organisms which trigger reactive arthritis. Clin. Exp. Immunol. 76:348, 1989.

104. Olhagen, B.: Post-infective or reactive arthritis. Scand. J. Rheumatol. 9:193, 1980.

105. Huette, G.: De l'arthrite dysenterique. Arch. Gen. Med. 2:129, 1869.

106. Reiter, H.: Über eine bisher unerkannte Spirochäten-infektion (Spirochätosis Artritica). Dtsch. Med. Wochenschr. 42:1535, 1916.

107. Fiessinger, N., and Leroy, M. E.: Contribution à l'étude d'une épidémie de dysenterie dans la Somme (Juillet-Octobre 1916). Bull. Mem. Soc. Hop. Paris 40:2030, 1916.

108. Schittenhelm, A., and Schlecht, H.: Uber Polyarthritis enteritica. Dtsch. Arch. Klin. Med. 126:329, 1918.

109. Paronen, J.: Reiter's disease. A study of 344 cases observed in Finland. Acta Med. Scand. 212 (suppl.):1, 1948.

110. Berglöf, F. E.: Arthritis and intestinal infection. Acta Rheum. Scand. 9:141, 1963.

111. Vairtiainen, J., and Hurri, L.: Arthritis due to Salmonella typhimurium. Report of 12 cases of migratory arthritis in association with Salmonella typhimurium infection. Acta Med. Scand. 175:771, 1964.

112. Åhvonen, P., Sievers, K., and Aho, K.: Arthritis associated with Yersinia enterocolitica infection. Acta Rheum. Scand. 15:232, 1969.

113. Skirrow, B. M.: Campylobacter enteritis: A "new" disease. Br. Med. J. 2:9, 1977.

114. Urmaen, J. D., Zurier, R. B., and Rothfield, N. F.: Reiter's syndrome associated with Campylobacter fetus infection. Ann. Intern. Med. 86:44, 1977.

115. Aho, K.: Bowel infection predisposing to reactive arthritis. Baillière's Clin. Rheumatol. 3:303, 1989.

116. Bjorkman, P. J., Saper, M. A., Samraoui, B., et al.: Structure of the human class I histocompatibility antigen HLA-A2. Nature 329:506, 1987.

117. Hammer, R. E., Maika, S. D., Richardson, J. A., et al.: Spontaneous inflammatory disease in transgenic rats expressing HLA-B27 and human β_2m: An animal model of HLA-B27–associated human disorders. Cell 63:1099, 1990.

118. Nickerson, C. L., Luthra, H. S., Savarirayan, S., et al.: Susceptibility of HLA-B27 transgenic mice to Yersinia enterocolitica infection. Hum. Immunol. 28:382, 1990.

119. Tarough, J. D.: Immunology, genetics, and animal models of the spondyloarthropathies. Curr. Opin. Rheumatol. 2:586, 1990.

120. Ivany, P.: Clinical consequences for a mouse to be HLA-B27 transgenic. In Reactive Arthritis Workshop, Berlin 10–11.6. Berlin, Deutsches RheumaForschungsZentrum, 1990, p. 40.

121. Geezy, A. F., Alexander, K., Bashir, H. V., et al.: HLA-B27, *Klebsiella* and ankylosing spondylitis: Biological and chemical studies. Immunol. Rev. 70:23, 1983.

122. Schwimmbeck, P. I., Yu, D. T., and Oldstone, M. B.: Autoantibodies to HLA-B27 in the sera of HLA-B27 patients with ankylosing spondylitis and Reiter's syndrome. Molecular mimicry with *Klebsiella pneumoniae* as potential mechanism of autoimmune disease. J. Exp. Med. 166:173, 1987.

123. Ogasaware, M., Kono, D. H., and Yu, D. T.: Mimicry of human histocompatibility HLA-B27 antigens by *Klebsiella pneumoniae*. Infect. Immunol. 51:901, 1986.

124. Ebringer, A.: The relationship between *Klebsiella* infection and ankylosing spondylitis. Baillière's Clin. Rheumatol. 3:321, 1989.

125. Steiglitz, H., Fosmire, S., and Lipsky, P.: Identification of a 2-Md plasmid from *Shigella flexneri* associated with reactive arthritis. Arthritis Rheum. 32:937, 1989.

126. Lahesmaa, R., Skurnik, M., Vaara, M., et al.: Amino acid sequences shared by HLA-B27 and arthritis triggering microbes are not recognized by the human immune system (abstract). Clin. Rheumatol. 9:586, 1990.

127. van Bohemen, C. G., Grumet, F. C., and Zanen, H. C.: Identification of HLA-B27 M1 and M2 cross-reactive antigens in *Klebsiella, Shigella,* and *Yersinia*. Immunology 52:607, 1984.

128. Robinson, S., Panayi, G. S., Marsal, L., and Wollheim, F. A.: The attachment of certain gram-negative bacteria to buccal epithelial cells from patients with *Yersinia* arthritis. Clin. Exp. Rheumatol. 1:207, 1983.

129. Robinson, S., and Panayi, G. S.: The binding to human lymphocytes of arthritogenic and non-arthritogenic bacteria. Clin. Exp. Rheumatol. 1:211, 1983.

130. Lauhio, A., Lähdevirta, J., Janes, R., et al.: Reactive arthritis associated with *Shigella sonnei* infection. Arthritis Rheum. 31:1190, 1988.

131. Wakefield, D., Stahlberg, T., Freston, J., and Buckley, R.: Seronegative arthritis associated with serological evidence of *Yersinia* infection in Australia. Aust. N. Z. J. Med. 19:331, 1989.

132. Abbott, W. G., and Caughey, D. E.: Reactive arthritis due to *Clostridium difficile*. Aust. N. Z. Med. J. 95:287, 1982.

133. Hannonen, P., Hakola, M., Möttönen, H., et al.: Reactive oligoarthritis associated with *Clostridium difficile* colitis. Scand. J. Rheumatol. 18:57, 1989.

134. Eastmond, C. J.: *Clostridium difficile* as possible cause of reactive arthritis. Scand. J. Rheumatol. 18:443, 1989.

135. Hughes, B. R., and Hind, C. R. K.: Reactive arthritis associated with *Staphylococcus epidermidis* peritonitis in patient undergoing continuous ambulatory peritoneal dialysis. Br. Med. J. 286:188, 1983.

136. McDonald, E. C., and Weisman, M. H.: Articular manifestations of rheumatic fever in adults. Ann. Intern. Med. 89:917, 1978.

137. Gabrielle, H., Hugonot, G., and Duval, M.: Syndrome uretroarticulaire au course d'une entérite à *lamblia*. Lyon Med. 162:299, 1938.

138. Woo, P., and Panayi, G. S.: Reactive arthritis due to infestation with *Giardia lamblia*. J. Rheumatol. 11:719, 1984.

139. Weyand, C., and Goronzy, J. J.: Immune response to *Borrelia burgdorferi* in patients with reactive arthritis. Arthritis Rheum. 32:1057, 1989.

140. Winter, R. J. D., Richardson, A., Lehner, M. J., and Hoffbrand, B. I.: Lung abscess and reactive arthritis: Rare complications of leptospirosis. Br. Med. J. 288:448, 1984.

141. Alarcon, G. S., Bocanegra, T. S., Gotuzzo, E., et al.: Reactive arthritis associated with brucellosis. HLA studies. J. Rheumatol. 8:621, 1981.

142. de Dios Colmenero, J., Reguera, J. M., Fernandez-Nebro, A., et al.: Osteoarticular complications of brucellosis. Ann. Rheum. Dis. 50:23, 1991.

143. Puddey, I. B.: Reiter's syndrome associated with *Salmonella muenchen* infection. Aust. N. Z. J. Med. 12:290, 1982.

144. Leirisalo, M., Skylv, G., Kousa, M., et al.: Follow-up study on patients with Reiter's disease and reactive arthritis with special reference to HLA-B27. Arthritis Rheum. 25:249, 1982.

145. Repo, H., Leirisalo-Repo, M., and Koivurunta-Vaara, P.: Exaggerated inflammatory responsiveness plays a part in the pathogenesis of HLA-B27–linked diseases—hypothesis. Ann. Clin. Research 16:47, 1984.

146. Sheldon, P.: Specific cell-mediated response to bacterial antigens and clinical correlations in reactive arthritis, Reiter's syndrome and ankylosing spondylitis. Immunol. Rev. 86:5, 1985.

147. Mäki-Ikola, O.: Reactive arthritis after unusual *Salmonella* infections. Lancet 336:1387, 1990.

148. Valtonen, V. V., Leirisalo, M., Pentikäinen, P. J., et al.: Triggering infections in reactive arthritis. Ann. Rheum. Dis. 44:399, 1985.

149. Keat, A.: Reiter's syndrome and reactive arthritis in perspective. N. Engl. J. Med. 309:1606, 1983.

150. Håakansson, U., Eitrem, R., Löw, B., and Winblad, S.: HLA antigen B27 in cases with joint affections in an outbreak of salmonellosis. Scand. J. Infect. Dis. 8:245, 1976.

151. Winblad, S.: Arthritis associated with *Yersinia enterocolitica* infections. Scand. J. Infect. Dis. 7:191, 1975.

152. Marsal, L., Winblad, S., Wollheim, F. A.: *Yersinia enterocolitica* arthritis in southern Sweden: A four-year follow-up study. Br. Med. J. 283:101, 1981.

153. Herrero-Beaumont, G., Elswood, J., Will, R., et al.: Postsalmonella reactive phenomena in 2 patients with ankylosing spondylitis: No modification of the underlying disease. J. Rheumatol. 17:250, 1990.

154. Arvastson, B., Damgaard, K., and Winblad, S.: Clinical symptoms of infection with *Yersinia enterocolitica*. Scand. J. Infect. Dis. 3:37, 1971.

155. Inman, R. D., Johnston, M. E. A., Hodge, M., et al.: Postdysenteric reactive arthritis. A clinical and immunogenic study following an outbreak of salmonellosis. Arthritis Rheum. 31:1377, 1988.

156. Ahvonen, P.: Human yersiniosis in Finland. II. Clinical features. Ann. Clin. Res. 4:39, 1972.

157. Sairanen, E., Paronen, I., and Mähönen, H.: Reiter's syndrome. A follow-up study. Acta Med. Scand. 185:57, 1969.

158. Hannu, T. J., and Leirisalo-Repo, M.: Clinical picture of reactive *Salmonella* arthritis. J. Rheumatol. 15:1668, 1988.

159. Good, A. E.: Long-term follow-up in relation to development of ankylosing spondylitis. Ann. Rheum. Dis. 38:(Suppl.) 39, 1979.

160. Larsen, H. J.: *Yersinia enterocolitica* infections and rheumatic diseases. Scand. J. Rheumatol. 9:129, 1980.

161. Christensen, K., and Sörensen, S. F.: *Yersinia enterocolitica* infections and chronic connective diseases. Scand. J. Rheumatol. 11:21, 1982.

162. Stein, H. B., Abdullah, A., Robinson, H. S., and Ford, D. K.: *Salmonella* reactive arthritis in British Columbia. Arthritis Rheum. 23:206, 1980.

163. Frydén, A., Bengtsson, A., Foberg, U., et al.: Early antibiotic treatment of reactive arthritis associated with enteric infections: Clinical and serological study. Br. Med. J. 301:1299, 1990.

164. Gripenberg, M., Miettinen, A., Kurki, P., and Linder, E.: Humoral immune stimulation and antiepithelial antibodies in *Yersinia* infection. Arthritis Rheum. 21:904, 1978.

165. Granfors, K., Viljanen, M., Tiilkainen, A., and Toivanen, A.: Persistence of IgM, IgG, and IgA antibodies in *Yersinia* arthritis. J. Infect. Dis. 141:424, 1980.

166. Granfors, K., Lahesmaa-Rantala, R., and Toivanen, A.: IgM, IgG and IgA antibodies in yersinia infection. J. Infect. Dis. 157:601, 1988.

167. Mäki-Ikola, O., Heesemann, J., Lahesmaa-Rantala, R., et al.: Combined use of released proteins and lipopolysaccharide in enzyme-linked immunosorbent assay for serological screening of *Yersinia* infections. Scand. J. Rheumatol. 85(Suppl.):45, 1990.

168. Granfors, K., Isomäki, H., van Essen, R., et al.: *Yersinia* antibodies in inflammatory joint diseases. Clin. Exp. Rheumatol. 1:215, 1983.

169. Granfors, K., and Toivanen, A.: IgA anti-*Yersinia* antibodies in *Yersinia*-triggered reactive arthritis. Ann. Rheum. Dis. 45:561, 1986.

170. Granfors, K., Lahesmaa-Rantala, R., Toivanen, A., et al.: Rheumatoid factors in *Yersinia*-triggered reactive arthritis. Scand. J. Rheumatol. 75(Suppl.):272, 1988.

171. Leirisalo, M., Gripenberg, M., Julkanen, I., and Repo, H.: Circulating immune complexes in *Yersinia* infection. J. Rheumatol. 11:365, 1984.

172. Lahesmaa-Rantala, R., Granfors, K., Kekomäki, R., and Toivanen, A.: Circulating *Yersinia*-specific immune complexes after yersiniosis: Follow-up study of patients with and without reactive arthritis. Ann. Rheum. Dis. 46:121, 1987.

173. Toivanen, A., Lahesmaa-Rantala, R., Vuento, R., et al.: Association of persisting IgA response with *Yersinia*-triggered reactive arthritis: A study of 104 patients. Ann. Rheum. Dis. 46:898, 1987.

174. Lahesmaa-Rantala, R., Granfors, K., Lehtonen, O. P., and Toivanen, A.: Characterization of circulating *Yersinia*-specific immune complexes in patients with yersiniosis. Clin. Immunol. Immunopathol. 42:202, 1987.

175. Lahesmaa-Rantala, R., Granfors, K., Isomäki, H., and Toivanen, A.: *Yersinia*-specific immune complexes in the synovial fluid of patients with *Yersinia*-triggered reactive arthritis. Ann. Rheum. Dis. 46:510, 1987.

176. Friedberg, M., Denneberg, T., Brun, C., et al.: Glomerulonephritis in infections with *Yersinia enterocolitica* O-serotype 3. Acta Med. Scand. 209:103, 1981.

177. Brenner, M. B., Kobayashi, S., Wiesenhatter, C. W., et al.: In vitro T-lymphocyte proliferative response to *Yersinia enterocolitica* in Reiter's syndrome. Lack of response in the HLA-B27–positive individuals. Arthritis Rheum. 27:250, 1984.

178. Vuento, R., Leino, R., Viander, M., and Toivanen, A.: In vitro lymphoproliferative response to *Yersinia*: Depressed response in arthritic patients years after *Yersinia* infection. Clin. Exp. Rheumatol. 1:219, 1983.

179. Ford, D. K.: Synovial lymphocyte responses in the spondyloarthropathies. *In* Ziff, M., and Cohen, S. B. (eds.): Advances in Inflammation Research. Vol. 9. The Spondyloarthropathies. New York, Raven Press, 1985.

180. Winchester, R., Bernstein, D. H., Fischer, H. D., et al.: The co-occurrence of Reiter's syndrome and acquired immune deficiency. Ann. Intern. Med. 106:19, 1987.

181. Henriksson, V.: Kan tunntarmsresektion försvaras som terapi mot fettsot. Nord. Med. 47:744, 1952.

182. Payne, J. H., DeWind, L. T., and Commons, R. R.: Metabolic observations in patients with jejunocolic shunts. Am. J. Surg. 106:273, 1963.

183. Ross, C. B., Scott, H. W., and Pincus, T.: Jejunal bypass arthritis. Baillière's Clin. Rheumatol. 3:339, 1989.

184. Shagin, J. W., Frame, B., and Duncan, H.: Polyarthritis in obese patients with intestinal bypass. Ann. Intern. Med. 75:377, 1971.
185. Buchanan, R. F., and Wilkens, R. F.: Arthritis after jejunoileostomy. Arthritis Rheum. 15:644, 972.
186. Stein, H. B., Schlappner, O. I. A., Boyko, W., et al.: The intestinal bypass arthritis-dermatitis syndrome. Arthritis Rheum. 24:684, 1981.
187. Clarke, J., Weiner, S. R., Bassett, L. W., et al.: Bypass disease. Clin. Exp. Rheumatol. 5:275, 1987.
188. Clegg, D. O., Samuelsson, C. O., Williams, H. J., and Ward, J. R.: Articular complications of jejunoileal bypass surgery. J. Rheumatol. 7:65, 1980.
189. Ginsberg, J. H., Quismorio, F. P., Mongan, E. S., et al.: Articular complications after jejuno-ileal shunt: Clinical and immunological studies. Arthritis Rheum. 19:797, 1976.
190. Utsinger, P. D.: Bypass arthritis: A bacterial antigen-antibody systemic immune complex disease (abstract). Arthritis Rheum. 23:758, 1980.
191. Jorizzu, J. L., Schmalstieg, F. C., Dinehart, S. M., et al.: Bowel-associated dermatosis-arthritis syndrome. Immune complexes mediated vessel damage and increased neutrofil migration. Arch. Intern. Med. 144:738, 1984.
192. Lichtman, S., Sherman, P., and Forstner, G.: Production of secretory immunoglobulin A in rat self-filling blind loops. Gastroenterology 91:1495, 1986.
193. Clegg, D. O., Zone, J. J., Samuelsson, Jr., C. O., and Warel, J. R.: Circulating immune complexes containing secretory IgA in jejunoileal bypass disease. Ann. Rheum. Dis. 44:239, 1985.
194. Klinkhoff, A. V., Stein, H. B., Schlappner, O. L. A., and Boyko, W. B.: Postgastrectomy blind loop syndrome and the arthritis dermatitis syndrome. Arthritis Rheum. 28:214, 1985.
195. Whipple, G. H.: A hitherto undescribed disease characterized anatomically by deposits of fat and fatty acids in the intestinal and mesenteric lymphatic tissues. Johns Hopkins Hosp. Bull. 18:382, 1907.
196. Maizel, H., Ruffin, J. M., and Dobbins, W. O.: Whipple's disease—review of 19 patients from one hospital and a review of the literature since 1950. Medicine 49:175, 1970.
197. Putte, R. H., and Tesluk, H.: Whipple's disease. Am. J. Med. 19:383, 1955.
198. McKinley, R., and Grace, C. S.: Whipple's disease in an HLA-B27–positive female. Aust. N. Z. J. Med. 15:758, 1985.
199. McMenemy, A.: Whipple's disease, familial Mediterranean fever, and adult-onset Still's disease. Curr. Opin. Rheumatol. 2:600, 1990.
200. Gupta, S., Pinching, A. J., Onwubalili, J., et al.: Whipple's disease with unusual clinical findings. Gastroenterology 90:1286, 1986.
201. Viteri, A. L., Stinson, J. C., Barnes, M. C., and Dyck, W. P.: Rod-shaped organism in the liver of a patient with Whipple's disease. Dig. Dis. Sci. 24:560, 1979.
202. Font, R. L., Rao, N. A., Issarescu, S., and McEntee, W. J.: Ocular involvement in Whipple's disease. Arch. Ophthalmol. 96:1431, 1978.
203. Good, A. E., Beals, T. F., Simmons, J. L., and Ibrahim, A. H.: A subcutaneous nodule with Whipple's disease: Key to early diagnosis? Arthritis Rheum. 23:856, 1980.
204. Bayless, T. M., and Knox, D. L.: Whipple's disease: A multisystem infection. N. Engl. J. Med. 300:920, 1979.
205. Caughey, D. E., and Bywaters, E. G. L.: The arthritis of Whipple's syndrome. Ann. Rheum. Dis. 22:327, 1963.
206. Kelly, J. J., III, and Weissiger, B. B.: The arthritis of Whipple's disease. Arthritis Rheum. 6:615, 1963.
207. Ayoub, W. T., David, D. E., Torretti, D., and Viozzi, F. J.: Bone destruction and ankylosis in Whipple's disease. J. Rheumatol. 9:6, 1982.
208. LeVine, M. E., and Dobbins, W. O., III: Joint changes in Whipple's disease. Semin. Arthritis Rheum. 3:79, 1973.
209. Canoso, J. J., Saini, M., and Hermos, J. A.: Whipple's disease and ankylosing spondylitis. Simultaneous occurrence in HLA-B27 male. J. Rheumatol. 5:79, 1978.
210. Hawkins, C. F., Farr, M., Morris, C. J., et al.: Detection by electron microscopy of rod-shaped organisms in synovial membrane from a patient with the arthritis of Whipple's disease. Ann. Rheum. Dis. 35:502, 1976.
211. Spapen, H. D. M., Severs, O., DeWit, N., et al.: Electron microscopic detection of Whipple's bacillus in sarcoid-like periodic acid–Schiff–negative granulomas. Dig. Dis. Sci. 34:640, 1989.
212. Southern, J. F., Moscicki, R. A., Magro, C., et al.: Lymphedema, lymphocytic myocarditis, and sarcoid-like granulomatosis: Manifestations of Whipple's disease. J.A.M.A. 261:1467, 1989.

213. Davis, S. J., and Patel, A.: Distinctive echogenic lymphadenopathy in Whipple's disease. Clin. Radiol. 42:60, 1990.
214. Rubinow, A., Canoso, J. J., Goldenberg, D. L., and Cohen, A. S.: Synovial fluid and synovial membrane pathology in Whipple's disease. Arthritis Rheum. 19:820, 1976.
215. Ryser, R. J., Locksley, R. M., Eng, S. C., et al.: Reversal of the dementia associated with Whipple's disease by antibiotics which penetrate the blood brain barrier. Gastroenterology 86:745, 1984.
216. Bowman, C., Dieppe, P., and Settas, L.: Remission of pseudospondylitis with treatment of Whipple's disease. Br. J. Rheumatol. 22:181, 1983.
217. Dobbins, W. O., III: Is there an immune deficit in Whipple's disease? Dig. Dis. Sci. 26:247, 1981.
218. Feurle, G. E., Dorken, B., Schopf, E., and Lenhard, V.: HLA-B27 defects in the T-cell system in Whipple's disease. Eur. J. Clin. Invest. 9:385, 1979.
219. Lindström, C. G.: "Collagenous colitis" with watery diarrhoea: A new entity? Pathol. Eur. 11:87, 1976.
220. Rams, H., Rogers, A. I., and Ghandur-Mnaymneh, I.: Collagenous colitis. Ann. Intern. Med. 106:108, 1987.
221. Erlendsson, J., Fengec, J., and Meinicke, J.: Arthritis and collagenous colitis. Scand. J. Rheumatol. 12:93, 1983.
222. Fausa, O., and Foerster, A.: Collagenous colitis (abstract). Scand. J. Gastroenterol. 18:15, 1983.
223. Tegelbjaerg, P. S., Thaysen, E. H., and Jensen, H. H.: Development of collagenous colitis in sequential biopsy specimens. Gastroenterology 87:703, 1984.
224. Farah, D. A., Mills, P. R., Lee, F. D., et al.: Collagenous colitis: Possible response to sulfasalazine and local steroid therapy. Gastroenterology 88:792, 1985.
225. Jessrun, J., Yardby, J. H., Giardiello, F. M., et al.: Chronic colitis with thickening of the subepithelial collagen layer (collagenous colitis): Histopathologic findings in 15 patients. Hum. Pathol. 18:839, 1987.
226. Giardiello, F. M., Bayless, T. M., Jessurun, J., et al.: Collagenous colitis: Physiologic and histopathologic studies in seven patients. Ann. Intern. Med. 106:46, 1987.
227. Roubenoff, R., Ratain, J., Giardiella, F., et al.: Collagenous colitis, enteropathic arthritis, and autoimmune diseases: Result of a patient survey. J. Rheumatol. 16:1229, 1989.
228. Rask-Madsen, J., Grove, O., Hansen, M. G. J., et al.: Colonic transport of water and electrolytes in a patient with secretory diarrhoea, due to collagenous colitis. Dig. Dis. Sci. 28:1141, 1983.
229. Eaves, E. R., Walls, P. L., McIntyre, R. L. E., and Korman, M. G.: Collagenous colitis: A recently recognized reversible clinicopathological entity. Aust. N. Z. J. Med. 13:630, 1983.
230. Yeshaya, C., Novis, B., Bernheim, J., et al.: Collagenous colitis. Dis. Colon Rectum 27:111, 1981.
231. Debongnie, J. C., DeGalocsy, C., Cahlolessur, M. O., and Haot, J.: Collagenous colitis: A transient condition? Report of two cases. Dis. Colon Rectum 27:672, 1984.
232. Giardello, F. M., Lazenby, A. J., Bayless, T. M., et al.: Lymphocytic (microscopic) colitis. Clinicopathological study of 18 patients and comparison to collagen colitis. Dig. Dis. Sci. 34:1730, 1989.
233. Adelizzi, R. A., Pecora, A. A., and Chiesa, J. C.: Celiac disease: Case report with an associated arthropathy. Am. J. Gastroenterol. 77:481, 1982.
234. Pinals, R. S.: Arthritis associated with gluten-sensitive enteropathy. J. Rheumatol. 13:201, 1986.
235. Bourne, J. T., Kumare, P., Huskisson, E. C., et al.: Arthritis and coeliac disease. Ann. Rheum. Dis. 44:592, 1985.
236. Zammit-Maepel, I., Adamson, A. R., and Halsey, J. P.: Sclerodactyly complicating coeliac disease. Br. J. Rheumatol. 25:396, 1986.
237. Poncet, A.: Rheumatism tuberculex abarticulaire. Lyon Medical 99:65, 1902.
238. Isaacs, A. J., and Sturrock, R. D.: Poncet's disease—fact or fiction? A reappraisal of tuberculous rheumatism. Tubercle 55:135, 1974.
239. Sattar, M. A., Guindi, R. T., and Tungekar, M. F.: Reactive arthritis: Yet another cause. Scand. J. Rheumatol. 18:239, 1989.
240. Ames, P. R. J., Capasso, G., Testa, V., et al.: Chronic tuberculous rheumatism (Poncet's disease) in a gymnast. Br. J. Rheumatol. 29:72, 1990.
241. van Eden, W., Holoshitz, J., Nero, Z., et al.: Arthritis induced by a T-lymphocyte clone that responds to *Mycobacterium tuberculosis* and to cartilage proteoglycan. Proc. Natl. Acad. Sci. U.S.A. 82:5717, 1985.

Index

Note: Page numbers in *italics* refer to illustrations; those followed by (t) indicate tables.